Textbook of

Oral and Maxillofacial Surgery

Textbook of Oral and Maxillofacial Surgery

Fourth Edition

SM Balaji, MDS, MFDS RCPS(Glasg.), FDS RCPS(Glasg.) PhD, DSc (Hons)

Director and Consultant Oral and Maxillofacial Surgeon
Balaji Dental, Craniofacial Hospital and Research Institute, Chennai, Tamil Nadu, India
Adjunct Professor, The Tamil Nadu Govt Dr MGR Medical University, Chennai, Tamil Nadu, India
Member, Dental Council, Government of India
Dr B C Roy National Awardee, Medical Council of India
Diplomate, International Council of Implantology, USA
Former Member of Senate, The Tamil Nadu Govt. Dr M G R Medical University, Chennai, Tamil Nadu, India
Former Member of Senate and Syndicate, Annamalai University, Chidambaram, Tamil Nadu, India
Former Executive Member, Dental Council, Government of India
Consultant Maxillofacial Surgeon
Indira Gandhi Memorial Hospital, Male, Republic of Maldives
Victoria Hospital, Mahe, Republic of Seychelles
Govt Jawaharlal Nehru Hospital, Port Louis, Republic of Mauritius
Formerly Apollo Hospital, Colombo, Sri Lanka

Padma Preetha Balaji, BDS, MDS

Consultant Oral and Maxillofacial Surgeon
Balaji Dental, Craniofacial Hospital and Research Institute,
Chennai, Tamil Nadu, India

ELSEVIER

ELSEVIER

RELX India Pvt. Ltd.
Registered Office: 818, 8th Floor, Indraprakash Building, 21, Barakhamba Road, New Delhi 110 001
Corporate Office: 14th Floor, Building No. 10B, DLF Cyber City, Phase II, Gurgaon-122 002, Haryana, India

Textbook of Oral and Maxillofacial Surgery, 4e, SM Balaji, Padma Preetha Balaji

Publisher's note: Elsevier takes a neutral position with respect to territorial disputes or jurisdictional claims in its published content, including in maps and institutional affiliations.

ISBN: 978-81-312-6469-0
eISBN: 978-81-312-6470-6

First Printed in India 2023, Reprinted 2024

Sr Content Strategist: Ruchi Mullick
Content Project Manager: Anand K Jha
Sr Production Executive: Dhan Singh Rana
Sr Graphic Designer: Gopal Venkatesan

Typeset by GW India

Printed and bound at Rajkamal Electric Press, Kundli, Haryana.

To
my mother for her incessant prayers
my father for making me what I am
Prof US Nayak for honing my skills
my wife for being my strength
my children, all the reasons of my life

FOREWORD

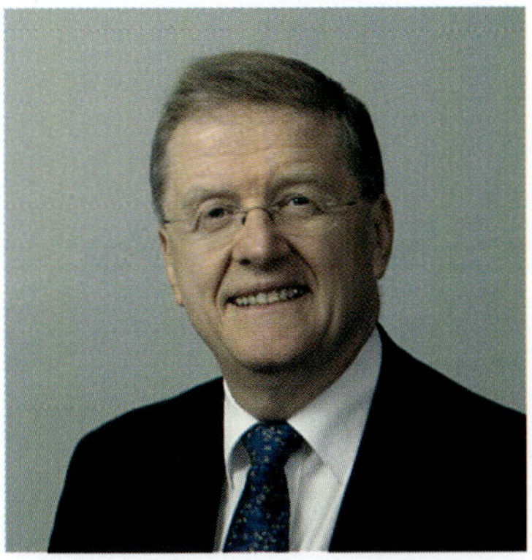

When a surgical textbook reaches its 4th edition, the reader knows that he is purchasing a proven winner. This latest version of the "Textbook of Oral & Maxillofacial Surgery" should actually be titled "**The** Textbook of Oral and Maxillofacial Surgery" as this book has become the standard reference text on the subject. This book has been updated at five-year intervals to incorporate all the changes that have occurred in the specialty with the passage of time. One thing that has never changed is the quality and the comprehensive nature of the knowledge that it contains. If you open the pages of any chapter, the first thing that you will appreciate is the sheer volume of data and detailed information that can be found in each section. The knowledge contained within the book is encyclopedic, however the reader is not overwhelmed by the quantity of information as the book has multiple clinical photographs to "walk" the reader through the text. In addition, there are numerous diagrams, illustrations and tables that concisely explain what the most important elements are in any clinical scenario.

Oral and Maxillofacial Surgery is a specialty which encompasses a wide range of techniques which range from relatively simple intraoral dental procedures to complex advanced craniofacial techniques. The specialty has expanded not only in its surgical scope but in the technological advances it has made in the last ten years, e.g. the use of computer planning and computer-generated 3-D models for procedures. To cover all this material in a single book is truly a monumental achievement and the authors should be very proud of what they have accomplished in their latest text. As was the case in previous editions the book is written so that it is simple to read and to grasp the essential concepts that are being described. This textbook was designed to be appreciated primarily by undergraduate students and residents, however, even clinicians with many years of experience can gain new knowledge and understanding from its pages. In keeping with the up-to-date educational learning techniques of the younger generation, this book also contains instructional videos which are aimed at explaining the more complicated surgical techniques.

The senior author, Professor S. M. Balaji is a surgeon who has an outstanding reputation both in his own country and internationally. This textbook will further enhance his standing and will be an essential part of his legacy. Even those of us who know him well, cannot fail to be amazed at how he found the time to produce such a complete work. If you had to choose just one book to read on oral and maxillofacial surgery, this would be the one.

Robert A. Ord BDS, MBBCh (Hons), FRCS, FACS, MS, MBA
Professor and Chairman Emeritus
Department of Oral and Maxillofacial Surgery
University of Maryland
Greenbaum Cancer Center
Baltimore MD, USA

PREFACE TO THE FOURTH EDITION

The *fourth edition* of the Textbook of Oral and Maxillofacial Surgery is out and we have thoroughly pruned the manuscript, making it a major revision over the previous editions. After 15 years, the book is still a leading oral and maxillofacial surgical reference. With worldwide appreciation from students, lecturers, and professors, we made this version more informative and comprehensive. Since the previous version of this book was published, both the art and science of oral and maxillofacial surgery have advanced. We are pleased to have contributed to the first comprehensive introduction to one of dentistry's most important subspecialties in the capacity of textbook authors.

This book is being launched at a time when dental practices and practitioners are receiving unprecedented attention for pandemic survival. The pandemic affected dental offices, but this encouraged us to review infection control in the chapter *Sterilization and disinfection*. Education and training are being promoted to avoid infectious illnesses and improve safety worldwide.

The whole manuscript has been revised and restructured. At the beginning of each chapter, an outline highlights key concepts to make the content more accessible. Tables allow learners to comprehend, compare, and apply facts across the textbook. Flowcharts for trauma, airway, and Ludwig's angina management help students prepare for test simulations. This textbook is structured to aid students in gaining a basic understanding of oral surgery by offering a detailed explanation of the first stage in patient care, which is diagnosis. This step is the most important phase in providing treatment for patients and a case study approach has been used in each of these chapters, *History taking and clinical examination, Radiodiagnosis, Diagnostic aid – hematological, biochemical, Microbiological investigations and Histopathological investigations*. The next most significant task a dentist must experience in his profession is medical and emergency management of a patient undergoing oral surgery. So, in this edition the chapters *Management of medically compromised patients, Haemorrhage and shock, Therapeutics in oral surgery, Medical Emergencies and their Management in Dental Office. An abstract on Premalignant lesions and conditions, Oral cancer and its management* and the sections on *TMJ, Reconstructive surgery, Neurogenic Disorders of Maxillofacial region and Maxillofacial Trauma* are a total rewrite, and all these chapters have been logically structured. Guidelines from various international organizations have been included where they were deemed to be of use. Painless surgical technique is explained in the section on anaesthesia for oral surgery with a new chapter on *Conscious sedation*. To facilitate learning, we have modernized all the images and added brand new ones to the chapter on *Local anaesthesia*. Students can master nerves and nerve blocks using flowcharts. The *Armamentarium* chapter has photos and explanations of each instrument. This approach helps students explore and learn the clinical instruments faster. *Dental implantology* is revamped in this edition. We included fresh illustrations, a table of clinical steps, and the latest dental implant advances. Oral surgery curriculum covers a wide range of subjects, including *maxillofacial pathologies, reconstructive surgery, abnormalities of the temporomandibular joint, neurogenic illnesses of the maxillofacial region, dentofacial deformities, and maxillofacial trauma* all of which are discussed in the subsequent chapters. A review of the most recent advancements in this discipline is presented as the last section of this textbook.

Oral and maxillofacial surgery will shift from treating basic facial disorders, deformities, and pathologies to reconstructing the maxillofacial and craniofacial regions utilizing tissue engineering and artificial intelligence. As this speciality transitions into the new age, this edition keeps and enhances its basic principles, focus, and depth to teach dental students and practitioners, even if it incorporates many major revisions.

S M Balaji
Padma Preetha Balaji

PREFACE TO THE FIRST EDITION

As an Oral and Maxillofacial Surgeon, I have explored that our students still lack a practical and concise textbook on oral and maxillofacial surgery and need to refer several textbooks to learn each aspect of Oral Surgery. When I was a student I found that there were no Indian authors for any book of oral and maxillofacial surgery. All these had motivated me to frame a specialised, aphoristic and updated book, based on my clinical and surgical experience for the past 18 years in the field of oral and maxillofacial surgery and that of my colleagues, accepted and published by peer reviewed journals. I intend to provide a lucid and comprehensive package of the pathologies encountered in the oral cavity demanding surgical treatment, their clinical detection, the use of modern technological advancement in the diagnosis, the various treatment options available, their advantages and limitations, the recent advances, application of the results of the research work undertaken and the possible vistas of improvements in the future. I have tried to present my knowledge in the subject adhering to the contemporary, accepted standards of proficiency and competence.

The line diagrams are an expressive interpretation of our surgical pictures which are worked upon and simplified to render them more comprehensible and comparable with the real photographs. Therefore, these illustrations are easy to remember and reproduce during examination. The practical and pictographic explanation of the procedures has an edge over the conventional method of learning.

The emphasis is laid upon the language that is simple, understandable and exclusively designed for the students whilst maintaining its international standards. Therefore I believe that this book would be very useful from examination point of view for both undergraduate and postgraduate students. My objective was to present this area of expertise of oral and maxillofacial surgery in its fullest scope by accumulating as inclusive a text as possible. I have made my first attempt and I hope that this text serves the requirements of the students. In the future I assure of enhanced endeavour to present an even broader scope of this field.

SM Balaji, 2007

CONTENTS

Contents

Section I

Introduction to Oral Surgery

Chapter 1

Definition and Scope of Oral Surgery

OUTLINE

DENTISTRY (ADA DEFINITION)

The evaluation, diagnosis, prevention and/or treatment (non-surgical, surgical or related procedures) of diseases, disorders and/or conditions of the oral cavity, maxillofacial area and/or the adjacent and associated structures and their impact on the human body; provided by a dentist, within the scope of his/her education, training and experience, in accordance with the ethics of the profession and the applicable law.

THE DENTIST ACT 1948

Scope of dentistry has been defined by the Dental Council of India (DCI), which, in turn, has been empowered by the Parliament to structure a course aimed at preventing, diagnosing and treating diseases of the mouth and teeth. According to the Dentist Act (1948), 'Dentistry' includes:

1. The performance of any operation on and the treatment on any disease, deficiency or lesion of the human teeth or jaws and the performance of radiography or in connection with human teeth or jaws or the oral cavity
2. The giving of any anaesthetic in connection with any such operation or treatment
3. The mechanical construction or the renewal of artificial dentures, or restorative dental appliances
4. The performance of any operation on, or the giving of any treatment, advice or attendance to any person preparatory to, or for the purpose of, or in connection with the fitting, inserting, fixing, constructing, repairing or renewing of artificial dentures or restorative dental appliances, and the performance of any such operation and the giving of any such treatment, advice or attendance, as is usually performed or given by dentists.

The Dentist Act is clear in its mandate and has entrusted approved universities all over the India to run courses to qualify individuals in the art and science of dentistry. With advances in the field of dentistry, postgraduate programmes were also started to develop focus in certain areas of dentistry, thus paving the way for specialists such as orthodontists, periodontists, prosthodontists, maxillofacial surgeons, etc.

The specialists are expected by implication to focus on their unique areas so as to impart concentrated information to dental students. The graduate dentist is therefore expected to fully evolve out of the united endeavour of many specialists who teach him/her the respective subjects.

ORAL SURGERY

The word 'Surgery' is derived from the Greek word *chir* meaning hand and *ergos* meaning work. Therefore, theoretically surgery means any work done with the hands; but the usage is generally limited to practical therapies such as those involving cutting, repairing and dressing living tissues.

Therefore, 'Oral Surgery' deals with the diagnosis and treatment of oral conditions of the jaw and mouth structures that require surgical intervention. This dental speciality is limited to the surgical removal of teeth and the treatment of diseases, deformities and defects of the jaws and associated structures.

Setting rigid limits to any speciality is likely to stifle development and enterprise and cannot satisfactorily account for variation in interest and ability among its practitioners. So, although oral surgery could be said to be an area of practice within dentistry, its limits are not well defined and it spreads somewhat towards other aspects of surgery. 'Maxillofacial surgery' is a term that implies a greater scope of surgical interest. 'Craniofacial surgery', on the other hand, is a more specific term relating to the specialised area dealing with disorders that affect both the cranial and the facial skeleton.

ORAL AND MAXILLOFACIAL SURGERY

Oral and maxillofacial surgery (OMS) is a speciality of dentistry concerned with the diagnosis and surgical treatment of congenital or acquired diseases, dysfunction, defects or injuries of the mouth, jaws, face, neck and adjacent craniofacial regions.

SCOPE OF PRACTICE OF A DENTIST AND ORAL AND MAXILLOFACIAL SURGEON

The word 'scope' is, as the Webster's dictionary would have it, 'the range of one's awareness, thoughts or actions'. The general dental practitioner, who acquires a registration to practice on finishing his/her undergraduate degree and 1 year of internship, is required to undertake surgical treatments beyond the tooth and its supporting ligament as well as to diagnose a range of disorders that may benefit from a surgical solution or may have to be distinguished from those that require surgery.

The scope of practice of a dentist and a maxillofacial surgeon are widely different. A postgraduate maxillofacial surgeon is trained to treat more complex disorders of the teeth and the facial structures. There is also an important distinction to be drawn between those conditions that a dentist should treat in the practice and those that are better treated by a specialist or in a hospital setting. Further distinction must be made between what is common practice in one country and what is not accepted in another. Some of these differences are cultural and some are historical.

ORAL SURGICAL PROCEDURES PERFORMED BY A GENERAL PRACTITIONER

- Extraction and simple impactions
- Management of complications arising due to minor surgical problems
- Endodontic surgeries
- Incision and drainage of abscess
- Alveoloplasty
- Traumatic injuries not involving severe bone fractures
- Management of pathological conditions of the oral mucosa and bone.

PROCEDURES THAT SHOULD BE PERFORMED ONLY BY SPECIALISTS

- Roots displaced into the maxillary sinus
- Orthognathic surgery
- Transplantation of tissues
- Oral oncology
- Complicated maxillofacial surgeries and space infections
- Difficult impactions such as distoangular impactions
- Temporomandibular joint problems
- Congenital malformations of the orofacial region
- Preprosthetic surgeries.

PURPOSE OF SPECIALISATION

Specialisation would essentially serve to equip one with a sharper focus on one of the areas within a broad speciality. It is also expected (though not mandated) that the specialist will not dilute his skills by performing general dental work. They may be considered as an authority in their subject with skills far beyond the requirement of legal competence. They would, as mandated by the Dental Council of India, be qualified to teach the subject in recognised dental institutions.

Over many decades dentistry and medicine have undergone a series of specialisations. The development of dentistry itself could be seen as a specialisation within medicine. The advantage of specialisation is increased skill among practitioners in that area of practice. The disadvantage is loss of some general and widely applicable abilities.

RELATIONSHIP OF ORAL SURGERY WITH OTHER DENTAL SPECIALITIES

Orthodontics are required for the correction of malocclusion and jaw deformities in cleft or other craniofacial defects. Preprosthetic surgery performed by the oral surgeon sometimes becomes mandatory for the better functioning of the prosthesis. The practice of conservative dentistry and periodontics requires application of oral surgery for the treatment of periapical pathology. Management of medically compromised patients and medical emergencies necessitates the understanding of medicine and physiology. The speciality also has a very close association with other branches of dentistry such as oral medicine and radiology, oral pathology and forensic odontology.

The relationship of oral surgery with plastic surgery, neurosurgery, ENT and orthopaedic surgery is well known in the treatment of various maxillofacial and craniofacial deformities. Each speciality substantiates its validity in fruitful coexistence, therefore, it is difficult to limit the professional interests of the specialities.

THE CURRICULUM

Undergraduate curriculum in oral and maxillofacial surgery is designed, based on its objectives, to expose students to the speciality and help them develop the knowledge, skills and values to become competent in performing minor oral surgery. The educational programme rests on two central elements: (1) A rigorous didactic programme that combines lectures with small-group learning and (2) A clinical programme that imparts proficiency in the basics of oral surgical practice. Beyond core surgical competencies, students completing the course should come away with a good understanding of the evaluation, diagnosis and perioperative management of the surgical patient. The blending of critical thinking and a humanistic approach to patient care with the latest techniques of surgical practice is a pervasive theme throughout the curriculum. The curriculum provides the students with a solid foundation that they will use for the rest of their professional lives, whether or not surgery is a career goal.

The 1-year senior internship programme is a period of expanded clinical experience in oral surgery. It gives ample exposure to a variety of minor oral surgical procedures. The internship is a demanding and time-intensive period in a student's professional education, but one that serves as a building block for acquisition of advanced knowledge in the field of surgery, regardless of a student's ultimate career goals.

WHAT A GRADUATE SHOULD KNOW

- Assess the general condition of the patients, be able to manage patients with medical illness in the general practice and make appropriate specialty referral
- Appropriately assess and diagnose oral and maxillofacial surgery conditions, order the proper investigations necessary at the general practice level and then to treat or refer the case
- Control pain and anxiety
- Basic surgical skills including exodontias, raising mucoperiosteal flaps, removal of retained roots and roots broken during extraction and simple removal of impacted wisdom teeth
- Assess facial fractures, oral neoplastic lesions, craniomaxillofacial deformities and facial infections
- Manage intraoperative and postoperative complications arising in a clinical practice, including medical and surgical complications and to provide necessary lifesaving and airway maintenance procedures.

DUAL DEGREE QUALIFICATION

In India, practice of oral and maxillofacial surgery as a clinical speciality requires a Masters in Dental Surgery (maxillofacial surgery) alone. But of late, in the United States and other nations, there has been an increased inclination towards making this speciality a dual degree one. There has been a rise of the dual degree (DDS/MD) programmes among American OMS residencies. Dual degree programmes have been embraced by about 40% of the existing OMS programmes in the United States.

Oral and maxillofacial surgery has a unique position, straddling the dental and medical professions, creating controversy over whether dual medical and dental qualifications are necessary.

Oral surgeons are the products of a unique style of hybrid professional education that includes areas of both dentistry and medicine. We are the 'surgeons' to our dental colleagues and the 'dentists' to our medical colleagues.

As the scope of oral and maxillofacial surgery continues to expand into areas that have traditionally been medical specialities, the educational and political advantages of membership in the medical fraternity will be important, as the number of dual qualified surgeons will continue to increase. At the same time, the scope of practice for OMS is not an issue of single or dual degree but must be related to the surgeon being trained to competence in the procedures performed. Future evolution will be based on continual advancements in the speciality and related areas, as well as the development of new techniques. While medical education may improve a core fund of general knowledge, surgical residency is the determinant of surgical competence and the scope of practice.

PROS AND CONS OF THE SPECIALITY

Rapid growth and development of the speciality provide a wide range of opportunities for the students and increase the scope of the speciality.

Unfortunately, due to the overlapping of the speciality with other specialities such as ENT, Ophthalmology and likewise, we are unable to achieve any kind of generalisation, which the other surgeons have achieved.

The goal of oral surgery is to provide the highest level of training in the full scope of oral and maxillofacial surgery and to ensure the development of skilled surgeons capable of providing continued comprehensive care. The curriculum should have a strong academic flavour with a high priority given to research.

Chapter 2

Medicolegal Considerations in Dentistry

OUTLINE

LAW

The function of law is primarily to maintain order in social relationship and protect the legitimate interest of members of a given society. This is achieved by laying down a variety of norms for social behaviour through the legislative process, ensuring its observance in social harmony through the administrative process and adjudicating disputes in enforcement through the judicial process. The law and its enforcement system have become complicated and diversified with the advancement of civilisation, consistent with the felt needs of the society, thus have emerged major branches of the legal system such as criminal law, commercial law, labour law, administrative law, consumer protection, etc. Tooth injury is considered as a grievous injury and is punishable under law according to the Indian Penal Code (IPC).

CRIME AND PENAL CODE

The word *crime* in its broad sense may be explained as an act of commission or omission that is baneful to the society in general.

Human beings are morally autonomous, with the basic faculty to understand reality and distinguish right from wrong, able to contribute to the developing social norms, to understand and internalise them, competent to decide how to act and capable of realising that decision. This concept dictates the boundaries of penal law and influences the principles of criminal responsibility.

The substantive criminal law of our country is found in the IPC, as well as in other local and special laws. With regard to the condition of criminal responsibility, the IPC is the sole authority. Medical negligence is predominantly a civil matter.

The moral and ethical responsibilities associated with the practice of dentistry are well recognised, but the legal obligations between the dentist and the patient are often less well understood. In recent years, the number of malpractice claims against dentists has been increasing swiftly.

MALPRACTICE

Malpractice is defined as negligent actions of professionals while performing their professional duties.

Although medical treatment is generally perceived as being beneficial, in some circumstances the administration of treatment can make a health care practitioner liable to criminal action. Medical malpractice may give rise to two common law actions in tort. The first, that of *trespass* to the person or battery, is of limited significance. The second, that of negligence, forms the basis of most malpractice claims. Battery is the unlawful application of force to another person without his consent and if done intentionally or recklessly, as opposed to negligently is a crime as well as tort at common law.

RASHNESS AND NEGLIGENCE

Criminal rashness is undertaking a dangerous or risky act with the knowledge that it is risky and that it may cause injury, but without the intention of causing injury. The criminality lies in running the risk of doing such an act with recklessness or indifference to the consequences. There is a distinction between a negligent act and a rash act.

A negligent act is not doing something that a reasonable man would have done or doing something that a prudent man would not do in the given circumstances. *Rashness* is a positive act committed by the accused and *negligence* is the wilful inaction on the part of the accused so as to drive him within the mischief of negligence. It is the criminal rashness and negligence, which endangers human life or the personal safety of others that renders an act of offence under the penal code.

Such an act is considered an offence if:

i. The act is the cause of the hurt
ii. The act is done with criminal rashness or negligence and is of such a degree as to endanger human life or personal safety of others.

This applies only if the grievous hurt caused is the direct result of the rash or negligent act, not a remote result of the act.

ELEMENTS OF A NEGLIGENCE CLAIM

Negligence is defined as a conduct that falls below the standard established by law for the protection of others against unreasonable risk of harm.

In order to establish a valid negligence claim, following elements must exist:

- A duty of care was owed by the dentist to the patient
- Dentist violated the applicable standard of care
- Patient suffered a compensable loss or injury
- Such an injury was caused in fact and proximately by the substandard care.

Duty of care means that the patient had accepted for treatment and therefore the dentist is obliged to provide a certain standard of accepted care to the patient. Duty does not prevent the dentist from refusing to prescribe treatment or to perform a procedure which the dentist does not believe is indicated, but the physician cannot refuse to provide care once the relationship is established.

A violation to provide an applicable standard of care must be demonstrated. *Standard of care* generally means that degree of care and skill, which is expected of a reasonably competent practitioner in the same class to which he belongs, acting in the same or similar circumstances.

It has to be proven that the patient had suffered loss or injury due to failure of the dentist to provide the applicable standard of care.

CONSENT–CONTRACT BETWEEN DOCTOR AND PATIENT

The object of consent in a medical treatment or a surgical procedure involving interference of human body is that every human being has a right vested with them to determine what should be and should not be done with their body. Any encroachment upon this right invites liability on the invader.

Responsibility of a doctor towards their patients begins the moment he/she agrees to examine the case. A doctor–patient relationship pertains to a legally binding contract wherein nowadays it has become obligatory as well as mandatory, to obtain a specific consent before the commencement of a treatment.

The *Indian Contract Act* defines consent: 'Two or more persons are said to consent when they agree upon the same thing in the same sense'.

INFORMED CONSENT

Consent may be written or implied. A patient approaching a medical practitioner for treatment impliedly gives their consent for medical procedures undertaken by the said doctor. Such a hypothetical consent when judged subjectively may expose the doctor to the danger of being accused by the patient, who by using the benefit of hindsight, would deny the fact of giving consent, even when full disclosure of methodology of treatment, risk involved in it and even side effects if any, had been clearly made aware beforehand. Therefore, to avoid accusations of this sort, it is always advisable to obtain a specifically written consent (i.e. an express consent) from the patient, which thereafter makes the contract unchallengeable on the grounds of 'lack of consent'. Express consent may compulsorily be obtained even in diagnostic procedures such as radiology, CT scan, etc. A legally valid consent is that obtained from the patient/his/her parent/guardian/attendant, as the situation warrants and not from a stranger to the scenario.

The goal of the informed consent is to provide patients with as much information as possible on any specific problems that the patient may have their relationship to overall health and methods of managing them.

Informed consent actually consists of three phases:

- Discussion
- Written consent
- Documentation in the patient's chart.

DISCUSSION

- Nature of the disease, injury or deformity
- Purpose, goals of treatment and consequences of not treating
- The proposed treatment
- Limitation of the treatment
- Anticipated or common side effects
- Possible complications of treatment and its frequency
- Type of anaesthesia to be used
- Treatment alternatives
- Uncertainties about final outcome, including a statement that the treatment has no absolute guarantees or warranties.

WRITTEN CONSENT

Once the discussion regarding the treatment is over, the dentist should get a written informed consent signed by the patient or the parent or legal guardian in case of children. This written consent includes all the discussions carried out between the doctor and the patient, described in easily understandable terms. Consents should be written in a language well understood by the patient. The consent form should not contain technical or medical terminologies. Consent must be obtained at a time when the patient is mentally capable of giving it.

Medical liability theory involves the concept of lack of consent to a procedure enabling a patient to recover damages, even if the medical procedure was successful. In a lawsuit for negligence, the patient needs only to prove that the treatment was in some way harmful and that was not disclosed by the doctor.

The written consent

1. Should be legible
2. Contains only those terms and abbreviations, which are comprehensible to similar licensees
3. Contains adequate identification of the patient
4. Indicates the date of all provided professional services
5. Contains pertinent and significant information concerning the patient's condition
6. Reflects what examinations, vital signs and tests were obtained, performed or ordered, findings and results of each
7. Indicates the initial diagnosis and the patient's initial reason for seeking the licensee's service
8. Indicates the medications prescribed, dispensed or administered and strength of each
9. Reflects the treatment performed or recommended
10. Documents the patient's progress during the course of treatment provided by the licensee.

DOCUMENTATION IN THE PATIENT'S CHART

The final phase of the informed consent procedure is to document in the patient's chart that an informed consent was obtained. The first documented information that is reviewed by the patient's attorney (in case if the patient sues the doctor) is this documented record. The document should include a note stating that the discussion took place. The written consent form should be included in the chart.

The following is the information that should be included in the chart:

1. Chief complaint
2. Clinical findings
3. Dental history
4. Medical history
5. Current medication
6. Drug allergies
7. Radiographic findings and interpretations
8. Recommended treatment
9. Informed consent
10. Therapy actually instituted
11. Suggested follow-up.

Other information often overlooked that should also be included in every chart are as follows:

1. Any medical prescriptions given to the patient
2. Date and time of appointments
3. Missed appointments
4. Any laboratory tests done and the results obtained
5. Postoperative instructions and care given
6. Discharge of the patient (with or without consent of the doctor).

Advantages of the informed consent

Apart from fulfilling the legal obligations, the informed consent has the following advantages:

- A patient who understands the nature of the problem well and has practical and sensible expectations is less likely to sue
- A documented informed consent prevents any claim based on misunderstanding or unrealistic expectations of the treatment by the patient.

Situations where informed consent is not taken

There are three special situations in which an informed consent may deviate from these guidelines:

- On the specific request of the patient, all the aspects of treatment and complications are not informed but this must be documented in the chart
- Sometimes it is not appropriate to provide all the information to the patient
- In case of an emergency or if the patient is unconscious, a doctor can lawfully operate on or give other treatment to the patient who is incapable of consenting to his doing so, provided that the operation or treatment is necessary to save life of the person or to save him from permanent disability or from unnecessary pain and sufferings.

Complications

Although the dentist takes extreme care and precision regarding the diagnosis, treatment planning and surgical technique, sometimes the final result is not satisfactory and desirable. In such cases, the dentist should make it a point to discuss the case frankly.

WHEN A PATIENT THREATENS TO SUE

Certain precautions have to be considered whenever a patient or his attorney threatens to sue the dentist against any malpractice.

- All such threats should be reported at once to the malpractice insurance carrier
- As far as possible, the dentist must not admit accountability or error. This is because admission or other information disclosed during discussions may ultimately be used against the dentist during lawsuit
- As a final point, it is very important that no alterations are made in the patient's dental record. Records must be handled carefully and should not be misplaced or destroyed.

PATIENT ABANDONMENT

Certain situation might arise wherein the dentist may be unable to complete a treatment plan scheduled for the patient.

Such problems include:

- Failure of the patient to return for the necessary appointments
- Failure of the patient to follow explicit instructions
- A total breakdown of communication and loss of rapport between the dentist and the patient.

To avoid being accused of patient abandonment, the dentist should follow certain steps before discontinuing.

1. A letter is sent to the patient, indicating the intention of the dentist to withdraw from the case and the unwillingness to provide further treatment
   a. The letter should be sent by certified mail and it should be made sure that it has been received by the patient
   b. The letter should be followed with a copy by regular mail
   c. Unless it is required by the state law, the dentist need not state a reason. Never offer incompatibility as justification
2. The patient's condition must be stable and not emergent. Care must be provided during the time frame (15–30 days) given to the patient to find a new provider.

CRIMINAL LIABILITY OF DOCTORS IN DEATH DURING MEDICAL PROCEDURES

A doctor is not criminally liable for his patient's death, unless his negligence or incompetence passes beyond a mere matter of compensation and shows such a disregard for the life and safety as to amount to an offence against the state.

Section 304-A deals with cases where a rash and negligent act results in the death of a person. Section 304-A reads 'Whoever causes death of a person by doing any rash or negligent act not amounting to culpable homicide shall be punished with imprisonment of either description for a term which may extend to 2 years or with fine or with both'. This section was added by an amendment of the IPC in 1870. Mere carelessness is not sufficient, but the act should result in the death of a person.

In order to impose a criminal liability on a doctor, it is necessary that the death should have been the direct result of a rash or negligent act of the accused and that act should be the proximate cause of the death.

An employer cannot be held guilty under the criminal law, where death or hurt (simple or grievous) has been caused by the rashness and negligence of his servant or employee. Hence, a doctor cannot be held liable under criminal law for any rash or negligent act done by their employee.

Section II

Diagnosis

Chapter 3

History Taking and Clinical Examination

OUTLINE

A CASE SHEET

The first step in treatment is the patient evaluation, it allows the development of a clinical diagnosis (Fig. 3.1).

Importance of case history:

a. For making correct diagnosis and treatment plan
b. Assessment of patient's mental and behavioural status
c. Awareness of any systemic diseases
d. To know the exact nature of medication the patient is taking
e. For research purposes
f. Expression of interest, warmth and compassion by clinicians, encourages patients to communicate their concerns.

In this chapter, we will see a brief note on history taking and clinical examination. It is important for the clinician to have the knowledge of various pathologic entities that involve the region before getting any information from history and clinical examination.

The information that we receive from the patient acts as the clinical database and helps during medicolegal issues, thus it is important that it be done in a sequential manner.

- Complete history taking
- Clinical examination
- Photographs
- Radiographic and other laboratory investigations
- Diagnosis
- Treatment plan.

HISTORY TAKING

It is important for the clinician to establish good communication with the patient to assess patient's need and best treatment to the clinical situation.

PERSONAL INFORMATION

a. Name: Doctor– patient communication becomes easier and better
b. Age: Age-related diseases, age-related dosage for drugs
c. Sex: Sex predominance in certain diseases
d. Address: Helps in communication; regional predominance in certain diseases
e. Occupation: Some diseases are occupational hazards

CHIEF COMPLAINTS

- Patient is asked to describe the problem or the reason for seeking treatment along with duration
- Should be recorded in patient's own words

HISTORY OF PRESENTING ILLNESS

History of presenting illness is a detailed account of the chief complaint. The clinician asks questions to receive more information *in chronological order* of the presenting complaint or illness. The history procured is taken down in the following order:

1) Mode of onset of the problem
2) Site along with duration of the complaint
3) Rate of growth
   a) Slowly growing (months to years) lesions are reactive hyperplasia, cysts, benign tumours
   b) Moderately growing masses (few weeks to months) are chronic infections, cysts, malignant tumours
   c) Rapidly growing masses (hours to days) are abscesses, infected cysts, aneurysms, salivary extravasation/retention phenomena, haematomas
4) Swellings
   a) Swelling recurring only during eating are usually sialolithiasis

CASE HISTORY SHEET

Personal Information:

Name: Age/Sex: Date:
Address:

Reg. No.:
Occupation:
Address: Religion/Race:

Chief Complaints:
History of present illness:
Past medical or injury history:
Family history:

Personal history:
Habits:
Income:
Diet:
Type of Work:

Drug/Allergies history:

General Physical Examination:

General appearance – conscious/apprehensive/lethargic/unconscious
Development
Built
Gait
General Condition: Fair/moderate/poor

Temperature:
Pulse (rate/rhythm/character):
Respiration (rate/character):
Blood Pressure:
Pallor:

Cyanosis: Central/Peripheral
Icterus:
Clubbing:
Edema feet:
Dyspnea:
Lymph nodes:
Peripheral pulsations: Present/Absent
Auscultation: HS:
RS:
Palpation abdomen: Soft/Tender/Non Tender/Guarding
Palpation liver & spleen:
Local Examination:
Extra oral:
Intra oral:
Provisional Diagnosis:
Radiographic Examination
Investigations:
Routine:
TLC:
DLC:
Hb%:
BT:
CT:
ESR:
Urine examination for Albumin:
Sugar:
Microscopic examination:
Plasma Sugar → Fasting:
→ Post prandial

Final Diagnosis:
Treatment plan:

Figure 3.1 Oral surgery case sheet for diagnosis and treatment plan.

   b) Swelling associated with fever are seen in infections, lymphomas
5) Associating factors
   a) Association with pain
   b) Any history of associated fever or rigors, if any, how long?
   c) Is it associated with the tooth?
   d) Any associated discharge or secondary changes
      i) Purulent discharge—infected cyst, abscess
      ii) Serosanguineous—carcinomatous ulcer
      iii) Bluish black discharge—actinomycosis
6) Aggravating factors
7) Relieving factors
8) Previous treatments.

PAST MEDICAL HISTORY

Past medical history must include details on the patient's medical illness in the past.

1) Serious significant illness pertaining to the system
   a) ***CVS:*** Myocardial infarction, angina pectoris, congestive cardiac failure, rheumatic heart disease, congenital heart diseases, valvular disease, infective endocarditis and hypertension
   b) ***RS:*** Bronchial asthma, bronchitis, chronic obstructive pulmonary disease (COPD)
   c) ***GI:*** Peptic ulcer, gastritis, cirrhosis, jaundice, hepatitis, diarrhoea, vomiting, loss of appetite
   d) ***GU:*** Pregnancy, postpartum, lactation, periodicity of menstrual cycle, oral contraceptives
   e) ***Endocrine:*** Hyperthyroidism, diabetes mellitus, Addison disease, Cushing syndrome, hyperparathyroidism—Brown's tumour (Fig. 3.2A)
   f) ***CNS:*** Seizures, hemiplegia, previous head injury, psychiatric disorders
   g) ***Bleeding/clotting disorders:*** Haemophilia, anticoagulant therapy, ITP
   h) ***Autoimmune disorders:*** SLE, scleroderma, long-term steroid therapy
   i) ***Infectious disease:*** Tuberculosis, acquired immunodeficiency syndrome (AIDS), herpes, hepatitis
   j) ***Psychiatric aliments:*** Stress/anxiety disorders, patient on antidepressants
   k) ***Renal disorders:*** Renal failure, dialysis
2) Previous hospitalisations
3) Blood transfusion history
4) Allergy to pharmacotherapeutic agents or other allergies: Local anaesthetics, penicillin, other antibiotics, metal allergy
5) Pregnancy

DRUG HISTORY

Medication history is elucidated with the patient. Any medication being taken for any systemic illness with dosage

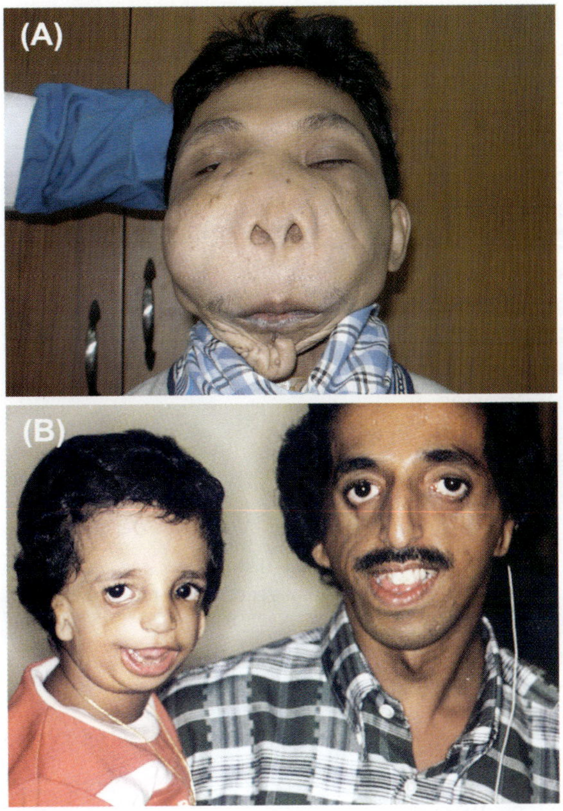

Figure 3.2 (A) Brown tumour of bilateral nasomaxillary complex in a known case of hyperparathyroidism. (B) Treacher Collins syndrome—father and son.

and duration is noted. Some diseases or lesions can be caused due to these drugs. Over-the-counter drugs such as nonsteroidal antiinflammatory drugs (NSAIDs) should also be noted down. Other important drugs such as corticosteroids, anticoagulants, antiepileptic drug and antidepressants should be recorded as they can interfere with the use of local anaesthetics and dental treatment.

PAST SURGICAL HISTORY

Detailed past surgical history with diagnosis, procedure and postsurgical details is mandatory.

Any history of blood transfusions, allergies, complications due to general anaesthetics/muscle relaxants/reversing agents used needs to be elicited. Any history of treatment of facial bone fractures and usage of rigid fixation implants.

PAST DENTAL HISTORY

History of past dental treatments undertaken should be elicited.

1. History of extraction, scaling, filling, root canal treatments, minor surgical procedures
2. History of any implants, prosthesis used
3. History of allergy, complication due to local anaesthetics
4. Eventful/uneventful postextraction period.

Any history of invasive dental treatments, conservative treatment and any prosthetic appliance should be noted.

FAMILY HISTORY

The family history gives details on diseases that may be influenced by genetic causes such as migraine, psychological disorders, immune related conditions and systemic illness such as endocrine disorders, cardiovascular disorders, etc. The clinician can receive the following information.

1. Age and health status of parents, siblings and children
2. Cause of death of deceased family members
3. History of parental consanguinity
4. Any history suggestive of hypertension, diabetes, neoplasia, bleeding disorders, facial deformities, infectious diseases
5. History of similar defect or disorder in the parent or immediate relative indicating inheritance (Fig. 3.2B).

SOCIAL AND OCCUPATIONAL HISTORY

1. ***Social:*** Identify psychosomatic disturbances, history of recent travel
2. ***Occupation:*** Physical and environmental factors with emotional strains and stresses may be reflected in the oral cavity.
   - Silicosis, berylliosis—Glass factory workers
   - Hepatitis and HIV risk—Commercial sex workers, health care workers and surgeons.

PERSONAL HISTORY

1. ***Diet:*** Vegetarian or non-vegetarian
2. ***Brushing habits***
3. ***Tobacco abuse:*** Which form of tobacco consumption, duration of habit and frequency of use
4. ***Alcohol abuse:*** Duration, quantity and frequency
5. ***Other habits:*** Cigarette, paan masala, gutkha.

CLINICAL EXAMINATION

Examination of the patient represents the second stage of diagnostic procedure. Under clinical examination, the first step will be general examination, followed by systemic and local examination. The systemic examination contains inspection, palpation, percussion and auscultation of the physiological systems.

GENERAL EXAMINATION

1. Patient's general state of mind, whether calm and quiet or any discomfort, restlessness
   - Level of consciousness
2. Ambulatory or nonambulatory
3. Gait disturbances (gait—patient's walk)
   - Types of gait—staggering, wadding, ataxic gait, shuffling, etc.

4. Built—well-built/moderately built/poorly built
5. Nourishment—well-nourished/undernourished
6. Pallor
   - It is the pale colour of the skin and mucous membranes. Seen at the palpebral part of the conjunctiva, tongue, soft palate, palm and nails
   - Causes—anaemia, shock, peripheral vascular disease
7. Icterus
   - It is the clinical sign to diagnose jaundice
   - Presents with yellowish discoloration of bulbar part of conjunctiva, nail, skin and mucosa
   - Caused by bile pigment load to the liver
8. Cyanosis
   - Bluish discoloration of the skin and mucosa (Hb less than 5 g%)
   - Types of cyanosis—central, peripheral, mixed, differential
9. Clubbing
   - Bulbous swelling of the nail bed of the fingers and toes
   - Grades—I, II and III
   - Common causes—bronchitis, interstitial lung disease, Chron's disease, cyanotic congenital heart disease, acromegaly, etc.
10. Ecchymosis and petechiae
    - Haemorrhagic discolouration on the skin or mucous membrane
    - Petechiae are less than 1 mm in diameter
11. Oedema—collection of fluid in the interstitial spaces
    - Pitting oedema
    - Non-pitting oedema
12. Structural deformities or alterations—for example, syndactyly, kyphosis, scoliosis, etc.
13. Psychological status
14. Vital signs
    - Temperature
    - Pulse rate
    - Respiratory rate
    - Blood pressure.

SYSTEMIC EXAMINATION

A systematic examination of the general body systems including cardiovascular, gastrointestinal, central nervous and genitourinary systems is carried out. Any relevant abnormalities are documented. This is not usually done in detail in a dental setup.

LOCAL EXAMINATION

EXTRAORAL EXAMINATION

Inspection

A close observation of the abnormal area (lesion) is made. Then the lesion is compared to the normal architecture of the structure giving consideration for age, gender and site. The spectrum of the change can range from complete absence as in aplasia to extensive overgrowth (neoplastic). This comparison of abnormal to normal tissues should be carefully performed taking into account the principles of facial growth, bone remodelling, development of facial musculatures, as well as the extent of muscle activity.

The structural alteration could be as a result of:

1) Congenital anomalies
   a) Agenesis
   b) Hypoplasia
   c) Hyperplasia
2) Developmental anomalies
   a) Hypotrophy
   b) Hypertrophy
3) Traumatic
   a) Abrasion
   b) Erosion
   c) Ulceration
   d) Laceration
   e) Fractures
      i) Simple fracture
      ii) Compound fracture
      iii) Comminuted or greenstick fractures
   f) Avulsion
   g) Denervation
4) Neoplastic
   a) Nodular
   b) Ulcerative
   c) Papillomatous
   d) Proliferative
5) Infective
   a) Swelling
   b) Redness
   c) Loss of function.

Skin

Changes in the colour, texture of the skin/surrounding structures as well as the anomalous shape of the structure are noted in the soft tissue examination.

1) *Pallor*—anaemia
2) *Discolouration*—inflammation, haemangioma, SLE, ecchymosis, naevi, melanoma, etc.
3) *Texture*—proliferative lesion such as squamous cell carcinoma

Eye

Though ophthalmic examination needs to be performed by a specialist, certain basic findings need to be elicited before arriving at a provisional diagnosis

1) Presence/absence of structures of the eye
2) Intercanthal distance: Increased—hypertelorism, decreased—hypotelorism
3) Interorbital distance
4) Interpupillary distance
5) Eye movements: Extraocular muscles
6) Asymmetry in movement and at rest: Strabismus
7) Proptosis, exophthalmos: Hyperthyroidism
8) Subconjunctival haemorrhage: Circumorbital oedema, enophthalmos.

External ear (pinna)

1) Anotia: Complete absence of external ear
2) Positional changes: Low set ears
3) Change in morphology of the external ear: Microtia, bat ears, cupped ears
4) Ear bleed: For example, condylar fracture
5) Discharge: For example, middle ear infection.

Nose

Changes in size, shape, symmetry of the nasal structures, such as the ala, columella, septum, dorsum and the nasion, should be examined and documented. Congenital deformities such as the cleft, hemiarhinia, hypertelorism, encephalocoele are accompanied by nasal deformities pathognomonic to the nature of the lesion.

1) Asymmetric ala, septum and dorsum: Unilateral cleft lip nose
2) Depressed nasal bridge, shortened columella and broad nasal base: Bilateral cleft lip nose
3) Discharge from the nose: Epistaxis, CSF rhinorrhoea (trauma)
4) Regurgitation of fluids: Oronasal fistula
5) Septal deviation.

Lips

The colour, contour, size, shape and symmetry of the lip are examined.

1) Colour change: Haemangiomas
2) Contour: Cleft, lip pits, tumours
3) Size: Macrostomia
4) Asymmetry: Facial palsy.

Palpation

Palpation is for the confirmation of inspectatory findings. Palpation of each region is described in detail in the following sections.

Jaw movements and mouth opening

1) Protrusion, retrusion and lateral movements are assessed to detect any deviation from midline (Fig 3.3A)
2) Mouth opening: It is assessed as maximal interincisal distance measured from maxillary to mandibular central incisors. In case of edentulous patient, alveolar ridge of both jaws (Fig 3.3B)
   - **Staging of functional mouth opening** (Fig. 3.3C–F)
     - M1—Interincisal mouth opening more than 35 mm
     - M2—Interincisal mouth opening between 25 and 35 mm
     - M3—Interincisal mouth opening between 15 and 25 mm
     - M4—Interincisal mouth opening less than 15 mm.

Temporomandibular joint (TMJ) examination

1. The TMJ is examined bilaterally in the preauricular area. Palpate directly over the joint with index finger when the mandibular movements are made. The joints can be palpable by two methods:
   a. Intra-aural (finger through the external auditory meatus)
   b. Preauricular (anterior to tragus).

The abnormalities such as tenderness, clicking or popping sounds are observed during opening, closing of the mouth and during both vertical and lateral movements.

2. The joint may also be auscultated for crepitus or popping sounds. Detailed description on examination and diagnosis of TMJ disorders has been explained in Chapter 37.

Lymph nodes examination

Lymph nodes are tissue aggregations that are a part of the adaptive immune system. These nodes are connected by the lymphatic system. It drains the lymph from different sites of the body to bigger lymph trunks that drain into the veins. The lymph nodes examined in the head drain into those of the neck called cervical nodes, which in turn drain into the jugular trunk. Clinical conditions like infection, malignancy can cause these regional nodes to swell. The nodes of the head have been described in Table 3.1.

1) ***Size***: Nodes are generally considered to be normal if they are up to 1 cm in diameter and become palpable only when enlarged
2) ***Pain/tenderness:*** When a lymph node increases in size, its capsule stretches and causes pain. Pain is usually the

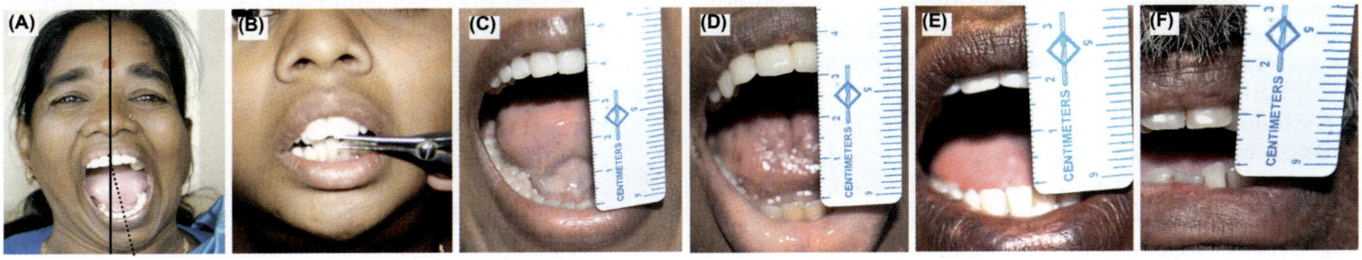

Figure 3.3 (A) Deviation on mouth opening due to TMJ internal derangement. (B) Limitation in mouth opening—trismus. (C–F): Staging of mouth opening (C) M1—Interincisal mouth opening more than 35 mm (D) M2—Interincisal mouth opening between 25 and 35 mm. (E) M3—Interincisal mouth opening between 15 and 25 mm. (F) M4—Interincisal mouth opening less than 15 mm.

TABLE 3.1 Lymph Nodes of the Head with the Areas of Drainage

Major lymph nodes of the head		Drainage
Ventral side (Face)	Submental lymph nodes	• Bilateral—From tip of tongue • Unilateral—Anterior 2/3rd of tongue • Anterior part of floor of mouth to submental nodes to the upper deep cervical nodes • Lower incisors to submental nodes to the submandibular and ends with lower deep cervical nodes
	Submandibular lymph nodes	• Posterior part of floor of mouth • Anterior part of hard palate • Maxillary sinus • All teeth either directly to submandibular nodes or may continue to upper deep cervical lymph nodes • Anterior 2/3rd of the tongue
	Buccal nodes	Anterior cheek, drains into the submandibular nodes
	Parotid lymph nodes or the preauricular lymph nodes	Conjunctiva, skin of the cheek, eyelids, and temporal region of the scalp
Dorsal side (back of the head)	Mastoid or the postauricular lymph nodes	Temporoparietal region, the upper part of the ear and the external auditory meatus. The lymph then drains into the deep cervical lymph nodes
	Occipital lymph nodes	From occipital region of the scalp, drains into the deep cervical lymph nodes

result of any inflammatory process or suppuration, but may also result from haemorrhage into the necrotic centre of a malignant node

3) **Consistency:**
   a) Soft nodes—infections or inflammatory conditions
      i) Tender, mobile, enlarged—Acute infection
      ii) Nontender, mobile, enlarged —Chronic infection.
   b) Stony hard, fixed, enlarged—carcinoma usually metastatic, squamous cell carcinoma
   c) Firm rubbery nodes, enlarged—lymphoma
   d) Suppurant nodes—fluctuant
   e) Shotty nodes—refers to small nodes that feel like buckshot under the skin, as found in the cervical nodes of children with viral illness
   f) Matted nodes, nontender—A group of nodes that feel connected and seem to move as a unit. Nodes that are matted could be benign like in tuberculosis, sarcoidosis, lymphogranuloma venereum or malignant such as metastatic carcinoma
4) ***Location:*** Localised lymphadenopathy is based on the infection or lesion in the node per se or in its drainage area
   - Oral infection: Submandibular/submental
   - Tonsillitis: Upper jugular nodes.

Lymphatic drainage of the scalp, face and oral cavity

- The lymph of the skin of the scalp drains into the occipital, mastoid and parotid nodes (Figs 3.4, 3.5)
- The lower eye lid and malar areas drain into the buccal nodes, which drain into the submandibular lymph nodes
- The posterior cheek area drains into the parotid, buccal and submandibular nodes
- The upper lip and area lateral to the lower lip drain into the submandibular nodes
- The medial middle third of the lower lip cross over and drains into the submental nodes
- The upper and lower gingivae drain into the submandibular, submental and upper deep cervical lymph nodes.
- The palatal lymph vessels primarily drain into the submandibular and then into the superior deep cervical nodes (level II)
- All teeth drain into the submandibular and deep cervical lymph nodes. The anterior floor of mouth drains into submental and upper deep cervical nodes, while the posterior part into submandibular and upper deep cervical.

To understand the lymphatic spread of oral cancer, it is important for the clinician to have a sound knowledge of the lymph nodes draining the head and neck region (refer Chapter 30, page 623)

Salivary glands examination

Parotid gland

Parotid gland swelling typically presents as preauricular swelling elevating the ear lobule. In case of glandular swelling, the location, size and shape of the swelling are assessed as for any other swelling. Motor nerve function of facial or

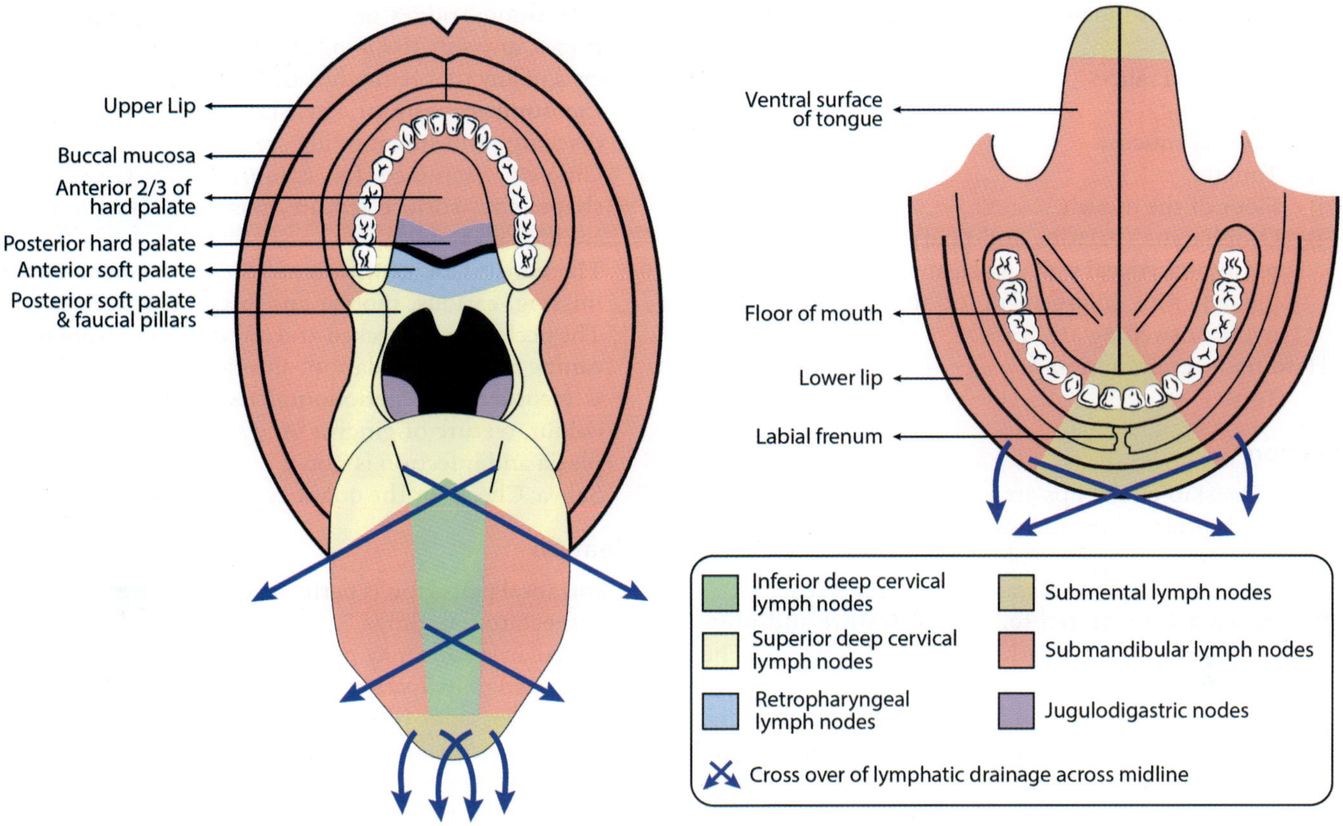

Figure 3.4 Lymphatic drainage of the oral cavity.

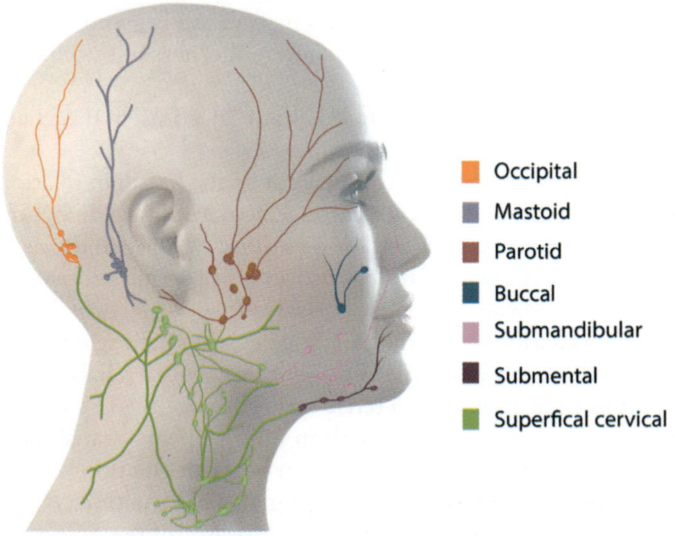

Figure 3.5 Lymph nodes of head and neck—lymphatic drainage of the scalp and face.

ipsilateral side should be assessed to rule out nerve compression or involvement. Intraorally, any inflammation or pus discharge from the duct opening is noted (Fig. 3.6A).

Sublingual and submandibular glands

Bimanual palpation of the gland is done with index fingers, one intraorally and the other extraorally, medial to the lower

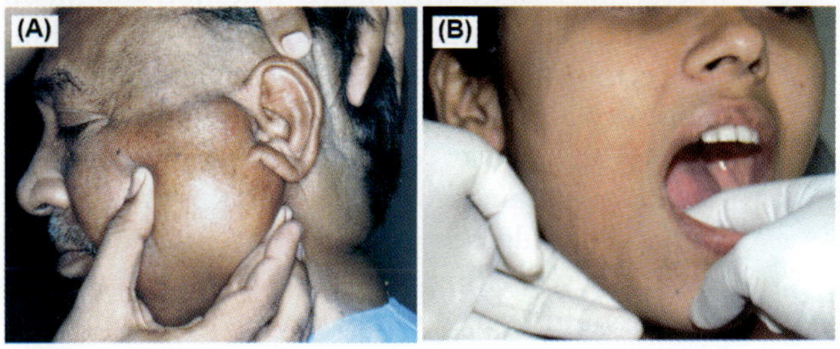

Figure 3.6 (A) Examination of parotid gland swelling. (B) Bimanual palpation.

border of the mandible (Fig. 3.6B). Intraorally, the openings of the duct are identified and any inflammation, quality of salivary flow and pus discharge are noted.

INTRAORAL EXAMINATION

After extraoral examination, intraoral examination is done. Intraoral examination is divided into the soft tissue examination and the hard tissue examination.

Oral cavity

1) Soft tissue examination
    a) Lips
    b) Labial mucosa
    c) Buccal mucosa

   d) Maxillary and mandibular mucobuccal and lingual sulcus
   e) Palate and fauces
   f) Gingiva
   g) Alveolar mucosa
   h) Tongue
   i) Floor of the mouth
   j) Oropharynx (palatine and pharyngeal tonsils, posterior pharyngeal wall, uvula, anterior and posterior pillars). Any enlargement of tonsil, deviation of uvula or swelling are noted.
2) Hard tissue examination
   a) Teeth

Inspection

1. Lips: The skin of the lips are examined, the colour, texture, and surface abnormalities are recorded. Angular or vertical fissures, lip pits, cold sores, ulcers, scabs, nodules, sclerotic plaque and scars are also recorded
2. The mucosa is inspected for colour, texture and presence of ulcerations, growth or draining sinuses. The size of the tongue, surface and mobility are inspected. Then the tongue is depressed to visualise the uvula, soft palate. Any deviation to the uvula, abnormal movement of soft palate, mass at the base of the tongue are identified
   a. Labial mucosa: The minor salivary glands and granules are examined and recorded
   b. Buccal mucosa: Change in pigmentation and mobility of the buccal mucosa is noted. Pronounced linea alba is a common finding. Other pathological lesions such as leukoedema, intraoral swellings, ulcers, nodules, scars, other red and white patches are noted
   c. Maxillary and mandibular mucobuccal and lingual sulcus: The sulcus is examined for mucosal colour, texture, any swelling or fistula. The labial and lingual frenulum are examined and the attachment level is recorded
   d. Palate and fauces are inspected for discoloration, swelling, fistula, hyperplasia, tori, ulcers, hyperkeratinisation, asymmetry of structure, function and anatomy
   e. Tongue: Dorsal and ventral aspect of the tongue are examined for any swelling, ulcer, and variations in colour, size and texture
   f. The floor of the mouth is examined for any inflammation. The Wharton's duct is examined for abnormalities. The mucosa is examined for presence of any slough or membrane, mass, hematoma is noted
   g. Oropharynx is examined for any pathologies on the tonsils and pharynx (note for colour, size and surface abnormalities)
3. The salivary gland orifices are examined for any signs of inflammation or pus discharge
4. Edentulous ridges are examined for the form of the ridges, any soft tissue or bony abnormalities, and presence of any root remnants. In cases of ulcer and swelling, the number, position, site, size, shape, the floor, edges, discharge and surrounding area are noted
5. Gingiva: Examined for colour, contour, consistency, shape, size, surface texture, position, sinuses, fistulas, swelling and ulcers
6. The hard tissue dentition are then examined, a note of missing, carious, mobile and malposed teeth is made. The occlusion is checked and any deviation from normal canine and molar relation, anterior open bite, deep bite is recorded. The periodontal tissues are examined for colour, texture of gingiva. Any sign of recession, hyperplasia and infection is noted
7. Saliva: Check for the quantity and quality of saliva.

Palpation

1. Intraoral palpation is performed for the confirmation of inspectatory findings
2. Vascular lesions may produce a bruit, which can be appreciated on palpation
   An extraosseous or intraosseous swelling is palpated to record the consistency and the extent of the swelling. By palpation, the swelling is noted if it is sessile or pedunculated. On palpation, the local temperature is always raised in all acute inflammatory swellings
3. Gingiva is examined for bleeding on probing and exudation on pressure
   Palpate the mucobuccal sulcus for swelling and tenderness over the roots of teeth and tenderness of buccinator insertion
4. In ulcers, tenderness, mobility and bleeding of ulcers are also appreciated on palpation
   - The size, position and extent of the lesion in relation to the underlying anatomic structures are of significance in diagnosis (e.g. a midline swelling in the neck that moves with deglutition and tongue protrusion is indicative of thyroglossal cyst)
5. Fluctuation is characteristic of cystic swellings, that is swelling which contains fluid. It is usually a reliable sign, but may be absent in tense cysts
6. Swelling that contains clear fluid appears translucent (e.g. Ranula-bluish translucent mass in the floor of the mouth due to submandibular gland obstruction)
7. Swelling arising from the skin, for example papilloma, cutaneous wart epithelioma, moves with the movement of skin. When the skin is fixed, it can neither be moved nor be pinched up. This occurs in inflammatory conditions and carcinomas. The skin over a rapidly growing mass as sarcomas may be stretched making it immobile though not fixed. Thrill is palpable murmur commonly found in arteriovenous malformation. Once the clinical examination is complete, the radiological

studies and biochemical investigations will support the final diagnosis.

Auscultation

- All pulsatile swellings as aneurysms or AV malformations should be auscultated
- Temporomandibular joint: Clicks, crepitus
- Neck: Carotid bruits.

Examination for pressure effects

1) Mandibular swelling compresses the inferior alveolar canal and can cause paraesthesia of the inferior alveolar nerve dermatome (e.g. ameloblastoma)
2) Parotid swelling compressing on the facial nerve can cause facial paralysis or palsy, as in malignant pleomorphic adenoma.

Examination of aspiration fluid

Aspiration is the last part of examination of the swelling as it is invasive. Aspiration is done only in cystic and fluid-filled masses. It should be performed only with large wide bore (18-gauge) needle. The aspirated content may contribute to the diagnosis of the lesion. In suspected vascular lesions, aspiration is contraindicated.

1) Straw coloured fluid: Dentigerous cyst, periapical cyst
2) Curdy white: Odontogenic keratocyst
3) Frank pus: Abscess or infected cyst
4) Negative aspiration: Stafne bone cyst (traumatic bone cyst)
5) Blood: AV malformations, haemangioma.

DIAGNOSIS

Diagnosis is defined as the identification of disease after clinical examination and proper investigation of the clinical signs and symptoms. Though diagnosis can be arrived at using clinical examination alone, some diseases require further investigation using special aids. Diagnosis is arrived at by a hypothetico-deductive process, which is refined in every stage of investigation performed on the patient. When the patient presents with a complaint, the clinician elicits the history and performs the preliminary clinical examination to arrive at a 'provisional diagnosis' and 'differential diagnosis'. Based on this provisional diagnosis, relevant investigations are advised to confirm the diagnosis. While an array of diagnostic tools is now available to the clinician, these investigative tools are expensive and sometimes invasive. Therefore, a good provisional diagnosis based on history and clinical examination will reduce the risk and economic burden. Sometimes definitive diagnosis may not precede treatment too. In many cases, the final diagnosis or 'definitive diagnosis' can only be arrived after removal of the lesion and by examining it under a microscope to determine its histopathology.

BOX 3.1 Provisional and Differential Diagnosis

- **Provisional Diagnosis** - To identify oral disease, process and to distinguish one disease from the other.
- **Differential Diagnosis** - It is the process of identifying a condition by differentiating it from all pathological processes that produce a similar lesion.

Based on the chief complaint and the preliminary clinical examination, the clinician arrives at the provisional diagnosis and differential diagnosis (Box 3.1).

DIAGNOSTIC TOOLS

The most commonly used diagnostic tools are broadly classified as follows:

- Radiological examination
- Haematological investigation
- Biochemical investigation
- Microbiological investigation
- Salivary diagnostics
- Histopathological examination.

RADIOGRAPHIC EXAMINATIONS

Though diagnosis can be arrived at using clinical examination alone, some diseases require further investigation using radiographic examination (refer Chapter 4).

INVESTIGATION

Most lesions of the oral and maxillofacial region can be diagnosed using clinical and radiological investigation alone. In lesions that require histopathological analysis, biopsy or FNAC is performed and histopathological diagnosis becomes the final diagnosis. In conditions where the cause is microbial, this is usually performed by haematological or biochemical analysis of the blood (refer Chapter 5).

FINAL DIAGNOSIS

Based on the provisional diagnosis, radiological studies and biochemical investigations, the final diagnosis is confirmed.

TREATMENT PLAN

A treatment plan is a sequential series of treatments by the concerned specialist or the clinician. It is designed to benefit the patient with the disease by evidence-based treatments. Prime importance is placed on eliminating or controlling the etiologic factor that has caused the disease. The secondary plan would be to repair all existing damage by the etiologic factor and the disease itself. The final plan would comprise of prevention and functional maintainability.

CASE FILES

CASE REPORTS ON EXTRAORAL FEATURES
(FIG. 3.7–3.15)

VARIOUS DEFORMITIES OF SKULL

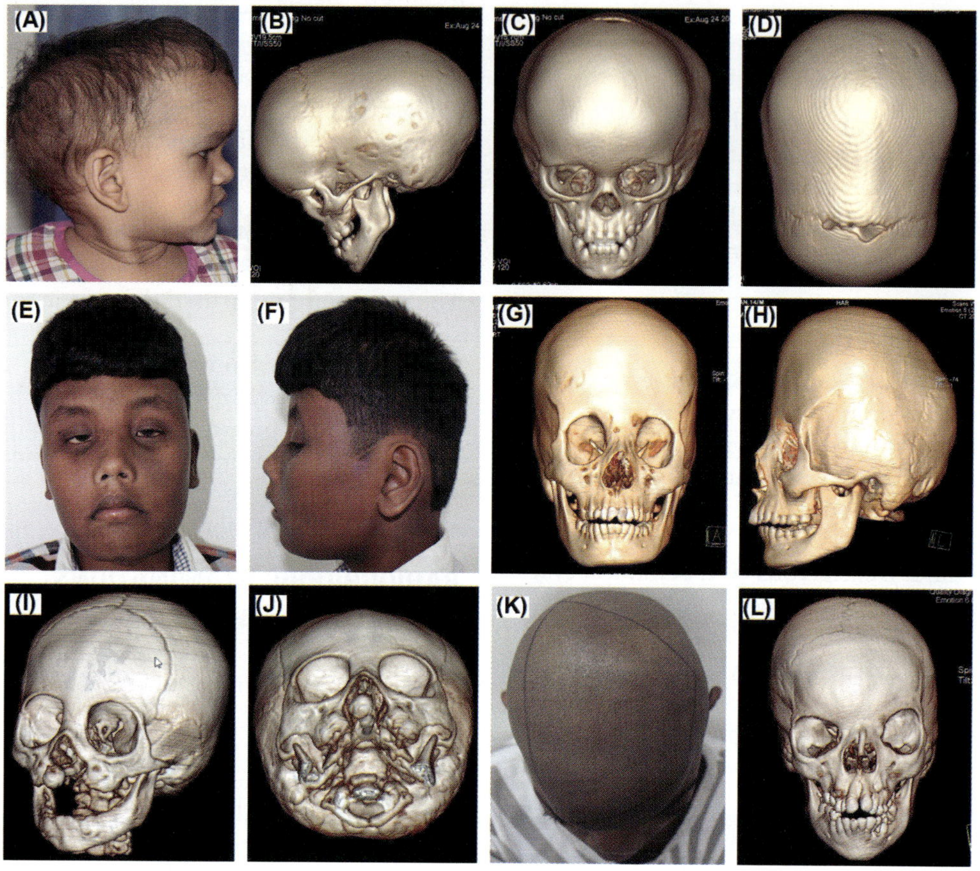

Figure 3.7 Various skull forms (A–D) Scaphocephaly–premature sagittal synostosis. (E–H) Turricephaly–tower head deformity–premature synostosis of bicoronal with other sutures. (I and J) Trigonocephaly–premature metopic suture synostosis. (K) Plagiocephaly showing flattened left forehead. (L) Premature fusion of left coronal suture.

DEFECTS AFFECTING THE LIPS

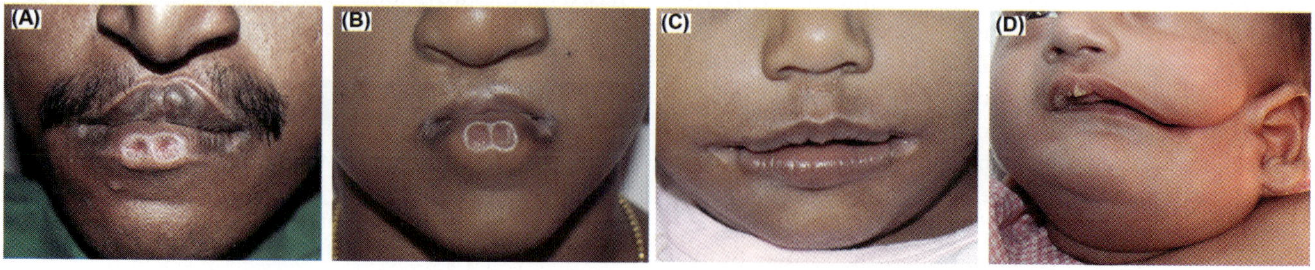

Figure 3.8 Defects affecting the lips. (A and B) Lip pits–lower lip (adult and child). (C) Macrostomia. (D) Lateral facial cleft.

DEFORMITIES ASSOCIATED WITH FACE

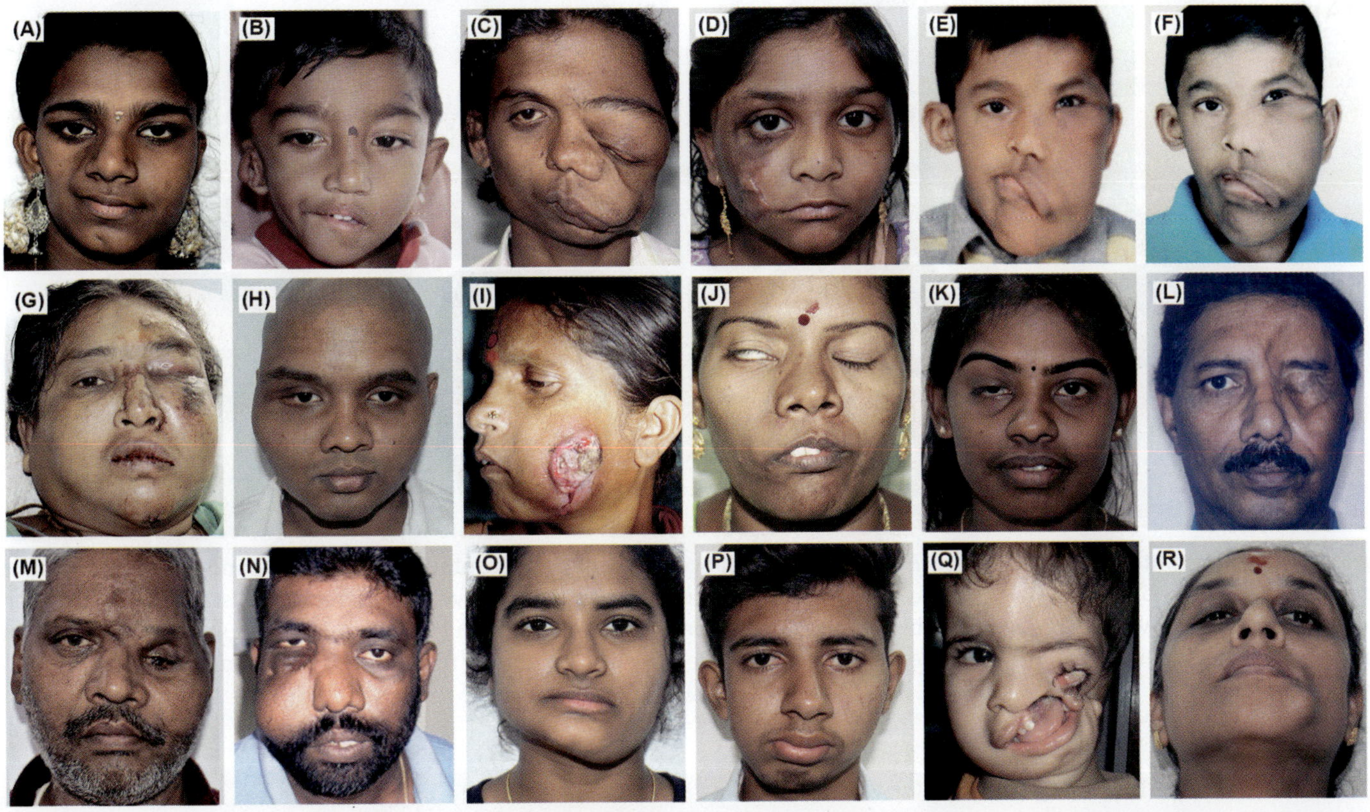

Figure 3.9 (A) Hemifacial atrophy (Parry Romberg syndrome). (B) Hemifacial microsomia (OMENS). (C) Plexiform neurofibromatosis. (D) Postburn scar. (E–F) Congenital facial lipomatosis involving left-sided face progressive with age. (G) Left canine space infection with orbital cellulitis. (H) Fibrous dysplasia. (I) Ulceroproliferative lesion—squamous cell carcinoma. (J) Complete facial palsy. Right lower motor neuron lesion (LMNL). (K) Ptosis of right upper eyelid. (L) Postsurgical ablation—loss of hard tissue-induced facial asymmetry. (M) Loss of hard tissue posttrauma. (N) Cementifying fibroma of right maxilla—superolateral displacement of right orbital contents. (O) Hemimandibular elongation. (P) Unilateral TMJ ankylosis with secondary deformity. (Q) Left orofacial cleft. (R) Facial asymmetry due to left mandibular osteoma.

SKIN CONDITIONS ON THE MAXILLOFACIAL REGION

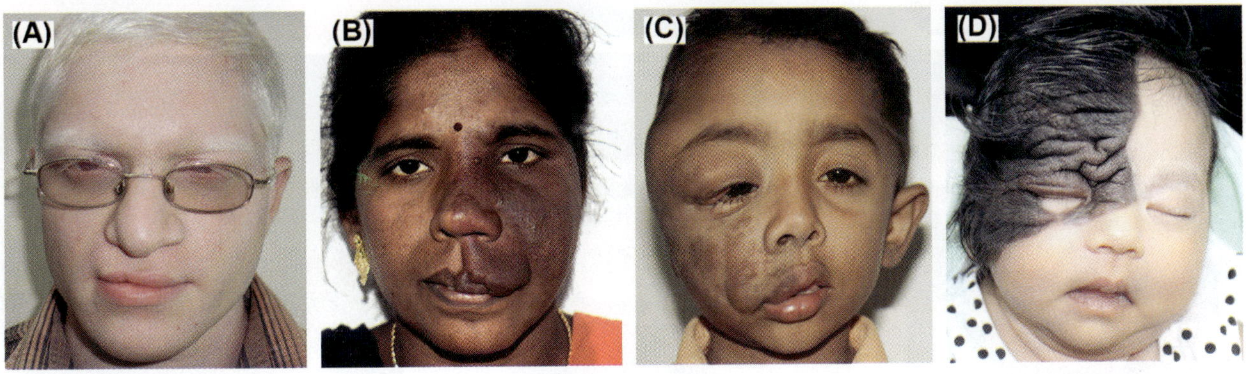

Figure 3.10 (A) Albinism. (B) Haemangioma. (C) Café-au-lait spots in neurofibromatosis. (D) Hairy naevus.

DEFECTS AFFECTING THE POSITION AND STRUCTURE OF THE EYES

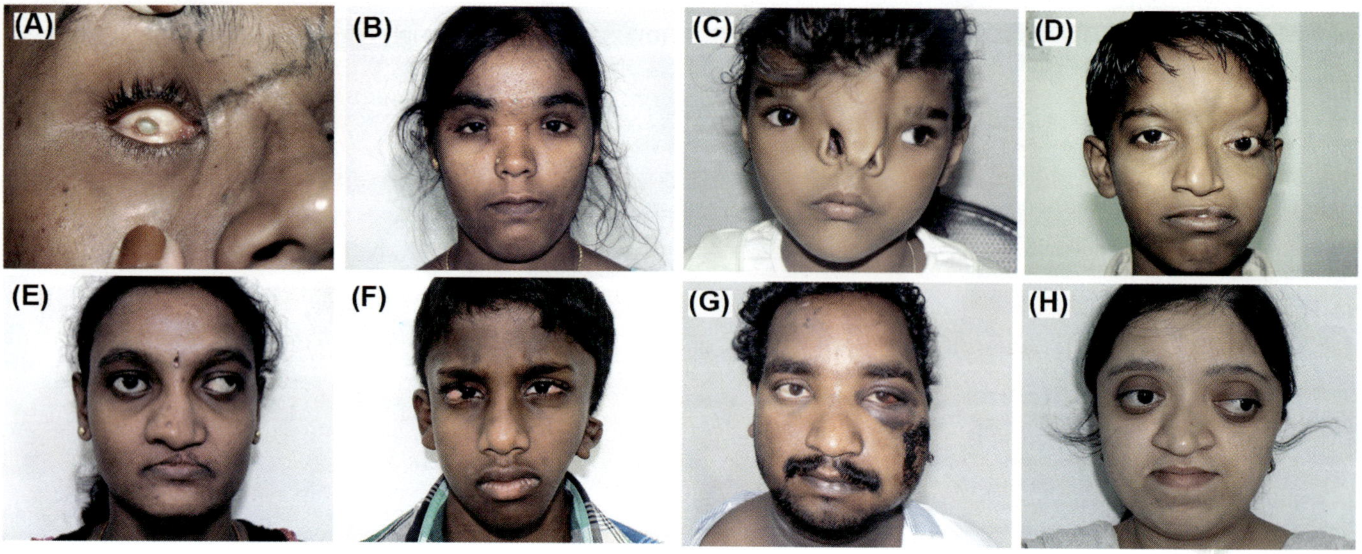

Figure 3.11 (A) Anophthalmia. (B) Increase in intercanthal distance—traumatic telecanthus (interpupillary and interorbital distance normal). (C) Increased interorbital distance—hypertelorism (increased interpupillary and interorbital distance). (D) Unilateral orbital hypertelorism with dystopia. (E) Strabismus. (F) Goldenhar syndrome—mandibular hypoplasia, epibulbar dermoid with ear deformity. (G) Subconjunctival haemorrhage, circumorbital oedema, swelling due to trauma with abrasion. (H) Exophthalmos—Crouzon's syndrome.

DEFECTS AFFECTING THE POSITION AND STRUCTURE OF THE EARS

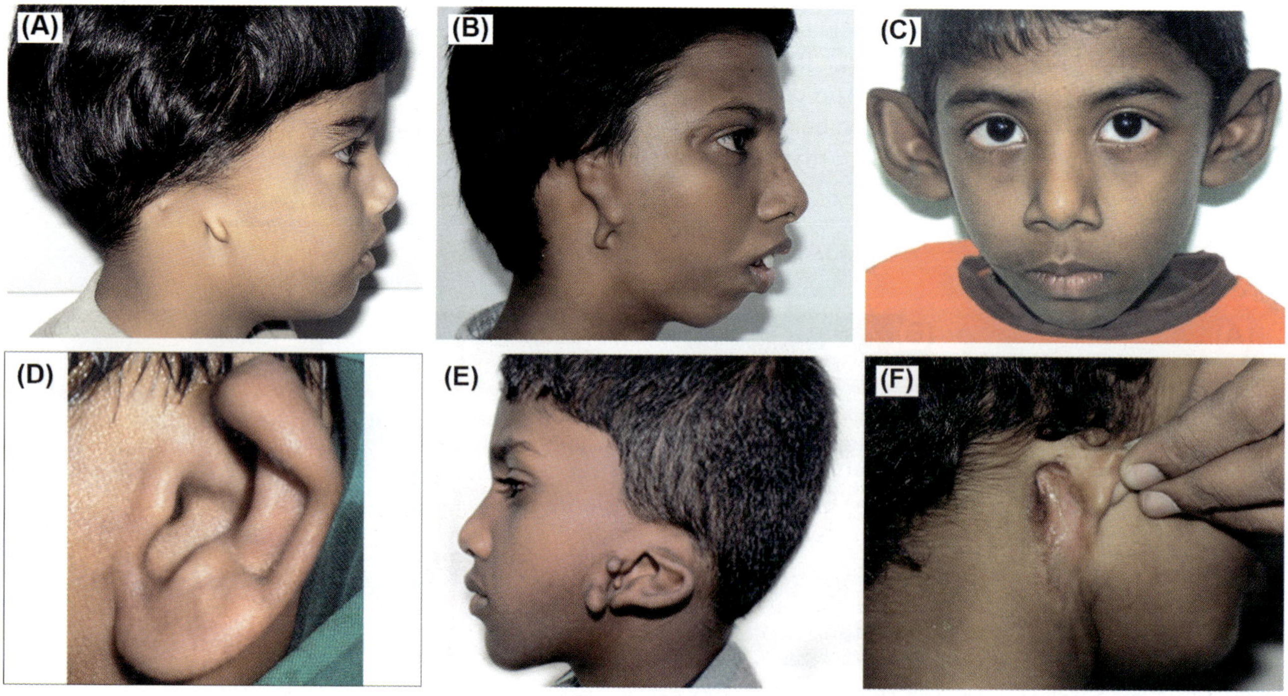

Figure 3.12 Defects affecting the position and structure of the ears (A) Anotia–absence of external ear. (B) Microtia. (C) Bat ear deformity. (D) Cup ear deformity. (E) Low set ear with pre-auricular skin tags. (F) First branchial cleft sinus.

DEFECTS AFFECTING THE POSITION AND STRUCTURE OF THE NOSE

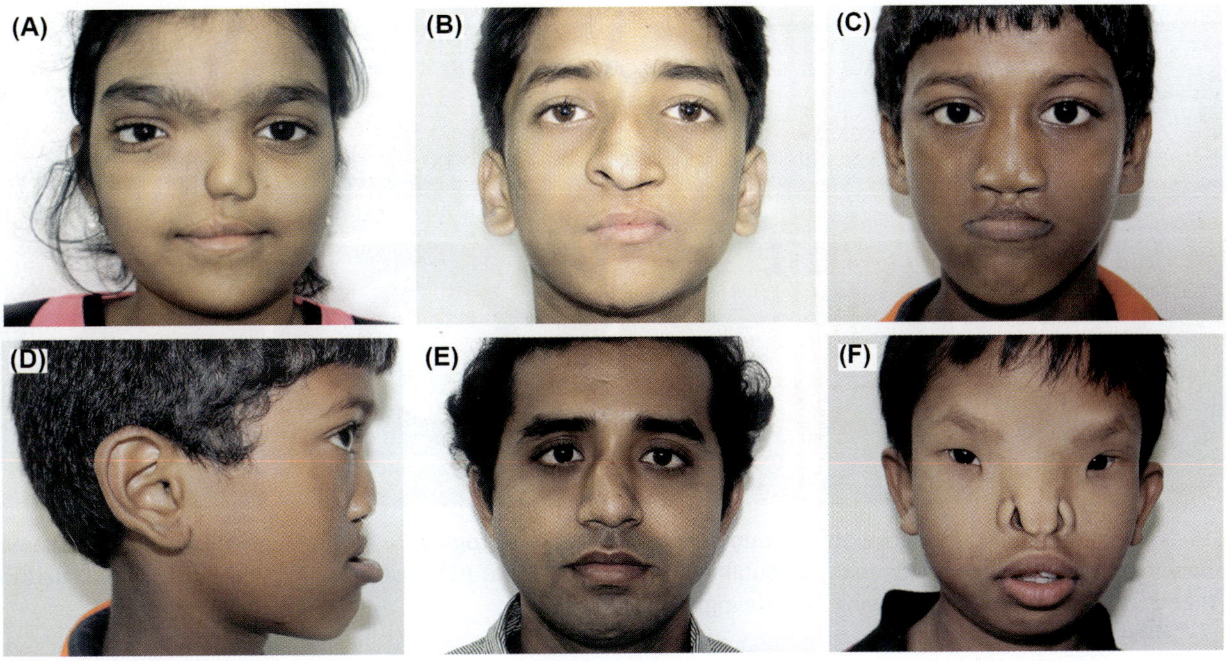

Figure 3.13 Defects affecting the position and structure of the nose. (A) Arhinia. (B) Asymmetric ala, septum and dorsum associated with unilateral cleft lip (operated). (C and D) Depressed nasal bridge, shortened columella and broad nasal base—bilateral cleft lip. (E) Deviated nasal septum. (F) Bilateral cleft ala.

CASE REPORTS ON INTRAORAL FEATURES

INTRAORAL PATHOLOGICAL LESIONS

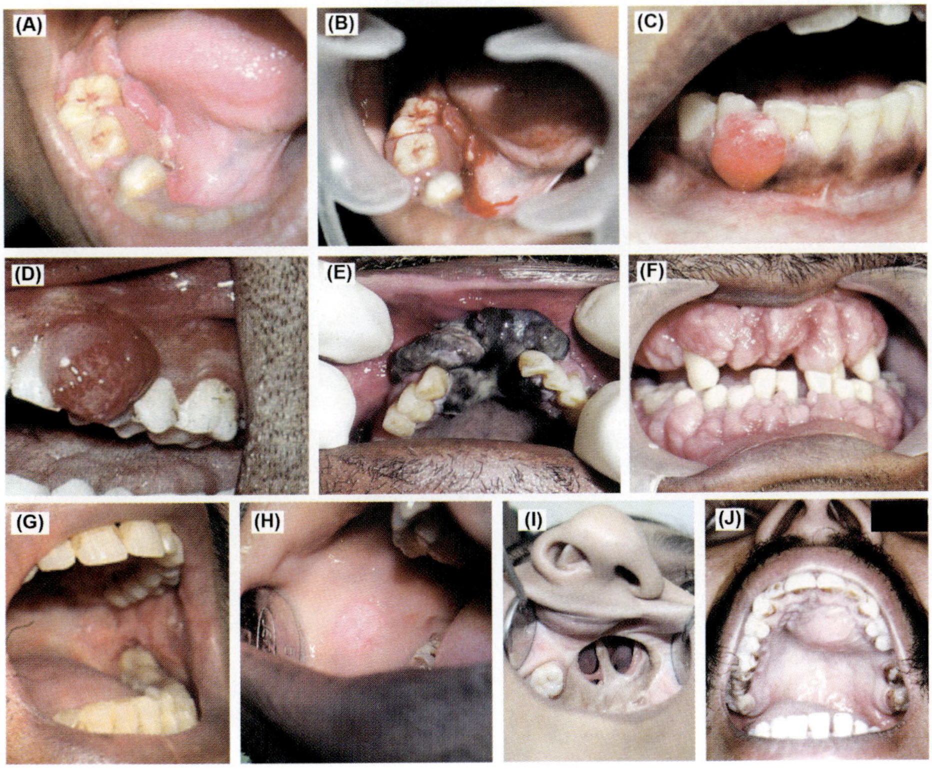

Figure 3.14 Intraoral pathological lesions. (A) Haemangioma—right retromolar region. (B) Bleeding on provocation. (C) Epulis. (D) Pyogenic granuloma. (E) Malignant melanoma. (F) Gingival fibromatosis. (G) Buccal mucosa showing alterations associated with submucous fibrosis. (H) Buccal mucosa showing altered texture in a white lesion. (I) Palatal fistula. (J) Palatal abscess due to fractured 22.

INTRAORAL PATHOLOGY OF THE TONGUE

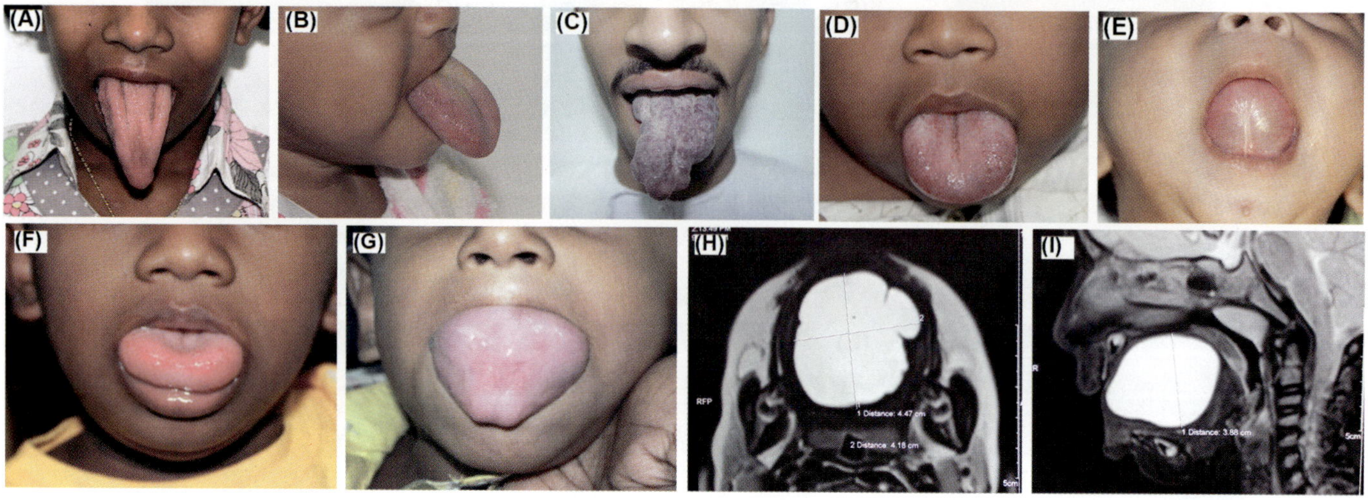

Figure 3.15 (A) Macroglossia. (B) Beckwith–Wiedemann syndrome—macroglossia. (C) Tongue enlargement—haemangioma. (D) Lymphangioma. (E) Sublingual dermoid. (F) Sublingual lymphangioma. (G) Cystic swelling within the musculature of the tongue. (H and I) MRI with contrast showing an intralingual cystic mass.

Chapter 4

Radiodiagnosis

OUTLINE

RADIATION-BASED IMAGING

RADIOGRAPHS

Radiographs or X-ray photographs are the most commonly employed diagnostic tools since they are usually available at the dental chair side or hospital itself. They are also faster, easy to acquire and much cheaper than the other diagnostic tools. The X-rays are captured in a film or a sensor. By processing the film or the sensor, a two-dimensional (2D) image of the structures through which the X-rays passed through can be obtained as a radiographic film or a digital image on the computer, which can be later printed out in any media as per requirement.

The radio opacity of the image is determined by the amount of X-ray beam attenuated by the structure:

- The radiopaque or white parts of the image show the dense structures, which have completely obstructed by the X-rays. Example: bone, metallic objects, such as implants, plates, embedded foreign particles, bullets, etc
- The radiolucent or black parts of the image show the areas where the X-ray beam has passed through the object without any hindrance. Example: air-filled maxillary sinus
- The grey parts show areas where the X-ray beam has been hindered to a varying degree. Example: soft tissues such as fat, muscle and glands have varying radio opacities. Cartilage is more radio opaque than fat but less than bone.

The radio opacity of the image obtained also depends on the intensity of the X-rays used, possibility of superimposition, distance from the X-ray source and sensitivity of the film. Depending on the *placement of the film,* the plain radiographs that are used in maxillofacial surgery are classified as *intraoral and extraoral.*

INTRAORAL RADIOGRAPHS

- Intraoral radiographs have been used due to their advantages:
  a. They have the best spatial resolution
  b. Minimal distortion
  c. Midline structures can be best visualised without superimposition
     i. The radiograph is clearer
     ii. A small area alone is targeted and requires lesser radiation
  d. Chair side availability—not required to move the patient
- Types: Depending upon the site of placement, they are classified as intraoral periapical (IOPA), occlusal or bitewing
- IOPA and occlusal radiographs are widely employed in oral and maxillofacial surgery
- Bitewing radiograph is used for detection of decay and periodontal lesions
- Procedure: The X-ray generator and the film are held close to the area being investigated. The size of the film or the sensor is reduced, in order to accommodate it easily within the mouth
- Disadvantages
  a. Cannot be used in patients with restricted mouth opening.
  b. Not useful for viewing large lesions.

Intraoral periapical (IOPA) radiograph

- The film or sensor is held parallel to the long axis of the tooth as this provides the best radiographic image. It should also be in close proximity and the rays should be perfectly perpendicular to the tooth and the film
- Size 2: 31 × 41 mm—standard size
- IOPA radiograph is an integral armamentarium of dental and oral surgery. It is used for basic investigations where

lesions are small and the patient is able to open the mouth adequately. A digital version of the same is called Radiovisuography (RVG) where the X-ray film is replaced with a sensor. When IOPA radiograph is not possible, an Orthopantomogram (OPG) is advised

- Radiographic localisation: Intraoral radiography technique for positioning an anatomical structure like palatal or buccal placement of a tooth can be done by the **Clark's technique** (described in Chapter 19, Fig. 19.31).

Techniques

Parallel cone technique

- Cone: Long cone to obtain parallel, non-divergent X-rays
- Film: Placed in a holder parallel to the long axis of the tooth, perpendicular to the X-rays
- Holder: A Rinn holder with a bite plane and a ring to direct the X-ray perpendicular to the film.

Bisecting cone technique

- Film: The film packet is placed as close to the tooth as possible without bending the film (Fig. 4.1)
- Cone: The angle formed between the long axis of the tooth and the long axis of the film packet is assessed and imaginarily bisected. The X-ray tube is placed at a right angle to this bisecting line with the central ray of the X-ray beam aimed through the long axis of the tooth. Using the geometrical principle of *Cieszynski's rule of isometry,* the actual length of the tooth in the mouth will be equal to the length of the image of the tooth on the film
- Structures viewed
  a. Teeth, periapical area, lamina dura, periodontal ligament space, alveolar bone, floor of maxillary sinus adjacent to the roots of the maxillary teeth
- Indications
  a. For detection and assessment of dental caries, periodontal lesions, alveolar fracture, periapical lesions, retained root fragments, foreign body and impacted teeth

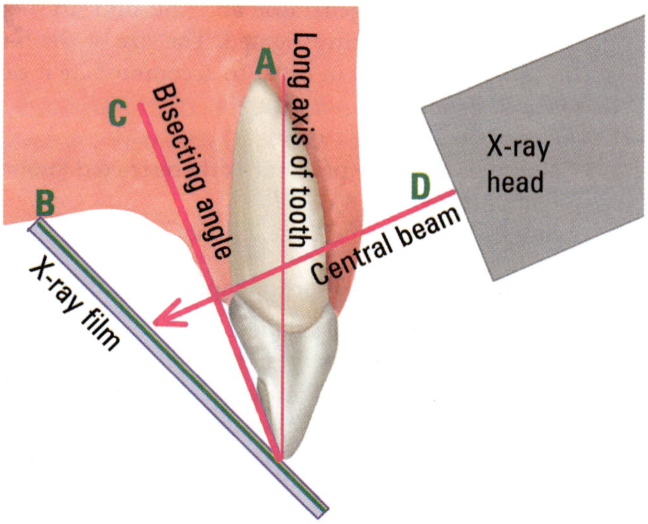

Figure 4.1 Bisecting angle technique.

  b. Evaluation of root apex formation
  c. During endodontic treatment
  d. Detecting fracture of teeth
  e. Study of crown and root length and their morphology.

Occlusal radiograph

Occlusal radiographs are those intraoral radiographs taken placing the film in the occlusal plane. The films are usually of size 5.7 × 7.6 cm.

Lateral mandibular occlusal projection

- Structures viewed
  a. Mandibular dental arch, floor of the mouth, buccolingual borders of the mandible and calcifications on the floor of the mouth
- Indications
  a. Sialolith/radiopaque calculi in the submandibular ducts
  b. Buccolingual position of the unerupted mandibular teeth
  c. Buccolingual expansion of the body of the mandible by cysts, tumours or osteodystrophies
  d. Assessment of displacement of fractures of the anterior mandible in the horizontal plane
- Advantages
  a. Identify the submandibular duct calculi
  b. Differentiate between buccal or lingual positioning of impacted tooth.

Lateral maxillary occlusal projection

- Structures viewed
  a. Maxillary dental arch, hard palate, greater palatine foramina and buccal cortex of the maxilla
- Indications for prescription
  a. Unerupted canines, supernumeraries and odontome
  b. Cleft alveolus and palatal swellings
  c. As midline view, to determine the buccopalatal position of unerupted canines
  d. Evaluation of size and extent of lesions, such as cysts and tumours in the anterior maxilla/palate
  e. Assessment of fracture of the anterior teeth and alveolar bone
- Advantages
  a. Periapical assessment of the maxillary anterior teeth, especially in children but also in adults unable to tolerate periapical films.

EXTRAORAL RADIOGRAPHS

Extraoral radiographs are most commonly used for detection of maxillofacial fractures and large lesions of the jaws. Lesions of the cranial bones can be detected on these radiographs such as Paget's disease and multiple myeloma. The sclerotic phase of Paget's disease in the skull shows a '***cotton-wool***' appearance (Fig. 4.2A) and multiple myeloma shows ***multiple punched out*** radiolucencies (Fig. 4.2B). However, unlike long bones, facial bones cannot be viewed without superimposition. Therefore, several angulations have been

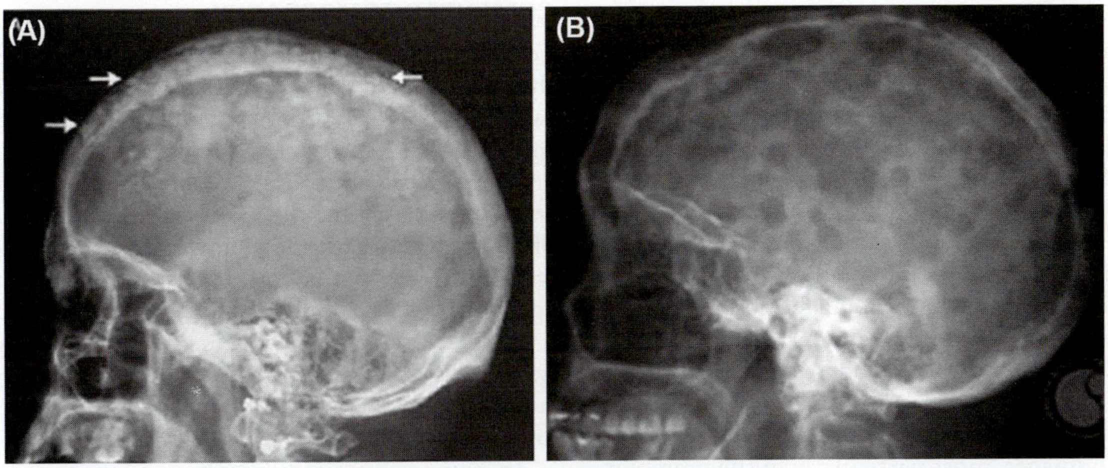

Figure 4.2 (A) Lateral view skull—Paget's disease. (B) Lateral view skull—Multiple myeloma.

standardised to view specific anatomic units of the maxillofacial skeleton. The most commonly used extraoral radiograph is the orthopantomograph (OPG).

Advantages

- Superior spatial resolution
- Low cost

Disadvantages

- 2D image of 3D structure
- Superimposition of structures

Orthopantomogram

Panoramic film size: 5 × 12 inch, 6 × 12 inch.

Structures viewed

Teeth, orbit, nasal cavity, nasal septum, inferior nasal concha, incisive foramen, nasal spine, maxillary sinus, palate, maxillary tuberosity, pterygoid processes, pterygopalatine fossa, zygomatic bone, articular tubercle, coronoid process, condyle, joint space, mandible, mandibular canal, mental foramen and hyoid bone (Fig. 4.3).

Indications

- Screening for pathologies such as cysts, tumours, fractures, impacted teeth in mandible
- Dental caries, periodontal and periapical lesions of maxillary and mandibular dentition
- Screening for osteoporosis
- TMJ ankylosis
- TMJ disorders and lesions
- Explain status of teeth.

Advantages

- Evaluation of maxilla and mandible in one film
- Useful in case of patients with the complaint of limited mouth opening, extreme gag reflex, fearful or uncooperative children.
- Less time is required to do OPG survey than intraoral survey
- Aids in patient education and case presentation. Conditions such as impactions, eruption pattern of teeth, growth and development, need for replacement of missing teeth and fractures are more easily illustrated on panoramic views

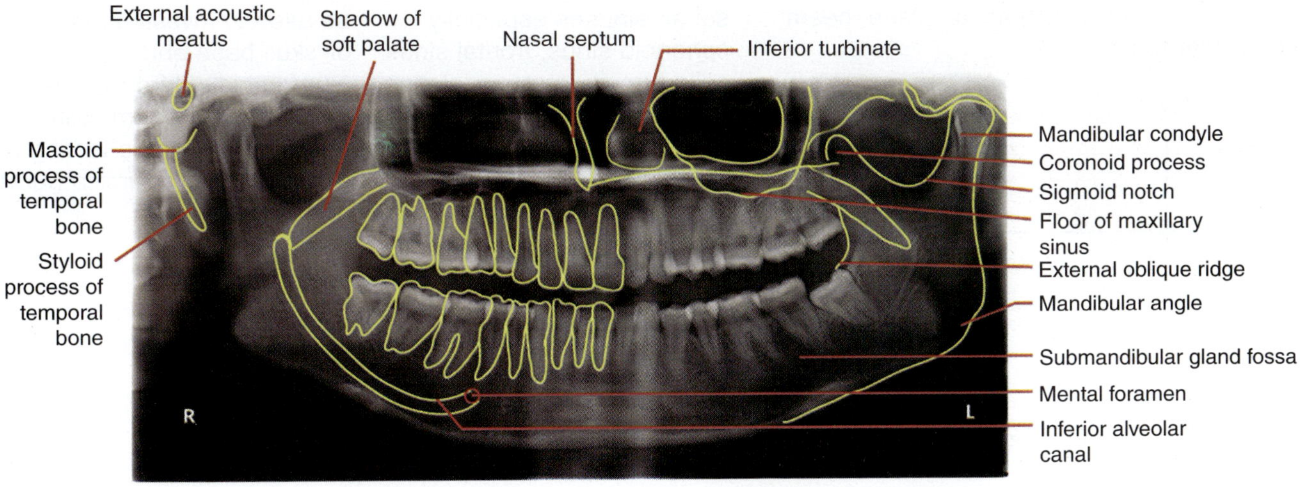

Figure 4.3 OPG showing normal anatomical landmarks.

- Reduces the risk of multiple exposures to radiation when compared with conventional full mouth intraoral radiography
- Relatively simple procedure to perform
- Requires minimal patient cooperation (patients are only required to stand still for 15–20 s of exposure).

Disadvantages

- Image quality: Tomograms inherently show magnification, geometric distortion and poor definition. Less effective in detecting early interproximal or recurrent caries, disruptions in lamina dura, loss of crestal alveolar bone and thickened periodontal membrane
- Overlap: OPG units have a tendency to produce overlapping of teeth images, most particularly in the premolar area
- Superimposition: There is often superimposition of the vertebral column on the anterior portion of the OPG (incisors region)
- Distortion: The amount of horizontal and vertical distortion varies from one part of the film to another. This results in an uneven magnification of the image. Some structures and spaces may appear larger than actual size
- Overuse: The ease and convenience in obtaining the OPG might lead to carelessness by substitution for other projection that might be adequate. This is one of the prime concerns in regard to patient's radiation dosage.

Other extraoral radiographs

The structures that can be viewed and the indications for prescription of other extraoral radiographs have been enumerated in Table 4.1 (Figs. 4.4-4.16).

COMPUTED TOMOGRAPHY

Tomography can be utilised to section or slice the object and thereby eliminating undesirable overlap. It is achieved by simultaneous movement of the X-ray tube and the film. The movement occurs around a point or fulcrum as the tube and the film are connected. The objects closest to the point or fulcrum are seen most sharply and the objects farthest away from the point of rotation are almost completely blurred. Thus, an image layer within the body is produced while the blurring makes the images of structures above and below that layer invisible.

In CT, the images are produced by an ionising radiation, which allows visualisation of greater variety of tissue structures; beyond the four basic densities (air, bone, soft tissue and fat) seen on the conventional radiograph.

In conventional radiograph, one projection is used to form an image while CT uses multiple small projections across the body and combines the information to form an image. A section or axial 'slices' refers to each individual picture of CT (Fig. 4.17).

The entire CT process is divided into three segments:

1. Data acquisition
2. Image reconstruction
3. Image display.

An image is reconstructed after the raw data is averaged and each pixel is assigned a Hounsfield number (quantified measurement of density). Each axial CT image is about 1.5 mm thick. The maxilla usually requires about 20–30 axial sections, whereas the mandible requires about 30–35 sections.

HOUNSFIELD UNITS

Hounsfield units (HU) or CT numbers are named after *Sir Godfrey Newbold Hounsfield*. It is a quantitative scale used to describe radio opacity.

TABLE 4.1 Comparison of Extraoral Radiographs

Extraoral radiograph	Structures viewed	Indications
True lateral skull Film placed parallel to midsagittal plane; beam perpendicular to film 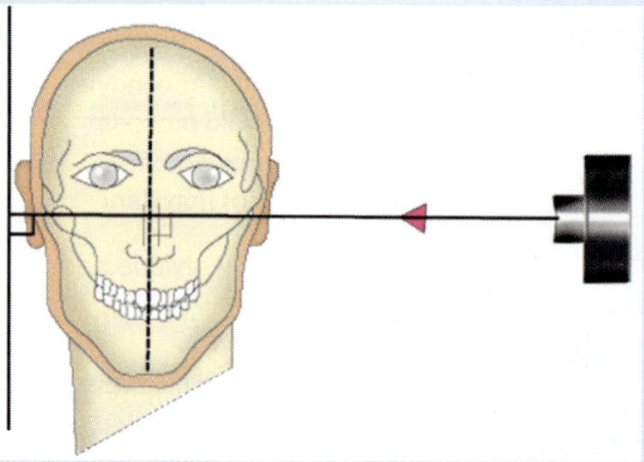 Figure 4.4 Technique of taking lateral view of skull.	Craniofacial bones paranasal air sinuses especially sphenoid sinus, frontal sinus, sella turcica, pterygopalatine fossa, maxillary antrum	True lateral skull radiograph can be used to investigate fractures of skull base and of the cranium, middle third fractures, frontal, sphenoid, maxillary sinuses, conditions affecting the skull vault, sella turcica (tumour of pituitary gland)

TABLE 4.1 Comparison of Extraoral Radiographs—cont'd

Extraoral radiograph	Structures viewed	Indications
Lateral view skull/cephalogram Film placed parallel to midsagittal plane; beam perpendicular to film (difference between true lateral skull and true cephalometric lateral skull is that the true lateral skull is not standardised or reproducible) 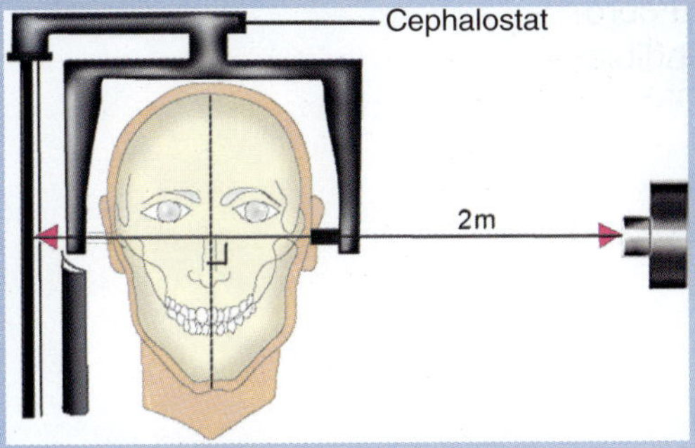 Figure 4.5 Technique of taking lateral cephalogram, using cephalostat and standardised beam distance.	Craniofacial bones, paranasal air sinuses especially sphenoid sinus, frontal sinus, sella turcica, pterygopalatine fossa, maxillary antrum	• Cephalometric radiograph is used for growth studies and orthognathic surgery • Asymmetry of the mandibular ramus and body can also be investigated
PA view skull/cephalogram Canthomeatal line at 90 degree to film; head tipped forward (forehead and nose touching the film) (forehead nose position); X-ray beam perpendicular to film 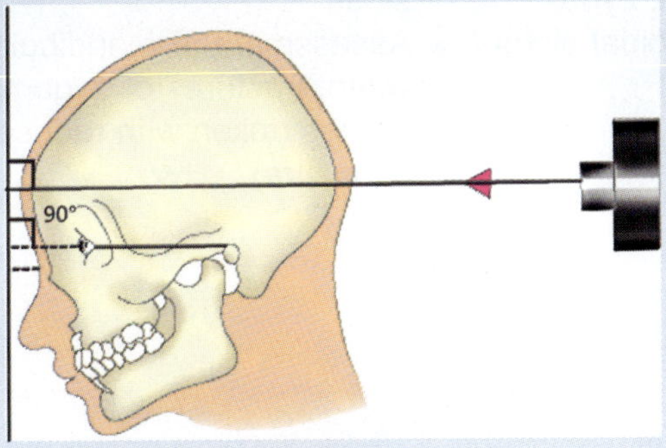 Figure 4.6 Technique of PA view.	Skull vault, orbit, frontal bone and the frontal sinus, nasal cavity, nasal septum, condylar neck, ramus and angle of the mandible, facial skeleton	• Investigation of frontal sinuses, fractures of skull vault • Conditions affecting the cranium (Paget disease, multiple myeloma, Brown's tumour) • Intracranial calcifications • Facial asymmetry
Standard occipitomental view—0-degree OM Film placed perpendicular to sagittal plane with canthomeatal line 45 degree to the film; (Nose chin position); X- ray beam centred through occiput at horizontal (0 degree) 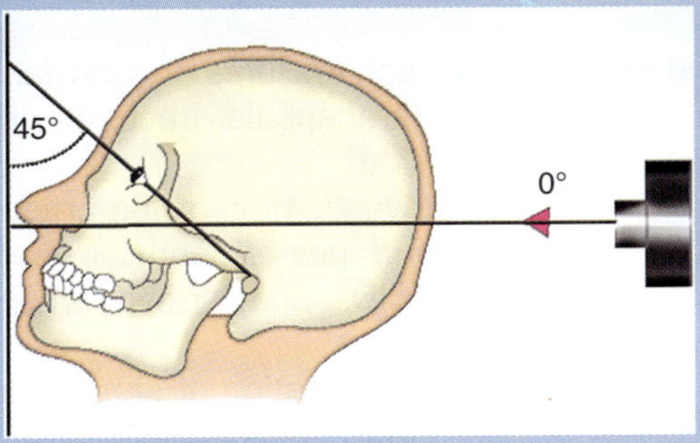 Figure 4.7 Technique of standard occipitomental view.	Frontal sinus, orbits, nasal bones, nasal septum, maxilla, zygoma, mandible, sphenoidal sinus	• Investigation of maxillary antrum, ethmoid and frontal sinuses • Detecting Le Fort I, Le Fort II, Le Fort III, zygomatic complex, nasoethmoid complex, orbital blow out, coronoid process fractures

Continued

<table>
<tr><th colspan="3">TABLE 4.1 Comparison of Extraoral Radiographs—cont'd</th></tr>
<tr><th>Extraoral radiograph</th><th>Structures viewed</th><th>Indications</th></tr>
<tr><td>Waters view (30-degree occipitomental view)
Same as standard except that beam directed 30 degree to horizontal from above the head
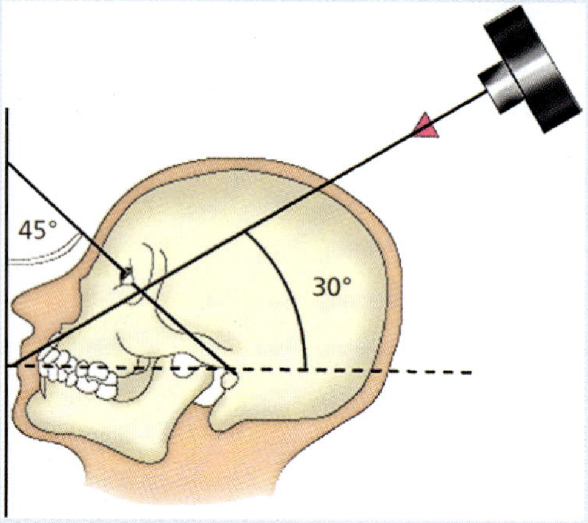

Figure 4.8 Technique of 30-degree occipitomental view (Waters view).</td><td>Orbits, maxillary sinus, zygoma, frontal sinus, nasal cavity, nasal septum, zygomatic arches, frontal, maxillary, temporal process of zygoma, zygomaticofrontal suture, condylar and coronoid process of mandible</td><td>To diagnose the infections and pathologies of paranasal sinuses.
To view orbitozygomatic fractures</td></tr>
<tr><td>Submentovertex view
Canthomeatal line parallel to film; the vertex of the skull touches the film; X-ray beam aimed upward at 5 degree to the horizontal.
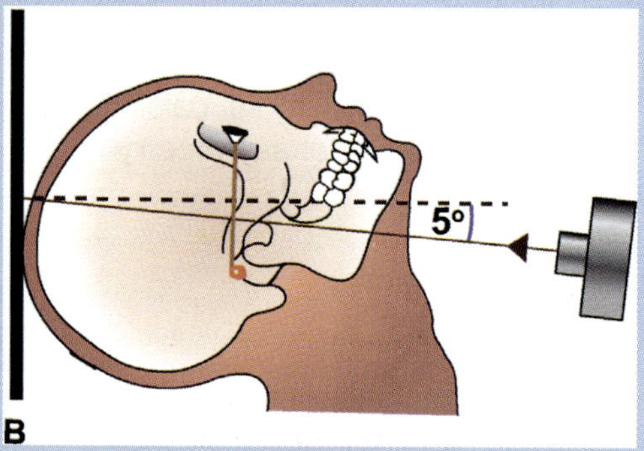

Figure 4.9 Technique of submentovertex view.
Submentovertex view is of two types:
• Base of skull projection
• Zygomatic arch projection (called as the jug-handle view)
Similar to base of the skull projection but radiation exposure is less</td><td>Base of mandible, base of skull, lateral wall of orbit, foramen magnum, condylar head, lateral pterygoid plate, articular eminence, zygomatic arch, sphenoidal sinus</td><td>• Destructive/expansive lesions affecting the palate, pterygoid region or base of skull
• Investigation of sphenoid sinus
• Assessment of mandibular width, fractures of zygomatic arches (taken with reduced exposure)</td></tr>
<tr><td>Reverse Townes view
Canthomeatal line at 90 degree to film; Head tipped forward (forehead nose position); X-ray beam perpendicular to film; mouth open</td><td>Condylar heads and necks</td><td>• High fractures of condylar neck
• Intracapsular fractures of the TMJ
• Investigation of the articular surfaces of condylar heads in TMD, condylar hyper-/hypoplasia
• Investigation of sphenoidal sinus</td></tr>
</table>

TABLE 4.1 Comparison of Extraoral Radiographs—cont'd

Extraoral radiograph	Structures viewed	Indications
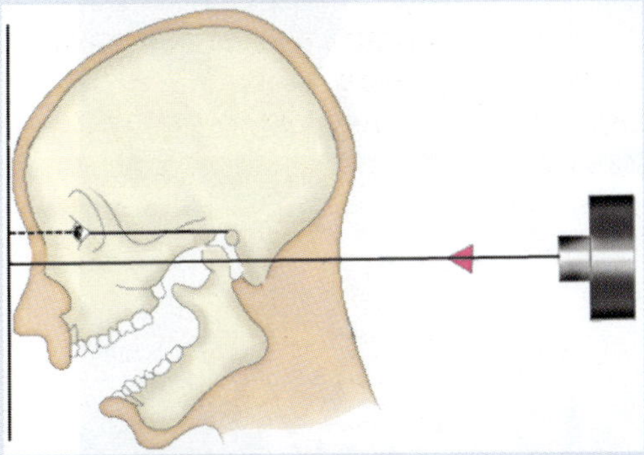 Figure 4.10 Technique of Reverse Townes view.		
Oblique lateral—body Film in contact with cheek at molar area; beam aims at molar–premolar area oblique to the sagittal plane of the patient. 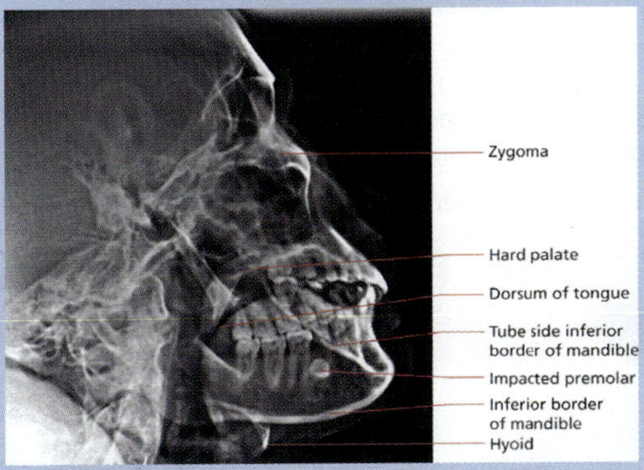 Figure 4.11 Oblique lateral projection of mandibular body.	Teeth, alveolar ridge and body of the mandible	• Assessment of the presence/position of the impacted teeth • Detect fractures of mandible • Osseous lesions of mandible
Oblique lateral—ramus Film in contact with cheek at the ramus area; beam aims at ramus area 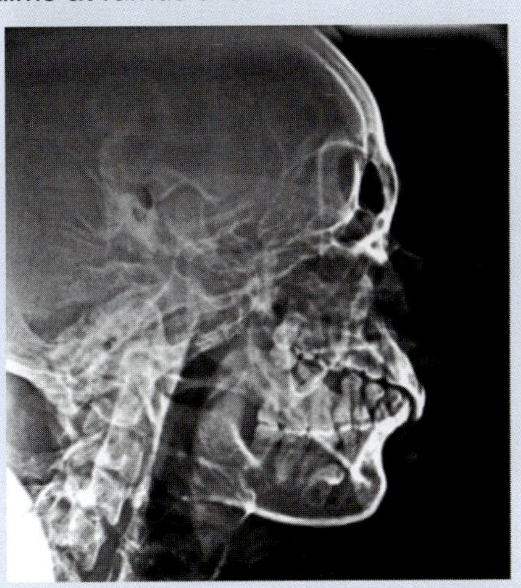 Figure 4.12 Oblique lateral projection of mandibular ramus.	Third molar–retromolar area, angle, ramus, condyle and coronoid process of the mandible	To diagnose the pathologies and fractures of the mandibular ramus and condyle

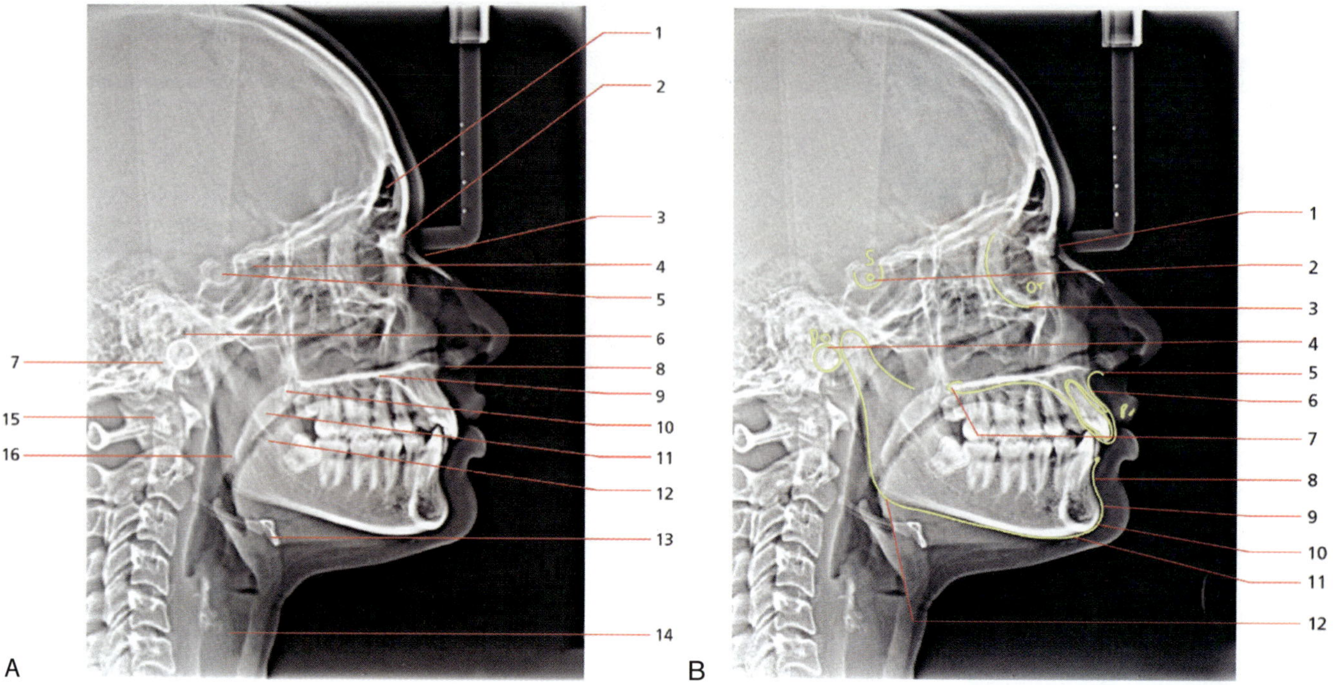

1. Frontal sinus, 2. Nasion, 3. Nasal bone, 4. Sphenoid sinus, 5. Sella, 6. External auditory meatus, 7. Mastoid, 8. Anterior nasal bone, 9. Hard palate, 10. Pterygoid, 11. Soft palate, 12. Dorsum of tongue, 13. Hyoid, 14. Trachea, 15. Atlas, 16. Posterior wall of pharynx.

1. Nasion (N), 2. Sella (S), 3. Orbitale (Or), 4. Porion (Po), 5. Anterior nasal spine (ANS), 6. Point A, 7. Posterior nasal spine (PNS), 8. Point B, 9. Pogonion (Pog), 10. Gnathion (Gn), 11. Menton (Me), 12. Gonion (Go).

Figure 4.13 (A) True lateral cephalogram showing anatomical landmarks. (B) True lateral cephalogram showing cephalometric landmarks.

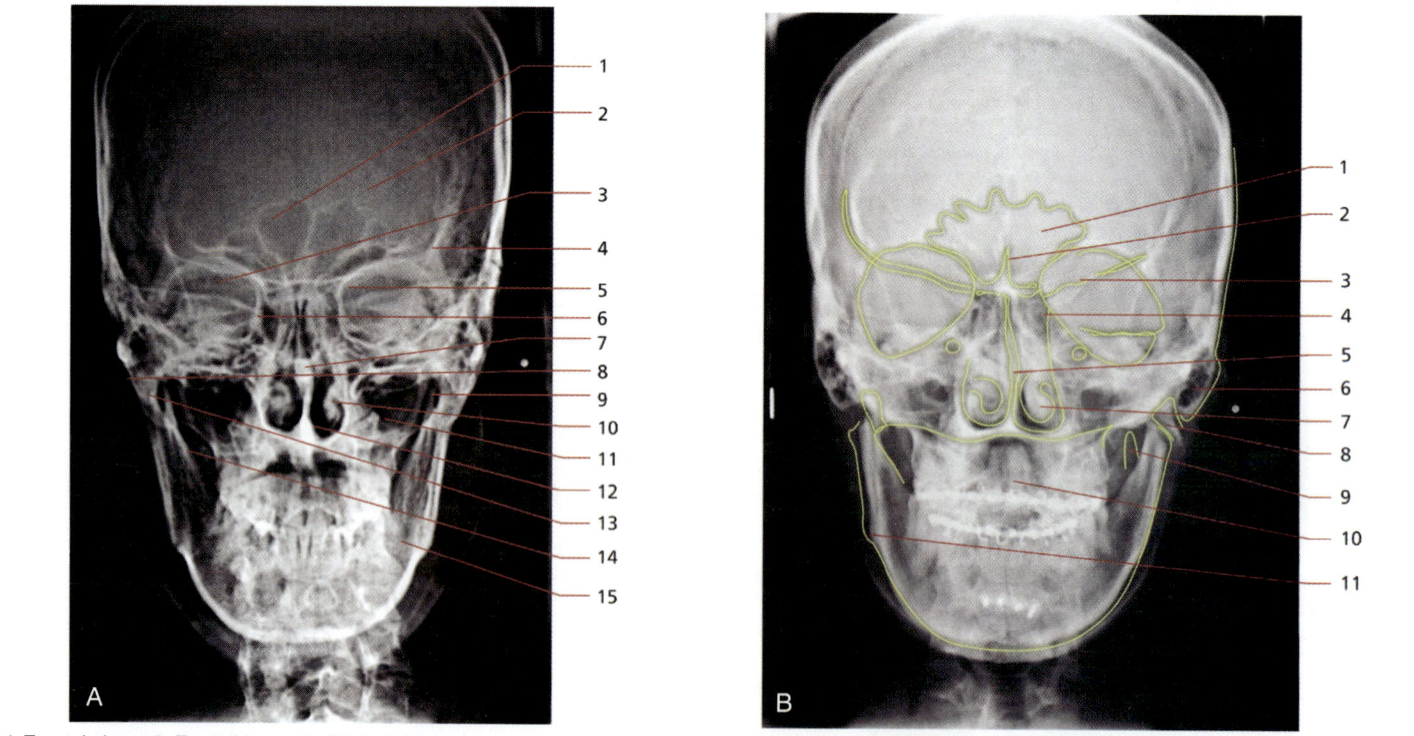

1. Frontal sinus, 2. Frontal bone, 3. Orbit, 4. Linea temporalis, 5. Sphenoid, 6. Ethmoid air cells, 7. Nasal septum, 8. Mastoid, 9. Coronoid, 10. Inferior turbinate, 11. Maxillary sinus, 12. Nasal cavity, 13. Condyle, 14. Transverse process of atlas, 15. Angle of mandible.

1. Frontal sinus, 2. Cribriform ethmoid/with crista galli, 3. Greater wing of sphenoid, 4. Sphenoidal sinus, 5. Nasal septum, 6. Mastoid process, 7. Inferior turbinate, 8. Fractured condyle, 9. Coronoid process, 10. Dens of axis vertebra, 11. Angle of mandible.

Figure 4.14 (A) PA skull showing anatomical landmarks. (B) PA view showing bicondylar fracture.

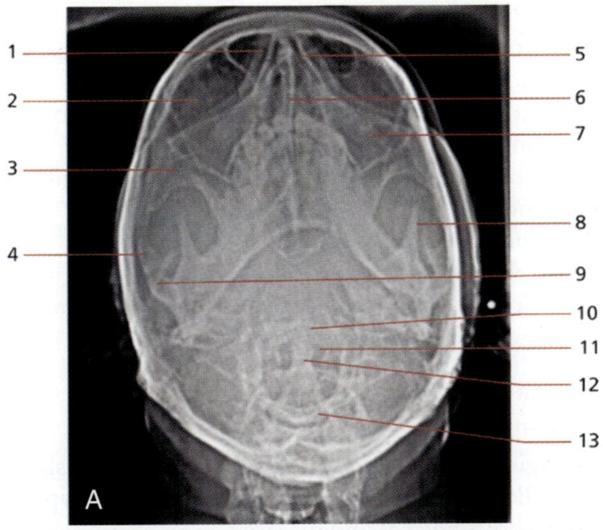

1. Frontal sinus, 2. Orbit, 3. Zygoma, 4. Zygomatic arch, 5. Nasal bone, 6. Nasal septum, 7. Maxillary sinus, 8. Coronoid process, 9. Condyle, 10. Anterior arch of atlas, 11. Foramen magnum, 12. Dens, 13. Posterior arch of atlas.

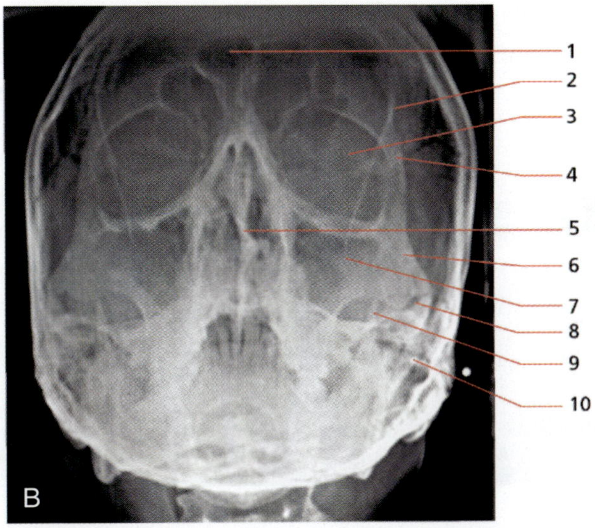

1. Frontal sinuses, 2. Linea temporalis, 3. Orbit, 4. Zygomatic frontal suture, 5. Nasal septum, 6. Zygoma, 7. Maxillary sinus, 8. Zygomatic arch, 9. Coronoid, 10. Condyle.

Figure 4.15 (A) Standard occipitomental view. (B) PNS view (Waters projection).

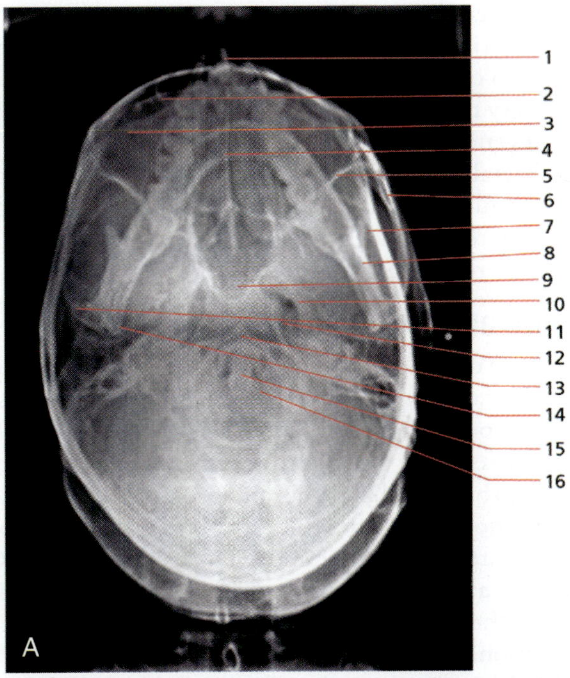

1. Nasal septum, 2. Medial wall of orbit, 3. Anterior wall of maxilla, 4. Nasal septum (vomer), 5. Lateral wall of orbit, 6. Zygomatic arch, 7. Coronoid process, 8. Ramus of mandible, 9. Sphenoid sinus, 10. Foramen ovale, 11. Condyle, 12. Foramen spinosum, 13. Anterior arch of atlas, 14. Angle of mandible, 15. Dens, 16. Foramen magnum.

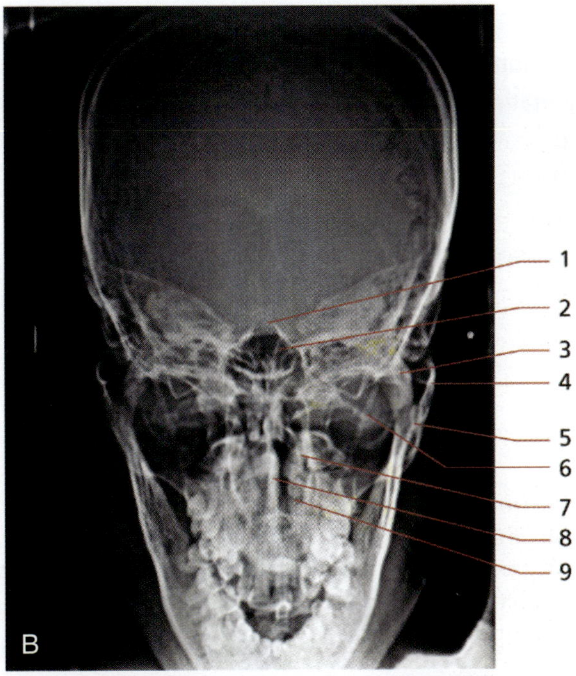

1. Arch of atlas, 2. Foramen magnum, 3. Condyle, 4. Zygomatic arch, 5. Neck of condyle, 6. Orbit, 7. Middle turbinate, 8. Nasal septum, 9. Inferior turbinate.

Figure 4.16 (A) True submentovertex view—basal view. (B) Reverse Townes projection.

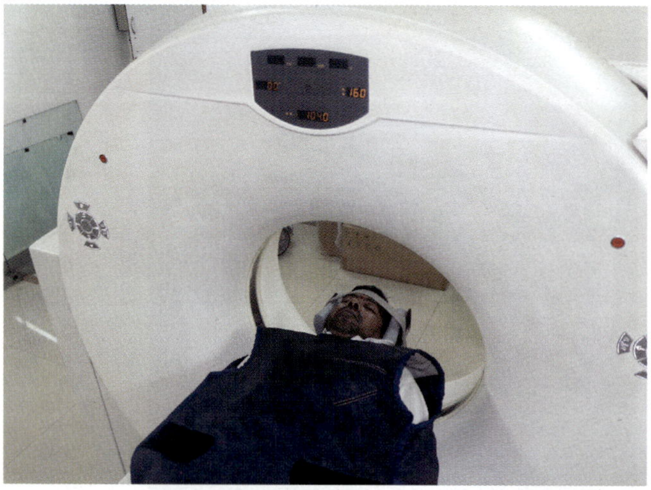

Figure 4.17 CT scanner.

TABLE 4.2 Hounsfield units Depicting the Density of Different Tissues of the Body

Tissue	Intensity value (HU)
Bone	1000
Liver	40–60
White matter in brain	46
Grey matter in brain	43
Blood	40
Muscle	10–40
Kidney	30
Cerebrospinal fluid	15
Water	0
Fat	−50 to 100
Air	−1000

HU denotes the amount of the X-ray beam that a particular voxel of tissue attenuates. In CT scan, HU is proportional to the degree of X-ray attenuation. It is allocated to each *pixel* (picture element) to represent the density of the tissue. HU for different tissues have been described in Table 4.2.

3D RECONSTRUCTION OF CT IMAGES (FIG. 4.18)

- The original 2D slices are used to create 3D images
- No additional scanning or radiation exposure is needed
- Artefacts may be produced in the reformation process
- The reconstructed 3D images assist in the visualisation of large comminuted, displaced and complex fractures involving multiple planes, easy to diagnose expansile lesions, useful in planning surgery, in the fabrication of stereolithographic models and patient education.

Indications of head and neck CT scan

- Investigation of intracranial disease including tumours, haemorrhage, and infarcts
- Assessment of fractures involving faciomaxillary skeleton.
- In tumour diagnosis and staging
- Investigation of bone and soft tissue pathologies of head and neck
- Malformations of skull
- Pathologies of paranasal sinuses
- Aneurysm, arteriovenous malformations or vascular pathology (CT angiography).

Advantages of CT scan

- Detailed imaging of intracranial lesions
- Imaging of hard and soft tissues simultaneously
- Excellent differentiation between different types of tissues, both normal and diseased
- Reconstructed images can be obtained
- Images can be enhanced by the use of IV contrast media and providing additional information
- Linear measurements, area, volume of structures can be calculated using built-in or added software.

Disadvantages of CT scan

- The equipment is very expensive
- Multiple exposure should be avoided to prevent radiation overdose
- Very thin, contiguous or overlapping slices may result in a generally high-dose investigation
- Metallic objects, such as stainless steel mini-plate and stainless-steel crown may produce marked artefacts such as streak or star across the CT image
- Inherent risks associated with i.v. contrast agents.

CONE-BEAM CT (CBCT)

It is one of the latest cutting-edge technologies in dental and maxillofacial imaging. The CBCT scanner rotates 360 degrees around the patient's head (Fig. 4.19A and B). It enables quick, fast, easy visualisation of patient's craniofacial structure with unparallel precision of 3D. It provides undistorted dimensional images of the jaws in cross-sectional, axial, coronal, sagittal, panoramic and 3D images (Fig. 4.20A–G). CBCT utilises a cone-shaped X-ray beam directed towards the patient's head, whereas a fan-shaped X-ray beam is used by traditional medical CT. The difference between CT scan and CBCT scan has been described in Table 4.3. It also uses less radiation compared to the CT scan. Multiple 2D projection images are acquired for a field of view selected according to the region of interest in CBCT. The degree of X-ray attenuation is shown by grey scale (voxel value) in CBCT while in CT, it is measured in pixels.

CBCT IMAGE FORMATION

- The object is placed between the source and the detector mechanism

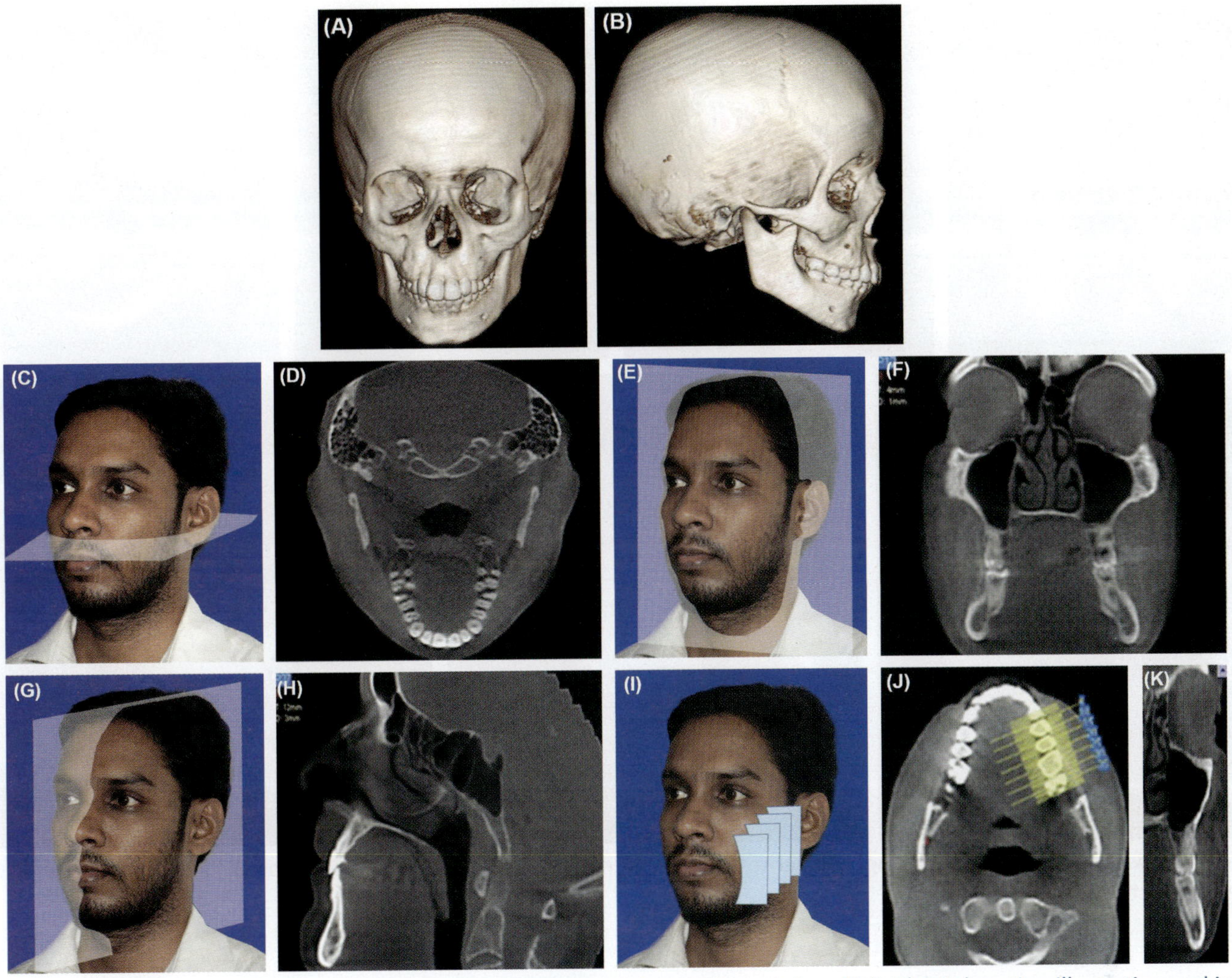

Figure 4.18 (A) 3D Reconstruction of normal skull straight view. (B) 3DCT lateral view. (C & D) Axial section illustration and image. (E & F) Coronal section. (G & H) Sagittal section. (I-K) Transaxial image.

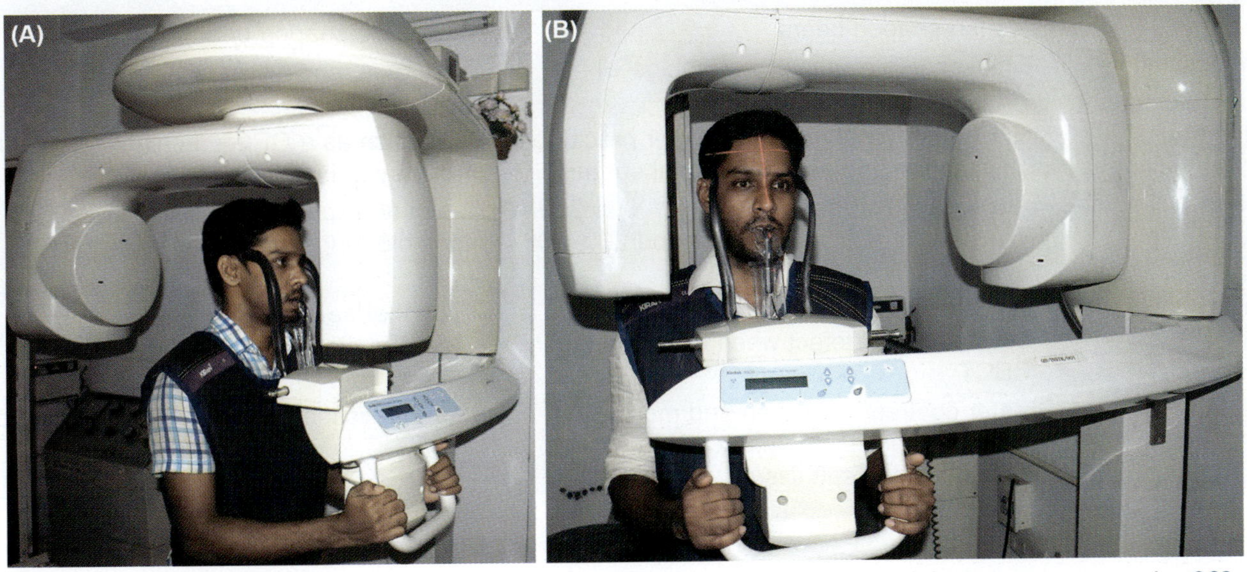

Figure 4.19 (A) Cone-beam CT scanner used for imaging in a patient in standing posture. (B) CBCT scanner rotating 360 degrees around the patient's head during scanning.

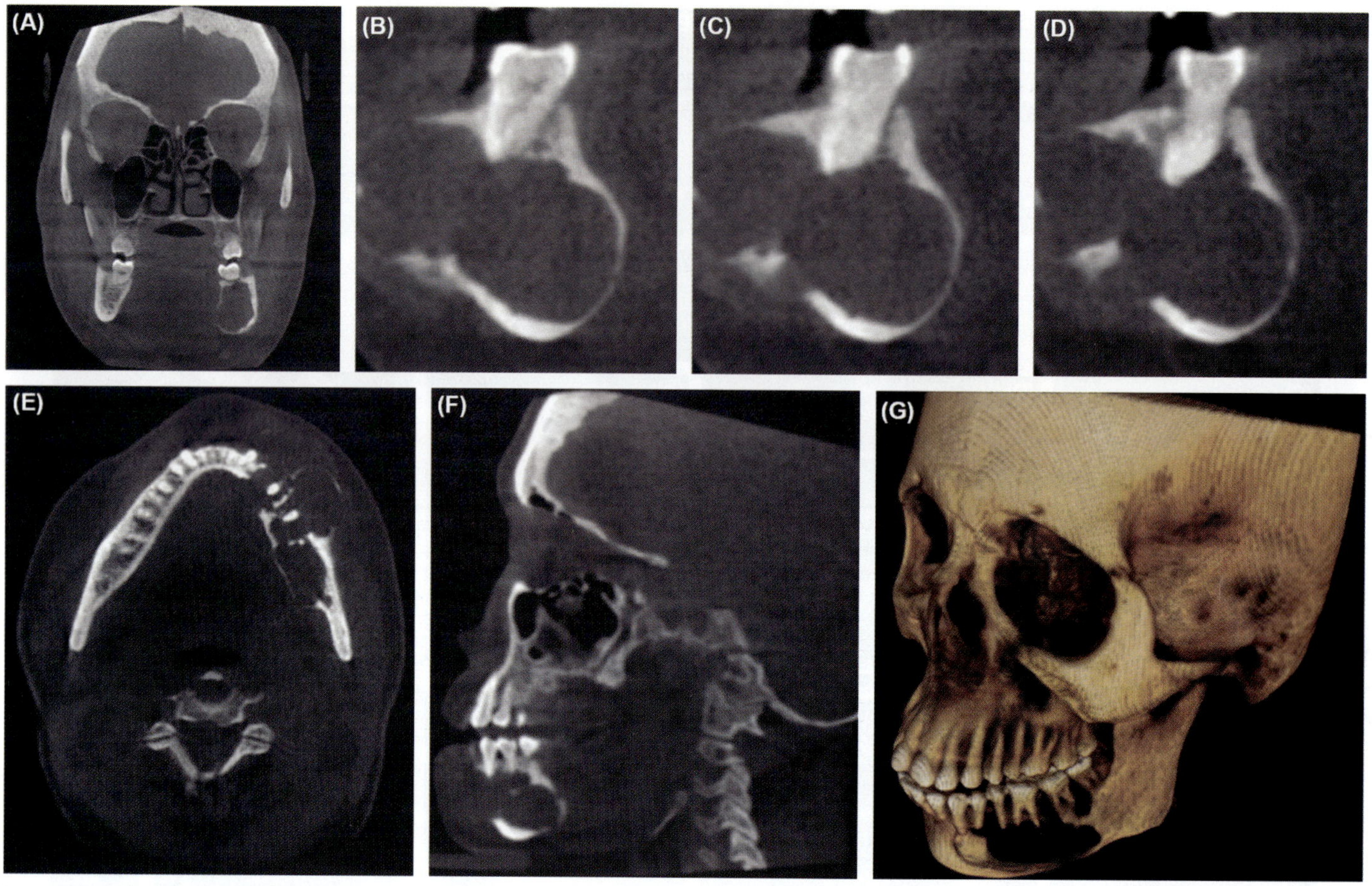

Figure 4.20 (A–D) Axial sections showing hypodense lesion in left mandible body. (E) Coronal section. (F) Sagittal section. (G) CBCT 3D reconstruction.

TABLE 4.3 Comparing CT and CBCT Scans

Entity	CT	CBCT
Technology	Uses fan-shaped beam	Uses cone-shaped beam
Patient positioning	CT makes use of a supine machine with a large gantry	Sitting up/standing machine of smaller dimensions
Machine size	Size of a conventional CT scanner precludes its installation and usage in dental surgery	Same size as a OPG machine—compact and easy to install
Radiation	Radiation exposure ranges from 100 to 300 micro sieverts (μSv) for maxilla and 200–500 (μSv) for the mandible	Radiation exposure for both maxilla and mandible ranges from 34–102 (μSv)
Artefacts	• Artefacts arising from metal are severe • Less motion artefact when compared to CBCT	• Not that severe • More motion
Image quality	Greater contrast resolution and more discrimination between different tissue types (bone, teeth and soft tissue)	Poor soft tissue contrast when compared to CT

- The X-ray imaging unit rotates around the object at a continuous rate
- X-ray source produces cone-shaped beam that radiates the patient's mouth and jaw as the arm rotates
- The images of the object are taken at a rate of 5–10 per second for about 30 seconds.

After 360-degree rotation, the image data is converted by a computer into 3D images.

INDICATIONS OF CBCT

- Oral and maxillofacial implants
- Impacted teeth, cystic and neoplastic lesions
- Maxillofacial trauma
- Orthodontic treatment planning and implant
- Anchorage
- Endodontic pathology
- Temporomandibular joint (TMJ) analysis
- Airway studies (sleep apnoea).

ADVANTAGES OF CBCT

- Low radiation than CT scan
- Unlimited 3D views
- Less discomfort
- Can be taken in sitting posture.

DISADVANTAGES OF CBCT

- High-speed scans (less than 30 s)
- Compact/Reduced size—feasible for use in dental office
- *High-spatial resolution* applicable for maxillofacial diagnosis
- *Low-radiation exposure* (10 times lesser than the regular CT scanner)
- Cost effective
- Safe for children.

DENTA SCAN

- The technique of dental CT was developed by Schwarz et al. in 1987
- They used curved multiplanar reconstruction of jaw. Dental CT involves the acquisition of axial scans of the jaw with the highest possible resolution with curved and orthogonal multiplanar reconstructions
- Best useful for dental implant procedure
- Reduced metal artefact when compared to CT
- Allows accurate display of the vertical and buccolingual dimensions of the jaw in actual 1:1 life size
- Indication: Implant-bone estimation (height and width).

DEXA SCAN

Bone density scanning, also called *dual-energy X-ray absorptiometry* (DEXA) or bone densitometry. It is an enhanced form of X-ray technology that is used to measure bone loss/bone mineral density. DEXA is most often done on the lower spine and hips. It is used primarily in the diagnosis and management of osteoporosis and other disease states characterised by abnormal bone metabolism disorder.

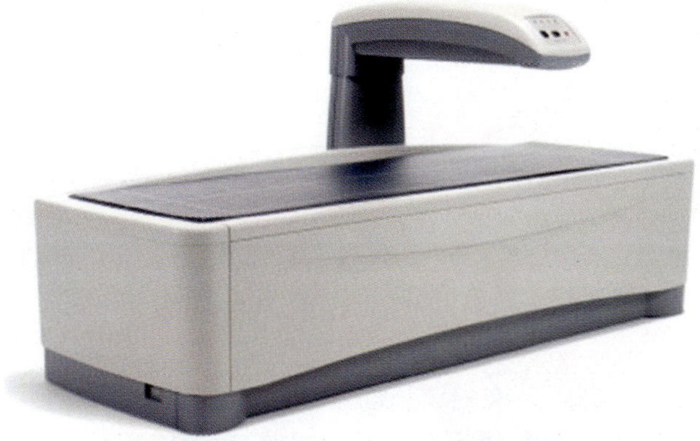

Figure 4.21 Bone density test.

- WHO osteoporosis classification (T score):
  Normal: >-1
  Osteopenia (low bone mass): -1 to -2.5
  Osteoporosis: <-2.5
  Severe osteoporosis <-2.5 plus fragility fractures (Fig. 4.21).

ARTHROGRAPHY

Arthrography involves injection of a radiopaque contrast material into the joint spaces. The space occupied by the disc can then be visualised lying between the layers of contrast material. Arthrography provides information regarding the soft tissue components, specifically the shape and position of the articular disc (Fig. 4.22A & B).

TYPES OF ARTHROGRAPHY

1. Single-contrast arthrography
2. Double-contrast radiography

COMPLICATIONS

- Joint sepsis
- Allergic reaction to the iodinated contrast medium
- Haemarthrosis
- Pain during and after the procedure
- Extravasation of the contrast medium
- Disc perforation
- Transient facial paralysis.

NONRADIATION-BASED IMAGING

ULTRASONOGRAPHY

Ultrasonography (USG) is a diagnostic tool that is widely available, relatively inexpensive, noninvasive and easily reproducible. It is valuable in identifying various orofacial swellings, such as inflammatory swellings due to dental or skin infections, diseases of the salivary glands, lymph node pathologies, soft tissue cysts and neoplasms.

Transducers with very high-pulsed frequencies (3.5–10 MHz) are used in USG to generate electrical impulses that are transmitted into the tissues being examined.

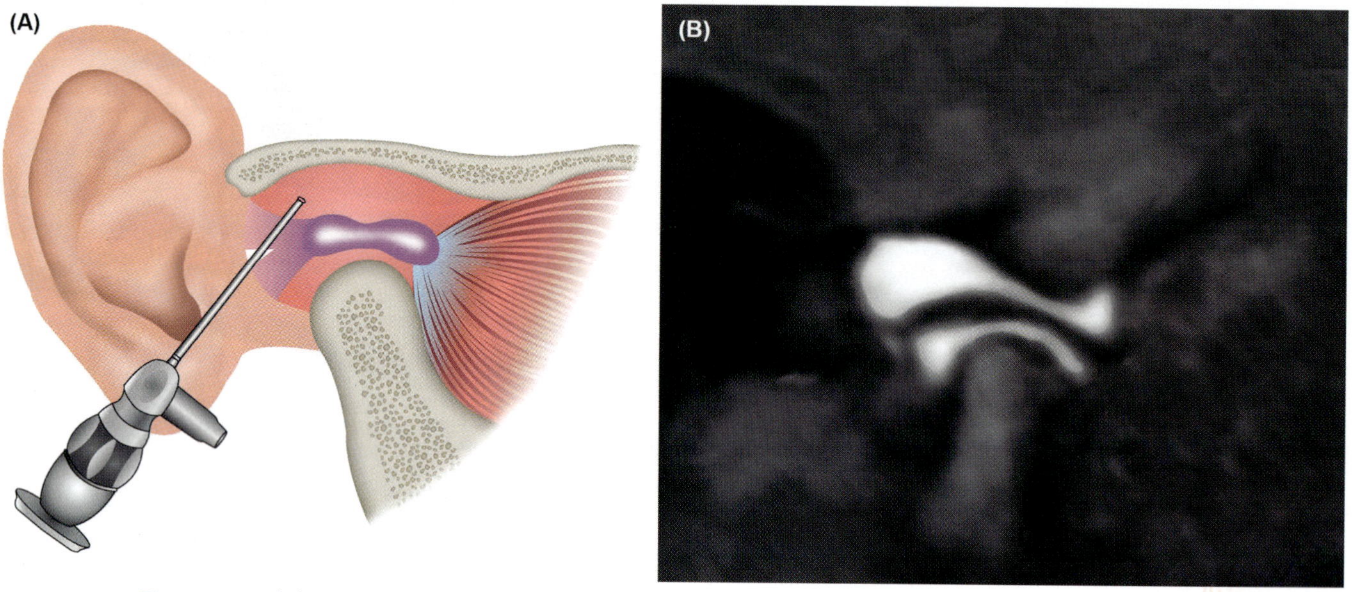

Figure 4.22 (A) Arthrography—insertion of needle into the joint space. (B) Arthrographic image.

As the sound passes through the tissues of different acoustic impedances, it is partly transferred to particles within the medium (as vibrational energy), part of it continues to penetrate, and part of it is reflected back towards the transducer.

The reflected echoes are reconverted into electrical energy, amplified, processed and displayed on a screen. The echoes of the sonographic images are termed as hypoechoic, hyperechoic and isoechoic images.

HYPOECHOIC IMAGES

A mass is hypoechoic if its intensity is lower than that of the adjacent tissue. Hypoechoic masses are darker.

HYPERECHOIC IMAGES

A mass is hyperechoic if its intensity is higher than that of the adjacent tissue. Hyperechoic masses are brighter.

ISOECHOIC IMAGES

A mass is isoechoic if its intensity is similar to that of the adjacent tissue. The appearances of isoechoic masses are also bright.

A calcified mass appears hyperechoic and a clear fluid or blood appears anechoic (free of echoic masses).

LIMITATIONS

- Limited use in hard tissue lesions
- The USG wave must be capable of travelling through the tissue to return to the transducer. If the tissue absorbs it, no image will result. Since air, bone and other calcified materials absorb nearly the entire ultrasonography beam; it is of limited use in diagnosing hard tissue lesions.

ADVANTAGES

- Sound waves are not ionising radiation
- No known harmful effects on any tissues by the present energies and doses used in diagnostic USG
- Images show good differentiation between different soft tissues and are very sensitive to detect focal disease in the salivary glands
- Technique is widely available and inexpensive. To assess the continuity of distracted soft callus before the commencement of consolidation period (distraction osteogenesis).

DISADVANTAGES

- USG has limited use in the head and neck region because sound waves are absorbed by bone. Its use is therefore restricted to the superficial structures. Technique is operator dependent
- Images can be difficult to interpret for inexperienced operators because image resolution is often poor
- Real-time imaging as the radiologist must be present during the investigation.

MAGNETIC RESONANCE IMAGING

Another imaging modality is MRI. It is based on the behaviour of protons (positively charged nuclear particles) in a magnetic field (Fig. 4.23). Hydrogen, the simplest atom consists of one proton in the nucleus and one orbiting electron. These hydrogen protons are used to create the magnetic resonance image.

INDICATIONS

- Soft tissue neoplasia—tongue, cheek, neck, etc
- TMJ—integrity and position of the disc
- Malignant involvement of the lymph nodes
- Perineural invasion by malignant neoplasia

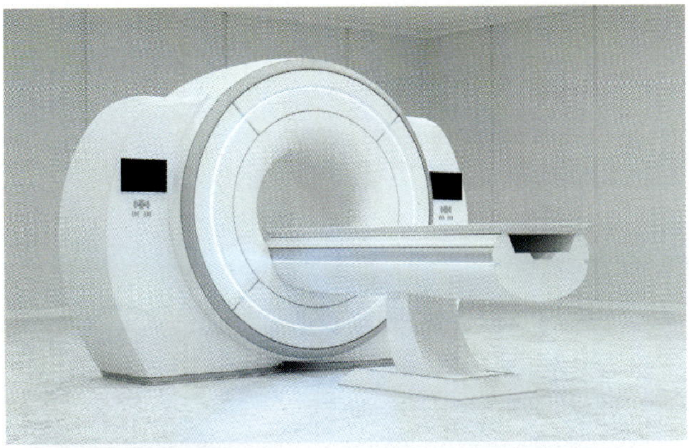

Figure 4.23 Magnetic resonance imaging machine.

- Soft tissue swelling—space infections, masseter hypertrophy, space occupying lesion, etc.

CONTRAINDICATIONS

- Ferromagnetic or electronically operated active devices, such as automatic cardioverter defibrillators
- Cardiac pacemakers and other pacemakers, for example for the carotid sinus
- Metallic splinters in the eye
- Ferromagnetic haemostatic clips in the central nervous system (CNS)
- Cochlear implants
- Insulin pumps and nerve stimulators
- Prosthetic heart valves (in high fields, if dehiscence is suspected)
- Haemostatic clips (body)
- Nonferromagnetic stapedial implants
- Claustrophobia
- Intraocular ferrous foreign bodies
- Bullets, pellets and shrapnel
- Orthopaedic implants, materials and devices.

ADVANTAGES

- Noninvasive
- Uses non-ionising radiation
- Produces high-quality images of soft tissue resolution in any imaging planes.

DISADVANTAGES

- Bone cannot be captured by MRI as bone does not give any MR signal; a signal is only obtainable from bone marrow, although this is of less importance
- Long scanning time and thus demanding on the patient.
- Contraindicated in patients with surgical clips, cardiac pacemakers, and cochlear implants and in the first trimester of pregnancy
- Equipment tends to be claustrophobic and noisy
- Equipment is more expensive
- Differentiation is difficult as bone, teeth, air and metallic objects all appear dark.

NUCLEAR MEDICINE

Nuclear medicine refers to the branch of medicine that uses radioactive substances in diagnosis and therapy. It consists of pharmaceutical substances labelled with radioisotopes—*radiopharmaceuticals*. They consist of chemical molecule, which determines the behaviour of the radiopharmaceutical in the body. The radiation emitted by the radionuclide may be detected from outside the body by a radionuclide-imaging device *(a gamma camera)* or may be detected in a sample of a body fluid *(e.g. plasma or urine)*.

RADIOISOTOPES

Radioisotopes are isotopes with unstable nuclei which undergo radioactive disintegration. This disintegration is often accompanied by the emission of radioactive particles or radiation (Table 4.4).

The important emissions are:

- Alpha particles
- Beta – (electron) and beta + (positron) particles
- Gamma radiation.

RADIOISOTOPE IMAGING

Radionuclide imaging is also called functional imaging. It assesses physiologic changes, which is a direct result of biochemical alteration. In the head and neck region, Hand-held gamma camera for static and dynamic imaging is used in sentinel node biopsy in the detection of cervical metastasis of malignancy (refer Chapter 30 page 625).

GAMMA CAMERA

It is an electronic device used in medical diagnosis for imaging the distribution of radioactive compounds in the tissues (after injection) (Fig. 4.24).

PROCEDURE

Radioactive compounds have an affinity for particular tissues. The doubtful target tissues are injected intravenously with these compounds. The compounds get concentrated in the target tissue and their radiation emissions are then detected and imaged, usually using a stationary gamma camera. It allows the function of the target tissue to be examined under both static and dynamic conditions.

TABLE 4.4 Common Isotopes Used in Head and Neck Region Imaging

Radionuclide	$t_{1/2}$	Target areas
^{99m}Tc-MDP (technetium-99m methylene diphosphonate)	6 h	• Salivary glands, thyroid, bone • Blood, liver, lung and heart
Gallium (^{67}Ga)	78 h	Tumours and inflammation
Iodine (^{131}I or ^{123}I)	8 days	Thyroid

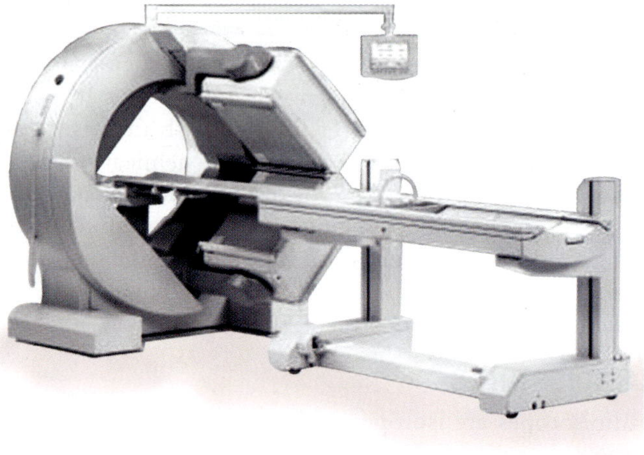

Figure 4.24 Static gamma camera.

INDICATIONS

- Tumour staging—assessment of the sites and extent of bone metastasis
- Assessment of continued growth in condylar hyperplasia.
- Investigation of salivary gland function, particularly in Sjogren syndrome
- Evaluation of bone grafts
- Evaluation in osteomyelitis of maxillofacial bones
- Investigation of the thyroid abnormalities (Table 4.5).

SINGLE-PHOTON EMISSION COMPUTERISED TOMOGRAPHY (SPECT)

The photons (gamma rays) are emitted from the patient and detected by a gamma camera rotating around the patient. A cross-sectional image or SPECT scan shows the distribution of radioactivity, thereby enabling the exact anatomical site of the source of the emissions to be determined. Produces image similar to CT and MRI in that a computer creates thin slices through a particular organ. Example: cardiac perfusion, brain, liver and bone studies (Fig. 4.25A and B).

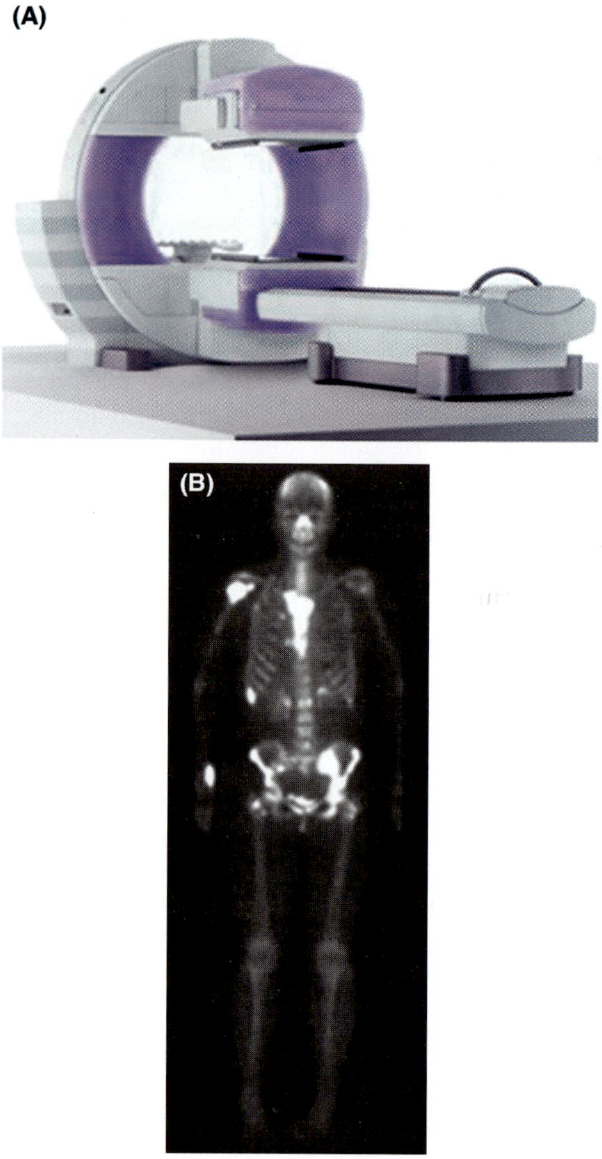

Figure 4.25 (A). SPECT machine. (B) SPECT image.

TABLE 4.5 Advantages and Disadvantages of Radioisotope Imaging

Advantages	Disadvantages
• Assessment of function of the target tissue • During one bone scan the whole skeleton can be imaged • Results can be enhanced	• Poor image resolution: minimal information about target tissue anatomy • High radiation dose • Images are not usually disease specific • Some investigations take several hours • Facilities are not widely available

POSITRON EMISSION TOMOGRAPHY (PET)

PET-CT is an advanced imaging modality, which depicts the metabolic or biochemical activity in the body correlated with anatomic imaging by CT scan. PET scan uses positron emission from particular radionuclides to produce detailed functional images within the body. PET is unique in that its images are of blood flow or metabolic processes at the cellular level rather than the more conventional anatomic image produced by X-ray, CT, MRI or even SPECT.

Useful in diagnosis of regions of increased metabolic activity as:

- Malignancies and distant metastasis
- Osteomyelitis of jaw
- Metastatic masses of unknown origin
- Acute inflammatory lesions (Fig. 4.26A–D).

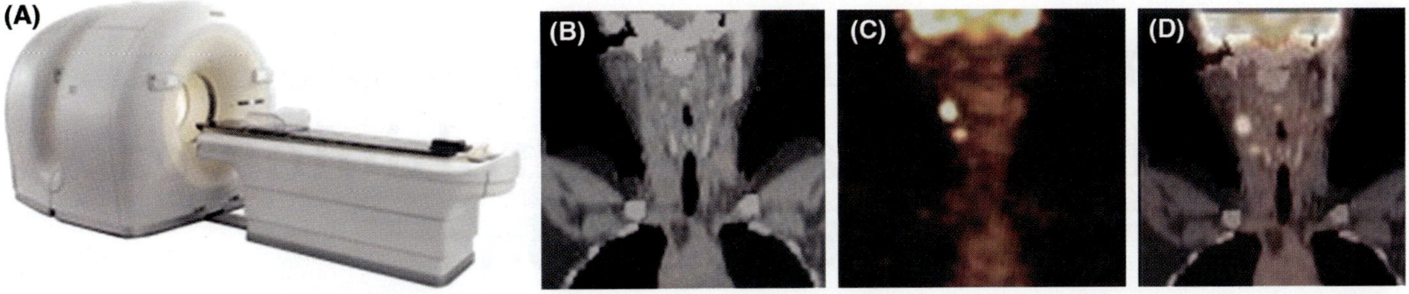

Figure 4.26 (A) PET machine. (B) CT image showing no significant neck mass. (C) PET image shows two lumpy abnormal radioactive concentration shadows on the right side of the neck. (D) PET/CT image shows two abnormal fluorodeoxyglucose hypermetabolism areas in the sternocleidomastoid region of the right side of the neck, which were considered lymph node metastases.

BONE SCAN

Bone scintigraphy is a diagnostic study used to evaluate the distribution of active bone formation in the body. Phosphate analogues can be labelled with ^{99m}Tc and are used for bone imaging because of their good localisation in the skeleton and rapid clearance from soft tissue. ^{99m}Tc-MDP (^{99m}Tc methylene di-phosphonate) uptake depends on osteoblast and osteoclast activity. Increased uptake denotes osteoblastic activity and decreased uptake signifies pure lytic lesion, osteoclast activity (Fig. 4.27). Abnormality in a bone scan is seen either as increase or decrease in radionuclide accumulation described as hot spot or cold spot. A hot spot is an area that appears black because bone growth is more active with increased accumulation of radionuclide (e.g. increased vascularity, bone formation, metastasis, new bone formation/growth, bone graft with positive vascularity). A cold spot is an area that appears lighter or white because bone growth (metabolic activity) is less active (e.g. malignant tumours such as lung and breast, bone ischaemia and necrosis, haemangiomas, radiation therapy and infection).

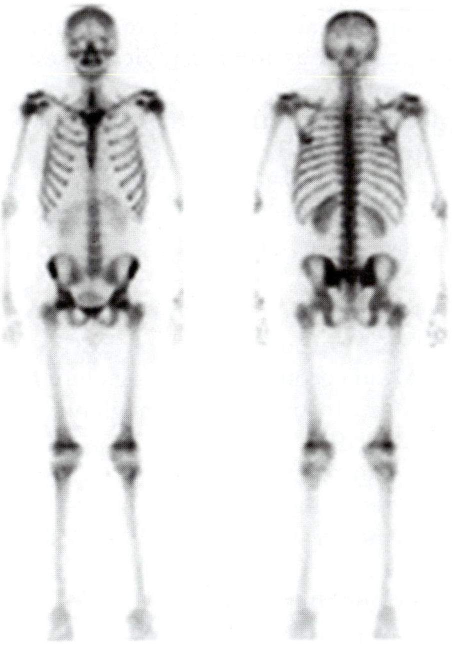

Figure 4.27 Normal bone scan.

THREE-PHASE BONE SCAN

It is done to see if there is soft tissue hyperaemia.
First phase: It is the perfusion phase or vascular phase.
Second phase: It is the blood pooling phase or soft tissue phase.
Third phase: It is the bony phase.

First phase

A total of 30–60 dynamic images are usually obtained over 1 minute immediately after injection. This is radionuclide angiography and gives an idea about the local vasculature. During the first minute after injection, injected dose is still intravascular.

Second phase

Static image is obtained in 5 minutes after dose injection. Within 5 min postinjection, the radiopharmaceutical moves from intravascular space to extravascular space (soft tissue). It shows details on soft tissue oedema.

Third phase

It is the bony phase image obtained in 2–4 h postinjection. It is the same as whole-body bone scan.

Chapter 5

Diagnostic Aid—Haematological, Biochemical and Microbiological Investigations

OUTLINE

Most lesions of the oral and maxillofacial region can be diagnosed using clinical and radiological investigations alone. However, when the cause of the lesion is beyond the oral cavity, like an oral manifestation of a systemic disease, investigations need to be broadened to assess the general health of the patient. This is usually performed by a 'haematological' or 'biochemical' analysis of the blood and other body fluids such as urine (Table 5.1). In the same way, in cases where the cause is microbial, investigation of the causative organism and its antibiotic sensitivity helps us in treating the disease more effectively rather than resorting to empirical antibiotics. Therefore, haematological, biochemical and microbiological investigations form a main part of the 'diagnostic' aids.

HAEMATOLOGICAL INVESTIGATIONS

Haematologists analyse and record the appearance of red blood cells (RBCs), white blood cells (WBCs) and platelets to predict, detect and diagnose diseases. These tests are essential in the diagnosis of oral diseases since conditions as severe as leukaemia can first manifest as an inflamed gingival lesion. While abnormalities in clotting and bleeding time may pinpoint a disease, it is also one of the mandatory presurgical tests for ensuring preparation of the oral surgeon to manage postsurgical complications.

VENUPUNCTURE FOR BLOOD COLLECTION

Blood collected for haematological investigations is collected in a tube containing potassium ethylenediamine tetraacetic acid (EDTA). The phlebotomist collects up to 4 mL of blood per tube. The tube is shaken gently, as EDTA prevents clotting of the blood sample. Consent for blood collection has become a mandatory procedure.

The haematological tests that are commonly done to elicit disease, as well as for presurgical assessment of the patient are:

I. **Complete blood count with differential count**
   1. Peripheral blood smear
   2. Haematocrit/Packed cell volume (Hct/PCV)
   3. Haemoglobin (Hb)
   4. Platelet count
   5. RBC count
   6. RBC indices
      i. Mean corpuscular volume (MCV)
      ii. Mean corpuscular haemoglobin (MCH)
      iii. Mean corpuscular haemoglobin concentration (MCHC)
   7. WBC count and differential
      i. Neutrophils
      ii. Lymphocytes
      iii. Monocytes
      iv. Eosinophils
      v. Basophils
   8. Erythrocyte sedimentation rate (ESR)

II. **Coagulation profile**
   1. Clotting time (CT)
   2. Bleeding time (BT)
   3. Prothrombin time (PT) and International Normalised Ratio (INR)
   4. Activated partial thromboplastin time (APTT)
   5. Clotting factors.

TABLE 5.1 The Most Important and Frequently used Haematological and Biochemical Investigations

Tests Frequently used by Dentists	Laboratory Tests Occasionally done	Test Rarely Used in the Dental Office
• CBC—Hb, Hct, WBC, differential WBC • Bleeding studies—PT, PTT, BT, platelet count • Peripheral blood smear • Fasting blood sugar	• Tests for disturbance of bone—Ca, P, alkaline phosphatase • Erythrocyte sedimentation rate • Urinalysis • Syphilis screening	• Enzymes—Creatinine phosphokinase, Serum Glutamic—Oxaloacetic transaminase (SGOT), Serum glutamic pyruvic transaminase (SGPT), Lactic dehydrogenase • Bilirubin • Reticulocyte count • Creatinine • Blood urea nitrogen • Acid phosphatase

COMPLETE BLOOD COUNT (CBC)

It is the most commonly performed test. The test consists of several individual tests of significance in understanding the patient's circulatory, immune and cardiovascular system (Fig. 5.1A and B).

ERYTHROCYTE SEDIMENTATION RATE (ESR)

The ESR is a simple, frequently performed haematology test, which measures the speed at which RBCs sediments in 1 h in a vertical column of anticoagulated blood under the influence of gravity (Fig. 5.1C and D). ESR, expressed in mm/h, would be increased in inflammatory and necrotic conditions.

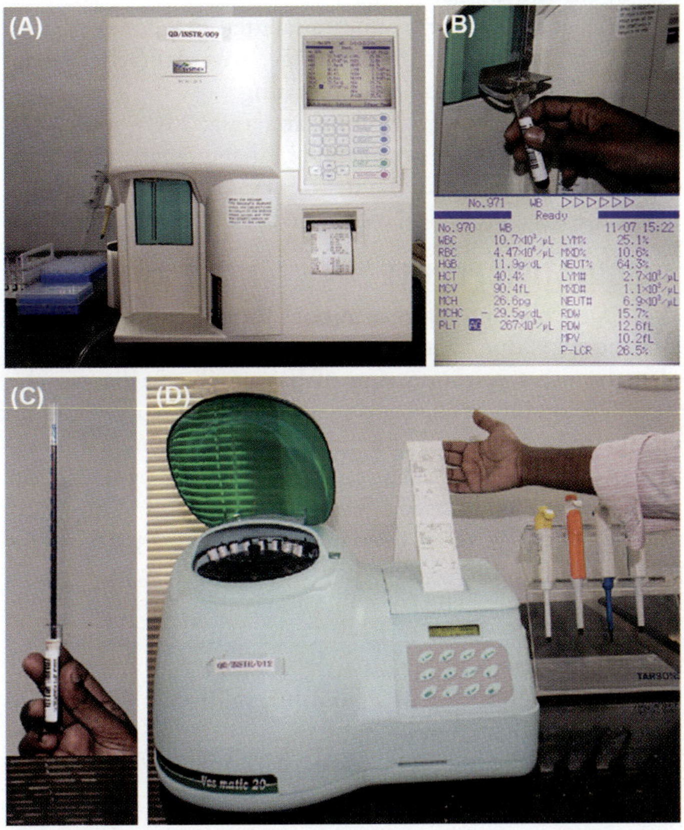

Figure 5.1 **(A & B)** Automated haematology analyser and result **(C)** ESR analysis—Wintrobe method. **(D)** Fully automated ESR analyser.

PERIPHERAL BLOOD SMEAR

Blood smear is a qualitative measure of blood cells that involves the preparation of a smear of peripheral blood drop on a slide. The smear is then microscopically examined to observe the morphology of RBCs, WBCs and platelets. Size, shape, colour and structure of the RBC are observed. WBC is measured for number and distribution. Number and appearance of platelets are observed for thrombocytopathy.

Abnormal RBC can be:

1. *Hyperchromic*—megaloblasticanaemia
2. *Hypochromic*—iron-deficiency anaemia
3. *Anisocytes*—vitamin B_{12} deficiency
4. *Macrocytes*—pernicious anaemia, folic acid deficiency
5. *Microcytes*—iron-deficiency anaemia and thalassaemia major (microcytic anaemia)
6. *Sickle cells*—sickle cell anaemia
7. *Target cells*—thalassaemia major, iron deficiency, liver disease, post splenectomy
8. *Ovalocytes/elliptocytes*—microcyticanaemias, megaloblastic anaemias
9. *Poikilocytes*—anaemia
10. *Schistocytes*–haemolytic anaemia, prosthetic valves, severe valvular disease and burns
11. *Heinz–Ehrlich bodies*—glucose-6-phosphate dehydrogenase deficiency, drug-induced haemolytic anaemia
12. *Howell–Jolly bodies*—severe haemolytic anaemia, pernicious anaemia, leukaemia, thalassaemia, myelodysplasias and in post splenectomy
13. *Rouleaux formation*—cryoglobulinaemia, giant cell arteritis, macroglobulinaemia and multiple myeloma

14. *Basophilic stippling*—heavy metal poisoning and thalassaemia
15. *Stomatocytes*—acute alcoholism, congenital stomatocytosis, drugs such as phenothiazines, hepatobiliary, cardiovascular and neoplastic diseases.

RED BLOOD CELL (RBC) INDICES

Tissue oxygenation depends on the number and function of RBCs and the concentration of Hb. RBC indices are used to measure if the RBCs are normal in size, have the appropriate amount of Hb and for the diagnosis of anaemia.

Diagnosis of anaemia using RBC indices

1. Normocytic, normochromic anaemia: MCV, MCHC normal, for example, haemolytic anaemia and anaemia of chronic disease
2. Microcytic/hypochromic anaemia: MCV decreases, MCHC decreases, for example, iron-deficiency anaemia, thalassaemia, lead poisoning
3. Macrocytic/normochromic anaemia: MCV decreases, MCHC—normal, for example, anaemia of folate deficiency and vitamin B_{12} deficiency

All the haematological tests have been briefed in Table 5.2.

COAGULATION PROFILE

Prolonged bleeding after a minor surgical procedure most commonly is due to a local cause or tissue injury, but it is also the most common sign of haemorrhagic disease and may develop into a haemorrhagic emergency. Sometimes investigations performed after encountering prolonged bleeding after a dental procedure may be the way by which the disease is first recognised.

The following tests are therefore, essential parts of the coagulation profile:

1. Bleeding time (BT)
2. Capillary fragility test
3. Clotting time (CT)
4. Prothrombin time (PT) and International Normalised Ratio (INR)
5. Activated partial thromboplastin time (APTT)
6. Clotting factors.

BLEEDING TIME (BT)

Bleeding time is the measure of the duration of bleeding after an injury, namely, a skin puncture. It is a screening test for diagnosis of platelet function and for vascular (peripheral capillary) defects. It can be determined by either Duke (1–3 min) or lvy method (2–9 min). BT is useful to differentiate Von Willebrand disease from haemophilia.

CAPILLARY FRAGILITY TEST

The capillary fragility or tourniquet test is based on the appearance of petechiae (small red bleeding spots) formation produced by an inflated blood pressure cuff over a 5-min period. It is also called as Hess test or Rumpel-Leede test. Normally less than 15 petechiae are seen. 15 or more petechiae indicate capillary fragility, which occur due to poor platelet function, bleeding diathesis or thrombocytopaenia, and can be seen in cases of scurvy and dengue fever.

CLOTTING TIME (CT)

CT is measured as the time taken for the blood to form fibrin bands or thrombus. The venous blood drawn is filled immediately into capillary tubes and the formation of bands checked by breaking the tubes at regular intervals and checking the formation of the strings of fibrin. Anticoagulants and tetracyclines may cause increased CT whereas corticosteroids and epinephrine cause decreased values. Prolonged coagulation times are associated with haemophilia, hypofibrinogenaemia and factor IX deficiency. Abnormalities in any of these tests indicate the requirement for further coagulation studies.

PROTHROMBIN TIME (PT)

- PT is used to assess efficient functioning of the coagulation process. The PT measures the amount of time it takes for a fibrin-clot to form in a plasma sample with added calcium and tissue thromboplastin. PT is also an index of the capacity of plasma to form thrombin. PT is reported either in seconds or as the percent of prothrombin calculated from a standard activity curve
- A normal range for PT is 8.8–11.6 s, but varies according to the norms established by individual laboratories (Fig. 5.2).

  USES:
  - Identifying bleeding disorders caused by either deficiency or inefficiency of coagulation factors
  - To monitor the effectiveness of anticoagulant therapy with warfarin sodium, which interferes with the production of vitamin K-dependent clotting factors such as prothrombin
  - To monitor oral anticoagulant therapy, which aims to maintain the PT at 1.5–2 times the control value (in seconds). Thus, a therapeutic goal, if receiving an anticoagulant, would be a PT of 24 seconds or 25% of normal activity.

PROTHROMBIN TIME (PT)—INTERNATIONAL NORMALISED RATIO (INR)

To provide standardisation of PT reporting among different laboratories, the WHO recommends the use of the INR to express the intensity of therapy. Most laboratories now report both the PT and the INR (Box 5.1).

$$INR = \frac{\text{Patient PT}}{\text{Lab PT}}$$

TABLE 5.2 Haematological Tests—The Complete Blood Count with Normal Values and Conditions that Increase and Decrease These Levels

Haematological Test	Normal Values	Increased Level	Decreased Level
Haemoglobin	Female: 12–16 g/dL Male: 13–18 g/dL Pregnancy: Decreased by haemodilution Elderly: Slightly decreased Newborn: Increased	Polycythaemia vera Myeloproliferative diseases Dehydration	Anaemia
PCV—Haematocrit	Female: 37%–48% Male: 42%–52% Pregnancy: Decreased due to haemodilution Elderly: Slightly decreased Newborn: Increased	Burns, cardiovascular disease, chronic lung disease, congenital cardiac defects, Cushing disease, dehydration, polycythaemia vera, liver cancer and shock.	Anaemia, haemorrhage, chronic infection, bone marrow suppression, leukaemia, malnutrition, lymphoma, multiple myeloma, cirrhosis, rheumatic fever and hypothyroidism.
Erythrocyte sedimentation rate (ESR)	Age below 50 years: Men 0–15 mm/h Women 0–20 mm/h Age above 50 years: Men 0–20 mm/h Women 0–30 mm/h	Polymyalgia rheumatica, temporal arteritis; rheumatoid arthritis; pregnancy; infections; anaemia; inflammation; trauma; diabetes mellitus, end-stage renal failure, heart disease, collagen vascular disease and malignancy	Polycythaemia, sickle cell anaemia
Platelet count	150,000–400,000 cells per cubic mm.	High altitudes, cold temperatures, exercise, excitement, drugs (cephalosporins, clindamycin, clozapine, corticosteroids, danazol, dipyridamole, donepezil, eptoin, gemfibrozil, lithium and oral contraceptives).	Hormones prior to menstruation, drugs (ACE inhibitors, acetaminophen, allopurinol, antiarrhythmics, barbiturates, chemotherapeutic agents, diuretics, donepezil, infliximab, NSAIDs and phenothiazines).
Red blood cell	*Adult male:* 4.7–6.1 × $10^6/mm^3$ *Female:* 4.2–5.4 × $10^6/mm^3$ *Newborn:* 3.5–5.1 × $10^6/mm^3$ *1–2 years:* 3.6–5.2 × $10^6/mm^3$ *3–7 years:* 4.1–5.5 × $10^6/mm^3$ *8–12 years:* 4.0–5.4 × $10^6/mm^3$	Polycythaemia is seen in smoking, polycythaemia vera, cardiovascular diseases, chronic hypoxia, chronic lung disease, Cushing disease, hepatic cancer, drugs (corticosteroids, danazol, gentamicin, thiazide diuretics).	Anaemia is seen in haemorrhage, vitamin B deficiency, leukaemia, multiple myeloma, alcohol abuse, bone marrow suppression, chronic infection, renal failure, haemodilution, Systemic lupus erythematosus (SLE), drugs (acetaminophen, acyclovir, allopurinol, amitriptyline, antimalarials, MAO inhibitors, phenytoin, captopril, chemotherapy).
RED BLOOD CELL INDICES			
$MCV = \frac{\text{Haematocrit (\%)} \times 10}{\text{RBC (millions/mm}^3\text{)}}$	*Male: 78–100 fL* *Female: 78–102 fL*	Large (macrocytic) RBC—macrocytic anaemia as in vitamin B_{12} or folic acid deficiency.	Smaller (microcytic) RBC—iron deficiency and thalassaemia.

Continued

TABLE 5.2 Haematological Tests—The Complete Blood Count with Normal Values and Conditions that Increase and Decrease These Levels—cont'd

Haematological Test	Normal Values	Increased Level	Decreased Level
$MCH = \frac{Haemoglobin\ (g/dL) \times 10}{RBC\ (millions/mm^3)}$	*Normal: 26–33 pg/cell*	-	-
$MCHC = \frac{Haemoglobin\ (g/dL) \times 100}{Haematocrit\ (\%)}$	*Normal: 32–36 pg/cell*	Hyperchromic RBC—hereditary spherocytosis	Hypochromic RBC—iron deficiency and thalassaemia
WHITE BLOOD CELL COUNT AND DIFFERENTIAL COUNT			
White blood count (total)	Adult: 4500–10,500/mm^3 Child 6–12 years: 4500–13,500/mm^3 Child 2–6 years: 5000–15,500/mm^3 Child <2 weeks: 5000–21,000/mm^3 Newborn: 9000–30,000/mm^3	Pregnancy; exercise; infection; trauma; leukaemia; uraemia	Idiopathic, bone marrow diseases, drugs, viral infections, early leukaemia
Neutrophils	40%–60%: 3000–7000 cells/mm^3	Exercise; pregnancy; infection; trauma; malignancy; leukaemia	Endocrinopathies, bone marrow diseases, SLE
Eosinophils	1%–4%: < 450 cells/mm^3	Allergic diseases; parasitic infestations; skin diseases	Cushing syndrome or corticosteroid administration
Basophils	0.5%–1%: 15–100 cells/mm^3	Chronic myelocyticleukaemia, splenectomy, infections, injection of foreign proteins	Stress, pregnancy hyperthyroidism, steroid intake
Lymphocytes	20%–40%: 1000–4000 cells/mm^3	Some infections; leukaemia; physiological; bowel disease	Drugs, viral infections, immune defects (e.g. HIV, AIDS)
Monocytes	2%–8%: < 850 cells/mm^3	Certain infections; tuberculosis; neutropaenia	HIV, rheumatoid arthritis steroid intake
OTHER TEST FOR THE DIAGNOSIS OF ANAEMIA			
Folic acid	2–20 ng/mL	Folic acid therapy	Alcoholism; dietary deficiency; haemolytic anaemias; malabsorption; myelodysplasia; phenytoin; methotrexate; trimethoprim; pyrimethamine; sulfasalazine; cycloserine; oral contraceptives; pregnancy
Vitamin B_{12}	200–600 pg/mL	Liver disease; leukaemia; polycythaemia rubra vera	Pernicious anaemia; gastrectomy; Crohn disease; ileal resection; vegans; metformin
Vitamin D	20–50 ng/mL	Vitamin D intoxication	Vitamin D deficiency, primary hyperparathyroidism

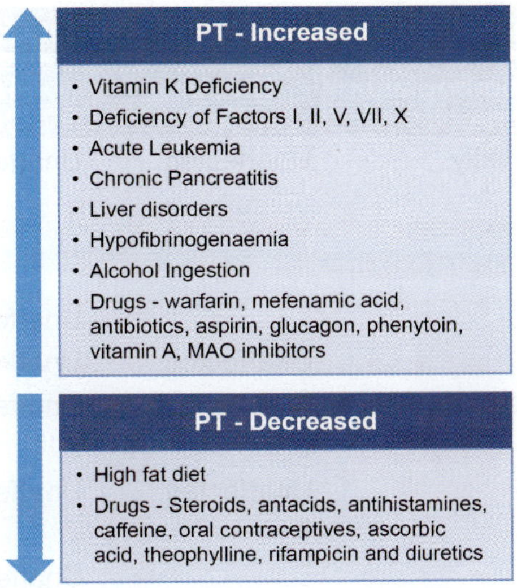

Figure 5.2 Prothrombin time (PT) is increased and decreased in the conditions listed.

BOX 5.1 PT–INR Treatment Guidelines

INR of 1.0 means patient is normal

- Normal range: 0.9–1.3

INR greater than 1.0 means clotting time is elevated (prophylactic anticoagulant therapy)

INR of 2.0–3.0 is advised for no change in drug dosage

- This is the target INR for patients on anticoagulant therapy (warfarin clopilet)

INR of 2.5–3.5 is recommended for higher doses of anticoagulant therapy in

- Cardiac valve replacement
- Antiphospholipid antibody syndrome

ACTIVATED PARTIAL THROMBOPLASTIN TIME (APTT) OR PARTIAL THROMBOPLASTIN TIME (PTT)

- The PTT is used to appraise the proper functioning of the coagulation cascade by measuring the time taken for a clot to form in a plasma sample to which calcium and partial thromboplastin have been added.
- If additional chemicals are added to standardise and accelerate the test, the result is reported as an APTT. Normal range for PTT is 60–90 s; APTT is 25–35 s.
- This test is helpful for diagnosing bleeding disorders that occur due to deficient or defective coagulation factors I, II, III, V, IX, X, XI and XII that form the intrinsic system.
- The PTT and APTT are used to monitor heparin therapy. If the APTT is higher than 100 s, the patient is at high risk for spontaneous bleeding wherein the dosage needs to be tapered.

COAGULATION FACTOR ASSAY

Coagulation factor assay is performed to diagnose congenital or acquired deficiency of haemostasis such as haemophilia, Von Willebrand disease, vitamin K deficiency, etc. For example, tests of factor VIII-related antigen are used in the differential diagnosis of classic haemophilia and Von Willebrand disease in cases in which there is no family history of bleeding and bleeding times are borderline or abnormal. A test for ristocetin cofactor is done to help diagnose Von Willebrand disease by determining the degree or rate of platelet aggregation that is taking place.

Bleeding and coagulation disorder should be investigated and diagnosed as shown in Flowchart 5.1 and Table 5.3.

Flowchart 5.1 depicts the way a bleeding disorder should be investigated and diagnosed.

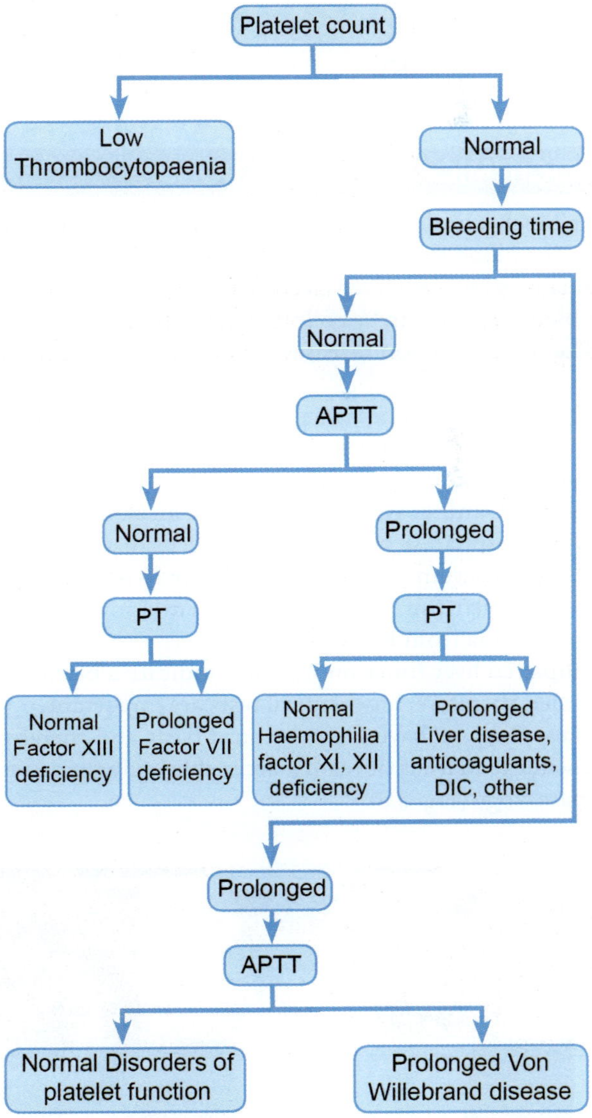

Flowchart 5.1 Bleeding disorder investigations.

TABLE 5.3 Diagnosis of Bleeding and Coagulation Disorders based on PT, PTT, BT and Platelet Count

Condition	Prothrombin Time	Partial Thromboplastin Time	Bleeding Time	Platelet Count
Vitamin K deficiency or warfarin	↑	Normal or mildly prolonged	Unaffected	Unaffected
Disseminated intravascular coagulation (DIC)	↑	↑	↑	↓
Von Willebrand disease	Unaffected	↑	↑	Unaffected
Haemophilia	Unaffected	↑	Unaffected	Unaffected
Aspirin	Unaffected	Unaffected	↑	Unaffected
Thrombocytopaenia	Unaffected	Unaffected	↑	↓
Liver failure, early stage	↑	Unaffected	Unaffected	Unaffected
Liver failure, end stage	↑	↑	↑	↓
Uraemia	Unaffected	Unaffected	↑	Unaffected
Congenital afibrinogenaemia	↑	↑	↑	Unaffected
Factor V deficiency	↑	↑	Unaffected	Unaffected
Factor XII deficiency	Unaffected	↑	Unaffected	Unaffected

BIOCHEMICAL INVESTIGATIONS

Most biochemical investigations can be carried out on serum. The blood sample can be collected in a plain container. Plasma may be needed for electrolytes, cortisol and proteins. The blood sample can be collected in a lithium heparin tube.

The most common diseases of the oral and maxillofacial region:

- Cotton wool appearance, multifocal radiodense conglomerates seen in osteitis deformans (Paget's disease) may also be encountered in florid cementosseous dysplasia and Gardner syndrome; however, an elevation of alkaline phosphatase occurs only in Paget's disease
- Elevated serum calcium can indicate hyperparathyroidism (Brown tumour). Thus, differentiating a giant cell granuloma from Brown tumour
- Impaired liver function may also indicate a bleeding disorder; therefore, biochemical tests are important.

Many diseases have a biochemical basis and therefore, a biochemical analysis of readily accessible body fluids reveals the pathology (Fig. 5.3).

In the dental surgical practice, oral manifestation of a systemic disease can be diagnosed by biochemical tests briefed in Table 5.4.

MICROBIOLOGIC TESTS

Diagnostic microbiology tests deal with the detection of the microbial agent of an infection. The microbe causing the infection in a host body can be identified by inducing the specimen taken from the host body to a number of laboratory procedures. The most common sample in a dental practice is exudate from a cyst or abscess or periodontal specimens. These should be collected before antibiotics are started. The sample should be collected and sent in a sterile container or by a sterile swab. If the microbiological specimen is not processed within 2 h, it should be placed in a transport medium and stored in low temperature at 4°C.

Methods of microbial diagnosis are:

1. Nonculture methods
2. Culture method
3. Culture media

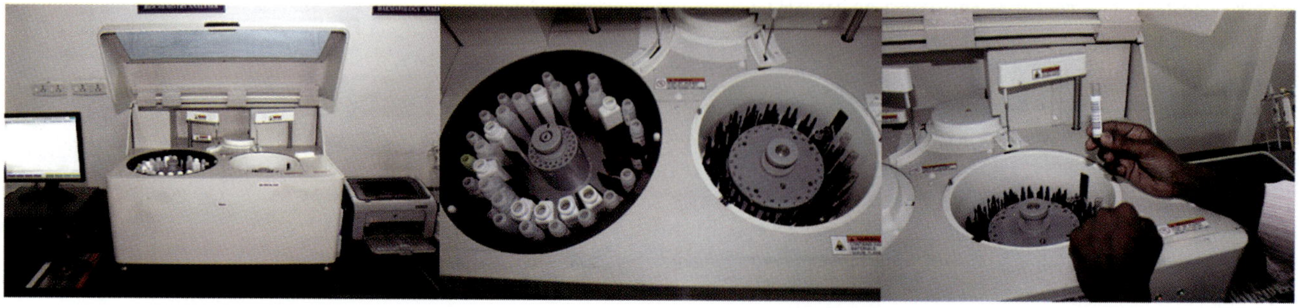

Figure 5.3 Automated biochemistry analyser.

TABLE 5.4 Biochemical Tests used for Diagnosis

Biochemical Tests	Normal Value	Elevated/Decreased
BLOOD GLUCOSE LEVELS		
Glucose	**Fasting – 70–100 mg/dL** **Post-prandial – 100–140 mg/dL**	Increased: Diabetes mellitus; pancreatitis; hyperthyroidism; hyperpituitarism; Cushing disease; liver disease; post head injury Decreased: Hypoglycaemic drugs; Addison disease; hypopituitarism; hyperinsulinism; severe liver disease
HbA1C (glucose attached to Hb)	**Normal: below 5.7 %** **Prediabetic: 5.7%–6.4%** **Diabetic: more than 6.4 %**	

METABOLIC BONE DISEASE TESTS

Systemic Jaw lesions such as Paget's disease, fibrous dysplasia, osteoporosis, multiple myeloma, osteogenic sarcoma or metastatic carcinoma can have changes in the following tests (N – Normal)

		Rickets	Osteomalacia	Paget's Disease	Hyperparathyroidism	Osteogenic Imperfecta	Metastatic Bone Cancers
Serum Calcium	**8.5–10.5 mg/dL**	**N**	↓	**N**	↑	**N**	↑
Serum Phosphorus	**2.5–4.9 mg/dL**	↓	↓	**N**	↓	**N**	**N**
Vitamin D **PTH**	**20–50 ng/mL** **14–65 pg/mL**	↑	↓	↑	↑	↑	**N/↑**
ALP	**Discussed below under liver function test**						

ESTIMATION OF ELECTROLYTES

The major electrolyte levels tested are the sodium, chloride, potassium and bicarbonate.
Electrolytes play a major role in maintaining fluid levels inside and outside the cells by Osmotic gradient. Electrolytes maintain pH and changes can cause protein denaturation and loss of enzyme functions. This can be life threatening and will require immediate intravenous substitution of electrolytes.

Sodium	**136–145 mEq/L**	**Increased:** Dehydration, CNS trauma or disease, hyperadrenocorticism, corticosteroid overdose, glycosuria, diabetes insipidus **Decreased:** Adrenal insufficiency, burns, chronic diarrhoea, hyperglycaemia
Chloride	**95–108 mEq/L**	**Increased:** Dehydration, hyperparathyroidism, renal insufficiency, nephrosis **Decreased:** GI disease, chronic renal failure, diabetic ketoacidosis, CHF
Potassium	**3.5–5.2 mEq/L**	**Inadequate intake:** Malabsorption, use of diuretics, amphotericin B
Bicarbonate	**24–30 mEq/L**	**Increased:** Metabolic alkalosis, respiratory acidosis, dehydration **Decreased:** Metabolic acidosis, respiratory alkalosis

LIVER FUNCTION TEST

ALKALINE PHOSPHATASE (ALP)

ALP is an enzyme found in the cells lining the biliary tract and in the **osteoblasts** involved in the **formation of new bone** and also in liver, bone, placenta, intestine and kidneys. Increased ALP levels are found most commonly during periods of **bone growth** (as in children), in various types of liver disease and in biliary obstruction. ALP is also a **tumour marker** that increases in the case of **osteogenic sarcoma** and in breast or prostate cancer that has **metastasised to the bone**.

GAMMA GLUTAMYL TRANSFERASE (GGT)

GGT is often measured in conjunction with ALP to determine whether the ALP is increased due to liver disease. While ALP may be increased with either hepatobiliary or bone disorders, the GGT is more specific for hepatobiliary problems such as alcoholic cirrhosis or hepatic carcinoma. GGT is more sensitive than ALP, the transaminases (ALT, AST) and leucine aminopeptidase in detecting obstructive jaundice, cholangitis and cholecystitis.

Continued

TABLE 5.4 Biochemical Tests used for Diagnosis—cont'd

Biochemical Tests	Normal Value	Elevated/Decreased
SGPT AND SGOT		
SGPT refers to alanine transaminase (ALT) and SGOT refers to aspartate transaminase (AST). ALT value is used mainly in the diagnosis of liver disease and to monitor the effects of hepatotoxic drugs. ALT is assessed along with AST in monitoring liver damage. AST is an enzyme present in the heart, liver and muscle. It is released into the circulation subsequent to damage or death of cells. AST levels usually increase within 12 h of the injury and remain elevated for 5 days. Thus, this test is performed along with creatine kinase (CK) isoenzymes, LDH, LD and troponin when there has been damage to the cardiac muscle as in myocardial infarction.		
Bilirubin	Total bilirubin: 0.3–1.0 mg/dL	**Drugs that increase total bilirubin:** Allopurinol, steroids, MAO inhibitors, oral contraceptives **Drugs that decrease total bilirubin:** Barbiturates, caffeine, penicillin
	Direct (conjugated) bilirubin: 0.0–0.4 mg/dL	**Elevated direct bilirubin:** Biliary obstruction (e.g. choledocholithiasis), cirrhosis, pregnancy
	Indirect (unconjugated) bilirubin: 0.1–1.0 mg/dL	**Increased indirect bilirubin:** Increased haemolysis, decreased hepatic uptake/conjugation (e.g. Gilbert syndrome), cirrhosis, erythroblastosisfoetalis, malaria
Prothrombin time	10–14 s	**Elevated:** Strong prognostic indicator of poor outcome and need for liver transplantation in acute liver failure, acetaminophen overdose
Total Protein	6.3–7.9 g/dL	**Increased:** Liver disease; multiple myeloma; sarcoid; connective tissue disease **Decreased:** Pregnancy; nephrotic syndrome; malnutrition; enteropathy; renal failure; lymphomas
Albumin	3.5–5.0 g/dL	**Increased:** Dehydration **Decreased:** Malnutrition, severe illness, renal losses (e.g. nephritic syndrome) and gut losses (protein-losing enteropathy)
AST or SGOT	Female: 7–30 U/L Male: 10–55 U/L Elderly: Slightly high	**Increased in:** Acute hepatocyte injury due to drugs (e.g. acetaminophen overdose), viruses (e.g. hepatitis A, hepatitis B), or ischaemia (e.g. myocardial infarction) AST >× 2 higher than ALT characteristic of alcoholic liver disease; also in cirrhosis, hepatitis, pancreatitis, liver CA
	Children: 2–3 times adult normal values ALT:AST = 1:1	**Decreased in:** Beriberi, diabetic ketoacidosis, haemolysis, pregnancy, uraemia **Drugs that increase:** Acetaminophen, allopurinol, antibiotics, chlorpropamide, cholinergic, methyldopa, vitamin A **Drugs that decrease:** Metronidazole
ALT or SGPT	Female: 7–30 U/L Male: 10–55 U/L ALT:AST = 1:1	**Increased in:** Hepatitis, cirrhosis, liver cancer, biliary obstruction (cholestasis), bone metastasis, congestive heart failure, muscle inflammation, infectious mononucleosis, shock, trauma **Drugs that increase:** ACE inhibitors, acetaminophen, anticonvulsants, antibiotics, heparin, NSAIDs
• **AST** > ALT infers alcohol-induced hepatitis, cirrhosis and metastatic cancer of the liver. • **AST** < ALT infers viral or drug-induced hepatitis and hepatic obstruction other than malignancy.		
ALP	Female: 30–100 U/L Male: 45–115 U/L Elderly: Slightly high	**Increased in:** Biliary obstruction, bone metastasis, calcium deficiency, CA pancreas, cirrhosis, eclampsia, fracture, hepatitis, high-fat intake, ***hyperparathyroidism***, infectious mononucleosis, leukaemia, CA liver, osteogenic sarcoma, ***Osteomalacia***, ***Paget's disease***, pancreatitis, pregnancy, RA, rickets, vitamin D deficiency

TABLE 5.4 Biochemical Tests used for Diagnosis—cont'd

Biochemical Tests	Normal Value	Elevated/Decreased
	Children: 1–3 times adult Puberty: 5–6 times adult norms	**Decreased in:** Cystic fibrosis, excessive vitamin D intake, hypophosphataemia, perniciousanaemia, celiac disease, chronic nephritis, scurvy, hypothyroidism **Drugs that increase:** ACE inhibitors, anticonvulsants, heparin, NSAIDs, oestrogens **Drugs that decrease:** Fluorides, propranolol
GGT	Female: 5–29 U/L Male: 5–38 U/L Child: 3–30 U/L Newborn: 156.7 ± 98.2 IU/L	**Increased in:** Acute pancreatitis, alcoholism, biliary obstruction, cholecystitis, cholelithiasis, cirrhosis, hepatitis, MI, renal cancer, SLE GGT is a sensitive marker of alcohol ingestion and certain hepatotoxic (liver toxic) drugs Marker of cholestasis, but may be due to alcohol and other drugs through enzyme induction **Drugs that increase:** Aminoglycosides, barbiturates, NSAIDs, phenobarbital, phenytoin **Drugs that decrease:** Oral contraceptives
RENAL FUNCTION TESTS		
BUN (blood urea nitrogen)	7–20 mg/dL	**The end product of protein metabolism is urea, which is excreted entirely by the kidneys; therefore, the BUN is an indication of liver and kidney function** **Increased:** Renal failure; dehydration; gastrointestinal bleed **Decreased:** Liver disease; nephrotic syndrome; pregnancy; malnutrition
Serum creatinine	0.7–1.3 mg/dL	**Increased:** Renal failure; urinary obstruction **Decreased:** Pregnancy
24-h urine collection for creatinine clearance	**Measures GFR and is dependent upon renal artery perfusion and glomerular filtration (GF)**	
Uric acid	4–8.5 mg/dL	**Increased:** Gout; leukaemia; renal failure; multiple myeloma **Decreased:** Liver disease; probenecid; allopurinol; salicylates
CHOLESTEROL AND LIPID TESTS		
Total Cholesterol	< 200 mg/dL	**Increased:** Hypercholesterolaemia; pregnancy; hypothyroidism; diabetes; nephrotic syndrome; liver or biliary disease **Decreased:** Malnutrition; hyperthyroidism
Lipids (triglycerides)	<150 mg/dL	**Increased:** Hyperlipidaemia; diabetes mellitus; hypothyroidism; hypervitaminosis D
CARDIAC BIOMARKERS		
Creatinine kinase	22–198 U/L	**Increased:** Myocardial infarction
CK—MB	<3–5% of total CK	**Increased:** Myocardial infarction
Lactate dehydrogenase (LDH)	<140–280 U/L	**Increased:** Myocardial infarction; trauma; liver disease; haemolytic anaemias; lymphoproliferative diseases **Decreased:** Radiotherapy
Myoglobin	17.4–105.7 ng/mL	Early marker of MI
Cardiac Troponin	0.01–25 ng/mL	**Increased:** Myocardial infarction
INDICATORS OF INFECTION AND INFLAMMATION		
C-reactive protein (CRP)	Less than 10 mg/L	Infection, trauma, chronic disease, risk of myocardial infarction
D-Dimer	< 250 ng/mL	Thrombotic disease, DVT; pulmonary embolism, DIC

Continued

TABLE 5.4 Biochemical Tests used for Diagnosis—cont'd

Biochemical Tests	Normal Value	Elevated/Decreased	
THYROID FUNCTION TEST			
Thyroid function test	Untreated hyperthyroidism	Untreated primary hypothyroidism	Normal values
TSH	Low	High	0.35–5.0 μIU/L
T3	High	Low or Normal	100–200 ng/dL
T4	High	Low	6–12 μg/dL
Free T3	High	Low	260–480 pg/dL
Free T4	High	Low	0.7–1.53 ng/dL
URINE ANALYSIS			
Cloudy, foul smelling, WBCs—urinary tract infection (UTI) Dark yellow—dehydration Acetone odour—diabetic ketoacidosis Presence of protein—injured glomerular membrane Glucose—diabetes mellitus Ketones—fatty acid metabolism Crystals—renal stone formation possible Many hyaline casts—proteinuria Cellular casts—nephrotic syndrome			

4. Molecular diagnostics
5. Immunologic methods.

NONCULTURE METHODS

i. *Bright field or standard microscopy* (Fig. 5.4A and B): Organisms from a specimen or colonies can be identified by the morphological features as viewed under microscope
ii. *Dark field microscopy* (Fig. 5.4C): The specimen is illuminated obliquely by a special condenser so that light rays do not enter the objective directly. The organisms look bright against a dark background, e.g. *Treponema pallidum*
iii. *Fluorescence microscopy* (Fig. 5.4D): Bacteria or cells are stained with fluorescent dyes such as auramine to detect microbial antigens in a specimen. The latter is 'stained' with specific antibodies tagged with fluorescent dyes. For example, Quantitative Buffy Coat (QBC) Malaria test tubes are internally coated with acridine orange stain and anticoagulant with specific antibodies tagged with fluorescent dyes. The specimen is collected in the tube and centrifuged, then examined under special fluorescence microscopes to detect the parasite. Fluorescence microscopy is used for tuberculosis bacilli also.

CULTURE METHODS

The pathogen is multiplied in a conducive environment and identified by viewing under a light or electron microscope. Their virulence and sensitivity to antibiotics can also be tested after their colonies are grown.

1. Solid or liquid media are used for bacterial and fungal growth (Fig. 5.5A)

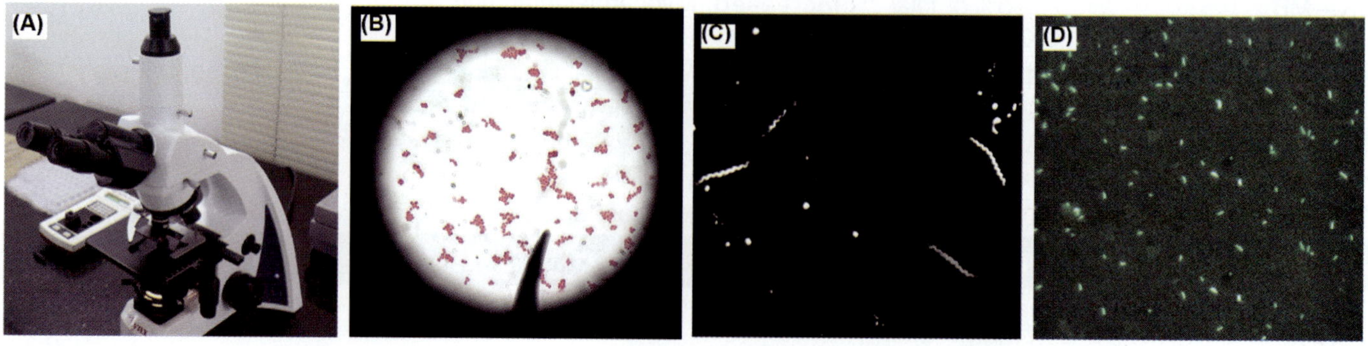

Figure 5.4 **(A)** Binocular bright field microscope. **(B)** Bright field microscopy showing streptococcus. **(C)** Dark field microscopy showing *Treponema pallidum*. **(D)** Fluorescence microscopy showing *Tuberculosis bacilli* stained by Ziehl–Neelsen dye.

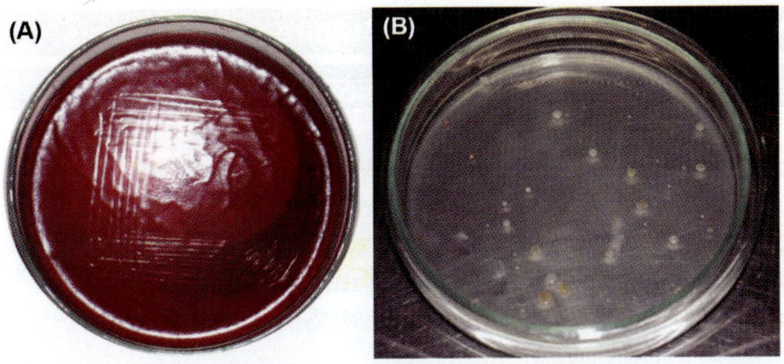

Figure 5.5 (**A**) Blood agar streaked with bacterial inoculum. (**B**) Gold colour—growth of *Staphylococcus aureus*, white colour—*Staphylococcus albus* in agar.

2. Cultured cells from animals/human beings are used for viral growth.

Bacteria can be identified by its morphological, physiological and biochemical characteristics:

1. The size, shape, elevation (flat, convex, umbonate), margin (entire, undulate, filamentous), colour, smell and texture; effect on blood (alpha, beta or nonhaemolytic) (Fig. 5.5B)
2. *Staining*
   a. Gram stain is performed routinely to reveal the shape and size of bacteria and to classify organisms into four categories: gram-positive cocci, gram-positive bacilli, gram-negative cocci, gram-negative bacilli. Gram stain gives clues to plan further diagnostic techniques and therapy
   b. Ziehl–Neelsen stain is performed on specimens of sputum, urine and pus when infections by mycobacteria are suspected
   c. Indian ink (negative staining) is used for capsulated bacteria
   d. Albert and Neisser stain can identify *Corynebacterium diphtheriae*. Spore staining is a technique for detecting sporulating bacteria
3. *Aerobic/anaerobic:* Bacteria can be identified depending on their growth in the presence or absence of air in the culture period. They are differentiated as aerobic, anaerobic, capnophilic (i.e. grows well in carbon dioxide excess) based on their growth requirements
4. *Biochemical tests:* Biochemical reactions of the bacteria are used to identify them. Sugar fermentation reactions, the fermentation of glucose, lactose, sucrose, mannitol and other sugars by pure culture are checked for the production of acid and gas or both
5. *Enzyme profile:* The organism is incubated with an appropriate, known enzyme substrate. If the enzyme is secreted by the organism, then this will react with the substrate and cause a colour change. Some bacteria can be identified primarily by production of a characteristic enzyme, e.g. coagulase produced by *Staphylococcus aureus*, lecithinase produced by *Clostridium perfringens*.

OBTAINING SAMPLE FOR CULTURE AND DETECTION

To achieve an accurate result and to interpret it clinically, following points should be considered while collecting the sample for culture and sensitivity:

1. The specimen collected should be of good quality and before commencement of antimicrobial therapy. Contamination by the normal microbiota of the surrounding areas misleads the diagnosis. For example, pus should be collected from the depth of the lesion and not from the surface
2. Vitality of the organism till it reaches the laboratory should be ensured
3. The timing of collection should be at the acute infectious phase
4. Label the specimen with at least two relevant details about the patient
5. Treatment should not be deferred until identification of pathogen since growth of pathogen in the culture may be delayed
6. Adequate quantity of specimen should be collected (Table 5.5).

CULTURE MEDIA

Majority of pathogenic bacteria grow on solid media, nutrient agar or blood agar (the most widely used culture media). Routinely, specimen is inoculated on blood agar and MacConkey agar. The culture media in which the bacteria are cultured or grown are chosen as per the organism under consideration.

CULTURE MEDIA USED FOR BACTERIA

1. **Blood agar** is a solid nutrient agar with 5%–10% horse or sheep blood, the most commonly used culture media
2. **Chocolate agar**, which is heated blood agar, is used for isolation of *Haemophilus influenzae, Neisseria* species
3. **Cysteine-lactose-electrolyte deficient (CLED) agar,** which contains peptone, L-cysteine, lactose, etc. is used to culture coliform bacteria
4. **Peptone and semisynthetic media** are used for antibiotic sensitivity tests
5. **Deoxycholate citrate agar, selenite F broth** are used for culturing *Salmonella* and *Shigellla* species
6. **Thiosulphate-citrate-bile salts-sucrose (TCBS) agar** for *Vibrio cholerae*
7. **Wilson and Blair's medium** for *Salmonella* species
8. **Thayer–Martin medium** for *Neisseria* species
9. **Lowenstein–Jensen (LJ) medium** for Mycobacteria
10. **Robertson's cooked meat liquid medium** is used mainly to culture anaerobes
11. **Liquid media containing peptone, sodium chloride and water** is used as base for sugar fermentation tests
12. **Liquid nutrient broth with meat extract** is used for general culture.

TABLE 5.5 The Common Diseases of the Oral Cavity for Microbial Isolation and Culture for Diagnosis

Disease	Specimen	Commonly Isolated Pathogens
Odontogenic infection	Pus	Polymicrobial Group A β-haemolytic streptococci, *S. aureus*
Wounds, tissues, bone, abscesses, fluids	The pus in closed, undrained soft tissue abscesses and osteomyelitis: mostly contains only one organism as the infecting agent. To diagnose anaerobic bacteria (bacteroides, pepto streptococci) anaerobic culture must be performed.	Anaerobes: *Bacteroides melaninogenicus, Eikinella corrodens*
Perioral abscess		Mixed flora of mouth and pharynx *Klebsiella pneumoniae*, *Streptococcus* sp., *Staphylococcus* sp.
Osteomyelitis	Pus or bone specimen obtained by aspiration or surgery	Multiple; often *S. aureus* Acute osteomyelitis: Organisms can often be cultured from blood before the infection has become chronic. Chronic osteomyelitis has deep suppurating lesions. The flora of the draining fistula should not be swabbed for culture. Instead, specimens should be aspirated from the primary lesion through uninfected tissue.
Cellulitis of skin, eroded skin and mucous membranes	Punch biopsy	Bacteria: Group A β-haemolytic streptococci, *S. aureus*
		Fungus: Yeast, Candida, Aspergillus and other fungi can be seen microscopically in smears or scrapings from suspicious areas and can be grown in cultures. KOH and calcofluor white greatly enhance the observation of yeasts and moulds in the specimen.
Impetigo	Swab	Group A β-haemolytic streptococci, *S. aureus*; rarely, *Corynebacterium diphtheria*
Ulcers	Punch biopsy; deep tissue aspirate or biopsy	Open wounds, mucosal surfaces have multiple microorganisms (Mixed flora).

CULTURE MEDIA USED FOR FUNGUS

Many types of yeast will grow on **blood agar**. Biphasic and mycelia phase fungi grow better on media designed specifically for fungi. **Brain–heart infusion agar**, with and without antibiotics and **inhibitory mould agar** have largely replaced the traditional use of **Sabouraud dextrose agar** to grow fungi. **Media made with plant and vegetable materials**, the natural habitats for many fungi, also grow many fungi that cause infections. Cultures for fungi are commonly done in paired sets, one set incubated at 25–30 °C and the other at 35–37 °C. Staining agents that are used for identifying fungal mycelium are KOH preparation, Indian ink preparation and calcofluor white stain.

LABORATORY AIDS IN THE SELECTION OF ANTIMICROBIAL THERAPY

Test for antibiotic susceptibility

1. The specimen is inoculated in two agar plates for culturing under aerobic and anaerobic conditions
2. The blood agar is then incubated for 2–3 days at 37 °C for 18 h
3. The plates are inspected for bacterial growth. The shapes and sizes of the colonies are identified. If the infections are monomicrobial, they are identified and can be cultured further for antibiotic sensitivity. If they are polymicrobial, the putative pathogens are isolated and subcultured on fresh blood agar plates to obtain single-organism cultures and incubate it at 37 °C for 24–48 h.
4. The pure culture is harvested and identified using biochemical reactions, selective media or specific antibody reactions
5. A filter paper disc impregnated with different antibiotics is applied onto a lawn of the organism seeded on an agar plate. After overnight incubation, the growth pattern of the colonies around the impregnated antibiotics shows the susceptibility of the organism to the antibiotic. Zones of growth indicate resistance and zones of inhibition indicate susceptibility.

Disc diffusion susceptibility test

Interpretation

1. The disc test measures the ability of drugs in inhibiting the growth of bacteria. The results correlate well with therapeutic response to eliminate infectious microorganisms
2. In general, only one member of each major class of drugs is represented in the disc test
   a. For *Staphylococci*, ***penicillin G, oxacillin, cefazolin, erythromycin, gentamicin and vancomycin*** are used
   b. For gram-negative rods, ***ampicillin, piperacillin, cefazolin, second- and third-generation cephalosporins and other 'antipseudomonal penicillins', trimethoprim-sulphamethoxazole, fluoroquinolones and the aminoglycosides (amikacin, tobramycin, gentamicin)*** are included
3. The diameter of *zones of growth inhibition* of one drug being larger than that of drug acting on the same organism does not mean higher susceptibility since the sizes depend on molecular size and diffusability of the drug and not on inhibitory action. Each drug has a specific and different minimum diameter of inhibition zone that denotes 'susceptibility' of an isolate by the disc diffusion technique (Fig. 5.6).

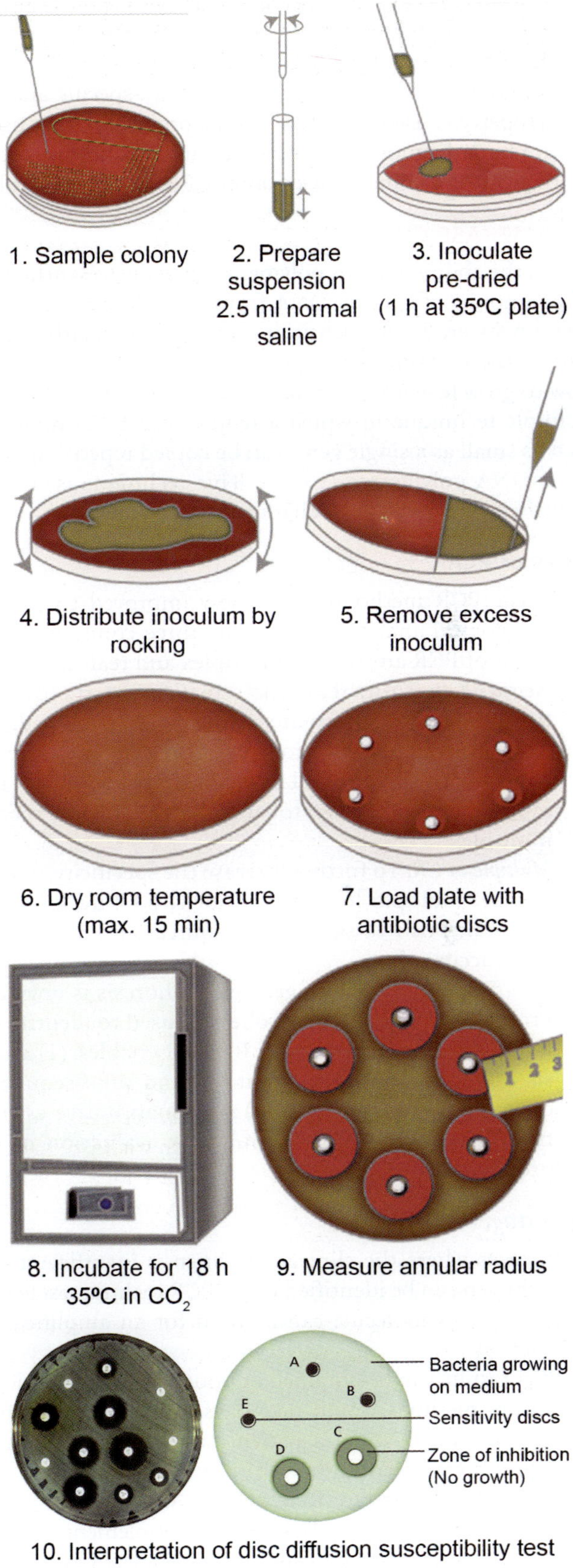

Figure 5.6 Disc diffusion susceptibility test.

MOLECULAR DIAGNOSTICS

Molecular diagnostics has two modalities:
1. Nucleic acid probe test
2. polymerase chain reaction (PCR).

NUCLEIC ACID PROBE TEST

It uses gene probes (cloned fragments of DNA) that recognise complimentary sequences of nucleic acid of microorganisms, based on which the infecting organism is identified. The test can be used for diagnosis of mycobacterial, chlamydial, neisserial and other bacterial infections.

GENE IDENTIFICATION PROBES

Every identified species of microbe has a unique DNA or RNA sequence somewhere on its genome that differentiates it from another species. In diagnostic microbiology, this character is used to detect microbes in the clinical samples from the infected patient by detecting the DNA sequence. The advantage of gene identification is that the swab samples could be simply sent by post to distant laboratories for identification, even in paper points, without the fear of death of organisms and the associated cumbersome culture procedures or transport media. Gene identification is done using probes. A few examples are:

1. *DNA gene probes* are pieces of DNA that are labelled radioactively or with a chemiluminescent marker. The probes carry a single strand of DNA analogous to the pathogen from the clinical sample

2. *Oligonucleotide probes* are based on the variable region of the 16 s ribosomal RNA genes, they are much more specific than the DNA probes
3. *Ribosomal RNA (rRNA)* is highly species-specific and this property is used to produce RNA probes that are useful for both diagnostic microbiology and taxonomic studies. The most commonly used are the 5, 16 and 23 S probes.

POLYMERASE CHAIN REACTION (PCR)

It uses the ability of DNA polymerase enzyme to synthesize a large amount of specific DNA from a single piece of DNA. These tests are highly sensitive and are particularly important in the identification of organisms that are difficult or slow to grow (e.g. *Mycobacterium, Neisseria, Chlamydia*). PCR is a simple technique in which a region of a DNA molecule, even as small as a single gene, can be copied repetitiously using a DNA polymerase enzyme. This technique is used to identify bacteria and virus that cannot be cultured.

Types of PCR

The basic PCR methodology is now improved to provide microbiological analytical tools. The three commonly used variations of PCR are: nested, multiplex and real-time PCR.

1. *Nested PCR*: To increase the sensitivity of the conventional PCR, two different sets of primers are used: one to begin the amplification primarily and the other to anneal with the internal sequence of the amplion in a more specific manner to obtain much more specific multiples
2. *Multiplex PCR*: To further increase the specificity, instead of one, multiple loci of the nucleotide are amplified simultaneously to save time, resources and to diagnose more accurately
3. *Real-time PCR*: Usage of gel electrophoresis is obviated. Probes or labelled fluoroprobes are used to identify the target sequence in real-time. RT-PCR enables: (1) analysis of multiple amplicons at specific time sequences during a reaction period; (2) semiquantitative estimation of the yield and (3) multiplex evaluation of the products.

Advantages

- In cases where the clinical specimen is insufficient, the pathogen can be identified using PCR techniques. Even a single DNA molecule can be used for an amplification reaction
- PCR results can be obtained in hours while conventional culture methods would take days to obtain. Amplification of viral DNA in a patient sample could be made within hours, even before the onset of symptoms
- It can be used even for RNA viruses. After the RNA molecule is converted into single-strand complementary DNA (cDNA) with an enzyme called reverse transcriptase, which transcribes the RNA code into DNA in a reverse manner, the PCR primers and Taq polymerase are added, followed by standard PCR techniques to obtain results.

IMMUNOLOGICAL METHODS

ANTIGEN TESTING

The microbe's antigenic property can be used for its detection.

a. ***Latex agglutination test***—used for detection of soluble antigen (Ag) in specimens such as urine, CSF, serum, etc. in infections due to *H. influenzae*, streptococci (Group A and B), Neisseria, etc
b. ***Co-agglutination test***—detection of Ag in streptococcal, pneumococcal, neisserial, salmonella, *H. influenzae* and other infections
c. ***Enzyme-linked immunosorbent assay (ELISA)***—detection of Ag in various bacterial infections
d. ***Slide agglutination test***—used for identification and confirmation of bacteria grown in culture
e. ***Commercial kits*** are available to detect antigenic property of many viruses, herpes simplex I and II, influenza A and B, CMV, etc
f. The advantages of these procedures are that they allow detection of viruses that do not readily grow in cell culture (e.g. rotaviruses, hepatitis A virus) or that grow very slowly (e.g. cytomegalovirus). In general, the antigen detection assays for viruses are less sensitive than the viral culture and nucleic acid amplification methods.

ANTIBODY TESTING

Antibody testing is performed for the identification of antibody or cell-mediated immune responses to the microbe in the host body. Serological tests are used in the diagnosis of infections in which causative agent is difficult to culture, e.g. *Treponema pallidum, Mycoplasma pneumoniae, Chlamydiae*, etc. Diagnosis is done on the basis of detection of specific antibody to the infectious agent. Active infection is diagnosed by demonstrating specific IgM or a fourfold increase in IgG antibodies taken 10–14 days apart.

The commonly used serological tests in different bacterial infections are:

a. *Agglutination test*, e.g. **Widal test** in enteric fever, **Brucella agglutination test** in brucellosis and **latex agglutination test**
b. *Indirect Coombs test*—for demonstration of incomplete antibodies in serum, e.g. brucellosis
c. *Complement fixation test*—for diagnosis of Q fever, syphilis, etc
d. *Flocculation test:* e.g. VDRL test for syphilis
e. *Indirect immunofluorescence test*—for antibody detection in syphilis, legionella, mycoplasma, borrelia and other infections
f. *Enzyme-linked immunosorbent assay* (ELISA) and radioimmunoassay (RIA) tests are used for detection of antibodies in a number of bacterial infections

g. *Immune electron microscopy (IEM):* Viruses not detectable by conventional techniques may be observed by immune electron microscopy (IEM). Antigen–antibody complexes or aggregates formed between virus particles in suspension are caused by the presence of antibodies in added antiserum and are detected more readily than individual virus particles. IEM is used to detect viruses that cause enteritis and diarrhoea; these viruses generally cannot be cultured by routine virus culture.

ELISA

Enzyme-linked immunosorbent assay (ELISA) systems involving use of antigens, haptens or antibodies labelled with an enzyme for measurement of substances in biological fluids. A capture antibody specific to the antigen in question is bound to the wells of plastic microdilution trays. Then the clinical specimen suspected to contain the microbe and therefore the antigen is incubated in the wells. The wells are then washed. A second antibody for the antigen, labelled with enzyme, is used to detect the antigen. The antigen is then detected colorimetrically by adding the substrate for the enzyme.

Western blot

Another form of enzyme-immunoassay (EIA) to detect antibody is immunoblotting (Western blot) whereby defined antigens are placed on strips of nitrocellulose paper. Following incubation with the test antibody-containing specimen, the strip is further treated with an enzyme-labelled antibody, usually from another animal, against the test antibody. Addition of the substrate for the enzyme allows detection of the antigen-specific bound antibody by colorimetric reaction. Western blot tests are used as the confirmatory tests for antibodies in HIV infection and Lyme disease.

ELISA and Western blot are diagnostic tests for HIV.

The viral infections and their corresponding detecting system have been briefed in Table 5.6.

Measuring the immune response to virus infection

A viral infection elicits both cellular and humoral immune responses. Measurement of either may be used to diagnose and quantify a viral infection.

Cellular immunity

1. This can be assessed by:
   a. Dermal hypersensitivity: When available, tests for dermal hypersensitivity to measure cellular immune responses offer certain advantages in easily and quickly determining prior exposure to infectious agents. The mumps skin test is often used (along with the candida skin test) as a positive control when tuberculin skin tests are applied. Most people have had mumps or mumps vaccine and those with normal immunologic systems have positive skin tests. The skin test may lead to an increase in antibodies, e.g. in the complement fixation test
   b. Lymphocyte transformation
   c. Cytotoxicity tests.

Humoral immunity

- IgM appears initially and is followed by IgG antibodies
- IgM antibodies disappear in several weeks
- IgG antibodies persist for many years.

TABLE 5.6 Viral Infections, Specimen Collected and Detecting System

Syndrome and Virus	Specimen	Detecting System
Infectious mononucleosis Epstein–Barr (EB) virus		
Cytomegalovirus	Blood, nasopharyngeal swab	Lymphoid cell culture, PCR; serologic testing
Hepatitis A virus	Blood, urine, throat swab	Cell culture; shell vial culture, antigen detection, PCR
	Serum, faeces	IEM, EIA, RT-PCR
Hepatitis B virus	Serum	EIA, PCR
Hepatitis C virus	Serum	EIA, PCR
Hepatitis D virus	Serum	EIA
Exanthemas		
Varicella-zoster virus	Vesicle fluid	Cell culture. Direct fluorescent antibody is most sensitive
Measles (rubeola) virus	Nasopharyngeal swab, blood, urine	Cell culture. Direct fluorescent antibody
Rubella virus	Nasopharyngeal swab, blood, urine	Cell culture
Herpes simplex virus	Vesicles, usually oral or genital	Cell culture
AIDS (Acquired immunodeficiency syndrome)		
Human immunodeficiency virus (HIV)	Blood, particularly leukocytes	Cell culture

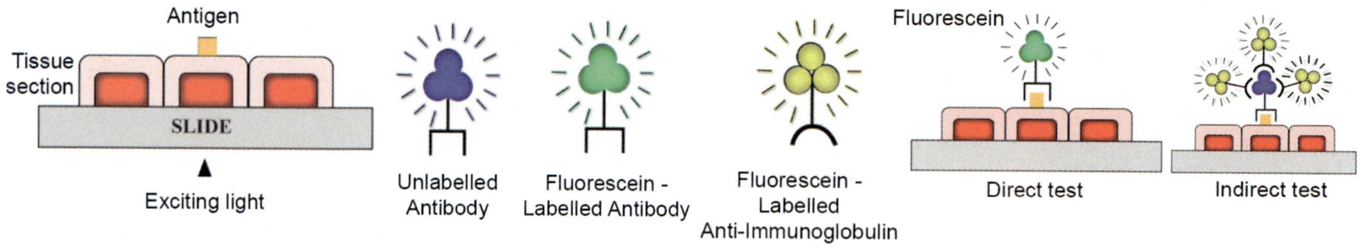

Figure 5.7 Immunofluorescence test.

Diagnosis of a viral infection is done serologically by demonstrating a rise in antibody titre to the virus or by demonstrating antiviral antibodies of the IgM class.

The methods used include:

a. The neutralisation (Nt) test
b. The complement fixation (CF) test
c. The haemagglutination inhibition (HI) test
d. The immunofluorescence (IF) test (Fig. 5.7)
e. Passive haemagglutination
f. Immunodiffusion.

Chapter 6

Histopathological Investigations

OUTLINE

Anaplasia/anaplastic: Any difference in the form or the arrangement of cells evident by the appearance of immature cells resulting from failure of differentiation. Anaplasia is the hallmark of malignant transformation.

Apoptosis: Programmed cell death. A type of cell death occurring in a cell causing cell shrinkage, chromatin condensation and cell fragmentation, which is removed by phagocytosis.

Atypia: Atypia is a nonspecific term referring to any change in a cell form that may be due to inflammation, precancerous condition or malignancy.

Biopsy: Biopsy is a method of removal of tissues from the living organism to determine the presence or extent of a disease. The tissues are analysed microscopically and chemically.

Cytopathology: Cytopathology is the study of cells under the microscope to analyse the features of the underlying disease.

Desmoplasia/desmoplastic: As the malignant cells penetrate the adjacent tissues, a connective tissue barrier of new collagen is formed as a host response in an effort to control the malignant cells. This host response is called desmoplasia and it is the characteristic feature of invasion and malignancy.

Differentiation: Described as the degree of resemblance of the malignant cells to their normal counterparts.

Well differentiated: Malignant cells that almost appear like normal cells of the tissue are termed as well differentiated. They do not advance aggressively.

Moderately differentiated: Intermediate in aggressiveness. Poorly differentiated or undifferentiated–the malignant cells whose appearance is primitive or bizarre. It advances aggressively.

Dysplasia: Irregularly arranged cellular variations that appear in epithelium, but shows no malignant growth. Although nonmalignant, it is recognised as an important risk factor for the development of malignancy.

Extravasation: Describes the process by which the cellular components of blood such as red or white blood cells pass through the walls of the blood vessel and enters the adjacent tissues.

Grade/grading: Grading is a measure of prognosis that generally depends on the extent of differentiation of the cancerous cells. Low-grade cancer is well differentiated and high-grade cancer is poorly differentiated. Each cancer has a specific grading system and standards. Numerical grading system is usually followed for most cancers. They are specified as grade I well-differentiated cancer to grade III–IV, high-grade poorly differentiated cancers. Usually, low-grade cancers are slowly progressive while the high-grade cancers are highly aggressive.

Hydropic degeneration: Blebbing of cells usually found in cell injury.

Hyperchromatic: Describes the dark staining of cell nucleus with routine H and E staining. It indicates the active growth phase, such as in cancer cells.

Immunohistochemistry: It is the process of identifying specific antigens from the samples, which comprises immunology (study of the immune response) and histology (study of the microscopic anatomy and chemistry).

Inflammation: It is the host response of the tissues to harmful stimuli such as irritation, injury or infection. The cardinal signs are pain, heat, redness, swelling and sometimes loss of function.

Invasion: One of the characteristic features of malignant tumour, describing growth pattern of cancer cells, invading the basement membrane and infiltrating the adjacent tissue.

Karyorrhexis: Describes the rupture and breakdown of a cell nucleus during cell death or necrosis.

Mesenchymal: Usually refers to soft tissue. The mesenchymal derivatives are collagen connective tissue, neural tissue, smooth and skeletal muscle, cartilage and sometimes bone.

Mitogen: Chemical substance that triggers mitosis in the cells.

Multifocal: Arising independently in several different places.

Myofibroblast: A variant fibroblast, which has the structural feature of both fibroblast and smooth muscle cell. It consists of a highly irregular nucleus, large amounts of rough endoplasmic reticulum and a dense cluster of filaments, which enable the muscle to contract.

Oncogene: A gene, which is capable of causing cancer.

Oncoprotein: A protein, which is related to cancer, either due to the decrease or increase of the chance or virulence of a tumour. Oncoproteins are synthesised when the oncogene is expressed.

Perineural invasion: Cancer cells penetrating in and around nerves, for example, adenoid cystic carcinoma.

Pleomorphic, pleomorphism: Alteration in size and shape of cell and/or their nuclei.

Stage/staging: A qualitative assessment of cancer prognosis. The four components of staging are tumour size, nodal status, grade and metastasis.

Stroma: Described as the connective tissue supporting matrix, which acts as a framework.

Vascular invasion/lymphatic invasion: Cancer cells penetrating into and localised within the blood or lymphatic vessels.

Histopathological investigation is described in Flowchart 6.1.

CYTOLOGY

Cytology refers to a branch of pathology that deals with making diagnosis of diseases and conditions through the examination of cell samples from the tissues of the body. Only cellular architecture can be studied using this technique. Cytologic examinations may be performed on body fluids like blood, urine and cerebrospinal fluid or on aspirated fluid (drawn out via suction into a syringe). Difference between biopsy and cytology is depicted in Table 6.1.

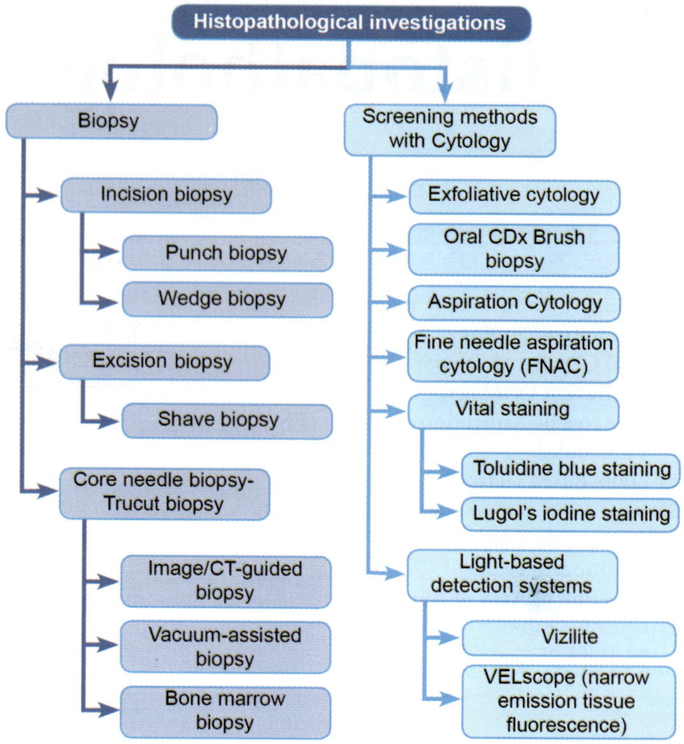

Flowchart 6.1 Histopathological investigations.

SCREENING METHODS WITH CYTOLOGY

Screening methods are required for quick diagnosis and to verify if a biopsy is required. Some lesions may be extensive and these screening methods will also help localise the best area to be biopsied. The various methods are classified as shown in Flowchart 6.2.

EXFOLIATIVE CYTOLOGY

- Using an orange wood spatula or a sterile plastic spatula, the superficial mucosal lesions are scrapped by a single powerful stroke
- The collected material is placed on glass slides and a thin smear is made
- The cells thus collected are then fixed using absolute alcohol or standard fixatives
- Ideally performed to identify suspected premalignant lesions, candidiasis and herpes zoster and very rarely for certain mucocutaneous lesions.
- The lesions are reported as:
  a. Class I (*Normal*)—Only normal cells were observed
  b. Class II (*Atypical*)—Presence of minor atypia, but no evidence of malignancy

TABLE 6.1 Difference Between Biopsy and Cytology

Biopsy	Cytology
A biopsy is the procedure that is used to extract tissue for microscopic or other types of investigation.	Cytopathology is the branch of pathology dealing with diagnosis of disease at the cellular level.
Biopsy may be diagnostic or therapeutic.	Cytology tests may be used for diagnosis or for screening.
Advantages: • It is easy to tell the difference between carcinoma in situ and invasive carcinoma. • Additional sections can be cut from the paraffin block and used for special stains or immuno-histochemistry. • Complete cure in case of excisional biopsy.	*Advantages:* • There is better microscopic detail of the cells. • It is often more convenient and less expensive than biopsy techniques. • A fine needle can reach anatomical areas where biopsy would be difficult—the head of the pancreas, retroperitoneum and the periphery of the lung. • Not as uncomfortable as a biopsy. • The diagnosis may be available within a few minutes (histologic diagnosis, other than frozen section diagnosis, normally takes 1 day).
Disadvantages: • Invasive • Patient discomfort	*Disadvantages:* • It is difficult to diagnose whether the malignancy is in situ or invasive. • Cytology preparations do not lend themselves to good immuno-histochemistry (with some exceptions).

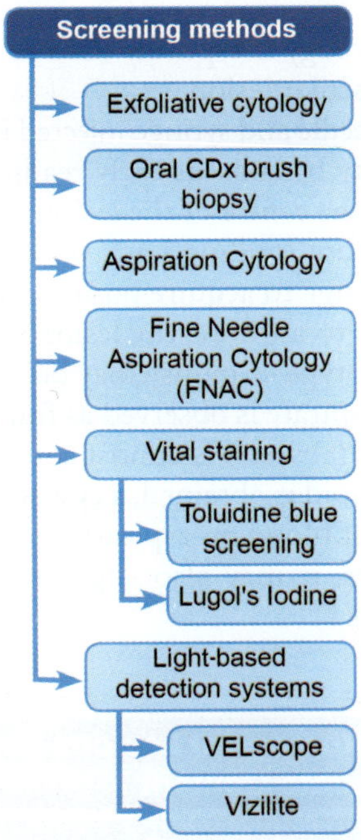

Flowchart 6.2 Classification of screening methods for quick diagnosis.

c. Class III (*Intermediate*)—The cells display wide atypia that may be suggestive of malignancy, precancerous lesions or carcinoma in situ

d. Class IV (*Suggestive of cancer*)—A few epithelial cells with malignant characteristics or cells with borderline characteristics

e. Class V—Positive cancer cells, that are obviously malignant

- Class I and II need not be followed up on a periodic basis depending on degree of clinical suspicion. However, for class III, an incisional biopsy is suggested while for classes IV and V, a definitive biopsy is indicated.

ORAL CDx BRUSH BIOPSY

- Brush biopsy is an easy, affordable and noninvasive technique of biopsy
- The purpose of the oral brush biopsy is to identify lesions that are clinically innocuous though histologically may exhibit atypical cells, dysplasia or frank carcinoma
- This is the latest diagnostic procedure that utilises a computer-assisted method of analysis developed by Oral CDx (Oral Scan Laboratories, Suffern, NY). It is a main tool in clinical assessment of oral lesions
- The Oral CDx is a diagnostic system that combines a painless oral brush biopsy (full transepithelial oral biopsy), which is taken in the dental office with advanced computer analysis
- A manufacturer-supplied brush biopsy kit includes a brush biopsy instrument (round stiff nylon brush), a barcoded glass slide, alcohol-based fixative, a protective plastic case and instruction page
- The nylon brush is designed to collect cells from all layers of epithelium, including basal cell layer (Fig. 6.1)
- This method of collection is in contrast to traditional exfoliative cytology where only superficial epithelial cells are usually collected and evaluated

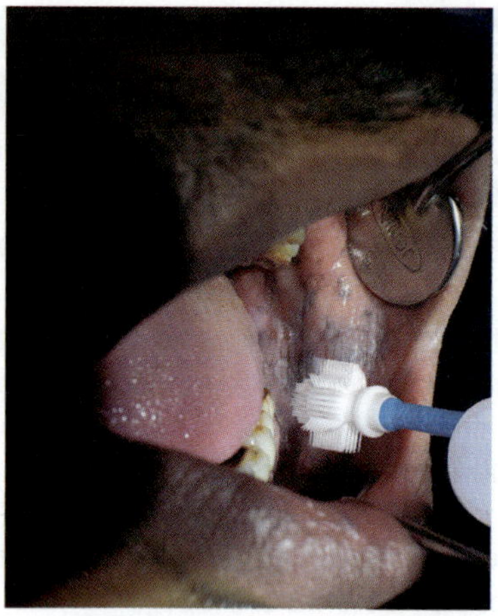

Figure 6.1 Brush biopsy.

- The procedure includes applying firm pressure on the lesion and rotating the brush 5–10 times
- Pinpoint bleeding or exposure of pinkish-red mucosa usually signals an adequate and successful sample collection
- Following cell extraction, the nylon brush is manipulated over the glass slide so that more cells are distributed evenly across the slide
- The slide is treated with the alcohol fixative in the kit. The slide is dried, transferred to a plastic container and mailed
- It is analysed by computerised programmes specifically designed for pathological review
- Results are given as negative, atypical or positive (Table 6.2)
- A biopsy returned with a result of atypical or positive requires an incisional or excisional biopsy to microscopically review the histological architecture of the lesion for definitive diagnosis.

Advantages of oral CDx and brush biopsy over exfoliative cytology

- The dysplastic or cancerous cells that are located deep to the keratin layer are included in the biopsy
- The procedure consists of microscopic screening of the cytological smear consisting of thousands of normal cells to identify abnormal cells because the exfoliating normal cells are in enormous numbers because of epithelial turnover.

TABLE 6.2 Classification of Oral CDx Specimen

Categories	Interpretation
Negative	No epithelial abnormality
Atypical	Abnormal epithelial changes of uncertain diagnostic significance
Positive	Definite evidence of dysplasia or carcinoma
Inadequate	Incomplete transepithelial biopsy

Advantages

- Helps in diagnosis of recurrent tumour in previous cancer site
- Noninvasive procedure compared to surgical biopsy
- Local anaesthesia is not required
- Reduced chairside time
- Simple procedure, which is easy to master
- Can be used as a screening tool for oral cancer.

Indications

- Precancerous lesions
- Oral squamous cell carcinoma
- Candidiasis
- Herpes simplex virus infection
- Human papilloma virus infection
- Pemphigus vulgaris.

ASPIRATION CYTOLOGY

Needle aspiration cytology refers to the procedure of removing contents of a lesion, usually a swelling for the purpose of analysis or quick observation by the clinician (Table 6.3).

- Aspiration cytology is typically used to rule out the possibility of a vascular lesion
- An 18-gauge needle and syringe injected into the exact area
- The needle may be subsequently readjusted so that it is placed within the centre of the lesion
- Negative pressure (pulling back on the plunger) is created in the syringe to acquire positive aspiration
- If it is difficult to aspirate, the lesion is most likely solid and a different type of biopsy may be needed
- If a purulent aspirate is observed as frank pus, possibility of an infection (abscess) is almost confirmatory
- If a straw-like fluid is obtained, a cyst should be suspected
- The presence of blood on aspiration indicates a vascular lesion; however, it may also suggest the presence of a bleeding lesion.

TABLE 6.3 Pathological Lesions and their Suspected Aspirate Content

Aspirate	Suspected Lesion
Air	Traumatic bone cyst, paranasal sinuses
Purulent (frank pus)	Abscess, infected cyst or lesions
Straw-coloured fluid	Cyst
Frank blood	Vascular lesion/bleeding lesion
Curdy white or cheesy white	Odontogenic keratocyst (OKC)

FINE NEEDLE ASPIRATION CYTOLOGY (FNAC)

FNAC uses a 23–24-gauge needle to aspirate the contents of a lesion through a puncture on the lesion.

After inserting the needle into the swelling, clumps of cell aggregates are aspirated into the syringe. These are smeared on a slide, stained and visualised under a microscope by the pathologist.

Indications

- Initial method of diagnosis for almost all solid or cystic swellings of the head and neck region (Fig. 6.2)
- This helps rule out vascular lesions prior to surgery
- Part of initial diagnostic work-up of lymphadenopathy, metastatic lesions or lymphomas
- Indicated in distinguishing benign from malignant and cystic lesions from inflammatory lesions
- Part of initial evaluation of swelling of major salivary gland
- Helps in distinguishing salivary gland neoplasm, soft tissue neoplasm, parotid lymph nodes, lymphoepithelial cells and sialadenitis with sensitivity and specificity
- Used for definitive diagnosis of odontogenic tumours like ameloblastoma, odontogenic keratocyst (OKC), etc.

Advantages

- Minimally invasive
- Safe, fast and cost-effective method
- Less time-consuming
- They do not spread the tumours or disrupt the field for surgical dissection
- Helps in differentiating benign and malignant lesions, thus helping in presurgical planning.

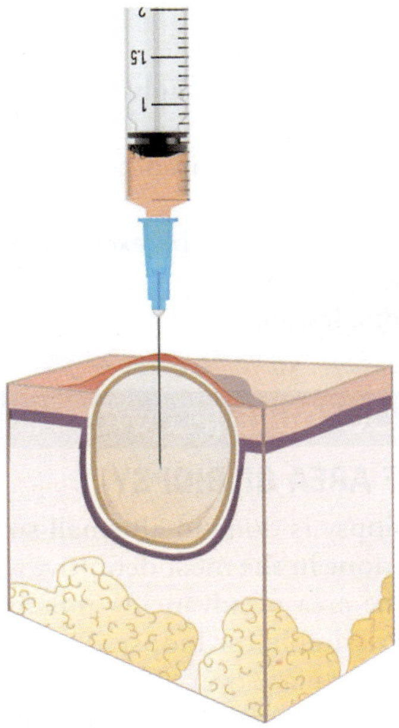

Figure 6.2 Fine needle aspiration cytology.

VITAL STAINING

TOLUIDINE BLUE STAINING

Toluidine blue staining is performed for diagnosis of the dysplastic areas in the oral cavity. It is a metachromatic vital dye of the thiazine group that increases visual detection of oral precancer and cancer lesion after negative clinical examination. It is effectively used as a nuclear stain because of its ability of DNA binding (Chapter 29, Fig. 29.2B).

Procedure

The patient is asked to rinse the mouth twice with water (20 s each time), followed by a rinse with 1% acetic acid (20 s). The suspicious area is dried with gauze. Toluidine blue solution 1% is applied over the dry mucosa. The patient is asked to rinse with 150 mL of acetic acid for 1 min, followed by a rinse with water. The positive stained mucosa is recorded. This procedure is repeated in 1 week. All areas that stained positive in both visits are subjected to biopsy.

Mechanism

The dysplastic and malignant cells contain quantitatively abundant nucleic acid as compared to normal cells. Since the toluidine blue stain is basically a nuclear dye, it stains these abnormal cells specifically and thus helps in diagnosis. Actively growing tissues contain high level of sulphated mucopolysaccharides; hence, the dyes will bind to the actively growing tissues like tumours, which is rich in sulphated mucopolysaccharides. Toluidine blue also binds to negatively charged mitochondrial membranes, which occurs more prominently in dysplastic and malignant cells.

Composition

100 mL of 1% toluidine blue consists of:

- 1 g Toluidine blue powder
- 10 mL of 1% acetic acid
- 4.19 mL absolute alcohol
- 86 mL distilled water.

Procedure

The patient is asked to rinse with:

1. Water for 20 s to remove debris
2. 1% acetic acid for 20 s
3. 1% Toluidine blue water solution for high-risk areas for 20 s
4. Mouthwash with 1% acetic acid should be applied to clear mechanically retained stain
5. A final rinse with water.

The sample should include healthy tissue at the margin of the lesion.

Advantages

- Vital stain with toluidine blue has been helpful in early diagnosis and treatment
- It is used to confirm clinical impressions regarding tissues at the risk of malignancy

- Helps in deciding the area of biopsy site within suspected lesions and surgical margins.

Disadvantage

False positive result may occur in case of dye retention by filiform papillae, ulcerations and mechanically in fissures.

LUGOL'S IODINE STAINING

Lugol's iodine staining is based on the principle of higher amount of glycogen in the normal mucosa compared to abnormal mucosa. It has greater specificity for the detection of oral squamous cell carcinoma. It produces a brown black staining (Chapter 29, Fig 29.2C).

Composition

- Iodine
- Potassium iodide
- Distilled water.

Lugol's iodine is retained in the normal squamous epithelial cells than in the dysplastic cells. Dysplastic or cancer cells have lower glycogen content owing to proliferation when compared to normal cells.

LIGHT-BASED DETECTION SYSTEMS

VIZILITE

It is a chemiluminescent light shined over areas in the oral cavity after an acetic acid rinse. The acetic acid changes the refractile properties of lesions like leukoplakia. When Vizilite is shown on the mucosa, the abnormal tissue shines brighter than the normal tissues.

VELscope (NARROW EMISSION TISSUE FLUORESCENCE)

- Approximately 30 years ago, it was discovered that cancer can be detected by using the autofluorescence property of tissues
- Consequently, the technology concerning fluorescence imaging and spectroscopy in cancer screening for a number of anatomic sites including the oral cavity has improved
- In fluorescence spectroscopy, the tissues are exposed to various excitation wavelengths so that subtle differences between normal and abnormal tissues are noted
- The fluorescence imaging involves the exposure of tissue to a specific wavelength of light, which results in the autofluorescence of cellular fluorophores after excitation
- When there is morphological alteration in the cells, the concentration of fluorophores is altered, which affects the scattering and absorption of light in the tissue. This leads to change in colour, which is observed visually
- VELscope is a portable tool used for direct visualisation of the oral cavity. It is available for commercial use for screening oral cancer
- The unit emits intense blue excitation light (400–460 nm) and a pale green autofluorescence is emitted by the normal mucosa, which is seen through the selective (narrow-band) filter incorporated within the instrument handpiece
- Filtration of the normal light beam is essential so that the narrow range of reflected blue-white light needed to cause the autofluorescent signal is visualised
- The areas of abnormal or suspected tissues are darker than the adjacent normal tissue due to decreased amounts of normal autofluorescence.

BIOPSY

Biopsy is a surgical procedure to obtain tissue from a living organism for its microscopical examination, usually to obtain a diagnosis. In maxillofacial surgery, a biopsy may be the only way to confirm the diagnosis of a lesion. There are various methods of obtaining the biopsy. Irrespective of the method used, the main objective is to give a sufficient amount of ideal sample for the pathologist to interpret. An improper uncharacteristic sample cannot be interpreted and should be avoided because the patient is unnecessarily subjected to an additional biopsy.

INDICATIONS FOR BIOPSY

A biopsy is mandatory for:

- An idiopathic lesion of more than 2 weeks duration
- Any inflammatory lesion that does not respond to topical treatment for 2 weeks
- Any persistent tumescence (swelling), either visible or palpable beneath relatively normal tissue without any clear diagnosis
- Lesions that is suggestive of malignancy (Fig. 6.3)
  a. Erythroplakia
  b. Speckled erythroplakia
  c. Nonhealing ulcer
  d. Rapidly growing lesion
  e. Lesions that bleed on slight pressure/manipulation
  f. Indurated lesions
  g. Lesions that feel fixated to the base or adjacent tissues
- Bone lesions that cannot be exclusively based on their radiographic appearance
- Hyperkeratotic lesions.

BIOPSY PROCEDURE (FLOWCHART 6.3)

SELECTION OF AREA OF BIOPSY

An excisional biopsy is done in all small-sized lesions. Incisional biopsy is done in the most definitive area of the lesion. Preferentially, the area of advancing inflammatory changes of the lesion is desirable for biopsy. This is because pathological changes take place over a period of time, hence a too early biopsy may be nonspecific. If the differential diagnosis is broad, obtaining biopsy samples from a variety of places can help to reduce the chance of a sampling error.

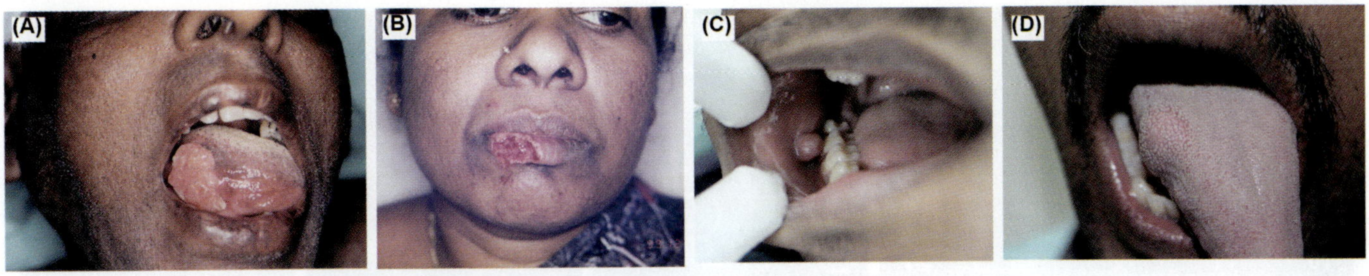

Figure 6.3 Lesions with characteristics that increase suspicion of cancer.

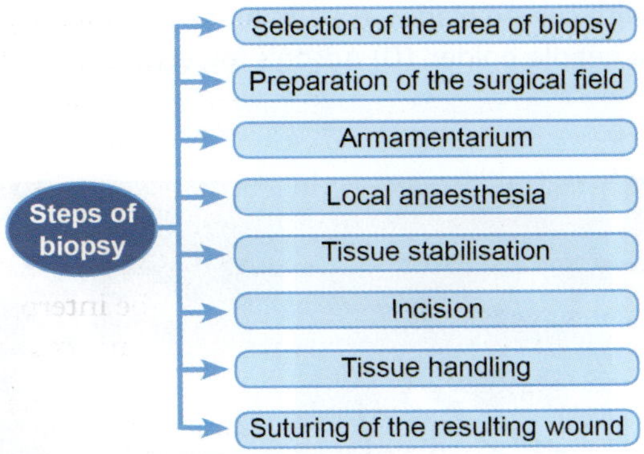

Flowchart 6.3 Illustration showing steps in biopsy as explained.

Older lesions showing secondary changes like crusts, fissures, erosions, excoriations and ulcerations are avoided since the characteristic feature of disease may not be clearly distinguished (Table 6.4). Important cosmetic areas such as the face should be approached with caution and areas with poor healing characteristics should be avoided if other sites are available for biopsy.

In case of doubtful malignant character of the lesion, the following aids can be used as an adjunct to select representative areas:

- Exfoliative cytology (explained under cytology)
- Vital staining
- Light-based detection systems.

Once the site of biopsy has been decided, the following steps follow:

1. **Preparation of the surgical field:**
   - Common skin antiseptics such as isopropyl alcohol, povidone iodine or chlorhexidine gluconate can be used to prepare the biopsy site
   - Mark the intended lesion with a surgical marker as it may be temporarily obliterated following injection of the anaesthetic solution
   - An amide-type local anaesthetic with vasoconstrictor is used. Infiltration should be given 1 cm away from the area to be biopsied.
2. **Armamentarium**
   - The tissue is incised with the scalpel, most commonly no. 15 B.P. blade. It may be available with a reusable handle or a disposable handle
   - The soft tissues are cut with curved sharp scissors. The two major tissue-cutting scissors are iris scissors and Metzenbaum scissors (Fig. 6.4). The iris scissors are small and allow fine and delicate work while the Metzenbaum scissors are used for undermining the soft tissue and cutting it
   - Sutures and needle holder
   - Tissue stabilising instruments.
3. **Tissue stabilisation:**
   - Oral soft tissues and mucosa require proper stabilisation for proper biopsy specimen. The most common technique is the utilisation of a surgical assistant (Fig. 6.5A).This allows accurate surgical incision and helps decrease bleeding during the procedure, especially in the lip, as the assistant compresses the vessels
   - The Adson's forceps and Allis tissue forceps are used to grasp and stabilise small lesions for excision biopsy. Holding the tissue allows a stable surface to incise (Fig. 6.5B and C)
   - Alternatively, chalazion type of device can also be used
   - Retraction sutures are mandatory on the tongue and other tissues as this helps prevent damage to the tissue specimen during biopsy (Fig. 6.5E).

TABLE 6.4 Lesions and Their Biopsy Sites

Pathological Lesion	Selection of area for biopsy
Infection	Avoided; however, a biopsy is indicated to rule out infection.
Vesicles	Vesicles should be biopsied with intact adjacent normal appearing skin, usually within 48 h of their appearance.
Bulla	At their edge, keeping the blister roof intact.
Nonbullous lesion	Maximal lesional skin and minimal normal skin.
Larger lesion	Edge, the thickest portion or the area with abnormal colouration, because these sites will most likely contain the distinctive pathology.

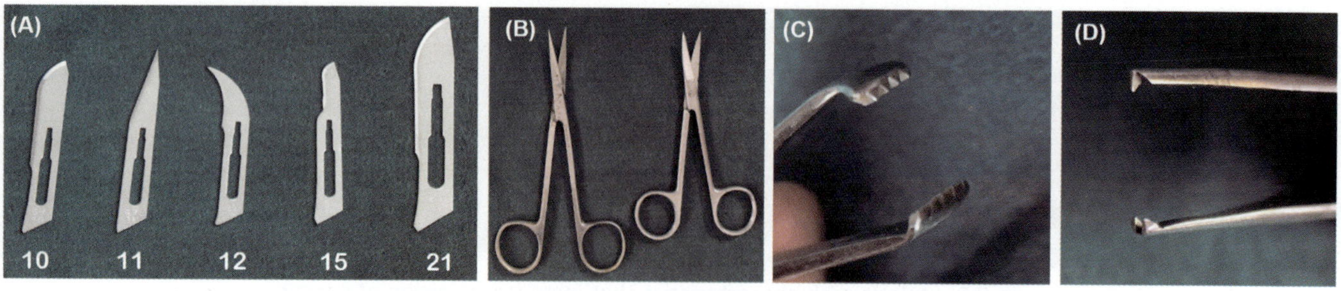

Figure 6.4 (**A**) Scalpel blades are available in a variety of forms and sizes. The most frequently used blade for oral surgery is the 15 blade. (**B**) Two forms of soft tissue scissors are available. Metzenbaum scissors are longer, more delicate scissors. Metzenbaum scissors are available with a sharp or blunt tip. Iris scissors are small, sharp with curved blades. (**C**) Allis tissue forceps are excellent for grasping and securing excised tissue. Allis forceps are held similarly to a needle holder. (**D**) Adson's forceps—a comparison of Adson and Allis beaks demonstrates the differences in their designs.

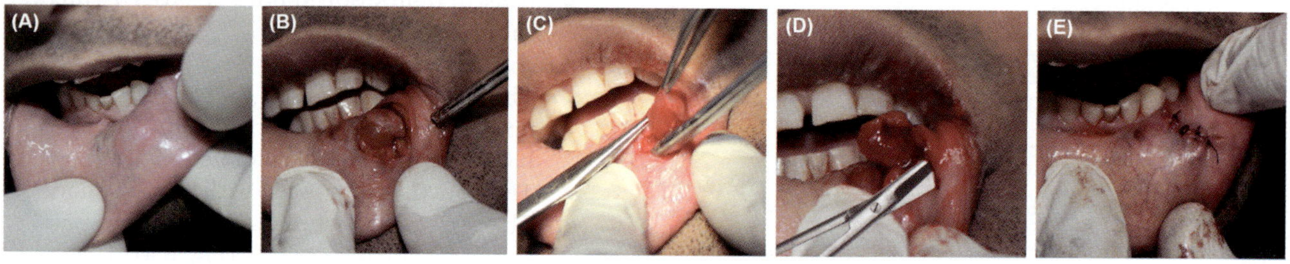

Figure 6.5 Examples of techniques for tissue stabilisation prior to biopsy (**A**) The assistant's fingers support the tissue prior to performing an excisional biopsy on a suspected mucocoele (**B**) An elliptical incision is created around the lesion while using Adson forceps to stabilise the tissue (**C** & **D**). Using soft tissue scissors, the surgeon dissects around the affected minor salivary gland E Undermining and closure of the consequent mucosal wound.

4. **Incision:**
   - A well-defined, delicate incision is made to remove a portion of the tissue during an incisional biopsy
   - Soft tissue incisions are elliptical in shape, and thus a V-wedged tissue comprising both the lesion and the healthy margins is obtained
   - In case of more than one lesion in the oral cavity, multiple biopsies are necessary.
5. **Biopsy tissue handling** (Fig. 6.6**):**
   - Tissue orientation: Before performing a complete excision, a short suture and a long suture are placed at the superior and lateral or medial margins of the lesion, respectively. This is done in order to properly orient the tissue. In order to facilitate the diagnosis of the margins, this information needs to be entered into the requisition form. During frozen section biopsies, accurate diagnosis of the margins is essential for determining malignancy. Before closing the wound, the surgeon waits for the pathologist to indicate that all the margins are clear.
   - The ***biopsy specimen*** should be meticulously handled to avoid crushing of tissues and placed in the fixing solution
   - Wash the specimen with copious running saline to remove traces of blood

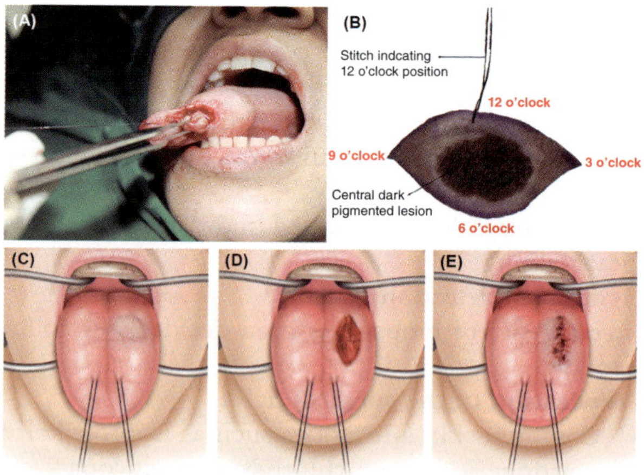

Figure 6.6 (**A**) Traction sutures are used to hold the tongue and the specimen is held with a forceps while the lesion is being incised. This allows the specimen to be lifted from the wound bed. The suture can then be knotted and left attached to the lesion to indicate the specimen's orientation. (**B**) An oriented specimen of melanoma. (**C–E**) Tongue stabilisation before biopsy. (**C**) To stabilise the tongue prior to excisional biopsy, two silk sutures are employed. They are inserted via the tongue's structure (mucosa and muscle) in order to avoid tearing through tissue. (**D**) The lesion is excised following an elliptical incision around it. (**E**) Sutures are used to approximate muscle and close the mucosa.

- ***10% formalin*** is the widely used fixing agent as it causes minimal histological alterations in the samples. Other reagents such as isopropyl or methyl alcohol, saline or distilled water should never be used as it severely alters the microstructure leading to misdiagnosis
- Surplus amount of fixing agent should be used about 10 to 20 fold the volume of the sample used
- For immunofluorescence or immunostaining, the specimens should not be fixed and should be sent immediately to the laboratory for freezing or placed in ***Michel's solution*** (Michel's transport media is not a fixative, it is merely a solution that maintains isotonicity and pH of the tissue [7.0–7.2]). It effectively stabilises the proteins for immunofluorescence. This solution is made up of citric acid, ammonium sulphate, *N*-ethylmaleimide and magnesium sulphate
- When the specimen is sent to the pathologist, it should also carry a summary containing identification of the patient, clinical records, clinical signs, radiographic features (if applicable), a provisional diagnosis and the orientation of the sample

6. **Suture and wound closure**
   - Undermining adjacent surface tissues with tissue scissors allows proper closure of the wound by decreasing the tension
   - The suture should achieve good haemostasis, facilitate healing and should be removed after 6–8 days
   - Contraindications to suturing include biopsies in infected or poorly healing skin; these wounds heal better by secondary intention. It is also contraindicated in susceptible cancerous lesions to avoid cell seeding in healthy tissue.
7. **Histopathology requisition**
   - The site of biopsy should be marked for proper record keeping. This helps with diagnosis in case of recurrence of the lesion (Fig. 6.7)
   - The lesion is also described in terms of anatomic location, physical characteristics, number of lesions, size,

Surgical Pathology Requisition Form
Dental Associates and Maxillofacial Pathology Biopsy Service

Date of Surgery: ____________
Date Specimen Received: ____________
Patient Name: ____________
Dental Record Number: ____________
Patient Address: ____________
____
Phone Number: ____________
Patient Age: ________ DOB: ____________
Gender : M / F
Referring Clinician: ____________
Practice Name and Address: ____________
____
____
Practice Phone: ____________
Fax: ________ E-mail: ____________
Clinical Description (Including size): ____________
Clinical HIstory: ____________
Clinical Impression: ____________
Previous Biopsy: Y or N (No. ____________)
Procedure: Excisional Biopsy ____________
Incisional Biopsy ____________
Other ____________

Location of Lesion (Please draw in anatomic location)

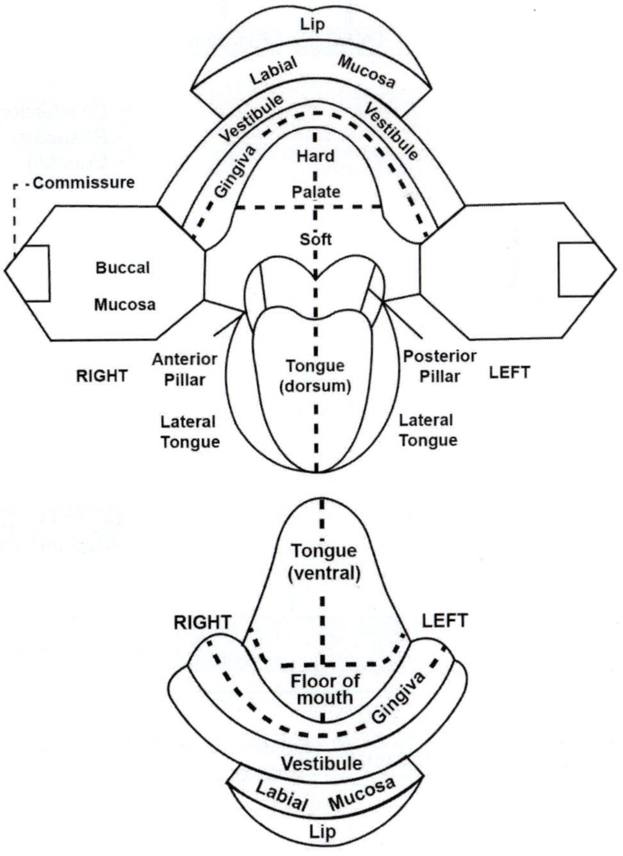

Radiograph Y/N or clinical photo sent Y/N

Figure 6.7 Surgical and histopathological requisition form.

shape, growth, surface appearance, colour, sharpness of borders, mobility, consistency when palpated, presence or absence of pulsation and positive regional lymph nodes
- Other clinical description and differential diagnoses are also enclosed in the histopathological requisition.

TYPES OF BIOPSIES

Biopsy can be classified as surgical and nonsurgical types. Nonsurgical type is primarily cytology where tissue sample is not taken but instead cell sample is used. The surgical type of biopsy further classifies as curative and diagnostic. Curative biopsy is performed when the biopsy itself becomes the treatment like excisional biopsy. Diagnostic type is when the tissue sample is used to diagnose the lesion to plan a treatment, like in the case of carcinoma (Flowchart 6.4).

Another classification is based on the exposure of the tissues during procedure. Open type of biopsy includes incisional and excisional biopsy, where the operative wound is open and requires suturing. The closed type is where the site of biopsy is accessed with a needle or instrument. This would not require suturing most of the time (Flowchart 6.5).

INCISIONAL BIOPSY

- It is the excision of a precise portion of the oral lesion for microscopic examination

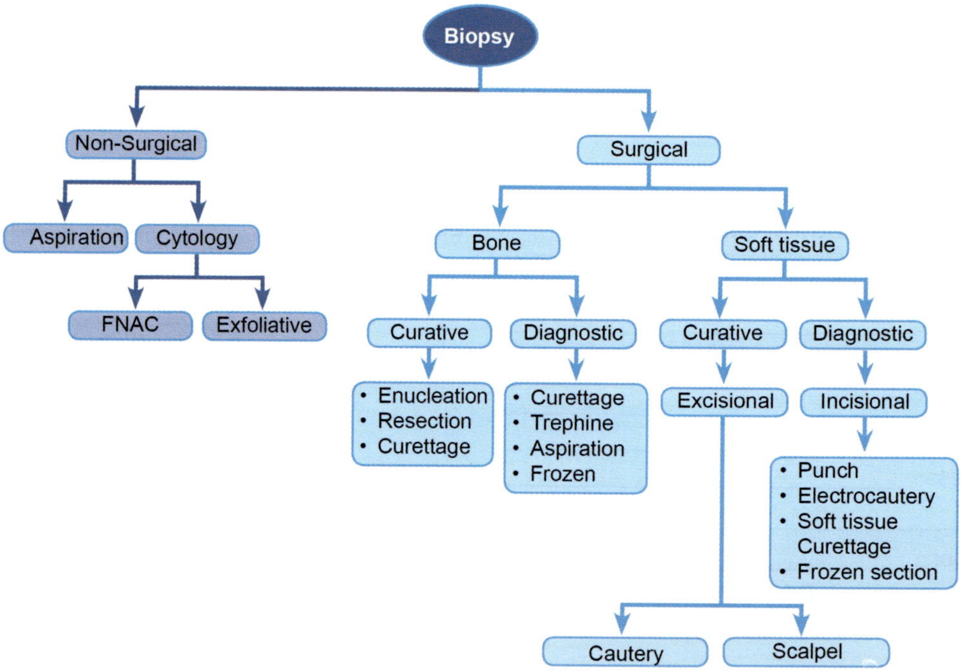

Flowchart 6.4 Classification of surgical and non-surgical biopsy techniques.

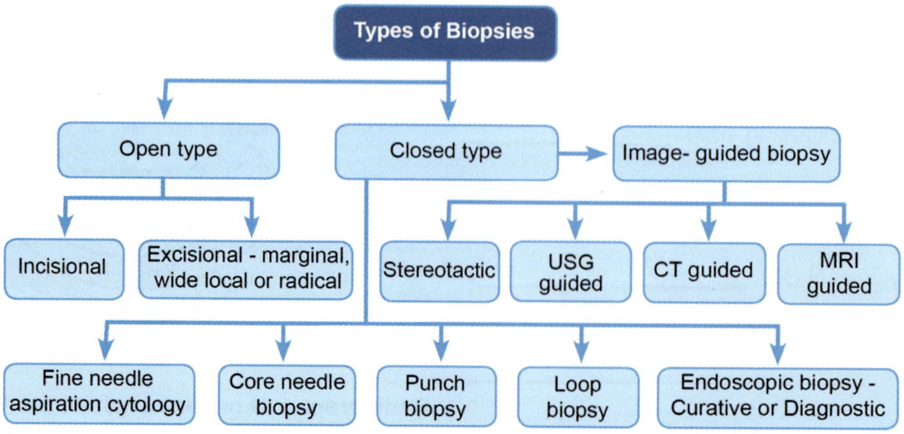

Flowchart 6.5 Open and closed techniques of biopsies classified.

- It is employed on large, diffuse lesions often above the size of 2 cm in its maximum dimension
- The biopsied tissue should be narrow and deep enough to involve the normal tissue. It should be taken at the border of the lesion involving the normal border (Fig. 6.8)
- It is also employed on lesions with suspected malignant potential
- The aim of the procedure will be to remove a portion of the lesional tissue in question along with a sample of normal adjacent tissue for comparison
- A wedge biopsy is made by a wedge-shaped incision, begins 2–3 mm from the normal tissue and penetrates into the region surrounding the abnormal tissue. It is always better to incise tissue narrow and deep than broad and shallow
- A punch biopsy is a type of incisional biopsy that is done using a surgical punch of diameter (usually 4/8/10 mm in diameter). This type of biopsy is usually done in mass screening programmes from representative areas.

Advantage

Incision biopsy is minimally invasive and generally very safe.

PUNCH BIOPSY (FIG. 6.9)

- A small cylindrical punch is applied into the lesion through the full thickness of the skin and a plug of tissue is removed

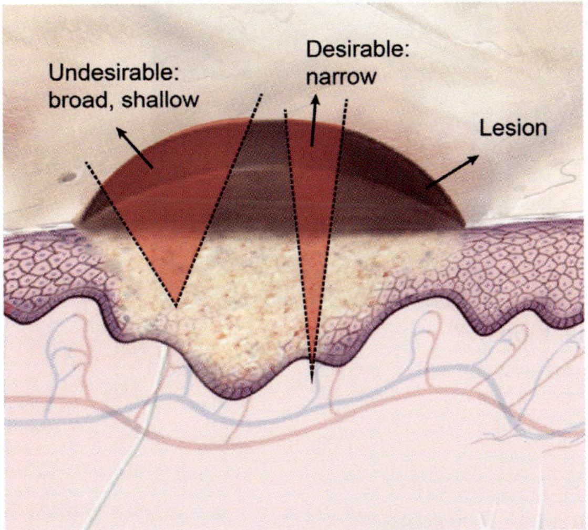

Figure 6.8 Obtaining a deep desirable specimen rather than a broad and shallow specimen when incisional biopsy is conducted. In cases where malignant cells are concentrated near the base of a lesion, a wide and shallow biopsy may not be able to obtain these cells for proper diagnosis. Incisional biopsy of the soft tissue lesion's margin is desirable. A biopsy specimen collected from the centre of the lesion may not provide as much diagnostic information as a specimen taken at the junction of the tumour with normal tissue. An ulcer biopsy necessitates the use of this precautionary measure.

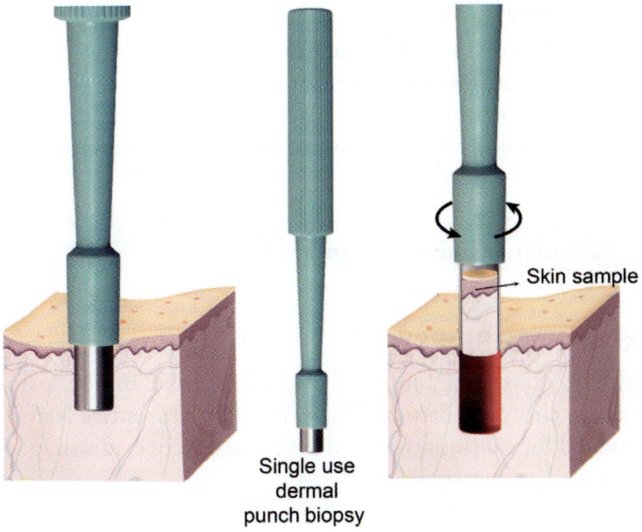

Figure 6.9 Punch biopsy.

- A small cylindrical plug is removed from the lesion. The plug comprises the full thickness of skin and the plug of tissue
- The plug of tissue comprises a cone-shaped core of tissue with its widest diameter at the skin surface and narrowest at the biopsy base
- It is the widely accepted procedure for diagnostic skin biopsy or removing small lesions.

Indications

- It is the method of choice for many flat lesions
- Interpretation of skin tumours like *basal cell carcinoma or Kaposi's sarcoma*
- Diagnosis of bullous kind of lesions like *Pemphigus vulgaris*
- Diagnosis of inflammatory skin disorders *like discoid lupus erythematoses*
- Removal of small skin lesions, such as *intradermal naevi*
- Diagnosis of atypical appearing lesions like atypical mycobacterial infections
- Evaluation of the lesions of uncertain origin
- Used to confirm or exclude the presence of malignancy.

Advantages

- Simple procedure
- Can be expedited by the physician
- Time conserving
- Low incidence of infection, bleeding or nonhealing
- Scarring is insignificant, hence it is cosmetic.

Disadvantage

Punch biopsy less than 3 mm heals by secondary intention. Punch biopsy greater than 3 mm needs one or two sutures to prevent unacceptable scarring.

WEDGE BIOPSY

- An incisional biopsy in which a lesion is removed with a wedge of normal surrounding tissue
- Elliptical skin incision is made using the scalpel
- A large wedge biopsy may require two-layered closure.

Indications

- Vesicular or bullous lesion
- Ulcerative lesion.

EXCISIONAL BIOPSY

Usually, excisional biopsy is done for small minor lesions that are clinically benign (Fig. 6.10A–C). The entire lesion is removed for examination and diagnosis. Hence, it is diagnostic as well as curative.

Application

These are performed for lesions that require complete removal for diagnostic or therapeutic purposes. Indicated for lesions diagnosed as benign, requiring complete removal. Generally, lesions less than 2 cm at their greatest dimension are least likely to be malignant.

Advantages

- An excisional biopsy allows for histopathologic examination of an entire lesion
- Another advantage of an excisional biopsy is the amount of tissue that can be removed from one biopsy site, ensuring adequate samples for various studies such as culture, histopathology, immuno-fluorescence and electron microscopy.

Disadvantages

- If the tumour is highly infiltrative, the margin of excision cannot be exactly elicited and further surgery will be needed
- Furthermore, cancerous cells actively multiply at the tumour margins, and debulking of the mass may result in residual cancerous cells left behind.
- Excision requires greater precision and skill from the surgeon.

SHAVE BIOPSY (FIG. 6.11)

- A scalpel or razor blade is used to shave off a thin layer of the lesion parallel to the skin
- Shave biopsies will normally provide information only about the epidermis and high dermis
- It may be both diagnostic and curative in case of keratoses, plane warts and benign pigmented lesions
- The shave biopsy may also be used to sample tumours such as basal and squamous cell carcinoma
- Indications for shave biopsies include lesions elevated above the skin, pathology confined to the epidermis
- Examples include *seborrhoeic or actinic keratoses, skin tags, warts and superficial basal or squamous cell carcinomas*

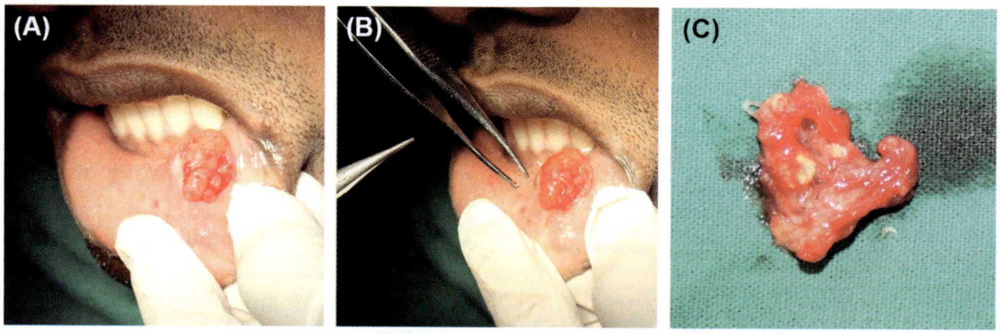

Figure 6.10 (A–C) Excisional biopsy.

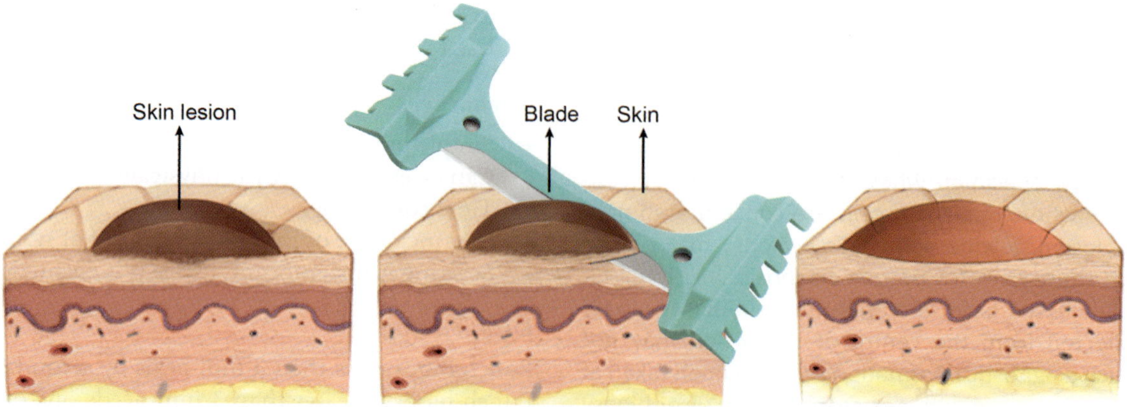

Figure 6.11 Shave biopsy.

TABLE 6.5 Differences between Superficial and Deep Shave Biopsy	
Superficial Shave Biopsy	**Deep Shave Biopsy**
• Superficial shave biopsies are done across or nearly parallel to the skin surface and extend into the epidermis and superficial dermis, for example, removal of skin tags and other small exophytic growths.	• The deeper shave biopsy (also known as 'saucerisation' biopsy) facilitates sampling of dermis and epidermis, which is important for assessing carcinomas, for example, basal cell and squamous cell carcinoma.

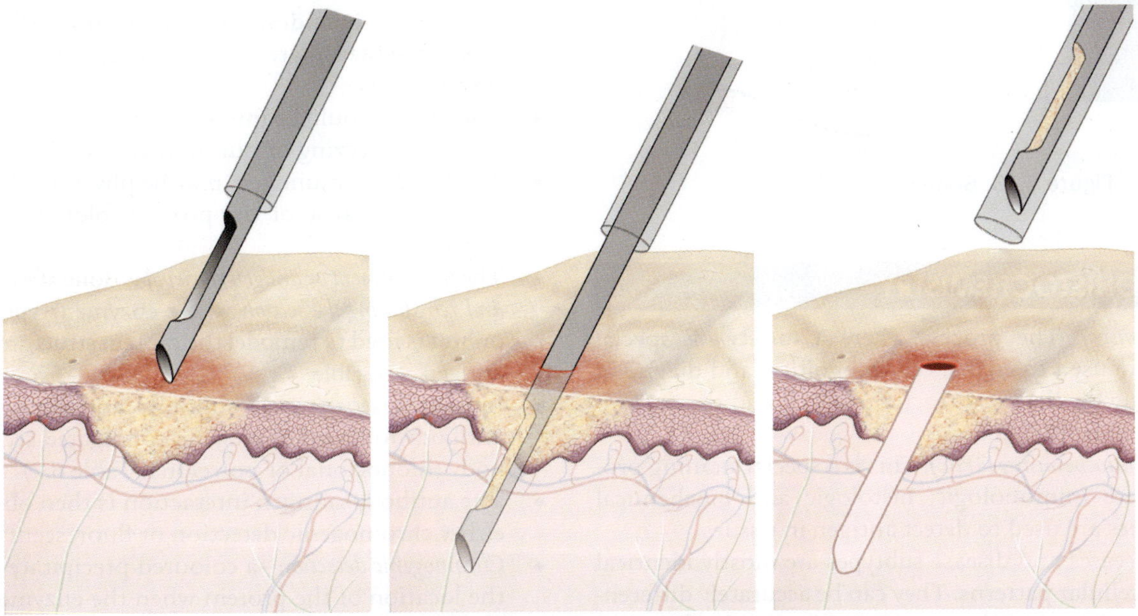

Figure 6.12 Core needle biopsy—trucut needle biopsy.

- Performing a shave biopsy is classified into superficial and deep (Table 6.5)
- ***Advantage:*** Shave biopsies are time conserving, need only little expertise and heal without the need of sutures
- ***Disadvantage:*** Shave biopsies should not be used for pigmented lesions since if unsuspected melanoma is partially removed, it cannot be properly staged.

CORE NEEDLE BIOPSY—TRUCUT BIOPSY

Core needle biopsy (CNB) involves the removal of a core of deep tissue usually using a Trucut needle (Fig. 6.12).

Advantages

- CNB allows for *accurate diagnosis* because of the large quantity of tissue that can be obtained
- The type and grade of the tumour, its invasiveness as well as hormone receptor status can be assessed. This is an advantage over FNAC, particularly in case of patients with large masses suggestive of cancer.

Image/CT-guided biopsy

- The procedure is comparable to core biopsy; it is conducted with a larger needle with assisted CT scan equipment
- The simultaneous CT scan allows identification and visualisation of the exact site of the tumour on the computer screen
- This advanced technology enables the operator to directly guide the needle into the tumour and obtain several samples of tissue. The tissue samples are later examined by the pathologist.

VACUUM-ASSISTED BIOPSY

It is a variant of the core biopsy. An automated suction device is attached to the lateral side of the needle. It increases the amount of fluid and cells aspirated through the needle. This ensures larger tissue sample and reduces the need for repuncture.

BONE MARROW BIOPSY

- Bone marrow is a spongy substance present in the core of large bones where blood cells are formed
- Bone marrow biopsy is indicated in patients with abnormal blood counts, as in case of unexplained anaemia, high white blood cell count and low platelet count (Fig. 6.13)
- Bone marrow is obtained from the red marrow of pelvic bone, mainly from the posterior superior iliac spine.

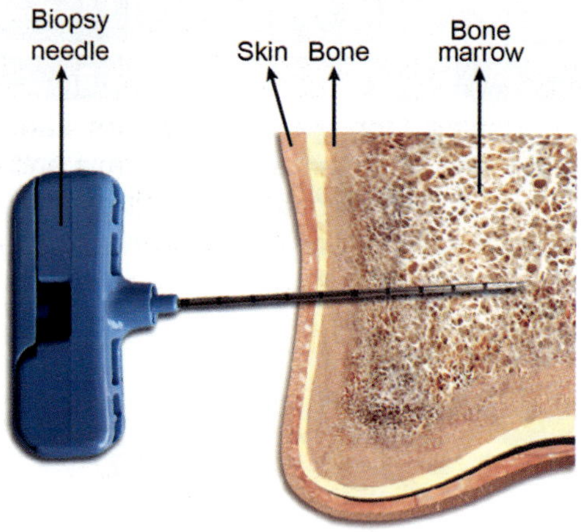

Figure 6.13 Bone marrow biopsy.

IMMUNOHISTOCHEMISTRY

- *Histochemistry:* The process where a variety of 'special stains' are used to enable cell recognition and diagnosis depending on chemical reactions of cell and tissue components in frozen section.
- *Immunohistochemistry (IHC)*: This is a special staining process where immunologic, histologic and biochemical techniques are used to detect antigen in tissues
- Many diseases and disease subtypes are mostly identical in their cellular patterns. They can be accurately differentiated by detecting the specific molecules in the cells. These specific molecules are called markers
- Immunohistochemistry is the immunological process of localising proteins in cells of a tissue section using the principle of antibody-antigen binding in biological tissues
- Distribution and localisation of specific cellular components within a cell or tissue is best visualised by IHC.

BASIC PRINCIPLE AND PROCEDURE

- The basic critical principle of IHC, as with any other special staining method, is the binding of the specific antibody to the target immunogen followed by the amplification and visualisation of the antigen–antibody link. Cytoplasmic, nuclear, cell membrane, lipids and proteins are the target cellular antigens in immunohistochemistry
- Immunohistochemical staining is done with the antibodies that identify the target protein (Table 6.6)
- Antibodies are highly specific and bind only with the target protein in the tissue section
- IHC can be carried out on different types of *cell and tissue preparation*, including routine formalin-fixed, paraffin wax-embedded material, frozen section and cytological preparations
- The tissue should be immediately transferred to the laboratory for freezing or put in Michel's solution
- The target 'immunogen' may be physically hidden by the antibody because of the protein folding caused during fixation
- The *pretreatment or antigen retrieval* is done after *deparaffinising and rehydrating the section* where enzyme (trypsin/proteases) or heat is used to remodel the protein structure, making the antigen accessible
- Immunohistochemical staining—application of primary antibody followed by enzyme-conjugated secondary antibody (monoclonal or polyclonal Table 6.7)
- The antibody-antigen interaction is then observed using either chromogenic detection or fluorescent detection
- *Chromogenic detection*—a coloured precipitate is formed at the location of the protein when the enzyme-conjugated antibody cleaves the substrate
- *Fluorescent detection*—after conjugation with the antibody, fluorophore can be seen under fluorescence microscopy (direct and indirect immunofluorescence Table 6.8).

APPLICATION

- Immunohistochemistry has been used in the field of cell and tissue biology, embryology and diagnostic pathology.
- Location of replicating, apoptotic and signaling cells
- Identification of activation states and different types of cells in tissues
- Examination of cytoskeletal structures.

TABLE 6.6 Cell Types and their Molecular Staining

Cell Type	Tumour	Molecular Staining
Epithelial	Papillomas, adenomas, carcinomas (squamous cell carcinoma, basal cell carcinoma, adenocarcinoma)	Cytokeratin, epithelial membrane antigen (EMA)
Plasma cells	Plasmacytomas	Monoclonal immunoglobulin light or heavy chains; plasma cell-associated antigens (PCA, PC, CD 38); EMA
Langerhans histiocytes	Langerhans cell histiocytosis (e.g. eosinophilic granuloma)	S-100 protein; CD1a

TABLE 6.7 Polyclonal and Monoclonal Antibodies

Polyclonal Antibodies	Monoclonal Antibodies
Polyclonal—a mixture of antibodies • Will recognise multiple epitopes and provide robust detection • Tolerant to changes in antigen, can work with denatured proteins • Can be used when the antigen is not fully characterised • Produced from intact living animals.	Monoclonal—only one type of antibody • Highly specific, as a primary antibody • Vulnerable to loss of epitope • Will attach to one antigen in a mixture • Less 'background' response • Produced from animals cell in culture.

TABLE 6.8 Direct and Indirect Immunofluorescence

Direct Immunofluorescence	Indirect Immunofluorescence
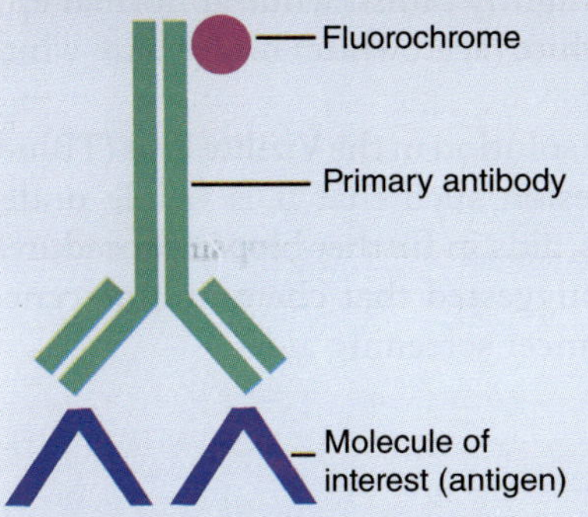	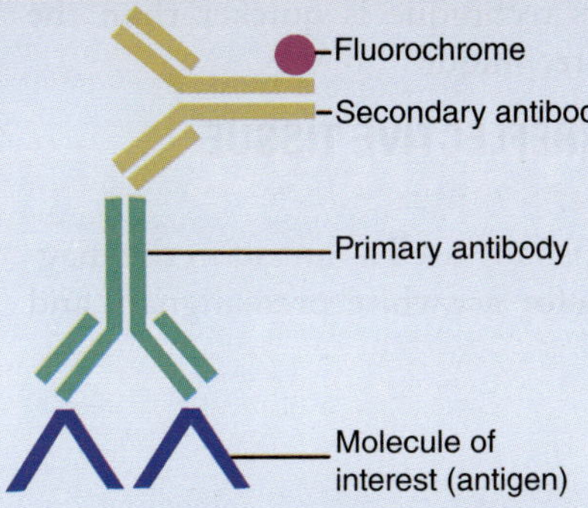
• Choose an antibody that attaches to the molecule of interest	• A second antibody is attached to the complex composed of the antigen and the primary antibody
• A fluorochrome is chemically attached to the antibody to form a 'conjugate'	• The fluorochrome is attached to the secondary antibody
• The molecule of interest is considered to exist wherever fluorescence from the attached fluorochrome is detected	• The secondary antibody must be generated against the immunoglobulins of the primary antibody source

• Advantage: Simplicity
• Disadvantages:
  • Expensive
  • The fluorescent signal could be too weak requiring amplification.
	• Advantage: Can result in greater fluorescence if more than one secondary antibody sticks to a primary antibody.

RECENT ADVANCES IN HISTOPATHOLOGICAL EVIDENCES

ENDOSCOPIC/ARTHROSCOPIC BIOPSY

- The endoscope or arthroscope can be used to view the TMJ and a biopsy of any joint lesion can be effectively done
- *Advantage:* It is possible to visualise the lesion directly and to take tissue samples through the scope for further analysis
- *Disadvantages:* Expensive and difficult to master.

SENTINEL LYMPH NODE BIOPSY

A sentinel lymph node is defined as the first lymph node to which cancer cells are most likely to spread from a primary tumour. Sometimes, there can be more than one sentinel lymph node. A sentinel lymph node biopsy (SLNB) is a procedure in which the sentinel lymph node is identified, removed and examined to determine whether cancer cells are present. This is done by injecting a radioactive substance, a blue dye or both near the tumour to locate the position of the sentinel lymph node. Once the sentinel lymph node is located, the surgeon makes a small incision (about 1/2 inch) in the overlying skin and removes the node. SLNB can also be performed prior to surgical excision of carcinoma as it may help in avoiding more extensive lymph node surgery. Removing additional nearby lymph nodes to look for cancer cells may not be necessary if the sentinel node is negative for cancer (Chapter 30, Figs. 30.27 & 30.28).

FROZEN SECTION

- During resection of malignant and huge benign tumours, it is required that the surgical margins are made free of tumour cells

- Hence, during surgery, bits of tissues along the surgical margin are taken and sent for rapid microscopic examination and opinion
- The bits of tissue are processed in a special instrument called cryostat, which is a microtome (a laboratory instrument used to cut the tissue into thin slices of thickness 1 μm) inside a freezer
- The tissue is loaded on a metallic cassette, and it is stabilised and rapidly frozen to −20°C to −300°C
- The specimen is blocked in a gel-like medium, usually a mixture of polyethylene glycol and polyvinyl alcohol
- Consecutively, it is cut frozen with the microtome. The sections are placed on a glass slide, stained with haemotoxylin and eosin. This technique is quicker than the conventional histology technique.

CHEMILUMINESCENCE (REFLECTIVE TISSUE FLUORESCENCE)

- Chemiluminescence is usually used as an aid in the diagnosis of cervical mucosa for 'ace white' premalignant and malignant lesions
- Nowadays, the same technology is adapted for use in the oral cavity and marketed as Vizilite Plus and MicroLux DL
- These systems aim for easy identification of oral mucosal abnormalities. The systems are used similarly; the patient should first rinse mouth with a 1% acetic acid solution and the oral cavity is directly visualised by a blue-white light source
- A disposable chemiluminescent light packet is present in Vizilite Plus, while a reusable battery-powered light source is present in Microlux DL
- 1% Acetic acid wash removes surface debris due to the mild cellular dehydration; visibility of epithelial cell nuclei is increased
- Normal epithelium is lightly bluish while abnormal epithelium is distinctly white (acetowhite) under blue-white illumination
- The tolonium chloride solution in the Vizilite Plus (TBlue) labels the ace white lesion such that it is visible under normal light, and thus, aids in further biopsy procedures
- Various studies have suggested that chemiluminescence is a dependable oral cancer screening aid.

Section III

Medical Management in Oral Surgery

Chapter 7

Management of the Medically Compromised

OUTLINE

INTRODUCTION

Dental consideration for the treatment of medically compromised patients requires a detailed medical history and a thorough knowledge of the medical condition for complete treatment for the patient. Chapter 3 on 'History taking and clinical examination' will give a complete medical history. This chapter is classified based on the various systems which present with diseases and the most common and important diseases for oral surgery will be explained in detail (Box 7.1).

CARDIOVASCULAR DISEASES

Cardiac diseases are not an absolute contraindication for oral and maxillofacial surgery. It is important for the surgeon to decide on the choice of anaesthesia and other drugs used in the treatment.

1. **Preoperative investigations for patients with cardiac diseases:**
   a. Posterior anterior view chest radiograph
   b. Echocardiograph
   c. Electrocardiograph (ECG)
   d. Stress test
   e. Lipid profile
   f. Bleeding time, Clotting time and Prothrombin time—International Normalised Ratio (PT-INR) for long-term anticoagulant/antiplatelet drug users.
2. **Antibiotic prophylaxis for patients with cardiac diseases like Coronary artery bypass graft surgery (CABG) or valve replacement.**

BOX 7.1 ASA Classification of Physical Status

- **ASA I:** A patient without systemic disease; a normal, healthy patient
- **ASA II:** A patient with mild systemic disease
- **ASA III:** A patient with severe systemic disease that limits activity, but is not incapacitating
- **ASA IV:** A patient with severe systemic disease which is incapacitating that is a constant threat to life
- **ASA V:** A moribund patient not expected to survive 24 h with or without surgery
- **ASA E:** Emergency operation of any kind, E precedes the ASA number, indicating the patient's physical status

3. **Intraoperative Considerations:**
   a. Continuous monitoring by ECG, pulse oximeter and arterial line
   b. Patient should continue the ongoing cardiac drugs by intravenous route until oral feeds are started
   c. Fluid volume should be monitored through CVP (Central Venous Pressure) and fluid overload should be avoided especially in congestive cardiac failure.

LONG-TERM ANTICOAGULANT DRUG USE

Oral anticoagulant drugs are classified under coumarins and indandiones. These drugs work by interfering with the synthesis of vitamin K-dependent clotting factors (Flowcharts 7.1 and 7.2).

Patients are advised long-term use of anticoagulant or antiplatelet drugs for the prevention of intravascular clots. When these drugs are withdrawn, this may precipitate a thromboembolic event. Conditions where anticoagulant drugs are prescribed: Deep Vein Thrombosis, Pulmonary Embolism, Rheumatic Heart Disease, Arterial Fibrillation, Prosthetic Valve Replacement, Coronary Artery disease (CAD), Myocardial Infarction, Unstable Angina and Stroke. Patients undergoing invasive procedures are required to discontinue the drug until after the procedure. Patients on

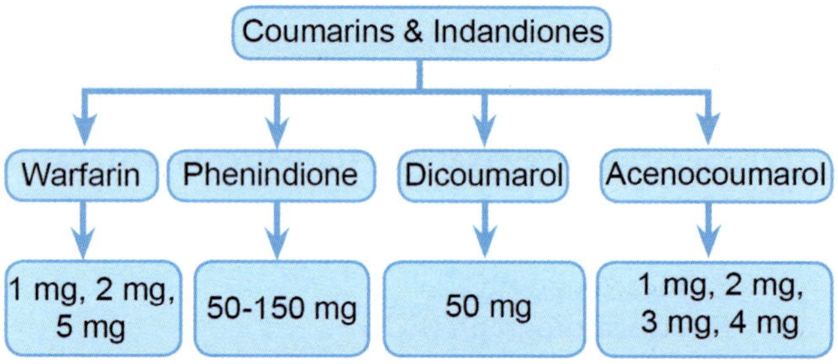

Flowchart 7.1 Oral anti-coagulation drugs with available dosage.

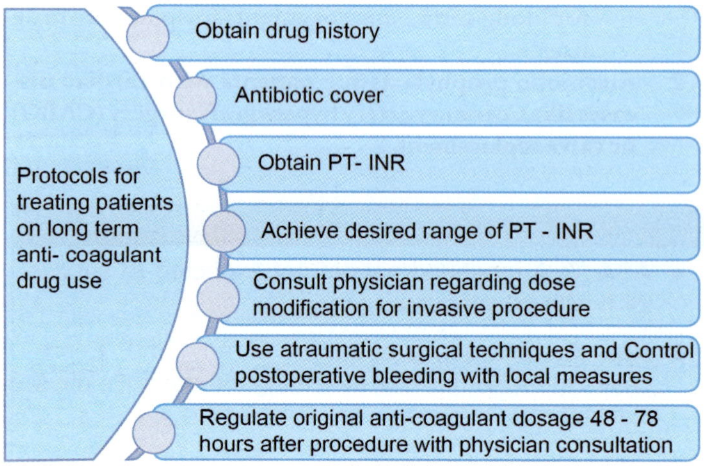

Flowchart 7.2 Protocols for treating patients on long-term anticoagulant drug use.

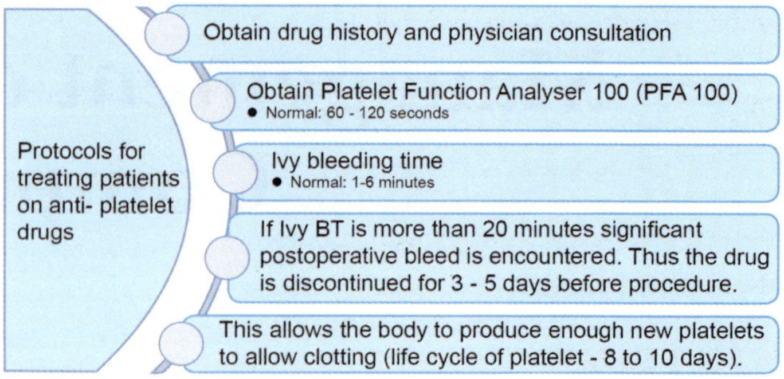

Flowchart 7.3 Protocols for treating patients on antiplatelet drugs.

long-term anticoagulants are required to take a PT-INR. (PT-INR range given in Box 7.3).

PATIENTS ON ANTIPLATELET DRUGS

Antiplatelet drugs irreversibly inhibit cyclooxygenase enzyme in the platelets. It prevents thromboxane A2 (TXA2) synthesis inhibiting platelet aggregation. These drugs are used in patients with Cerebrovascular accident (CVA), CABG and Coronary Artery Disease (CAD) after an MI episode and CAD with unstable angina as platelet plug formation is inhibited by antiplatelet drugs. Antiplatelet drugs are aspirin (Colisprin, Ecosprin)–75–150 mg; Dipyridamole, Clopidogrel–75 mg; and Ticlopidine–250 mg (Flowchart 7.3).

CONGENITAL HEART DISEASE (CHD)

Invasive procedures for patients with CHD can cause

1. Infective endocarditis–Antibiotic prophylaxis is given to prevent it
2. Postoperative bleeding (seen in patients with right to left shunting of blood due to thrombocytopaenia, coagulation factor deficiency due to thrombosis and anticoagulation drugs)–BT and PT-INR should be tested before surgical procedures
3. Congestive Cardiac Failure.

RHEUMATIC HEART DISEASE (RHD)

Infective endocarditis can be prevented with antibiotic prophylaxis using amoxicillin 2 g one hour before the procedure. RHD patients are usually on daily low dose of penicillin to prevent rheumatic fever. The patient need not discontinue penicillin for other invasive procedures.

INFECTIVE ENDOCARDITIS

Infective endocarditis (IE) is an infection of the lining of heart chambers and heart valves caused by bacteria, viruses, fungi or other infectious agents. The infection may be due to bacteria in the blood stream, which occurs after dental and surgical procedures causing bacterial growth on the heart valves, lining of the heart or lining of the blood vessels. This bacterial growth can dislodge, forming emboli to the brain, lungs, kidneys or spleen. *Streptococcus viridans*, an organism commonly found in the mouth, is responsible for approximately half of all bacterial endocarditis. Other common organisms include *Staphylococcus* and *Enterococcus*.

From the purely dental standpoint, it is obligatory to prevent the onset of infective endocarditis in view of the high morbidity and mortality. This depends on:

- Identification of patients at risk
- Planned preventive dental care
- Deciding which treatments require antimicrobial cover
- Giving the appropriate antibiotic(s) at the appropriate time.

Pre-existing conditions that increase the likelihood of developing endocarditis

- Congenital heart disease (tetralogy of Fallot, atrial septal defect, patent ductus arteriosus and others)
- Rheumatic heart disease
- Cardiac valve anomalies (such as mitral valve prolapse)
- Prosthetic heart valves
- Previous infective endocarditis
- Scar tissue or prosthetic coverings in the cardiovascular system.

MANAGEMENT

Prophylactic antibiotics must be prescribed for patients with degenerative cardiac or atherosclerotic valvular defects as dental procedures are likely to produce a bacteraemia. The purpose of prophylactic antibiotics is to prevent the colonisation of bacteria in these areas of susceptibility. Gram-positive cocci, which predominate the oral aerobic microflora, are implicated in most cases of bacterial endocarditis (Tables 7.1–7.3).

TABLE 7.1 Cardiac Conditions where Antibiotics are Indicated and Not Indicated are Presented

Prophylaxis Indicated	Prophylaxis not Indicated
1. Prosthetic cardiac valves	1. Atrial septa defects
2. Previous infective endocarditis	2. Ventricular septal defects
3. Unrepaired cyanotic congenital heart disease, including palliative shunts and conduits	3. Patent ductus arteriosus
4. Completely repaired congenital heart defect with prosthetic material or device, during the first six months after the procedure	4. Mitral valve prolapse
5. Repaired congenital heart disease with residual defects at the site or adjacent to the site of a prosthetic patch or prosthetic device (which inhibit endothelialisation)	5. Previous Kawasaki disease
6. Cardiac transplant recipients with cardiac valvulopathy	6. Hypertrophic cardiomyopathy
7. Rheumatic heart disease if prosthetic valves or prosthetic material used in valve repair.	7. Previous CABG surgery
	8. Cardiac pacemakers (intravascular and epicardial) and implanted defibrillators
	9. Bicuspid aortic valves
	10. Coarctation of the aorta
	11. Calcified aortic stenosis
	12. Pulmonic stenosis.

TABLE 7.2 Prophylaxis Recommended & Not Recommended for Dental Procedures

Dental Procedures for which Prophylaxis is Recommended	Dental Procedures for which Prophylaxis is not Recommended
• Extractions	• Restorative dentistry (operative and prosthetic) with or without the use of retraction cord (clinical judgment may indicate use of prophylaxis if significant bleeding is anticipated)
• Periodontal procedures	• Local anaesthetic injections (other than intraligamentary)
• Subgingival placement of antibiotic strips	• Intracanal endodontic or restorative treatments
• Scaling	• Placement of rubber dams
• Root planing	• Postoperative suture removal
• Probing	• Placement of removable prosthodontic/orthodontic appliances
	• Taking of oral impressions
	• Fluoride treatments
	• Taking of oral radiographs
	• Orthodontic appliance adjustment
	• Shedding of primary teeth.

TABLE 7.3 Suggested Antibiotic Prophylaxis Regimens for Preventing Infective Endocarditis

Patient Group	Antibiotic	DOSE (single, 30-60 mins before procedure)	
		Adults	Children
LA procedure	Amoxicillin	2 g	50 mg/kg
LA procedure Allergic to penicillins or ampicillin	Cephalexin	2 g	50 mg/kg
	Clindamycin	600 mg	20 mg/kg
	Azithromycin or Clarithromycin	500 mg	15 mg/kg
GA procedure	Amoxicillin	2 g i.m. or i.v.	50 mg/kg i.m. or i.v.
	Cefazolin or Ceftriaxone	1 g i.m. or i.v.	50 mg/kg i.m. or i.v.
GA procedure Allergic to penicillins or ampicillin	Cefazolin or Ceftriaxone	1 g i.m. or i.v.	50 mg/kg i.m. or i.v.
	Clindamycin	600 mg i.m. or i.v.	20 mg/kg i.m. or i.v.

BOX 7.2 Stress Reduction Protocol Based on ASA Physical Status

Stress reduction protocol for normal, healthy and anxious patient (ASA I)

1. Recognise the patient's level of anxiety by proper communication
2. Premedicate the evening and immediately before the dental appointment, as needed—short-acting benzodiazepines—Diazepam dosage
3. Triazolam 0.125–0.25 mg night before and 1 h prior to the appointment
4. Conscious sedation or GA are indicated for longer procedures
5. Schedule the appointment late in the morning
6. Minimise the patient's waiting time
7. Use adequate pain control with local anaesthetics during procedure
8. Follow up with postoperative pain/anxiety control

Stress reduction protocol for patients with medical risk (ASA II, III, IV)

1. Recognise the patient's degree of medical risk and receive complete medical consultation before dental therapy
2. Schedule the patient's appointment late mornings
3. Monitor and record preoperative and postoperative vital signs
4. Use of anxiolytics for stress reduction based on the medical condition
5. Use adequate pain control during therapy
6. Length of appointment—variable; do not exceed the patient's limits of tolerance
7. Follow up with postoperative pain/anxiety control

ISCHAEMIC HEART DISEASE (IHD) OR CORONARY ARTERY DISEASE (CAD)

Angina Pectoris

Patients with angina pectoris can present with a series of risks during the procedure, as follows:

1. Stress and anxiety can lead to an angina attack during procedure
2. Myocardial infarction
3. Cardiac arrest–death.

DENTAL CONSIDERATIONS

Obtain a detailed medical history and physician consultation. Stress reduction protocol should be followed (Box 7.2). Premedication for reducing anxiety can be given (Diazepam 5-10 mg). Prophylactic Nitroglycerine (NTG) should be given preoperatively. Limit the administration of epinephrine to 0.04 mg. Avoid use of vasopressors anytime for treatment except 1:100,000 or 1:200,000 epinephrine local anaesthetic solution. Aspirate to avoid positive aspiration and injecting into the circulation. If angina pectoris occurs, stop the treatment, administer oxygen, minimise stress and wait till the pain resolves, follow the emergency protocol (Flowchart 7.4).

ACUTE MYOCARDIAL INFARCTION (MI)

Patients within 6 months of an MI (recent MI) have been considered at greatest risk of further MI. Chest pain, dysrhythmias and other complications have generally been classified as ASA Class IV. A level of reinfarction of 50% has

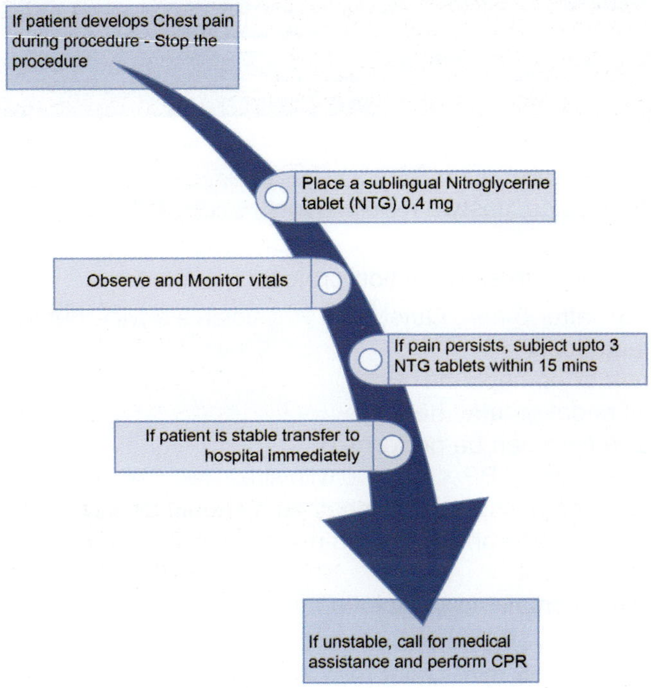

Flowchart 7.4 Steps to follow when patient presents with anginal pain during procedure.

been reported in major surgery done during this period. Therefore, in recent MI:

- Higher risk procedures such as elective surgery should be deferred
- Elective dental care should be deferred
- Simple emergency dental treatment under local anaesthesia may be given during the first 6 months after an MI, but the opinion of a physician should be sought first.

Asymptomatic patients with previous older MI (more than 6 months and below 12 months) can normally have elective dental care carried out safely under stress reduction protocol (Box 7.2). Higher risk procedures such as elective surgery may need to be deferred.

Symptomatic previous but older MI (more than 12 months) can normally have elective dental care carried out safely under stress reduction protocol. Patients present with a series of risks during the procedure, as follows:

1. Cardiac arrest—death
2. Congestive cardiac failure
3. Postoperative bleeding when on prophylactic anticoagulant or antiplatelet drugs
4. Infective endocarditis can occur in implanted pacemaker
5. Electrical interference for patients with pacemaker.

DENTAL CONSIDERATIONS

1. Follow stress reduction protocol
2. Continuous monitoring of the vitals should be done. If patient is on antihypertensive medication, BP should be monitored
3. All emergency drugs, basic life support kit and medical assistance should be available
4. Premedicate with Diazepam 5–10 mg
5. Anticoagulant dosage should be adjusted based on PT-INR, which should be within the desired range (Box 7.3)
6. Short appointments are made. If patient feels fatigued, terminate procedure
7. Patients on drugs like digitalis, quinidine and procainamide can present with nausea and vomiting. The surgeon should avoid stimulating the gag reflex
8. Manipulation of the neck, carotid sinus or eyes (vagal reflex) should be avoided
9. Drugs that cause tachycardia used in general anaesthesia should be used carefully (antisialogogues—atropine methantheline)
10. Avoid use of Cavitron and electrocautery for patients with pacemaker.

HYPERTENSION (HTN)

Hypertension (HTN) refers to blood pressure that is consistently above 140/90 mmHg (for more than 6 months). HTN may have no cause (essential or idiopathic) or may be associated with any primary disease (secondary hypertension). Uncontrolled HTN can lead to excessive bleeding postoperatively and can have ill effects on the heart, thereby posing an anaesthetic risk. Complications due to elevated blood pressure are:

1. Stress and anxiety
2. MI or CVA may be precipitated
3. Excessive intraoperative and postoperative bleeding may occur
4. Postural hypotension
5. Hypotension due to sedative action of antihypertensives.

DENTAL ASPECTS AND TREATMENT MODIFICATIONS

1. Preoperative investigations:
   - Chest x-ray—to view cardiac enlargement, ECG, USG of the kidneys, ophthalmic evaluation—papilloedema and retinal haemorrhage, renal function test - blood urea nitrogen (RFT-BUN), serum creatinine, serum electrolytes
   - Complete medical and drug history is recorded
   - Blood pressure should be controlled before elective dental treatment or the opinion of a physician should be sought first (Table 7.4).
2. Preoperative considerations
   - Follow stress reduction protocol. It is essential to avoid anxiety and pain, since endogenous epinephrine released in response to pain or fear may induce dysrhythmias
   - Patients are best treated in the late morning as adverse cardiac events are most likely to occur early in the morning. Endogenous epinephrine levels are highest in the morning hours
   - Regular antihypertensive drugs should be consumed before the procedure with sips of water

TABLE 7.4 Hypertension; ASA (American Society of Anaesthesiologists) Grading and Dental Management

Systolic mmHg	Diastolic mmHg	ASA grade	Hypertension Stage	Dental Management
<120	<80	I	Normal	• Routine dental care.
120–139	80–89	I	Prehypertension	• Routine dental care • BP monitoring and lifestyle modification.
140–159	90–99	II	Stage I HTN	• Physicians consult • Dental care with stress reduction protocol.
≥160	≥100	III	Stage II HTN	• Recheck BP after 5 min. Quiet rest. Physician's advice before routine dental care • Restrict use of epinephrine • Conscious sedation may help • Noninvasive care can be performed • Invasive procedures if BP <180/110 with stress reduction protocol • Epinephrine containing local anaesthesia should be used cautiously. The epinephrine should not exceed 0.04 mg during a single visit • Avoid sodium-containing i.v. solution; also avoid rapid posture changes.
>220	>120	IV	Stage III HTN—Hypertensive crisis	• Recheck BP after 5 min. Quiet rest. Avoid extraction until the BP is under control • Emergency procedure managed with antibiotics and analgesics till BP is controlled • Emergency BP reduction to prevent organ damage • Medical advice before routine dental care • Avoid vasoconstrictors.

BOX 7.3 PT-INR Range for Reference

PT 1.5–2 and INR 2.0–3.0—do not stop or alter the drug dosage

PT 2.0–2.5 and INR 2.5–3.5—dosage may be altered

PT >2.5 and INR >3.5—delay invasive procedure, until dosage is decreased

*If the value is within the recommended range, minor bleeding with local measures can be managed. When the value is not within the recommended range, patient should be given intravenous anticoagulants

3. Intraoperative and postoperative considerations
   - Continuous blood pressure, ECG and pulse oximeter monitoring are indicated
   - Regular antihypertensive drugs should be continued during the procedure and after the procedure
   - Changing the patient's position suddenly from the supine position can cause postural hypotension. If the patient is on antihypertensive drugs like thiazides, furosemide or a calcium-channel blocker, it may cause loss of consciousness also
   - Avoid adrenaline in local anaesthetic. Bupivacaine has no effect on the cardiac status
   - Postoperative supplements of potassium for patients on diuretics
4. The management of hypertensive patients may also be complicated by diseases such as cardiac or renal failure
5. Drug interactions
   - Systemic corticosteroids may raise the blood pressure—adjust anti-HTN drug dosage
   - Some nonsteroidal anti-inflammatory drugs (indomethacin, ibuprofen and naproxen) can reduce the efficacy of antihypertensive agents
   - Reduce dosage of barbiturates as their sedative effect is enhanced when on anti-HTN drugs
   - Patients on monoamine oxidase inhibitors (MAOIs) should avoid CNS depressants, sedatives, hypertensives and narcotics
   - Avoid epinephrine in patients on MAOI or Paryline.

Local anaesthesia and HTN

- An aspirating syringe should be used to give a local anaesthetic, since epinephrine (adrenaline) in the anaesthetic given intravenously may increase HTN and precipitate dysrhythmias. Blood pressure tends to rise

during oral surgery under local anaesthesia and epinephrine can contribute to this
- Epinephrine in combination with local anaesthetics is contraindicated in a hypertensive patient with blood pressure of more than 200/115 mmHg. Large doses for patients on nonselective beta-blockers may induce HTN and cardiovascular complications
- Conscious sedation may be advisable to control anxiety.

General anaesthesia and HTN

- All antihypertensive drugs are potentiated by general anaesthetic agents and can induce hypotension. This is especially the case with barbiturates and opioids
- Intravenous barbiturates in particular can be dangerous in patients on antihypertensive therapy, but halothane, enflurane and isoflurane may also cause hypotension in patients on beta-blockers
- However, antihypertensive drugs should not be stopped, since rebound HTN can result
- HTN may be a contraindication to general anaesthesia if complicated by cardiac failure, coronary or cerebral artery insufficiency and renal insufficiency.

RESPIRATORY SYSTEM

BRONCHIAL ASTHMA

An asthmatic attack involves narrowing of the smaller airways, wheezing and dyspnoea. It may be triggered by immunological, chemical, infections or emotional causes. Proper medical history should be taken regarding precipitating factors, frequency and severity of the attacks, medication used, etc. It is treated immediately with corticosteroid inhalers, bronchodilators and β adrenergic stimulators.

Dental consideration and management

- Preoperative medical consultation
  a. Postpone the treatment until the disease is well controlled
  b. Asthmatic patients should be asked to bring their usual medications with them when coming for dental treatment
- Use stress reduction protocol
- Check for any wheezing at the time of surgery
- A bronchodilator inhaler should be easily available
- Adrenal insufficiency should be considered in patients on long-term corticosteroid therapy
- Avoid NSAIDs and morphine
- Ask patient to continue the medication.

Drug aspects

- **Interactions of theophylline** with epinephrine, erythromycin, clindamycin, azithromycin, clarithromycin or ciprofloxacin may result in dangerously high levels of theophylline
- **Patients on leukotriene–modifying drugs** may have a prolonged INR and bleeding tendency because of impaired liver metabolism
- Patients on **systemic corticosteroid treatment**–provide prophylaxis for adrenal insufficiency
- Occasionally, patients with asthma may react to the sulphites present as preservatives in vasoconstrictor-containing **local anaesthetics**. It may be better to avoid solutions containing vasoconstrictors.

Conscious sedation in asthmatics

Relative analgesia with nitrous oxide and oxygen is preferable to intravenous sedation and gives more immediate control of the asthmatic patient. Sedatives are avoided during an acute asthmatic attack, even benzodiazepines can precipitate respiratory failure.

General anaesthesia in asthmatics

General anaesthesia is best avoided. General anaesthesia may be complicated by hypoxia and hypercapnia, which can cause pulmonary oedema even if cardiac function is normal and cardiac failure if there is cardiac disease. The risk of postoperative collapse of the lung or pneumothorax is also increased. Halothane, or better enflurane, isoflurane, desflurane or sevoflurane are the preferred anaesthetics, but ketamine may be useful in children. An asthmatic attack may be precipitated by drugs causing direct release of histamine; therefore, morphine, methohexitone, thiopentone, suxamethonium, tubocurarine and pancuronium should be avoided.

RENAL DISEASES

DENTAL MANAGEMENT OF THE PATIENT RECEIVING HAEMODIALYSIS

- Accurate medical history (medication prescribed) in consultation with the nephrologist
- Investigations required before invasive procedures: Renal Function Profile–blood urea and nitrogen, serum creatinine and serum electrolytes, serum calcium, serum phosphorus, creatinine clearance test, urine analysis, ultrasound of both kidneys, renal doppler studies and radionucleotide scanning for renal clearance time
- Monitorisation of fluid balance, acid–base balance and electrolyte balance intraoperatively and postoperative blood pressure as they have a high prevalence of arterial HTN
- Take proper local haemostatic measures and blood replacement is done by washed packed cells
- If patient is on heparin anticoagulation, perform dental treatment on the day when not receiving dialysis to be sure that there is no heparin in the blood (mean life of 4 h)
- Renal osteodystrophy due to secondary hyperparathyroidism (late sign of chronic renal insufficiency)
- Bone more susceptible to fractures
- Careful dental extraction technique to avoid fractures

TABLE 7.5 Dose Adjustment According to Creatinine Clearance of the Drugs More Frequently Prescribed in Dentistry

Drugs	DOSE ADJUSTMENT ACCORDING TO CREATININE CLEARANCE (CC)		
	Normal Dose	Dose with CC 10–50 mL/min	Dose with CC <10 mL/min
ANTIBIOTIC			
Amoxicillin	500/1000 mg/8 h	500/1000 mg/8–12 h	500/1000 mg/12–24 h
Augmentin	625 mg/8 h	625 mg/8 h	625 mg/12–24 h
Penicillin G	0.3–1.2 million IU/6–12 h	50%–100% of the dose every 8–12 h	25%–50% of the dose every 12 h
Clindamycin	300 mg/8 h	300 mg/8 h	300 mg/8 h
Doxycycline	100 mg/24 h	100 mg/24 h	100 mg/24 h
Erythromycin	250–500 mg/6 h	250–500 mg/6 h	250–500 mg/6 h
Metronidazole	250–500 mg/6 h	Every 8–12 h	Every 12–14 h
Azithromycin	500 mg/24 h, 3 days	500 mg/24 h, 3 days	500 mg/24 h, 3 days
ANTIFUNGALS			
Amphotericin	0.3–1 mg/kg/24 h	0.3–1 mg/kg/24 h	0.3–1 mg/kg/24–48 h
Fluconazole	100–200 mg/24 h	50–200 every 24 h	50–100 every 24 h
ANALGESICS			
Paracetamol	500–1000 mg/4–6 h	500–1000 mg/4–6 h	500–1000 mg/4–6 h
Aspirin	Contraindicated (produces water retention, deterioration of renal function and risk of gastric haemorrhage)		
Ibuprofen	200–600 mg/4–6 h	200–600 mg/4–6 h	200–600 mg/4–6 h

- The patient should be covered with broad-spectrum antibiotics to prevent sepsis. As most antibiotics are excreted through the kidneys, only a few have been proven to be safe for use (Table 7.5).

ENDOCRINE SYSTEM

DIABETES MELLITUS

Diabetes mellitus (DM) is commonly divided into two types:

- **Type I diabetes (insulin-dependent diabetes mellitus—IDDM)** is an autoimmune disease resulting in the loss of pancreatic insulin-producing beta cells with absolute lack of insulin and is associated with episodes of ketoacidosis. The condition usually begins at an early age and insulin has to be administered from an outside source
- **Type II diabetes (noninsulin-dependent diabetes mellitus—NIDDM)** is a condition where pancreatic beta cells continue to produce insulin, but glucose level in the blood remains high because of decreased insulin activity, insulin receptor resistance or both. Long-term complications include autonomic and peripheral neuropathies as well as ocular, renal and cardiovascular manifestations. Acute complications include hypoglycaemia and coma from either ketoacidosis or a nonketotic hyperglycaemic hyperosmolar state.

INVESTIGATIONS FOR ASSESSING DIABETIC PATIENTS BEFORE INVASIVE TREATMENT

- Urine analysis for sugar and acetone
- Oral glucose tolerance test (GTT)
  a. Traditional GTT—for diabetic individuals
    i. Patient has to be on an 8-12-h period of fasting
    ii. First, a fasting sample (zero sample) of blood and urine is collected
    iii. The patient is given oral glucose solution of 75 g of glucose in 250 mL of water
    iv. The next samples are collected at 30, 60, 90, 120, 150 and 180 min from zero sample (normal values are shown in Table 7.6)
    v. The GTT curve is plotted on a graph
  b. Modern or Mini GTT
    i. It is similar to the traditional GTT, but only two samples are collected, one as zero sample (fasting) and another at 2 h
- Fasting blood glucose, postprandial blood glucose

TABLE 7.6 Showing Normal Values in Glucose Tolerance Test

Sample	Fasting (Zero Sample)	30 min	60 min	90 min	120 min	150 min	180 min
Blood glucose (mg/dL)	90	100	150	120	110	80	70
Urinary glucose	Nil	Nil	Nil	Nil	Nil	Nil	Nil

- Random plasma glucose
- Renal profile: blood urea nitrogen, serum creatinine and serum electrolyte.

DENTAL CONSIDERATIONS

ASA physical status and treatment considerations

- ASA II—Eat normal breakfast and take usual insulin dose in the morning; avoid missing meals before and after surgery; if unavoidable, consult physician or decrease insulin dose by half
- ASA III—Monitor blood glucose levels more frequently for several days following surgery and modify insulin accordingly; Consider medical consultation
- ASA IV—Consult physician before treatment
- Uncontrolled diabetes patient can present with oral candidiasis and angular stomatitis
- Uncontrolled DM with ketoacidosis—mucormycosis in paranasal sinus, dentoalveolar abscess that can lead to Ludwig's angina
- Diabetics on insulin: Neuropathy, sialosis, temporary lingual and labial nerve paraesthesia after 3rd molar removal due to neuropathy, burning mouth syndrome, Grinspan syndrome (DM, lichen planus, HTN)
- Patients with diabetes are more prone to infections, hence pre- and postoperative antibiotics are necessary for prevention of infection
- Also, in case of long-standing diabetics, they may have additional systemic complications like renal failure, cardiac disorders, ophthalmic problems and vascular diseases.

MINOR AND MAJOR SURGICAL PROCEDURE

Diabetics on insulin (IDDM—Type I) and uncontrolled NIDDM (Type II)

- Simple invasive procedures (extraction of one tooth)
  a. Procedures should be done within 2 h after breakfast and morning insulin dose
- Minor surgical procedure (multiple extractions)—done as inpatient
  a. Early morning procedure
  b. Preoperative assessment—Before 2 days from day of procedure, stabilise patient with twice daily dose of insulin
  c. Monitor blood glucose level on chart at fasting, midday and before night meal done till discharge
  d. Intraoperative:
     i. Glucose level checked at 8–9 am
     ii. GIK infusion started: Glucose 10 g, insulin 2 units and K (potassium) 2 mmol/h
  e. Postoperative: Insulin sliding scale till patient resumes normal feeding
  f. Return to preoperative insulin dosage after normal feeding
- Major Surgery
  a. Preoperative assessment—Two days from day of procedure, stabilise patient with twice daily dose of insulin. One day before major surgery, use short-acting insulin
  b. On day of surgery:
     i. Estimate blood glucose level
     ii. I.V infusion of GIK at 8 am for 4 h
     iii. Adjust insulin and potassium to keep blood glucose 100–180 mg/dL
  c. Postoperative:
     i. Continue GIK infusion 4 hourly
     ii. Blood glucose monitored 4 hourly
     iii. Potassium monitored 8 hourly
  d. Return to preoperative insulin dosage after normal feeding resumes.

Diabetics on oral hypoglycaemics—NIDDM (Type II DM)

Well-controlled diabetics—minor procedures under LA or GA

- Procedures can be done safely without insulin
- Glucose is monitored every 2 h.

Well-controlled diabetics—Major procedures under GA

- Preoperative assessment—Two days from day of procedure, stabilise patient with twice daily dose of insulin
- On day of surgery:
  a. Estimate blood glucose level
  b. i.v. infusion of GIK (10% glucose, insulin 5 units and K (potassium) 10 mmol/L)
  c. Adjust insulin based on blood glucose as follows:
  d. Sugar levels and insulin doses
     i. 80–120 mg/dL—plain 5% dextrose
     ii. 120–180 mg/dL—4 units in 5% dextrose
     iii. 180–250 mg/dL—8 units in 5% dextrose
     iv. 250–300 mg/dL—14 units in 5% dextrose
     v. 300 mg/dL and above—14 units in normal saline
- Postoperative:
  a. Infusion is stopped
  b. Oral hypoglycaemics started.

PREVENTION OF PATIENT GOING TO KETOACIDOSIS OR HYPOGLYCAEMIA

- To prevent hypoglycaemia, diabetic patients should have consumed their medication and meals at correct times and procedures should be done within 2 h after breakfast. The blood glucose level can be checked by a glucometer before and after the procedure. If lower than 180 mg/dL, oral glucose can be administered
- Signs of diabetic ketoacidosis: vomiting, tachypnoea, Kussmaul breathing (deep, rapid breathing at regular intervals), dehydration, circulatory collapse. Summon medical assistance and shift to emergency room. Management of diabetic ketoacidosis includes administration of insulin to normalise body metabolism and restoration of body fluids and electrolytes.

HYPERPARATHYROIDISM

There are three types of hyperparathyroidism:

Primary hyperparathyroidism—caused by parathyroid adenoma or rarely carcinoma of parathyroid gland. It is treated by 1,25-dihydroxycholecalciferol (1, 25-DHCC) for severe bone involvement and by parathyroidectomy

Secondary hyperparathyroidism—caused as a response to chronic renal failure due to low calcium levels. It is treated by 1,25-DHCC and parathyroidectomy

Tertiary hyperparathyroidism—due to autonomous secondary hyperparathyroidism. It is treated by parathyroidectomy.

DENTAL CONSIDERATIONS

- Formation of giant cell tumour due to hyperparathyroidism is called Brown's tumour. When the skull is involved, patient presents with ***Leontiasis osse***
- Dental changes—Loss of lamina dura, bone rarefaction and long-standing hyperparathyroidism can cause Brown's tumour (Table 7.7)
- Dental treatments can become complicated due to subsequent bone fragility and other systemic complications of the renal system, cardiac complications and GI system. General anaesthesia also becomes complicated for the same reasons
- Local anaesthesia is a safer treatment protocol for these patients, especially if they present with HTN and arrhythmia.

THYROID DISORDERS

Thyroid disorders can be classified as hypothyroid, euthyroid and hyperthyroid states. Hypo and hyperthyroid states pose risks for elective surgery. These patients are brought to euthyroid state for any surgical procedures. The patients diagnosed with thyroid disorders are subjected to investigations as follows: T3, T4 and TSH hormone levels, serum electrolytes, serum protein and radionuclide thyroid scan to study the gland.

Intraoperative and postoperative management:

- Continuous monitoring of the vitals—BP, pulse, temperature, signs and symptoms of hypo/hyperthyroidism, respiratory and cardiac functions in case of thyroid crisis or thyroid storm (Flowchart 7.5)
- Hypothyroid patients can present with depressing effect, which can be prevented with proper use of narcotic and anaesthetic agents.

ADRENAL DISORDERS

Overproduction of the hormones can cause Cushing's syndrome presenting with diabetes, sodium retention, water retention, potassium excretion, HTN, fat redistribution, osteoporosis, poor wound healing and purpura on the skin. During surgical procedures, blood pressure, carbohydrate

TABLE 7.7 Oral Manifestations of Parathyroid Disorders

Hyperparathyroidism	Hypoparathyroidism

• Dental abnormalities
  • Obliteration of pulp chamber by pulp stone
  • Alterations in dental eruption
  • Loosening and drifting of teeth
  • Malocclusions
  • Spacing of teeth
  • Partial loss of lamina dura
  • Periodontal ligament widening
  • Teeth become sensitive to percussion and mastication
  • Floating teeth
• Brown tumour
• Generalised bone rarification of jaw
• Soft tissue calcifications
• Hypercalcemia may result in sialolithiasis
• Mandibular tori
• Complaint of vague jaw bone pain
	• Dental abnormalities
	  • Enamel hypoplasia
	  • Delayed eruption
	  • Hypodontia and microdontia
	  • Poorly calcified dentin
	  • Widened pulp chambers
	  • Dental pulp calcifications
	  • Shortened roots with blunt apex
	  • Malformed roots
	  • Delay or cessation of dental development
	  • Dental malocclusion
	  • Ankylosis
	  • Caries
	• Chronic candidiasis
	• Paresthesia of the tongue or lips
	• Alteration in facial muscles

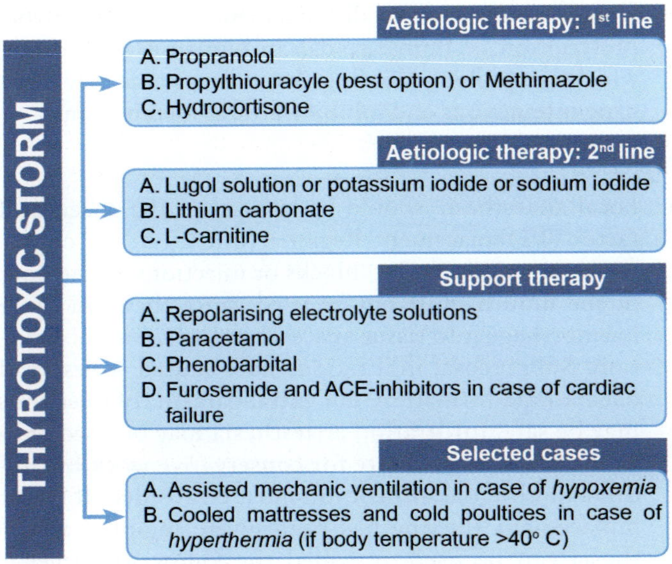

Flowchart 7.5 Management of thyroid storm.

level, sodium and potassium ion levels should be maintained. Postoperative bleeding and delayed wound healing may be encountered.

Underproduction of the hormones causes Addison's disease. The patient is on long-term use of corticosteroid for the disease. Patients who have received steroids for more than 2 weeks within a year prior to surgery can precipitate adrenal insufficiency.

Preoperative considerations: Regular check of renal profile test, serum electrolyte, blood glucose, platelet count and coagulation profile. For long-term use of corticosteroids, supplement steroids prior to procedure to combat stress in adrenal insufficiency (Table 7.8).

Intra- and postoperative considerations: Continuous monitoring of vital signs, i.v. corticosteroid supplementation to prevent adrenal crisis, maintain fluid and electrolyte balance and monitor blood sugar levels.

LONG-TERM USE OF CORTICOSTEROIDS

The rule of twos

Adrenal suppression can be precipitated when a patient is on 20 mg of cortisone or its equivalent every day for 2 weeks within 2 years of dental treatment. General anaesthesia, infection and pain can increase the risk of adrenal crisis in susceptible patients (Table 7.8).

NEUROLOGICAL DISORDERS

- Relative contraindication: Cerebrovascular disorders, epilepsy, patients with head injury
- Absolute contraindication: Cerebellar infarcts, aneurysm, arteriovenous malformations
- Preoperative investigations: PA view and lateral view radiographs, CT Brain, MRI Brain, Electroencephalogram (EEG) and Liver function test (LFT)
- Epilepsy should be controlled prior to the surgery and the morning dose of antiepileptic should be consumed with sips of water before the surgical procedure
- Intra and postoperative investigations: Intraoperative intravenous dose of antiepileptic should be given and postoperative normal dose should be consumed. Hypotension, that is, hypoxia, is to be avoided during procedure for optimal cerebral perfusion
- Seizure disorder with status asthmaticus can be life-threatening.

HAEMOPOIETIC SYSTEM

HAEMOPHILIA A

- Haemophilia A is due to defective **factor VIII** (antihaemophilia factor, AHF). Factor VIII is a glycoprotein of several components including,
  a. **factor VIII C** (procoagulant that participates in the clotting cascade),

TABLE 7.8 Dental Procedures and Recommended Corticosteroid Supplementation in Patients with Adrenal Insufficiency

Procedure	No Steroids for Previous 12 Months	Steroids Taken During Previous 12 Months	Steroids to be Taken
Conservative dentistry or dentoalveolar surgery ↓ LA	No cover required	Give usual oral steroids dose in morning or hydrocortisone 25–50 mg i.v. preop	Double oral steroids dose in morning or hydrocortisone 25–50 mg i.v. preop, continue normal steroid medication postop
Intermediate surgery (multiple extractions, or surgery ↓ GA)	Consider cover if large doses of steroids were given	Give usual steroids dose in morning + hydrocortisone 25–50 mg i.v. preop + i.m. 6 hourly for 24 h	Double oral steroid dose in morning + hydrocortisone 25–50 mg i.v. preop + i.m. 6 hourly for 24 h, then continue normal medication
Maxillofacial surgery or trauma	Consider cover if large doses were given	Same + i.m. 6 hourly for 72 h	Same + i.m. 6 hourly for 72 h + normal thereafter

   b. **VIII R: Ag** (von Willebrand factor, which binds to platelets and is the carrier for factor VIII C) and
   c. **VIII R: RCo** (ristocetin cofactor, which supports platelet aggregation).
   d. In haemophilia A, only factor VIII C is reduced.
- Haemophilia typically becomes apparent in childhood when bleeding into muscles or joints (haemarthroses) occurs following injuries. Haemarthroses can cause joint damage and cripple the patient, but bleeding after dental extractions is sometimes the first or only sign of mild disease
- Dental extractions or deep lacerations are followed by persistent oozing for days or weeks and can be fatal as the haemorrhage cannot be controlled by pressure or local measures
- The characteristic feature of bleeding in haemophilia is that it seems to stop immediately after the injury (as a result of normal vascular and platelet response) but, after an hour or more, intractable oozing or rapid blood loss starts and persists.

Diagnosis and management of haemophilia A

The typical findings in haemophilia can be summarised as follows:

1. Prolonged activated partial thromboplastin time (APTT)
2. Normal prothrombin time (PT)
3. Normal bleeding time
4. Evaluation of clotting factors and time: Low factor VIII C, but normal VIII R:Ag (von Willebrand factor) and VIIIR: RCo (Ristocetin cofactor)
   a. Factor VIII assay is required as even the APTT may be normal in mild haemophilia
   b. If bleeding starts or is expected, treatment consists of replacement of the missing clotting factor, rest and often the use of antifibrinolytic agents
   c. Rarely, von Willebrand disease may mimic haemophilia. Recording of medical history will distinguish between them, but laboratory testing is required
   d. Porcine factor VIII and genetically engineered factor VIII; considerably replaced them with *desmopressin and tranexamic* acid.

Management of haemophiliac requiring oral surgery

Replacement therapy

- Human freeze-dried factor VIII concentrate (factor VIII fraction, dried) is used when the deficiency is sufficiently severe. This preparation is stable for 1 year at 4°C, but once reconstituted, it should be used without delay. New recombinant factor VIII can also be used as replacement agent. In milder cases (factor VIII levels within 5%–25% of normal), *desmopressin and tranexamic* acid may be used satisfactorily. Once the clot has been formed, instruct the patient not to do any activity like blowing, gargling, etc., which would result in dislodgement of the clot. Avoid prescription of non-steroidal anti-inflammatory drugs, which can prolong bleeding. Avoid drugs that may cause drug interactions and inhibit warfarin metabolism.

Injections

- Local anaesthesia should be avoided in the absence of factor VIII replacement. Regional (inferior dental or posterior superior alveolar) blocks or injections in the floor of the mouth must not be used, since they can cause haemorrhage into tissue spaces, causing airway obstruction. Submucosal infiltrations have caused widespread haematoma formation, but intraligamentary injections may be safe. Infiltration anaesthesia may be used with caution and is adequate for conservative work in children, but lingual infiltration must be avoided. If factor replacement therapy has been given, regional anaesthesia can be used, provided the factor VIII level is maintained above 30%, but infiltration is preferable. Intravenous midazolam or relative analgesia can be used. Intramuscular injections should be avoided unless replacement therapy is being given, as they can cause large haematomas.

Minor surgery

- Endotracheal intubation for general anaesthesia may cause bleeding from nasal trauma and is dangerous in unprepared patients. Since replacement therapy has to be given for surgical procedures, intubation can be carried out. An oral latex cuffed endotracheal tube is recommended to minimise trauma to the nasal and tracheal lining
- A factor VIII level of between 50% and 75% is required for dental extractions (Table 7.9)
- ***Antihaemophilic factor*** **(AHF)** to be given postoperatively, but many patients can be managed with antifibrinolytic agents given during the subsequent 10 days. If oral bleeding recurs postoperatively, factor VIII must be given. ***Antifibrinolytics*** significantly reduce factor VIII requirements
- ***Tranexamic acid*** is used in a dose of 1 g (30 mg/kg) orally, 4 times daily starting 24 h preoperatively. *Tranexamic* acid used topically reduces bleeding significantly. Ten millilitres of a 5% solution used as a mouth rinse for 2 min, 4 times daily for 7 days, is recommended. This solution can be made up by diluting 10% tranexamic acid solution with sterile water
- ***Desmopressin***, a synthetic analogue of vasopressin allows the release of factor VIII C, Von Willebrand factor and tissue plasminogen activator from their storage sites. Given as an intravenous infusion, it can temporarily correct the haemostatic defect in mild haemophilia. It can cause facial flushing and slight tachycardia, but more commonly tachyphylaxis—declining response on repeated injection

TABLE 7.9 Factor VIII Dose Schedule

Operation	Factor VIII Level Required	Preoperatively Given	Postoperative Schedule
Dental extraction, dentoalveolar or periodontal surgery	Minimum of 50% at operation	Factor VIIIa i.v. Tranexamic acid 1 g i.v. (or by mouth starting 24 h preoperative)	Soft diet. For 10 days, give tranexamic acid 1 g q.i.d. If there is bleeding during this period, repeat dose of Factor VIIIa i.v.
Maxillofacial surgery	100% at operation; 50% for 7 days postoperative	Factor VIIIb i.v.	Soft diet. Factor VIIIb i.v. BD (twice daily) for 7–10 days

[a]Factor VIII dose in units = weight in kg × 25 given 1 h preoperatively (for dental extraction).
[b]Factor VIII dose in units = weight in kg × 50 given 1 h preoperatively (for maxillofacial surgery).

- ***Impacted lower third molar removal by*** the buccal approach is safer. Minimal bone should be removed and the teeth should be sectioned for removal where possible
- ***Local haemostasis:*** The packing of extraction sockets is unnecessary if replacement therapy has been adequate but an oxidised cellulose pack soaked in tranexamic acid will give better result. Acrylic protective splints have a liability to cause mucosal trauma leading to sepsis, but are needed for the palate. Local haemostasis can be aided by collagen, gelfoam or surgicel, cyanoacrylate or fibrin glues
- ***Antibiotics:*** Infection induces fibrinolysis, so to avoid secondary haemorrhage, antibiotics are administered
- ***Postoperatively***, a diet of cold liquid and minced solids should be taken for up to 10 days. Care should be taken to detect haematoma formation, which may manifest itself by swelling, dysphagia or hoarseness. The patency of the airway must always be ensured.

CHRISTMAS DISEASE (HAEMOPHILIA B)

- Christmas disease (Factor IX deficiency) is clinically identical to haemophilia A and inherited in the same way
- Human dried factor IX concentrate is supplied as a powder to be reconstituted with sterile distilled water for intravenous administration. A dose of 20 units factor IX per kg body weight is used intravenously 1 h preoperatively
- The standard preparation may also contain factors II, VII and X. Factor IX is more stable than factor VIII. Its half-life is often up to 2 days, so that replacement therapy can sometimes be given at longer intervals than in haemophilia A.

INFECTIOUS DISEASES

HUMAN IMMUNODEFICIENCY VIRUS

Human immunodeficiency virus (HIV) is a human retrovirus, which depends upon the enzyme reverse transcriptase (RNA-directed DNA polymerase) to replicate itself within the host cells. HIV has a short latency period, after which clinical symptoms become evident with eventual progression to acquired immunodeficiency syndrome (AIDS). HIV is transmitted via direct absorption (by needle puncture or break in the skin or mucous membrane) of body fluids, including blood, semen, vaginal secretions, cerebrospinal fluid, synovial fluid, pleural fluid, pericardial fluid, peritoneal fluid, saliva, as well as unfixed tissues.

Patients with positive HIV serology and CD4 count below 200 cells/μL are considered to have AIDS. Compared with other health care providers, dental professionals have a lower risk of being infected with HIV due to the decreased amount of viral load in saliva. Pure saliva does not contain viruses unless contaminated by blood. It has been estimated that the risk of transmission from patients to health care providers is higher than transmission from health care providers to patients. Due to the social stigma attached to the infection, the laboratory diagnosis must be established precisely, with no possibility whatsoever of a false positive result.

Factors which increase the risk for HIV transmission include

- Donor source from a patient with terminal AIDS
- Injury with a sharp device with visible blood
- Injury with hollow bore needles—has higher rate of transmission of disease, since it contains an inoculum of blood and virus.

PROTOCOL FOR DENTAL MANAGEMENT OF HIV POSITIVE INDIVIDUALS

1. An annual routine dental check-up
2. Oral prophylaxis (plaque control, supra/subgingival scaling) every 6–12 months
3. Annual radiographic assessment
4. ***Oral surgical procedures***: Assess the risk of septicaemia (institute antibiotic prophylaxis). Estimate the haemostasis status (in the event of history of thrombocytopaenia purpura or hepatic problems, postpone the surgery). Estimate CD4, CD8 counts, platelets and red blood cell counts
5. Institute an appropriate treatment schedule based on the patient's requirements:
   a. Identify, diagnose and manage fungal, bacterial, viral and other oral lesions (biopsy appropriate)
   b. Manage xerostomia: Patients should be instructed to avoid tobacco and alcohol, greater liquid intake is recommended, xylitol chewing gum can be prescribed to stimulate salivation
   c. Cellulitis and osteomyelitis can be treated with penicillin V 2 g/day for 5–10 days + metronidazole 400 mg at 8-h intervals

d. Periodontal treatment: Scaling, root planing, periodontal surgery if indicated (Irrigate with 0.1% chlorhexidine gluconate). Complex periodontal surgeries (bone regenerative procedures) can be postponed in individuals with CD4 count less than 200
e. Conservative and endodontic treatment: Regular fluoride applications, caries removal and restoration. Asymptomatic and symptomatic periapical lesions should be treated with endodontic treatment and periapical surgery (if indicated)
f. Prosthodontic treatment: Complex prosthodontic rehabilitation (fixed denture prosthesis, implants) can be planned in individuals with CD4 count more than 200. Simple prosthodontic work such as removable partial dentures or complete denture can be planned for patients with CD4 count. Patients can be instructed to clean their removable dentures with 0.1% chlorhexidine gluconate or with 1 part benzal chloride in 7.5 parts of water + antiseptic soap + 1% hypochloride.

ORAL MANIFESTATIONS OF HIV (Table 7.10)

Post-HIV exposure prophylaxis

Management of occupational exposure and post-exposure prophylaxis:

1. Basic regimen
   - Zidovudin 300 mg twice a day for 4 weeks
   - Lamivudine 150 mg twice a day for 4 weeks
2. Extended regimen
   - Basic regimen + Indinavir 500 mg/thrice
   - Basic regimen + Protease inhibitor.

TABLE 7.10 Oral Manifestations with Treatment

Oral Opportunistic Diseases	Treatment Considerations
Pseudomembranous candidiasis (thrush) or erythematous/atrophic candidiasis	• Candidiasis treatment should be considered for 2–3 days after the disappearance of clinical signs (typically 10–14 days of therapy) • Topical administration is useful until CD4 cell count drops below 150–200 • Azole-resistant strains may develop.
Angular cheilitis	Topical application (Ketoconazole 2%, Nystatin) usually 3 times daily for 2 weeks
Human papilloma virus (condyloma acuminatum, venereal wart)	High recurrence rate with all forms of treatment; surgical removal
Epstein–Barr virus infection (oral hairy leukoplakia)	Treatment is not necessary and instituted only upon patient's request, can be surgically removed or treated with acyclovir
Recurrent herpes simplex virus infection	Rapid institution of therapy will reduce lesion severity
Varicella zoster virus infection (herpes zoster, shingles)	Involvement of ophthalmic division requires ophthalmologist consultation; treatment may prevent postherpetic neuralgia
Cytomegalovirus infection	• Referral for evaluation of systematic and ocular cytomegalovirus involvement and intravenous or oral ganciclovir • Scaling of affected areas.
Linear gingival erythema (formerly HIV-G), necrotising ulcerative gingivitis, necrotising ulcerative periodontitis (formerly HIV-P) and necrotising stomatitis	Debridement and dental prophylaxis
Kaposi's sarcoma	• Debridement and dental prophylaxis in area of gingival involvement • Radiation therapy treatment surgical debulking for aesthetics • Carbon dioxide laser excision.
HIV-salivary gland disease	• Chewing or sucking sugarless candy • Commercial artificial saliva substitutes • Avoid products containing caffeine and alcohol • Topical fluoride patients with persistent xerostomia.
Major aphthous ulcerations	Systemic steroids for severe cases

HEPATITIS B

Exposed health care workers are at risk for main types of viral hepatitis like hepatitis B. The chance of transmitting hepatitis B virus (HBV) is about 30% per encounter. The risk of transmission is directly related to the extent of contact with contaminated body fluids. HBV is a highly infectious agent capable of being transmitted sexually, perinatally and parenterally. Transmission usually occurs via blood and blood products in volumes of even less than 0.0001 mL. Risk groups for HBV include parenteral drug users, health care workers who have frequent exposure to blood, haemodialysis patients and infants born to infected mothers. Risk of hepatitis B in health care workers is high due to high carrier state (unknown) in the patients. Immunisation against hepatitis B is acquired via recombinant and yeast-derived vaccinations that are very effective. Poor responders to vaccinations are patients on haemodialysis, immunosuppressed patients, elderly and obese patients, smokers and those with HIV-related disease. All health care workers should be immunised against hepatitis B.

PREGNANCY AND LACTATION

- **First trimester:** No dental treatment except in emergencies
- **Second trimester:** This is the appropriate time for all dental procedures
- **Third trimester:** No dental treatment except in emergencies. Due to risk of supine hypotensive syndrome in the third trimester, the patient is turned to one side (left lateral position) during treatment
- In all the cases, avoid unnecessary exposure to radiation and use proper protection
- Avoid using drugs with teratogenic potential
- **Postpartum**—Avoid administering drugs secreted in breast milk.

Chapter 8

Medical Emergencies and their Management in Dental Office

OUTLINE

Oral surgical procedures being elective and outpatient procedures are not prone to many emergency situations. However, if encountered, the patient would anticipate the practitioner to be equipped to handle the same. Some life-threatening emergencies require split-second decisions and immediate treatment. A delay may prove fatal. This chapter discusses the most common emergencies that may be encountered, the equipment and the medications that must be readily accessible, basic life support measures and means of anticipating (and avoiding) such situations.

IMPORTANCE OF MEDICAL HISTORY

Knowledge of medical and drug history of the patient would prepare the oral surgeon to handle an exacerbation of the medical problem. The procedure may be duly modified to suit the patient. Scoring systems like the one designed by American Society of Anesthesiologists (ASA) assess a patient at risk of such emergencies.

AMERICAN SOCIETY OF ANESTHESIOLOGISTS PHYSICAL STATUS CLASSIFICATION SYSTEM

- ASA physical status 1—A normal healthy patient
- ASA physical status 2—A patient with mild systemic disease
- ASA physical status 3—A patient with severe systemic disease that limits activity but is not incapacitating
- ASA physical status 4—A patient with incapacitating severe systemic disease that is a constant threat to life
- ASA physical status 5—A moribund patient who is not expected to survive without an operation
- ASA physical status 6—A declared brain-dead patient whose organs may be removed for donor purposes.

The classification of the patient helps us decide if the patient can be treated as an outpatient. A patient with a higher risk of medical emergencies must be treated in a hospital with adequate facilities to handle emergencies. If the patient is under treatment for a systemic disease, is pregnant, has undergone a recent surgery or has undergone an immunity modifying treatment, due opinion, concurrence and consent should be obtained from the treating specialist before embarking on any oral surgery.

EMERGENCY DRUGS AND EQUIPMENT

The emergency drugs used in the oral surgery practice can be classified based on the size of the clinical practice. The minimal drugs suggested to be placed in a dental practice for emergency, drugs and equipment used in a hospital set up have been briefed in the table (Table 8.1, Fig. 8.1A–E).

BASIC LIFE SUPPORT

The most commonly encountered emergency in oral surgical practice is the patient fainting. Unconsciousness or syncope can be caused by a myriad of reasons ranging from fear to a

TABLE 8.1 Emergency Equipment and Drugs Used in Dental and Oral Surgical Practice

Emergency Equipment Used in Dental and Oral Surgical Practice	
1.	Oxygen cylinder with regulator suitable for delivering high flow oxygen (two cylinders)
2.	Oxygen face mask with tube
3.	Portable oxygen apparatus
4.	Pocket mask with oxygen port
5.	Oropharyngeal and nasopharyngeal airways (size 1, 2, 3 and 4)
6.	Ambu bag—Bag valve mask with trained staff
7.	Face masks for adults and children
8.	Basic airway adjuncts (Laryngeal mask airways (LMA) oropharyngeal and nasopharyngeal airways)
9.	Automated external defibrillator (AED) to be accessible to all clinical areas
10.	Portable suction with suction catheters
11.	Bag-mask device with oxygen reservoir
12.	Basic airway adjuncts (LMA oropharyngeal and nasopharyngeal airways)
13.	Equipment for recording blood pressure
14.	Spacer device to deliver salbutamol or any bronchodilator
15.	Disposable sterile syringes—2, 5 and 10 mL
16.	Paper bag

Emergency Drugs Used in Dental and Oral Surgical Practice			
Emergency Drugs Kept in Outpatient Clinics		**Emergency Drugs Kept in Hospital-Based Practices**	
1.	Oxygen	1.	Dextrose 50%
2.	Adrenaline/epinephrine (1:1000, 1:10.000)	2.	Glucagon
3.	Glyceryl trinitrate (nitroglycerine)	3.	Normal saline
4.	Aspirin tablets	4.	Haemaccel
5.	Salbutamol inhaler	5.	Promethazine
6.	Prednisone tablets	6.	Midazolam
7.	Hydrocortisone i.v.	7.	If equipped with defibrillator: amiodarone and atropine
8.	Chlorpheniramine tablets	8.	Morphine (with due narcotic drug license)
9.	Pheniramine maleate i.v.	9.	Sodium bicarbonate
		10.	Calcium gluconate
		11.	Potassium chloride
		12.	i.v. Lignocaine
		13.	Diazepam
		14.	Theophylline

Emergency Drugs Kept in the Operation Theatre (OT)		
Parenteral Preparations		
1.	Anticonvulsant—status epilepticus	Diazepam, 5 mg per minute i.v. (up to 10 mg) or Midazolam 3 mg per minute i.v./i.m. (up to 6 mg)
2.	Antihistamine	Diphenhydramine Chlorpheniramine
3.	Antihypoglycaemic	30% Dextrose in water, Glucagon inj. 1 mg i.m.
4.	Corticosteroid	Methylprednisolone Dexamethasone Hydrocortisone

Continued

TABLE 8.1 Emergency Equipments and Drugs Used in Dental and Oral Surgical Practice—cont'd

5.	Narcotic antagonist	Naloxone
6.	Vagolytic	Atropine
7.	Sympathomimetic	Epinephrine/Adrenaline—1:1000, 1 mg/mL In case of anaphylaxis 0.5 mL of 1:1000 adrenaline given as i.m. (Repeat at 5 min if needed)
8.	Hydrating agent	Normal saline
Oral Preparations		
9.	Antihistamine	Diphenhydramine
10.	Antihypoglycaemics	Candy, sugar, Glucose powder 5 g in water Oral glucose solution
11.	Vasodilator	Nitroglycerine
12.	Antiplatelet aggregator	Aspirin
13.	Steroid	Prednisolone
Inhaled Preparations		
14.	Bronchodilator—acute exacerbation of asthma	Epinephrine bitartrate, salbutamol aerosol—100 mcg/activation
15.	Respiratory stimulant	Aromatic ammonia
16.	Oxygen	

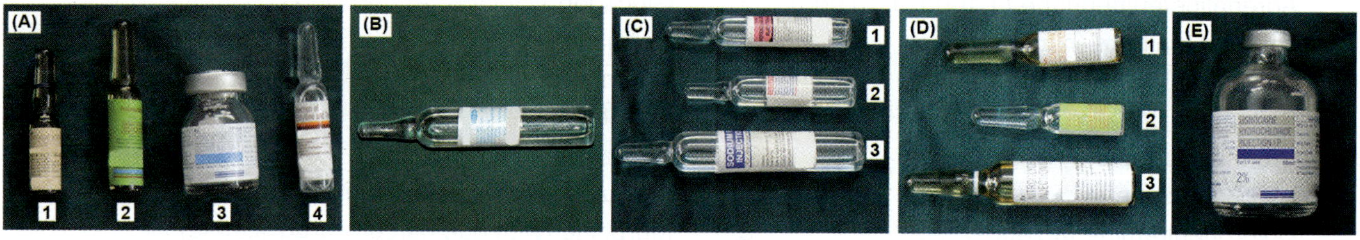

Figure 8.1 Emergency Drugs **(A)** 1. Adrenaline, 2. Avil, 3.Hydrocortisone, 4. Deriphyllin **(B)** 25% Dextrose **(C)** 1. Potassium chloride 2. Calcium gluconate, 3. Sodium bicarbonate **(D)** 1. Diazepam, 2. Atropine, 3. Nitroglycerine **(E)** Lignocaine Hydrochloride

complication caused by an existing medical condition. An oral surgeon can also be called to handle an emergency on the roadside or at a community. In such instances, emergency management precedes diagnosis of the condition. The diagnosis of the condition can follow next. No other aspect of emergency care is as important.

RECOGNITION OF MEDICAL EMERGENCY

Make sure that you are safe and then ensure the safety of the patient. The patient must be moved to a safer place where he/she may not injure himself/herself or be injured by any other external factors. The dental chair may be surrounded by sharp, rotary instruments that can potentially harm the patient. It might be safer to shift the patient to the floor in case there is a chance he/she may roll or fall from the chair. The supine position is preferred.

RESPONSIVENESS

Responsiveness of the patient will determine the mental alertness of the patient. A verbal response will ensure the patency of airway. Responsiveness of the patient may be classified as '**AVPU**'.

A = Alert
V = Response to verbal stimulus
P = Response to pain
U = Unresponsive

CALL FOR HELP

Summon medical assistance (ambulance).

STEPS IN BASIC LIFE SUPPORT

If there is no pulse, chest compressions should be started immediately. If there is a bleeding and loss of blood volume, direct compression to injured area may be employed to arrest the bleeding as well as CPR should be initiated at the earliest (*CPR: 2010 American Heart Association cardiopulmonary resuscitation (CPR) and emergency cardiac care (ECC)*).

Basic life support (BLS) is the foundation for saving lives following cardiac arrest. Fundamental aspects of adult BLS include immediate **recognition** of sudden cardiac arrest and **activation** of the emergency response system, early performance of **high-quality CPR**.

- However, the conventional teaching for many years was that initiating the effort to maintain a patent airway and ventilation was the priority. Thus following:
  A. *Airway*
  B. *Breathing*
  C. *Circulation*
- The newest development in the *2010 AHA Guidelines for CPR and ECC* is a change in the BLS sequence of steps from 'A-B-C' (Airway, Breathing, Circulation) to 'C-A-B' (Circulation, Airway, Breathing) for adults and pediatric patients (children and infants, excluding newborns).

CIRCULATION (C)

The Circulation is assessed by checking the carotid pulse. If no pulse is felt, CPR should be started immediately. Positioning the head, attaining a seal for mouth-to-mouth rescue breathing or obtaining or assembling a bag-mask device for rescue breathing, all take time and should be done simultaneously while chest compressions are going on.

CHEST COMPRESSIONS AND VENTILATION (CPR)

- Heel of one hand to be positioned over the junction of the lower and middle third of the sternum, between the nipples and the other hand is placed on top of the fist
- Chest to be compressed hard and fast at a rate of 100 per minute
- Depth of compression should be 2 inches (5 cm) at least. Wait for chest recoil
- Release pressure and repeat cycles of 30 compressions, followed by two attempted rescue breaths (ratio of compressions:breaths = 30:2)
- By changing the sequence to C-A-B, chest compressions will be initiated sooner and ventilation only minimally delayed until completion of the first cycle of chest compressions (30 compressions should be accomplished in approximately 18 s) (Fig. 8.2A–G).

For a victim of asphyxial arrest, the priority would be to provide about five cycles (about 2 min) of conventional CPR (including rescue breathing) before activating the emergency response system. Also, in newly born infants, arrest is more likely to be of a respiratory aetiology and resuscitation should be attempted with the A-B-C sequence unless there is a known cardiac aetiology. 'Look, listen and feel' has been removed from the algorithm. Performance of these steps has been considered inconsistent and time consuming. The recommended compression-ventilation ratio is 3:1 in infants because ventilation is critical to reversal of newborn asphyxial arrest, and higher ratio may decrease minute ventilation. If the arrest is known to be of cardiac aetiology, a higher ratio (15:2) should be considered. If no circulation is present, if you are unsure or in infants, if the pulse rate is less than 60 per minute, start external **chest compressions at the rate of 100 compressions per minute**. Minimise interruptions in effective chest compressions until return of spontaneous circulation or termination of resuscitative efforts. Any unnecessary interruptions in chest compressions (including longer than necessary pauses for rescue breathing) decrease CPR effectiveness.

Electrical therapies (defibrillators and automated external defibrillators (AED))

- To give the victim the best chance of survival, three actions must occur within the first moments of a cardiac arrest: activation of the emergency medical services (EMS) system, provision of CPR and operation of a defibrillator (Fig. 8.2H–I)
- Rescuers should minimise the interval between stopping compressions and delivering shocks and should resume CPR immediately after shock delivery
- If more than two rescuers are present, CPR should be performed while a defibrillator is being obtained and readied for use (Fig. 8.2M)
- In an out-patient setup, the AED should be placed at a place where all clinical areas can access it (Stroke ischaemia to brain time is only 3 min) (Fig. 8.2H)
- When two rescuers are present, the rescuer operating the AED should be prepared to deliver a shock as soon as the compressor removes his or her hands from the victim's chest and all rescuers are 'clear' of contact with the victim. Rescue breathing prior to the shock will increase the time from compression to shock, and thus it is reasonable to proceed immediately to shock without rescue breathing (Fig. 8.2I)
- Cardioversion of adult atrial flutter and other supraventricular tachycardias generally requires less energy; an initial energy of 50–100 J is often sufficient. If the initial shock fails, providers should increase the dose in a stepwise fashion
- After shock delivery, the rescuer should not delay resumption of chest compressions to recheck the rhythm or pulse. After about five cycles of CPR (about 2 min, although this time is not firm), ideally ending with compressions, the AED should then analyse the cardiac rhythm and deliver another shock if indicated.

AIRWAY (A)

In an unconscious patient, if the pulse can be felt then the airway is analysed, objects obstructing airway are removed. If an external agent is not present blocking the airway (as in case of an aspirated object), the tongue could be posteriorly displaced causing a partial or total airway block at the level of the larynx. To prevent hypoxia, airway needs to be cleared, obstruction removed and free flow of air to lungs ensured. If

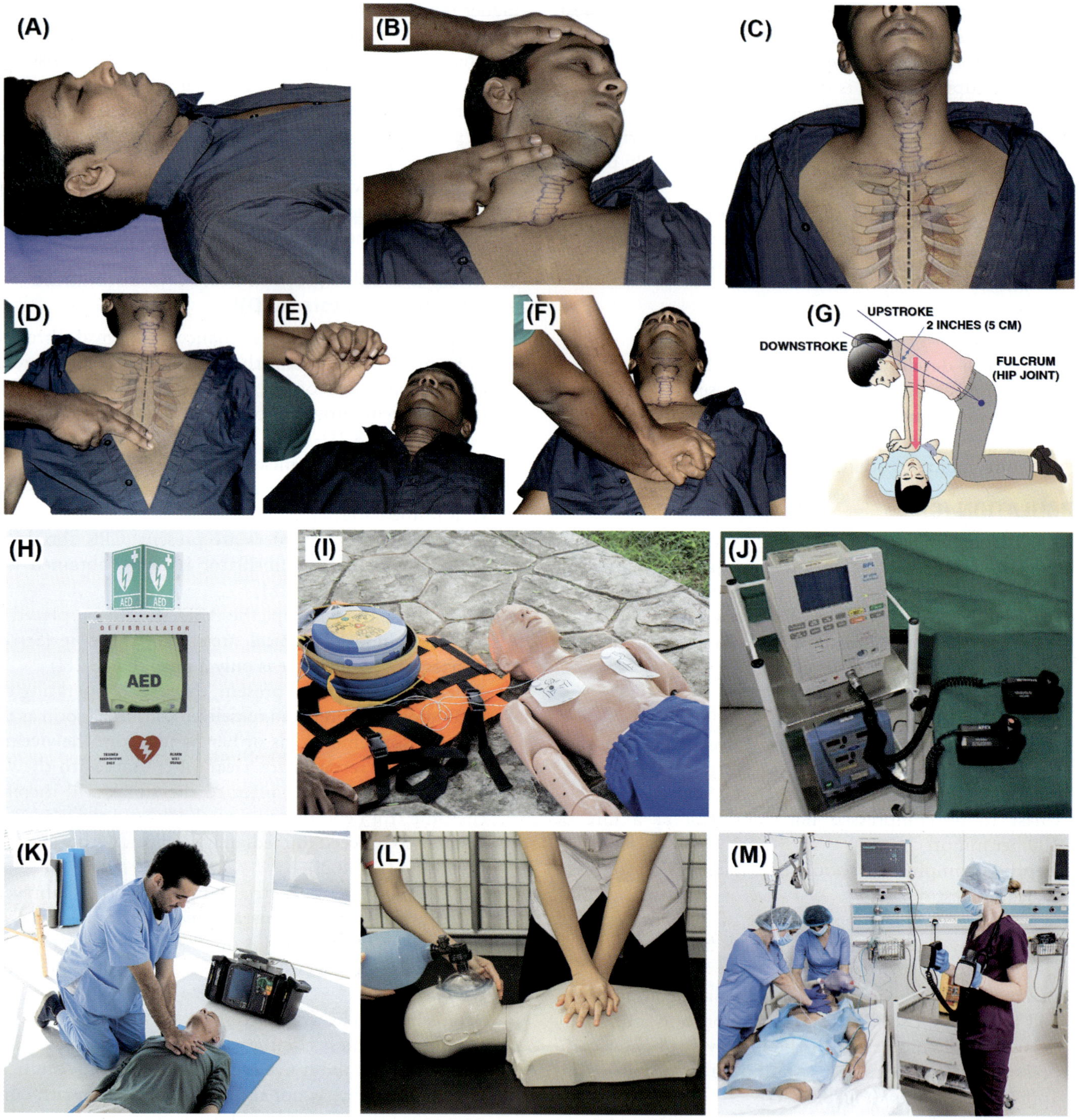

Figure 8.2 (**A**) Patient made to lie on a flat surface away from danger. (**B**) Check for carotid pulse. (**C**) Anatomical landmarks of the chest—sternum, ribs, heart within the rib cage. (**D & E**) The heel of one hand is placed over the junction of middle and lower third of sternum between the nipples. The other hand is placed on top of the fist. (**F**) Compression is made to a depth of 2 inches (5 cm). (**G**) Chest compression is done with the arm unflexed at elbow. (**H**) Automated External Defibrillator should be accessible to all clinical areas. (**I**) Automated External Defibrillator at a basic life support training event. It is brought by the emergency medical service during emergencies. (**J**) Defibrillator in a hospital set up. (**K**) Single rescuer—does CPR and breaths at 30:2. (**L**) Two rescuers for CPR and ventilation at 15:1 breaths. (**M**) CPR, ventilation and use of defibrillator by emergency team.

required, ensuring a patent airway is followed by oxygenation with rescuer (mouth-to-mouth respiration/rescuer exhaled air), Ambu bag (atmospheric air) (Fig. 8.3D) or 100% oxygen if available.

Head tilt/chin lift procedure

Patient should be in supine position.
Lift the chin forward to move the mandible anteriorly while tilting the head backwards.
Neck is hyperextended (Fig. 8.3A–C).

Jaw thrust/chin lift manoeuvre (for neck injury patients)

Jaw thrust manoeuvre: Lift the mandible forward with your index fingers while pushing against the zygomatic arches with your thumbs. Your thumbs provide the counterpressure to prevent movement of the head when the mandible is pushed forward.

Chin lift manoeuvre: Place one hand on the forehead to stabilise the head and neck. Grab the mandible between the thumb and the index finger of the other hand. Lift the mandible forward.

Hold the head to keep the head and neck still and in alignment with the rest of the body.

Cannot be used in mandibular fracture or dislocation patients.

Securing the airway (refer to Chapter 12)

- *Supraglottic devices*
  a. Oropharyngeal airway (Fig. 8.3E–G)
  b. Nasopharyngeal airway
  c. Laryngeal mask airway
- *Intubation-endotracheal tube*
- *Cricothyrotomy*
  a. Needle cricothyrotomy
  b. Surgical cricothyrotomy.

BREATHING (B)

- Once airway is secured, breaths are given
- To give breaths to a child, use a mouth-to-mouth technique
- Make sure the breaths are effective (i.e. the chest rises). Each breath should take about 1 s. If the chest does not rise, then reposition the head, make a better seal and try again
- It may be necessary to move the child's head through a range of positions to provide optimal airway patency and effective rescue breathing
- In an infant, if there is difficulty making an effective seal over the mouth and nose, then try either mouth-to-mouth or mouth-to-nose ventilation. When the mouth-to-mouth technique is used, pinch the nose closed. When using the mouth-to-nose technique, close the mouth.

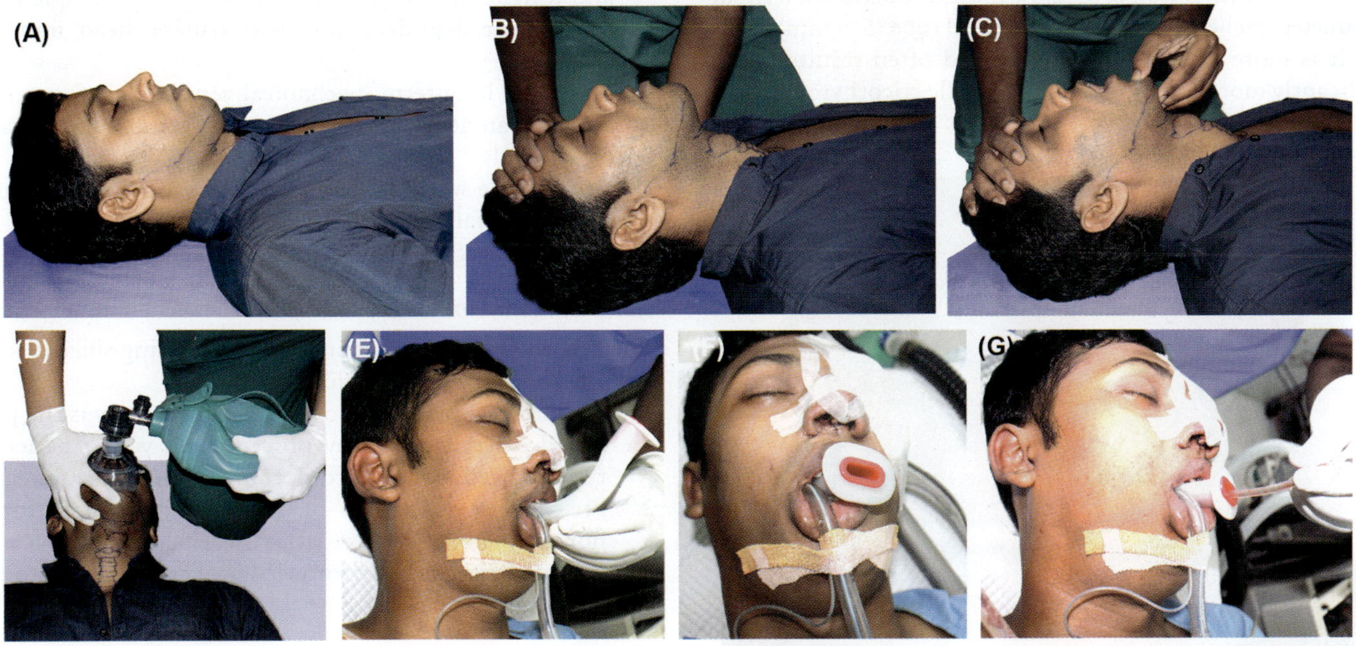

Figure 8.3 **(A–C)** Head tilt chin lift manoeuvre in an unconscious patient. **(A)** Patient at rest. **(B)** Pressure at forehead tilting the head and extending the neck creating a patent straight airway. **(C)** Head tilted at forehead. Extending the neck with chin lifted opening the jaw and hence a patent airway. **(D)** Oxygenation using Ambu bag. **(E & F)** Placement of oropharyngeal airway to secure the airway. **(G)** Airway secure for emergency access. Through the anterior flange, suction is introduced to clear upper airway or oropharynx.

- In either case, make sure the chest rises when you give a breath. In case of one rescuer, provide two effective ventilations using as short a pause in chest compressions as possible after each set of 30 compressions
- One cycle of CPR consists of 30 compressions and 2 breaths (Fig. 8.2K). When compressions are delivered at a rate of about 100 per minute, five cycles of CPR should take roughly 2 min (range: about 1.5–3 min)
- In case of two rescuers, 15 compressions 1 breath per rescuer (Fig. 8.2L).

METHODS OF SECURING THE AIRWAY (A)

NEEDLE CRICOTHYROTOMY

The cricothyroid membrane is identified and punctured using a large-bore cannula (12–14 gauges) attached to a syringe. Aspiration of air confirms that the cannula lies within the trachea. The cannula is then angled to about 45 degrees caudally and advanced off the needle into the trachea. A high-flow oxygen supply is then attached to the cannula and insufflated for 1 s followed by a 4 s rest. Expiration occurs via the upper airway as normal. This technique only oxygenates the patient and does not eliminate carbon dioxide. It is therefore limited to about 30-min use while a definitive airway is created (Fig. 8.4A and B).

SURGICAL CRICOTHYROTOMY

This involves making an incision through the cricothyroid membrane with a scalpel to allow the introduction of a small-diameter tracheostomy tube or tracheal tube (5–6 mm).

It is more difficult to perform and often results in significantly more bleeding than the needle cricothyroidotomy.

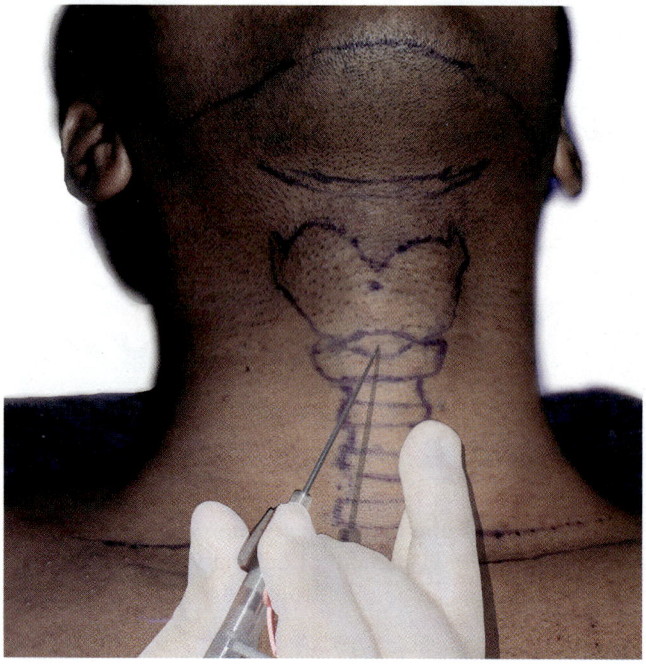

Figure 8.4 Location and position of the needle for cricothyrotomy.

The advantage, however, is that once a tube of this diameter has been inserted, the patient can be adequately ventilated, thereby ensuring oxygenation and elimination of carbon dioxide and the airway suctioned to remove any blood or debris.

TRACHEOSTOMY

Tracheostomy or tracheotomy (though different procedures, terms used interchangeable) refers to surgical/nonsurgical (percutaneous) entry into trachea through the anterior wall to secure airway for oxygenation. The surgical tracheostomy techniques were standardised in 1909 by Chevalier Jackson. Recently, due to increased complications and morbidity of surgical tracheostomy, percutaneous tracheostomy or cricothyrotomy is preferred.

Indications of tracheostomy

- To secure and clear the airway in upper respiratory tract obstruction (actual or potential)
- To secure and maintain a safe airway in patients with injuries to the face, head or neck and following certain types of surgery to the head and neck in unstable cervical spine fracture
- To facilitate the removal of bronchial secretions where there is poor cough effort with sputum retention
- To protect the airway of patients who are at high risk of aspiration, that is patients with incompetent laryngeal and tongue movement on swallowing, for example neuromuscular disorders, unconsciousness, head injuries, stroke, etc.
- To enable long-term mechanical ventilation of patients, either in an acute ICU setting or sometimes chronically in hospitals
- To facilitate weaning from artificial ventilation in acute respiratory failure and prolonged ventilation
- Facilitate long-term airway management.

Contraindications

There is no absolute contraindications existing since it is an emergency lifesaving procedure.

1. Children under 5 years of age. Tracheostomy is the preferred emergency airway procedure in young patients, though needle cricothyroidotomy is more desirable
2. Pre-existing pathology of larynx—for example carcinoma, epiglottitis
3. Lack of experience and knowledge of cricothyroidotomy.
4. Cervical trauma.

Classification of tracheostomy

1. Depending on the method of initial insertion
   a. Surgical
   b. Percutaneous (needle)
2. Depending on the intended duration
   a. *Temporary tracheostomy,* when the patient requires long-/short-term respiratory support or cannot

maintain the patency of their airway due to existent or anticipated upper airway obstruction. These tubes will be removed when the patient recovers

b. *Long-term/permanent tracheostomy* is usually performed due to carcinoma of the naso-oropharynx or larynx. Dependent on the stage of the disease, either a tracheostomy or a laryngectomy will be performed

3. Depending on the situation demanding the procedure as
   a. *Emergent tracheostomy* is performed within 2–3 min in an emergency situation when patient is anoxic and requires immediate oxygenation and verification to avoid cerebral hypoxia
   b. *Urgent tracheostomy or timely tracheostomy* procedure is performed in 5–10 min where patient is not severely anoxic maybe from partial upper airway obstruction but has high potential to become completely anoxic in short duration
   c. *Elective tracheostomy* is performed in the operating room with adequate equipment, assistance, hyperextended neck as planned earlier.

Surgical tracheostomy: procedure

Step 1 The skin from the chin to below the clavicles is sterilely prepared.

Step 2 Local anaesthesia with a vasoconstrictor is usually infiltrated into the skin and deeper tissues to reduce the amount of bleeding during the procedure (*Steps 1 and 2* will not be performed in emergency and urgent tracheostomy).

Step 3 The skin of the neck over the second tracheal ring is identified (Fig. 8.5A).

a. A vertical incision about 2–3 cm in length is created in emergencies (Fig. 8.5C)
   i. If incision is placed superior or inferior to intended location, it can be extended accordingly without wasting time
   ii. Though incision crosses the aesthetic Langer's line of tension with potential unaesthetic scar, aesthetics is not a consideration in emergency

b. For elective tracheostomy, incision is placed horizontally along natural cervical skin crease (Fig. 8.5B).

Step 4 Sharp dissection following the skin incision is done to cut across the platysma muscle.

Step 5 Blunt dissection parallel to the long axis of the trachea is done to spread the submuscular tissues (sternohyoid, sternothyroid and other strap muscles until the thyroid isthmus is identified). If the gland lies superior to the third tracheal ring, it can be bluntly undermined and retracted superiorly to gain access to the trachea. If the isthmus overlies the second and third ring of the trachea, either the gland is mobilised or complete transection of the isthmus must be made.

Step 6 A cricoid hook engages the space between cricoids and first tracheal ring pulling the trachea upward. Blunt dissection is continued longitudinally through the pretracheal fascia.

Step 7 Entry into trachea.

a. *Linear incision:* A linear incision is the simplest choice and least traumatic to the cartilage. Typically, it is made through the interspace between the second and third tracheal rings. This can also be done as vertical with guide sutures placed on either side

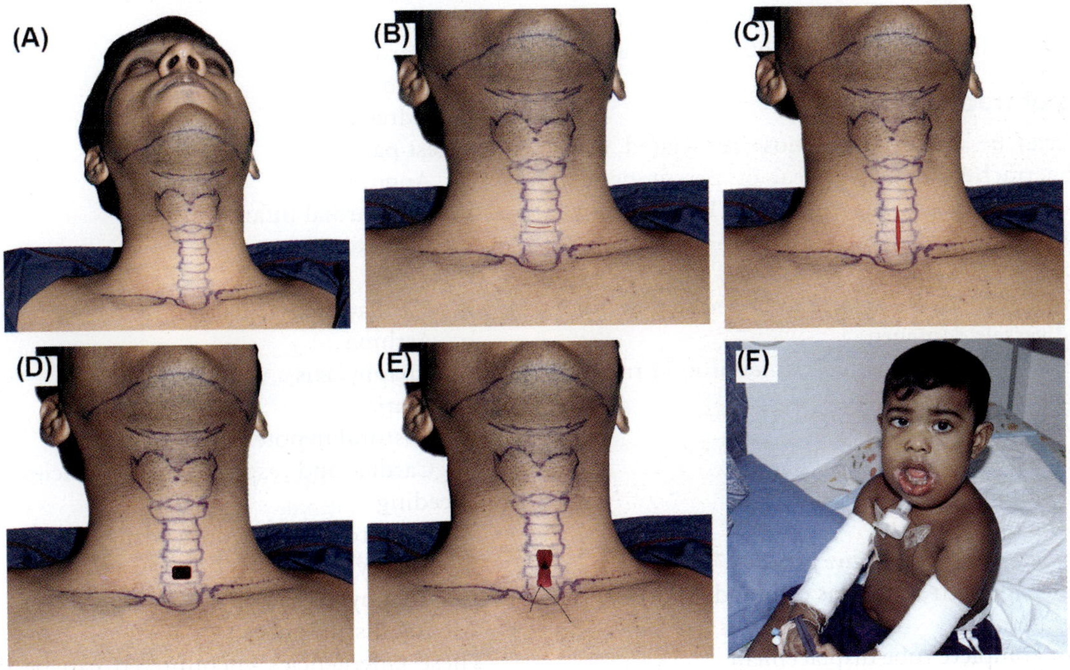

Figure 8.5 (**A**) Anatomical landmarks of the neck. (**B**) Horizontal incision for elective tracheostomy. (**C**) Vertical incision for emergency tracheostomy. (**D**) Entry into the trachea—tracheal window. (**E**) Entry into the trachea—Bjork flap. (**F**) Tracheostomy tube in situ in a child with potential upper airway compromise.

b. *Tracheal window* removes the midportion of the third or fourth tracheal ring to create a window. This minimises trauma to the remaining cartilage resulting from passage of the tracheostomy tube (Fig. 8.5D)
c. *Bjork flap* an inferiorly based U-shaped flap that incorporates the ring below the tracheal incision is raised and sutured to the skin at the inferior margin of the tracheotomy. This helps to keep the tracheal incision close to the skin edge and facilitates tube replacement if the tube is accidentally dislodged. During removal of tube, the flap can be resutured. This fistula is truly a 'stoma' with tracheal mucosa approximated to the skin. The stability of this tract is believed to be superior to the ring resection-removal technique (Fig. 8.5E).

Step 8 Placement of the tube and securing to the neck. The tube is inserted vertically downward into the trachea avoiding damage to the tracheal mucosa of posterior wall. The tube is secured by suturing the flanges to the neck skin. This is followed by tying the flanges of tube with thread encircling the neck taking care to avoid strangulation (Fig. 8.5F).

Percutaneous tracheostomy

This is the most commonly used technique in critical care as it is simple and quick. It can be performed at the bedside using anaesthetic sedation and local anaesthetic and therefore is often the technique of choice in the critically ill. The procedure involves the insertion of a needle through the neck into the trachea followed by a guide wire through the needle. The needle is removed and the tract made gradually larger by inserting a series of progressively larger dilators over the wire until the stoma is large enough to fit a suitable tube (Seldinger technique). This is then secured by cloth ties or a holder.

Complications of tracheostomy

Complications can be divided into those associated with insertion of the tracheostomy (surgical or percutaneous) or those which arise following the procedure. These complications are grouped as follows:

1. *Immediate complications (perioperative period)*
   a. Haemorrhage (usually minor, can be severe if thyroid or blood vessels damaged)
   b. Misplacement of tube—within tissues around trachea or to main bronchus
   c. Pneumothorax
   d. Tube occlusion
   e. Surgical emphysema
   f. Loss of the upper airway
2. *Delayed complications (postoperative period <7 days)*
   a. Tube blockage with secretions or blood. May be sudden or gradual
   b. Partial or complete tube displacement
   c. Infection of the stoma site
   d. Infection of the bronchial tree (pneumonia)
   e. Ulceration and/or necrosis of trachea
   f. Mucosal ulceration by tube migration (due to loose tapes or patient intervention)
   g. Risk of occlusion of the tracheostomy tube in obese or fatigued patients who have difficulty extending their neck
   h. Tracheoesophageal fistula formation
   i. Haemorrhage (local tissue trauma or erosion through blood vessels)
3. *Late complications (late postoperative period >7 days)*
   a. Granulomata of the trachea may cause respiratory difficulty when the tracheostomy tube is removed
   b. Tracheal dilation, stenosis, persistent sinus or collapse (tracheomalacia)
   c. Scar formation requiring revision
   d. Blocked tubes may occur at any time, especially if secretions become thick, the secretions are not managed appropriately (suction) and humidification is not used
   e. Haemorrhage.

COMMON MEDICAL EMERGENCIES IN DENTAL PRACTICE

The common medical emergencies faced by the dental practitioners are:

- Loss of consciousness—collapse
  a. Syncope
  b. Diabetic collapse
     i. Hypoglycaemia
     ii. Diabetic ketoacidosis
  c. Epilepsy—Seizures
  d. Anaphylaxis
  e. Cardiac arrest
  f. Stroke
  g. Adrenal crisis
- Chest pain
  a. Angina
  b. Myocardial infarction
  c. Cardiac arrest
- Shortness of breath
  a. Cardiac emergencies
  b. Asthma
  c. Anaphylaxis
- Palpitation
  a. Postural hypotension
  b. Cardiac and respiratory emergencies
- Bleeding
- Reaction to the procedure—drugs
  a. Allergy
  b. Anaphylaxis
- Mental disturbances

These emergencies encountered can be due to anxiety, medical condition, drugs the patient has been subjected under during treatment, due to an accident during the procedure and can be a postsurgical sequela (Table 8.2).

TABLE 8.2 A Comparison of various Medical Emergencies and their Clinical Features

Medical Emergencies in Dental Practice		Clinical Features	PR	BP	RR
	Syncope (Fainting)				
Due to anxiety	**Vasovagal Syncope**	Giddiness, feeling weak, paleness, sweating	↑ ↓	↓	↓
	Postural Hypotension	Palpitations	=	↓	
	Hyperventilation (may be mistaken as syncope)	Gasping, rapid breathing, giddiness, numbness of fingers and toes, palpitations	↑		↑
	Respiratory Emergencies				
Due to the prior medical condition of the patient	**Status asthmaticus**	Breathlessness, blue extremities, audible wheeze	↑	↑	↑
	Cardiac emergencies				
	Angina pectoris	Moderate to severe crushing central chest pain radiating to left arm. Neck or mandible, bounding pulse, dyspnoea	↑	↑	↑
	Acute myocardial infarction (previous history of angina pectoris, acute myocardial infarction hypertension, diabetes)	Chest pain will be similar to angina but not relieved by glyceryl trinitrate tablets over 10 min. Suspect infarction in anginal patient who says pain is much worse than usual or if this is first episode of chest pain. Shallow breathing	↑	↓	↓
	Cardiac arrest (previous history especially angina and acute myocardial infarction)	Sudden unconsciousness, no breathing. Irregular to nonpalpable pulse	No PR	No BP	No RR
	Status epilepticus; epilepsy (grand mal) (inquire as to control of condition, missing medication, previous episode)	Sudden unconsciousness, temporary apnoea and cyanosis in tonic phase, involuntary movement of body in clonic phase. Status epileptics: when a convulsion lasts longer than 30 min or when a tonic-clonic seizure occurs repeatedly	↑	±	↑
	Diabetic Complications				
	Hypoglycaemia (history of insulin-dependent diabetes mellitus)	Slurred speech, altered behaviour, confusion. sweating, hunger, tremor, apprehension, drowsiness, then loss of consciousness, bounding pulse. Rapid fall in BP if treatment is not initiated	↑	↑ ↓	↑
	Hyperglycaemia— diabetic ketoacidosis	Thirst, increased urine output and dehydration. A progressive reduction in conscious level may progress to coma and cessation of urine output in severe cases. The patient has to be shifted for emergency care as soon as possible.		↓	
	Endocrinal Emergencies				
	Adrenal crisis (adrenal insufficiency—Addison's disease)	Sudden loss of consciousness, rapid weak or impalpable pulse, rapid fall of blood pressure	↓	↓	

Continued

TABLE 8.2 A Comparison of various Medical Emergencies and their Clinical Features—cont'd

Medical Emergencies in Dental Practice		Clinical Features	PR	BP	RR
Due to the anaesthetic/drugs used by the oral surgeon	**Anaphylaxis**— a potentially life-threatening immune reaction to foreign material. History of allergies	Asthma-like symptoms (sneezing and breathlessness), circulatory collapse, cardiac arrest, following drug administration. Urticaria, angioedema, bronchospasm, tachycardia, rapid fall may go in for cardiac arrest	↑	↓	
	LA toxicity (refer to Chapter 11)				
An accident during the procedure	Needle breakage (refer to Chapter 11)				
	Choking and aspiration **Acute airway obstruction** (choking)	Sudden apnoea or dyspnoea, cyanosis, violent coughing spasms, inability to breathe, loss of consciousness, complete obstruction may lead to cardiac arrest			
Postsurgical sequelae	**Haemorrhage (**refer to Chapter 9)				
	Haematoma (refer to Chapter 11)				
	Surgical emphysema				

VASOVAGAL SYNCOPE

Vasovagal syncope is usually defined as a transient loss of consciousness due to cerebral ischaemia caused by a reduction in blood supply to the brain. Vasodilatation causes pooling of blood in peripheries and vagal stimulation causes slowing of the heart; this combination causes a dramatic fall in blood pressure.

Causes

- Psychologic factor—pain or fear
- Postural changes
- Anoxia
- Carotid sinus syndrome

Pathophysiology of vasovagal syncope

Anxiety causes increased release of catecholamines, which cause decreased peripheral vascular resistance, resulting in pooling of blood in the peripheries and fall in arterial blood pressure. Compensatory mechanisms come into play and cause increased heart rate, rapid breathing, pallor and perspiration. Decompensation occurs soon which results in hypotension and reduced cerebral blood flow and eventually syncope.

Three phases of vasovagal syncope are:

- Presyncope
- Syncope
- Postsyncope (Flowchart 8.1)

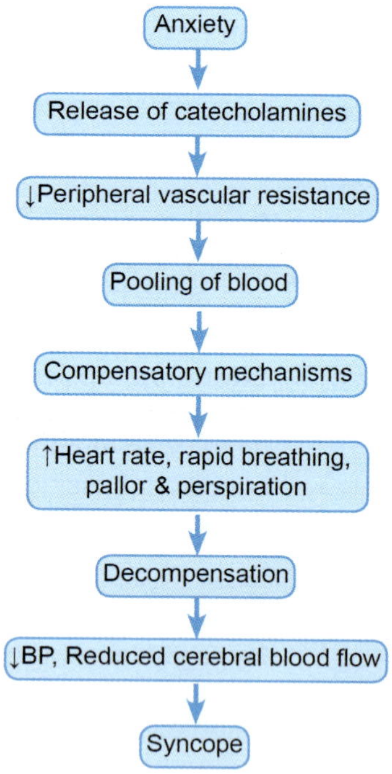

Flowchart 8.1 Syncope—pathogenesis.

Dental consideration

Follow anxiety reduction protocol to prevent syncope in anxious patients. Follow adequate postoperative pain and anxiety control technique. In case of a syncope, recognise it (Tables 8.3 and 8.4).

STRESS-REDUCTION PROTOCOL

- Premedicate the patient with hypnotics for a relaxed sleep the night before the surgery
- Premedicate the patient with sedatives on the day of surgery
- Schedule the surgery in the morning
- Minimise the patient waiting time
- Consider psycho-sedation during surgery
- Administer adequate pain control measures during surgery

TABLE 8.3 Clinical Finding and Pathophysiology of Syncope

	Clinical Finding	Pathophysiology
Presyncope		
Early	Feeling of warmth in the neck and face	Fear/pain: Release of catecholamines
	Pallor and BP decreased	Decreased peripheral vascular resistance, pooling of blood in peripheries (skeletal muscles), decreased cardiac return
	HR increased	Compensatory carotid and aortic reflex
	Perspiration (forehead)	Fatigue
	Patient complains of feeling dizzy or nauseous	Decreased vascular perfusion to brain (normotensive patient requires diastolic of 50 mmHg at upright position and 30 mmHg in supine position to maintain cerebral perfusion)
Late	Yawning	Cerebral hypoxia
	Coldness of hand and feet	Compensatory peripheral vasoconstriction
	HR decreased	Reflex bradycardia
	Dilated pupils Disturbed vision	Decreased cerebral perfusion
	Loss of consciousness	BP falls by 30/15 mmHg
Syncope		
	Breathing irregular, jerky, gasping/quiet shallow barely perceptible/apnea	CNS depression
	Dilated pupils	
	Convulsive twitching	
	HR decreased < 50 per minute pulse weak and thread, severe cases: ventricular systole	Reflex bradycardia
	Incontinence	Muscle relaxation
	Airway obstruction	Tongue fall back
	If not recovered with 5 min with proper management—it is not just a vasovagal syncope	
Postsyncope (Recovery)		
	Consciousness regained	Increase in BP after proper positioning Consciousness regained by increase in BP after change of posture
	Pallor, nausea, weakness, sweating	Can persist up to 24 h due to autonomic disturbances
	HR, BP normalises	Restored cerebral perfusion

TABLE 8.4 Differentiating Clinical Findings Between Syncope and Seizure

Symptoms or Signs	Syncope	Seizure
Tongue biting	Anterior tongue	Lateral tongue
Duration	<5 min	>5 min
Aura	No	Yes
Postictal state	Seconds	Minutes or longer
Incontinence	No	Yes
Tonic–clonic jerks	Occasional	Frequent
Metabolic acidosis	Occasional	Frequent

- Reduce the length of the appointment
- Avoid any anxiety during surgery
- Follow-up postoperative pain and anxiety control
- Effective postoperative analgesics.

Management

Vasovagal syncope in a fit, healthy young patient:

- Stop all the treatment; make the patient in supine position
- Relieve any compression on the neck and maintain an airway
- Raise patient's legs
- Give supplemental oxygen
- Monitor vital signs, check for breathing. Perform BLS if breathing is absent, summon for medical assistance
- If breathing is present, then crush and make the patient smell the fumes of some ammonia salts. By irritating the mucous membrane, the ammonia excites the circulatory system
- When consciousness is regained, patient should be kept flat and reassured.
- Once pulse and blood pressure recover, slowly raise patient to seated position
- Patients with significant medical problems, or when syncope is prolonged or complicated by seizure activity, should be transferred to a hospital environment for further assessment as indicated. Have the patient escorted home.

POSTURAL HYPOTENSION

Postural hypotension or orthostatic hypotension is defined as a disorder of the autonomic nervous syndrome in which syncope occurs when patient assumes an upright position. Orthostatic (postural) hypotension differs from vasodepressor syncope in that there is only reduction in the blood pressure, whereas in syncope, peripheral circulatory failure is also present.

Predisposing factors

- Chances of postural hypotension increase with age
- If we suddenly change the position of the dental chair after a long period of recumbency to upright position, the risk of postural hypotension increases
- It is more common in pregnant women in the first and third trimester
- Patients who are receiving drugs that produce vasodilatation (antihypertensives, narcotics and many psychiatric drugs) have a predisposition to orthostatic hypotension.

Pathophysiology

Due to the failure of one or more normal adaptive mechanisms, body's response to gravity is inadequate in case of postural hypotension. When the patient moves into upright position, the systolic pressure drops to less than 60 mmHg. However, the heart rate changes slightly or remains the same. The combination of rapid decrease in BP, but no change in heart rate is pathognomonic of postural hypotension. When the cerebral blood flow drops below the critical level of approximately 30 mL of blood per minute per 100 mg of brain, the patient loses consciousness.

Clinical features

Patient usually complains of palpitations and generalised weakness.

Dental consideration

Patients undergoing treatment in supine or semisupine position should not rise rapidly. By changing the patient's chair position 2–3 times within a minute or by uprighting the chair position gradually after the treatment, postural hypotension can be prevented.

Management

The unconscious patients should be placed in a supine position with the legs elevated. This helps in cerebral perfusion. If the patient does not regain consciousness, treat patient as for syncope.

HYPERVENTILATION

Hyperventilation is often caused by anxiety which is most commonly seen in patients in their adolescence and early adulthood and can frequently be prevented through anxiety control. Males are often affected.

Hyperventilation may lead to profound metabolic changes that include a fall in arterial CO_2 concentration. This causes cerebral vasoconstriction and respiratory alkalosis, resulting in loss of consciousness.

The patient may notice tingling of fingers or lips, muscular tremor, tetanic spasm of the peripheries and dizziness. These symptoms tend to increase anxiety, respiratory rate and depth. Eventually the patient will become unconscious due to cerebral hypoxia. The patient may be apnoeic for a period due to reduced respiratory drive with low arterial CO_2 concentration. As the arterial CO_2 level rises and cerebral vasoconstriction reverses, the patient starts breathing and regains consciousness. Hyperventilation recommences and the cycle continues with further loss of consciousness.

Manifestations of hyperventilation

- Dizziness
- Weakness
- Disturbed consciousness
- Tingling or numbness of fingers, toes and lips
- Increased rate and depth of breathing
- Shortness of breath
- Angina
- Xerostomia
- Palpitations
- Tachycardia

- Myalgia
- Tremor
- Tetanic spasm
- Extreme anxiety.

Management

Stop the treatment as soon as you notice the symptoms and reassure the patient. Make the patient lie in semierect position. If the patient is conscious, ask him/her to re-breath into paper bags to increase inspired CO_2 and to overcome alkalisation. Do not prescribe this for diabetics since Kussmaul's respirations during ketoacidosis may mimic hyperventilation. If the patient is unconscious, maintain proper airway until he/she regains consciousness. This condition is a self-limiting one and will settle. If the previously discussed steps fail to terminate an episode of hyperventilation, parenteral drugs may have to be administered to reduce the patient's anxiety and to slow the rate of breathing. The drugs of choice in this situation are parenteral (i.v.) diazepam or midazolam. Diazepam 10–15 mg or midazolam 3–5 mg for the average adult or titrated until the patient exhibits clinical recovery.

ASTHMA

Asthma described by American Thoracic Society is a disease characterised by an increased responsiveness of the trachea and bronchus to various stimuli and is manifested by undispersed narrowing of the airways that changes in severity either spontaneously or as a result of therapy. In case of asthmatic patients, respiratory problems are easily triggered by emotional stress or through a variety of pharmacological agents. So, it is a challenge to manage these patients safely if there is no known history of asthma, but in most cases, patient will give a history of asthma and would be carrying medications for the same.

Clinical features

- Respiratory distress (patient will complain of shortness of breath and want to sit erect—orthopnoea)
- Audible wheezing
- Coughing
- Dyspnoea
- Tachycardia
- Difficulty with expiration.

If the patient has severe bronchospasm, he/she might become cyanotic and hypoxic with eventual loss of consciousness.

Dental consideration

By strictly adhering to anxiety reduction protocol, acute episodes of asthma precipitated by emotional stress can be minimised or eliminated. Patients should be asked to bring their regular medication with them. Care should be taken while administering local anaesthesia (LA) with vasodepressors due to sulpha-containing agents (preservative) which can trigger. Barbiturates, opioids and non-steroidal anti-inflammatory drugs (NSAIDs) should not be used since these groups increase the risk of bronchospasm by histamine release.

Management

- Terminate all dental treatment and position the patient in an erect or semierect position. Before proceeding further, we should assess the severity of asthma
- If the patient is in acute severe phase, he/she cannot speak in complete sentences. His/her pulse rate (PR) will be greater than 110 per minute, respiratory rate (RR) will be greater than 45 per minute
- If the patient has severe life-threatening asthma, then he/she will have a silent chest, cyanosis, sweating, hypercarbic flush, bradycardia, confusion and agitation
- Administer the antiasthmatic drug normally used by the patient, use up to 4 metered doses of aerosol bronchodilator (patient's own), followed immediately by hydrocortisone 200 mg intravenously along with oxygen
- If there is no response within 2–3 min, give salbutamol or terbutaline by slow intravenous injection or 1 mL of 1 in 1000 adrenaline intramuscularly. Summon for medical assistance
- Life-threatening asthma
  a. 'Silent chest', cyanosis, sweating, hypercarbic flush, bradycardia/hypertension, confusion, agitation
  b. High flow oxygen
  c. Salbutamol—one puff into large volume spacer and allow six breaths to be repeated up to six times
  d. Prednisone 30–60 mg orally
  e. Repeat spacer bronchodilator treatment every 15 min.

ANGINA PECTORIS

Angina is a Latin word describing a spasmodic, cramp-like, choking and suffocating pain in the chest. Angina indicates the presence of significant degree of coronary artery disease or ischaemic heart disease. The discomfort from cardiac ischaemia is described as squeezing sensation, which begins in the retrosternal location radiating to the left shoulder and arm.

Types

The two types of angina are stable and unstable angina.

Stable angina

Stable angina occurs only on exertion and is relieved by rest with no changes in precipitating factors within the previous 60 days.

Unstable angina

Unstable angina describes a syndrome that is intermediate between stable angina and myocardial infarction (MI). There are changes in the pattern, frequency and duration of precipitating factors. Sudden onset is considered unstable.

Management

If patient complains of chest pain:

- Stop the dental procedure (remove all foreign body including cotton/gauze)
- Change chair position to patient's comfort (mostly upright)
- Administer 0.6 mg glyceryl trinitrate (GTN) sublingually
- Monitor vitals. Repeat dose in 5 min after first checking BP and again after another 5 min if pain persists
- If pain relieved in 2–3 min and vitals remain stable, postpone the dental treatment
- If no pain relief, if no improvement after 15 min, treat as acute MI, medical management and hospital care is required.

MYOCARDIAL INFARCTION (MI)

MI is a clinical condition caused by necrosis of a region of myocardium due to decrease in the coronary artery blood supply. This condition is usually characterised by severe and prolonged substernal pain which simulates angina pectoris but is of more intense and of longer duration.

Predisposing factors

Similar to that of angina pectoris.

Clinical features

The patient complains of severe pain, usually described as pressing, squeezing, bursting, burning, choking or crushing sensation within the chest not relieved by rest or nitroglycerine and can persist for a long time. It is most commonly located over the middle to upper third of the sternum.

Signs and symptoms

- Cold sweat
- Levine sign (characterised by the patient's fist clenched over the sternum describing the discomfort)
- Dyspnoea
- Orthopnoea
- Nausea
- Vomiting
- Giddiness
- Light-headedness.

Signs include pale appearance of face and mucous membranes, peripheral cyanosis, tachycardia and tachypnoea. The patient is usually very restless with cool, pale and moist skin.

Dental consideration

Patients with recent episode of MI within 6 months are usually on oral anticoagulant and are at increased risk of another episode. Delaying any dental treatment for 6 months post-MI is advisable. The risk:benefit ratio of temporarily stopping the anticoagulant is assessed before initiating the dental treatment (invasive).

Patient with an episode of MI >6 months earlier

- Anxiety reduction protocol should be followed
- Proper history should be taken for evaluation and identification of the patients who are at an increased risk of another episode
- Dental treatment should be carried out with effective LA, less anxiety and oxygen saturation, pulse and BP monitoring. The dose of LA should be limited. Gingival retraction cords containing adrenaline should be avoided.

An episode of MI on dental chair

- Terminate all dental treatment and position the patient in a semireclined posture if he/she is unconscious
- If the patient is conscious and breathless, reassure and change posture to sitting posture
- Give GTN tablets or spray under the tongue.

Repeat this after 5 min if pain is not relieved, patient requires emergency hospital care.

Acute MI may occur on dental chair or patient may have a previous history of angina pectoris and acute MI hypertension. Summon ambulance. Monitor BP, PR, RR, 100% oxygen. Dissolved aspirin tablet 300 mg and 1 GTN dose stat and one repeat in 5 min.

Cardiac arrest

Previous history: Angina and acute MI. Possibility of irreversible hypoxic brain damage in 3–5 min.

- Summon ambulance. Initiate cardiopulmonary resuscitation, early defibrillation, oxygen. Further medical management with appropriate drugs. (It is wise to have stock of cardiac emergency drugs, namely sodium bicarbonate, calcium gluconate and potassium chloride in close proximity—for use by certified professionals when in need).

EPILEPSY

Epilepsy is a group of disorders of brain function causing episodic disturbances of consciousness and motor or sensory function. There are several types of epilepsies. In major seizures, there is a sudden spasm of muscles producing rigidity (tonic phase). Jerky movements of the head, arms and legs may occur (tonic–clonic phase). The victim becomes unconscious, may have noisy or spasmodic breathing, salivation and urinary incontinence.

Status epilepticus refers to a type of seizure that continues for more than 5 min or a repeated seizure that begins before the individual recovers from the initial episode and is a true medical emergency. A common precipitating factor for status epilepticus is failure of the epileptic patients to take antiepileptic drugs, other factors being trauma and tumour.

Causes of seizures in dental office

1. Hypoxia secondary to syncope
2. Hypoglycaemia
3. Local anaesthetic overdose

4. Failure of epileptic patients to take antiepileptic drugs
5. Head injury

Triggering factors

1. Flashing lights
2. Alcohol ingestion
3. Physical or emotional stress
4. Decreased physical health
5. Missed meal
6. Infection
7. Epileptogenic drugs
8. Withdrawal of anticonvulsant medication

Clinical manifestations

There may be involuntary movement of one part of the body before the loss of consciousness or a generalised convulsion. This is known as aura. The aura consists of mood changes, irritability, brief hallucination or headaches. Clinical manifestations are characterised by sudden loss of consciousness, continued spasm of respiratory muscles, which makes breathing impossible. The skin colour and mucous membrane become dusty or cyanotic. Bladder and bowel control may be lost.

Dental considerations of an epileptic patient

- Adequate history regarding the disease should be obtained with specific reference to its duration and predisposing factors, types of drugs taken and duration of medication
- Treatment should be undertaken only if the patient is under good control, with no recent episodes
- Premedication with antianxiety drugs and stress reduction protocol should be followed
- Optimal dosage of local anaesthesia.

Management

- Terminate the dental treatment. Place the patient in the supine position, loosen any tight clothes and avoid restraining the patient. The mouth should not be forced open nor attempts made to insert any object into the mouth. Turn the victim into a stable side position as soon the seizures stops, open and maintain clear airway to avoid aspiration and check for breathing
- If the patient is conscious after the seizure, monitor vital signs, administer oxygen and consult a physician. Have the patient escorted to the hospital by attendant
- If the patient is unconscious with no response to management, get medical assistance as early as possible, maintain airway, monitor vital signs, initiate basic life support and transfer the patient to hospital care facility
- If the seizure lasts for more than 5 min (status epilepticus) or if repeated seizure occurs, then the following protocol must be followed:
    a. Administer **diazepam 5 mg** per minute i.v. (up to 10 mg) or **midazolam 3 mg** per minute i.v./i.m. (up to 6 mg) titrate until seizure stops. Once the seizure stops, monitor the vital signs, administer oxygen and transport to emergency care facility.

HYPOGLYCAEMIA

A common emergency situation encountered in a diabetic patient is hypoglycaemia resulting from mismatch of insulin dose and serum glucose. Usually it results from failure to take food or over dosage of insulin, hypoglycaemic drugs or alcohol.

Clinical manifestations

Hypoglycaemia is of rapid onset; with varied clinical presentation as lethargy, sweating, tachycardia, nausea, anxiety, irritability, disorientation, unconsciousness, hypotension, hypothermia and seizure.

Dental considerations

1. Stress reduction protocol is of paramount importance in managing these patients
2. Appointments should be of short duration and early in the morning
3. Routine dental procedures and minor surgical procedures under local anaesthesia can be carried out just after a meal (preferably breakfast) and routine antidiabetic medication with no special precautions
4. Glucose drinks should be available in the dental clinic while dealing with diabetic patients
5. It is advisable to use local anaesthesia without epinephrine because minimal doses of epinephrine have been shown to elevate blood glucose concentration. However, it has also been shown that the dose used in dental local anaesthetic solution is unlikely to cause any danger. The use of appropriate local anaesthetic of shorter duration minimises the complication
6. Antibiotic cover prior to dental surgery is advised to prevent infection
7. Complicated oral surgical procedures should be avoided in such patients until blood glucose levels are stabilised.

Management

- In case of known diabetic, when the patient loses consciousness or altered level of consciousness, the first suspicion of hypoglycaemia is made, unless otherwise proven.
- If conscious, oral sugar sources such as candy or glucose solutions can be given.
- If patient is unconscious, 20 mL of 50% dextrose i.v. or 1 mg glucagon i.m. can be given.

ACUTE ADRENAL INSUFFICIENCY

A rarely encountered factor, which may result in unconsciousness, is adrenal crisis or acute adrenal insufficiency. Cortisol is considered to be the most important hormone of the adrenal cortex, which helps the body to adapt to stress and is essential for survival. Primary adrenal insufficiency owing to destruction of adrenal cortex is extremely rare.

Adrenal insufficiency secondary to exogenous corticosteroid administration is becoming relatively common due to the extensive use of therapeutic corticosteroids. Most significant complication of long-term corticosteroid therapy is suppression of adrenocorticotropic hormone secretion, leading to adrenal atrophy and failure to respond to stress.

Prevention of acute adrenal insufficiency

Based on history and questionnaire, acute adrenal insufficiency can be prevented. Adrenocortical suppression should be considered if the patient has had glucocorticosteroid therapy:

- In a dose of 20 mg or more of cortisone
- Via oral or parenteral route for a continuous period of 2 weeks or longer
- Within 2 years of dental therapy.

Clinical manifestations

Nausea, fatigue, vomiting, hypotension, mental confusion, pain in the back, abdomen, legs, which may ultimately lead to coma and death.

Dental consideration

Acute adrenal insufficiency patients are unable to adapt to stress, therefore their blood steroid level should be increased by administration of exogenous steroids. Stress-reduction protocol should be strictly followed. Minor operations under LA may be performed by giving steroids (double the usual dose) 2 h pre- and postoperatively. Aspirin and other NSAIDs should be avoided as they may increase the risk of peptic ulceration in those on corticosteroids. Susceptibility to infection is increased by systemic steroid use; no prophylactic antibiotic may be indicated.

Management (Flowchart 8.2)

- Terminate all dental procedures
- Monitor vital signs
- Summon medical assistance
- Administer glucocorticoid (200 mg hydrocortisone i.v.)
- Provide BLS
- Transport to hospital for emergency medical care
- Check blood level for glucose and give glucose (oral or i.v.), if hypoglycaemic. Repeat 200 mg hydrocortisone at 4–6 h interval as required and monitor BP.

Step 1: Terminate dental therapy

As soon as signs and symptoms of possible acute adrenal insufficiency are noted, dental treatment must be interrupted immediately. Acute adrenal insufficiency should be suspected in patients who develop symptoms of mental confusion, nausea, vomiting and abdominal pain and who are currently receiving glucocorticosteroids or have received 20 mg or more of cortisone (or its equivalent) by oral or parenteral administration for a period of 2 weeks or longer within the past 2 years.

Criteria for determining adrenal insufficiency

1. History of current or recent long-term steroid use
2. Mental confusion
3. Nausea and vomiting
4. Abdominal pain
5. Hypotension.

MANAGEMENT OF ADRENAL INSUFFICIENCY

Step 2: Position the patient

If the patient appears mentally confused, the patient is placed in supine position with the legs elevated slightly or in a comfortable position.

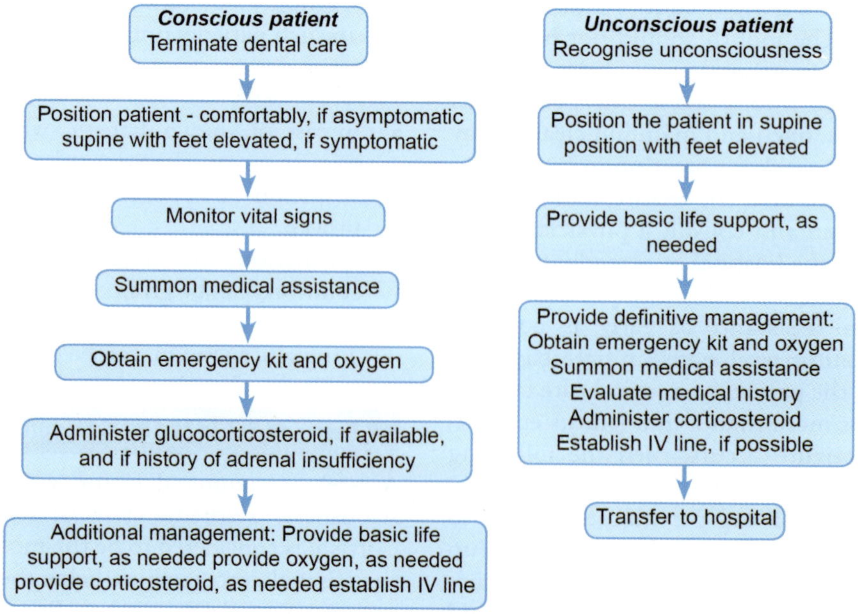

Flowchart 8.2 Management protocol for conscious patient and unconscious patient.

Step 3: Monitor vital signs

Blood pressure and heart rate should be monitored every 5 min during the episode. Hypertension and tachycardia are common.

Step 4: Summon medical assistance

Medical assistance with emergency kit and oxygen should be summoned as early as possible. Oxygen may be administered by means of a full face mask or nasal hood. A flow of approximately 5–10 L/min will be adequate.

Step 5: Administer glucocorticosteroid

Step 6:

In a patient known to have chronic adrenal insufficiency, the immediate administration of 100 mg of hydrocortisone sodium succinate is suggested and should be re-administered every 6–8 h.

If possible, the 100 mg of hydrocortisone should be administered intravenously over 30 s. The intramuscular route may be employed instead of intravenous administration, with 100 mg (2 mL) injected into the vastus lateralis or mid-deltoid area.

Step 7: Additional management

Additional drugs include intravenous fluids to counteract the volume depletion and hypotension that are usually present. An Addisonian patient may be up to 20% volume depleted. Hypoglycaemia is also treated immediately and aggressively with intravenous administration of (to check) or 1–2 mg glucagon administered i.m.

ANAPHYLAXIS

Anaphylaxis is a potentially life-threatening immune reaction. Anaphylactic reactions may occur after a single and first-time exposure to certain substances such as drugs. Anaphylaxis is a clinical syndrome of severe hypersensitivity reaction characterised by cardiovascular system (CVS) collapse, respiratory system depression, skin reactions and smooth muscle contractions.

Pathophysiology

Whenever a foreign body (antigen) enters into the host, defence mechanism comes into play, like phagocytes and nonspecific clinical substance assisting the removal of the foreign substance. The combination of antigen with circulating antibody on sensitised cells apparently results in the release of histamine, which causes the spasmodic contraction of smooth muscles of bronchioles, pulmonary arteries and gastrointestinal tract (GI) tract. Increased capillary permeability with resulting oedema occurs, particularly in the tracheolaryngeal mucosa, which is life-threatening and a common cause of death in anaphylaxis.

Clinical features

Cutaneous manifestations

- Pruritus
- Urticaria
- Angioedema
- Generalised erythema.

Respiratory manifestations

- Wheezing
- Coughing
- Stridor
- Dyspnoea
- Laryngeal oedema
- Respiratory arrest.

CVS manifestations

- Tachycardia
- Shock
- Light-headedness
- Hypotension
- Cardiac dysrhythmia
- Cardiac arrest.

GIT manifestations

- Nausea
- Vomiting
- Abdominal cramps
- Urinary incontinence
- Diarrhoea
- Tenesmus.

Dental consideration

A proper history should be taken and patient should be questioned about the drugs to which he/she is allergic and manifestations of the allergies. When a drug allergy is suspected, precaution must be taken to prevent the administration of the drug and alternative should be considered. In a patient with a history of allergy, LA is avoided and pain is controlled through the administration of oral analgesics. Equipment, drugs and assistance needed for the management of anaphylaxis should always be available when allergy testing is carried out. If the allergy is confirmed, the patient should be sent to physician for hypersensitivity testing and information should be recorded permanently in his/her case sheet.

Management

- Terminate the dental treatment. Summon ambulance
- If the allergic reaction is confined to the skin, an antihistamine is administered either intravenously or intramuscularly
- Always check whether respiratory distress is due to other causes. Assess the degree of cardiovascular collapse (pulse and blood pressure). Assess the degree of airway obstruction (upper—angioedema, lower—bronchospasm)
- Position the patient in supine position with the legs elevated, ensure a clear upper airway

- Give oxygen
- Administer 0.5 mL of 1:1000 epinephrine by establishing intramuscular access. Adrenaline should be followed by an antihistamine like chlorpheniramine 10 mg i.v. and 20 mg i.v. of hydrocortisone
- Repeat this every 5 min, if needed as guided by BP, pulse, until the patient gets better. Continue oxygen at the rate of 5–6 L/min. Adrenaline is given i.m. and not i.v. unless the patient is severely ill or has no pulse
  a. In case of bronchospasm, administer salbutamol, initiate BLS and monitor vital signs. Consider cricothyrotomy by specialist if the laryngospasm is not relieved with epinephrine. Administer 100% oxygen. CPR, if cardiac arrest occurs. If BP fall is rapid, 1:10,000 adrenalin may be infused i.v. slowly (refer to Chapter 11, Flowchart no. 11.5).

CHOKING/FOREIGN BODY ASPIRATION

During oral surgical procedures, aspiration of foreign bodies into the airway is always a serious problem, which might cause severe airway obstruction. This is much more common if the patient is positioned in a supine or semierect position or when there is absence of gag reflex (when the patient is sedated). The aspirated foreign body can either obstruct the airway or might be swallowed and pass through the gastrointestinal tract harmlessly. However, this should be confirmed by a chest radiograph to rule out foreign body in the respiratory tract. When a foreign body is aspirated into the larynx, violent coughing may expel the aspirated material if it is small, but in case of larger objects, it might obstruct the airway and coughing cannot expel the aspirated material. Small materials like burs, reamers, files, inlays, tooth structure, etc. may dislodge into the oropharynx of patients who may swallow or aspirate them. Objects swallowed into the GI tract can produce peritoneal abscess, perforation and peritonitis. Objects aspirated into the bronchus can produce lung abscess, pneumonia, atelectasis and infection.

Prevention

A rubber dam is very effective during any operative procedure in preventing the swallowing of objects. Therefore, it is recommended for most procedures except for periodontics and oral surgery where it is not feasible to use a rubber dam. Oral packing using gauze creates a pharyngeal curtain, which effectively prevents the entry of small instruments or fluids like blood into the airway (under GA).

Clinical features

- Coughing
- Choking sensation
- Dyspnoea
- Stridorous breathing
- Cyanosis

Management (Table 8.5, Flowchart 8.3)

- Once a foreign body aspiration is suspected, stop the dental procedure
- Ask the patient to cough out the obstruction
- If the patient is unable to cough out the object, becomes apprehensive and gasps for breath, perform Heimlich manoeuvre (Fig. 8.6A–E)
- If patient losses consciousness during these unsuccessful attempts, shift the patient to the floor and perform the Heimlich manoeuvre again and inspect the oral cavity for object. Perform 'finger sweep' or use Magill forceps to remove the object if visible (Fig. 8.6 F)
- If successful in retrieval, BLS is done based on vitals

TABLE 8.5 Management of Foreign Body Obstruction

Types of Obstruction	Management
1. Partial-adequate air exchange	Encourage patient of cough and clear the airway
2. Partial-inadequate exchange	If poor air entry, increasing high pitched stridor, increased respiratory distress, manage as for complete airway obstruction
3. Complete obstruction and conscious patient	• Patient unable to talk, breathe or cough • If patient is in the dental chair sit them up, turn patient side on in chair, support chest with one hand deliver five sharp back blows between the shoulder blades with the heel of the other hand • If back blows fail, five abdominal thrusts-Heimlich manoeuvre • Repeat till object dislodged
4. Complete obstruction and unconscious patient	• Open airway and activate BLS with four manual thrusts and two finger sweeps • Cricothyroidotomy, if no air entry • Administer oxygen, arrange transfer to hospital for bronchoscopy

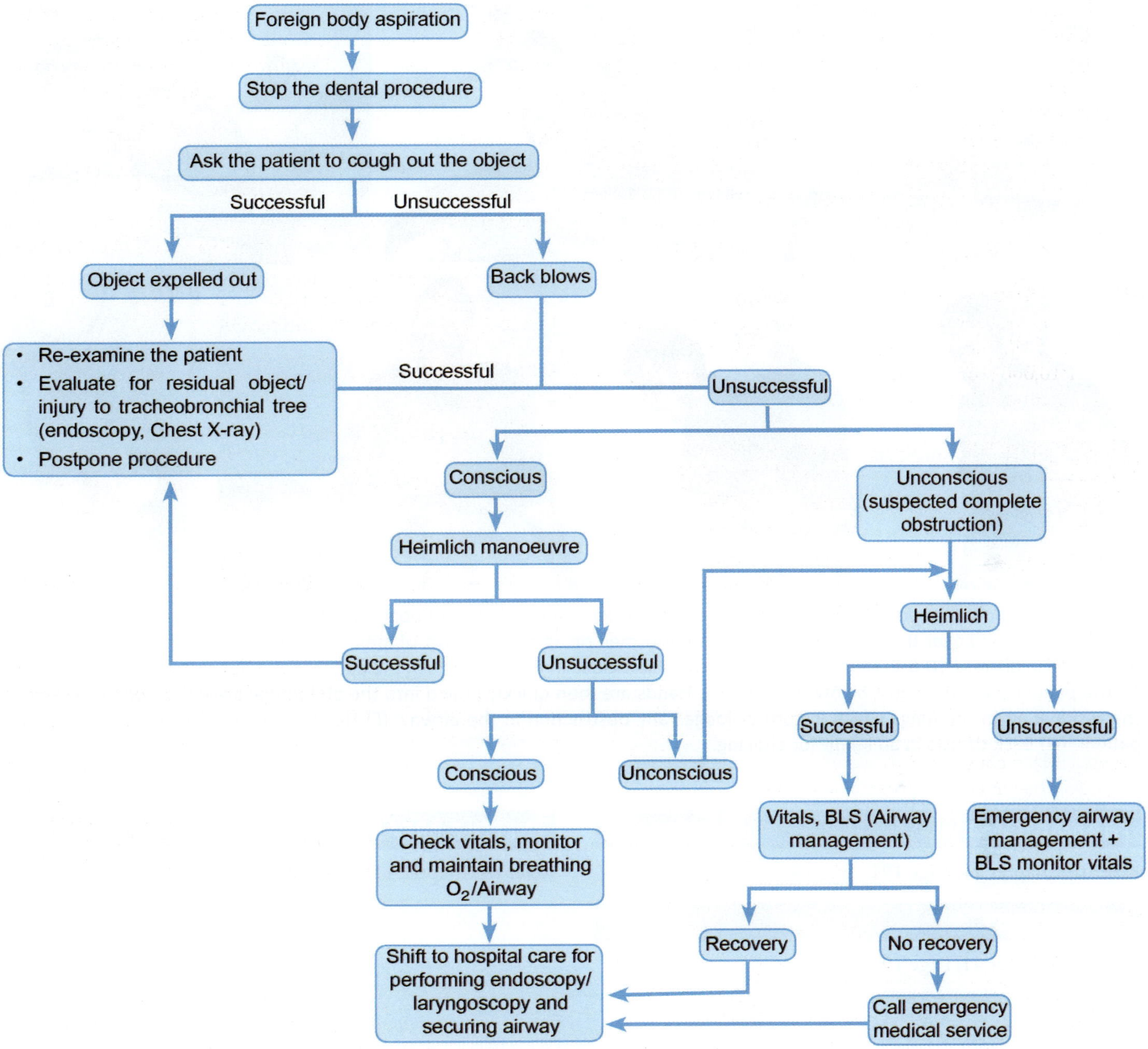

Flowchart 8.3 Management of foreign body aspiration.

- If unsuccessful in retrieval, then look, listen and feel for breathing. If the patient is breathing with adequate ventilation, then monitor vitals and shift for hospital care
- If the patient shows no signs of breathing, it is indicative of airway obstruction, emergency airway management should be initiated followed by hospital-based care
- Choking in infants is managed by back blows and chest thrusts (Fig. 8.6G).

HAEMORRHAGE

Refer to Chapter 9, Page 115.

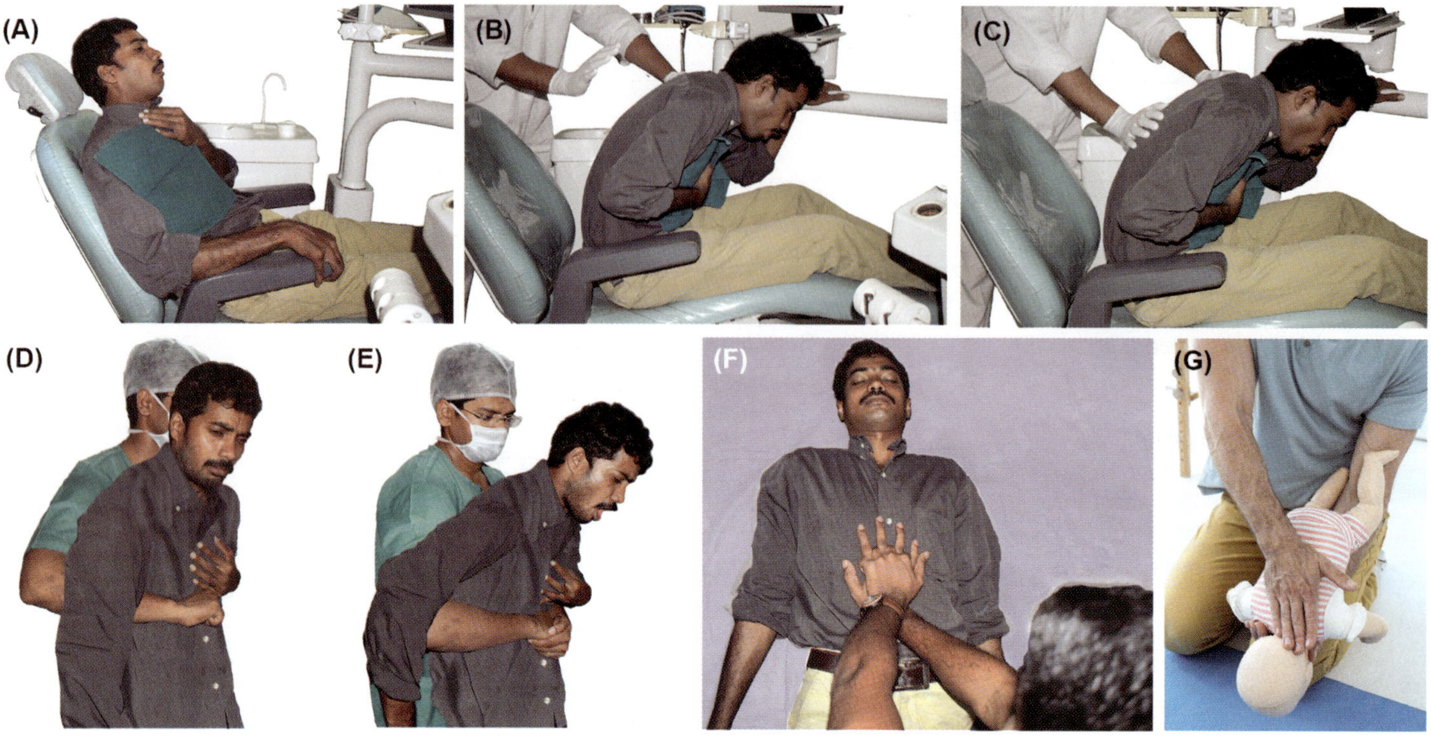

Figure 8.6 Method of performing Heimlich manoeuvre. (**A**) Patient choking from upper airway obstruction typically showing distress signal of hand over the chest. (**B**) Back blows performed on an adult as part of initial airway management. (**C**) Note the patient is still in distress. (**D & E**) Heimlich manoeuvre in a conscious patient. Approach the patient from behind and keep your hands on the patient's abdomen just below the rib cage. Hands are then quickly pulled into the abdominal area attempting to remove the residual air in the lungs which in turn dislodges any obstruction in the airway. (**F**) Heimlich manoeuvre in an unconscious patient. (**G**) Back thrusts in an infant for choking.

HAEMATOMA

Refer to Chapter 11, Page 191.

LA TOXICITY

Refer to Chapter 11, Page 195–196.

NEEDLE BREAKAGE

Refer to Chapter 11, Page 190.

Chapter
9

Haemorrhage and Shock

OUTLINE

HAEMORRHAGE

Haemorrhage is the escape of blood from the cardiovascular system to the surface of the body or into the body tissues or cavities. Haemorrhage can be classified in several ways for ease of identification and treatment as discussed in Table 9.1.

CAUSES OF HAEMORRHAGE

1. Trauma
2. Infections
3. Local irritants
4. Congenital malformations
5. Surgical (intraoperative/postoperative)
6. Haemorrhage due to abnormalities in clotting factors
7. Clotting factor deficiencies
   a. Hereditary–haemophilia A, haemophilia B, thrombocytopaenia
   b. Anticoagulant, antiplatelet or fibrinolytic therapy–warfarin, coumarin, heparin, enoxaparin, aspirin, clopidogrel, argatroban, alteplase, tirofiban, dipyridamole, eptifibatide, fondaparinux
   c. Liver disease (Factor II, VII, IX, X deficiencies)
8. Dysfunction of clotting–multiple myeloma
9. Haemorrhage due to abnormalities in platelets
   a. Deficiencies
   b. Idiopathic thrombocytopenia purpura
   c. Secondary thrombocytopenia purpura
   d. Leukaemia
   e. Thrombocytosis
   f. Dysfunction–thrombocytopaenia
10. Haemorrhage due to systemic disease
11. Viral infection
12. Scurvy
13. Allergy.

CLINICAL FEATURES OF ACUTE BLOOD LOSS

1. Increasing pallor
2. Increasing pulse rate
3. Restlessness
4. Air hunger (deep respiration)
5. Cold, clammy skin
6. Thirst
7. Tinnitus
8. Blindness
9. Blood pressure (BP) - falling of BP is not a sign of acute blood loss. A normal or slightly raised BP can be recorded. Collapse and death can occur suddenly
10. Urinary output–can be reduced in case of acute blood loss
11. Haemoglobin level–not immediately, but after a few hours, it may fall.

HAEMATOLOGICAL INVESTIGATIONS

The bleeding tendency of any patient can be assessed by means of haematological investigations. These lists of tests are termed the 'coagulation profile'. Patients with liver disease, a previous history of haemorrhage, under an anticoagulant therapy, a familial history of blood dyscrasias may be advised to be subjected to an investigation prior to any oral surgical procedure. The coagulation profile includes:

- Clotting time (CT)
- Bleeding time (BT)
- Prothrombin time (PT) and international normalised ratio (INR)
- Activated partial thromboplastin time (APTT)
- Factors assay.

Refer page 44—Chapter 5 on Diagnostic Aid—Haematological, Biochemical and Microbial Investigations for detailed description and interpretation of these tests.

TABLE 9.1 Classifications of Haemorrhage

CLASSIFICATION	CLASSIFICATION SUBTYPES		
Based on Source of Blood Loss	**Arterial Haemorrhage**	**Venous Haemorrhage**	**Capillary Haemorrhage**
Colour	Bright red	Dark red	Intermediate red
Pulsating character	Positive	Negative	Capillary bleeding may be quite aggressive in the maxillofacial region as a result of the strong pulse on one side of the capillaries
Vigor of flow	Increased	Less rapid flow	Oozing type
Spurt	Blood will spurt with each heartbeat from the cut end of the artery	It does not spurt	Ooze from raw surface
Based on time of occurrence	**Primary haemorrhage**	**Secondary haemorrhage**	**Reactionary (intermediate) haemorrhage**
	• The bleeding that happens as a result of an injury or operation is known as primary haemorrhage	• Secondary haemorrhage is recurrence of bleeding, it occurs weeks after injury or even later than that • Infection is the cause for reopening of the bleeder vessel in most cases • It is typically seen in patients with retained root tips or foreign materials in extracted socked	• The reappearance of bleeding within 24 h of the injury or operation is known as reactionary haemorrhage. It is produced by the clot dislodging as a result of a spike in blood pressure following the injury • Restlessness in the postinjury or postoperative period can also lead to either dislodging of the clot or slipping of the ligature • Coughing and vomiting increases the venous pressure, especially in the neck veins and this is often the cause for bleeding from extraction site or thyroidectomy wounds in the immediate postoperative period • This can also happen once the local anaesthetic's vasoconstrictive effect wears off. By acting on the alpha receptors in the smooth muscles of the vasoconstriction. However, as the alpha stimulation wears off, its action on β2 receptors causes a rebound vasodilation. When epinephrine concentrations of 1:50,000 or 1:100,000 are employed, this rebound beta effect can occur. Even after the patient has been discharged from the hospital following surgical treatment, this could occur
Based on visualisation of blood loss	**External haemorrhage**		**Internal haemorrhage**
	Bleeding onto the exterior as in skin laceration or bleeding through an orifice as epistaxis or otorrhoea bleeding		• Internal or concealed haemorrhage occurs in injuries to abdominal viscera • It is typically seen in rupture of the spleen
			• The diagnosis has to be made from history and clinical signs of blood loss like pallor, rising pulse rate and falling BP

TABLE 9.1 Classifications of Haemorrhage—cont'd

CLASSIFICATION	CLASSIFICATION SUBTYPES			
Based on volume of blood loss	Mild haemorrhage—less than 500 mL	Moderate haemorrhage—500 mL to 1 L of blood loss	Severe haemorrhage— more than 1 L	
Based on speed of blood loss	Acute haemorrhage—massive bleeding in a short span of time		Chronic haemorrhage—slow bleeding with a small quantity over a long period of time	
Based on percentage volume of blood loss	Class I Up to 15%	Class II 15%–30%	Class III 30%–40%	Class IV more than 40%
Based on clinical signs of haemorrhage	Petechial haemorrhage	Ecchymosis-haemorrhage	Haematoma-haemorrhage	

MECHANISM OF HAEMOSTASIS

The mechanism of cessation of extravasation of blood is called Haemostasis. Coagulation is a process during which, the injured blood vessel wall components trigger a series of reactions to counteract and reduce the extravasation of blood by transforming the cells and the components of blood into an insoluble gel (clot or thrombus) to plug and seal the injury site (Flowchart 9.1). When there is a tissue injury leading to extravasation of blood, the body aims to stem the bleed by initiating steps as depicted in Fig. 9.1.

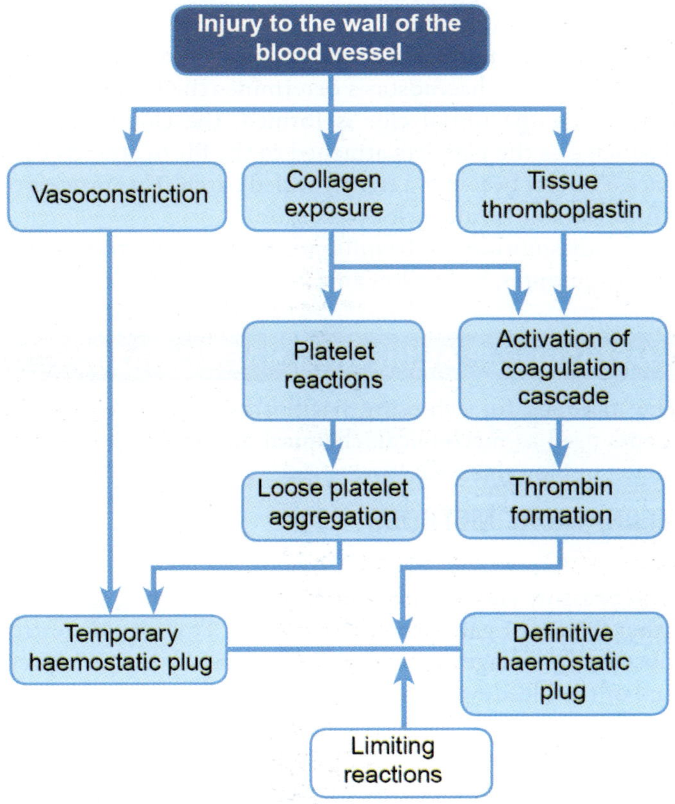

Flowchart 9.1 Summary of reactions involved in haemostasis.

1. Vasoconstriction
2. Primary haemostasis by platelet plug formation
3. Initiation of the coagulation cascade for secondary haemostasis
4. Tertiary haemostasis by consolidation of the fibrin clot.

VASOCONSTRICTION

The damaged blood vessel helps to limit blood loss by slowing down the flow by narrowing the lumen. This is controlled by

- *Local control factors:* Vasoconstrictors such as thromboxane A2, serotonin, fibrinopeptide B are released at the site of the injury
- *Systemic control factors:* Epinephrine from the adrenal glands stimulates general vasoconstriction.

PRIMARY HAEMOSTASIS BY PLATELET PLUG FORMATION

A physical barrier that plugs the tear in the wall of the blood vessel is the immediate goal of haemostasis, and this is accomplished by the platelets.

- *Platelet adhesion:* Damage to blood vessels causes exposure of collagen fibres to which platelets adhere to form a one-cell-thick carpet. Integrins, von Willebrand factor promote the adherence of platelets to the endothelial cells of the blood vessels
- *Platelet activation or secretion:* On activation, platelets release local factors, such as adenosine diphosphate, thromboxane that causes more platelets to aggregate
- *Platelet aggregation:* A platelet plug is formed by self-association of the platelets. Platelet aggregation can be inhibited naturally by the absence of calcium, presence of prostacyclins or by administrations of drugs like aspirin. The platelet plug thus formed is still weak and therefore

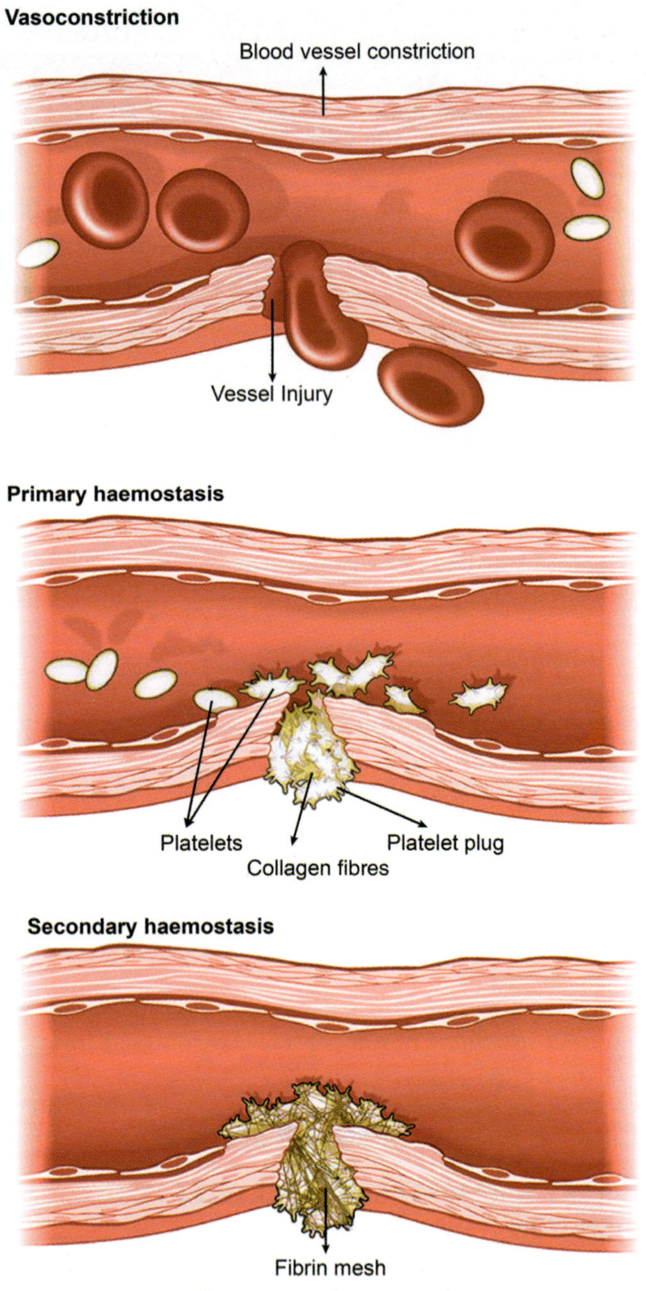

Figure 9.1 Illustration of stages in haemostasis.

a bleed should not be 'wiped' but 'dabbed' using the capillary action of a dry towel.

SECONDARY HAEMOSTASIS OR THE COAGULATION CASCADE

Tissue injury or injury to blood vessels prompts platelets to aggregate at the site of injury. These platelets release factors that begin secondary haemostasis (coagulation cascade) wherein the weak, soluble platelet aggregate matures to form the insoluble 'clot'. This cascade is mediated by a number of factors (Table 9.2). When the injury causes the blood to come in contact with the collagen in the walls of the traumatised blood vessels, the intrinsic pathway or contact activation pathway is initiated, which involves the sequential activation of factor XII (Hageman factor), factor XI (plasma thromboplastin antecedent), factor IX (Christmas factor) and factor VIII (antihaemophilic haemoglobin). Tissue injury or vascular wall injury launches the extrinsic factor which is triggered by the release of tissue thromboplastin (factor III) from the damaged vascular or tissue cells. The extrinsic pathway is stimulated when the factor III meets factor VII (stable factor). Both pathways activate coagulation factor X (Stuart-Prower factor), which leads to the conversion of pro-thrombin (factor II) to thrombin (activated factor IIa). Thrombin then stimulates the formation of fibrin (factor Ia) from fibrinogen (factor I) (Table 9.2). Fibrin in combination with fibrin-stabilising factor (factor XIII) forms a stable fibrin clot at the site of injury. This also initiates a thrombus-resolving cascade where the fibrinolytic agents, such as plasmin form fibrin-degrading products (Table 9.2). Any excess amounts of clotting factors which are formed are inactivated by fibrin inhibitors, such as antiplasmin, antithrombin III and protein C, limits clot formation. Clot formation or coagulation can be inhibited in states of hypercoagulability using drugs like warfarin, heparin, coumadin, etc.

TERTIARY HAEMOSTASIS CONSOLIDATION OF FIBRIN CLOT

Tertiary haemostasis comprises of:

1. Maturation of the clot
2. Cross-linking of fibrin monomers within the clot
3. Controlled activation of the fibrinolytic system.

This phase of haemostasis determines the lifespan of the clot. When the initial clot is formed, the clot undergoes shrinkage as the platelets attached to the fibrin strands contract. The clot becomes a tightly sealed patch. This process of reinforcement is called clot retraction.

Clot dissolution can be inhibited by drugs like tranexamic acid, desmopressin, epsilon amino caproic acid, etc.

METHODS OF ACHIEVING HAEMOSTASIS

The methods for achieving haemostasis are based on the agents used as mechanical, chemical and thermal agents as shown in Flowchart 9.2.

MECHANICAL METHODS

PRESSURE

Firm pressure should be applied over the bleeding site using either fingers or gauze for at least 5 min. This would control most haemorrhages by counteracting the hydrostatic pressure of the bleeding vessel.

HAEMOSTAT

Application of haemostat at the bleeding points helps in direct occlusion of the bleeding vessel.

TABLE 9.2 Pathway of Coagulation, Activation of Plasmin, Factors of the Coagulation Cascade

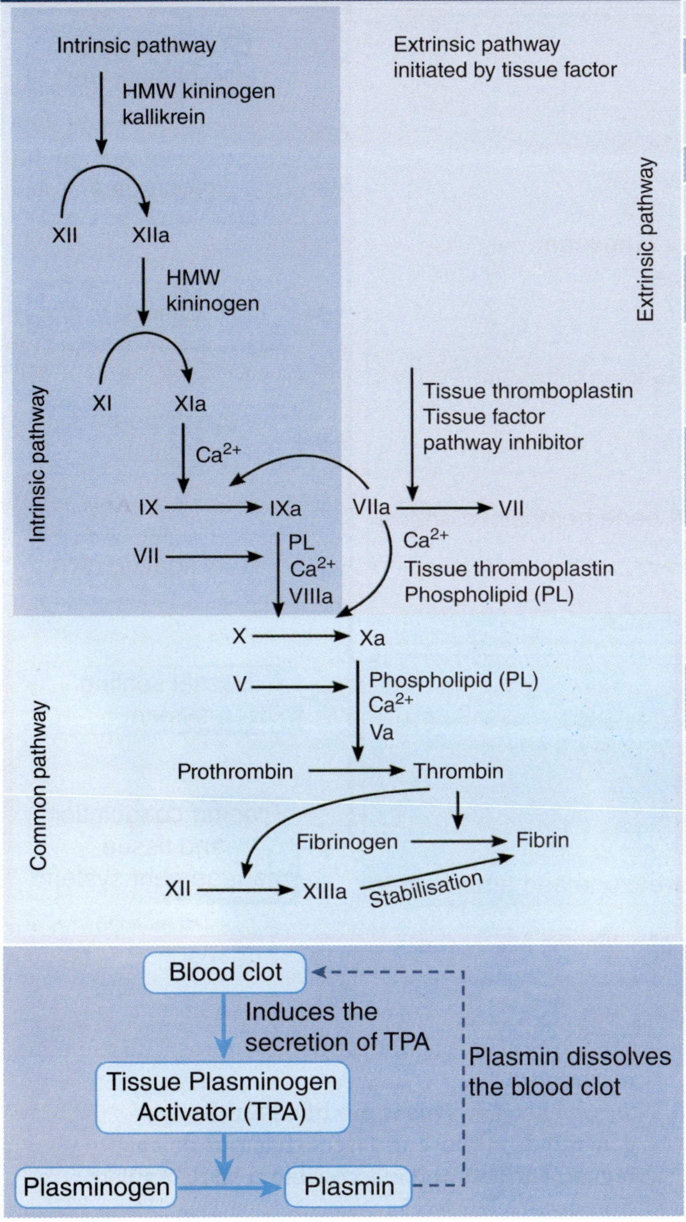

Factor	Another Name	Pathway
Factor I	Fibrinogen	Both
Factor II	Prothrombin	Both
Factor III	Tissue factor, tissue thromboplastin	Extrinsic
Factor IV	Calcium	Both
Factor V	Proaccelerin, labile factor, accelerator (Ac) globulin	Both
Factor VI (Va)	Accelerin	
Factor VII	Proconvertin, serum prothrombin conversion accelerator (SPCA)	Extrinsic
Factor VIII	Antihaemophilic factor A, platelet cofactor 1, antihaemophilic globulin (AHG)	Intrinsic
Factor IX	Christmas factor, platelet thromboplastin component (PTC), antihaemophilic factor B	Intrinsic
Factor X	Prothrombinase, Stuart–Prower factor	Both
Factor XI	Plasma thromboplastin antecedent (PTA)	Intrinsic
Factor XII	Hageman factor, contact factor, glass factor	Intrinsic
Factor XIII	Fibrin-stabilising factor (FSF), protransglutaminase, fibrinoligase, fibrinase	Both

EMBOLISATION OF THE VESSEL

The facial artery, lingual artery, internal maxillary artery and other branches of the external carotid artery can be embolised for lesions like arteriovenous malformation, epistaxis and preoperative tumor embolisation—for vascular tumors like juvenile nasopharyngeal angiofibroma, paraganglioma of the carotid body, jugular bulb, tympanic plexus and vagal nerve. This makes these tumors smaller, less vascular, easier to manipulate and remove surgically. Thus, shortening the operative time, reduce blood loss, and lower the risk of complications. The lesion is first assessed with angiography followed by embolisation with micro coils. Polyvinyl alcohol foam, gel foam, silicone spheres and methyl methacrylate through the femoral artery by catheterisation under careful mapping angiographically.

SUTURES AND LIGATION

Ligatures can be used to bind severed blood arteries. The haemostat is replaced by a ligature as a permanent means of successful haemostasis. For large pulsatile artery, a transfixation suture to prevent slipping is indicated. Nonresorbable sutures such as silk and polyethylene are used

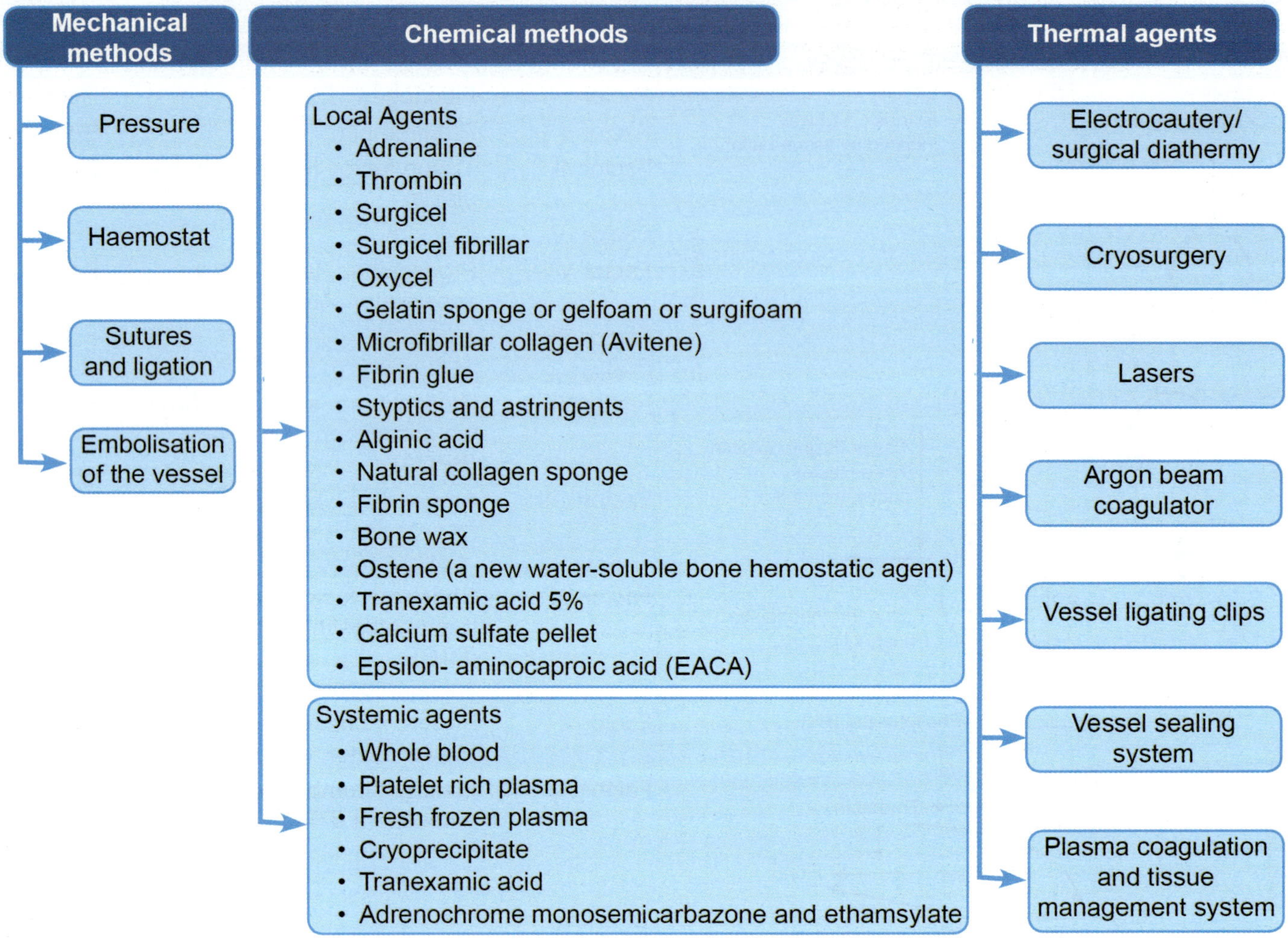

Flowchart 9.2 Various methods of achieving haemostasis.

as they evoke less tissue reaction. The arteries that are prone to haemorrhage in the head and neck region are briefly explained in Table 9.3.

CHEMICAL METHODS

LOCAL AGENTS

1. *Adrenaline:* Topical administration of adrenaline induces bleeding capillaries to constrict. Adrenaline is available in ampoule, which is applied with the help of gauze. The concentration of 1 in 10,000 is used for haemostasis over the oozing site
2. *Thrombin:* Thrombin helps in converting fibrinogen into fibrous clot and acts as haemostat
3. *Surgicel:* Surgicel was introduced in 1940 as an oxidised cellulose polymer obtained by dissolving pure alpha-cellulose in an alkaline solution (Fig. 9.2A and B). It acts by forming acid products from partial dissolution that coagulates the plasma proteins to form a black or brown sticky gelatinous clot. The applied Surgicel resorbs from the site in 4–8 weeks. However, the disadvantage is that the Surgicel clot is not formed by normal physiological mechanism
4. *Surgicel fibrillar:* This is modified Surgicel or oxidised regenerated cellulose in layers that can be adapted to irregular surfaces and inaccessible areas. Complete resorption occurs in 2 weeks
5. *Oxycel:* Oxycel is an oxidised cellulose polymer product. The controlled oxidation of cellulose with nitrous dioxide produces this absorbable haemostatic compound. The cellulosic acid (cytotoxic acid) present in Oxycel has affinity for haemoglobin, which leads to the formation of artificial clot. It should be applied on the dry surface as the acid formed during the wetting process inactivates the thrombin. The platelets plug into its meshwork-like surface and helps in clot formation. In addition, the pressure of the mass itself enhances the coagulation. It has bacteriostatic property because of its relatively low pH. At this pH, few bacterial proteins are deactivated and denatured, making the bacteria more sensitive for antibiotics. It favorably attaches to bone in

TABLE 9.3 Techniques of Haemostasis and Ligation of Arteries Encountered in the Head and Neck Regions

Artery	Anatomy and Technique of Haemostasis
Greater palatine artery	The artery exits the greater palatine foramen and runs parallel to the inner plate of the alveolar process.
	An incision parallel to the artery is made, the mucosal flaps are raised to expose the artery and clamped. Copious bleeding can be controlled with a pressure pack—a round bolus of gauze is sutures over the site for 24 h.
Sublingual artery	It is a branch of the lingual artery, and is present on the mucosal surface of the floor of the mouth. The anatomic variation is that it may be a branch of the submental artery which is a branch of the facial artery.
	As it is a small artery, local clamping and electrocautery usually controls the haemorrhage. But if that does not control the bleeding, the lingual artery is ligated. With anatomical variations, this would not suffice and ligating the facial artery would stop the bleeding.
Lingual artery ligation	It is a branch of the ECA, as it emerges close to the tip of the greater cornu of the hyoid, it lies on the middle pharyngeal constrictor muscle. The suprahyoid artery is its first branch, which branches upwards and anteriorly. It then travels deep to the hyoglossus muscle, where it gives off the dorsal lingual arteries. Then continues into the floor of the mouth, passing lateral to the genioglossus muscle. At the anterior border of the hyoglossus muscle, the lingual artery takes an upward turn and bifurcates into the deep lingual and sublingual arteries.
	A submandibular incision is made from the gonial angle to the mental region. The skin, platysma and fascia are incised, lower pole of submandibular gland is lifted upwards. The lesser triangle formed by the digastric tendon, posterior border of mylohyoid and hypoglossal nerve is identified. The hyoglossus muscle inside the triangle is separated and lingual artery is identified and ligated. Expanding haematoma from the lingual artery can obstruct airway, which can require tracheostomy.
Facial artery ligation	It is the third branch of the ECA. The artery passes just anterior to the anterior border of the masseter at the lower border of the mandible.
	It can be ligated easily through a submandibular incision 1–2 cm below the lower border of the mandible. The skin, platysma and deep fascia are incised and retracted superiorly. The artery lies anterior to the masseter muscle, it is ligated.
Internal maxillary artery (IMA) ligation	It is the terminal branch of the ECA. The IMA arises posterior to the mandibular condyle. It traverses the parotid gland and passes anteriorly between the sphenomandibular ligament and the ramus of the mandible. It runs a superficial course after this, which is lateral to the lateral pterygoid muscle.
	IMA ligation has a higher success rate than ECA ligation with three techniques Transantrally via a Caldwell-Luc approach and using operating microscope, the posterior maxillary sinus wall is removed and the internal maxillary artery and its terminal branches are elevated with nerve hooks, then ligated. The sinus wall is packed with Gelfoam, and the buccal sulcular incision is closed. The transoral approach—through a gingivobuccal incision, buccal fat pad is removed, and the coronoid process is identified. The vessel is lateral to the lateral pterygoid muscle which is medial to the coronoid process. The vessel is exposed, it is doubly clipped and divided. This procedure has a higher failure rate as the vessel is too deep to access. In transnasal endoscopic method, a large middle meatal antrostomy is made and middle turbinate is partially resected to expose the posterior sinus wall. The subsequent processes are the same as in the conventional transantral method.
Superficial temporal artery ligation	The superficial temporal artery is the smaller of two terminal branches of the ECA. It originates in the parotid gland, at the level of the condyle. It runs superiorly over the zygomatic process in front of the tragus of the auricle accompanied by the superficial temporal vein and auriculotemporal nerve. This is the clinical landmark for palpating pulse in temporal region. When in the calvaria, 3 cm superior to the zygomatic process, it gives off two branches (anterior and posterior).

Continued

TABLE 9.3 Techniques of Haemostasis and Ligation of Arteries Encountered in the Head and Neck Regions—con'td

Artery	Anatomy and Technique of Haemostasis
	The artery can be exposed by the preauricular incision (TMJ approach). The artery can be directly identified and ligated below the skin and subcutaneous tissue layers.
External carotid artery (ECA)	The ECA is a division of the common carotid artery, which is from the aortic arch on the left side and from the brachiocephalic trunk on the right side. It runs on the side of the neck within the carotid sheath, which is posterior to the sternocleidomastoid muscle.
Carotid triangle ligation of ECA	Through an incision at the level of the hyoid, the skin, platysma, superficial layer of deep fascia are incised to enter the carotid triangle. The sternocleidomastoid muscle is retracted and the carotid sheath is blunt dissected. The ECA is identified below the IJV with the pulsations. The vagus nerve below the vessels should not be disturbed. The ligatures are passed around the ECA superior to the superior thyroid artery and ligated if needed.
Retromandibular fossa ECA ligation	A retromandibular incision extending inferiorly along the anterior border of the sternocleidomastoid muscle was made. The parotid capsule's attachment to the sternomastoid's anterior edge was separated with a scalpel. Parotid gland is retracted and postbelly of digastric, stylohyoid muscle is visible, above this stylo-mandibular ligament can be palpated if lower jaw of the patient is pulled forward. This movement widens the entrance into the retromandibular fossa and tenses the stylomandibular ligament. Pulsations of ECA are felt, isolated and then ligated with silk sutures immediately after the bifurcation. To minimise collateral flow, the superior thyroid, ascending pharyngeal and lingual arteries were also ligated.

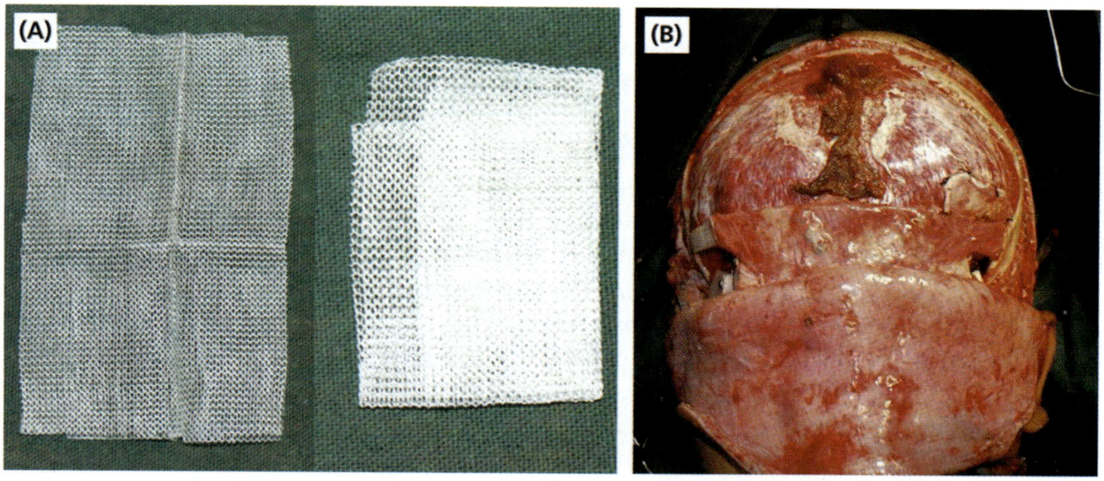

Figure 9.2 (**A**) Surgicel. (**B**) Surgicel in use for craniofacial surgery.

extraction socket with satisfactory haemostasis. It is available in gauze form or pellet form. Oxycel is composed of hollow 'twisted tubule' fibres in comparison to the irregular solid fibres of Surgicel

6. *Gelatin sponge or gelfoam or surgifoam:* Gelfoam is manufactured from purified pork skin gelatin (Fig. 9.3A). This is a nonantigenic and completely absorbable material. It has the capacity to absorb 45 times its weight in blood. It resorbs completely in 4–6 weeks
7. *Microfibrillar collagen (Avitene):* Collagen derived from bovine skin causes contact activation in addition to direct platelet aggregation. In spite of its advantage of causing minimal swelling, it tends to reduce platelet count in normal individuals and ineffective in thrombocytopenia. Its absorption time is 3 months
8. *Fibrin glue:* It is a biological adhesive which contains thrombin, fibrinogen, factor VII, aprotinin
9. *Styptics and astringents:* Precipitates protein and arrests bleeding. Commonly used styptics and astringents are Monsel's solution containing ferric subsulphate and tannic acid. Thrombin and gelatin sponge are now widely used
10. *Alginic acid:* This is available in powder form in special 5-mg packages. It is placed over the bleeding sites, a protective film is formed over the bleeding site, this film compresses the capillaries and stabilises the blood clot in place

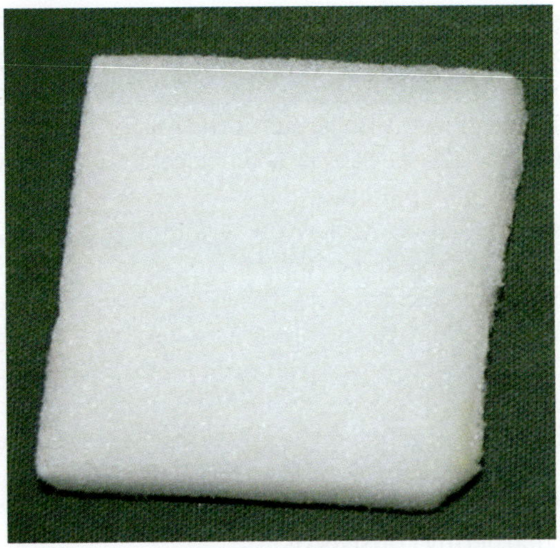

Figure 9.3 Gelfoam.

11. *Natural collagen sponge:* This is a white sponge material, nonantigenic and fully absorbable. It promotes platelet aggregation, which improves haemostasis. It activates coagulation factors XI and XIII. It is preferred in patients who are susceptible for haemorrhage after dental surgical procedures
12. *Fibrin sponge:* The fibrin sponge is nonantigenic and is obtained from bovine material. It is chemically treated to avoid allergic reactions. It is applied on the bleeding site especially in postextraction socket. It stimulates coagulation thereby forming a normal clot; it also acts as a temporary plug over the small injured blood vessels. The fibrin sponge is fully absorbed by the tissues within 4–6 weeks
13. *Bone wax:* Bone wax is a sterilised, nonabsorbable mix of waxes. Bone wax consists of seven parts by weight of wax (white bees wax, paraffin wax and an isopropyl ester of palmitic acid), two parts of olive oil and one part of phenol. It is white and available as a solid rectangular plate weighing 2.5 g. It is indicated in cases of bleeding from the bone or from chipped edges of bone. The bone wax is softened with the fingers to a desirable consistency and then applied over the bleeding site. Its haemostatic mechanism is through mechanical obstruction of the osseous cavity containing the bleeding vessels. Frequent use may lead to the formation of wax granuloma (foreign body)
14. *Ostene (a new water-soluble bone haemostatic agent):* Earlier, the formulations containing naturally obtained bees wax were used as bone wax which interfered with the normal healing process and caused inflammatory reactions. Ostene is a new bone haemostatic agent, made of water-soluble alkylene oxide copolymers. Ostene showed no incidence of adverse response in the cortical defect site, medullary cavity or the surrounding tissue. With the use of the conventional bone wax, foreign body response including fibrous tissue infiltration by macrophages, giant cells and lymphocytes at the sites of the bone defects are not uncommon. Further bone wax also displaced the bone marrow and interfered with bone ingrowth into the defects. Ostene, a water-soluble bone haemostatic agent has shown no adverse tissue response or the interference with bone healing as seen with the use of bone wax
15. *Tranexamic acid 5%:* Used to prevent excessive blood loss from major trauma, surgery, extraction of tooth, postpartum bleeding. It is an antifibrinolytic. It helps in clotting of blood
    It decreases blood flow during menstruation and is used to control bleeding in pregnancy
    Side effects caused by tranexamic acid are nausea, diarrhea, vomiting, fever, chills, etc.
    Adult dosage for bleeding:
    Initial dose: 10 mg/kg i.v., immediately before dental extraction
    Maintenance dose: 10 mg/kg i.v. 3–4 times daily
    Duration of therapy: 2–8 days
    In haemophilia patient, it is used for short term in order to prevent haemorrhage and also to reduce the requirement for replacement therapy during and following a tooth extraction
16. *Calcium sulphate pellet:* The pellets mechanically block the open vessels in bone, used in osteotomies larger than 7–10 mm. It is a bone inductive agent and resorbs in 3 weeks
17. *Epsilon-aminocaproic acid (EACA).*

SYSTEMIC AGENTS

1. Whole blood
2. Platelet rich plasma
3. Fresh frozen plasma
4. Cryoprecipitate
5. Tranexamic acid
6. Adrenochrome monosemicarbazone and ethamsylate.

THERMAL AGENTS

Surgical cutting instruments have been modified using thermal agents in order to achieve haemostasis during surgery. Delivery of heat or cold during the cutting can be done by electric current (electrocautery), laser beam (like argon), liquid nitrogen (cryosurgery), radio frequency energy, etc. These thermal agents coagulate and seal the blood vessels as they cut achieving haemostasis and a bloodless field during surgery. These instruments are also useful in the surgery of vascular lesions like haemangiomas that can potentially cause life-threatening intraoperative bleeding.

ELECTROCAUTERY/SURGICAL DIATHERMY

Electrocautery is a surgical technique that depends on thermal effect of electric current. In electrocautery/surgical diathermy, a high-frequency current is applied to a specific area of the body for the purpose of removal of unwanted tissue, coagulation or to create a surgical incision. The frequency of current used in surgical diathermy units are in the range of 1–3 MHz. Electrocautery is cleaner, safer and more efficient than many of the alternatives. The instrument used to perform this procedure is also known as an electrocautery.

Properties of surgical diathermy

Diathermy uses high-frequency electrical current to produce coagulation.

It can also be used to cut as well as cauterise tissue. Electrical frequency used by diathermy is in the range of 300 kHz to 3 MHz.

In this procedure, the electro conductivity of the human body is used and the patient's body forms part of the electrical circuit, the electric current used usually has no effect on muscles.

Types of diathermy

- Monopolar
- Bipolar

Monopolar diathermy

Monopolar diathermy consists of (Fig. 9.4):

a. *High-frequency AC generator (over 20,000 Hz)*—generates alternating current at a very high frequency
b. *Regulator*—controls the current generated by the AC
c. *Foot control*—the passage of current is controlled by the foot control
d. *Active electrode*—it is the tip of the instrument
e. *Indifferent electrode*—it is a flat electrical plate which is placed on the patient.

When the foot control is pressed, the current passes between the instrument tip (active electrode) and indifferent electrode. As the surface area of the instrument tip is less than that of the indifferent electrode (the electrical plate), high-current density is produced around the active electrode, which results in localised heating around the tip of the instrument and minimal heating is produced at the indifferent electrode.

Bipolar diathermy

Bipolar diathermy consists of:

i. Low power AC generator
ii. Foot control
iii. Two electrodes combined in an instrument (e.g. forceps).

When the foot control is pressed, a low power AC is generated and passes through the two tips of the same instrument. When the tips are brought together, a circuit is created producing a localised current. As the current produced is of small power, the instrument is used only for coagulation and not for cutting.

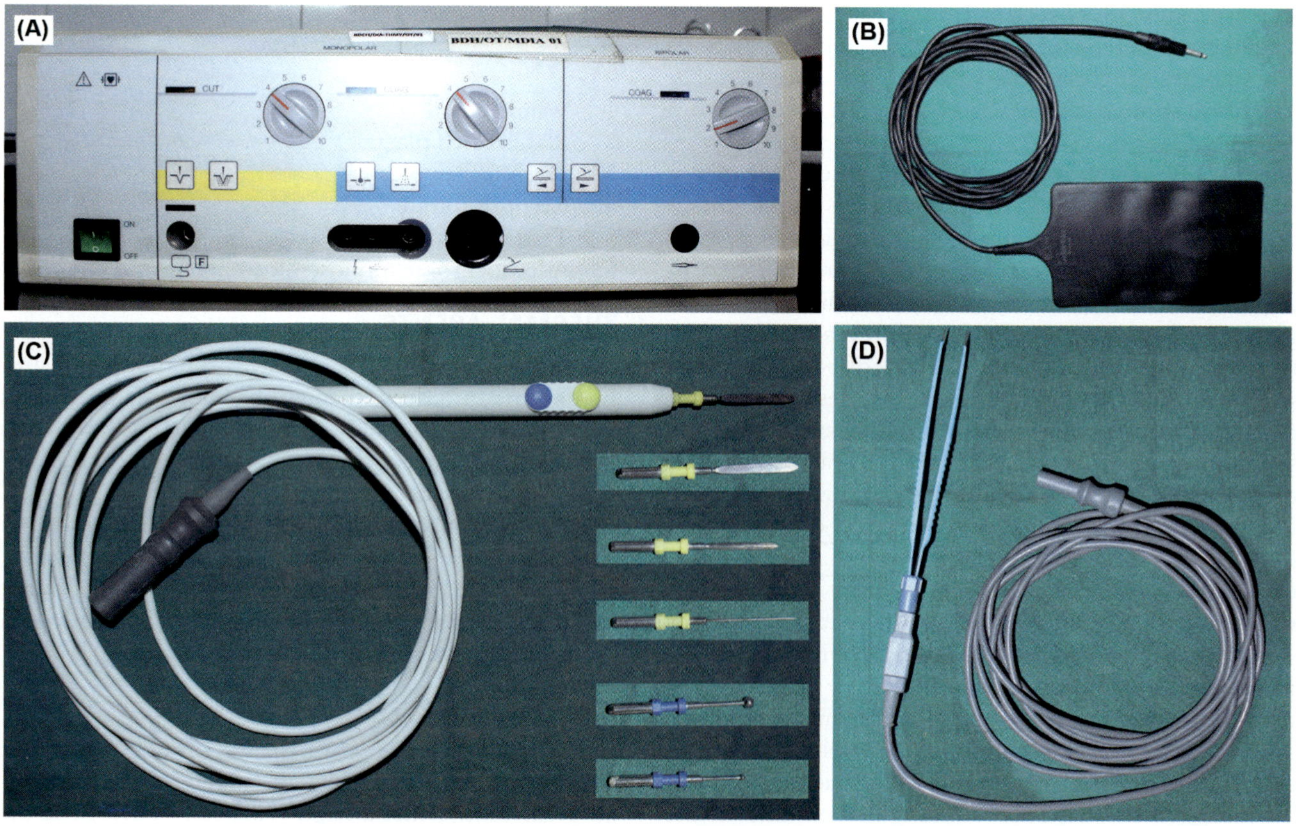

Figure 9.4 **(A)** Diathermy equipment. **(B)** Diathermy indifferent electrode. **(C)** Monopolar diathermy tips (active electrode). **(D)** Bipolar diathermy tip.

Advantages

Diathermy reduces the risk of spark ignition of the anaesthetic gases. The effect produced by the diathermy depends upon the current intensity and waveform used. By changing the intensity of the current, various functions are possible.
Coagulation—small bleeding vessels and capillaries can be coagulated with the help of this instrument.
Cutting—soft tissues with diffuse capillary network can be incised using diathermy.
Fulguration—destruction of tissue using an electric current is known as fulguration. Small growths like papilloma, leukoplakia, etc. can be removed using diathermy.

Risk and caution

- Can interfere with pacemaker function
- Arcing can occur when the tip contacts other metal instruments or implants
- Superficial burns can occur in spirit-based skin preparation
- Diathermy burns can occur under indifferent electrode if plate is improperly applied
- The indifferent electrode should not be placed near bony ridges
- The operator should use rubber footwear so as to avoid accidental burn
- Should not be used near isolated vascular pedicles or nerves.

CRYOSURGERY

Cryosurgery is the process of rapidly freezing tissue by exposing it to intensely low temperatures. Usually a probe containing liquid nitrogen is used. While it is not an ideal coagulating method, cryosurgery does minimise the extent of blood loss in extensive ablative surgeries.

Effects of rapid freezing

- Increased concentration of intracellular solutes
- Reduction in intracellular water
- Cell shrinkage
- Cell membrane damage
- Formation of intracellular ice crystals
- Formation of extracellular ice crystals.

Technique of application

1. Spray technique
2. Probe technique
3. Forceps technique.

General clinical uses

- Solar keratoses
- Seborrheic keratoses
- Viral warts
- Skin tags
- Xanthelasmas
- Lentiginous macules
- Actinic cheilitis
- Erosive lichen planus.

There are also reports of successful treatment of basal cell carcinoma of skin, tongue carcinoma and other aggressive jaw lesions.

Cryosurgery is not useful in controlling active bleeding. Since the properties of lasers were more beneficial and user friendly, laser has replaced cryosurgery in many surgical applications.

Apparatus

The apparatus consists of a container in which the pressurised refrigerant media (gases) are stored as liquid gases. The refrigerant media generally used are liquid nitrogen at a temperature of –196 °C. Other refrigerants are carbon dioxide, nitrous oxide and freon, which may reach a temperature of –20°C to –90°C. A probe is connected to the container through a tube. This probe is applied on the region of the abnormal tissue. The time required for destruction of the tissue by the probe depends upon the temperature reached, size of the lesion and type of the tissue. Freezing and thawing are done alternatively as many times as necessary for the lesion. This process destroys the tissues.

Disadvantages

1. Delayed bleeding
2. Paraesthesia
3. Neuropathy
4. Nitrogen gas insufflation (nitrogen gas bubbles in skin)
5. Alopecia
6. Cartilage necrosis.

Lasers

Laser helps in coagulating small blood vessels. Refer to Chapter 57 for further reading.

SHOCK

Shock is a clinical condition characterised by inadequate tissue perfusion and hence cellular hypoxia.

CLASSIFICATION

Shock can be classified based on the aetiology as:

1. Hypovolaemic shock
2. Vasogenic shock
   a. Anaphylactic shock
   b. Hypoadrenal shock
   c. Systemic inflammatory response syndrome
   d. Traumatic shock
3. Cardiogenic shock
4. Septic shock
5. Neurogenic shock.

PATHOGENESIS

Obstruction in the cycle of oxygen delivery to the cell due to failure or malfunction in any system results in cellular hypoxia leading to vicious cycles that result in shock. The basic pathology in all forms of shock is impairment of microcirculation and deranged cell metabolism.

HYPOVOLAEMIC SHOCK

ENDOGENOUS COMPENSATORY MECHANISMS

Mild to moderate hypovolaemia is usually compensated by endogenous mechanisms. They aim to restore circulating blood volume and adequate blood pressure for vital organ perfusion. When there is severe hypovolaemia, these endogenous mechanisms fail leading to a state called hypovolaemic shock that leads to multiorgan failure (Flowchart 9.3).

CLASSIFICATION OF RESPONSE TO HYPOVOLAEMIA

1. Class I: Up to 15% (750 mL)
   a. Physiological response—BP, Pulse rate, Respiratory rate, Tissue perfusion, Mild tachycardia are all normally compensated by body
2. Class II: 15%–30% (800–1500 mL)
   a. Physiological response–Tachycardia, Tachypnoea, ↑ Diastolic BP [← Peripheral vascular constriction ← catecholamines ← hypovolaemia], ↑ Pulse pressure, ↑ Capillary refill time and skin is cold and moist
3. Class III: 30%–40% (1500–2000 mL)
   a. Detrimental to survival of vital organs
   b. Classic signs of inadequate tissue perfusion
      i. Marked tachycardia (120–140 beats/min)
      ii. Tachypnoea
      iii. ↓ Systolic BP
      iv. Marked vasoconstriction
      v. Diaphoresis
      vi. Anxiety
      vii. Restlessness
      viii. ↓ Urinary output
4. Class IV: >40% Immediate life-threatening situation
   a. Marked tachycardia
   b. ↓ Systolic BP <60 mmHg
   c. Very narrow pulse pressure
   d. Marked diaphoresis
   e. Obtunded mental state
   f. No urinary output.

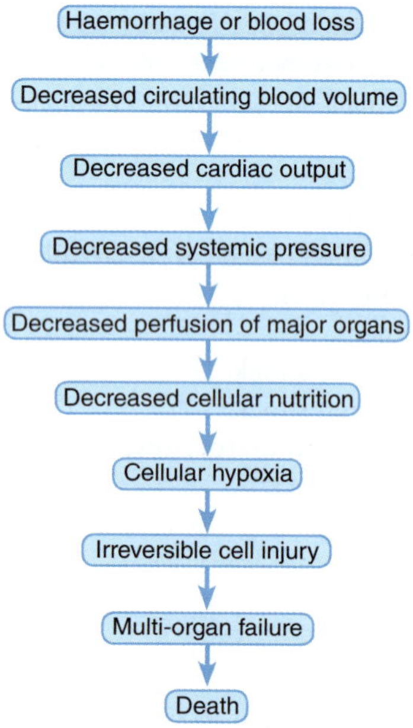

Flowchart 9.3 The chain of reactions that lead to hypovolaemic shock.

Microcirculation

Peripheral vasoconstriction occurs during hypovolaemia, leading to redirection of major volume of blood to the essential organs. This maintains the critical blood pressure for tissue perfusion in the vital organs like kidney, brain and heart at the expense of gastrointestinal tract and skin. This mechanism fails when systolic blood pressure drops to the critical level of less than 60 mmHg.

Neuroendocrine mechanism

Hypovolaemia- and hypotension-induced hypoxia detected by chemoreceptors and baroreceptors induce an autonomic response. This is characterised by decreased vagal activity and decreased adrenergic activity, resulting in compensatory tachycardia and thus increased cardiac output. In addition, epinephrine and ACTH induced cortisol secretion increases glycogenolysis, gluconeogenesis with decreased peripheral glucose uptake.

Renal mechanism

The kidney helps to maintain circulatory blood volume by renal shut down or acute renal failure, a complication of hypovolaemic shock. This mechanism aims to conserve body electrolytes and water.

MANAGEMENT OF HYPOVOLAEMIC SHOCK

1. Monitoring of vitals: Pulse, blood pressure (both arterial and venous)
2. Assessment of state of shock by haemodynamic parameters such as cardiac output, oxygen saturation, etc.
3. Attempt to restore circulating blood volume immediately through intravenous fluid administration (Flowchart 9.4)
4. Identify the cause of blood loss and treat the cause.

CARDIOGENIC SHOCK

Cardiogenic shock is the result of diminished myocardial contractility, which results in inadequate cardiac output, decreased oxygen delivery and decreased tissue perfusion.

HAEMODYNAMICALLY

- Persistent hypotension—systolic blood pressure <90 mmHg or mean arterial pressure is less <60 mg
- Increased peripheral vascular resistance with reduction in cardiac output—cardiac index (<2.0 L/min/m^2)
- Increased pulmonary artery wedge pressure (18 mmHg).

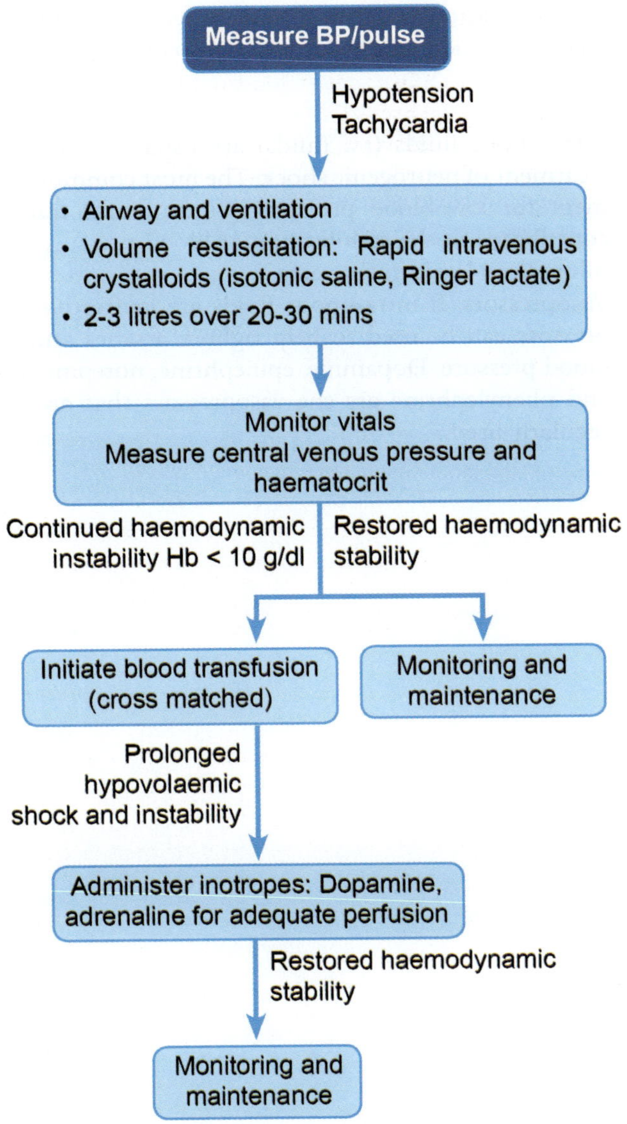

Flowchart 9.4 Management of hypovolaemic shock.

SYMPTOMS

Chest pain, heavy perspiration, coma, dizziness, restlessness, tachypnea and shortness of breath are all possible symptoms.

DIAGNOSIS

In most cases, cardiogenic shock is discovered in an emergency room environment. The tests that may be administered are:

1. Measurement and monitoring of blood pressure (Extremely low blood pressure levels)
2. Chest X-ray
3. Angiogram—cardiac catheterisation: This examination can indicate arteries that are obstructed or constricted. A long thin tube (catheter) is sent through the femoral or radial artery. Dye is injected into the catheter and imaging is performed
4. Coronary angiography
5. Echocardiogram
6. Electrocardiogram (ECG or EKG): Using electrodes linked to the skin, this rapid, noninvasive test monitors the electrical activity. Shows abnormal electrical signals in case of cardiac injury or fluid build-up around the heart (pericardial effusion).

TREATMENT

Emergency medical therapy may involve the administration of enriched oxygen through a tube or mask, breathing assistance (ventilator), intravenous (i.v.) fluids and drugs to raise blood pressure or improve cardiac performance. A number of medications, including dopamine, epinephrine, dobutamine and norepinephrine, are used to treat the condition.

SEPTIC SHOCK

Septic shock is a terrible condition that develops as a result of sepsis and it is a severe consequence. In addition, it is connected with a high mortality rate. Septic shock is most typically caused by Gram-negative bacteria, but it can also be caused by fungi, viruses and parasites. Paediatric patients, immunocompromised persons and the elderly are the most frequently affected by septic shock.

Changes in mental status, arterial hypotension (mean arterial pressure less than 60 mmHg or systolic blood pressure less than 90 mmHg), changes in organ perfusion and other indications of organ failure are all signs and symptoms of organ failure.

SYMPTOMS

Low blood pressure, chills, decreased mental status, lightheadedness, palpitations, tachycardia, tachypnea, breath shortness, restlessness, agitation, confusion.

PATHOGENESIS

Major factors contributing to the pathophysiology include:

- Inflammatory mediators
- Endothelial activation and injury
- Induction of procoagulant state
- Metabolic abnormalities
- Organ dysfunction
- Immune suppression.

MANAGEMENT

1) Antibiotic therapy and control of infection
2) Effective and early volume replacement
3) Adequate oxygen supply to cells
4) Restoration of tissue perfusion.

In minor cases, simply administering fluids is sufficient to restore haemodynamic stability. In contrast, in the vast majority of cases, the use of vasopressors is required to raise arterial pressure. It is necessary to choose between dopamine and noradrenaline. Dopamine is the drug of choice because it aids in the preservation of mesenteric and renal circulation, as well as the preservation of organ blood flow and oxygenation. It is recommended that noradrenaline be added to the regimen if hypotension persists even after dopamine administration.

NEUROGENIC SHOCK

Neurogenic shock is caused due to a loss of vasomotor tone and a decrease of sympathetic tone, along with unopposed parasympathetic control and eventual development of cardiovascular instability. The most prevalent reason for this is an acute spinal injury. Hypotension, bradycardia and autonomic dysfunction are the hallmarks of this condition.

SYMPTOMS

The following symptoms of neurogenic shock are present: hypotension, bradycardia, pale skin, nausea, tachycardia, heavy perspiration, dizziness, anxiety, visual disturbance, pupillary dilatation and hyperpnea (hyperventilation).

TREATMENT

- Intravenous fluids (i.v. fluids) are usually used in the treatment of neurogenic shock. The most common treatment for low blood pressure is intravenous fluids. It contributes to the stabilisation of blood pressure by refilling fluid levels in the veins.
- Vasopressors: If intravenous fluids are ineffective, vasopressors can be used to help tighten arteries and raise blood pressure. Dopamine, epinephrine, norepinephrine and phenylephrine are the vasopressors that are most regularly used.

Chapter 10

Therapeutics in Oral Surgery

OUTLINE

INTRODUCTION

Drugs are of utmost significance in the control of infections, pain and postoperative consequences. With trends towards increasing outpatient care, an increasing number of medically compromised patients can be expected to be seen in a typical dental clinic. The mechanism of action and potential interactions of various commonly used drugs are important to the clinician treating the medically compromised patient to provide optimal care and prevent iatrogenic damages.

ANTIBIOTICS

Antibiotics are chemical substances, which either kill or inhibit the growth of microorganisms. One of the most difficult problems to manage in dentistry is an odontogenic infection. These infections may range from low-grade, well-localised infections requiring minimal treatment to a severe, life-threatening facial space infection. Antibiotics are used for three reasons in dentistry:

- To treat infections of the oral cavity
- As preoperative prophylaxis to prevent bacterial endocarditis and other systemic complications in susceptible patients due to bacteraemia caused by dental procedures
- To prevent postoperative infections and improve healing at the operative site.

CLASSIFICATION OF ANTIBIOTICS

Antibiotics are classified on the basis of chemical structure, effect, type of organism and spectrum of activity (Table 10.1). Antibiotic administration regimens for oral infection is described in Table 10.2.

CONSIDERATION BEFORE ADMINISTRATION OF ANTIBIOTICS

Antibiotic efficacy, toxicity, cost, dosage, method of administration, duration of antibiotic treatment and usage of combination therapy are some factors to consider.

Aetiology of the underlying disease

The underlying aetiology of the disease should be confirmed as being microbial.

Culture sensitivity

Whenever possible, the pus, blood, saliva, urine or other secretions should be collected for the microorganism culture and should be tested against different antibiotics for maximum sensitivity.

Efficiency

If the drug can reach the site of infection and be active against the pathogenic organisms, it has good efficacy.

Toxicity

This relates to idiosyncratic reactions and dose-dependent organ damage. The antibiotics should maintain broad effect of antimicrobial action with minimal risk to the patient.

Age of the patient

Certain drugs are not recommended for infants like chloramphenicol, which can cause *'grey baby syndrome'*.

Pregnancy

Certain drugs are considered to be teratogenic and should not be administered in pregnant women.

TABLE 10.1 Classification of Antibiotics

On the basis of the chemical structure	
• Sulphonamides • β-lactam antibiotics • Aminoglycosides • Imidazole derivatives • Polypeptide antibiotics • Diaminopyrimidines	• Quinolones • Tetracyclines • Macrolides • Polyene antibiotics • Nitrobenzene derivatives
On the basis of effect	
• *Bacteriostatic:* Tetracyclines, chloramphenicol, erythromycin, ethambutol, sulphonamides • *Bactericidal:* Penicillins, aminoglycosides, ciprofloxacin, rifampin, cotrimoxazole, polypeptides, cephalosporins, vancomycin, nalidixic acid	
On the basis of action against the type of organism	
• Antibacterial • Antiviral • Antihelmintic	• Antifungal • Antiprotozoal
On the basis of spectrum of activity	
• *Narrow-spectrum:* Penicillin, erythromycin, streptomycin • *Broad-spectrum:* Tetracyclines, chloramphenicol	
On the basis of origin	
• *From fungi:* Cephalosporin, griseofulvin, penicillin • *From bacteria:* Bacitracin, polymyxin B, colistin • *From actinomycetes:* Aminoglycosides, tetracyclines, chloramphenicol, macrolides, polyenes	
Mechanisms of action	
• *Inhibition of cell wall synthesis:* Penicillins, cephalosporins, bacitracin, vancomycin • *Destruction of cell membrane:* Colistin, bacitracin, amphotericin, polymyxins • *Inhibition of protein synthesis:* Chloramphenicol, erythromycin, clindamycin, tetracyclines • *Interfere with DNA functioning:* Rifampicin, metronidazole • *Interfere with DNA synthesis:* Acyclovir, zidovudine • *Interfere with DNA gyrase:* Ciprofloxacin • *Interfere with RNA functioning:* Streptomycin, gentamycin • *Antimetabolite:* Sulphonamides, ethambutol, trimethoprim, pyrimethamine	

Drug resistance

Drug resistance refers to the emergence of resistant strains of bacteria. It results most commonly due to mutation. These resistant strains survive in spite of the antibiotic therapy.

Drug allergy

If the patient gives a history of allergy to any particular drug, an alternative should be considered.

Agents that inhibit cell wall synthesis

Antibiotics require growing cells (cells synthesising new cell wall material) to exert a bactericidal effect. Likewise, if little growth is occurring, a bacteriostatic agent has little to no effect (e.g. penicillins and cephalosporins).

Cost

This involves price of the agent, frequency of the doses and duration of treatment. Newer drugs may be available in the market, which may be more costly but not necessarily more effective.

Dosages

This should maintain serum levels within wide or narrow margins between therapeutic and toxic levels. Usually, drugs with narrow margins of safety are calculated on the basis of the patient's condition and severity of the infection. Oral therapy is indicated for low to moderate grade infections, whereas parenteral therapy should be considered in compromised patients or in more serious infections as blood serum and tissue levels are achieved more rapidly. Duration

TABLE 10.2 Antibiotic Administration Regimens for Oral Infections

Antibiotic	Route	Mechanism	Dosage and Frequency	Indication
Aminoglycosides Gentamicin	i.m. or i.v.	Bactericidal	3 mg/kg/day in equal doses q 8 h	Component of bacterial endocarditis prophylaxis for patients at high risk
Cephalosporins Cefaclor	PO	Bactericidal	250–500 mg q 8 h	Useful when broader spectrum is needed
Cefadroxil			500 mg to 1 g q 12 to 24 h	
Cephalexin	PO		250–500 mg q 6 h	
Pencillin G	i.m. or i.v.	Bactericidal	600,000–120,000 units q 12–24 h	Drug of choice for most infections
Penicillin V	PO		500 mg initially, then 250–500 mg q 6 h	Drug of choice for most infections
Amoxicillin			1 g initially, then 250–500 mg q 6 h	Bacterial endocarditis prophylaxis
Cloxacillin	PO		25–500 mg q 6 h	Staphylococcus infection
Dicloxacillin	PO		125–250 mg q 6 h	Drug of choice of serious infections
Erythromycin	PO	Bacteriostatic	250–500 mg q 6 h	Useful for mild infection and bacterial endocarditis prophylaxis if patient is penicillin allergic
Azithromycin	PO		10 mg/kg up to 500 mg initially followed by 5 mg/kg up to 250 mg qd to complete 5 days	
Clarithromycin	PO		250–500 mg PO b.i.d. Peds: 7.5 mg/kg PO b.i.d	
Doxycycline	PO	Bacteriostatic	Initially 100 mg q 24 h or 50 mg q 12 h	Mild infections when need broad-spectrum, periodontal disease
Oxytetracycline	i.m.		250 mg q 24 h	
Tetracycline	PO		500 mg q 6 h	
Clindamycin	i.v. or PO	Bactericidal and bacteriostatic	150 mg q 6 h	Instead of metronidazole for penicillin-allergic patients with serious infections or endocarditis prophylaxis if cannot use penicillin or erythromycin
Metronidazole	i.v. or PO	Bactericidal	500 mg q 6 h	Second line of therapy for odontogenic infections, ANUG, HIV periodontitis
Vancomycin	i.v.	Bactericidal	1 g infused over 1 h before procedure	Component of bacterial endocarditis prophylaxis for patients at high risk

of treatment is dependent on type and severity of infection, organism sensitivity, patient's clinical improvement and is typically continued for 5–14 days.

COMBINATION THERAPY

This is usually indicated for more severe life-threatening infections to achieve appropriate antibiotic therapy. The advantage of multiple antibiotic therapy results from the synergistic nature among antibiotics. Combinations of antibiotics are indicated in infections caused by Pseudomonas, enterococcal group D streptococci, resistant pathogens and life-threatening infections.

Advantages

- It helps in achieving additive synergistic activity of the antibiotics

- Due to synergistic combination, the doses of individual drugs are reduced, which in turn reduces adverse effects of the individual drug
- It reduces the development of drug resistance
- It widens the spectrum of activity of the drugs and hence can be used against many mixed infections and in other infections where the bacterial diagnosis is unknown.

Disadvantages

- Increased cost of therapy
- Increased risk of adverse effects when both the drugs have adverse effects
- Increased risk of super infection by the resistant organisms.
- Alteration of the normal flora.

FACTORS INVOLVED IN THERAPEUTIC EFFECTIVENESS

Incision and drainage of abscesses

- The avascular nature of the abscess hinders the distribution of an antibiotic to the centre of the infectious foci
- Abscesses are usually caused by anaerobic bacteria, which grow slowly and produce an infection that is difficult to treat
- Proper incision and drainage helps in removing a number of causative bacteria; it allows the killing of strict anaerobes by exposure to oxygen.

Age and extent of infection

Chronic and well-established abscess consists mainly of a large number of slowly growing bacteria against which both bactericidal and bacteriostatic agents may be relatively ineffective. A higher concentration of antibiotic may be required for an infection with a large number of bacteria.

Bactericidal versus bacteriostatic antibiotics

In a patient with impaired immune function, a bactericidal antibiotic is preferable to a bacteriostatic agent. By killing the bacteria, less reliance is placed on host defence processes, which are ultimately responsible for the eradication of the infection.

Antibacterial spectrum

Narrow-spectrum antibiotics are preferred if the antibacterial activity includes the aetiologic agents because: (1) they are often more effective when compared to broad-spectrum agents against a specific group of microorganisms and (2) the likelihood of superinfection is reduced as they have less effect on the normal microflora.

Route of administration and timing of dosage

Most antibiotics are given orally and usually on an empty stomach to prevent destruction by gastric acidity.

Dosage regimen

Adequate concentration of the antibiotic must be attained at the infection site as inadequate concentration leads to destruction of less-susceptible bacteria and the development of a resistant infection. An average of 5–7 days of therapy is required; however, with severe infections or lowered host resistance, a longer duration may be required.

Distribution of antibiotic in the body

In order to be effective, an antibiotic must gain access to the infected site, whether it is in bone, soft tissue or an area with a poor blood supply. Most antibiotics gain ready access to oral soft tissues.

Metabolism and excretion of antibiotics

When choosing an antibiotic, the dentist should have a thorough knowledge of the patient's medical history, such as in case of a renal insufficiency, avoid a drug that is excreted by the kidney or at least mandate a reduction in dosage.

Patient factors (pregnancy) (Tables 10.3–10.4)

The use of antimicrobial agents during pregnancy is associated with varying degrees of risk; utmost care is required when antibiotic administration is contemplated, especially during the first trimester:

- Streptomycin, one of the first drugs to be linked to fetotoxicity, has been associated with damage to the cranial nerve VIII and skeletal defects
- Tetracyclines used during the last trimester of pregnancy cause hypoplasia of teeth and bones of the foetus and have been associated with the occurrence of congenital cataracts
- Maternal hepatic toxicity can be caused with tetracycline use during pregnancy
- Other antibiotics like sulphonamides and chloramphenicol cross the placenta and are contraindicated
- Some antibiotics are secreted into milk and may present problems for the nursing infant.

PENICILLIN

Penicillin remains the first-choice antibiotic for the initial treatment of most acute odontogenic infections. Penicillin compounds may be divided into two groups:

i. Natural penicillins
ii. Semisynthetic penicillins.

Naturally occurring penicillins

Penicillin G and Penicillin V are the most commonly used.

Semisynthetic penicillins

These penicillins are produced by chemically combining specific side chains or by incorporating specific precursors in the mould cultures.

TABLE 10.3 Drugs Usage in the Pregnant Patient

Drugs	Safe to use in the pregnant patient	Minimal foetal risk—possibly safe to use, but no accurate studies are available	Evidence of foetal risk—should not use	Drugs to avoid in pregnancy—Significant foetal risk
Analgesics	Acetaminophen	Fentanyl Hydrocodone Ibuprofen Meperidine Naproxen Oxycodone	Aspirin Codeine Propoxyphene	
Antimicrobials	Amoxicillin Amoxicillin-clavulanic acid Ampicillin Ampicillin-sulbactam Cefazolin Cephalexin Erythromycin Nystatin Penicillin	Acyclovir Azithromycin Clarithromycin Clindamycin Vancomycin		Ciprofloxacin Doxycycline Tetracycline
Anti-inflammatory		Ibuprofen Naproxen	Glucocorticoids	

TABLE 10.4 Drugs to avoid in the Nursing Mother

Drug	Effect on Nursing Infant
Metronidazole	Potential for tumourigenicity Nursing may be resumed 48 h after drug has been stopped
Antihistamines	Antihistamine sensitivity is higher in newborns and infants
Benzodiazepines	These drugs can cause sedation in infants

Oxacillin and methicillin have relatively narrow ranges of antibacterial activity but are effective against Staphylococci resistant to the other types of penicillin. Now strains resistant to methicillin (MRSA—methicillin-resistant *Staphylococcus aureus*) and Vancomycin (VRSA—vancomycin-resistant *S. aureus*) are being treated by Linezolid, quinupristin/dalfopristin and daptomycin.

PENICILLIN V

Spectrum

The antibacterial spectrum of penicillin V includes:

- Gram-positive cocci (streptococci, some nonresistant staphylococci and pneumococci)
- Gram-positive rods (*Bacillus*, *Corynebacterium*, *Clostridium* and other genera)
- Most oral anaerobes such as *Bacteroides, Porphyromonas, Prevotella, peptococci, peptostreptococci, Actinomyces, Veillonella, Eubacterium, Eikenella, Capnocytophaga, Campylobacter, Fusobacterium* and others
- Penicillin V is also effective against *Treponema pallidum* and some other spirochetes.

Many of the microorganisms listed above are involved in odontogenic infections. The semisynthetic compounds are effective against many strains of penicillinase-producing staphylococci and their use generally should be confined to this area.

Action

They are bactericidal in action. They are effective only against organisms that are actively reproducing.

Dosage

The average adult dosage is 600,000 to 1200,000 units daily. When necessary, much larger doses may be given with little danger of toxicity. The average adult dosage of phenoxymethyl penicillin (penicillin V) is 125–250 mg, four times daily. This dosage also applies to the semisynthetic penicillins.

Administration

Penicillin may be administered orally, intramuscularly or intravenously. Adequate blood levels can be achieved with penicillin V via the oral route. For most patients who are not critically ill, this is probably the most desirable method of administration.

Precautions

Penicillin is the antibiotic most frequently involved in untoward reactions.

1. Avoid penicillins in patients with a history of allergy or one who has reacted unfavourably to the drug. Patients with a history of asthma, hay fever or other allergy are more prone to have a sensitivity reaction to penicillin. Patients may have cross-sensitivity to penicillin
2. Injectable penicillinase may be used to neutralise penicillin. This must be used with care, since some severe allergic responses have been reported to penicillinase itself. Theoretically, penicillinase will have no neutralising effect on the semisynthetic penicillin compounds.

Adverse effects

These include allergic reactions and gastrointestinal disturbances. Patients allergic to one penicillin derivative should be considered allergic to all derivatives unless proven otherwise.

AMOXICILLIN

- It is a semisynthetic penicillin, effective against Gram-negative bacteria as well as Gram-positive bacteria and most oral anaerobes
- It is slightly less active than penicillin V against Gram-positive cocci, except enterococci for which it is more active
- Amoxicillin has been shown to be active in vitro against *Actinobacillus actinomycetemcomitans*
- Its broader spectrum has advantages in those situations where extended-spectrum penicillin is important
- Amoxicillin yields effective concentration that are higher than equivalent dose of penicillin V because of its better oral absorption and lower binding to plasma protein (20% for amoxicillin vs 80% for penicillin V)
- Amoxicillin, in fact, would be the drug of choice for treatment of orodental infection
- It has greater potential to produce superinfection of the gastrointestinal tract and vagina (because of its broader spectrum of activity against Gram-negative aerobes) and its tendency to produce skin rash (9%), a possible consequence of allergic reactions to the 6-amino side chain of amoxicillin
- Amoxicillin is currently indicated for the treatment of mixed Gram-positive and Gram-negative aerobic infections (e.g. some periodontal infections)
- It may also be useful in treating early onset periodontitis and refractory periodontitis. Amoxicillin may retain clinical efficacy against infections involving streptococci or other species resistant to penicillin V by a mechanism other than beta-lactamase production.

Dosage

500 mg 8 hourly—oral.

AMOXICILLIN WITH CLAVULANIC ACID (AUGMENTIN)

- The addition of clavulanic acid, which has essentially no antibacterial activity of its own, but beta-lactamase enzymes makes amoxicillin more effective against many bacteria (e.g. *Bacteroides, Haemophilus, Peptococcus, Peptostreptococcus* and *Staphylococcus*) that have become resistant to amoxicillin by elaboration of beta-lactamase enzymes
- When treating infection where beta-lactamase production is a problem, amoxicillin with clavulanic acid may be a useful choice while awaiting culture and sensitivity tests (it should be noted again that both anaerobic, as well as aerobic culture and sensitivity tests should be obtained).

Dosage

Available in dosages as 375 mg (Amox 250 mg + Clavulanic acid 125 mg), 625 mg (Amox 500 mg + Clavulanic acid 125 mg), 1 g (Amox 875 mg + Clavulanic acid 125 mg). Used according to the severity and the site of the infection.

CLOXACILLIN AND DICLOXACILLIN

- These are penicillin derivatives that are resistant to beta-lactamase enzyme inactivation
- They are less effective than penicillin V against most Gram-positive cocci and their use is reserved for the treatment of infections caused by nonmethicillin-resistant penicillinase-producing *S. aureus*.

AMPICILLIN

Ampicillin is active against both Gram-positive and Gram-negative organisms, including *Escherichia coli*.

CARBENICILLIN

It is active against Pseudomonas; these agents have very specific usage indications and should not be substituted for the natural penicillins.

CEPHALOSPORINS

The cephalosporins comprise a group of beta-lactamase antibiotics that resemble penicillins in structure.

- There are more than 20 cephalosporins, of which 8 can be given orally
- The mechanism of action of cephalosporins is almost identical to that of the penicillins
- Of the orally active cephalosporins, only cefaclor, cefuroxime and cefprozil (second generation) have significant activity against anaerobes, Gram-positive and Gram-negative organisms and are therefore preferred for orodental infections
- Some first-generation cephalosporins, despite poor anaerobic activity, are used to treat dental infections such as dentoalveolar abscess
- Their clinical effectiveness may be due to their activity in killing aerobes that deplete oxygen in the local environment and facilitate the growth of anaerobes
- A number of cephalosporins may reach therapeutic concentrations in osseous tissues (bone concentrations) after

administration of usual doses and are useful for bone and joint infections caused by susceptible microorganisms (e.g. cephalexin, cefoperazone, have been shown in alveolar bone and are active against various Gram-positive aerobic bacteria found in dental infections)

- The bactericidal action of cephalosporins is beneficial for patients with a compromised immune system
- The restricted activity of the orally active first-generation and second-generation cephalosporins against anaerobes limits their usefulness in treating orodental infections of anaerobic aetiology (e.g. periapical abscesses)
- Cephalosporins can be cross-allergenic with the penicillins. They may be used cautiously only if the patient's reaction to penicillin was not of the immediate type. Cephalosporins cannot be used in patients who have exhibited anaphylactic reactions to any penicillin derivative
  Orally active second-generation cephalosporins are considerably more expensive than erythromycin or clindamycin, which usually would be effective in treating such anaerobic orodental infections
- Third- and fourth-generation cephalosporins have antipseudomonal activity, extended activity against Gram-negative and anaerobes than first and second generations
- All third- and fourth-generation cephalosporins cross the blood–brain barrier except cefoperazone.

Dosage

- Cefaclor 250 mg 8 hourly—oral
- Cefuroxime 500 mg 12 hourly—oral
- Ceproxil 500 mg 24 hourly—oral.

MACROLIDES

- The macrolide antibiotics effective for treating dental infections are *erythromycin (various dosage formulations), clarithromycin and azithromycin*
- The use of *erythromycin* for treatment of common orodental infections of bacterial origin is second only to that of the penicillin derivatives, but it should be borne in mind that resistance develops rapidly
- Erythromycin is effective against most of the aerobic Gram-positive microorganisms that cause orodental infections and it also exhibits good activity against many oral anaerobic bacteria
- The drug has been used successfully for treating oral infections, such as pericoronitis, periapical abscesses, periodontal abscesses, cellulitis, infected cysts, purulent osteitis, various forms of infectious stomatitis and necrotising ulcerative gingivitis (NUG)
- The average adult dose is 250 mg every 6 h
- *Clarithromycin* and *azithromycin* are useful in treating susceptible orodental infections in patients in whom erythromycin causes gastrointestinal disturbances
- Clarithromycin is also more active than erythromycin (2–4 times) against streptococci, staphylococci and anaerobic bacteria. There may be cross-resistance between erythromycin and new macrolides, particularly among streptococci and staphylococci.

CLINDAMYCIN

- Clindamycin is well suited to treat certain orodental infections
- Its spectrum encompasses most aerobic and anaerobic microorganisms encountered in orodental infections, but its antibacterial spectrum is not so broad as to cause significant superinfection
- An important exception is *pseudomembranous colitis* caused by overgrowth of Clostridium difficile
- Clindamycin is bacteriostatic
- It is well absorbed after oral administration, has minimal adverse effects (except diarrhoea and pseudomembranous colitis), gives high active concentrations in bone and soft tissues and exhibits few problems of resistance development by microorganisms
- Clindamycin is usually taken orally but can also be given parenterally if patients cannot tolerate oral administration. It should be considered as an alternative for treatment of orodental infections caused by susceptible Gram-positive cocci or Gram-positive or Gram-negative anaerobes
- Clindamycin is indicated for *purulent osteitis or* other *bone infection and infections caused by anaerobic organisms, such as Bacteroides species* or by other pathogens that cannot be eradicated by penicillin or one of the macrolide antibiotics
- Clindamycin is useful in treating *dentoalveolar abscesses and chronic infections.*

TETRACYCLINE

The broad-spectrum bacteriostatic tetracycline antibiotics have been employed extensively in the treatment of infections. Tetracyclines used for treatment of orodental infections are tetracycline, minocycline and doxycycline.

- Tetracyclines may be useful in treating certain types of periodontal disease. A 2-week course of tetracycline therapy has been found to be effective in patients with advanced periodontitis unresponsive to conventional therapy alone
- Tetracyclines are also useful in treating *juvenile periodontitis and early onset periodontitis*
- In humans, tetracycline is used as bone growth marker for biopsies
- It is also useful as a biomarker in wildlife to detect consumption of medicine or vaccine containing baits
- Higher concentration of tetracyclines, especially minocycline, in gingival fluids may help eradicate bacteria resistant to concentrations that can normally be achieved in the plasma
- Studies of tetracycline and doxycycline have indicated enhanced repair and tissue regeneration of the periodontium and prevention of *recurrent periodontitis* in high-risk patients. The tissue collagenase-inhibiting effect of the

tetracyclines is relatively marked in the gingival crevice because the drugs are concentrated several folds in sulcular fluid.

Tetracyclines may have a role in preventing endocarditis after dental therapy.

Dosage

Tetracycline: 250–500 mg, four times daily.

Doxycycline

50–100 mg once or twice daily.

METRONIDAZOLE

Metronidazole is used for strict anaerobic infections, ciprofloxacin for oral treatment of Pseudomonas infection and penicillinase-resistant penicillins for infections caused by penicillinase-producing strains of Staphylococcus.

- Metronidazole is active only against obligate anaerobic bacteria, but within this range, it is highly efficacious against the groups most responsible for clinical diseases: Bacteroides, Prevotella, Porphyromonas, Eubacterium, Fusobacterium, Veillonella, Campylobacter, Capnocytophaga, Clostridium, Treponema, Peptococcus and Peptostreptococcus
- Metronidazole has been shown to be an effective drug for the treatment of ANUG, but its use in the majority of dental infections, at least as a single agent, will probably be limited by its lack of effectiveness against aerobic and facultative bacteria
- Metronidazole can also be used in localised juvenile periodontitis and in chronic destructive periodontal disease
- When given along with alcohol, it produces a disulfiram-like reaction.

Dosage

400–800 mg 8 hourly depending on disease severity.

FLUOROQUINOLONES

Ciprofloxacin and ofloxacin are of potential use in dentistry.

- At present, the only therapeutic application for ***ciprofloxacin*** is as an orally active agent for an orodental infection caused by a susceptible species of Pseudomonas
- Nevertheless, the drug is active against a variety of aerobic and facultative organisms implicated in infections involving oral structures and its use is being explored
- Because ***ofloxacin*** has a broader spectrum of activity against oral anaerobes, it may be preferred for orodental infections.

Dosage: 400 mg 8 hourly.

ANTIFUNGAL AGENTS

NYSTATIN

- Topical nystatin is the most commonly used drug for treatment of candidal infections of the oral cavity (oral moniliasis, thrush, denture stomatitis)
- The adult dosage is 3 mL (300,000 units) of suspension in each side of the mouth (600,000 units), which is swished and held in the mouth for 5 min before swallowing
- This treatment should be repeated every 4 h for at least 10 days or 48 h after disappearance of all clinical symptoms
- For nystatin pastilles (200,000 units each), one or two may be dissolved in the mouth 4–5 times daily
- Denture stomatitis may be treated by lining the tissue surface of the denture with the ointment form (100,000 units/g).

CLOTRIMAZOLE

- Clotrimazole is a highly effective, more palatable alternative to nystatin that is administered topically for treatment of oral candidiasis in the form of a troche (lozenge)
- Slow dissolution allows binding to the oral mucosa from which it is gradually released to exert its antifungal activity
- The swallowed drug is variably but poorly absorbed, therefore it is considered a topically applied antifungal agent
- Clotrimazole is not used systemically
- The dosage regimen is a 10 mg troche dissolved in the mouth, five times daily, for at least 14 days
- 1% cream or lotion is available for cutaneous candidiasis and dermatophytoses.

KETOCONAZOLE

- Ketoconazole is useful in treating chronic mucocutaneous candidiasis
- Although very effective against oral candidiasis, it should be reserved for cases refractory to other antifungal agents
- Ketoconazole given orally interacts with a number of drugs, including terfenadine and astemizole (may cause serious cardiac arrhythmias)
- When ketoconazole is given systemically, the daily dosage regimen is 200–400 mg orally; it is also applied topically as a 2% cream.

FLUCONAZOLE

- Fluconazole is the drug of choice for systemic management of candidiasis
- Studies have shown a 96% and 79% cure rate in oropharyngeal candidal infections with fluconazole and clotrimazole, respectively
- Drug interactions are less of a problem than with ketoconazole; however, fluconazole can inhibit the metabolism of cyclosporine, phenytoin, oral anticoagulants, sulphonylureas and zidovudine
- The daily dose of fluconazole is 100–200 mg orally.

NEOMYCIN

- Bactericidal
- Effective against Gram-positive and Gram-negative organisms at the dosage of 5 mg per gram of soluble base

- The route of choice is topical
- The drug may also be administered orally and intramuscularly
- Systemic administration may cause renal damage and possible damage to the cranial nerve VIII.

ANALGESICS

Analgesics are the drugs that relieve pain regardless of its source and type. Control of postoperative pain following oral surgery involves choosing the analgesic regime that is appropriate for each patient. It is divided into two groups based on their site of action:

i. Peripherally acting analgesics—nonsteroidal antiinflammatory drugs (NSAIDs)
ii. Centrally acting analgesics—opioid.

NONSTEROIDAL ANTIINFLAMMATORY DRUGS

Management of acute postsurgical pain is essential to adequately treat oral and maxillofacial surgery patients. Postsurgical pain can be managed effectively by using specific treatment methods like

- Use of long-acting local anaesthesia
- Administration of an oral analgesic prior to the time of surgery
- Meticulous and careful surgery
- Administration of a perioperative glucocorticoid
- A regularly administered analgesic for 48–72 h.

Use of such strategies gives the clinician the greatest probability of effective pain management. Pain control by the use of opioids and NSAIDs are the most common therapies (Flowchart 10.1).

Mechanism of action

NSAIDs interfere with the production of prostaglandins in the surgical wound. Specifically, the conversion of arachidonic acid into prostaglandins by cyclooxygenase is inhibited. Prostaglandins are nociceptive compounds that enhance pain by sensitising primary afferent nerves, that is they reduce the threshold at which these nerves are activated to send pain signals to the central nervous system (CNS). Reduction of prostaglandins in the surgical wound results in a diminished intensity of pain by essentially elevating the threshold at which pain afferent nerves discharge.

Advantages associated with use of NSAIDs

- NSAIDs are effective and useful analgesics for postsurgical pain and can be administered in a variety of formulations (oral, tablet and liquid) and dosages
- A major advantage to the use of these agents is that there is no risk of addiction and abuse potential is low
- The adverse effects associated with NSAIDs occurs, especially when the patient is monitored postsurgically for unanticipated or continuing pain
- Moreover, the cyclooxygenase-2 pathway inhibitors may prove to have fewer adverse effects
- NSAIDs have a topical effect when applied to a surgical wound and a local effect when injected in or around an area of wounded tissue. If this route of administration proves to be feasible, it is possible that many of the adverse effects associated with NSAIDs might be avoided.

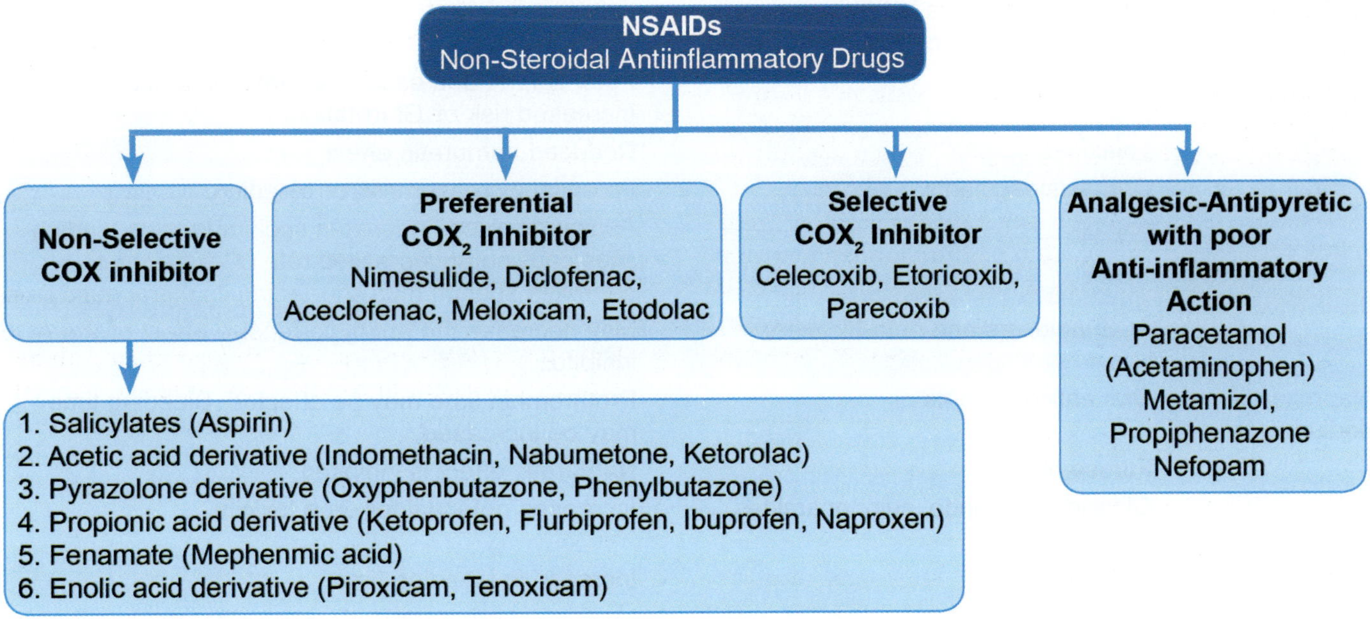

Flowchart 10.1 Classification of NSAIDs.

Adverse drug reaction (Table 10.5)

NSAIDs are usually taken orally. While side effects are rare when used properly, they act systemically, causing negative effects. NSAIDs reduce the formation of thromboxane A2, a powerful platelet aggregating agent, increasing the risk of bleeding. A decrease in gastric prostaglandins, especially prostaglandin E2 and prostacyclin, increases the risk of gastrointestinal (GI) bleeding. The main NSAID risk is spontaneous GI haemorrhage, which increases when an NSAID is taken alongside an anticoagulant. NSAIDs also harm the genitourinary system. Chronic renal disease patients have lower renal blood flow and glomerular filtration rates. As a result, NSAIDs may be contraindicated in diuretic users and definitely in those with severe renal illness. Chronic or combination NSAID use is linked to nephrotoxicity along with dyspepsia, peptic ulcer, dysphagia and abdominal pain. NSAIDs should be taken with or after meals to reduce the risk of these side effects. NSAIDs should be used with caution in patients with GI illness. Caution is advised in patients with a history of alcoholism or peptic ulcer disease. NSAIDs and aspirin pose a greater risk of severe allergic reactions or anaphylaxis. Patients having a history of aspirin sensitivity, multiple drug allergies or asthma are at risk. In addition, hepatic adverse effects (increased liver enzymes) have been recorded less frequently.

TABLE 10.5 Drug Interactions with Commonly Used Pain Medications

Pain Control Medication	Drugs Interacting	Reaction
Aspirin	Aluminium carbonate, aluminium hydroxide, sodium bicarbonate, magnesium oxide	Concurrent administration delays the rate of absorption as aspirin.
	Oral hypoglycaemic	May cause hypoglycaemia by competing with the hypoglycaemic agent for binding sites in the plasma causing an increased level of the free hypoglycaemic agent available in the circulation.
	Warfarin/oral anticoagulants	Aspirin will potentiate the anticoagulation effects by inhibiting platelet clumping and by displacing oral anticoagulants from plasma protein to increase its activity in preventing synthesis of pro-thrombin.
Acetaminophen	Rifampin—barbiturates	Decreases the analgesic effect of acetaminophen. Increased risk of acetaminophen-induced hepatotoxicity
	Chronic use of Ethyl alcohol	Increased potential for hepatotoxicity even with normal doses of acetaminophen.
Oxycodone Hydrocodeine Codeine	CNS depressants, anxiolytic hypnotics, narcotic analgesics, sedatives, MAO inhibitors, tricyclic antidepressants	Increased CNS depression.
Ibuprofen	Aspirin	Potential net decrease in antiinflammatory activity. Increased risk of GI irritation.
	Thiazides	Reduced natriuretic effect
	Oral anticoagulants	Potential increased risk of bleeding.
	Aspirin	Aspirin displaces naproxen sodium from its binding sites causing an increased rate of excretion of naproxen sodium thus shortening its therapeutic time.
	ACE inhibitors and beta-blockers	May decrease the antihypertensive effect of the ACE inhibitor.
Naproxen sodium	Oral anticoagulants	Prothrombin time may be affected. Bleeding time may be increased
	Furosemide	Natriuretic effect is inhibited.
	Glipiside, glyburide, sulphonamides, anticonvulsants	Increased potential for drug toxicity.
	Warfarin	Increase in bleeding time.

IBUPROFEN

Mode of action

Nonsteroidal antiinflammatory agent which reduces prostaglandin activity by inhibiting prostaglandin synthesis.

Indications

Control postsurgical pain. Peak blood levels obtained within 1–2 h stays active as an analgesic for 4–6 h.

Side effects

Gastrointestinal problems like nausea, dyspepsia, heartburn, vomiting and abdominal pain can occur. Gastric ulceration and bleeding can occur in patients using ibuprofen for prolonged period of up to 1 year. Changes in vision, tinnitus, aseptic meningitis, increased fluid retention and skin disorders have also rarely been reported with ibuprofen.

Contraindications

History of allergic reactions to ibuprofen, other NSAIDs and aspirin. Not recommended for pregnant or nursing women.

Precautions

Ibuprofen inhibits platelet aggregation, but this effect usually causes small changes in bleeding time in normal patients. This is less than that seen with aspirin. Patients on anticoagulant therapy or with intrinsic bleeding disorders can be at risk for haemostatic problems with the concurrent use of ibuprofen.

Patients with decreased renal or liver function, heart failure or under diuretic therapy can be at risk for liver dysfunction, renal failure and fluid retention while taking ibuprofen.

Dosage

200–400 mg; 4–6 hourly.

ACETYL SALICYLIC ACID (ASPIRIN)

Mode of action

Its analgesic action is explained by synergism between prostaglandins and pain-producing substances like bradykinins released by the inflammatory process. The inhibition of prostaglandin synthesis leads to analgesia by raising the threshold of pain. The antipyretic action results from inhibition of prostaglandin synthesis in hypothalamus.

Antiinflammatory effects are also derived from their ability to inhibit prostaglandin synthesis. Since prostaglandins are potent vasodilator agents, aspirin provides symptomatic relief from inflammatory effects.

Indication

It is an effective analgesic for mild to moderate degrees of pain.

Side effects

Rashes, swelling, asthma and rarely anaphylaxis. Ingestion can promote nausea, vomiting, bronchospasm and gastrointestinal bleeding due to erosion of mucous membrane.

Precautions

Young children are highly susceptible to aspirin poisoning (therapeutic overdose).

Dosage

325–650 mg 4–6 hourly as an analgesic.

PHENYLBUTAZONE AND OXYPHENBUTAZONE

Mode of action

Same as aspirin.

Indication

These drugs are potent antiinflammatory and poor analgesics.

Side effects

These drugs have been proved to cause agranulocytosis and leukopaenia. They are also known for causing gastric irritation.

Precautions

Retention of sodium and water may aggravate hypertension and congestive cardiac failure.
Precautions to be taken for any dental procedure if the patient is in aspirin.
However, their judicious use is advocated for pronounced antiinflammatory effect.

NAPROXEN

Mode of action

Nonsteroidal antiinflammatory agent, which reduces prostaglandin activity. It has antiinflammatory, analgesic and some antipyretic activity.

Contraindication

History of allergic reactions to naproxen, other NSAIDs and aspirin.

Precautions

Naproxen inhibits platelet aggregation, but this effect usually causes small changes in bleeding time in normal patients. This is less than that seen with aspirin.

Patients on anticoagulant therapy or with intrinsic bleeding disorders can be at risk for haemostatic problems with the concurrent use of naproxen. Patients with decreased renal or liver function, heart failure or under diuretic therapy can be at risk for liver dysfunction, renal failure and fluid retention while taking naproxen.

Dosage

500 mg 8 hourly.

ACETAMINOPHEN (PARACETAMOL)

Mode of action

Peripheral and centrally active analgesic and antipyretic, minimal antiinflammatory activity. Hence, it is not categorised as NSAIDs.

Indications

Control of postsurgical pain. Peak blood levels obtained within 30 min to 1 h stays active as an analgesic for 4–6 h.

Side effects

Minimal side effects.

Contraindication

History of allergic reaction to acetaminophen.

Dosage: 500 mg 8 hourly, maximum of 4 g/day

CENTRALLY ACTING ANALGESICS—OPIOIDS

Centrally acting analgesics include the opiates (morphine and codeine) and opiate-like analgesics (methadone and meperidine).

Advantages

- Opioids are used for the management of moderate to severe acute pain.
- Opioid receptors are present in the CNS but have also been discovered in peripheral primary afferent nerve fibres.
- Opioids can be administered via many more routes than NSAIDs, including transdermal, oral, intramuscular, intravenous, transmucosal, intranasal and other routes.
- As a medication to control acute pain caused by oral and maxillofacial surgical procedures, opioids are prescribed in combination with acetaminophen or NSAIDs (including aspirin) administered orally.

Risks associated with the use of opioids

- Universal fear of *patient abuse and dependence.*
- Opioids when used in the management of postoperative pain have been associated with nausea and vomiting.
- Gastric intolerance is a significant adverse drug reaction.
- Because of the respiratory depressive effect associated with opioids, they are contraindicated in patients with chronic respiratory impairment, for example chronic bronchitis or chronic obstructive pulmonary disease (COPD), head injury.
- Other adverse effects are genitourinary system (urine retention), the CNS (hallucinations, psychomimetic effect) and the GI system (hepatic toxicity).

MORPHINE

Mode of action

Depresses the cerebral cortex and raises the threshold to afferent pain stimuli.

Indications

Pain relief, sedation sleep and as preanaesthetic medication.

Side effects

Nausea, vomiting and constipation.

Contraindications

Morphine releases histamine from the tissues, resulting in mucosal oedema, bronchospasm and consequently difficulty in breathing. So, it is contraindicated in patients with respiratory distress, acute head injury.

Precautions

- Because of its depressant action on respiratory centre and pupillary constriction, it should not be administered in head injuries and lung diseases.
- Due to the drug dependence, withdrawal symptoms begin with a sense of craving for this drug. Later, the patient develops anxiety, agitation and restlessness followed by depression.

CODEINE

- Codeine is the methyl ether of morphine.
- This is a naturally occurring analgesic.
- It is considerably more potent than the antipyretic analgesics.
- It is nonaddictive.
- Produces no disturbing side effects except constipation and dryness of mouth.

ANTIINFLAMMATORY DRUGS

STEROIDAL ANTIINFLAMMATORY DRUGS

CORTICOSTEROIDS

Corticosteroids are naturally occurring substances produced by the adrenal cortex. Synthetic corticosteroids are used extensively in all aspects of clinical medicine as they possess potent antiinflammatory and immunosuppressive properties.

Perioperative use of corticosteroids has been advocated for reduction of pain, oedema and trismus following oral surgical procedures. The potency of short-acting products is the lowest. Hydrocortisone is one example. Prednisolone and methylprednisolone, which are intermediate-acting products are four to five times more potent than hydrocortisone. Dexamethasone is a long-acting, systemic corticosteroid; its potency is about 25 times greater than the short-acting products.

Systemic steroids can be used as adjuvant analgesics in the treatment of neuropathic and cancer-related pain.

Classification

Duration of action

Short-acting

- Cortisol (hydrocortisone)
- Cortisone
- Prednisone
- Prednisolone
- Methyl prednisolone.

Intermediate-acting

- Triamcinolone

Long-acting

- Betamethasone
- Dexamethasone.

Antiinflammatory action of corticosteroids

- Corticosteroids inhibit many of the processes associated with inflammation, which include decreased production of prostanoids owing to decreased expression of cycloxygenase-2, decreased generation of cytokines [interleukin (IL)-1 to IL-8 and tumour necrosis factor-alpha (TNF-α)], reduction in the concentration of complement proteins in the plasma, decreased histamine release from mast cells
- At the cellular level, corticosteroids reduce polymorphonuclear leukocyte (PMN) chemotaxis and phagocytosis.

HYDROCORTISONE

Uses

The antiinflammatory and immunosuppressive effects of hydrocortisone are utilised in the treatment of:

1. Inflammatory ocular, dermatological and bowel conditions
2. Asthma
3. Allergic reactions and shock
4. Rheumatoid diseases
5. Immunosuppression and organ transplantation
6. Malignancies, particularly leukaemia
7. Cerebral oedema.

Hydrocortisone can also be used as replacement therapy in

1. Adrenal insufficiency
2. Congenital adrenal hyperplasia.

Mechanism of action

- Hydrocortisone is the endogenous glucocorticoid cortisol, which is released at times of stress and disease
- Hydrocortisone increases the synthesis of lipocortin-1, which in turn inhibits the activity of phospholipase A2, leading to a decrease in synthesis of prostaglandins, thromboxane and leukotriene
- This is essential for preparation of the body for assault, as well as dampening the immune response to disease, which can be potentially self-destructive in the absence of cortisol
- Hydrocortisone exerts its effects by regulating gene expression in target tissues, which generally leads to a delay of hours between its administration and any observed clinical effects
- Antiinflammatory and immunosuppressive properties of hydrocortisone are very complex and are brought about by effect on blood vessels, inflammatory cells (lymphocytes, monocytes and granulocytes) and inflammatory mediators
- Hydrocortisone decreases the synthesis of vasoactive chemicals such as histamine, cytokines, lysosomal enzymes and various components of the complement system
- The exact mechanism by which this inhabitation takes place may involve the inhibition of arachidonic acid release.

Perioperative corticosteroid use

- Perioperative use of corticosteroids has been advocated for reduction of pain, oedema and trismus following oral surgical procedures
- Corticosteroids reduce the amount of inflammation associated with oral surgery, especially oedema
- Corticosteroid doses ranging from 80 to 625 mg hydrocortisone equivalent antiinflammatory dosage. No significant adverse reactions were noted
- The potential for complications induced by perioperative corticosteroid use such as adrenal suppression and delayed wound healing should also be considered
- In patients with prolonged steroid therapy, the adrenocortical activity is suppressed; in such patients, supplementary hydrocortisone should be given
- Prolonged presence of steroid in blood results in decreased output of ACTH. This results in decreased function and atrophy of the adrenal cortex. Rapid withdrawal of hydrocortisone results in adrenal crisis
- For routine activities, level of secretion may be sufficient, but in case of stress as in any minor or major dental surgical procedure, the adrenal cortex may be unable to secrete more to cope with the stress
- Even minor surgery may prove disastrous. Therefore, such patients should be hospitalised and supplemented with double the usual dose 2 days before surgery and 2 days after surgery. Later on, the dose is gradually tapered.

Implications in dentistry

- Recurrent oral ulceration may be treated with topical steroids, but maintaining long enough contact between the steroid and the oral lesion is often difficult
- Systemic corticosteroids are utilised for treatment of severe oral lesions like pemphigus, erosive lichen planus, etc.
- Intraarticular hydrocortisone may be injected in the temporomandibular joint to relieve refractory pain and stiffness from joint inflammation
- Sometimes, a corticosteroid is needed to suppress pain and swelling due to dental surgery (e.g. impacted third molar extraction)
- In case of patients who are/have been, in the recent past, on long-term corticosteroid therapy, consideration has to be given to the need for supplementary prophylactic corticosteroids to cover a dental procedure
- In general, simple extractions and other mildly traumatic surgeries do not warrant additional steroid dose
- For traumatic procedures and those to be performed under general anaesthesia, supplementary steroids may be needed, particularly if the dose and duration of steroid therapy are such as to have caused significant adrenal suppression or the patient is excessively anxious.

ANTIINFLAMMATORY ACTIONS OF CORTICOSTEROIDS APPLICABLE TO DENTISTRY

Oral ulceration and oral mucosal lesion

- Corticosteroids are widely used in the treatment of recurrent aphthous ulceration and other oral mucosal lesions such as lichen planus, mucous membrane, pemphigoid and pemphigus
- Many of these conditions are treated by topical applications and examples of such preparations include hydrocortisone sodium succinate oromucosal tablets (2.5 mg), triamcinolone acetonide 0.1% in an adhesive base (Orabase), betamethasone spray (50–100 μg) and betamethasone-soluble tablets (500 μg) dissolved in water and used as a mouthwash
- Applying any topical medication to the oral mucosa is difficult and often the best results are achieved when there is maximal contact time between the lesion and the medication
- For severe cases of oral ulceration, systemic corticosteroids may be necessary and the drug of choice is prednisolone.

Bell's palsy

- This is unilateral facial paralysis affecting one or more branches of the facial nerve
- Bell's palsy is of unknown aetiology but may be subsequent to a viral infection
- Systemic prednisolone is the treatment of choice and therapy must be started within 5–6 days of onset of the paralysis
- It is usual to start the treatment with high-dose prednisolone, reducing this over a period of 10 days.

Postoperative pain and swelling after dental surgery

- There has been much interest in the use of systemic corticosteroids to reduce pain and swelling after removal of impacted lower third molars and after orthognathic surgery
- Methyl prednisolone and betamethasone are the corticosteroids used for this purpose, usually administered intramuscularly just before surgery or dexamethasone intravenously
- The efficacy of corticosteroids for reducing postoperative pain after dental surgical procedures remains uncertain and such pain may respond better to an NSAID.

Steroid drug and antiinflammatory dosage

Cortisol (hydrocortisone)—100 mg
Prednisolone—5 to 10 mg for postoperative swelling, used up to 30 mg tapering dosage in case of acute neural inflammation as in Bell palsy.
Methyl prednisolone—4 to 48 mg/day orally (adult dose).

Intermediate-acting

Triamcinolone—topical.

Long-acting

Betamethasone—adult: 0.5–5 mg daily.
Dexamethasone—8 mg B.D. or T.D.S. according to the need.

DEXAMETHASONE

- It is a synthetic corticosteroid that is extremely selective and powerful at the glucocorticoid receptor
- It is used to treat allergy and inflammatory disorders, as well as cerebral oedema and shock
- It helps to minimise swelling and pain after an oral surgical procedure is performed
- It is typically provided before or immediately after the extraction of the third molar
- It has the potential to be ulcerogenic
- Patients suffering from peptic ulcer disease should avoid taking this medication.

Dosage: Dexamethasone—8 mg B.D. or T.D.S. as needed, depending on the situation.

NONSTEROIDAL ANTIINFLAMMATORY DRUGS

Refer to NSAIDs on Page 137.

ANTIOEDEMATOUS SUBSTANCES

For the prevention of traumatic oedema and the treatment of postoperative and traumatic oedema, certain enzymes and antihistamines may be used.

HYALURONIDASE

Hyaluronidase is an enzyme prepared from mammalian testes and acts by depolymerising hyaluronic acid, an essential component of intracellular ground substance, which determines the permeability of tissues.

Mechanism of action

It causes breakdown of the intercellular cement by hydrolysing hyaluronic acid, mucoitin acid and chondroitic sulphuric acid, leading to the permeability of connective tissues. Hyaluronidase helps in:

- Resorption of persistent swelling from injuries or operative procedures
- Elimination of muscular trismus
- Providing better nutrition to flaps and skin grafts
- Treatment of temporomandibular joint disturbances.

The injection of a few drops of a local anaesthetic into the surface is recommended, but deep infiltration should be avoided since epinephrine constricts the blood vessels. Pressure applied after the injection is beneficial. Inserting a gauze pack intraorally or an ice bandage to apply a pressure pack extraorally can accomplish this. No pain or other untoward effects should result. Hyaluronidase (for injection)—Vial contains 150 turbidity reducing units (TRU). Dissolve in 1–5 mL sterile saline solution.

STREPTOKINASE

Streptokinase tablets contain 10,000 units of streptokinase and at least 2500 units of streptodornase, a concentrated combination of enzymes elaborated by haemolytic streptococci.

Mechanism of action

- Streptokinase brings about lysis by removing the barrier and limiting membrane in areas of oedema
- It improves circulation, which facilitates the action of body defence and the effect of antibiotics
- It activates plasminogen, a component of blood plasmin, which acts on the fibrin present in large amounts in oedema fluids and prevents ecchymosis.

Uses

- Antiinflammatory effect
- Postoperative oedema
- Swelling
- Abscesses
- Haematomas associated with fractures or operative procedures
- Prevent ecchymosis caused by extravasation of blood.

The tablets are placed into the buccal pouch and allowed to dissolve slowly so that absorption can take place from the mucosa. The swallowed enzymes are destroyed by gastric acidity. Results are obtained in 24–48 h. In case of infections, antibiotics should be given simultaneously.

Dose: Streptokinase tablets use one quarterly (6 h)

SERRATIOPEPTIDASE

- Serratiopeptidase is a proteolytic enzyme
- It hydrolyses bradykinin, histamine and serotonin responsible for oedemic status
- It reduces swelling, improves microcirculation, etc.

It has antiinflammatory, antioedemic and fibrinolytic activity and acts rapidly on localised inflammation. It acts by binding to alpha-2-macroglobulin in the blood in the ratio of 1:1, which helps to mask its antigenicity but retains its enzymatic activity and is slowly transferred to the site of inflammation. Serratiopeptidase when consumed in unprotected form is destroyed by acid in the stomach.

Adverse effects

Hypersensitivity reactions, such as rash or redness, may infrequently occur.

Anorexia, gastric discomfort, nausea or vomiting may infrequently occur. These can be minimised if the tablets are taken after meals.

Dose

10–20 mg one quarterly (6 h).

ANTIALLERGIC DRUGS

ADRENALINE

- Adrenalin is the drug of choice for anaphylactic shock from any cause in addition to oxygen, which should be administered promptly
- This drug is important in the treatment of allergic diseases since it will quickly relieve the patient in acute attacks of angioneurotic oedema and urticaria
- Other types of allergic reactions are overcome by direct competitive action with histamine due to a physiologic antagonism
- It is administered through the subcutaneous route because through its local vasoconstrictor action, it is absorbed so slowly that excessive action is avoided
- Intravenous injections are used in emergency only. 0.15 mL of a 1:1000 solution is drawn into the syringe and is diluted with water to make 1 mL
- 0.05 mL of the diluted solution is injected slowly. Repeat at the rate of 0.1 mL every 30 s until the syringe is empty. In severe emergency, as much as 1–2 mL of adrenalin 1:1000 may have to be administered.

HYDROCORTISONE

Classification

Corticosteroid (short-acting).

Hydrocortisone (Cortisol) is a steroid of the glucocorticoid class. Its antiinflammatory and immunosuppression property is used in emergency management of allergies as anaphylaxis. It is the second drug of choice to adrenaline. It mainly acts by:

1. Antiinflammatory—decreases laryngeal oedema thereby life saving
2. Bronchodilation
3. Immunosuppression.

Emergency indications and actions

- To prevent further deterioration in patients severely affected by an anaphylactic reaction
- Acute asthma exacerbations
- Acute adrenal crisis
- Life-threatening reactions require large doses of hydrocortisone as well. Inj. hydrocortisone takes several hours to exert its effect
- Naturally it is not so useful in acute anaphylactic reactions, but it can prevent the relapse of symptoms when the effect of adrenaline is over
- In acute asthma exacerbations or status asthmaticus, patients cannot inhale inhalational glucocorticoids properly. These patients may require i.v. hydrocortisone along with other measures like O_2 inhalation, i.v. fluid therapy and nebulised or SC salbutamol

- Hydrocortisone inhibits the synthesis of prostaglandins and leukotrienes and reduces the inflammation of bronchial tree and alveoli.

Dosage

In anaphylactic reaction, Inj. hydrocortisone sodium succinate (100–200 mg) is administered i.v. after adrenaline.

In asthma exacerbations, 200 mg (children 100 mg) is administered i.v. every 6 h.

Intravenous therapy with hydrocortisone is soon replaced by oral prednisolone once clinical improvement is evident.
Adult: 100–500 mg i.v.
Paediatric: 1–2 mg/kg i.v.

Contraindications

Hydrocortisone should not be used in patients with active untreated infections or in patients with known alcohol or bisulphate hypersensitivity.

Precautions

Chronic treatment may lead to adrenal suppression. Therefore, the lowest dose for the shortest period of time must be used. Hydrocortisone should be used with caution in patients with hypothyroidism or cirrhosis.

Adverse reactions and side effects

Adverse reactions and side effects are more common when hydrocortisone is used at high doses and for long-term therapy.
CVS: hypertension
CNS: headache, restlessness, depression, personality changes
Eyes: increased intraocular pressure
GI: anorexia, nausea, vomiting, peptic ulcer formation

Drug interactions

Hydrocortisone may cause an increased risk of hypokalaemia with the use of diuretics. Hypokalaemia may increase the risk of digoxin toxicity. Hydrocortisone may increase the risk of GI effects with the concurrent use with NSAIDs, including aspirin.

SEDATIVES AND HYPNOTICS

Goals of sedatives and hypnotics in oral surgery

- Alleviate patient's fear and anxiety
- Sedate and calm the patient intraoperatively
- Minimise spontaneous movements intraoperatively
- Alter patient's recall (anterograde amnesia)
- Maintain protective reflexes (conscious sedation)
- Allow rapid and complete recovery in outpatient settings
- Achieve safe and effective pain and anxiety control (intraoperatively and postoperatively).

BARBITURATES

These drugs are derived from barbituric acid. They are used for simple insomnia, neurosis and hysteria. Also used to prevent excitation, convulsions and sometimes after local anaesthesia and postoperative struggling, nausea and vomiting.

PENTOBARBITAL SODIUM

Pentobarbital sodium is a sedative. Its action is of short duration and has a more prolonged hypnotic effect. It is used orally as premedication the night before an operation and shortly before an anaesthetic is used.

Dose

For sedation

Pentobarbital sodium, 0.1 g per orally. If deep hypnosis is desired, a double dose may be given—0.2 g per orally.

PHENOBARBITAL

Phenobarbital is the slowest acting barbiturate. Phenobarbital sodium has a greater solubility and acts more rapidly. Used orally before an operation under local anaesthesia, it gives excellent sedation.

Dose

Sedation: Phenobarbital sodium, 0.03 g PO
Hypnosis: Phenobarbital, 0.1 g PO

NONBARBITURATE SEDATIVES

These are recent drugs that are nonhabit forming and have none of the disadvantages of barbiturates, which in large doses produce depression and coma.

These are excellent for the management of neurotic, refractory patients and nervous and apprehensive children.

BENZODIAZEPINES

These are well suited for moderate and deep sedation. These drugs provide sedation and retrograde amnesia with minimal effect on cardiovascular and respiratory systems in healthy patients. They do not provide analgesia.

Commonly used drugs are:

- Midazolam (Versed)
- Diazepam (Valium)
- Lorazepam (Ativan).

Mechanism of action

They act by facilitating the gamma aminobutyric acid (GABA) receptors in the brain. GABA is the chief inhibitory neuropeptide in the brain. They are highly lipid soluble and rapidly enter the CNS and bind to GABA receptors. This results in the opening of the chloride channels and hence reduces excitability.

Clinical effects

- Moderate to deep sedation
- Anxiolysis
- Hypnosis
- Anterograde amnesia
- Anticonvulsant
- Spinal cord mediated skeletal muscle relaxation.

The clinical effects of each benzodiazepine are due to binding to GABA receptors at different sites.

Adverse effects

- Cardiovascular, haemodynamic changes and respiratory depression becomes more significant when given in combination with steroid
- Longer elimination and greater anxiety in elder patients
- Venoirritation may occur in case of diazepam and lorazepam.

DIAZEPAM

- Water insoluble and highly lipid soluble and hence enter the brain rapidly
- Used as sedative, anxiolytics, amnesic and anticonvulsant drug
- Highly protein bound
- Metabolised in liver producing oxazepam and dimethyl diazepam as two active metabolite.

Dosage

- Adult—2.5–10 mg slowly over 2 min, titrate: 2–5 mg every 5–10 min, maximum—20 mg
- Paediatric—0.1–0.3 mg/kg increment over minimum of 3 min, maximum 0.6 mg/kg
- Premedication oral dose—0.2–0.4 mg/kg.

Contraindications

Decreased albumin concentrations like burns, malnutrition, liver disease, sepsis and renal dysfunction may increases its effects.

Side effects

- Painful on injection—(since it is dissolved in propylene glycol and sodium benzoate)
- Withdrawal effect—(due to abrupt discontinuation of drug after prolonged use) causing anxiety, hyperexcitability and seizures.

MIDAZOLAM

- Short-acting
- Water-soluble benzodiazepine
- Used as sedative, anxiolytic, amnesic and anticonvulsant drug
- Two to three times more potent than diazepam, commonly used in procedural sedation
- Binds strongly to plasma proteins
- Metabolism is by hydroxylation in liver
- Excretion is by kidney after conjugation.

Dosage

- Adult—0.5–2.5 mg slowly over 2 min, titrate 0.5 mg increments, maximum 5 mg
- Paediatric—0.05–0.1 mg/kg, titrate 0.25 mg/kg every 5 min, maximum 0.2 mg/kg
- Premedication oral dose—0.5 mg/kg.

Contraindication

Obese patient—due to increase volume of distribution and prolonged half-life of drug.

LORAZEPAM

- Long-acting benzodiazepine
- Similar properties of midazolam and diazepam
- Potent amnesic property
- Metabolised in liver to inactive metabolites
- Slower onset of action with slower metabolic clearance compared to midazolam
- Used for longer procedures requiring amnesia, sedation and anxiolysis.

Dosage

- Adult—0.02–0.05 mg/kg slowly over 2 min, may repeat 1/2 dose every 10–15 min, maximum 2 mg
- Paediatric—0.05 mg/kg over 2 min, may repeat 1/2 dose every 10–15 min, maximum 2 mg
- Premedication oral dose—0.05 mg/kg.

ANTICOAGULANTS

WARFARIN

One of the most widely used oral anticoagulants, warfarin, works by counteracting vitamin K's action to prevent thromboembolism. It is entirely absorbed and reaches its peak in 1 h. It has a half-life of approximately 36 h in circulating albumin and is metabolised in the liver and eliminated largely in the urine. The risk of postoperative bleeding in patients taking warfarin for tooth extractions was observed to be very low when the INR was within acceptable ranges; however, significant haemorrhage can be controlled with local haemostatic agents, suturing and tranexamic acid.

NEWER DRUGS

Daptomycin
Linezolid
Tigecyclin (Tetracyclines group)
Dalfopristin–Quinupristin
Newer fluoroquinolones (Trovafloxacin)
Newer beta lactum antibiotics
  - Cephalosporins—Ceftaroline, ceftabiprole

Newer macrolides
  - Fidaxomicin.

Section IV

Anaesthesia in Oral Surgery

Chapter 11

Local Anaesthesia

OUTLINE

INTRODUCTION

'Local anaesthesia (LA) is defined as a transient and completely reversible loss of sensation in a circumscribed area of the body caused by a depression of excitation in nerve endings, or an inhibition of the conduction process in peripheral nerves'.

METHODS TO INDUCE LOCAL ANAESTHESIA

1. Mechanical trauma
2. Low temperature anoxia
3. Chemical irritants
4. Neurolytic agents such as alcohol and phenol
5. Chemical agents such as local anaesthetics.

COMPOSITION OF LOCAL ANAESTHETICS

Composition of local anaesthetics is described in Table 11.1.

BASIC PHYSIOLOGY OF LOCAL ANAESTHESIA

PERIPHERAL NERVES

The functional unit of a nerve is an individual nerve fibre. The size of an individual nerve fibre is between 0.5 μm and 20 μm in diameter. The fibres that are larger than 2 μm are the myelinated nerves and those that are smaller than 2 μm are the unmyelinated nerves (Table 11.2). All of these nerve fibres lie in a bundle, thus being exposed to stimuli or local anaesthetic agents simultaneously. When the nerve fibre is stimulated, there is a change in electric potential, which proceeds as waves or jumps depending on the type of nerve fibre. The threshold for the speed of conduction of impulses is based on the diameter of the axon. The speed of conduction of impulses can be calculated by the formula:

$$\text{Diameter of fibre } (\mu m) \times 6 = \text{speed of impulse } (m/s)$$

NERVE FIBRE CLASSIFICATION

The most popular nerve fibre classification is the Erlanger and Gasser classification, which is depicted in Table 11.3.

The nerve fibres are broadly classified as groups A, B and C elevations. The A group is further subdivided into groups Alpha (α), Beta (β), Gamma (γ) and Delta (δ) on the basis of diameter, conduction velocity and threshold. The Aα fibres are the largest and fastest, perceiving motor and proprioception and are the most easily excited. The Aβ fibres are the next largest and perceive touch, pressure, motor and proprioception. The Aγ-fibres perceive only touch and pressure. The Aδ-fibres are the smallest and least sensitive to stimulation of the group and perceive temperature and pain.

1st PAIN AND 2nd PAIN

Aδ-fibres transmit the 1st pain impulses faster than non-myelinated C-fibres, which transmit the 2nd pain. 1st pain is perceived within seconds after the injury and the characteristic sharp localised pain is felt at the site of stimulus. The 2nd pain is slower to develop, and the characteristic dull, throbbing/gnawing pain is felt and lasts longer than the 1st pain. An Aδ-fibre transmits impulses along its axon at a rate of 5–25 m/s. Impulse transmission is slower in unmyelinated C-fibres as they transmit impulses at approximately 1 m/s.

TABLE 11.1 Composition of Local Anaesthetics in a Multidose Vial

	Constituent and Function	Composition	Quantity
1.	Local anaesthetic agent	Lignocaine hydrochloride	2% (i.e. 20 mg/mL)
2.	Isotonic solution maintains isotonicity of the solution	Sodium chloride or Ringer's solution	6 mg
3.	Diluting agent	Distilled water	
4.	Vasoconstrictor increases depth and duration of anaesthesia	Adrenaline	1:80,000 (0.0125 mg) 1:100,000 (0.01 mg) 1:200,000 (0.005 mg)
5.	Reducing agent (antioxidant)	Sodium metabisulphite	0.5 mg
6.	Bacteriostatic agent	Methylparaben	0.1% (1 mg)
7.	Fungicide	Thymol	
8.	To adjust pH	Sodium hydroxide	
9.	Present oxygen from being trapped in the cartridge and potentially destroying the vasopressor	Nitrogen bubble	1.2 mm in diameter

Methylparaben was removed from cartridges as it causes allergy; however, it is added in multidose vials because a cartridge is used for one patient and discarded (single use), but multidose vials are used multiple times.

TABLE 11.2 Major Differences Between Myelinated Nerve and Unmyelinated Nerve Fibres

	Myelinated Nerve Fibres	Unmyelinated Nerve Fibres
Myelin sheath	Present	Absent
Nerve impulse transmission	Faster	Slower
Nodes of Ranvier	Present	Absent
Colour	White	Grey

MODE OF IMPULSE CONDUCTION

Nociception (pain awareness) is mediated by nerve ending receptors called nociceptors in the peripheral tissues. The stimuli are transmitted by the nociceptors to the CNS by intramembranous transfer of particles like sodium and potassium. The constant change in the membranous potential allows the impulses to be conducted through the nerves. The resting potential inside the nerve is usually −70 mV and any impulse initiations that fail to reach the threshold potential (−55 mV) dies without progressing.

TABLE 11.3 Erlanger and Gasser Classification Based on Axon Size

Fibre (Type/Group)	Sub-group	Myelinated	Function	Nerve Fibre Affected	Sensitivity to Lidocaine
A group	Aα	Myelinated Motor neurons	Motor Proprioception	3rd affected nerve fibres are the large myelinated nerves. These include Aα (motor) and Aβ (touch) fibres	+
	Aβ	Myelinated Skin touch afferents	Motor Proprioception Touch Pressure		++
	Aγ	Myelinated Motor to muscle spindles	Touch (Proprioception) Pressure	First	++++
	Aδ	**Myelinated Skin temperature afferents**	**Temperature (cold) First pain (sharp pain)**	**Second**	**++++**
B group		Lightly myelinated pain afferents	Preganglionic fibres		+++
C group		**Unmyelinated autonomic postganglionic neurons**	**Second pain (dull pain)**	**Last**	**++**

The most important fibres for local anaesthesia are the Aδ-fibres and C-fibres, which have been highlighted.

DEJONG'S PRINCIPLE

DeJong described impulse conduction as 'the active progress of spark along a fuse of gunpowder; once lit, the fuse burns along its length by distributing to neighbour and reaches gunpowder'. Impulse generation is similar to this, as transmission and propagation take place through the nerves until the stimulus reaches the brain.

ELECTROPHYSIOLOGY OF NERVE CONDUCTION (FIG. 11.1A & B)

STEP 1: Slow depolarisation is the development of the potential to reach threshold potential (-55 mV). A few Na^+ ions move into the nerve membrane at this stage to increase the membrane potential.

STEP 2: The threshold potential is a critical level to which a membrane potential must be depolarised, and is usually between −50 and −55 mV. At this threshold potential, the cell's voltage-gated sodium channels open to begin a cascade of events involving other ion channels for conduction of the nerve impulse.

ELECTROCHEMISTRY OF NERVE CONDUCTION

STEP 3: A sudden sodium influx occurring inside the membrane is called as rapid depolarisation. The potential reaches a maximum of +40 mV, which is called peak action potential.

STEP 4: This is followed by repolarisation, which occurs due to potassium efflux. Steps 1–4 take 1 ms to complete and reach resting potential. Hyperpolarisation is the event of undershooting of the membrane potential below the resting potential up to -90 mV.

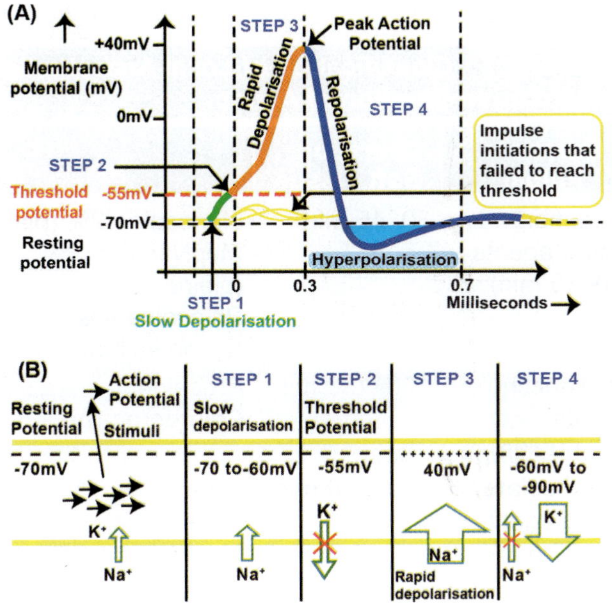

Figure 11.1 **(A)** The graph depicts Steps 1 to 4 of nerve conduction. **(B)** The sequence of events that occur in Steps 1 to 4 of nerve conduction.

CONDUCTION BLOCK (PHYSIOLOGY OF LA AGENT)

The principle of the Local Anaesthetic Agent (LAA) is that it prevents both impulse generation and nerve conduction by setting up a chemical block between the source of impulse and the brain. LAA prevents the increase in membrane permeability to sodium ions that leads to formation of a nerve impulse, thereby blocking nerve conduction. This is called conduction block.

THEORIES FOR PHYSIOLOGICAL MODE OF ACTION OF LOCAL ANAESTHESIA

Acetylcholine theory (Dett Barn-1967)

Acetylcholine is involved in nerve conduction as a neurotransmitter at nerve synapses. Local anaesthesia prevents acetylcholine at the synapse to alter the cell permeability. This theory is less accepted as there is no evidence of involvement of acetylcholine in neural transmission along the body of the neuron, and it is not always present at the synapse.

Calcium displacement theory (Goldman-1966)

According to this theory, local anaesthesia blocks calcium channels and prevents the displacement of calcium from some membrane sites that control sodium permeability needed for depolarisation. This theory is also less accepted as local anaesthesia acts well even in the abundance of calcium.

Surface charge theory (Wei-1969)

Local anaesthetics bind to the nerve membrane and change the electrical potential at the membrane surface. For example, LA molecules carrying a positive charge make the electrical potential at the membrane surface more positive, thereby increasing the threshold potential, but evidence shows that there is no change in the resting potential by local anaesthetics and they act within the nerve membrane channels rather than at the surface. This theory also could not explain the action of uncharged anaesthetic agents like benzocaine.

Membrane expansion theory (Lee-1976)

For LAA like benzocaine that do not have a cationic form, this theory explains its potent action as a topical anaesthetic. Local anaesthetics diffuse to hydrophobic regions and expand the membrane preventing sodium permeability. Lipid soluble molecules alter the lipoprotein matrix of the nerve membrane and decrease the diameter of sodium channels. There is no direct evidence to support this theory.

Specific receptor hypothesis (Strichartz-1987)

Specific receptor hypothesis is the most favoured theory. Local anaesthetics act by attaching themselves to specific receptors in the nerve membrane. The local anaesthetics receptor is located at or near the sodium channel in the nerve membrane either on its external surface or on the internal axoplasmic surface. Once the receptor access is gained, sodium ion permeability is decreased or eliminated and nerve conduction interrupted.

PHARMACOLOGY OF LOCAL ANAESTHETICS

CLASSIFICATION

LAA are classified based on different features like chemical structure, site of action, duration of action and mode of administration.

CLASSIFICATION OF LOCAL ANAESTHETICS BASED ON CHEMICAL STRUCTURE (TABLES 11.4–11.6)

LAA are classified into two main types defined by the linkage between the hydrophilic and lipophilic groups (chemical structure). Amides seem more beneficial and more commonly used, as they are heat stable and have lesser allergic reactions. The two most important factors that the chemical structure determines are the lipid solubility and ionisation constant (pKa).

Ester-linked local anaesthetics are readily hydrolysed in aqueous solution whereas amide-linked local anaesthetics are relatively resistant to hydrolysis.

TABLE 11.4 Classification of Local Anaesthetics Based on Chemical Structure

Esters	Amides	Quinoline
Benzoic acid esters	Prilocaine	Centbucridine
Butacaine	Bupivacaine	
Cocaine	Mepivacaine	
Benzocaine	Etidocaine	
Hexylcaine	Articaine	
Piperocaine	Lidocaine	
Tetracaine		
Para-aminobenzoic acid (PABA) esters		
Procaine		
Chloroprocaine		
Propoxycaine		

TABLE 11.5 Important Difference Between Ester and Amide Groups

Esters	Amides
Rapid metabolism of ester LAA is done by the enzyme plasma cholinesterase. They are short acting drugs.	Hepatic metabolism—the metabolites can cause sedation.
Patients may present with allergic reaction as it is similar to para-aminobenzoic acid (PABA) structure.	Patients can present with malignant hyperthermia. Allergies are rare with amides.
Poor shelf life-unstable in solution as it degrades faster.	Longer shelf life-stable in solution.
pKa dissociation constant: 8.5–8.9.	pKa dissociation constant: 7.6–8.1.

TABLE 11.6 Classification of Local Anaesthetics According to Biologic Site and Mode of Action

Class A	Agent acting at receptor site—external surface of nerve membrane
Class B	Agent acting at receptor site—internal surface of nerve membrane
Class C	Agent acting by a receptor independent physico-chemical mechanism eg., Benzocaine
Class D	Combination of receptor dependent and receptor independent mechanism (mostly LA, e.g., lignocaine, mepivacaine)

The ester type anaesthetics are metabolised by the hepatic pseudocholinesterase and plasmatic esterase, producing para-amino benzoic acid (PABA), which is excreted in urine. The ester type is 100% metabolised and the amide type is 90% metabolised, the remainder being unmetabolised anaesthetics.

Apart from these differences, amides will contain an 'I' in the generic name prior to '-caine', for example, lidocaine, mepivacaine, prilocaine, bupivacaine while esters do not contain an 'I' in the generic name prior to '-caine', for example, procaine, chloroprocaine, cocaine, benzocaine.

CLASSIFICATION OF LOCAL ANAESTHETICS BASED ON DURATION OF ACTION (TABLES 11.7 AND 11.8)

Duration of action of a LAA is dependent on the ability to bind to plasma proteins; LA molecules, which bind easily to plasma proteins have a longer duration of action and lower

TABLE 11.7 Classification of Local Anaesthetics According to Duration of Action

Duration: Pulpal	Duration: Soft Tissue	LA
Ultrashort acting agents (10–15 min)	30–45 min	Lignocaine 2% (plain) Mepivacaine 3% (plain) Prilocaine 4% (as an infiltration)
Short-acting agents (45–60 min)	120–180 min	Procaine Chloroprocaine
Intermediate acting agents (60–90 min)	180–270 min	Lignocaine, Prilocaine (as a block) Mepivacaine 2% (pulpal)
Long-acting agents (>90 min)	>270 min	Bupivacaine Etidocaine Tetracaine

TABLE 11.8 Classification of LA Based on Mode of Administration

Injectable Anaesthetics	Surface Anaesthetics
a. Low potency, short duration i. Procaine ii. Chloroprocaine	a. Soluble i. Cocaine ii. Lidocaine iii. Tetracaine
b. Intermediate potency and intermediate duration i. Lidocaine ii. Prilocaine	b. Insoluble i. Benzocaine ii. Butyl aminobenzoate (Butamben) iii. Oxethazaine
c. High potency, long duration i. Tetracaine ii. Bupivacaine iii. Ropivacaine iv. Dibucaine	

risk of toxicity. Lower pH can reduce protein binding capacity and increase risk of toxicity.

MECHANISM OF ACTION OF CONDUCTION BLOCK (FIG. 11.2)

CHEMICAL REACTION OF LOCAL ANAESTHETICS (FIG. 11.3)

The LAA can dissociate into the membrane only in the nonionic form. It exists at a lower pH than pKa as a more stable solution. Thus, depending on the environmental pH, the LAA can dissociate into the required form as shown below.

$RNHCL \rightarrow RNH^+ + Cl^-$

A stable LA solution contains a weak base (LAA) and a strong acid.

RNHOH (weak base) + HCl (strong acid) → RNHCl (acid salt) + water.

Role of the aromatic group—lipid solubility (Fig. 11.4)

The benzene ring forms the lipophilic part or the hydrophobic part of the LAA. It allows the LA molecule to diffuse into

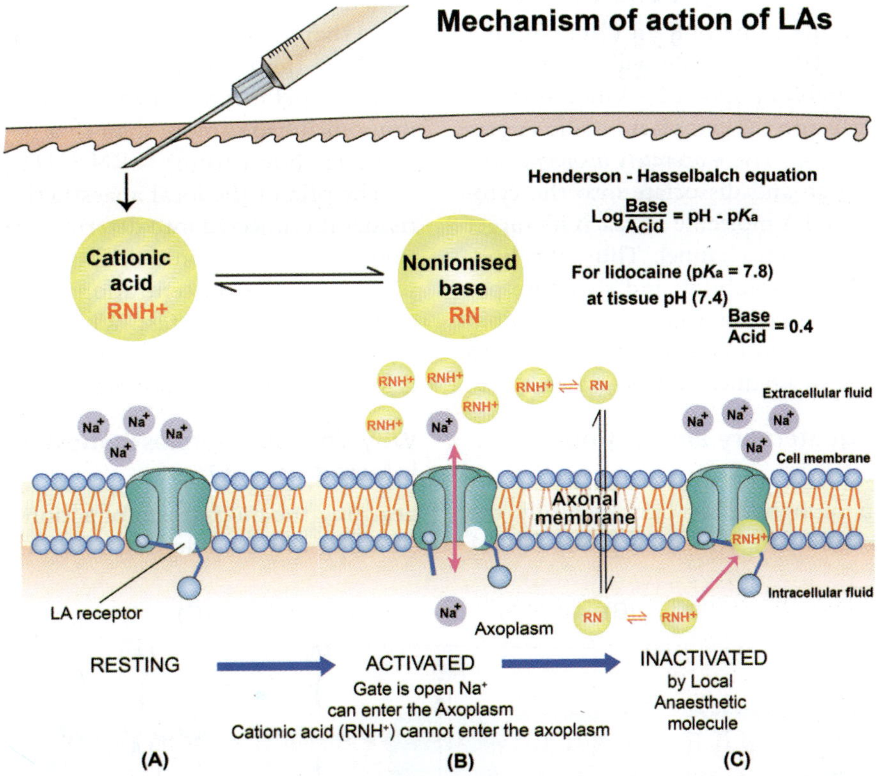

Figure 11.2 Injection of the local anaesthetic solution containing cationic acid (RNH^+) into the tissues, the cationic acid gets converted into nonionised base (RN). This nonionised base can enter the lipoid barriers (bi-lipid layer). Once inside the axoplasm, the nonionised base (RN) gets converted into cationic acid (ionised form—RNH^+). The pH and pKa play an important role in this conversion and is determined by the Henderson–Hasselbalch equation. (**A**) Resting state of a sodium channel gate, sodium cannot enter the gated channel as it is closed in the resting state (does not reach threshold). There is no stimuli or nerve conduction in this resting phase. (**B**) Activated state—sodium can enter and exit the opened channel in this state. It can be noted that the LAA molecule cannot enter the bi-lipid layer in the ionic form (RNH^+). There is stimuli and pain is felt. (**C**) Inactivated state—sodium cannot enter the channel as the LA molecule has reached the target site causing the gate to be closed. The stimuli is present and pain is not felt as LA is working by inactivating the sodium channel.

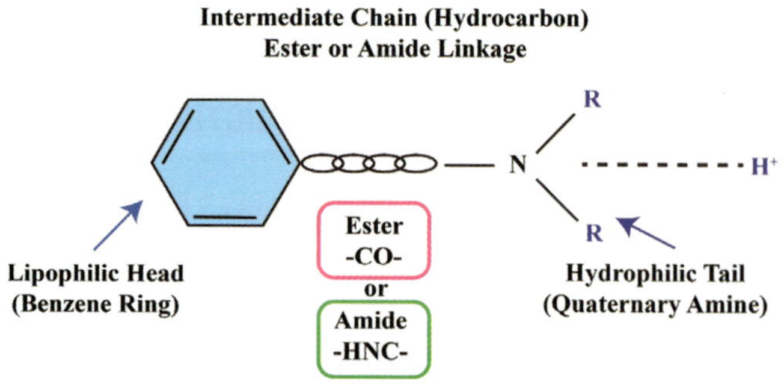

Figure 11.3 The chemical structure of the LA molecule has been illustrated. It is important for us to understand the aromatic group that helps in lipid solubility of the molecule to enter the nerve cell through the bi-lipid layer, and the amine group that is responsible for the protein bindability (i.e. the attachability of the LA molecule at the target site on the voltage-gated sodium channel).

the nerve cell. All LAA contains the aromatic group (benzene ring) that gives this lipophilic character, and adding an amino nitrogen or alkyl substitute increases this character. The bi-lipid layer of the biological membrane allows this diffusion. It is important for the molecule to be only moderately lipophilic, as poorly lipophilic LAA molecule will not perfuse through the layer whereas highly lipophilic LAA molecule will diffuse out extremely slowly into the cytoplasmic side or gets trapped inside the bi-lipid layer. The *moderately lipophilic LAA* molecule will diffuse through and dissociate into the cytoplasmic side. This allows the LA molecule to reach its target site on the voltage-gated sodium channel. Thus, the lipophilic portion determines lipid solubility and therefore potency, toxicity and duration of action. Clinically, more lipid soluble agents are administered in lower doses according to *Bowman's principle*, resulting in a reduced rate of onset.

Role of the tertiary or quaternary amine group—protein bindability

The hydrophilic portion or lipophobic part, typically the amine group determines ionisation. The amine group of LAA can exist in either the acid form or the base form. The acid form is the ionic form or the positively charged or the protonated form (RNH^+). The base form is the nonionic form or the deprotonated form or the neutrally charged form (RN).

pH and pKa—onset of conduction block

Ionisation constant (pKa) determines the onset of the drug. At physiologic pH of 7.4, the pKa values of LA is between 8 and 10. The pKa of a LA molecule is the pH at which 50% of the agent exists in the protonated form and 50% in the deprotonated form. Only ionic form of LA molecules will bind to the target binding sites. Therefore, the weak LA base forms (nonionic forms) are effective as they diffuse rapidly across the membrane. Once the drug enters the cytoplasm, it will gain a proton (H^+) becoming an ionic form that binds with much higher affinity to the drug's target binding site. Higher pKa results in a longer duration of block.

This is expressed in the **Henderson–Hasselbalch equation:**

$pKa - pH = \log [RNH^+]/[RN]$; where [RN] is the concentration of nonionised form and $[RNH^+]$ is the concentration of ionised drug.

When the pH is higher, concentration of the ionic form is more than that of the nonionic form.

RNH^+ (ionic form) $>$ $RN + H^+$ (nonionic form)

When pH is lower (acidic environment), concentration of nonionic form is more than that of the ionic form.

RNH^+ (ionic form) $<$ $RN + H^+$ (nonionic form)

The pKa of the local anaesthetic agent and the pH of the tissues it is injected into determine the percentage concentration of ionic and nonionic forms that are present. When the pKa is low, the concentration of the nonionic form is high and speed of onset is fast. When the pKa is high, the percentage of nonionic form of the molecules present in the solution is low. Thus, the speed of onset of the LAA is slow (Box 11.1).

Why does local anaesthetic agent not work in infected tissues?

Learning the mechanism of action of a LAA helps in understanding why LAA do not work in an area of low tissue pH,

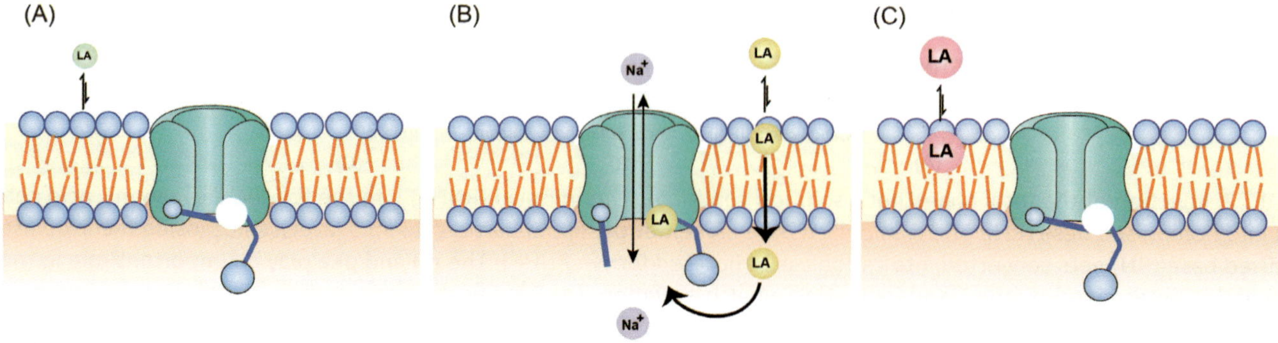

Figure 11.4 The above figure illustrates the role of the lipophilic part of the LA drug. (**A**) A poorly lipophilic LAA molecule does not perfuse through the layer. (**B**) A moderately lipophilic LAA molecule will diffuse through and dissociate into the cytoplasmic side. The LA molecule then undergoes ionisation and binds to the target molecule. (**C**) A highly lipophilic LAA will diffuse out extremely slowly into the cytoplasmic side or gets trapped inside the bi-lipid layer.

BOX 11.1 Ideal Properties of a Local Anaesthetic

1. It should not be irritating to the tissues to which it is applied.
2. It should not cause any permanent alteration in the nerve structure.
3. Its systemic toxicity should be low.
4. It must be effective regardless of whether it is injected into the tissues or applied locally to the mucous membranes.
5. Time of onset of anaesthesia should be as short as possible.

Rate of onset is dependent on:

Drug Factors		Patient Factors	
↑ Rate of Onset	↓ Rate of Onset	↑ Rate of Onset	↓ Rate of Onset
Fick's law: Increasing the dose increases the rate of onset Increased concentration of drug also increases the rate of onset	Increased volume by diluting will decrease rate of onset	Nerve activity Local anaesthetics produce a frequency dependent blockade, meaning nerves firing frequently will be blocked more rapidly than quiescent nerves	Hyperkalaemia

6. Duration of action must be long enough to permit completion of the procedure yet not so long as to require an extended recovery.

Duration of action is dependent on:

Drug Factors		Patient Factors	
↑ Duration of action	↓ Duration of action (DOA)	↑ DOA	↓ DOA
1. LAA causing vasoconstriction (cocaine) 2. Addition of epinephrine 3. ↑ Lipid solubility (LAA remains in the nerve for longer) this ↑ potency 4. ↑ Protein binding capacity	1. LAA that cause vasodilatation 2. ↓ pH—↓ protein binding capacity—↓ DOA	1. Metabolic impairment like hepatic failure and butyl cholinesterase deficiency 2. Site of administration—well-vascularised tissue like the intercostal area will have increased systemic uptake of the drug	1. ↓ Tissue pH

7. It should have potency sufficient to give complete anaesthesia without the use of harmful concentrated solutions.

   i. Potency is demonstrated with the use of a minimum effective concentration of the local anaesthetic drug (Cm). In a healthy individual, at this concentration, the drug can cause complete block of a nerve fibre. More potent LAA have a lower Cm.
   ii. Potency is dependent on two factors (Fig. 11.5):
      a. Lipid solubility:
         i. Potency increases with higher lipid solubility.
      b. Vasodilator effect of LA.

8. It should be relatively free from producing allergic reactions.
9. It should be stable in solution and readily undergo biotransformation.
10. It should either be sterile or capable of being sterilised by heat without deterioration.

Drug	pKa 36° C	Onset time	Protein binding (%)	Duration	Lipid solubility	Potency
Amides						
Prilocaine	7.7	Fast 3-5 mins	55%	Moderate		Medium
Lidocaine	7.8	Rapid 2-4 mins	64%	Moderate	4	Medium
Mepivacaine	7.7	Rapid 2-4 mins	75%	Moderate	1	Medium
Articaine	7.8	Rapid 2-4 mins	95%	Moderate	17	
Etidocaine	7.9	Rapid 2-4 mins	94%	Long	140	High
Bupivacaine	8.1	Moderate 5-8 mins	95%	Long	340	High
Ropivacaine	8.1	Rapid 2-4 mins	94%	Long	2.8	Medium
Esters						
Tetracaine	8.4	Slow 10-15 mins	85%	Long	80	
Amethocaine	8.5	Slow	76%	Moderate		Medium
Cocaine	8.7	Slow	98%			High
Procaine	8.9	Slow 14-18 mins	6%	Short	<1	Low
Chloroprocaine	9.1	Moderate 6-12 mins (Hydrolyses 4 times faster than Procaine)	7%	Short	>1	

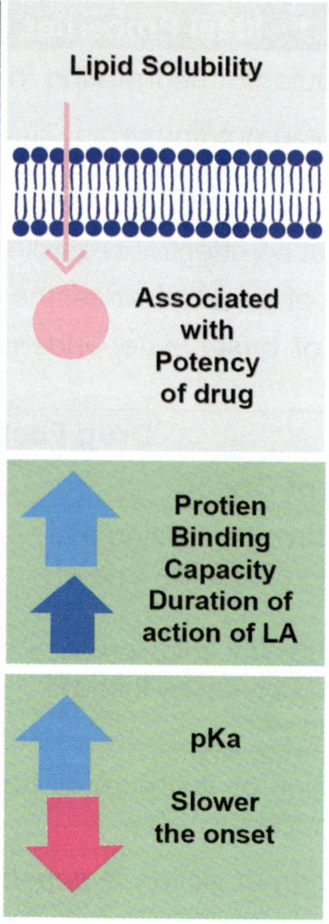

Figure 11.5 The relationships between the properties of LA agents.

that is in the presence of infections. It is important to understand that the LAA is available as acid salts of weak bases, which means the local anaesthetic weak base (RNHOH) should be combined with a strong acid (HCL) to make an acid salt. For this acid salt (RNHCL) to act as an anaesthetic agent, it requires a basic environment to dissociate into a free base, which is unlikely in infections. At an infected site, the pH is approximately 5 to 6 and lower than the normal physiologic pH (7.4). At low pH, the pKa increases–which means the ionic form of LA is higher. This does not diffuse into the cell membrane with inability to reach the target site on the cytoplasmic side. Sodium bicarbonate can be added to the LA solutions to raise the pH of the infected tissue, which can increase the speed of onset.

Why does bupivacaine have a long duration of action?

The pKa of bupivacaine is 8.1. The higher the pKa, the higher the percentage of the ionic form of the molecule present in the solution. Hence, the lower the concentration of the nonionic form, the slower the speed of onset of the drug. Agents that bind poorly to the protein (target site on the sodium channel) such as procaine and chloroprocaine are immediately washed out. This reduces the duration of the local anaesthetic block compared to those, which are highly protein-bound such as bupivacaine and etidocaine. Bupivacaine is not easily washed out. Conduction blockade is active for a longer period of time.

PHARMACOKINETICS—MOVEMENT OF THE DRUG WITHIN THE BODY

ABSORPTION—UPTAKE

ORAL ROUTE

The LAA is poorly absorbed by the oral route. When taken orally, it gets metabolised by the 'hepatic 1st pass metabolism'. After this, the remaining drug is carried to the liver where 72% of the dose is biotransformed into inactive metabolites. This is why lidocaine could not be an effective oral antidysrhythmic drug.

TOPICAL ROUTE

The absorption rate of topical anaesthesia is depicted in the Fig. 11.6. It takes approximately 5 min to achieve peak blood level through topical route. LAA does not get absorbed through intact skin, eutectic mixture of local anaesthetics (EMLA) cream with prilocaine and lidocaine has been developed that can anaesthetise skin. Eutectic mixture means lowering of the melting point of two solids when combined (emulsified). Lidocaine and prilocaine are emulsified with water to form a cream, which is called EMLA. 20% topical benzocaine (flavoured) is a topical mucosal gel, which has a duration of action of 12–15 min and a quick onset of 2 to 3 min (indicated for children).

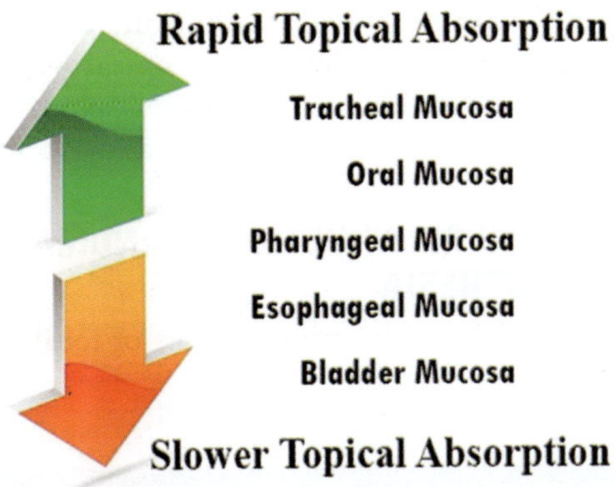

Figure 11.6 Illustrates the rate of topical LAA absorption from the various mucosa of the body (rapid to slow absorption).

INJECTION (INTRAVENOUS) ROUTE

Rate of uptake of drug after injection is completely dependent on two important factors, the vascularity of the site of injection and the vasoactivity of the local anaesthetic drug. While i.v. administration is suggested only for prefatal ventricular dysrhythmias, it is important for the clinician to understand the toxic effects of administering it through the i.v. route.

WHAT HAPPENS TO THE LOCAL ANAESTHETIC DRUG ONCE IT HAS BEEN INJECTED?

It is important for the clinician to understand that vasodilatation causes an increase in the rate of absorption of the drug but there is a decrease in the depth of anaesthesia. When injected into the soft tissues, all LAA cause vasodilatation except cocaine which causes vasoconstriction.

DISTRIBUTION

Once the drug enters the circulatory system, the blood vessels transmit the drug throughout the body. The distribution percentage of the drug is dependent on the percentage of cardiac output received by the organ. Higher perfusion of blood is seen in areas such as the brain, head, liver, kidneys, lungs and spleen while there are other organs that have less blood perfusion. It has been observed that LAA that are distributed to the skeletal muscles having lower blood perfusion contain the maximum concentration of drug compared to these organs. This is because it constitutes the larger proportion of the body. Level of concentration of the drug in blood depends on:

1. Rate at which the drug is absorbed into cardiovascular system (CVS)
2. Rate at which the drug is distributed from vasculature to tissue
3. Elimination of the drug through excretion. 'Elimination half-life (t1/2)'.

All LAA can cross the blood–brain barrier and the placenta to the growing foetus.

BIOTRANSFORMATION

BIOTRANSFORMATION OF ESTERS

Esters are hydrolysed in the plasma by pseudo-cholinesterase enzyme and in the liver by the esterase enzyme. The clinician should consider patients with *plasma pseudo-cholinesterase enzyme deficiency* (1 out of 2500) as they can have high toxic blood levels, if injected with ester-linked local anaesthetics. In normal patients, the rate of hydrolysis of the drug can influence the toxic levels of the drug. Slower hydrolysis can increase drug level toxicity.

BIOTRANSFORMATION OF AMIDES

The liver is the primary site of metabolism of amide local anaesthetic drug by hepatic microsomal enzymes. The entire metabolic process occurs in the liver for lidocaine, mepivacaine, articaine, bupivacaine and etidocaine. Prilocaine is metabolised in the liver and lung. Articaine is metabolised in the blood and liver. Liver function and perfusion play an important role and the clinician must consider those with hypotension, Congestive heart failure (CHF), liver cirrhosis and conditions where hepatic blood flow is compromised as the intermediate products of metabolism can cause complications. Prilocaine metabolite, *orthotoluidine* can cause *methaemoglobinaemia* by inducing formation of *methaemoglobin*. Lidocaine metabolites, monoethyl glycine xylidide, and *xylidide* can cause *sedation* by accumulating in the system.

EXCRETION

Kidneys are the primary excretory organs for all the metabolites and an unchanged proportion of the local anaesthetic agent. Smaller percentage of parent molecules of ester anaesthetics are excreted unchanged, and a larger percentage of unchanged form of amide drugs are excreted. Renal impairment causes accumulation of the drug and its metabolites causing toxicity.

PHARMACODYNAMICS—EFFECTS OF THE LOCAL ANAESTHETIC AGENT

SYSTEMIC EFFECTS OF LOCAL ANAESTHETIC SOLUTION

CARDIOVASCULAR SYSTEM

Local anaesthetics decrease electrical excitability of the myocardium, conduction rate and force of contraction. All these factors combined can result in myocardial depression (more than 2 μg/mL). At a dose of 1.5–5 μg/mL, it has antiarrhythmic activity. It can be used as a potent drug for ventricular tachycardia, ventricular premature contractions and in cardiac arrest from ventricular fibrillation.

BLOOD VESSELS

Local anaesthetics at the site of injection cause vasodilatation of the blood vessels except for cocaine, which produces vasoconstriction. Vasodilation decreases the duration of action of the local anaesthetic and prolongs the onset time. Thus, decreasing the depth of anaesthesia. It primarily produces hypotension (at a level approaching overdose) due to depression of the myocardium and smooth muscle relaxation of the vessel wall. At lethal levels, it causes cardiovascular collapse.

CENTRAL NERVOUS SYSTEM (CNS)

At low levels, there is no significant effect. Further increase in the dose causes CNS depression, and respiratory arrest as a result of respiratory depression. Lidocaine causes CNS depression at toxic levels (Table 11.9).

RESPIRATORY SYSTEM

At nonoverdose levels, it has a relaxant effect on bronchial smooth muscles, suppresses the cough reflex during laryngoscopy, endotracheal intubation, extubation and bronchoscopy. Overdose leads to respiratory arrest as a result of respiratory centre depression (CNS depression).

Refer page number 194 for overdose and 195 for toxicity.

ABSOLUTE AND RELATIVE CONTRAINDICATIONS OF LOCAL ANAESTHESIA

Absolute and relative contraindications of local anaesthesia is described in Table 11.10.

CLINICAL ACTION OF SPECIFIC AGENTS

Most common local anaesthetic agents (lidocaine, bupivacaine, mepivacaine, cocaine) and newer agents (articaine, centbucridine, ropivacaine, etidocaine) with improved efficacy and safety are discussed below.

TABLE 11.9 CNS Effects of LAA at Normal and Toxic Dosages

Below 0.5 µg/mL	No CNS Effects
At 0.5–4 µg/mL—anticonvulsive action	Due to their depressant action on the CNS, local anaesthetics raise the seizure threshold by decreasing the hyperexcitability of the cortical neurons from where the convulsive episodes originate.
At 4.5–7 µg/mL—preseizure signs and symptoms	Preseizure signs and symptoms include slurred speech, shivering, tremor, warm flushed feeling of the skin, light headedness, dizziness, drowsiness, visual disturbance, auditory disturbance, etc.
At 7.5–10 µg/mL—convulsive action	At this dose, lidocaine causes tonic–clonic seizure. Seizure continues as long as the drug is present in the blood. The duration of presence of local anaesthesia in blood is further increased by increased blood flow to the brain. Increased cerebral metabolism also leads to progressive metabolic acidosis, which prolongs the seizure activity.

TABLE 11.10 Absolute and Relative Contraindications of LA Drugs

Absolute Contraindications of LA		
Medical contraindication	Avoid	Replace with
Ether allergy	Ether LAA	Amide LAA
Amide allergy	Amide LAA	Ether LAA
Bisulphite allergy	LA + vasoconstrictor	Plain LA
Sulphur allergy	Articaine	Nonsulphur types
Relative Contraindications of LA		
Atypical cholinesterase	Ether	Amide
Methaemoglobinaemia	Prilocaine and articaine	Lidocaine, etc.
Severe liver disease and congestive heart failure (ASA III–IV)	Amides	Either esters or amides (reduce the dose)
Severe kidney disease (ASA III–IV)	Amides and esters	Either esters or amides (reduce the dose)
Severe cardiovascular disease (ASA III–IV)	Excess vasoconstrictors	Plain anaesthesia or with vasoconstrictor (low dose)
Severe thyrotoxicosis (ASA III–IV)	Excess vasoconstrictors	Plain anaesthesia or with vasoconstrictors (low dose)

LIDOCAINE HYDROCHLORIDE (HCL) (NILS LÖFGREN, 1943)

OTHER NAMES: Octacaine, dentocaine.

BRAND NAMES: Xylocaine, lignocaine, biocaine, LOX solution.

POTENCY: 1 (gold standard for comparison) (in the past, lidocaine = 2, procaine = 1, was used in the past before discovery of lidocaine).

It was the 1st nonester type of LAA used in dentistry, as it can be stored in room temperature with a long shelf life. It has replaced procaine in the past and is the most common amide type of LAA used in dental practice. Thus, becoming the gold standard drug with which all new anaesthetics are compared. It is heat stable and can withstand autoclaving. It is used in treating operative pain and diagnosing neurologic pain. In India, 2% lidocaine plain and with 1:80,000 or 1:200,000 concentrations with adrenaline are most commonly available.

MECHANISM OF ACTION: Lidocaine causes conduction blockade by blocking the voltage-gated sodium (Na^+) channels in the cell membrane. With sufficient blockade, the membrane of the presynaptic neuron will not undergo depolarisation, that is lidocaine blocks the sodium channel preventing sodium influx into the cell. This fails to transmit an action potential. Loss of formation of an action potential prevents the stimulus from travelling to the brain through the nerve cell. Thus, the pain stimulus fails to reach the thalamus and the subsequent somatosensory cortex where pain is processed from the trigeminal nerve.

BIOTRANSFORMATION: The half-life of lidocaine is 90–120 min in most patients. This may be prolonged in patients with hepatic impairment because lidocaine metabolises in the liver (p450 system). These metabolites can cause sedation when it accumulates in the blood. It is completely eliminated by the kidney after about 9 h, of which, 10% of the drug remains in an unchanged form and 80% is eliminated in the form of the aforementioned metabolites.

PHARMACOLOGY: The pH is 6.5, while the pH of the solution with vasoconstrictor is ~3.5. It has a dissociation constant of 7.85 (pKa) and a rapid onset as it diffuses through the bi-lipid layer of the nerve easily. It has a rapid onset of action (3–5 min). Half-life of lidocaine is 90 min.

PHARMACOKINETICS:

Lidocaine on CNS: At adequate drug levels, lidocaine blocks conduction around the targeted nerve, but higher doses can initially cause drowsiness and lethargy followed by excitation and then depression.

Lidocaine on CVS: Decreases electrical excitability of myocardium, conduction rate and force of contraction. Used to treat dysrhythmias.

Lidocaine on blood vessels: Vasodilation occurs at the injected area.

DURATION OF ACTION: The duration of action of various forms of lidocaine is described in Table 11.11.

CLINICAL USES:

In general anaesthesia, to blunt the stress response to intubation, prior to laryngoscopy, 2% lidocaine can be sprayed into the trachea. During induction of G.A., 2 mL of 2% lidocaine in 10 mL of propofol can be added to reduce the pain during intravenous injection of propofol. Plain lidocaine is used in these settings.

In invasive dental procedures and oral surgery: Deep fillings, RCT, extraction, flap surgery, other minor surgical procedures and major surgeries under G.A., 2% lidocaine is used topically or as infiltrations or as nerve

TABLE 11.11 Duration of Action of Lidocaine Based on the Route of Administration

Agent/Route	Duration of Action	Comments
i.v. injection	15–30 min (for arrythmias)	
i.v. regional anaesthesia (limbs)	Tourniquet time (Bier's block)	25% less drug used
Peripheral nerve block	1 h without epinephrine/3 h with epinephrine	
Pulpal anaesthesia—2% lignocaine without vasoconstrictor	Provides 5–10 min	Increased adverse reactions seen
2% Lignocaine with 1: 50,000 concentration of adrenaline	Provides 60 min of pulpal and 3–5 h of soft tissue anaesthesia	Primarily used for haemostasis at the surgical site
2% Lignocaine with 1:200,000 adrenaline	Provides 60 min of pulpal and 3–5 h of soft tissue anaesthesia	Recommended formulation used for dental practice
Topical mucosal gel 2% lidocaine (LOX)	10–15 min	The onset of action is 3–5 min. It is ineffective when applied to intact skin.
EMLA (eutectic mixture of local anaesthesia)—it is a mixture of lignocaine and prilocaine formed into an ointment	Variable in each individual approximately 5–45 min	It is applied 60 min prior to insertion of cannula, needle, anaesthetising intact skin or under occlusive dressing

blocks. Topical lidocaine is used to numb pain of ulcers and to reduce pain before injecting into the soft tissues. The commonly used concentration in the dental setting is 1:200,000 ratios with adrenaline.

As an antiarrhythmic drug: When amiodarone is not available or is contraindicated, lidocaine (i.v.) is used intravenously for the treatment of ventricular arrhythmias. It should be given only after defibrillation, CPR and vasopressors have already been initiated.

MAXIMUM RECOMMENDED DOSAGE OF ADULTS BY ADA: 4.4 mg/kg body weight.

CONCENTRATION OF LIDOCAINE:

Lidocaine solutions are available in 0.5%, 1%, 1.5% and 2%. These contain lidocaine hydrochloride at 5, 10, 15 and 20 mg/mL, respectively. Solutions with epinephrine contain 1:100,000 or 1:200,000 concentration of epinephrine.

LIDOCAINE CONTRAINDICATIONS:

- Second or 3rd degree heart block (without pacemaker)
- Serious adverse drug reaction to lidocaine or amide local anaesthetics
- When patient is under treatment with class I antiarrhythmic agents. These drugs can inhibit the enzyme—cytochrome P450 leading to an increase in blood levels of lidocaine.

MRD WITH AND WITHOUT ADRENALINE

MRD with and without adrenaline are depicted in Table 11.12

TABLE 11.12 MRD with and without Adrenaline for all Important Anaesthetic Agents

Agent	MRD Calculation	Maximum Cartridge and mL Calculation	
	Facts to be memorised have been typed in bold	To calculate number of cartridges (multiply mg/mL by 1.8)	
Plain 2% lidocaine	Plain 2% lidocaine (2% means that there is 2 g of lidocaine in 100 mL of solution) = 2 g in 100 mL = 2000 mg in 100 mL = 20 mg/mL	**1 cartridge = 1.8 mL** (Per cartridge contains 20 × 1.8 = 36 mg) = 36 mg/cartridge	
	Maximum dosage of lidocaine = 4.4 mg/kg	How many cartridges can be used? (300/36) = 8.3 cartridges	What is the MRD in mL that can be given? (300/20) = 15 mL
	(A normal healthy male weight (70 kg) (4.4 × 70) = 300 mg is the maximum recommended dose of lignocaine		
2% Lidocaine with 1:200,000 concentration epinephrine	2% Lidocaine with 1:200,000 concentration epinephrine **Maximum dosage of lidocaine with adrenaline = 7 mg/kg**	How many cartridges can be used? (490/36) = 13.6 cartridges	What is the MRD in mL that can be given? (490/20) = 24.5 mL
	A normal healthy male weight (70 kgs) (7 mg × 70) = 490 mg		
	Safe dose of adrenaline for ASA I (healthy individual) = 0.2 mg/visit	Maximum volume of plain adrenaline at 1:200,000 is 40 mL (~15 mL is a buffer). The MRD of epinephrine will not be exhausted when we use only 24.5 mL of lidocaine with adrenaline at 1:200,000 concentration	
	Safe dose in cardiac disease ASA III or ASA IV (one-fifth dosage of ASA I, i.e. healthy individual) (0.2/5) **= 0.04 mg/visit**	Maximum volume of plain adrenaline at 1:200,000 is 8 mL (~15 mL is a buffer). The MRD of epinephrine will not be exhausted when we use only 24.5 mL of lidocaine with adrenaline at 1:200,000 concentration	
3% Mepivacaine	**5.5 mg/kg**	**400 mg maximum for a person**	
0.5% Bupivacaine with adrenaline	**1.3 mg/kg**	**90 mg maximum for a person**	
4% Articaine	**7 mg/kg**	**500 mg maximum for a person**	

The technique to calculate has also been explained in steps. (The facts to be memorised have been highlighted in bold)

MRD FOR VARIOUS BODY WEIGHT

The dosage of lidocaine for adults is 4.4 mg/kg (plain) and 7 mg/kg (with adrenaline).

But for paediatric patients, the dosage should be calculated using Young's formula, which is based on age or using Clark's rule, which is based on weight. For infants up to 2 years old (24 months), Fried's rule can be followed.

Clark's Rule:

$$\frac{\text{Weight (lb)} \times \text{adult dose}}{150}$$

Young's Rule:

(For children 2 years and above):

$$\frac{\left(\text{Age}\left(\text{yr}\right)\right) \times \text{adult dose}}{\text{Age}\left(\text{yr}\right) + 12}$$

Fried's Rule:

(For infants up to 2 years old):

$$\frac{\left(\text{Age}\left(\text{month}\right)\right) \times \text{adult dose}}{150}$$

TOXICITY OF LIGNOCAINE: Toxicity of local anaesthetics will be discussed in detail in systemic complications of local anaesthesia (page number 201).

Toxicity of lidocaine can be remembered with the pneumonic **'SAMS'**.

S—Slurred speech; difficulty to talk due to paraesthesia of lips and tongue.

A—Altered CNS; patient presents with drowsiness, dizziness, restlessness, confusion and arrythmias.

M—Muscle twitching; tremors.

S—Siezures; convulsions, respiratory depression, respiratory and cardiac arrest (Fig. 11.7).

OTHER LOCAL ANAESTHETIC AGENTS (TABLE 11.13)

PHARMACOLOGY OF VASOCONSTRICTORS

WHY DO WE NEED TO ADD A VASOCONSTRICTOR TO THE LOCAL ANAESTHETIC AGENT?

LAA are vasodilators. This results in increased and fast absorption of the solution into the bloodstream, thereby increasing its toxicity and reducing the duration of local anaesthetic effect. The duration of local anaesthetics activity is also decreased and bleeding at the site of administration is increased. The addition of epinephrine in the LAA overcomes all these drawbacks as it causes vasoconstriction of the local blood vessels, but local anaesthesia without epinephrine is more active than the same agent with epinephrine because the pH of solutions with epinephrine is less (3.3), when compared to the pH of solutions without epinephrine (5.5) (Table 11.14).

CLASSIFICATION OF VASOCONSTRICTORS

Vasoconstrictors used in local anaesthetics can be classified based on chemical structure and mode of action (Tables 11.15 and 11.16). Catecholamines are chemically identical to

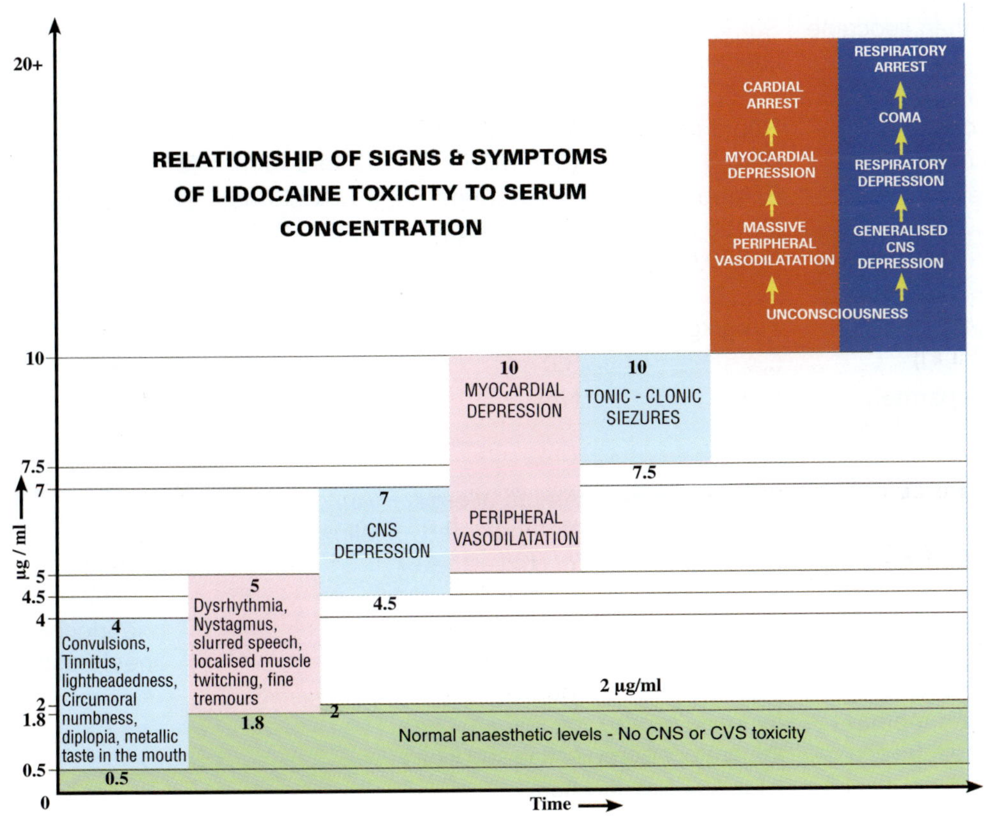

Figure 11.7 The dose related progressive symptoms and systemic effect of local anaesthetics have been illustrated in the graph. Dose up to 2 µg/mL is normal dose shown in green. Doses above this are shown in pink and blue colours. Pink depicts CVS symptoms and blue depicts CNS symptoms. The dark red shows the CVS effect of doses above 20 µg/mL and dark blue shows CNS effect of the same leading to respiratory arrest.

TABLE 11.13 Various Local Anaesthetic Agents and their Properties

Feature	Mepivacaine	Prilocaine	Articaine	Bupivacaine	Etidocaine	Procaine
Salient features	Best for short procedures as it is the least vasodilating	Used in dentistry combined with lidocaine as a dermal anaesthetic (EMLA). Used for intravenous regional anaesthesia (IVRA) as it has low cardiac toxicity. Since it comes in combination with a dilute form of epinephrine (1:200,000) ASA III and IV patients can receive up to four cartridges.	Articaine is able to diffuse through soft and hard tissues more reliably than other local anaesthetics. So maxillary buccal infiltration for one tooth can provide palatal anaesthesia also.	Bupivacaine is indicated for long dental procedures for which deep anaesthesia more than 90 min is necessary. It is also used for the management of postoperative pain following a surgical procedure providing a pain free period of up to 12 h.	Etidocaine is an injectable LAA used in general surgery and OB/GYN. It has a long duration of action, but has the disadvantage of increased bleeding during **oral surgery**.	Procaine is used with penicillin to reduce the pain of intramuscular injection of penicillin. Used as intraarticular injection to stop arteriospasm. Not used in dentistry after introduction of lidocaine.
Type of LAA	Amide	Amide	Amide	Amide	Amide	Ester
Potency	Same as lidocaine	Same as lidocaine	It is 1.5 times that of lidocaine	Four times potent than lidocaine	Four times potent than lidocaine	Potency = one weak anaesthetic agent
Metabolism	Liver	Liver, kidney and lung	Plasma	Liver	Liver	Plasma pseudocholinesterase
Excretion	Kidneys	Kidneys, faster than any amides	Kidneys	Kidneys	Kidneys	Kidney
Vasodilating properties	Less than lidocaine	Less than lidocaine	Same as lidocaine	More than lidocaine	More than lidocaine	Highest vasodilatation of all agents
Onset of action	Rapid (1.5–2 min)	Fast onset (3–5 min)	Rapid onset (2 to 3 min)	Moderate (5–8 min)	Rapid onset (2 to 3 min)	Moderate (6–10 min)
Vasoconstrictor used	Levonordephrin (1:20,000) or epinephrine (1:100,000)	Epinephrine (1:200,000)	Epinephrine (1:100,000) (1:200,000)	Epinephrine (1:200,000)	Epinephrine (1:200,000)	Epinephrine (1:50,000)
MRD mg/kg	4.4 mg/kg	6 mg/kg	7 mg/kg	1.3 mg/kg	8 mg/kg	
pH (with VC)	3.5	4.0	5.4	3.0	3.0	3.5–5.5
Topical	N/A	N/A separately EMLA with lidocaine	N/A	N/A	N/A	N/A
Contraindication	Amide allergy	Idiopathic or congenital methaemoglobinaemia, sickle cell anaemia, cardiac or respiratory failure due to elevated methaemoglobin levels	Should not be used in pt. with para group (sulphur containing drug) allergy, because it contains hydroxyl group. In para position.	Amide allergy Not indicated for children below 12 and for mentally handicapped due to increased risk of self-inflicted soft tissue injury	Amide allergy	1. Ester allergy 2. Patients with altered pseudocholinesterase

N/A- not available, VC- vasoconstrictor. Refer to Chapter 12 for ASA classification.

TABLE 11.14 Effects of LA without Vasoconstrictor versus with Vasoconstrictor

Effects	Local Anaesthetic without Vasoconstrictor	Local Anaesthetic with Vasoconstrictor
Absorption rate	↑ absorption of LA into CVS → faster removal from injection site	Constriction of blood vessels → slower removal from injection site
Duration of action and depth of anaesthesia	Rapid diffusion of LA from injection site ↓ ↓ duration of action and depth of anaesthesia	Higher volume of LA around nerve ↓ ↑ duration of action
Risk of toxicity	Higher plasma level of LA → ↑ risk of toxicity	Slow absorption into CVS → low anaesthetic blood level → ↓ risk of toxicity
Bleeding	↑ bleeding at injection site	↓ bleeding at injection site
Pain control	No difference in pain control	
Wound healing	No changes in wound healing seen	Delayed wound healing is seen in some patients who underwent treatment with LA + adrenaline

TABLE 11.15 Classification of Vasoconstrictors based on Chemical Structure

Catecholamines	Noncatecholamines
Epinephrine (natural)	Amphetamine
Norepinephrine (natural)	Methamphetamine
Levonordefrin (synthetic)	Ephedrine
Isoproterenol (synthetic)	Mephentermine
Dopamine (natural)	Hydroxyamphetamine, metaraminol, methoxamine, phenylephrine

TABLE 11.16 Classification of Vasoconstrictors Based on Mode of Action

Direct-Acting Drugs	Indirect-Acting Drugs	Mixed-Acting Drugs
Epinephrine Norepinephrine Levonordefrin Isoproterenol Dopamine Methoxamine Phenylephrine	Tyramine Amphetamine Methamphetamine Hydroxyamphetamine	Metaraminol Ephedrine

sympathetic nervous system mediators (neurotransmitters). Chemical structure is related to catechol nucleus, if an amine group is attached to the aliphatic side, it is classified as a catecholamine. They are either naturally occurring or synthetic catecholamines.

Based on mode of action, the vasoconstrictors can be classified as direct acting drugs that act directly on the adrenergic receptors, the indirect acting drugs that act by releasing norepinephrine from adrenergic nerve terminals and the mixed acting drugs that act in both ways, directly on receptors and through release of norepinephrine.

Amphetamine or tyramine act indirectly and causes release of norepinephrine from storage in nerve terminals. Repeated doses of drug are less effective due to depletion of norepinephrine, this state is called tachyphylaxis.

SYSTEMIC EFFECTS OF VASOCONSTRICTORS

CARDIOVASCULAR SYSTEM

It increases cardiac output, stroke volume, systolic and diastolic blood pressure, heart rate, myocardial oxygen consumption and force of myocardial contraction (leads to decreased cardiac efficiency).

BLOOD VESSELS

Small capillaries contain α receptors. Vasoconstrictors can cause vasoconstriction when it binds with α receptors (Box 11.2). However, in large blood vessels supplying skeletal muscles (which contain both alpha and beta receptors), β-2-receptor activity predominates in small doses and alpha receptor activity predominates in larger doses.

RESPIRATORY SYSTEM

It causes bronchodilation of smooth muscles of the bronchioles (β 2 effect).

CENTRAL NERVOUS SYSTEM

In therapeutic doses, vasoconstrictors have no effect on the CNS, but in excessive dose, it acts as a CNS stimulant.

METABOLISMS

It stimulates glycogenolysis in the liver and skeletal muscles, thereby increasing blood sugar level. It increases oxygen consumption in the tissues.

BOX 11.2 Adrenergic Receptors

These receptors are found in most tissues of the body, they are the Alpha (α) and Beta (β) receptors.

Alpha receptors: Alpha receptors are activated by sympathomimetic drug. It causes vasoconstriction by contraction of smooth muscle in the blood vessel.

Two types of α receptors:

- α1 receptors
- α2 receptors

Beta receptors:

- β1-Found in heart and intestines → increased heart rate and strength of contraction.
- β2-Found in bronchi, vascular beds, uterus → bronchodilation and vasodilation.

Rebound Vasodilatation

The action of epinephrine on α receptors is vasoconstriction, this occurs when an optimal dose of adrenaline is present as this dosage can only stimulate the α receptors. But when the plasma level of adrenaline decreases, the lower dose stimulates β2 receptors that cause vasodilatation. This phenomenon is called rebound vasodilatation. This reverse dilation can cause increased bleeding. The rebound vasodilatation causes postoperative bleeding 6 h after injection.

DILUTION OF VASOCONSTRICTORS

The concentration of vasoconstrictor is expressed in ratios. The concentration of vasoconstrictor in 1:1000 means that there is 1 g (1000 mg) of vasoconstrictor in 1000 mL (1 L) of solution, or in other words 1 mg/mL or 1000 μg/mL. 1:1000 is more concentrated than 1:100,000, which contains only 0.01 mg/mL or 10 μg/mL. The dosage of epinephrine in various concentrations are depicted in Fig. 11.8. Vasoconstrictors need to be used in much diluted forms for dental anaesthesia. To produce these dilutions, the illustration in Fig. 11.9A and B can be followed.

The 1:80,000 concentration contains 12.5 μg/mL (0.0123 mg/mL) as shown in Fig. 11.9. It was used for dentistry in the past, but studies have shown the efficacy of 1:200,000 concentration and this is preferred now. The 1:200,000 concentration contains 0.005 mg/mL of epinephrine (i.e. 5 μg/mL). This concentration has provided comparable results and with fewer systemic side effects, thus, it is widely used and accepted in dentistry.

SELECTION OF VASOCONSTRICTOR

Factors for selection of vasoconstrictor:

- Length of dental appointment—need to prolong duration and depth of anaesthesia.
- Requirement for haemostasis.

Concentration ↑		Dosage ↓
1:1000	1 mg/ml	1000 μg/ml
1:10,000	0.1 mg/ml	100 μg/ml
1:50,000	0.02 mg/ml	20 μg/ml
1:80,000	0.0125 mg/ml	12.5 μg/ml
1:1,00,000	0.01 mg/ml	10 μg/ml
1:2,00,000	0.005 mg/ml	5 μg/ml
1:10,00,000	0.001 mg/ml	1 μg/ml

Figure 11.8 The concentration of dilution of vasoconstrictors and their subsequent dosage in mg/mL and μg/mL have been illustrated. The relationship between concentration and dosage has been depicted by the direction of the arrows.

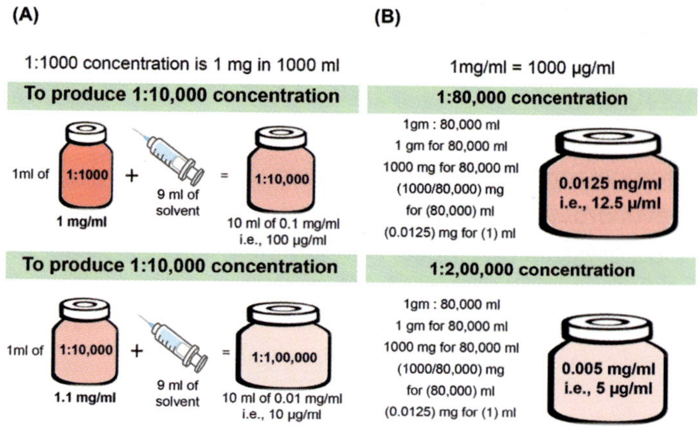

Figure 11.9 (**A**) The illustration shows how 1:10,000 and 1:100,000 dilutions of vasoconstrictor is obtained from 1:1000 dilution of vasoconstrictor. (**B**) The commonly used concentrations of vasoconstrictors in dentistry are shown with calculation of dose/mL according to the concentration.

- Vasoconstriction with rebound vasodilation.
- Medical status of patient—risk versus benefit must be evaluated.

EPINEPHRINE OR ADRENALINE

The drug has been summarised in Table 11.17.

OTHER VASOCONSTRICTORS USED WITH LOCAL ANAESTHETIC AGENTS (TABLE 11.18)

MAXIMUM SAFE DOSAGE OF VASOCONSTRICTORS

The most commonly accepted concentration of adrenaline 1:200,000 in LA. A concentration of 1:100,000 is acceptable in certain countries. The maximum dosage of epinephrine in a healthy adult weighing 70 kg is 0.2 mg/mL, that is 200 μg/mL.

TABLE 11.17 The Most Commonly Used Vasoconstrictor, Epinephrine, in Dental LA has been Summarised

	Epinephrine
Proprietary name	Adrenaline
Biosynthesis in the human body	In the chromaffin cells of adrenal medulla and postganglionic nerve fibres
Source of drug	Natural form and synthetic form
Chemical properties	Available as a HCL acid salt Highly soluble in water They are stable when they do not come in contact with air or metal ions Sodium bisulphite is added as a preservative to increase the shelf-life
Mode of action	Powerful stimulant of both α and β adrenergic receptors
Sympathomimetic reactions	Apprehension, tachycardia, sweating, heart palpitation
Reaction to intravascular injection (positive aspiration)	Increase in heart rate of 25–70 beats per minute Elevation in BP 2 to 70 mmHg Rhythm disturbances Premature ventricular contractions (PVCs)
Cardiovascular dynamics	↑ Systolic BP ↑ diastolic BP ↑ Cardiac output ↑ Stroke volume ↑ Heart rate ↑ Strength of contraction ↑ Myocardial demand for oxygen ↓ ↓ Overall efficiency of cardiac function
Vasculature	α Receptor stimulation—vasoconstriction of vessels in skin, mucous membranes, kidneys β2 Receptors—vasodilation α1 Receptors—vasoconstriction
Haemostasis	Epinephrine is used for vasoconstriction
Respiratory system	Potent beta 2 stimulation—bronchodilation—bronchiolar smooth muscles get relaxed
CNS	Epinephrine is not a potent CNS stimulant Overdose: CNS stimulation: Increasing fear, tension and anxiety Muscle tension, tremors, weakness Dizziness, pallor, palpitation and respiratory difficulty
MRD	Typical concentrations of LA + epinephrine is not contraindicated The clinician has to adhere to the following: • Aspiration is mandatory • Inject slowly • Smallest effective dose administered • Maximum dose limited to 0.2 mg per appointment

Therefore various dilutions will have different maximum volumes that can be injected into the patient. This has been summarised in Table 11.19.

CONTRAINDICATIONS OF LA WITH ADRENALINE

1. It should not be used in proximity to end arteries in the following locations: Fingers, toes, penis, nose tip, ear lobules
2. In patients with allergy to sulphites. Sulphite sensitivity can be caused by the antioxidant added to the solution to preserve epinephrine
3. During general anaesthesia (GA), with agents such as cyclopropane or halothane as these may sensitise the heart to arrhythmic action of sympathomimetic drugs
4. Pregnancy:
   a. Vasoconstrictors can stimulate uterine contractions

TABLE 11.18 The Other Vasoconstrictors that are Used With LA have been Compared and Summarised

Generic Name	Norepinephrine or Noradrenalin	Levonordephrin	Felypressin
Systemic actions	CVS: ↑ Systolic BP ↑ Diastolic BP ↑ Mean arterial pressure ↓ Heart rate Stimulates the pacemaker cells Blood vessels: Coronary arteries—vasodilatation Cutaneous vessels—vasoconstriction Respiratory system: α induced constriction of lung arterioles (not used for management of bronchospasm) CNS: Normal doses—no action on CNS Overdose—stimulates CNS	Resembles norepinephrine but to a lesser degree	CVS: No effect on myocardium No effect on pacemaker cells Blood vessels: High dose impairs blood flow through coronary arteries Cutaneous vessels—high doses—vasoconstriction CNS: No effect on CNS Pregnancy: Antidiuretic and oxytocic action (contraindicated in pregnancy)
Clinical action	As vasoconstrictor for LA To manage hypotension	As vasoconstrictor for LA	As vasoconstrictor for LA
Maximum dose	ASA I—0.34 mg/visit ASA III or IV—0.14 mg/visit	ASA I—1 mg/visit ASA III or IV—0.2 mg/visit	ASA III or IV—0.03 IU (0.54µg/ml)

TABLE 11.19 The Maximum Volume in mL, the Maximum Number of Cartridges, the Maximum Dosage in mg/mL and µg/mL of Epinephrine and Levonordefrin

Vasoconstrictor		Epinephrine/adrenaline		
Dilution with distilled water		1:80,000	1:100,000	1:200,000
Maximum dosage in **ASA I** (healthy individual)	Max. volume (mL)	16 mL	20 mL	40 mL
	Max. no. of cartridges (1 cartridge = 1.8 mL)	8 cartridges	11 cartridges	22 cartridges
	mg/visit	0.2 mg/visit		
	µg/visit	200 µg/visit		
Maximum dosage in **ASA II** (1/2 the dosage of ASA I, i.e. healthy individual)	Max. volume (mL)	8 mL	10 mL	20 mL
	Max. no. of cartridges (1 cartridge = 1.8 mL)	4 cartridges	5.5 cartridges	11 cartridges
	mg/visit	0.1 mg/visit		
	µg/visit	100 µg/visit		
Maximum dosage in cardiac disease **ASA III or ASA IV** (one-fifth dosage of ASA I, i.e. healthy individual)	Max. volume (mL)	3.2 mL	4 mL	8 mL
	Max. no. of Cartridges (1 cartridge = 1.8 mL)	1.6 cartridges	2 cartridges	4 cartridges
	mg/visit	0.04 mg/visit		
	µg/visit	40 µg/visit		

The maximum volumes and cartridges in dilutions with **distilled water** at 1:80 k, 1:1 lac and 1:2 lac have also been added as they are the most commonly used dilutions in dentistry. It is important to understand that the maximum volume or cartridge mentioned in this table is only for plain epinephrine in solution without a local anaesthetic. The maximum dosage of LA with adrenaline will be much lesser than the volumes mentioned in this table. Maximum volume of plain adrenaline at 1:200,000 concentration with distilled water is 40 mL. The MRD of lidocaine with adrenaline (1:200,000) is 24.5 mL. The MRD of epinephrine will not be exhausted when we use only 24.5 mL of lidocaine with adrenaline at 1:200,000 concentration.

5. Antidepressant drugs:
   a. Patient on tricyclic antidepressants have greater risk of dysrhythmias
   b. Patients on monoamine oxidase inhibitors
   c. Patient on phenothiazines with epinephrine may cause postural hypotension
6. Uncontrolled endocrine disorders:
   a. Patient with unstable diabetes (epinephrine causes glycogenolysis, hyperglycaemia and ketoacidosis)
   b. Thyrotoxicosis
   c. Hyperthyroid state
7. CVS and vascular disorders:
   a. Patient on nonselective beta blockers
   b. Patient is unstable—active angina
   c. Patient with recent Myocardial infarction (MI)/ Coronary artery bypass graft (CABG)
   d. Patient with severe hypertension (HTN) or untreated HTN [contraindicated if uncontrolled (over 170 systolic)]
   e. Patient with uncontrolled CHF, strokes and ischaemic heart disease.

LOCAL ANAESTHETICS AND VASOCONSTRICTOR—DRUG INTERACTIONS

Drug interactions of local anaesthetics and vasoconstrictor is described in Table 11.20.

TABLE 11.20 LA and Vasoconstrictor With Other Drugs

LA/vasoconstrictor—Drug Interaction	Clinical Symptoms and Significance	Caution or Treatment
Combination interaction with other LAA (**combination of LAA**)	Combined dose if excess can cause toxicity	MRD of each drug should be calculated
Vasoconstrictor and tricyclic antidepressants **Levonordefrin—amitriptyline**	In patients with major depression who take TCA enhances cardiovascular action of levonordefrin	Avoid using vasoconstrictors
Vasoconstrictors and β blocker **Propranolol—epinephrine**	↑ BP Reflexive bradycardia	Monitor BP and other vitals. Shift to ER. Use LA without adrenaline
Vasoconstrictor with hydrocarbon inhalation anaesthetic **Halothane or enflurane—epinephrine**	Cardiac dysrhythmias	Discuss with anaesthetist before administration of LA
Vasoconstrictor with cocaine	Can result in cardiac arrest	Avoid using vasoconstrictors in cocaine users
CNS depressants like **Alcohol** **Antidepressants** **Antihistamines** **Benzodiazepines** **Opioids** **Antipsychotics**	Overdose effects of CNS Respiratory depression	Limit dosage of LA
Methaemoglobianemia **Prilocaine overdose**	Patient presents with cyanosis that does not reverse on presentation of O_2	Use minimal dose of prilocaine. Patients shows symptoms only after 3 to 4 h. i.v. Methylene blue or intravenous (i.v.) or intramuscular (i.m.) ascorbic acid
Congenital methaemoglobianemia **Prilocaine normal dose**	Brown colour arterial blood Chocolate brown colour gingival venous blood	
Vasoconstrictor with antipsychotic (α—adrenoceptor blocker) **Phenoxybenzamine, haloperidol, thioridazine**	Hypotension	Use vasoconstrictors with caution
Inhibitors of metabolism—amide LAA **Cimetidine—lidocaine**	Cimetidine is a H_2 receptor blocker that can modify biotransformation of lidocaine	Use LA cautiously, ASA III patients—toxicity. Use minimum dose of LA

Continued

TABLE 11.20 LA and Vasoconstrictor With Other Drugs—cont'd

LA/vasoconstrictor—Drug Interaction	Clinical Symptoms and Significance	Caution or Treatment
Sulfonamides—esters	Esters inhibit sulfonamides action. Infection will not subside	Avoid ester anaesthetics in patients taking sulfonamides
Vasoconstrictor—**monoamine oxidase inhibitor (MAOI)**	MAOI are used in major depression, phobic-anxiety, OCDs Increases the vasoconstrictor action	Avoid or use vasoconstrictors minimally

Interaction, clinical symptoms and caution or treatment have been discussed in the order of significance. Clinical significance score is higher for the drug interactions mentioned above compared to below.

ARMAMENTARIUM USED IN LOCAL ANAESTHESIA

SYRINGE

STANDARD OF A SYRINGE

The gold standard syringes are the aspirating dental syringes. Their ability to aspirate blood if the tip of the needle is located intravascularly is crucial as we administer LA agent, which can have systemic effects.

ADA GUIDELINES FOR INJECTION SYRINGES

1. It should be made with a durable material and can withstand repeated sterilisation without damage
2. It should be compatible with cartridges and needles from different manufacturers
3. It should allow repeated use
4. It should be inexpensive
5. It should be lightweight and simple to use with one hand
6. It should have a simple aspiration technique
7. It should allow visibility of cartridge, so blood can be seen through the glass cartridge.

TYPES

1. Nondisposable or reusable syringes
2. Disposable syringes
3. Safety syringes.

NONDISPOSABLE TYPES OF SYRINGES (FIG. 11.10)

1. Breech-loading, metallic, cartridge, aspirating-type

This is the most widely used syringe for dentistry in the United States, United Kingdom, European countries. In breech-loading syringes, the dental cartridge is loaded from the side of the syringe. To inject the solution, a needle is attached to the barrel of the syringe at the needle adaptor. This needle passes into the barrel and pierces the diaphragm of the local anaesthetic cartridge. The harpoon is a sharp tip that is attached to the piston or plunger. It penetrates the cartridge's thick silicon rubber stopper, known as the bung at the back of the cartridge. To aspirate, negative pressure is applied to the thumb ring. If blood enters the glass local anaesthetic cartridge, it is called a positive aspiration. The tip of the needle has entered into the lumen of a blood vessel. The needle should be removed from the tissues and the cartridge must be discarded. The clinician must try again with a new cartridge. These syringes use the elasticity of the rubber diaphragm in the anaesthetic cartridge to obtain the necessary negative pressure for aspiration.

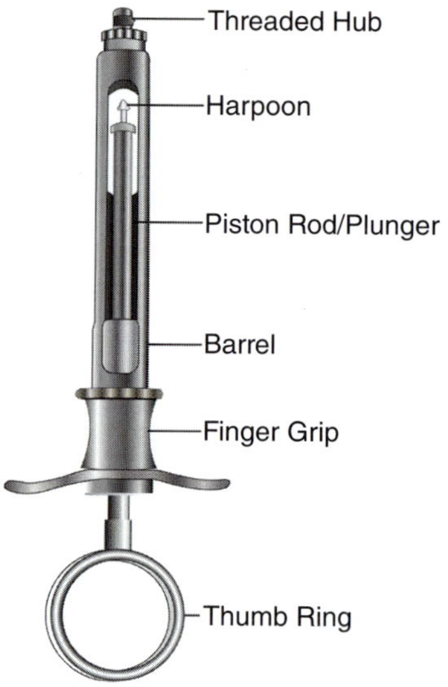

Figure 11.10 Parts of a nondisposable syringe.

2. Self-aspirating syringes

The major factor for the mechanism of aspiration in this type of syringe is the gauge of the needle being used.

First-generation self-aspirating syringes

These syringes have a thumb disc, which forces the operator to the thumb disc to aspirate.

Second-generation self-aspirating syringes

These syringes do not have thumb disc. Once the operator stops applying pressure to the thumb ring, the syringe aspirates by itself.

3. Pressure syringes

Periodontal ligament (PDL) (intraligamentary) injections are made possible with pressure syringes for mandibular single tooth pulpal anaesthesia. In the past, complete inferior alveolar nerve block (IANB) was necessary. These syringes are expensive. When too much pressure is applied too quickly for PDL injection, it can shatter the glass cartridge.

4. 2000 psi jet syringes

These syringes are more expensive. It has a needleless injection technique where the local anaesthesia solution is forced through very small openings called jets. This is done at very high-pressure of 2000 psi. Thus penetrating skin or intact mucous membrane (traditional syringes—600 psi). Syrijet is the most popular jet syringe used today. It can hold any 1.8 mL cartridge of local anaesthetic.

5. Computer-controlled local anaesthetic delivery

Computer-controlled local anaesthetic delivery (C-CLAD) was designed to improve the ergonomics and precision of LA injection technique. It has a foot activated delivery of solution and fingertip precision is provided with a pen-like grasp on the wand; this offers increased tactile sensation. The flow rates of solution delivery are computer controlled and is consistent. It has reported a threefold decrease in the interpretation of pain. The wand is also less threatening to the patients visually.

It allows two rates of delivery: (1) Slow: 0.5 mL/min; (2) fast: 1.8 mL/min.

To aspirate, the clinician has to release the foot peddle and the machine will aspirate automatically; the aspiration cycle is approximately 4.5 s.

DISPOSABLE TYPE OF SYRINGE

Disposable plastic syringes are widely used for dentistry in the Asian countries. They are sterile until opened, disposable and are available in various sizes. The solution can be loaded directly into the barrel of the syringe from a multidose vial or a single dose vial. Cartridges cannot be used with these syringes. They are lightweight and provides better tactile sensation. Aspiration with one hand is possible with practice.

SAFETY SYRINGE

These syringes are used to minimise accidental needle prick injury, but they are more expensive than nondisposable syringes.

NEEDLE

PARTS OF THE NEEDLE

1. *The bevel:* It is the point or tip of the needle. The angle of bevel is 12 degrees. The angle of bevel influences the deflection of the needle as it passes through the tissues. The three types of bevel available are as follows:
   - Long
   - Medium
   - Short

   Short bevelled needles are better as they have lesser tendency to deflect. Long bevelled needles deflect more and can lead to breakage of needle. There have been innovations with bevel design like large bore needles, where the inner diameter is more compared to the traditional needles. An innovative scalpel designed bevel has been introduced for easier penetration. The standard bevel design is the *triple bevelled design.*
2. *The shank (shaft):* The shank is from the bevel to the hub. The diameter of the lumen of the shank is the needle gauge
3. *The hub:* It is the plastic or metallic piece that attaches to the syringe
4. *The cartridge penetrating end:* It is placed into the needle adaptor and perforates the rubber diaphragm of the cartridge.

SELECTION OF NEEDLE

Needle selection is done based on the length and gauge. They are determined by the technique of anaesthesia (Table 11.21).

Gauge

The diameter of needle lumen (inner hallow) determines the gauge of the needle. 25 or 27 gauges are most commonly used. The smaller the gauge, the greater the lumen diameter. It has been described in Table 11.22.

Length

The length of the needle is measured from the hub to the tip. It is available in various lengths, most commonly used are the long or short needles. The length of the needle provides different depth penetration of the needle into the tissue for different techniques. It also allows leaving a safety length of ~5 mm of the needle during use. The weakest portion of the needle is at the hub. If the needle breaks, the excess 5 mm helps the clinician to remove the needle with a haemostat. Clinician should never insert the needle up to the hub.

1. *Long:* It is about 32 mm

   Used for Vazirani–Akinosi mandibular nerve block, Gow-Gates nerve block, IANB, maxillary nerve block (through palatine foramen)
2. *Short:* It is about 25 mm

   Used for maxillary segmental anaesthesia [posterior superior alveolar (PSA), middle superior alveolar (MSA), anterior superior alveolar (ASA) nerve block], infiltrations, mental nerve block, lower anterior anaesthesia.
3. *Ultra-short:* Palatal approach for ASA nerve block.

SAFE NEEDLE MANAGEMENT

One hand recapping method or plastic housing.

THE PREPARATION

CARTRIDGE

The cartridge is a glass tube sealed with a rubber stopper or plunger on one end, and a rubber diaphragm sealed with

TABLE 11.21 Selection of Needle Gauge and Length Based on Depth of Penetration and Technique

Gauge	Length		Depth of Penetration	Technique
30	Ultra-short	16 mm	6–10 mm	Palatal approach-anterior superior alveolar (P-ASA)
27	Short	25 mm	~4–6 mm	Supraperiosteal infiltration
27	Short	25 mm	16 mm	Posterior superior alveolar (PSA)
27	Short	25 mm	~5–7 mm	Middle superior alveolar (MSA)
27	Short	25 mm	3–4 mm	Anterior middle superior alveolar (AMSA)
27	Short	25 mm	5 mm	Greater (anterior) palatine
27	Short	25 mm	5 mm	Nasopalatine
27	Short	25 mm	3–5 mm	Palatal infiltration
25 or 27	Long	32 mm	16 mm	Anterior superior alveolar (ASA, infraorbital)
25	Long	32 or 40 mm needle	30 mm	Maxillary (V2) nerve block
25 or 27	Long	32 mm	20–25 mm	Inferior alveolar nerve block
25 or 27	Long	32 mm	25 mm	Gow-Gates
25 or 27	Long	32 mm	25 mm	Vazirani–Akinosi
25 or 27	Short	25 mm	5 to 6 mm	Mental
27	Short	25 mm	2–4 mm	Long buccal
27	Short	25 mm	5–6 mm	Incisive

TABLE 11.22 The Needle Gauge and Diameter are Shown, with their Relationship Illustrated by Arrows

Gauge	Diameter in mm	Needle Deflection		Needle Breakage	Patient Comfort
20	0.81	Lesser deflection	Greater accuracy	Lesser chance to break	Decreased
21	0.72				
22	0.64				
23	0.57				
24	0.51				
25	0.45				
27	0.40				
30	0.30	Greater deflection	Lesser accuracy	Higher chance to break	Increased, easier to penetrate tissues

aluminium cap on the other end. The rubber stopper is forced into the tube when loaded into a syringe with the plunger. The rubber diaphragm is pierced by the needle once attached to the hub. It is available in presterilised conditions, vacuum sealed, blister packed and disposable. The volume of a cartridge in the United States and France is 1.8 mL, in United Kingdom and Australia it is 2.2 mL.

MULTIDOSE VIAL

They are available in 30 mL vials with different dilutions, like 1:80,000, 1:100,000, 1:200,000.

ADDITIONAL ARMAMENTARIUM

1. Topical anaesthetic (strongly recommended)—ointments, gels, pastes, sprays
2. Applicator sticks
3. Cotton gauze
4. Topical antiseptic.

ANATOMIC CONSIDERATIONS (APPLIED ANATOMY)

Pain sensation in the orofacial region is carried by the trigeminal pathway to the brain.

The trigeminal nerve—cranial nerve V (CN V)

The trigeminal or V cranial nerve is the sensory nerve of the face and consists largely of somatic afferent fibres, but it also contains motor afferent fibres. It is the nerve of the

1st branchial arch and is the largest of the cranial nerves. The larger sensory and smaller motor root of this nerve leaves the bone about halfway up its ventrolateral surface. The cell bodies of the sensory root form the Gasserian (trigeminal or semilunar) ganglion, which lies in an invagination of the dura mater near the apex of the petrous temporal bone. The three divisions of the nerve leave the ganglion and exit the skull via the superior orbital fissure, foramen rotundum and foramen ovale. The innervation of the maxillary teeth and adjacent soft tissues comes from the following branches of the 2nd division, that is the maxillary nerve (Fig. 11.11).

Maxillary nerve (Fig. 11.12)

The nerves anaesthetised by the dental practitioner have been described below. The maxillary nerve branches that are anaesthetised for intraoral procedures are as follows:

a. *The posterior superior alveolar (or dental) nerves*, usually two or three in number, leave the maxillary nerve in the pterygopalatine fossa to course downwards on the surface of the maxillary tuberosity, which they enter through small foramina to supply the roots of all molar teeth except the mesiobuccal root of 1st molar
b. *The middle superior alveolar nerve* arises from the infraorbital nerve and supplies the premolar teeth and the mesiobuccal root of 1st molar
c. *The anterior superior alveolar nerve* arises further anterior in the infraorbital canal and supplies the anterior teeth
d. *The greater palatine nerve* travels via the greater palatine canal from the sphenopalatine ganglion to the hard palate. It supplies tissues on the palate posterior to the canine teeth
e. *The long sphenopalatine nerve* (or nasopalatine nerve), after leaving the sphenopalatine ganglion passes medially through the sphenopalatine foramen, crosses the root of the nose to travel along the nasal septum and enter the oral cavity via the incisive canal. It supplies palatal tissues adjacent to the anterior teeth and anastomoses with the greater palatine nerve in the region of the canine tooth. These branches may be seen as two nerve loops: (1) the outer loop lies deep to the cortical bone of the maxilla, and consists of the superior alveolar nerves and their parent nerve (the maxillary infraorbital nerve); (2) the inner loop consists of the greater palatine nerve only and the long sphenopalatine nerve, which leave the sphenopalatine ganglion and anastomose near the maxillary canine tooth.

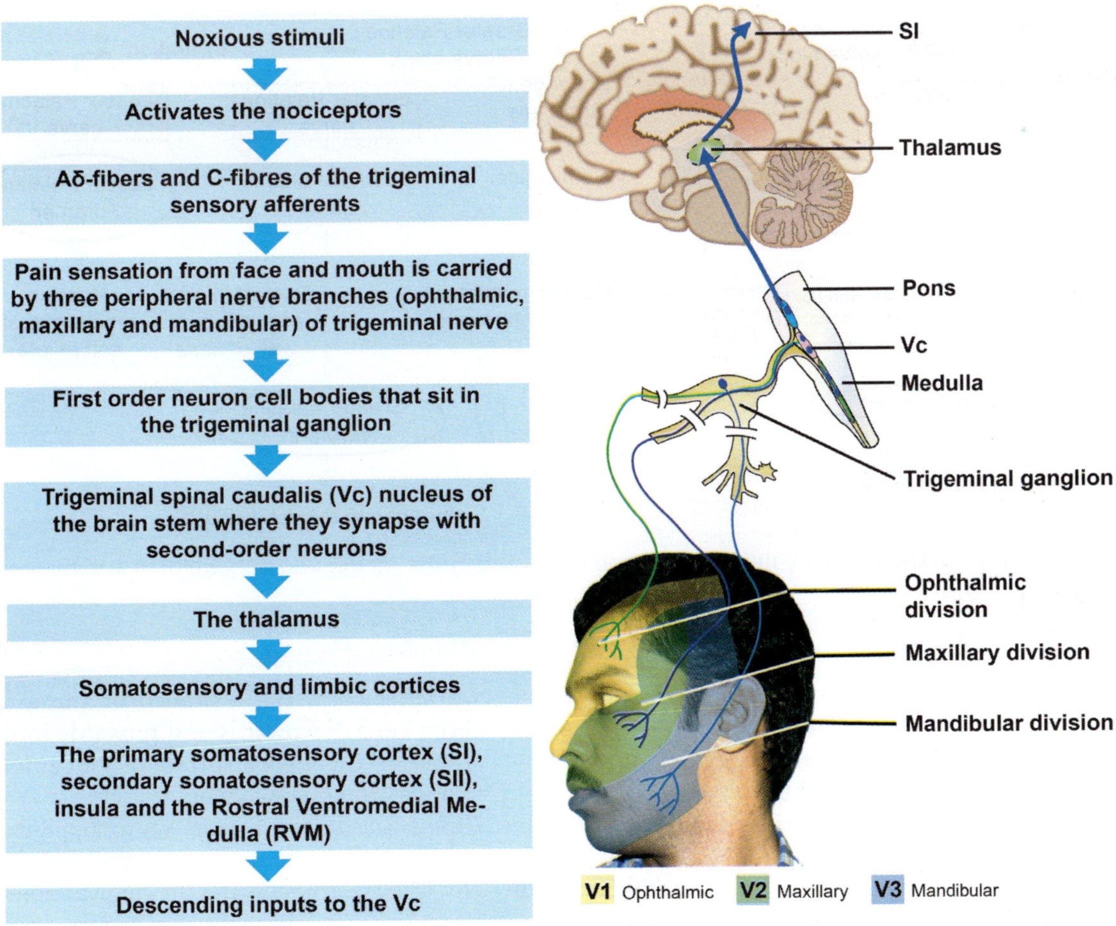

Figure 11.11 Flowchart illustrating trigeminal nerve pain pathway.

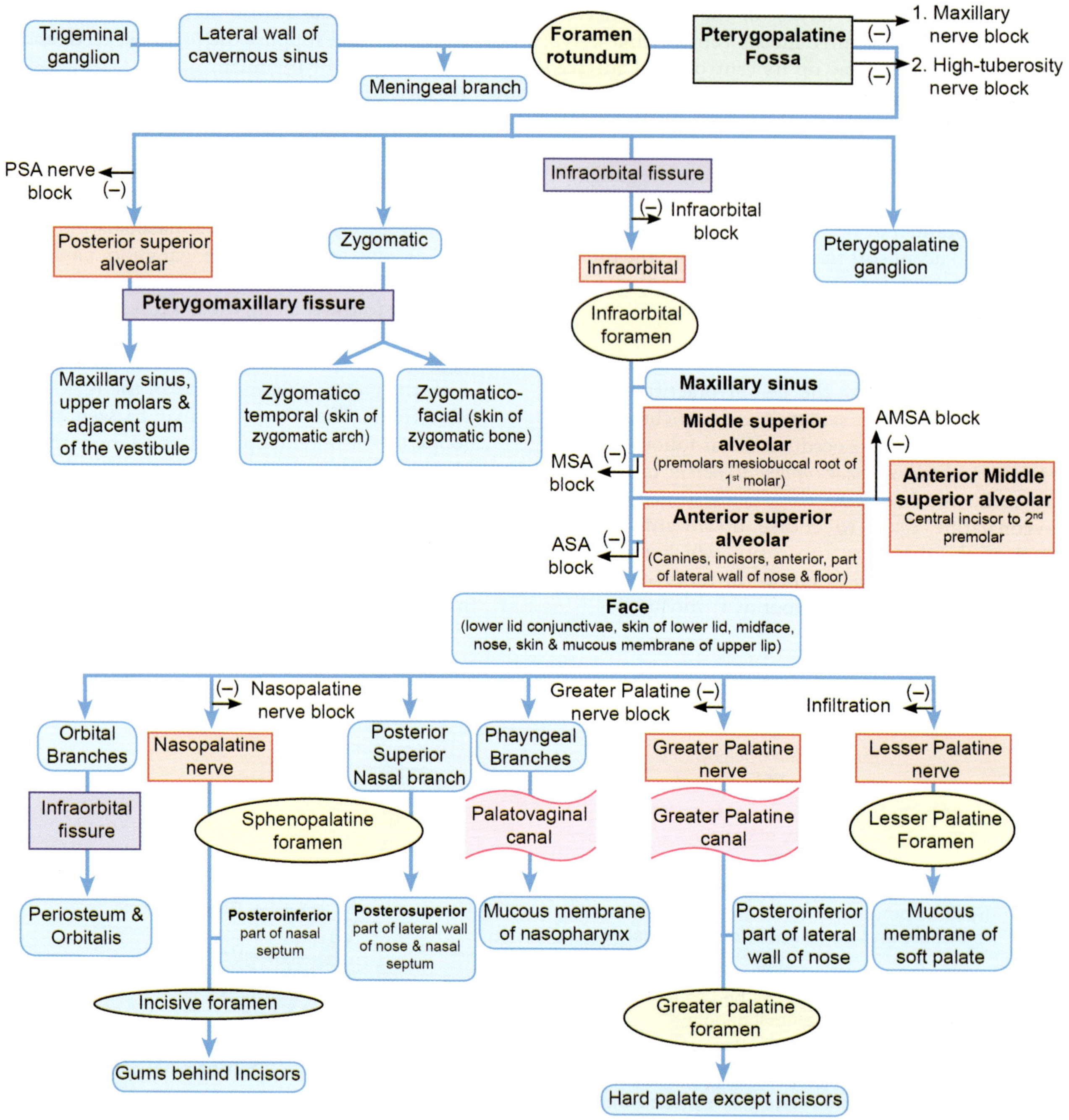

Figure 11.12 The branches of the maxillary nerve have been illustrated in the figure. The nerve blocks and the nerves have also been highlighted in the figure.

Mandibular nerve (Fig. 11.13)

The motor root runs with the 3rd or mandibular division and supplies four masticatory muscles, two tensors (tympani and palati), anterior belly of the digastric and mylohyoid.

The innervation of the mandibular teeth and contiguous tissues arises from the following branches of the 3rd division:

a. *The inferior alveolar nerve*, which enters the mandible at the mandibular foramen and together with its terminal branches and incisive nerve, supplies all the teeth
b. *The mylohyoid nerve*, a branch of the inferior alveolar nerve, runs downwards and forwards in the mylohyoid groove on the medial surface of the ramus of mandible to innervate the mylohyoid muscle
c. *The lingual nerve*, which on its way to supply the anterior two-thirds of the tongue also supplies the lingual gingival tissues
d. *The mental nerve* innervates the gingiva anterior to the mental foramen, as well as the skin and mucous membrane of the lower lip and chin approximately to the midline.

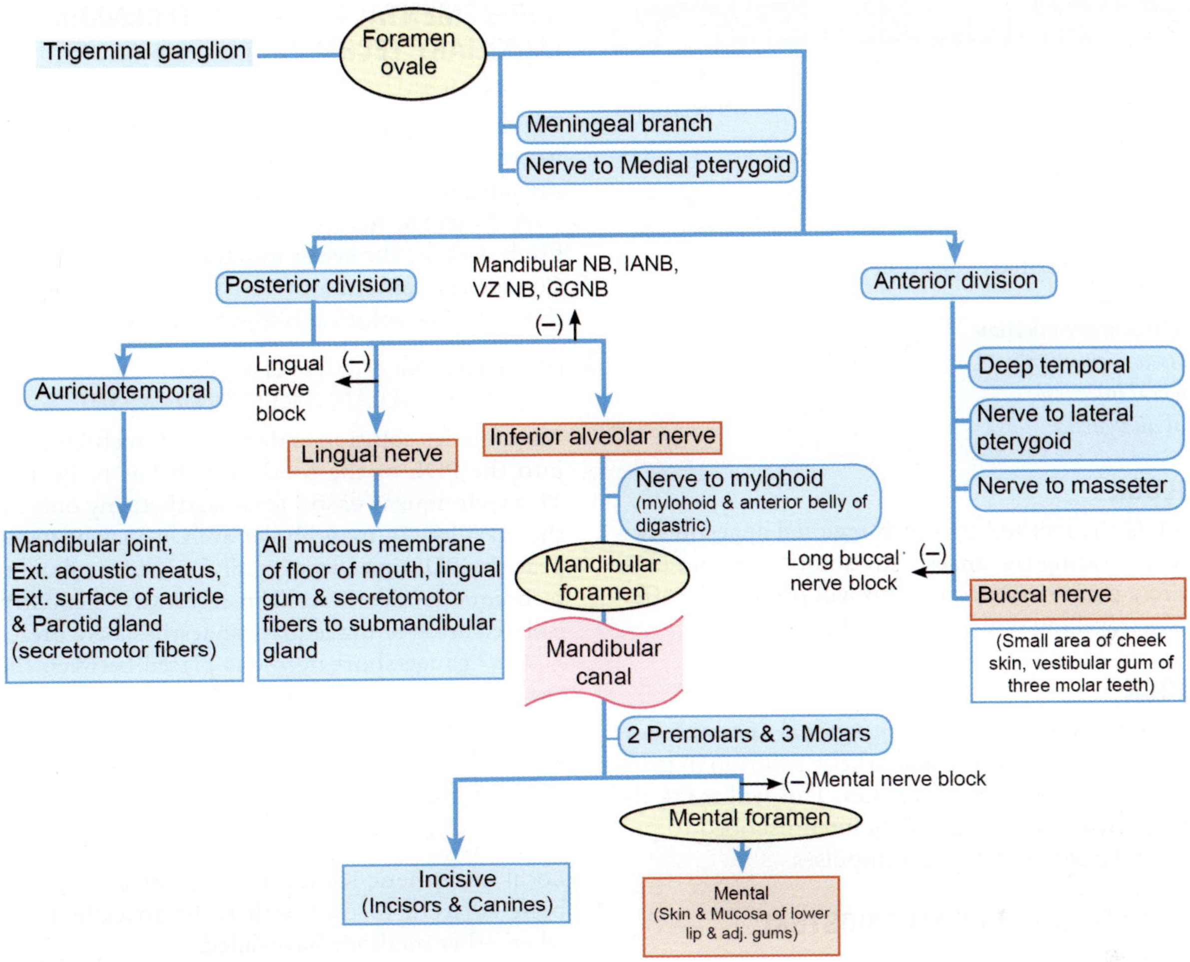

Figure 11.13 The branches of the mandibular nerve have been illustrated in the figure. The nerve blocks and the nerves have also been highlighted in the figure.

PREOPERATIVE ASSESSMENT OF THE PATIENT

Pain control is important as it leads to increased stress and the release of endogenous catecholamines, which can result in an unexpected cardiovascular response. Obtain a thorough medical history: (1) Any drug allergy? (2) Have you ever had a reaction to local anaesthesia? (3) If yes, describe what happened? (4) What was the treatment given? Drug history: Substance abuse, insulin for diabetes, hypertensive drugs. Classify patient according to ASA classification. Mental status including emotional state and level of consciousness should be evaluated. Explanation of local anaesthetics and the procedure should be given to the patient.

PREOPERATIVE ASSESSMENT:

1. Baseline vital signs
2. Check all laboratory values
3. Results of ECG monitoring
4. Weight, height and age
5. Dosage of LA is calculated on the basis of body weight in kilograms (mg/kg).

STRESS REDUCTION PROTOCOL

1. Morning appointments are usually best
2. Keep appointments as short as possible
3. Freely discuss any questions, concerns or fears that the patient has
4. Establish an honest, supportive relationship with the patient
5. Maintain a calm, quiet, professional environment
6. Provide clear explanations of what the patient should expect and feel
7. Premedicate with benzodiazepines if patient seems anxious in the prior visits
8. Lorazepam 1 mg the night before the procedure and 90 min before the procedure
9. Ensure good pain control intraoperative and post-operatively
10. Use gradual position changes to avoid postural hypotension
11. End the appointment if the patient appears over-stressed.

BASIC INJECTION TECHNIQUES

Depending upon the site of injecting the local anaesthetic solutions in relation to the nerve, there are three major techniques of LA as:

- *Nerve block*
- *Field block*
- *Local infiltration*

There are other auxiliary injection techniques as:

1. *Intrapulpal injection*
2. *Intraligamentary injection*
3. *Intraosseous injection*
4. *Intraseptal injection*
5. *Topical analgaesia.*

NERVE BLOCK

Nerve block is the method by which regional anaesthesia is secured by depositing the anaesthetic solution within close proximity to a main nerve trunk. This will prevent the afferent impulses travelling centrally beyond this point.

FIELD BLOCK

Field block is the method by which regional anaesthesia is secured by depositing the local anaesthetic solution in proximity to larger terminal nerve branches. This will make the anaesthetised area to be walled off or circumscribed to prevent the central passage of afferent impulses.

LOCAL INFILTRATION (SUPRAPERIOSTEAL INFILTRATION)

In this technique, small terminal nerve endings in the area of surgery are flooded with anaesthetic solution so that the area becomes insensible to pain, or prevent them from becoming stimulated and creating an impulse. Buccal and palatal infiltration is used for single tooth anaesthesia in the maxilla (Fig. 11.14).

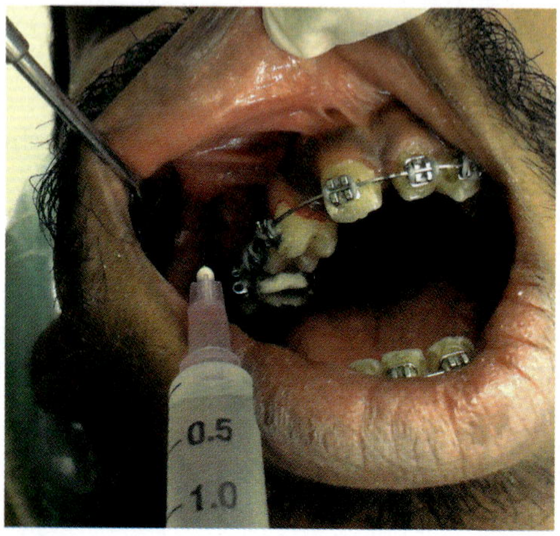

Figure 11.14 Local infiltration.

SUPPLEMENTAL INJECTION TECHNIQUES (AUXILIARY TECHNIQUE)

INTRAPULPAL INJECTION

This technique is utilised in procedures, which require direct instrumentation of the pulpal tissue. Intrapulpal injection can adequately control pain arising from pulpal exposure.

A 25-gauge needle is inserted into the pulp chamber; firmly wedging the needle into the chamber or canal (Fig. 11.15). Considerable amount of resistance might be encountered; therefore, the solution is injected under pressure.

INTRALIGAMENTARY INJECTION (PERIODONTAL LIGAMENT INJECTION)

Anaesthetics solution is deposited forcefully under pressure into the PDL of the tooth, which has to be anaesthetised. This technique is useful for anaesthetising only one tooth of the maxillary or mandibular arch. It may be necessary to repeat the PDL injection on all four sides of the tooth. This technique is mostly used in restorative dentistry whenever isolated areas of inadequate anaesthesia are present.

A 27-gauge short needle is placed between the PDL and the tooth such that bevel of the needle faces the tooth to be anaesthetised. The needle may need to be bent for gaining access. A 0.2 mL of the local anaesthetic is deposited under pressure (Fig. 11.16).

INTRAOSSEOUS INJECTION

Local anaesthetic solution is deposited into the cancellous bone adjacent to the tooth to be anaesthetised. It is used when other methods have failed.

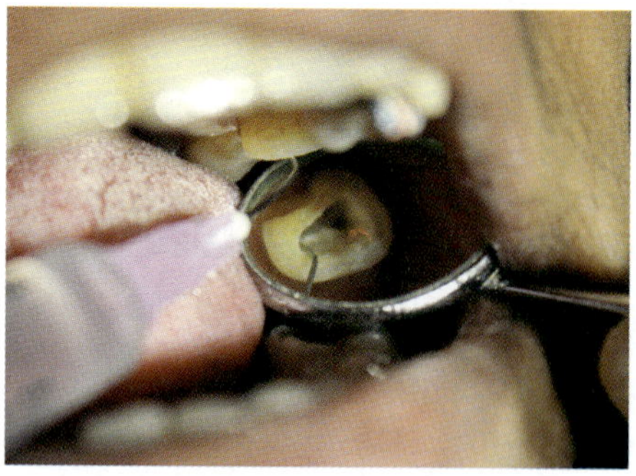

Figure 11.15 Intrapulpal injection.

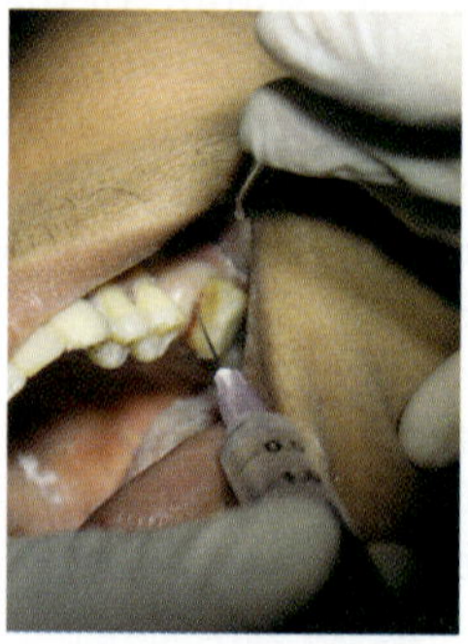

Figure 11.16 Intraligamentary injection.

The soft tissues are anaesthetised using a local infiltration. A small incision is made in the apical region of the tooth to be anaesthetised and a hole is drilled through the dense cortical plate to reach the cancellous bone. A 25-gauge needle is inserted to this hole and approximately 1 mL of local anaesthetics solution is deposited under pressure.

INTRASEPTAL INJECTION

The intraseptal injection is a variation of the intraosseous and PDL injections. This injection may be effective where the condition of the periodontal tissues in the gingival sulcus precludes the use of PDL injection. It is useful in achieving osseous soft tissue anaesthesia and haemostasis for periodontal curettage and surgical flap procedures.

The soft tissue over the area is anaesthetised through local infiltration and a 27-gauge short needle is inserted distal to the tooth in the porous intraseptal bone. A total of 0.2 mL of the local anaesthetics is deposited under pressure. This technique is more effective in children and younger adults.

TOPICAL LOCAL ANAESTHESIA

Topical local anaesthesia renders the free nerve endings in accessible structures incapable of stimulation by application of a suitable solution directly over the surface.

TECHNIQUES OF MAXILLARY ANAESTHESIA (BLOCK ANAESTHESIA FOR THE MAXILLA) (FLOWCHART 11.1)

Volumes of local anaesthetic solution for maxillary injection techniques are summerised in Table 11.23.

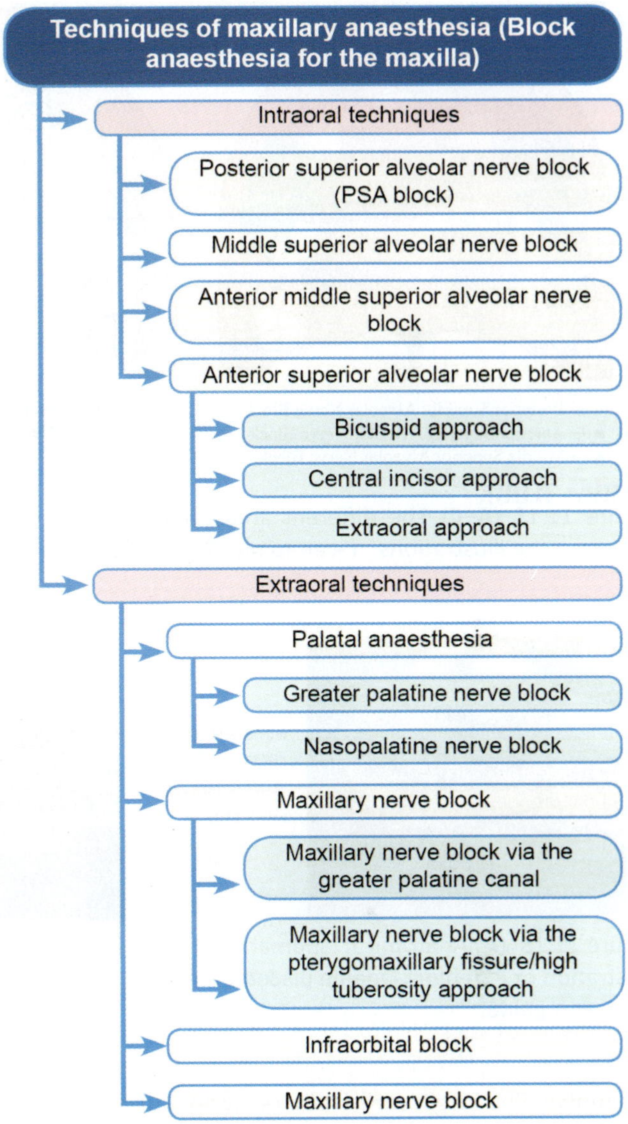

Flowchart 11.1 Techniques of maxillary anaesthesia.

TABLE 11.23 Volumes of Local Anaesthetic Solution (in mL) for Maxillary Injection Techniques

Technique	Volume (mL)
Supraperiosteal infiltration	0.6
Posterior superior alveolar (PSA)	0.9–1.8
Middle superior alveolar (MSA)	0.9–1.2
Anterior superior alveolar (ASA, infraorbital)	0.9–1.2
Anterior middle superior alveolar (AMSA)	1.4–1.8
Palatal approach-anterior superior alveolar (P-ASA)	1.4–1.8
Greater (anterior) palatine	0.45–0.6
Nasopalatine	0.45
Palatal infiltration	0.2–0.3
Maxillary (V2) nerve block	1.8

INTRAORAL TECHNIQUES (FIG. 11.17)

POSTERIOR SUPERIOR ALVEOLAR NERVE BLOCK (PSA BLOCK)

Other names: Tuberosity block, zygomatic block.

Areas anaesthetised

In this technique, the area supplied by the posterior superior alveolar nerve is anaesthetised. They are: pulpal anaesthesia of 3rd, 2nd and 1st maxillary molars (with the exception of the mesiobuccal root of the maxillary 1st molar), buccal periodontium and bone overlying these teeth.

Landmarks

Mucobuccal fold, maxillary tuberosity and zygomatic process of maxilla.

Technique (Fig. 11.18A–C)

Position the patient such that the occlusal plane of the maxilla is at a 45-degree angle to the floor. A 25-gauge short needle is used. The needle should be inserted at the height of the mucobuccal fold in the region distal to the maxillary

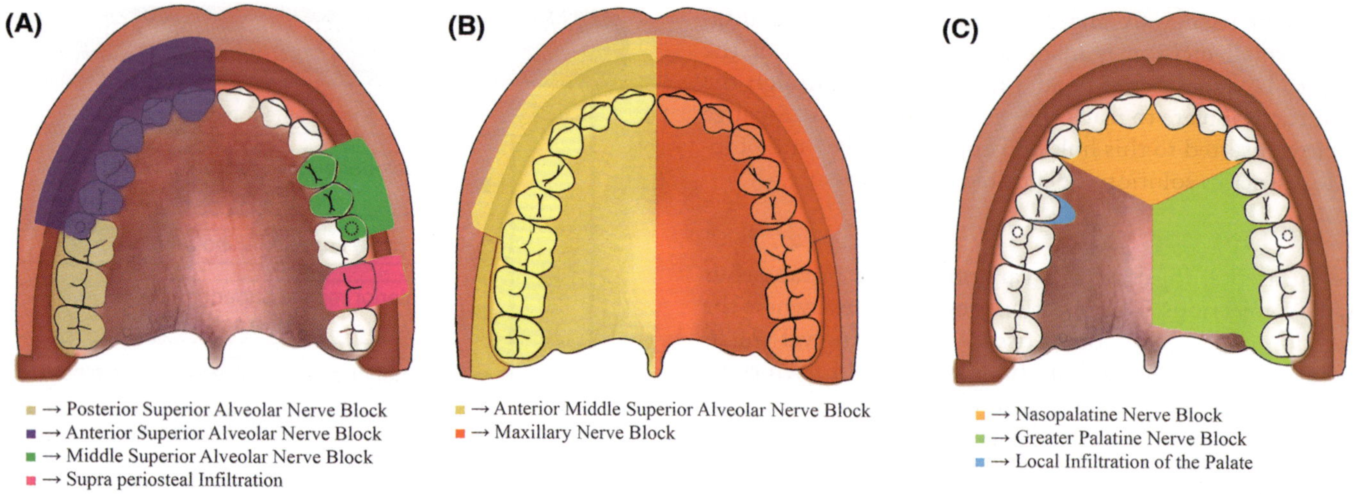

Figure 11.17 (**A–C**) The different areas anaesthetised—intraoral nerve block techniques and supraperiosteal infiltration are shown in the illustrations. (Scan to play Maxillary Local Anaesthesia techniques.)

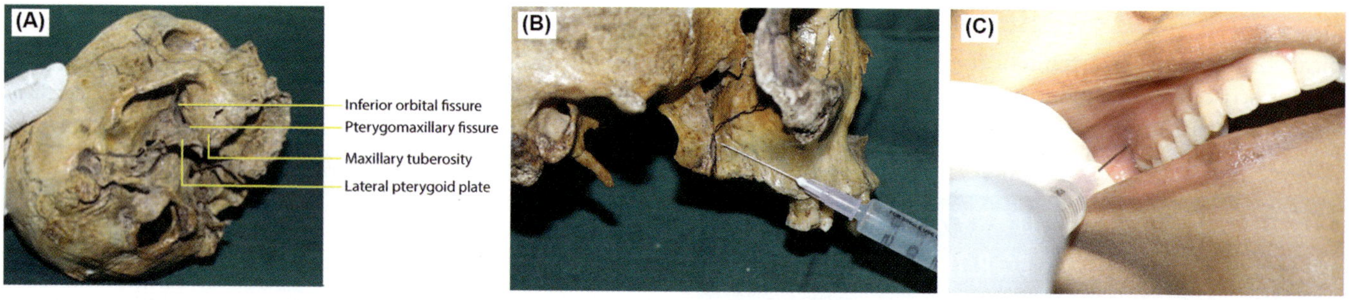

Figure 11.18 (**A**) Anatomical landmarks for PSA block shown in a skull. (**B**) Demonstration of PSA block in a skull. (**C**) Clinical demonstration of PSA block-needle placed distal to 2nd molar and directed 45 degrees to the sagittal and occlusal plane with the buttress as a guide.

2nd molar. The target area is the posterior superior alveolar nerve as it enters the posterior surface of the maxilla. This necessitates that the patient's mouth be opened just to a comfortable extent, as excessive opening brings the coronoid process of the mandible forwards and prevents the needle from being advanced from the lateral aspect. This nerve is located posterosuperior and medial to the maxillary tuberosity.

The index finger is placed in the mucobuccal fold of the bicuspid area and moved posteriorly until the prominence of the zygomatic buttress is reached. This is approximately in the region above the 1st molar area. Here the fingertip is rotated so that the finger nail is facing the attached gingiva. The finger is passed posteriorly over this buttress until it dips in a sulcus posterior to the buttress. The finger is kept such that it is at a 90-degree angle to the occlusal surface of the maxillary teeth and at a 45-degree angle to the sagittal plane. The needle is positioned in the depth of the sulcus close to the pterygomaxillary fissure, high in the mucobuccal fold above the distobuccal root of the 2nd molar, bisecting the fingernail.

MIDDLE SUPERIOR ALVEOLAR NERVE BLOCK (FIG. 11.19)

Middle superior alveolar nerve is not always present, and when absent, the posterior superior alveolar nerve supplies the molars and premolars.

Nerves anaesthetised

Middle superior alveolar nerve and terminal branches.

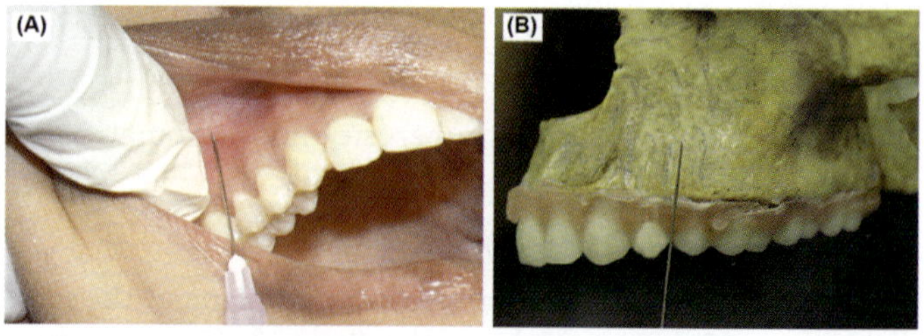

Figure 11.19 (**A** and **B**) The needle is inserted at the height of the mucobuccal fold above the maxillary 2nd premolar with the orientation of the bevel towards the bone.

Area anaesthetised

Maxillary 1st and 2nd premolars with mesiobuccal root of the 1st molar with the adjacent buccal mucosa and bone over the tooth.

Indications

It is given when ASA nerve block fails to anaesthetise the 1st and 2nd premolar and PSA nerve block fails to anaesthetise the mesiobuccal root of 1st molar.

Technique

The upper lip is retracted to make the tissue taut and to gain visibility, and a 27-gauge needle is inserted at the height of the mucobuccal fold above the maxillary 2nd premolar with orientation of the bevel towards the bone. The needle is penetrated till the needle tip is located above the apex of the 2nd premolar. After negative aspiration, 0.9–1.2 mL of solution is deposited over 30–40 s.

ANTERIOR MIDDLE SUPERIOR ALVEOLAR NERVE BLOCK (FIG. 11.20)

Area anaesthetised

The anterior and middle superior alveolar (AMSA) nerve block achieves pulpal anaesthesia from the central incisor to 2nd premolar through the palatal approach with a single injection. The palatal mucosa from midline raphe to the cervical region of the maxillary teeth and the gingival and buccal mucosa of all the maxillary teeth of the corresponding side.

Technique

This technique was 1st reported by Freidman and Hochman in 1997 with the development of C-CLAD system. It provides pulpal anaesthesia to multiple teeth from a single injection site. The site of penetration with C-CLAD on the palatal side of the premolars at the intersection of the horizontal and vertical aspects of the palate opposite the apices of the premolars, a point midway between the gingival crest bisecting the premolars and the median palatine raphe.

Disadvantage

This technique has an unpredictable anaesthetic success of the teeth and variable duration of action for clinical use as the 1st choice when compared to the other techniques that have greater efficacy in the maxilla.

Advantage

In the maxilla, most dental procedures require multiple injections that anaesthetise facial structures and affect the smile line. Anaesthetising the teeth without numbing the facial muscles is usually useful in restorative dentistry.

ANTERIOR SUPERIOR ALVEOLAR NERVE BLOCK

Other names: Infraorbital nerve block, anterior superior and middle superior alveolar nerve block.

Areas anaesthetised

In this technique, the areas supplied by the anterior superior alveolar nerve, middle superior alveolar nerve, infraorbital nerve along with its branches, the lateral nasal nerve, inferior palpebral nerve and superior labial nerves are anaesthetised. Areas anaesthetised are maxillary incisors, canine, premolars and mesiobuccal root of maxillary 1st molar on the injected side, buccal periodontium and bone of the same teeth, lower eyelid along with lateral aspect of nose and the upper lip.

Landmarks

Supraorbital notch, infraorbital notch, pupil of the eye, infraorbital foramen, bicuspid teeth and mental foramen.

Techniques (Fig. 11.21)

There are basically three techniques for infraorbital nerve block:

i. **Bicuspid approach**
ii. **Central incisor approach**
iii. **Extraoral approach.**

Patient is positioned in such that the maxillary occlusal plane is at an angle of 45 degrees to the floor. The target is

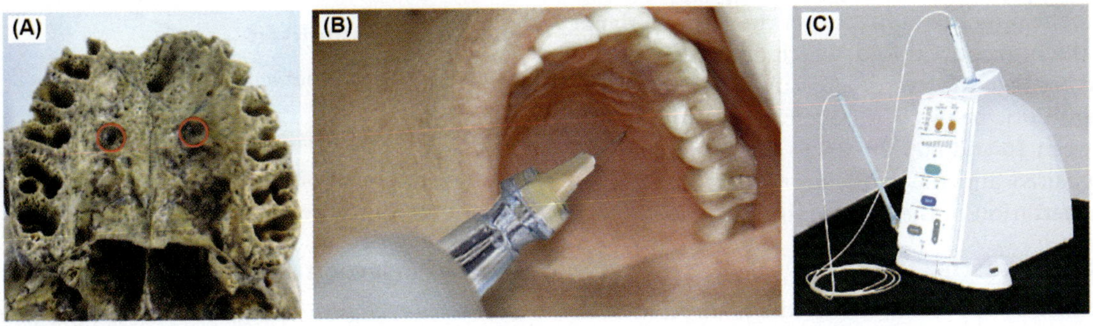

Figure 11.20 **(A)** Anterior middle superior alveolar foramen through which the corresponding nerve exits to supply the palatal soft tissue, buccal gingival tissue and the pulps of the incisors, canines, premolars and the mesiobuccal root of the 1st molar. **(B)** The site of deposition of the anaesthetic agent into the foramen by the wand of a computer-controlled local anaesthetic delivery (C-CLAD). **(C)** C-CLAD system.

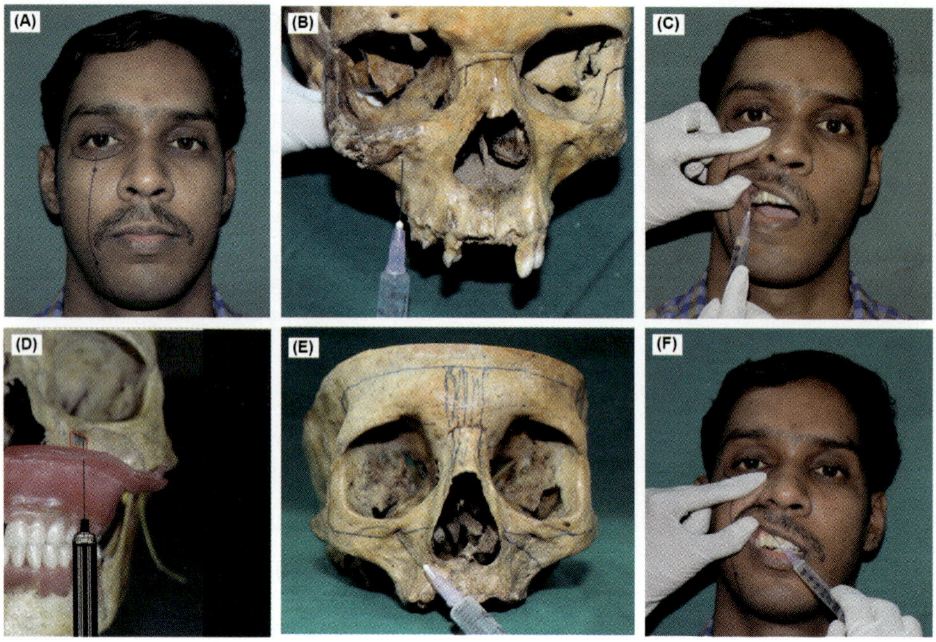

Figure 11.21 (**A**) Surface anatomical landmarks. A vertical imaginary line connecting pupil, infraorbital rim, infraorbital notch, infraorbital foramen and mental foramen. (**B**) Bicuspid approach demonstration in a skull. (**C** and **D**) Bicuspid approach. Needle oriented parallel to the bicuspids towards the infraorbital foramen with the index finger over the infraorbital rim acting as the guide. (**E**) Demonstration of central incisor approach in a skull. (**F**) Central incisor approach—needle bisects the central incisor from mesial to distal penetrating the vestibular mucosa with the index finger over the infraorbital rim.

determined by palpating the supraorbital and infraorbital notches. A vertical imaginary line is drawn through these landmarks, which will pass through pupil of the eye, infraorbital foramen, bicuspid teeth and mental foramen. After palpating the infraorbital margin, the finger is moved downwards from it where a concavity will be felt. This is the infraorbital depression and the infraorbital foramen is in its deepest part. Maintaining the index finger on this foramen externally, retract the lip using the thumb to expose the mucobuccal fold or vice versa.

Bicuspid approach

In the bicuspid approach, the needle is held parallel to the bicuspid teeth. The puncture is made over the 1st premolar at the height of the mucobuccal fold, which allows the needle to be advanced between the levator labii superioris above and the levator anguli oris below. The penetration of the needle should be between 16 and 20 mm; 0.9 to 1.2 mL of solution should be deposited and the overlying tissues gently massaged to aid penetration of the solution into the canal.

Central incisor approach

In the central incisor approach, the needle is directed such that it bisects the crown of the central incisor of the same side from the mesioincisal angle to the distoincisal angle. The needle is inserted for about 5 mm from the mucobuccal fold and 0.9 to 1.2 mL of anaesthetic solution deposited.

Extraoral approach

A 27- or 30-gauge needle is used to approach the infraorbital foramen percutaneously by injecting between the ala of the nose and the upper part of the nasolabial fold, directing the needle laterally towards the infraorbital foramen.

PALATAL ANAESTHESIA

Palatal injection proves to be a very traumatic experience for many dental patients.

GREATER PALATINE NERVE BLOCK

Other names: Anterior palatine nerve block.

Nerves anaesthetised

Anterior palatine nerve.

Areas anaesthetised

Posterior portion of hard palate and its overlying soft tissues, anteriorly up to the 1st premolar and medially to midline.

Area of insertion

Soft tissues slightly anterior to the greater palatine foramen.

Landmarks

Greater palatine foramen and junction of maxillary alveolar process and palatine bone.

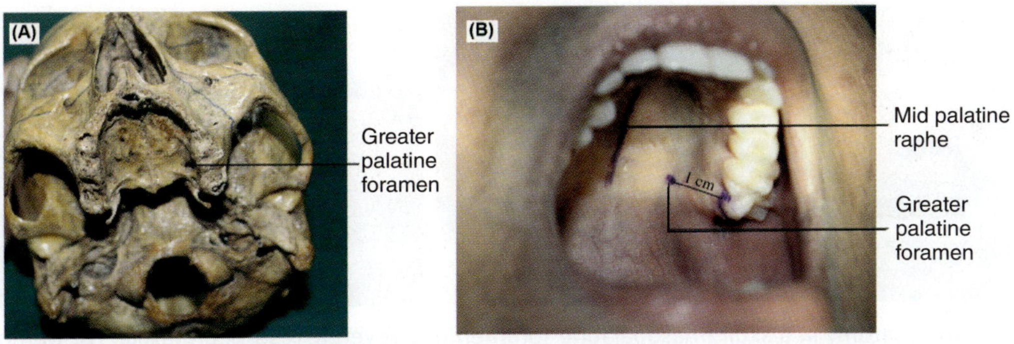

Figure 11.22 (**A**) Landmarks in the skull. (**B**) Surface anatomical landmarks. Midpalatine raphe, palatal gingival margin of 2nd molar and the half way between the two landmarks is the greater palatine foramen.

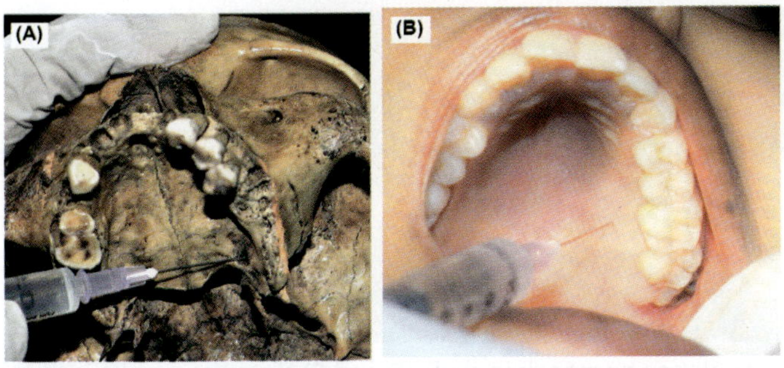

Figure 11.23 (**A**) Demonstration of greater palatine nerve block in a skull. (**B**) Clinical demonstration of greater palatine nerve block—needle directed from opposite side just anterior to the foramen located 1 cm medial to the palatal gingival margin of 2nd molar.

Technique (Figs 11.22 & 11.23)

The greater palatine foramen is located about 4 mm anterior to the termination of the hard palate, so that it is normally situated opposite the 2nd molar about halfway between the gingival margin and midline. A 27- or 25-gauge needle is used. The greater palatine foramen, is approached from the opposite side at a right angle to the curvature of the palatal bone. The needle is inserted anterior to the foramen halfway between the palatal aspect of the gingival margin of the second molar and the midline of the palate. Approximately 0.25 mL of solution is deposited here.

NASOPALATINE NERVE BLOCK

Other names: Incisive canal nerve block, sphenopalatine nerve block.

Nerves anaesthetised

Right and left nasopalatine nerves.

Areas anaesthetised

Hard and soft tissues in the area between canine to canine.

Area of insertion

Tissue lateral to incisive papilla.

Target area

Incisive foramen located beneath incisive papilla.

Landmark

Central incisors and incisive papilla.

Technique (Fig. 11.24A–C)

This procedure is extremely painful. Therefore, a preparatory anaesthesia is secured before insertion of the needle into the incisive papilla.

Preparatory anaesthesia

A 0.25 mL of local anaesthetics solution is deposited by inserting the needle at a right angle to the labial plate into the labial intraseptal tissues in between the two maxillary central incisors.

Procedure

The position of the nasopalatine canal is marked by the papilla situated just behind the central incisors. The needle is withdrawn and reinserted slowly into the groove surrounding the papilla. The bevel is best placed so that it faces distally and the needle is advanced through the canal. Up to 0.25 mL of anaesthetic solution is deposited.

MAXILLARY NERVE BLOCK

Maxillary nerve block is useful for profound anaesthesia of the maxilla. Two approaches are usually employed: (1) greater palatine canal approach–difficulty in locating and negotiating the canal; (2) high tuberosity approach–higher incidence of haematoma.

Other names: 2nd division nerve block, V2 nerve block.

AREAS ANAESTHETISED

1. Pulpal anaesthesia of maxillary teeth on the side of nerve block (central incisor to last molar)
2. Buccal periodontium and bone overlying these teeth
3. Soft tissues and bone of hard palate and part of soft palate medial to the midline
4. Skin of lower eyelid, side of nose, cheek and upper lip.

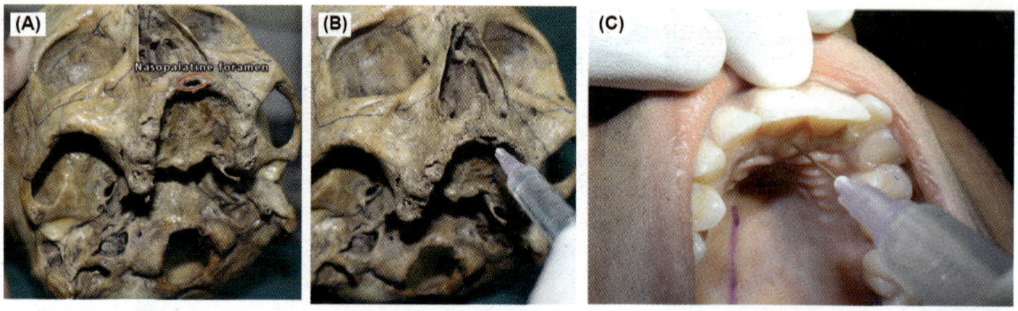

Figure 11.24 (**A**) Surface anatomy in a skull—nasopalatine foramen in a severely resorbed maxilla. (**B**) Demonstration of nasopalatine nerve block in skull. (**C**) Clinical demonstration—of nasopalatine nerve block—needle insertion into the incisive papilla directed parallel to the inclination of the central incisors.

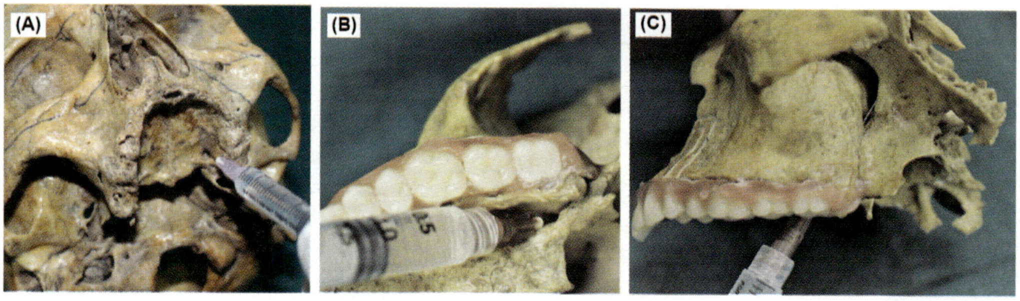

Figure 11.25 (**A**) Demonstration of maxillary nerve block through greater palatine approach in skull. (**B and C**) Note the needle inserted into greater palatine foramen ends in the pterygopalatine fossa anaesthetising the trunk of maxillary branch of trigeminal nerve (V2). Greater palatine foramen in the horizontal plate of palatine bone continues as a canal that opens into pterygopalatine fossa.

TECHNIQUES

MAXILLARY NERVE BLOCK VIA THE GREATER PALATINE CANAL (FIG. 11.25)

The puncture point for this injection is about 4 to 5 mm anterior to the greater palatine foramen, the needle having to pass through soft tissue before entering the foramen. The foramen opens into the greater palatine canal, which is situated between the 2nd and 3rd maxillary molars about 1 cm towards the midline of the palate from the palatal gingival margin.

Occasionally, a slight depression may be noted overlying the foramen. A 42 mm needle is passed upwards and backwards about 45–60 degrees to the upper occlusal plane and slightly laterally (less than 10 degrees) to almost its full depth.

About 2 mL of solution is deposited and this usually diffuses adequately through the superior end of the canal to reach the maxillary nerve. The patient's head is tilted back with wide mouth opening to give good access and possibility. Aspirate immediately as the needle enters a tissue space, as inadvertent penetration into the nasopharynx may be demonstrated by aspiration of air.

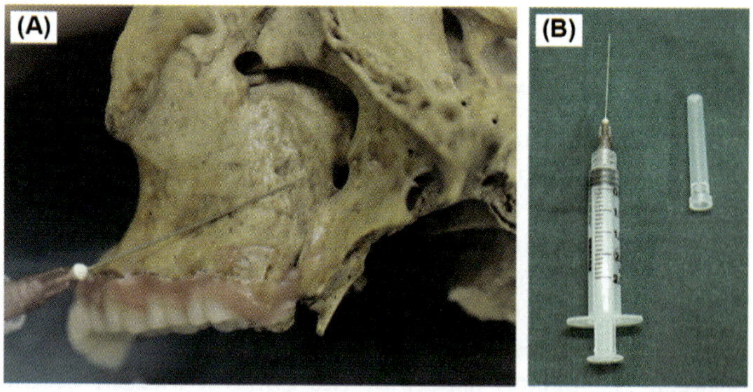

Figure 11.26 (**A**) The needle inserted at the height of the mucobuccal fold distal to the maxillary 2nd molar ends in the pterygopalatine fossa anaesthetising the trunk of maxillary branch of trigeminal nerve (V2). (**B**) A 42 mm needle is used for both techniques.

MAXILLARY NERVE BLOCK VIA THE PTERYGOMAXILLARY FISSURE/HIGH TUBEROSITY APPROACH (FIG. 11.26)

A 25-gauge long needle is inserted high on the mucobuccal fold above the distal aspect of maxillary 2nd molar. The bevel should be oriented towards the bone. To make it easier, the patient is asked to open the mouth partially and the mandible is retracted towards the side of injection. Advance the needle slowly in an upward, inward and backward direction for approximately 30 mm. No resistance should be felt while advancing the needle; the presence of any resistance indicates that the angle of the needle towards midline is too far. The tip of the needle is now in the pterygopalatine fossa

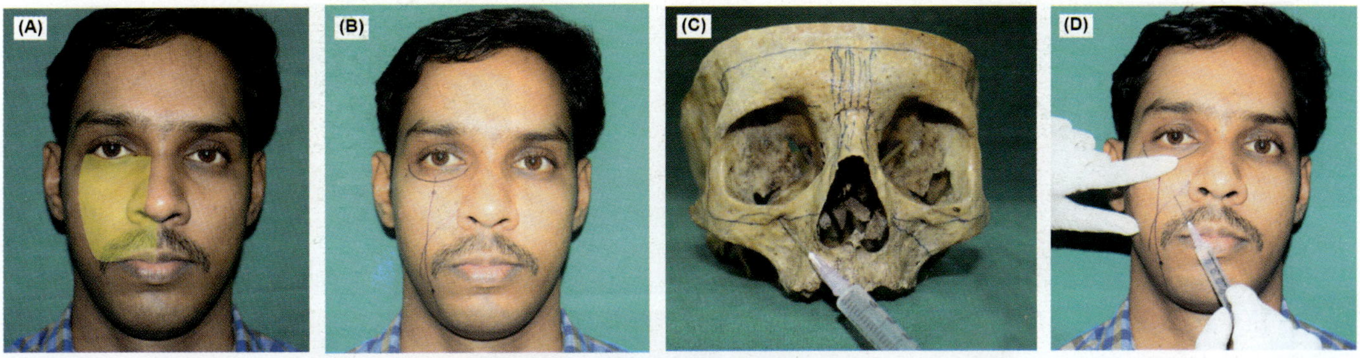

Figure 11.27 (**A**) Illustration of infraorbital nerve dermatome. (**B**) Surface anatomical landmarks for infraorbital nerve block. Nasolabial fold, infraorbital rim, vertical imaginary line through pupil connecting infraorbital foramen and mental foramen, as a straight line. (**C**) Surface anatomy of infraorbital foramen in a skull showing the orientation of needle. Note the foramen opens inferiorly and medially. (**D**) Clinical demonstration of infraorbital nerve block (extraoral)—needle directed superiorly and medio-laterally towards the infraorbital foramen just lateral to the nasolabial fold. This direction is in accordance with the infraorbital foramen which opens inferomedially.

in proximity of maxillary nerve. About 2 mL of solution is deposited following negative aspiration.

EXTRAORAL TECHNIQUES

INFRAORBITAL NERVE BLOCK (FIG. 11.27)

Nerves anaesthetised

- Infraorbital nerve and its branches: Inferior palpebral, lateral nasal and superior labial
- Anterior middle and superior alveolar nerve.

Areas anaesthetised

Incisors and bicuspids on the injected side, alveolar bone and overlying tissues, upper lip, side of the nose, lower eyelid.

Landmarks

Pupil of the eye, infraorbital notch, infraorbital ridge, infra-orbital depression.

Technique

Using the landmarks mentioned for the intraoral approach, the infraorbital foramen is located, and the foramen is marked. The overlying skin and subcutaneous tissues are anaesthetised by local infiltration. A 27-gauge needle is inserted through the marked area between ala of the nose and upper part of the nasolabial fold and directed slightly upward and laterally and entered into the foramen. It should not exceed a depth of 0.3 mm into the foramen. After negative aspiration, 1 mL of anaesthetics solution is deposited slowly.

MAXILLARY NERVE BLOCK (FIG. 11.28)

Nerves anaesthetised

Maxillary teeth, hard and soft palate, tonsils, maxillary alveolar bone and overlying tissues, nasal septum and floor of the nose, anterior cheek, upper lip, side of the nose, lower eyelid, anterior temporal and zygomatic regions.

Technique

The midpoint of the zygomatic process and the depression in its inferior surface are marked. A 22-gauge needle of 4.5 cm is marked with a rubber marker. The syringe is directed perpendicular to the sagittal plane until it contacts the lateral pterygoid plate. The insertion of the needle should not exceed the rubber marker. The needle is then withdrawn and redirected in a slightly forward direction and anaesthetic solution is slowly deposited.

TECHNIQUES OF MANDIBULAR ANAESTHESIA (BLOCK ANAESTHESIA FOR THE MANDIBLE)

The nerves, which supply the teeth and associated tissues of the mandible are the inferior alveolar nerve with its mental and incisive branches, the lingual nerve and the long buccal nerve. The inferior alveolar nerve and its two branches can be blocked at the mandibular and mental foramina, respectively. The lingual and long buccal nerves are blocked at very definite locations (Fig. 11.29A and B).

Volumes of local anaesthetic solution for mandibular injection and techniques of mandibular anaesthesia are summarised in Table 11.24 and Flowchart 11.2..

INTRAORAL TECHNIQUES

MENTAL NERVE BLOCK

Nerves anaesthetised: Mental nerve and terminal branch of inferior alveolar nerve.

Areas anaesthetised: Buccal mucous membrane anterior to the mental foramen, that is from 1st molar to midline, lower lip and skin of chin.

Target area: Mental nerve when it exits from the mental foramen, located between the apices of the 1st and 2nd premolars.

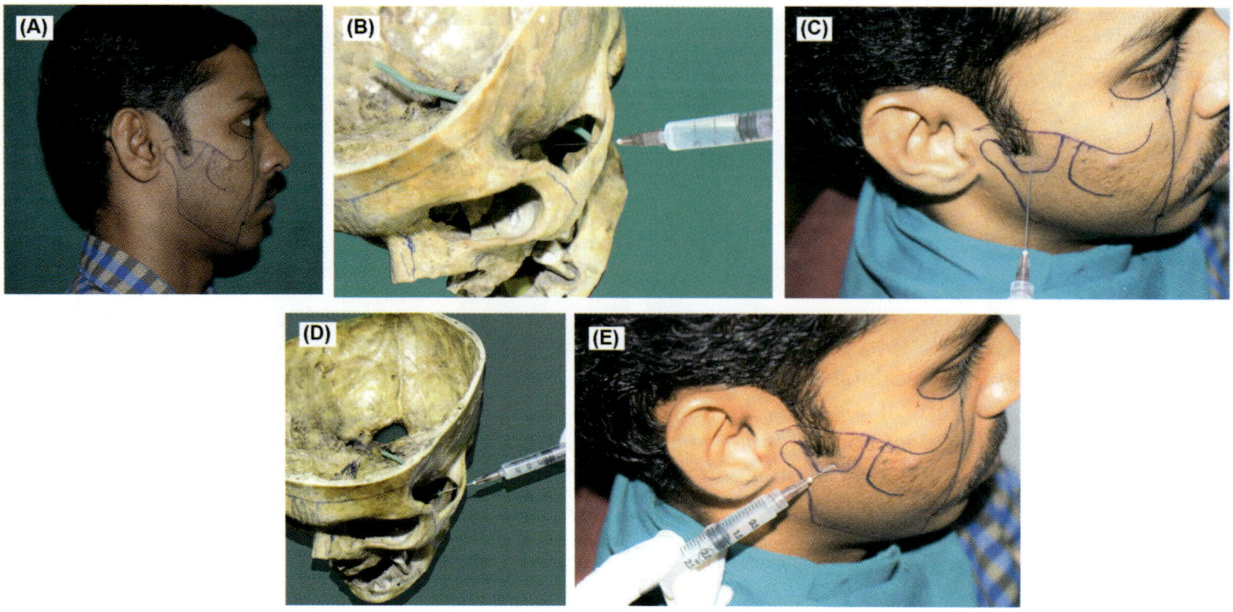

Figure 11.28 (**A**) Surface anatomical landmarks for extraoral maxillary nerve block—sigmoid notch, inferior border of zygomatic arch. (**B**) Demonstration in skull—position 1. (**C**) Clinical demonstration—position 1: needle penetrates perpendicular to the skin through the centre of the sigmoid notch and hits the lateral pterygoid plate. (**D**) Demonstration of position 2 in skull. (**E**) Clinical demonstration—position 2. Needle withdrawn slightly and redirected anteriorly to the pterygomaxillary fissure.

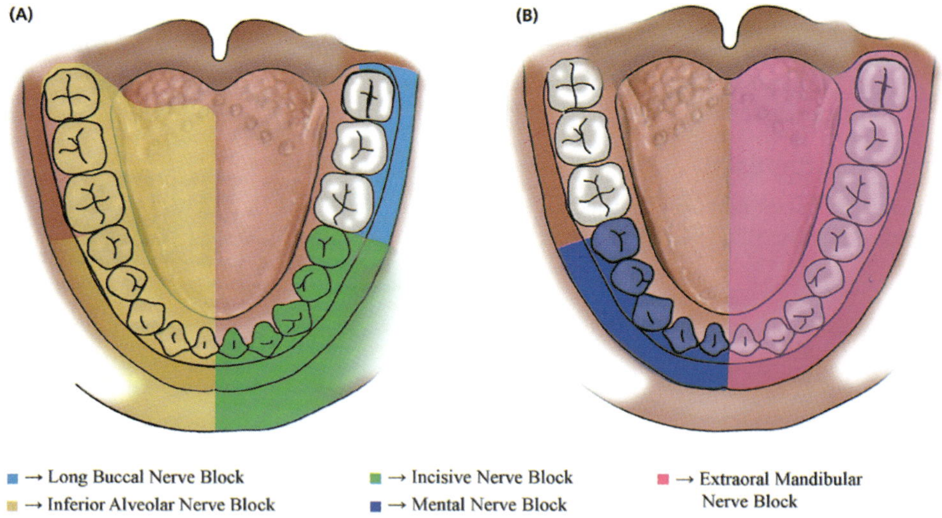

Figure 11.29 (**A** and **B**) The different areas anaesthetised by intraoral and extraoral nerve block techniques are shown in the illustrations.

Technique (Fig. 11.30A–D)

The apices of the two premolars are estimated and 1 inch, 25-gauge needle is used to puncture at a point just behind the mental foramen and somewhat lateral to the depth of the labial sulcus (the cheek being retracted), so that about 1 cm of tissue is penetrated. The needle is advanced to a position beneath the fingertip where gentle palpation should allow the foramen to be found. The needle travels mainly downwards, but also slightly anteriorly and medially until the periosteum of the mandible is gently contacted. About 0.6–1 mL of solution is deposited and the fingertip is used to help massage it into the canal.

TABLE 11.24 Volumes of Local Anaesthetic Solution for Mandibular Injection

Technique	Volume (mL)
Inferior alveolar	1.5
Buccal	0.3
Gow-Gates	1.8–3.0
Vazirani–Akinosi	1.5–1.8
Mental	0.6
Incisive	0.6–0.9

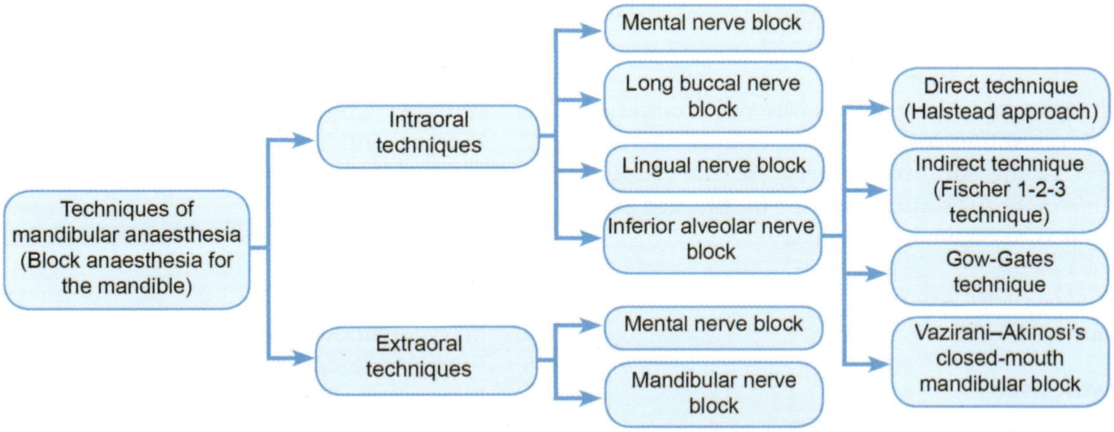

Flowchart 11.2 Technique of mandibular anaesthesia.

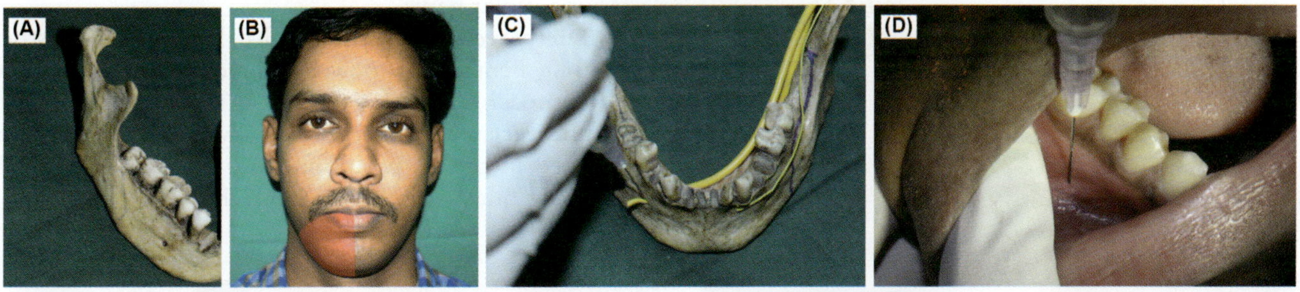

Figure 11.30 (**A**) Surface anatomy of mental foramen in a mandible at the apex of premolars directed posterosuperiorly. (**B**) Illustration of mental nerve block dermatome. (**C**) Demonstration of mental block in a skull—note the direction of needle anteroinferiorly in accordance with the foramen anatomy. (**D**) Clinical demonstration of mental nerve block.

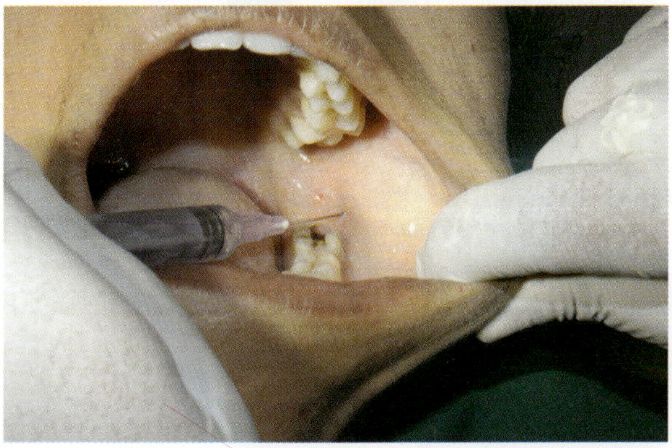

Figure 11.31 Long buccal nerve block. Also, the position 3 of the Fischer's 1,2,3, technique—clinical demonstration—position 3: anaesthetising the long buccal nerve.

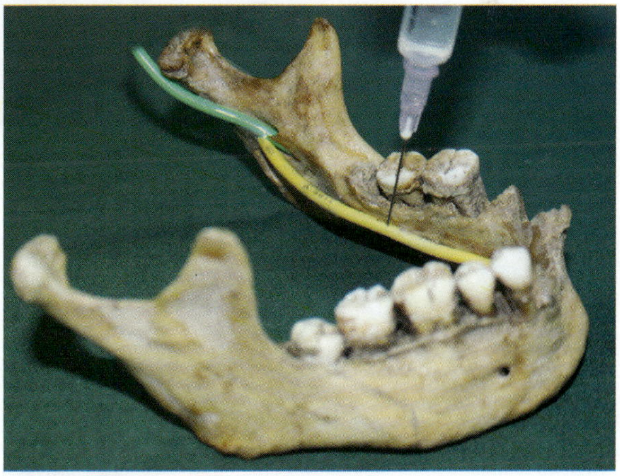

Figure 11.32 Demonstration of lingual nerve block in a mandible. Note the nerve can be anaesthetised anywhere along its course.

LONG BUCCAL NERVE BLOCK (FIG. 11.31)

Alternative names: Buccal nerve block, buccinator nerve block.

Target area: Buccal nerve as it passes over the anterior border of ramus.

Landmarks: Mandibular molars and mucobuccal fold.

Technique:

1. Buccal soft tissue is retracted with the index finger of the left hand
2. Syringe is directed towards injection site parallel to the occlusal plane on the side of injection
3. Penetrate needle distal and buccal to last molar
4. With negative aspiration, deposit 0.3–0.5 mL of solution.

LINGUAL NERVE BLOCK (FIG. 11.32)

The lingual nerve is usually blocked in the pterygomandibular space where it lies anteromedial to the inferior alveolar nerve, about 1 cm or slightly less from the mucosal surface. It is possible to inject this nerve either before or after the inferior alveolar nerve is anaesthetised.

The lingual nerve can be blocked at a site posteroinferior to the 3rd molar by a submucosal injection, or anaesthetised by infiltration at the site of surgery in the lingual sulcus. Up to 0.5 mL of the solution is used for blocked side. An aspiration test is normally not necessary.

INFERIOR ALVEOLAR NERVE BLOCK (IANB) (FIG. 11.33)

Alternative name: Mandibular block.

Nerves anaesthetised

1. Inferior alveolar nerve
2. Incisive nerve
3. Mental nerve
4. Lingual nerve
5. Long buccal (occasionally).

Areas anaesthetised

1. Mandibular teeth to midline
2. Body of mandible
3. Inferior portion of ramus
4. Buccal mucoperiosteum and mucous membrane anterior to mandibular 1st molar
5. Lingual soft tissues and periosteum
6. Anterior two-thirds of tongue and floor of oral cavity
7. External and internal oblique ridge.

Landmarks

1. External oblique ridge
2. Coronoid notch
3. Buccal pad of fat
4. Pterygomandibular raphe
5. Pterygotemporal depression
6. Pterygomandibular space.

Technique

There are basically two techniques for anaesthetising the inferior alveolar nerve.

- **Direct technique:** Inferior alveolar nerve is anaesthetised first, hence it is known as direct technique (Halstead's approach) (Fig. 11.33A–D)
- **Indirect technique:** Inferior alveolar nerve is anaesthetised in the 3rd position; hence it is known as indirect technique or 'Fischer's 1-2-3 technique.'

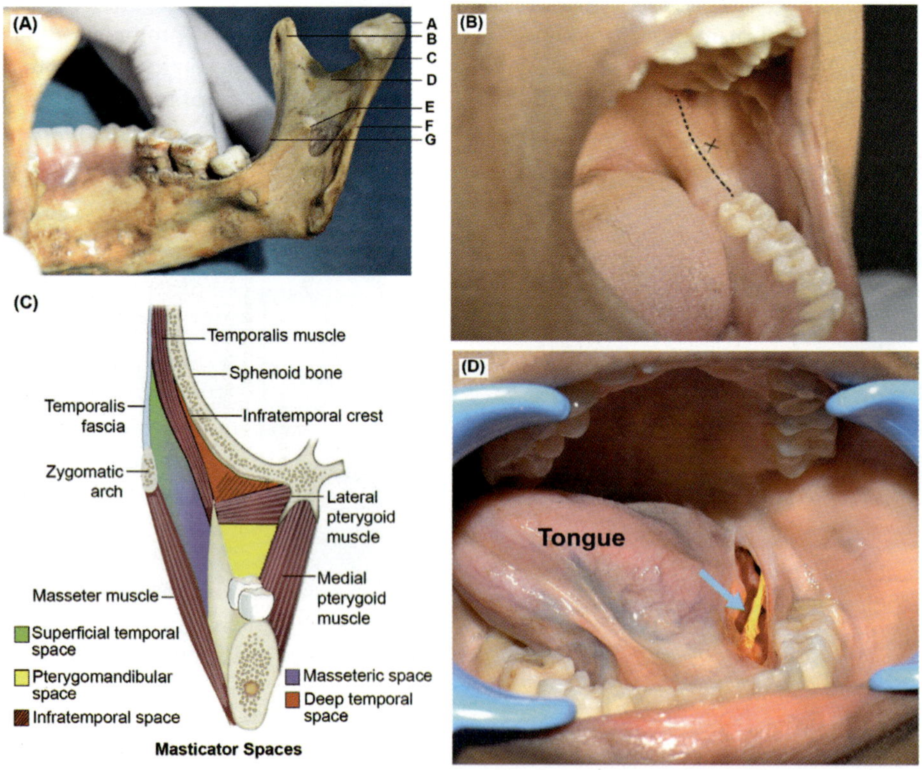

Figure 11.33 (**A**) Osseous anatomy of the medial aspect of the mandible, this is the site where the local anaesthetic drug is deposited (A—head of condyle, B—coronoid process, C—neck of condyle, D—sigmoid (mandibular) notch, E—lingula, F—distal border of ramus, G—coronoid notch). (**B**) Soft tissue anatomy and point of insertion of the needle has been marked. (**C**) The pterygomandibular space consisting the inferior alveolar nerve and vessels, this is the site where the local anaesthetic solution is deposited for an inferior alveolar nerve block. The space is bounded medially by the medial pterygoid and laterally the ramus of the mandible. (**D**) Lingual nerve dissected intraorally. The arrow points to the lingual nerve.

Direct technique (Halstead's approach) (Fig. 11.34A–E)

Needle position

- First position: Inferior alveolar nerve is anaesthetised from the opposite side
- Second position: Lingual nerve is anaesthetised from the opposite side
- 3rd position: Long buccal nerve is anaesthetised separate.

Technique

Patient is positioned in supine or semi supine position with mouth wide open such that the mandibular plane is parallel to the floor. Using index finger or thumb of the left hand, palpate the external oblique ridge and move the finger posteriorly till the coronoid notch (greatest depth of the anterior border of the ramus of the mandible) is contacted. The palpating finger is moved across the retromolar triangle and onto the internal oblique; pterygomandibular raphe and pterygotemporal depression can be seen clearly. Now place the index finger or thumb behind the mandible extraorally to assess the width of the mandible. A 25-gauge needle is inserted from the opposite side parallel to the mandibular plane bisecting the thumb or index finger up to half the distance between the palpating finger intraorally, and the finger behind the ramus of the mandible extraorally until the needle contacts the bone. After negative aspiration, 1.8 mL of solution is deposited slowly. The needle is now withdrawn about half the inserted depth and the remaining local anaesthetics solution is injected to anaesthetise the lingual nerve. The long buccal nerve is anaesthetised using a separate insertion between the external and internal oblique ridges.

The tissue in the mucobuccal fold is entered with the help of a 25-gauge needle at an angle of 45 degrees to the body of mandible just distal to the most posterior tooth.

Indirect technique (Fischer's 1-2-3 technique)

Indirect technique (Fischer's 1-2-3 technique) (Fig. 11.35).

Needle position

- First position: Long buccal nerve is anaesthetised from the opposite side
- Second position: Lingual nerve is anaesthetised from the same side
- 3rd position: Inferior alveolar nerve is anaesthetised from the opposite side.

Technique

The position of the patient and identification of landmarks are similar to that of the direct technique.

First position (long buccal nerve)

Once the tip of the finger is on the internal oblique ridge, the patient is asked to open the mouth wide and a 15/8-inch needle is held in a pen grasp and inserted from the opposite side's bicuspid area into the mucous membrane bisecting the index finger nail. The clinician should not attempt to contact the bone. Six millimetres of the needle should have penetrated the tissues. A total of 0.5 mL of local anaesthetic drug is deposited here to anaesthetise the long buccal nerve, but usually this nerve does not get anaesthetised.

2nd position (lingual nerve)

The syringe is withdrawn slightly and shifted on the same side so that it glides over the temporalis tendon on the

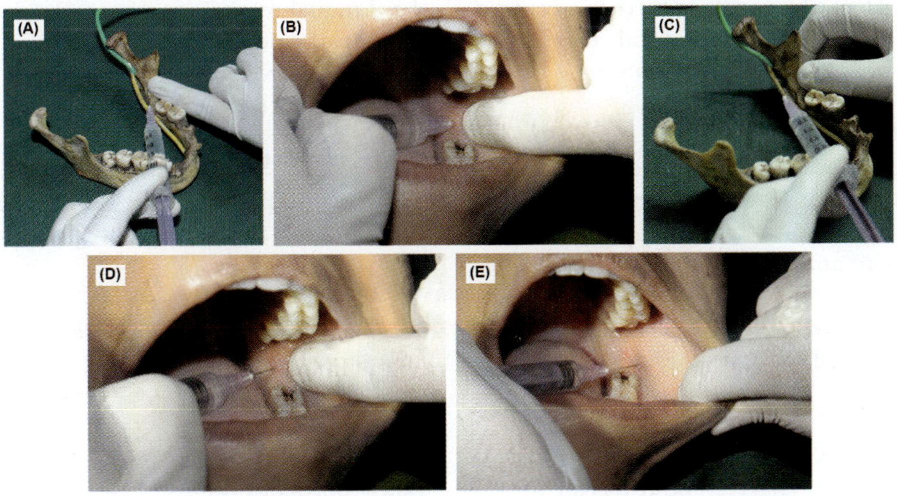

Figure 11.34 **(A)** Demonstration of direct inferior alveolar nerve block in skull-position 1. Needle is directed from the contralateral premolars just behind the lingual nerve anaesthetising the inferior alveolar nerve directly. **(B)** Clinical demonstration—position 1: anaesthetising inferior alveolar nerve. Note the index finger placed along the deepest portion of anterior ascending ramus and needle bisecting it. **(C)** Demonstration of position 2 in skull: needle is withdrawn from position 1 along the same direction with simultaneous injection of LA to anaesthetise the lingual nerve. **(D)** Clinical demonstration—position 2: anaesthetising lingual nerve. **(E)** Clinical demonstration—position 3: anaesthetising long buccal nerve.

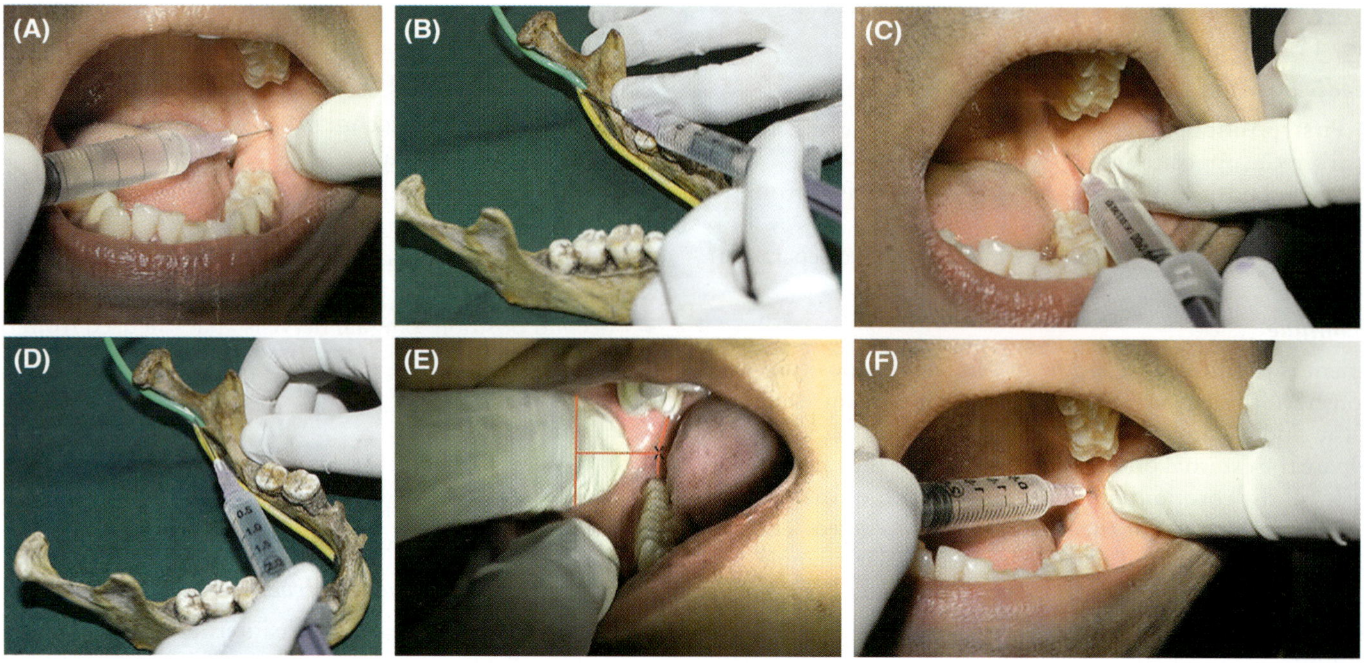

Figure 11.35 (**A**) The 1st step in the indirect technique is anaesthetising the long buccal nerve, this is the position 1 where the syringe barrel will be placed on the opposite side premolars and the depth of penetration of the needle is ~3 to 4 mm after which the retromolar bone will be hit. The clinician will deposit the solution supraperiosteally to anaesthetise the long buccal nerve. (**B**) The 2nd nerve to be anaesthetised is the lingual nerve from the same side of the nerve. The demonstration has been shown on the mandible. The green wire represents the IAN and the yellow wire represents the lingual nerve. (**C**) Clinical demonstration of lingual nerve block position 2. (**D**) Position 3, inferior alveolar nerve block demonstration on a mandible. The syringe barrel is placed on the opposite side premolars, penetrated into the tissues ~20–25 mm, and then deposited. At this point, we can appreciate the needle very close to the nerve and the lingula. The solution will be deposited at the point where the nerve enters the canal. (**E**) The clinician must identify the point of insertion of the needle by using the thumb as a guide. (**F**) Clinical demonstration of position 3. The inferior alveolar nerve block is given once the needle penetrates 20–25 mm into the tissues.

internal oblique ridge. Here, the needle is further advanced to a depth of 6-9 mm and 0.5 mL of local anaesthesia should be deposited.

3rd position (inferior alveolar nerve)

The syringe is again returned to the opposite side and further advanced to a distance of 12-15 mm until bony resistance is felt. After negative aspiration, 1.8 mL of the solution is deposited slowly to anaesthetise the inferior alveolar nerve.

A tingling sensation in the lower lip and one-half of the tongue indicates the effects of the anaesthesia.

GOW-GATES' TECHNIQUE

Devised by Dr. George Gow-Gates, a general practitioner of dentistry, in Australia in 1973. This technique has an advantage of higher success rate than IANB.

Nerves anaesthetised

1. Inferior alveolar nerve
2. Mental nerve
3. Incisive nerve
4. Lingual nerve
5. Mylohyoid nerve
6. Auriculotemporal nerve
7. Buccal nerve.

Areas anaesthetised

Same as IANB along with skin over zygoma, posterior portion of cheek and temporal regions.

Target area

Lateral region of condyle neck, just below the insertion of lateral pterygoid muscle.

Landmarks

Extraoral

Lower border of tragus of ear, which corresponds to the centre of the external auditory meatus and the corner of the patient's mouth.

Intraoral

Tip of the needle is placed just below mesiopalatal cusp of maxillary 2nd molar.

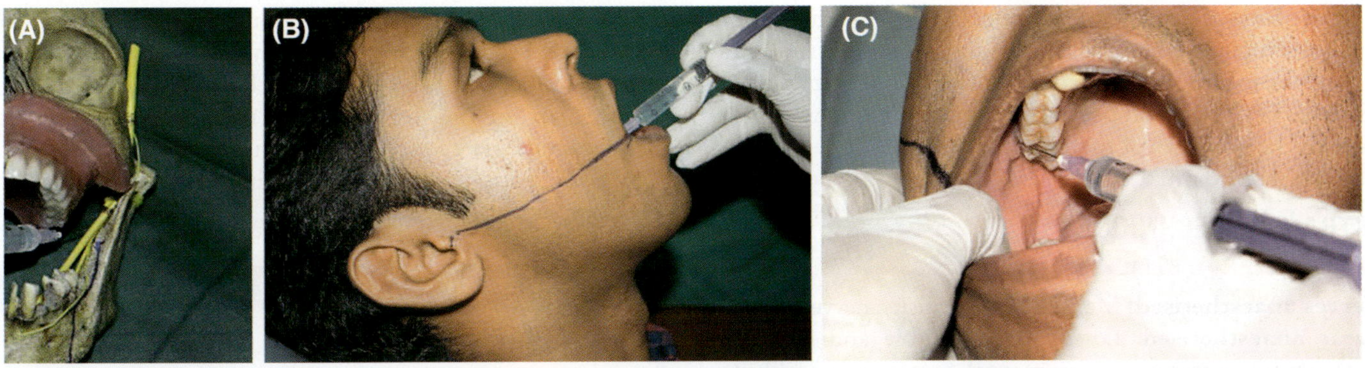

Figure 11.36 (**A**) Demonstration of Gow-Gates' technique in skull. (**B**) Clinical demonstration of Gow-Gates' technique: mouth wide open and needle is directed parallel to the intertragic notch line drawn from the corner of the mouth to intertragic notch. (**C**) The needle is angulated parallel to the divergence of ear to face.

Technique (Fig. 11.36)

Patient is positioned in supine posture with neck extended and mouth wide open. This position facilitates the injection by moving the condyle anteriorly. Now palpate the anterior border of the ramus of the mandible and identify the tendon of temporalis muscle. Penetrate the needle gently into the tissues just distal to the maxillary 2nd molar tooth at the height of mesiopalatal cusp of the 2nd molar. The needle should be just medial to the temporal tendon and directed in the direction parallel to an imaginary line drawn from the corner of the mouth to the intertragic notch of the ear and advanced until the fovea region of the condylar neck is contacted. With negative aspiration, deposit 1.8 mL of solution over 60–90 s. The patient is asked to keep the mouth wide open for 20–30 s after the injection to allow bathing of the nerve with the solution.

VAZIRANI–AKINOSI CLOSED-MOUTH MANDIBULAR BLOCK

This technique was originally proposed by Dr. Joseph Akinosi in 1977, and later gained importance since the landmarks are easily identified and the technique is simple to master (Fig. 11.37).

Nerves anaesthetised

1. Inferior alveolar nerve
2. Mental nerve
3. Incisive nerve
4. Lingual nerve
5. Buccinator
6. Mylohyoid nerve.

Areas anaesthetised: Same as IANB.

Target area

- Soft tissue on the medial border of ramus of the mandible in the region of the inferior alveolar nerve, lingual and mylohyoid nerves
- Height of injection is below that of Gow-Gates' technique.

Landmarks

1. Mucogingival junction of maxillary 2nd or 3rd molar
2. Maxillary tuberosity
3. Coronoid notch of ramus of the mandible.

Technique: Patient is positioned in the supine posture with the teeth occluded.

Retract the lip to expose the maxillary and mandibular teeth. The syringe is directed parallel to the occlusal and

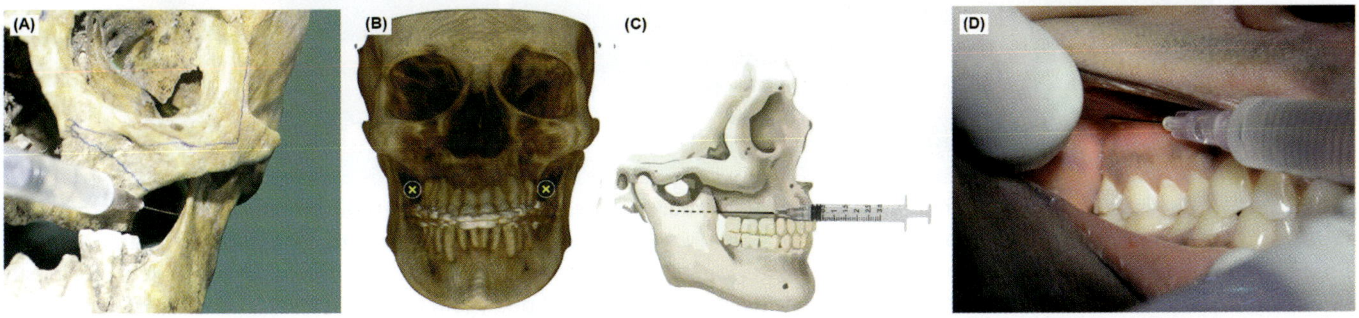

Figure 11.37 (**A**) Demonstration of Akinosi's technique in skull. Note the needle in contact with the green wire (indicating inferior alveolar nerve). (**B and C**) Illustration depicting the site of needle insertion in Vazirani–Akinosi technique. (**D**) Clinical demonstration of Vazirani–Akinosi technique: needle insertion medial to ramus at the height of maxillary molar mucogingival junction.

sagittal planes at the level of the mucogingival junction of the maxillary molars. Penetrate the needle just medial to the ramus of the mandible 25–30 mm into the tissues. Now the tip of needle lies in the mid portion of pterygomandibular space, close to the branches of mandibular nerve. With negative aspiration, 1.5–1.8 mL of anaesthetics solution is deposited.

EXTRAORAL TECHNIQUES

MENTAL NERVE BLOCK

Nerves anaesthetised: Mental nerve, incisive nerve.

Areas anaesthetised: Lower lip, mandible and overlying structures anterior to the mental foramen, mandibular teeth anterior to the mental foramen.

Landmarks: Bicuspid teeth, lower border of the mandible, supraorbital notch, infraorbital notch, pupil of the eye.

Techniques: The supraorbital and infraorbital notches are located by palpation. An imaginary line is drawn through the supraorbital notch, pupil of the eye and the infraorbital notch, which continues down to pass through the mental foramen. A point which is midway between the lower border of the mandible and gingival margin is estimated, and marked on the imaginary line to locate the mental foramen. A 22-gauge needle is directed slightly anteroinferiorly towards the mental foramen that opens in a posterosuperior direction. After negative aspiration, 1 mL of anaesthetic solution is deposited slowly into the foramen.

MANDIBULAR NERVE BLOCK (FIG. 11.38A–G)

Nerves anaesthetised: Mandibular nerve and its subdivision.

Areas anaesthetised: Temporal region, auricle of the ear, external auditory meatus, temporomandibular joint, salivary glands and lower portion of the face except the angle of the jaw.

Landmarks: Same as that for extraoral maxillary nerve block.

Technique: The technique is same as that for maxillary nerve block with the exception that the marker is placed at 5 cm on the needle. When the needle contacts the pterygoid plate, it is withdrawn and redirected slightly upwards and posterior, so that it passes posterior to the lateral pterygoid plate.

COMPLICATION OF LOCAL ANAESTHESIA

LOCAL COMPLICATIONS

The causes of local complications of LA can be iatrogenic (wrong technique), due to the vasoconstrictor or the LA, needle or the patient (Fig. 11.39).

A) COMPLICATIONS ARISING FROM DRUGS OR CHEMICAL USED (TABLE 11.25)

1. Soft tissue injury
2. Toxicity of the drug
3. Allergy to the drug
4. Burning sensation
5. Tissue ischaemia and necrosis
6. Lip chewing.

B) COMPLICATIONS ARISING FROM INJECTION TECHNIQUES (TABLE 11.26)

1. Needle breakage
2. Haematoma
3. Failure to obtain LA
4. Postinjection intraoral lesions
5. Needle stick injury

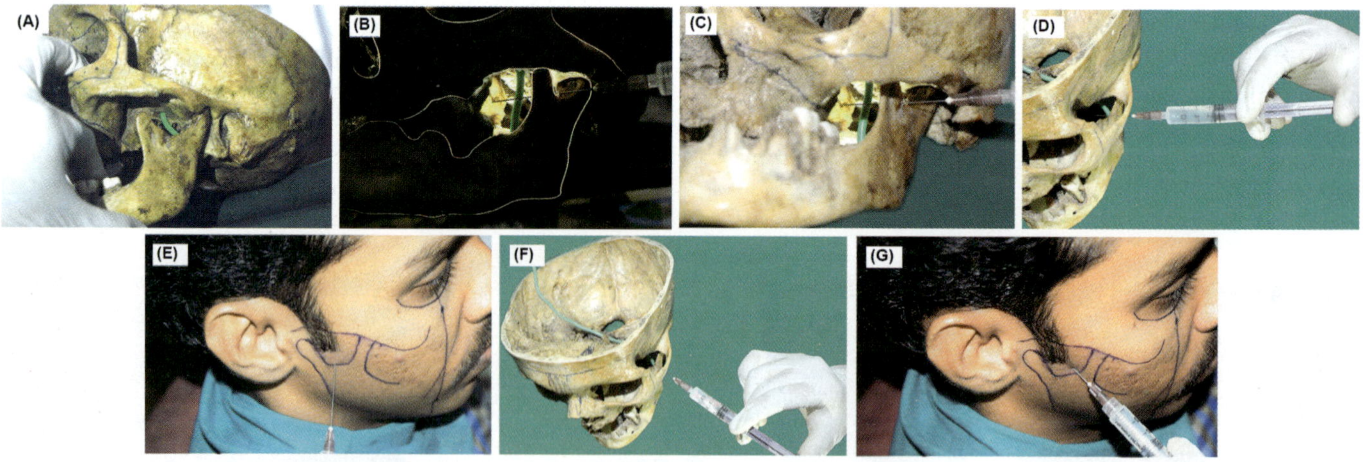

Figure 11.38 (**A**) Surface anatomical landmarks for extraoral mandibular nerve block—sigmoid notch, inferior zygomatic arch, lateral pterygoid plate. Note the mandibular nerve exiting the foramen ovale directed towards the mandibular foramen. (**B**) Note the mandibular nerve (V3) exiting the foramen ovale posterior to the lateral pterygoid plate. (**C**) Demonstration in skull—position 1. Needle directed perpendicular through the sigmoid notch hitting the lateral pterygoid plate. (**D**) Demonstration of same in skull. (**E**) Clinical demonstration—position 1. Needle penetrates perpendicular to the skin through the centre of the sigmoid notch. (**F**) Demonstration in skull—position 2. Needle withdrawn slightly and directed posterior to the lateral pterygoid plate and LA deposited close to the mandibular nerve (V3). (**G**) Clinical demonstration of position 2 of mandibular nerve block.

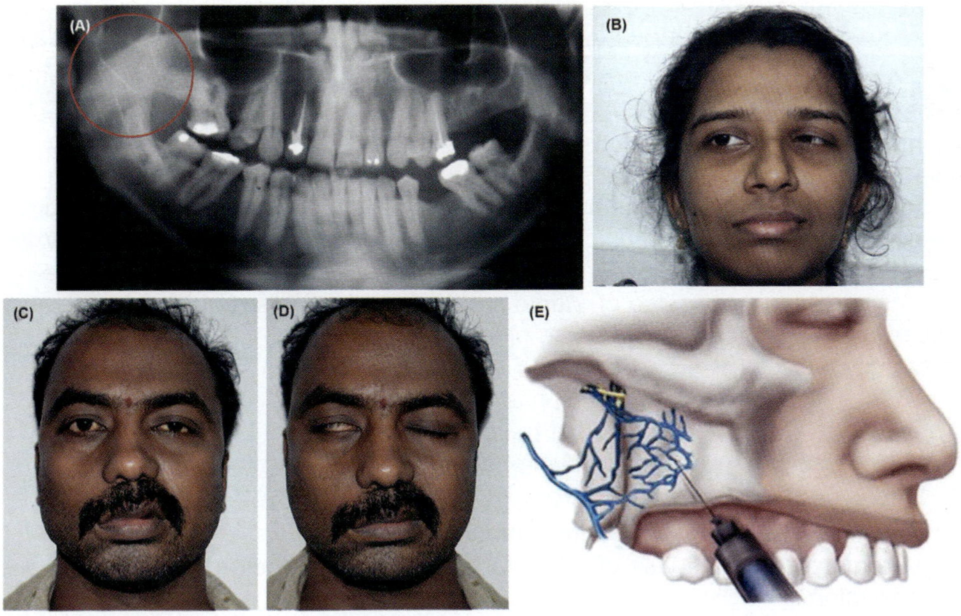

Figure 11.39 Local complications of local anaesthesia. (**A**) Needle breakage in the pterygomandibular raphe area. (**B**) Diplopia—due to paralysis of lateral rectus muscle (abducent nerve). (**C**) Transient facial palsy of right side at rest. (**D**) Transient facial palsy of right-side during action. (**E**) Figure illustrating needle penetration into the pterygoid venous plexus, damage to which can cause haematoma. This commonly occurs during the high tuberosity nerve block.

TABLE 11.25 Complications Arising from Drugs or Chemical Used

Complications Arising from Drugs or Chemical Used	Causes	Prevention	Management
Soft tissue injury	Can occur in patients eating very hot food when the tongue and oral mucosa are numb	Use minimum effective dose Warn patients to avoid hot food while they are numb.	
Toxicity of the drug Clinical presentation of extended systemic effects as a result of overdosage or excessive administration of a drug. Clinically, the patient demonstrates talkativeness, excitability, restlessness, lethargy, increased blood pressure, tachypnoea, unconsciousness, etc.	Accidental intravascular injection High dosage Rapid absorption into the bloodstream	A thorough medical history of the patient prior to administration of LA Administration of minimal effective volume of drug sufficient to achieve the desired anaesthesia Aspiration should be done before depositing the solution Slow administration of the anaesthetic solution	Depending on the degree of clinical presentation, it is treated by: Symptomatic treatment Discontinue any further administration of the LA Adequate ventilation must be maintained BLS is performed if patient loses conscious
Allergy to the drug Allergy is defined as a hypersensitive state due to exposure to a particular allergen, for example, LA solution. The clinical manifestations may include angioedema, urticaria, dermatitis, fever, asthma, rhinitis and anaphylaxis.	Specific antigen–antibody reaction in a patient who has been previously sensitised to a particular drug or chemical derivative.	Intradermal test dose No drugs should be administered if the patient gives a history of allergy	Depending on the degree of clinical presentation, it is treated by: Antihistamine agents Oxygen Steroids BLS administration if required In case of anaphylaxis, management varies (refer to Chapter 8, page number 111)

Continued

TABLE 11.25 Complications Arising From Drugs or Chemical Used—cont'd

Complications Arising from Drugs or Chemical Used	Causes	Prevention	Management
Burning sensation Usually, a transient symptom	Nonisotonic LA solution Decreased pH of the injected solution Rapid injection Contamination of local anaesthetics cartridges LA solution with vasoconstrictor	Sodium chloride or Ringer's solution is added by manufacturers for isotonicity Slow administration of LA Use of sterile cartridges Avoid using older cartridges—if sodium metabisulphite gets oxidised, it becomes sodium bisulphate which has a lower pH	In the majority of cases, the patient may not even be aware of the sensation and since it lasts for only a few seconds, no management is required.
Tissue ischaemia and necrosis Can occur in the hard palate, prolonged vasoconstriction can cause ischaemia of tissues and cause a sterile abscess, ulceration or necrosis of palatal tissue.	This usually occurs when larger than required volume of solution is deposited Rapid deposition with excessive pressure High concentration of vasoconstrictors	Slow administration of LA Use of dilute forms of vasoconstrictors	
Lip or tongue chewing When the patient cannot understand that chewing numb lip/buccal mucosa/ tongue can cause pain later	Seen in children or mental retardation	They must be cautiously monitored	Analgaesics Antibiotics if infected Saline irrigation Petroleum jelly to cover the mucosal trauma—reduces irritation

TABLE 11.26 Complications Arising from Injection Techniques

Complications Arising from Injection Techniques	Causes	Prevention	Management
Needle breakage	Sudden and unexpected movement by the patient in the opposite direction of the needle insertion Reuse of needles Defective manufacturing	Use larger gauge needles Do not insert the needle till its hub Do not redirect the needle in multiple directions inside the tissues	Remove the needle if it is visible, with the help of a haemostat If not visible, take appropriate radiographs of the region. Localise the needle and if in accessible region removal can be done surgically If the needle is lost into the tissue spaces, for example, pterygomandibular space, infratemporal space, assure the patient and review regularly. Unless complicated by pain or infection, fibrous capsule forms and the foreign body, requires no management

TABLE 11.26 Complications Arising from Injection Techniques—cont'd

Complications Arising from Injection Techniques	Causes	Prevention	Management
Haematoma Haematoma is effusion of blood into the extravascular space	Damage of blood vessel by the needle during penetration of soft tissues	Use an appropriate technique Lower the number of needle penetrations Use techniques with lesser risk of haematoma The surgeon should use shorter needles for posterior superior alveolar nerve block	Apply direct pressure over the bleeding site for a few minutes Apply ice-pack (2 to 3 min) locally Prescribe analgaesics, antibiotics and muscle relaxants
Failure to obtain local anaesthesia	Faulty technique Expired LA cartridge Intravascular or intramuscular administration of entire dose of LA solution Infection Anatomical barriers Additional innervation from nutritional canal	Good knowledge of anatomy and surgical technique Aspirate	Repeat injection Give supplementary injections like PDL, pulpal, intraosseous If infection is present, consider reappointment Anaesthetise additional nerves
Postinjection iintraoral lesions Trauma to the oral tissues caused by the needle or any other instrument reactivates the dormant disease	Recurrent aphthous ulcer or herpes simplex sometimes develops after intraoral injection of local anaesthetics *Herpes simplex* develops on oral mucosa attached to the bone, for example palate, attached gingiva *Recurrent aphthous stomatitis* develops on oral mucosa not attached to the bone, for example, buccal mucosa *Pain* is the major symptom and may last for 7–10 days	Gentle handling of tissues	Topical anaesthetics Reassurance to the patient Avoid steroidal antiinflammatory drugs
Needle stick injury Accidental injuries caused by needle already used in a patient. Refer to Chapter 15 page number 273.	Careless technique causes needle stick injury These injuries become serious when patients present with infections like Hepatitis B, Hepatitis C and HIV	Careful handling of sharp objects Prophylactic vaccines	**Hepatitis B** check antibody titer Hepatitis B Immunoglobulins within 48 h of exposure If titre more than 100 μg/mL—no treatment required If titre is low—booster dose of vaccine given **Hepatitis C** Monitor liver function, Interferon α HIV HIV prophylaxis

Continued

TABLE 11.26 Complications Arising from Injection Techniques—cont'd

Complications Arising from Injection Techniques	Causes	Prevention	Management
Mucosal blanching Arteriospasm due to vasoconstrictor	Excessive concentration of vasoconstrictor in LA Depositing more volume of LA in firm mucosa	Avoid intraarterial administration of LA Adhere to LA protocols	Usually, transient will reverse back

6. Failure to obtain anaesthesia
7. Mucosal blanching.

C) COMPLICATIONS ARISING FROM BOTH (TABLE 11.27)

1. Pain on injection
2. Trismus
3. Oedema
4. Persistent paraesthesia or anaesthesia
5. Infection
6. Persistent pain
7. Facial nerve paralysis
8. Visual disturbances—diplopia.

SYSTEMIC COMPLICATIONS (SYSTEMIC EFFECTS OF LOCAL ANAESTHETIC SOLUTION)

ADVERSE DRUG REACTIONS (ADRs):

ADR caused by the drug itself:

(1) Side effects; (2) overdose; (3) toxicity; (4) methaemoglobinaemia.

ADR caused due to the recipient of the drug:

(1) Systemic illness; (2) emotional disturbance; (3) genetic aberrations (malignant hyperthermia); (4) idiosyncrasy.

ADR caused by allergy:

(1) Allergy; (2) anaphylaxis; (3) local toxic effects.

TABLE 11.27 Complications Arising from Both Drug and Injection Technique

Complications Arising from Both	Causes	Prevention	Management
Pain on injection Pain on injection can increase anxiety and may lead to sudden unexpected movement that can cause needle breakage	Dull needles Rapid deposition of solution is painful Barbed needles—when the operator uses same needle for penetration into the vial or when the needle hits the bone on injection, the needle's bevel may bend forming a barb. Patient presents with pain on withdrawal Extremes of temperature of the solution can cause discomfort during injection. Temperature between 15°C and 37°C is not detected by the patient When the soft tissues are not reflected properly—not taut	Slow administration of LA Sharp needle Avoid multiple penetration into the tissues or into the vial to prevent barbs Keep vial at room temperature Reflect the tissue properly so the site of injection is taut	

TABLE 11.27 Complications Arising from Both Drug and Injection Technique—cont'd

Complications Arising from Both	Causes	Prevention	Management
Trismus Muscle spasm resulting in defective mouth opening	Trauma to the muscles and blood vessels in the infratemporal space Trauma to the muscle caused by repeated needle insertion especially medial pterygoid in inferior alveolar nerve block Low grade infection Excessive haemorrhage or haematoma which produces irritation of the tissues and muscle dysfunction Solutions which contain alcohol or other cold sterilising solutions irritate the tissues and produce trismus	Use sharp, sterile, disposable needles as the trauma and infection caused by them is less The injection technique should cause as less trauma as possible Clean the area of needle insertion with an antiseptic solution before injection Avoid repeated insertion A barbed needle is one where the needle tip is deflected upon impact with bone, as occurs during an injection (like IANB). It's preferable not to reuse the needle. When a needle with this barb at the tip is inserted into the muscle, it can cause significant damage.	Moist heat therapy wherein hot towels are applied for 20 min an hour Analgaesics for managing pain Muscle relaxants (chlorzoxazone—250 mg) Physiotherapy involving dynamic jaw exercise If trismus is caused by infection Low grade infection—antibiotics and reappointment High grade infection—check if pus accumulation is present. Incision and drainage
Oedema Oedema (also known as dropsy or fluid retention) is swelling caused by the accumulation of abnormally large amounts of fluid in the spaces between the body's cells or in the circulatory system	Trauma Allergy (angioedema is most common) Haematoma Infection Injection of irritating solution	Asepsis: Avoid injecting into abscess or infection site and reinjecting—area of the oral cavity Use atraumatic techniques and gentle handling of tissues Proper medical history of the patient	Assess the type of oedema, cause and check for airway (no risk of obstruction) and vital signs Traumatic oedema resulting from inflammation resolves in 1–3 days with antiinflammatory drugs Allergic oedema: Requires immediate assessment to avoid risk of anaphylaxis; treated with antihistamines and steroidal antiinflammatory drugs
Persistent paraesthesia or anaesthesia It refers to altered sensation in the area of skin or mucosa	Trauma to the nerve by inadvertent needle penetration Injection of local anaesthetic solution with alcohol or cold sterilising solution near a nerve produces irritation and oedema of the tissues and subsequent pressure on the nerve Haemorrhage around the neural sheath also causes pressure on the nerve, leading to paraesthesia	Proper injection technique	Most cases resolve within 8 weeks Reassurance to the patient Vitamin B complex supplements Review regularly to check for Tinel's sign If it persists for more than 1 year, it requires neurosurgical intervention If no recovery after 1 year, microneurosurgery may be advocated

Continued

TABLE 11.27 Complications Arising from Both Drug and Injection Technique—cont'd

Complications Arising from Both	Causes	Prevention	Management
Infection Use of unsterilised, contaminated needles can induce infection	Commonly involved pathogens include *Pseudomonas, Escherichia coli, Staphylococcus aureus, Mycobacterium*	Use of disposable syringes and needles Use of appropriately sterilised needles Avoid cross contamination between different sites within the oral cavity	Treat the infection with appropriate antibiotics Needle stick injury Failure to obtain anaesthesia Mucosal blanching Persistent paraesthesia
Persistent pain	Subperiosteal infiltration of the LA solution—tears periosteum	Supraperiosteal or para periosteal infiltration	Analgaesics
Facial nerve paralysis Usually occurs in inferior alveolar nerve block. Facial nerve is the motor supply to muscles of facial expression.	Injection of local anaesthetic agents in the parotid capsule or within the substance of the parotid gland The patient suffers unilateral paralysis of the facial muscles.	Ensure that the needle tip contacts the bone before the solution is injected	Reassure the patient and explain that it is transient Remove contact lenses if the patient is wearing Avoid further dental therapy and reassess for recovery Loss of motor action of the muscles of facial expression produced by local anaesthesia lasts for 1–3 hours.
Visual disturbances—diplopia Diplopia refers to double vision	It is caused by the paralysis of the lateral rectus due to diffusion of anaesthetic solution directly from the pterygomaxillary fossa to the inferior orbital tissue in the orbit. This will, in turn, affect the ciliary ganglion located between the optic nerve and the lateral rectus muscle of the eye	Proper injection technique	Reassure the patient by explaining the situation. The diplopia lasts only for a few hours and will resolve without any residual effect

OVERDOSE

Overdose reactions are those clinical signs and symptoms that manifest as a result of an overadministration of a drug. When the drug reaches the systemic circulation in concentrations that are more than normal (maximum recommended dose), the patient presents with a series of symptoms and signs depending on the severity. Three types of overdose are (1) mild, (2) moderate and (3) severe. Overdose of LA drug depends on various factors like:

a) Patient factors: Age, sex, BMI, use of other drugs, presence of systemic diseases, genetics and environment
b) Drug factors: Vasoactivity, concentration, dose, route of administration, rate of injection, vascularity of injection site, presence of vasoconstrictors.

According to literature, overdose is a serious and more common complication in children. It is important to restrict the number of procedures and quadrants requiring LA for children. The surgeon also should calculate the MRD for the child previous to the appointment and plan the procedure accordingly. The symptoms of minimal to moderate overdose is between 2 and 10 μg/mL and the severe symptoms are above 10 μg/mL, these symptoms have been illustrated in Fig. 11.7 for easy understanding.

CAUSES: The plasma levels have an unusually slow biotransformation and is slowly eliminated as biotransformed and unbiotransformed drug through the kidneys. Overdose of LA agents also have an unusually rapid absorption and inadvertent intravascular administration.

MANAGEMENT: Depending on the rate of onset of symptoms the treatment will vary (Table 11.28).

TABLE 11.28 Management of Mild and Severe Overdose

Mild Overdose		Severe Overdose	
After 15 min	After/within 5 min	After 5–15 min	Immediate within 1 min
Patient is conscious and talking	Patient is either conscious and is progressive to convulsions	Patient is conscious and talking	Patient is unconscious
Caused by Large total dose Rapid absorption	Caused by Large total dose Rapid absorption Abnormal biotransformation Renal dysfunction	Caused by abnormal biotransformation, renal dysfunction	Due to intravascular injection of LA
Call for help (emergency medical assistance)			
BLS—position, airway, breathing, circulation			
Definitive care			
Administer O_2			
Monitor vitals			
Establish i.v. line		Establish i.v. line to administer anticonvulsant	
Assess	Administer i.v. midazolam 1 mg/min	i.v. midazolam 1 mg/mL	i.v. midazolam 1 mg/mL i.m. midazolam 5 mg/mL
If patient attains normal vitals Send patient with an attender	Examination by physician and follow medical advice	Examination by physician for managing hypotension and follow medical advice	Examination by physician for managing hypotension and follow medical advice

TABLE 11.29 Factors Affecting Toxicity

Drug Factors	Administration Factors	Patient Factors
1. Drug – CVS/CNS toxicity ratio for each drug is different 2. Dose – Continuous infusions or multiple procedures can cause delayed toxicity	1. Site of administration Intravascular—the most common cause of LA toxicity. Followed by intercostal, caudal, epidural, regional blocks and subcutaneous 2. Use of adjuncts (vasoconstrictor reduces systemic absorption of LA) 3. Technique—frequent aspiration	1. Blood flow to the site of administration 2. α1-Acid glycoprotein (neonates and infants have half the level of AAG than adults) 3. Hepatic disease 4. Age (both children and the elderly have reduced clearance of LA) 5. Acidosis (increases unionised portion) 6. Hypercarbia (increases cerebral blood flow)

TOXICITY

Local anaesthetics are toxic to both the CNS and CVS. This occurs when the rate of the drug entering the circulation is higher than the drug excreted from circulation. Toxicity is related to three factors (Table 11.29):

1. Drug factors
2. Administration factors
3. Patient factors.

Cardiac toxicity

Cardiac toxicity due to LA overdose causes direct myocardial depressant effects by blocking of the cardiac Na^+ channels. Severity of the toxicity depends on the time it takes for a drug to be bound to the sodium channels. Lidocaine is bound to the channel for the shortest amount of time and so causes the least amount of toxicity. This is also why lignocaine can be used as an antiarrhythmic, but other agents cannot. Bupivacaine takes 10 times longer to dissociate compared to lidocaine. Cardiac toxicity is triphasic; the three phases have been illustrated in flowchart 11.3 for easier understanding.

Central nervous system toxicity

LAA in their unionised form can cross the blood-brain barrier (BBB) and interfere with CNS conduction. CNS toxicity

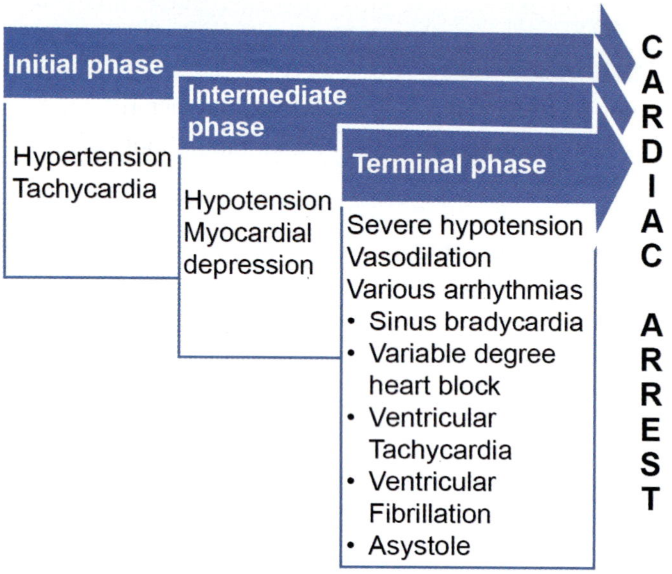

Flowchart 11.3 Phases of Cardiac toxicity.

is biphasic; the two phases have been illustrated for easier understanding.

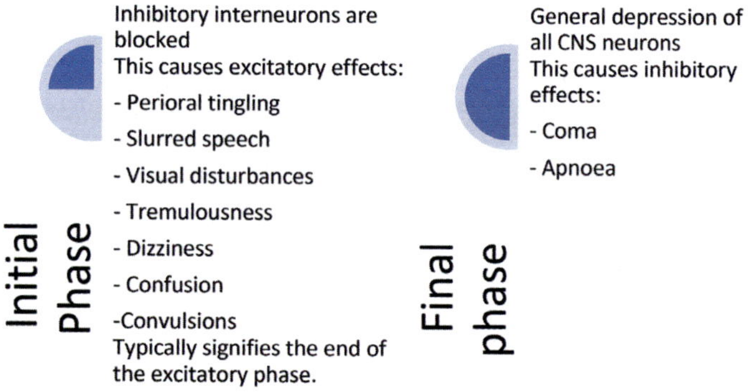

Treatment

Toxicity is managed initially with circulation, airway and breathing (CAB) approach in the dental office. The steps to be followed by a dental practitioner has been illustrated in the flowchart 11.4; the definitive management is injection of intralipid emulsion (ILE). ILE is a sterile, fat emulsion prepared for intravenous administration. It is made up of 10% soybean oil, 1.2% egg yolk phospholipids and 2.25% glycerin. Mechanism of action is uncertain, but theories include: ILE binds with unionised LA molecule, causing it to distribute off receptor sites and competitive antagonism—ILE may directly inhibit LA binding. Dose of ILE 20% is either as a bolus dose of 1.5 mL/kg over 1 min or by infusion at 15 mL/kg/h.

METHAEMOGLOBINAEMIA

After administration of amide local anaesthetics, methaemoglobinaemia can occur in some patients. In dentistry, prilocaine and benzocaine, which are quite commonly

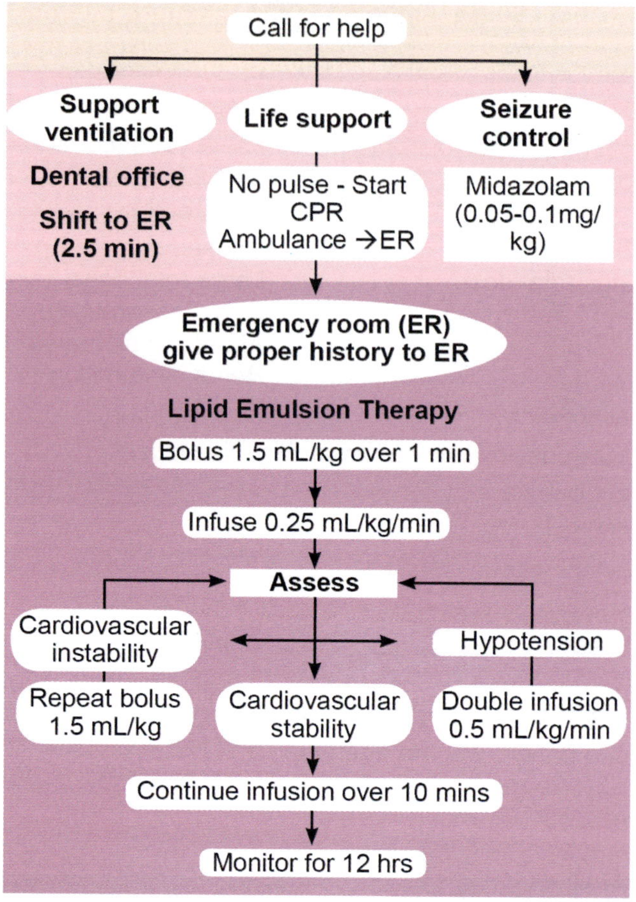

Flowchart 11.4 The steps of handling LA systemic toxicity.

used by some practitioners may induce methaemoglobinaemia. It occurs when the iron within the haemoglobin molecule gets oxidised from a ferrous state to ferric state. This state is called methaemoglobin. Methaemoglobin cannot deliver as much oxygen as haemoglobin due to its affinity for its bound oxygen and its decreased affinity for unbound oxygen.

Signs and symptoms usually do not appear until 3–4 h after the administration of overdose of local anaesthesia. Clinical signs of cyanosis are seen when blood levels of methaemoglobin reach 10%–20% followed by dyspnoea and tachycardia at levels 35%–40%. The diagnosis is confirmed by a blood sample and a cooximetry test.

ALLERGY

Allergy is when a patient presents with a hypersensitive state caused by exposure to an allergen. Reexposure to this allergen can cause a heightened reaction.

CAUSES: The patient who has been previously sensitised to a particular drug or a chemical agent (allergen) produces an allergic reaction. This is called antigen-antibody reaction.

SIGNS and SYMPTOMS: Skin rashes, utricaria, pruritis, oedema, erythema and wheezing.

PREVENTION: Proper personal history, past dental history and drug history.

MANAGEMENT: Antihistamines—diphenhydramine (benadryl) 20–50 mg, epinephrine 0.5 mL, administer O_2, if necessary.

ANAPHYLAXIS

Anaphylaxis is a life-threatening allergic reaction that can occur due to local anaesthetic drug. Patient presents with skin reactions, smooth muscles spasm, respiratory distress, cardiovascular collapse and loss of consciousness.

MANAGEMENT (FLOWCHART 11.5)

IDIOSYNCRASY

Idiosyncrasy is an unpredictable reaction to a LA agent that cannot be classified as allergic or toxic reaction.

PREVENTION:

Preanaesthetic evaluation, avoid combining drugs, mostly unpredictable and unpreventable.

Precautions to the patients under CNS depressant drugs can cause stimulation in some patients.

MANAGEMENT: Initially CAB (basic life support). Place the patient in the supine position with legs slightly elevated. Maintenance of airway, supply adequate O_2. Evaluate circulation—administer parenteral fluids. Treat symptomatically.

MALIGNANT HYPERTHERMIA

Malignant hyperthermia (MH; hyperpyrexia) is a pharmacogenic disorder caused by an autosomal dominant gene. This variant alters the individual's response to certain drugs that act as triggering agents. It does not cause any impediment in the dental practice, as studies from the 1980s proved that amide local anaesthetics do not trigger MH, but MH can occur in these genetically predisposed individuals when they undergo GA. Studies have shown that the most common drugs that triggers are succinylcholine and halothane. Lidocaine with or without epinephrine seem to be safe in these patients, however, it is preferable to do any invasive procedures for these patients under medical support (with emergency physicians or anaesthetist) to manage any ADRs. Acute symptoms of malignant hyperthermia are fever (above 104°F i.e., 40°C), cyanosis, tachycardia, tachypnoea, variable blood pressure, respiratory acidosis, metabolic acidosis, muscle rigidity and death.

RECENT ADVANCES IN LOCAL ANAESTHESIA

CENTBUCRIDINE

This drug belongs to quinolone group of drugs. Though it was formulated in 1983 (Central Drug Research Institute, Lucknow by Patnaik et al.), the drug has not been widely used in dentistry. The onset of action of centbucridine is slower than lignocaine + adrenaline, but the duration and depth of anaesthesia were similar. The advantages of this drug are its property of vasoconstriction; hence adrenaline need not be added with it. Theoretically, it has no cardiovascular interference. This allows the drug to be used for patients with CVS instability where adrenaline cannot be used. Centbucridine can be effectively used for patients who have ester and amide allergy.

3% TETRACAINE OXYMETAZOLINE NASAL MIST

This was formulated for upper anterior teeth and premolars. This nasal mist is used to anaesthetise ASA and MSA nerves, which are branches of the infraorbital nerve. The duration of action is approximately 5–45 min. This formula was also successful for paediatric patients. This composition was successful for incisive nerve supplying the anterior palatal mucosa for 15 min.

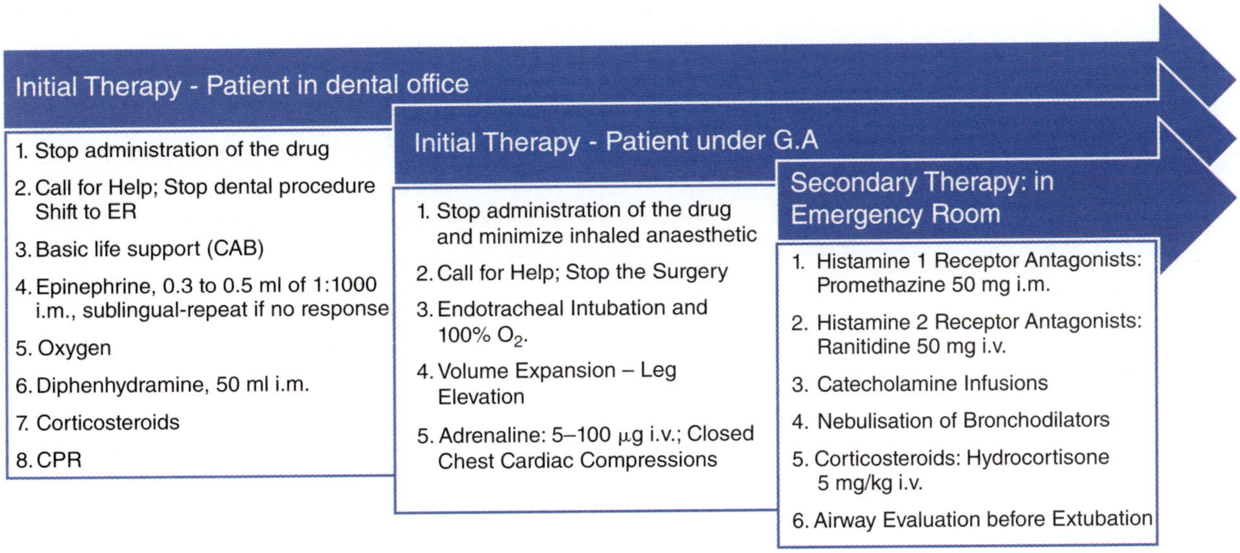

Flowchart 11.5 Management of Anaphylaxis.

ULTRA—LONG-ACTING LOCAL ANAESTHETIC AGENTS

SYNERGISTIC TOXINS (TETRODOTOXIN, SAXITOXIN, NEOSAXITOXIN)

The synergistic effects of toxins have been studied on animals. Tetrodotoxin from puffer fish and saxitoxin from dinoflagellates (marine plankton) and freshwater cyanobacteria (blue-green algae) are toxins that block a specific site on the extracellular side of the sodium channel blockers. Another compound neosaxitoxin also blocks the same site. These three compounds have a *synergistic effect* when used with a LAA (lidocaine + epinephrine). This can drastically increase the duration of action of the drug. Overdose of these compounds can result in respiratory distress. Studies on animals show that combining tetrodotoxin and bupivacaine can increase the duration of action to 9 h and 30 min.

LIPOSOMAL CARRIERS (DEPOFOAM)

To increase the duration of action, LAA are encapsulated in lipid-based particles. When injected into the site of action, the lipid matrix begins releasing bupivacaine in a sustained manner. Thus increasing the duration of action to approximately 72 h. Any local anaesthetic drug can be encapsulated into these liposomal carriers.

MAGNESIUM AS AN ADJUVANT FOR LOCAL ANAESTHESIA

In clinical trials, magnesium (150 mg) with bupivacaine increased the duration of action to 9.5 h. No magnesium related toxicity was observed.

OPTOGENETICS AND LOCAL ANAESTHESIA

A photo-isomerisable molecule, **quaternary ammonium–azobenzene–quaternary ammonium** (QAQ) was developed, that resembles lidocaine. It has two forms, cis and trans. The cis form converts to trans form when exposed to 500 nm of light activating pain control and the trans form to cis form at 380 nm of light inactivating pain control. The trans form blocks the ion channels and the cis form inactivates the molecule's function. Thus, the molecule is active in trans form and inactive in cis form. The 380 nm light acts as an 'off switch' and 500 nm acts as an 'on switch'. The researchers have not yet found a way to inject the QAQ into a living subject.

General Anaesthesia

OUTLINE

General anaesthesia (GA) is a drug-induced, reversible loss of consciousness during which patients are not arousable, even by painful stimulus. The ability to independently maintain ventilatory function is often impaired. Patients require assistance in maintaining a patent airway and positive pressure ventilation may be required because of depressed spontaneous ventilation or drug-induced depression of neuromuscular functions.

PREANAESTHETIC EVALUATION

Preanaesthetic evaluation consists of the consideration of information from multiple sources that may include the patient's medical records, interview, physical examination and findings from medical tests and evaluations. To avoid any complications, it is mandatory to elicit the required history from the patient including current medical/systemic/surgical problems.

PAST MEDICAL HISTORY

The aspects relating to the cardiovascular system (CVS) and respiratory system are the most important in a patient's medical history. The questions and details required will vary depending upon the disease present, its severity, anticipated anaesthesia and the planned operation. History of previous blood transfusions is important.

PREVIOUS ANAESTHESIA HISTORY

- History of any difficulties with previous anaesthetics, for example, nausea, vomiting, dreams, awareness, postoperative jaundice, etc. The records of previous anaesthetic exposure are noted to rule out or clarify problems such as difficulties with intubation, drugs administered or adverse drug reactions
- Idiosyncratic drug-induced liver injury (DILI) may result from repeated exposure to halothane. Hence, to avoid this risk, the approximate date of previous administration of anaesthetics, particularly if recent, is noted.

DRUGS AND ALLERGIES

Dose and duration of medication, prescribed as well as over-the-counter self-medication, herbal products, natural supplements, etc. Compared to any other group, the geriatric population consumes more systemic medications. Special attention must be paid to drug interactions and complications that arise in this population.

Medications that may have an interaction with anaesthetic agents should be discontinued. Other drugs that have to be adjusted, continued and discontinued are briefed in Table 12.1.

FAMILY HISTORY

A history of prolonged apnoea after anaesthesia may suggest pseudocholinesterase deficiency. History of any inherited or 'family' diseases, for example, sickle cell disease, porphyria, malignant hyperpyrexia, etc. Malignant hyperthermia is a rare inherited disorder with high mortality rate that occurs following GA administration.

SOCIAL HISTORY

Smoking

Avoiding smoking for 8 weeks improves the airways, for 2 weeks reduces their irritability. Carboxyhaemoglobin levels drop 24 hours before anaesthesia.

TABLE 12.1 Concurrent Drug Therapy: Drugs that have to be Adjusted, Continued or Discontinued

Drugs that Require Adjustment in Dosage	Drugs Continued on the Morning of Operation and Perioperatively	Preoperatively Drugs need to be Discontinued
1. **Angiotensin converting enzyme (ACE) inhibitors:** Captopril, enalapril—discontinued but replaced with other drugs 2. **Anticoagulants:** **Oral:** Warfarin, nicoumalone **Intravenous:** Heparin 3. **Insulin sliding scale** 4. **Steroids**	1. **Antibiotics:** Aminoglycosides, polymyxins 2. As selective **cyclooxygenase-2 (COX-2) inhibitors** do not potentiate bleeding they can be continued until surgery 3. **β-Blockers:** Atenolol, metoprolol, oxprenolol, propranolol, sotalol 4. **Calcium antagonists:** Diltiazem, nifedipine, verapamil, digoxin 5. **Anticonvulsants:** Barbiturates, phenytoin, carbamazepine 6. **Diuretics:** Thiazides, loop diuretics	1. **Monoamine oxidase inhibitors (MAOIs):** 2. Due to the increased risk of venous thrombosis, the **oral contraceptive pill** should be discontinued at least 6 weeks before elective surgery 3. To avoid excessive bleeding, **aspirin** should be discontinued 7–10 days before surgery and thienopyridines (such as clopidogrel) for 2 weeks before surgery 4. 4–5 days prior to invasive procedures **oral anticoagulants** should be stopped, allowing INR to reach a level of 1.5 before surgery

Alcohol

Induction of liver enzymes and tolerance to anaesthetic drugs are the result of excessive alcohol consumption. The risk of postoperative alcohol withdrawal syndrome should be considered.

Drugs

The use of drugs for recreational purposes needs to be determined specifically including type, frequency and route of administration. These groups of patients are at risk of infection with hepatitis B and human immunodeficiency virus (HIV). In patients using an intravenous (i.v.) route due to widespread thrombosis of veins, there can be difficulty with venous access.

Pregnancy

In all women of childbearing age, the date of the last menstrual period (LMP) should be noted. In early pregnancy, the risk of inducing a spontaneous abortion is increased by anaesthesia, while in late pregnancy, the risk of regurgitation and aspiration is increased.

REVIEW OF SYSTEMS

A complete review of systems to look for undiagnosed disease or inadequately controlled chronic disease should be included in the history. The most relevant with respect to fitness for anaesthesia and surgery are the diseases of the CVS and respiratory system.

CARDIOVASCULAR SYSTEM

Specific enquiries must be made about:

- Angina: Its incidence, precipitating factors, duration and use of antianginal medications such as glyceryl trinitrate (GTN) tablets or spray
- Previous myocardial infarction (MI) and subsequent medical care
- History of palpitations, cough, shortness of breath and syncope
- History of orthopnoea, paroxysmal nocturnal dyspnoea and ankle swelling
- Patients with a history of ischaemic heart disease (IHD), MI, hypertension, heart failure and valvular heart disease are important to be identified
- Before performing noncardiac surgery after MI or revascularisation, a 3-month minimum delay is indicated. Recent studies have demonstrated a marked benefit of reduced cardiac complication rate by operating under the protection of β_1-adrenergic antagonism
- Greater risk of perioperative reinfarction, the incidence of which is related to the time interval between the infarct and the surgery in patients with a proven history of MI
- Exaggerated cardiovascular responses during anaesthesia may result from untreated or poorly controlled hypertension **(diastolic consistently > 110 mmHg)**. The risk of myocardial ischaemia is increased by both hypertension and hypotension. Blood pressure should not exceed 180/110 mmHg before general anaesthesia
- Anaesthetic drugs have depressant effects on the heart, which will worsen heart failure, thereby impairing the perfusion of vital organs
- Anticoagulants may be taken by patients with valvular heart disease or prosthetic valves. Before surgery, they may need to be discontinued or changed. During certain types of surgery, antibiotic prophylaxis will be required.

RESPIRATORY SYSTEM

Enquire specifically about these symptoms:

- Cough and production of sputum (volume and colour)
- Dyspnoea

- Wheeze and precipitating factors
- Identify patients who have a history of chronic obstructive pulmonary disease (COPD), emphysema, bronchiectasis and asthma
- Patients with preexisting lung disease, particularly if they are also obese, are more prone to positive chest infections. Unless it is for a life-threatening condition, a patient with an acute upper respiratory tract infection should have anaesthesia and surgery postponed
- A very useful indication of both cardiac reserve and respiratory reserve is the patient's ability to perform everyday physical activities before having to stop because of symptoms (e.g. chest pain, shortness of breath).

OTHER CONDITIONS THAT ARE IMPORTANT IF IDENTIFIED IN THE MEDICAL HISTORY

Diabetes

- When a diabetic patient needs surgery, *neglect of the long-term complications does more harm than short-term control of blood glucose levels.* The majority of long-standing diabetics develop compromise in one or more organs. Careful preoperative assessment of symptoms and signs of peripheral vascular, cerebrovascular and coronary artery disease is essential in a diabetic patient planned for elective surgery. It is important to identify and manage the coexisting pathologies perioperatively
- Postoperatively, patients may develop *hypoglycaemia* (glucose level <50 mg/dL [2.8 mmol/L] in adults and <40 mg/dL [2.2 mmol/L] in children) due to residual effects of long-acting oral hypoglycaemic agents or insulin preparations given preoperatively in addition to perioperative fasting, anaesthetics, analgesics, sedatives and sympatholytic agents alter the usual presenting symptoms of hypoglycaemia, thereby delaying the recognition of hypoglycaemia in the perioperative period. In addition, blunting of the adrenergic symptoms associated with hypoglycaemia is found in diabetics with autonomic neuropathy. Confusion, irritability, fatigue, headache and somnolence are the initial symptoms, which may progress to seizures, focal neurologic deficits, coma and death
- Generally, in diabetic patients, there is an increased incidence of IHD, renal dysfunction, postoperative infection, autonomic and peripheral neuropathy. The incidence of intraoperative and postoperative complications increase.

Neuromuscular disorders

In these patients, care must be taken when administering muscle relaxants.

Chronic renal failure

Anaemia, electrolyte abnormalities and altered drug excretion are some of the problems seen in these patients. The choice of anaesthetic agents is restricted due to altered drug excretion.

Jaundice

This is usually indicative of infective or obstructive liver disease. Alteration in drug metabolism may be present. Preoperatively, the patient's coagulation must be checked.

Epilepsy

- Perioperatively, in patients with a history of well-controlled epilepsy, measures should be taken to avoid disruption of antiepileptic medication. On the morning of surgery, regular medications should be continued and regular dosing should be reestablished as early as possible after surgery
- In case of day-case surgeries, if a single dose is missed, it should be taken as soon as possible after surgery. Antiepileptic drugs (AEDs) should be administered parenterally when multiple doses are likely to be missed. i.v. forms of phenytoin, sodium valproate and levetiracetam are available (where i.v. doses are equivalent to oral doses) and carbamazepine is available as a suppository
- Serum concentrations of phenytoin are checked daily in patients admitted to ICU. It serves as a guide for adjusting the dose.

GENERAL EXAMINATION

- **Physical examination**
- **Vital signs**
- **Airways:** Examination of airway is important as various causes related to dental, mandible or cervical spine may cause difficulty during endotracheal intubation. Especially in case of trauma, cervical spine examination is mandatory. Various causes related to difficult laryngoscopy are as follows:

1. Anatomical causes associated with difficult laryngoscopy
   a. Proclined incisors
   b. Long and high-arched palate
   c. Retrognathic mandible
   d. Restricted mandibular movement
   e. Decreased atlanto-occipital distance (causes reduced neck extension)
   f. Short muscular neck
   g. Gross obesity
   h. Large breasts in females
2. Conditions associated with difficult laryngoscope
3. Congenital deformities
   Down syndrome, Pierre Robin syndrome, Treacher Collins syndrome, Marfan's syndrome (associated with small mouth/large tongue/cleft palate)
4. Trauma and infection
   Dental abscess, fracture of mandible (causes reflex spasm of masseter and medial pterygoid relieved by anaesthesia)
5. Temporomandibular joint (TMJ) ankylosis
   Restricted/immobility of mandible (not relieved after anaesthesia)

6. Soft tissue oedema/swelling/mass
   Infections, trauma, tumours
7. Miscellaneous
   Foreign bodies, scarring after infection/radiotherapy/burns

AIRWAY ASSESSMENT

Assessment is often made in three stages: (1) observation of patient's anatomy, (2) simple bedside tests and (3) X-rays.

Observation of patient's anatomy

1. Amount of mouth opening (interincisal distance), a receding mandible
2. Teeth: position, number and health
3. Tongue size
4. Soft tissue swellings of the neck
5. Deviated larynx or trachea
6. Mobility of the cervical spine in both flexion and extension.

Simple bedside tests

Wilson score: Five factors are assessed and scored based on a set of criteria. A score greater than five suggests difficult intubation. Rarely used now.

Thyromental distance: With the head fully extended; on the neck, the distance between the bony point of the chin and the prominence of the thyroid cartilage is measured. A distance less than 7 cm indicates difficult intubation (Table 12.2).

Mallampati criteria: The patient is asked to open the mouth and maximally protrude the tongue while sitting upright. The view of the pharyngeal structures is noted and graded I–IV. Grades III and IV suggest difficult intubation (Table 12.3).

X-rays (not used routinely)

Measurements can be made on a lateral X-ray of the head and neck, which can be used to help predict an impaired view at laryngoscopy. These include a decreased distance between the occiput and the spinous process of C1 (<5 mm) and an increase in the posterior depth of the mandible (>2.5 cm). Allowance for any magnification should be taken into account for X-ray.

SYSTEMIC EXAMINATION

Cardiovascular system

Arrhythmias, for example, atrial fibrillation need to be determined. Auscultation should be done to rule out valvular heart disease, which may need further investigations. The patient's blood pressure should be taken. Finally, any potential problem with intravenous access can be identified by inspecting the peripheral veins.

TABLE 12.2 Difficulty Level Depicted by Thyromental Distance

	Thyromental Distance (Patil's Test)	
	Tip of the thyroid to mentum distance	**Difficulty level**
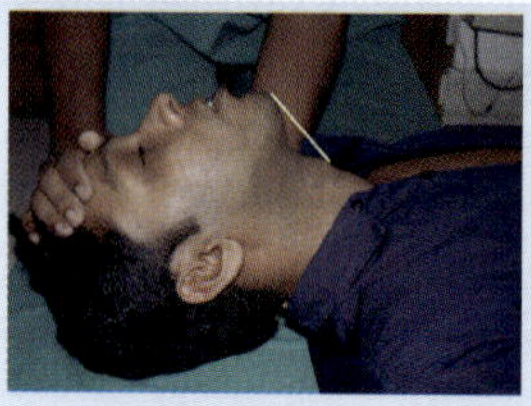	6.5 mm	No problem for laryngoscopy
	6–6.5 mm	Difficult, but laryngoscopy possible
	<6 mm	Very difficult/impossible laryngoscopy

TABLE 12.3 Modified Mallampati Classification

Grade I	Grade II	Grade III	Grade IV
Structures visualised			
Posterior pharyngeal wall, soft palate and uvula, faucial pillars, tongue base	Soft palate and uvula, faucial pillars, tongue base	Soft palate, faucial pillars, tongue base, base of uvula	Hard palate and tongue base. Only hard palate visible
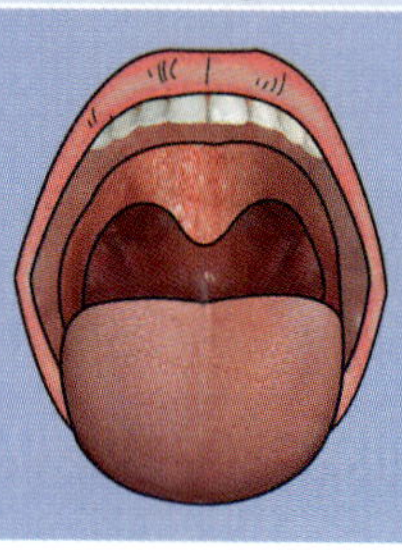	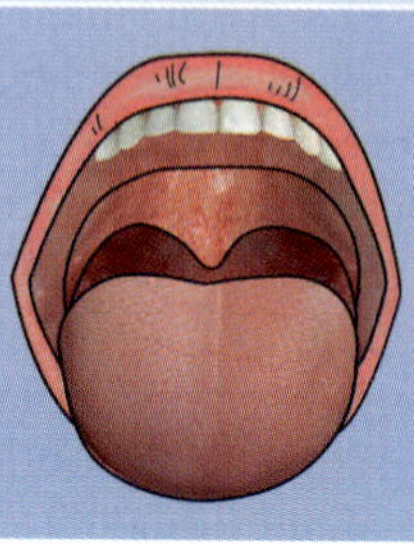	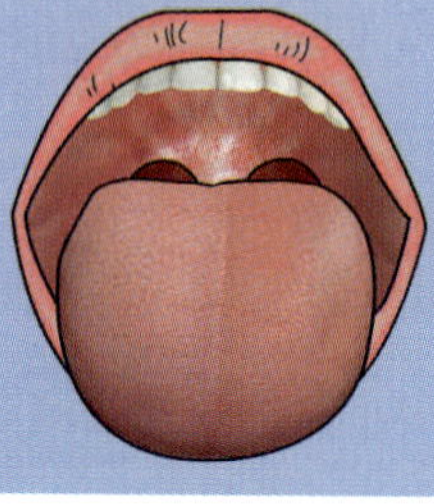	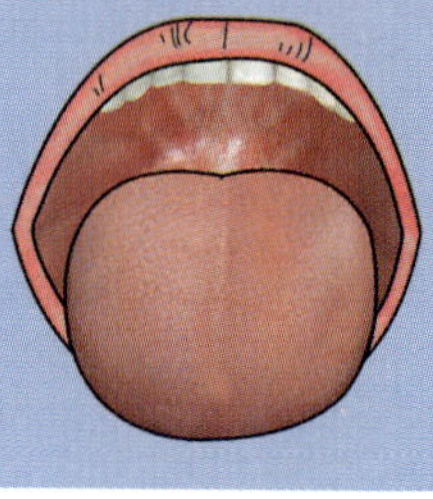

Respiratory system

Identify signs such as dyspnoea, wheezing, signs of collapse, consolidation and effusion. The presence and degree of pulsus paradoxus serves as a useful indicator of the severity of airway obstruction.

Nervous system

Identify chronic disease of the peripheral nervous system and central nervous system (CNS) and record any evidence of motor or sensory impairment.

Musculoskeletal system

Restriction of movement and deformities are seen in patients with connective tissue disorders. Patient's cervical and temporomandibular joints need specific attention—special investigations.

In patients with no evidence of concurrent disease, investigations can be limited (Table 12.4).

ADDITIONAL INVESTIGATIONS

Ultimately, the need for investigations is dictated by the presence of other diseases. Investigations depend on type of surgery, comorbid illness and patient's present medical condition.

Complete blood count (CBC), Haemoglobin (Hb), Haematocrit (HCT)

History of increased bleeding, haematologic disorders, renal disease, chemotherapy or radiation treatment.

Urea and electrolytes

Patients taking digoxin, diuretics, steroids.
Those with diabetes mellitus, hypertension, renal disease, vomiting, diarrhoea.

Liver function tests (LFT)

Patients with known hepatic diseases.
A history of a high alcohol intake (>50 units/week).
Evidence of malnutrition.
Patients with metastatic disease.

TABLE 12.4 Baseline Investigations for Otherwise Healthy Patients

Age	Sex	Investigations
<40	Male Female	Nil Hb and haematocrit values
41–60	Male Female	ECG, blood sugar, serum creatinine, Hb ECG, blood sugar, creatinine
>61	Both	Hb, ECG, blood sugar, creatinine

Hb—haemoglobin; ECG—electrocardiograph.

Blood sugar

Diabetes mellitus.
Patients with severe peripheral arterial disease.
Patients taking long-term steroids.

Electrocardiogram (ECG)

Patients known to be or found to be hypertensive or with a history of coronary artery disease (CAD), MI, diabetes, congestive heart failure (CHF) chest pain, palpitations, murmurs, peripheral oedema, syncope, dizziness, dyspnoea, shortness of breath, stroke.

Those patients with symptoms or signs of heart disease.

Chest X-ray

History or signs of cardiac or respiratory disease.
Patients with suspected or known malignancy.
Patients from areas of endemic tuberculosis who have not had a chest X-ray in the previous year.

Pulmonary function tests

Patients with dyspnoea on mild exertion and asthmatics require measurement of peak expiratory flow rate (PEFR); forced expiratory volume in 1 s (FEV 1); forced vital capacity (FVC).

Factors prompting preoperative pulmonary evaluation:

- Age >70
- Morbid obesity
- Thoracic surgery
- Upper abdominal surgery
- History of smoking, cough
- Any pulmonary disease.

Coagulation screening

Patients with history of bleeding diathesis or patients on anticoagulants or previous excessive intraoperative bleeding, hepatic disease, poor nutritional status.

Those with known history of liver disease or jaundice.

Sickle cell screen (Sickledex)

Patients with a family history of sickle cell disease.
Patients whose ethnic origin has risk of sickle cell disease.
If positive, electrophoresis may be required for definitive diagnosis.

Cervical spine X-ray

Patients with rheumatoid arthritis.
Patients with a history of major trauma or surgery to the neck.

Echocardiograph

Presence of any congenital disease, abnormal ECG, poor functional reserve, history or signs of cardiac disease.
History of cardiac illness in the family.

ANAESTHETIC RISK ASSESSMENT

General indicators of risk

Factors associated with increased risk of mortality:

- Increasing age: >60 years
- Sex: Male > female
- Worsening physical status
- Increasing number of concurrent medical conditions, in particular
  - MI
  - Diabetes mellitus
  - Renal disease
- Increasing complexity of surgery
  - Intracranial abnormalities
  - Major vascular disease
  - Intrathoracic disease
- Increasing length of surgery (>2 h)
  - Emergency operations.

Special indicators of risk

One system used to predict the risk of a cardiac event is the Goldman index. Points are awarded as shown in Table 12.5. Another risk indicator is classifying the patient based on ASA classification in Table 12.6.

TABLE 12.5 Goldman Index

History	Points
>70 years	5
Myocardial infarction in prior 6 months	10
Examination	
3rd heart sound (gallop rhythm) or raised jugular venous pressure (JVP)	11
Significant stenosis	3
ECG	
Rhythm other than sinus or presence of premature atrial complexes	7
More than five ventricular ectopics per minute	7
General	
PaO_2 < 60 mmHg; $PaCO_2$ > 50 mmHg	
K′ < 3 mmol/L	
Urea > 8.5 mmol/L; creatinine > 200 mmol/L	
Chronic liver disease	
Bedridden for noncardiac disease for one or more criteria	3
Operation	
Intrathoracic, intraperitoneal or aortic operation	3
Emergency surgery	4

Goldman index point scale showing risk of associated cardiac event or death

Points %	Risk Cardiac Event	% Risk Death
0–5	0.7	0.2
6–12	5	2
13–25	11	2
>26	22	56

PREANAESTHETIC PREPARATION OF THE PATIENT (Table 12.7)

PREMEDICATION

Premedication originally referred to those drugs administered to facilitate the induction and maintenance of anaesthesia, literally preliminary medication. Commonly used premedication for major oral and maxillofacial surgeries:

- Atropine 0.12 mg/kg or glycopyrrolate 0.044 mg/kg
- Pethidine 50 mg or pentazocine or buprenorphine 3-6 mg/kg or fentanyl
- Promethazine 25 mg.

The properties of the premedication drugs can be remembered as the 10 A's of premedication

1. Anxiolysis
2. Amnesia
3. Anaesthetic sedation
4. Antiemetic
5. Antacid
6. Antiautonomic effect
7. Antisialagogues
8. Analgesics
9. Antibiotic prophylaxis
10. Allergy prophylaxis.

THE DRUGS USED AS PREMEDICATION FOR ANAESTHESIA

ANXIOLYSIS, AMNESIA, SEDATIVES, HYPNOTICS

Many patients awaiting surgery are anxious. The drugs should also provide anterograde amnesia and reduce risk of awareness during surgery. Benzodiazepines are the most commonly prescribed among the anaesthetic drugs. A degree of sedation and amnesia is produced. Orally administered 45–90 min preoperatively, it is well absorbed from the gastrointestinal tract. Large doses may cause hypnosis and unconsciousness. It may cause moderate depression of circulation and respiration and also cause agitation/restlessness. Other agents that are useful as anxiolytics such as barbiturates, butyrophenones (droperidol) and phenothiazines (promethazine, trimeprazine, diphenhydramine). In addition, they produce sedation and are mildly antiemetic. Sometimes, phenothiazines are associated with extrapyramidal symptoms and hypotension, secondary to their α-blocking actions. β-Blockers may occasionally be of use in patients with excessive somatic manifestations of anxiety, for example, tachycardia.

TABLE 12.6 ASA (American Society of Anesthesiologists) Physical Status Scale and the Relationship Between ASA Status and Postoperative Mortality

ASA Physical Status Classification System	Absolute Mortality (%)	Guide Mortality per 10,000 Anaesthetics
ASA Physical Status 1—A normal healthy patient	0.1	7.2
ASA Physical Status 2—A patient with mild systemic disease	0.2	19.7
ASA Physical Status 3—A patient with severe systemic disease that limits activity and is not incapacitating	1.8	115.1
ASA Physical Status 4—A patient with incapacitating severe systemic disease that is a constant threat to life	7.8	766.2
ASA Physical Status 5—A moribund patient who is not expected to survive with or without an operation	9.4	3358
ASA Physical Status 6—A declared brain-dead patient whose organs may be removed for donor purposes		
ASA Class E—Added as a suffix for emergency operation E—Emergency operation of any variety (used to modify one of the above classifications [I–IV], i.e. ASA III–E)		

- The classification of the patient helps us decide if the patient can be treated as an outpatient
- A patient with a higher risk of medical emergencies must be treated in a hospital with adequate facilities to handle emergencies
- If the patient under treatment for a systemic disease, is pregnant, has undergone a recent surgery or has undergone an immunity modifying treatment, due opinion, concurrence and consent should be obtained from the treating specialist before embarking on any oral surgery

TABLE 12.7 Steps in Preanaesthetic Preparation of the Patient

Psychological counselling before procedure	Helps with anxiety and apprehension before the procedure	
Hypersensitivity reaction to local anaesthetic agents	Skin sensitivity test: Test is conducted 3 h before the procedure or in the previous visits. An erythematous wheal of greater than 1 cm depicts a positive test.	
Consent	Consent for undergoing general anaesthesia should contain consent for emergency procedures like tracheostomy	
Premedication	Premedication can be given through sublingual, i.v., i.m., oral and rectal routes	
	1. Anxiolysis	Temazepam 20–30 mg
	2. Amnesia	Diazepam 10–20 mg
	3. Anaesthetic sedation	Lorazepam 2–4 mg
	4. Antiemetic	Metoclopramide, ondansetron 4 mg i.v.
	5. Antacid—aspiration prophylaxis	Cimetidine 150–300 mg or Ranitidine 50–100 mg
	6. Antiautonomic drugs	Atropine 0.12 mg/kg
	7. Antisialagogues	Glycopyrrolate 0.044 mg/kg
	8. Analgesics	Fentanyl 1–2 μg/kg or Pethidine 50 mg or Pentazocine or Buprenorphine 3–6 mg/kg
	9. Antibiotic prophylaxis	
	10. Allergy prophylaxis	

Continued

TABLE 12.7 Steps in Preanaesthetic Preparation of the Patient—cont'd

The drugs and the properties of the premedication		
Preoperative instructions	Fasting guidelines before a GA procedure (NPO—nil per oral)	
	Clear fluids	Nonclear fluids and solid food
	For child less than 6 months	
	2 h NPO	4–6 h NPO
	For child 6 months to 3 years of age	
	2–3 h NPO	6 h NPO
	For child above 3 years of age	
	2–3 h NPO	6–8 h NPO
	For adults	
	2–3 h NPO	6–8 h NPO
	Concurrent drug therapy	
	Medications that may have an interaction with anaesthetic agents should be stopped. Other drugs that require to be modified, continued or discontinued have been described in Table 12.1.	
Other preanaesthetic instructions	Smoking	
	• Ideal to stop before 6 weeks • Should be stopped at least 1–2 weeks prior as this helps the health of the respiratory mucosa and decrease sputum volume • Ceased 12–24 h prior to procedure to remove circulation of nicotine and carbon monoxide from the blood	
	Removal of prosthesis	
	• Dentures can cause airway obstruction. • Prosthetic eye can cause dislodgement. • Contact lens can cause corneal abrasion. • Prosthetic limbs: The metal part can cause burns when electrocautery is used.	
	Hearing aid	
	• Patient must wear hearing aid to follow anaesthetist's instructions prior to induction and during extubation.	
	All jewellery	
	• Should be removed and presurgical disinfection of the surgical site should be done	
	Emptying bladder before procedure	

Those most commonly used include:

- Temazepam 20–30 mg
- Diazepam 10–20 mg
- Lorazepam 2–4 mg.

Diazepam: It is considered as the 'gold standard' drug with excellent anxiolytic, amnestic and sedative effect. It is dissolved in organic solvents and hence causes pain on i.v. and i.m. injection. It has a long duration of action, hence is not suitable for day-care surgical procedures. Preadministration of diazepam is given on the night before surgery for anxiolysis. It is contraindicated in cirrhosis, liver and renal dysfunction patients.

Midazolam: It is a rapidly metabolising drug with sedative, anxiolytic and excellent amnestic properties. Rapid onset of action and more potent than diazepam. Major advantage is that it does not cause phlebitis as it is water-soluble.

Barbiturates: It was previously used for preoperative sedation before benzodiazepines. They do not produce analgesia and may sometimes cause antianalgesic effects. It also causes cardiovascular and respiratory depression. It is contraindicated in porphyria patients. Due to its various side effects, it has been largely replaced by benzodiazepines.

ANALGESIA AND SEDATION

Although the oldest form of premedication, now generally reserved for patients in pain preoperatively. Intramuscular (i.m.) form is the best route of administration. The most commonly used are:

- Morphine
- Pethidine
- Fentanyl.

Morphine, Pethidine and Papaveretum were widely used due to their sedative effects, but are relatively poor as anxiolytics. Benzodiazepines have largely replaced them. In addition, opiates have side effects such as nausea, vomiting, respiratory depression and delayed gastric emptying. In patients receiving opioids preoperatively, these drugs may be continued with a watch on respiration. In patients with acute pain, paracetamol and nonsteroidal anti-inflammatory drugs (NSAIDs) are recommended as these are nonsedating and do not cause respiratory depression.

ANTIAUTONOMIC/ANTICHOLINERGIC DRUGS

Parasympathetic reflexes

Profound bradycardia resulting from excessive vagal activity may be seen following the use of certain anaesthetic agents:

- Use of halothane, especially for induction
- Repeated doses of suxamethonium
- Techniques using alfentanil, particularly if combined with vecuronium.

Surgical stimuli also have the same effect

- During traction on the extraocular muscles (squint corrections)—oculomotor reflex
- Elevation of a fractured zygoma
- Periorbital surgery.

In neonates and infants, atropine is given preoperatively before induction to prevent bradycardia intraoperatively.

Bradycardia is prevented by the administration of anticholinergic agents such as atropine and glycopyrrolate. Though used preoperatively, they are most effective when administered intravenously at induction.

Antisialagogues effect

In conjunction with hyoscine, they also prevent excessive secretion of saliva induced by the presence of objects in the mouth, for example, an oropharyngeal airway or the use of the anaesthetic agents such as ketamine and ether.

Sympathetic reflexes

Tachycardia and hypertension at the time of intubation indicate increased sympathetic activity. This is undesirable in certain patients, for example, IHD or raised intracranial pressure and hypertensive patients. Attenuation of these responses can be done by the use of β-blockers. They can be administered either orally preoperatively (atenolol, propranolol) or intravenously at induction (esmolol). Administration of potent analgesics at induction of anaesthesia (fentanyl, alfentanil) serves as an alternative.

ANTIEMETIC

Antiemetic drugs are often used as part of the premedication in an attempt to reduce the nausea and vomiting induced by the administration of opioids. Most commonly used drugs are metoclopramide and ondansetron. A wide variety of drugs have antiemetic properties and many of these can be used for premedication:

- Dopamine antagonists, for example, metoclopramide, domperidone, droperidol
- Antihistamines, for example, cyclizine, promethazine
- Anticholinergics, for example, atropine, hyoscine
- Phenothiazines, for example, promazine
- 5-Hydroxytryptamine antagonists, for example, ondansetron.

ANTACID

To reduce the risk of regurgitation and aspiration of gastric acid, patients who are about to be anaesthetised must have an empty stomach. This is usually achieved by a period of starvation preoperatively. It may be difficult to guarantee in patients who have hiatus hernias and those who are very anxious. Delayed gastric emptying is seen in patients who have received opiates preoperatively or present as emergencies, particularly if in pain. An alternative is using a nasogastric or orogastric tube for aspiration of gastric contents: only in pregnant or full stomach cases in emergency. Oral or intravenous formulations of ranitidine or pantoprazole are used preoperatively in mostly full stomach patients. To increase the pH and to reduce the volume, a variety of drug combinations are used:

- Oral sodium citrate: Chemically neutralises residual acid
- Cimetidine, ranitidine (H_2 antagonists): Reduce acid secretion
- Metoclopramide: Increases gastric emptying and lowers oesophageal sphincter tone. Potential for regurgitation is reduced.

OTHER PREMEDICANTS

Premedicants are a variety of other drugs that are commonly administered prophylactically prior to anaesthesia and surgery. The following are the most common:

- Steroids: To patients on long-term treatment or who have received them within the past 3 months
- Antibiotic prophylaxis: To patients with prosthetic or diseased heart valves
- Anticoagulants: As prophylaxis against deep venous thrombosis
- Transdermal GTN: Administered as patch or a paste (percutol) in patients with IHD to reduce the risk of coronary ischaemia
- Eutectic Mixture of Local Anaesthetics (EMLA): A topically applied local anaesthetic cream. It is used to reduce the pain of inserting an intravenous cannula.

Stage		Eyes: Reflexes abolished	Eyes: Pupil Size	Eyes: Ocular Movement	Respiration: Rate	Respiration: Muscle tone – Intercostal	Respiration: Muscle tone – Diaphragm	Airway reflexes abolished	CVS: Heart rate	CVS: Blood pressure	Muscle tone	Respiratory response to skin incision	Remarks
I. Analgesia		N	N	Voluntary control	N	N	N	None	↑	N	N	N	Good for venipuncture, labour pains, dental analgesia
II. Excitement		Lid		Divergent	Irregular			Swallowing	↑↑	↑	↑↑		Tachycardia, tachypnoea, risk of aspiration is present
III. Surgical Planes	Plane 1	Corneal			N			Vomiting and pharyngeal	↑	N			Risk of aspiration is present
	Plane 2			N	↓			Laryngeal	N	↓		No response to skin incision	Risk of aspiration is present, airway obstruction due to tongue fall
	Plane 3	Pupillary light		None	↓↓			Carinal	↓	↓↓			Ideal to intubate, surgical stage needs IPPR
	Plane 4	No light reflex		None	Nil			All	↑ or ↓	↓↓↓			Respiratory arrest and CVS collapse
IV. Imminent Death		Respiratory arrest Medullary paralysis (Due to overdosage of an anesthetic drug)				Apnea					Flaccid		Active cardiopulmonary resuscitation

N-Normal, ↑-Increase, ↑↑-Moderate increase, ↑↑↑- Significant increase, ↓-Decrease, ↓↓-Moderate decrease, ↓↓↓-Significant decrease

Abbreviations: CVS-Cardiovascular system, IPPR-Intermittent Positive Pressure Respiration

Figure 12.1 Stages of General Anaesthesia (GA) (especially with ether).

STAGES OF GENERAL ANAESTHESIA (Fig. 12.1)

1. **Stage I (stage of analgesia or disorientation)**: From the beginning of induction of general anaesthesia to loss of consciousness
2. **Stage II (stage of excitement or delirium):** From loss of consciousness to onset of automatic breathing. Only eyelash reflex disappears while other reflexes remain intact and coughing, vomiting and struggling may occur; respiration can be irregular with breath holding
3. **Stage III (stage of surgical anaesthesia):** From onset of automatic respiration to respiratory paralysis. It is divided into four planes:
   a. **Plane I**—from onset of automatic respiration to cessation of eyeball movements. Eyelid reflex is lost, swallowing reflex disappears, marked eyeball movement may occur, but conjunctival reflex is lost at the bottom of the plane
   b. **Plane II**—from cessation of eyeball movements to beginning of paralysis of intercostal muscles. Laryngeal reflex is lost although inflammation of the upper respiratory tract increases reflex irritability, corneal reflex disappears, secretion of tears increases (a useful sign of light anaesthesia), respiration is automatic and regular, and movement and deep breathing as a response to skin stimulation disappears
   c. **Plane III**—from beginning to completion of intercostal muscle paralysis. Diaphragmatic respiration persists, but there is progressive intercostal paralysis, pupils dilated and light reflex is abolished. The laryngeal reflex lost in plane II can still be initiated by painful stimuli arising from the dilatation of anus or cervix. This is the desired plane for surgery when muscle relaxants are not used
   d. **Plane IV**—from complete intercostal paralysis to diaphragmatic paralysis (apnoea)
4. **Stage IV: From stoppage of respiration till death.** Anaesthetic overdose causes medullary paralysis with respiratory arrest and vasomotor collapse. Pupils are widely dilated and muscles are relaxed.

PHASES OF GENERAL ANAESTHESIA

1. **Induction:** Induction time begins with the onset of administration of general anaesthesia to the development of surgical anaesthesia. Intravenous anaesthetic injection is used for the induction and then gases and vapours are administered for maintenance
2. **Maintenance:** Sustaining the state of general anaesthesia
3. **Recovery:** Administration of anaesthetic agent is stopped and consciousness is regained.

DRUGS USED FOR THE INDUCTION OF ANAESTHESIA

The classification of the drugs used to induce anaesthesia has been described in Flowchart 12.1. They are classified based on the route of administration.

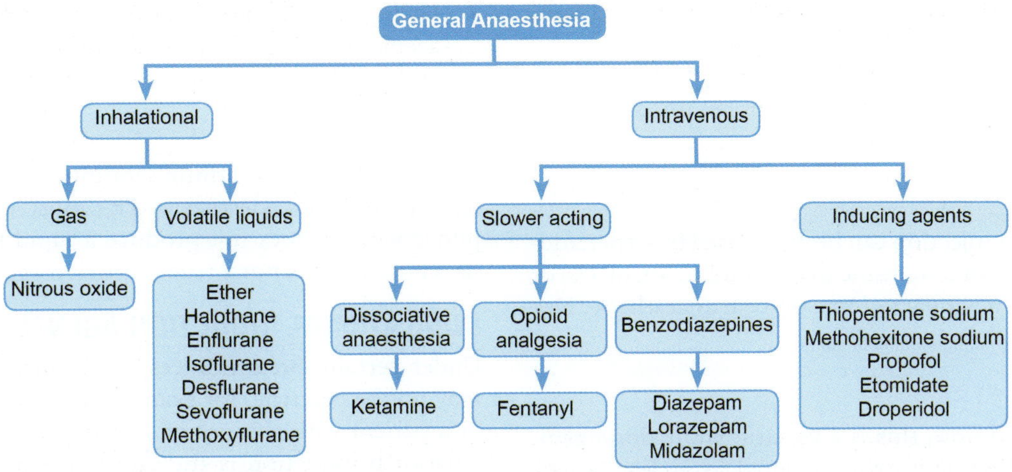

Flowchart 12.1 Classification of general anaesthesia.

INTRAVENOUS INDUCTION AGENTS

Induction agents are those drugs, which are used to start (induce) anaesthesia. Generally, consciousness is regained as these drugs are redistributed from the brain to other tissues. Alternatively, anaesthesia can be induced by the inhalation of an increasing concentration of a volatile agent. Of the i.v. agents currently in use, only propofol is used subsequently to maintain anaesthesia.

1. SODIUM THIOPENTONE

Sodium thiopentone is most commonly used water-soluble barbiturate induction agent. It is a yellow powder with a faint smell of garlic due to the presence of sulphur in the molecule. It is dissolved in water to make a 0.5% solution (500 mg in 20 mL), which is very alkaline (pH 12.5) and inhibits bacterial growth. The ampoules contain a small amount of sodium carbonate to maintain solubility. Thiopentone is incompatible with any other drug and precipitation follows mixing.

Induction

- Dose: 2–7 mg/kg
- Dose varies according to age: for adults 3–4 mg/kg
- Induction of anaesthesia is rapid and smooth
- Consciousness usually returns after 4–10 min.

Systemic effects

1. CNS: Sedation, loss of consciousness and anaesthesia, potent anticonvulsant property
2. CVS: Hypotension, fall in cardiac output, vasodilatation
3. Respiratory system: A short period of breath holding, hypercapnia and ultimately apnoea
4. Miscellaneous: Muscle relaxation, hepatic enzymes are induced and urine output is reduced.

Advantages

Induction is rapid with minimal excitation effects and good initial recovery. It is painless on i.v. injection.

Disadvantages

- Alkaline solution is an irritant to tissues and can cause necrosis if the injection extravasates. Respiratory depression and loss of protective laryngeal reflexes can both lead to the development of hypoxia and can cause hypotension and circulatory collapse in overdose
- Accidental intraarterial injection causes acute, severe pain with loss of the distal circulation due to intense vascular spasm. If untreated, this can cause gas gangrene.

2. PROPOFOL

Propofol is an i.v. anaesthetic agent, a phenolic derivative, which is not water-soluble. It is prepared as an emulsion (hence white in colour) in soybean oil and egg phosphatide. Ampoules contain a 1% solution (200 mg in 20 mL) with no bactericidal agent. Once opened, the contents must either be used or discarded.

Induction

- Dose is usually between 1.5 and 2.5 mg/kg
- Either pain or a burning sensation on injection can occur
- Induction of anaesthesia is rapid
- After 4–7 min, there is a rapid, full recovery of consciousness.

Systemic effects

1. CNS: Sedation, loss of consciousness and anaesthesia, may reduce the seizure threshold in epileptic patients
2. CVS: Hypotension, vasodilatation, inhibits baroreceptor reflex, hence no reflex tachycardia occurs
3. Respiratory system: Apnoea, ventilation and the response to carbon dioxide are depressed
4. Miscellaneous: Muscle relaxation is more pronounced after propofol.

Advantages

- Quality of recovery following propofol is better than any other agent, which has made it the drug of choice for day-care surgery

- Significant reduction in postoperative nausea and vomiting
- Nonirritant to veins
- Hypersensitivity and allergic reactions are uncommon
- Allergies can occur to propofol.

Disadvantage

The discomfort on injection can be minimised by either adding a small amount of lignocaine to propofol (2 mL of 1%) or by preinjection of a similar volume of local anaesthetic. Not used in patients below 1 year of age.

3. KETAMINE

Although less used now, this is a versatile induction agent. It is a phencyclidine derivative presented as a clear, water-soluble solution in three different concentrations: 10, 50 and 100 mg/mL. The multidose ampoules have a long shelf life. Unlike other agents, it can be administered either intravenously or intramuscularly to induce anaesthesia.

Induction

- i.v. dose is 1–2 mg/kg
- The i.m. dose is 5–10 mg/kg and it may take 8–10 min to lose consciousness and the subsequent duration of action is variable.

Systemic effects

1. CNS: Ketamine produces 'dissociative anaesthesia', the most important features of which are anterograde amnesia and intense analgesia. Intracranial pressure may be increased due to increased cerebral blood flow. It is strongly associated with vivid hallucinations during recovery
2. CVS: Tachycardia, increase in both systolic and diastolic blood pressure and increase in cardiac output. High doses cause direct cardiac depression
3. Respiratory system: Ventilation is minimally depressed and the response to carbon dioxide is maintained, bronchodilatation
4. Miscellaneous: Increased muscle tone, increase in salivation.

Advantages

- In cases of difficult venous access, i.m. injections are useful
- Used in repeated minor painful procedures, especially in children, for example, burns dressings.

Disadvantages

- Hallucinations and unpleasant dreaming during recovery, particularly in females
- The increase in intracranial pressure makes it potentially dangerous for use in patients with head injuries
- May exacerbate preexisting hypertension
- Hallucinations can be minimised by the use of benzodiazepines, either as premedication or given concurrently and by allowing a quiet, slow recovery.

4. MIDAZOLAM

Occasionally, the i.v. administration of a benzodiazepine is used to induce anaesthesia. The most commonly used is midazolam. It does not produce a rapid loss of consciousness and hence is not a true induction agent.

INHALATIONAL INDUCTION AGENTS

Under certain circumstances, i.v. induction of anaesthesia may not be practical, for example, in an uncooperative child or a patient with absence of suitable veins. Furthermore, inhalational induction is the safe technique in patients with airway compromise. The administration of an i.v. agent will cause the patient to become apnoeic, leading to a failure in securing the airway, thus causing failure of ventilation and oxygenation. The alternative is to use inhalational agents that are normally used to maintain anaesthesia. Preoxygenation is performed, which increases concentration of the inhalational agent (if there is airway compromise) or in a mixture of oxygen and nitrous oxide. Unlike when using the i.v. agents, anaesthesia is induced more slowly and respiration is preserved.

Earlier with the use of ether, four stages of anaesthesia (Guedel stages) were recognised, but this staging is not applicable to the present-day general anaesthesia (Fig. 12.2).

DRUGS AND INHALATIONAL AGENTS USED FOR THE MAINTENANCE OF ANAESTHESIA

After induction, anaesthesia is most commonly maintained by the administration of a combination of nitrous oxide and an anaesthetic vapour in oxygen, which the patient breathes spontaneously or which is delivered to the lungs by a ventilator. The amount of anaesthetic delivered is expressed as the percentage by volume, the concentration usually reflecting the potency of the agent used. An inspired concentration of 1%–2% of the halogenated agents will anaesthetise most patients, whereas 70% nitrous oxide alone may not be sufficient to guarantee unconsciousness.

NITROUS OXIDE

- Colourless, inorganic gas
- Sweet smelling
- Nonirritant gas
- Neither flammable nor explosive
- Supports combustion
- Available in cylinders coloured French blue.

Anaesthesia

- Good analgesic, but a poor anaesthetic
- 70% is the maximum safe concentration administered as an inspired oxygen concentration of 30% is required to provide adequate oxygenation during anaesthesia

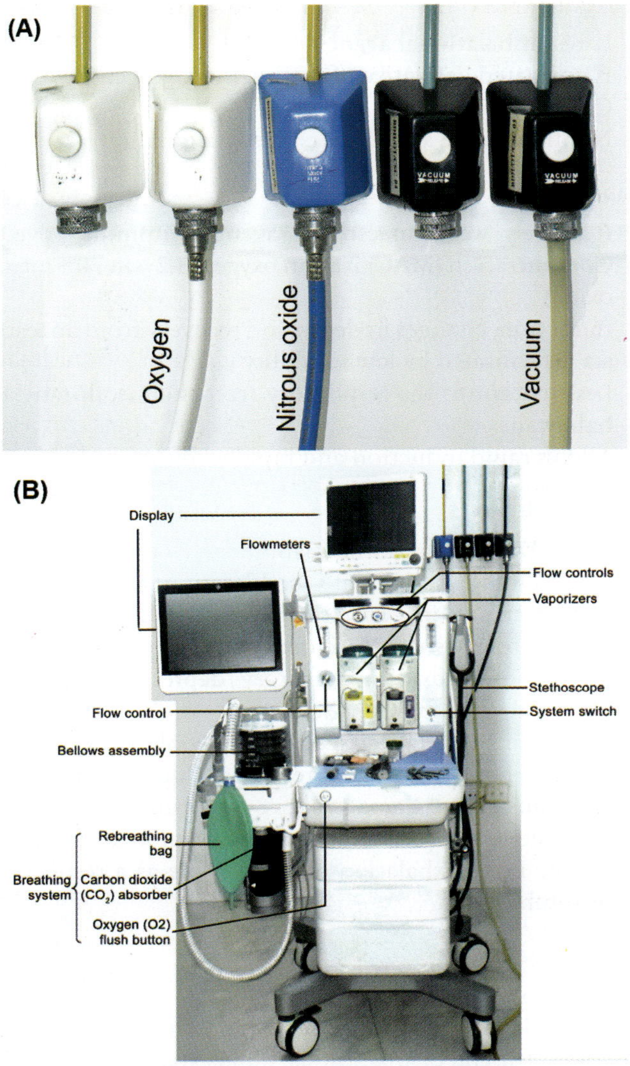

Figure 12.2 (**A**) PMGV system. Delivers anaesthetic gases and vacuum to the operation theatre through pipes. White: Oxygen, Blue: Nitrous oxide, Black: Vacuum. (**B**) Anaesthetic breathing system.

- Mainly serves as the vehicle for other potent volatile agents, at the same time reducing the concentration of volatile agent required.

Systemic effects

1. CNS: Increases cerebral blood flow, raises the intracranial pressure
2. CVS: It can increase catecholamine levels and causes epinephrine-induced arrhythmias. Cardiac output and blood pressure is slightly elevated or unchanged
3. Respiratory system: Causes a decrease in the tidal volume and slight increase in the respiratory rate. No muscle relaxation occurs with nitrous oxide.

Advantages

- Good analgesic
- Nitrous oxide has an excellent long-term record.

Disadvantages

- Nitrous oxide diffuses rapidly into air-filled cavities and causes a rise in pressure where expansion cannot take place, for example, in the middle ear or within the skull (pneumocephalus)
- Rapid excretion of nitrous oxide into the alveoli dilutes remaining oxygen present, thereby producing a transient hypoxia called as diffusion hypoxia or Fink effect at the end of anaesthesia
- Bone marrow suppression by interfering with the production of factors necessary for DNA synthesis.

HALOTHANE

- Colourless, volatile
- Pleasant odour
- Nonflammable and nonexplosive at clinical concentrations, even when mixed with oxygen
- Decomposition occurs on exposure to light. This is retarded by storing it in amber bottles with the addition of 0.01% thymol.

Anaesthesia

- Very potent anaesthetic
- It is administered via a calibrated vapouriser to prevent overdose. Induction can be achieved with 2%–4%
- Maintenance with 0.5%–1.5% inspired concentration when administered with 70% nitrous oxide and 30% oxygen
- No analgesic actions
- In spontaneously breathing patients, it is commonly used with nitrous oxide and oxygen or in the same combination as part of a balanced technique along with a muscle relaxant and an analgesic in a ventilated patient.

Systemic effects

1. CNS: Cerebral blood flow is increased causing a rise in intracranial pressure
2. CVS: Cardiac output and blood pressure falls, myocardial depression and vasodilatation, dysrhythmias, sinus bradycardia, increased vagal tone, ventricular extrasystoles are associated with increased circulating levels of adrenaline
3. Respiratory system: Respiratory depressant
4. Metabolism: Significant amount of halothane is metabolised in the liver (>20%) and gets excreted over many days.

Advantages

- Potent anaesthetic
- Rapid induction and recovery
- Recovery is slower with halothane as compared to other inhalational agents
- Potentiates the effects of nondepolarising muscle relaxants.

Disadvantages

- Significant rise in cerebral blood flow raising intracranial pressure

- One of the more potent triggers of malignant hyperthermia
- Hepatotoxicity
- Halothane hepatitis
- Has no analgesic action.

ISOFLURANE

- A colourless liquid
- Nonflammable at clinical concentrations
- Pungent smell
- Mild irritant upon breathing
- Isoflurane is a very stable molecule and hence does not require any preservative and has a long shelf life.

Anaesthesia

- More potent than halothane
- It is the least soluble, allowing very rapid changes in the depth of anaesthesia and recovery. Its use as an induction agent is limited by its pungency and tendency to cause coughing
- It does not have least solubility: Desflurane is least soluble
- 5% is required for induction
- 1%–1.5% for the maintenance of anaesthesia when used with 70% nitrous oxide and 30% oxygen.

Systemic effects

1. CNS: Isoflurane causes dose-dependent depression, with cerebral blood flow being affected minimally and intracranial pressure at low concentrations
2. CVS: Fall in blood pressure mainly due to peripheral vasodilatation. Minimal myocardial depression. Tachycardia in young patients due to the maintenance of the baroreceptor reflexes
3. Respiratory system: Depression of ventilation, tidal volume is affected greater than respiratory rate, response to hypoxia and hypercapnia is also reduced, good relaxation of skeletal muscle.

Advantages

- Rapid recovery
- Minimal hangover effects
- Popularly used in day-care surgery
- No apparent renal or hepatic toxicity and isoflurane can be repeated at short intervals
  - Widely used during operations requiring induced hypotension, as this effect is achieved mainly by vasodilatation rather than myocardial depression
  - Isoflurane is a preferred maintenance inhalation agent because it is cheaper and more cardio stable than halothane.

Disadvantages

- Pungency of isoflurane limits its use for inhalation induction of anaesthesia
- May worsen myocardial ischaemia in patients with severe coronary artery stenosis.

SEVOFLURANE

- Latest inhalational agent
- Fluorinated derivative of methyl isopropyl ether
- Colourless liquid
- Nonflammable at clinical concentrations.

Anaesthesia

- Relatively weak anaesthetic agent (Minimum Alveolar Concentration (MAC) 2.5% in oxygen, 1.2% in 70% nitrous oxide)
- Induction, changes in depth and recovery from anaesthesia is facilitated by low solubility
- Less irritant to the respiratory tract than isoflurane and halothane
- Allows rapid induction and rapid recovery.

Systemic effects

1. CNS: Depression of the CNS
2. CVS: Due to peripheral vasodilatation, the blood pressure decreases in a dose-related manner
3. Respiratory system: With decrease in ventilator response to carbon dioxide, ventilatory depression occurs. It causes reversal of bronchospasm
4. Miscellaneous: The effects of nondepolarising relaxants are potentiated. Minimal release of fluoride ions (which can cause renal damage above a certain concentration) and the levels quickly fall at the end of anaesthesia due to the rapid exhalation of sevoflurane as a result of its insolubility.

Advantages

Ease of inhalation and lack of solubility make sevoflurane useful in short cases, for example, anaesthesia for day-care surgery, at the end of anaesthesia, rapid exhalation of sevoflurane with minimal release of fluoride ion (nephrotoxic above certain level).

Disadvantages

Contact between sevoflurane and carbon dioxide absorbing agents, for example, soda lime in a circle system, results in the formation of a number of toxic compounds including formaldehyde, hydrofluoric acid and an alkene, termed Compound A. Initial investigations suggest that the concentrations produced in the clinical situation are below the level causing renal damage in humans.

The slow induction and recovery, frequent nausea and vomiting and profuse salivation requiring the use of an anticholinergic premedicant, are the main clinical disadvantages.

Ether predisposes to an unacceptable risk of fires and explosions due to its flammability considering the increasing use of electrical apparatus in the modern operating theatre.

PROPOFOL (2,6-DIISOPROPYLPHENOL)

The rate of infusion of propofol will vary between patients and will depend upon the concurrent administration of other drugs, for example, opioids or nitrous oxide, used in conjunction to provide analgesia and help prevent the risk of awareness. A typical infusion regimen in conjunction with oxygen-enriched air and an intravenous analgesic (alfentanil) would be 50–150 μg/kg/min with nitrous oxide or an opiate is a recommended dosage.

Advantages

- Total avoidance of all inhalational agents
- Risks such as malignant hyperpyrexia, hepatitis and the problems associated with nitrous oxide, particularly during long procedures can be eliminated.

Disadvantages

If an inadequate rate of infusion was used in a patient given muscle relaxants, it could potentially lead to them being conscious and paralysed (it must be remembered that this situation is not unique to infusions, the same can still happen if inadequate concentrations of an inhalational agent are used). Accurate devices are also required to deliver constant infusions (e.g. electronic syringe pumps), a situation analogous to the vaporisers required for inhalational agents.

ETHER (DIETHYL ETHER)

- Ether was the 1st agent used successfully to produce surgical anaesthesia
- Rarely used nowadays
- Inflammable.

Anaesthesia

- Moderately potent anaesthetic agent
- Irritant, causing coughing, breath holding and laryngeal spasm if the inspired concentration is increased rapidly
- High concentrations need to be given if ether is used for induction (15%–25%), with 3%–5% required for maintenance, increasing to 10%–12% for muscle relaxation.

Advantages

- In contrast to other volatile agents, ether causes a degree of respiratory and cardiovascular stimulation, until deep levels of anaesthesia are produced
- Muscle tone is reduced in proportion to the depth of anaesthesia, bronchial smooth muscle tone useful in asthmatics.

Disadvantages

The slow induction and recovery, frequent nausea and vomiting and profuse salivation requiring the use of an anticholinergic premedicant are the main clinical disadvantages. However, unacceptable risk of fires and explosions due to the increasing use of electrical apparatus in the modern operating theatre.

MUSCLE RELAXATION DURING ANAESTHESIA

Before the introduction of neuromuscular blocking drugs, high concentrations of inhalational anaesthetic agents or regional anaesthesia was used to achieve relaxation of skeletal muscles to facilitate surgical access. Both techniques are associated with hypotension, respiratory depression and delayed recovery. The neuromuscular blocking drugs or muscle relaxants work by interfering with the normal action of acetylcholine by blocking the receptors on the postsynaptic muscle membrane.

CLASSIFICATION OF SKELETAL MUSCLE RELAXANT

Muscle relaxants are classified based on the mode of action, duration of action and their site of action (Flowchart 12.2).

Peripherally acting muscle relaxant

Drugs acting peripherally at neuromuscular junction (NMJ) by causing nondepolarisation or depolarisation block.

1. ***Drugs acting on NMJ***
   a. ***Drugs causing nondepolarising block (competitive)***
      i. Long acting: d-Tubocurarine, metocurine, alcuronium chloride, pancuronium bromide, gallamine triethiodide, pipercuronium chloride, doxacurium hydrochloride
      ii. Intermediate acting: Vecuronium bromide, atracurium besylate, cisatracurium besylate, rocuronium bromide

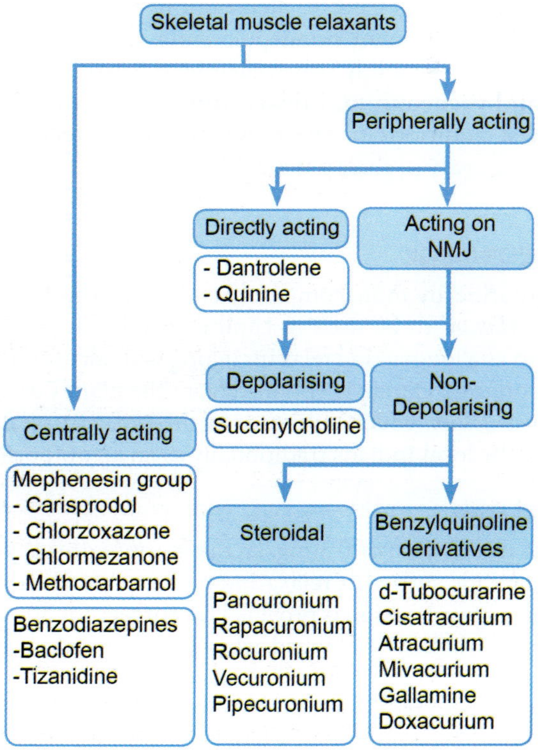

Flowchart 12.2 Classification of skeletal muscle relaxants.

iii. Short acting: Mivacurium chloride, rapacuronium bromide

b. ***Drugs causing depolarising block***

i. Decamethonium

ii. Succinylcholine (suxamethonium chloride)

2. ***Drugs acting directly on muscle***

a. Dantrolene sodium

b. Quinine.

Centrally acting muscle relaxant

- Barbiturates: Phenobarbitone
- Glycerol ethers: Mephenesin, carisoprodol, methocarbamol, chlormezanone, chlorzoxazone
- Benzodiazepines: Diazepam
- GABA derivatives: Baclofen.

NONDEPOLARISING MUSCLE RELAXANTS

These drugs compete with acetylcholine and block its access to the postsynaptic receptor sites on the muscle, but do not cause depolarisation. As increasing the concentration of acetylcholine will overcome their action, they are sometimes referred to as competitive relaxants. All of the nondepolarising relaxants are administered intravenously and the time of onset to maximum effect is relatively slow (1.5–3 min). Nondepolarising relaxants are used in two ways: along with **suxamethonium** in order to maintain relaxation during surgery or as the sole agent to provide relaxation for tracheal intubation and surgery. Although recovery of normal neuromuscular function occurs spontaneously after the use of these drugs, it is usually accelerated by the administration of an anticholinesterase. Curare, alcuronium and pancuronium were the predominant nondepolarising relaxants until the 1980s, but were rapidly superseded by the arrival of **atracurium and vecuronium. Mivacurium and rocuronium** are the latest additions to the range of muscle relaxants. All these drugs vary in their potency, duration of action and side effects.

TUBOCURARINE

Tubocurarine are more commonly curare was the 1st *nondepolarising relaxant* to be used in clinical practice. It is often referred to as a long-acting relaxant (along with alcuronium and pancuronium). Curare is obtained from the plant *Chondrodendron tomentosum,* which cultivates in the Amazon area and is used by the local Indians traditionally as an arrow poison.

Clinical uses

- The initial dose of 0.5 mg/kg takes approximately 3 min to provide sufficient relaxation to allow intubation
- Adequate relaxation is provided for surgery for 30–40 min. This is slightly prolonged when inhalational agents are used
- Supplementary doses of 0.15 mg/kg can be administered to extend the duration of block. It is supplied in 1.5 mL ampoules containing 10 mg/mL.

ALCURONIUM

Alcuronium is synthesised from a curare alkaloid and therefore has properties similar to curare. It is supplied in 2 mL ampoules containing 5 mg/mL. The amber-coloured ampoules deteriorate on exposure to sunlight.

PANCURONIUM

A synthetic muscle relaxant, pancuronium was the 1st one introduced into clinical practice, with a chemical structure based upon the steroid ring nucleus. **Clinical use:** It is not recommended for use in patients with renal failure.

ATRACURIUM

1st of the modern generation of intermediate duration nondepolarising relaxants, stored at 4°C to reduce the rate of spontaneous degradation.

Clinical uses

- Profound relaxation is produced by an initial dose of 0.5 mg/kg allowing intubation after 1.5–2 min. This lasts for 20–25 min and once spontaneous recovery starts, it proceeds very rapidly
- When used during prolonged procedures, the administration of an infusion (0.5 mg/kg/h) is preferable to intermittent increments in order to maintain a steady degree of relaxation
- In patients with either renal or hepatic dysfunction, it is the relaxant of choice. In hypothermic patients, its actions will be prolonged, for example, during cardiac surgery.

VECURONIUM

Vecuronium is related to pancuronium in that it has a steroid ring nucleus. It is supplied as a white, freeze-dried powder (10 mg), which is reconstituted for use with 5 mL of sterile water to give a solution containing 2 mg/mL.

Clinical uses

- Profound relaxation results with an initial dose of 0.1 mg/kg in 1.5–2 min. This will provide adequate relaxation for 15–20 min. This can be extended by increasing the dose to 0.15–0.2 mg/kg with few side effects
- More common to use an infusion of 50–80 µg/kg/h in case of longer procedures
- As with atracurium, recovery is rapid once it commences.

MIVACURIUM

The 1st of the two newest relaxants, mivacurium is structurally related to atracurium. It is regarded as a short acting nondepolarising relaxant. It is supplied in solution containing 2 mg/mL.

Clinical uses

- The initial dose of 0.15 mg/kg provides relaxation, allowing intubation in 2 min. However, the duration of action is only 10–15 min, after which time recovery is sufficiently rapid and does not require the routine administration of an anticholinesterase.

- Although it can be used to maintain relaxation, its use in day-care surgery for short procedures serves as a great advantage.

DEPOLARISING MUSCLE RELAXANTS

As their name suggests, following administration, they cause depolarisation of the motor end plate. Currently, only suxamethonium is in regular clinical use.

SUXAMETHONIUM CHLORIDE (SUCCINYLCHOLINE—SCh)

A quaternary amine ester, suxamethonium consists of two molecules of acetylcholine joined together 'back-to-back' (via their nonquaternary ends). On administration, it mimics the action of acetylcholine at the receptors on the motor end plate producing depolarisation of the muscle membrane followed by uncoordinated muscle contractions. Depolarisation continues for several minutes, thereby preventing further muscle activity, as suxamethonium is not broken down by acetyl cholinesterase. Ultimately, plasma cholinesterase hydrolyses it with the restoration of normal neuromuscular transmission.

Suxamethonium is available in 2 mL ampoules, containing 50 mg/mL. It hydrolyses at room temperature and therefore has to be stored at 4°C.

Clinical uses

- Suxamethonium can be administered intravenously, intramuscularly or subcutaneously
- Profound relaxation in 40–60 s, lasting 4–6 min is achieved with the dose of 1.5 mg/kg in adults
- Infants and neonates require a slightly higher dose, 1.5–2 mg, respectively.

Advantages

Suxamethonium produces profound, short-lived muscle relaxation that is more rapid in onset than any of the other currently available relaxants. Facilitation of tracheal intubation in an emergency makes it the drug of choice, for example, in a patient likely to regurgitate and aspirate.

Disadvantages

- Suxamethonium has to be stored at 4°C to prevent breakdown
- Administration may cause:
  a. *Hyperkalaemia*
  b. Malignant hyperpyrexia in susceptible patients
  c. Loss of vitreous exacerbating the damage in penetrating eye injuries may result from increased intraocular pressure
  d. Muscular pain around the limb girdles, which is most common 24 h after administration in young adults due the fasciculations damaging muscle fibres.
  e. Prolonged apnoea in patients with pseudocholinesterase deficiency, which may be secondary to liver dysfunction. Of greater importance is the presence in the population of individuals with genetically determined pseudocholinesterase deficiency, for example, Arya Vysya Chettiars of South India.

PSEUDOCHOLINESTERASE DEFICIENCY

A variety of genes have been identified, which are involved in pseudocholinesterase production. The most significant of these are as follows:

- *Normal homozygotes with sufficient enzyme:* Hydrolyse suxamethonium in 4–6 min (950 per 1000 population)
- *A typical homozygote with slightly reduced enzyme levels:* Suxamethonium lasts 10–20 min (50 per 1000)
- *A typical homozygote with marked deficiency of enzyme*: This group is apnoeic for up to 2 h after suxamethonium (<1 per 1000).

Treatment of this group consists of ventilatory support with maintenance of anaesthesia or sedation until recovery occurs. The patient should subsequently be warned, given a card with details, and because of its inherited nature, the remainder of the family should be examined appropriately.

PROLONGATION OF NEUROMUSCULAR BLOCKADE

- Occasionally, certain factors may prolong the effects of these drugs. For nondepolarising relaxants, this involves concurrent use of those drugs that affect calcium flux, most notably verapamil, nifedipine (calcium antagonists and also aminoglycoside antibiotics [e.g. gentamicin])
- Apart from the pseudocholinesterase deficiency, the length of action of suxamethonium will be prolonged in patients with liver failure, in the puerperium (reduced plasma cholinesterase) and in those using echothiophate eye drops, an anticholinesterase for the management of glaucoma
- Monitoring the degree of neuromuscular blockade in these patients and adjusting the dose of drug accordingly will overcome any potential problems of unanticipated prolonged paralysis.

MONITORING NEUROMUSCULAR BLOCKADE

This can be done either clinically or by the use of a peripheral nerve stimulator.

CLINICAL MONITORING

1. This method relies on having a conscious, cooperative patient and is therefore limited in its application to those patients recovering from anaesthesia. The NMJ in certain muscle groups is stressed by asking the patient to perform a sustained activity, in other words, to produce a tetanic contraction
2. Commonly used tests include:
   a. Lift the head off the pillow for 5 s.
   b. A handgrip for 5 s.
   c. The ability to produce a vital capacity breath, >10 mL/kg.

3. In a patient who has not completely recovered from anaesthesia and has a reduced level of consciousness, residual neuromuscular block can be indicated by the presence of 'see-sawing' or paradoxical respiration.

PERIPHERAL NERVE STIMULATION

One of the most common arrangements is stimulation of the ulnar nerve at the wrist while monitoring the contractions of the adductor pollicis.

ANTICHOLINESTERASES

- The administration of these drugs blocks the actions of the enzyme acetylcholinesterase, which destroys acetylcholine at cholinergic synapses and results in an increase in its concentration. This action is used to reverse neuromuscular block induced by the administration of nondepolarising relaxants
- The speed of action of these drugs in reversing neuromuscular block depends upon the intensity of the block when they are administered; the more the intensity of the block, the slower the reversal
- Anticholinesterases will work at the NMJ to increase acetylcholine levels (nicotinic effects) and also at parasympathetic nerve endings (muscarinic effects) to cause bradycardia, spasm of the bowel, bladder and bronchi, increased bronchial secretions, etc. Therefore, they are always administered with a suitable dose of atropine or glycopyrrolate, to block the unwanted muscarinic effects.

NEOSTIGMINE

This is the most commonly used anticholinesterase and a fixed dose of 2.5 mg intravenously is used in adults to reverse residual neuromuscular block. After approximately 5 min, its maximal effect is seen, which lasts for 20–30 min. It is usually administered concurrently with either atropine 1.2 mg or glycopyrrolate 0.5 mg. An ampoule containing 2.5 mg neostigmine premixed with 0.5 mg glycopyrrolate is available.

DELIVERY OF ANAESTHETIC GASES AND VAPOURS TO THE OPERATION THEATRE

PIPED MEDICAL GAS AND VACUUM (PMGV) SYSTEM

Delivery of gases to the operating theatre is achieved either by piped distribution (along with medical vacuum) known as 'piped medical gas and vacuum' (PMGV) (Fig. 12.2), or from bulk storage of the gas or by the use of small cylinders attached directly to the anaesthetic machine. This is used for the delivery of oxygen, nitrous oxide and vacuum. The gases are delivered via a specially made system with copper piping (to reduce degradation), which carries labels at regular intervals. These pipelines end in outlets, which serve as self-closing sockets, each specifically coloured and labelled for one gas. The gases are delivered at a pressure of 4 bar (400 kPa, 60 pounds per square inch [psi]), except for medical air, which is delivered at 7 bar (700 kPa, 75 psi) to power medical tools. Flexible reinforced hoses, colour-coded throughout their length, are used for onward delivery to the anaesthetic machine.

OXYGEN

A liquid oxygen reserve supplies the oxygen. It is the most often and most economical means to supply it. It is stored under pressure (10–12 bar, 1200 kPa) at approximately -180°C, in what is effectively a thermos flask or more correctly a vacuum insulated evaporator (VIE). From the VIE to the pipeline system, the gas is warmed to ambient air temperature (Fig. 12.2A). To manage possible failures of the main system, a reserve bank of cylinders of compressed oxygen is present.

NITROUS OXIDE AND MEDICAL AIR

These are supplied from multiple large cylinders. A bank is formed to a common manifold. There are usually two banks: one that is running (duty bank) with all cylinders turned on and a 2nd or reserve bank. An additional small emergency supply is also available. Switching between banks is carried out automatically and accompanied by audible and visual signals to indicate that replacement is required. A compressor is used to supply medical air, which delivers air to the central reservoir to meet the desired quality before distribution. It is delivered at a necessary pressure, as well as dried and filtered here (Fig. 12.2A).

VACUUM

Two pumps are connected to a system capable of generating a vacuum of at least 400 mmHg below atmospheric pressure. It is delivered to the anaesthetic rooms, operating theatre and other appropriate sites. Bacterial filters are present at several stages between the outlets and the pumps in order to prevent contamination by aspirated fluids (Fig. 12.2A).

ROLE OF THE ANAESTHETIC MACHINE

The precursor to the modern anaesthetic machine was the Boyle's machine, named after H.E.G. Boyle who commissioned the 1st British machine in 1917 having seen one in the USA. Its main functions are:

- To reduce the pressure of the gases from the pipelines or cylinders to a level that is safe to be used in patients
- For the accurate delivery of varying flows of gases to a patient's breathing system
- To permit additional anaesthetic vapours to be added to the gas stream (Fig. 12.2B).

In a spontaneously breathing patient, delivery of gases to the patient is achieved by using what is commonly referred to as an anaesthetic circuit or an '***anaesthetic breathing system***'. Only one true circuit is in common use, the '**circle system**'. There are five systems available and they are classified by Mapleson as **Mapleson A, B, C, D and E**. Final delivery of gas to the patient is via a facemask or by attaching the system to a laryngeal mask or tracheal tube. A low-resistance, disposable, bacterial filter at the patient end of the system is used as several patients in succession may breathe through the same system. In order to reduce the risk of cross-infection, this is changed between patients.

COMPONENTS OF A BREATHING SYSTEM

A connection for fresh gas input

On the anaesthetic machine, this may be a direct connection to the common gas outlet.

A reservoir bag (usually of 2 L capacity)

As its name suggests, this acts as a gas reservoir. Its presence overcomes the problems of having a constant flow from the machine and using relatively low flows. During expiration, fresh gas flow is diverted into the bag, which is then used to meet the patient's peak inspiratory flow (30–40 L/min), which exceeds the flow rate used for anaesthesia (usually <10 L/min). The reservoir can also be used to monitor ventilation by watching its movements, and by compressing it, the patient can be manually ventilated. Finally, the bag acts as a safety device wherein should an obstruction develop distally, it easily distends to accommodate the flow of fresh gas while maintaining a low pressure. This protects the lungs against barotrauma.

An inspiratory valve and an expiratory valve

The inspiratory one-way valve opens to allow inspiration of anaesthetic gases and vapours with oxygen. The 'inspiratory tubing' from the inspiratory valve to the patient carries only inspiratory gases. An expiratory valve is one, which opens during expiration to allow the elimination of gas containing carbon dioxide and prevent its accumulation within the system.

The circle system

The anaesthetic breathing systems relied on a combination of the opening of an expiratory valve and the inflow of fresh anaesthetic gas to eliminate carbon dioxide based on the patient's inspiration and expiration. The circle system is passed through a container of soda lime (the absorber), which chemically removes carbon dioxide and allows the other gases to reenter the circle system. The patient rebreathes the supplementary oxygen and anaesthetic agents that are added to maintain the required concentrations. In an ideal system, only enough oxygen and anaesthetic agent would be added to replace what is removed. This would consist of 250–300 mL oxygen, the body's basal requirement and the amount of anaesthetic required. More of both oxygen and agent will be required initially, gradually reducing as the tissues became saturated. In such a system, the volume of gas would remain constant. This is referred to as a closed system. In practice, such low flows are difficult to achieve and are potentially dangerous as hypoxia can rapidly occur. Consequently, totally closed systems are not commonly used, and more often, the circle is used with an excess fresh gas flow to allow for any leaks and to ensure adequate concentrations of oxygen and anaesthetic.

Soda lime

Soda lime helps the gases in the circle system to be heated and humidified. The gases usually are dry and cold and this can cause the respiratory mucosa to dry out causing other complications. Soda lime also absorbs the carbon dioxide from the circle system. Soda lime consists of a mixture of calcium hydroxide (90%), sodium hydroxide (5%) and potassium hydroxide (1%). Water is also present in the granules. Sodium carbonate is produced as a result of a reaction between carbon dioxide and sodium hydroxide. This in turn reacts with calcium hydroxide to form calcium carbonate. Important by-products of the reactions are water and heat. As a result, the gases within the circle are heated and humidified, which help prevent their loss from the patient. Eventually, the soda lime will become exhausted and unable to absorb any more carbon dioxide. This is indicated by an indicator, which results in a change in the colour of the granules. Transition from pink to white is seen in one of the commonly used preparations.

MECHANICAL VENTILATION

When a patient is rendered apnoeic, he/she becomes dependent upon the anaesthetist to support his/her ventilation. Apnoea is usually a deliberate occurrence following the administration of a muscle relaxant or a potent opioid analgesic. Ventilation of the lungs with oxygen and anaesthetic gases is achieved using a mechanical ventilator in conjunction with tracheal intubation. In the short term, ventilation is achieved by closing the expiratory valve and 'squeezing the bag' to increase the pressure in an anaesthetic breathing system, thereby forcing gas into the lungs. Such a technique is inefficient for all, but a short period of time and can lead to hypoxaemia and hypercarbia. It is most commonly used after the use of nondepolarising relaxant to maintain oxygenation via a face mask prior to intubation or following intubation using suxamethonium while waiting for the return of spontaneous ventilation. Whenever mechanical ventilation is employed as part of the anaesthetic technique, a gas-tight system is required to ensure that the lungs are ventilated and this is usually provided by the use of a cuffed tracheal tube. The patient is totally dependent upon the function of the ventilator and close clinical observation of the patient is essential, coupled with monitoring of, at least, expired volume, inspired oxygen concentration, airway pressure and pulse oximetry. Due to the risk of accidental disconnection at many places, a dedicated alarm capable of detecting is used.

PRINCIPLES OF MECHANICAL VENTILATION

During spontaneous ventilation, descent of the diaphragm and expansion of the chest wall causes the intrapulmonary pressure to fall 1–2 cm H_2O below atmospheric pressure. Air flows into the lungs, and at the end of inspiration, the pressure in the alveoli is atmospheric. Intermittent positive pressure ventilation (IPPV) is the technique where during mechanical ventilation, a positive pressure is applied to the anaesthetic gas by the ventilator so that it flows into the lungs. As these ventilators are very powerful and capable of generating high inspiratory pressures, they are usually pressure limited to reduce the risk of pulmonary barotrauma.

MANAGING THE AIRWAY

An essential prerequisite for safe and successful conduct of anaesthesia is maintenance of the patient's airway. During resuscitation, patients often have an obstructed airway either as the cause or result of their loss of consciousness.

Face masks

A face mask is used to maintain the airway when the patient is breathing spontaneously, to deliver the anaesthetic gases or for ventilating a patient prior to intubation. Loss of the airway as a result of muscle relaxation is most easily restored by a combination of a head tilt and a jaw thrust. The jaw thrust is provided by the anaesthetist's 4th and 5th fingers (of one or both hands) lifting the angle of the mandible. Patient's mandible is 'lifted' into the mask rather than the mask being pushed into the face for achieving the desired effect. In adults, anatomical face mask is the most commonly used (Fig. 12.3). Leakage of anaesthetic gases is prevented by its design, which fits the facial contours with minimal pressure. An air-filled cuff around the edge facilitates this. Different sizes of the mask are available. The smallest size provides a good seal and should be used (dead space that occurs is minimised by it). Ambu face mask is an alternative with a transparent body, permitting easy identification of vomit, thereby making it popular for use in resuscitation. In between use, all masks must be disinfected adequately.

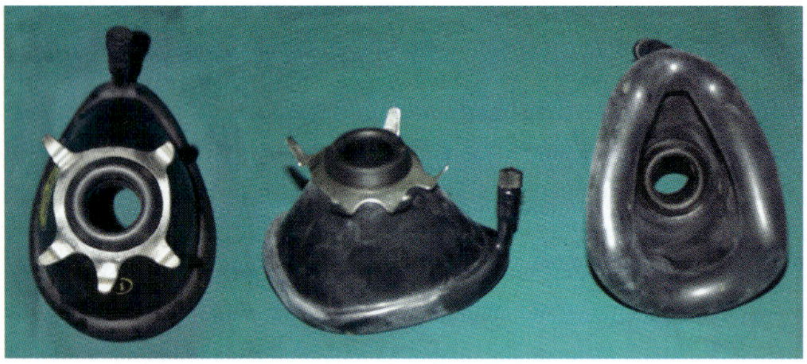

Figure 12.3 Adult anatomical face mask.

Airways

These are often used to help maintain the airway in conjunction with the techniques described above. After the induction of anaesthesia, most commonly used airway adjuncts are the oropharyngeal (Guedel airway) and nasopharyngeal airways, which are inserted to prevent stimulation of reflex activity, for example, coughing, vomiting and laryngeal spasm.

Oropharyngeal airway (Guedel airway)

Oropharyngeal airway is a curved plastic tube, flattened in cross-section and flanged at the oral end. The tongue is prevented from falling back by the design of the oropharyngeal airways, which lie over the tongue, preventing it from falling back into the pharynx. The sizes range from neonates to large adults. By comparing the airway length to the vertical distance from the corner of the patient's mouth to the angle of the mandible, the correct size is determined. In adults, the most common sizes are 2–4 for small to large adults, respectively (Fig. 12.4).

The oropharyngeal airway is inserted 'upside down' as far as the back of the hard palate. It is then rotated through 180 degrees and fully inserted until the flange lies in front of the teeth (or gums in an edentulous patient). This technique is used to try and reduce the risk of pushing the tongue back into the pharynx and causing obstruction.

Nasopharyngeal airway

Nasopharyngeal airway is an alternative to the oropharyngeal airway, and as the name suggests, it is inserted via the nose. They are round, malleable plastic tubes, bevelled at the pharyngeal end and flanged at the nasal end. They are sized on their internal diameter in millimetres, the length increasing with diameter. The most common sizes in adults are 6–8 mm for small to large adults, respectively (Fig. 12.5).

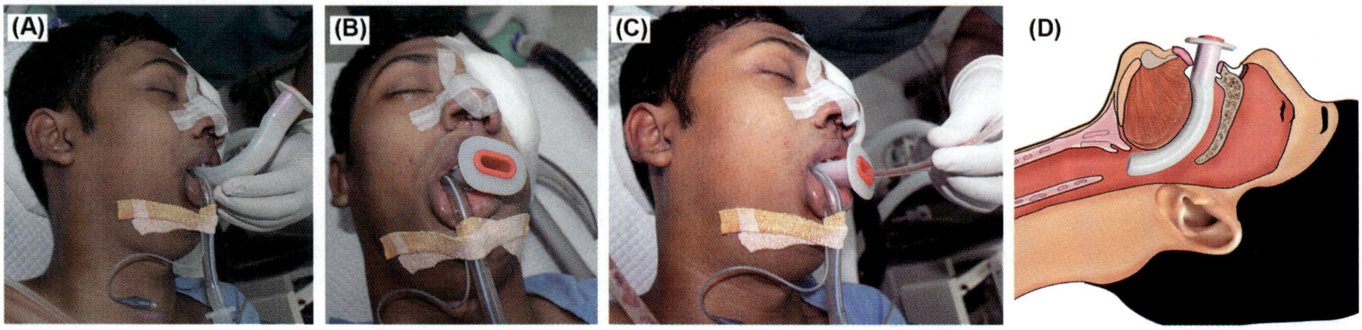

Figure 12.4 (**A** and **B**) Oropharyngeal airway insertion just before extubation. (**C**) Oropharyngeal airway in place, through the anterior flange suction is introduced to clear upper airway or oropharynx. (**D**) Illustration of oropharyngeal airway in position.

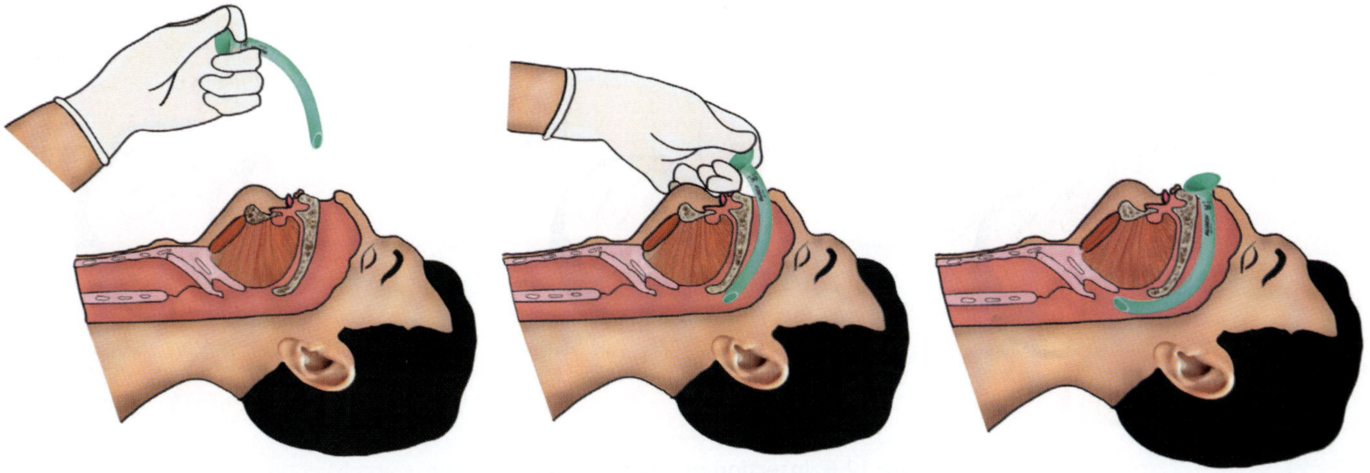

Figure 12.5 Insertion of nasopharyngeal airway. (Size of nasopharyngeal airway is measured from tip of the nose to tragus.)

The patency of both nostrils should be checked and the airway is lubricated before inserting a nasopharyngeal airway (usually the right). The airway is then inserted using a twisting action with the bevel facing medially to avoid traumatising the turbinates, along the floor of the nose. The tip should lie in the pharynx and the flange at the nostril when it is fully inserted. To prevent inhalation of the airway, a large safety pin may be inserted through the flange. Force should not be used if obstruction is encountered, as severe bleeding may be provoked. The other nostril can instead be tried.

Signs of airway obstruction

Indications that the methods above are failing to maintain the airway are as follows:

- Snoring sounds, usually as a result of the tongue partially obstructing the pharynx secondary to the mandible falling back
- Indrawing of the supraclavicular, suprasternal and intercostal spaces during obstructed inspiration
- Use of the accessory muscles; sternomastoid and scalene in an attempt to try and overcome the obstruction
- Paradoxical respiratory movement (see-saw respiration); indrawing of the thorax and expansion of the abdomen as the diaphragm contracts vigorously, usually in the face of complete obstruction

Common problems arising using these techniques along with a face mask during anaesthesia are:

- Absence of a good seal between the patient's face and the mask, particularly in patients without teeth
- For prolonged periods, fatigue when holding the mask
- Due to the loss of upper airway reflexes, the risk of aspiration remains.

Traditionally these problems were overcome by resorting to tracheal intubation. However, there is now an intermediate option - the laryngeal mask airway (LMA).

LARYNGEAL MASK AIRWAY (SUPRAGLOTTIC AIRWAY DEVICE)

Introduced in 1987, the LMA has substantially changed airway management in anaesthetic practice. Over the laryngeal opening, a mask is present. An inflatable cuff on the perimeter of the mask creates a seal and helps to stabilise it. A tube is attached to the mask, which protrudes from the mouth and directly connects to the anaesthetic breathing system. The LMA is available in a variety of sizes suitable for all patients. It ranges from neonates to adults. Sizes 3 and 4 are the most commonly used in female and male, respectively. Although it was designed to be used in spontaneously breathing patients, the LMA can be used to ventilate patients too. High inflation pressure must be avoided, else leakage occurs past the cuff, which reduces the ventilation and may cause gastric inflation. A version with a reinforced tube is also available.

TECHNIQUE FOR INSERTION OF LMA

To prevent coughing or laryngospasm, the patient's reflexes must be suppressed to a level similar to that needed for the insertion of an oropharyngeal airway.

- Deflate the cuff and lubricate the mask lightly
- A head tilt is performed, the patient's mouth is opened fully and the tip of the mask inserted along the hard palate with the open side facing, but not touching the tongue
- Using the index finger, the mask is then further inserted to provide support for the tube. Eventually, the tip of the mask lies at the upper oesophageal sphincter where resistance is felt
- Now the cuff is fully inflated using an air-filled syringe attached to the valve at the end of the pilot tube
- Either by a length of bandage or adhesive strapping attached to the protruding tube, the laryngeal mask is secured
- Some of the problems of the previous techniques are overcome by laryngeal mask. It is unaffected by the shape of the patient's face or the absence of teeth and provides a

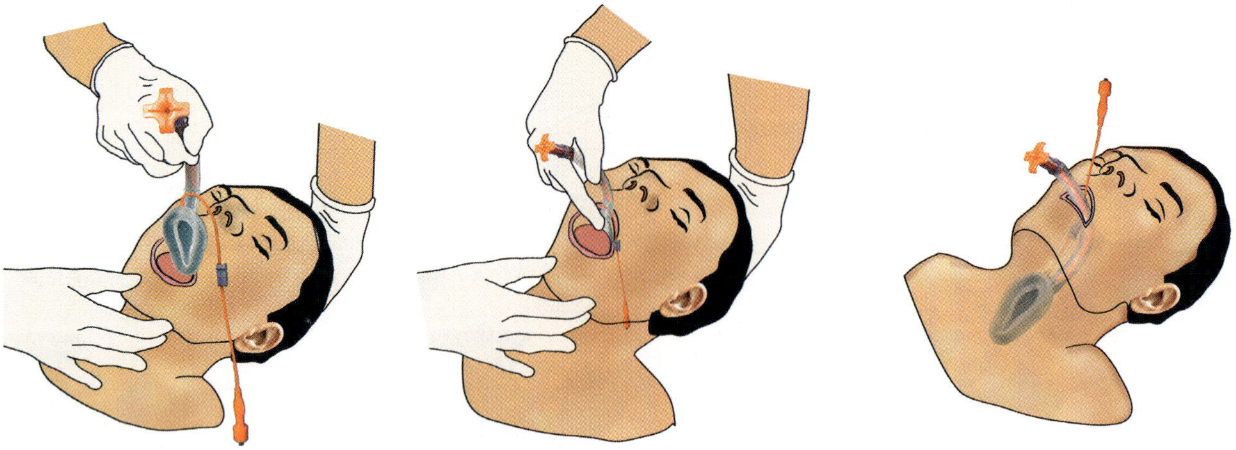

Figure 12.6 Insertion of laryngeal mask airway.

good seal. It avoids fatigue and other associated problems by not requiring the anaesthetist to hold it in position. Finally, it does not eliminate the risk of aspiration of regurgitated gastric contents (Fig. 12.6).

Relative contraindication to use LMA is in case of increased risk of regurgitation, for example, in emergency cases, pregnancy.

Recently, the laryngeal mask has been found to be useful in two other areas:

- Allows maintenance of the airway in a difficult tracheal intubation. Alternatively, via the LMA, a small-diameter tracheal tube or introducer can be passed into the larynx
- LMA can be inserted more rapidly and successfully during cardiopulmonary resuscitation by nonanaesthetists than a tracheal tube and can achieve more effective ventilation than by using a self-inflating bag and face mask. In the future, the LMA will find a role in airway management during resuscitation.

Unlike most modern equipment, the LMA is reusable if it is sterilised between patients.

TRACHEAL INTUBATION

The best method of securing a clear airway in the anaesthetised patient and during resuscitation is the tracheal intubation. The technique should be performed by a trained anaesthetist or emergency physician. It consists of inserting a tube via mouth (oral) or nose, through the larynx, so that the tip lies in the upper trachea, usually facilitated by direct laryngoscopy. In addition, abolition of laryngeal reflexes is required and this is achieved in anaesthesia most commonly by the administration of muscle relaxants. It is important to remember that at this point, the patient will also become apnoeic and is dependent upon the anaesthetist to maintain ventilation and oxygenation.

INDICATIONS FOR TRACHEAL INTUBATION

- Use of muscle relaxants as a part of the anaesthetic technique, thereby necessitating the use of mechanical ventilation
- In patients with a full stomach, usually those requiring emergency surgery, the presence of a cuffed tracheal tube protects from aspiration of regurgitated gastric contents
- Patient position which makes maintenance of the airway difficult, for example, the lateral or prone position
- During surgeries on the head and neck, to secure the airway, tracheal intubation protects against the aspiration of blood into the lungs
- Ventilation with 100% oxygen without leaks
- Suction clearance of inhaled debris
- A route for drug administration.

EQUIPMENT FOR TRACHEAL INTUBATION

The following is a list of the basic needs for adult oral intubation:

1. Laryngoscope with a curved blade (Macintosh)
2. Tracheal tubes, inflated and cuffed, available in a variety of sizes. The most important details are the internal diameter expressed in millimetres and the length in centimetres
    a. For males: **7.5–8 mm** internal diameter, 22–24 cm length
    b. For females: **7–7.5 mm** internal diameter, 20–22 cm length
3. Cuff inflation syringe: Once the tube is in place, use syringe to inflate the cuff
4. Catheter mount: Connect the tube to the anaesthetic system or ventilator tubing with a catheter mount or 'elbow'
5. Suction to remove excess secretions. For emergency patients, it must be switched on and kept ready for conditions where the patient vomits or regurgitates
6. Stethoscope: Listening for breath sounds during ventilation via stethoscope to check correct placement of the tube
7. A semirigid introducer (gum elastic bougie—60 cm) to assist with intubation

8. Magill's forceps, designed to remove debris or direct the tip of a tube
9. Throat pack: A length of bandage or tape to secure the tube by its reach into the pharynx.

LARYNGOSCOPES

The laryngoscope was designed to allow direct visualisation of the larynx to facilitate the insertion of a tracheal tube and consists of a handle and blade. The blade is placed into the mouth to sweep the tongue to the left and elevate the epiglottis to reveal the larynx. Illumination is provided by a light source close to the tip, powered by batteries situated within the handle. The most popular design in use today is the curved blade developed by Sir Robert Macintosh, which bears his name. There is a wide selection of laryngoscopes available for use in paediatric anaesthesia, which carries the names of their inventors, for example, Soper, Seward, Miller, Robert Shaw, Sheila Anderson.

ENDOTRACHEAL TUBES (Fig. 12.7)

These were earlier manufactured from red rubber and could be sterilised for reuse. They have now been largely superseded by disposable plastic (PVC) tubes. Apart from eliminating the risk of cross-infection, plastic tubes are chemically less irritating to the larynx, less likely to kink and require a lower pressure in the cuff to achieve a seal. Tracheal tube sizes are according to their internal diameter in millimetres and manufactured in 0.5 mm intervals. A standard 15 mm connector permits connection to the breathing system. A tracheal tube with an inflatable cuff is used for anaesthetic procedures in adults. This is necessary because once past the narrowest part of the airway (vocal cords), the tube lies in the trachea that has a much larger diameter. A seal prevents leakage of anaesthetic gases back past the tube when positive-pressure ventilation is provided. The cuff also helps prevent the risk of any foreign material, for example, gastric acid, food or blood being aspirated into the lungs. A syringe is used to inflate the cuff by injecting air, which runs part way either within or attached to the tracheal tube. At the distal end of the tube is a one-way valve in order to prevent deflation and a small pilot balloon indicating the cuff is inflated with caution to ensure that the cuff is not over-inflated as high pressure can be generated, which may compress the tracheal mucosa, rendering it ischaemic. During positive-pressure ventilation, the cuff is slowly inflated until there is no audible evidence of a leak. Tracheal tubes are connected to the appropriate breathing system or ventilator tubing via a catheter mount. This is simply a short piece of corrugated tubing with a 15 mm connection at one end and 22 mm connection at the other.

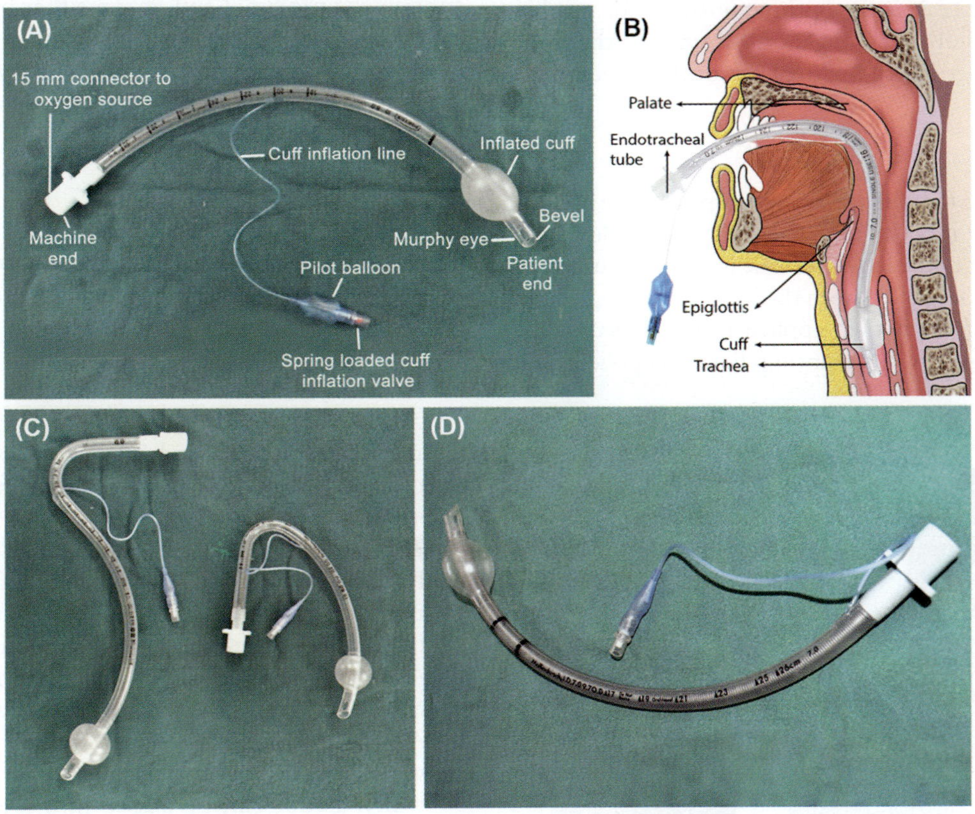

Figure 12.7 (**A**) Parts of an endotracheal tube. (**B**) Endotracheal tube in position. (**C**) Nasotracheal tube and orotracheal tube. (**D**) Flexometallic tube.

FLEXOMETALLIC TUBE

Flexometallic tubes are also called armoured endotracheal tubes. They are mainly in use for surgeries of the head and neck due to the resistance it has to kinking and compression of the tube. Flexometallic tubes also exert less pressure on the interarytenoid cartilages and the trachea. It can be used for nasal and oral routes of tracheal intubation.

Advantages

1. Nontraumatic to the septum, turbinates, cartilages, posterior pharyngeal wall and trachea
2. Easy to negotiate flexometallic tubes nasally and a smooth path through the oropharynx
3. No pharyngeal mucosal trauma and bleeding thus making reintubation easier due to better visibility. The tip of the flexometallic tube is softer compared to Ring-Adair-Elwyn (RAE) endotracheal tube. It also has a greater bevel angle
4. Flexometallic tubes can be positioned away from the surgical field easily.

TECHNIQUE OF ORAL INTUBATION

Abolition of the laryngeal reflexes required intubation. During the procedure the patient must be monitored appropriately.

Positioning

Patient's neck flexed and the head extended at the atlanto-occipital joint (Fig. 12.8) is the optimal position for intubation. With the help of index finger and thumb of the right hand in a scissor action, the patient's mouth is then fully opened.

Laryngoscopy

The left hand is used to hold the laryngoscope and the blade is introduced into the mouth along the right-hand side of the tongue, displacing it to the left. The blade is advanced until the tip lies in the vallecula, gap between the base of the tongue and the epiglottis. The force is then applied in the direction the handle of the laryngoscope is pointing. Force is applied such that the effort comes from the upper arm and not the wrist. The larynx gets exposed by lifting the tongue and the epiglottis. This should be seen as a triangular opening with the apex anteriorly and the true cords laterally (Refer Fig. 14.45).

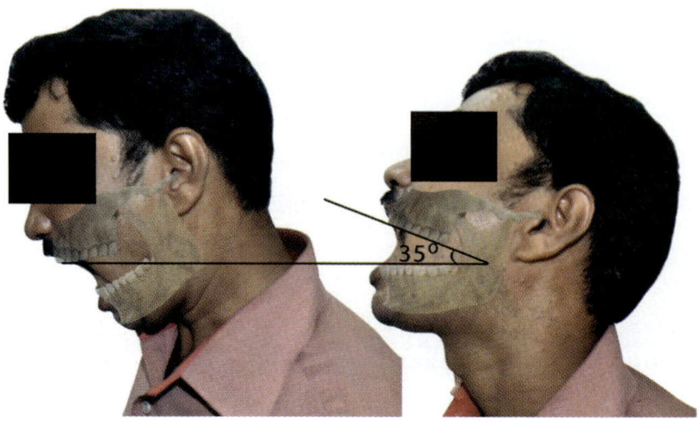

Figure 12.8 Atlanto-occipital extension.

Intubation

The tracheal tube is introduced through the right side of the mouth. It is then advanced and seen to pass through the cords until the cuff lies just below the cords following which it is further advanced. The right hand firmly holds the tube and the laryngoscope is carefully removed. The cuff is inflated sufficiently to prevent any leak during ventilation. Finally, by listening for breath sounds in both axillae, the position of the tube is confirmed and it is then secured in place.

Five-point auscultation is done

- Listen over the epigastrium (expect to hear nothing)
- Listen 4 points over the lungs
- Listen anteriorly just under the clavicles on either side of the sternum
- Listen in the axillary line approximately 5th intercostal space.

For nasotracheal intubation, through the right nostril along the floor of the nose with the bevel pointing medially, a well-lubricated tube is introduced to avoid damage to the turbinate. In the manner described above, it is visualised using a laryngoscope after advancing into the pharynx. By pressure on the proximal end, it can either be advanced directly into the larynx or the tip picked up with Magill's forceps (designed not to impair the view of the larynx) and directed into the larynx. As for oral intubation, the procedure is continued (Fig. 12.9).

Submental intubation

When both oral and nasal intubations are deemed unsuitable, control of the airway can be achieved by submental intubation. Major advantage is that it eliminates the risk associated with complication of tracheostomy (Fig. 12.9).

DIFFICULT INTUBATION

Tracheal intubation is usually not straightforward when the larynx cannot be visualised. This can be predicted at the preoperative assessment or may be unexpected. Many different techniques have been described to help solve this problem. These include:

- Pressure by an assistant in a downward and upward direction during the manipulation of the thyroid cartilage to try and bring the larynx or the posterior aspect into view
- A 60 cm long gum-elastic bougie is inserted into the trachea, and over this, a tracheal tube is 'railroaded' into place
- A fibreoptic bronchoscope is introduced into the trachea via either the mouth or the nose. It is used as a guide over which a tube can be passed into the trachea. It can be used in both anaesthetised and awake patients and hence is advantageous.

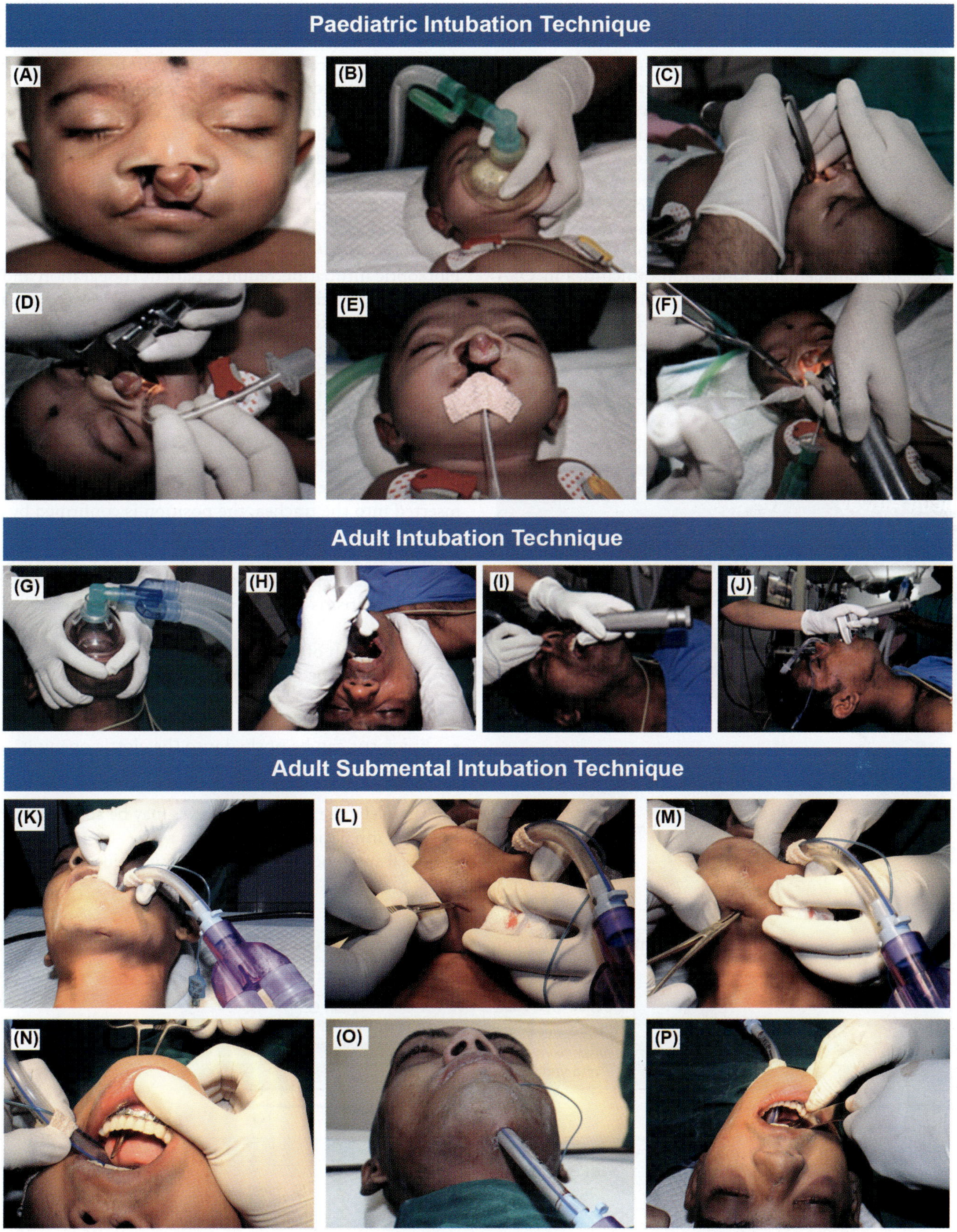

Figure 12.9 (**A–F**) Steps in oral intubation in a paediatric patient. (**G–J**) Step-by-step demonstration of intubation in an adult patient. (Scan to play an overview of General Anaesthesia.) (**K–P**) Adult submental intubation.

Causes for difficult airway (Table 12.8)

TMJ ankylosis: There is an anatomical modification in the path of the upper airway due to the failure of growth centre causing TMJ ankylosis. The trachea is placed at a more anterior position than normal. Blind awake intubation is the most commonly followed technique. Intubation by fibreoptic bronchoscopy is also being used. The management protocol is illustrated in Flowchart 12.3.

Obstructive sleep apnoea (OSA): Obstructive sleep apnoea syndrome is the development of upper airway obstruction during sleep and it poses considerable problems for anaesthetic management. Intubation difficulties in OSA are assessed by BMI, Mallampati grading, laryngoscopic grading (Cormack and Lehane), a line joining the angle of the mouth and tragus of the ear with the horizontal, sternomental distance and thyromental distance. Difficulty index ratio of OSA patients is higher than that of non-OSA patients.

TABLE 12.8 Congenital and Acquired Causes for Difficult Airway

Congenital	Acquired
Pierre Robin syndrome	Morbid obesity
Treacher Collins syndrome	Acromegaly
Goldenhar syndrome	Infections involving the airway (Ludwig's angina)
Mucopolysaccharidoses	Rheumatoid arthritis
Achondroplasia	Obstructive sleep apnoea
Micrognathia	Ankylosing spondylitis
Down's syndrome	Tumours involving the airway Trauma (airway, cervical spine)

MANAGEMENT OF DIFFICULT AIRWAY

During difficult intubation, whether predicted or not, hypoxia must be prevented. The LMA can be used as a temporary measure, and if intubation is essential, then a tracheostomy may have to be performed. If the patient cannot be oxygenated via the upper airway, then it may be necessary to resort to the creation of a surgical airway (Flowchart 12.4). Other techniques used when faced with difficult airway are blind nasotracheal intubation and awake intubation.

BLIND TRACHEAL INTUBATION

Fibreoptic intubation requires patient cooperation and cannot be performed on upper airways with preexisting narrowing pathology like a high Mallampati grade and a thick neck. If bronchoscope-guided intubation becomes unsuccessful, blind nasal intubation is performed by flexing the neck and pressure on the tracheal cartilage (optimal external laryngeal manipulation). The patient's head is placed in the sniffing position. The endotracheal tube is lubricated with a local anaesthetic gel and passed into the nasal cavity along the floor of the nose beneath the inferior turbinate. Once it is inserted into the trachea, the position is confirmed by bilateral lung auscultation and capnography. It is an alternative for difficult airway management and can be a lifesaving technique in emergencies. It is important to note that the skill of the anaesthetist is the main determinant for success.

Risks:

- Subluxation of the cricoarytenoid cartilage
- Damage to the glottic opening
- It is a 'nonvisualising' intubating technique
- Oesophageal intubation
- Epiglottis can be pushed into the glottic opening.

AWAKE INTUBATION

Alternatively, the laryngeal reflexes may be abolished by:

- Deep inhalational anaesthesia
- Local anaesthesia of the larynx, usually in an awake patient.

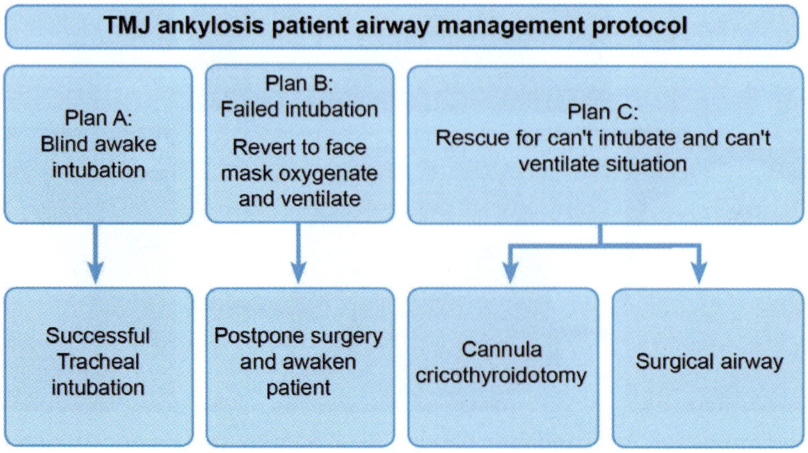

Flowchart 12.3 The management protocol for airway of a patient with TMJ ankylosis.

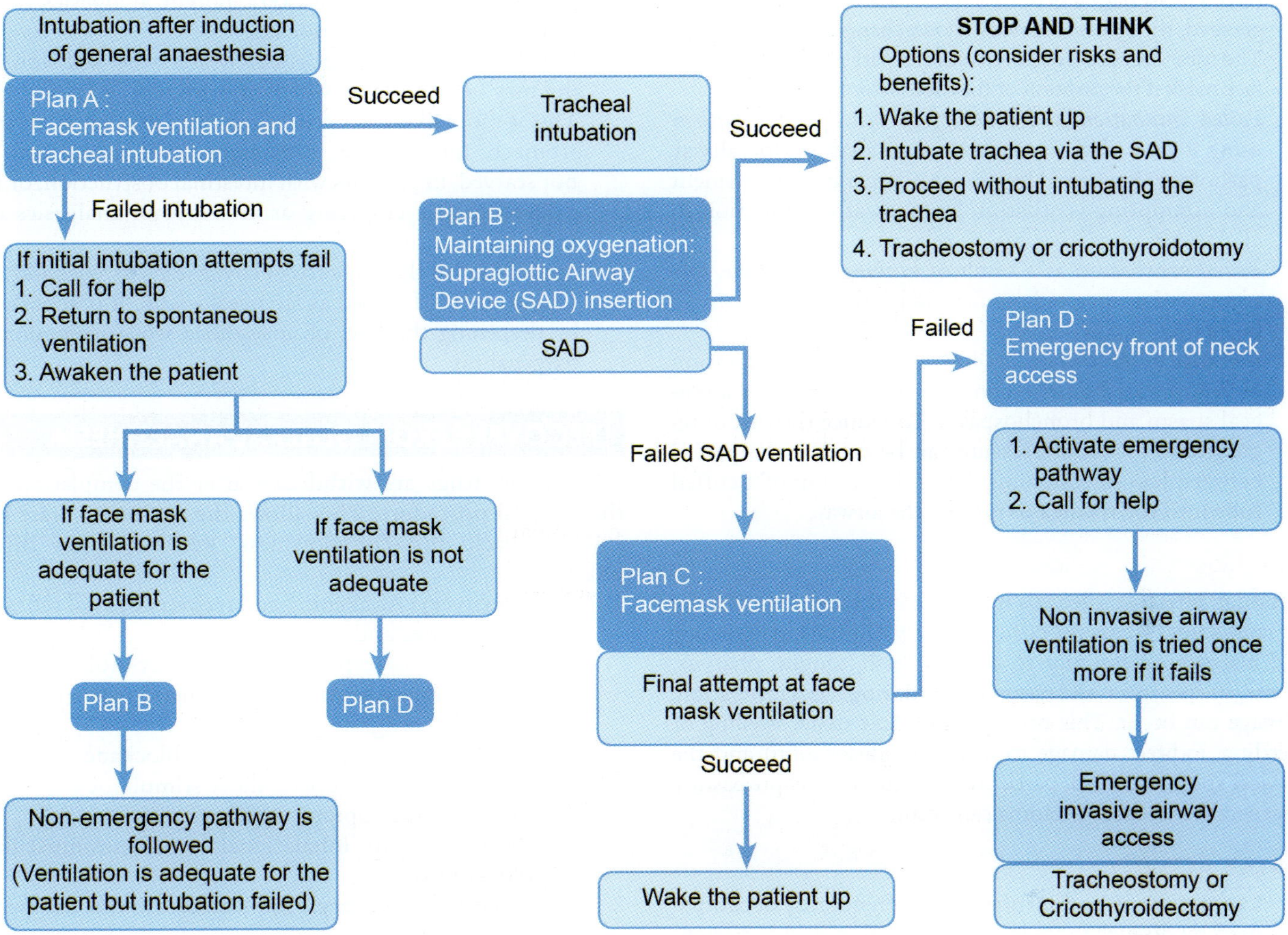

Flowchart 12.4 Guidelines to follow for tracheal intubation with or without difficulty in securing the airway.

These techniques are reserved for the patients with anticipated difficult intubation, when problems in ventilating the patient after the administration of a muscle relaxant, like in airway tumours, panfacial trauma, immobility of the cervical spine, TMJ ankylosis and trismus. In such circumstances, awake intubation is preferred. The patient is induced only after securing the airway (Flowchart 12.5).

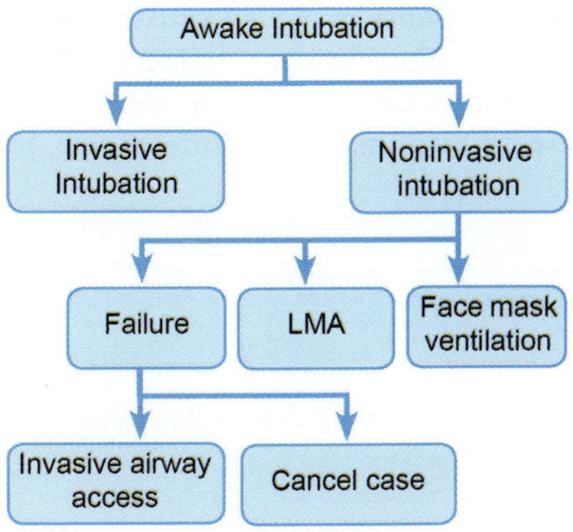

Flowchart 12.5 Awake intubation options for difficult intubation.

COMPLICATIONS OF TRACHEAL INTUBATION

HYPOXIA

Hypoxia can result from many causes.

1. ***Unrecognised oesophageal intubation:*** Oxygen and anaesthetic gases are delivered into the stomach. The best method for detecting this is to measure the carbon dioxide in expired gas; less than 0.2% is indicative of oesophageal intubation. The most reliable indicator is the monitoring of end-tidal carbon dioxide (ETCO_2) monitoring. Other less reliable signs are burping sounds as gas escapes, large volume of air required to fill the cuff, on auscultation, diminished breath sounds are heard, on ventilation, decreased chest movements are seen, gurgling sounds are heard over the epigastrium. An alternative is to withdraw the plunger rapidly of a 50 mL bladder syringe attached to the tracheal tube. If the tracheal tube is in the oesophagus, the walls collapse over the end of the tube, resistance is felt and air cannot be aspirated

(Wee's oesophageal detector). If the patient has been preoxygenated, then pulse oximetry shows changes at a later stage. The tube should be removed and the patient ventilated via a face mask if the position of the tube is doubtful

2. ***Failed intubation and inability to ventilate the patient using a face mask*** *due to* abnormal anatomy or airway pathology. Prevented by proper preoperative assessment and attempting ventilation by mask after induction in all patients to receive muscle relaxants
3. Failed ventilation as a result of ***kinking of the tube***, disconnected or inserted too far and passing into one main bronchus
4. ***Blockage of the airway*** directly resulting from aspiration of regurgitated gastric contents or secondary to laryngeal spasm and bronchospasm. To reduce the risk of regurgitation, cricoid pressure can be used in the period between loss of consciousness and insertion of a cuffed tube into the trachea to protect the airway.

TRAUMA

Although often regarded as a minor event, it is a common cause for complaint by patients postoperatively. During laryngoscopy and insertion of the tube to the lips, teeth, tongue, pharynx, larynx, trachea, nose and nasopharynx during nasal intubation, damage can occur. This usually causes soft tissue swelling or bleeding, indirect damage to mandible (dislocation) and the cervical spine and cord, particularly where there is preexisting degenerative disease or trauma can occur.

REFLEX ACTIVITY

1. Laryngoscopy and intubation are frequently accompanied by disturbances in cardiac rhythm and hypertension, which may jeopardise patients with coronary artery disease (CAD), aortic or intracranial aneurysms. These responses are exaggerated in hypertensive patients. These events may also cause a rise in intracranial pressure secondary to increased cerebral blood flow. Specific action is usually taken to reduce the hypertensive response in patients at risk, for example, pretreatment with β-blockers, potent analgesics (fentanyl, alfentanil) or lignocaine
2. In patients who are inadequately anaesthetised, vomiting may be stimulated when laryngoscopy is attempted. This is more likely to occur when there is material in the stomach, for example, in emergencies if the patient is not starved, in patients with intestinal obstruction, or in delayed gastric emptying as after opiate analgesics or following trauma
3. Stimulation of the epiglottis or larynx leads to reflex adduction of the cords called as laryngeal spasm. It is abolished by deepening the level of anaesthesia while maintaining oxygenation.

RECOVERY FROM GENERAL ANAESTHESIA

Anaesthetic drugs are withdrawn after the completion of the surgical procedure. This allows the patient to start recovering back into consciousness. Recovery is in three phases.

1. **Early recovery:** Awakening and recovery of vital reflexes like airway reflex and motor activity
   a. Patient starts responding to verbal stimuli
   b. Ventilation reduces the anaesthetic concentration thus hastening the recovery
   c. Recovery from neuromuscular blockade occurs—monitored by peripheral nerve stimulator
   d. Recovery from opioids and hypnotics
   e. Recovery from inhalational and neuromuscular blocking agents
2. **Intermediate recovery:** Immediate clinical recovery and home readiness
   a. Patient is shifted to the postanaesthesia care unit (PACU)
   b. Patient is placed in a 45-degree head-up position
   c. Vitals are monitored every 15 min
   d. Discharge from PACU is done after complete postanaesthesia discharge scoring system
3. **Late recovery:** Full recovery and psychological recovery

Chapter 13

Conscious Sedation

OUTLINE

INTRODUCTION

Sedation is decreasing the aggressive or anxiety response by administration of drugs, for the diagnostic, interventional, medical or surgical intervention by producing a degree of impaired response with or without the loss of consciousness. Conscious sedation is defined as 'minimally depressed level of consciousness that retains the patient's ability to independently and continuously maintain an airway and respond appropriately to physical stimulation or verbal command and that is produced by a pharmacological or nonpharmacological method or a combination'. The term conscious sedation refers to the '"administration of medication (an oral, intravenous or inhaled sedative) for the purpose of placing a patient in a relaxed state" for their dental procedure. In comparison to general anaesthesia, however, the patient remains conscious' (Table 13.1). The levels of sedation have been depicted in Flowchart 13.1.

INDICATIONS OF CONSCIOUS SEDATION

The decision for conscious sedation is based on the American Society of Anesthesiologists (ASA) classification (Table 13.2).

The need for conscious sedation is as follows:

- Only classes ASA I and II are considered for sedation in dental care settings
- To allay apprehension, anxiety or fear—dental anxiety and phobia—usually, children and people with high fear susceptibility
- To decrease stress associated with traumatic or prolonged procedures
- To stabilise the blood pressure for patients with hypertension or a history of cardiovascular disease
- Medical conditions causing the patient to impede the procedure
- Patient lacking psychological or emotional maturity
- Those patients with movement disorders with physical/mental issues
- For patients with severe gag reflex
- To enable prolonged unpleasant procedures to be carried out without distress to the patient, for example, surgical extraction of 3rd molars
- To avoid risks related to general anaesthesia (GA). Conscious sedation is used as intermediary between local anaesthesia (LA) and GA
- Medical conditions potentially aggravated by stress
- Conscious sedation for children with special needs
  a. Attention-deficit hyperactivity disorder (ADHD): Anaesthetic management is dependent on the level of cooperation of the child. Intravenous (i.v.) sedation technique can be followed

TABLE 13.1 Difference Between Conscious Sedation and General Anaesthesia

Conscious Sedation	General Anaesthesia
Purposeful response to verbal or tactile stimulation	Patient is completely unconscious
No premedication is required	Premedication is required
Airway is maintained	Ventilation is required
Nil per oral (NPO) is not required (NPO—patient cannot consume any food or fluids till the procedure)	NPO is required
Recovery period is 1–2 min	Recovery period can extend up to 2–3 h

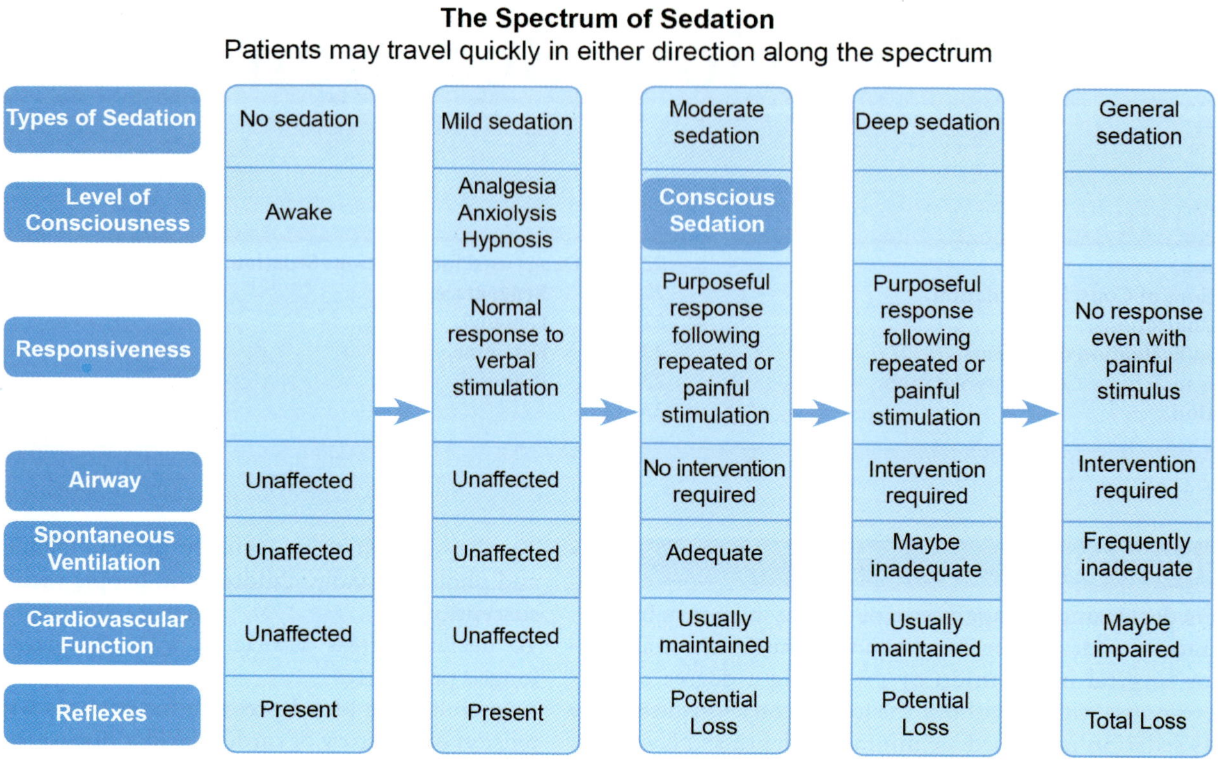

Flowchart 13.1 Spectrum of sedation.

TABLE 13.2 Indication of Conscious Sedation based on the ASA classification

ASA	Description	Example	Indication of Sedation
ASA class I	Healthy individual	No disease in medical history	Indicated when required
ASA class II	Mild systemic disease	Mild asthma Diabetes (under control with medication, good glucose control with lifestyle modifications) Controlled epilepsy Acyanotic congenital heart defects (CHDs)	Indicated when required
ASA class III	Severe systemic disease with functional limitation	Severe asthma Uncontrolled diabetes Uncontrolled epilepsy CHD with cyanosis and congestive heart failure (CHF)	Should be decided based on the modification of diseased state in elective cases. In case of emergency benefits, outweigh risks.
ASA class IV	Severe systemic disease with threat to life	Advanced respiratory, cardiac, hepatic, renal insufficiency	Benefits rarely outweigh risks
ASA class V	Moribund	Septic shock, severe trauma	Not indicated. Extremely poor response to safety during sedation.

b. Autism: As they present with ritualistic behaviours, benzodiazepines are drugs of choice. i.v. access is difficult to obtain and so potent inhalational or intramuscular ketamine can be used
c. Down's syndrome: They present with craniofacial features like macroglossia, micrognathia and short neck. These features can increase the risk of airway obstruction during sedation.

CONTRAINDICATIONS

- Chronic obstructive pulmonary disease (COPD)
- Uncontrolled epilepsy

- Bleeding disorders
- Uncooperative or unwilling patients
- Unaccompanied patients
- Prolonged surgery
- Lack of equipment or inadequate personnel
- Patients in ASA class III and class IV should be referred to hospital care
- Paediatric patients with:
  a. Congenital heart diseases (CHDs) associated with CHF or cyanosis
  b. Neurological impairment with poor pharyngeal coordination
  c. Severe obesity
  d. Airway abnormalities inclusive of upper respiratory tract infection (URTI)
  e. Obstructive sleep apnoea
  f. Raised intracranial pressure
  g. Cerebral palsy: Conscious sedation may be contraindicated due to the inability to clear oral secretions

While administering conscious sedation, it is imperative to have access to all resuscitative measures, as certain catastrophic complications may arise.

CLINICAL EFFECTS

- For 20–30 min acute detachment and later a state of relaxation
- Anterograde amnesia (loss of memory following administration of the drug) for the same period
- Cardiovascular depression is minimal (the relative hypotension and bradycardia due to the relief of hypertension and tachycardia caused by anxiety)
- In most cases, minimal respiratory depression is seen. The exception is in patients with impaired respiratory function or in those who have taken other depressants such as opiates and alcohol, where the effect may be more marked. However, excessively rapid intravenous injections have the potential to cause respiratory depression leading to apnoea and respiratory arrest, which is life-threatening if not diagnosed and treated promptly
- Additional properties of benzodiazepines:
  a. Muscle relaxant
  b. Anticonvulsant (used to treat status epilepticus).

CHARACTERISTICS OF CONSCIOUS SEDATION

- Retains the patient's ability to maintain a patent airway independently and continuously and the patient remains awake
- Permits appropriate response by the patient to physical stimulation or verbal command ('open your mouth', 'close down')
- They are responsive to sensation of pain except in the area where LA is used
- If the patient does happen to doze off, they can be easily awaken
- Patient's protective reflexes like breathing or coughing will remain functional
- The patient's cognitive functions (perception, reasoning, comprehension) may be modestly impaired
- But patient will lose all sensations and consciousness.

RISKS INVOLVED IN SEDATION

- Unintentional loss of consciousness (i.e. loss of verbal contact with the patient)
- Reduced intensity of protective airway and pain reflexes
- Depression of respiratory and cardiovascular systems
- Drug interaction with combination of wide variety of drugs used
- Nausea
- Hypoxia—decreased oxygen in the blood or bodily tissues
- Hyperactivity (inability to pay attention).

PRESEDATION EVALUATION OF PATIENTS

Patient history

1. Acute illness/injury
2. Prior illness
3. Medications
4. Psychological assessment
5. Drug allergies
6. Weight
7. Previous sedation experiences and if so, drugs used for it.

Following physical examination must be performed before sedation

1. Airway evaluation—note all abnormalities
2. Respiratory rate and oxygen saturation
3. Heart rate
4. Blood pressure
5. Determine ASA physical health status
6. Level of consciousness/baseline sedation score.

Patient preparations

1. Patient must receive verbal and written instructions regarding effects of sedation and their responsibilities before and after treatment
2. Fasting before sedation is not normally required unless patient presents with a gag reflex to prevent risk for vomiting and aspiration during treatment
3. Preoperative fasting is controversial. For elective procedures, the 2-4-6 fasting rule can be applied (2 hrs for clear fluids, 4 hrs for breast milk, and 6 hrs for solids).
4. Advised to avoid smoking, alcohol and large meals on the day of operation
5. There must be someone to accompany the patient for postsedation care of the patient
6. An informed consent is taken in written form for sedation and for the treatment planned. Other important preparations have been briefed in Table 13.3.

TABLE 13.3 Requirements for Conscious Sedation

Preparation for sedation procedure	
Operator: Anaesthetist and personnel skilled in advanced life support	
Suction	Functioning suction apparatus, age/size-appropriate suction catheters
Oxygen and nitrogen	Adequate oxygen supply and flowmeters Continuous flow design equipment with flowmeters for safe delivery of O_2 and N_2O (fail safe mechanism), pin-indexed yoke system—efficient scavenger
Nasal mask	Selected according to age and size of the patient—appropriately sized nasal hood should be selected. A flow rate of 5–6 L/min generally is acceptable to most patients.
Airway	Age/size-appropriate airway equipment (e.g. endotracheal (ET) tubes, laryngeal mask airways (LMA), oral and nasal airways, laryngoscope blades, stylets, bag mask)
Drugs	All required sedation medication—midazolam, fentanyl, pethidine, propofol, ketamine, thiopentone; emergency drugs, reversal agents for opioids or benzodiazepines (e.g. naloxone, flumazenil)
Intravenous access	For intravenous sedation is administered and for emergencies during light sedation and other techniques.
Monitors	Pulse oximeter, BP monitor, ECG, stethoscope, thermometer, cardiac monitor, end-tidal carbon dioxide ($EtCO_2$) monitor/detector
Equipment	Special equipment/drugs for particular patient (e.g. defibrillator, respiratory box, IV access equipment) should be readily available, resuscitation medications and equipment, Ambu bag—adult and paediatric, crash cart with automated external defibrillator (AED)

TECHNIQUES TO ACHIEVE CONSCIOUS SEDATION

There are various techniques to achieve conscious sedation such as inhalation sedation, oral (enteral) sedation, intramuscular sedation, submucosal sedation, intravenous sedation and rectal sedation. The most commonly used are as follows:

1. i.v. sedation or **deep conscious sedation** is a type of sedation involving administration of medications directly into the bloodstream through intravenous route. The greatest advantage of i.v. sedation is that the surgeon or anaesthesiologist has complete control of the entire procedure. In case of inadequate sedation, patient can be fully sedated or reversed. The i.v. sedation drugs are more effective than the same given orally, with a more profound amnesia associated with the i.v. technique. Drugs used are **diazepam, midazolam and other benzodiazepine groups**
2. **Enteral conscious sedation**, 'orally administered sedation', sometimes called 'sedation dentistry', is administered by taking an oral sedation. The body functions are normal and the patient is able to breathe on their own. The patient will often fall asleep. Some degree of amnesia is common. The disadvantage with this method of sedation is that the level of sedation for each person is not predictable. Drugs used are **midazolam, diazepam, lorazepam, triazolam and zaleplon**
3. **Inhalation conscious sedation, nitrous oxide/oxygen** sedation. This is the most frequently used sedation method in dentistry. All bodily functions remain normal and the person is able to breathe on their own. The patient will often sleep and experience some degree of amnesia of the dental appointment (Flowchart 13.2)

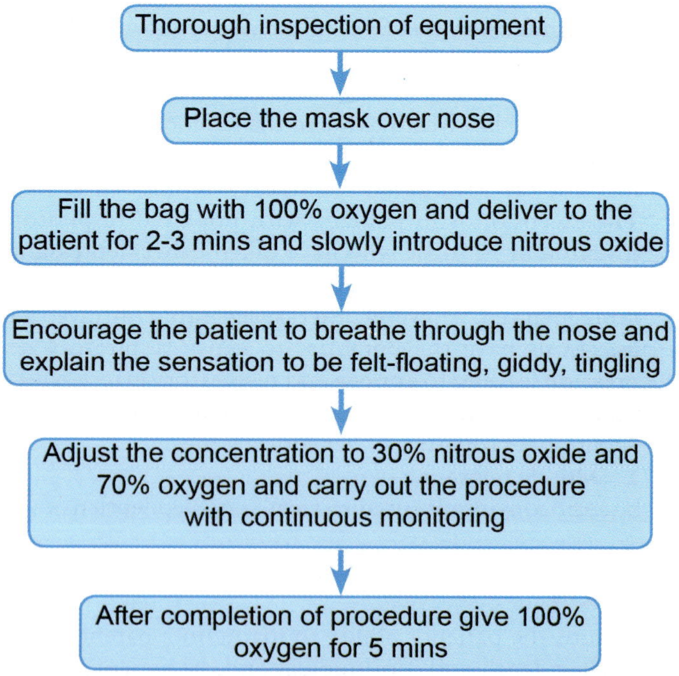

Flowchart 13.2 Procedure followed in inhalation conscious sedation technique.

4. **Combination of the above techniques.**

The procedure followed in inhalation technique of conscious sedation has been described in Flowchart 13.2.

ORAL SEDATION

Advantages

- Easily administered
- Less sensitive
- Noninvasive
- Good patient acceptance.

Disadvantages

- Inability to titrate reliability
- Variable onset of action
- Variable duration of action
- Limited use in young children.

Dosage for oral sedation (Table 13.4)

Commonly used pharmacological agents for conscious sedation.

DRUGS USED FOR CONSCIOUS SEDATION

BENZODIAZEPINES

Benzodiazepines have antianxiety, anticonvulsant, sedative, muscle relaxant and amnesic properties. Midazolam and diazepam are the medications used in the dental operating setup.

MIDAZOLAM

Midazolam is a short-acting benzodiazepine central nervous system (CNS) depressant. Conscious sedation prior to short diagnostic or surgical procedures is an indication, either alone or with a narcotic:

- Water-soluble
- Nonirritating to veins
- Faster and shorter acting
- Three times more potent than diazepam
- It may be administered i.v. (most common route), Intramuscular (i.m.), Per Oral (PO), rectally or nasally.

Midazolam is a potent sedative agent that should be administered slowly over 2 min for a single large bolus dose. Rapid or excessive i.v. doses may result in respiratory depression or arrest. If not recognised and treated promptly, death or hypoxic encephalopathy may result.

The initial i.v. dose may be as little as 0.5–1 mg, but should not exceed 2.5 mg in a healthy adult. It should be titrated to the desired effect. An excellent indicator of an adequate dose is slurred speech. For patients over 60 years of age, debilitated patients or patients receiving narcotics, lower doses should be used.

Onset of sedation after i.v. injection is achieved within 3–5 min. The duration of effect ranges from 1 to 6 h after i.v. injection, but patients should not do any activity that require fine motor or cognition skills (i.e. driving, cooking). The half-life ranges from 1.2 to 12.3 h.

Midazolam should not be used on patients with known benzodiazepine hypersensitivity or acute narrow-angle glaucoma. Adverse reactions from i.v. administration include hiccups, nausea, vomiting, over sedation, headache, coughing and pain at the injection site.

DIAZEPAM

Diazepam has been replaced for the most part by midazolam but is still used occasionally for conscious sedation and as a premedication for nonpainful procedures. Like midazolam, diazepam is indicated for conscious sedation prior to short diagnostic or surgical procedures, either alone or with a narcotic. It may be administered i.v., i.m. or PO, although i.m. administration is very painful and hence not recommended. A large vein should be used to inject diazepam. It cannot be mixed with other medications or diluted as it carries the risk of precipitation.

Adverse reactions

- Extremely irritating to the tissues
- Venous thrombosis
- Phlebitis
- Apnoea
- Hypotension
- Diazepam can be given orally as a premedication prior to many nonpainful surgical procedures
- Effective anxiolytic.

FENTANYL

Fentanyl is a synthetic opioid. It is indicated for analgesic action short duration procedures. If given alone, dosage should begin at 1–2 μg/kg, which is about 75–150 μg for an average size adult. If given in conjunction with a benzodiazepine, a smaller dose should be used. The average patient usually requires 50–100 μg. Fentanyl has an immediate response and effective excellent analgesia. It has a half-life of 2–4 h, but patients should not do any activities that require fine motor or cognition skills (i.e. driving, cooking).

Rapid i.v. administration can lead to a rigid chest wall and difficulty in breathing. This effect may be reversed with

TABLE 13.4 Dosage of Oral Sedation Based on Duration and Depth of Sedation

Appointment Time	Minimal Sedation	Moderate Sedation
2 h or less	Triazolam 0.125–0.25 mg	Triazolam 0.375–0.50 mg
Longer than 2 h	Triazolam 0.25 mg (or) diazepam 10–15 mg (or) temazepam 15 mg (or) oxazepam 10–15 mg	Triazolam 0.50 mg (or) diazepam 20–30 mg (or) temazepam 30 mg (or) oxazepam 20–30 mg
Longer than 3 h	Lorazepam 0.5–1 mg (or) alprazolam 0.25 mg	Lorazepam 2–3 mg (or) alprazolam 0.50 mg

naloxone (Narcan) or may require a depolarising muscle relaxant and intubation.

This short-acting (30–50 min) potent opioid analgesic related to pethidine is generally given i.v. at the beginning of painful surgical procedures. Reflex effects of painful stimuli are abolished.

Dose

2–4 mg/kg

After i.v. fentanyl, the patient becomes drowsy yet conscious and his/her cooperation can be commanded. Respiratory depression is marked, but predictable; patient may be encouraged to breathe and assistance may be provided.

Supplemental doses of fentanyl are required approximately every 30 min, but recovery gets prolonged after repeated doses.

1. Fentanyl is used effectively as sedation, adjunct to regional/local anaesthetics. It is also used as supplement anaesthetics in balanced anaesthesia. This permits use of lower anaesthetic concentrations with better haemodynamic stability
2. Combined with benzodiazepines, it can obviate the need for inhaled anaesthetics for diagnostic, endoscopic, angiographic and other minor procedures in poor risk patients, as well as for burn dressing.

KETAMINE

Ketamine is a nonbarbiturate hypnotic with very high margin of safety. It has good tissue compatibility (no irritation to veins). Ketamine produces a so-called '**dissociative anaesthesia'**—profound analgesia, immobility, amnesia with light sleep and feelings of dissociation from one's own body and the surroundings.

Dose

A dose of **1–3 mg/kg i.v.** (average 1.5 mg/kg) or **6.5–13 mg/kg i.m.** (average 10 mg/kg).

Ketamine produces the above effects within a minute and recovery starts after 10–15 min, but patient remains amnesic for 1–2 h. It does not cause relaxation of tongue, so it does not interfere with airways thus, making it ideal for dentistry.

Emergence delirium, hallucinations and involuntary movements occur in up to 50% patients.

1. Ketamine is effective for short procedures such as operations on head and neck especially in asthmatics
2. It is also useful for repeated use particularly for burn dressings
3. Combined with diazepam, it is useful in angiography, cardiac catheterisation and trauma surgery
4. Avoided in hypertensive and ischaemic heart disease patients
5. Major disadvantage is increased intracranial and intraocular pressure with increased occurrence of nausea and vomiting.

PROPOFOL

It is the recent i.v. anaesthetic agent, used for induction/maintenance of anaesthesia and also for sedation during short dental procedures done under LA. Major advantage of propofol is rapid recovery irrespective of the duration of infusion.

Dose

1–2 mg/kg/min (for sedation)

- Possess significant antiemetic property at low doses
- Rapid recovery without hangover effect
- Full orientation returns within 5–10 min.

Section | V |

Principles of Practising Oral Surgery

Chapter 14

Armamentarium

OUTLINE

The advancements in oral and maxillofacial surgery and the refinements in surgical technique have complimented the evolution of the surgical armamentarium. Armamentaria have evolved to ease surgery, shortening on-table time, widening the surgical field, increasing visibility, minimising trauma to surgical area, etc. A surgical instrument is a specially designed tool or device for performing specific actions and carrying out desired effects during a surgery or operation. Most of the surgical instruments are made of high-grade steel, either stainless steel, tungsten carbide or chrome-plated. Each instrument has a particular purpose and should be handled accordingly. Inclusion of rotary and power-driven tools in bone cutting procedures has greatly influenced the hard tissue surgeries. Armamentarium used in oral and maxillofacial surgery can be categorised as depicted in Table 14.1.

TABLE 14.1 Armamentarium in Oral and Maxillofacial Surgery

i. **Instruments used for handling sterile instrument**
1. Cheatle forceps
2. Cheatle forceps container

ii. **Presurgical draping and asepsis**
1. Swab holder
2. Towel clips
   - Pincher
   - Backhaus

iii. **Soft tissue handling instruments**
1. Scalpel
2. Scissors
3. Dissecting forceps
4. Tissue forceps
   - Allis forceps
   - Babcock forceps
   - Lane forceps
   - Kocher—Ochsner artery forceps
   - Haemostat (artery forceps)
5. Instruments used for reflecting the mucoperiosteal flap
   - Moon's probe
   - Periosteal elevators
   - Cleft palate raspatory
6. Needle holders
7. Retractors
   - Tongue and cheek retractor
   - Langenbeck retractor
   - Austin retractor
   - Cat's paw retractor
   - Obwegeser ramus retractor
   - Weider retractor
   - Seldin retractor
   - Minnesota retractor
   - Copper malleable retractor
   - Skin hook
   - Channel retractor
   - Alar retractor
   - Nasal speculum
   - Tongue depressor
8. Mechanical devices
   - Stapling devices
   - Haemostatic clips
9. Lister's sinus forceps

iv. **Hard tissue handling instruments**
1. Chisel
2. Periosteal elevator
3. Pterygoid chisel
4. Gigli saw
5. Mallet
6. Osteotome
7. Bone file
8. Bone gouge
9. Surgical curette
10. Bone rongeur
11. Bone scoop
12. Bone grasping forceps
13. Smith bone spreader
14. Rotary and power devices—burs/microsaws

v. **Airway maintenance/anaesthesia**
1. Laryngoscope
2. Face mask
3. Oral/nasal pharyngeal airway
4. Laryngeal mask airway
5. Endotracheal tube—oral/nasal
6. Tracheostomy tube

vi. **Special instruments in fracture management**
1. Hayton William forceps
2. Rowe maxillary disimpaction forceps
3. Rowe zygomatic elevator
4. Walsham forceps
5. Asch forceps
6. Awl—long/short
7. Wire pusher
8. Wire twister
9. Wire cutter
10. Plates—titanium/stainless steel

vii. **Miscellaneous instruments**
1. Mouth gag
2. Mouth prop
3. Trocar and cannula
4. Suction apparatus
5. Foley catheter
6. Operating microscope
7. Ryles tube
8. Surgical loupes
9. Diathermy
10. Surgical drain

INSTRUMENTS USED FOR HANDLING STERILE INSTRUMENTS

CHEATLE FORCEPS

- It is also called as transfer forceps
- The Cheatle sterilizer forceps is a long instrument having a curved shaft without a lock, used to remove sponges, gauze pieces or other sterilised instruments from boilers and formalin cabinets
- This ensures that each item is removed and the others are not infected (Fig. 14.1).

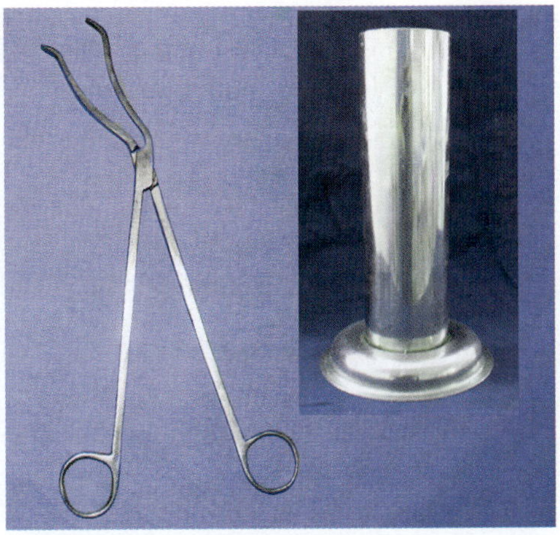

Figure 14.1 Cheatle forceps and container.

CHEATLE FORCEPS CONTAINER

- Forceps are placed in a container of methylated spirits when not in use
- It should be washed thoroughly and autoclaved once in a week.

PRESURGICAL DRAPING AND ASEPSIS

SWAB HOLDER

- The swab holder has a ratchet and two long blades, which has fenestrations and serrations at the operating end
- It is used to hold the swab and paint the surgical area with an antiseptic preoperatively
- It can also be used by the surgeons to hold soft tissue without causing much damage to the tissues
- To arrest haemorrhage by pressing on the tonsillar bed
- To hold the tongue and also to pick up gauge (Fig. 14.2).

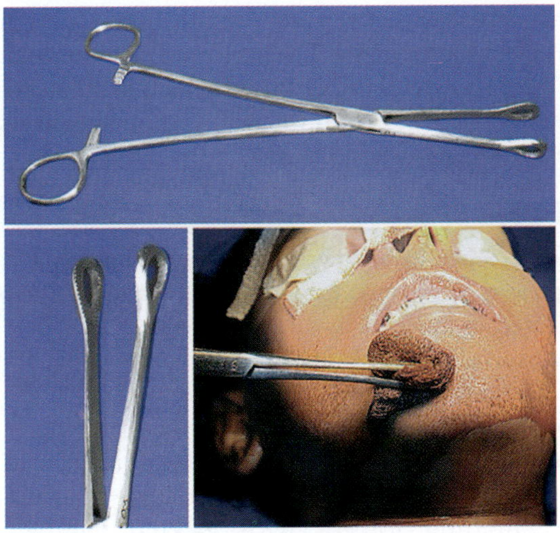

Figure 14.2 Swab holder. Swab holder being used for holding the betadine soaked swab as a part of preoperative asepsis.

TOWEL CLIPS

- The towel clips can be of forceps type (Backhaus towel clip) or Pincher type. The difference lies in the joints
- The Backhaus towel clip has a box joint and the Pincher type has a spring joint. The working ends may have either sharp points or blunt flat tips that overlap in the closed position (Fig. 14.3)

  Uses:
  - Towel clips are used to maintain surgical towels and drapes in the correct position during an operation, thereby creating a sterile surgical field
  - To stabilise suction tubes, motor cables and other cables to the sterile field
  - It is also used to hold the tongue while performing biopsy procedure in the posterior part of the tongue.

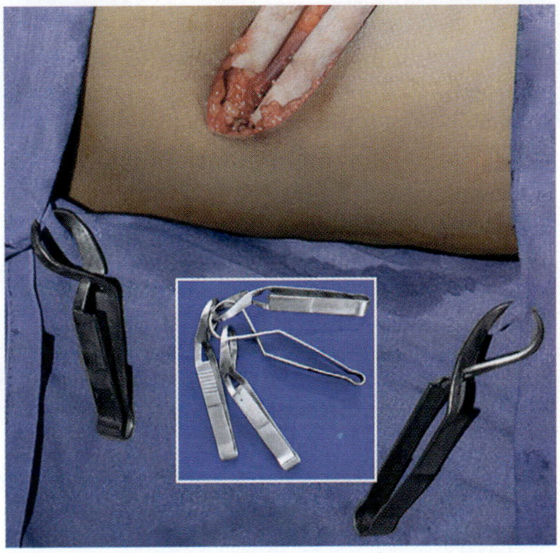

Figure 14.3 Towel clips.

SOFT TISSUE HANDLING INSTRUMENTS

SCALPEL

The scalpel *(scalpere = to cut, Latin)* is the traditional instrument of surgeons used to make incision or excise soft tissues. Scalpels are composed of a handle and a disposable blade.

BLADE

- The most commonly used blades are Bard-Parker (BP) blades.
- The blades come in presterilised packages and should be discarded after using once. They are attached and removed from the handles with haemostatic forceps
- This prevents accidental cuts and any possible infection
- The four blades most often used with this handle are the **no. 10, no. 11, no. 12 and no. 15**. Blades no. 10 and no. 15 have similar working ends. The difference is that

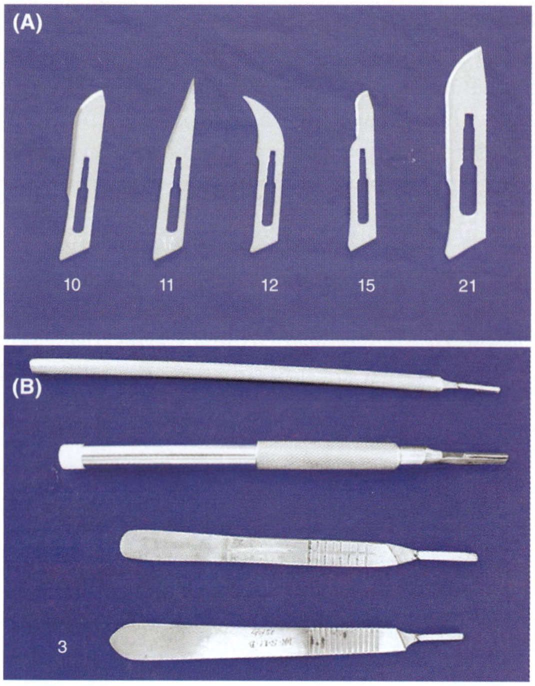

Figure 14.4 **(A)** Bard–Parker blades. **(B)** Scalpel handles (Bard–Parker).

the no. 10 blade is longer. The cutting edge on both the blades is on the curved part of the blade (Fig. 14.4A)

Uses of the different blades

- No. 10–for making skin incisions
- No. 11–for making stab incisions as in case of draining pus from an abscess cavity and drain placement
- No. 12 and no. 15–for carrying out surgeries in the mucogingival areas and other areas of the oral cavity.
- No. 21–It is used for procedures where you need to cut tissues or make a puncture.

BLADE HANDLE

- The two commonly used surgical scalpel handles are the no. 3 and beaver style.
- Each handle uses a different kind of blade and attachment method. The handle has a receiving slot for the blade. The no. 3 handle is short and wide; it uses a slotted blade that slides onto the handle
- Controlled pen grasp with the dominant hand is the common technique followed in placing incisions, though palm and thumb grasp may be used sometimes (Fig. 14.4B).

SCISSORS

(Latincisorium = a cutting instrument)

- Scissors are cutting instruments, used primarily for cutting soft tissues, dissecting through the tissue planes, excision of soft tissue and for cutting suture material
- It may be straight, curved or angled; blunt or sharp tipped. Choosing the correct scissors for the task is crucial in performing the procedure, for example, Mayo, Goldman Fox, Iris (Fig. 14.5).

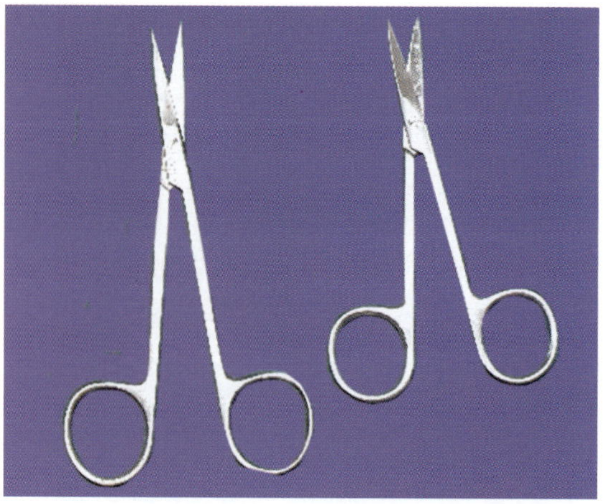

Figure 14.5 Straight and curved surgical scissors.

DISSECTING FORCEPS

Dissecting forceps or thumb forceps are the forceps that grip when compressed between thumb and fingers while the blades separate on releasing, as they are made of springing steel. They are excellent multipurpose instrument.

- As a rule, they are to be held like a pen
- They have no locking mechanism, as they intend to provide temporary grip to hold tissues
- Commonest types are toothed and nontoothed, available in various shapes (Fig.14.6A&B).

Toothed forceps: They have one tooth on one tip interdigitates with two teeth on opposing tip. The teeth puncture the tissue surface, tether and prevent it from slippage, rather than crushing it from compression of holding. It is best used to hold tough tissue as skin, fascia, cartilage and bone, for example, Adson tissue holding forceps (Fig. 14.6C).

Nontoothed forceps: They exert the grip through serrations on opposing tips. They are used to manipulate delicate tissue as small ducts, blood vessels and for suture removal. Sometimes round nosed nontooth forceps make excellent dissecting tool.

TISSUE FORCEPS

These forceps are instruments to grasp tissues that rely on the shape and opposing surfaces of the blades for grip. They are indicated for use in conditions where:

- A traction suture or hook may cut out
- Tissues tend to slip with smooth retractors

Types of tissue forceps

- Tissue holding forceps–Allis forceps and other forceps. **Allis forceps:** These are toothed tissue holding forceps with locking handle and a ratchet with triangular expansion at the tip where serrations are present. It is indicated for

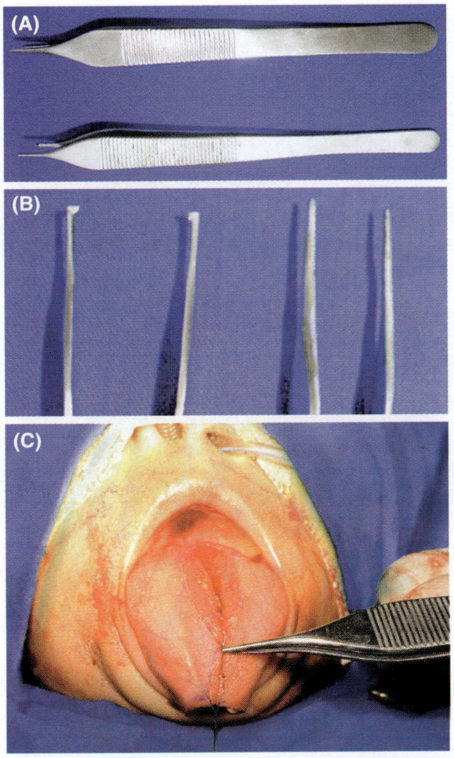

Figure 14.6 (**A and B**) Dissecting forceps Adson—toothed and nontoothed. (**C**) Adson toothed forceps used for suturing following partial glossectomy.

use to hold or grasp tough tissue and where fibrous tissue layers are planned for excision. It cannot be used on small excisions of histopathological importance as the sharp teeth can cause damage (Fig. 14.7A&B).

Other forceps: Lane forceps, Babcock forceps, Ring forceps (Haemostat), and Kocher–Ochsner artery forceps. They are used to grasp heavy tissue and may be used as clamp. They may have straight or curved jaws.

1. **Babcock tissue holding forceps**
   - It causes less trauma than the Allis forceps as they are nonperforating forceps used to grasp soft tissue (Fig. 14.7C)
   - It has a ratchet and triangular expansion with fenestrations at the end without teeth
   - It is used during head and neck dissection surgeries to hold thick flaps and the thyroid gland
2. **Lane tissue holding forceps**
   - Lane tissue forceps are nonratcheted thumb forceps The tip is broad and expanded with a wide opening
   - It is used for holding tough tissue such as fascia and cartilage (Fig. 14.7D)
3. **Kocher—Ochsner artery forceps**
   - It is ideally used on tough structures such as fascia, salivary gland and to divide strap muscles during thyroidectomy or tracheostomy
   - The forceps can also be used to catch the structure that is bleeding causing the bleeders to clog and provide haemostasis. The toothed tip grips the structure firmly, so that it will not slip (Fig. 14.7E)
4. **Haemostat** *(Haema—blood, stasis—stoppage—Greek)*
   - A haemostat, also called a haemostatic clamp, is a surgical tool which resembles a set of scissors with a locking clamp replacing the blade (Fig. 14.7F&G)
   - There are many types of haemostats namely Kelly, Crile and Halstead
   - A haemostat is commonly used to control bleeding, especially from a torn or punctured blood vessel,

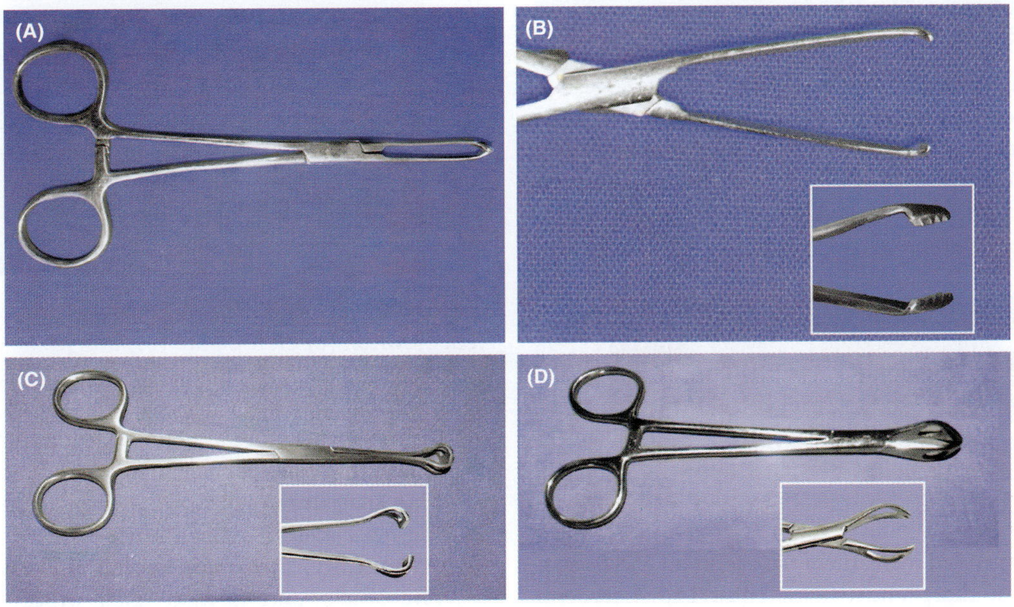

Figure 14.7 (**A**) Allis tissue holding forceps. (**B**) Working portion of the Allis tissue holding forceps with teethed serrations to hold tough tissues. (**C**) Babcock tissue holding forceps.

Continued

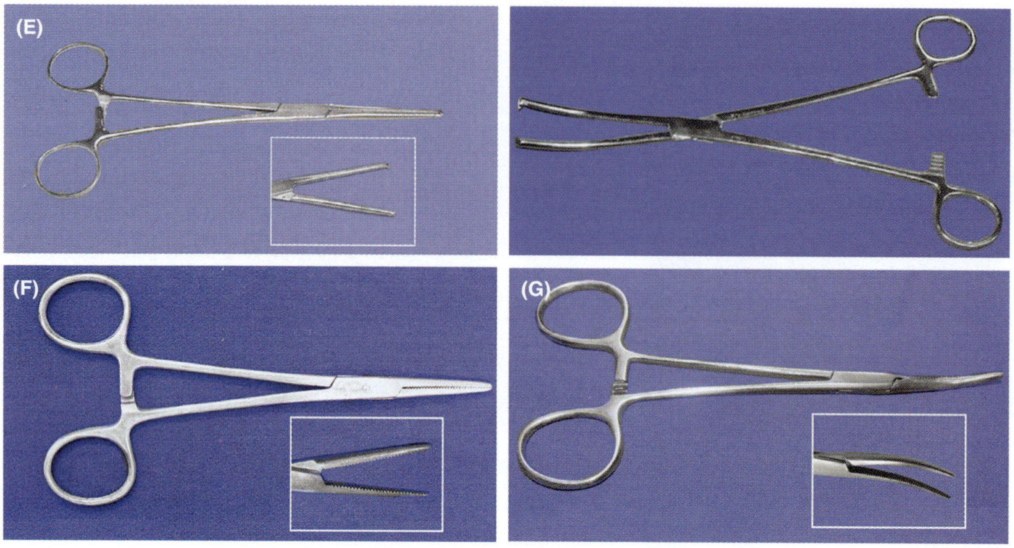

Figure 14.7, cont'd (**D**) Lane tissue holding forceps. (**E**) Kocher—Ochsner artery forceps. (**F**) Haemostat. (**G**) Straight artery forceps and curved artery forceps.

until the bleeding can be repaired by sutures or other surgical techniques

- The handle has a lock and thus the vessel may be held clamped. Small vessels may simply be crushed to attain haemostasis whereas larger vessels have to be ligated or cauterised
- Used to hold the ligatures end and help in easier ligature placement around the forceps
- Used for abscess drainage using Hilton's method.

INSTRUMENTS USED FOR REFLECTING THE MUCOPERIOSTEAL FLAP

MOON'S PROBE

- It is a right-angled probe with a narrow working edge, flat handle and blade, which is blunt and a rounded tip (Fig. 14.8)
- It helps in retracting the mucosa without traumatisation and used for elevation of the mucoperiosteum prior to extraction.

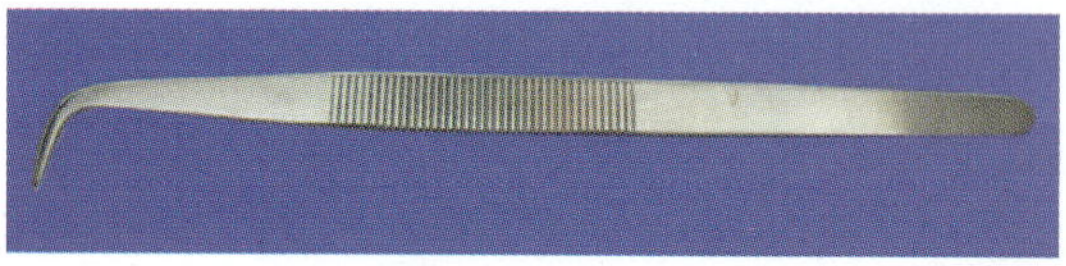

Figure 14.8 Moon's probe.

PERIOSTEAL ELEVATOR

- This is a double-ended instrument with a broad end (raspatory end) and a sharp end (rugine end). The sharp end should be maintained sharp to prevent shredding of the flap (Fig. 14.9)

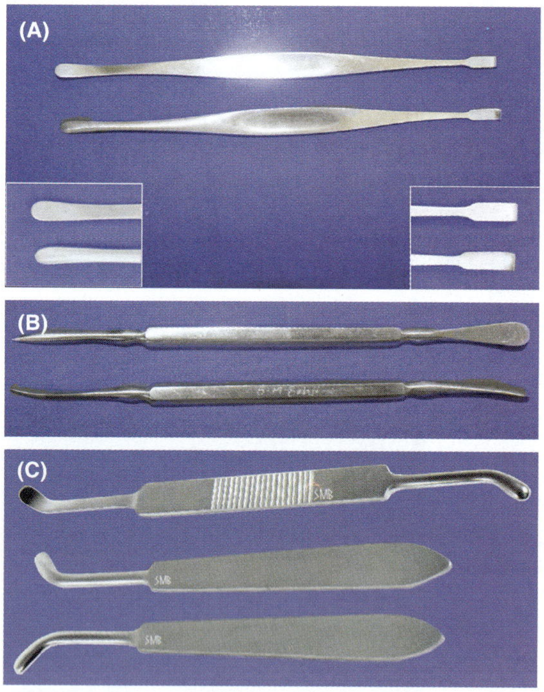

Figure 14.9 (**A**) Howarth periosteal elevator. (**B**) Molt periosteal elevator. (**C**) Cleft palate raspatory.

- Commonest in use are No. 9 Molt and No. 23 Seldin and Howarth periosteal elevator
- This instrument is used to expose the bone elevating the periosteum off the bone as a mucoperiosteal flap (intraorally) or separately (e.g. harvesting a rib graft). The sharp end is also used in tooth extraction to initially elevate the gingiva (prying motion) as well as aid in extraction by wedge principle

- The raspatory end is used to gently elevate the soft tissue flaps from the underlying bone without tearing
- It is used to retract flaps to visualise the area of interest during multiple extractions and surgical procedures
- Periosteal elevators are mainly used to lift full thickness soft tissue flaps.

NEEDLE HOLDER

- Needle holders are forceps with locking mechanism to hold needles during suturing procedures
- The typical needle holder has two short, rather blunt, serrated beaks with a distinct groove in each beak (Fig. 14.10). The grooves provide space for the placement and retention of the needle
- At the end of handles, there is a graduated, notched-locking device that lets the surgeon secure the suture needle in the desired position as if the needle were an extension of the needle holder
- A modification of this is Gillies needle holder that is a combination of needle holder and scissors.

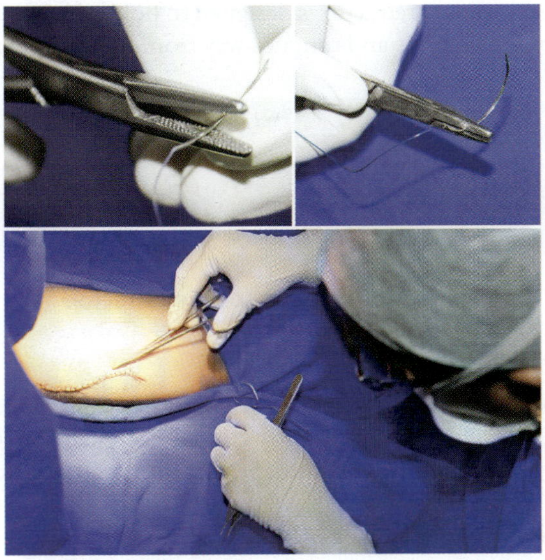

Figure 14.10 Needle holder.

RETRACTORS

- Retracting and exposing instruments are used to hold back or retract organs or tissue to gain exposure to the operative site. They are either 'self-retaining' (stay open on their own) or 'manual' (held by hand). While identifying retractors, look at the blade not the handle
- Retractors are also used to hold back structures in the oral cavity
- In oral surgery, tissue retractors hold tissues and flaps away from the surgical field to provide better visibility. Some retractors have blunt fork-like prongs that effectively allow handling of the tissues without causing excessive damage.

CHEEK RETRACTOR

- These retractors are designed to hold and retract the cheeks, tongue or a portion of the mucosa during surgical procedures
- The retractors are made of metal or plastic and may be large, curved or angled (Fig. 14.11).

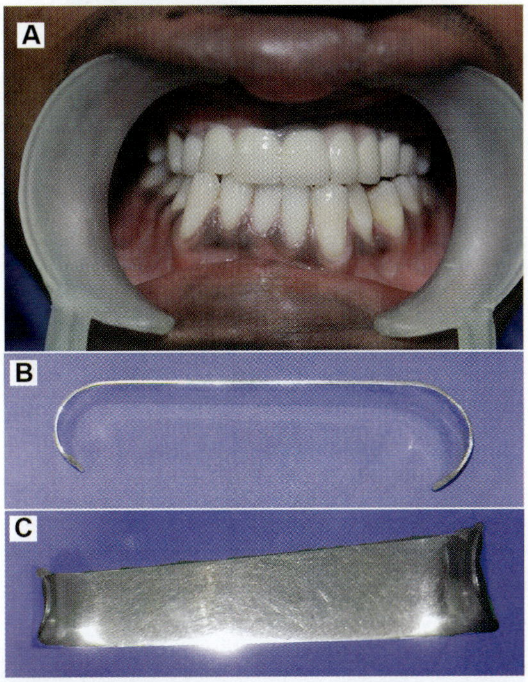

Figure 14.11 (**A**) Cheek retractor (**B** and **C**) Metal cheek retractor.

LANGENBECK RETRACTOR

- These are used for retraction of soft tissues and incision edges to have a better visibility of deeper structures
- This is the most commonly used retractor in oral surgery which has a long handle and an L-shaped blade on one or both the ends
- They are available in various sizes of blade width (Fig. 14.12).

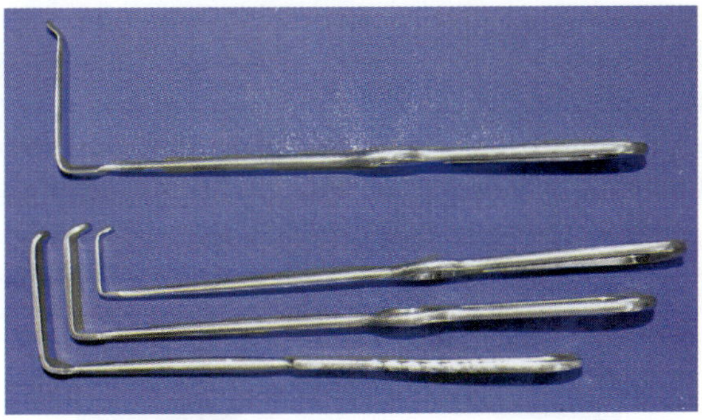

Figure 14.12 Langenbeck retractor.

AUSTIN RETRACTOR

- This is the most commonly used instrument in the removal of impacted 3rd molars

- It is a short right-angled instrument which is helpful in retracting the mucoperiosteal flap and to a lesser extent, the cheek (Fig. 14.13).

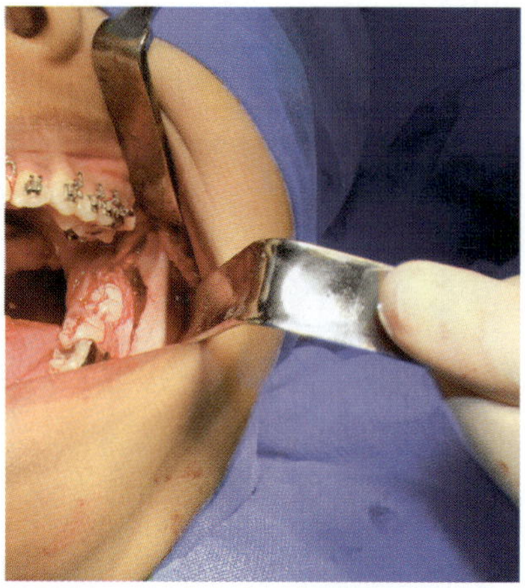

Figure 14.13 Austin retractor used in retracting buccal flap in bilateral sagittal split osteotomy (BSSO) procedure.

CAT'S PAW RETRACTOR

- The retractor end resembles a cat's paw
- It is most commonly used for gentle retraction of soft tissues
- Care should be taken not to apply excessive force which might lead to soft tissue damage (Fig. 14.14).

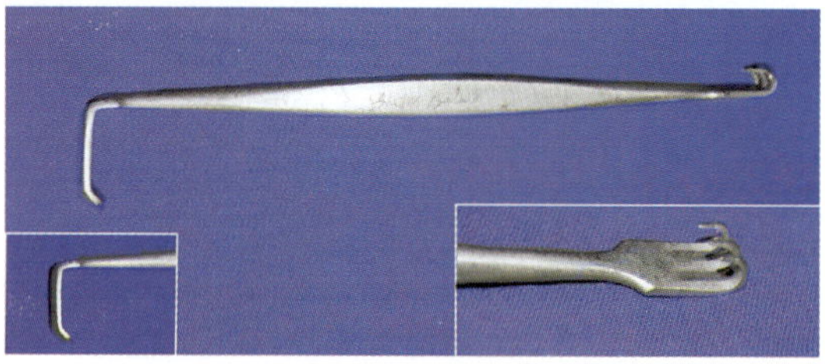

Figure 14.14 Cat's paw retractor.

OBWEGESER CORONOID/RAMUS RETRACTOR - NOTCHED RIGHT ANGLE RETRACTOR

It is used in retraction of the soft tissues and in surgeries involving the anterior border of the ramus of mandible (such as sagittal split osteotomy, coronoidectomy, angle fracture fixation, etc.). It has a V-shaped notch on the retracting end (Fig. 14.15 & 45.16).

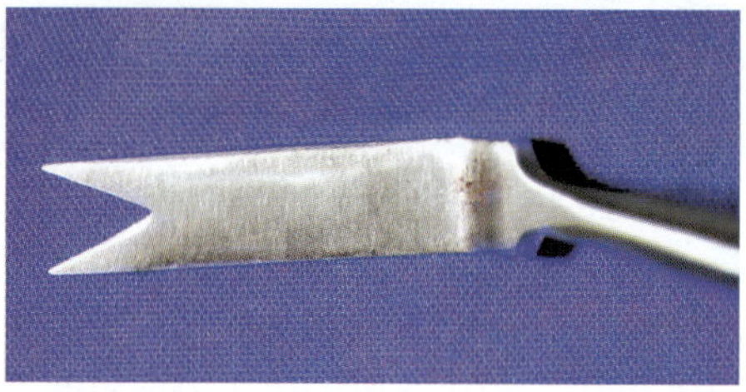

Figure 14.15 Obwegeser right angle retractor designed to engage anterior border of ramus and coronoid process retracting soft tissues.

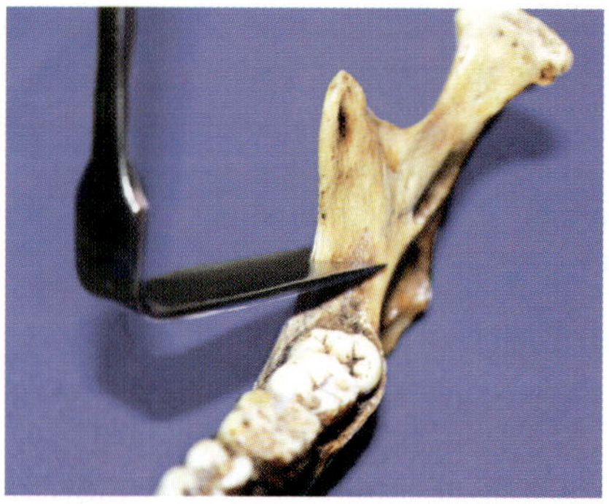

Figure 14.16 Demonstration of using coronoid retractor in mandible.

WEIDER TONGUE RETRACTOR

- Wieder retractor has a right-angled serrated blade, specifically designed to protect the tongue during lower jaw procedures, where the tongue must be removed from covering the occlusal surface of the teeth (Fig. 14.17).
- It is available in two sizes (small and large). The end of the handle is curved for better control
- Weider tongue retractor is designed to hold mucoperiosteal flaps, cheeks, lips and tongue away from the surgical area.

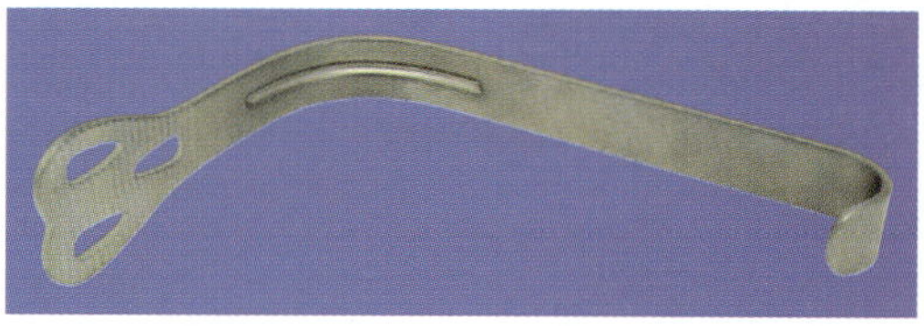

Figure 14.17 Weider tongue retractor.

SELDIN'S RETRACTOR

- It is a straight instrument with broad tip and a flat handle, the larger end is slightly curved designed for reflecting and retracting the mucoperiosteum after incisions of the gingival tissue
- It is a noncutting blade (Fig. 14.18).

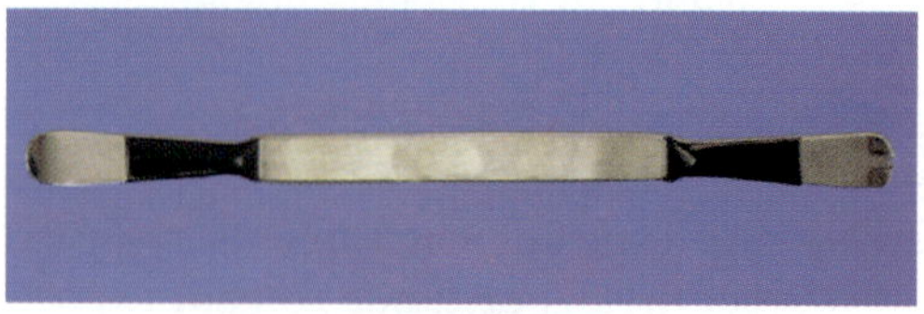

Figure 14.18 Seldin's retractor.

MINNESOTA RETRACTOR

- Both Austin and Minnesota retractors are used to retract cheek and the mucoperiosteum simultaneously.
- It consists of a handle and a rounded and slightly pointed working part. It is used for holding and retracting the lip or cheek (Fig. 14.19)
- It is suitable for retracting tissue edges and opening the cheek wide and can also be used as a lip retractor during an oral procedure.

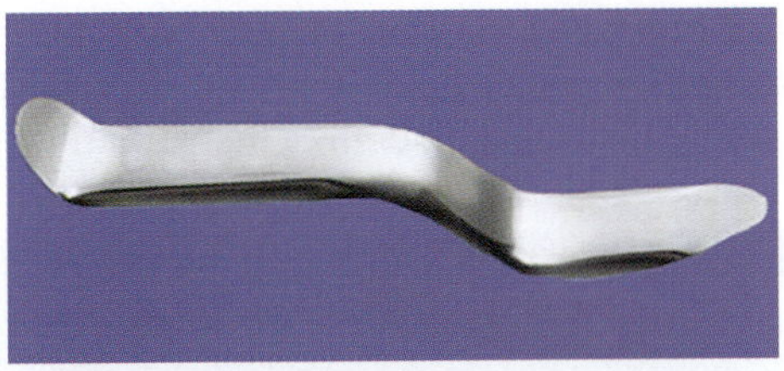

Figure 14.19 Minnesota retractor.

COPPER MALLEABLE RETRACTOR

- Copper malleable retractor is a flattened instrument that can be bent to the desired direction
- It is used in bicoronal flap and craniosynostosis surgeries, to retract the parenchyma while doing craniotomies and also to retract the eyeball during orbital floor reconstruction surgeries (Fig. 14.20).

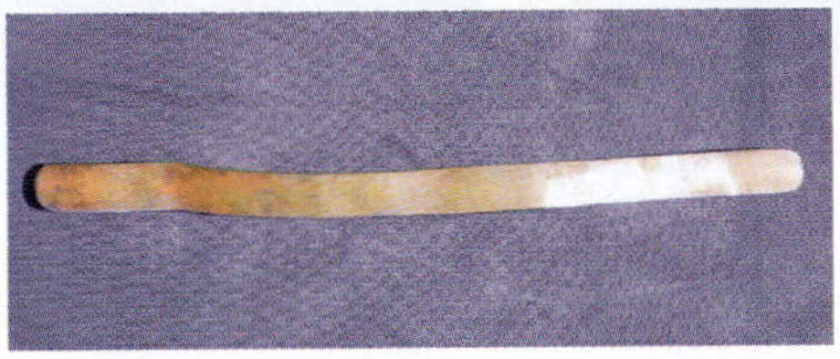

Figure 14.20 Copper malleable retractor.

SKIN HOOK

- Skin hook is a long narrow instrument with a curved tip to engage soft tissues
- It is used for retracting skin following the incision placement (Fig. 14.21).

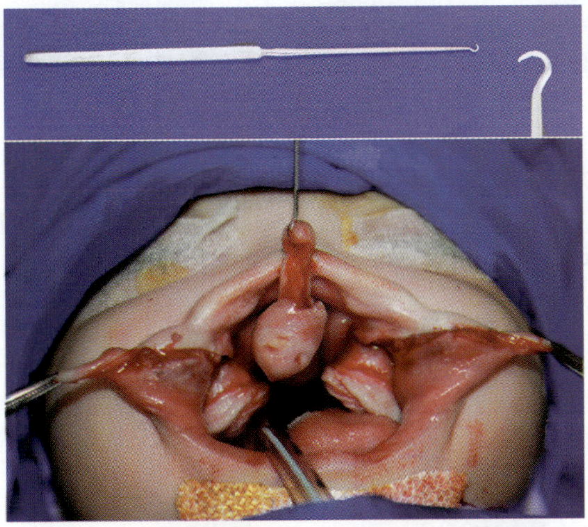

Figure 14.21 Skin hook. Skin hook in use during primary cleft lip repair.

OBWEGESER CHANNEL RETRACTOR

It is an effective lower border retractor useful in sagittal split osteotomy and mandibular body osteotomies. It is used to retract soft tissues and protect vascular structures (Fig. 14.22).

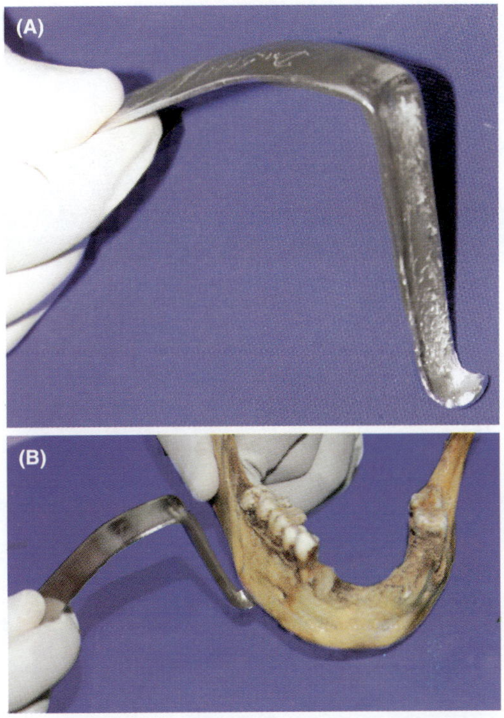

Figure 14.22 (**A & B**) Demonstration of using channel retractor in mandible engaging mandibular lower border.

OBWEGESER CHANNEL RETRACTOR WITH LIGHT SOURCE

Some retractors are designed to be enabled with external light source that facilitate good visual field and illumination, for example, Langenbeck, nasal speculum, etc (Fig. 14.23).

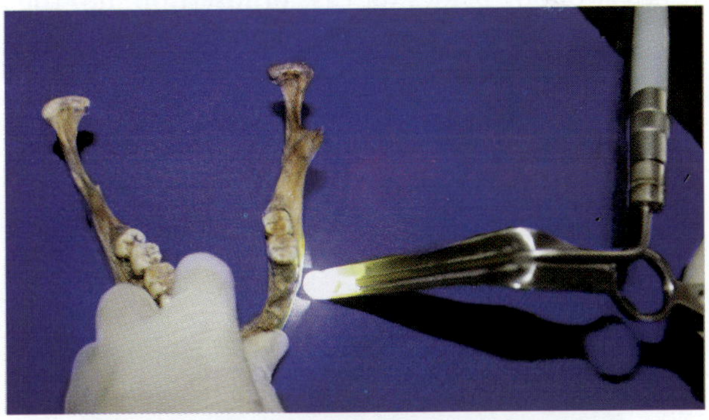

Figure 14.23 Channel retractor with light source.

SIGMOID NOTCH RETRACTOR

- It is a curved mandibular retractor used in vertical subsigmoid (vertical ramus) osteotomy
- Retraction of the masseter muscle during vertical ramus osteotomy (VRO) by inserting a sigmoid notch retractor into the sigmoid notch (Fig. 14.24)
- Another type of sigmoid notch retractor is called Bauer retractor which is used in VRO and bilateral sagittal split osteotomy (BSSO), it is placed to protect the contents of the sigmoid notch.

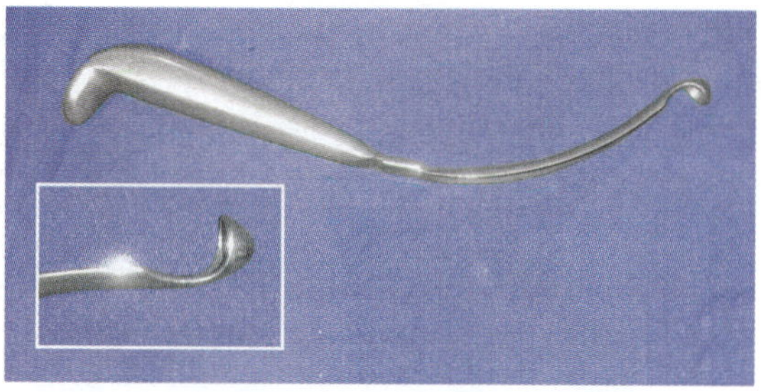

Figure 14.24 Sigmoid notch retractor.

ALAR RETRACTOR

It is used to retract the ala of the nose during rhinoplasty (Fig. 14.25).

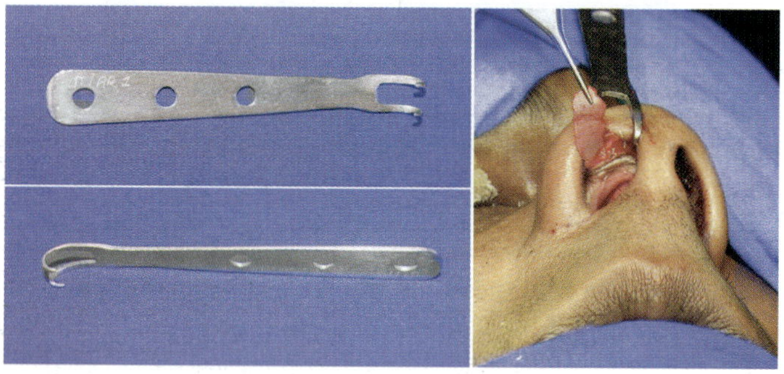

Figure 14.25 Alar retractor.

NASAL SPECULUM

- Nasal speculum is used to widen the nasal cavity and to examine the nasal and internal structures and is widely used in rhinoplasties (Fig. 14.26)
- It has two long blades for ease of insertion into the nostrils which are separated by a spring in between them when the handle is compressed.

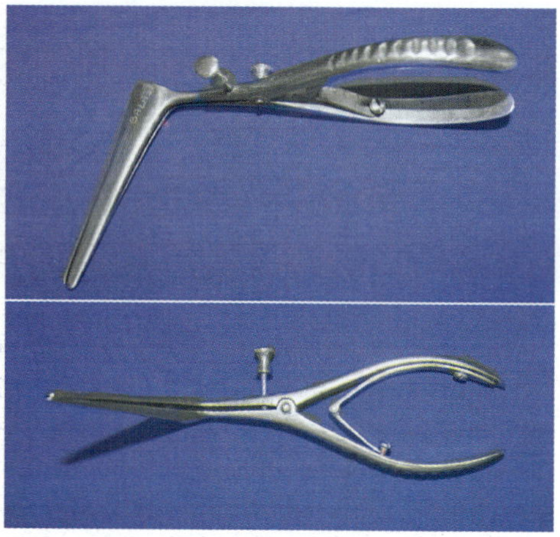

Figure 14.26 Nasal speculum.

TONGUE DEPRESSOR

- It is a retractor used for depressing the tongue for better examination of the oral cavity and in case of surgeries of posterior oral cavity and oropharynx that effectively displace tongue from the field of view of surgery (Fig. 14.27)
- It is a single L-shaped blade-like instrument.

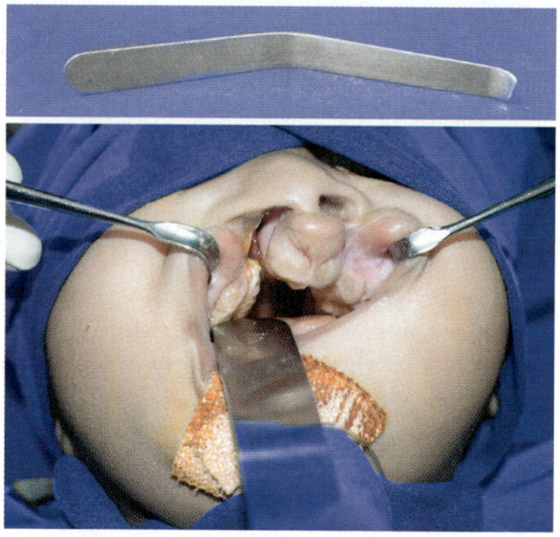

Figure 14.27 Tongue depressor.

MECHANICAL DEVICES

STAPLING DEVICES

These are devices similar to paper stapling machines used for skin approximation instead of sutures (Fig. 14.28).

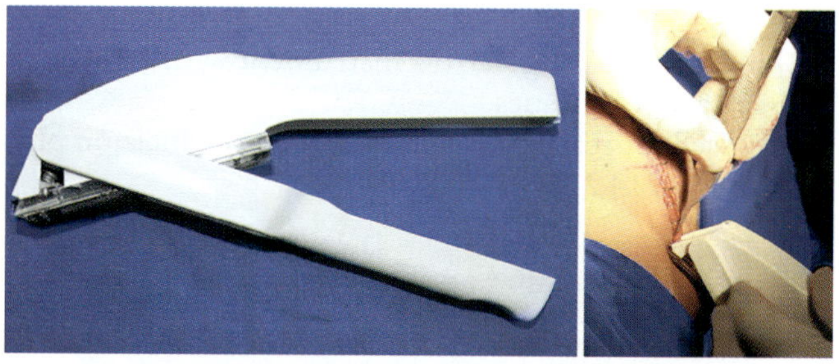

Figure 14.28 Stapling devices.

HAEMOSTATIC CLIPS

These are metal clips that can be applied across blood vessel and ducts to occlude by special forceps (Fig. 14.29).

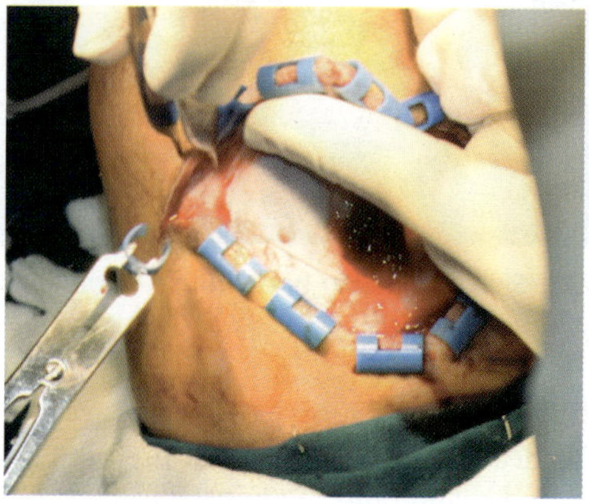

Figure 14.29 Haemostatic clips.

LISTER'S SINUS FORCEPS

- Lister's sinus forceps–long beaks with no ratchet–are used for probing and forcing an entry into an abscess sac (cavity) or for creating an opening into an abscess by Hilton's operation (Fig. 14.30)
- Forceps has gripping surfaces which are long and thin with slightly bulbous points. This helps in draining of the abscess
- This involves entering the sinus with jaw closed and exiting with the forceps opened
- This enlarges the wound, facilitates, drainage as well as avoids damage to the vital structures if any.

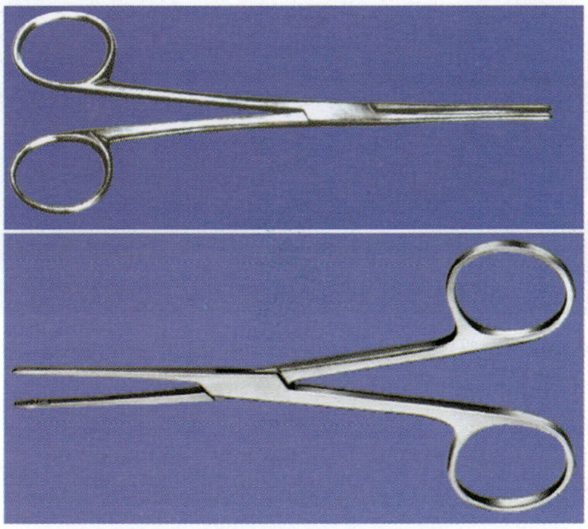

Figure 14.30 Lister's sinus forceps.

HARD TISSUE HANDLING INSTRUMENTS

CHISEL

- Chisel is a mono-bevelled instrument used for the removal of bone
- It has a heavy metal or fibre handle. The bevel has to be sharp for efficient chipping or cutting of bone (Fig. 14.31)

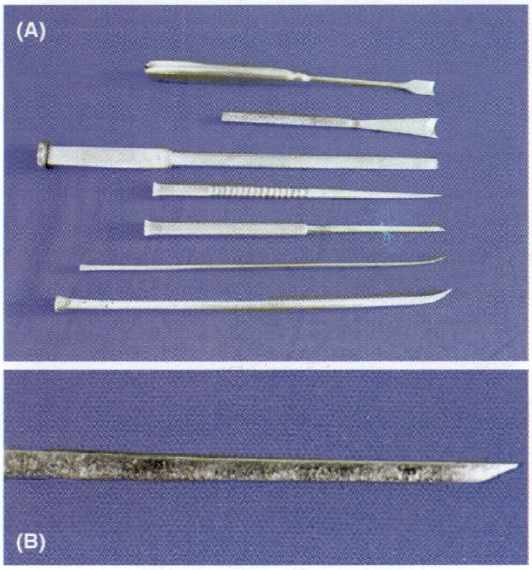

Figure 14.31 Chisel.

- For cutting or removal of the bone, the bevel is placed facing away from the bone or the bevel towards the bone to be removed

  Advantage: Clear cut is created with no bone dust

  Disadvantages:
  - Risk of uncontrolled force delivery that can be dangerous
  - Uncomfortable to use in awake patient (under LA).

PTERYGOID CHISEL

- This is an angled chisel available in sizes of 8, 10 and 12 mm
- The handle is usually long and made of heavy metal or fibre (Fig. 14.32)
- It is specifically indicated for pterygomaxillary dysjunction in Le Fort osteotomies of maxilla.

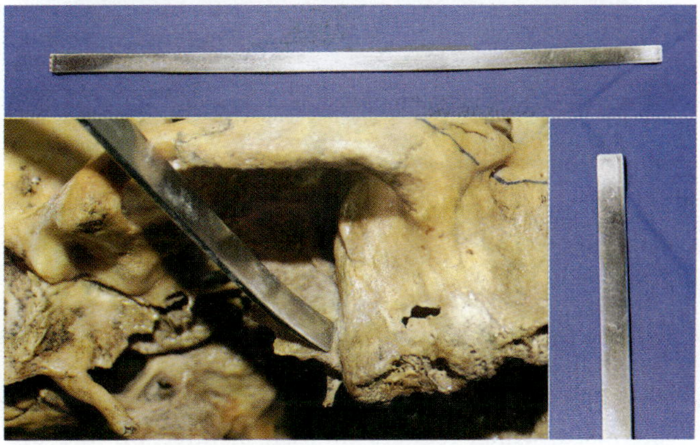

Figure 14.32 Pterygoid chisel.

PERIOSTEAL ELEVATOR

This instrument is used to expose the bone elevating the periosteum off the bone as a mucoperiosteal flap (intraorally) or separately (e.g., harvesting a rib graft) (Fig. 14.33).

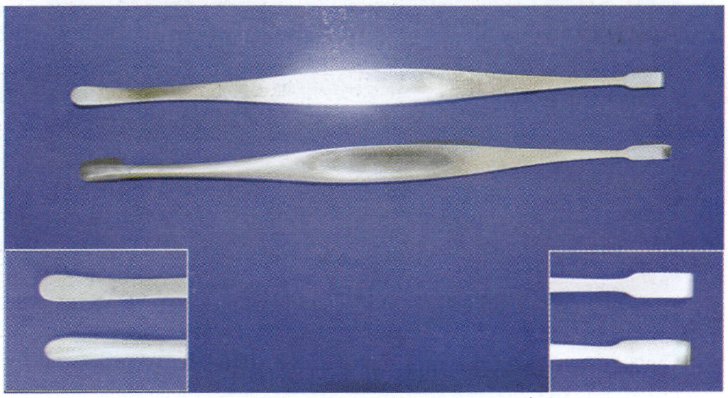

Figure 14.33 Howarth periosteal elevator.

GIGLI SAW

- A Gigli saw is a flexible wire with handled handles used in the cutting of bone manually
- It is generally used in segmental resection of the mandible and in craniotomies (Fig. 14.34)
- The bone cuts were smoother and predictable than the use of chisel and mallet.

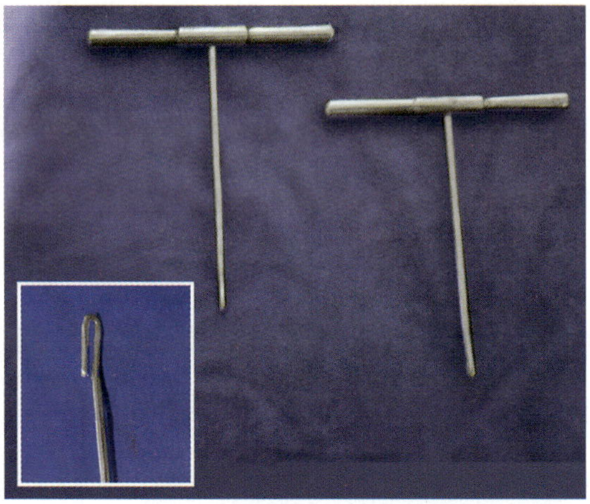

Figure 14.34 Gigli saw.

MALLET

- The mallet is made up of wood, rubber, nylon or stainless steel
- Stainless steel mallets are preferred because they can be sterilised, which reduces the risk of infection and prolongs its use (Fig. 14.35)
- The mallet is designed to weigh 8 oz for delivering controlled force on the chisel and the osteotome, for example, Gardner mallet.

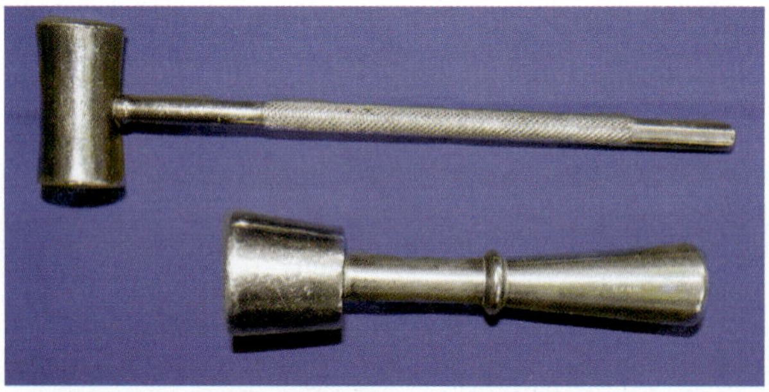

Figure 14.35 Mallet.

OSTEOTOME

- Osteotome is similar to chisel, but it is bibevelled (Fig. 14.36)
- Used for splitting of the bone as well as tooth (odontectomy).

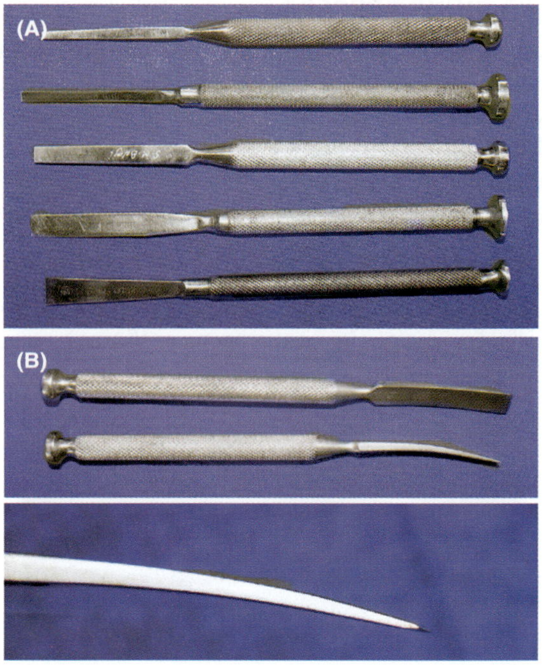

Figure 14.36 (**A**) Straight osteotomes of varying sizes. (**B**) Curved osteotomes-curved bibevelled instrument.

BONE FILE

- Used for smoothening of bone after extraction or during alveoloplasty (Fig. 14.37).

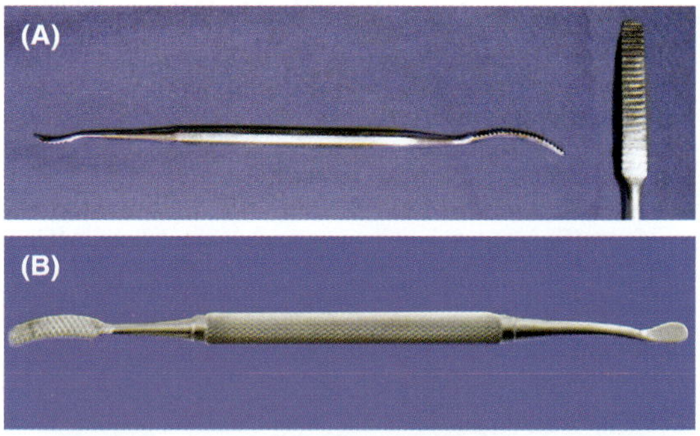

Figure 14.37 (**A** & **B**) Miller and Colburn bone file.

BONE GOUGE

- It is use to cut cortical bone tissue or to scoop the soft, cancellous bone collected for bone graftings.
- It is used in alveoloplasty (Fig. 14.38).

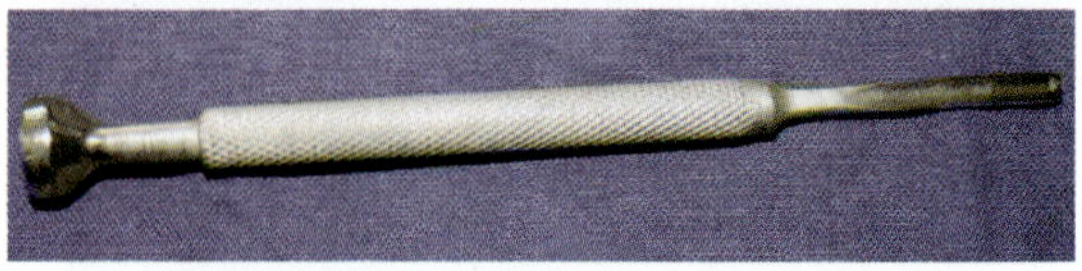

Figure 14.38 Bone gouge.

SURGICAL CURETTES

- To remove debris from the extraction site, for example, periapical granuloma
- To remove granulation tissues from the periapical lesions in apicoectomy
- To remove equestrum which develops in nonhealing sockets (Fig. 14.39)
- To debride small periapical cyst and other cysts.

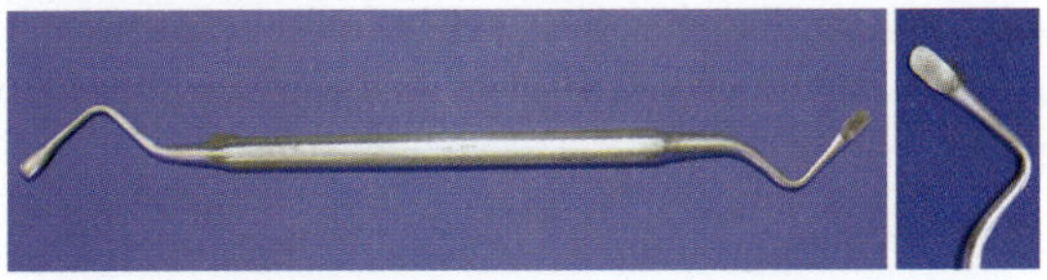

Figure 14.39 Surgical curettes.

BONE RONGEUR

- To remove sharp bony projections during alveoloplasty and after extraction
- To trim harvested bone graft (Fig. 14.40).

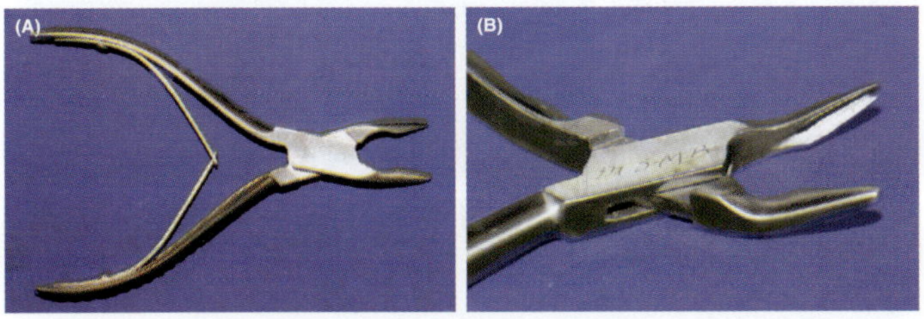

Figure 14.40 Bone rongeur.

BONE SCOOP

- Bone scoop has a working end similar to that of curette (e.g. Volkmann scoop) (Fig. 14.41)
- It is primarily used for debriding contents from an intraosseous abscess cavity or cyst
- Since it has sharper margins, it can also be used to scoop out periphery of the cavity bone
- It is also used to harvest cancellous bone during bone grafting, for example, iliac.

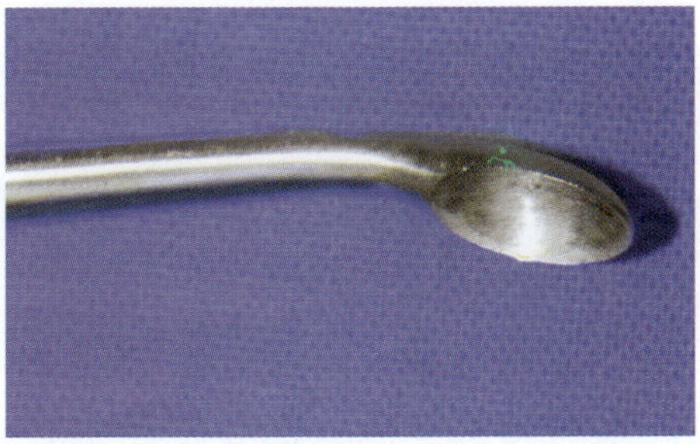

Figure 14.41 Bone scoop—working end.

BONE GRASPING FORCEPS

It is used to remove sharp edges of the alveolar crest of the bone following tooth extraction (Fig. 14.42).

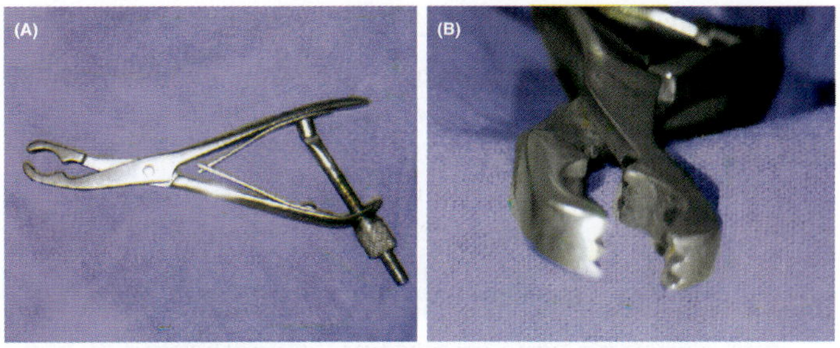

Figure 14.42 (**A** & **B**) Bone grasping forceps.

SMITH BONE SPREADER

- Spreader is an instrument with three blades (Fig. 14.43)
- It is activated by a spring mechanism
- Mainly used to separate the osteotomised fragments as in case of sagittal split osteotomy (e.g. Smith spreader).

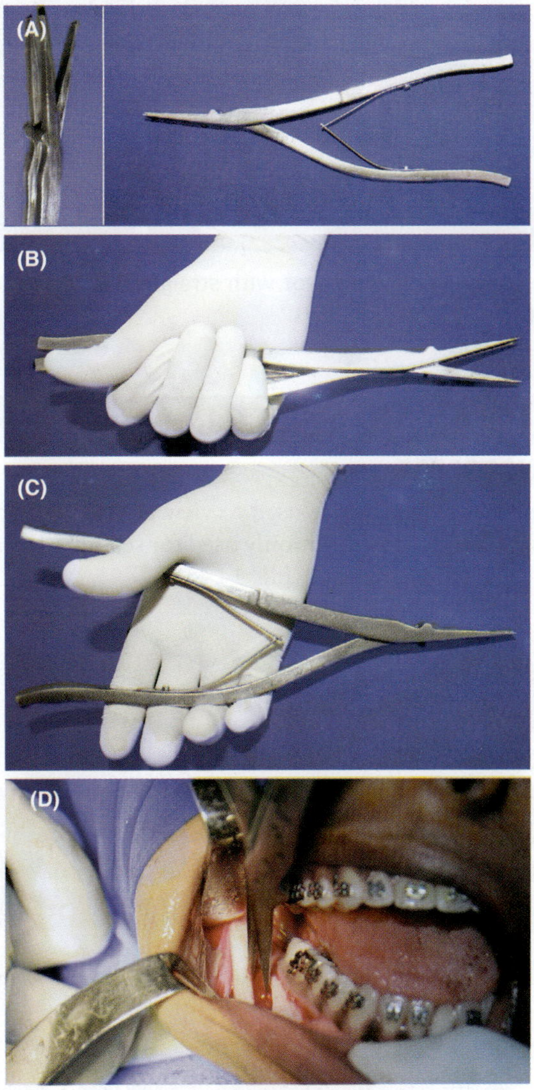

Figure 14.43 (**A**) Smith spreader—three blades. (**B**) Smith spreader in open position. (**C**) Smith spreader in closed position. (**D**) Smith spreader used to separate osteotomised segments in BSSO—position between the segments to be osteotomised.

ROTARY AND POWER DRILL INSTRUMENT

- Handpiece and burs are rotary instruments that remove bone most efficiently and quickly (Fig. 14.44A)
- The burs are available in various sizes and shapes and made up of carbide or stainless steel
- The bur is attached to the head of the handpiece, which has a cartridge driven by air pressure
- This drilling instrument is used for making osteotomy cuts, removing bone (osteotomy), smoothening of bone (osteoplasty), splitting of teeth (odontectomy) or drilling a hole in the bone for wiring or plate fixation.

BURS

These are stainless steel or tungsten carbide rotary cutting instruments used extensively in hard tissue surgeries as osteotomy, fracture fixation, etc (Fig. 14.44B).

MICROSAWS

- The microsaws are instruments used to cut bone (Fig. 14.44C)
- Due to their high speed and thin blade design they help in quick cutting of bone with minimal bone loss.
- Useful in maxillary and mandibular osteotomies.
- The main three types are oscillating, reciprocating and sagittal.

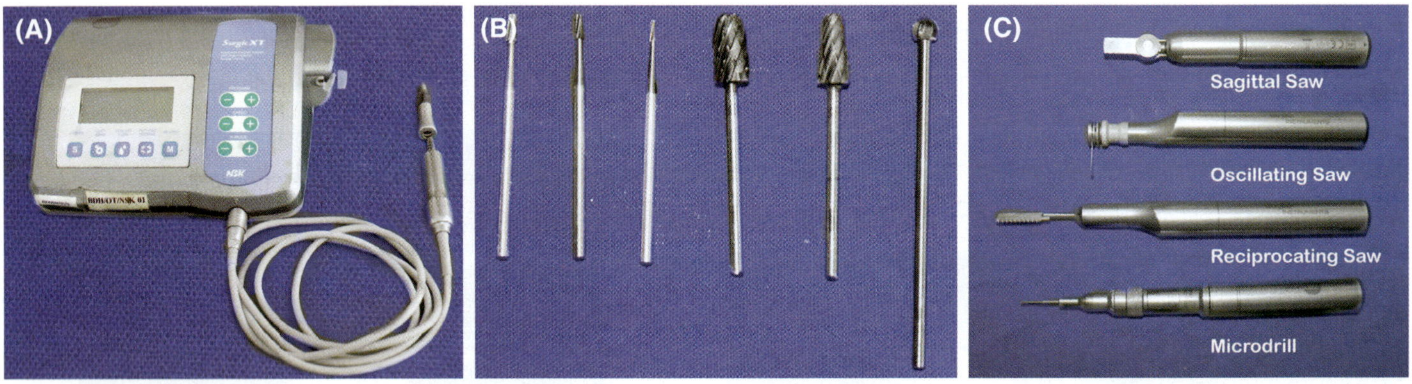

Figure 14.44 (**A**) Micromotor with straight handpiece. (**B**) Rotary power drill instruments—stainless steel and tungsten carbide burs. (**C**) Microdrill and saws.

AIRWAY MAINTENANCE/ANAESTHESIA

LARYNGOSCOPE

A laryngoscope is a device used to view the larynx and adjacent structures, most commonly used for securing the airway with a tube (endotracheal) (Fig. 14.45).

PARTS

- Detachable blade
- Handle unit with light source

FLEXIBLE FIBREOPTIC ENDOSCOPE

The fibreoptic endoscope is a flexible endoscope composed of the following parts (Fig. 14.46):

I. **Light source**
   - High intensity xenon light source is provided with a fibreoptic cable (light cord) connected to handle
   - Alternative light source–halogen light source or handle with batteries

II. **Handle**
   - Handle or body is the part held in the hand

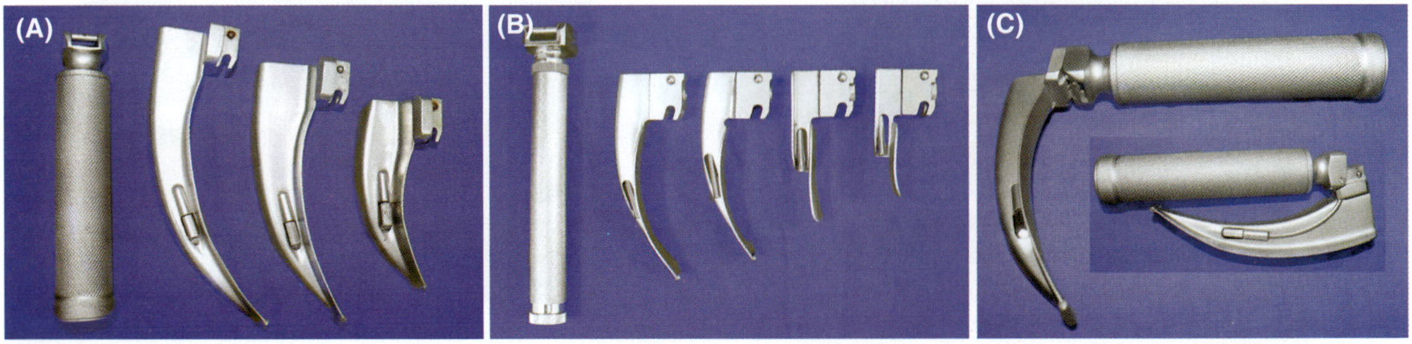

Figure 14.45 (**A**) Rigid laryngoscope—handle with curved blades of three different sizes for adults. (**B**) Paediatric rigid laryngoscope with short blades and long handle. (**C**) Laryngoscope in inactivated position and in working position—blade attached to the handle.

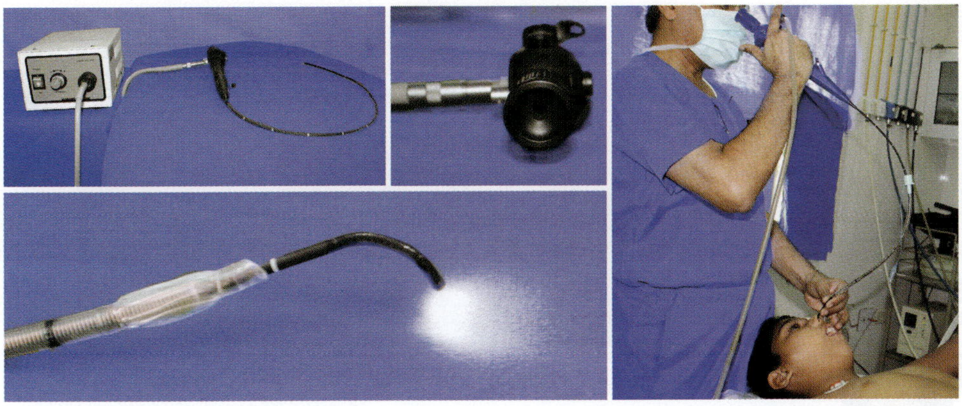

Figure 14.46 (A) Fibreoptic endoscope with the light source connected—external xenon light source. (B) Eyepiece and focusing ring. (C) Fibreoptic cable from the xenon light source illuminating the endoscope tip. (D). Under fibreoptic guidance nasotracheal intubation.

- Handle includes:
  - Eyepiece
  - Focusing ring
  - Working channel port
  - Tip control knob or lever (bending or angulations controls).

III. **Insertion portion or tube:** The portion of endoscope over which the tracheal tube is passed during intubation. It contains an image transmitting bundle and light conducting bundles

IV. **Accessories:** Suction.

TRACHEOSTOMY TUBE

- It is used to provide a patent airway, and access to the lower respiratory tract for airway clearance.
- Mostly used in case of emergency airway management
- It is sometimes used electively, for example, postlaryngectomy (Fig. 14.47).

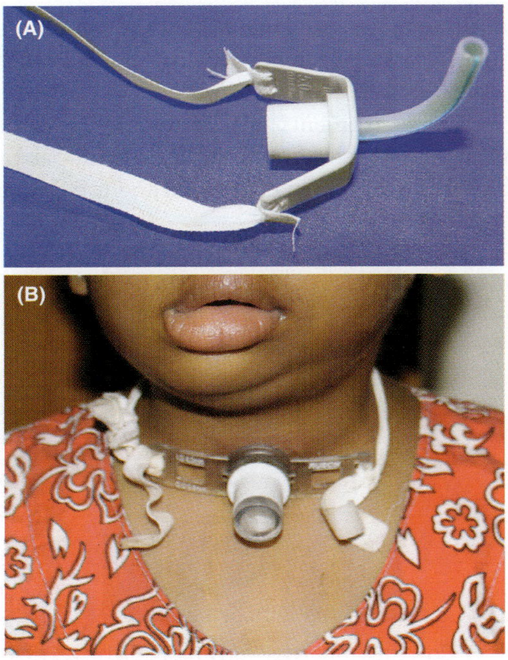

Figure 14.47 Tracheostomy tube.

FACE MASK

Face mask or piece allows administration of gases from external breathing system. It consists of mask body, face seal and a connector (Fig. 14.48).

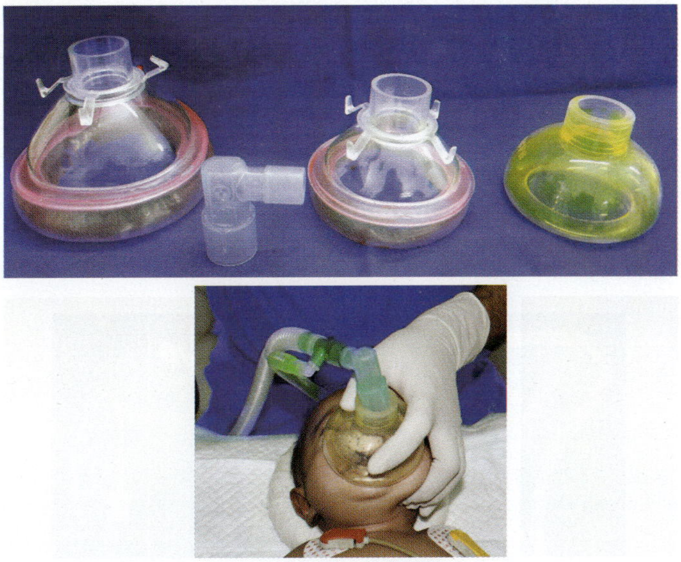

Figure 14.48 Face mask.

ORAL/NASAL PHARYNGEAL AIRWAY

OROPHARYNGEAL AIRWAY

- It is a rubber or plastic device that extends from the lip to the pharynx with the bite portion between the teeth and the flanges outside the lips (Fig. 14.49)
- It helps to maintain an open airway, prevent patient biting and occluding the tracheal tube, protect tongue from biting and facilitate suctioning, for example, Guedel airway.

NASOPHARYNGEAL AIRWAY

- A nasopharyngeal airway is also called nasal airway or nasal trumpet
- It resembles a shortened tracheal tube with flanged end made of rubber or plastic

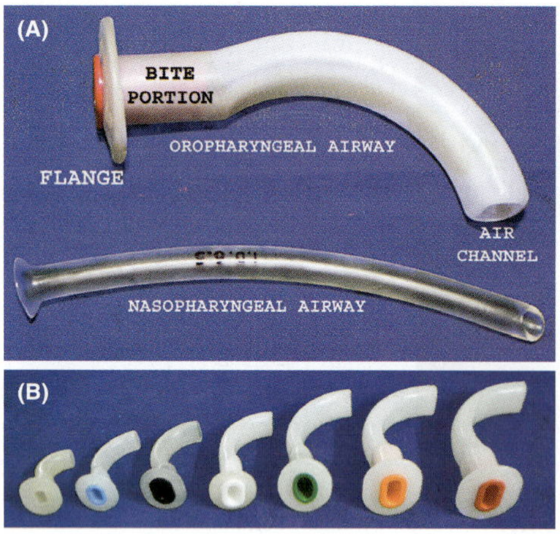

Figure 14.49 Oral/nasal pharyngeal airway.

- It is used as an alternative to oral airway, for example, Bardex nasopharyngeal airway.

ENDOTRACHEAL TUBE

- Endotracheal tube is a flexible tube which is placed in the trachea through mouth and nose (Fig. 14.50).
- This tube is inserted into the trachea and used to conduct gases and vapours to and from the lungs.
- The tube is usually connected to a a ventilator, which pushes oxygenated air into the lungs.

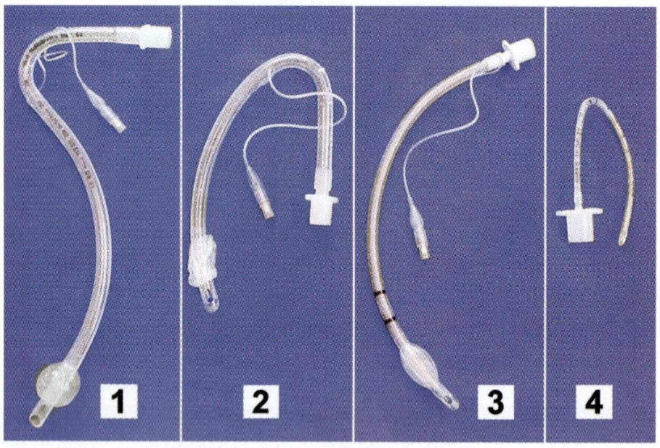

Figure 14.50 Endotracheal tube. PVC endotracheal tubes: (1) Inflated cuffed Ring–Adair–Elwyn (RAE) nasal tube. (2) Noninflated cuffed RAE oral tube. (3) Inflated cuffed flexometallic tube. (4) Uncuffed paediatric oral tube.

LARYNGEAL MASK AIRWAY

- Laryngeal mask is an alternative to both face mask and tracheal tube (Fig. 14.51)
- It is used to secure the airway by a low-pressure seal around laryngeal inlet; using inflatable cuff.
- It is also called brain mask, laryngeal mask airway or brain mask airway (BMA).

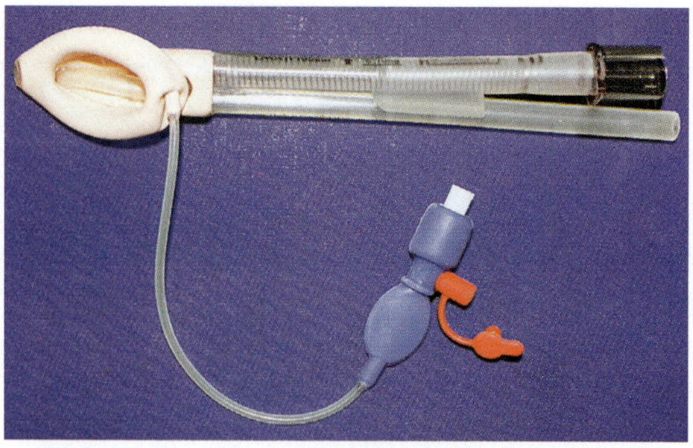

Figure 14.51 Laryngeal mask airway.

SPECIAL INSTRUMENTS IN FRACTURE MANAGEMENT

HAYTON WILLIAM FORCEPS

- It is used to hold both maxillae (R&L) as single segment before initiating disimpaction with Rowe forceps (Fig. 14.52).

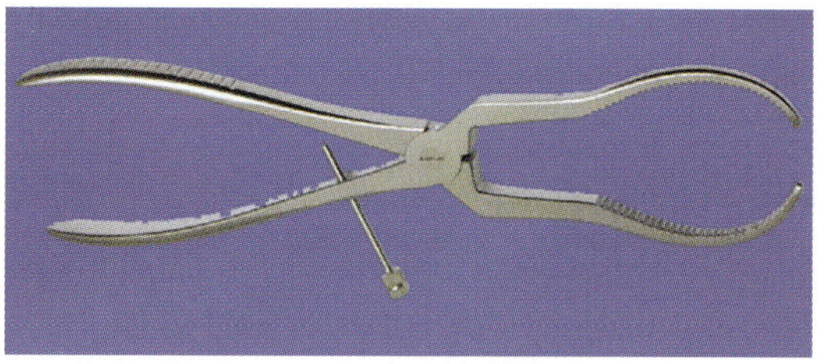

Figure 14.52 Hayton William forceps.

ROWE DISIMPACTION FORCEPS

- This instrument is used in pairs for the reduction of maxilla in Le Fort fractures where the maxilla is impacted (Fig. 14.53)
- The paired instruments are always used together along with Hayton-William forceps in case of mid-palatal split to disimpact the maxilla in downward and forward direction.

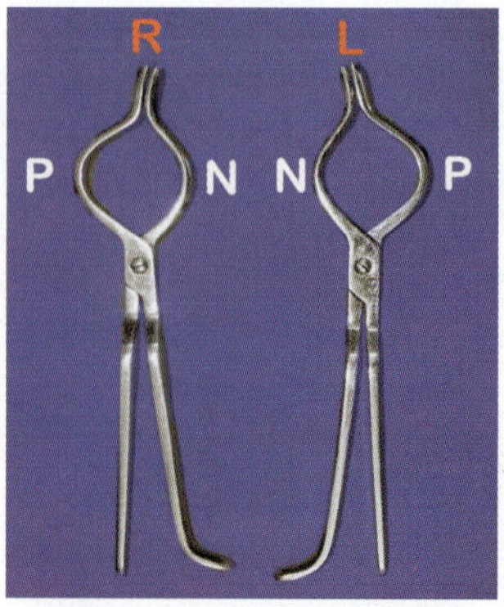

Figure 14.53 Rowe disimpaction forceps. R, Right; L, Left; P, Palatal; N, Nasal.

- It has two blades—straight and curved. The straight one is padded and used to pass through the nostrils.The curved one is unpadded and is used to pass into the oral cavity to grip the palate.

ROWE ZYGOMATIC ELEVATORS

- It is used to reduce the fractured zygoma through the Gillies temporal approach (Fig. 14.54)
- They work by 3rd order of lever principle with fulcrum at one end.

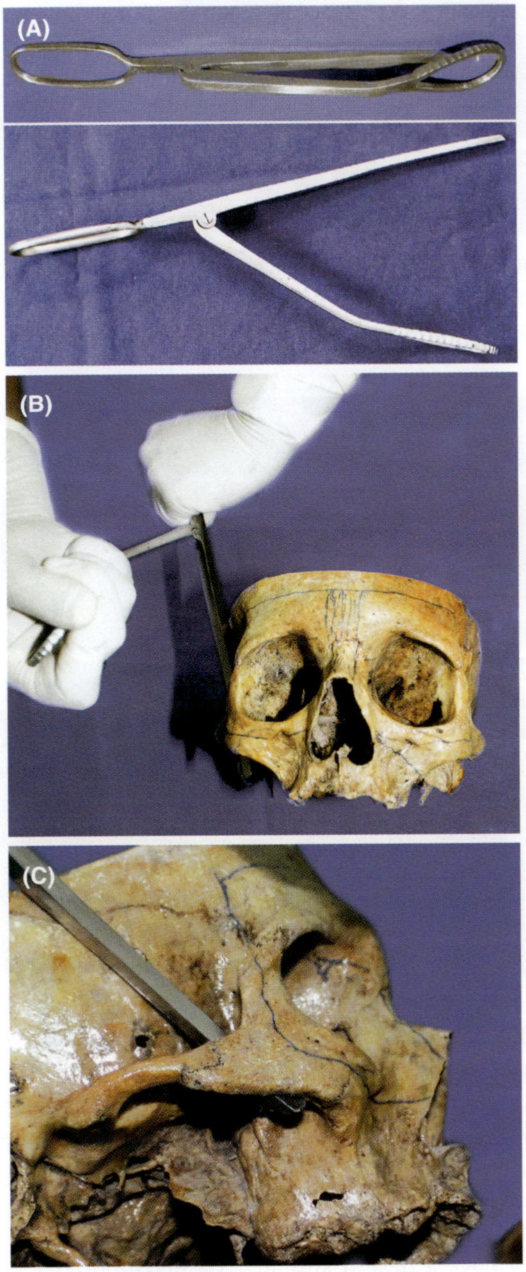

Figure 14.54 (**A**) Rowe zygoma elevator. (**B**) Rowe zygoma elevator to reduce fractured zygoma. Demonstration in a dry skull model. (**C**) Position of the working end of Rowe zygomatic elevator, posterior to the buttress.

WALSHAM FORCEPS

- This paired forceps is used for the reduction of nasal fractures (Fig. 14.55)
- It has two curved blades—one is padded and the other unpadded. The padded blade is inserted internally into the nostril and the unpadded blade is placed externally over the nasal bone and manipulated for the reduction of the nasal fracture.

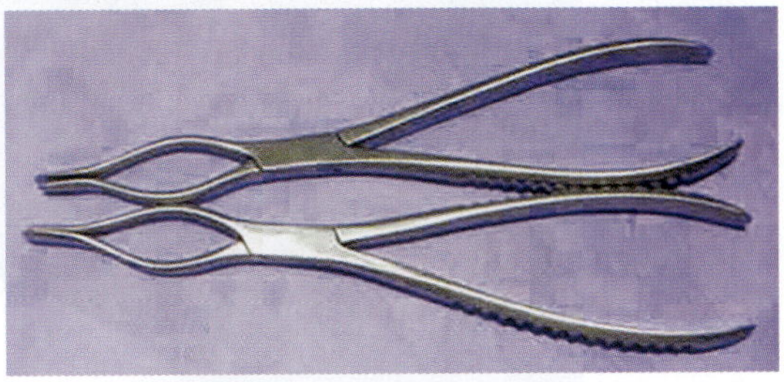

Figure 14.55 Walsham forceps.

ASCH FORCEPS

- These forceps are used for the reduction of nasal fractures and also to align the nasal septum (Fig. 14.56)
- When reducing the nasal septum, both the blades are inserted internally one on each side of the septum
- In case of nasal bone fracture reduction, one blade is inserted internally and the other is placed externally to hold the nasal bone laterally and medially, respectively.

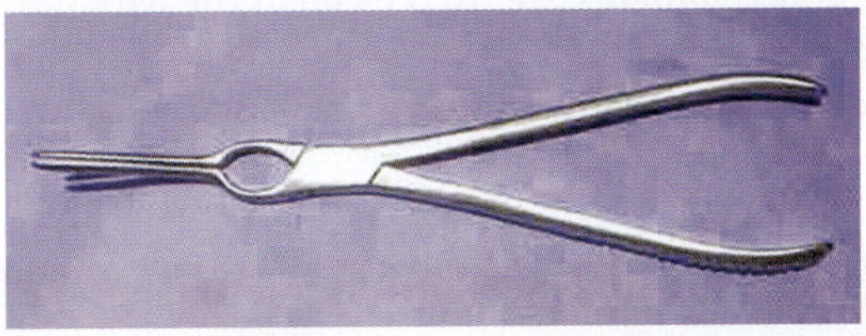

Figure 14.56 Asch forceps.

AWL

Awls are long slender instruments provided with an eyelet at the tip through which the wire or suture material is passed (Fig. 14.57).

LONG (OBWEGESER ZYGOMATIC ARCH AWL)

Used in

- Circumzygomatic suspension of Le Fort II fracture of maxilla
- Adam wire suspension for Le Fort III
- Circumzygomatic static suspension for facial palsy.

SHORT (KELSEY FRY BONE AWL)

Used in

- Per alveolar wiring by boring action on the alveolar ridge in circummandibular wire for cap splint or gunning splint placement

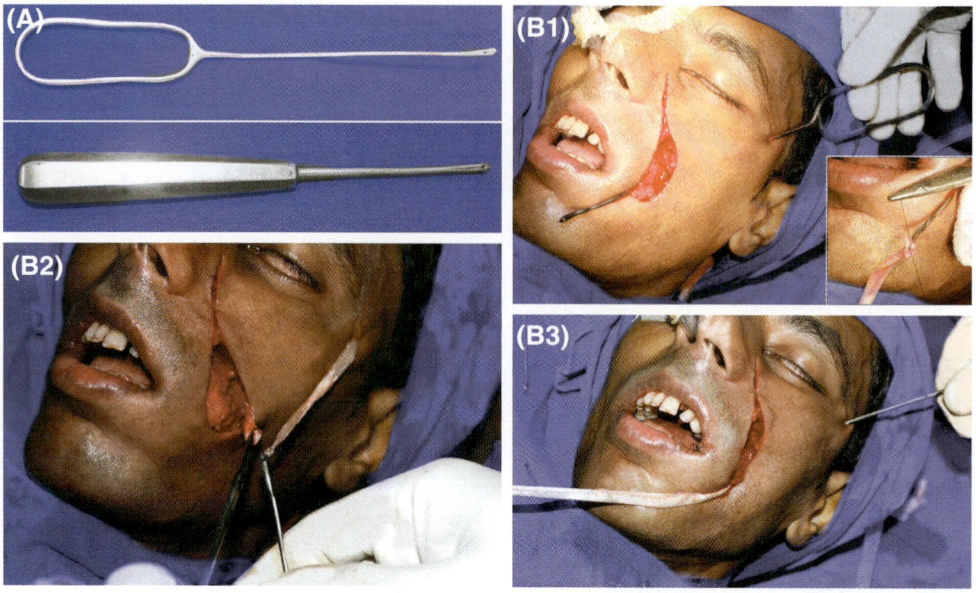

Figure 14.57 (**A**) Awl—long (Obwegeser) and short rigid. (**B**) Awl for circumzygomatic static suspension in facial palsy using tensor fascia lata. (**B1**) Awl introduced medial to the arch. Insert showing securing of harvested fascia lata to the eyelet of the awl. (**B2**) Fascia lata guided medial to the zygomatic arch using the awl. (**B3**) Checking for the length of the fascia lata before guiding it lateral to the zygomatic arch using the awl.

- Kelsey Fry bone awl is available as a straight type or in a curved pattern which is used in Obwegeser's method of circummandibular wiring.

WIRE PUSHERS

- These instruments are used to push the wire into the interdental space during intermaxillary fixation (Fig. 14.58)
- They are also useful in adapting the wires tightly around the teeth.

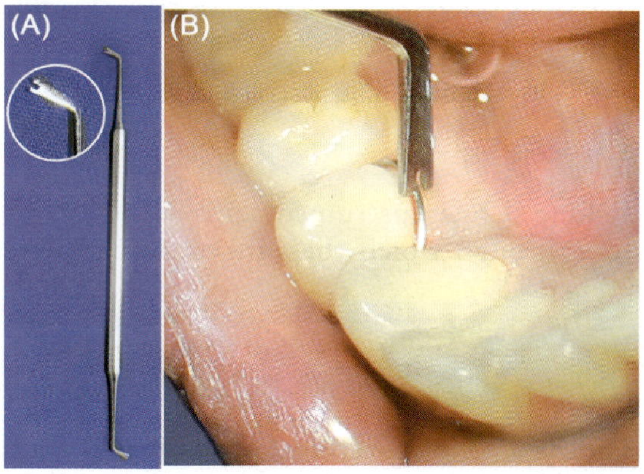

Figure 14.58 (**A**) Wire pusher. (**B**) Wire pusher being used for adapting the interdental wire.

WIRES, WIRE TWISTERS AND WIRE CUTTERS

- Thin stainless steel wires (26 gauge) are used in oral surgery for the fixation of fractures, osteotomy cuts and the intermaxillary fixation. These wires are available in different lengths and sizes (Fig. 14.59)

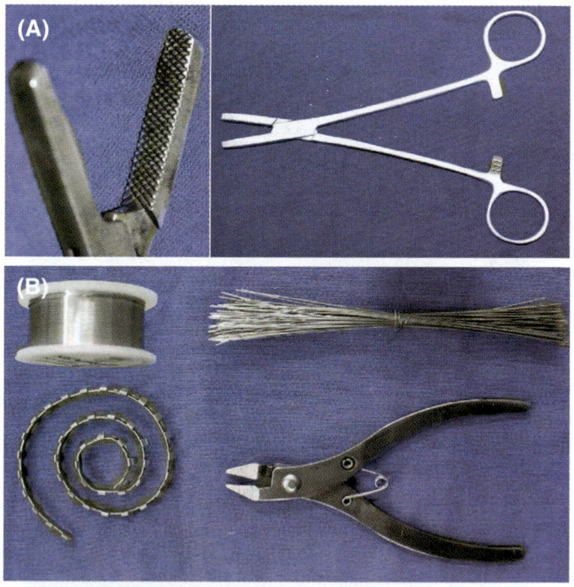

Figure 14.59 (**A**) Wire twister, note the short broad blades with crisscross grooves to prevent wire slippage. (**B**) Stainless steel wire, Erich arch bar and wire cutter.

- The 26-gauge wires are most commonly used for maxillofacial trauma
- A wire twister is an instrument used to hold the wire as well as for twisting it
- They have a design similar to a needle holder but with shorter broader blades and cross wire grooves that avoid wire slippage
- Wire cutters are used to cut off the excess wires after securing the wiring in place.

PLATES—TITANIUM AND STAINLESS STEEL

Bone plates and screws used to surgically fix the bone fractures, osteotomies, maxillary and mandibular reconstruction with on lay grafts. It is made up of titanium or stainless steel (Fig. 14.60).

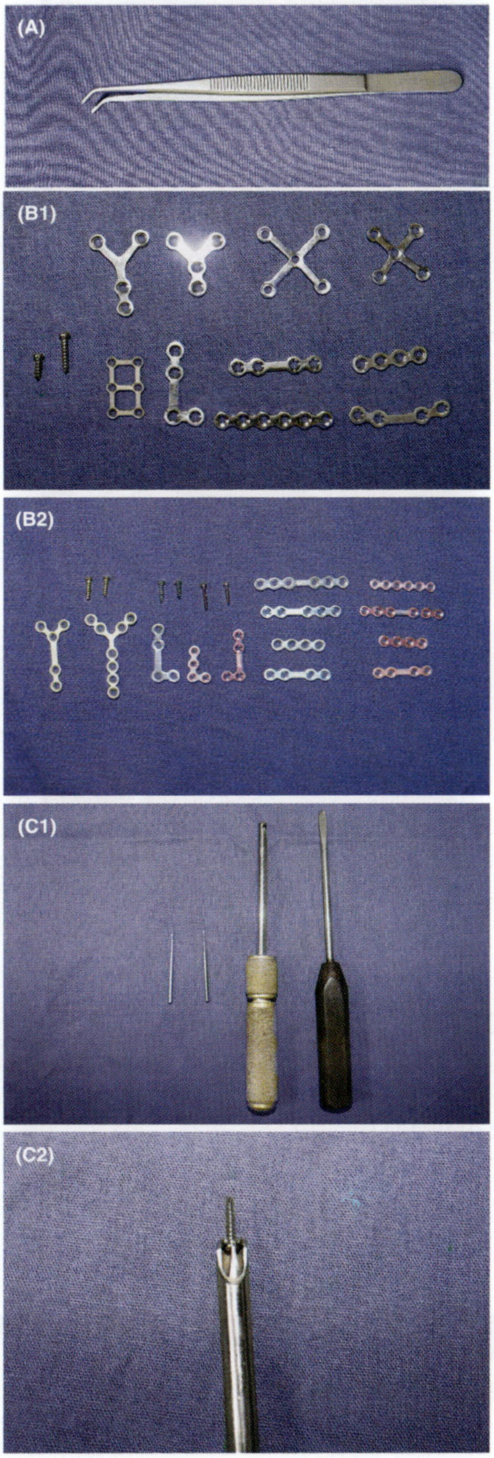

Figure 14.60 (**A**) Plate holder. (**B**) Plates—titanium and stainless steel. (**C**) Screw carrier and driver with 703 and 701 burs.

MISCELLANEOUS INSTRUMENTS

MOUTH GAG

- **Ferguson mouth gag**: This is a ratchet type gag with a long handle and box joint (Fig. 14.61A). It is used to improve mouth opening in patients with acute onset trismus, e.g. post surgery and infections.
- **Heister mouth gag**: It is a T-shaped mouth gag with 2 blades separated by an adjustable knob at the joint similar to Ferguson mouth gag (Fig. 14.61B&C).

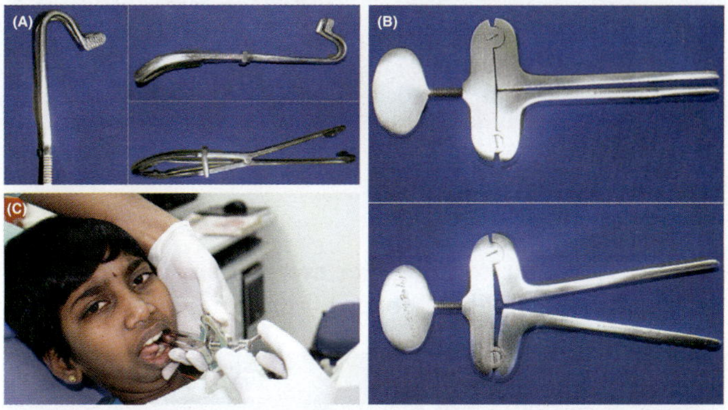

Figure 14.61 (**A**) Ferguson mouth gag—ratchet type gag with long handles and box joint. (**B**) Heister mouth gag—T-shaped gag with adjustable knob. (**C**) Heister jaw opener in clinical use—postgap arthroplasty physiotherapy.

DINGMAN

- It has two clamps on either side for adjusting the opposite pair of alveolar retractors. These alveolar retractors coact with the tongue retractors to retain the jaws in desired open position (Fig. 14.62)
- The alveolar retractors can be adjusted both for axial rotation and longitudinal sliding
- In addition, it has two self-retractory cheek retractors on either side to retract the cheek.

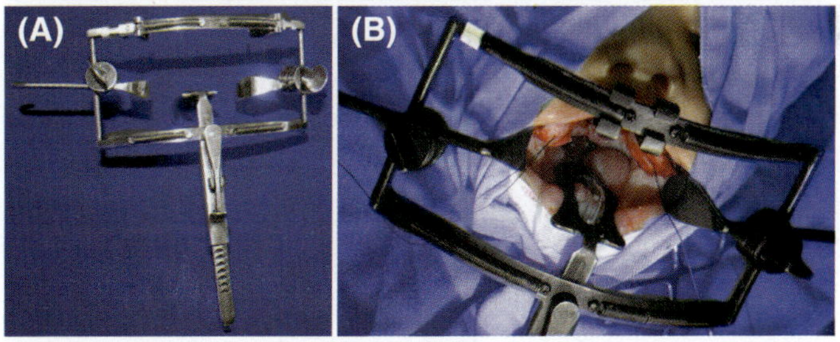

Figure 14.62 (**A**) Dingman mouth gag. (**B**) Dingman mouth gag for cleft surgery.

MOUTH PROP

- It is a device for maintaining the maxilla and mandible apart during the surgical procedure.

- It consists of a vertical rubber block having a concave surface on either of its ends to fit the maxillary and mandibular teeth (Fig. 14.63).
- Blocks of different sizes are available attached to a chain and the operator can choose the required amount of mouth opening.

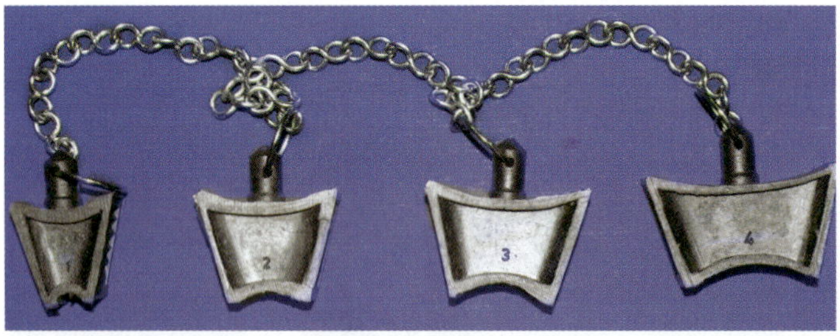

Figure 14.63 Mouth prop.

DOTT–KILNER

- This is similar to Dingman except that it lacks cheek retractors and has a C-shaped frame (Fig. 14.64).

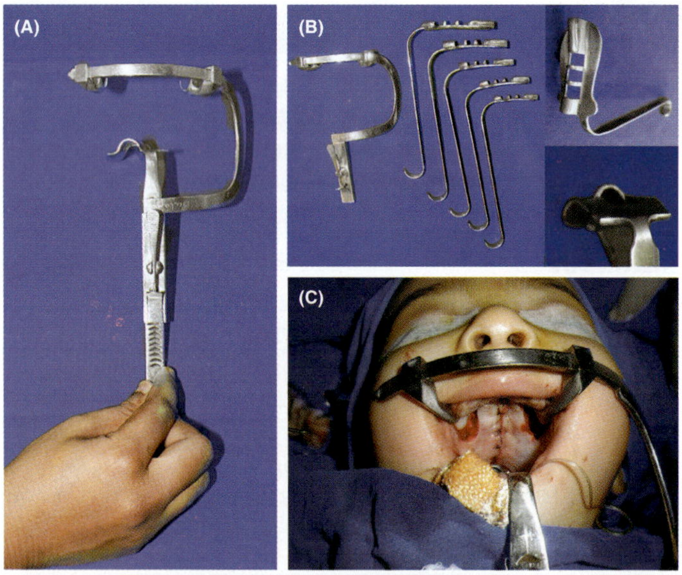

Figure 14.64 **(A)** Dott–Kilner mouth gag. **(B)** Dott–Kilner mouth gag C-shaped frame and tongue blades of different sizes. Note the tongue blade is designed to accommodate the oroendotracheal tube. **(C)** Dott–Kilner retractor used as mouth gag for cleft palate repair.

TROCAR AND CANNULA

- A trocar is a sharp cylinder pointed instrument with a sleeve or a cannula (Fig. 14.65)
- It is used to gain entry into the surgical site through a stab incision on the skin to avoid an incision, wide opening or scar
- In oral surgery, it is used for transbuccal approach to the ramus of the mandible.

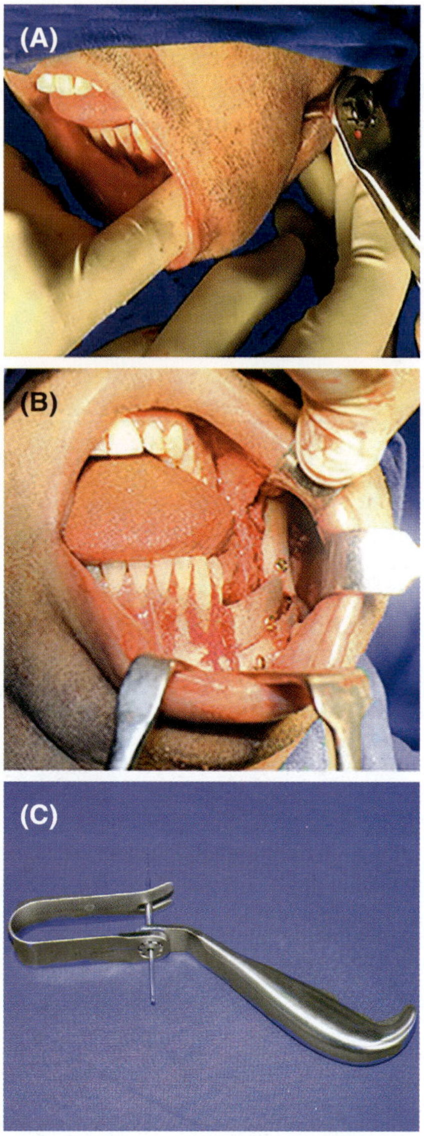

Figure 14.65 Trocar and cannula.

FOLEY CATHETER

- Foley catheter is a self-retaining disposable tube placed through the urethra into the bladder for continuous urine drainage (Fig. 14.66)
- A self-retaining catheter is one which can remain in the bladder and is held in by a balloon, which prevents it from displacement.

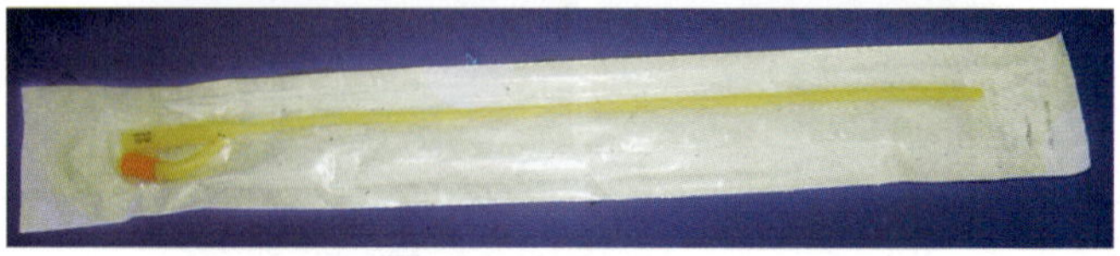

Figure 14.66 Foley catheter.

SUCTION APPARATUS

Components:

- Hose
- Handle
- Tip

Hose: The hose is used to connect the handle to the suction apparatus (Fig. 14.67)

Handle: The handle has a bulbous portion on one end and a chuck on the other end. The bulbous portion is slipped into one end of the hose and the chuck holds the tip

Tip:

- The tips are introduced into the surgical field to remove away blood, secretions, cystic fluid, etc. and create a clear visual field for surgery
- The tips may be straight or angulated. Sometimes styles are provided along with the tips to remove any debris if it gets lodged in the lumen.

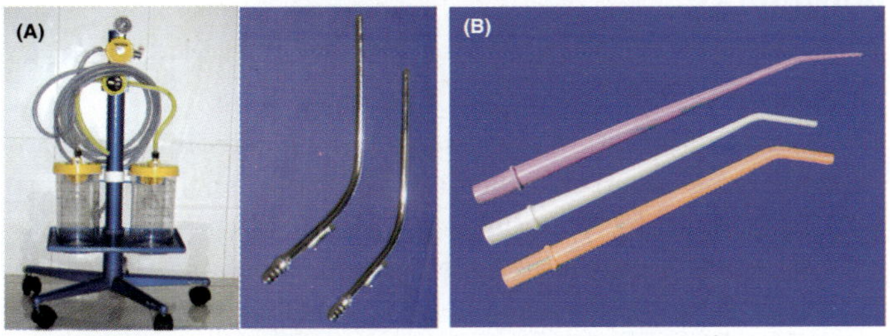

Figure 14.67 **(A)** Suction apparatus and suction tip. **(B)** Disposable suction tips.

OPERATING MICROSCOPE

- The microscope offers multiple flexibilities, magnification optics and comfort (Fig. 14.68)
- Surgical operating microscopes are used mainly during microsurgeries
- A compact optical unit delivers clear and sharply focused images. The magnification typically ranges from 4X to 40X

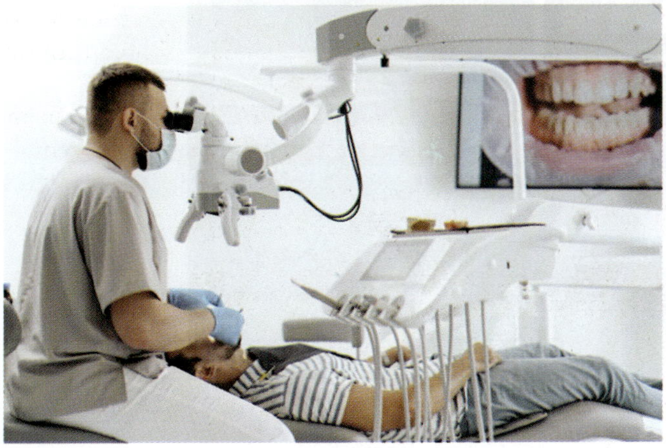

Figure 14.68 Operating microscope.

- It is used in microvascular surgery for reconstruction of the maxilla or mandible with free fibula graft
- Operating microscope is also used for direct neurorrhaphy of severed nerves.

RYLES TUBE

- Ryles tube is a specially designed tube made up of red rubber or nontoxic, nonirritant polyvinyl chloride (PVC) for nasogastric introduction of nutrition and aspiration of intestinal secretion.
- It measures about 105 cm (Fig. 14.69A).
- It may have three lead shots in the tip, which appears radiopaque in radiographic examination and assists the passage of tubing during intubation.
- Super smooth low friction surface facilitates easy intubation is provided with an X-ray opaque strip throughout the length.

USES

- For the purpose of feeding debilitated patients for long-term gastrointestinal feeding in patients who cannot take oral feed, for aspiration of intestinal secretions and for gastric lavage in case of poisoning (Fig. 14.69A).

INFANT FEEDING TUBE

Infant feeding tubes often incorporates a 1 cm depth markings used in infants with faciomaxillary injuries and anorexia (Fig. 14.69B).

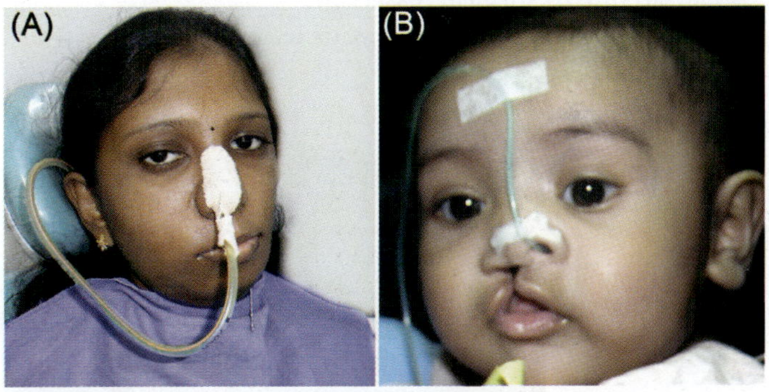

Figure 14.69 **(A)** Ryles tube in a patient on maxillomandibular fixation (MMF). **(B)** Ryles tube—infant feeding.

SURGICAL LOUPES

- Surgical loupes are optical magnification system used widely in surgical procedures requiring fineness (Fig. 14.70).
- These loupes may be simple, compound or prism type.
- Most maxillofacial, dental and periodontal procedures can be done with more preciseness.
- With either compound or prism loupes of ×4 to ×5 magnification.

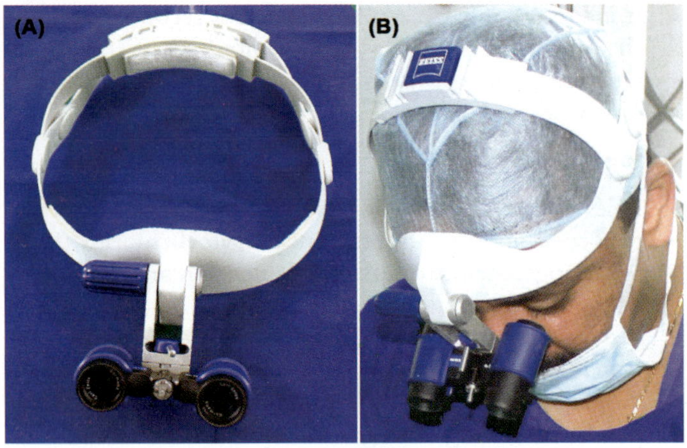

Figure 14.70 (**A** & **B**) Surgical loupes.

DIATHERMY

Surgical diathermy is electrically induced generation of local heat in body tissues by high-frequency electromagnetic currents been used in medical, dental surgeries for decades (Fig. 14.71).

USES

- To achieve haemostasis by thermal or electrical methods
- To cut through the tissues in an avascular surgical field
- To reduce blood loss in procedures where blood loss is caused due to surgical dissection
- Used to remove small cutaneous lesions.

SURGICAL DRAIN

Surgical drain is a channel or tube used to remove pus, blood or other fluids from a wound.

INDICATIONS

- Clean wounds with potential of inadequate haemostasis (e.g. exposed medullary bone)
- Contaminated or infected wounds
- Following incision of an abscess
- To obliterate postsurgical dead space that may fill with blood, serum (haematoma and seroma) and get subsequently infected.
- Treatment of osteomyelitis of mandible (drainage and irrigation)
- Drainage of maxillary antrum through nasal antrostomy
- To maintain graft in close relation to the recipient bed.

PRINCIPLES

- Insert the drain into the most dependent part of the cavity
- In cases of infections as abscess and/or osteomyelitis non-collapsible drain that facilitate irrigation shall be chosen
- Drain should preferably exit the wound through a separate stab incision away from the necrotic unhealthy tissue
- Fix it with a suture or any other device to prevent the drain from getting dislodged into or away from the wound
- Check regularly for the patency of the drains
- Drain removal: When the discharge ceases drain can be removed at 48 h or earlier if drainage becomes minimal

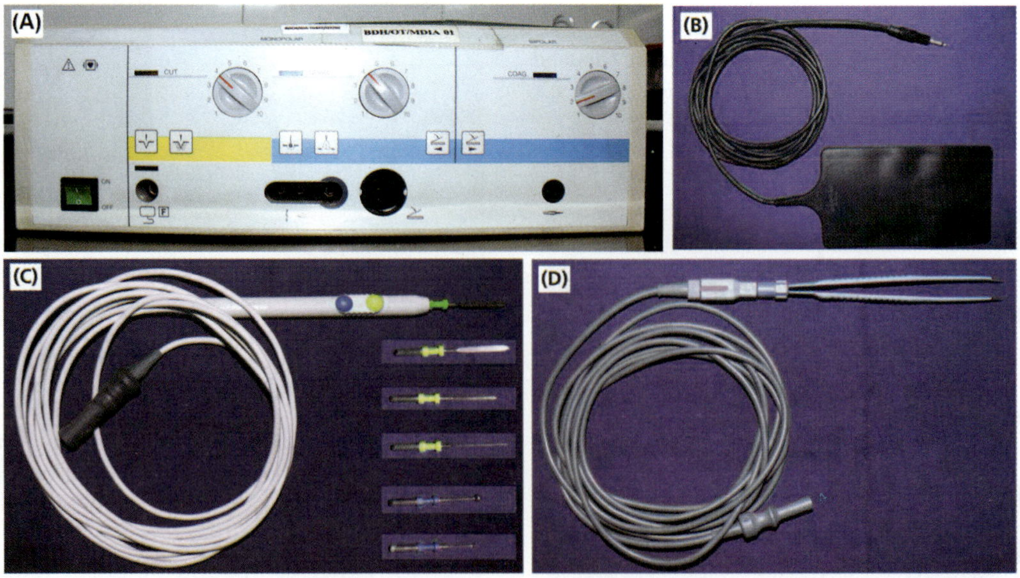

Figure 14.71 (**A**) Diathermy equipment. (**B**) Diathermy indifferent electrode. (**C**) Monopolar diathermy tips (active electrode). (**D**) Bipolar diathermy tip.

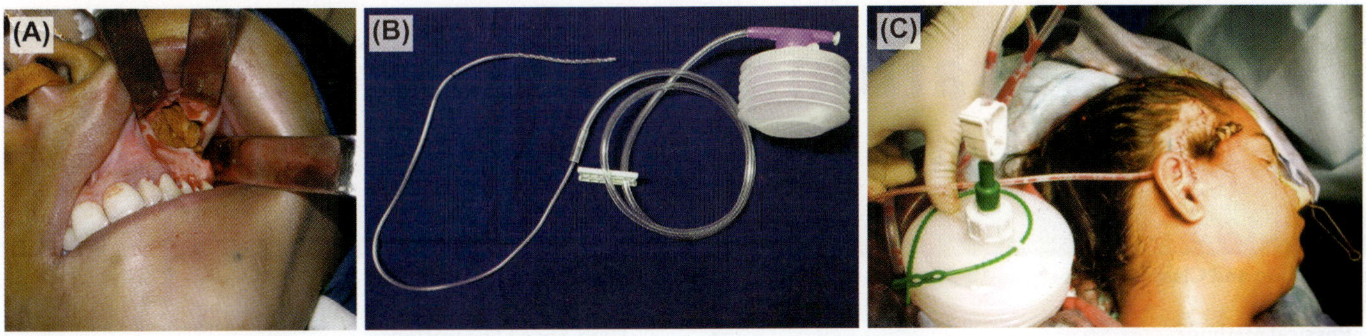

Figure 14.72 (**A**) Gauze drain for maxillary sinus exiting through nasal antrostomy. (**B**) Suction drain (Hemovac). (**C**) Vacuum drain in place after TMJ surgery.

- Drains are also used in clean wound, when there is significant potential for dead space formation with resultant haematoma or seroma.

TYPES OF DRAINS

1. Gauze drains (open passive drains)
2. Simple rubber drains (open passive drains)
3. Suction drains (closed active drains).

1. GAUZE DRAINS

- Nonmedicated or medicated (iodoform) (Fig. 14.72)
- Promote clotting of blood and plasma and act as plug rather than drains.

2. SIMPLE RUBBER DRAINS

It includes:

- Red rubber catheter
- Rubber dam material
- Latex Penrose drain
- Corrugated rubber drain, etc.

Functions

- Evacuates pooled blood, infected materials thus eliminating dead space
- Maintain patency of wound
- Provide a channel for movement of pus/blood by pressure or gravity

  Advantages: Adaptable, soft, inexpensive

  Disadvantages: Require a bulky external dressing to absorb the drainage that potentiates infection.

3. SUCTION DRAINS

- It acts by eliminating pooled blood, serum from the wound cavity as well as dead space, thus drawing separated tissue surfaces together
- It consists of polyethylene tubing (perforated/nonperforated) attached to a closed suction system (sterile container)
- Example: Hemovac, Jackson–Pratt drain system (J–P system).

Jackson–Pratt drain system

This type of drain system was introduced by Frederick E. Jackson and Richard A. Pratt, III in 1971. In maxillofacial facial surgery, this drain is commonly used after neck dissections, temporal bone resections and sialadenectomies. This system also plays a major role in the drainage and irrigation of facial abscess, osteomyelitis of mandible, elimination of dead space and prevention of haematoma formation. The J–P drain system consists of flat and round perforated drain made of high tensile strength silicone rubber, suction reservoir, extension tubing, T tubes, etc.

Advantages

- Soft nature of silicone rubber resists intraluminal clotting
- Does not cause erosion of adjacent vessels or compress nerves
- It can also be used as an irrigating drain in case of abscess or osteomyelitis
- Reliable aerobic culture can be obtained
- No need of separate puncture wound, as the flat shaped drain can be brought out through the same incision line.

Disadvantage

Bulkier than simple rubber or Hemovac drain.

Chapter 15

Sterilisation and Disinfection

OUTLINE

INTRODUCTION AND CLASSIFICATION

The 1st step in asepsis is cleanliness, a concept already adopted by Hippocrates. Modern concept of asepsis evolved in the 19th century. *Ignaz Semmelweis* showed that washing the hands prior to delivery reduced puerperal fever. After the suggestion by *Louis Pasteur*, Joseph Lister introduced the use of carbolic acid as antiseptic and reduced surgical infection rates. Trend went from antiseptics to asepsis, introducing principles and practices that have remained valid unto this day. Von Bergmann introduced the autoclave, a device used for sterilisation of surgical instruments.

- **Asepsis:** Asepsis is the practice to reduce or eliminate contaminants (such as bacteria, viruses, fungi and parasites) from entering the operating field in surgery to prevent infection. Ideally, a sterile field means free of contaminants, which is difficult to attain. However, the goal is elimination of infection, not sterility
- **Antiseptic:** A chemical that is applied to living tissues such as skin or mucous membrane to prevent infection by inhibiting the growth of bacteria
- **Disinfectant:** A chemical used on nonvital objects to kill surface vegetative pathogenic organisms, but not spores or viruses
- **Disinfection:** It is a process of complete elimination of vegetative forms of microorganisms, except the bacterial spores from inanimate objects.
- **Sterilisation:** It is a process of complete elimination or destruction of all forms of microbial life (both vegetative and spore forms).
- The agents used in sterilisation or disinfection are classified based on the mechanism as shown in Flowchart 15.1 and the classification of the agents that are in practical use are shown in Flowchart 15.2.

STERILISATION

Sterilisation is a process by which an object, surface or medium is freed of all microorganisms either in the vegetative or spore state. It is performed on all instruments and surfaces that will come in contact with the hard and soft tissues of a patient so that they are not contaminated by bacteria, spore, fungi or viruses. Sterilisation is done only after thorough cleaning of the instruments.

PHYSICAL METHODS

1. **Sunlight:** Sunlight possesses appreciable bactericidal activity and plays an important role in the spontaneous sterilisation that occurs under natural conditions. The action is primarily due to its content of ultraviolet rays
2. **Heat:** The lethal effect of heat on microorganisms has long been known. Heat is fast, reliable and relatively inexpensive. Above maximum growth temperatures, biochemical changes in the cell's organic molecules result in its death. These changes arise from alterations in enzyme molecules or chemical breakdown of structural molecules, especially in cell membranes. Heat also evaporates water and since all organisms depend on water, this loss may be fatal. The two types of heat are dry heat and moist heat
   i. *Dry heat:* The lethal effect of dry heat is due to protein denaturation, coagulation, oxidative damage and the toxic effect of elevated levels of electrolytes. Instruments with a sharp cutting edge, such as chisels are preferably sterilised by exposure to dry heat at 160°C for 1 h since autoclaving might reduce their sharpness and promote rusting
   Application of dry heat: Flaming, incineration and hot air oven

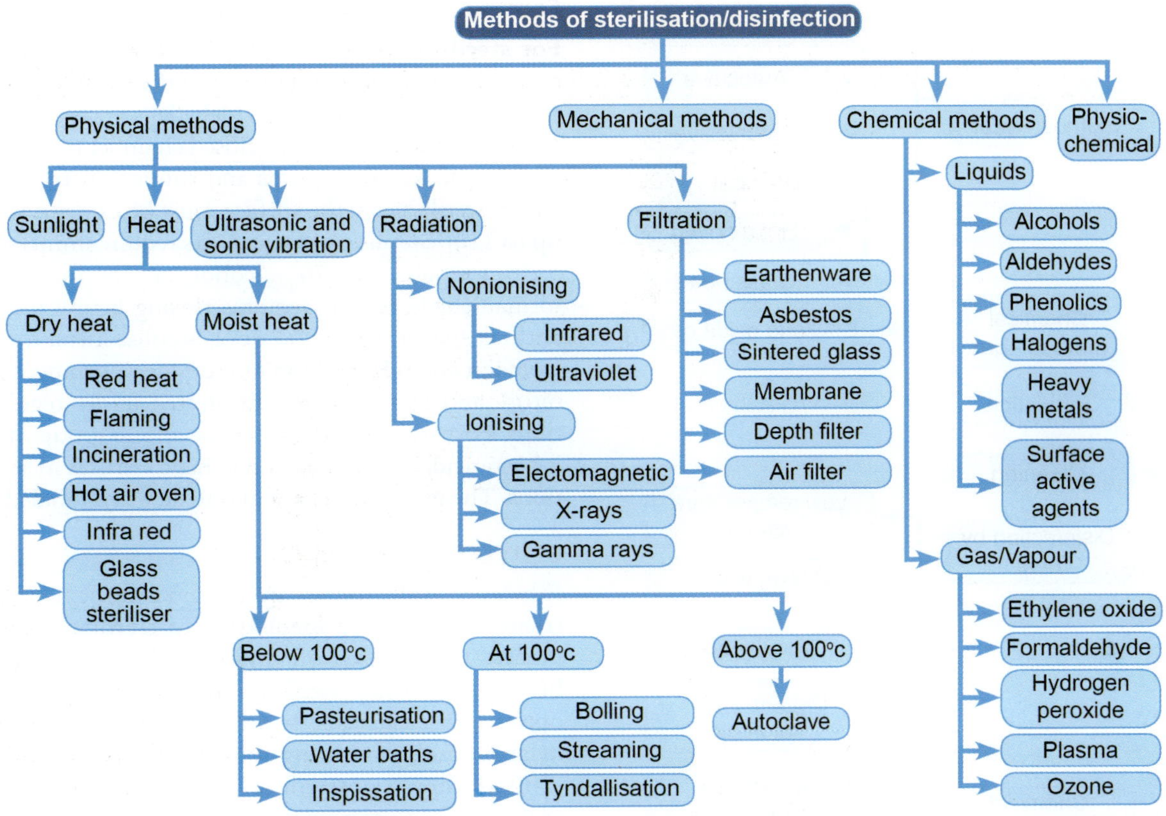

Flowchart 15.1 Methods of sterilisation/disinfection.

ii. *Moist heat:* Moist heat kills microorganisms by denaturing their proteins with ***latent heat***. Denaturation is a change in the chemical or physical property of a protein. It includes structural alterations due to destruction of the chemical bonds holding proteins in a three-dimensional form. As proteins revert to a two-dimensional structure, they coagulate (denature) and become nonfunctional. The coagulation of proteins requires less energy than oxidation and therefore less heat needs to be applied. Moist heat or steam sterilisation can penetrate better than dry heat, hence kills the microorganisms rapidly at a lower temperature than dry heat. Saturated steam is used under pressure for a quick sterilisation technique with an autoclave

Application of moist heat: Boiling, pasteurisation and autoclave

Types of steam sterilisers

a. Laboratory autoclaves
b. Hospital dressing sterilisers
c. Bowl and instrument sterilisers
d. Rapid cooling sterilisers.

CHEMICAL METHODS

Physical agents used to manage microorganisms aim to sterilise all organisms, especially bacterial spores. Chemicals rarely sterilise objects. Instead, they may only destroy pathogenic organisms on an object. Disinfection is the process of eliminating pathogens. A **disinfectant** is used on a lifeless surface, such as a tabletop. If the object is living, such as a human tissue, the chemical used is called an **antiseptic**. Antiseptics and disinfectants are usually bactericidal, but occasionally they may be bacteriostatic. A bactericidal agent kills microorganisms, while a bacteriostatic agent temporarily prevents their further multiplication without necessarily killing them. None of the chemicals used for cold sterilisation satisfy all of the criteria for effective sterilisation.

Application of chemical solutions in chemical method for sterilisation: 2% glutaraldehyde.

Application of gases in chemical method for sterilisation: Ethylene oxide gas.

ALDEHYDE

Glutaraldehyde—for sterilisation (Fig. 15.1A & B)

Glutaraldehyde (Cidex) is a potent chemical substance that can kill vegetative cells in 10–30 min and spores in 10 h. It is an alkylating agent, commonly used at 2% solution. Articles must be precleaned, immersed for 10 h, rinsed thoroughly with sterile water, dried in a dedicated cabinet with sterile air and stored in a sterile container. Materials may only be disinfected but not sterile if any of these parameters change. It kills tuberculosis bacilli, fungus and viruses. It is safe to use on rubber, anaesthesia tubes, plastic endotracheal tubes, metal equipment and polythene tubing.

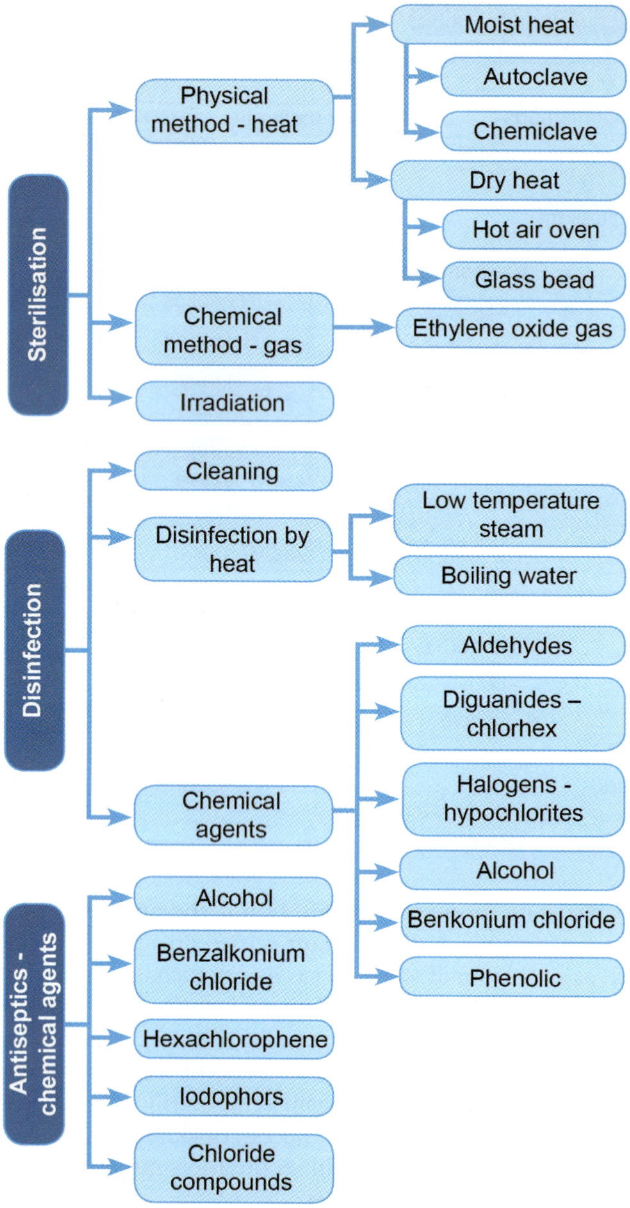

Flowchart 15.2 Classification of the agents.

Formaldehyde (Fig. 15.1C–E)

For sterilisation: Formaldehyde (HCHO) is a solid at room temperature. An amount of 37 g of the substance in 100 mL of water yields formalin. Formaldehyde is a gas at high temperatures, it is discharged into a closed chamber to sterilise surgical equipment, hospital gowns and surgical instruments. For effective sterilisation, the surface must be exposed to the gas for up to 12 h. Sterilising instruments require immersing them in a 20% formaldehyde/70% alcohol solution for 18 h. However, formaldehyde residue requires rinsing before use. It can kill anthrax spores in hair and wool. Sterilise metal tools with 10% formalin and 0.5% sodium tetraborate. Clothing, bedding, furniture and books can be disinfected under regulated conditions. Formaldehyde degrades the amino group in proteins. It is bactericidal, sporicidal and lethal to viruses in aqueous solutions. The gas is an irritant and toxic when inhaled.

ETHYLENE OXIDE GAS

Ethylene oxide gas is an alkaline, noncorrosive and extremely penetrative agent used to sterilise medical instruments. This is used on products that can be damaged by high temperature sterilisation methods such as plastics, optics and electricals. It kills microorganisms through alkylation and denaturing their nucleic acids. It is not to be utilised when heat sterilisation is possible due to its toxicity and irritating properties. It is highly flammable, but is less so when coupled with CO_2.

It is perfect for heat sensitive items. It is appropriate for electric, photographic and fiber endoscopes. It causes blisters when exposed to skin or mucous membrane. The contact time between the gas and the material to be sterilised depends on temperature, humidity, pressure and quantity of items. Certain materials such as plastic take 1–7 days to degas. Warming the objects during degassing speeds up the process. Commonly used for presterilising single use medical devices after manufacture. It has the added advantage of excellent penetration into plastics also, low temperature use and leaves no residue. It is a deodoriser, relatively harmless and can sterilise various heat sensitive items. On the other

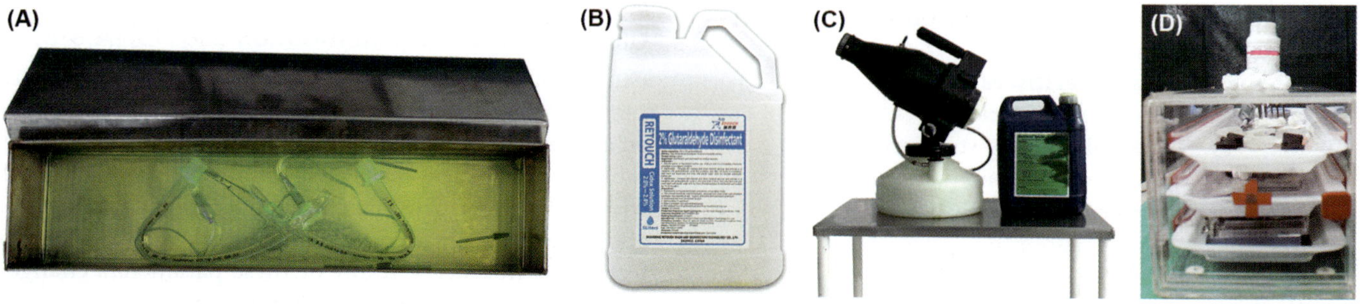

Figure 15.1 (**A** and **B**) Glutaraldehyde 2% solution. (**C**) Fumigators—formaldehyde for sterilising operating theatres and closed chambers. (**D**) Formalin chamber.

hand, the gas is hazardous and must be vented due to its high explosive/inflammable content.

FILTRATION

The filter is a mechanical device for removing microorganisms from a solution. As fluid passes through the filter, organisms are trapped in the pores of the filtering material. The solution that drips into the receiving container is decontaminated, or in some cases, sterilised. Filters are used to purify beverages, intravenous solutions, bacteriological media, toxoids and many pharmaceuticals.

Several types of filters are available for use in the microbiology laboratory:

1. Inorganic filters are typified by the Seitz filter, which consists of a pad of porcelain or ground glass mounted in a filter flask
2. Organic filters are advantageous because the organic molecules of the filter attract organic components in microorganisms. Example, the Berkefeld filter, utilises a substance called diatomaceous earth
3. Membrane filter is a 3rd type of filter that has received broad acceptance. It consists of a pad of organic compounds such as cellulose acetate or polycarbonate mounted in a holding device
4. Air can also be filtered to remove microorganisms. The filter generally used is a high-efficiency particulate air filter (**HEPA filter**). This apparatus can remove over 99% of all particles, including microorganisms with a diameter larger than 0.3 μm. The air entering surgical units and specialised treatment facilities, such as burn units, are filtered to exclude microorganisms. In some hospital wards, as pulmonary wards and in certain pharmaceutical filling rooms, the air is recirculated through HEPA filters to ensure its purity.

RADIATION

Two types of radiation are used for sterilising purposes: (1) nonionising and (2) ionising.

Infrared and ultraviolet rays are of the nonionising low energy type while γ-rays and high-energy electrons are of the high energy ionising type.

Nonionising radiation

In nonionising radiation, electromagnetic rays with wavelengths longer than those of visible light are used and these are to a large extent absorbed as heat.

1. Infrared radiation—can be considered as a form of hot air sterilisation. Infrared radiation is used for rapid mass sterilisation of syringes. It can also be used to purify air
2. Ultraviolet (UV) radiation—UV light disinfects enclosed environments like hospital wards, operating rooms and virus research laboratories. After exposure to it, DNA absorbs the energy and undergoes molecular modifications. This alters the production of important proteins via mRNA. Also, chromosomal replication by binary fission is hampered. Direct UV exposure lowers the microbial population. UV prevents airborne or surface contamination in a hospital or food service operation. Notably, UV radiation from the sun may be efficient in suppressing microorganisms in the air and top soil layers, but not all bacterial spores.

Ionising radiation

The spectrum of energies includes two forms of radiation useful for destroying microorganisms. These are (1) X-ray and (2) γ-rays.

Both have wavelengths shorter than ultraviolet rays. X-rays, gamma (γ) rays and cosmic rays all damage DNA and other cellular components. They have very high penetrative power. X-rays and γ-rays force electrons out of microbial molecules, generating ions. So, they are termed ionising radiations. The ions interact with proteins and nucleic acids, killing them. Gram-positive bacteria are more vulnerable to ionising radiation. Radiation is now utilised to sterilise heat-sensitive medications such as vitamins, hormones and antibiotics. Gamma radiation is used to sterilise swabs, culture plates, catheters, rubber, cardboard, oils, greases, textiles and metal foils.

FLAMING

The flame of the Bunsen burner is employed for a few seconds to sterilise the bacteriological loop before removing a sample from a culture tube and after preparing a smear. Flaming the tip of the tube also destroys organisms that happen to contact the tip, while burning away lint and dust. Scalpels and needles could be passed a few times through the Bunsen flame without allowing them to become red-hot (Fig. 15.2A and B).

INCINERATION

Incineration is an excellent method for rapidly destroying materials such as soiled dressings, animal carcasses, bedding and pathological material. Disposable hospital gowns and certain plastics are examples of materials that may be

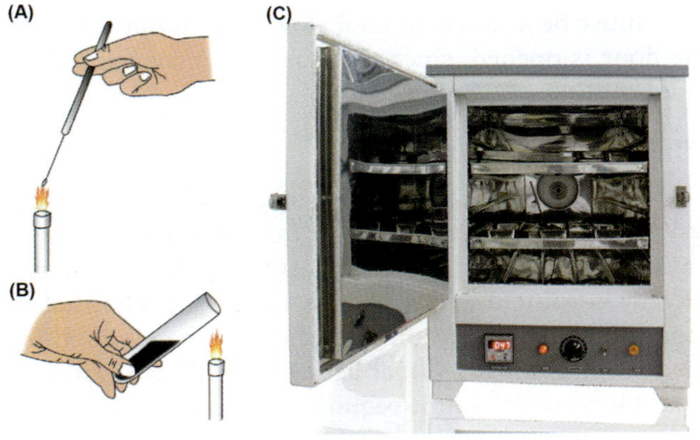

Figure 15.2 (**A** and **B**) Sterilisation by dry heat method: flaming. (**C**) Hot air oven.

incinerated. Incineration is a high-temperature dry oxidation process that reduces organic and combustible waste to inorganic, incombustible matter and results in a significant reduction of waste volume and weight. This process is usually selected to treat wastes that cannot be recycled, reused or disposed off in a landfill site. The combustion of organic compounds produces mainly gaseous emissions, including steam, carbon dioxide, nitrogen oxide, certain toxic substances (e.g. metals, halogenic acids) and particulate matter, plus solid residues in the form of ashes.

GLASS BEADS STERILISER

This method employs a heat transfer device. The media used are glass beads, molten metal and salt. The temperature achieved is 425°F–475°F or 218°C–246°C. The method employs submersion of small instruments, such as endodontic files and burs, into the beads; they are sterilised in 10 s provided they are clean.

HOT AIR OVEN

The hot air oven utilises radiating dry heat for sterilisation. This type of energy does not penetrate materials easily and therefore, long periods of exposure to high temperatures are necessary. For example, at a temperature of 160°C (320°F), a period of 2 h is required for the destruction of bacterial spores. Higher temperatures are not recommended because the wrapping used for the equipment tends to char at 180°C. The hot air method is useful for sterilising dry powders and water-free oily substances, as well as for many types of glassware, such as pipettes, flasks, forceps, scissors, scalpels and glass syringes. Dry heat neither corrodes sharp instruments as steam often does, nor does it erode the ground glass surfaces of nondisposable syringes (Fig. 15.2C and D).

Placing instruments inside the hot air oven

The material should be arranged so as to allow free circulation of air in between the objects. Glassware should be perfectly dry before being placed in the oven. Cutting instruments should ideally be sterilised for 2 h at 150°C. The oven must be allowed to cool slowly for about 2 h before the door is opened, since the glassware may crack due to rapid cooling.

Effect on microorganisms

The effect of dry heat on microorganisms is equivalent to that of baking. The heat changes microbial proteins by oxidation reactions and creates an arid internal environment, thereby burning microorganisms slowly. It is essential that organic matter such as oil or grease films be removed from the materials because organic matter insulates against dry heat. Moreover, the time required for heat to reach sterilising temperatures varies according to the materials. This factor must be considered in determining the total exposure time.

AUTOCLAVE (Fig. 15.3)

Types of autoclaves

1. Downward displacement steriliser—based on gravity
2. Steam steriliser with prevacuum and postvacuum processes

   Recently, two types of autoclaves available:

   i. Porous load autoclaves - a temperature of 121°C at 20 psi is maintained for 20 min to accomplish full sterilisation of drape clothes, suture supplies, cotton rolls and rubber gloves
   ii. Portable bench model autoclaves—for full sterilisation, as a temperature of 136°C at 32 psi is maintained for 5 min. The steam that enters the chamber from the top penetrates the material in a top-to-bottom flow. Used for unwrapped and solid instruments that must be used immediately. It always leaves leftover air in the autoclave chamber.

The use of dicyclohexylammonium nitrate or cyclohexylamine and decylamine, ammonia-based agents or 2% sodium nitrate into the autoclave has been reported to avoid or limit the corrosive impact of steam on metals.

Mechanism of autoclave

Autoclave includes boiling water to produce steam in a closed chamber, in which drums and trays containing the goods to be sterilised are kept. The resulting moist heat kills microbes quickly. A basic principle of chemistry is that when the pressure of a gas increases, its temperature increases proportionally. It is because steam is a gas, increasing its pressure in a closed system increases its temperature. As the water molecules in steam become more energised, their penetration increases substantially.

Pressure, temperature and time

As steam flows from the steam jacket into the sterilising chamber, cool air is forced out and a special valve increases the pressure to 15 psi, that is 15 pounds/square inch (lb/in^2) above the normal atmospheric pressure. To reach the required pressure, the temperature should be maintained at 121°C or 250°F. Sterilisation by steam under pressure is best carried at temperatures between 108°C and 147°C. A variety of materials like dressings, instruments, culture, media and pharmaceutical products can be sterilised by steam under pressure. The temperature for sterilising aqueous solutions is between 108°C and 126°C. Increasing temperature and pressure decreases the time taken to complete the sterilisation. The temperature of steam may reach 121°C at 15 psi pressure. At this temperature, it takes 15 min to destroy all microorganisms. Sterilisation can be performed at 126°C for 10 min and 134°C for 3 min. The amount of material and the thickness of the wrap also affect the time necessary for sterilising a specific object.

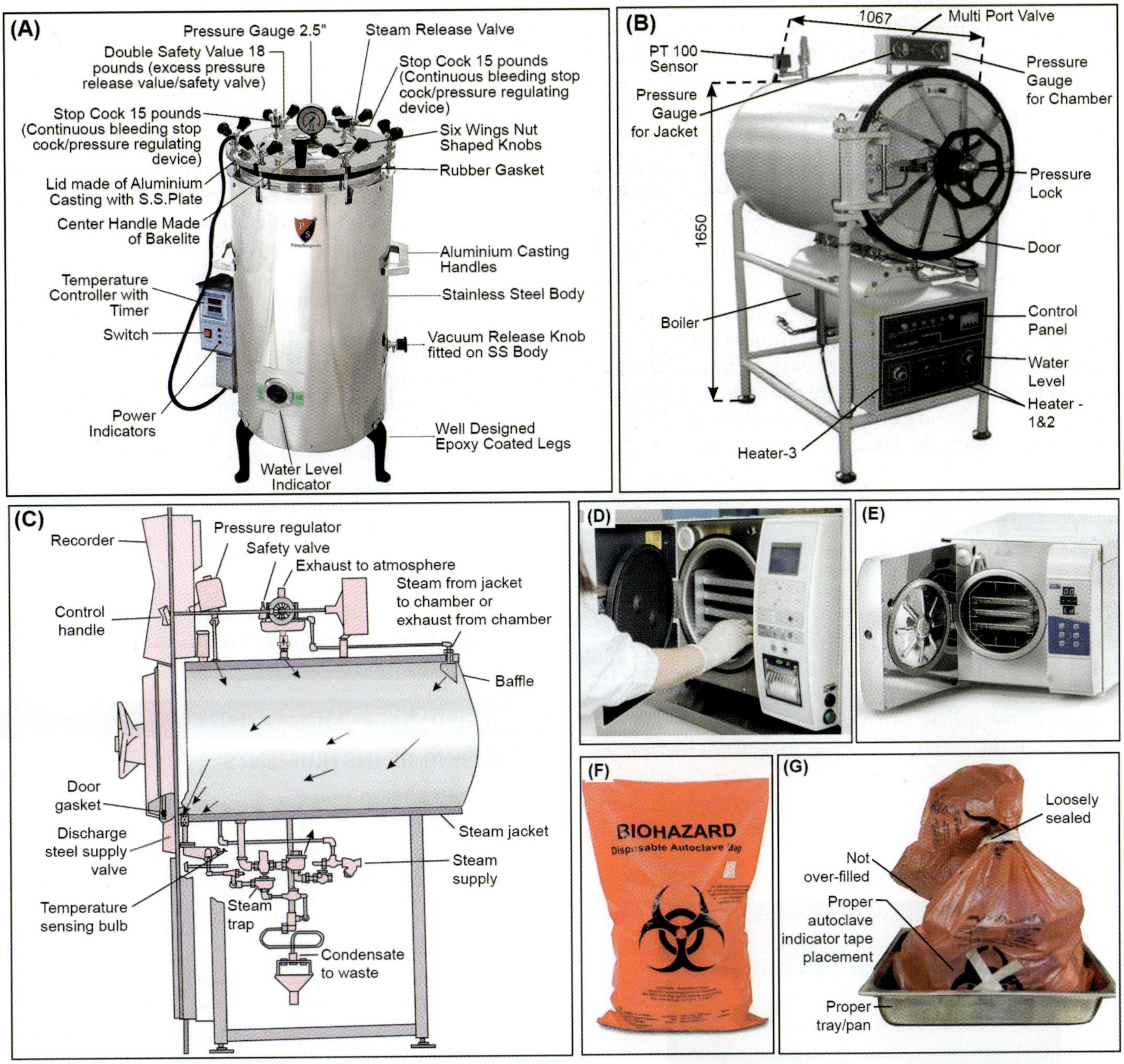

Figure 15.3 **(A)** Vertical autoclave. **(B)** Horizontal autoclave. **(C)** Mechanism of autoclave. **(D)** Modern tabletop autoclave. **(E)** Harvey chemiclave. **(F)** Biohazard bags used for autoclaves. **(G)** Instruments in surgical pack after autoclave.

Phases of autoclave

1. *Pretreatment heat up cycle:* After at least three vacuum pulses, the autoclave expels all air in the chamber outside, after which steam is pushed inside. This allows the saturated steam to effectively touch the articles during the 2nd phase
2. *Sterilisation cycle:* The temperature rises sufficiently to the point when sterilisation can take place. When the temperature in all regions of the autoclave chamber and its load reaches the sterilising temperature, the actual sterilising period, also known as 'holding time', begins. Throughout the holding period, this should remain consistent within the stipulated range of temperature
3. *Depressurisation cycle/drying phase:* To guarantee that the items are dried quickly, either the steam or the revaporised condensed water are evacuated by vacuum.

Parts of an autoclave

Autoclave is a vertical or horizontal cylinder of gunmetal or stainless steel supported by a sheet of iron casing. The lid or door is secured with screw clamps and sealed with an asbestos washer. The autoclave contains discharge taps for air and steam on its lid or upper side, as well as a pressure gauge and a safety valve that may be adjusted to blow out at any desired pressure. Heating is provided by either gas or electricity.

Tests for efficiency for heat sterilisation

Spore testing

Microbial indicator—should be conducted once in a week to ensure appropriate autoclave operation using *Geobacillus stearothermophilus* strips or vials.

Thermocouple

Thermocouple is used for thermometric testing and is a reliable gauge of efficiency. One recording is taken from a thermocouple placed inside a test pack of towels and a 2nd one from the chamber drain. Comparison between the two recordings gives a good guide regarding the speed at which the steam penetrates the load.

Brown's test

These are ampoules that contain a chemical indicator, which change colour from red through amber to green at a specific temperature.

Autoclave tape

This is a tape printed with sensitive ink that undergoes a colour change at a specific temperature. This test forms the basis of the Bowie–Dick test for high vacuum autoclaves. Two pieces of strips are struck onto a piece of square paper and placed in the middle of the test pack. With the application of temperature of 134°C for 3.5 min, there is a uniform development of bars throughout the length of the strips. This shows that the steam has passed freely and rapidly to the centre of the load (Fig. 15.4A and B).

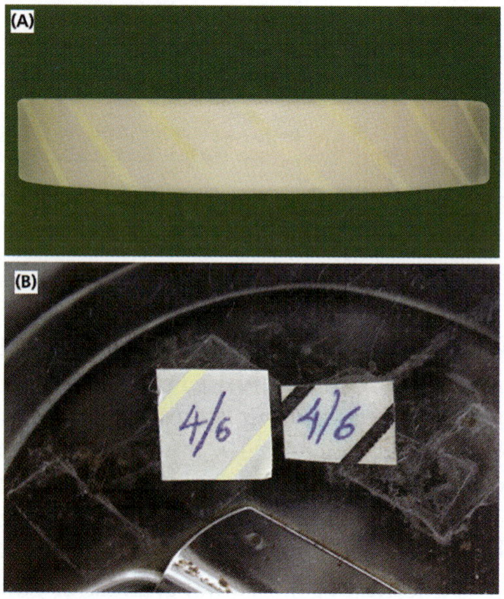

Figure 15.4 **(A)** Autoclave tape. **(B)** Autoclave tape—before and after sterilisation. Note the colour change.

CHEMICLAVE

The Harvey chemiclave, developed by Barnstead Thermolyne Corporation (Dubuque, IA), is used as a model to research certain phenomena linked with gaseous chemical sterilisation systems. Although, formaldehyde sterilisation is a unique and complex system, the current technique kills bacteria, spores and most viruses by employing dry saturated steam and formaldehyde. Microbes are destroyed by the heat and chemical action (formaldehyde). Formaldehyde alkylates nucleic acids, which synthesise proteins. Though working time is longer than autoclave, it is shorter than a hot air oven. Temperature combinations necessary are 127°C–132°C or 270°F at 20–40 psi for 30 min. This method's benefits include no instrument corrosion, shorter cycle and sterilisation at 73°C (a low temperature compared to autoclave), thus allows sterilisation of delicate plastic equipment, which other processes may damage. The downside is that it necessitates ventilation to remove chemical vapours from the end-of-cycle chamber. It employs 0.23% formaldehyde chemical solution, 72.38% ethanol or acetone or ketone. Burs—carbon steel and diamond, braces, bands, pliers, scalers, explorers and other hinged devices can be easily sterilised. Lethality rates of the microbes increase with time during the chemiclave sterilisation procedure and varies by load site.

Comparison of various sterilisation methods is described in Table 15.1.

METHODS OF DISINFECTION

CLEANSING OF INSTRUMENTS

1. Cleaning or removal of debris from instruments in the field is done to:
   - Reduce the number of microorganisms on the device
   - Reduce the nutrient material that might support pathogenic growth
   - Minimise the risk of environmental exposure from aerosolisation or spillage
   - Decrease the possibility of device damage from organic debris: blood, saline, iodine or radiologic dyes
   - Decreases the need to vigorously clean a device to remove encrusted debris
2. Cleaning of instruments is a very important *critical preparatory step* for effective sterilisation
3. Without adequate cleaning, many disinfection and sterilisation processes are ineffective. Cleaning is critical in removal of gross debris, *prevention of cross-contamination* and protection of the healthcare worker (HCW) in the processing area. Cleaning is considered to be the removal of visible dirt, soil, organic matter or other foreign material from an instrument or object. Cleaning generally means the removal of, rather than the killing of, microorganisms
4. *Soaps and detergents* are used for cleaning purposes. They reduce the surface tension along the instrument surface allowing emulsification of the contaminants, which are

TABLE 15.1 Comparison of Various Methods of Sterilisation

Autoclave	Hot Air Oven	Chemiclave
Economical	Economical	Expensive
Good penetration: Moist heat operates on enzymes and proteins by denaturing and coagulating them, whereas dry heat acts on cell elements via destructive oxidation	Slow penetration	Good penetration at a low temperature compared to autoclave
Short cycle time: Moist heat kills faster and at a lower temperature than dry heat	Longer cycle for complete sterilisation	Short time cycles
Easily monitored	Easily monitored	Easily monitored
No special chemicals or exhaust required	Comfortable working environment by maintaining temperature and ventilation	Good ventilation required as chemical vapours with unpleasant odour are released out
Carbon steel gets damaged	Does not rust metals	Limits rust on high carbon steel
Moisture retention	No moisture retention Difficult to control temperature	Instruments undergo a dry cycle
Compatible materials: Textiles, culture dishes and medium, contaminated glass equipment, vaccines, polypropylene (PP), polycarbonate (PC), plastics, borosilicate glass and all stainless steel instruments	Used for anhydrous oils and powders	Metal instruments, delicate plastic equipment
Incompatible materials: Materials contaminated with solvents, flammable chemicals, chemotherapeutic agents or cytotoxic drugs, bleach, phenol and trizol polystyrene (**PS**), polyethylene (**PE**), and high-density polyethylene (**HDPE**), plastics and household glassware	Cannot be used on textiles, rubber or metal solder joints	Damages textiles and liquids

then removed by rinsing. Other solvents like acetone, ether and xylene are used for cleaning
   a. *Mechanism of action: Coagulation of bacterial proteins*
   b. *Alteration of bacterial cell wall*
   c. *Sulfhydryl group binding*
   d. *Competition with substrates in bacterial cell wall*
5. Choose a detergent *compatible* with the type of the surgical instrument
6. *Hand cleaning* of dental instruments should be carried out using warm water and detergent using puncture resistant latex gloves
7. Dried fat or protein sediments and debris over the instrument surface may require an *enzyme detergent soak*
   a. Chemical fat solvent solutions: Acetone, xylene and ether
   b. Mechanical methods: Manual washing with stiff wire brush
   c. Ultrasonic cleaning device
8. Cleaning of instruments can also be done using *ultrasonic bath*. The liquid in the ultrasonic bath should be changed at least twice each day as it often becomes heavily contaminated. At the end of each day, the ultrasonic bath should be emptied, cleaned and dried
9. After ultrasonic cleaning, the instruments should be thoroughly rinsed with water to remove the cleaning solution and examined for any *residual debris*; if any is found, it should be removed manually
10. ***Cavitation*** is a process in which microscopic bubbles rapidly form and then collapse on the instrument surfaces creating suction that removes the debris. Ultrasonic cleaning is achieved by cavitation. To minimise organic build-up or reduce bioburden on the instruments, best practices in the preoperative setting would include keeping the instruments as free as possible of blood and organic debris during the surgical procedure
11. *Lumen of suction or cannulae* should be flushed with water to remove blood/fluids, which may dry and adhere to the surface
12. A *nonfibrous sponge* should be used to wipe off microsurgical and other delicate tips
13. Once the procedure has ended, *hinged instruments* should be opened and placed in a splash basin of sterile water to soak
14. Sharp, cutting, delicate or power instruments are managed separately to avoid damage to the surgical tools
15. Instruments that are too large to be contained in a basin may be covered with a towel soaked in water to keep the organic

debris and blood from drying on the instrument surface

16. Drying: Moisture is an essential prerequisite for bacterial growth. Drying creates an environment unsuitable for bacterial growth, but this method is unreliable and has no effect on spores
17. Ultrasonic and sonic vibration: Ultrasonic and sonic waves are credited with bactericidal powers, but the results are variable. Microorganisms vary in their sensitivity to them and survivors are found after such treatment. Hence, this method is of no practical value in sterilisation and disinfection (Fig. 15.5A–B).

CHEMICALS USED AS DISINFECTANTS

BENZALKONIUM CHLORIDE

Cationic surfactants, such as benzalkonium chloride, have actions and purposes that are identical to those of other quaternary ammonium antiseptics and disinfectants. It is used in 1:1000 solution and requires an antirust additive (sodium nitrate) and long periods of immersion (18 h) for the disinfectant action.

HEXACHLOROPHENE

The more recently introduced cold sterilising chemicals employ **hexachlorophene** compounds as the active base. These chemicals claim adequate sterilisation of heat-sensitive instruments in 3 h. Fundamentally, most of the cold sterilising media that may be safely used probably kill vegetative bacteria, but there is doubt of their effectiveness against spores and fungus.

PHENOLIC COMPOUNDS

Phenol is harmful to the skin and bone marrow on its own. Although phenolic compounds (Dettol) have been produced to minimise their adverse effects, they remain poisonous to living tissues. When present in high concentrations, these chemicals operate as protoplasmic poisons, precipitating proteins and destroying the cell wall. Their spectrum of activity extends to lipophilic viruses, fungi and bacteria, but not to spores. Because the newer synthetic combinations appear to be active against hydrophilic viruses, they have been recommended for use as a surface and immersion disinfectant. These substances are applied to inanimate items such as walls, floors and furniture to disinfect them. They might cause damage to certain plastics, but do not corrode several metals including brass, aluminium and carbon steel. Its activity is unique in that it continues to work for an extended length of time after the 1st application, often referred to as 'residual action'.

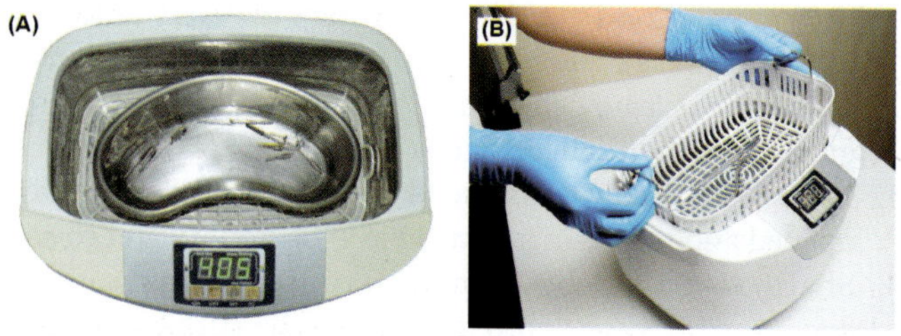

Figure 15.5 (**A**) Ultrasonic cleaning of implant drills. (**B**) Cleaning bigger drills and suction tips.

ALCOHOLS

Generally, ethyl alcohol is recommended as it kills vegetative bacterial cells such as *Mycobacterium tuberculosis* bacillus, but not spores. It denatures proteins and lipids, causing membrane disintegration. Ethanol is a powerful dehydrator. Medicinal equipment and thermometers must be thoroughly cleaned to remove organic matter before exposure to ethyl alcohol. Water slows the evaporation and aids penetration into tissues; therefore, a 50% to 80% alcohol solution is usually recommended. A 10-min soak in 70% ethyl alcohol disinfects a thermometer or other delicate instruments. Methyl alcohol is hazardous to tissues and is only used as a disinfectant for cabinets and incubators.

ALDEHYDES

As a disinfectant: Surfaces treated with this agent may emit an irritant vapour for a short period after disinfection, which can be neutralised by disinfecting with ammonia vapour. Formaldehyde is commonly used to disinfect operating rooms. It is also available in tablet form.

HALOGENS

Chlorine disinfectant: The halogens are a reactive group of elements. Chlorine and iodine are the two most common halogen disinfectants. Chlorine is a gas and an inorganic chemical. It is commonly utilised in municipal water systems to control bacterial populations. Chloramines are organic molecules that include chlorine. They help with basic wound care and root canal therapy. Chlorine kills most Gram-positive and Gram-negative bacteria, as well as numerous viruses, fungi and protozoa, but it is not sporicidal. Halogen releases atomic oxygen, which interacts with and inactivates some cytoplasmic proteins, such as enzymes. Another theory is that chlorine alters cell membrane structure, causing leaking. There are two types: sodium hypochlorite (bleach) and chlorine dioxide. **Sodium hypochlorite**—surface disinfectant with rapid action (3 min) and has a strong odour. One part 5% sodium hypochlorite to nine parts water is used. Alongside iodophors, these are the most popular surface disinfectants. **Chlorine dioxide or acid** can disinfect in 3 min.

GAS

Formaldehyde gas

Formaldehyde gas is widely used in operation theatres and other rooms. 1st, all windows and outlets are sealed. Following that, for every 1000 cu ft (28.3 m^3) of room volume, 150 g of $KMnO_4$ is added to 280 mL of formalin to produce formaldehyde gas.

The reaction produces considerable heat; therefore, heat resistant vessels should be used. After starting generation of formaldehyde vapour, the doors should be sealed and left unopened for 48 h.

Beta-propiolactone (BPL)

Beta-propiolactone is a condensation product of ketone and formaldehyde with a boiling point of 163°C. It is said to be more efficient for fumigating purposes than formaldehyde. It has a rapid biocide action, but unfortunately has carcinogenic activity.

CHLORHEXIDINE AS A DISINFECTANT

Interaction periods might vary from 30 s to 2 min, although this is the normal range for most concentrations of chlorhexidine and kill levels. It kills all microorganisms; however, its efficacy depends on the concentration. When it comes to cleaning, certain studies have shown that chlorhexidine is not the best choice. Problems regarding aquatic toxicity are raised because it combines with other compounds to produce more dangerous by-products, raising environmental concerns. Chlorhexidine is a cost-effective disinfectant.

TESTING OF DISINFECTANTS

In the Rideal–Walker test, suspensions containing equal numbers of typhoid bacilli are submitted to the action of varying concentrations of phenol and the disinfectant to be tested. The dilution of the test disinfectant that sterilises the suspension in a given time, divided by the corresponding dilution of phenol, is stated as the phenol coefficient (phenol = 1) of the disinfectant. This test does not reflect natural conditions as the bacteria and the disinfectant react directly without any organic matter being present. Modifications have therefore been suggested. In the Chick–Martin test, the disinfectant acts in the presence of organic matter. Even this modification falls short of simulating natural conditions. Various other modifications have been introduced, but no test is entirely satisfactory.

$$\text{Phenol coefficient} = \frac{\text{Dilution of test disinfectant}}{\text{Dilution of phenol}}$$

ANTISEPTICS

1. **Alcohol** is expensive, they are excellent skin antiseptics and medical instrument disinfectants. It evaporates readily and also rusts instruments. Many popular hand sanitizers contain **ethanol** as it is an alcohol-based skin antiseptic and is the most commonly used. It mechanically eliminates germs and lipids from the skin. **Isopropyl alcohol** (rubbing alcohol) has antibacterial activity up to 99%
2. **Chlorhexidine** is active against a number of bacteria. It can be prepared in alcohol or with cetrimide 0.5% chlorhexidine in 70% alcohol or cetrimide can be used as an antiseptic and 4% chlorhexidine with detergent can be used as a preoperative scrub. Chlorhexidine is lethal against bacteria including *Staphylococcus aureus* and some Gram-negative bacteria but not spores, fungi or viruses. It is always prepared with alcohol or cetrimide. Soap, pus, plastics, etc. inactivate it. It is being used as an antiseptic to clean the skin and mucous membranes; 0.2% aqueous solution or a 1% gel can be used to treat plaque and postoperative infection. At the concentrations used in oral rinses and skin cleansers, it is safe for humans to ingest. In contrast, anaphylactic responses are well documented
3. **Iodophor** compounds: The iodine atom is more reactive and germicidal than the chlorine atom. Iodine works by halogenating protein tyrosine portions. Tincture of iodine is made up of 2% iodine and sodium iodide dissolved in ethyl alcohol. Iodophors are the most effective antiseptics and is used as surgical scrubs and soaps. It stains surfaces and clothing. Usually works in 5–10 min. Iodine with **polyvinylpyrrolidone** (surface agents) becomes a stable organic complex (Betadine). Their activity is dependent on the complex releasing iodine. The surface agent forms a film, preventing stains on garments or skin. These substances kill bacteria, spores, viruses and fungi. Concentrates have less free iodine and diluting the fluid releases iodine. Dilute iodine, povidone-iodine and distilled water in 1:2:3 ratio. The benefits are minimal toxicity, extended residual effect, low cost and no odour. Repeated scrubbing accumulates these compounds on the skin, providing long-lasting antibacterial activity.

OPERATING ROOM DECORUM

Attainment of complete asepsis in surgery may never be fully possible. The air contamination of wounds is a ubiquitous problem.

- The ceiling, walls and floors should be disinfected on a regular basis
- Admission inside the operating room must be restricted to operating personnel
- Contemporary operating rooms are built with conductive flooring
- Autoclavable sterile light handles, disposable nasal cannula and nasal mask should be used to avoid cross-contamination.

OPERATOR'S PREPARATION

1. ***Conductive footwear:*** Operating room personnel and visitors must wear conductive footwear
2. ***Scrub suit:*** Street clothes are replaced with a scrub suit. The scrub suit comprises a pair of clean linen trousers and a short-sleeved shirt
3. ***Surgical head caps:*** A surgical cap is used to cover the hair completely. A head covering or cap protects the hair and head against splashes from the patient's vomit, blood or other body fluids. Use disposable or cotton caps
4. ***Eyewear:*** Protective clear eyeglasses or nonfogging goggles are used to protect the eyes from splashes or spills of infectious body fluids

5. ***Mask:*** A mask is used to cover the nose and mouth of the surgeon. It can be high efficiency particulate air (HEPA)-filter mask or surgical mask
   a. ***HEPA-filter or biosafety mask:*** A HEPA-filter mask filters the air to prevent breathing in small particles and harmful microorganisms. It provides protection from airborne transmission of microorganisms. A HEPA-filter or biosafety mask is lightweight and easy to use. It can be reused by the same HCW as long as it continues to fit comfortably and the mask does not become contaminated, crushed or splattered with body fluids
   b. ***Surgical masks*** will not filter out small particles, but they will protect the HCW from droplets or splashing of body fluids. A surgical mask consists of three layers: (1) inner layer facing the wearer absorbs water, (2) middle layer is the cotton filter and (3) outer layer is water resistant. Wearing surgical mask is a way to prevent the spread of droplet and respiratory tract infections
      i. The surgical mask should fit snugly over the face
      ii. The folds should face downward on the outside, with metallic strip uppermost
      iii. Tie all the strings that keep the surgical mask in place or fix the rubber bands of the surgical mask round the ears properly
      iv. The surgical mask should fully cover the nose, mouth as well as the chin
      v. The metallic wire part of the surgical mask should be moulded securely to the bridge of the nose and along both sides of the face beneath the eyes to prevent leakage
      vi. Once in position, one should not fiddle with the mask as this could transfer any contamination from the hands to the face
      vii. Always wash the hands before and after taking off the mask
6. ***Hand scrub technique:*** The surgeon's hands should be appropriately scrubbed. The suitable preparations for hand scrub are 4% chlorhexidine gluconate and 7.5% povidone-iodine (Betadine). Presently, highly detergent soaps containing hexachlorophene are commonly utilised in prescribed scrub techniques. Nails should be cut short and all jewellery removed before washing and the nails should be scrubbed 1st, thoroughly with a brush. The surgical scrubbing is done in the following manner. Brush, soap (or hexachlorophene detergents) and water are used to scrub the hands and forearms till the elbows. A 2-min scrub between operations is acceptable. The fingernails must be adequately cleansed. Sterile orangewood sticks are conveniently provided for this purpose. If nondetergent soap is used for the scrub, a longer scrub period is required and a postscrub rinse with a low-surface tension antiseptic such as alcohol or hexachlorophene is recommended. After the scrub, hands are dried in the operating room with a sterile hand towel. At this stage, the hands are considered surgically clean but not sterile (Fig. 15.6A–D)
7. ***Surgical gowns*** are available in disposable forms and as surgical cotton gowns. The surgeon's back as well as the

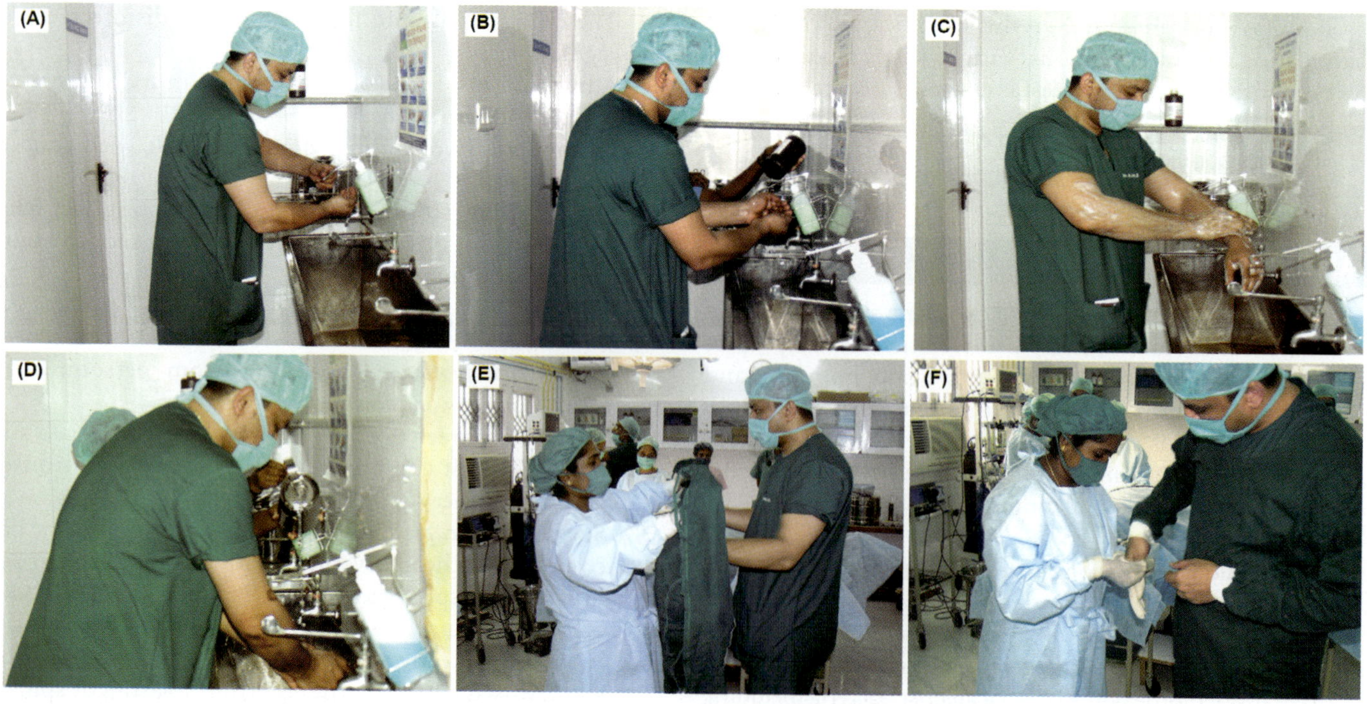

Figure 15.6 (**A–D**) Hand scrub technique. (**E**) Donning of surgical gown. (**F**) Gloving.

gown below the level of the waist are considered unsterile (Fig. 15.6E)

8. ***Gloving:*** Gloves are manufactured with natural rubber latex or synthetic rubber materials, such as vinyl, neoprene, nitrile, polyurethane or other synthetic compounds. Surgical gloves are generally latex gloves only, though synthetic ones are also available. Latex surgical gloves or sterile gloves are used to prevent cross-infection during surgery. They are flexible, durable and allow the required sensitivity during the procedures. During the gloving technique, only the interior of the glove should be touched by hands because the exterior surface is considered as sterile. The hand to glove and glove-to-glove technique of donning is used. Double gloving provides extra protection but reduced sensitivity, dexterity and possible discomfort (Fig. 15.6F). Modified starch powder has replaced talcum as the dusting agent of choice. However, sterile creams are being used for this purpose more than dusting agents. While selecting the type of examination glove, the material properties should be taken into consideration. Vinyl gloves can be used for short duration tasks where the stress on the gloves and exposure to body fluids is less. On the contrary, latex gloves can be used when the exposure to the body fluids is more
    a. Apart from their categorisation as natural latex or synthetic, they are further classified as specific use or specialty gloves. The choice is based on personal preference and procedure:
        1. Powdered surgical gloves
        2. Powder-free surgical gloves
        3. Synthetic surgical gloves
    b. These are available in different sizes, as:
        1. Small, medium, large or extra-large
        2. Number coded (eg., 6, $6^1/_2$ and 7)
    c. Ideally a glove should be:
        1. Soft
        2. Comfortable
        3. Elastic
        4. Sensitive
        5. Resistant to tearing or puncture
        6. Less allergenic potential
        7. Low levels of residual process chemicals
        8. Low levels of latex proteins.

INFECTION CONTROL

Infection:
The lodgement and multiplication of a parasite in or on the tissues of a host constitutes infection.

Infectious disease:
Infectious disease or **communicable disease** is a disease caused by a biological agent such as by a virus, bacterium or parasite.

Primary infection:
Initial infection with a parasite in a host is termed as primary infection.

Reinfection:
Subsequent infections by the same parasite in the host are termed reinfection.

Secondary infection:
When resistance of the host is lowered by a preexisting infectious disease and a new parasite sets up an infection, this is termed secondary infection.

Focal infection (focal sepsis):
Due to infection or sepsis at a localised site such as appendix or tonsils, generalised effects are produced.

Cross-infection:
When a patient is already suffering from a disease, a new infection is set up from another host or another external source.

Nosocomial infection:
Cross-infections occurring in hospitals.

Iatrogenic infections:
These are physician-induced infections resulting from investigative, therapeutic or other procedures.

Endogenous infections:
If the source of infection is from within the host's body, then it is termed as endogenous infection.

Exogenous infections:
If the source of infection is from outside the host's body, then it is termed as exogenous infection.

Atypical infections:
It is characterised by an absence of characteristic clinical manifestation of the particular infectious disease.

Latent infection:
Following infection, some parasites may remain in the tissues in a latent or hidden form, proliferating and producing clinical disease when the host resistance is lowered.

Carrier:
A person who harbours the pathogenic microorganisms without suffering any ill effects from it.

Healthy carriers:
A healthy carrier is one who harbours a pathogen, but has never suffered from any disease due to the pathogen.

Convalescent carrier:
A convalescent carrier is one who has recovered from the disease and continues to harbour the pathogen in his/her body.

Contact carrier:
These are persons who acquire the pathogen from the patients.

Paradoxical carrier:
These are patients who acquire the pathogens from another carrier.

Vector:
A living entity (animal, insect or plant) that transmits the aetiological agent.

Vehicle:
A nonliving entity that is contaminated with an aetiologic agent and as such is the mode of transmission for that agent.

Mode of transmission:
Means by which aetiological agents are brought in contact with the human host (e.g. infected blood, contaminated water, insect bite).

Direct contact:
Spread of infection through contaminated food or intravenous solutions.

Indirect contact:
Spread of infection from a patient to patient through the hands of HCW (Methicillin-Resistant Staphylococcus Aureus (MRSA), rotavirus).

Vector-borne contact:
Diseases that spread by vector such as mosquitoes (malaria) or rats (Leptospirosis).

Droplet contact:
Spread of infection by inhalation of droplets (>5 μm diameter) that cannot travel more than 3 feet (pertussis).

AIRBORNE CONTACT

Spread of infection by inhalation of droplets (≤5 μm in diameter) that can travel large distances on air currents (tuberculosis).

The severe acute respiratory syndrome (SARS), which was caused by the new Coronavirus Beta-2 (CoV-2), was responsible for starting the worldwide COVID-19 pandemic in the final weeks of 2019 and affecting the entire world beginning in early 2020. It was necessary for the dental practitioners to promptly review the standard operating protocols for infection control, which are typically carried out. Personal protective equipment (PPE) was used extensively throughout the delivery of oral health care to ensure the safety of both the staff and the patients. The goal was to reduce the number of times dentists were exposed to the virus for the 1st time through patients. Later research revealed that the SARS-CoV-2 virus was primarily transmitted through direct contact, droplets and fomites. After that, new research revealed that the virus might also spread airborne. Oral surgery operatives have a legitimate reason to be concerned about these modes of transmission because the practice includes the production of a significant quantity of droplets and aerosols, which can include the patient's saliva and even their blood at some points throughout the procedure. It is possible for the virus to spread through the air if a person breathes in contaminated spatter, droplets or aerosols. It is necessary to have a solid understanding of droplets as well as aerosol particles in order to elucidate further definitions of spatter.

Splatter is defined as a mixture of air, water and/or solid particles with a diameter more than or equal to 50 μm that are visible to the human eye and behave in a ballistic or projectile fashion.

Droplets are inspirable particles with a diameter greater than 5 μm that have the potential to deposit themselves on the levels of the upper respiratory tract and the mucosa.

An aerosol is described as a suspension of liquid or solid in the air. Some researchers characterise suspensions with particles of up to 50 m diameter as aerosols; however, the recognised use of the term 'aerosol' in infectious disease research includes only particles 5 m in diameter.

Bioaerosols, also known as infectious aerosols, are defined as aerosols that contain particles of biological origin or activity and have the potential to infect, poison or otherwise adversely influence living beings.

Oral surgery is frequently required to be performed in an environment that is polluted with blood and saliva. When providing basic dental care, those working in the field are expected to adhere to strict sanitation and disinfection protocols. It has been established that universal precautions can prevent the transmission of infectious diseases that are disseminated by droplets (particles with a diameter more than 5 μm). However, the risk of infection through droplets and aerosol (particles smaller than 5 μm) is becoming more widely recognised, and the methods for infection prevention have been reviewed.

Dentists, rather than merely relying on universal precautions, have been routinely using standard surgical barriers such as double gloves, masks and PPE in cases where it is anticipated that blood will splatter since the 1990s. This is done to reduce the risk of transmission of blood-borne diseases such as HIV, hepatitis B and hepatitis C. You can get further information about standard universal precautions, such as the barrier technique.

When addressing COVID-19 patients or dealing with an outbreak in the local area, all procedures that are considered conventional must be followed. Elective operations can be delayed, and conventional triage processes must be adhered to while providing emergency oral health care. These procedures include the measurement of temperature, the need for patients to have a seronegative status and the requirement that patients' temperatures be taken.

The dental operating area needs to have adequate ventilation with fresh air. In the event that this is not the case, the recirculation of air should be documented, as should the existence of any type of filter or disinfection system, such as HEPA. It is important to measure the number of air changes that occur per hour and adhere to the criteria that have been set. Suction devices and equipment that generates aerosols should be utilised with extreme caution, and the former should be used as little as possible. 2nd, it is important to provide a detailed description of the apparatus that is used for the procedures themselves, paying particular attention to the configurations that influence the generation of aerosols, such as the mixing of liquids and air. It is important to keep a record of the many types of suction devices that are used, as well as the amount of air that is drawn in while they are in operation. If it is determined to be required, sampling of the air may be performed. It is possible to disinfect the tools and the operatory after each treatment and patient visit in accordance with the standards that have been established. There is no question that this would lead to a rise in expenses; however, the advantages of implementing such a procedure would be enormously advantageous.

UNIVERSAL PRECAUTIONS

ASEPTIC PRECAUTIONS IN THE OPERATING ROOM

1. The operating room must have a negative bacterial culture, hence it should be fumigated
2. A strong disinfectant should be used to clean the floor.
3. Impervious packed paper, aluminium foil or clear plastic wraps may be used to cover surfaces that can be contaminated by blood or saliva and are difficult or impossible to disinfect. The coverings should be removed, discarded and then replaced with clean material between the patients
4. Light handles, switches, tabletops, etc. are liable to accumulate infective material. Surfaces should be cleaned and dried with a solution of 70% isopropyl alcohol that helps in preventing infection. Blood, pus stains should be removed and disposable clothes should be used
5. Hypochlorite solution containing 1% chlorine or 2% glutaraldehyde is used as disinfectant in cases of metallic surfaces. The solution left for minimum of 3 min in drying will help to prevent spread of infection
6. Clear plastic disposable sleeves may be used to cover tubes and hoses
7. Good ventilation will help in maintaining clean atmosphere.

HIGH-SPEED EVACUATION

High-speed evacuation tips not only take up excess saliva and water, but they also remove excess droplets and aerosolised pathogens that spray from high-speed handpiece. They are available in disposable and autoclavable forms.

HANDLING AND DISPOSAL OF SHARP INSTRUMENTS

Sharp instruments like scalpel blades should be handled carefully. Recapping of a needle increases the risk of unintentional needlestick injury. Needles should not be recapped and should be bent or broken before disposing. When multiple injections are required, it is more prudent to place the unsheathed needle into a sterile field between injections rather than recapping the needle. Disposable hypodermic syringes, scalpel blades and other sharp items must be placed into puncture-resistant containers located as close as practically possible to the area in which they are used (Fig. 15.7).

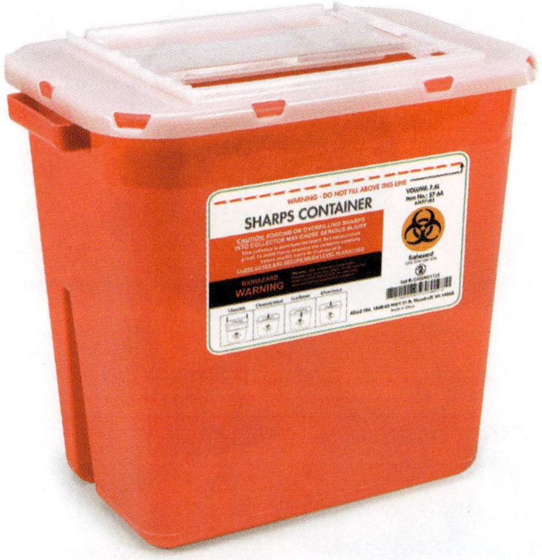

Figure 15.7 Sharps container.

BARRIER TECHNIQUE

Use of gloves

Gloves are used during both examination and treatment, wherein contact with skin, mucosa or body fluid is encountered. Changing gloves between patients or when they are torn or punctured is mandatory.

Gowns

The use of gowns, aprons or laboratory coats is required when splashes of fluids on the skin or clothing with body fluids are likely to occur. They should be made of or lined with fluid proof material and should protect all areas of exposed skin of the operator and the patient.

Masks and head caps

The procedure of drying the teeth with air during an examination aerosolises a higher concentration of bacteria than cough. There is a possibility of bacteria-loaded aerosols caused by airotor and ultrasonic scalers colonising the nasal flora. A well-fitting mask, which has efficient filtering capacity not only prevents aerosols from coming in contact with the operator's face, but also protects the patient from the droplets falling from the mouth and nose of the operator, but a mask that is worn for a prolonged period of time can act as a nidus of potentially pathogenic bacteria rather than as a barrier to the transmission of nasal, oral and skin organisms.

Head caps/cover: Head hair must be properly tied and covered with head caps.

It should be disposable and made of soft, nonporous cloth like material.

Protective eyewear

Human eyes are particularly susceptible to infection and injury because of poor vascularity and decrease in immune capacities. Glasses or a face shield should be worn while working on a patient to prevent trauma to the eye tissue from spattering droplets or aerosols containing infectious microbe-laden debris. However, these can become a source of infection and cross-contamination if used continuously for different patients without disinfection. 2% glutaraldehyde is used as a disinfectant.

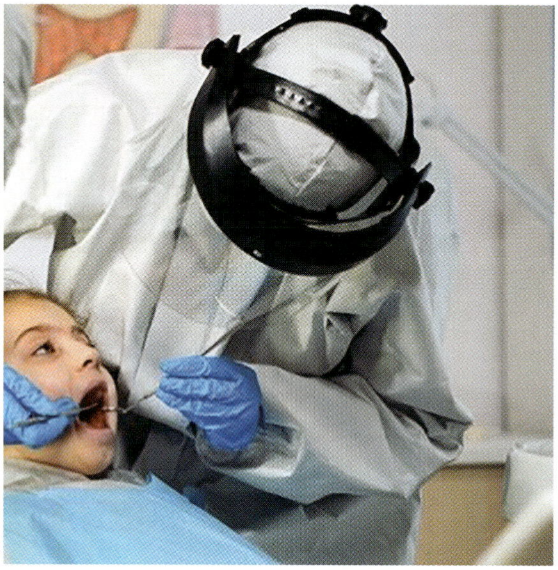

Figure 15.8 Face Shield.

Scrub suits

It is a pair of garments generally worn over or instead of regular clothing. It should be comfortable, loose-fitting and easy to clean and wash.

Face shields

It should be used when splattering of fluids is expected (Fig. 15.8).

STERILISATION PROCEDURES

1. Drop off: The contaminated instruments are dropped off at the vestibule. The staff wear PPEs before handling these instruments and sort them into separate sinks for the prewash soak (Fig. 15.9)
2. Decontamination
   a. The instruments are 1st sorted into separate sinks for those that require ultrasonic cleaning like burs—bone cutting instruments that contain minute grooves and those that require washing in the automatic cleaning machine
   b. Placing the instrument in a presoaking solution (phenolic compounds) prevents drying of debris, helps to dissolve or soften organic debris and sometimes helps in microbial killing
3. Cleaning
   a. It facilitates sterilisation. Cleaning can be done either by hand scrubbing or with the use of ultrasonic devices
4. Corrosion control and lubrication
   a. Instruments must be dried prior to sterilisation to decrease chances of corrosion. The nonstainless steel instruments should be coated with a rust inhibitor
5. Packaging
   a. The instruments can be packed individually or in small groups and distributed on sterile or disposable disinfected trays for use at chair side. For wrapping,

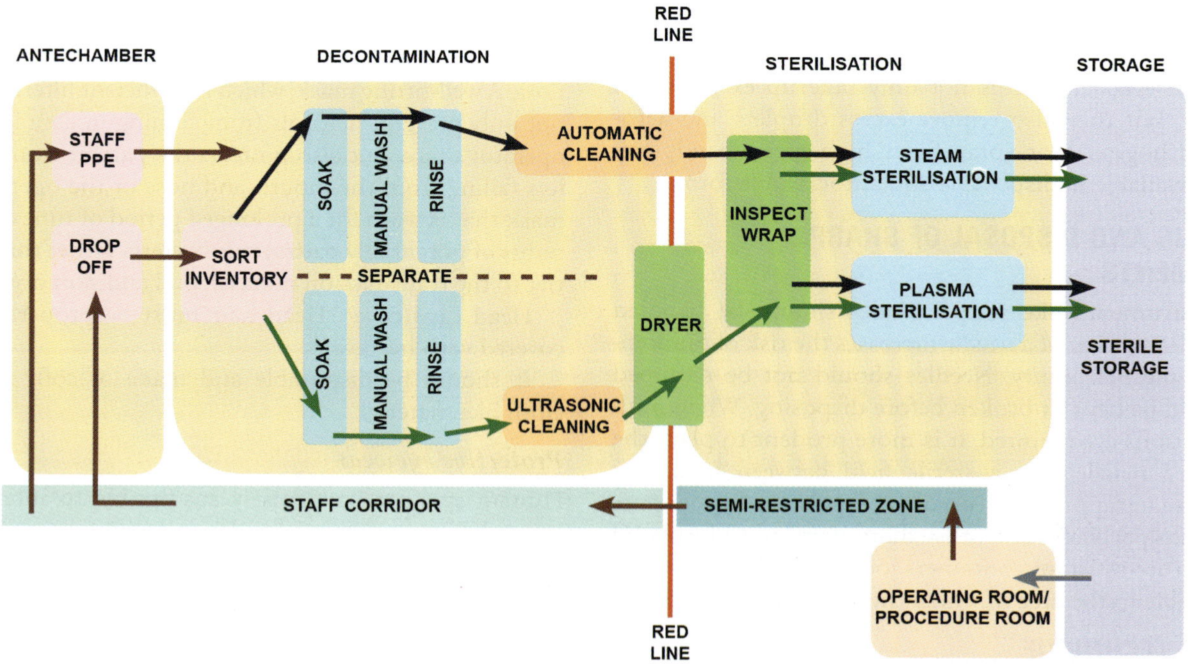

Figure 15.9 Procedure of sterilisation. Arrows depicted as: *Brown*—contaminated instruments, *Green*—instruments require ultrasonic cleaning like burs, *Black*—regular instruments, *Grey*—sterile instruments, *Red line* differentiates instruments that are contaminated and sterilised.

thin paper bags should be avoided as they will permit sharp and pointed instruments such as sickle scalers to protrude and may cause injury during handling. See through poly-film bags or pouches facilitate instrument identification

6. Sterilisation
   a. Autoclaving is the most accepted method of sterilisation of surgical instruments as it eliminates bacteria, viruses, fungi and spores. It works on the principle of steam under pressure of 15 lbs at 121°C for 20 min or 30 lbs at 134°C for 3 min. It has excellent penetration, facilitating exposure of all instrument surfaces to the steam. It has a relatively short cycle time and can sterilise water-based liquids. Dry heat ovens or the unsaturated chemical vapour sterilisers are the other means of sterilisation. Ultraviolet light may kill microorganisms that are directly exposed to the light; however, the light may not reach all the surfaces of an instrument. A temperature of 160°C–170°C maintained for 1 h is capable of sterilisation. This method is acceptable for cloth and paper items
7. Handling sterile instruments
   a. Poststerilisation procedures involve drying, cooling, storage and distribution. As far as possible, the sterile packages or trays should not be handled until required for use to reduce recontamination
8. Storage
   a. Sterile packs and trays should be kept in dry, low dust, low traffic areas away from sinks and water pipes, at least a few inches above the floor
   b. All sterilised instruments and materials must be placed in covered drawers
9. Distribution
   a. Sterilised packs containing functional sets or individual items can be placed on sterile, disposable trays for use at chair side. The instruments, which are disinfected in a liquid germicide should be handled aseptically with sterile tongs, kept on sterile trays and then covered. Placing unwrapped or wrapped instruments in drawers for direct use at chair side is not recommended
10. Expiry of sterilised instruments
    a. Expiry of sterilised instruments and materials depends on type, time and efficacy of sterilisation process
    b. Sterilised instruments and materials are considered to be safe and sterilised for a maximum of 4 weeks.

PROTECTIVE MEASURES

Vaccination against hepatitis B is highly effective, safe and stable for oral surgeons and dental staff. These injections do not give lifelong immunity and booster dose after 5 years is recommended.

a. Prevention of needlestick injuries
b. Disposal of waste.

NEEDLESTICK INJURY

Needlestick injuries are wounds caused by needles that accidentally puncture the skin. Needlestick injuries are a hazard for people who work with hypodermic syringes and other needle equipment. These injuries can occur at any time; during use, disassembling or disposal. Needlestick injuries transmit infectious diseases, especially blood-borne viruses. In recent years, concerns about AIDS, hepatitis B and hepatitis C has prompted research to find out the causes of these injuries and develop measures to prevent them. Despite published guidelines and training programmes, needlestick injuries remain an ongoing problem.

Accidental punctures by contaminated needles can inject hazardous fluids into the body through the skin. There is potential for injection of hazardous drugs, but injection of infectious fluids, especially blood, is by far the greatest concern. Even small amounts of infectious fluid can spread certain diseases effectively. Accidental injection of blood-borne viruses is the major hazard of needlestick injuries, especially the viruses that cause AIDS (HIV), hepatitis B and hepatitis C. The risk of infection after exposure to infected blood varies by blood-borne pathogen. The risk of transmission after exposure to HIV-infected blood is about 0.3%, whereas it is estimated to be around 100 times greater for hepatitis B virus (30%) and as high as 10% for hepatitis C virus.

Nursing and laboratory staff usually experience 30% to 50% of all injuries during clinical procedures.

CAUSES

EQUIPMENT DESIGN

Safer innovative devices using protected needle devices or needle-free systems with self-sealing ports would alleviate many of these injuries. Syringes with safety features reduce needlestick injuries.

RECAPPING

Recapping can account for 25% to 30% of all needlestick injuries. Often, it is the single most common cause.

It is extremely dangerous to hold a needle in one hand and attempt to cover it with a small cap held in the other hand. Injuries occur in three different ways:

Improper disposal

Virtually all needlestick injuries are from needles that have either been lost in the workplace or thrown into regular garbage. Janitors and garbage handlers can also experience needlestick injuries or cuts from ‘sharps’ when handling waste that contains needles or scalpels.

Prevention

Preventing needlestick injuries is the most effective way to protect workers from the infectious diseases that needlestick accidents transmit. A comprehensive needlestick injury prevention programme would include:

- Employee training
- Safe recapping procedures
- Effective disposal systems
- Improved equipment design.

Employee training

To reduce needlestick injuries, an effective programme must include employee training. Specifically, the training programmes should address:

- Risk of injury
- Potential hazards
- Recommended precautions for use and disposal of needles
- Procedures for reporting injuries
- The importance of hepatitis B vaccination where appropriate.

Single-handed scooping

Recapping can be safe when people lay the cap on a flat surface and scoop it onto the tip of a syringe held in one hand. They must keep the free hand away from the sheath and well behind the exposed needle.

DISPOSAL

Workers should place needles in wide mouth, puncture-proof containers. Place disposal containers specifically where needles are used to make safe disposal possible without recapping. Replace the containers before they are completely filled. Make sure that they are sealed, collected and disposed in accordance with local regulations for biomedical waste.

MANAGEMENT OF NEEDLESTICK INJURY

- Stop all operative procedures
- Identify and examine the wound
- Immediately wash, but do not scrub the injury
- Encourage bleeding
- Blood specimen of both the patient and the HCW should be taken for testing.

MANAGEMENT OF NEEDLESTICK INJURY WITH KNOWN INFECTION

HEPATITIS B

Source

HBsAg negative

- No further action necessary.

HBsAg positive or unknown

Exposed person already received a full course of hepatitis B vaccine

- If hepatitis B antibody (anti-HBs) level is known to be >100 IU/mL and a booster dose has been given 5 years after the primary course, no further action is needed (long-term immunity can be assumed). If it is more than 2 years since the primary course was given, but the 5-year dose has not been given, it should be given now
- If the postprimary vaccination course anti-HBs level is unknown or <100 IU/mL, take a 10 mL clotted blood sample for the level to be measured
    - Level >100 IU/mL: No treatment
    - Level <100 IU/mL: Give vaccine booster.

Exposed person not vaccinated

- Start the course of hepatitis B vaccine.
- Hepatitis B immunoglobulin (HBIG) will also be required. It is given intramuscularly at a different site to the vaccine if the exposure is considerable. Seek advice from medical microbiologists. HBIG should be given as soon as possible after exposure and certainly within 48 h. It is of no value if given later than 1 week after exposure.

Exposed person vaccinated but not completed full course

- Take 10 mL clotted blood and measure antibody level
- Level >100 IU/mL: No further action necessary, but vaccine course should be completed at recommended intervals
- Level <100 IU/mL: Give further dose and complete vaccine course. Seek advice from medical microbiologists regarding intervals. HBIG will also be required if exposure is considerable.

HEPATITIS C

There is no specific prophylaxis or vaccination available against hepatitis C. Therefore, no immediate action that needs to be taken following exposure to a possible hepatitis C source.

Exposed HCWs should be managed as follows:

1. ***Known hepatitis C infected source***
    - Obtain baseline serum for storage from HCW
    - Obtain clotted blood sample (serum) for hepatitis C virus RNA testing at 6 and 12 weeks
    - Obtain serum for hepatitis C Virus antibody (anti-HCV) at 12th and 24th week.
2. ***Source known to be uninfected with hepatitis C following testing at time of incident***
    - Obtain baseline serum for storage from HCW.
    - Obtain follow-up serum if symptoms or signs of liver disease develop.
3. ***Hepatitis C status of source unknown***
    - Obtain baseline serum for storage from HCW.
    - A risk assessment should be performed of the likelihood that the source is hepatitis C positive (assessed by clinician in charge of patient or occupational health or consultant microbiologist).
      High risk—manage as known infected source.
      Low risk—obtain serum for anti-HCV testing at 24 weeks.

HCWs found to have acquired hepatitis C infection following occupational exposure should be referred immediately for specialist assessment. Chronic hepatitis C infection can be prevented if acute hepatitis C infection is treated early.

HUMAN IMMUNODEFICIENCY VIRUS (HIV)

- This procedure applies to all possible exposures, whether they involve staff, patients or members of the public
- If there is a risk of HIV exposure, individuals must be dealt with urgently to obtain prophylaxis as soon as possible and preferably within 1 h
- If the source is in a high-risk group or exposure is considerable, the source patient should be tested for HIV antibody. This requires informed consent to be given. For this indication, these tests are not performed after hours. The decision to begin preventive medication should not be made simply on the basis of the results of an HIV antibody test, and any prophylaxis should be administered within an hour of exposure
- For any exposure incident when the source patient is known, it is recommended that hepatitis B, hepatitis C and HIV tests are carried out as a routine from that patient. These tests should be scheduled as soon as possible for high-risk sources or exposures
- A blood sample must be taken from the injured or exposed person and sent to the microbiology laboratory to be stored. This will be used for future testing, if necessary.
- The risk of seroconversion following a single percutaneous exposure to HIV is only 0.3%; and following mucous membrane and skin exposure, 0.1% and <0.1% respectively.

Three types of exposure pose a risk

- Percutaneous exposure, for example, needlestick
- Exposure of broken skin
- Mucous membrane exposure.

The risk of transmission is increased with

- Hollow bore needles
- Needles/sharps that are visibly blood stained
- Needles that have been in an artery or vein
- A high viral load in the source, for example, patient with AIDS/terminally ill.

Postexposure prophylaxis

- Postexposure prophylaxis (PEP) should be considered whenever there has been exposure to material known to be or strongly suspected to be infected with HIV
- High-risk body fluids are blood, amniotic fluid, vaginal secretions, semen, breast milk, CSF, peritoneal fluid, pericardial fluid, synovial fluid, unfixed tissues and organs and saliva in association with dental surgery
- PEP should not be offered following contact through any route with urine, vomitus, saliva and faeces unless they are visibly blood stained

The following should be recommended:

- Zidovudine 300 mg and lamivudine 150 mg BD
- Nelfinavir 1.25 g BD.

Management of needlestick injuries and accidents involving exposure to blood and body fluids is depicted (Fig. 15.7).

Refer to Chapter 7 page number 91.

DISPOSAL OF WASTE

Proper disposal of hospital waste is of paramount importance because of its infectious and hazardous characteristics (Tables 15.2 and 15.3).

WHO classified waste in the following manner:

- General nonhazardous
- Sharps
- Chemical
- Infectious

Types of waste materials

i. Biohazardous
ii. Non-biohazardous

Biohazardous materials

- Blood soaked waste materials or other body fluids
- Surgically extracted human tissues
- Waste susceptible of transmitting infections
- Bloodstained gloves
- Cotton roll, gauze soaked in blood
- Toxic waste materials

TABLE 15.2 Colour Coding and Type of Container for Disposal of Biomedical Wastes

Colour Coding	Type of Container	Waste Category	Treatment Options as per Schedule I
Yellow	Plastic bag	Cat. 1, Cat. 2, Cat. 3 and Cat. 6	Incineration/deep burial
Red	Disinfected container/ plastic bag	Cat. 3, Cat. 6 and Cat. 7	Autoclaving/microwaving/chemical treatment
Blue/white translucent	Plastic bag/puncture-proof container	Cat. 4 and Cat. 7	Autoclaving/microwaving/chemical treatment and destruction/shredding
Black	Plastic bag	Cat. 5, Cat. 9 and Cat. 10 (solid)	Disposal in secured landfill

Notes: (1) Colour coding of waste categories with multiple treatment options as defined in Schedule I, shall be selected depending on the treatment option chosen, which shall be as specified in Schedule I. (2) Chlorinated plastics should never be utilised for the fabrication of waste collection bags that are used for collecting wastes that need incineration. (3) Category 3 if disinfected locally need not be in containers/bags.

TABLE 15.3 Categories of Biomedical Waste in India

Option	Waste Category	Treatment and Disposal
Category No. 1	Human anatomical waste (Human tissues, organs, body parts)	Incineration[a]/deep burial
Category No. 2	Animal waste (Animal tissues, organs, body parts carcasses, bleeding parts, fluids, veterinary hospitals and colleges, discharge from hospital, animal house)	Incineration[a]/deep burial
Category No. 3	Microbiology and biotechnology waste (Waste from laboratory cultures, stocks or specimens of microorganisms, live or attenuated vaccines, human and animal cell culture used in research and infectious agents from research and industrial laboratories, waste from production of biological, toxins, dishes and devices and for transfer of cultures)	Local autoclaving/microwaving/ incineration[a]
Category No. 4	Waste sharps (Needles, syringes, scalpels, blades, glass, etc. that may cause puncture and cuts. This includes both used and unused sharps).	Disinfection (chemical treatment[b]/autoclaving/microwaving and mutilation shredding)
Category No. 5	Discarded medicines and cytotoxic drugs (Wastes comprising of outdated, contaminated and discarded medicines)	Incineration[b] destruction and drugs disposal in secured landfills
Category No. 6	Solid waste (Items contaminated with blood and fluids including cotton, dressings, soiled plaster casts, lines, beddings, other material contaminated with blood)	Incineration[b] autoclaving/ microwaving
Category No. 7	Solid waste (Wastes generated from disposable items other than the waste sharps such as tubings, catheters, intravenous sets, etc.)	Disinfection by chemical treatment[c] autoclaving/microwaving and mutilation/shredding[d]
Category No. 8	Liquid waste (Waste generated from laboratory and washing, cleaning, house-keeping and disinfecting activities)	Disinfection by chemical treatment[c] and discharge into drains
Category No. 9	Incineration ash (Ash from incineration of any biomedical waste)	Disposal in municipal landfill
Category No. 10	Chemicals used in production of biological, chemicals used in disinfection, as insecticides, etc.	Chemical treatment[c] and discharge into drains for liquids and secured landfill for solids

[a]Deep burial shall be an option available only in towns with population less than 5 lakhs and in rural areas.
[b]There will be no chemical pretreatment before incineration. Chlorinated plastics shall not be incinerated.
[c]Chemical treatment using least 1% hypochlorite solution or any equipment chemical reagent. It is necessary to ensure that chemical treatment disinfects.
[d]Mutilation/shredding must be such so as to prevent unauthorised reuse.

Non-biohazardous materials

- Head caps, masks
- X-ray films, and impression materials
- Matrix bands, dental plaster casts, Alginate

Sharps

Objects such as needles, syringes, lancets (sharps) and other sharp objects used for medical purposes should be placed in medical sharps container or a heavy plastic or metal container. The sharps container should be puncture-proof with a tight-fitting lid.

Infectious waste

Infectious wastes are collected in metallic containers, decontaminated and then disposed. The metallic container is autoclaved for reuse.

Chapter 16

Suture Materials and Suturing Techniques

OUTLINE

INTRODUCTION

The purpose of a suture is to hold tissues in apposition until the wound has healed sufficiently to be self-supportive. The art of suturing wounds is by no means a recent endeavour. Unique methods of closing wounds have existed in many ancient cultures. Galen (AD 75) was the first to experiment with catgut. In 1869, Lord Joseph Lister developed the concept of both impregnating chromic acid in catgut and sterilising suture materials. Halsted proclaimed the advantages of silk over catgut in the early part of the 20th century and, as a result, silk soon became the most common suture material in surgical practice. Today, a wide array of suture materials and needles are available and it is essential to be aware of the basic properties in conjunction with proper suturing techniques to maximise the outcome of any oral surgical procedure.

Sutures function primarily to maintain wound closure and to promote wound healing during the time when the wound is most vulnerable. The wound healing process can be affected by the amount of suture material used, suture type, the suturing technique and amount of tension in the suture.

IDEAL REQUIREMENTS FOR SUTURE MATERIALS

1. It should have high tensile strength to hold the wound margins appropriately till the healing is complete
   a. Tensile strength of the suture material is the tension it can withstand without breaking. It is directly proportional to the diameter of the suture
2. It should not be allergic or cause any tissue inflammation
3. It should have the least capillarity to avoid retaining the inflammatory transudate at the wound
4. It should have good knot stability
5. It should be easily sterilised
6. It should be visible in the surgical field
7. It should be affordable.

BIOLOGICAL RESPONSE OF TISSUES TO SUTURE MATERIALS

A cellular response occurs whenever a foreign object is implanted in living tissue. This response is generally very mild with most surgical sutures, though marked if complicated by infection or trauma. If uncomplicated, the acute response usually changes in about 3 days and the original population of neutrophils is replaced by predominantly monocytes, plasma cells and lymphocytes.

SIZE OF THE SUTURE MATERIALS

The suture materials are available in various sizes depending upon its tensile strength. The standard for identifying varying tensile strengths of a given suture material is determined by the number of zeros. The smaller the cross-sectional diameter, the more zeros the suture has. Sizes start with zero and the diameter decreases with increasing number (1-0, 2-0,... 10-0). Thus, 4-0 nylon has a greater diameter than 6-0 nylon and therefore, a greater tensile strength.

CLASSIFICATION

Sutures can be conveniently classified into the following groups (Table 16.1):
- Natural, metallic and synthetic
- Absorbable and nonabsorbable
- Monofilament and multifilament
- Coated and noncoated
- Knotting of the sutures.

ABSORBABLE SUTURES

These are suture materials that are digested or hydrolysed by the enzymes present in the body or by other mechanisms. Thus, they require no removal from the surgical site. The actual dissolution time of the suture material depends on material type, tissue blood supply, tissue structure and degree of fluid accumulation on suture material.
- Natural
- Synthetic

TABLE 16.1 Suturing Materials—Monofilament and Multifilament

Suture Material	Absorbable	Nonabsorbable
Monofilament	Surgical gut (plain and chromic)	Nylon/polyamide
	Collagen (plain and chromic)	Polypropylene
	Monocryl	Stainless steel
	Polydioxanone II (PDS II)	Polyester
	Polyglactin 910	Polyvinylidene fluoride (PVDF)
Multifilament	Polyglycolic acid	Surgical silk
		Surgical linen
	Polyglactin 910-Rapide	Cotton
		Nylon/polyamide braided
	Polyglactin 910	Polyester braided
		Stainless steel

NONABSORBABLE SUTURES

These materials cannot be metabolised by the body's natural mechanism. Therefore, they should be removed by the surgeon at the end of healing or not removed and left in place if used for repair of vascular/neural structures.
- Natural
- Metallic—gold, silver, titanium, and stainless steel
- Synthetic

MONOFILAMENT SUTURES

- This consists of a single strand of suture material
- Advantages: Monofilament sutures are smoother and stronger. They do not allow any bacteria to survive
- Disadvantages: Monofilament sutures cannot be handled like multifilament sutures. They have to be handled properly and delicately without any damage to the strand during surgical procedures to avoid any breakage postoperatively.

MULTIFILAMENT SUTURES

This consists of several filaments twisted or braided together, can be coated to allow smooth movement into tissues. Multifilament sutures are generally easier to tie and handle than monofilament sutures, but they can harbour bacteria and are not suitable in the presence of contamination and infection. This transfer of microbes from the oral cavity through the multiple filaments into deeper tissue is known as the ***'wicking effect'***.

COATED SUTURES

Polyester sutures are coated with biologically inert compounds. These nonresorbable layers can lubricate the braids, allowing smooth movement of the suture through the tissues, but cause difficulty in knotting, thus requiring multiple knots.

ABSORBABLE SUTURE MATERIALS

NATURAL ABSORBABLE SUTURE MATERIALS

CATGUT

Types: Fast absorbing gut, plain gut, chromic gut

This natural product, also called surgical gut, is made of collagen harvested from the submucosal layer of the small intestine of sheep and the serosal layer of cattle's small intestine (cattle intima). Although used for centuries, it is gradually fading from use because gut suture material has poor tensile strength, poor in vivo knot stability and high tissue reactivity. However, gut that is soaked in chromic acid salts will usually have a delayed absorption time, better tensile strength and a reduction in tissue reactivity compared with untreated catgut. Gut usually retains its strength for 2–3 weeks. Fast absorbing gut is a newer form of catgut not treated with chromic salts. This can also be used as a percutaneous suture in split-thickness skin grafts or in children where it is difficult to remove sutures. One can usually find a synthetic material preferable to catgut. This is because the newer synthetic materials have substantially decreased tissue reactions and have more predictable absorption. Catgut undergoes resorption by proteolysis (proteolytic enzymes). It is not recommended to be used for mucosal intraoral suturing (Fig. 16.1A).

SYNTHETIC ABSORBABLE MATERIALS

POLYGLYCOLIC ACID—DEXON

This polymer of glycolic acid, introduced in 1970, was the first synthetic absorbable suture material to become available. It was renowned for its excellent tensile strength and knot stability. In addition, it has delayed absorption and diminished tissue reactivity compared to catgut. The absorption of polyglycolic acid is by hydrolysis when compared to the proteolytic absorption of catgut.

COATED POLYGLACTIN 910—VICRYL

- Vicryl, introduced in 1974, was the next synthetic material to be marketed
- Composition: 90% glycolide, 10% lactide, coating with 35% glycolide and 65% lactide. Polyglactin 910 suture is a copolymer of lactide and glycolide, manufactured with a coating of polyglactin 370 and calcium stearate. This lubricant coating provides Vicryl its excellent handling and smooth tie down properties
- Vicryl is degraded by hydrolysis like all synthetic polyesters and thus, causes minimal tissue reaction
- Vicryl is braided and comes in either a clear undyed or violet-dyed form (Fig. 16.1B)
- Vicryl plus: It is an antibacterial suture with Triclosan. Contraindicated in ophthalmic, cardiovascular and neural tissues
- Vicryl Rapide: The Vicryl suture is exposed to gamma radiation, which reduces the molecular weight to less than that of coated Vicryl. It is available only in the undyed natural form. It loses its tensile strength by the 12th day and gets absorbed within 42 days. Indicated for mucosal and skin wounds where healing is complete within 10 days.

POLIGLECAPRONE 25—MONOCRYL

- Composition: 75% glycolide and 25% caprolactone
- Very pliable, flexible and outstanding handling properties. Tensile strength is lost by 3 weeks and resorbs by 120 days. It is best for subcutaneous suturing.

POLYDIOXANONE—PDS II

Polydioxanone is a polymer made from paradioxanone and was marketed as having prolonged tensile strength in vivo compared with Vicryl or Dexon. Therefore, PDS can prove useful in situations where extended wound tensile strength is required. Polydioxanone is hydrolysed more slowly than other synthetic absorbables. Complete absorption occurs about 180 days after implantation, but its foreign body reactions were found to be minimal. A disadvantage of using PDS is that it is more difficult to use than the braided synthetics because of intrinsic stiffness. Polydioxanone II is a newer product that has decreased stiffness and smoother handling characteristics than PDS while keeping the original tensile strength qualities (Fig. 16.1C).

POLYTRIMETHYLENE CARBONATE—MAXON

This synthetic monofilament is the newest absorbable material prepared from polyglyconate, a copolymer of glycolic acid and trimethylene carbonate. It was developed to combine the

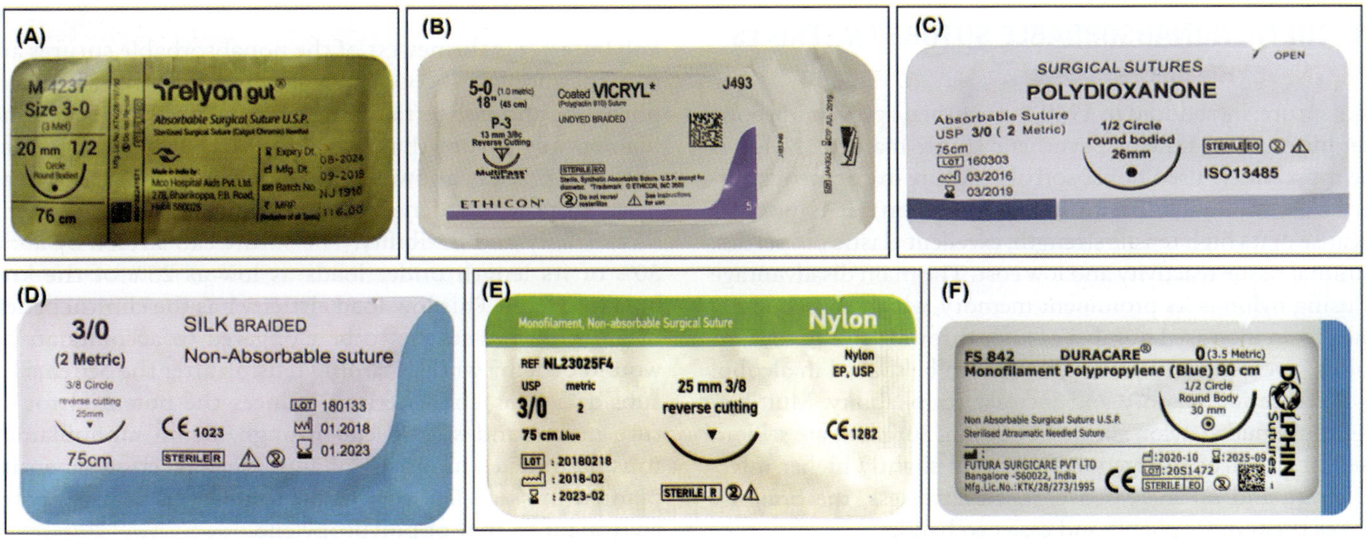

Figure 16.1 (A) Chromic gut. (B) Polyglactic acid (Vicryl). (C) Polydioxanone (PDS). (D) Silk. (E) Nylon. (F) Polypropylene.

excellent tensile strength knot stability of PDS with improved handling properties. Maxon provides wound support over an extended period of time. Maxon is much more supple and manageable than PDS with 60% less rigidity and minimal memory. Although the cost of Maxon is more than Vicryl or Dexon, its improved strength and handling characteristics make it the absorbable suture material of choice.

NONABSORBABLE SUTURE MATERIALS

Nonabsorbable sutures are generally defined as filamentous materials that are resistant to the degradation mechanisms of living mammalian tissue. However, the term nonabsorbable is relative because many of these sutures are eventually degraded.

NATURAL NONABSORBABLE SUTURE MATERIALS

SILK

Silk is created from natural protein filaments spun by the silkworm larva as it builds a cocoon. Modern silk is braided, soft and perhaps the easiest suture material to handle and tie. Unfortunately, it has the lowest tensile strength of any material tested. It elicits more inflammatory reaction than any other suture except catgut. Silk also has a high capillary quality due to its braiding pattern and should be avoided in areas prone to infection (i.e., distal extremities). In cutaneous surgery, it can be used around the eyelids and lips, where it lies flat, causes minimal irritation and has a low potential for infection (Fig. 16.1D).

LINEN

Linen is a cellulose material made from flax. It is twisted to form a fibre to make a suture. Tissue reaction is similar to silk and the material has good knot stability. It gains 10% tensile strength when wet and is fairly unique in this respect. It is widely used for tying pedicles and as ligatures. It has excellent knotting properties.

SYNTHETIC NONABSORBABLE SUTURE MATERIALS

NYLON—ETHILON

This suture, introduced in 1940, is a synthetic polyamide polymer fibre and was the first synthetic suture material. Nylon is the most widely used nonabsorbable suture in cutaneous surgery as a monofilament (Ethilon, Dermalon). It is popular because of its high tensile strength, excellent elastic properties, minimal tissue reactivity and low cost. The main disadvantage of using nylon is its prominent memory, which subsequently leads to an increased number of knot throws (three to four) to hold a given stitch in place. Ethilon can be soaked in alcohol to decrease its memory and increase its pliability. Multifilamentous braided nylon sutures (Nurolon, Surgilon) are seldom used in cutaneous surgery because of a slightly higher infection rate and an increased cost. Nevertheless, the braiding makes them more pliable and easier to handle.

Although nylon is classified as a nonabsorbable suture, it still encounters partial degradation through hydrolysis at a very slow rate. Thus, nylon would be more appropriately classified as a slowly absorbable suture than as a nonabsorbable suture. A study comparing clear monofilament nylon and polyglycolic acid in buried sutures demonstrated less clinical inflammatory response with nylon (Fig. 16.1E).

POLYPROPYLENE (PROLENE, SURGILENE)

Polypropylene is a plastic suture formed by the polymerisation of propylene by means of a catalyst. Prolene is an extremely inert suture whose tissue reactivity and tensile strength are comparable to that of nylon. It has a very smooth surface with low adherence to tissue, which is ideal for a subcuticular intradermal suture because it tends to slide out smoothly at the time of suture removal. Its extreme smoothness does compromise knot security and extra throws are required to compensate for this drawback. Prolene is especially noted for its plasticity. When swelling occurs, this suture will stretch to accommodate the wound, thus there will be little cutting through the tissue. When wound swelling recedes, the suture will remain loose (Fig. 16.1F).

BRAIDED POLYESTERS (MERSILENE, DACRON)

Polyester fibres are polymers that are formed as nylon by condensation polymerisation. Braided polyesters were manufactured to provide the same high tensile strength and low tissue reactivity as the monofilaments, but with improved qualities in handling and knot security. Polyester sutures are either coated or uncoated. Mersilene and Dacron are uncoated braided polyesters with a rough surface that produces drag when pulled through tissues and when knots are set. In order to ameliorate this problem, coated polyesters such as Ethibond were developed. They are not commonly used as they are expensive and the coating susceptibility to "cracking" after knots are tied.

POLYBUTESTER

Polybutester is the newest of the nonabsorbable sutures and is a thermoplastic copolymer composed of butylene terephthalate and polytetramethylene ether glycol. It is a monofilamentous suture that was designed to be stronger, less stiff and possess a lower coefficient of friction than either nylon or polypropylene. A unique feature of polybutester is its elasticity and flexibility. The suture can stretch by about 50% of its length under loads as low as 25% of the knot breaking level. This low-load elsticity has the clinical benefit of allowing the suture to be elongated to accomodate for wound oedema while retaining tension after the oedema has subsided. This characteristic reduces the potential for suture marks and suture cut-through. Being monofilamentous, it induces minimal inflammatory reaction when implanted in skin. The cost of polybutester is approximately equivalent to that of polypropylene.

A comparison of all suture materials is elaborated in Tables 16.2 and 16.3.

TABLE 16.2 Comparison of Resorbable Suture Materials (Popular Brand Name Given in UPPERCASE)

Sutures	Material	Natural/ Synthetic	Construction	Material Colour		Absorption Time	Absorption Process
FAST ABSORBING GUT suture	Beef serosa or sheep submucosa	Natural	Monofilament (virtual)	Yellowish tan	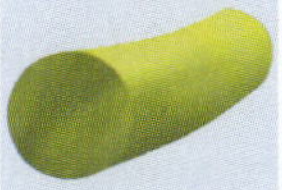	21–45 days	Proteolytic enzymatic digestion
PLAIN GUT suture				Yellowish tan		70 days	
CHROMIC GUT suture				Brown or blue	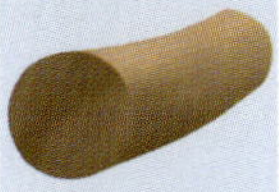 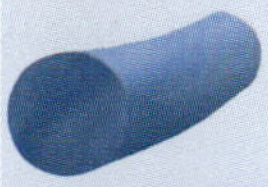	90 days	
Coated VICRYL RAPIDE suture	Polyglactin 910	Synthetic	Braided	Violet or undyed (natural beige)	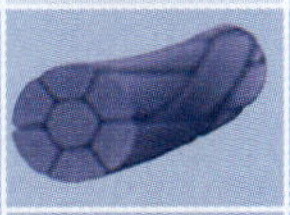	42 days	Hydrolysis
Coated VICRYL suture			Braided		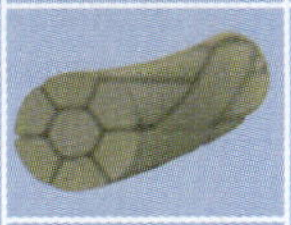	56–70 days (63-days avg.)	
Coated VICRYL PLUS suture					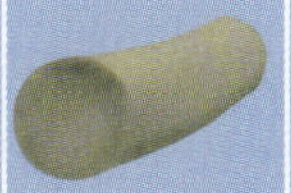		
Coated VICRYL suture			Monofilament				
Undyed Poliglecaprone 25 suture MONOCRYL	Poliglecaprone 25-75% glycolide and 25% caprolactone	Synthetic	Monofilament	Undyed (natural)	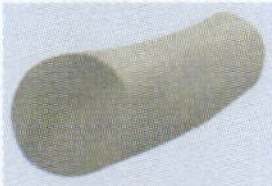	91–119 days	Hydrolysis
Dyed Poliglecaprone 25 suture MONOCRYL				Violet	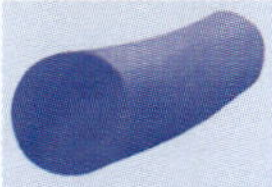		
PDS II suture	Polydioxanone	Synthetic	Monofilament	Violet or clear	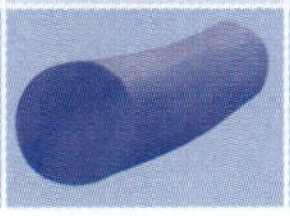	180–210 days	Slow hydrolysis

NEEDLES

Needles are made of either stainless steel or carbon steel. There are basically two shapes of needles—straight and curved needles (Fig. 16.2B and C).

1. **Straight needles**
   a. Types
      i. Round bodied—circular or oblong in cross-section and gradually tapers to a point
      ii. Taper cut—triangular in cross-section and are sharp enough to finely pass through keratinised mucosa
   b. Uses
      i. For closure of thoracic, iliac or abdominal region
      ii. In maxillofacial surgery, the needle is used for the passage of circummandibular or circumzygomatic wires
2. **Curved needles**
   a. Curved needle is usually used for skin and mucous membrane surgery. The curvatures come in various types such as 1/4, 3/8, 1/2 and 5/8 (Fig. 16.2D)
   b. Types (Fig. 16.2E)
      i. Round bodied
      ii. Taper cut
      iii. Conventional cutting—has one of the three cutting edges on the internal surface of the needle
      iv. Reverse cutting—the internal surface is flat. It is the most popularly used needle
   c. Uses
      i. Tapered needles are used for closing muscle or fascia
      ii. Cutting needle is used for keratinised mucosa, skin or subcuticular layers where the tissue is difficult to penetrate

TABLE 16.3 Comparison of Nonresorbable Suture Materials (Popular Brand Name Given in UPPERCASE)

Sutures	Material	Natural/ Synthetic	Construction	Material Colour	
SURGICAL STEEL suture	316 L Stainless steel	Natural alloy	Monofilament	Metallic silver	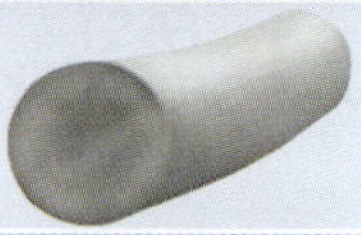
Nylon suture ETHILON	Polyamide 6	Synthetic	Monofilament	Black or green or clear	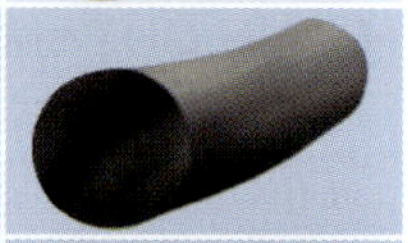
Braided nylon suture NUROLON	Polyamide 6	Synthetic	Braided	Black	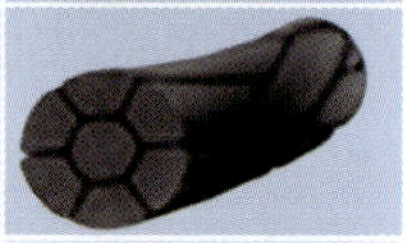
Silk suture MERSILK, PERMA-HAND, SUTUPAK	Silk filaments spun from cocoon of silkworm	Natural	Braided	Black or white	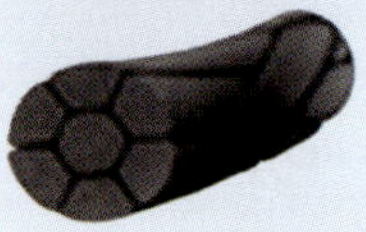 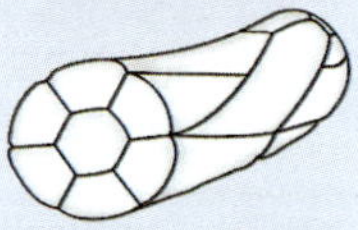
Polyester fibre suture MERSILENE	Polyester/Dacron	Synthetic	Braided	Green or white	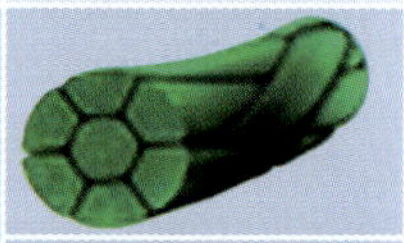 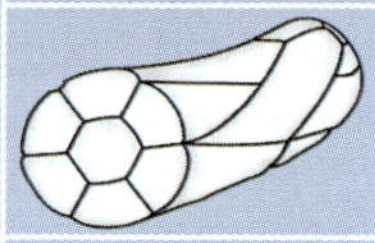
Polyester fibre suture ETHIBOND EXCEL	Polyester/Dacron	Synthetic	Monofilament	Green	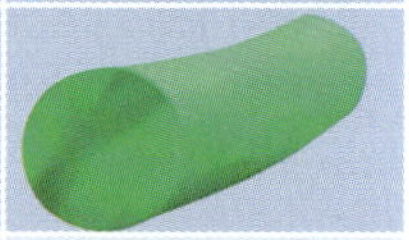
Polypropylene suture PROLENE	Polypropylene	Synthetic	Monofilament	Blue or clear	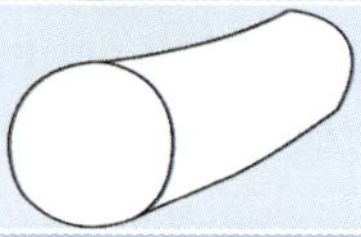
Poly-hexafluoropropylene-VDF PRONOVA	Polymer blend of polyvinylidene fluoride and polyvinylidene fluoride-co-hexafluoro polypropylene	Synthetic	Monofilament	Blue or clear	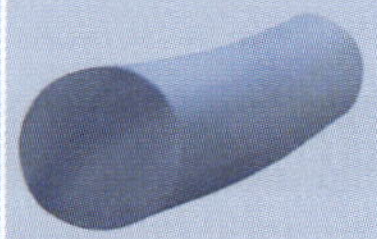

3. Another type of classification that is commonly used (Fig. 16.2A)
   a. Eyed needles: These needles can be reused. The suture material is tied in the eye of the needle and passed through the tissue. Since the eye is larger than the diameter of the suture material, the needle causes tissue trauma. Split-eyed needle used for easy threading and release of suture is also available
   b. Eyeless (swaged) needles: In this type of needle, the suture material is inserted into the needle hollow during manufacturing and the metal is compressed to seal around the suture material. These needles cannot be reused. Eyeless needles are ideal for use in surgery as they cause minimal tissue trauma. Different shapes and types of eyeless needles are available and are required for various surgical procedures
4. Advantages of eyeless needles
   a. They are also called atraumatic needles since they cause minimal trauma to the tissue during suturing (single strand of thread throughout the surgical tissues causing minimal tissue disruption compared to the double strands of the eyed needle)
   b. No need of prior sterilisation, since it is supplied as a presterilised pack

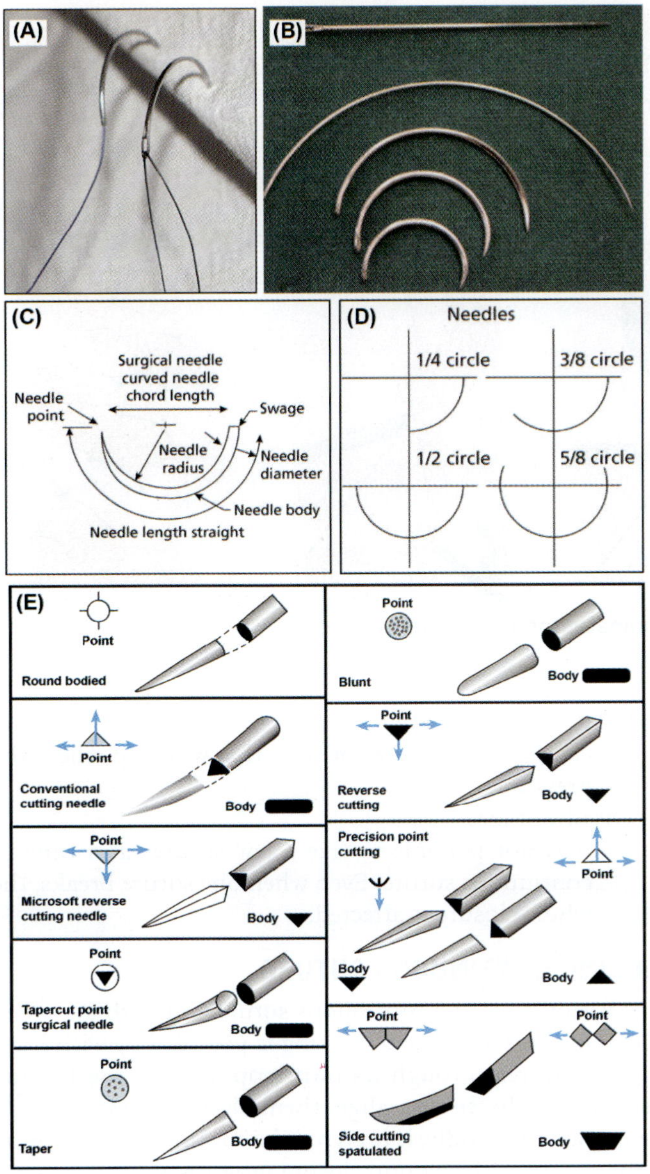

Figure 16.2 **(A)** Eyed and eyeless (swaged) needles. **(B)** Surgical needles. **(C)** Parts of a surgical needle. **(D** and **E)** Types of curved needle.

c. Disposable after single use, hence hygienic and no issues of loss of sharpness
d. Sharp tip helps in precise and efficient completion of suturing
e. Less time-consuming when compared to eyed needles, no need of sterilising and threading the needle
f. No issue of accidental unthreading of the needle during surgery.

PRINCIPLES OF SUTURING

1. The needle should be grasped with the help of needle holders at approximately three-fourths of its distance from the tip of the needle
2. The needle should never be held at the swage as it is the weakest point of the needle and grasping at this point results in either bending or breakage of the needle
3. The needle should pierce the tissue perpendicular to its surface, as piercing the tissue obliquely may result in a tear
4. The curved needles should be passed through the tissues following the curvature of the needle to prevent tearing of the tissues
5. The suture should be placed equidistant (2–3 mm) from the incision line. The depth of penetration should also be equal on both sides of the line
6. The needle should be passed from mobile tissue to the fixed tissue
7. When one side of the tissue is thinner than the other side, then the needle should pass from the thinner to the thicker side
8. Similarly, when one side is deeper and the other side is superficial, the needle should pass through the deeper to the superficial side
9. The distance from the incision point to the needle penetration should be less than the depth to which the needle penetrates into the tissues in order to cause eversion of wound margin when the suture is tied
10. The suture should not be tied so tightly that it results in blanching of the tissues. The suture should just approximate the wound margins
11. The knot should not be placed over the wound margins
12. Each suture should be placed 3–4 mm apart. The spacing between the sutures depends upon the type of the tissues, which are approximated. When the sutures are placed upon areas of underlying muscular activity, they should be close to each other
13. When the length of tissue on one side of the wound is longer than the other, suturing it would result in dog-ear formation. In order to eliminate this, the excessive tissue should be undermined and an incision at approximately 30 degrees to the original incision is directed at the undermined tissue. The extra tissue is pulled over the incision, the appropriate amount is excised and the wound is closed (Fig. 16.3)
14. The choice of suture material, needle and type of suturing depends on:
    a. Location of the wound
    b. Thickness of the wound edges
    c. Tension exerted on the wound
    d. Approximation of the wound edges
    e. Any additional requirements such as haemostasis, cosmetic needs, etc.

SUTURING TECHNIQUES

SIMPLE INTERRUPTED SUTURE

Simple interrupted suture is the most commonly used suturing technique. The sutures are placed independently. The

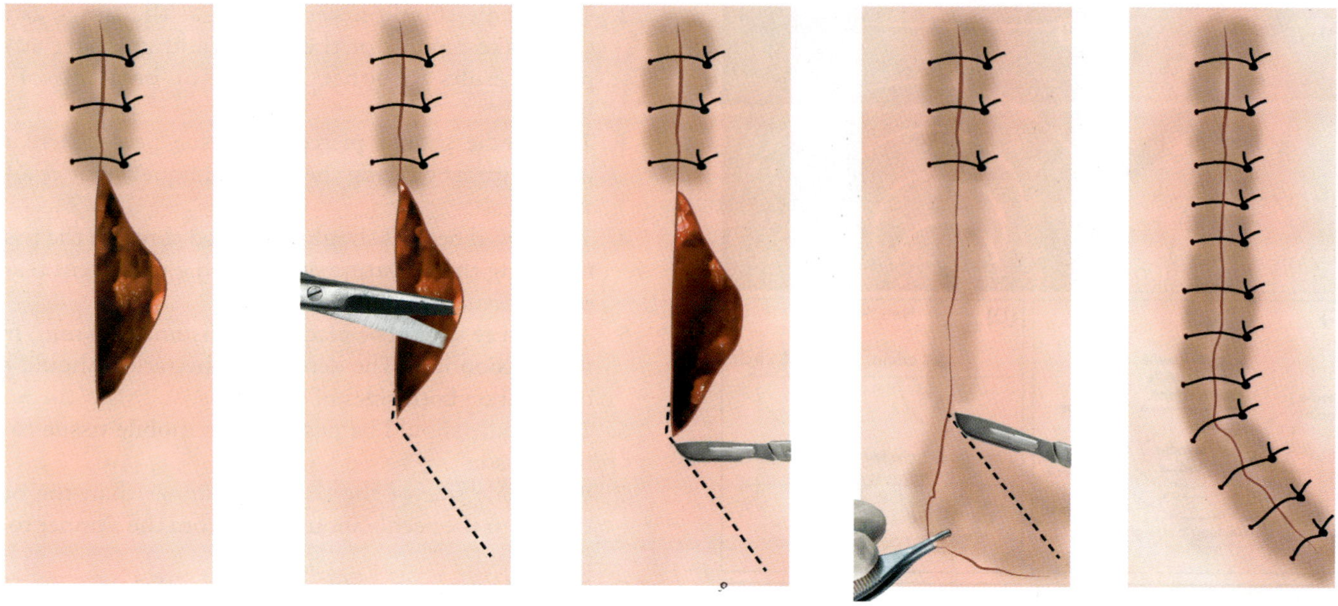

Figure 16.3 Suturing method to eliminate dog-ear formation.

distance between each suture and the incision line can be varied according to necessity and convenience. This suture provides great strength (Fig. 16.4A).

- **Advantages:**
  a. Selective adjustments of wound edges can be made
  b. Failure of one suture does not necessarily prejudice the others
- **Disadvantages:**
  a. Suture marks (rail road track scar appearance on the cutaneous surfaces) after postoperative oedema occurs
  b. Increased knots reduce 50% of the strength of the suture.

SIMPLE CONTINUOUS SUTURE

The simple continuous suture provides rapid secure closure with an even distribution of tension along the length of the wound, preventing excess tightness in any one area. This technique also provides additional wound eversion, accomplished by everting the wound edges with fingers or an instrument as the needle enters and exits the skin surface. It provides more watertight closure as required by intraoral bone grafting. It should not be used in areas where there is already existing tension (Fig. 16.4B and C).

- Indications:
  a. Long wounds with minimal wound tension and good wound approximation
  b. To secure split or full thickness grafts
  c. Areas of cosmetic importance as less scarring occurs
  d. Well-approximated wounds with minimal tension that have been initially created by well-placed buried sutures
- Advantages:
  a. The advantage of this method is that it is quick and has fewer knots
  b. If the tissues swell in one area, the remaining suture can provide a degree of slack that will help relieve the pressure
- Disadvantages:
  a. It is not possible to free a few sutures at a time in continuous suture. Even when one suture breaks, the whole closure is affected.

LOCKING CONTINUOUS SUTURE

This is similar to the continuous suture, but with an added advantage that a degree of locking is provided by withdrawing the sutures through its own loop. Due to the locking mechanism, the tissues align themselves perpendicular to the incision. Secondly, it prevents the continuous tightening of the suture as the wound closure progresses.

- Indicated in areas of moderate wound tension with good vascularisation, but requiring additional haemostasis, for example, scalp, postauricular, alveoloplasty (Fig. 16.4D).

MATTRESS SUTURES

Mattress sutures are commonly used in the region of the abdomen or hip and not in the head and neck. Hence, it is useful in closing the wound of iliac and rib bone graft. It provides more tissue eversion than the simple interrupted sutures. Mattress sutures are of two types:

- **Vertical mattress**
- **Horizontal mattress.**

VERTICAL MATTRESS (FIG. 16.4E-G)

Vertical mattress sutures are similar to simple interrupted sutures, but an additional bite through the wound edge is used to ensure edge eversion. This suture is placed by first taking a large bite of the tissue from the wound edge and

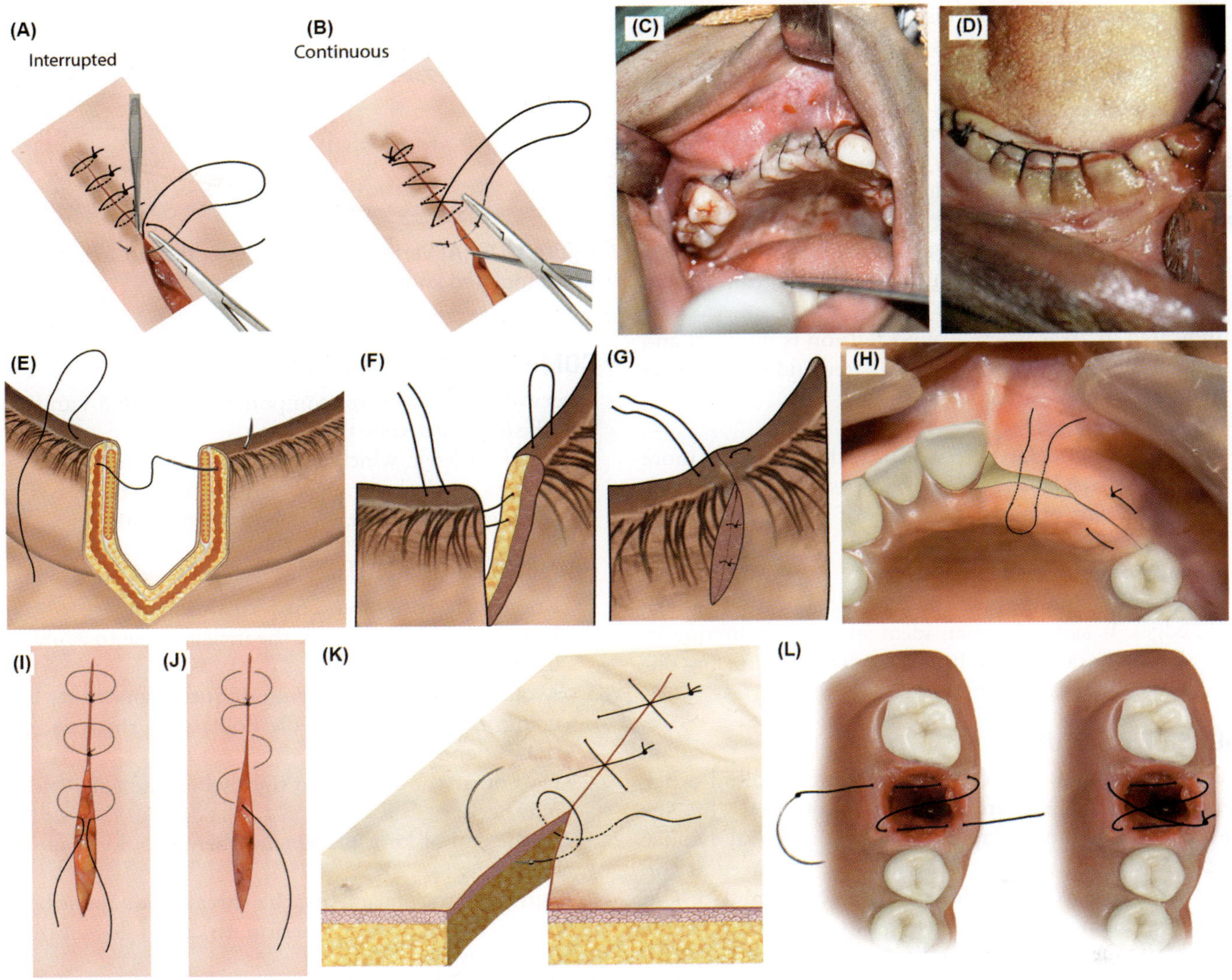

Figure 16.4 Types of suturing—**(A)** Simple interrupted suture. **(B)** Simple continuous suture on a linear incision. **(C)** Simple continuous suturing of an intraoral crestal incision. **(D)** Locking continuous suture for an incision on the alveolar ridge postalveoloplasty. **(E–G)** Vertical mattress suture on the eyelid. **(H)** Horizontal mattress suture on an intraoral incision with some tension. **(I and J)** Subcuticular suture—interrupted and continuous. **(K)** Figure of 8 suture on a laceration. **(L)** Figure of 8 suture on an extracted socket.

crossing through the tissue to an equal distance on opposite side of the wound. The needle is then reversed and returned with a very small bite at the epidermal/dermal edge in order to closely approximate the wound edge.

- Indicated for areas that require wound eversion and to reduce wound tension and to eliminate the dead space
- **Advantages:**
  a. Decreases the dead space and providing increased strength across a wound
  b. Does not interfere with healing as the suture runs parallel to the blood supply
- **Disadvantages:**
  a. Fine wound edge approximation is difficult
  b. Prominent suture marks can form if the sutures are not taken out earlier than in other suturing techniques.

HORIZONTAL MATTRESS

In this technique, eversion and the continuity provide a very versatile closure. Hence, it is often used for intraoral bone grafting. The needle is passed from one edge of the incision to the other and again from the latter to the first edge. The procedure is continued till the entire length of the incision and a knot is then tied which provides strength and wound eversion and hence used in wounds under high tension (Fig. 16.4H).

- **Disadvantages:**
  a. Blood supply to the flap edge may be diminished and can cause necrosis and dehiscence if not used properly.

SUBCUTICULAR SUTURES

This procedure was popularised by Halsted in 1893, who explained that the procedure may be used with no knots by having the ends exit a short distance from the wound and taping them to the skin. In this procedure, the needle penetrates the skin ahead of incision and exits within the wound. Needle is then inserted on the opposite side of the incision in a continuous pattern. At the end of incision, the suture is brought out at a distance from the wound. By pulling both ends of the suture, incision is closed and the suture ends are taped to the skin. For better retention of the sutures, it can be performed with two knots at the beginning and the end of the stitch or interrupted subcuticular sutures can also be given (Fig. 16.4I and J).

- Indicated in areas where wound tension is minimal and dead space has already been eliminated and in areas that require cosmetic correction.
- **Advantages:**
  a. The subcuticular suture can be left in place more than 1 week in areas of wound tension or underneath a cast with minimal problems of suture marks and skin irritation.
- **Disadvantages:**
  a. Time consuming method that does not evert wound edges. It can still be an ideal suturing technique in certain locations of the body where minimising suture marks can be appreciated.

FIGURE OF 8 SUTURES

It is used for the closure of the extraction sites and other intraoral sites that require papillary adaptation. This suture provides a good adaptation of the gingival papilla along the adjacent teeth. For the knot to be placed at the buccal side, the suture should begin at the buccal flap. The first bite is taken at the mesial side of the buccal flap followed by the mesial side of the lingual or palatal flap. The next bite is taken on the distal side of the buccal flap followed by the distal side of the lingual flap. Now the suture ends are knotted with a surgeon's knot. This forms an X shape over the socket, which also acts as a barrier for the socket (Fig. 16.4K and L).

KNOT

A knot is an intertwining of threads for the purpose of joining them. Suture security is the ability of the knot and material to maintain tissue approximation during the healing process. Failure is generally the result of untying due to knot slippage or breakage. Since the knot strength is always less than the tensile strength of the material, the site of disruption is always the knot when force is applied. This is because shear forces produced in the knot lead to breakage. Knot slippage is determined by the nature of the material, suture diameter and type of knot. Monofilament and coated sutures (Teflon, silicone) have a low coefficient of friction and a high degree of slippage whereas braided sutures such as uncoated dacron and catgut have greater knot security because of their coefficient of friction.

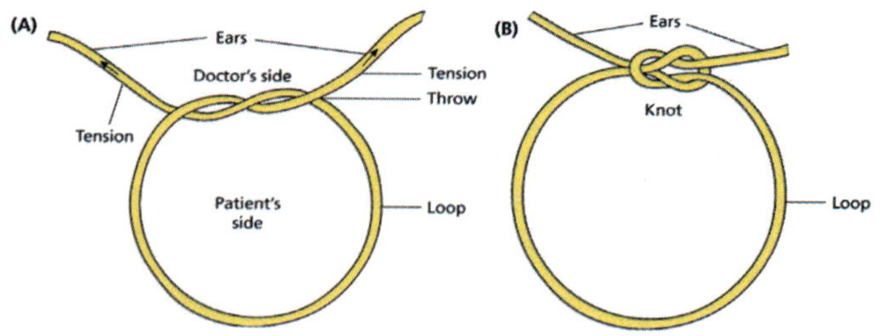

Figure 16.5 **(A)** Various knot components prior to completion. **(B)** Completed knot anatomy.

COMPONENTS OF A KNOT

A sutured knot has three components (Fig. 16.5A and B):

1. The *loop* created by the knot
2. The *knot* itself, which is composed of a number of tight 'throws', each throw represents a weave of the two strands
3. The *ears*, which are the cut ends of the suture.

PRINCIPLES OF KNOT

1. Knot must be tight and firm to avoid slippage
2. Knots should not lie over the incision line to avoid wicking of bacteria
3. Avoid crushing or crimping of suture materials by not using haemostats or needle holders on them except on the free end for tying
4. Do not tie the suture too tightly because tissue necrosis may occur
5. At the end of knot placement, there should be no tissue blanching
6. During knot placement, the thread ends must be kept taut with adequate traction to avoid loosening the first loop
7. Coated and monofilament sutures require additional throws for knot security and to prevent slippage.

TYPES OF KNOTS

- Square knot
- Half-hitch knot
- Granny knot
- Reef knot
- Triple throw knot
- Surgeon's knot
- Buried knot

1. Square knot (Fig. 16.6C): Single loop formed by a clockwise or counterclockwise throw of one thread over the other
2. Half-hitch/slip knot: It is an alternative to the square knot. It is frequently created by incorrect knotting technique, causing a knot that readily slips. The surgeon uses it to remove tension by using it as a slip knot (Fig. 16.6C). However, it is followed by several square knots to prevent slippage of knot
3. Granny knot (Fig. 16.6C): A single loop formed by two throws, both in same direction (clockwise or counterclockwise). It has more holding power than a square knot

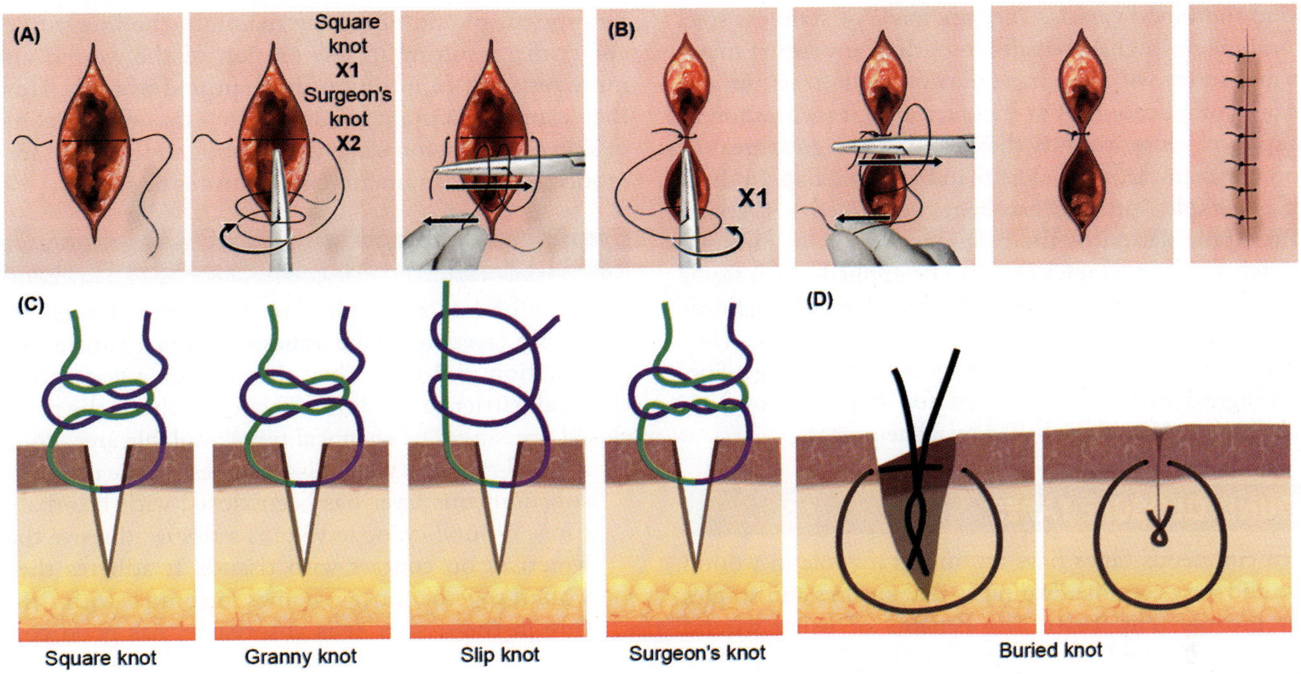

Figure 16.6 (**A** and **B**) Technique of a complete knot, with a needle holder has been illustrated in detail. (**C**) Other sutures have been illustrated—square knot, granny's knot, slip knot or half-hitch knot and surgeon's knot. (**D**) Buried knot.

4. Reef knot (reef = fold, knot used to gather a ship's sail to reef in a strong wind): Loop formed by two throws; first clockwise and second counterclockwise or vice versa
5. Triple throw knot: As the name says, three throws; first two similar to reef knot as a clockwise and counterclockwise throw followed by a third throw similar to the second. This is a more reliable and standard method in surgery
6. The surgeon's knot is a square knot with an extra throw (two clockwise followed by one anticlockwise).

REMOVAL OF SUTURES

Sutures should be removed as atraumatically and cleanly as possible. Principles of suture removal are as follows:

1. The area should be swabbed with hydrogen peroxide for the removal of encrusted necrotic debris, blood and serum from the sutures
2. A sharp suture cutting scissor should be used to cut the loops of individual or continuous sutures. It is often helpful to use a No. 23 explorer to lift the sutures if they are within the sulcus or in close opposition to the tissue. This will avoid tissue damage and unnecessary pain
3. During removal, the cut end of the knot is held gently and the suture is removed towards the incision line. This is to prevent the tension across the wound.

MECHANICAL WOUND CLOSURE METHODS

STAPLES

The principle of using staples in surgery is similar to the paper stapling device (Fig. 16.7). Even though not regularly used in oral and maxillofacial region, staples are often very effective for closing wounds that are at least 5 mm away from

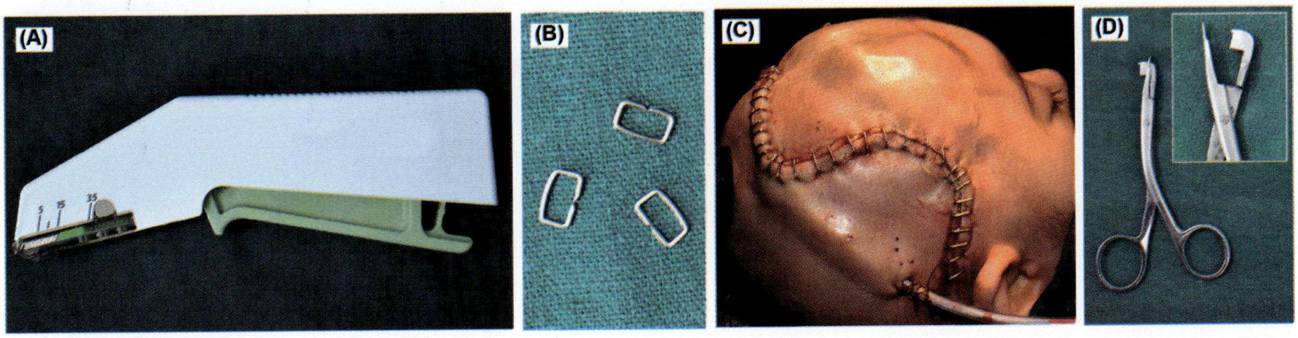

Figure 16.7 (**A**) Stapler-easy to grip cartridge for delivering staples. (**B**) Staple pin. (**C**) Staples used for the closure of bicoronal flap. (**D**) Specially designed extractor for staple removal.

the bone and blood vessels. They are made of stainless steel and combine the highest tensile strength of any suture material in use today with low incidence of tissue reaction and infectious complications. For these reasons, it is common to use staples to close wounds that are under a great deal of tension, for example, scalp closure in bicoronal flap. In these instances, staples provide excellent wound edge eversion without strangulation of the tissue and result in minimal crosshatch scarring. Staples can also be applied much faster than the sutures, which is an advantage in closing long linear wounds. Staples come in two sizes: regular and wide. They are dispensed from a lightweight, easy to grip cartridge. Specially designed extractors are used for staple removal although this can be accomplished by a haemostat.

WOUND CLOSURE TAPES

Modern cutaneous tapes have an important role in wound closure and have certain advantages that sutures and staples cannot provide (Fig. 16.8). The benefits of using wound closure to hold wound edges together is that the skin surface is not penetrated with a needle and iatrogenic trauma is thus minimised. In addition, they maintain the integrity of the epidermis, resulting in less tension to the wound and are more resistant to infection than sutured wounds. However, they cannot maintain adequate deep tissue approximation or skin edge eversion when used alone and therefore are commonly used in conjunction with sutures or staples.

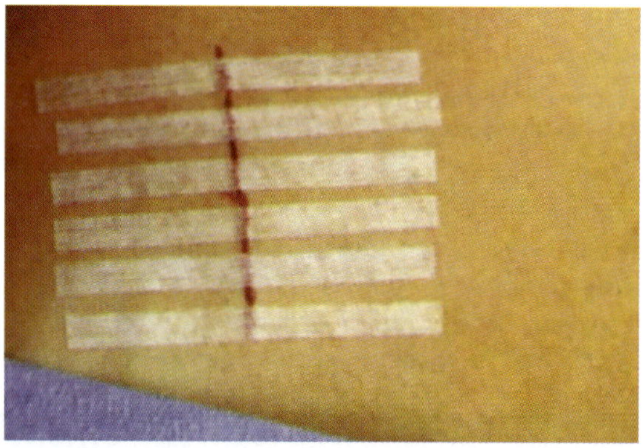

Figure 16.8 Wound closure tapes used at the incision sites.

TISSUE ADHESIVES

Tissue adhesives are applied to dry skin in layers. At least three thin layers of tissue adhesive offers a suture—free approximation in 3 min. They also provide a waterproof mechanical barrier to ward off infection without the need for a closed dressing. The chemical types available are:

1. n-Butyl-cyanoacrylate: Tissue adhesives are used after the subcutaneous layer has been closed with resorbable sutures. n-Butyl-cyanoacrylate is a tissue adhesive that polymerises on contact with tissues. It adheres the open wound together once it comes in contact with the moisture in the tissues. It is absorbable, has good cosmetic results and acts as a haemostatic agent also
2. 2-Octyl cyanoacrylate: It has a long carbon chain and has a three-dimensional strength. It is stronger than n-butyl-cyanoacrylate, but both adhesives have a plasticiser and a nontoxic transparent bond
3. Silicone tissue adhesives with silicone elastomers are being prepared for the same use.

THIN FILM POLYMER SPRAY (LIQUID BANDAGE)

Frequently called as liquid bandage, it consists of a polymer dissolved in alcohol or water, antiseptic and local anaesthetic. It is packed in an airtight container with high air pressure, as this allows the formation of a thin film over abrasions. It cannot be used over lacerations. Polyvinylpyrrolidone, ethyl cellulose, pyroxylin/nitrocellulose or poly methyl acrylate-isobutene-monoisopropyl maleate and acrylate are used.

Section VI

Minor Oral Surgery

Principles of Minor Oral Surgery

OUTLINE

INTRODUCTION

Minor oral surgery definition: A surgical procedure that can be comfortably done by a competent nonspecialised dental surgeon within 30 min under local anaesthesia with or without sedation. Minor oral surgery includes hard tissue procedures such as removal of tooth or root piece, impacted tooth and cysts of the upper and lower jaws as well as soft tissue procedures such as removal of high labial or lingual frenum, mucocele, ranula, etc. in the oral cavity.

The decision to ensure surgery should be the result of several diagnostic processes. The 1st step towards treating any patient is making a correct diagnosis. The diagnostic sequence is divided into five steps:

1. History taking
2. Clinical examination
3. Radiological analysis
4. Laboratory investigations, interpretation
5. Final diagnosis.

The 1st four steps aid in attaining a clinical database, which is interpreted by the clinician to arrive at a final diagnosis (refer to Chapter 3 for steps in history taking). Therefore, the decision of whether surgery is indicated or not is only made after a complete logical analysis of all the available data.

In the modern era, it is accepted that all surgeries should be painless. The most important aspect of patient care is pain management. The advancement in anaesthetic agents and techniques is probably the most significant progress that has occurred in dental science, enabling the profession to make remarkable therapeutic advances that would otherwise not be possible.

The choice between general and local anaesthesia will depend on surgical as well as medical considerations and the decision should be made jointly with the anaesthetist when doubt persists (Boxes 17.1–17.2). The anaesthetist and the patient may regularly have to be guided as to which is better in particular circumstances. For the convenience of the patient, the surgeon must strive to achieve local anaesthesia using block anaesthesia wherever possible. Various techniques of dental anaesthesia are illustrated in Fig. 17.1. A variety of novel anaesthetic agents comprising eutectic mixtures of anaesthetics, anaesthetic delivery devices, which use pressure and vibration and supplemental anaesthesia into the osseous tissue have been introduced to lessen the pain and reduce the area to be anaesthetised. Thus, decreasing the failure rates of achieving local anaesthesia and the unwanted residual effects of the anaesthesia (refer to chapter 57 page number 1053–1055).

BOX 17.1 Factors influencing the choice of Local Anaesthetic Technique

1. The area to be anaesthetised
2. Extent of the surgical procedures
3. Duration of the anaesthesia required
4. Haemostasis
5. Presence of infection
6. Age of the patient

BOX 17.2 Indications of General Anaesthesia

- Acute and subacute infections
- <4 years old patient
- Surgery involving several quadrants of the mouth
- Long surgical procedures
- Emergency treatment
- Patient with special safety needs
- Patient with extreme phobia and anxiety
- ASA III patients

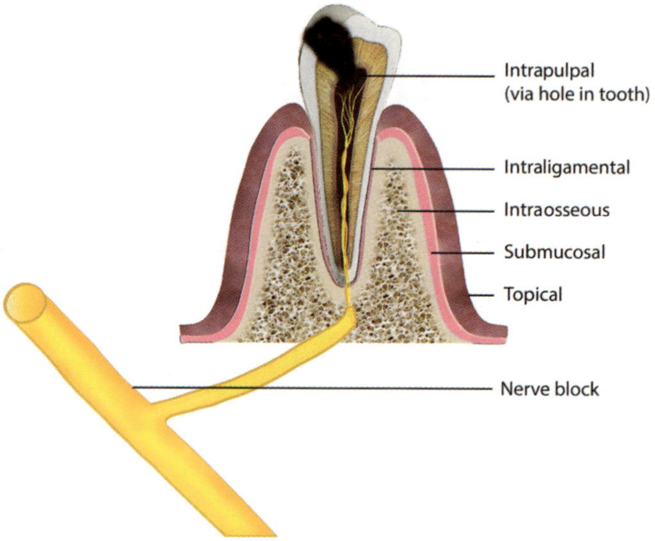

Figure 17.1 Dental anaesthesia techniques.

ASEPSIS

Asepsis is the elimination of microorganisms from the operative field to prevent them from entering the wound. Various measures are taken to maintain asepsis prior to minor surgical procedures such as preoperative scaling, preparing the patient skin and oral cavity with antiseptic solution to eliminate the bacterial load. Sterilised instruments used in the surgical field must be handled under complete aseptic techniques. Aseptic techniques to be followed under minor surgical procedures are described in Chapter 15 page number 267.

ADEQUATE ACCESS

Efficient surgery depends on (1) adequate access, (2) adequate visibility, (3) proper lighting, (4) effective evacuation device and (5) well-trained assistant.

Adequate access is achieved by:

- Surgically created exposure (incision)
- Patient's mouth opening
- An incision is a cut or wound made intentionally by an operator in the skin or mucosa using a sharp instrument, such as surgical blade/electrocautery, to expose the underlying structure tissue so that a surgical procedure can be performed
- Proper access to the site is gained via proper planning of incision. Thorough anatomical knowledge is required before placing an incision.

PRINCIPLES OF WOUND INCISION

1. The surgical site has to be maintained in a sterile and aseptic condition
2. The length and direction of incision
   a. To permit sufficient operating space and optimum exposure
   b. The direction of wound healing naturally is from side-to-side, not end-to-end
   c. The arrangement of tissue fibres in the area to be dissected varies with tissue type
   d. The best cosmetic results when incision is made in the direction of the tissue fibres
3. The incision should be placed along the **relaxed skin tension lines (Langer's line)** (Fig. 17.2)
   a. These are the skin lines that are oriented perpendicular to the direction of the underlying muscle fibres
   b. It is determined by the examination of patient's natural skin creases at rest
4. Fusiform excision
   a. Performed with longitudinal axis running parallel to the Langer's lines
   b. The length should be four times the width of the defect to produce an accurate approximation of skin edges without **dog-ear** formation
   c. **Dog ears** refer to the areas of redundant skin and subcutaneous tissue resulting from a wound margin being longer on one side than the other; it can be corrected by
      i. Incremental oblique placement of sutures
      ii. Fusiform excision of the dog ear, which lengthens the scar considerably
5. Basic surgical skills of wound incision
   a. Marking of important landmarks
   b. Application of a gentle traction to the skin to avoid wrinkles
   c. The operator should not direct the incision in an outward direction
   d. A single firm continuous stroke through the subcutaneous fat should be used with cross hatches with ink or marking pen for accurate wound closure
   e. Cuts in different planes should be avoided.

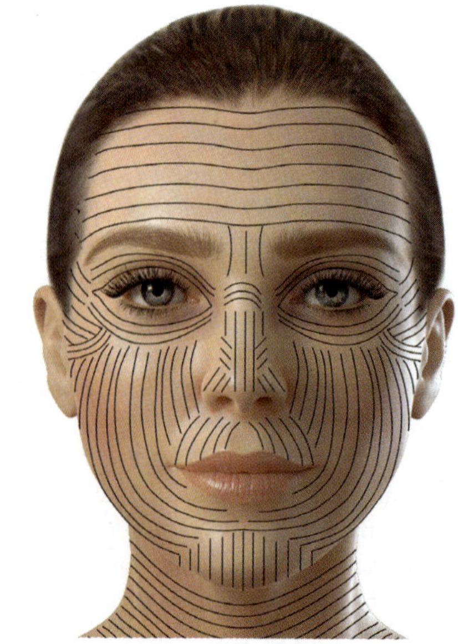

Figure 17.2 Langer lines—relaxed skin crease line.

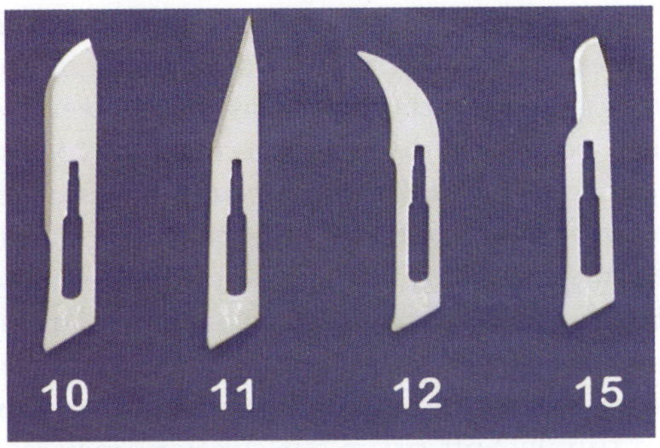

Figure 17.3 Common surgical blades used in oral surgery.

Common surgical blades used in oral surgery (Fig. 17.3)**:**

- No. 15: Most commonly used for intraoral procedures. It is used to make incisions around teeth and through soft tissue
- No. 12: Hooked blade, designed especially for incisions performed distal to posterior teeth (retromolar, tuberosity)
- No. 11: Sharp and pointed, best for stab incisions such as incision and drainage
- No. 10: Used for extraoral skin incisions.

TYPES OF BLADE GRASP

Palmar grip: Scalpel is held with the index finger over the upper border of the handle between the thumb, middle, ring and fifth fingers with the handle grabbed in the palm. This grip is used for making incisions through tough tissues. The periosteal elevator is also held in a similar manner (Fig. 17.4).

Pen grip: Scalpel is held as a pen and used in making small, precision cuts where the handle lies over the palm. The movement is given from the fingers to make fine cuts (Fig. 17.5).

Fingertip grip: The scalpel is held with the fingertips and the handle lies under the palm. It is a modification of the palmar grip and used in making long incisions, usually on the skin as large length of blade lies in contact with the skin (Fig. 17.6).

Stab grip: The scalpel is held at a 90-degree angle to the skin surface and is a modification of the pencil grip. This position allows maximum control over penetration into the surface. Used for incision and drainage.

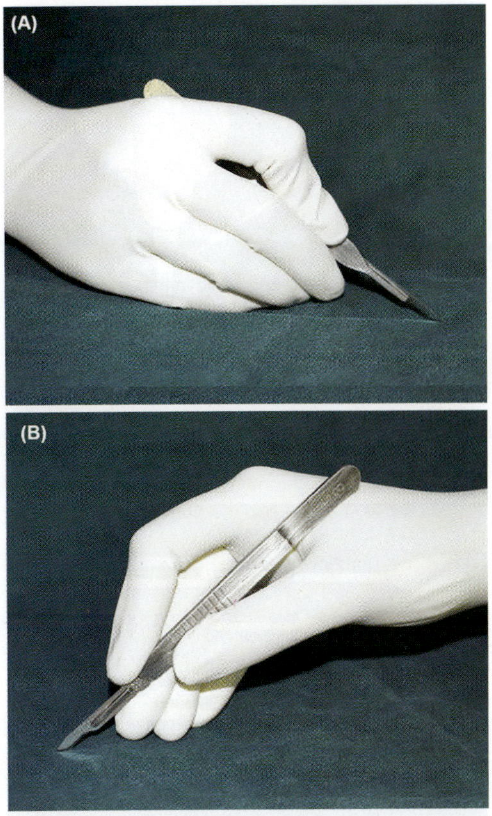

Figure 17.5 (**A** & **B**) Pen grip.

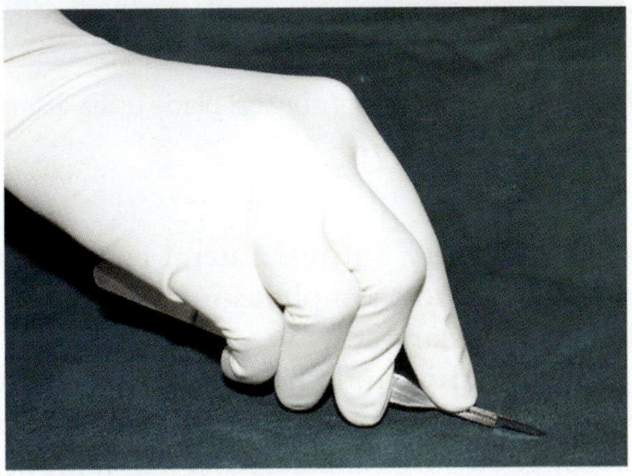
Figure 17.6 Fingertip grip.

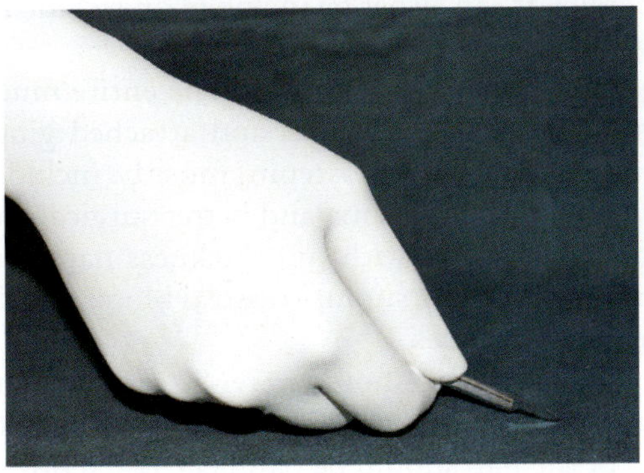
Figure 17.4 Palmar grip.

Technique of removal of surgical blade (Fig. 17.7).

Insertion of surgical blade (Fig. 17.8).

INTRAORAL INCISIONS

Intraoral incisions and transoral incisions are made to gain access predominantly to the dentoalveolar structures as in endodontic surgery, ridge augmentation, dental implants, sinus lift, extraction of impacted teeth, etc. In addition, they play an important role in surgical access to various sites such

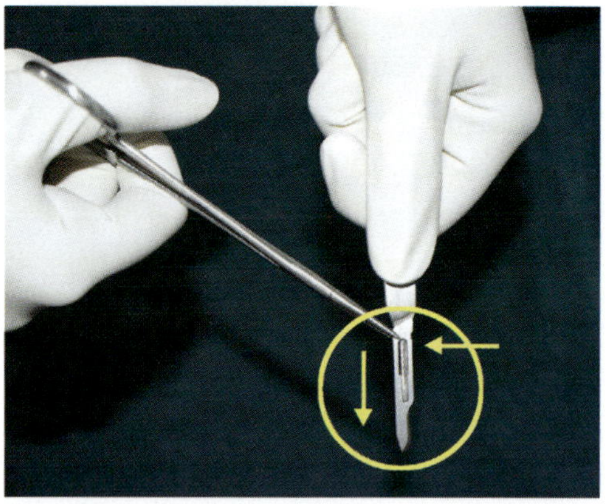

Figure 17.7 Removal of surgical blade using artery forceps.

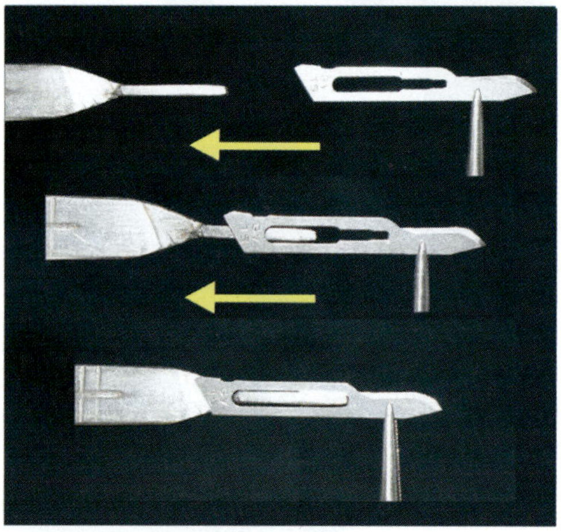

Figure 17.8 Steps in insertion of surgical blade using artery forceps.

as zygomaticomaxillary buttress, lateral pyriform aperture, mandibular angle, body, symphysis in case of fracture fixation and bone graft harvest.

Though intraoral wounds heal uneventfully with minimal scar and complications, the choice of the flap design is important for good surgical access and less complications.

PRINCIPLES AND GUIDELINES FOR FLAP DESIGNS

1. All surgical instruments used for cutting or incising should be sharp and of appropriate size
2. While incising the tissues, firm and continuous strokes should be used
3. Avoid cutting vital structures such as the nerves and vessels
4. Instruments should be perpendicular to the epithelial tissue. This angle creates sharp wound edges that heal with minimal scar tissue formation
5. Long incisions not only give better access and ease in tissue separation but also heal faster
6. *Avoid horizontal and severely angled vertical incisions:* Horizontal and severely angled incisions sever more collagen fibres and gingival blood vessels as the blood vessels and collagen fibres, which attach to the periosteum in the gingiva course parallel to the long axis of the teeth. The flap shrinks excessively during surgery due to contraction of the cut collagen fibres. As a result, extensive tension is placed on the soft tissues leading to tearing of sutures followed by subsequent scar formation
7. *Avoid incisions over bony eminences:* Radicular eminences such as the canine often fenestrate through the cortical bone or are covered with very thin bone with a poor blood supply. Soft tissue fenestrations may result from these bony defects if incisions are made over them. Vertical incisions must be made parallel to the long axis of the teeth and always made over solid interdental bone
8. *Incisions should be placed and flaps repositioned over solid bone:* Incision must never be placed over areas of periodontal loss or periradicular lesions. In the absence of good bone support to the repositioned edges of the mucoperiosteal flap, inadequate blood supply results, which in turn leads to necrosis and sloughing of the soft tissue
9. *Avoid incisions across major muscle attachments:* Difficult repositioning of the flap and healing by secondary intention resulting in scar tissue formation if incisions are made across major muscle attachments. This is avoided by including the muscle attachment within the flap
10. *Tissue retractor must rest on solid bone:* The extension of the vertical incision must be sufficient to allow the tissue retractor to sit on bone, thereby leaving the site of surgery well exposed. Inadequately extended vertical incision will produce a possibility of traumatising the mucosal tissue at the base from the retractor, which in turn affects the blood supply of the tissue
11. *Provide adequate visual and operative access with minimal soft tissue trauma:* Horizontal incision for mucoperiosteal flaps usually extend lateral to one or two teeth, which is to be treated. This is helpful in providing adequate access, minimal tension and soft tissue stretching
12. *Never split the involved interdental papilla:* Vertical incision must intersect the horizontal incision and terminate in the intrasulcular area at the mesial or distal line angle of the tooth. A vertical incision or intersection of the horizontal incision should never split the involved interdental papilla. It can either be included or excluded in a flap design
13. *Involve the entire mucoperiosteum:* The entire mucoperiosteum (marginal, interdental and attached gingivae, alveolar mucosa and periosteum) must be included in the flap. Less surgical trauma and better surgical haemostasis can be achieved with full thickness flaps due to the maintenance of the supraperiosteal blood vessels, which supply these tissues
14. The apex of the flap should never be wider than the base. Exception is when a major artery is present in the base. Sides of the flap should be parallel to each other or convergent from the base (Fig. 17.9)

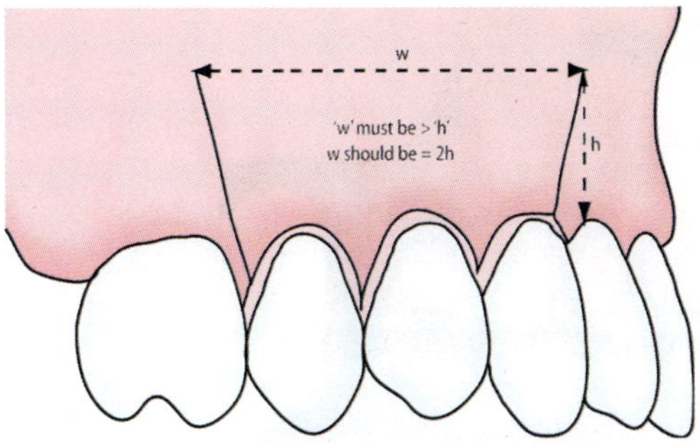

Figure 17.9 Flap design—base wider than apex.

15. The length of the flap must not exceed twice the width of the base
16. An axial blood supply must be included in the base of the flap
17. The base of the flap should not be stretched or twisted excessively since this will compromise the supplying vessels.

FLAP DESIGN

Flap design selection varies with each surgical procedure and various other factors to dictate the selection on an individual case basis. The factors to be considered are (1) anatomy, (2) good access (3) types of restorations at the surgical site, (4) width of attached gingiva, (5) bone thickness and (6) muscle attachment.

CLASSIFICATION OF INTRAORAL SURGICAL FLAPS

There are two major categories of flap design depending on the location of the horizontal component of the incision. Further, the flap designs are classified based on geometric terms (triangular, rectangular and trapezoidal) for easy identification.

1. **Sulcular full thickness flaps** (full mucoperiosteal flap)
   The sulcular full thickness flap design involves an intrasulcular horizontal incision along with the reflection of the marginal and interdental gingival tissues as part of the flap (Fig. 17.10A and B)
   a. Triangular (one vertical releasing incision)
   b. Rectangular (two vertical releasing incisions)

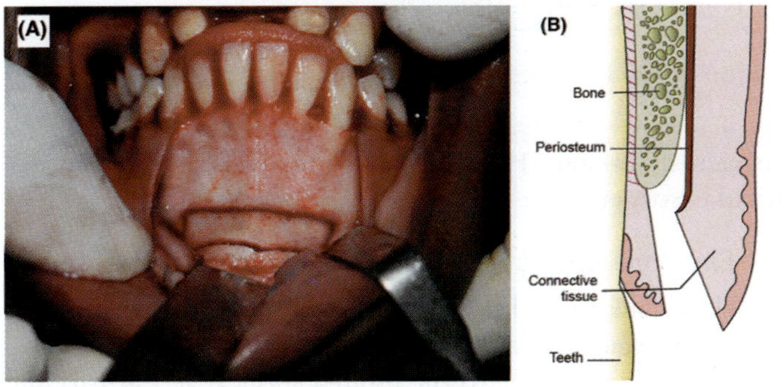

Figure 17.10 **(A)** Full thickness mucoperiosteal flap exposing mandibular symphysis for grafting. **(B)** Cross-sectional view showing full thickness mucoperiosteal flap.

   c. Trapezoidal (broad-based rectangular)
   d. Horizontal (no vertical releasing incision)
2. **Mucogingival flaps** (limited mucoperiosteal flap)
   The mucogingival flap design has a submarginal horizontal or horizontally oriented incision and the marginal or interdental papilla is not included in the flap
   a. Submarginal curved (semilunar)
   b. Submarginal scalloped rectangular (Luebke–Ochsenbein)
3. **Locoregional flaps**
   Some local flaps can be used for smaller defects in the maxillofacial region as tongue flap for oral submucous fibrosis and palatal flaps for oroantral fistulae.

1. SULCULAR FULL THICKNESS FLAPS (FULL MUCOPERIOSTEAL FLAP)

(a) Triangular flap (Fig. 17.11A–C)

Triangular flap is created by a horizontal, intrasulcular incision and a vertical releasing incision.

Advantage: There is minimal disruption of vascularity to the flap tissue with satisfactory wound healing and sutures need for flap reapproximation is minimal.

Disadvantage: Limited surgical access due to the single vertical releasing incision. Exposure of the root apices of long teeth is difficult due to the limited surgical access.

Distal relaxing incision provides an additional access in a reflected-triangular flap. A relaxing incision is a short vertical incision placed in the marginal and attached gingivae. It is located to the extent of the horizontal incision opposite to the vertical releasing incision. This also relieves the flap retraction tension while achieving adequate surgical access.

It is recommended for posterior teeth as it provides favourable surgical access and excellent wound healing. Due to the anatomic structures contraindicating other flap designs, only the triangular flap with mesial vertical incision is recommended for mandibular posterior teeth.

(b) Rectangular flap (Fig. 17.14)

Rectangular flap is formed by an intrasulcular, horizontal incision and two vertical releasing incisions.

Advantage: Increase in surgical access to the root apex.

Disadvantages: (1) Difficult reapproximation of the flap margins and wound closure. (2) Difficult postsurgical stabilisation as only the sutures hold the flap tissues in position. (3) Greater chance for postsurgical flap dislodgement.

It is especially useful for mandibular anterior teeth, multiple teeth and teeth with long roots such as maxillary canines. For posterior teeth, this flap design is not recommended due to the distal vertical incision that causes suturing problems due to extremely limited space in that area.

(c) Trapezoidal flap (Fig. 17.12A–C)

Trapezoidal flap is similar to the *rectangular* flap except that the two vertical releasing incisions intersecting the horizontal

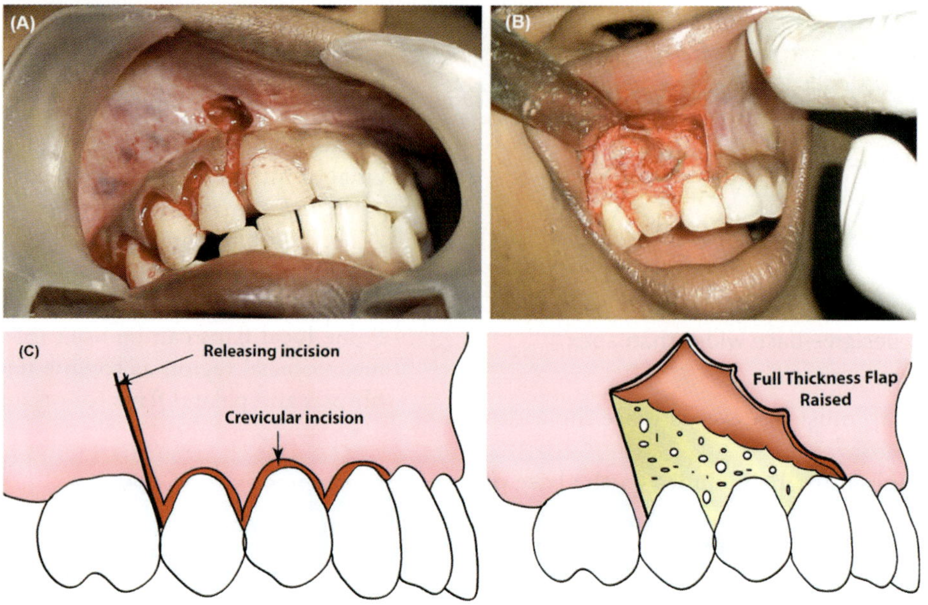

Figure 17.11 (**A**) Triangular flap. (**B**) Triangular flap exposing periapical lesion. (**C**) Exposing periapical triangular flap.

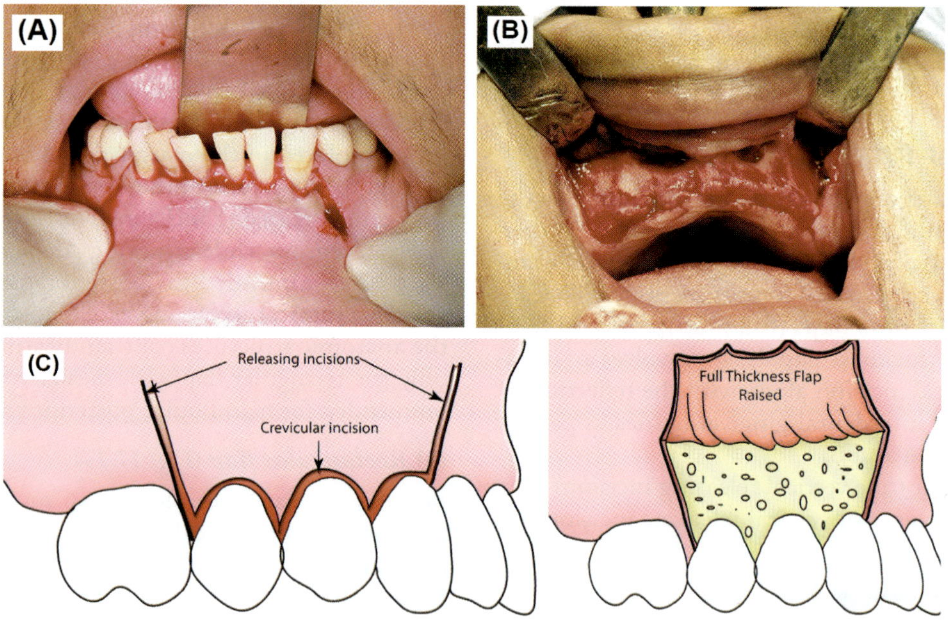

Figure 17.12 (**A** and **B**) Trapezoidal flap. (**C**) Illustration of full thickness mucoperiosteal flap.

intrasulcular incision are at an obtuse angle. A broad-based flap with the vestibular portion wider than the sulcular portion is obtained by the angled vertical releasing incisions. This flap is desirable based on the assumption of providing a better blood supply to the flapped tissues.

However, blood vessels and collagen fibres in the mucoperiosteal flap are oriented in a vertical direction and the angled vertical releasing incisions may damage the vital structures. This results in more bleeding, disruption of the vascular supply to the unflapped tissues and flapped tissues shrinkage. Hence, it is contraindicated in periradicular surgery.

(d) Envelope flap (horizontal flap) (Fig. 17.13A–C)

Envelope flap is also known as horizontal flap and is made by a horizontal, intrasulcular (crevicular) incision with no vertical releasing incision. Due to the limited surgical access, this flap has limited use in periradicular surgery. Its application is limited to repair of cervical defects, root perforations, resorption, caries, etc.

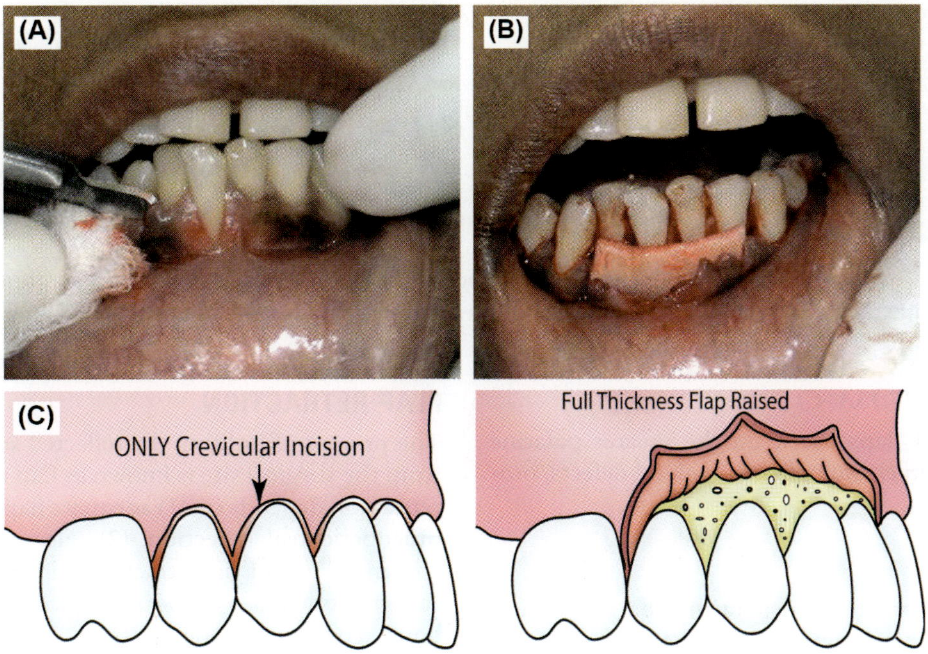

Figure 17.13 (**A**) Crevicular incision. (**B**) Envelope flap. (**C**) Illustration showing envelope flap.

2. MUCOGINGIVAL FLAPS (LIMITED MUCOPERIOSTEAL FLAP)

(a) Semilunar flap (Fig. 17.14)

This is a horizontal incision with a dip towards the incisal aspect in the centre of the flap, resembling a *half-moon*.

Advantage:

- Small incision suitable for upper canine surgery
- Utilised for incision and drainage procedure.

Disadvantages:

- Limited surgical access to the root apex
- Difficulty in suturing as the flap tension is high due to the presence of muscle fibres, and also risk of suture dehiscence is high
- Flap design leaves a noticeable scar.

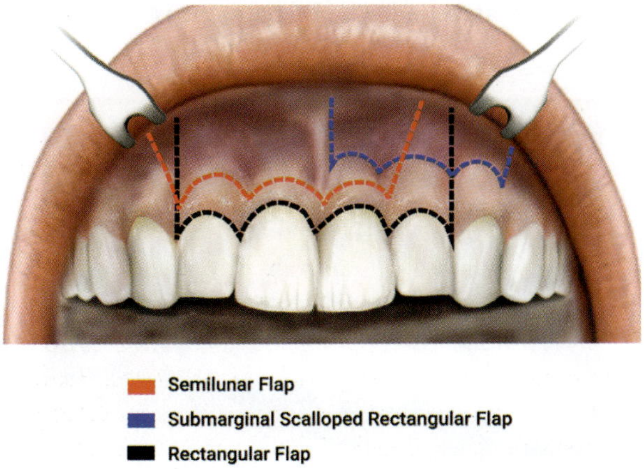

Figure 17.14 Dotted lines representing various flap design.

(b) Submarginal scalloped rectangular flap (Luebke–Ochsenbein) (Fig. 17.14)

The flap design calls for a scalloped incision in the middle of the attached gingiva. The angle of the incision in relation to the cortical plate is 45 degrees because this angle provides the widest cut surface, allowing for better adaptation once the flap is repositioned. The purpose of the scalloped horizontal incision is to provide a guide for the correct repositioning of the elevated flap for suturing. Therefore, it is important to scallop the incision, precisely tracing the gingival margin. Thus, attached gingiva around the crown margin will remain intact.

Mesial or mesiodistal vertical releasing incisions permit adequate access to the surgical site without violating the integrity of the attached gingiva around the tooth or crown. The vertical incision of the mucogingival flap should be parallel, rounded at the junction of intersection of the horizontal scalloped incision to promote smoother and faster healing. When the intersection of these two incisions is made at a sharp 90-degree angle, it heals very slowly and leaves a small, hard, knobby scar. This design is most suitable for crowned teeth, where there is an aesthetic concern for open crown margins as a result of the surgery.

Advantages: (1) The marginal or interdental gingiva is not involved, (2) It does not expose the crestal bone.

Disadvantages: (1) Excessive bleeding, (2) risk of flap shrinkage, and (3) delayed healing and scar formation.

3. INTRAORAL LOCOREGIONAL FLAPS

(a) Tongue flap

Tongue flaps are commonly used in anterior palatal fistula and oral submucous fibrosis.

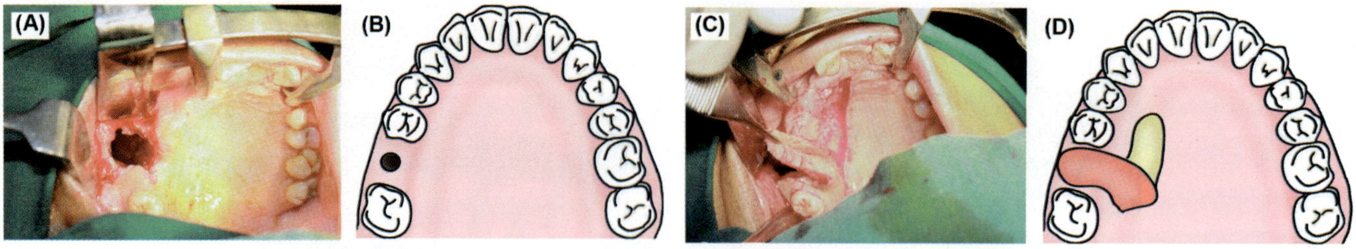

Figure 17.15 (**A**) A large oroantral fistula (**B**) Illustration of oroantral fistula. (**C**) Palatal flap based on greater palatine artery for closure of fistula. (**D**) Illustration of palatal pedicle flap based on greater artery for closure of fistula.

(b) Palatal flap (Fig. 17.15A–C)

Palatal flaps are axial flaps based on the greater palatine artery and are useful in closure of small palatal defects, oroantral fistulae.

FLAP REFLECTION

Flap reflection is the process of separating the soft tissues (gingiva, mucosa and periosteum) from the surface of the alveolar bone. This process must begin in the *vertical incision* a few millimetres apical to the junction of the horizontal and vertical incisions. The periosteum and its superficial tissues from the cortical plate are elevated gently with the help of periosteal elevator (Fig. 17.16). The marginal and interdental gingivae are separated from the underlying bone and the opposing incisional wound edge by directing the elevator coronally without applying a dissectional force.

This approach is referred to as *undermining elevation* and it allows all the reflective forces to be directed to the periosteum and the bone. The sharp pointed end of the elevator, 1st pries the interdental papilla free from the underlying bone as well as the attached gingiva. The broad end of the elevator continues to reflect the attached gingiva and alveolar mucosa more apically along with periosteum until adequate surgical access is obtained. On complete flap reflection, small tissue tags, *cortical retained periosteal tissues* can be noted, which should not be damaged or removed as they play an important role in reattaching the flap.

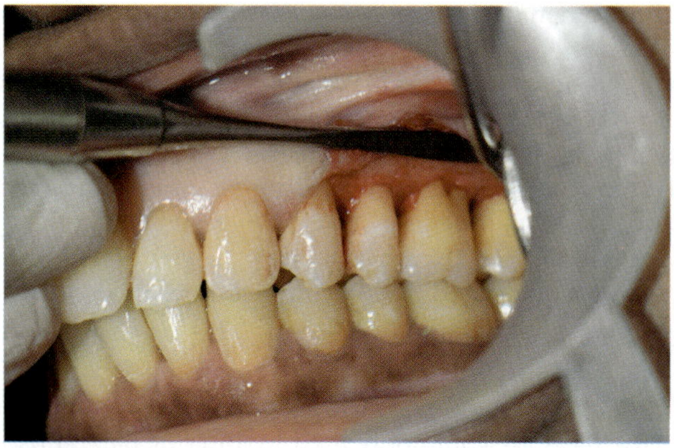

Figure 17.16 Flap reflection using periosteal elevator.

FLAP RETRACTION

The process of holding the reflected soft tissues in position from the surgical site is known as flap retraction. Proper flap retraction depends on (1) adequate flap extension and proper mucoperiosteal reflection, (2) selection of the appropriate size and shape of the retractor and (3) position of the retractor—must act as a *passive mechanical barrier* resting on solid bone. The type of the retractor should be appropriate for the size of the flap. For small flaps, periosteal elevators are used whereas for large flaps, Minnesota retractors are used (Fig. 17.17). Improper retraction will result in soft tissue trauma and an extended surgical time. This may delay the wound healing. Frequent saline irrigation of the periosteal surface prevents dehydration.

TISSUE HANDLING

To minimise postoperative pain and to promote satisfactory wound healing, gentle handling of tissues must be done. Thus, tissues must be retracted passively, avoiding excessive use of force by surgeon/assistant. Minimal use of electrocautery and chemical agents must be done. Continuous saline irrigation must be done while cutting the bone by using handpiece and bur. All these factors will contribute to minimising the tissue trauma.

DISSECTION

Using a periosteal elevator, the mucoperiosteal flap must be reflected, primarily in the buccal sulcus where the periosteum is loosely attached. The instrument is 1st inserted into

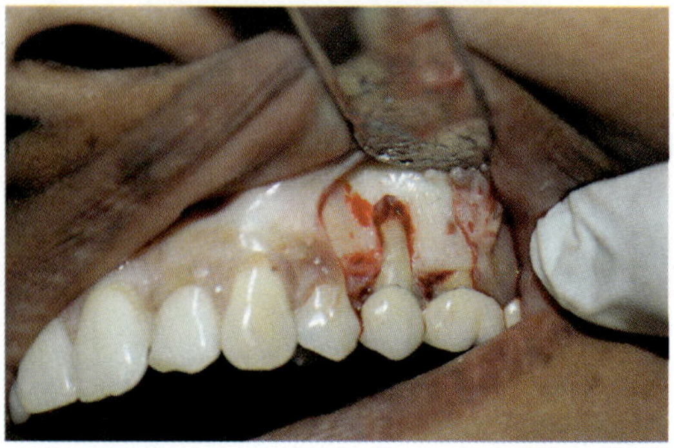

Figure 17.17 Flap retraction.

the incision and the 1st few millimetres at the edge of the flap are gently freed along its periphery. Then, with the end of the instrument pressed and kept firmly against the bone, it is reflected evenly along its whole length. Buttonholing the flap is avoided and adequate blood supply is to be maintained.

Applied aspect: Great care must be taken to avoid stripping the mentalis muscle from the symphysis. In general, to avoid chin laxity, a minimal of 10 mm of mentalis muscle should be left attached to the mandible, otherwise known as a witch's chin.

BONE CUTTING

The purpose of bone removal is to (1) gain access to the tooth structure, (2) reduce resistance around the tooth structure, (3) provide point of application for elevator or forceps and (4) create space into which the tooth may be displaced by manipulation. This is done commonly using burs in oral surgery, the efficiency of dental handpieces and sharp burrs giving superlative control. Novel equipment such as piezo saws give excellent properties of minimal damage. On occasion, chisels, files, rongeurs and gouges may also be used, but is declining.

CHISELS AND OSTEOTOMES

Chisels are monobevelled instruments used for cutting the bone. These are used in younger patients under 40 years of age where natural lines of cleavage along the 'grain' of the bone are present. In older patients over 40 years of age, as the bone is brittle and the mandible may shatter along unpredictable planes, the use of chisels is contraindicated. Chisels are used either by hand or more usually with a mallet. In either case, they must be supported firmly against slipping. The osteotome is similar to a chisel. Unlike a chisel, it is a bibevelled instrument used for splitting the bone.

RONGEURS AND FILES

These instruments are mostly used for smoothing and trimming bone edges when the operation has been completed.

SAWS

Saws are attached to either an electric motor or air engine and can be used to divide the jaw in osteotomies or remove blocks of bone for grafting.

Burs (Fig. 17.18)

The burs commonly used for the removal of bone are the round bur and fissure bur. When the surgical procedure involves greater bone surface area (torus) or smoothing of bone edges, a large bone bur similar to an acrylic bur may be used. Adequate cutting with fine control can only be achieved using high speeds and minimal pressure. Sterile saline irrigation must be done to avoid overheating of the tissues and clogging of the bur.

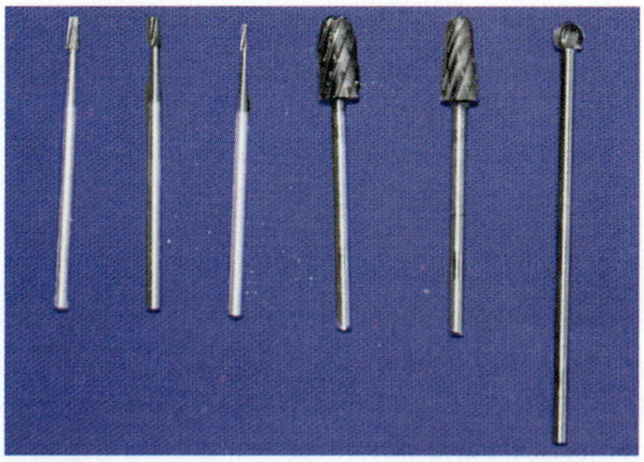

Figure 17.18 Rotary power drill instruments—stainless steel and tungsten carbide burs.

Piezosurgery

Piezosurgery uses modulated ultrasonic vibration to allow precise cutting of bony structures. Delicate bony structures can be cut simply and with great accuracy without destruction of teeth and soft tissues. In addition, with the so-called cavitation effect, a blood-free surgical site can be attained using peizosurgery device.

CLEANSING THE FIELD OF OPERATION

In the field of operation, fluids (blood, saline) and loose debris (from cutting hard tissues) might obscure the surgeon's view or remain in the wound to become foreign bodies. The assistant must do intermittent suctioning. The tip of the sucker should be kept at the single point of dependent drainage, as moving it frequently can interfere with the surgeon's instrumentation. Forceps are used to lift large bone fragments or tags of tissue.

ARREST OF HAEMORRHAGE

Various procedures can be used to achieve haemostasis. The arrest of primary haemorrhage at the surgical field may be achieved by the application of *intermittent pressure* to the vessel walls. For small vessels, 20–30 s and for larger vessels 5–10 min of continuous pressure must be maintained for effective blood clotting. *Ligation* of larger vessels that are difficult to manage by mere pressure can be done with the help of sutures. In major haemorrhage from the jaws, which cannot be controlled by local measures, the external carotid artery is to be ligated. When a vessel is cut during operation, it must be found quickly and secured with artery forceps. In case of persistent haemorrhage, *electrocautery* (thermal coagulation) or ligation with ties or metal clips can be used in soft tissue surgery. *Absorbable haemostatic packs* such as Surgicel and Gelfoam are packed in the surgical site to control bleeding.

Bleeding from bone can be controlled by burnishing the bone with a small instrument. Application of bone wax over the surface of the bone is also very effective in occluding small vessels, but must be removed prior to closure as it can cause foreign body reactions.

DECONTAMINATION AND DEBRIDEMENT

Decontamination is done to reduce bacterial count and hence to reduce risk of infection. This can be done by irrigating the field by saline or antiseptic solutions under pressure to remove any particles or debris.

Debridement is the careful removal from injured tissue of necrotic, severely ischaemic and foreign materials that would impede wound healing. To remove any loose fragments from the socket and the area of surgery, bone curettes are used. Rongeurs or bone cutting forceps are used to trim sharp bony edges or bony projections and bone files for smoothing of edges.

PRINCIPLES OF DRAINAGE

Infected and contaminated wounds need to be drained freely after the operation. Dead space must be eliminated by proper drainage. Any area that remains devoid of tissue after closure of wound is referred as dead space and it usually fills in with blood or serum and subsequently become infected. It can be eliminated by:

A. Multilayer suturing together to minimise postoperative void
B. Place a pressure dressing. This brings the tissue planes together until either they are bound by fibrin or pressed by oedema or both (takes up to 12–18 h)
C. Place a surgical packing in the void
D. With the use of drains with or without pressure packs.

Fine superficial drains: It is made of pieces of rubber gloves and is used to allow tissue exudates to escape from the wounds of the face. It must be usually removed after 48 h.

Larger superficial drains: Yeates drain or a corrugated rubber drain used in a dental abscess to keep the wound edges apart and allow thick pus to flow freely. Mainly used for extraoral incisions and drainage and also used for large collections of pus drained intraorally (Fig. 17.19).

Vacuum drains: They are inserted into a cavity at its most dependent point away from the operation wound and fixed with a suture to prevent them from falling out or being drawn into the wound. The negative pressure developed assists in removal of fluid. They should be examined daily and are removed usually between the 3rd and seventh days (Fig. 17.20).

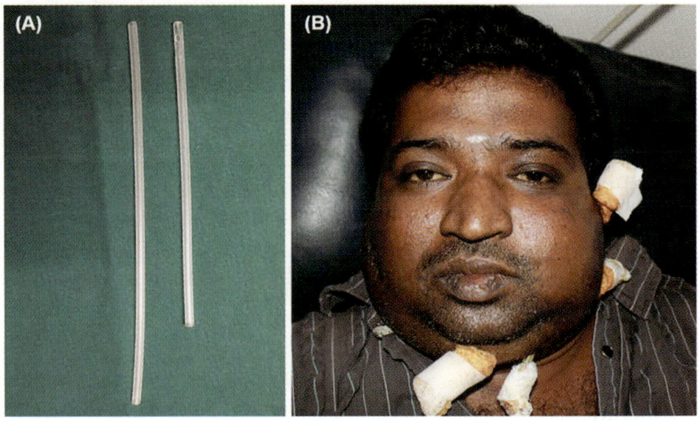

Figure 17.19 (**A**) Simple drain—perforated and nonperforated. (**B**) Simple drain placed for draining Ludwig's angina.

SUTURING

Suturing is the final step in most surgical procedures and also an important step that prepares the wound for healing. Different suture material and suturing techniques are discussed in detail in Chapter 16.

POSTOPERATIVE CARE

PATIENT GENERAL HEALTH AND NUTRITION

Proper healing of wounds depends on the patient's ability to:

1. Resist infection
2. Provide essential nutrients for use as building materials
3. Carry out reparative cellular processes.

Postoperative instructions must be clearly explained to the patient. Analgesics and antibiotics are prescribed as needed. Oral hygiene must be emphasised after minor surgical procedures to prevent chances of reinfection.

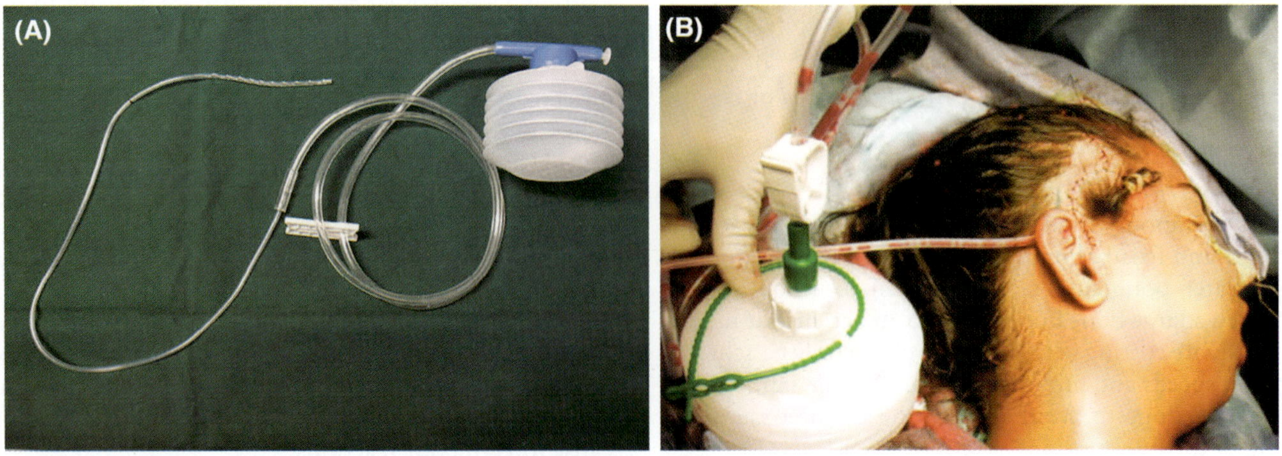

Figure 17.20 (**A**) Suction drain (Hemovac). (**B**) Vacuum drain in place after Temporomandibular Joint (TMJ) surgery.

Chapter 18

Exodontia

OUTLINE

INTRODUCTION

Exodontia or extraction is a minor oral surgical procedure performed for the therapeutic removal of teeth from the oral cavity, using proven techniques and specialised instruments, causing minimal trauma to the attaching apparatus and least injury to the surrounding tissues, in a pattern conducive to uneventful healing in order to achieve best possible prosthetic rehabilitation.

Ideal tooth extraction is—***The painless removal of the whole tooth or root with minimal trauma to the investing tissues, so that the wound heals uneventfully and no postoperative prosthetic problem is created (Geoffrey L Howe).***

METHODS OF EXTRACTION

Intraalveolar (closed) extraction of teeth is the wrenched removal of an erupted tooth by expansion of the bony alveolar socket alone using principles of lever, wedge and wheel.

Transalveolar (open) extraction is a minor surgical procedure performed for the therapeutic removal of impacted, partially erupted and unerupted teeth that includes access through a surgical flap for visualisation and appropriate bone removal to create a path for delivery and facilitate extraction.

INDICATIONS FOR EXTRACTION

- ***Deeply carious tooth with pulpal pathology:*** Either acute or chronic pulpitis where successful endodontic therapy is not possible or patient is unwilling
- ***Teeth with apical pathology:*** A tooth with apical pathology should be extracted if it fails to respond to conservative treatment. Such teeth are extracted before they involve the adjacent teeth
- ***Periodontitis:*** Periodontally compromised teeth, which are not salvageable by periodontal therapy and teeth with guarded prognosis
- ***Malpositioned and overerupted teeth:*** Should be extracted if they disturb the occlusal harmony
- ***Impacted:*** If the impacted tooth is found to be responsible for facial pain, periodontal disturbance of the adjacent tooth, temporomandibular joint (TMJ) problems or bony pathology like cyst
- ***Retained deciduous teeth:*** If the primary tooth is retained beyond its chronological age of shedding, it should be extracted to prevent the malocclusion of the permanent dentition
- ***Tooth in the line of fracture:*** Teeth which are in the line of fracture should be extracted if
  - There is a potential source of infection (dental caries, fractured teeth)
  - Their retention interferes with the reduction of the fractured segments

- ***Teeth with fractured root:*** Teeth with a vertical fracture extending into the root of the tooth cannot be treated conservatively
- ***Orthodontic purpose:*** For the purpose of orthodontic treatment, certain permanent molars or premolars are extracted (therapeutic extraction). Serial extraction is also one of the entities wherein judicious extraction of certain deciduous teeth is done to provide enough space for the proper eruption of the permanent teeth
- ***Prosthetic purpose:*** Extraction of one or two teeth is justified if it aids in better design or stability of the prosthesis.
- ***Before radiation therapy (teeth in line of fire):*** Patients who have to undergo radiation therapy for malignant tumours should undergo extraction of those teeth, which have poor prognosis and are prone to get infected. This is done to prevent the incidence of osteoradionecrosis
- ***Prophylactic extraction:*** This procedure is done as a presurgical prophylaxis for patients who have a higher risk of bacterial endocarditis or rheumatic fever. It may require the removal of all nonvital teeth as well as those of questionable vitality in an effort to eradicate all foci and potential *foci of infection*. Richards in 1932 presented bacteraemia in patients after infected tooth extraction, Okell and Elliott (1935) showed in a study that *Streptococcus viridans* was present in the bloodstream in 75% of the 40 patients after extraction. The use of local anaesthetic solution due to the presence of a vasoconstrictor has shown a decrease in the rate of spread of infection
- ***Root fragments:*** Fragments of roots should be removed as soon as they are found. However, small pieces of roots may be left as such in the socket as long as it does not cause any problem, but with advancing age, it is always risky to leave the fragments, hence should be removed. In edentulous patients, fractured segments present under the mucosa constantly get irritated from the overlying denture resulting in chronic ulcers, which may sometimes undergo neoplastic changes. The root fragment may themselves undergo cystic or other pathological changes.

CONTRAINDICATIONS FOR EXTRACTION

All contraindications whether local or systemic can be relative or absolute depending upon the general condition of the patient. Whenever the contraindication is absolute, extreme care must be taken before the extraction to avoid any risk to the patients. The absolute and relative contraindications for extraction have been briefed in Table 18.1.

TABLE 18.1 Absolute and Relative Contraindications for Extractions

Absolute Contraindications	Relative Contraindications
• Uncontrolled diabetes • Leukaemia • Renal failure • Cirrhosis of liver • Cardiac failure	• Diabetes • Hypertension • Cardiac disease • Patients on steroid therapy • Pregnancy • Blood dyscrasias • Patients on anticoagulant therapy • Toxic goitre • Jaundice/hepatitis • Renal disorders • Medically compromised patients • Recently irradiated patients

RELATIVE CONTRAINDICATIONS

Diabetes

If extraction is carried out in an uncontrolled diabetic patient, he/she would be more prone to develop infection in the extraction wound extending into the surrounding tissues. This is due to the deposition of cholesterol in the peripheral circulation (thinning of arterioles) and secondly, the chemotactic mechanism, which helps in wound healing is impaired in diabetic patients.

Diabetic patients undergoing minor surgical procedures may precipitate into diabetic ketoacidosis due to stress. The stress response leads to a chain of metabolic and neurohormonal changes, which creates a mechanism for coping up with stress. The hyperglycaemia induced by stress is attributed to hypersecretion of counterregulatory hormones such as catecholamines, glucagon, cortisol and growth hormones that antagonise the effect of insulin by increasing glucose production. This causes a spike in circulating glucose from glycogenolysis and impaired glucose utilisation. (hyperglycaemia impairs glucose use and residual insulin secretion).

Hypertension (Table 18.2)

Hypertension can be of mainly two types:

- Primary—unknown cause (essential hypertension)
- Secondary—which occurs secondary to any other systemic disease.

Extraction can be carried out in mild or moderate hypertension, that is when the systolic pressure is less than 200 mmHg and the diastolic pressure less than 110 mmHg. Extraction is contraindicated when the blood pressure exceeds the aforementioned values.

Cardiac disease

The cardiac conditions that most frequently complicate exodontia are myocardial infarction, angina pectoris and cardiac decompensation. The surgeon has to follow a few preventive measures such as:

- Obtaining a detailed history preoperatively
- Always obtain the treating physician's consent

TABLE 18.2 Guidelines for Extraction Considering Blood Pressure in Adults

Blood Pressure (mmHg)	ASA Classification	Dental Therapy Considerations
<140 and <90	I	• Observe routine dental management • Recheck in 6 months.
140–159 and/or 90–94	II	• Recheck blood pressure before dental treatment for three consecutive appointments; if all measurements exceed these guidelines, medical consultation is recommended • Observe routine dental management • Implement stress reduction protocol as indicated.
160–199 and/or 95–114	III	• Recheck blood pressure in 5 min • If still elevated, perform medical consultation before beginning dental therapy • Observe routine dental therapy • Implement stress reduction protocol.
>200 and/or >115	IV	• Recheck blood pressure in 5 min • If elevated, do not perform dental therapy, routine or emergency, until elevated blood pressure is corrected • Refer to hospital if immediate dental therapy indicated.

- In the indicated pathologies, administer antibiotics to avoid bacterial endocarditis due to *S. viridans* that invades the bloodstream following an extraction
- Stress reduction protocol should be followed.

Patients on steroid therapy

Patients on steroids may have suppression in the output of adrenocorticotrophic hormone from the pituitary gland. Even patients for whom the steroid therapy had ceased years ago show insufficient adrenal secretion to withstand the stress of an extraction. A physician's opinion should be sought and steroids should be prescribed a day or 2 before and after the extraction. A detailed history of the systemic complications should be obtained preoperatively to avoid any adrenal crisis due to stress.

Pregnancy

Special consideration before an extraction in pregnant patient.

- A detailed history about the patient ruling out other related systemic complications
- If any other complication is foreseen, an expert opinion from a gynaecologist should be obtained
- If the procedures are elective, then the treatment should be scheduled during the ***2nd trimester***, which is considered as the optimum time
- Patient should be positioned comfortably in supine position or left lateral if feasible
- Local anaesthetics such as lignocaine, bupivacaine and codeine are believed least likely to harm a foetus
- Emergencies because of pain, infection or other acute problems can be accomplished under general anaesthesia (GA), bearing the safety norms. If GA is necessary, combination of an intravenous short-acting barbiturate (pentothal), muscle relaxant (succinylcholine) and nitrous oxide is the method of choice
- Drugs to be avoided in a pregnant patient are as follows
  - **Aspirin and other nonsteroidal antiinflammatory drugs (NSAIDs), Carbamazepine, Chloral hydrate (if chronically used), Chlordiazepoxide, Corticosteroids, Diazepam and other benzodiazepines, Diphenhydramine hydrochloride (if chronically used), Morphine, Pentazocine hydrochloride, Phenobarbital, Promethazine hydrochloride, Propoxyphene, Tetracycline, Metronidazole**.

Blood dyscrasias

- Anaemia, haemorrhagic diseases such as haemophilia and leukaemia are blood dyscrasias cause many problems during extraction
- Profuse bleeding complications should be dealt with careful evaluation. A preoperative laboratory investigation confirming the integrity of coagulation cascade avoids complications
- An expert opinion from a haematologist can be acquired to avoid complications during recovery of the patient. Refer to Chapter 7 page number 89.

Patients on anticoagulant therapy

Patients on anticoagulant therapy who are to undergo oral surgical procedure may face prolonged postoperative haemorrhage and/or fatal thromboembolic accidents within 6 months of myocardial infarction. Preoperative assessment of the blood clotting and profile including BT, CT, PT and INR is mandatory. Refer to Chapter 7 page number 80.

Toxic goitre

Extraction can precipitate a thyroid crisis in known hypertensive patients. The symptoms manifested by a patient with thyroid crisis are altered consciousness, restlessness (which is uncontrollable even with heavy sedation), cyanosis and delirium with an extremely rapid, thready pulse and high temperature. Under these conditions, no surgical procedures should be performed and the patient requires medical attention.

Jaundice/hepatitis

The postoperative complication of this condition is haemorrhage. If extraction is imperative, prophylactic doses of vitamin K should be administered before operation. Care is taken in use of local anaesthesia (LA) and drugs that metabolise in the liver in order to avoid workload on the liver.

Renal disorders

Nephrotic patients pose a challenge during exodontia as extraction of chronically infected teeth often provokes an acute nephritis. Nephrotic patients should always undergo dental procedures after due consent from the concerned physician.

Patient on renal dialysis and heparination can undergo extraction, following certain protocols. Refer to Chapter 7 page number 85.

Medically compromised patients

Treatment for this group of patients is the most challenging and risky task, and hence preoperative evaluation of these patients' general condition is must. Any associated systemic condition can interfere with the dental treatment. Iatrogenic effects due to drug interaction should be avoided.

Extraction of teeth in recently irradiated patients

This group of patients need special attention as the blood supply to the jaws is reduced due to radiation therapy. Osteoradionecrosis is the condition of the jaws, which occurs as a result of trauma added with infection, and hence, it is advisable to avoid extraction in these conditions.

ASSESSMENT OF TEETH FOR EXTRACTION

A tooth can be atraumatically and successfully extracted out of the socket depending upon the technique used, morphology of the tooth, its position in the dental arch and condition of the surrounding bone.

Before the removal of the tooth, preoperative radiographs are taken for assessment of the tooth to be removed.

The preoperative assessment should cover the following points:

- Morphology of the crown:
  - Normal
  - Macroform/microform
  - Abnormal/deformed
- Morphology of the roots (dilacerated, fused, impacted, ankylosed, hypercementosed or divergent roots)
- The density of the bone surrounding the tooth
- The relationship of the tooth to adjacent teeth and other important anatomical structures such as inferior alveolar canal
- Presence of any pathology of the tooth or the bone surrounding it
- Conditions indicating dental or dentoalveolar deformities such as osteitis deformans, hypercementosis, cleidocranial dysostosis—hooked root, therapeutic irradiation, osteopetrosis, etc.

PREOPERATIVE RADIOGRAPHS

INDICATIONS

1. Previous difficulty with extractions and attempted extractions
2. Close approximation with important anatomical structures
3. Abnormal root pattern—3rd molars, misplaced canine
4. Tooth having periodontal problem and some sclerosis—hypercementosis
5. Trauma to tooth—fracture of tooth, roots and alveolar bone
6. Isolated and unopposed maxillary molars
7. Partially erupted, unerupted tooth and retained roots
8. Delayed erupting or having abnormal crown.

ARMAMENTARIUM

Forceps or elevators are the main instruments used in the extraction of teeth. Forceps help in dilatation of the alveolar socket, luxation of the tooth and its removal.

EXTRACTION FORCEPS

Parts of the forceps:

- Pair of handles
- Pair of beaks
- A hinge.

The upper jaw forceps have beaks, which are parallel to the long axis of the handle; the beaks of the lower jaw forceps are at right angle to the long axis of the handles (Fig. 18.1A–K).

FORCEPS DESIGN STYLE

- American pattern—hinge is directed in a horizontal direction with the handles of the forceps
- English pattern—hinge is directed in a vertical direction with the handles of the forceps.

Elevators

Elevators are used primarily as levers. A lever is a mechanism for transmitting a modest force with the mechanical advantage

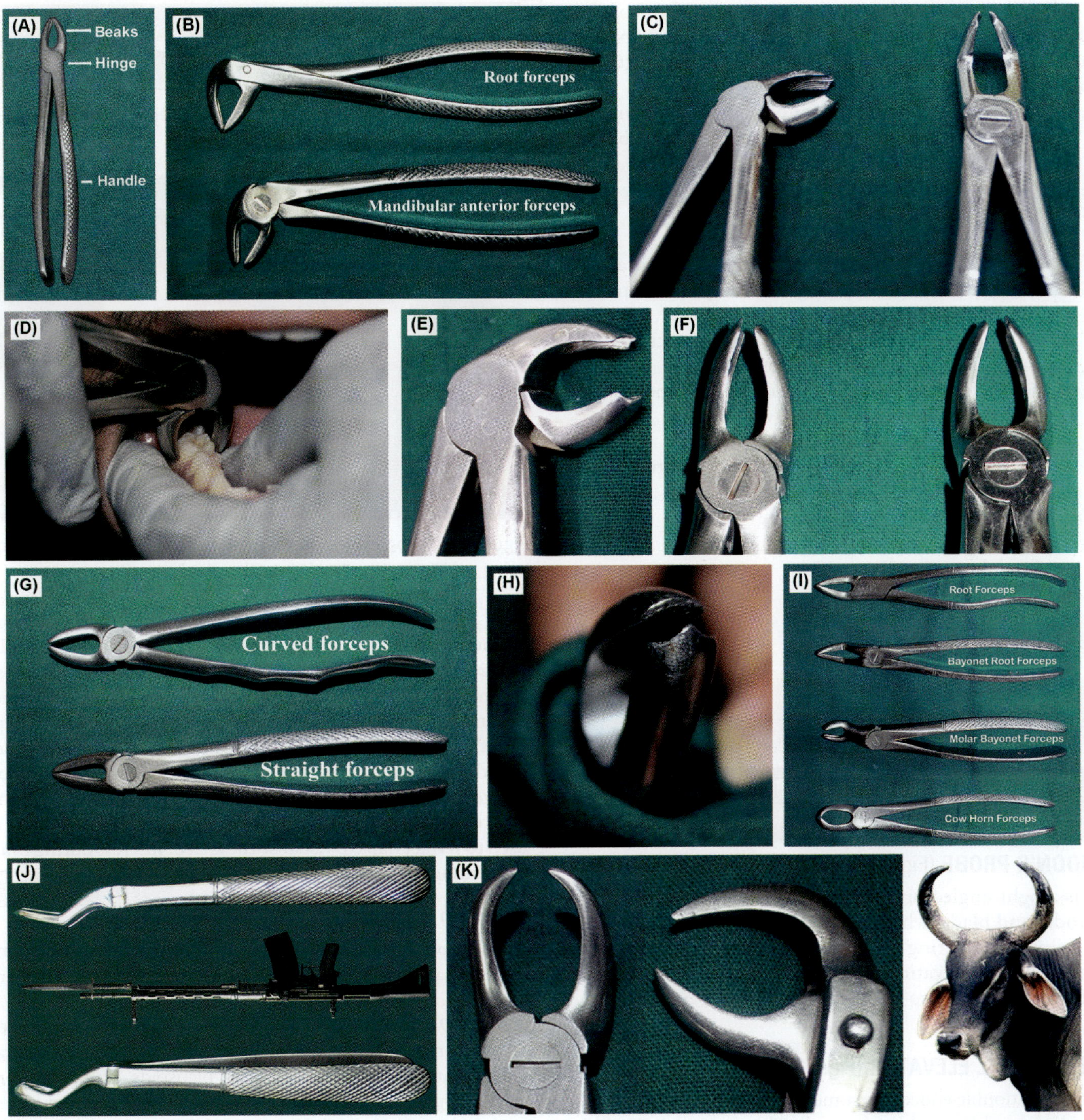

Figure 18.1 **(A)** Parts of a forceps. **(B)** Forceps for extraction of mandibular anterior teeth and roots. Note approximation of beaks in root forceps whereas beaks do not meet in the other. **(C)** Forceps for extraction of mandibular molars. Two types based on axis of working end in relation to handle. **(D)** Application of beaks of forceps for extracting mandibular molar. **(E)** Buccal and lingual beaks of mandibular molar forceps designed to engage the furcation between the mesial and distal roots. **(F)** Forceps for extraction of maxillary molars, right and left. **(G)** Forceps for extraction of maxillary anterior teeth. **(H)** Right maxillary molar forceps—buccal beak is pointed to engage the furcation between MB and DB roots; palatal beak is rounded to engage the single palatal root. **(I)** Special armamentarium for extraction of maxillary teeth. **(J)** Maxillary bayonet forceps with angled beaks facilitating extraction of last molar. Implication of the name is from bayonet gun. **(K)** Maxillary cow horn forceps, mandibular cow horn forceps, implication of the name cow horn.

of a long lever arm and a short effector arm. When correctly used, they are very safe and efficient, but when misapplied, it may cause damage to the tissues, bones and other structures.

Parts of an elevator:

- *Handle*—this part is used for holding the instrument
- *Shank*—this part connects the handle with the blade
- *Blade*—this part of the instrument engages the crown or the root to be removed.

Indications for the use of elevators:

- To reflect mucoperiosteum
- Elevators can be used to widen the periodontal ligament space before applying the forceps for extraction (wedge/lever principle)
- To luxate and remove the tooth from its socket, which cannot be engaged with forceps
- To remove a fractured or carious tooth or roots, which might fracture when engaged with beaks
- To remove interradicular bone
- To remove a fractured root when the fracture line is below the cervical margin of alveolar bone.

Classification of elevators:

According to the form:

- Straight
- Angular
- Crossbar

Commonly used elevators are as follows:

- Periosteal elevators
- Crossbar elevators
- Apexo elevators

INSTRUMENTS USED FOR REFLECTING THE MUCOPERIOSTEAL FLAP

MOON'S PROBE (Fig. 18.2)

It is a right-angled probe with a narrow working edge, flat handle and blade, which is blunt and with a rounded tip. It helps in retracting the mucosa without traumatisation and used for elevation of the mucoperiosteum prior to extraction. It is also used to test the area anaesthetised after injecting LA.

PERIOSTEAL ELEVATOR (Figs. 18.3 and 18.4)

This is a double-ended instrument with a broad end (raspatory) and a sharp end (rugine end). The sharp end should be

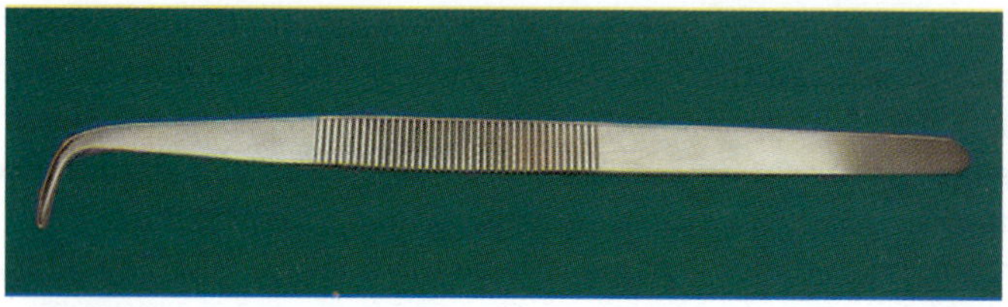

Figure 18.2 Moon's probe used for elevation of the mucoperiosteum.

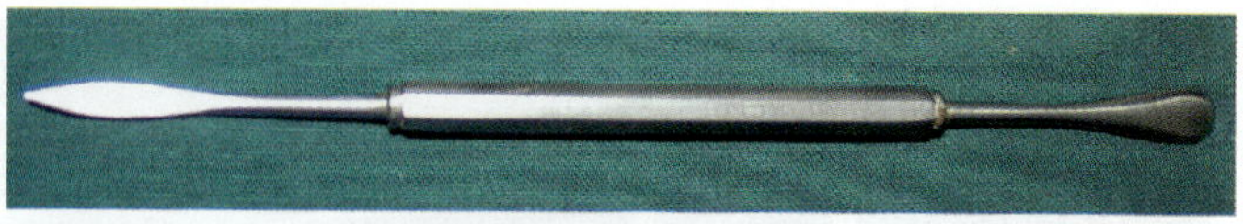

Figure 18.3 *Molt periosteal elevator no 9.*

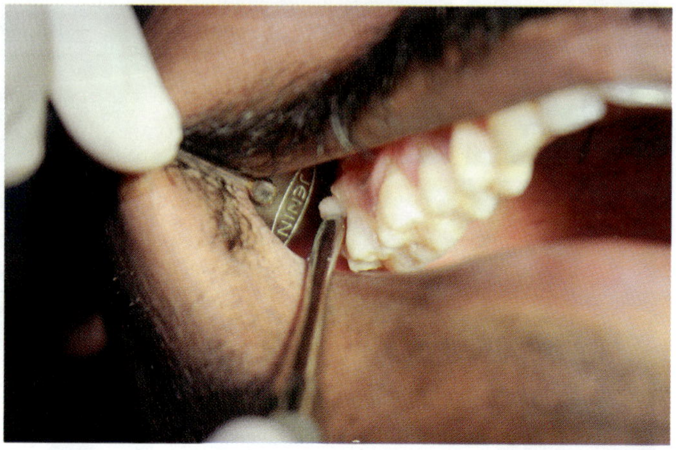

Figure 18.4 Application of sharp end of the periosteal elevator using prying motion to elevate the gingiva.

maintained sharp to prevent shredding of the flap. No: 9 Molt, No: 23 Seldin, and Howarth periosteal elevator are the most commonly used. This instrument is used to expose the bone, elevating the periosteum off the bone as a mucoperiosteal flap. The sharp end is also used in tooth extraction to initially elevate the gingiva (prying motion) as well as aid in extraction by wedge principle. The raspatory end is used to gently elevate the soft tissue flaps from the underlying bone without tearing. It is used to retract flaps to visualise the area of interest during multiple extractions and surgical procedures.

1. Apexo elevators (Fig. 18.5A–C)

Apexo elevators are used for removal of fractured roots, impacted maxillary 3rd molars and impacted cuspids. They are available in various numbers.

- ***No. 301 straight Apexo elevators*** are used for the removal of fractured roots (at the gingival line) of maxillary central and lateral incisors, cuspids and bicuspids. These elevators are applied on the mesial and distal sides of the root by using the wedge principle to expand the socket. Finally, when the socket has expanded sufficiently, rotary motion is applied to remove the root from the socket (Fig. 18.6A–E)
- ***No. 73 and 74 elevators*** are used for removing the impacted maxillary 3rd molars
- ***No. 4 (302) and 5 (303) Apexo elevators*** are used when the mandibular root has fractured below the gingival line. In these elevators, the blade is at a 90-degree angle to the handle (Fig. 18.7). These are used in a similar manner as that of the straight Apexo elevators. The No. 4 elevators can be applied on the mesial aspect of the left

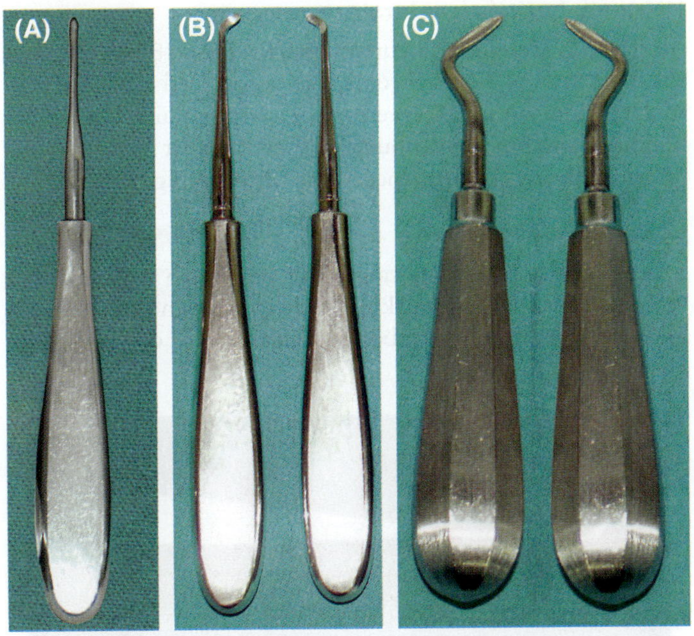

Figure 18.5 (**A**) No. 301 straight Apexo elevators remove the root tips in both jaws and for the extraction of impacted 3rd molars of the upper jaw. (**B**) No. 73 and No. 74 Apexo elevators. (**C**) No. 302 Apexo elevators and No. 303 Apexo elevator.

lower fractured roots, as well as on the distal aspect of the fractured root in the right lower side. Similarly, the No. 5 Apexo elevators can be used on the distal side of the fractured roots in the left lower side, as well as on the mesial side of the fractured roots in the right lower side. After applying these forceps on the respective sides of the fractured root, apical and rotary pressure is applied to achieve a depth of 2–3 mm in between the fractured tooth root and the bone to expand the socket. If this depth is not obtained, a purchase point can be drilled before inserting the elevator. Alternatively, this pressure is applied on the mesial and distal side of the root until it luxates out of the socket.

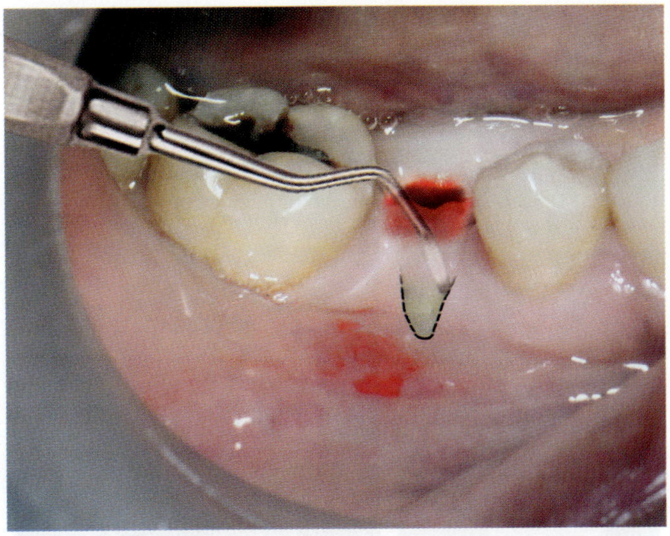

Figure 18.7 Removal of root tip using No. 302 Apexo elevator.

2. Crossbar elevators

Crossbar elevators are used particularly for removal of mandibular molar roots and impacted mandibular 3rd molars (Fig. 18.8). It is also known as Winter's crossbar elevator. It is available in various numbers such as 11L and 11R, 14L and 14R, 1L and 1R.

They work on the principle of the wheel and axle and can extract with extreme forces.

No. 11L and 11R: No. 11L crossbar elevator is used for removing right lower 3rd molars wherein the thick buccal plate acts as fulcrum. The elevator is inserted from the buccal aspect of the right lower 3rd molar to engage between the bifurcation of the molar, and the elevator is rotated to lift the tooth out of the socket.

Similarly, No. 11R is used for removing the left lower 3rd molar. These elevators can also be used to remove the vertically impacted 3rd molars and roots of horizontally impacted 3rd molars.

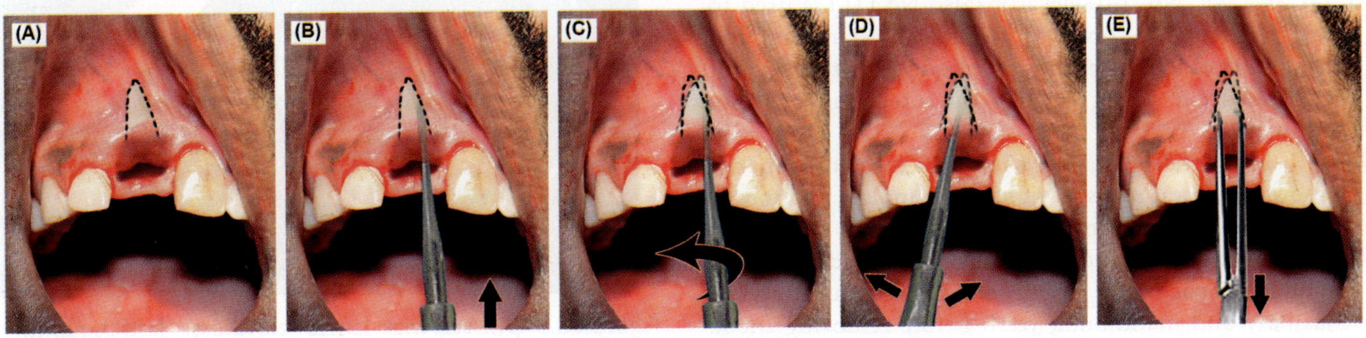

Figure 18.6 Removal of root using No. 301 Apexo elevator. (**A**) Retained maxillary central incisor root tip at the level of gingiva. (**B**) Application of straight Apexo elevator no 301. (**C and D**) Using wedge principle, application on the mesial and distal sides of root for expansion of socket. (**E**) Removal of root using rotatory motion.

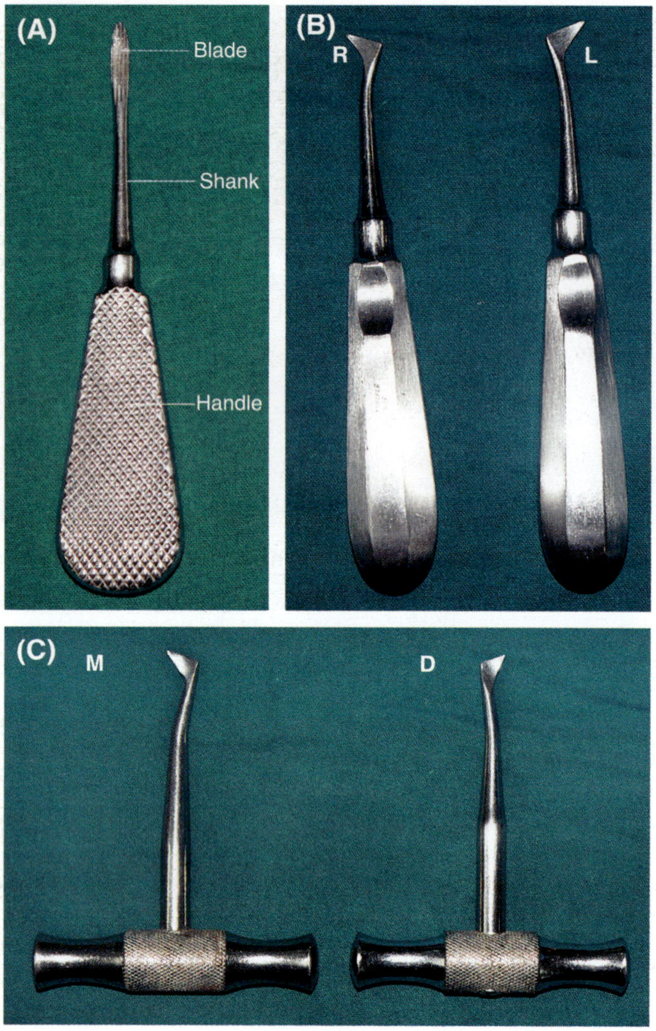

Figure 18.8 (**A**) Parts of an elevator. (**B**) Cryer's paired—right (R) and left (L) used to luxate mandibular molar roots and upper 3rd molar tooth. (**C**) Winter's cross bar—working end similar to Cryer's but its handle is at a right angle to the shank, paired instrument—mesial (M) and distal (D) used only in the mandible, for removal of root of a molar after the other root has already been removed.

No. 14L and 14R: No. 14L elevator (also No.11L) is used to remove the mesial roots of the right lower molars and distal roots of left lower molars, by engaging the elevator in the adjacent socket wherein the intervening septum is thin.

No. 14R elevator (also No.14R) is used in a similar manner to remove the distal roots of right lower molars and mesial roots of left lower 3rd molars.

No. 1L and 1R: No. 1L and 1R elevators are used to extract vertically impacted 3rd molars and also for luxating the maxillary and mandibular teeth before removing them. The elevator is wedged in between the teeth and antero-posterior force is applied to loosen them, which are then removed with forceps.

Warwick James' elevators

Available as straight and curved (paired) (Fig. 18.9A), used for the extraction of retained roots, deciduous teeth, maxillary 3rd molars and teeth with less resistance in the maxilla. It has a flat handle, therefore the amount of force against bone will decrease, reducing the incidence of the fracture (Fig. 18.9B).

Coupland elevator

Most commonly used elevator. It is similar to a straight elevator, except that the working end is sharp and straight cut and used for chiselling of bone to create point of application

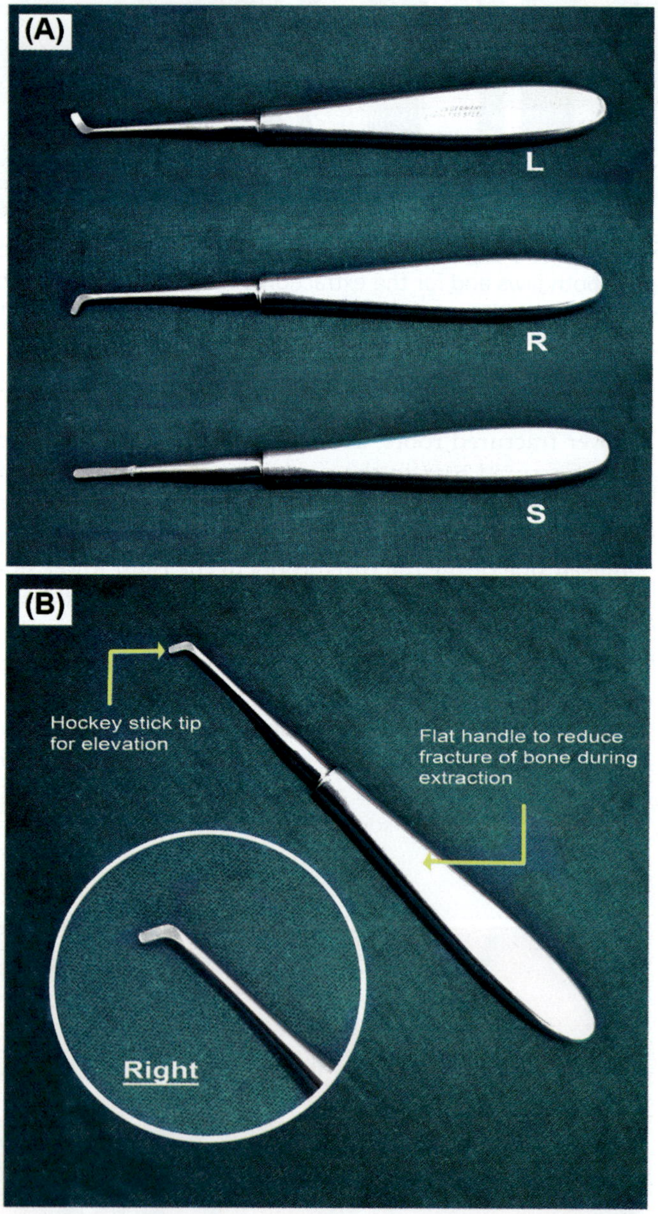

Figure 18.9 (**A**): Warwick James' elevators - left(L), right(R) & straight (S) (**B**) Note the hockey stick-shaped working end of the Warwick James' elevator and flat handle designed to reduce the amount of the force against the bone during extraction.

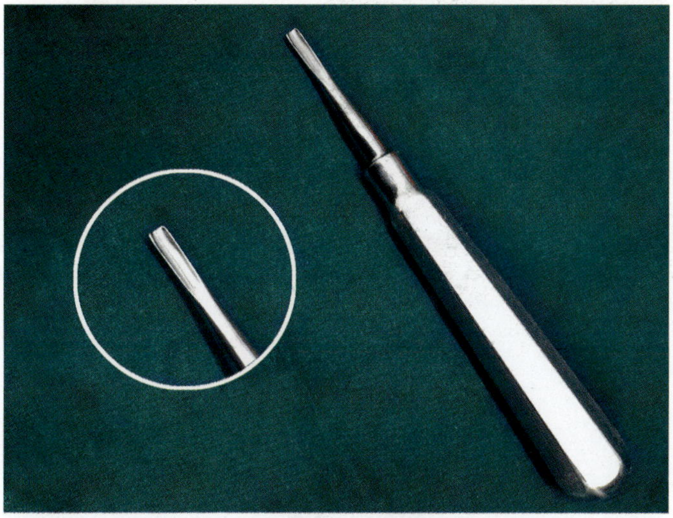

Figure 18.10 Working end of Coupland elevator showing one convex side inserted towards the bone and concave side inserted towards the root surface with flat end.

or to split the tooth. It has one concave working surface and another convex surface (Fig. 18.10). It is available in sizes 1, 2 and 3—working end gets larger with increase in size number. No. 1 (narrow), No. 2 (moderate), No. 3 (broad).

PRINCIPLES OF TOOTH EXTRACTION

Access and visual field

Good access and clear visual field is important for successful tooth extraction.

Use of controlled force

The forces applied for tooth extraction should always be kept under control. Elevators help in widening the periodontal ligament (PDL) space, thus loosening the teeth before its removal. Forceps help in the removal of the teeth by applying rotatory forces and buccal and lingual movements.

Unimpeded path of removal

Whenever there is any resistance to the removal, sectioning of the teeth (odontectomy) should be considered. Malposed, impacted and deeply carious teeth do not have a clear path of exit and therefore must be sectioned before removal.

Expansion of bony socket

Forceps extraction requires and cause bony socket expansion. Expanding the bony socket cause the force to slowly separate the periodontal ligament from the bone.

MECHANICAL PRINCIPLES IN TOOTH EXTRACTION

Once adaptation and securing the grip of the instrument over the tooth is done, the forces to be applied should be in a predetermined direction, which depends on certain mechanical principles. A clear understanding of these principles is necessary to carry out the extraction successfully.

The following mechanical principles used in tooth extractions are:

- Lever principle of 1st order
- Wedge principle
- Wheel and axle.

Lever principle of 1st order

The lever principle has three basic components: fulcrum, effort and load. In a lever of 1st order, the position of the fulcrum is between the effort and the load. In this principle, to gain a mechanical advantage, the effort arm on one side of the fulcrum should be longer than the load arm on the other side of the fulcrum. The force is transmitted at the long effort arm and a mechanical advantage is gained at the short load arm (Fig. 18.11). The mechanical advantage (MA) of a lever is calculated using the *formula:* **MA = effort arm/load arm**.

The effort arm is the distance between the point of effort and the fulcrum; whereas the load arm is the distance between the point of resistance and the fulcrum.

Application

Forceps (Fig. 18.12)

This principle is not particularly useful when applied alone to forceps. However, when combined with a wheel and axle, it functions well. The hinge of the forceps acts as a fulcrum while the two arms represent each component of the lever. The length of the handle in relation to the blade represents the mechanical advantage. To gain a mechanical advantage, the grip should be farther from the fulcrum and the blade should be shorter.

Elevators (Fig. 18.13)

This principle is used in elevators wherein the handle of the elevator represents the effort and the working end, which engages the tooth represents the load.

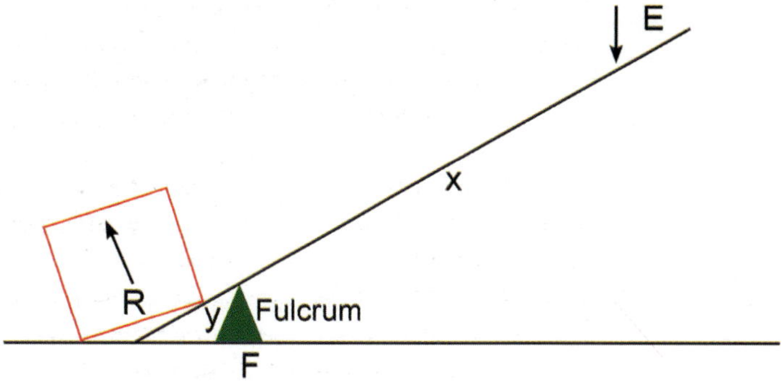

Figure 18.11 Lever principle. *x*-Long arm; *y*-short arm; E = Effort (handle, hand), R = Resistance (tooth), F = Fulcrum (alveolar crestal bone).

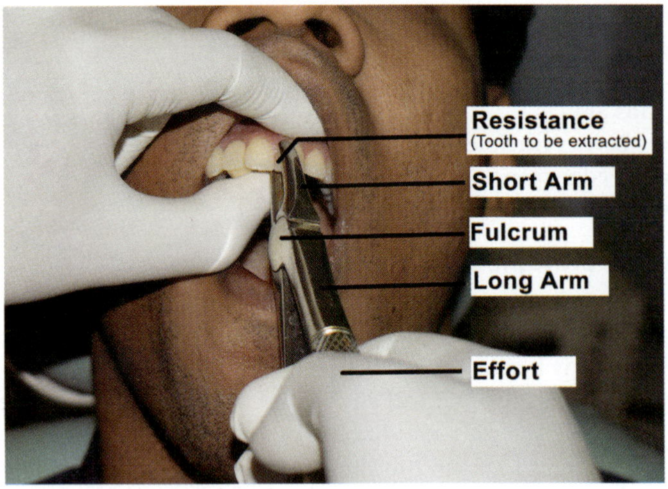

Figure 18.12 Lever principle in forceps. Hinge = fulcrum, beaks = short arm, handles = long arm, teeth = resistance, hand = effort. To gain a mechanical advantage, the effort arm must be longer than the resistance arm, therefore the grip should be farther from the fulcrum.

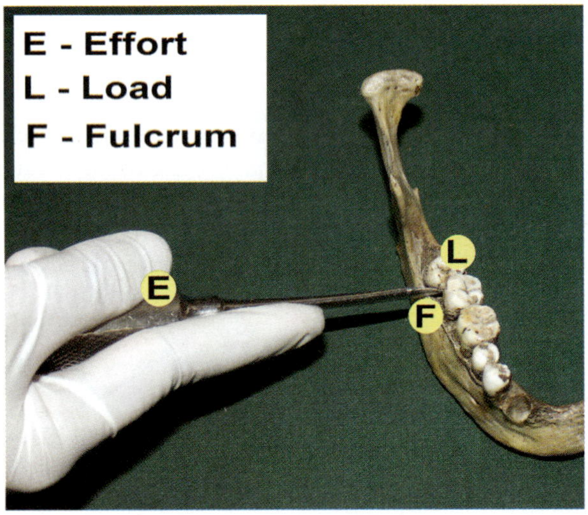

Figure 18.13 Lever principle in elevators. Tooth and working tip = load, handle = effort, external oblique ridge (buccal bone) = fulcrum. When the elevator working tip (load) is applied at a point and the handle (effort) forces apically, the tooth is elevated occlusally out of socket with buccoalveolar bone used as fulcrum.

Wedge principle

The wedge consists of two movable inclined planes with a base on one end and a blade on the other end, which overcomes a large resistance at right angles to the applied force. The effort is applied to the base of the plane and the resistance has its effect on the slant side (Fig. 18.11). The mechanical advantage is calculated by *formula = length of the slope/width of the wedge*. The mechanical advantage of a wedge is 2.5.

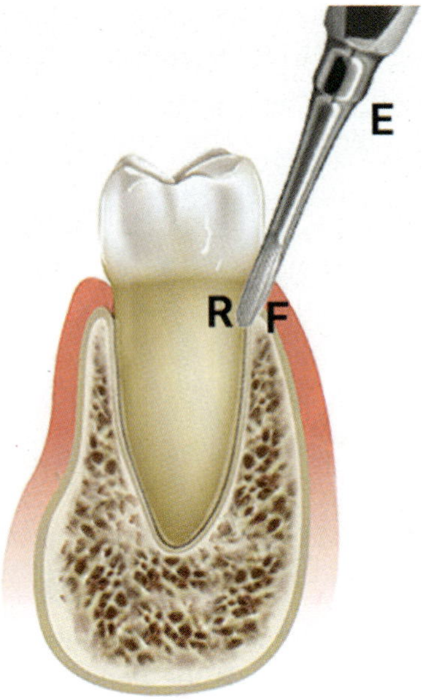

Figure 18.14 Wedge principle: insertion of straight elevator between the tooth and the alveolar bone along the long axis of the tooth, expanding the PDL space. *E = Effort, R = Resistance, F = Fulcrum.*

Application (Fig. 18.14)

Wedge principle can be used as a sole principle in extracting a tooth. However, it is more frequently used in conjunction with lever principle. According to this principle, a wedge can be used to split, expand or displace the portion of the substance that receives it.

Elevators (Fig. 18.15)

Elevators can also be used based on this principle, for example, when luxating a tooth from its socket, a straight elevator is applied between the tooth and the bone to separate the attachment of the periodontal ligament from the bone as described previously.

Extraction forceps (Fig. 18.16)

The forceps is applied using this principle. For carrying out extraction, the tip of the forceps is inserted in between the mucoperiosteum and surface of the tooth. When the beaks are inserted further, the mucoperiosteum gets displaced, the bony sockets are expanded which results in slow separation of the periodontal ligament from the bone.

Wheel and axle

Wheel and axle is a simple machine being a modified form of lever. The effort is applied to the circumference of the wheel, which turns the axle so as to raise the weight. Greater the diameter of the wheel, more is the MA (Fig. 18.17). *Formula = (Effort × radius of wheel = resistance × radius of axle)(R/E=Rw/Ra)*. MA of this principle is 4.6.

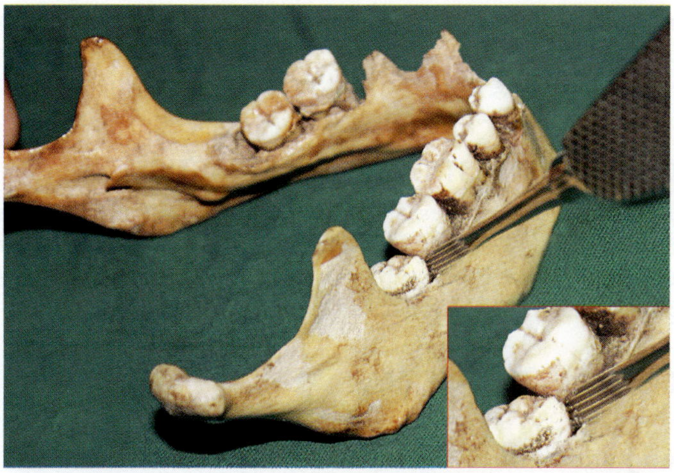

Figure 18.15 Wedge principle in elevators—the blade of the elevator is used as a wedge to displace the tooth root out of the socket.

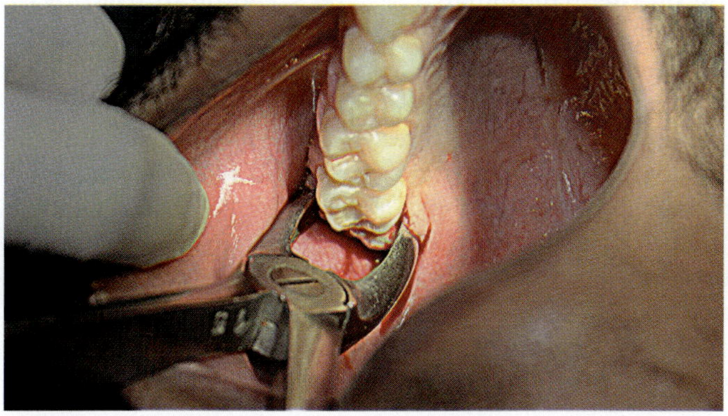

Figure 18.16 Wedge principle in forceps—expansion of bony socket by the use of wedge-shaped beaks of forceps inserted between the mucoperiosteum and tooth, further into PDL space displacing the tooth out of socket.

Application

Applied to elevators (Fig. 18.18A–D)

Winter's crossbar elevators are used for removing the mandibular roots based on this principle. The working point of this elevator is engaged deep into the space between the tooth root and the bone and the handle (compared to the wheel) is rotated. The root is removed from its socket by moving about a circumference of the circle (compared to the axle), which the roots would have made if they continued on around.

Extraction forceps (Fig. 18.19A and B)

To remove a tooth, the beaks of the forceps are applied firmly on either side of the tooth and force is applied in the form of an arc. According to the principle of wheel and axle, when the force is applied on the handle of the forceps, it results in a bodily rotation of the tooth in the socket, which is ultimately delivered out.

To gain a mechanical advantage, always hold the forceps handle (compared to the wheel) as farther away as possible to increase the effort arm (compared to the axle). When using this principle with forceps, the periodontal attachment gets ruptured due to the bodily rotation of the tooth. This principle can be used separately or in conjunction with wedge or lever principle in removing the teeth.

CHOICE OF ANAESTHESIA

Most of the minor surgical procedures can be performed under LA successfully; however, in certain situations, GA may be necessary, for example, when the patient is allergic to local anaesthetic, uncooperative patient. Choice is determined by a group of factors such as type or extent of the operation, patient's preference (physical or mental condition), age of the patient, condition of the operative site (presence of infection) and place of operation (dental setup/hospital setup).

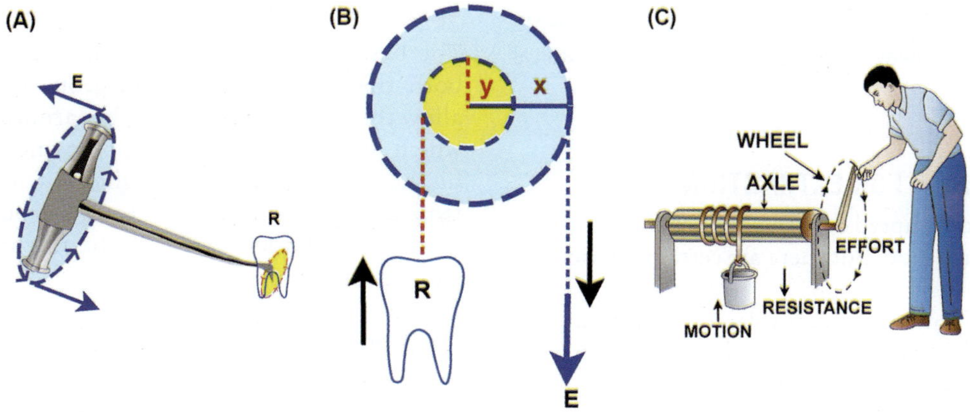

Figure 18.17 (A-C) Wheel and axle. x = Radius of wheel; y = radius of the axle, E = effort, R = resistance, mechanical advantage of crossbar is 4.6.

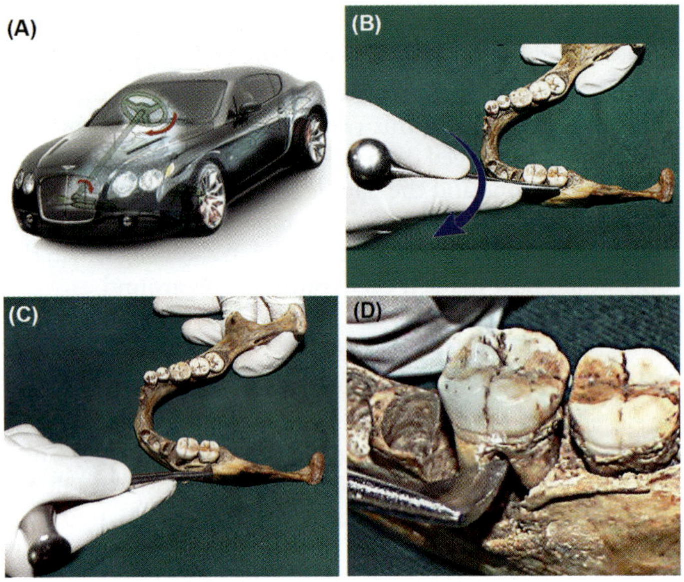

Figure 18.18 (**A**) Illustration of wheel and axle in a car. (**B**) Wheel and axle principle in elevators. Position 1—the working point of crossbar engages the space between the tooth and bone at the furcation. Note the hand in pronation. (**C**) Position 2—the working tip and handle rotates around its axis (axle) with handle acting as wheel. Note supination of the hand. (**D**) Demonstration in skull model application of elevator tip into the buccal furcation.

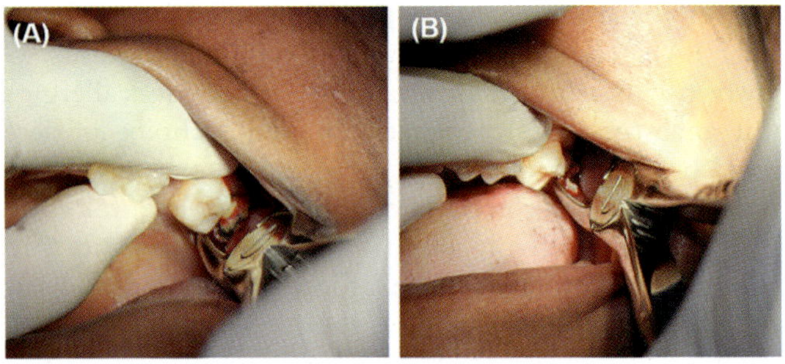

Figure 18.19 (**A and B**) Wheel and axle principle. Forces applied from forceps in the form of an arc and the periodontal attachment gets ruptured due to the bodily rotation of the tooth. Note the position of the hand away from the axle to gain a mechanical advantage.

LOCAL ANAESTHESIA FOR EXTRACTION

For the extraction of erupted and the impacted teeth, LA is the safest available method, but there are certain restrictions of LA such as:

- Some conscious patients cannot tolerate lengthy surgical procedures carried out under LA
- Children under the age of 8 years cannot differentiate between the sensation of pain and pressure, and hence they perceive pressure as pain and become uncooperative. Even an older individual who is nervous can have the same problem
- If there is an area of acute infection, it is not advisable to inject the local anaesthetic solution in that area for risk of spreading infection and failure of anaesthetic effect due to acidic environment.

GENERAL ANAESTHESIA FOR EXTRACTION

For shorter procedures lasting less than 10 min, intravenous injection followed by inhalation anaesthesia is suitable, but if the procedure is beyond this time, an endotracheal intubation should be used. Refer to Chapter 12.

GENERAL ARRANGEMENT

DENTAL CHAIR POSITION

Angulation of the chair

When the mouth is open, the chair is angulated in such a way that the operative field is in the most visible and accessible position. The chair should be angulated in such a way that the occlusal surface of the mandibular teeth are parallel or at 10 degrees to the floor, when the operator is working on the mandibular teeth and standing in front of the patient.

When the operator is standing behind the patient, the angle of the occlusal plane of the mandibular teeth is increased until the tooth or teeth can be grasped without positioning the dentist or his/her arm and hand in an uncomfortable position.

When working on the maxilla, the chair should be angulated so that the occlusal plane of the maxillary teeth is between an angle of 45 and 60 degrees to the floor.

Height of the chair

Procedures on the mandible (Fig. 18.20): The occlusal plane of the mandibular teeth should be at or slightly below the level of surgeon's elbow.

Procedures on the maxilla (Fig. 18.21): The occlusal plane of the maxillary teeth should be above the level of the surgeon's elbow towards his/her shoulders.

1) POSITION OF THE PATIENT

The best possible position is one that is comfortable for both the patient and the surgeon. This position should allow the surgeon to keep his/her arm close to his/her body, which lends stability and support and also allows to keep his/her wrist straight enough to deliver maximum controlled force to the patient's tooth through the forceps. The force should be delivered with the arm and shoulder but not with the hand.

Position of the patient's head, neck and trunk (Fig. 18.22)

The chair is adjusted in such a way that the head, neck and trunk are in one line. This will nullify any strain caused by stretching it backward or pushing it forward.

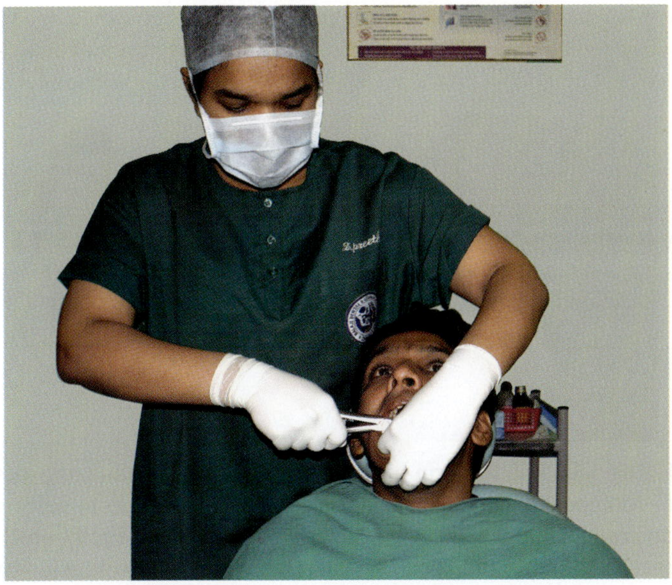

Figure 18.20 Position of operator during extraction of 4th quadrant teeth. The operator should stand behind the patient. Note the dominant hand of operator's elbow above the mandibular occlusal plane, holding the forceps and the nondominant hand retracting cheek and tongue in addition to supporting the mandible. (Scan to play extraction of 48).

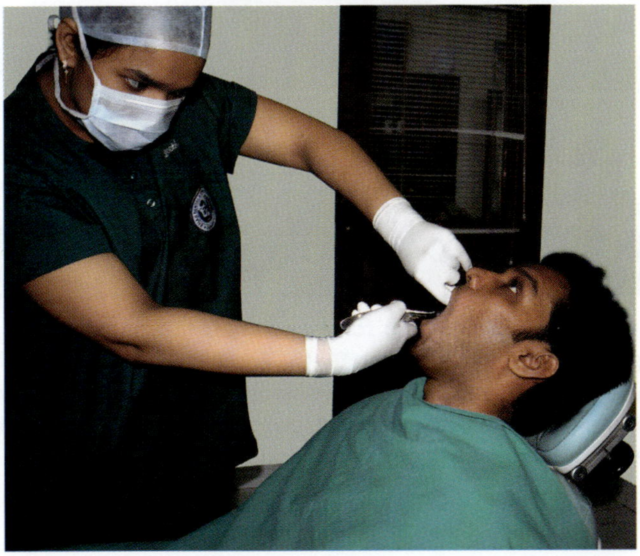

Figure 18.21 Position of the operator during extraction of maxillary teeth. The operator should stand in front of the patient. Note the dominant hand of surgeon's elbow below the maxillary occlusal plane. (Scan to play extraction of 28).

2) POSITION OF THE OPERATOR DURING EXTRACTION

The surgeon should position himself/herself in such a way that he/she can apply the forces necessary for extraction without any stress to his/her own back or shoulders. The dentist should stand as erect as possible with his/her weight

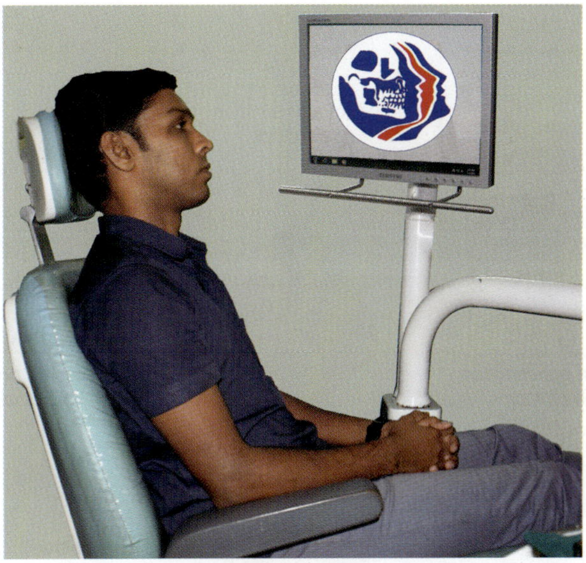

Figure 18.22 Chair adjusted in such a way that the position of patient's head, neck and trunk in one line.

equally distributed on each foot. Operator's arms must be close to body and delivery of force must be with arm and shoulder, not with hand, while performing extractions. For performing extractions in 1st, 2nd and 3rd quadrants, the right handed operator should stand at 7 o'clock to 8 o'clock position whereas for 4th quadrant, he should stand at 11 o'clock position. Standing position for right and left handed operator for extraction is shown in Table 18.3. Pictorial presentation to describe operator positions in exodontia is shown in Fig. 18.23.

For the extraction of maxillary teeth (Figs. 18.24–18.25)

The surgeon should stand on the right side and in front of the patient with the bent elbow for posterior and straight for anterior teeth, and should apply the forceps onto the tooth while the other hand holds the alveolus with the finger and thumb on either side of the involved tooth.

TABLE 18.3 Operator's Standing Position for Extraction

Teeth	Position for Right-Handed Operator	Position for Left-Handed Operator
All maxillary teeth and mandibular anterior teeth	7 o'clock to 8 o'clock	4 o'clock to 5 o'clock
Mandibular left posterior teeth	7 o'clock to 8 o'clock	1 o'clock
Mandibular right posterior teeth	11 o'clock	4 o'clock to 5 o'clock

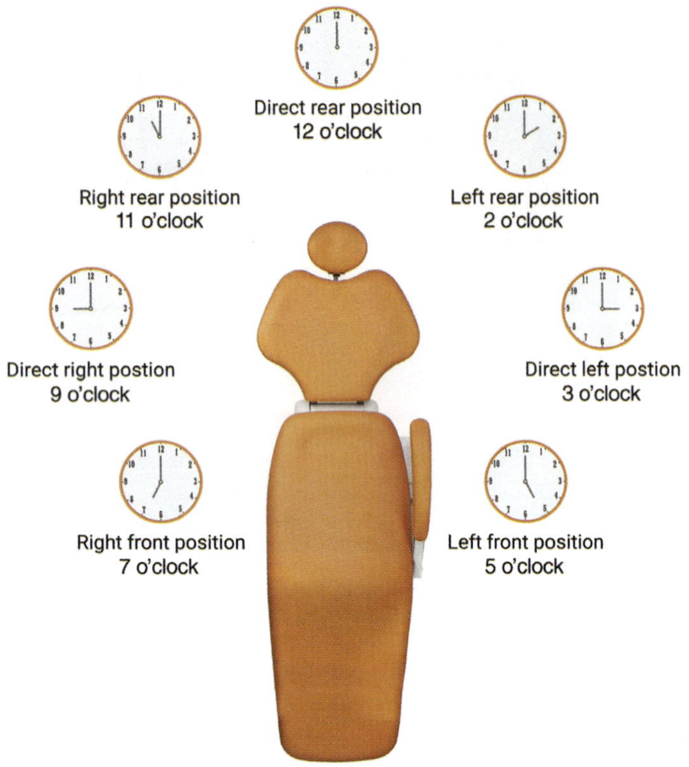

Figure 18.23 Pictorial presentation to describe operator positions in exodontia. 7 o'clock position for extractions in 1st, 2nd and 3rd quadrants, whereas, for 4th quadrant operator should stand at 11 o'clock position for a right-handed operator.

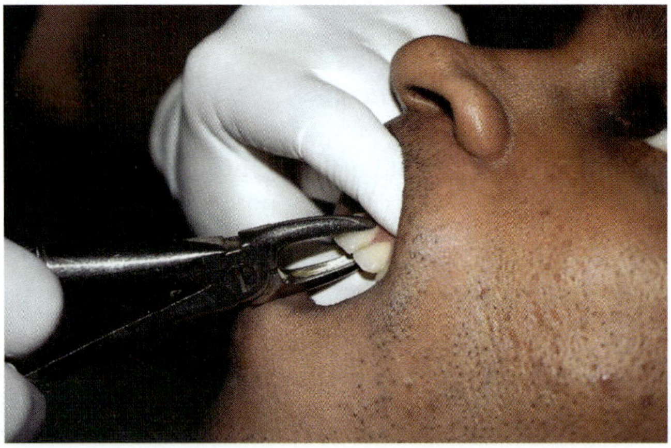

Figure 18.24 Extraction of maxillary anterior teeth—dominant (right) hand holds the forceps while nondominant (left) hand supports the alveolus. Scan to play exodontia extraction of 23.

For the extraction of mandibular teeth (Figs. 18.26–18.27)

The surgeon should stand on the right side of the patient for both the quadrants. For the extraction of the left lower side, the operator should stand in front of the patient; and for the right lower side, the operator should stand behind the patient. Apart from supporting the alveolus on each side by the thumb and forefinger, the left hand should also support the mandible.

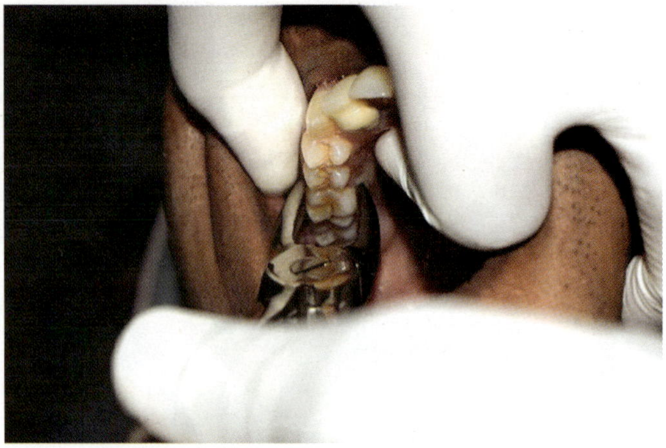

Figure 18.25 Extraction of maxillary posterior teeth. Long axis of forceps beak should engage the neck of the tooth, resting on cementum and must be parallel to that of the tooth which results in minimum tooth apical movement and expansion of the socket. Note-Dominant hand holds the forceps while non-dominant hand supports the alveolus.

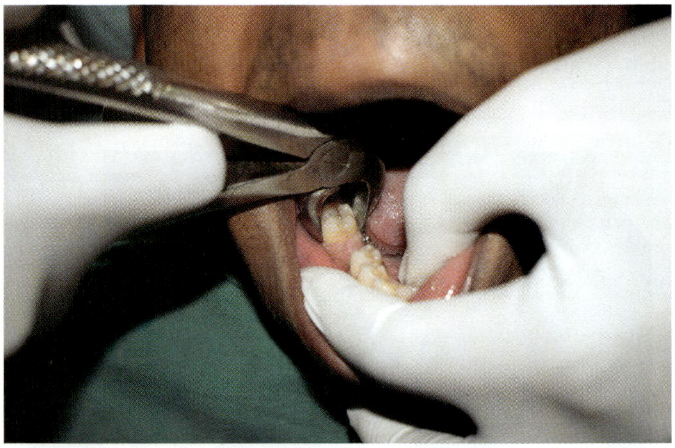

Figure 18.26 Sling grasp for mandibular teeth. Extraction of right mandibular posterior teeth. Forceps beaks engage the buccal and lingual furcation. Nondominant hand, thumb and forefinger retract and support alveolus while the palm and remaining fingers support the mandible.

Extractions with the surgeon seated

The surgeon seated on a mobile chair capable of moving in an arc about the patient's head and the chair is adjusted such that patient is placed in supine position. Principles of extraction are similar to the normal technique. When working on the upper jaw, some slight modification of the supporting hand is necessary. Operating on a supine position, patient has

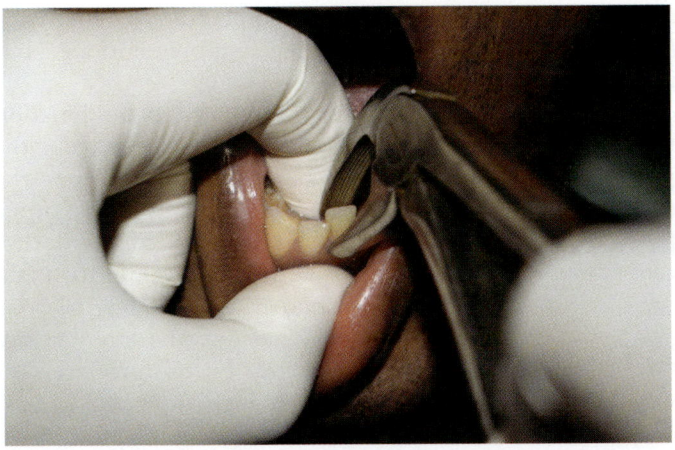

Figure 18.27 Extraction of mandibular anterior teeth. Long axis of forceps beak must be parallel to that of the tooth without impinging the adjacent teeth and must grasp the tooth firmly on sound root structure and not on the enamel of the tooth crown. Nondominant hand thumb and forefinger retracts and support the alveolus.

some hazards as the displaced teeth, roots or fillings may fall back into the pharynx, and to prevent this, adequate steps must be taken. Placement of gauze prior to extraction, use of high volume suction can help in preventing displacement of the tooth. During the operation, the conscious patient can be asked to cooperate by turning their head well to one side.

LIGHT

Must provide good illumination.

ROLE OF OPPOSITE HAND

a. Reflection of the soft tissue
b. Protection of the other teeth
c. Stabilising patient's head
d. Supporting and stabilising the mandible
e. Supports alveolar bone
f. Tactile information
g. Compression of the socket
   Pinch grasp: The operator pinch grasps the alveolar bone around the tooth to be extracted while extracting maxillary teeth (Fig. 18.25)
   Sling grasp: The operator sling grasps the alveolar bone around the tooth to be extracted while extracting mandibular teeth (Fig. 18.26).

ROLE OF ASSISTANT

a. Assistant helps the surgeon to gain access and visualise the field
b. Suction
c. Protect the teeth of opposite arch
d. Support the head
e. Support the mandible
f. Psychological and emotional support.

AMBIDEXTEROUS EXTRACTIONS

To facilitate extractions from only one position, techniques can be extrapolated with other hand (less dominant hand), once the techniques have been well acquired with one hand. All the forces applied are similar regardless of hand used. For example, for extraction of all the teeth in both upper and lower jaws, some operators may favour the use of only one pattern of lower right-angled premolar forceps sitting behind the patient using both hands. For the upper and lower teeth, right hand is used for extraction of teeth on right and those on the patient's left with left hand.

ORDER OF EXTRACTION OF TEETH

Extraction of the teeth in the maxillary arch should be performed before mandibular arch as the upper arch gets anaesthetised earlier than the lower arch. Moreover, extraction of upper arch prior to the lower arch prevents any inadvertent fall of enamel or amalgam debris into the extraction socket in the lower arch. This rule can be applied in all cases except for the removal of impacted teeth.

- Extraction of the most posterior tooth in the dental arch is done 1st; this causes haemorrhage to collect in the posterior region so that the vision to the surgical field is not affected in the anterior region
- If complete extraction has to be done in a patient with complete set of teeth or in whom it results in a better purchase on the tooth and also has the advantage of earlier plate expansion resulting from adjacent extractions. These two teeth are encased in the so-called bony pillar of the face
- Following the above rules, the order of extraction in an arch of a jaw is as follows:
  - 3rd molar
  - 2nd molar
  - 2nd premolar
  - 1st molar
  - 1st premolar
  - Lateral incisor
  - Canine
  - Central incisor

TECHNIQUES OF EXTRACTION

1. Intraalveolar extraction (closed technique) (Flowchart 18.1).
   - Forceps technique
   - Elevator technique
2. Transalveolar extraction (open method).

FORCEPS TECHNIQUE

It is the most commonly used technique. This technique is contraindicated in case of root deformities, grossly decayed crown and root, brittle root and hypercementosis.

Principles of use (*Fig. 18.28*)

The forceps is applied with an apical pressure by inserting the beaks on the buccal/labial and lingual/palatal aspect of the tooth, in between the bone and the surface of the tooth so

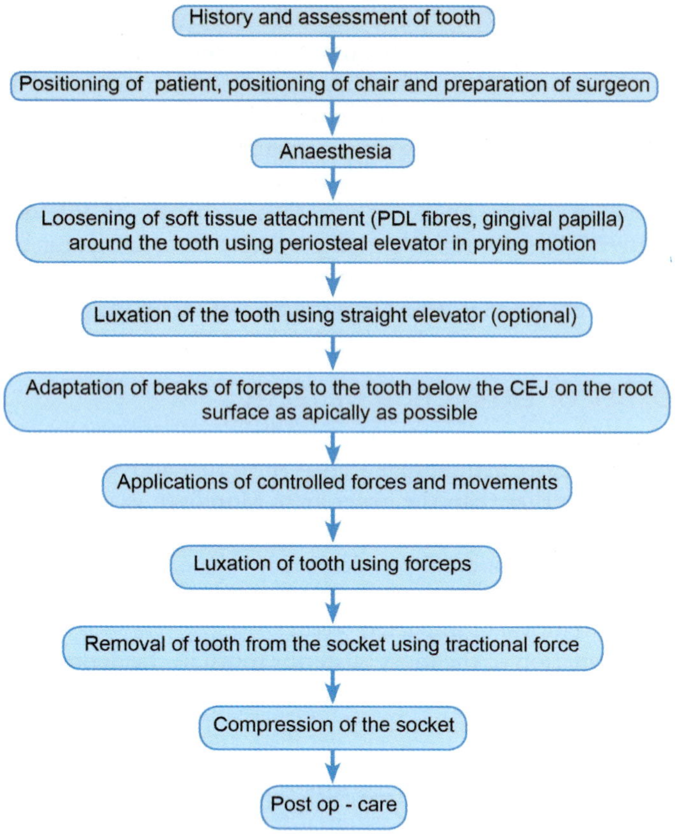

Flowchart 18.1 Steps in intraalveolar/closed extraction technique.

that the beaks rest on the root/roots of the tooth. The beaks of the forceps should be parallel to the long axis of the tooth. This results in a minimum apical movement of the tooth and expansion of the socket.

Force application

When *buccal force* is applied, it results in the expansion of the buccal plate. This movement causes the pressure to be concentrated on the crest of the alveolar ridge on the buccal aspect and also causes lingual apical pressure. Then, *lingual force* is applied with a similar concept as aforementioned, but in a lingual direction.

The buccal and lingual forces are applied in combination for the removal of most of the teeth. As in the maxilla, the palatal bone is thicker when compared to the buccal bone, the teeth are removed via strong buccal force and less vigorous palatal force (if stronger palatal force is applied, the palatal root tip may fracture, which is hard to retrieve). In the mandible also, the buccal bone is thinner than the lingual bone particularly in the anterior teeth. Therefore, the anteriors and the premolars are removed via strong buccal force and less vigorous lingual force. However, in the molar region, the buccal plate of bone is thicker; hence, strong lingual force should be applied and the tooth is removed through the buccal force.

Then, *rotational force* is applied on the tooth, which causes expansion of the socket and rotation of the tooth around its fulcrum, which usually lies near the apical tip of the tooth root. If the roots of the tooth are very long or if they are curved or multiplied, then root fracture is more likely when using rotational force. Applied for conical single rooted which are circular in cross-section with cylindrical root, for example, maxillary central incisors and mandibular premolars.

The 1st force is always applied on less accessible side of the tooth, in case of cervical caries, 1st movement is directed towards carious side of tooth.

Rules to be observed in the application of forceps (Figs. 18.29–18.30)

1. The correct forceps for the particular tooth to be extracted must be selected
2. Grasp the forceps at the far end of the handles so that they are almost covered by the palm of the hand. Do not grasp the forceps near the beaks
3. The long axis of the forceps beaks must be parallel to the long axis of the tooth
4. Forceps beaks must be grasped firmly on sound root structure and not on the enamel of the tooth crown
5. Make certain that the beaks of the forceps do not impinge on adjacent teeth during the luxation.

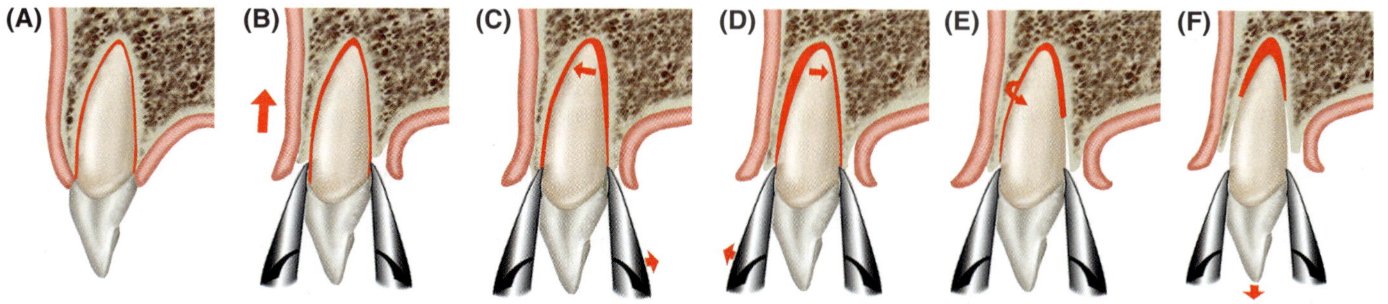

Figure 18.28 Method of usage of forceps for extraction of teeth. **(A)** Before extraction. **(B)** Apical pressure applied with forceps. **(C)** Application of lingual pressure. **(D)** Application of buccal pressure. **(E)** Rotational force applied. **(F)** Tractional force applied and tooth removed by the buccal aspect.

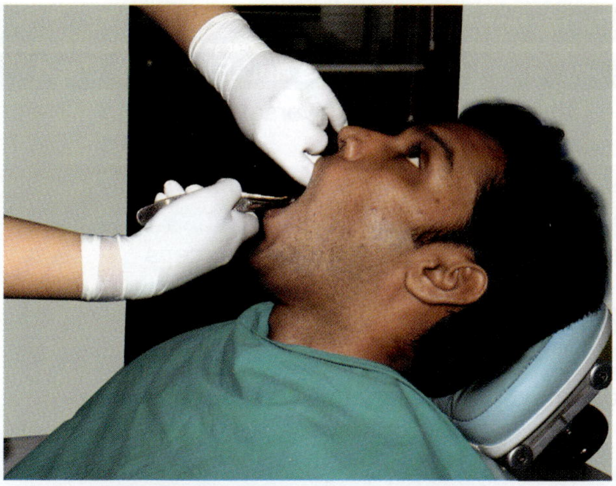

Figure 18.29 Forceps should be grasped at the far end of the handle away from the beaks for maximal mechanical advantage.

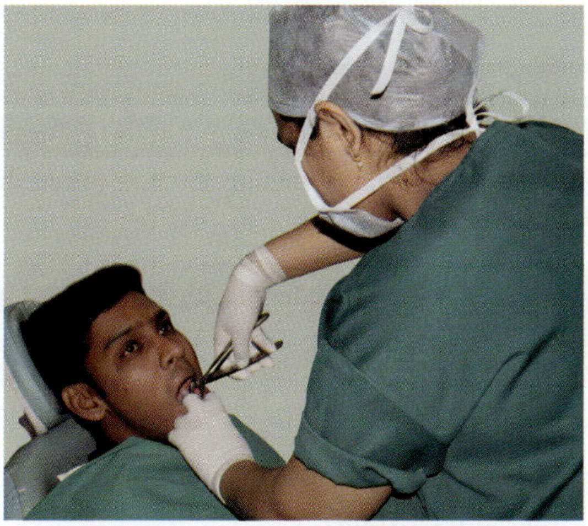

Figure 18.30 Figure showing the holding of forceps for extraction. Note: The 1st three fingers are placed around the handles below the joint and the little finger is placed in between handles and the handles are held apart by the little finger initially. Once the forceps are thoroughly applied, the little finger can be brought around the handle.

Forces applied for different teeth

Basic forces exerted in extraction of maxillary teeth in normal position in the arch (Table 18.4)

As already mentioned, the 1st pressure applied for the extraction of all maxillary teeth is apical force. The beaks of the forceps should engage the neck of the tooth, resting on cementum. Then, apply pressure as follows.

Basic forces exerted in extraction of mandibular teeth in normal position in the arch (Table 18.5)

Similar to the maxillary teeth, the 1st force is the apical force so that the beaks of the forceps rest on the cementum. Then, apply pressure as follows.

Holding the forceps

The 1st three fingers are placed around the handles below the joint and the little finger is placed in between the handles initially, which helps in holding the handles apart. The little finger can be brought around the handle once the forceps are thoroughly applied. The thumb should not be placed between the handles as this also misaligns the instrument and also can lead to tooth breakage during extraction.

ELEVATOR TECHNIQUE

It works on lever and fulcrum principle, it forces the tooth/root from their bony socket along the line of withdrawal. *Line of withdrawal* is the path along which the tooth or root will move out of its socket with the application, and this line is primarily determined by root pattern (long axis of the tooth). *Point of application* is the force applied on the site of root for effective delivery and is in turn determined by the line of withdrawal. The point of application can be buccal point, mesial point and distal point (Fig. 18.31). The application of elevator must be at 45 degrees to long axis of tooth in periodontal space.

Stobie's technique—extraction of multiple mandibular anteriors by using elevators between teeth. In this technique, the adjacent teeth are used as fulcrum.

Precautions to be followed in using elevators:

- We should never use the adjacent tooth as a fulcrum as this will damage or even luxate the adjacent tooth
- We should always use finger guard to protect the patient's tissue, as slipping of the instrument tip into the soft tissue might cause tissue damage
- The forces applied through the instrument should be under control; failing to do so would cause fracture of the maxilla, mandible or the alveolar process. Thus, control of the instrument with index finger on the shank is mandatory (Fig. 18.32)
- The instrument tip should deliver the force in the correct direction to avoid the accidental forcing of the tooth into the maxillary antrum.

TRANSALVEOLAR EXTRACTION (OPEN METHOD)

Transalveolar extraction refers to surgical removal of a tooth or root that involves bone removal.

INDICATIONS

- Any tooth or root, which cannot be removed using elevators or forceps
- Unerupted teeth, impacted teeth
- Tooth with extensively curved or dilacerated roots
- Endodontically treated teeth or grossly carious teeth
- Hypercementosed or ankylosed teeth
- Retained root fragments.

The principles and surgical procedures of transalveolar extraction (open method) are explained in detail in Chapter 19 on, Page no. 345 and Fig. 19.32.

TABLE 18.4 Basic Forces Applied for the Maxillary Teeth Extraction

Teeth	Steps in the Procedure	Forceps and Elevators Used
Central incisors	Labial pressure, then lingual pressure, then labial pressure with mesial rotation	Maxillary universal forceps
Lateral incisors	Labial pressure, then lingual pressure, then labial pressure with mesial rotation	Maxillary universal forceps
Cuspids	Labial pressure, then lingual pressure, then labial pressure with mesial rotation	Maxillary universal forceps
1st bicuspids	Buccal pressure, lingual pressure and removal in the buccal direction	Maxillary universal forceps or no. 150 forceps
2nd bicuspids	Buccal pressure, lingual pressure and removal in the lingual or buccal direction	Maxillary universal forceps or no. 150 forceps
1st and 2nd molars	Buccal pressure, slight palatal pressure and distal rotation	Maxillary right or left molar forceps for the respective side
3rd molar		Maxillary right or left 3rd molar forceps Cryer's paired—right (R) and left (L)

TABLE 18.5 Basic Forces Applied for the Mandibular Teeth Extraction

Teeth	Steps in the Procedure	Forceps and Elevators Used
Central, lateral incisors and cuspids	Labial pressure, lingual pressure; slight mesial to distal force and removal in the labial direction	Vertical hinge mandibular forceps (mandibular anterior forceps)
1st and 2nd bicuspids	Buccal pressure, with slight mesiodistal rotation	Vertical hinge mandibular forceps (mandibular anterior forceps)
1st and 2nd molars	Buccal pressure, lingual pressure and removal in the buccal direction.	Mandibular molar forceps (vertical or horizontal hinge forceps) Mandibular cow horn forceps
3rd molar	Buccal pressure and removal in the buccal or lingual direction	Mandibular right or left 3rd molar forceps (straight elevator) Straight Bein elevator (Coupland elevator)

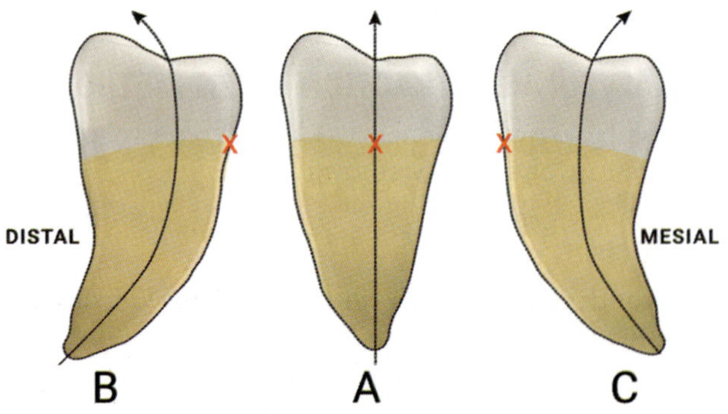

Figure 18.31 Figure showing various root pattern and the point of application of elevator on the root for effective delivery of the tooth. Line of withdrawal is the path along which the tooth or root will move out of its socket with the application, and this line is primarily determined by root pattern (long axis of the tooth).

FRACTURE OF TOOTH ROOT

Fracture of the tooth root is a common complication encountered during extraction. There are many factors responsible for root fracture.

Causes

- Improper technique
- Application of incorrect instrument and force
- Ankylosed teeth or hypercementosed teeth
- Condensing osteitis
- Excessively curved roots
- Endodontically treated teeth
- Teeth with gross filling
- Extensively carious teeth
- Uncooperative patient.

Methods for retrieval of fractured root

Using appropriate elevators, roots fractured at various levels can be removed.

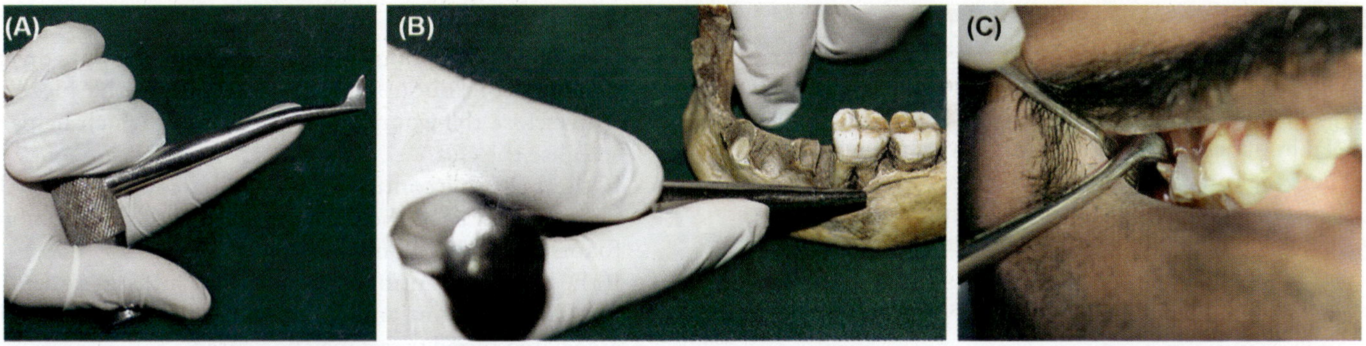

Figure 18.32 (**A**) Crossbar–palm grasp with the index finger placed over the shank for delivery of controlled force. (**B**) Application of elevator demonstrated in a skull model. (**C**) Application of Cryer's elevator in extraction of maxillary 3rd molar.

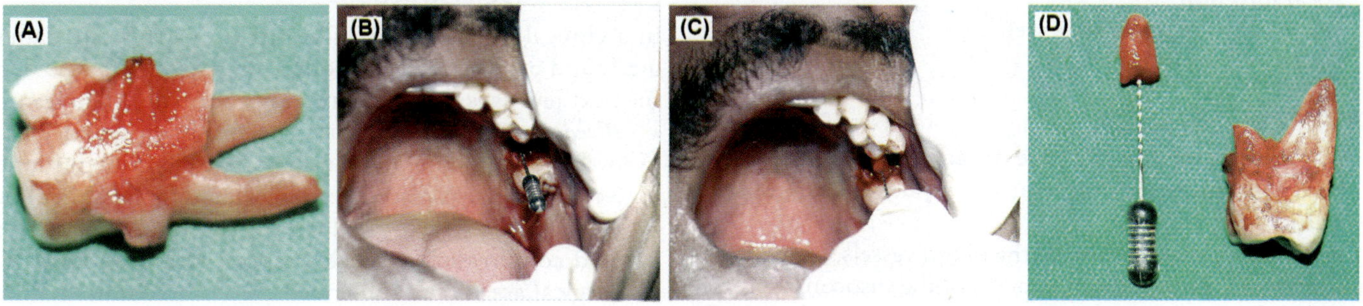

Figure 18.33 Removal of fractured root using reamer. (**A**) Fractured palatal root in relation to 26. (**B**) Reamer used to engage the root. (**C**) Fractured root removed with reamer. (**D**) Figure showing the extracted tooth and its fractured root.

Forceps with slender beaks can be used to remove certain roots. Reamers can also be used to retrieve roots. The technique is shown in Fig. 18.33. If the aforementioned methods fail, transalveolar extraction should be attempted.

Consequences of retained roots

Retained roots may act as a source of infection. They might be a chronic source of irritation giving rise to neuralgic pain. When large retained roots are lying in the submucosa just beneath the denture, the overlying mucosa constantly gets inflamed and may interfere with the proper functioning of the denture.

Root removal after healing of the socket

As a preparation for dentures, the dental surgeon may be required to extract buried roots as they are believed to be a source of pain or sepsis.

Localising roots

To inflict minimal damage onto the alveolar bone, once again diagnosis and assessment is important. Localisation of root accurately is the 1st step. Sometimes two radiographs at right angles to each other are required, either an orthopantomogram (OPG) or long cone periapical and occlusal views would be appropriate.

Removal of roots

The removal of old retained roots is similar to that of removal of newly fractured teeth. The horizontal incision is placed just buccal to the alveolar crest, where the mucous membrane is less tightly bound down in the edentulous jaw. A curved incision is placed in the alveolus away from the crest of the ridge where root apices are deeply placed, and the fragment is removed through this incision.

Policy for leaving root fragments

When a root tip has fractured, the surgeon may consider leaving the root in place when closed approaches of removal have been unsuccessful and when the open approach may be excessively traumatic. The surgeon must balance the benefits of surgery against the risks of surgery as with any surgical approach. Three conditions exist where tooth root can be left in the alveolar process.

1st, smaller root fragment, that is length not more than 4 to 5 mm. 2nd, the root fragment must not be superficial. It must be deeply embedded in bone, to prevent interfering with the prosthesis with subsequent bone resorption from exposing the tooth root in edentulous area. 3rd, there must be no radiolucency around the root apex, that is the involved tooth must not be infected. In these three conditions, consideration can be given to leaving the root tip.

MANAGEMENT OF HAEMORRHAGE

Bleeding is a common sequela of oral surgery. Refer to Chapter 9 page number 118 for the management. This may be seen in patients with or without any systemic cause.

There are three type of postoperative bleeding:

- **Primary**—occurs continuously after the surgery
- **Reactionary**—haemorrhage restarts after a period of about 3 h
- **Secondary**—occurs after a few days.

Causes

I. **In patients without any systemic cause:**

Primary

- Local infection
- Tear of any major blood vessel
- Punctured wound.

Reactionary

- Disturbance of the clot due to activities like chewing hard substances, gargling, consuming alcohol and taking warm food
- Reactionary vasodilation of the blood vessels, which had contracted during administration of the vasoconstrictors along with LA.

Secondary

- Blood clot may be infected by certain bacteria like streptococci, which may dissolve the clot and result in bleeding
- Acute ulcerative necrotising bleeding.

II. **In patients with a systemic cause:**

Hereditary

- Haemophilia

Acquired

- Hypertension
- Anticoagulant therapy
- Vitamin K deficiency
- Thrombocytopaenia
- Liver disorders.

Prevention

- A proper medical history of the patient should be taken to detect any systemic disorders
- The necessary investigations, that is prothrombin time (PT), partial thromboplastin time (PTT), bleeding time (BT), clotting time (CT), test for detection of clotting factors, etc. should be performed in suspected cases
- In such cases, the extraction should be carried out taking due precautions
- Avoid unnecessary incision or flap elevation or any other trauma to the tissues
- In haemophilic patients, the lacking clotting factor should be administered before the extraction.

Management

- As soon as continuous bleeding is detected, apply digital pressure continuously for 2 to 3 min. If the bleeding stops, close the wound by using sutures, which helps to stabilise the clot
- If the bleeding continues, it may be coming from the bony socket. Pack the bony socket with Gelfoam, fibrin foam, Surgicel or bone wax
- If the bleeding continues despite these measures, identify the bleeding point and cauterise it with diathermy. The associated blood vessel may be ligated
- A sample of blood may be sent for testing to find out any systemic involvement. Appropriate treatment for the cause can then be given.

Postoperative instructions

In a clinical practice, it is judicious to instruct the patient orally and in a written form concerning exactly what to do in the next few days. These instructions normally include:

- ***Bleeding***: The patient must bite firmly on gauze placed over the wound for 30–45 min. In case bleeding continues, another gauze is placed over the wound for a further hour
- ***Oedema***: After the procedure, the extraoral placement of cold compresses (ice pack wrapped in a towel) over the surgical area is recommended every 15–20 min at a time and repeated every half hour for at least 4–6 h
- ***Oral hygiene***: The patient should be advised to brush and floss, but should avoid the surgical area. Rinsing the mouth is not allowed for the 1st 24 h. After this, the mouth may be rinsed with salt water, three to five times a day for 3 to 4 days
- ***Antibiotics and analgesics***: Antibiotics are mandatory for patients who undergo any invasive procedure. Many studies show evidence that antibiotics administered preoperatively or postoperatively reduce the risk of infection, pain and dry socket after tooth extraction. Analgesics advised (e.g. NSAIDS and opioids but not salicylates, aspirin) should be consumed, as long as the pain persists
- ***Diet***: The patient's diet on the day of the surgical procedure must consist of cold, liquid foods (pudding, yogurt, milk, cold soup, orange juice, etc.)
- ***Removal of sutures***: Intraoral sutures are usually removed in a week.

COMPLICATIONS OF EXTRACTION

1. INTRAOPERATIVE COMPLICATIONS (IMMEDIATE)

- Soft tissue injury
- Extraction of the wrong teeth
- Fracture of the teeth and its root during extraction
- Fracture of the alveolus, tuberosity, and the mandible
- Displacement of the tooth into the maxillary sinus
- Creation of oroantral fistula
- Breakage of instrument
- Luxation of adjacent tooth
- Injury to inferior alveolar and lingual nerve

- Swallowing of teeth
- Aspiration of teeth
- Dislocation of condyle.

2. POSTOPERATIVE COMPLICATIONS (DELAYED)

- Presence of bony spicules and haemorrhage
- Postoperative oedema/swelling and dry socket
- Infection and Trismus.

SOFT TISSUE INJURY (FIGS. 18.34–18.36)

Types and causes

Abrasion: These injuries are caused by careless use of rotary instruments.

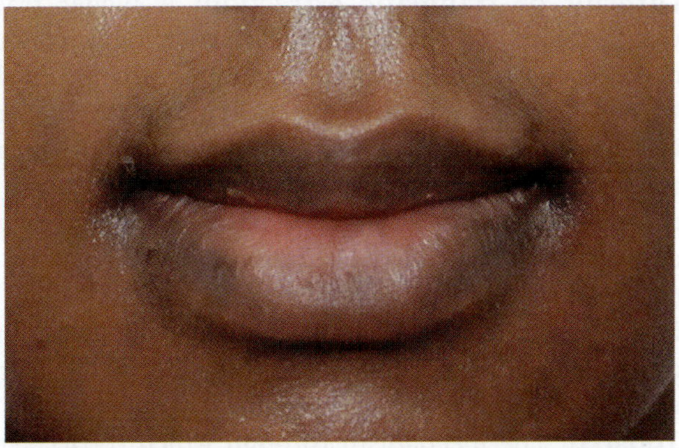

Figure 18.34 Soft tissue injury—abrasion of corners of mouth caused by careless use of rotary instruments.

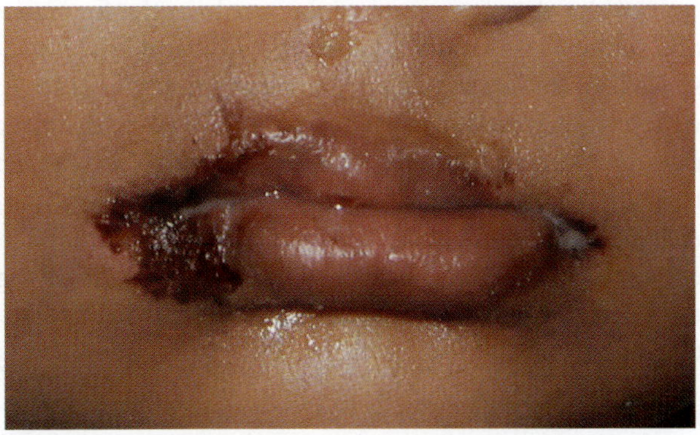

Figure 18.35 Soft tissue injury—thermal injury from heated rotary instruments.

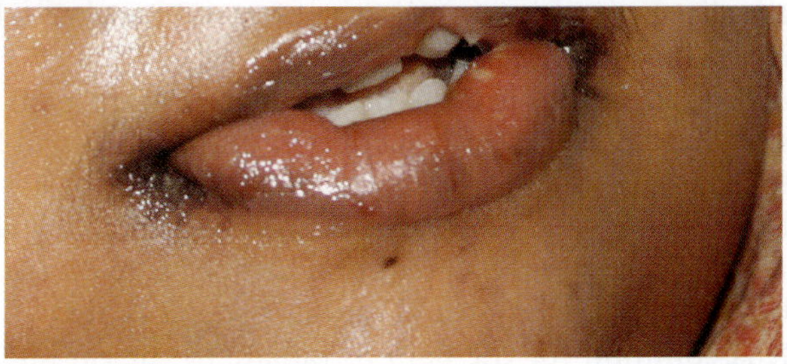

Figure 18.36 Soft tissue injury—oedema and mucosal injury caused by improper instrumentation and flap elevation.

Thermal injuries: These are caused when instruments taken out from autoclave or hot air oven are used immediately intraorally.

Mucosal tears: These are caused due to injudicious use of instruments, improper elevation of flap or the use of excessive force.

Prevention

- Take extreme care during the handling of the rotary or other hand instruments
- Cool the instruments properly before using to prevent thermal injuries. Mucosal tears can be prevented by proper designing and elevation of the flap, by proper handling of the flap and by gentle and effective manipulation of the elevators
- Retract the cheek and lips properly during dental treatments to prevent trauma from dental instruments.

Management

- If the tear or abrasion is large, suturing should be done for closure
- Scars produced due to thermal injuries can be managed by the application of petroleum jelly or topical antiseptic/analgesic.

OROANTRAL FISTULA (Fig. 18.37)

Causes

- Close proximity of the posterior teeth to the sinus predisposes to an oroantral fistula during the extraction of these teeth
- Injudicious instrumentation to remove a broken root tip.

Prevention

Application of appropriate force, which effectively removes the teeth without any fracture of bone or teeth.

- Avoid injudicious instrumentation to remove a broken root tip
- Proper radiographs should be taken before the extraction to assess the proximity of the root tip to the sinus

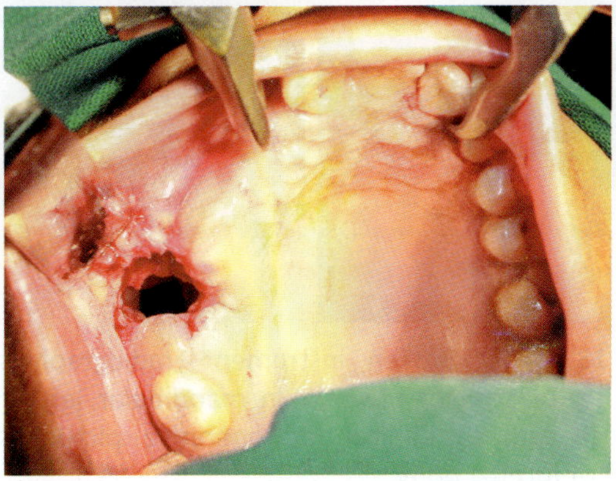

Figure 18.37 Oroantral fistula in right maxillary molar region.

- Support the jaw and the alveolus adequately before extraction.

Management

- As far as possible, leave the clot as it is and do not disturb it
- Prescribe antibiotics, analgesics, nasal drops and nasal decongestants to control any infection
- For large defects, surgical closure is done. Refer to Chapter 25.

BREAKAGE OF INSTRUMENTS (Fig. 18.38)

Causes

- Application of excessive force
- Improper technique
- Defect in manufacturing
- Old and worn out instruments.

Prevention

- Proper selection of the instrument
- Proper handling and usage.

Management

- Remove the burs or elevator tips with a haemostat if it is visible
- If impacted deeply, surgical removal of the instrument is advised unless contraindicated as in close proximity to vital structures.

POSTOPERATIVE COMPLICATIONS (DELAYED)

Dry socket

Crawford used the term "dry socket" for the 1st time in the literature in 1896. Dry socket is a postoperative complication that occurs after a dental extraction. It has been defined as a '*postoperative pain in and around the dental alveolus, which increases in severity at some moment between the 1st and 3rd day after a dental extraction, accompanied by partial or total disintegration of the intraalveolar clot, causing a foul smell*'.

Many terms have been used as synonyms of dry socket that includes *painful dry socket, necrotic alveolar socket, alveolagia, delayed extraction, localised osteomyelitis, fibrinolytic osteitis, alveolar osteitis, osteomyelitis postextraction syndrome, fibrinolytic alveolitis and localised alveolar osteitis*.

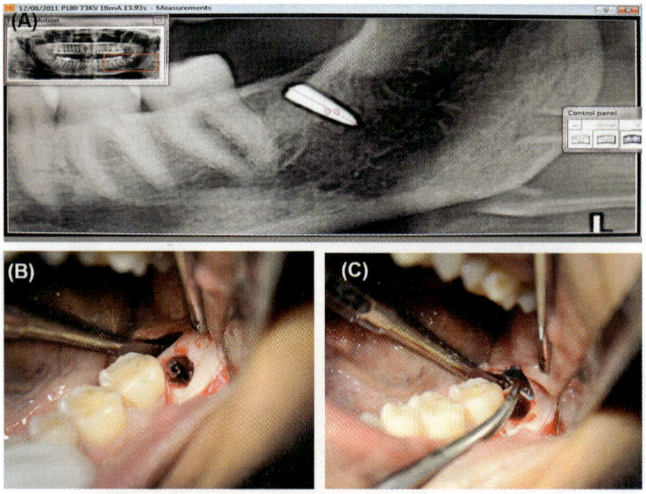

Figure 18.38 (**A**) Broken instrument—radiograph showing broken tip of straight elevator in mandibular left 3rd molar region. (**B** and **C**) Clinical intraoperative picture showing removal of foreign body.

Aetiology

The following factors are considered as possible aetiology in the development of dry socket:

- **Difficult or traumatic extraction:** A bigger trauma would produce a delay in the alveolar healing and it could provoke a thrombosis of the underlying vessels as well as lesser resistance to infection in the alveolar bone
- **Use of oral contraceptives:** Oestrogens and other drugs activate the fibrinolytic system in an indirect way (increasing the factors II, VII, VIII, X and the plasminogen), contributing to premature destruction of the clot and the development of dry socket
- **Hormonal changes:** The changing levels of endogenous oestrogens during the menstrual cycle could also influence the healing process
- **Tobacco:** The mechanism through which tobacco interferes in alveolar healing is the incorporation of pollutants in the wound or the suction effect on the clot in formation
- **Inadequate intraoperatory irrigation:** Inadequate irrigation of the alveolus can also play a role in the formation of dry socket. Use of an anaesthetic solution with vasoconstrictor or an intraligamentous technique of anaesthetic in which the anaesthetic is deposited very near to the alveolus, mainly if the anaesthetic is colder than the body temperature, increases the incidence of dry socket in these patients
- **Advanced age** of patients, immunocompromised state, extraction site in the mandible and excessive or exaggerated irrigation of the socket can all contribute to the formation of dry socket.

Clinical features

- Pain typically appears on the 2nd or 3rd day after the extraction and it usually lasts either with or without treatment for about 10 to 15 days
- Localised pain is present in the extraction socket, which is sensitive to even light probing
- Although suppuration is not evident, a sharp pain persists that increases with suction or mastication and lasts for few days
- Halitosis is invariably present. The condition probably arises as a result of complex interaction between surgical trauma, local bacterial infection and various systemic factors
- It is common for the pain to radiate to the ear and the ipsilateral side of the head. There is usually absence of a

normal healthy postextraction blood clot in the socket, which may be empty or contain fragments of disintegrating blood clot
- Radiological studies do not show important alterations and in advanced phases, rarefaction areas can be detected.

Aetiopathogenesis

After tooth extraction, an orderly sequence of events causes normal tissue healing. The alveolar socket fills with blood that undergoes coagulation and contraction. Angioblastic ingrowth occurs into the clot while epithelium covers the clot. Fibroplasia into the clot then ensues with cellular elimination of fibrin and blood debris. A variable amount of osteoid is then produced by induced mesenchymal cells. Woven bone is formed, followed by osteoblastic and osteoclastic activity that ends in mature bone, often with some loss of total bone volume.

This sequence of normal healing does not always occur. In some instances, early clot formation in the socket is followed by premature clot necrosis, accompanied by pain and fetor oris (Halitosis). The characteristic triad of pain, fetor oris, and early extraction socket clot loss/necrosis has been referred to as dry socket or alveolitis sicca dolorosa. Intense pain in the extraction site may radiate and be accompanied by a low-grade fever and ipsilateral lymphadenopathy. Histologically, this syndrome shows an intense focal osteomyelitis with healing in 1–4 weeks by sequestration or resorption of the necrotic socket wall bone and delayed secondary intention.

Theories of dry socket:
- Birn's fibrinolytic theory
- Bacterial theory

According to ***Birn's fibrinolytic theory***, after the extraction of a tooth, an inflammatory process begins that could affect the formation and retention of the clot. Laboratory and clinical studies have shown an increase of fibrinolytic activity in the pathogenesis of dry socket. The fibrin would disintegrate due to the effect of kinase liberated in the inflammation process or due to direct or indirect activation of the plasminogen, which affects the stability of the clot and facilitates the development of dry socket.

Plasminogen is a single-chain glycoprotein, which is synthesised in the liver and released into the circulation. Plasminogen is then activated by proteolytic cleavage into the active form, plasmin, which in turn acts proteolytically on fibrinogen and fibrin, causing clot dissolution and forming a number of fibrin degradation products. The plasminogen is cleaved into plasmin by one or more plasminogen activator substances.

The plasminogen activator factors can be direct or indirect (not physiologic) and are also classified as extrinsic or intrinsic activators. Intrinsic direct activators include factor XII and the urokinase, mediated by leukocytes whereas the extrinsic direct activators include tissue plasminogen activator (TPA) and the endothelial plasminogen activator (EPA). The indirect activators are produced by bacteria and include Streptokinase and Staphylokinase. The aetiopathogenesis of dry socket is shown in Fig. 18.39.

Bacterial theory is endorsed by the existence of a high count of bacteria around the extraction site in patients who suffered from alveolar osteitis as compared to those who did not suffer from it. Anaerobic microorganisms are generally found and the alveolar pain is due to the effect of the bacterial toxins on the nerve endings in the alveolus. Dry socket is also more frequent in patients with poor oral hygiene or in previously existing pericoronitis or concomitant periodontal illness.

Actinomyces viscosus and *Streptococcus mutans* have been related to dry socket because it has been demonstrated that they retard the alveolar postextraction healing in an animal model. Additionally, a fibrinolytic activity has been observed, which increases with *Treponema denticola*, a periodontopathogenic microorganism. This infection never appears in children before colonisation of the mouth by *T. denticola*.

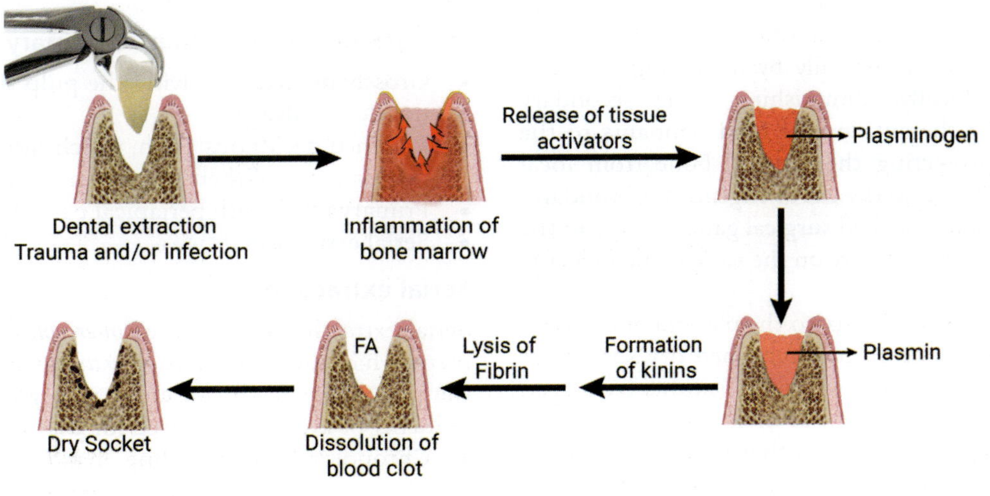

Figure 18.39 Birn's hypothesis—aetiology and pathogenesis of fibrinolytic alveolitis (FA) (dry socket).

Preventive measures

- A comprehensive history with identification of risk factors should be taken
- Preoperative oral hygiene measures to reduce plaque levels to a minimum should be instituted
- Where the clinical history and/or radiographic examination suggest a particularly difficult extraction, consideration should be given to an elective transalveolar approach
- All extractions should be completed with the minimum amount of trauma, the maximum amount of care and as rapidly as possible depending upon the experience of the operator
- Avoid extracting lower 3rd molars in the presence of active infection or ulcerative gingivitis
- Appropriate antibiotic prophylaxis should be administered for difficult lower 3rd molar bony impactions for immunocompromised patients and for patients with a history of previous pericoronitis or ulcerative gingivitis.
- Patients who smoke should be advised to cease smoking preoperatively and for at least 2 weeks postoperatively while the socket heals
- Wherever possible, in female patients using oral contraceptives, extractions should be performed during days 23 through 28 of the tablet cycle when the fibrinolytic system is suppressed
- Patients should be advised to avoid vigorous mouth rinsing for the 1st 24 h postextraction and to use gentle tooth brushing and mouth rinses for 7 days postextraction.

Management

- Patients should be radiographed to exclude the possibility of retained fragments of tooth or foreign bodies
- The affected socket should be gently irrigated with 0.12% warmed chlorhexidine and all debris dislodged and aspirated. In extremely painful cases, LA may be required, and in this instance, regional nerve blocks should be employed wherever possible
- Intraalveolar pastes consisting of zinc oxide eugenol paste, anaesthetic and an antibiotic (metronidazole) can be placed. They act principally by increasing the drug concentration locally, diminishing their secondary effects, avoiding the entrance of food remnants to the alveolus and protecting the exposed bone from local irritation in addition to the use of eugenol as obtundant. Place a strip of paste-soaked surgical gauze loosely in the socket. Do not exert pressure on the socket when placing the strip
- The complications secondary to the placement of dressings in the treatment of an established dry socket are ignored, although some local complications have been described after the placement of these dressings
- Despite the logical supposition that topical steroid use may decrease the intense local inflammation and hence decrease postextraction clot breakdown, the literature does not support the use of topical steroid antiinflammatory medications in extraction sites. However, the topical application of an emulsion of oxytetracycline and hydrocortisone has been shown to significantly decrease alveolar osteitis after impacted mandibular 3rd molar removal. Unfortunately, contribution of the antibiotic cannot be separated from that of the steroid in these studies
- Earlier investigations into the fibrinolytic nature of alveolar osteitis indicated that the topical use of parahydroxybenzoic acid (PHBA) in extraction wounds significantly decreased the incidence of mandibular 3rd molar dry socket in a dose-dependent fashion. However, antibacterial nature of PHBA may have contributed to these findings
- Appropriate analgesics as nonsteroidal antiinflammatory drugs are useful in managing pain
- When it is considered that socket dressings are no longer required, the patient can be instructed in home socket irrigation techniques using 0.12% chlorhexidine
- Patients should be kept under review until they are pain free and socket healing is ensured
- Inadequate aseptic preparation.

LATE COMPLICATIONS

- Nerve damage—anaesthesia/paraesthesia
- Chronic osteomyelitis/osteoradionecrosis.

SYSTEMIC COMPLICATIONS

- Syncope
- Seizures
- Respiratory obstruction
- Hyperventilation
- Myocardial infraction

Refer to Chapter 8 for Management.

EXTRACTION OF DECIDUOUS TEETH

Extraction of deciduous teeth differs slightly from the normal extraction method used for the permanent teeth. Unlike the permanent teeth, dental radiographs are essential before the extraction of any tooth.

Indications for extraction of primary teeth

- Grossly decayed involving the pulp that cannot or does not deem salvage
- Retained deciduous teeth, which interfere with the normal eruption of their permanent successor
- Primary tooth with periapical pathology & root fracture.
- Serial extraction.

Serial extraction

Serial extraction is a form of *interceptive* orthodontic treatment, which aims to relieve *crowding* at an early stage so that the permanent teeth can erupt into good alignment, thus reducing or avoiding the need for *later orthodontic therapy*.

- Chronologically, crowding may become manifested at *7 years* of age on eruption of the incisors, at *10–12 years* on eruption of the canines, premolars or during the *adolescence* in the form of late labial segment imbrications.

Indications

- The patient should be between *8–9 years* of age with crowding of incisors
- The fundamental arch relationship should be normal (*Angle class I*) showing harmony between skeletal and muscular system
- *Arch length deficiency as compared to tooth material is the most important indication for serial extraction*
  This is indicated by:
  - Absence of physiological spacing
  - Unilateral or bilateral premature loss of deciduous canines with midline shift
  - Malpositioned or impacted lateral incisor that erupt palatally out of the arch
  - Markedly irregular or crowded upper or lower anteriors
  - Localised gingival recession in the lower anterior region is a diagnostic feature of *arch length deficiency*
  - *Ectopic eruption* of teeth
  - Mesial migration of buccal segment
  - Abnormal eruption pattern and sequence
  - Lower anterior flaring
  - *Ankylosis* of one or more teeth
- There should be a normal or reduced overbite and all the teeth should be seen on radiograph and in good position to erupt
- There should be a large arch perimeter deficiency of *10 mm* or more.

Contraindications

Serial extraction is contraindicated in a number of conditions:

- *Class II and III* malocclusion with skeletal abnormalities
- Spaced dentition
- Anodontia/oligodontia
- Open bite and deep bite
- Class I malocclusion with minimal spaced efficiency
- Unerupted malformed teeth, for example, dilaceration
- Extensive caries or heavily filled 1st permanent molars
- Mild disproportion between arch length and tooth material that can be treated by proximal striping.

Methods

Different procedures have been described by different authors such as:

- Dewel's method (1978); $8^1/_2$ years [CD4]
- Tweed's method (1966); 8 years [DC4]
- Nance's method (1940); [D4C].

Extraction technique

Young children have very elastic bone, which expands rapidly when pressure is applied. The permanent successor of deciduous teeth usually lies below them and may be closely related to the roots of the deciduous teeth; therefore, extreme care must be taken while extracting the deciduous teeth. During extraction, if the root is broken, it can be left as such because though not always, it will get naturally resorbed. Secondly, inadvertent removal of the root may jeopardise the permanent tooth bud lying below it.

The forceps used for extraction are comparatively smaller than those used for extraction of the permanent teeth. For extracting mandibular and maxillary anteriors, labial pressure with mesial rotation is applied and removed to the labial side. For removing the maxillary and mandibular molars, buccal pressure is applied followed by lingual pressure and is removed to the lingual side. The forces required to remove the teeth are very less and the forceps need not be inserted too deep along the root. The elevators can be used for the removal of deciduous roots. In case of molars, they should be applied distally for the removal of distal root and mesially for the removal of mesial roots.

If by accident, the unerupted or partially erupted permanent tooth is removed during extraction, it should be carefully replaced into the crypt or socket and the wound should be closed. The patient should be instructed not to disturb that area. The use of curettes should be avoided to remove the granulation tissue after the extraction of the primary tooth.

Extraction of submerged deciduous teeth

When a deciduous molar undergoes ankylosis of the roots during replacement resorption, the alveolar bone envelopes this deciduous teeth, which seems to have partially or fully submerged. These teeth are usually identified during regular radiographs. Occasionally, they might be a source of infection leading to sinus formation.

The roots of the submerged tooth are often very slim and have a very thin periodontal membrane covering or are in direct contact with the bone. It is extremely important to ensure that all the roots are removed during extraction. Removal of submerged deciduous teeth is similar to removal of impacted teeth.

TECHNOLOGICAL ADVANCEMENT IN EXTRACTION TECHNIQUES

- **Physics forceps**
- **Piezosurgery**
- **Lasers**
- **Periotome**
- **Vertical extraction system**
- **Easy X-trac system**
- **Benex technique (refer to chapter 57).**

PHYSICS FORCEPS (Fig. 18.40)

The physics forceps uses 1st class level mechanics to extract a tooth atraumatically from its socket by placing a bumper in the buccal vestibule and a thin beak on the lingual aspect of the tooth. One handle of the device is attached to a bumper, which acts as a fulcrum during the extraction. Later, constant pressure must be applied to the tooth, which elevates the root from the socket 1 to 3 mm. Once the tooth is loosened, it can be removed with conventional forceps. This forceps minimises root or alveolar bone fractures and preserves

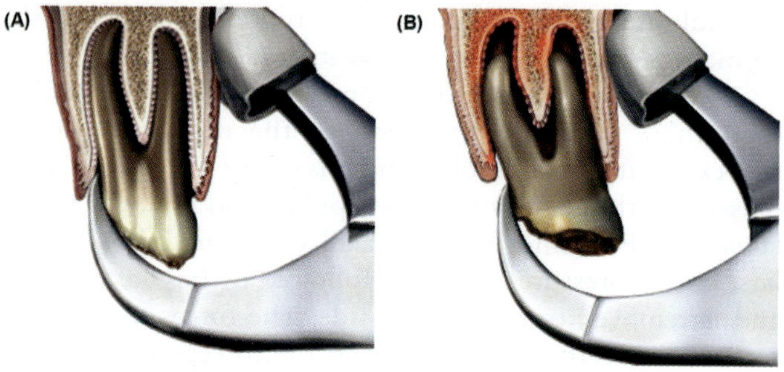

Figure 18.40 Diagrammatic illustration showing (**A**) placement of beak on the palatal root of the tooth into the gingival sulcus and the bumper end on the buccal aspect. (**B**) Application of constant steady force using wrist alone and the bumper as fulcrum.

surrounding bone providing atraumatic extraction (refer to chapter 57 page number 1066).

PIEZOSURGERY

Piezosurgery uses modulated ultrasonic vibration to allow precise cutting of bony structures. Delicate bony structures can be cut simply and with great accuracy without destruction of teeth and soft tissues. In addition, with the so-called cavitation effect, blood-free surgical site can be attained using piezo. It also reduces postoperative facial swelling and trismus.

LASER

Using Er:YAG laser, the covering bone is 1st ablated layer by layer for the surgical extraction of the teeth. The advantages of laser therapy include the creation of a bloodless surgical field and thus, better visualisation during surgery, decreased postoperative pain, and limited scarring and contraction.

PERIOTOMES

Periotomes are extremely thin and sharp instruments, such as the luxator periotome. It transects the periodontal ligament by inserting the extremely thin edge between the root surface and the alveolar bone and also simultaneously expands the bone acting as a wedge. Periotomes have important role in preserving bone and gingival architecture.

VERTICAL EXTRACTION SYSTEM

Vertical extraction system includes placement of a pin into the tooth canal followed by placement of the extractor apparatus. Using a traction wire, vertical traction is applied to the tooth, which is attached from the pin to the extraction apparatus. Until the extraction is completely successful, the traction is increased. The system is highly successful in single-rooted, and teeth with no root canal therapy. Advantages of this system include successful extraction of severely decayed teeth without having to elevate a flap or remove buccal/interproximal bone.

Chapter 19

Impaction

OUTLINE

INTRODUCTION

AETIOLOGY OF IMPACTION

Berger lists the following local and systemic causes of impaction.

I. LOCAL CAUSES

- Irregularity in the position and pressure of the adjacent tooth
- Density of the overlying or surrounding bone
- Localised chronic inflammation with resultant increase in density of the overlying mucous membrane
- Lack of space due to underdeveloped jaws, arch length and tooth size discrepancy
- *Obstructions*: It can be a soft or hard tissue obstruction caused by retained deciduous teeth, thick fibrous alveolar mucosa or chronically inflamed mucosa, dense bone with inflammatory changes due to odontome, cyst or odontogenic tumour that prevents eruption at the chronological age
- *Dilacerations:* Abnormal path of eruption of the tooth due to traumatic forces during the eruption period
- Overretained deciduous teeth
- Alveolar cleft, dental trauma, and odontoma are the causes of ectopic tooth bud.

II. SYSTEMIC CAUSES

General causes

A. ***Prenatal causes:*** Heredity
B. ***Postnatal causes:*** All those conditions that may interfere with the development of the child, such as:
   1. Rickets
   2. Anaemia
   3. Congenital syphilis
   4. Tuberculosis
   5. Endocrine dysfunctions
   6. Malnutrition
C. ***Rare conditions:***
   1. Cleidocranial dysostosis
   2. Oxycephaly
   3. Progeria
   4. Osteopetrosis
   5. Cleft palate

III. GENETIC FACTORS

Hereditary factors such as the presence of an alveolar cleft and malposed tooth germ.

Impacted tooth: A tooth which is completely or partially unerupted, is positioned against another tooth, bone or soft tissue so that its further eruption is unlikely and described according to its anatomic position (Fig. 19.1).
Partially erupted: When the tooth has failed to erupt into a normal functional position but has crossed the bone barrier and has not reached the occlusal line. The terms unerupted and partially erupted are commonly applied to normally developing as well as impacted teeth, the two states being separated by the event of clinical emergence. It is important that impaction is clearly distinguished from normal development.

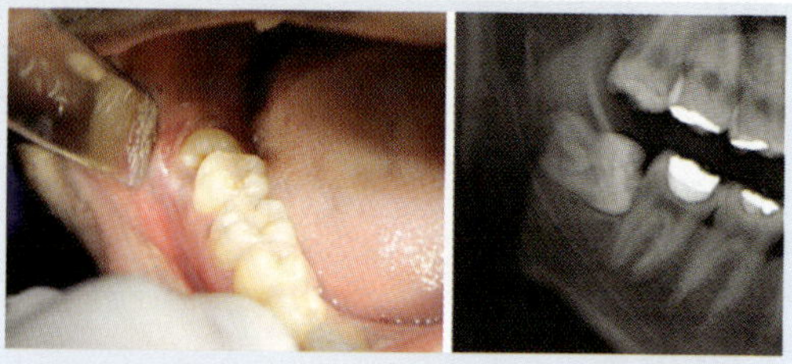

Figure 19.1 (**A**) Impacted partially erupted tooth 48. (**B**) Impacted tooth (48) in close relation to IAN.

Unerupted tooth: A tooth that has not perforated the oral mucosa (includes both teeth with and without apex closure). Unerupted teeth may or may not be impacted (Fig. 19.2).

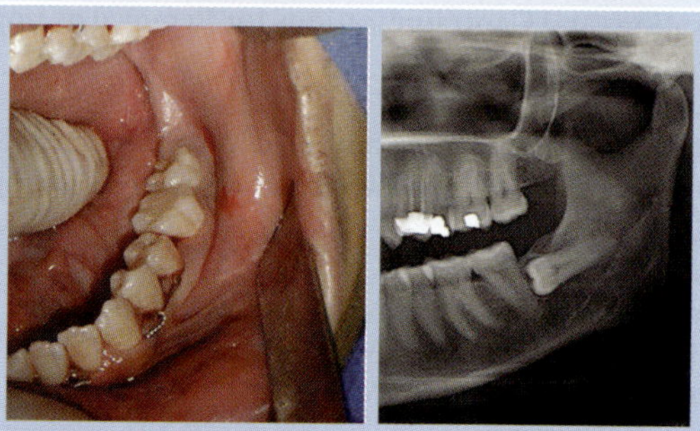

Figure 19.2 (**A**) Clinically unerupted and impacted tooth (38). (**B**) Unerupted and impacted teeth 38.

Ankylosed tooth: When the cementum of the tooth is fused to the alveolar bone and there is no periodontal ligament in between, a tooth is considered to be ankylosed (Fig. 19.3).

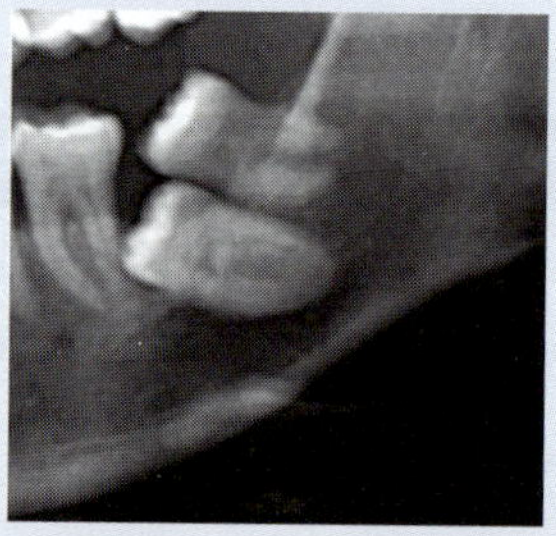

Figure 19.3 Ankylosed tooth (37) with obliteration of periodontal ligament space and malposed in position.

Malposed tooth: A tooth, unerupted or erupted, that is in an abnormal position in the maxilla or mandible. An impacted tooth may be malposed or unerupted. However, the reverse does not apply (Fig. 19.4).

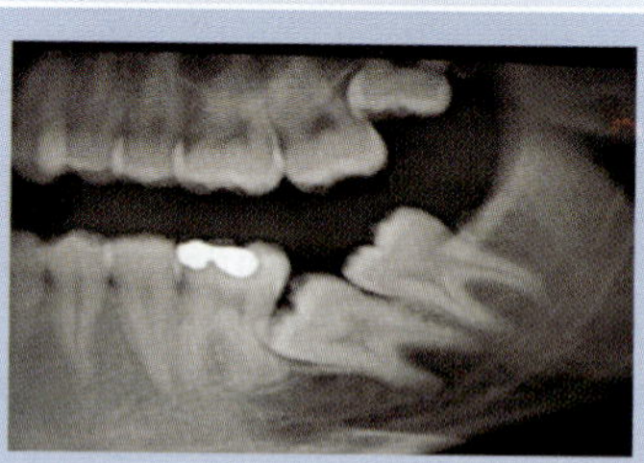

Figure 19.4 Malposed tooth in abnormal position (37).

Ectopic/displaced teeth: A tooth is ectopic if malpositioned due to congenital factors or displaced by the presence of pathology (Fig. 19.5).
While diseased erupted teeth can be removed by simple intraalveolar extraction using forceps, some teeth require surgical transalveolar extraction techniques. These teeth are usually impacted, unerupted, partially erupted, submerged, fractured below the cementoenamel junction (CEJ), endodontically treated, ankylosed teeth, etc. These teeth may require bone removal and a different set of armamentarium for removal. Since they require bone removal, these treatments are minor surgical procedures requiring aseptic environment and patient preparation.

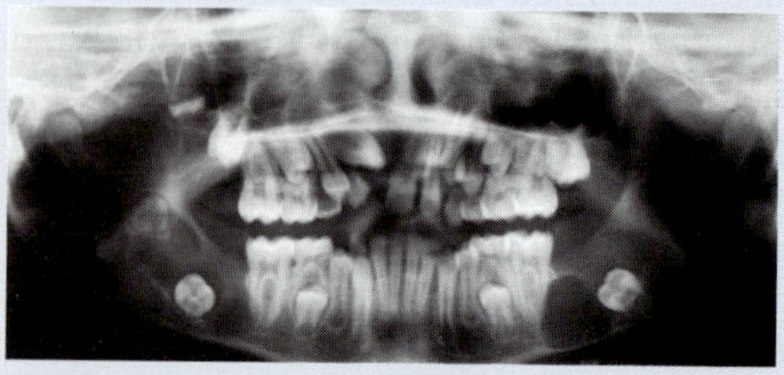

Figure 19.5 Multiple impacted teeth displaced due to odontogenic keratocyst evident as multilocular radiolucencies.

IMPACTED TEETH OCCUR FREQUENTLY IN THE FOLLOWING ORDER:

1. Mandibular 3rd molars
2. Maxillary 3rd molars
3. Maxillary canines
4. Mandibular premolars
5. Mandibular canines
6. Maxillary premolars
7. Maxillary central incisors
8. Maxillary lateral incisors.

SURGICAL ANATOMY OF MANDIBULAR 3rd MOLAR

The mandibular lower 3rd molar tooth is located at the distal end of the body of the mandible where it meets a relatively thin ramus. This meeting point constitutes a line of weakness and if undue force is exerted during elevation of an impacted 3rd molar fracture may occur. The lower 3rd molar is embedded between the thick buccal alveolar bone buttressed by the external oblique ridge and the narrow inner cortical plate (Fig. 19.6A). The apices of the lower 3rd molar frequently perforate the lingual plate as the lingual plate is extremely thin. Attempts to elevate fractured roots might inadvertently lead to their displacement through the thin lingual cortex into the 'lingual pouch' below the mylohyoid muscle (Fig. 19.6B). The thicker buccal bone is predominantly formed by the buccal cortical plate and the external oblique ridge of mandible

Neurovascular bundle

The mandibular canal is located below and alongside the roots of the 3rd molar. It is usually situated apically and slightly buccal to the roots of the 3rd molar and also there can be variations from the usual position. The neurovascular bundle is enclosed within the mandibular canal, which contains the inferior alveolar artery, vein and nerve enclosed in a fascial sheath. Before the formation of roots of the 3rd molar, the calcification of mandibular canal is completed. The growing roots might cause a deflection of the canal by its impingement (Fig. 19.7). Sometimes the root apices might protrude into the superior wall of the canal. In such cases,

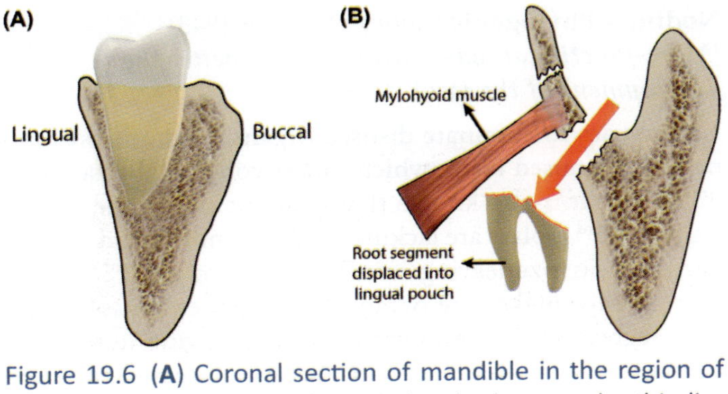

Figure 19.6 (**A**) Coronal section of mandible in the region of 3rd molar showing a thick buccal alveolar bone and a thin lingual plate. (**B**) Tooth root displaced into lingual pouch beneath the mylohyoid muscle.

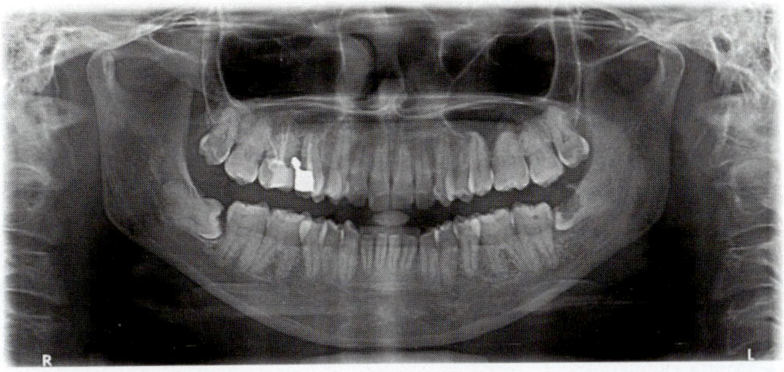

Figure 19.7 Radiograph showing close relationship of right impacted 3rd molar roots to the mandibular canal.

attempts to elevate small fractured root tip might displace it into the mandibular canal. Moreover, profuse bleeding can be encountered due to injury of the artery or vein by penetration of the mandibular canal by instrumentation or forceful intrusion of 3rd molar roots.

Retromolar triangle

Retromolar triangle is a depressed roughened area, which is bounded by the lingual and buccal crests of the alveolar ridge behind the 3rd molar. The retromolar fossa is a shallow depression, lying lateral to the retromolar triangle. Branches of the mandibular vessel emerge either in the retromolar triangle or in the fossa and supply the temporalis tendon, buccinator muscle and adjacent alveolus. During surgical exposure of the 3rd molar, brisk haemorrhage can occur if the distal incision is carried up the ramus and not taken laterally towards the cheek. There is a tendinous insertion of temporalis muscle at the borders of the retromolar triangle. Therefore, excessive stripping of these fibres during the removal of 3rd molar can result in postoperative pain and trismus.

Facial artery and vein

The facial artery and facial vein lie in close relationship with the lower 2nd molar near the anterior border of masseter. When making a buccal cut in that region, it is possible to cut these vessels if the BP blade slips. Henceforth, it is advised to commence the incision in the depth of the sulcus and direct the blade upwards towards the tooth.

Lingual nerve

The lingual nerve lies on the medial aspect submucosally in contact with the periosteum covering the lingual wall of the 3rd molar socket. During surgical removal of wisdom teeth, great care must be taken to protect it. Injury to the lingual nerve can lead to prolonged anaesthesia of the anterior two-thirds of the tongue. The lingual nerve is found to be about 0.6 mm medial to the mandible and about 2.3 mm below the alveolar crest on an average.

Mylohyoid nerve

Just before entering the mandibular foramen, the nerve branches off from the inferior alveolar nerve and penetrates the sphenomandibular ligament. The nerve lies enclosed in the canal in 16% of cases.

Damage to the nerve is likely during lingual approach for the removal of impacted mandibular 3rd molar.

Long buccal nerve

The nerve emerges and passes anteriorly on the outer surface of buccinator muscle. Injury to this nerve is most unlikely but can occur when the posterior incision is placed too laterally.

Musculature

The muscles surrounding the 3rd molar region are:

- Buccinator—anteriorly
- Temporalis—distally
- Medial pterygoid and mylohyoid—medially
- Masseter—laterally.

Buccinator muscle

This horseshoe-shaped muscle is inserted along the external oblique ridge and continues along the pterygomandibular raphae in the mandible. In the maxilla, it is attached at the level of the apices of molar roots. Marked postoperative swelling, trismus and pain result as the muscle is severed during surgical removal of deeply impacted 3rd molars.

Temporalis muscle

This fan-shaped muscle with two tendons is inserted on the anterior border of the coronoid process and the temporal crest of mandible. In between these two tendons lies the retromolar fossa. To enable flap reflection, the outer tendon needs to be sectioned during the removal of 3rd molar.

Masseter muscle

On the lateral side of the ramus, the muscle is inserted from the coronoid process up to the angle. During 3rd molar surgery, this muscle is rarely involved. Postoperative oedema may extend posteriorly to involve the submasseteric space and an abscess can develop from preoperative or postoperative infections.

Medial pterygoid muscle

Insertion of the medial pterygoid muscle is on the medial aspect of the mandible in the angle region.

The lingual technique may produce postoperative oedema that predisposes to trismus due to secondary muscle involvement.

Mylohyoid muscle

Mylohyoid muscle is inserted on the medial aspect of the mylohyoid line from canine to 3rd molar region. This muscle is partly severed during lingual approach.

SURGICAL ANATOMY OF MAXILLARY 3rd MOLAR

The maxillary 3rd molar is situated distal to the 2nd molar, in the tuberosity region of the maxilla. The upper 3rd molar

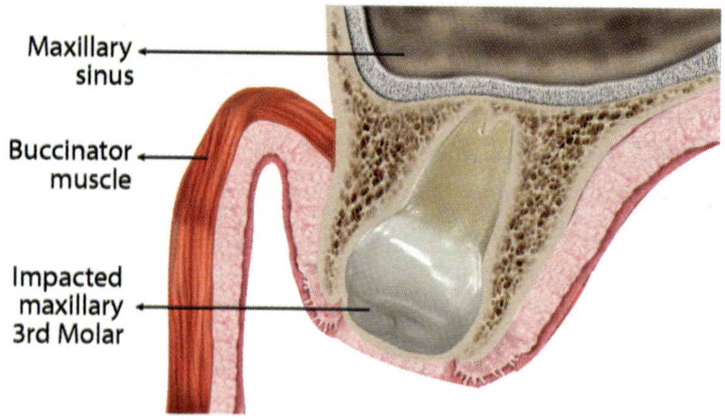

Figure 19.8 Diagrammatic illustration of maxillary 3rd molar region showing relationship of impacted 3rd molar to the maxillary sinus and buccinator muscle.

roots are frequently in close proximity to the floor of the maxillary sinus (Fig. 19.8). Roots of these might protrude into the sinus when the sinus is large, resulting in the development of oroantral fistula following its removal. Usually a thin layer of buccal cortical plate covers the impacted upper 3rd molar. Fracture of the tuberosity might result during the removal of 3rd molar as the unerupted 3rd molar constitutes an area of weakness.

THEORIES OF IMPACTION

Orthodontic theory (small jaw-decreased space)

Jaws develop in a downward and forward direction, while teeth move in a forward direction; the presence of dense bone decreases the movement of teeth in a forward direction. As growth of the jaw and movement of teeth occur in forward direction, anything that interferes with such moment will cause an impaction. Dense bone decreases the movement of teeth in a forward direction. Causes for increased density of bone are (1) Acute infection, (2) Local inflammation of periodontal ligament (PDL), (3) Malocclusion, (4) Trauma, (5) Early loss of primary teeth and arrested growth of the jaw, leading to insufficient space available for normal eruption. Without a doubt, this condition contributes to impaction.

Nodine's Phylogenic theory (Nodine 1943) *[More-functional masticatory force—better the development of the jaw]*

Nature tries to eliminate disused organs. This causes elimination of unused teeth, which causes congenital absence of 3rd molars. It is also known that in about 10% of the Caucasian race, 3rd molars are lacking, as the mandible and maxilla decreased in size leaving insufficient room for 3rd molars, that is usage makes the organ develop better, disuse causes slow regression of the organ. Due to changing nutritional habits, our civilisation has practically eliminated the need for large powerful jaws, and over the centuries, the mandible and maxilla have decreased in size leaving insufficient room for 3rd molars.

Mendelian theory

Heredity is the most common cause. An individual may inherit small jaws from one parent and a complement of large teeth from the other, that is hereditary transmission of small jaws and large teeth from parents to children. This may be an important aetiological factor in the occurrence of impactions, that is small mandible with impaction of 2nd and 3rd molars.

Pathological theory

Osteosclerosis in the 3rd molar area, caused by early disease and chronic infections in adjacent molars, may produce osseous tissue condensation, inhibiting jaw growth and development.

Endocrinal theory

Increase or decrease in growth hormone secretion may affect the size of jaws. An imbalance of endocrine activity could lead to a lack of growth of the jaws and could cause impactions.

Nature and nurture theory

Described by A. J. MacGregor, this explains that impaction can occur due to a mismatch in size and shape of teeth and jaws. This can be due to the following: Primate evolution owing to the increase in brain size with sacrifice of jaw size without reduction in teeth size. Softer consistency of diet in the modern age leading to underutilisation of teeth.

AETIOLOGY OF IMPACTED CANINE

The most common impacted tooth after maxillary 3rd molars is the maxillary canine. The factors that have been suggested for the failure of eruption of maxillary canines as described by Dewel are:

1. Hard palatal bone offers more resistance to eruption than alveolar bone on the ridge
2. Thick mucoperiosteal soft tissue covering the anterior part of hard palate is dense and resistant than other soft tissues of the oral cavity
3. Eruption of teeth depends to some extent on an associated increase in apical development. This aid to eruption is minimised in maxillary canine as root formation completes at the time of eruption
4. Greater the distance a tooth must travel from its point of development, greater the possibility of deflection and resultant impaction. This is true for maxillary canines
5. During development, the crown of the permanent cuspid lies immediately lingual to the apex of the primary canine root. Any pathological change in primary canine thereby easily causes deviation in the position and direction of growth of the permanent canine tooth bud
6. Delayed resorption of primary canine root can affect eruption of permanent canine
7. The canines are the last of permanent tooth to erupt and hence are vulnerable for a long period of time to any unfavourable environmental influences
8. The canines erupt between teeth already in occlusion and are usually competing for space
9. Primary canine has a lesser mesiodistal diameter than that of the permanent canines, thus providing less space.

INDICATIONS AND CONTRAINDICATIONS FOR REMOVAL OF IMPACTED MANDIBULAR MOLAR

INDICATIONS

- ***Infections:*** Removal of any symptomatic impacted tooth should be considered with food impaction causing halitosis, especially where there have been one or more episodes of infection such as pericoronitis (75%–80% of patients with impacted mandibular 3rd molar develop pericoronitis), cellulitis, abscess formation; or untreatable pulpal/periapical pathology (Fig. 19.9A and B)
- ***Unrestorable caries:*** Removal should be considered when there is caries in the impacted tooth or when there is caries in the adjacent 2nd molar tooth which cannot be satisfactorily treated without removal of the 3rd molar (Fig. 19.9C)
- ***Periodontal diseases:*** When there is periodontal disease between the 3rd and 2nd molars, early removal of the impacted 3rd molar will result in repair of the injured periodontium and is therefore beneficial. Untreated impacted teeth are particularly prone to cause bone loss distal to the adjacent teeth due to pressure effect
- ***Dentigerous cyst formation:*** Other related pathologies which expand the bone and results in pathological fracture (Fig. 19.9D)
- ***External resorption of the 2nd molar:*** Caused by the pressure of the 3rd molar on 2nd molar (Fig. 19.9E)
- ***Buccoverted impacted molars:*** May cause cheek bite, frictional keratosis or traumatic fibroma mandating extraction (Fig. 19.9F)
- Third molar removal may occasionally be indicated for ***orthodontic reasons***
- Removal of the 3rd molar may be indicated ***prior to orthognathic surgery***, for example, when a sagittal split osteotomy is planned, removal of the 3rd molar diminishes the risk of surgical complications with regard to that of osteotomy
- ***Prophylactic removal*** in presence of specific medical and surgical conditions
- ***Fracture of the mandible*** in the 3rd molar region or when a tooth is involved in tumour resection
- ***Atypical pain*** from an unerupted 3rd molar is an unusual situation. It is crucial to rule out any connection to temporomandibular joint (TMJ) or muscle dysfunction before considering removal
- Impacted teeth in edentulous ridge that cause ulcerations in the mucosa under a *denture*
- Third molar removal may be considered for ***autogenous transplantation to a 1st molar socket***.

CONTRAINDICATIONS

- Impacted teeth which are likely to erupt successfully and have a functional role in the dentition should not be removed

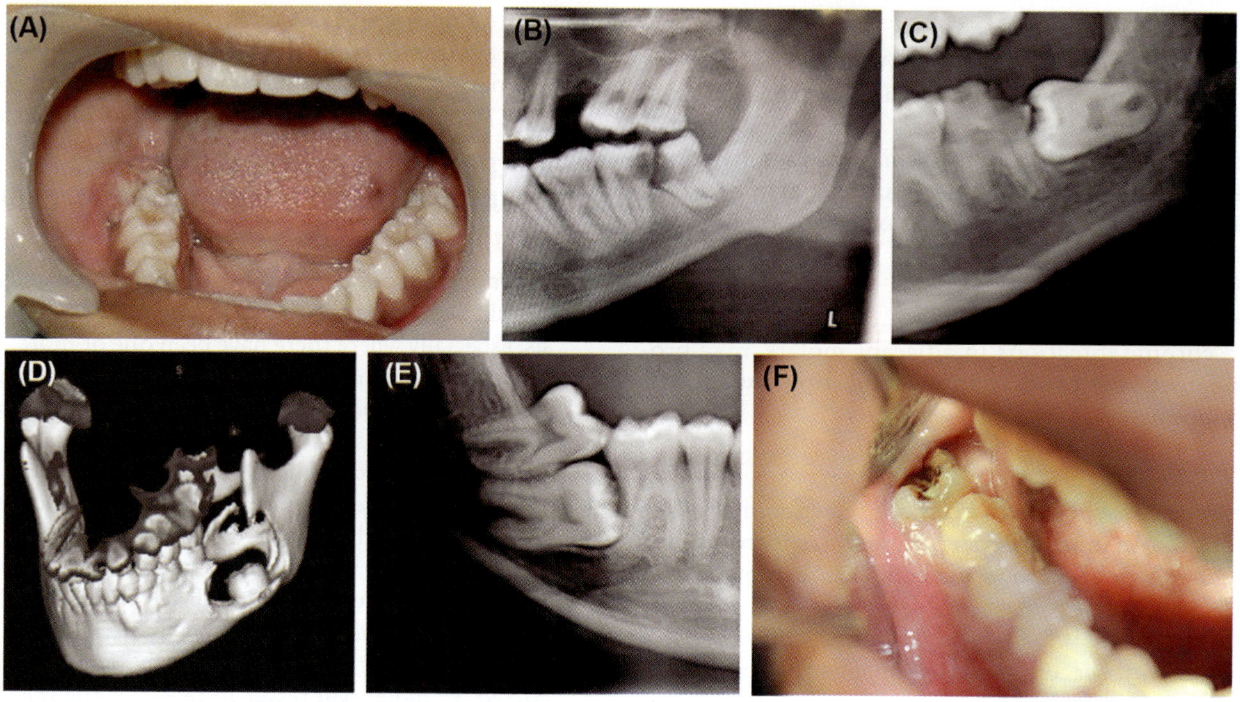

Figure 19.9 Indications for removal of mandibular 3rd molar. (**A**) Pericoronitis in relation to 48. (**B**) OPG showing grossly decayed left lower 2nd and 3rd molar with periapical radiolucency. (**C**) Dental caries in 37 (unrestorable) with horizontal impacted 38. (**D**) Displaced tooth (37) from pathologic dentigerous cyst. (**E**) External resorption of 46 from impacted 47 and 48. (**F**) Buccally placed 48 causing ulceration from cheek bite.

- Partially impacted teeth which can be used as an abutment in the construction of fixed partial denture
- Medical history contraindicates surgical procedure
- Deeply impacted 3rd molars in patients with no history of any bony pathology to avoid damage to the vital structures
- Third molars should not be removed in patients where the risk of surgical complications is judged to be unacceptably high or where fracture of an atrophic mandible may occur.

PERICORONITIS

Pericoronitis refers to inflammation of soft tissues covering around the partially or completely erupted 3rd molar.

CAUSES

- Bacterial growth beneath the soft tissue flap covering the partially or completely erupted 3rd molar
- Trauma caused to the soft tissue flap overlying the mandibular 3rd molar by the cusps of the opposing maxillary 3rd molar. This is mainly due to supraerupted maxillary 3rd molars opposing an unerupted or partially erupted mandibular 3rd molar. This inflammation along with bacterial colonisation causes pericoronitis.

SYMPTOMS

- The overlying soft tissues show the four cardinal signs of inflammation namely, pain, redness, swelling and warmth
- Trismus is a condition when the soft tissues underlying the partially or fully erupted 3rd molar are affected. The temporalis, medial pterygoid, and pterygomandibular raphae are affected causing inability to open the mouth
- Chills, fever, malaise and halitosis are present
- Regional lymph nodes may be enlarged, tender and indurated.

TREATMENT

When the condition is due to supraeruption of the maxillary 3rd molar, it should be extracted. The significance of removal of the maxillary 3rd molar should be explained to the patient. Due to the overeruption, normal contact between the maxillary 2nd and 3rd molar is lost, which facilitates food impaction, bacterial growth and loss of interseptal bone and subsequent loss of the 2nd and 3rd molar. Hence, removal should be considered.

Pericoronitis can be treated in the following manner:

- Conservative method
- Surgical excision of the overlying flap and the tooth.

Conservative method

Irrigation with warm saline should be done beneath the flap. A 10 cc syringe with a 20 gauge needle, which can be bent slightly to gain better access can be used.

Alternatively, 1 cc iodine solution can also be used to irrigate beneath the flap. The usually used irrigating solution consists of:

- Phenol 5%, 6 cc
- Tincture of aconite, 12 cc
- Tincture of iodine, 18 cc
- Glycerine, 24 cc.

Patient should be instructed to irrigate the area every hour and appropriate antibiotics should be prescribed. Irrigation is carried out until the acute symptoms subside following which the tooth can be extracted. If the tooth can erupt into a normal functioning position, the overlying flap should be removed.

Surgical removal of the overlying flap

Operculectomy

Operculum is the dense fibrous flap, which covers about 50% of the occlusal surface of a completely or partially erupted mandibular 3rd molar. The removal of this flap is known as operculectomy. It is not easy to remove this flap as the tissues are freely movable and slides away beneath the usual scalpel or scissors.

This flap can be best removed with the help of electrosurgical scalpel or radiosurgical loop.

Electrosurgical scalpel

The advantages of using electrosurgical scalpel are that the tissues can be cut precisely since there is no lateral or sliding movement of the flap and there is no need to apply pressure as with a traditional scalpel. The small capillaries begin to coagulate, which lessens bleeding and improves sight.

Radiosurgical loop

However, the most efficient method for removing this dense fibrous mucoperiosteal tissue is to use a radiosurgical loop. The radiosurgical loop is placed beneath the flap as far posteriorly as possible. Now the current is applied and the loop moved superiorly resulting in the cutting of the bulk of the tissue. Once the flap is removed, the tissue distal to the tooth is excised to remove the distal crypt. This helps in the proper eruption of the tooth if it is properly positioned.

INDICATIONS FOR REMOVAL OF IMPACTED MAXILLARY 3RD MOLAR

1. **Pain**
   May be due to pericoronitis, dental caries exposure or close location of adjacent surface of maxillary 2nd molar. Pericoronitis is rare in the upper jaw and seldom gives rise to those extensive infection that is seen in lower 3rd molar.
2. **Supraeruption of the upper 3rd molar**
   This could happen after the lower 3rd molar has been extracted, impinging on the retromolar soft tissue and causing ulceration. Unopposed 3rd molars on the maxilla also have a tendency to trap food and develop caries.

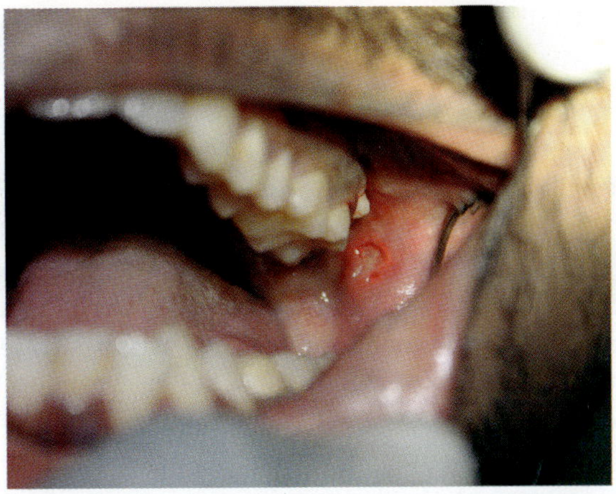

Figure 19.10 Buccoverted 28 impinging on buccal mucosa causing ulceration.

3. **Upper wisdom teeth erupting towards cheek** (Fig. 19.10)
   This will lead to inflammation and oedema of the mucosal tissue of the cheek. It may also impinge on coronoid process and cause a bite of convenience causing jaw deviation.
4. **Exacerbation of pericoronitis of lower 3rd molar**
   Due to upper 3rd molar impingement on the overlying gum pad.
5. **Before construction of full upper denture**
   It is necessary to extract an upper unerupted 3rd molar tooth, before construction of full upper denture, which will fit over that area. However, asymptomatic maxillary 3rd molar which are completely embedded in bone need not be removed unless the patient is to be fitted with a full upper denture.

INDICATIONS AND CONTRAINDICATIONS FOR REMOVAL OF IMPACTED CANINE

Indications

1. Impacted canine is located very far from the occlusal plane
2. No other methods are possible to retain the tooth
3. Patient is not willing to undergo orthodontic treatment for longer duration
4. Retention may result in resorption of adjacent dental structures
5. Pathological changes in the crypt like infection, cyst formation, etc
6. Required space does not exist for the canine tooth in functional position
7. Because of unfavourable anatomy of the tooth, other methods like repositioning is not likely to be successful.

The prognosis of the retained deciduous canine must be assessed and the patient must be informed regarding further treatment.

Contraindications

1. When the canine can be brought into normal position surgically or orthodontically

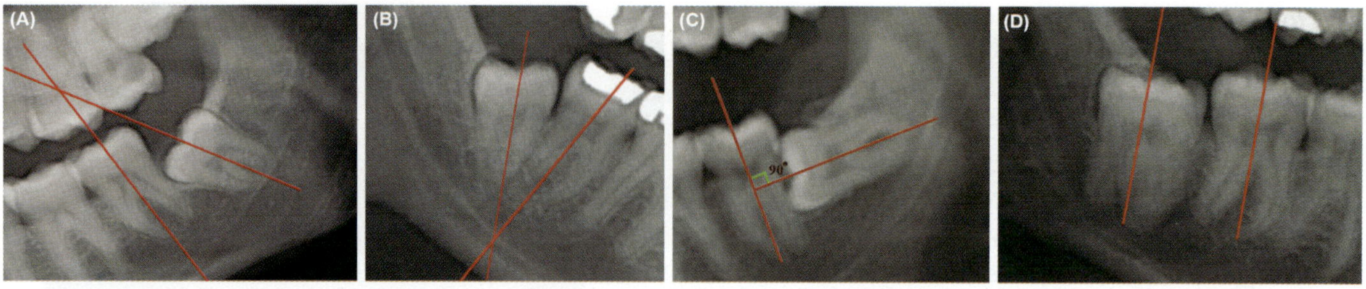

Figure 19.11 (**A**) **Mesioangular** 38—long axis of 38 bisects the long axis of 37 above the occlusal plane. (**B**) **Distoangular**—long axis of 48 is away from long axis of 47 at the level of occlusal plane. (**C**) **Horizontal**—long axis of 38 bisects long axis of 37 at right angle. (**D**) **Vertical**—long axis of the impacted 48 runs parallel to the long axis of the 47.

2. Medically compromised patients, presenting with impacted canines.

CLASSIFICATION

Systematic and meticulous classification of the position of the impacted teeth helps in assessing the best possible path of removal of the impacted teeth and also in determining the amount of difficulty, which would be encountered during removal.

CLASSIFICATION OF IMPACTED MANDIBULAR 3rd MOLARS

1) Based on the nature of the overlying tissue
2) Winter's classification—1929
3) Pell and Gregory's classification—1933.

BASED ON THE NATURE OF THE OVERLYING TISSUE

Based on the nature of overlying tissue, impacted mandibular 3rd molar can be classified as:

1. **Soft tissue impaction**
   The presence of dense fibrous tissues overlying the teeth sometimes prevents its normal eruption. This is frequently seen in cases of permanent central incisors, in which early loss of primary teeth with subsequent masticatory trauma to the ridge results in fibrosis.
2. **Hard tissue impaction**
   When the teeth fail to erupt due to obstruction caused by the overlying bone, it is known as hard tissue impaction. Here the impacted tooth is completely engaged into the bone so that, when the soft tissue flap is reflected, the tooth is not visible. Extensive amount of bone must be removed and the tooth may require sectioning before removal (odontectomy).

WINTER'S CLASSIFICATION

It is based on the inclination of the impacted 3rd molar tooth to the long axis of the 2nd molar

Mesioangular: Long axis of 3rd molar bisects the long axis 2nd molar at or above occlusal plane (Fig. 19.11A)

Distoangular: Long axis of 3rd molar away from long axis of 2nd molar at the level of occlusal plane (Fig. 19.11B)

Horizontal: Long axis of 3rd molar bisect long axis of 2nd molar at right angle (Fig. 19.11C)

Vertical: The long axis of the impacted tooth runs parallel to the long axis of the 2nd molar (Fig.19.11D)

Buccal or lingual: In combination to the above described impaction, the tooth can also be buccally or lingually impacted (Fig. 19.12)

Transverse: Tooth completely impacted in the bucco-lingual direction.

This is the most commonly used classification since it classifies the teeth according to inclination, and each inclination has some definite path of withdrawal of the teeth. The classification also assesses the difficulty of removal to some measure. For example, mesioangular impactions are the easiest to remove, but distoangular impactions are the most challenging.

PELL AND GREGORY'S CLASSIFICATION

(A) Based on their relationship with the anterior border of the mandible:

Class I: The anteroposterior diameter of the tooth is equal to the space between the anterior border of ramus of the mandible and distal surface of the 2nd molar tooth (Fig. 19.13A).

Class II: A small amount of bone covers the distal surface of the tooth and the space is inadequate for eruption of the tooth, that is mesiodistal diameter of the tooth is greater than the space available (Fig. 19.13B).

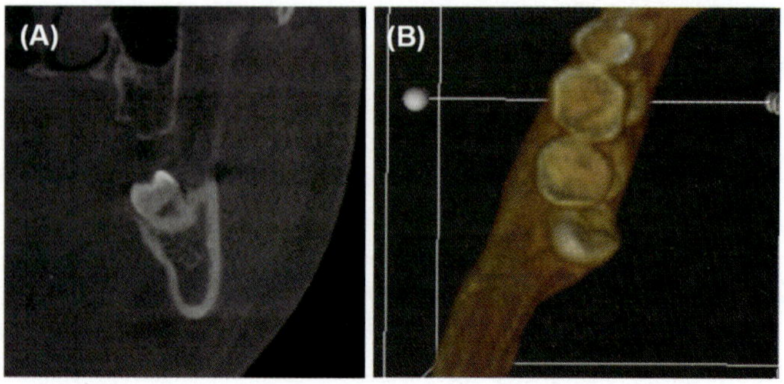

Figure 19.12 (**A**) CBCT-coronal view and (**B**) 3D CBCT showing linguoversion of mesioangular impacted tooth.

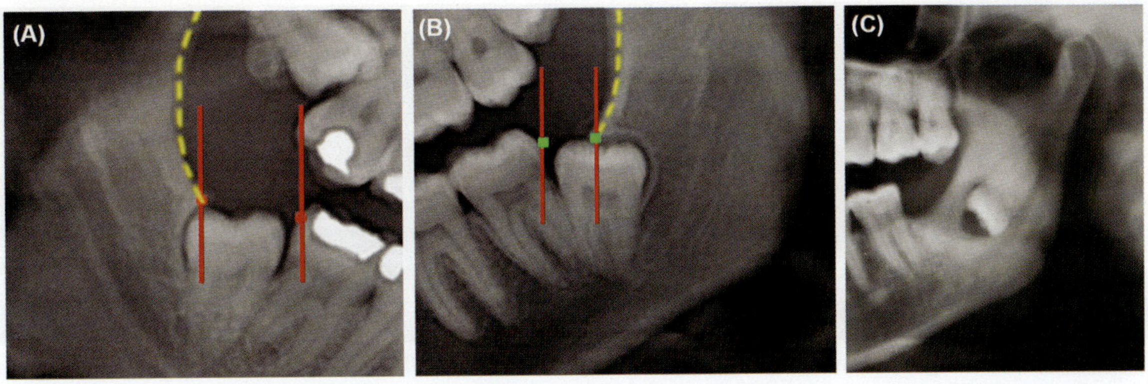

Figure 19.13 Pell and Gregory classification (**A**) Class I: The diameter of the 48 is equal to the space between the anterior border of ramus and distal surface of the 2nd molar. (**B**) Class II: Distal crown of 38 is covered by anterior border of ramus. (**C**) Class III: 38 located completely within mandibular ramus.

Class III: Tooth is located completely within the ramus of the mandible—least accessible (Fig. 19.13C).

(B) Based upon the amount of bone covering the impacted tooth and relation to occlusal plane:

Position A: Occlusal plane of the impacted tooth is nearly in the same level as the occlusal level of the adjacent 2nd molar tooth (Fig. 19.14A).

Position B: Occlusal plane of the impacted tooth is in the midway between the cervical line and the occlusal plane of the adjacent 2nd molar tooth (Fig. 19.14B).

Position C: Occlusal plane of the impacted tooth below the level of cervical line of the 2nd molar tooth (Fig. 19.14C). This can be applied for the maxillary teeth also.

(C) Based on long axis of the impacted tooth:

It is similar to the one as proposed in the Winter's classification (Fig. 19.16).

CLASSIFICATION OF IMPACTED MAXILLARY 3RD MOLARS

The classification of impacted maxillary teeth is similar to mandibular teeth but variations do exist. The following are the classifications which are commonly used.

CLASSIFICATION BASED ON ANATOMIC POSITION

I. Relative depth of the impacted maxillary 3rd molar in bone (Pell and Gregory)

Class A: The lowest portion of the crown of the impacted maxillary 3rd molar is on a line with the occlusal plane of the 2nd molar (Fig. 19.15A).

Class B: The lowest portion of the crown of the impacted maxillary 3rd molar is between the occlusal plane of the 2nd molar and the cervical line (Fig. 19.15B).

Class C: The lowest portion of the crown of the impacted maxillary 3rd molar is at or above the cervical line of the 2nd molar (Fig. 19.15C).

II. The position of the long axis of the impacted maxillary 3rd molar in relation to the long axis of the 2nd molar

1. Vertical (Fig. 19.16A)
2. Horizontal (Fig. 19.16B)

These may also occur:

- Mesioangular (Fig. 19.16C)
- Distoangular (Fig. 19.16D)
- Inverted

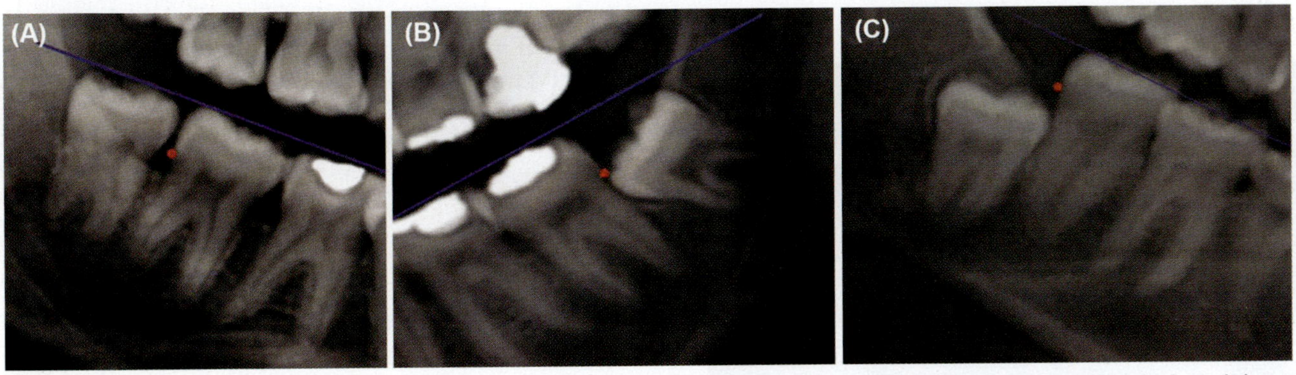

Figure 19.14 Pell and Gregory classification (**A**) Position A—Occlusal plane of 48 is at same level as occlusal level of 47. (**B**) Position-B—Occlusal plane of the impacted 38 is in the midway between the cervical line and the occlusal plane of 37. (**C**) Position-C—Occlusal plane of the impacted 48 is below the level of cervical line of 47.

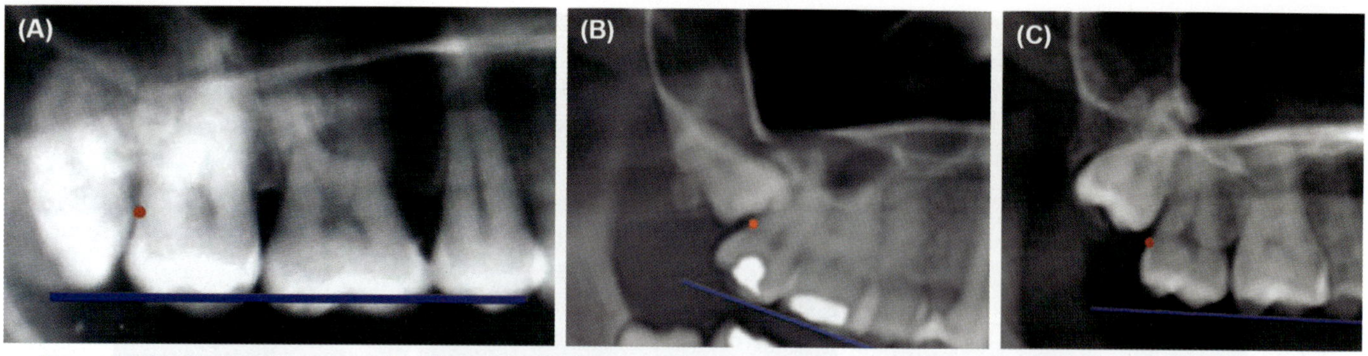

Figure 19.15 Pell and Gregory classification (**A**) Class A impacted 18. (**B**) Class B impacted 18. (**C**) Class C impacted 18.

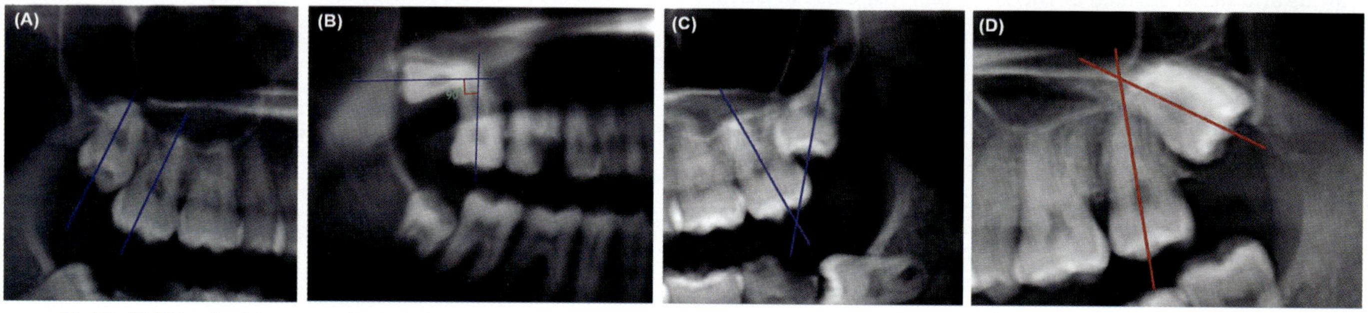

Figure 19.16 (**A**) Vertical impacted 18. (**B**) Horizontal impacted 18. (**C**) Mesioangular impacted 28—long axis of 2nd and 3rd molars meeting occlusally. (**D**) Distoangular impacted 28.

- Buccoangular
- Linguoangular.

III. Relationship of the impacted maxillary 3rd molar to the maxillary sinus (Fig. 19.17)

1. Sinus Approximation (SA): No bone or a thin partition of bone between the impacted maxillary 3rd molar and the maxillary sinus is known as 'maxillary sinus approximation'
2. No Sinus Approximation (NSA): 2 mm or more of bone between the impacted maxillary 3rd molar and the maxillary sinus is known as 'no maxillary sinus approximation'

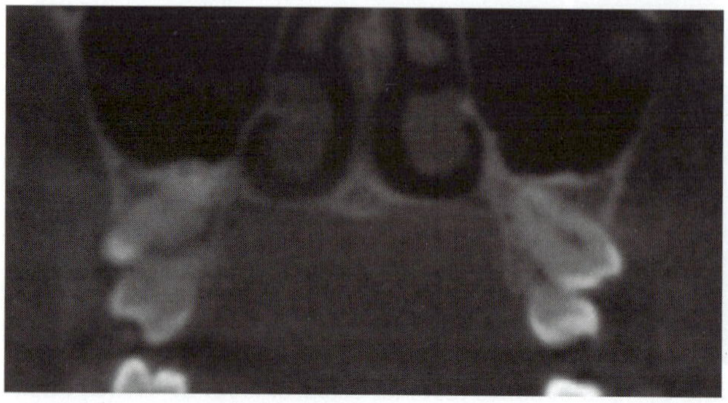

Figure 19.17 Tooth 18 showing sinus approximation and 28 showing no sinus approximation.

CLASSIFICATION OF IMPACTED MAXILLARY CANINES

BASED ON POSITION IN THE DENTAL ARCH

Class I: Impacted canine in palate
1. Horizontal
2. Vertical
3. Semivertical

Class II: Impacted canine on buccal surface
1. Horizontal
2. Vertical
3. Semivertical.

Class III: Impacted canine located both in the palatal process and labial maxillary bone (e.g. crown on the palate and the root passes through between the roots of adjacent teeth in the alveolar process and ends in the labial or buccal surface of maxilla).

Class IV: Impacted canine located in the alveolar process usually vertically between the incisor and premolar.

Class V: Impacted canine located in an edentulous maxilla.

FIELD AND ACKERMAN'S CLASSIFICATION (1935)

1. Maxillary canines

a. Labial position (Fig. 19.18)
   i. Crown in intimate relationship with incisors
   ii. Crown well above the apices of incisors

b. Palatal position (Fig. 19.19)
   i. Crown near the surface, in close relationship to roots of incisors

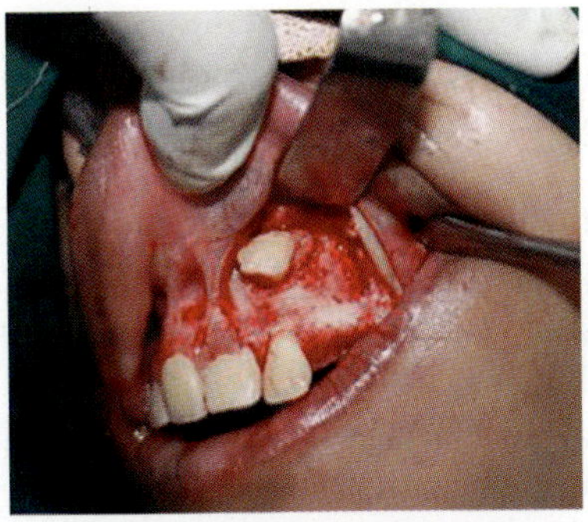

Figure 19.18 Buccal impacted maxillary canine.

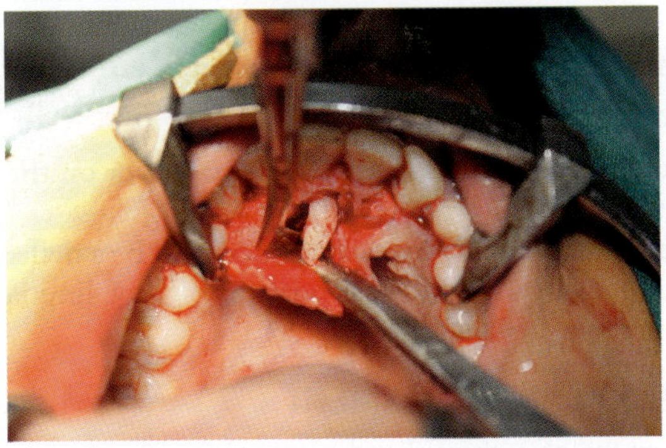

Figure 19.19 Palatally impacted maxillary canine.

ii. Crown deeply embedded in close relationship to apices of incisors

c. Intermediate position
   i. Crown between lateral incisors and 1st premolar roots
   ii. Crown above these teeth with crown labially placed and root palatally placed or vice versa

d. Unusual positions
   i. In nasal or antral wall
   ii. In infraorbital region.

2. Mandibular canines

a. Labial position
   i. Vertical (Fig. 19.20)
   ii. Oblique
   iii. Horizontal

b. Unusual positions
   i. At inferior border
   ii. In mental protuberance
   iii. Migrated to the opposite side along with the original nerve supply.

PREOPERATIVE PLANNING

CLINICAL EVALUATION

A thorough medical and dental history should be obtained, followed by an extraoral and intraoral clinical examination. Positive examination results should include radiographic evaluation in determining whether removal is necessary.

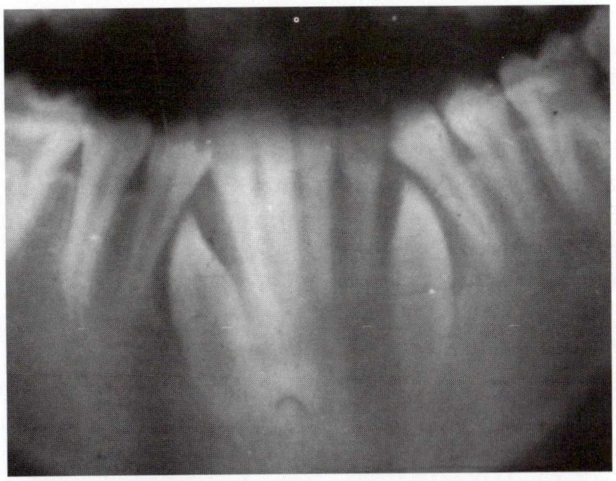

Figure 19.20 Bilateral mandibular impacted canine in vertical labial position.

GENERAL EXAMINATION

The general examination should be done in a similar manner as for any other surgical procedure. The presence of any systemic disorders or diseases should be detected and precautions should be taken accordingly before surgery. Patients should also be assessed for undergoing certain therapies like irradiation and organ transplantation.

- Age and general fitness are important. Increasing age adds to the difficulty of the removal
- The presence of facial swellings and enlarged, tender lymph nodes indicates presence of active infection and treatment should be deferred till it is treated.

LOCAL EXAMINATION OF IMPACTED MANDIBULAR 3rd MOLAR MANDIBULAR

- **The eruption status of the impacted tooth:** The amount of visibility of the 3rd molar crown is assessed. Completely or partially visible teeth are less difficult to extract than completely impacted teeth
- **Occlusal relationship:** The occlusal relationship of the maxillary 3rd molars to the mandibular 3rd molars should be assessed
- **The presence of local infection like pericoronitis:** The inflammation of the soft tissues covering the crown of the erupting tooth, increases vascularity making the procedure difficult
- **Periodontal status:** The presence of pocket around the impacted 3rd molar or the 2nd molar tooth should be assessed
- **Caries or resorption of the 3rd molar and the adjacent tooth:** Due to lack of space, there may be food impaction in the area distal or mesial to the impacted tooth leading to dental caries. This factor may/may not facilitate extraction
- **Resorption of the 2nd molars:** Due to lack of space, the impacted 3rd molar might impinge on the 2nd molar root resulting in resorption. Following removal of the impacted 3rd molar, the 2nd molar should be assessed for

both endodontic and periodontic intervention depending upon the degree of resorption and pulpal involvement.

- **External oblique ridge:** The external oblique ridge buccal to the 3rd molar is palpated to identify its position. If it is low, vertical and posterior to the tooth, it indicates the presence of thin bone buccal to the 3rd molar. If it is high and forward, it indicates a thick cortex of ridge present buccal to the 3rd molar, which makes extraction difficult
- **Internal oblique ridge:** The internal oblique ridge lingual to the 3rd molar is palpated to identify its position. If it is posterior to 3rd molar, it indicates thin bone lingually. If it is anteriorly placed, the lingual cortex in relation to the 3rd molar is anticipated to be nonyielding
- **Upper 3rd molar:** Position of upper 3rd molar and its relation to lower 3rd molar is checked. The indentations of the upper 3rd molar on the mandibular pericoronal flap indicate extraction of upper 3rd molar also
- **Soft tissue assessment:** Thickness of the buccal soft tissue indicates the retractability of the cheek. Difficulty in retraction is encountered in well-built patients and also in submucous fibrosis
- ***Regional lymph nodes:*** Swelling and tenderness of the regional lymph nodes may be indicative of infection of the 3rd molar
- **TMJ function:** Preoperative assessment of the TMJ function is done to:
    1. Assess mouth opening: To gauge the degree of difficulty in surgery
    2. Identify preexisting TMJ pathology: To avoid prolonged mouth opening and excessive forces on the joint, thereby preventing worsening of the condition.
    Factors complicating the removal of mandibular 3rd molar:
        - Preexisting joint problem: Preexisting joint problem creates a risk of dislocation or derangement during procedure. Restriction in joint motion causes reduced mouth opening and difficulty in surgical procedure
        - Position of the impacted 3rd molar: Deeper the impacted tooth is buried inside the hard tissues, the more difficult it is to remove it
        - Thickness of the oblique ridge: The presence of a thick oblique ridge poses difficulty in buccal traction of the impacted tooth during removal
        - Surrounding bone: Dense surrounding bony socket resists the easy removal of the tooth. In young age, the bone is expandable and as age advances, the bone becomes sclerosed and brittle.

LOCAL EXAMINATION OF IMPACTED MAXILLARY 3rd MOLAR

This must establish:

1. The state of eruption
2. Any buccolingual displacement
3. Tooth impaction against 2nd molar
4. Size of the mouth and mouth opening
5. Space around the 3rd molar—when mouth open/closed.

Local examination of impacted canines

- In maxilla, the malposed canines are found three times as frequently on the palatal side of the arch than on the labial side
- They are almost always rotated upon the longitudinal axis and are usually in an oblique position
- In mandible, the canines are rarely found in a horizontal position or on the lingual side of the dental ridge, being located most often on the lateral surface of mandible.

Localising impacted maxillary canines

Clinical signs

1. Presence of distinct bulge in the palate or on the buccal aspect of the maxilla
2. If canine is labially impacted, there will be a deflection of the lateral incisor (apical portion of root lingually and the crown labially).

RADIOLOGICAL ASSESSMENT

The purpose of a careful radiological evaluation is to complement the clinical examination by providing additional information about the 3rd molar, the related teeth and anatomical features and the surrounding bone. This is necessary in order to make a sound decision about the proposed surgical procedure, the most appropriate location for this to take place and to highlight aspects of management which may require specific mention to the patient.

Types of radiographs used for impacted mandibular 3rd molar

- Intraoral periapical (IOPA) radiograph
- Bitewing radiograph
- Occlusal radiograph
- Lateral oblique radiograph
- Orthopantomogram (OPG)
- Cone beam computed tomography (CBCT) (in indicated cases).

Intraoral periapical radiograph (Fig. 19.21)

An IOPA radiograph is a simple and most suitable radiograph for assessment of the lower molar. An ideal IOPA radiograph should show whole of 2nd and 3rd molar, bone surrounding 3rd molar and inferior alveolar canal.

Disadvantages

- Gagging of the patient
- Deflection of the film by the soft tissues lying in the floor of the mouth
- The deeply impacted tooth may not be visible in the radiograph

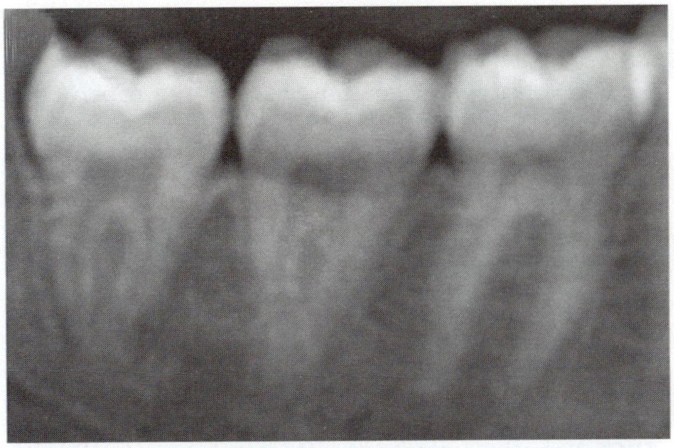

Figure 19.21 An ideal IOPA radiograph showing whole of 46, 47 and 48, bone surrounding 48 and IAC.

- It cannot completely reveal the buccal-lingual version of the impacted tooth
- Two-dimensional image of three-dimensional structure.

Frank's technique of localising mandibular canal

Frank suggested that a modification of the 'tube-shift' method can be used to determine whether the mandibular canal is medial to, lateral to or below an impacted mandibular 3rd molar. The principle involved is the same as that of the 'Clark shift' to localise a maxillary impacted canine. In this technique, an IOPA radiograph of the 3rd molar is taken by conventional method with the X-rays directed perpendicular to the tooth. In the 2nd step, a 2nd IOPA radiograph is taken by directing the X-rays 25 degrees below the plane of occlusion. This will make a distant object move downward in relation to the nearest object. If the canal lies lingual to impaction, it will move downward in relation to the roots of the 3rd molar. If the canal lies on the buccal side of roots, it will appear to move upward in relation to the roots. If the canal remains in the same position, it is directly below the roots or passes between the roots or is in a groove in the root substance apically, lingually or buccally.

Bitewing radiograph

In Class I–II impacted mandibular 3rd molars, the actual relationship of the 2nd and 3rd molars is made by correctly angled bitewing film. Central ray is directed through the crown of the 2nd molar at right angle to the film with 0 degree vertical angulations.

Occlusal radiograph

Occlusal radiograph for mandibular 3rd molar assessment is done by placing the film over the occlusal surface of lower molar and positioned till the distal edge of the film is in contact with the anterior border of ramus. It helps in visualising the buccal or lingual version of the impacted tooth.

- Should be taken for all difficult teeth and particularly when tooth is completely unerupted
- Provides an alternative view to the periapical film of the roots of horizontal teeth, especially in the presence of a 3rd root
- Essential for buccolingually placed teeth to identify the position of crown and shape of the roots
- Shows the thickness of lingual alveolar plate in a buccally placed molar.

Lateral oblique view

It is useful in assessing:

- Deeply buried teeth
- Grossly misplaced teeth
- Impacted teeth involved in secondary pathology.

Disadvantages

- Distance between film and tooth is greater, resulting in less definition
- Angulation of central ray is such that the relationship between 2nd and 3rd molars is not accurately shown
- Because of inevitable distortion, it is of limited value in the diagnosis.

Orthopantomogram (OPG)

Indications

a. In patient with exaggerated gag reflex where IOPA radiograph may not be possible
b. Tooth cannot be projected onto the IOPA film because of its position
c. Pathological lesions larger than that of the film such as cysts, tumours and fracture
d. The 3rd molar is in close relationship to lower border of mandible.

Advantages

- Viewing both the upper and lower jaw in one radiograph (Fig. 19.22)
- Detailed description of the anatomy of the hard tissues surrounding the impacted tooth
- Position of the tooth in relation to the canal
- Details of the bone surrounding the tooth.

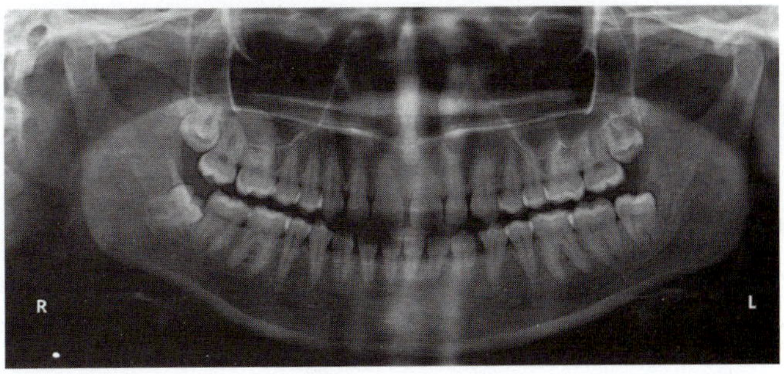

Figure 19.22 OPG showing impacted teeth of both jaws in single film.

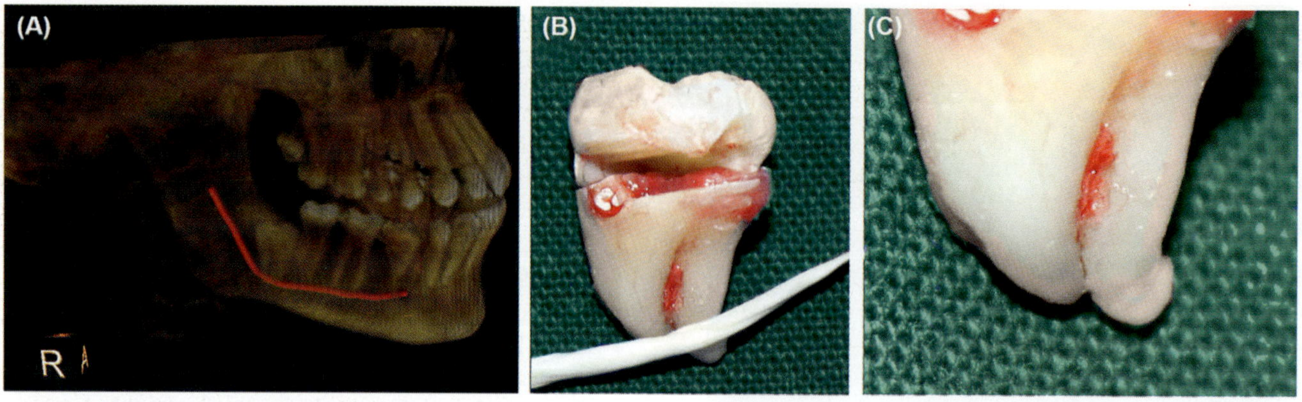

Figure 19.23 (**A–C**) Demonstration of nerve root relationship traced in CBCT. Note the extracted tooth root demonstrating grooving of root by canal.

Cone beam computed tomography (CBCT)

CBCT is indicated in:

- Completely impacted teeth in abnormal position
- Relationship of the impacted tooth to the canal is questionable using other radiographs (Fig. 19.23)
- Ectopic presentations
- Multiple impacted teeth
- Pathologies like dentigerous cyst, odontoma, etc.

INTERPRETATION OF THE RADIOGRAPH

Assessment of access

Easy access to the impacted teeth is determined by the inclination of the radiopaque line caused by the external oblique ridge

- When the radiopaque line is more horizontal, access is easy; when it is more vertical, access is poor
- If the radiopaque line is situated behind the impacted tooth, the access is good; if it is situated in front of the tooth, the access is poor.

Assessment of position and depth

- The orientation of the impacted mandibular 3rd molars may be mesioangular, distoangular, vertical or horizontal
- When a vertical impaction is present, the anteroposterior width of the interdental septum between the 2nd and 3rd molars is similar to that of the septum between the 1st and 2nd molars. Whereas, when distoangular impaction is present, the interdental septum between the 2nd and 3rd molars is narrower than between the 1st and 2nd molars
- They may be present at varied depth inside the mandibular jaw bone. Ectopic positions (in the coronoid or condylar process), though rare, do exist.

WAR lines

Position and depth of the impacted mandibular 3rd molar can be determined by means of George Winter's WAR lines. George Winter described three imaginary lines drawn on the standard radiograph with different colours such as White, Amber and Red.

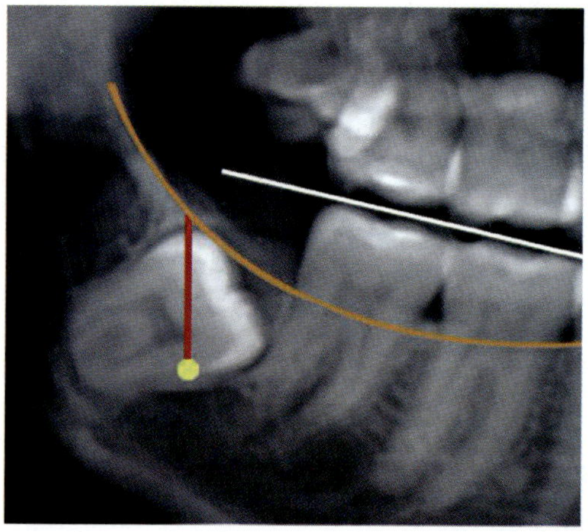

Figure 19.24 WAR lines - White (W) line, Amber (A) line, Red (R) lIne.

White line

White line is drawn along the occlusal surfaces of the erupted mandibular molars and extended over the 3rd molar region posteriorly. The axial inclination of the impacted tooth can be seen apparently (Fig. 19.24).

- The occlusal surface of the vertically impacted 3rd molar is parallel to the white line
- The occlusal surface of the 3rd molar with distoangular impaction meets the white line in front of the 3rd molar
- The occlusal surface of the 3rd molar with mesioangular impaction meets the white line behind the 3rd molar
- The occlusal surface of horizontally impacted 3rd molar meets the white line in a perpendicular direction
- Indicates
  a. The depth of the tooth within the mandible
  b. Relationship of occlusal surface of impacted tooth with the erupted molars.

Amber line

Amber line is drawn from the surface of the bone on the distal aspect of the 3rd molar to the crest of the interdental septum between the 1st and 2nd mandibular molars. This line represents the margin of the alveolar bone covering the 3rd molar (Fig. 19.24).

Red line

Red line is an imaginary line drawn perpendicular from the amber line to an imaginary point of application of the elevator. Usually this point is the CEJ on the mesial surface of the impacted tooth (exception is the distoangular impaction where the point of application of the elevator is on the CEJ on the distal aspect). The length of the red line indicates depth of the impacted tooth (Table 19.1). With each increase in length of the red line by 1 mm, the impacted tooth becomes three times more difficult to remove (Fig. 19.24).

Assessment of the roots of the impacted mandibular 3rd molar

The position and root pattern of the impacted as well as the adjacent tooth may create difficulty while removing the impacted tooth. The eruption status of the impacted tooth should be assessed as the status of formation of root determines the time of removal.

Length of the root

The ideal time of removal of impacted tooth is when two-thirds of the root is formed. In this stage, the roots will be blunt and removal is very easy (Fig. 19.25). When the root is one-third formed, the tooth tends to roll in its crypt like ball in a socket, which prevents easy elevation.

Fusion of root

The roots may be fused into a single, conical root or as separate distinct roots (Fig. 19.26A and B). The fused, conical roots are easier to remove than widely separated roots.

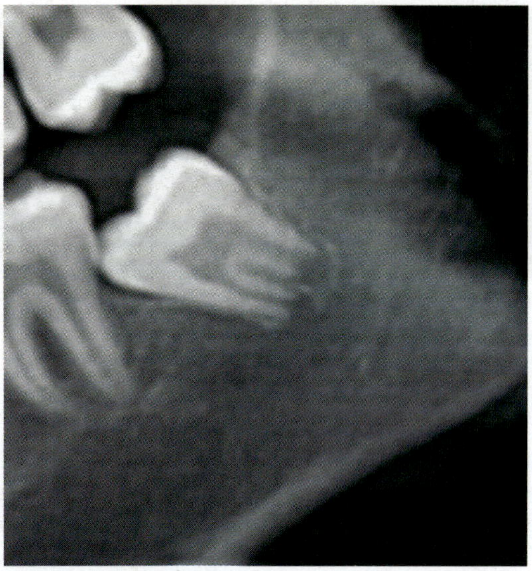

Figure 19.25 X-ray showing impacted tooth with two-thirds formed root—ideal time for extraction.

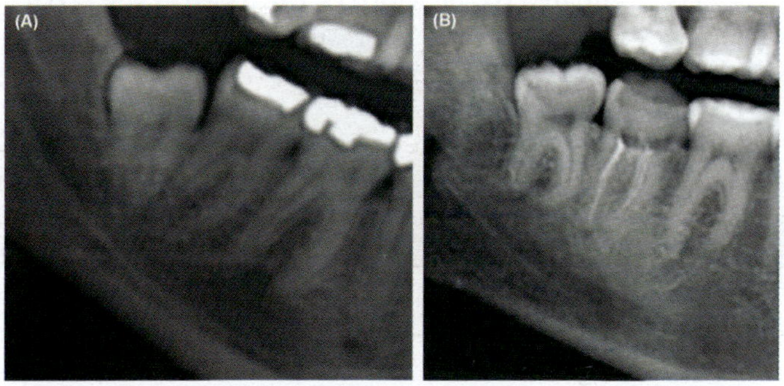

Figure 19.26 Impacted 3rd molar tooth showing **(A)** fused conical root and **(B)** distinct separate roots.

TABLE 19.1 WAR Line and its Implications

WAR Line	Line Extension	Significance
W-White line	Drawn along the occlusal surfaces of the erupted mandibular molars and extends posteriorly over the 3rd molar region	Indicates the depth of the tooth within the mandible relationship of occlusal surface of impacted tooth with the erupted molars.
A-Amber line	Drawn from surface of the bone distal to the 3rd molar and to the crest of the interdental septum between the 1st and 2nd molars	Indicates the height of the margin of the alveolar bone enclosing the tooth. Indicates the amount of vertical bone that requires removal for the extraction of the 3rd molar.
R-Red line	It is the perpendicular line drawn from the amber line to the imaginary point of application of the elevator. For all types of impacted teeth, the red line is drawn on the mesial side, except for distoangular, where it is drawn on the distal side.	Longer the red line, more difficult the extraction. <5 mm—less difficult. For every 1 mm increase after 5 mm difficulty increases by three times. >5 mm—advised under GA. ≥ 9 mm—very difficult, denuding of distal root of 2nd molar may mandate the removal of 2nd molar also.

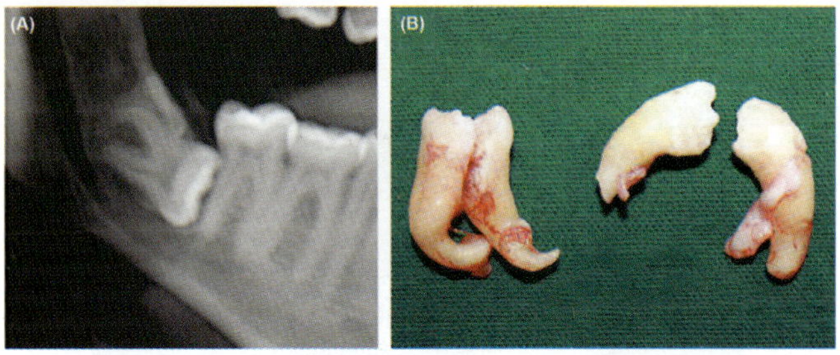

Figure 19.27 **(A)** Unfavourable dilacerated tooth—difficult to remove. **(B)** Dilacerated roots.

Curvature of the root (Fig. 19.27)

The curvature of the tooth roots also plays a role in the difficulty of extraction. Severely curved or dilacerated roots are more difficult to remove than straight or slightly curved roots. The apex area of the radiograph should be carefully assessed for the presence of small, abnormal and sharply hooked roots that would fracture during removal.

Width of the root

The total width of the roots in the mesiodistal direction should be compared to the width of the tooth at the cervical line. If the tooth root width is greater or has hypercementosis, the extraction will be more difficult (Fig. 19.28).

Root of the 2nd molar

If the 2nd molar roots are smaller in relation to the impacted tooth or are fused and conical, care must be taken not to luxate the 2nd molar during the elevation. Similarly, absence of 1st molar leaves the 2nd molar unsupported. During elevation, inadvertent luxation or dislodgement of 2nd molar should be avoided.

Assessment of bone texture

Texture of the bone varies between individuals, with age and site within the same individual. In younger age group, the

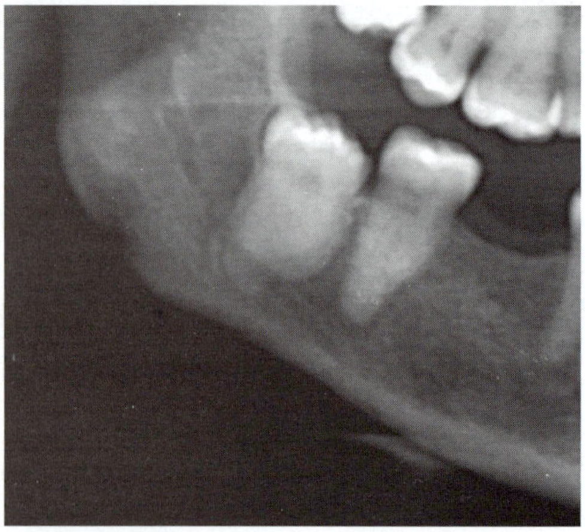

Figure 19.28 Mesiodistal root width greater than cervical width indicative of difficulty in removal (tooth must be sectioned before extraction).

bone is cancellous and elastic, whereas it becomes dense and sclerosed as the age advances. The nature of the bone is the factor, which decides the choice of bur or chisel used to remove bone. If the bone is less dense as in younger individuals, it is easier to cut with bur than the chisel.

Assessment of relationship with inferior alveolar nerve

Sometimes the inferior alveolar canal can be seen crossing the roots of the mandibular 3rd molar. When it is very obvious in the radiograph, the patient should be informed about the possible postoperative impairment of sensation over the area supplied by the inferior alveolar nerve.

Changes related to the tooth root

Normally, a tooth will be of uniform radiopacity throughout. When there is any darkening or decrease in the radiopacity of the tooth, it indicates that the density of the tooth structure and cortical lining of the inferior alveolar canal is decreased in that area, due to the grooving of the tooth by the canal and its contents. When the canal crosses only the apex of the tooth, apical notching or bifid root apex may be seen.

Changes related to the canal

The inferior alveolar canal is represented by two radiopaque lines and disruption or interruption in continuity of these lines indicates that a deep grooving of the tooth root by the canal is present. When there is a break in continuity of only the upper radiopaque line, an apical notch is present, which indicates that only the tooth apex is grooved by the canal. The canal may sometimes appear to be diverting when it perforates the tooth root completely. This is due to eruption of the tooth which drags the contents of the canal along with it.

SEVEN RADIOLOGICAL SIGNS HAD BEEN SUGGESTED BY HOWE AND POYTON (1960)

The relationship between the mandibular 3rd molar tooth and the inferior alveolar canal is indicated by the seven radiological signs. Four of these signs are related to the root of the tooth, and the other three are changes in the appearance of the inferior alveolar canal.

1. Darkening of the root

- The density of the root is not altered by the overlapping of the tooth and inferior alveolar canal
- Impingement of the canal on the tooth root results in the loss of root density, resulting in darkening of the root (Fig. 19.29A).

2. Deflected root

- Deflected roots or roots hooked around the canal are seen
- There will be abrupt deviation of the root, when the root reaches the inferior alveolar canal
- The root being deflected to the buccal, lingual or both sides in order to completely enclose the canal

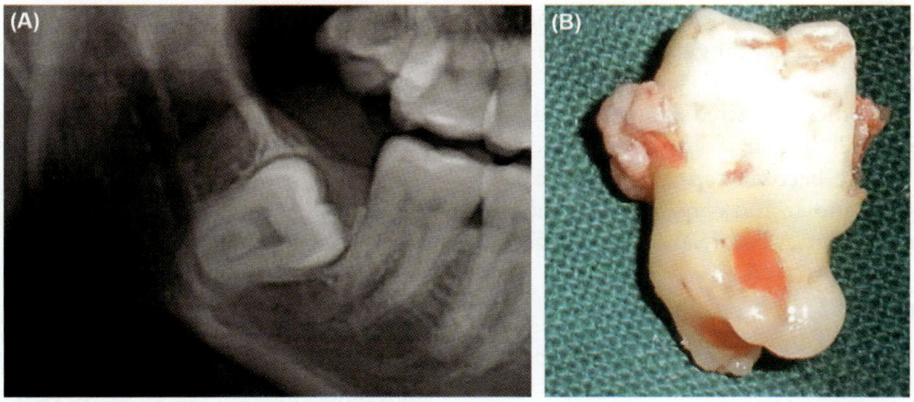

Figure 19.29 (**A**) X-ray showing darkening of the roots-loss of density of the root. (**B**) Extracted 48 showing grooving of the root apex by canal.

- It may also be deflected to the mesial or distal aspect (Fig. 19.29B).

3. Narrowing of the root

- Narrowing of the root on crossing the canal implies that the greatest diameter of the root has been involved by the canal
- It may also be associated with deep grooving or perforation of the root.

4. Dark and bifid root

- Dark and bifid root appears when the inferior alveolar canal crosses the apex
- It is identified by the double periodontal membrane shadow of the bifid apex.

5. Interruption of the white line(s)

- Radiologically, the inferior alveolar canal appears as the two radiopaque lines (the 'roof' and 'floor' of the inferior alveolar canal)
- Disappearance of this white line (either one or both) immediately before it reaches the tooth structure is considered to be interrupted
- The interruption of the white line(s) indicates deep grooving of the root
- Narrowing of the inferior alveolar canal indicates the perforation of the root
- The interruption of the white line is considered to be a 'danger sign' indicating the true relationship between tooth root and canal.

6. Diversion of the inferior alveolar canal

- The canal changes its direction when it crosses the mandibular 3rd molar and is considered to be diverted
- There will be upward displacement of the canal along with its contents, during the eruption of the 3rd molar.

7. Narrowing of the inferior alveolar canal

- Narrowing of the inferior alveolar canal is appreciated when the canal crosses the root of the mandibular 3rd molar

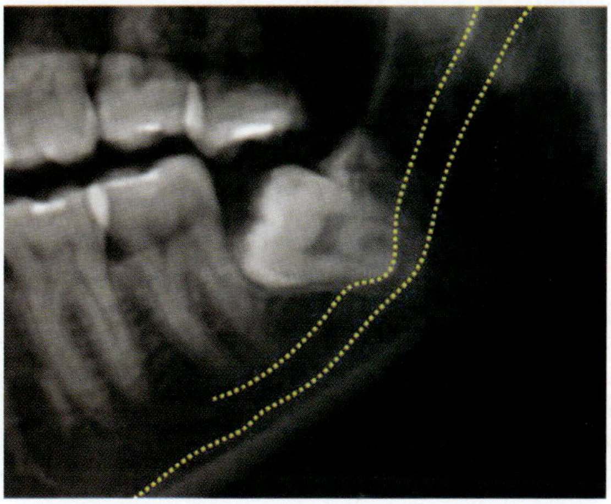

Figure 19.30 X-ray showing narrowing of the inferior alveolar canal in relation to 38.

- Diameter of the canal is reduced
- Narrowing of the canal may be due to:
  a. Downward displacement of the upper border of the canal
  b. Displacement of the upper and lower borders towards each other resulting in hourglass appearance
- The hourglass shape may indicate partial or complete encirclement (Fig. 19.30).

RADIOGRAPHIC EXAMINATION OF IMPACTED MAXILLARY MOLAR

IOPA film ideally should show the 2nd molar and whole of 3rd molar

Lateral oblique and OPG indicated when the 3rd molar is high in the maxilla or when the patient will not tolerate an IOPA radiograph.

Interpretation of the radiograph

(a) Position of tooth

i. **Vertical:** It will erupt normally unless it is lying apical to the 2nd molar

ii. **Distovertical:** When the tooth erupts, it may traumatise the mucosa overlying the ascending ramus as it is directed distally
iii. **Mesioangular:** It becomes impacted against the distal aspect of the maxillary 2nd molar
iv. **Partially erupted:** May become carious or can cause pocket around the 2nd molar and consideration should be given to prognosis of latter before and after surgery.

(b) Morphology of the tooth

Morphology of upper 3rd molars is very variable, particularly in the number of roots. These are often multiple and fine. Divergent fine roots present a problem in extraction because they may fracture during surgical removal.

Assessment of bone texture

While removing a maxillary 3rd molar, a buccal approach is preferred than palatal approach since it is surrounded by spongy, egg-shell thin cortical bone on the buccal and distal aspect, whereas more bone is present on the palatal aspect.

RADIOGRAPHIC LOCALISATION OF CANINE

The position of the upper canine is assessed from radiographs, which are taken in two planes to give three-dimensional impressions of the tooth and associated structures. They are:

1. IOPA films
2. Vertex occlusal film

These are supplemented with:

i. Oblique occlusal films
ii. Anterior occlusal films
iii. True lateral films
iv. Tangential views films
v. CBCT.

Intraoral periapical film

More than one IOPA may be necessary to cover the whole length of the tooth adequately and to show the vertical and anteroposterior relationship to adjacent teeth, antrum and nose. Parallax method of *Clarks (1909) or tube shift technique* is useful in identifying the buccopalatal position of the tooth.

RADIOGRAPHIC LOCALISATION

Principle of Parallax by Charles A. Clark:

By changing the angulation of the X-ray beam, an apparent displacement of the object to be localised was seen. When the reference object is considered as the tooth closest to the object to be localised, the image of the object that is farther (palatally or lingually placed object) from the X-ray tube moves in the same direction as the tube, whereas the image of the object closer to the X-ray tube (buccally placed object) moves in the opposite direction. This technique was introduced by *Clark*. He used a horizontal shift of the tube; *Richards* introduced the concept of a vertical shift (Fig. 19.31).

Vertex occlusal film

This shows the buccopalatal relationship of canine to the roots of adjacent teeth.

Supplementary films

- True lateral film shows the vertical height of a canine and its relationship to the nose and antrum
- Tangential view will show a canine erupting buccal to incisor teeth
- Oblique and anterior occlusal film shows the whole of the canine where it cannot be seen on periapical films. These films should only be used to examine the morphology of the canines.

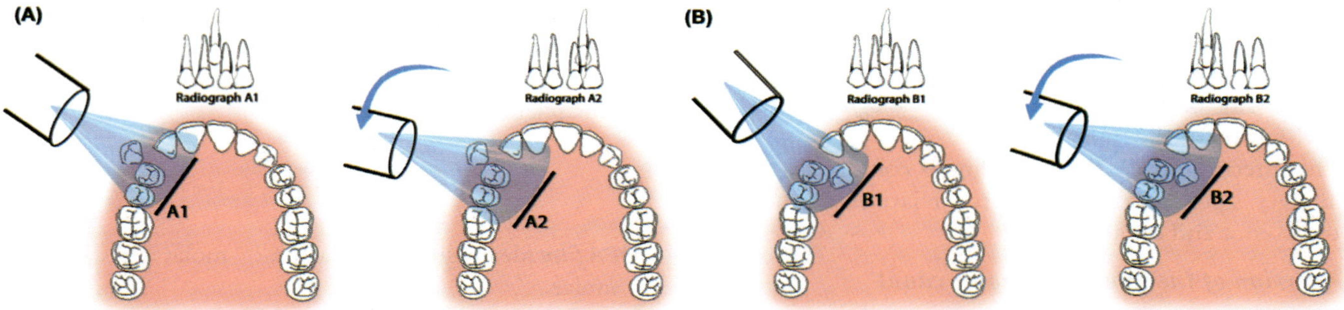

Figure 19.31 This image illustrates the 1st step of Clark's tube shift technique for the localisation of the canine in a buccolingual plane. (**A**) A bucally impacted 13 has been illustrated. The corresponding radiographs A1 shows similar position of the canine due to the central X-ray perpendicular through the objects. In the 2nd step, the X-ray tube has been shifted distally. The radiograph A2 shows a shift of the canine towards the incisors (mesial-shift), which is opposite to the position of the X-ray tube (Opposite side—Buccal). (**B**) Illustration of palatally impacted 13, the corresponding radiographs B1 shows similar position of the canine. In the 2nd step of clarks technique, the X-ray tube is shifted distally. Radiograph B2 shows a shift of the canine towards the premolars (distal-shift), which is the same side of the X-ray tube (Same side—Lingual or Palatal).

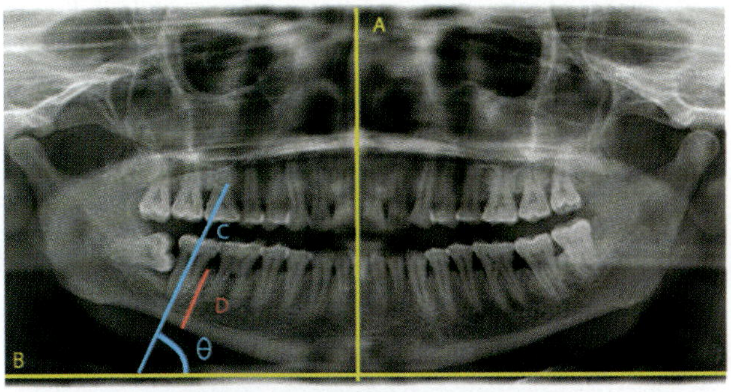

Figure 19.32 Wharfe's assessment.

CBCT

CBCT is a low radiation CT scan useful in localising canine position preoperatively.

Assessment of difficulty of removal

Wharfe's assessment (Fig. 19.32)

Scoring details for Wharfe's assessment are depicted in Table 19.2.

Crown of the impacted tooth

Teeth with large bulbous crown and prominent cusps are difficult to remove when compared to small conical crowns and flat cusps. In cases of tooth impaction wherein the withdrawal of the 3rd molar is obstructed by the presence of the 2nd molar, the cusps of the 3rd molar may impinge on the 2nd molar and cause root resorption of the 2nd molar. In such cases, the impacted tooth will have to be sectioned for removal.

Pederson's scale

Pederson proposed a modification of the *Pell–Gregory* scale that included a 3rd factor, the angulation of the molar (*mesioangular*, *horizontal*, *vertical* or *distoangular*) (Table 19.3). The *Pederson* scale is designed for evaluation in *OPG*.

Armamentarium for surgical removal of impacted teeth is shown in Fig. 19.33

TABLE 19.2 Scoring Details for Wharfe's Assessment

Criteria	CATEGORY	Score
1. Winter's classification	Horizontal Mesioangular Vertical Distoangular	2 1 0 2
2. Height of the mandible	1–30 mm 31–34 mm 35–39 mm	0 1 2
3. Angulation of II molar	1–59° 60–69° 70–79° 80–89° 90°+	0 1 2 3 4
4. Root shape and development a) Less than 1/3rd complete b) 1/3rd to 2/3rd complete c) More than 2/3rd complete:	 Complex Favourable curvature Unfavourable curvature	 2 1 3 2 1
5. Follicles	Normal Possibly enlarged Enlarged Impaction relieved	0 −1 −2 −3
6. Path of exit	Space available Distal cusp covered Mesial cusp covered Both covered	0 1 2 3
Total		33

SURGICAL REMOVAL OF IMPACTED 3RD MOLAR

Procedure for surgical removal of the tooth (Fig. 19.34A and B) varies depending upon the following factors:

- The type and degree of impaction (local or general anaesthesia)
- Amount of soft tissue exposure to aid in removal of bone (type of flap)
- Amount and technique of bone removal (chisel or bur)
- Odentectomy—need to divide the tooth prior to delivery.

PATIENT POSITION

The dental chair is positioned in such a way, which is comfortable for the patient and at the same time allows the operator and the assistant to have a clear view of the surgical site. During mandibular surgical procedure, the occlusal plane of lower teeth must be parallel to the floor, and for maxillary procedures, occlusal plane of upper teeth should be at 45° angle to the floor.

ASEPSIS AND ISOLATION

The instruments are arranged in a rational order of their intended use over a separate instrument trolley or over the instrument tray of the dental chair on a sterile towel. To maintain the sterility of the instruments and avoid contamination, the instruments must be covered with another sterile towel, if there is any delay in starting the surgery. Head cap and face mask are worn by surgeon and the assistant, which is followed by scrubbing the hands till the elbow level. Minimum of 3–5 min is the ideal time for scrubbing. A sterile gown must be worn by surgeon and the assistant, which is followed by donning sterile gloves. To maintain complete asepsis, the patient's head and front part of body must be draped using sterile towel or disposable cap, exposing the face. The preparation of surgical site is

TABLE 19.3 Pederson's Scale

Classification	Value
Spatial relationship	
Mesioangular	1
Horizontal transverse	2
Vertical	3
Distoangular	4
Depth	
Level A: High occlusal level	1
Level B: Medium occlusal level	2
Level C: Deep occlusal level	3
Ramus relationship space available	
Class 1: Sufficient space	1
Class 2: Reduced space	2
Class 3: No space	3
Difficulty index	
Very difficult	7–10
Moderately difficult	5–6
Slightly difficult	3–4

done by wiping the patient's face using antiseptic solution like povidone iodine (Betadine), followed by swabbing the 3rd molar area using 0.5% solution of chlorhexidine or betadine.

ANAESTHESIA

Mostly the procedure is performed under local anaesthesia, which is obtained by nerve block of the inferior alveolar nerve, lingual nerve and long buccal nerve.

General anaesthesia is indicated when the impacted tooth is situated deep in the jaw bone (when the red line is more than 5 mm) and when more than two impacted molars have to be removed at a time.

INCISION

Most commonly used are:

- Ward's
- Modified Ward's (for horizontal lower 3rd molar impaction).

MUCOPERIOSTEAL FLAP

Ideal requirements of the flap

- It should provide adequate exposure of the operative site
- The base of the flap should be wide so that the soft tissues get adequate blood supply after wound closure
- To avoid soft tissue trauma during surgical procedures, the flap should expose the entire site of operation
- The flap should not be extended too far distobuccally in which case it might injure the buccal vessels, cause postoperative trismus (due to the trauma to the temporalis muscle) or herniation of the buccal pad of fat into the operating field
- The incision should be designed so that the flap can be primarily closed over solid bone
- The incision should not damage any of the vital anatomic structures
- The following are the different types of the flaps employed (Fig. 19.35):
    - Envelope flap
    - L-shaped flap
    - Bayonet flap
    - Triangular (Three cornered) flap.

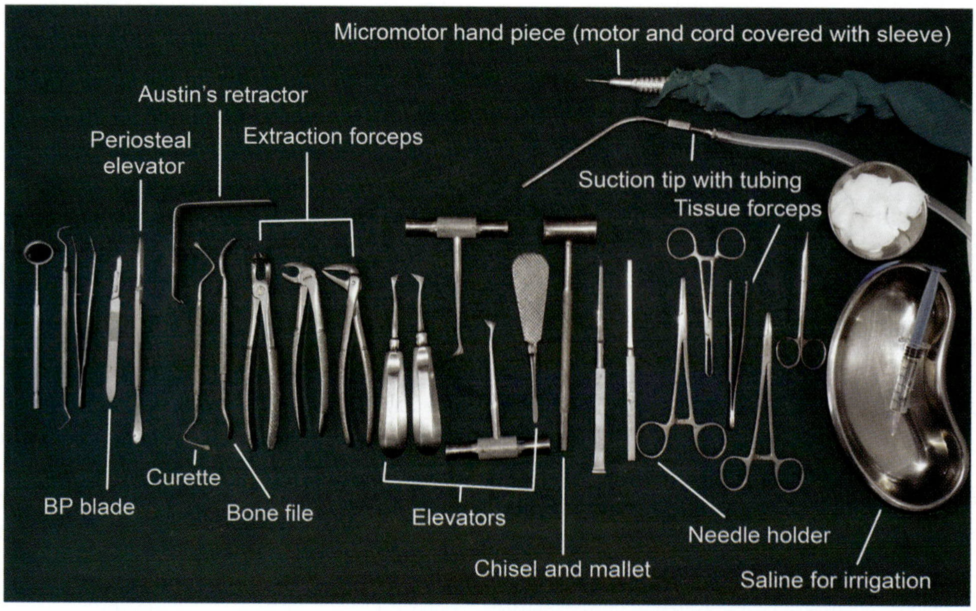

Figure 19.33 Armamentarium for surgical removal of impacted teeth.

Steps in surgical removal impacted teeth

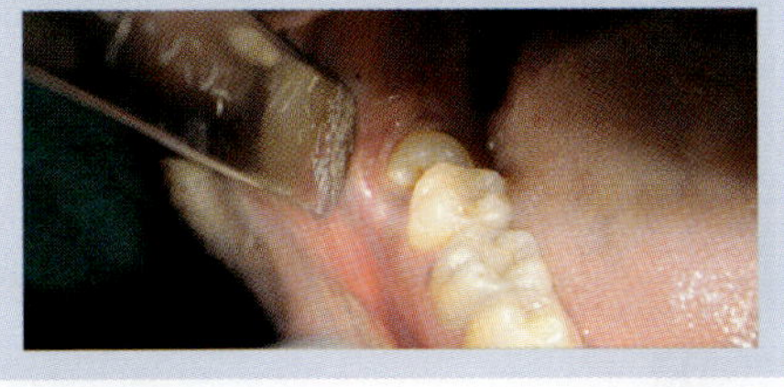

Step 1: Clinical assessment of the impacted, mesioangular 48.

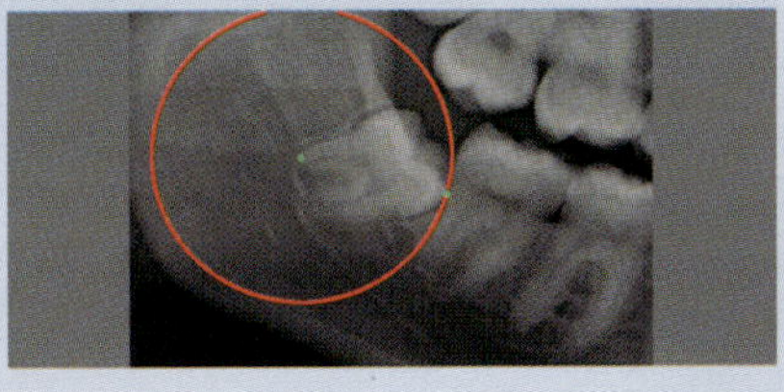

Step 2: Radiographic assessment of the impacted 48. Arc of rotation is drawn with centre of circle at distal root tip and periphery at mesial cusp tip. As the arc crosses the distal half of 47, it indicates need for odontectomy (splitting of the tooth) since the path of withdrawal of 48, in toto, is not favourable.

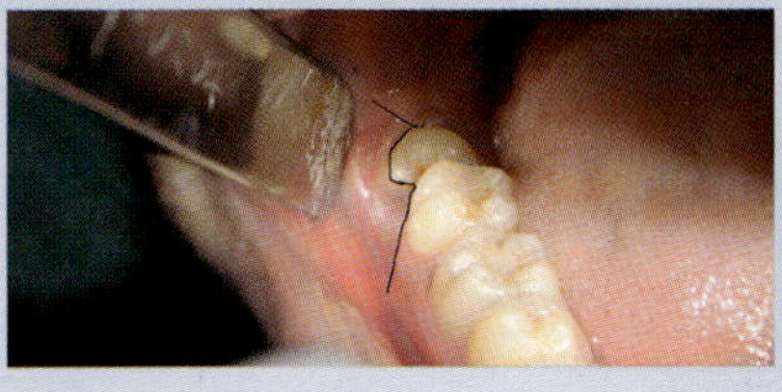

Step 3: Pictorial representation of the planned Ward's incision.

(anterior limit of the incision should not cross the mesial line angle of 47 to avoid encountering the facial artery)

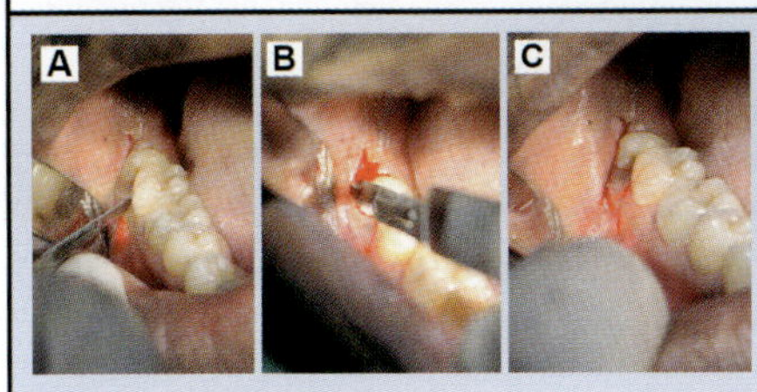

Step 4A: Anterior releasing incision is made including the interdental papilla distal of 47 extending downwards at 45 ° to the long axis of 47.

Step 4B: Crevicular incision around 48 is given.

Step 4C: Distal release incision is made buccolaterally to avoid encountering the lingual nerve

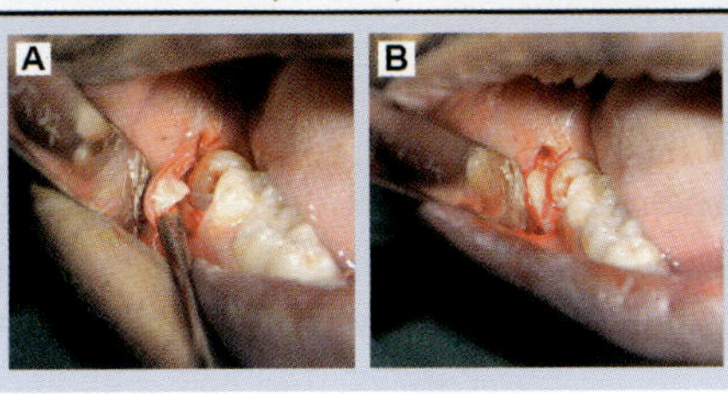

Step 5A: Buccal mucoperiosteal flap is raised including the interdental papilla.

Step 5B: complete elevation of the buccal mucoperiosteal flap exposing the impacted 48. Note the Austin retractor placed over the external oblique ridge retracting the buccal flap.

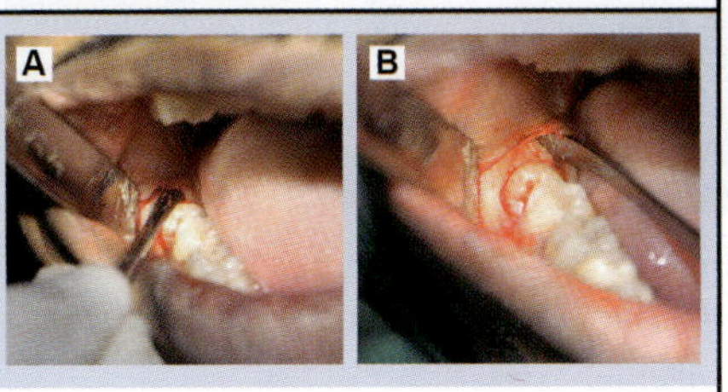

Step 6A: Raising of the lingual mucoperiosteal flap.

Step 6B: complete exposure of the impacted 48 and surrounding bone. Note the Howarth periosteal elevator placed subperiosteally retracting lingual flap and protecting lingual nerve.

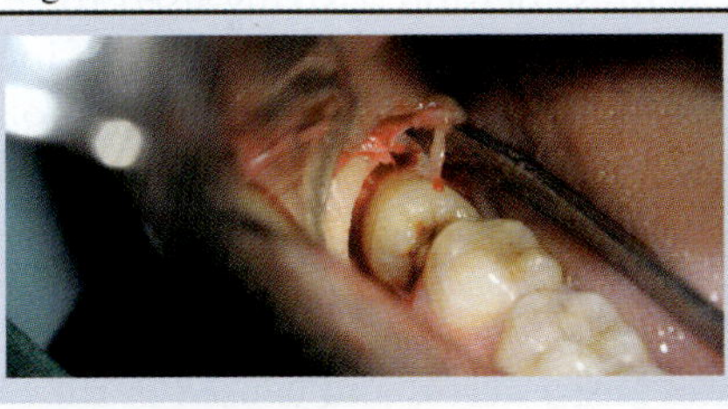

Step 7: Guttering of the mesial, buccal and distal bone of 48 closest to the tooth (Moore-Gillbe collar technique).

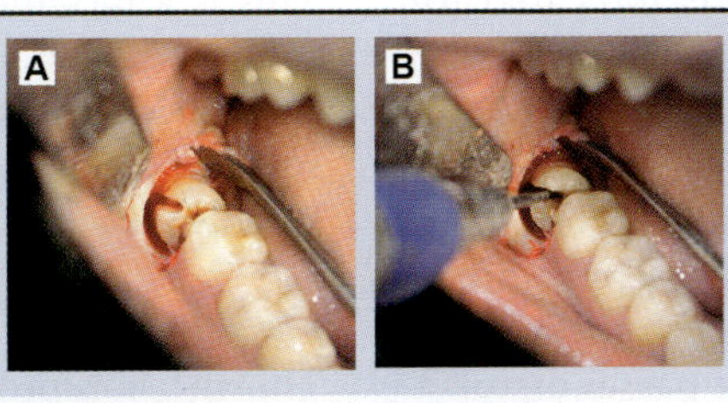

Step 8A: Initiation of odontectomy along the long axis of tooth midway at the bifurcation.

Step 8B: Odontectomy performed until two-third of the buccolingual width of the tooth using rotary instrument.

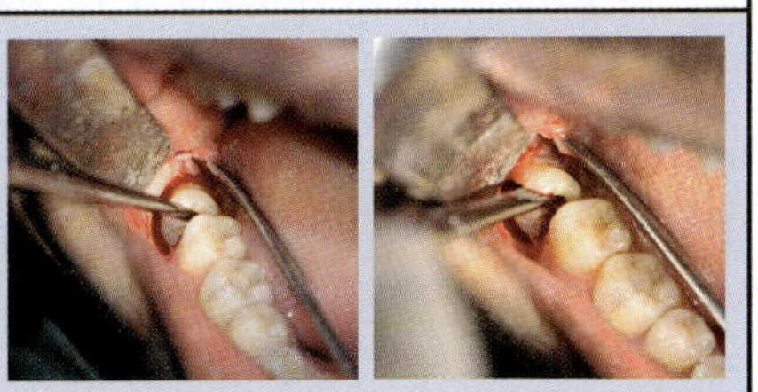

Step 9: Completion of odontectomy using straight elevator. The working end of the elevator is engaged into the created groove and rotated clockwise to complete the odontectomy.

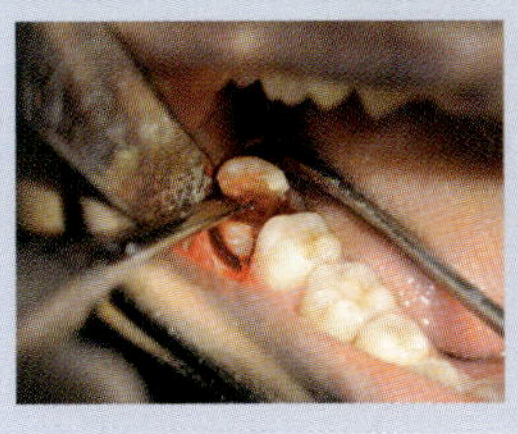

Step 10: Removal of the distal segment of 48.

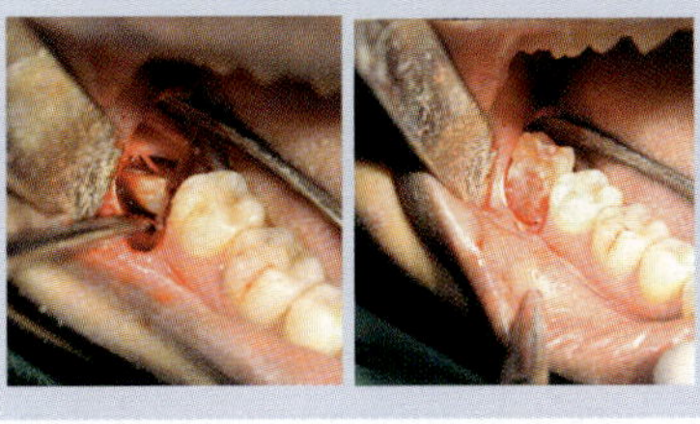

Step 11: Removal of the mesial segment of 48 into the distally created space using mesial point of elevation.

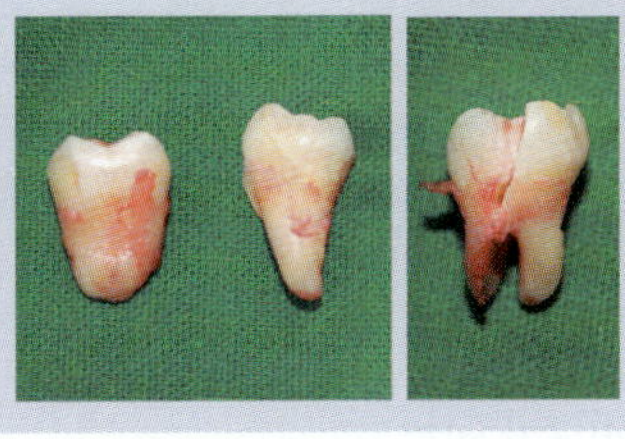

Step 12: Extraoral reorientation of the extracted tooth fragments and confirmation of complete tooth extraction.

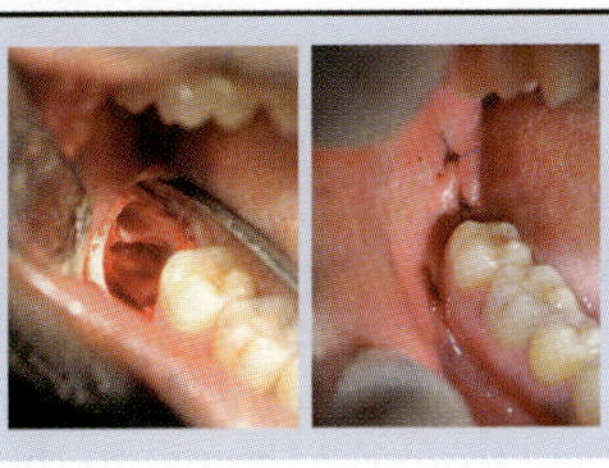

Step 13: Wound debridement and primary closure.

Figure 19.34 Clinical demonstration of surgical removal of mesioangular impacted 48.

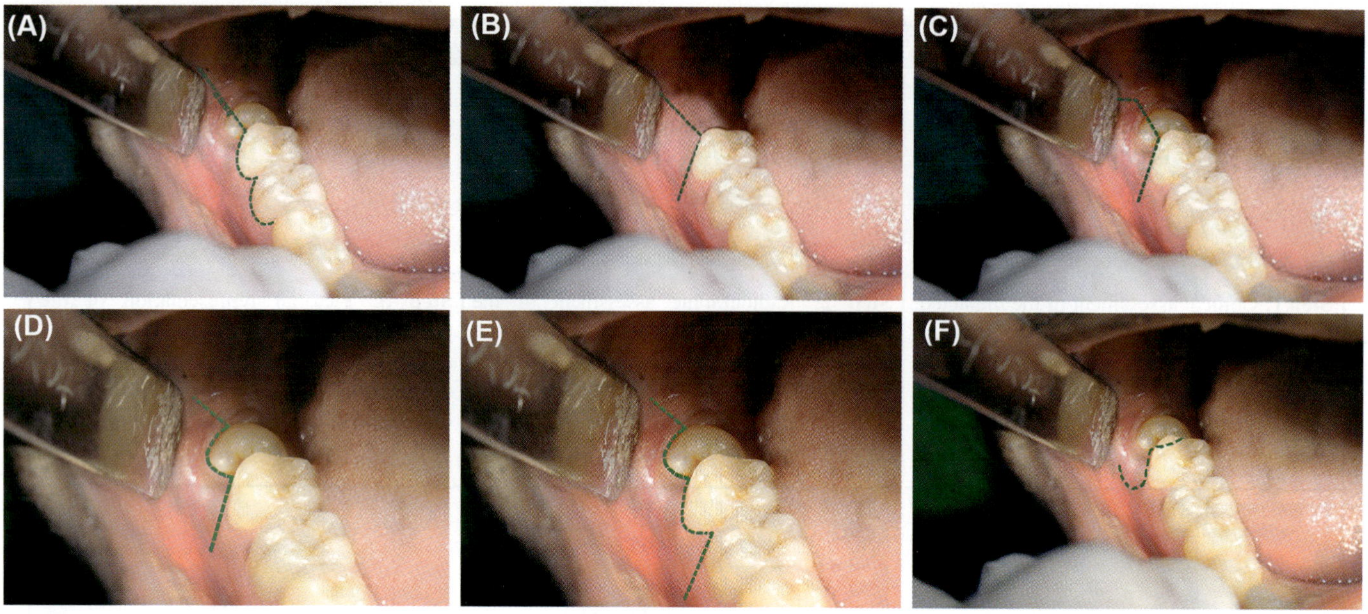

Figure 19.35 Different types of flaps and incision for surgical removal of 3rd molar. **(A)** Envelope flap. **(B)** L-shaped flap. **(C)** Trapezoidal flap. **(D)** Bayonet flap with Ward's incision. **(E)** Modified Ward's incision. **(F)** Comma-shaped incision.

Envelope flap (Fig. 19.35A)

The flap extends from the mesial papilla of the mandibular 1st molar and passes around the neck of the teeth to the distobuccal line angle of the 2nd molar.

Now the incision line extends posteriorly and laterally up to the anterior border of the mandible. Care should be taken not to damage the lingual nerve. The advantage of this flap is that the wound heals quickly. This flap is indicated for mesioangular/soft tissue impactions.

L-shaped flap (Fig. 19.35B)

This flap suits only the buccal approach since it is difficult to raise a lingual flap from this approach. The posterior limb of the incision extends from a point just lateral to the ascending ramus of the mandible into the sulcus. It passes distolateral to the periodontium by avoiding or including it, depending upon the proximity of the 3rd molar with the 2nd molar. The junction between the limbs may be curved and the incision made in one sweep or it may be angled.

Bayonet flap (Fig. 19.35D)

This incision has three parts: distal or posterior, intermediate or gingival and an anterior part. Also known as Ward's incision, the posterior part of the incision goes around the gingival margin of the 2nd and even the 1st molar, before turning into the sulcus. It joins the gingival margin of the 2nd molar anywhere from the lingual to the buccal side.

The intermediate part of the incision can be carried forward to a variable extent. It extends entirely around the buccal margin of the 2nd molar to end at the papilla in between the 1st and 2nd molars. The anterior part of the incision is angled from the gingival margin in a forward and downward direction towards the sulcus. The disadvantage of this flap is that overextension of the incision into the sulcus may cause brisk oozing of blood from the venous plexus. This can be avoided by making the anterior part of the incision more oblique in direction.

Triangular (Three cornered) flap (Fig. 19.35E)

This is a modified Ward's incision. Usually used for deeply impacted teeth. In this incision, the anterior part of incision should commence at the distobuccal corner of 1st molar instead of 2nd molar and the distal incision is given similar to Ward's incision.

Comma-shaped incision (Fig. 19.35F)

This incision provides larger access and is used in the case of deep horizontal impaction. Beginning at the depth of the extended vestibule, the incision moves in an anterior direction. Posterior to the 2nd molar at it's distobuccal line angle, the incision is made, gently curving up to meet the gingival crest. The incision is carried on as a crevicular incision around the distal half of the 2nd molar as a distolingually based flap. This incision exposes the entire 3rd molar area, allowing reflection of a distolingually based flap.

ELEVATION OF THE FLAP

To allow adequate exposure of bone and the tooth, a full thickness mucoperiosteal flap should be elevated. Periosteal elevator can be used to elevate this flap. After the elevation of the buccal flap, the lingual soft tissue must be reflected. This is accomplished by means of a periosteal elevator which is inserted under the periosteum and passed in a distolingual direction to reach the lingual border of the mandible. The flap is then elevated very carefully, avoiding any damage to the lingual and mylohyoid nerves.

Once the flap has been raised adequately, appropriate retractors (Bowdler-Henry, Austin, etc.) are used to retract the flap.

Bone removal

The amber line determines the amount of bone covering the impacted tooth, which has to be removed for applying the elevator to remove the tooth. The red line determines the depth of the 'point of application' of the elevator. When the entire crown lies above and in front of the amber line, there is no necessity to remove the bone. In other cases, bone can be removed with the help of chisel or burs.

Removal of bone with bur

Adequate amount of bone is removed using high speed headpiece and straight bur no. 702 or 703 carbide fissure burs under copious saline irrigation. By sectioning of the tooth, extensive bone removal can be minimised.

TECHNIQUES

Postage stamp technique (Fig. 19.36)

In this technique, holes in the form of postage stamp are created using round bur on the buccal aspect of the tooth. These holes are then connected and a disc or postage stamp piece of bone is removed permitting adequate access for application of elevator in the surgical area. This technique helps in controlled removal of bone, preventing uncontrolled fracture of the alveolar process and allows judicious use of elevators and forceps.

Moore–Gillbe's collar technique (Fig. 19.37)

The bur is used to create a gutter around the neck of the impacted tooth. On the buccal and the distal aspect, the bone must be removed to expose the entire crown till the CEJ. When the bone is removed around the distolingual region, care must be taken by the operator to avoid any damage to the lingual flap and lingual nerve (Fig. 19.37B). When point of application of the elevator is on the mesial side, adequate bone must be removed so that the elevator stands up at an angle of 45° to the mandible without any support. The area should be irrigated constantly with saline during the drilling procedure to avoid bone necrosis. The tooth should not be removed unless enough space exists where the tooth can be displaced. When the tooth has been removed using appropriate elevator, sharp bony edges should be removed and smoothened.

REMOVAL OF BONE WITH CHISEL (Fig. 19.38)

Mandibular grains

The bone trajectories of the mandible must be borne in mind before using the chisel. This method depends upon the mandible having grains similar to wood. The grains are

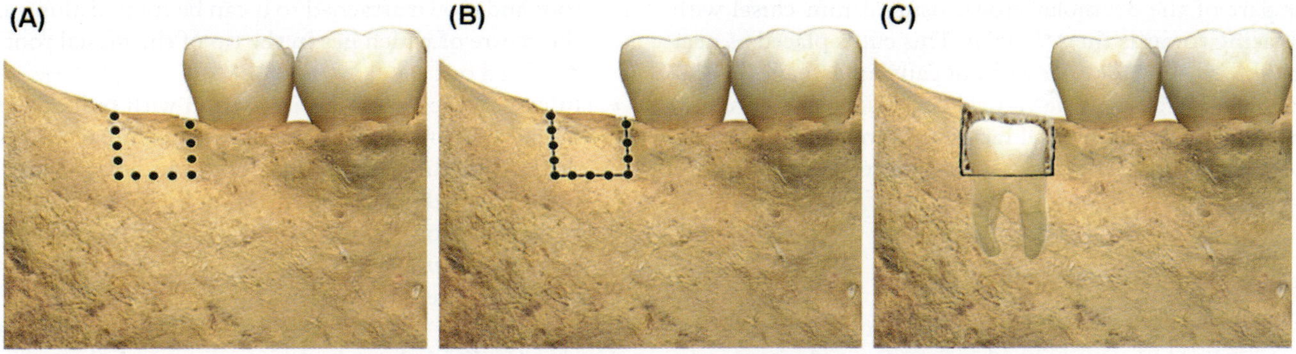

Figure 19.36 Postage stamp technique. (**A**) Bur holes are made on the buccal aspect. (**B**) Bur holes are connected together creating a window which provides access for the application of elevator. (**C**) Impacted tooth exposed.

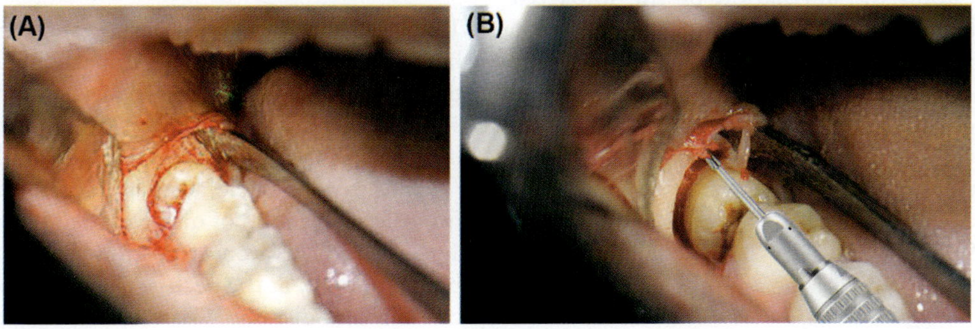

Figure 19.37 Moore–Gillbe's collar technique. (**A**) Elevation of flap and exposure of horizontally impacted tooth. (**B**) Using bur buccal and distal aspect of bone is removed till the CEJ (Note the periosteal elevator is used to retract the lingual flap to protect the lingual nerve from damage).

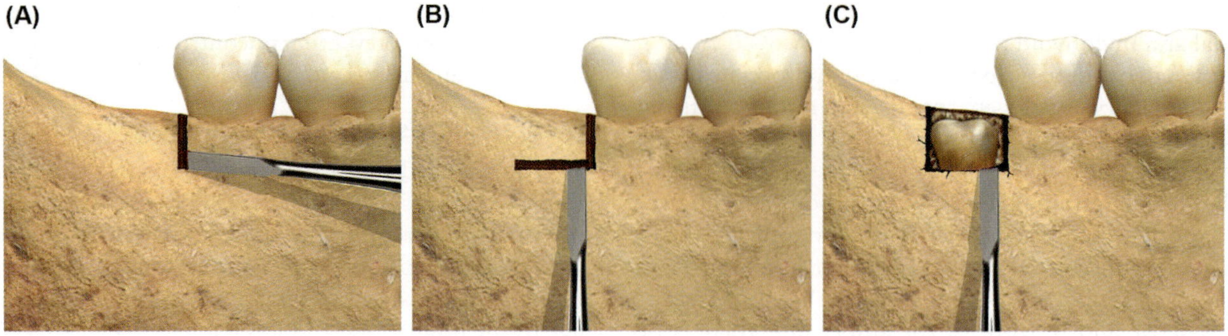

Figure 19.38 (**A–C**) Removal of lower 3rd molar by **Chisel and mallet technique**.

related to the direction of the fibres, which in turn are related to haversian systems and the blood supply. In the 3rd molar region, the bone trajectories run parallel to the oblique ridge. The use of chisel parallel to the grains may cause the cut to extend towards the 1st molar the ramus distally and cause a fracture. To prevent this phenomenon, mesial and distal vertical stop cuts are made initially before using the chisel on the buccal aspect.

Buccal bone may also be carved away by chiselling. When using chisel for removing the bone in the mandibular 3rd molar region, the mandible should be adequately supported. In this technique, bone is removed buccally, distally and superiorly. A vertical step cut is made down to the level of the lower part of the 3rd molar crown using 3 mm chisel with bevel facing towards the 2nd molar. This cut is placed as near as possible to the 2nd molar without causing damage. 2nd cut is placed at the base of the vertical cut, using a 5 mm chisel at an angle of 45° with bevel facing upwards, and the cut is made till the distal point of the 3rd molar tooth to allow for delivery of the tooth. The disadvantage of this technique is that it cannot be used for older patients.

TOOTH SECTIONING

In some situations, sectioning of the tooth in multiple segments should be considered before removal, due to the difficulty that is predicted to be encountered in the path of removal of the tooth. The direction of the tooth sectioning primarily depends upon the angulation of the impacted tooth. Care must be taken not to injure the lingual nerve while sectioning the tooth. Sectioning of tooth reduces the amount of bone to be removed before elevation and thus reduces postoperative oedema. It also reduces the risk of damage to neighbouring teeth and inadvertent luxation. Copious saline irrigation must be done while sectioning the tooth.

Advantages of odontectomy

Pell and Gregory stated the following advantages of splitting technique:

- Amount of bone to be removed is reduced
- The time of operation is reduced
- The field of operation is small and therefore damage to adjacent teeth and bone is reduced
- Risk of jaw fracture is reduced
- Risk of damage to the inferior alveolar nerve is reduced.

Disadvantages of odontectomy

- In elderly patients, splitting of the tooth is difficult due to the sclerosis of the tooth structure
- Sometimes due to the presence of shallow grooves on the tooth structure, splitting is difficult
- Vertically impacted tooth with bulbous crown and prominent cusps are usually impacted below the distal convexity of the 2nd molars. Vertical splitting of the 3rd molar is indicated here, which permits removal of the distal root and portion of the crown attached to it. Then the mesial root and crown attached to it can be rotated along an arc, the centre of which lies in the tip of the mesial root to be delivered out
- In case of mesioangular impaction with bulbous crown, mesial portion of the crown, which is impacted beneath distal convexity of the 2nd molar, can be split at the cementoenamel margin by means of bur or osteotome. The crown can now be moved distally into the space created earlier and removed. The roots are then elevated into the space occupied by the crown and removed
- If the roots are unfavourably curved, the roots can also be divided at the bifurcation and then removed separately.

TOOTH ELEVATION

The bone removal should establish sufficient space between the height of the contour of the impacted tooth and the bone to permit the application of an elevator. Similarly, sufficient bone should be removed distal to the impacted tooth to make a space into which the impacted tooth can be displaced while removal.

The direction of elevation is determined by curvature of the roots. Disimpaction of mesioangular teeth is done using a no. 1 Coupland elevator or a straight Warwick James elevator placed mesially at the neck of the tooth and rotated to move it buccally and distally. Whereas, in case of distoangular impaction, there is lack of space between the impacted tooth and the 2nd molar, therefore the elevation on the mesial aspect is compromised. Division of roots is done in case of horizontally impacted tooth, which are then elevated individually.

DEBRIDEMENT OF WOUND AND WOUND CLOSURE

The wound should be debrided to eliminate particulate bone chips and debris which might have accumulated during the surgery. Periapical curettes can be used to debride the socket mechanically. The sharp margins of the bone should be smoothened using a bone file. Following this, careful irrigation with sterile saline should be carried out thoroughly under the reflected tissue flaps.

The wound should now be closed with sutures. The initial suture is placed on the distal aspect of the 2nd molar. Additional sutures are placed in the anterior and posterior limbs of the incision. Sometimes the wound may be left to heal by granulation tissue formation wherein no sutures are placed, but it is packed with gauze soaked with Whitehead's varnish. Oral and written postoperative instructions are given to the patients following the procedure which can greatly help the patient and also ensure better patient compliance.

INSTRUCTIONS TO PATIENT FOLLOWING SURGICAL REMOVAL OF IMPACTED TOOTH

For the overall success of the surgical procedure and also for a smooth postoperative period, proper written or oral instruction is essential.

1. Following the surgery, the patient is asked to bite on gauze pad for at least 1 h
2. Advise application of ice packs for the 1st 24 h to decrease the postoperative oedema
3. Advise soft diet for the 1st day
4. Advise avoidance of warm saline gargles, smoking, spitting and sucking from straw in the 1st 24 h
5. From the surgical site, mild bleeding/oozing of blood can be expected for one to two days. In case of excessive bleeding, the patient is asked to bite on a fresh piece of sterile gauze and inform the doctor
6. Patient is advised to take the drugs prescribed by the doctor at regular intervals
7. Advice brushing of teeth from the night of surgery onwards to maintain oral hygiene
8. Advised to avoid disturbance of the surgical site in order to prevent loosening or removal the blood clot
9. Review the patient for suture removal.

Complications

- Swelling
- Trismus
- Bleeding
- Neurologic
    a) Lingual nerve damage–paraesthesia of tongue
    b) Inferior alveolar nerve damage–paraesthesia lower lip
- Fractured lingual plate (Fig. 19.39)
- Loss of tooth into submandibular and sublingual space
- Mandibular fracture
- 2nd molar
    a) Hypersensitivity
    b) Distal periodontal pocket
    c) Gingival recession.

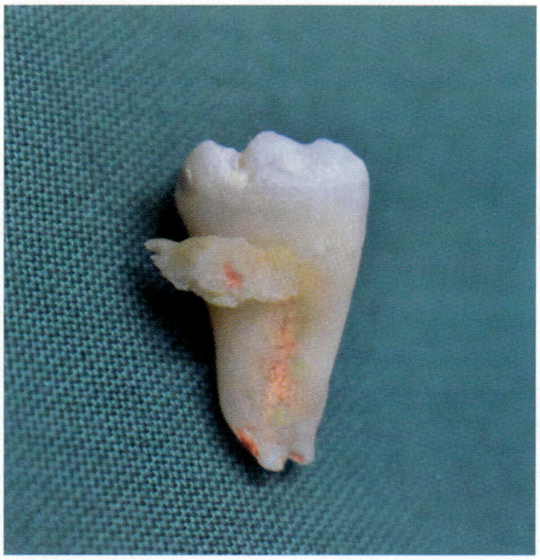

Figure 19.39 Lingual plate fracture in ankylosed 3rd molar.

OTHER METHODS OF REMOVAL OF IMPACTED MANDIBULAR 3rd MOLAR

LINGUAL SPLIT TECHNIQUE (KELSEY FRY'S TECHNIQUE) (Fig. 19.40)

This method was introduced by Sir William Kelsey Fry. It takes advantage of the thinness of the lingual cortical plate, avoids and preserves plate and hence preserves the buccal plate and external oblique ridge.

Procedure

- The incision is made on the 3rd molar region exposing the tooth surrounding bone. A mucoperiosteal flap is elevated on the buccal side to expose the bone enclosing the impacted tooth. A vertical stop cut is made in the anterior end of the impacted tooth using a chisel
- The chisel is placed horizontally with the bevel facing downwards just below the vertical stop cut and a horizontal cut is made extending backwards
- A point of application for an elevator is made with a chisel by excising the triangular piece of bone bounded anteriorly by the lower end of the stop cut and above by the anterior end of the horizontal cut
- The distolingual bone is now fractured inward by using chisel. The chisel is held at an angle of 45° to the bone surface and pointing in the direction of 2nd premolar on the contralateral side. The cutting edge of the chisel is kept parallel to the external oblique ridge and a few light taps are given with the mallet that separates the lingual plate from the alveolar bone and hinges it inward on the soft tissue attached to it. At this point, care must be taken that the cutting edge of the chisel is not held parallel to the internal oblique ridge as this may lead to the extension of the lingual split to the coronoid process.
- The 'peninsula' of bone which then remains distal to the tooth and between the buccal and lingual cuts is excised
- A sharp, pointed, fine-bladed straight elevator is then applied to the mesial surface of the tooth and minimum

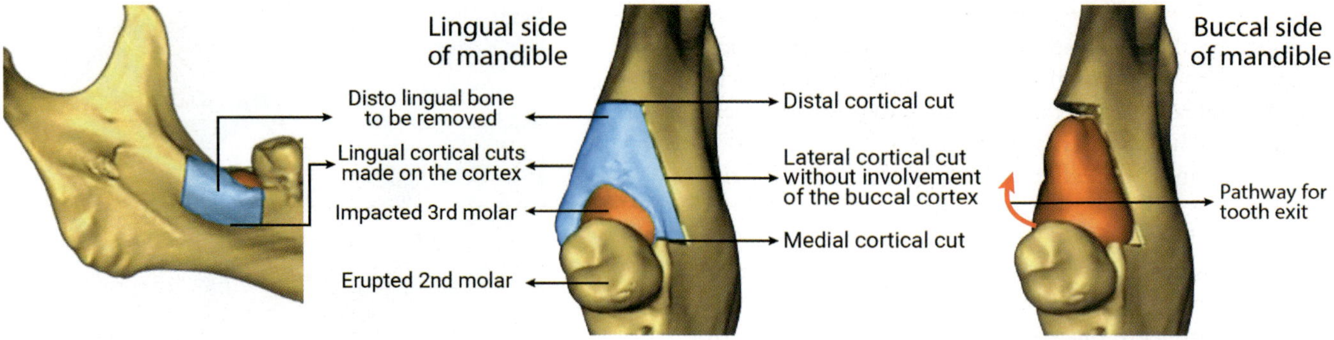

Figure 19.40 Diagrammatic illustration of lingual split technique—showing horizontally impacted 3rd and erupted 2nd molar tooth. The medial, lateral and distal cortical cuts are made using chisel fracturing the buccal and disto-lingual bone facilitating removal of impacted tooth.

force is used to displace the tooth upward and backward out of its socket

- As the tooth moves backward, the fractured lingual plate is displaced from its path of withdrawal, thus facilitating delivery of the tooth. After the tooth has been removed from its socket, the lingual plate is grasped in fine haemostats and the soft tissues are freed from it by blunt dissection
- The fractured lingual plate is then lifted from the wound, thus completing the saucerisation of the bony cavity
- The bone edges are smoothened with bone files; the wound is irrigated with saline and closed with sutures.

Advantages

- It is a quick technique
- Helps in removal of lingually impacted 3rd molar without much of buccal bone removal
- This technique helps in reduction of the size of the residual blood clot by means of saucerisation of the socket.

It is mostly indicated in children in whom the bone is very elastic. General anaesthesia is preferred.

LATERAL TREPHINATION

Technique (Fig. 19.41)

This procedure was first described by Bowdler-Henry to remove any partially formed and unerupted 3rd molar in the age group of 9–16 years. The advantage of this technique is that the bone healing is excellent without any loss of alveolar bone around the 2nd molar.

- Under anaesthesia, the external oblique ridge is palpated and an S-shaped incision is made
- The incision line starts from the retro molar fossa and extends across the external oblique ridge curving down along the reflection of the mucous membrane above the vestibule and ends anterior to the 1st permanent molar
- A full thickness mucoperiosteal flap is elevated and retracted using a Bowdler-Henry retractor
- Using a round bur, the buccal cortical plate over the 3rd molar crypt is trephined till it covers the entire anteroposterior length of the crypt. Following this, a vertical cut is made on the external plate at its anterior margin

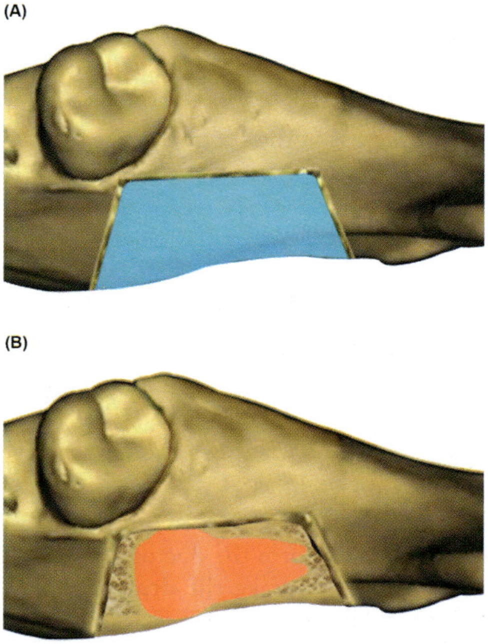

Figure 19.41 **(A)** Use of bur and chisel to remove the buccal bone overlying the tooth bud. **(B)** Exposure of tooth bud and its removal.

- At the posterior end of the crypt, a 2nd cut is made through the outer plate at an angle of 45° from the trephine holes
- Now the buccal plate is fractured to expose the 3rd molar crypt using a chisel vertically over the trephine holes. The fractured buccal plate can be removed using a curved haemostat
- Using an elevator, the impacted tooth is delivered out of the crypt
- Care should be taken not to leave any follicular remnants and also not to injure inferior alveolar canal while debriding the follicular sac
- The bony margins are smoothened, the wound irrigated and closed.

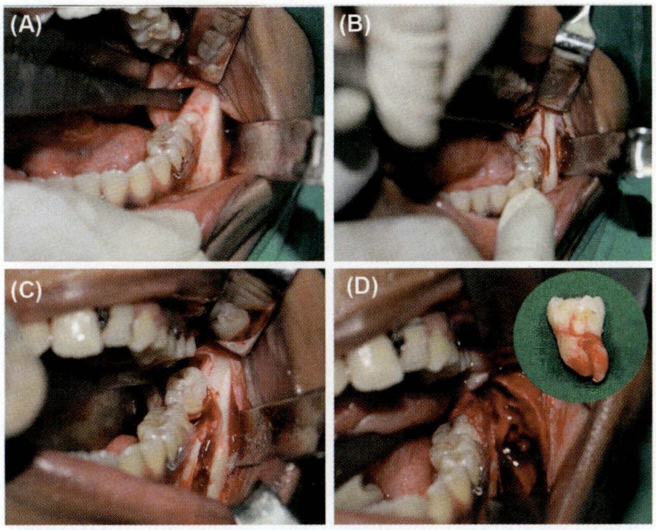

Figure 19.42 Surgical removal of impacted mandibular 3rd molar by sagittal split ramus osteotomy. (**A**) Incision is given starting from retromolar region and extending to canine tooth, and the full thickness flap was raised exposing the ramus. (**B**) Sagittal splitting of the ramus. (**C**) Removal of impacted tooth. (**D**) Extracted tooth.

SAGITTAL SPLIT TECHNIQUE (FIG. 19.42)

Amin (1995), Toffanin (2003) and Jones (2004) reported sagittal spit technique for the removal of impacted tooth. Conventionally this technique has been used for the surgical correction of mandibular deficiency (advancement) and for mandibular excess (push back). Although not a standard procedure for removal of impacted teeth, this technique is performed when the 3rd molar is deeply impacted when they are in close proximity to the inferior alveolar nerve. This procedure is involved with disadvantages, which include greater extent of removal of bone, compromised visibility, malocclusion and risk of injury to the nerve and chances of fracture of mandible. On contrast, the advantages of this technique includes good access, conservation of bone that would otherwise be removed and visibility of nerve.

BUCCAL CORTICOTOMY (FIG. 19.43)

Buccal corticotomy is an alternative approach that offers access to deeply impacted mandibular teeth. This technique includes raising a trapezoidal mucoperiosteal flap in the mandibular molar region and placing a rectangular window using a narrow fissure bur over the deeply impacted tooth, with mesial and distal cuts almost reaching lower border of mandible. An osteotome is used to remove the buccal cortical plate and the impacted tooth is then sectioned using a bur and removed. The buccal bony fragment is positioned back and secured using plates or wire and screws. The site is irrigated and wound closure is done.

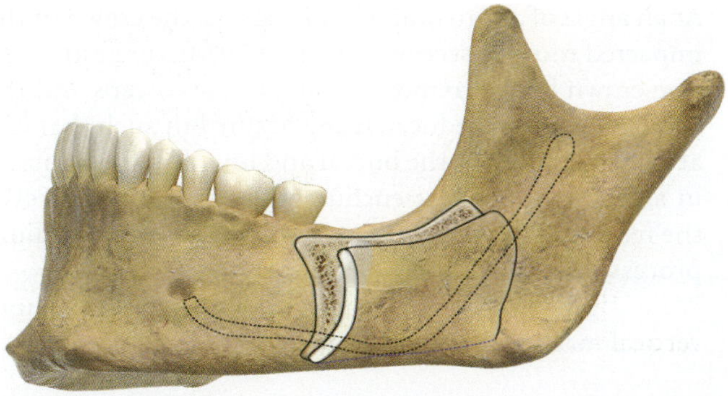

Figure 19.43 Diagrammatic illustration of the buccal corticotomy technique showing mesial and distal bony cuts reaching lower border of the mandible. When the buccal cortical bone is removed, the impacted tooth is exposed.

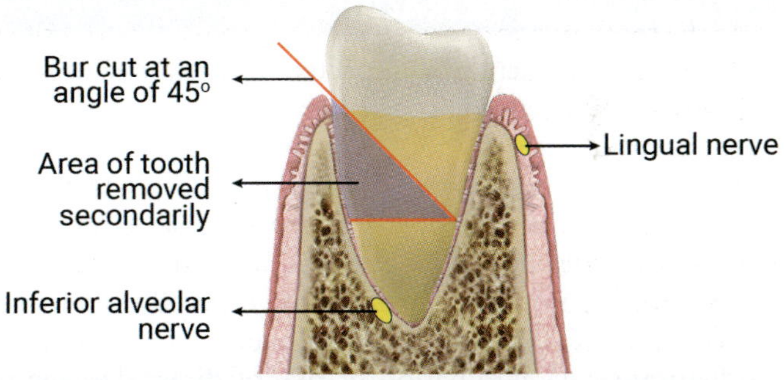

Figure 19.44 Diagrammatic representation of coronectomy technique. The bur is directed at an angle of 45° to section the crown. Following this, the area marked is removed to place the remaining root portion of the tooth 2–3 mm below the crest of bone. Note the position of inferior alveolar nerve and lingual nerve.

PARTIAL ODONTECTOMY (FIG. 19.44)

One of the most common complication following surgical removal of 3rd molar is inferior alveolar nerve injury. Partial odontectomy (coronectomy, deliberate root retention) is a technique that may reduce the possibility of nerve injury. The risk of nerve injury is estimated to be 14% when there is intimate relationship between roots of teeth and inferior alveolar nerve (IAN). This intimate relation to the nerve can be studied using OPG. Assessment of relationship with inferior alveolar nerve and the changes related to the root and nerve are already discussed. According to current recommendation, CBCT scanning should be advised if there is any close relationship between the roots of 3rd molar and the IAN assessed by an OPG. In this technique, the part of root related to IAN is intentionally left undisturbed.

Technique

- After prophylactic antibiotic administration, the conventional incision is placed and elevation of mucoperiosteal flap is done

- At an angle of approximately 45 degrees, the crown of the impacted tooth is sectioned using #701 fissure bur
- The crown is then removed using tissue forceps and the remaining root is reduced using fissure bur such that it is at least 3 mm below the buccal and lingual cortical plates in all dimensions as it encourages bone formation over the retained root fragments as part of the normal healing process
- Water tight closure of wound is done using one or more vertical mattress sutures.

CONTRAINDICATIONS

This technique is contraindicated when the tooth is mobile, horizontally impacted or in case of active infection in the radicular portion of tooth.

ORTHODONTIC EXTRACTION

This procedure is useful for impacted 3rd molars with close proximity to the inferior alveolar nerve.

Treatment phase includes 1) preparation for orthodontic device, 2) surgical exposure of the crown of deeply impacted tooth under local anaesthesia, 3) placement of orthodontic device, 4) uprightment of mesially or horizontally impacted molars, 5) assessment of extrusion level clinically and radiographically and 6) extraction of 3rd molar.

Advantages: 1) elimination of risk of direct damage to the nerve, 2) lesser instrumentation, 3) favourable position of tooth for surgical extraction, 4) lesser postoperative oedema, pain and trismus, 5) avoidance of possibility of mandibular fracture related to removal of deeply impacted tooth and 6) prevention of development of an infrabony defect on distal side of adjacent 2nd molar.

Disadvantages: 1) intraoral orthodontic appliance might cause discomfort due to impingement on the soft tissues, 2) time-consuming procedure, 3) expensive procedure and 4) cooperation between surgeon and orthodontist is required. Thus, this approach cannot be used on a routine basis and can be carefully chosen.

SURGICAL REMOVAL OF IMPACTED MAXILLARY 3rd MOLAR

SURGICAL PROCEDURE

ANAESTHESIA

Posterior superior alveolar nerve block and greater palatine nerve blocks are given.

INCISION AND FLAP

Incision is made starting beyond the tuberosity in the hamular notch with a no. 12 or 15 blade. The mucous membrane overlying the tuberosity is incised from the distal most portion of the tuberosity forward (anteriorly) until the midpoint of distal surface of the upper 2nd molar.

The incision is continued buccally around the neck of 2nd molar to the interproximal space of 1st molar and then towards the mucobuccal fold at 45° angle. This last incision is made with no. 15 BP blade. The mucoperiosteal flap is raised with Howarth periosteal elevator and is retracted by a broad periosteal elevator. The palatal portion of mucoperiosteum over the tuberosity is loosened and held by sutures, thus providing adequate access to remove the overlying bone (Fig. 19.45).

ELEVATION AND BONE REMOVAL

The overlying bone is usually not dense and can be readily removed with chisel or rongeurs to expose the crown. Bone surrounding the height of contours should be removed providing sufficient space between the height of contour of the impacted tooth and the bone to permit an elevator. Appropriate elevator is inserted above the height of contour and using the buccal plate as a fulcrum; the tooth is elevated buccally and distally from the alveolus. Extreme care is taken to avoid driving the tooth inadvertently into the maxillary sinus or pterygomaxillary space.

WOUND TOILET (IRRIGATION) AND CLOSURE

Debridement of the socket and smoothing of bone margins is carried out before the wound is closed. Sutures are placed to hold the wound edges securely together.

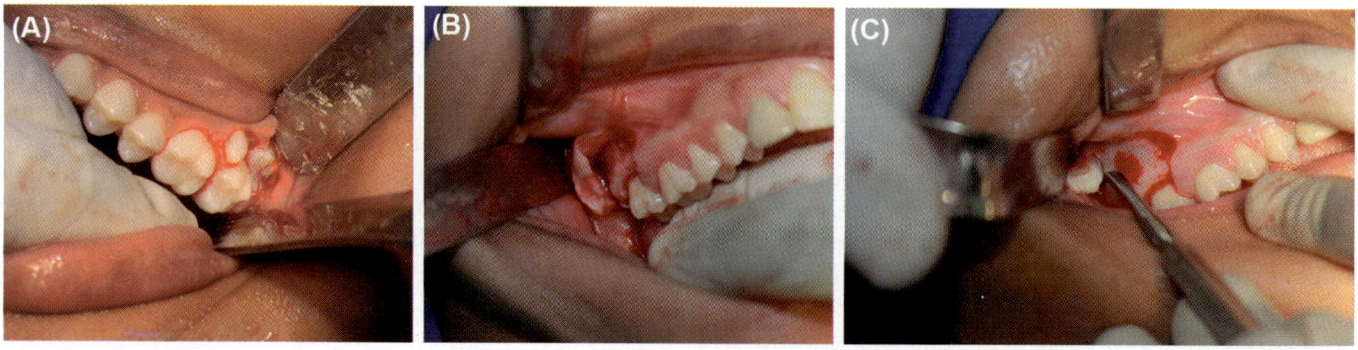

Figure 19.45 **(A)** Envelope flap for exposing impacted supernumerary and 28. **(B)** Triangular mucoperiosteal flap was raised to expose the impacted tooth in 18. **(C)** Impacted 18 extracted using mesial point of elevation.

COMPLICATIONS

Intraoperative complications

1. Fracture of tuberosity
2. Dislodgement of tooth into maxillary antrum
3. Dislodgement of tooth into soft tissues
4. Damage to adjacent 2nd molar.

1. Fracture of tuberosity

This is the most common complication occurring during 3rd molar surgery.

This problem does not occur in completely unerupted 3rd molars as the tooth itself constitutes most of the tuberosity. Fracture of tuberosity is more likely to occur when forceps are used in the extraction of tooth.

If the fractured tuberosity has periosteal attachment indicative of vascularity, then the wound is closed primarily.

2. Dislodgement into maxillary sinus

This occurs most commonly when the tooth is partially erupted with a conical root and extraction is attempted with an extraction forceps. It may also occur when the elevator is incorrectly applied. If entire tooth is dislodged into the antrum, removal is done through '*Caldwell Luc approach*'.

3. Dislodgement into the soft tissue

Usually this occurs when an inadequate flap is raised. The tooth should be localised by radiographs followed by early surgical removal to avoid infection.

4. Damage to adjacent molar

This occurs due to uncontrolled use of burs or chisel.

Accidental subluxation of the 2nd molar occurs during elevation of the 3rd molar, if the 2nd molar has conical root or is unsupported mesially by 1st molar.

Postoperative complications

1. Infection
2. Dry socket
3. Oroantral fistula.

SURGICAL REMOVAL OF CANINE IMPACTION

IMPACTED CANINE

The most common impacted tooth after maxillary 3rd molars is maxillary canine. Since these impactions are asymptomatic, they are incidentally found on radiographic examinations. However, impaction of mandibular canines is less common. Unerupted canines occur 20 times more frequently in the maxilla than in the mandible. They are almost always rotated from 60 to 90 degrees on their longitudinal axis (Figs. 19.46 and 19.47).

TREATMENT

FACTORS DETERMINING TREATMENT

a. Age of the patient
b. Stage of tooth development
c. Position of impacted tooth
d. Evidence of root resorption of adjacent permanent teeth.

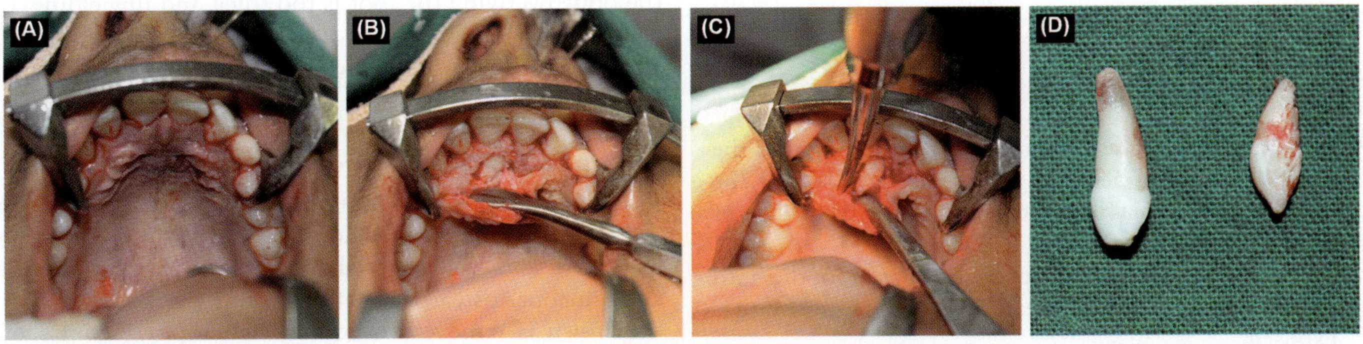

Figure 19.46 (**A–D**) Maxillary bilateral palatal impacted canines removed by surgical transpalatal approach.

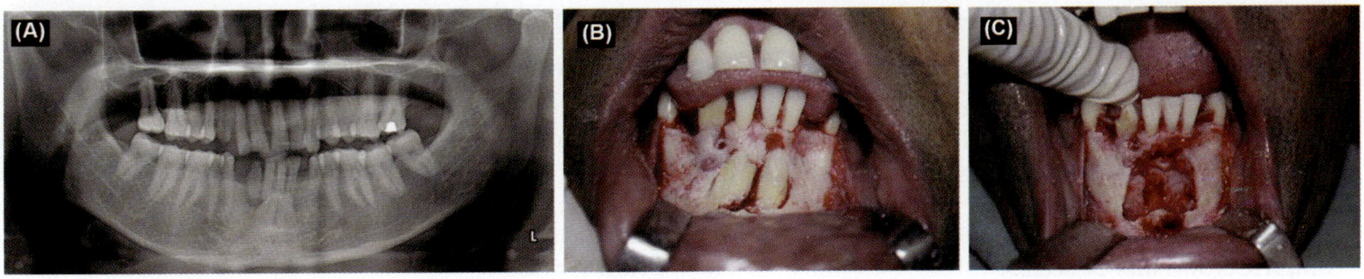

Figure 19.47 (**A** and **B**) Mandible canines—unusually impacted in mental protuberance removed surgically.

TREATMENT OPTIONS

i. No treatment
ii. Surgical removal of unerupted canine and exposure of the crown with or without orthodontic treatment
iii. Surgical repositioning and transplantation.

No treatment (to leave the tooth in situ)

The patient may not be willing to undergo any type of treatment if there is no occlusal disharmony and in case there is a persistent deciduous canine. But the patient must be educated regarding the possible complication of leaving behind the impacted canine in situ.

Surgical removal

Techniques

Operative plan:
a. Study radiographs
b. Classify impaction
c. Plan the type of soft tissue flap
d. Decide whether sectioning of tooth is needed.

Factors complicating the surgical removal

1. Proximity to the adjacent teeth
2. Proximity to the antral and nasal cavities
3. Formation of oroantral fistula leading to acute sinusitis.

SURGICAL PROCEDURE

ANAESTHESIA

Infraorbital and palatal infiltration of incisive canal and bilateral palatal nerve blocks are given.

REMOVAL OF IMPACTED CANINE IN CLASS I POSITION

Soft tissue flap

1. No. 12 BP blade is used to incise the tissues around the neck of the teeth, beginning on the lingual side of the maxillary central incisor and extending to distal side of 2nd premolar
2. The flap is raised as a mucoperiosteal flap from the hard palate by means of periosteal elevator until the bone is exposed.

Bone removal

- After reflecting the flap, it can be retracted with the help of a flat-bladed instrument such as the Austin retractor or Howarth periosteal elevator
- Alternatively, the flap can be retracted with the help of tie sutures, tied around the necks of opposite side teeth
- Bone is removed circumferentially 3 mm around the crown of the impacted tooth being careful not to damage the roots of adjacent teeth
- Enlarge the size of the opening with burs so that the complete crown may be seen.

Elevation of tooth

- An appropriate elevator is placed on one side of the crown and with the palatal bone as the fulcrum; the impacted tooth is lifted from its crypt in the palate. Extreme care should be taken to prevent injury to the adjacent teeth
- If this does not remove the impacted tooth, the opening should be enlarged and the procedure should be repeated. using two elevators in the same way
- If the tooth is still not luxated, the tooth requires crown root sectioning and extraction.

Wound irrigation and closure

- All the debris, spicules are removed and bony margins trimmed
- Tooth follicle is removed, if present and the flap is sutured back into position
- The flap is compressed onto the palatal bone with a gauze palatal packing placed for 4 h. Alternatively, a compound stent or clear acrylic plate (prepared preoperatively) may be used to prevent haematoma collection and to maintain sustained pressure.

REMOVAL OF IMPACTED CANINE IN CLASS II POSITION

Labially placed impacted canine can be exposed by using:
1. Trapezoidal flap—two vertical limbs
2. Semilunar flap—no vertical limb
3. Triangular flap—only one vertical limb.

After the mucoperiosteal flap is raised, bone is removed by using a chisel or bur to expose the crown. Using the labial cortical plate as a fulcrum, the elevator is inserted into the space between the bone and the tooth, to luxate the tooth. If the bone overlying the root is too thick and unyielding, the tooth is divided to remove the crown and root separately. Wound is debrided and closed primarily.

REMOVAL OF IMPACTED CANINE IN CLASS III POSITION

(A) Crown in the palatal bone and root on buccal side

A semicircular flap is raised to expose the root apex. Circumferential bone removal is done exposing the root. Root is sectioned and delivered labially. Palatal flap is outlined and mucoperiosteal flap reflected and the bone overlying the crown is removed to expose the periphery completely. A blunt instrument is placed in contact with the root end of the crown through the buccal crypt and tapped with a mallet, driving the crown out of its crypt palatally. The flap is replaced and the wound closed primarily.

(B) Maxillary canine lying in the line of arch—along alveolar crest

When an impacted maxillary canine occurs in an edentulous jaw and lies in the line of arch along the alveolar crest, every effort must be made to retain as much bone as possible since they provide part of hard tissue of denture bearing area.

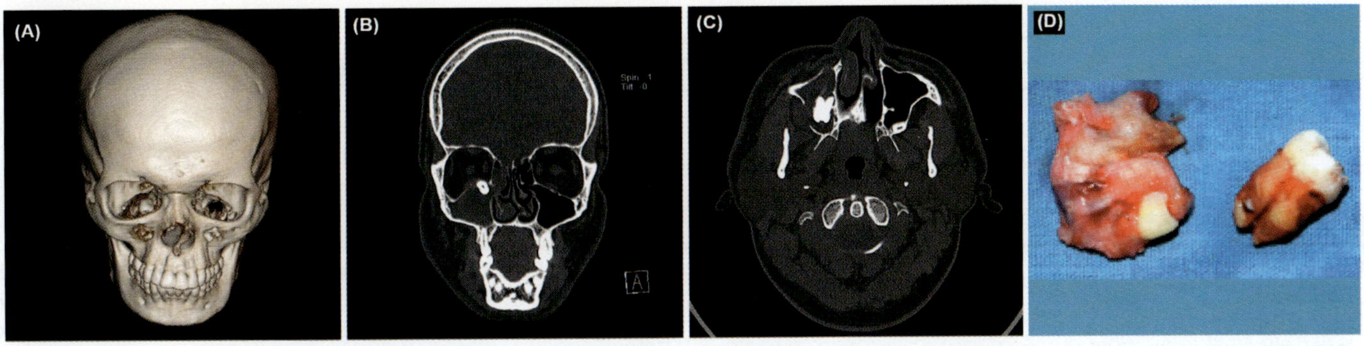

Figure 19.48 (**A–C**) Preoperative CT scan showing impacted 3rd molar and distomolar tooth in close approximation to the floor of the orbit. (**D**) Extracted 3rd molar and distomolar tooth with cystic lining.

Osteoplastic flap

A trapezoidal flap, slightly longer than the total width of the canine, is designed in relation to the impacted canine. The bone is osteotomised along the incision line using chisel and mallet. A buccal osteomucoperiosteal flap is raised exposing the canine. The impacted canine is removed in toto or in sections accordingly with minimal bone loss. After tooth removal, the osteomucoperiosteal flap is replaced and primary closure is performed.

Ectopic teeth

The process of tooth eruption involves migration of the tooth structure to its functional position within the oral cavity from its intraosseous location in the jaw. Ectopic tooth eruption is the disruption in the usual course of the tooth due to bone or soft tissue impediment. These ectopic teeth are formed and/or erupted into nonoral areas such as mandibular condyle, coronoid process, palate, chin, maxillary sinus, nasal septum and rarely, near the orbit. Prolonged retention of the impacted tooth or abnormal cell signals may also result in acute infections, inflammation, sinus formation and complicate to form cyst which would necessitate the removal of impacted tooth. The surgical approaches for the removal of ectopic teeth are intra- or trans-oral, extraoral and endoscope assisted.

This is a case of impacted maxillary 3rd molar associated with maxillary sinus and a distomolar in association with the floor of orbit medially to the inferior-orbital canal is presented. The surgical management of the condition is as follows (Fig. 19.48).

The impacted right 3rd molar and distomolar were planned to be surgically removed along with follicular tissues. Via intraoral access, with standard Caldwell Luc procedure, the maxillary sinus was reached carefully to locate both the right 3rd molar and distomolar. By careful manipulation, the teeth were removed. The sinus was drained and closed in layers with a drain placed. Histopathological examination revealed the follicular tissues to have features suggestive of a dentigerous cyst.

Chapter 20

Endodontic Surgery

OUTLINE

INTRODUCTION

Endodontic surgery encompasses surgical procedures performed to remove the causative agents of periradicular pathosis and to restore the periodontium to a state of biologic and functional health. A tooth that has failed endodontic treatment, but needs to be retained can be salvaged through surgical intervention. Failure of an endodontic treatment can be due to poor access cavity preparation, inadequate instrumentation, faulty obturation, missed canals and coronal leakage. So, in these cases, surgical endodontics is needed to save the tooth. Surgical endodontics can be defined as *'a surgical procedure related to the problem of a pulpless or periodontally involved tooth, requiring root amputation and endodontic therapy'*.—John I. Ingle. The objective of endodontic surgery is to remove the causative agents of the periradicular pathology, to restore the periodontium to a state of biologic and functional health and to provide a barrier between the periodontium and root canal foramina.

Apical surgery is done to surgically maintain a tooth that has an endodontic lesion, which cannot be resolved by conventional endodontic (re-)treatment. This goal should be achieved by **root-end resection, root-end cavity preparation and closure of the root canal system at the cut root-end with a retrograde filling.** Additionally, curettage should ensure complete debridement of pathological tissue from the periapical region such that there is complete removal of any extra radicular infection, foreign body material or cystic contents. The 1st step at the root-end of a tooth in apical surgery has greatly benefited from introduction of new diagnostic tools, surgical instruments and materials. Success rates approaching 90% or above have been documented in several clinical studies.

According to Kim and Kratchman (2006), the surgical approach to certain apical pathologies tends to be more conservative than nonsurgical treatment. Contraindications for apical surgery include the following: The tooth has no function, inadequate periodontal support, cannot be restored, or has a vertical root fracture, uncooperative patient or a patient with a compromised medical history for an oral surgical intervention.

INDICATIONS

1. Need for surgical drainage (Fig. 20.1B)
2. Failed nonsurgical endodontic treatment due to (Fig. 20.1A)
   a. Irretrievable (root canal filling material and Intraradicular post)
   b. Retreatment (treatment has been rendered atleast 2 times and not feasible)
3. Calcific metamorphosis of pulp space
4. Iatrogenic error
5. Corrective surgery
6. Procedural errors
   a. Instrument fragmentation
   b. Nonnegotiable ledging
   c. Root dilacerations
   d. Symptomatic overfilling
7. Anatomic variations
   a. Root perforation
   b. Apical root fenestration
8. For periapical biopsy due to
   a. Formation of periapical granuloma or cyst
   b. Presence of a draining sinus tract
   c. Nonresponsive to root canal treatment (RCT)
9. Conservative procedures require endodontic surgery for
   a. Root resorptive defects
   b. Root caries
   c. Root resection
   d. Hemisection
   e. Bicuspidisation
   f. Teeth with ceramic crowns

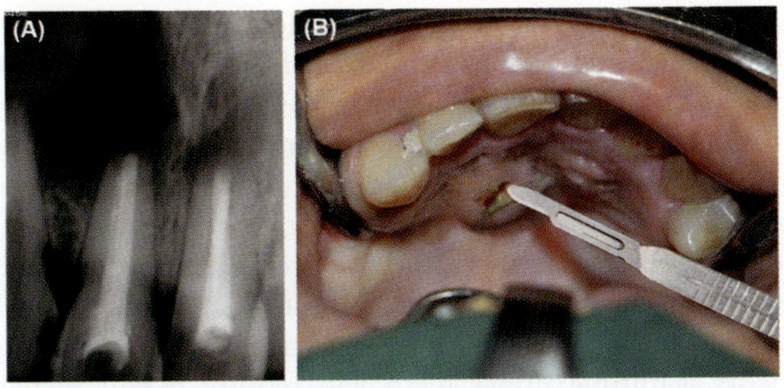

Figure 20.1 **(A)** Radiograph showing failure of nonsurgical treatment. **(B)** Surgical drainage.

10. For replacement surgery such as in
    a. Intentional (Extraction/Replantation)
    b. Posttraumatic reimplantation.

CONTRAINDICATIONS

1. Poor periodontal health of the tooth with grade III mobility (bone loss)
2. Local anatomical factors
    a. Proximity to nerve bundles
    b. 2nd mandibular molar to the maxillary sinus
    c. Proximity to nasal floor
    d. Maxillary sinus
    e. Mandibular canal and its neurovascular bundle
    f. Mental foramen
3. Traumatic occlusion, which cannot be corrected
4. Short root length
5. Poor patient's medical status
    a. Systemic diseases
    b. Leukaemia
    c. Uncontrolled diabetes
    d. Anaemia
    e. Thyrotoxicosis
    f. Bleeding disorders
    g. Recent heart surgery
    h. Cancer
    i. Old/ill patient
6. If the periodontal status is inadequate
7. Active uncontrollable periodontal disease
8. Poor restorability with a post
9. Dormant or successful endodontic restoration.

CLASSIFICATION OF ENDODONTIC SURGERY

INGLE'S CLASSIFICATION

1. Fistulative surgery
    a. Incision and drainage
    b. Cortical trephination
    c. Decompression procedures
2. Periradicular surgery (primary focus of this chapter)
    a. Curettage
    b. Root-end preparation, filling & resection
3. Corrective surgery
    a. Perforation repair
        i. Mechanical (iatrogenic)
        ii. Resorptive
    b. Periodontal management
        i. Tooth & root resection
    c. Intentional replantation.

ARMAMENTARIUM FOR PERIRADICULAR SURGERY (FIG. 20.2)

1. Sterile towels & gauze
2. Local anaesthetic & Aspiration equipments
3. Irrigating syringes with sterile saline or Stropko irrigator

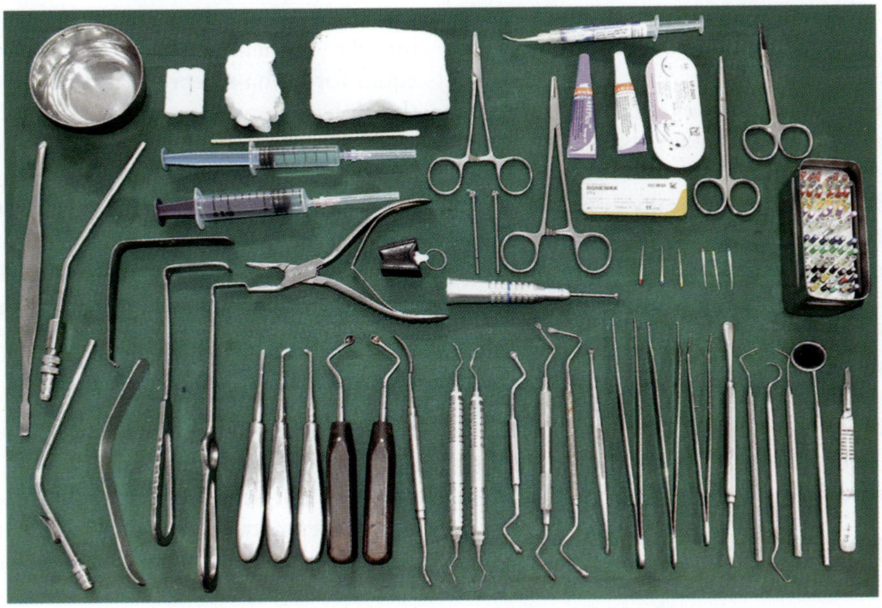

Figure 20.2 Armamentarium used for periapical surgery.

4. Tweezers and tissue forceps
5. Scalpel blades
6. Front surface mouth mirror
7. Probes: hooked, curved, angled
8. Locking cotton pliers
9. Periosteal and root-tip elevators
10. Flap retractors
11. Bone and periodontal curettes
12. Low or high-speed handpiece
13. Surgical length carbide burs
14. Ultrasonic unit and surgical tips
15. Root-end filling materials, carrier and condenser
16. Suture materials, needles and surgical scissor
17. Surgical operating microscope
18. Endodontic instruments for canal preparation and obturation may also be required.

PRESURGICAL PATIENT MANAGEMENT

Proper history taking is mandatory for the complete diagnosis and treatment plan. The patient should be evaluated for major systemic disorders through the medical history (cardiovascular, renal, hepatic, digestive, immune and skeletal muscle), which may contraindicate or compromise invasive procedures such as endodontic surgery. Periodontal evaluation helps in determining the prognosis of the tooth and helps in finalising the treatment plan.

PREMEDICATION

The following drugs are used in endodontic practices and are recommended before and after endodontic surgery.

- *Antiinflammatory analgesics:* It is recommended that the patient (average weight of 150lb/60kgs) take ibuprofen (400 mg) *just before* surgery to minimise the postsurgical inflammatory response. To minimise bleeding problems during surgery, the dose should not be taken sooner. With this regimen, most patients will not require narcotic pain medication
- *Tranquilisers:* If a patient is very anxious about the surgery, sublingual triazolam or 10 mg diazepam taken 15–30 min before the surgery provides relief
- *Antibiotics:* As stated previously, medically compromised patients (e.g. with advanced diabetes, heart valve disease) must be premedicated in accordance with the most recent American Heart Association (AHA) recommendations
- *Antibacterial rinses:* To reduce oral microflora, the patient should be instructed to use a 0.12% chlorhexidine gluconate mouth rinse the night before surgery, the morning of surgery and 1 h before surgery. Rinsing after the surgery for 1 week reduces microorganisms in the oral cavity and promotes better healing.

ANAESTHESIA AND HAEMOSTASIS

Use of local anaesthesia should be evaluated based on medical history. Maxillary and mandibular anaesthesia are given based on the tooth/teeth that require endodontic surgery. If the supraperiosteal infiltration technique of anaesthesia is too extensive, then the posterior superior alveolar nerve block is administered to anaesthetise the buccal mucosa adjacent to and for the 1st molar except mesiobuccal root, 2nd and 3rd molars; the middle superior alveolar nerve block for anaesthesia of the buccal mucosa adjacent to and the premolars and mesiobuccal root of the 1st molar and the anterior superior alveolar nerve block for the buccal mucosa adjacent to and canine and incisors. Multiple upper teeth will require maxillary nerve block with greater palatine nerve block or nasopalatine nerve block. A single upper tooth can be anaesthetised by supraperiosteal infiltration. Anterior mandibular teeth will require incisive block or mental nerve block. Multiple teeth extending from anteriors to posteriors or only posterior mandibular teeth will require inferior alveolar nerve block for complete anaesthesia. It is important to anaesthetise the long buccal nerve for the posterior teeth to place the incision. Further pain can be managed by periodontal ligament (intraligamentary) injection, intraseptal injection or intraosseous (IO) injections depending on the placement of the lesion.

HAEMOSTASIS

Haemostasis in periradicular surgery can be considered in three phases:

1. Presurgical haemostasis

The vasoconstrictor used in the local anaesthetic solution will influence both the duration of anaesthesia and the quality of haemorrhage control at the surgical site. These agents include epinephrine (adrenaline), levonordefrin and levarterenol (noradrenaline). The action of a vasopressor drug on the microvasculature depends on: (1) predominant receptor type and (2) receptor selectivity of vasopressor drug.

Alpha-receptors predominate in the oral mucosa and gingival tissues, whereas beta-receptors predominate in the skeletal muscle. Epinephrine receptor selectivity is approximately equal for alpha-receptors and beta-receptors. Stimulation of the alpha-adrenergic receptors will result in contraction of the smooth muscle cells in the microvasculature with a subsequent reduction of blood flow through the vascular bed. Stimulation of beta-adrenergic receptors will result in relaxation of the smooth muscle cells in the microvasculature with a subsequent increase in blood flow. Epinephrine is the most effective and most widely used vasoconstrictor agent in dental anaesthetics.

Haemostatic technique of LA deposition

Nerve block anaesthesia involves injection in close proximity to a main nerve trunk that is usually located some distance from the surgical site. Thus, the vasopressor agent will not cause haemostasis at the surgical site. Haemostasis can be accomplished by local *infiltration at the surgical site.*

Following block anaesthesia, using a 30-gauge needle with the bevel towards the bone, a small amount of solution

(0.25–0.50 mL) should be slowly deposited throughout the entire surgical field in the alveolar mucosa just superficial to the periosteum at the level of the root apices. Rate of injection in the target sites directly affects the degree of haemostasis. Recommended injection rate is 1 mL/min, with a maximum safe rate of 2 mL/min. Rapid injection produces localised pooling of solution in the injected tissues, resulting in delayed and limited diffusion into adjacent tissues. This results in minimal surface contact with the microvascular bed and less than optimal haemostasis.

2. Surgical haemostasis

Local haemostasis can be achieved by pressure technique of pressing cotton pellets or gauze in the bony crypt for a few minutes. However, if bleeding persists, topical haemostats are to be considered. Topical haemostats are classified based on their mode of action (Box 20.1).

3. Postsurgical haemostasis

After the flap is sutured, haemostasis is achieved by an ice-cold wet sterilised gauze placed over the sutures to stabilise the flap and control oozing of the blood from the surgical sites. The gauze should be placed into the mucobuccal fold for about 1 h and an ice pack should be applied to the cheek for 10 min on and 5 min off for 1–2 h.

BOX 20.1 Haemostatic agents

A. Mechanical agents
- Bone wax

B. Chemical agents
- Epinephrine saturated cotton pellets
- Other vasoconstrictors
- Ferric sulphate solution

C. Biological agents
- Thrombin USP

D. Absorbable haemostatic agents
- i. Intrinsic action
  - Gelfoam
  - Absorbable collagen
  - Microfibrillar collagen haemostats
- ii. Extrinsic action
  - Surgicel
- iii. Mechanical action
  - Calcium sulphate

PRINCIPLES OF ENDODONTIC SURGERY

PERIRADICULAR VERSUS PERIAPICAL SURGERY

As endodontic surgery encompasses all the surgical procedures that are not strictly limited to apical procedures, the use of the term 'periradicular' is more rational as opposed to periapical. Periradicular curettage was thought to be the definitive treatment in endodontic surgery without root-end resection. Their rationale was to maintain the cemental covering of the root surface and root length as much as possible for tooth stability, but studies showed the importance of the ablation of the apical portion of root-end and the attached soft tissue.

STEPS IN PERIRADICULAR SURGERY

1. **Need for profound local anaesthesia and haemostasis**
2. **Management of soft tissues**
3. **Management of hard tissues**
4. **Surgical access, both visual and operative**
5. **Access to root structure**
6. **Periradicular curettage**
7. **Root-end resection**
8. **Root-end preparation**
9. **Root-end filling**
10. **Soft tissue repositioning and suturing**
11. **Postsurgical care.**

MANAGEMENT OF SOFT TISSUES

Incisions and blade used

- No. 15: Most commonly used for intraoral incisions around tooth structures and incising through soft tissue
- Microblade No. 15c: The blade size allows better access to the gingival sulcus for the incision in full mucoperiosteal flap
- No. 11: Sharp and pointed, best for stab incisions for incision and drainage.

Flap design

The general principles of flap design and reflection have been explained in detail in Chapter 17, pages 295–298, Figs 17.10–17.15.

Sulcular full thickness flaps (full mucoperiosteal flap)

The sulcular full thickness flap design involves an intrasulcular horizontal incision along with the reflection of the marginal and interdental gingival tissues as part of the flap (Fig. 17.10A and B).

a. Triangular (one vertical releasing incision):
   - It is recommended for maxillary incisors and posterior teeth (Fig. 17.11)
b. Rectangular (two vertical releasing incisions) (Fig. 17.14)
   - Mandibular anteriors

- Multiple teeth
- Teeth with long roots, such as maxillary canines

c. Trapezoidal (broad-based rectangular) (Fig. 17.12)
d. Horizontal (no vertical releasing incision) (Fig. 17.13)
  - For the repair of cervical defects (root perforations, resorption, caries)
  - For hemisections and root amputation.

Mucogingival flaps (limited mucoperiosteal flap)

The mucogingival flap is designed with a submarginal horizontal or horizontally oriented incision and does not contain the marginal or interdental papilla.

1. Submarginal curved (semilunar) (Fig. 17.14)
   - Used when aesthetic crown is present
   - For trephination
2. Submarginal scalloped rectangular (Luebke–Ochsenbein) (Fig. 17.14)
   - Used when prosthetic crowns are present
   - For periradicular surgery of anterior region
   - For longer roots.

Flap reflection

Flap reflection is the process of separating the soft tissues, the gingival mucosa and periosteum from the surface of the alveolar bone. The commonly used instruments for flap reflection are traditional periosteal elevators, microsurgical elevators, soft tissue elevators, Molt curette and most commonly used is periosteal elevator No. 9.

Flap retraction

- Flap retraction is the process of holding the reflected soft tissues in position
- Proper retraction depends on adequate extension of the flap incisions and proper reflection of the mucoperiosteum
- The tissue retractor should be placed over solid cortical bone with gentle but firm pressure.

Commonly used retractors are the Austin retractor and the cat's paw retractor. Some types of endodontic tissue retractors are Arens tissue retractor, Selden retractor and University of Minnesota retractor.

Anatomical consideration

Anatomical structures that may be of importance during endodontic surgery include the neurovascular bundles associated with

- The greater palatine foramen
- The mandibular canal
- The mental foramen
- The maxillary sinus
- The floor of the nose and any other anatomical structures that limit or compromise visualisation and access to the surgical site.

MANAGEMENT OF HARD TISSUE (SURGICAL ACCESS)

Stages of hard tissue management

Hard tissue management in endodontic surgery involves four stages:

1. **Locating the root-end**
2. **Osteotomy (for periapical cyst or granuloma that has not involved the buccal cortical plate)**
3. **Periradicular curettage**
4. **Periradicular surgery**
   a. Root-end resection
      i. Instrumentation
      ii. Extent of root-end resection
      iii. Angle of root-end resection
   b. Root-end preparation and filling.

Locating the root-end

A number of factors are considered in locating the root-end for the bony window.

1. The **angle of the crown to the root** should be assessed to determine the height and depth of the bony window
2. **Root prominence or eminence** helps in the identification of the root angulation and position easily
3. **Measurement of the entire tooth length** by the use of a sterile millimetre ruler on the radiograph can be transferred to the surgical site
4. The **bone covering the root** is thinner
5. **Periapical radiographs** imaged perpendicular to the roots from two different horizontal angles are done to ascertain the length and curvature of the roots, position of the apices in relation to the crown and number of roots
6. The exact location of the apex can be determined by **two methods**:
   a. Using the tooth length measurement obtained from a well-angled radiograph, a small surgical defect is created on the surface. A small amount of radiopaque material such as gutta-percha is placed and a direct radiograph exposed. The radiopaque material provides guidance for the position of the root apex
   b. Locate the body of the root coronal to the apex where bony covering is thinner. Then working in an apical direction, bone covering the root is slowly removed with light brush strokes until root apex is identified.

Clinician should superimpose the virtual image gained from the radiographs and clinical examination onto the cortical plate to precisely locate the root-end. Once the root has been located and identified, the bone covering the root is slowly and carefully removed with light brush strokes (using a surgical handpiece) and this process should be continued in an apical direction until the root apex is identified. The root surface can be distinguished from the surrounding osseous tissue using the following criteria:

i. Root structure generally has a yellowish colour
ii. Roots do not bleed when probed

iii. Root texture is smooth and hard when compared to the granular and porous nature of bone
iv. The root is surrounded by the periodontal ligament.

Osteotomy

Once reflection and retraction of the mucoperiosteal flap is completed to expose the bone, surgical access to the periapical lesion is made through the cortical bone. This procedure of removal of a portion of the cortical bone to expose the root-end is called osteotomy (Fig. 20.3A and B). The instruments used to make the cortical trephination or osteotomy are the straight handpiece, microhead handpiece or the Impact Air 45-degree handpiece with H161 Lindemann bone cutting bur. There are vast ranges of burs that can be used for this procedure with a surgical straight handpiece. Most commonly used burs are the round burs of various sizes and the tapered fissure burs such as the 701, 702 or the 703 bur depending on the surgeon's choice (Fig. 20.3C). Generation of heat is of major importance during osseous tissue removal by bur as heating bone tissue above 60°C results in interruption of blood flow and tissue necrosis. The heat production can be minimised by the use of:

1. **Liquid coolant** during bone removal. The coolant functions by: (1) dissipating the heat generated and (2) keeping the cutting flutes of the instruments free of debris
2. **Light brush strokes** with short, intermittent cutting.
   Visual and operative accesses are the factors that determine the osteotomy size. Failure to achieve sufficient visual and operative access results in increased time required for the surgical procedure, increasing the stress level of the surgeon and trauma to adjacent tissues.

PERIRADICULAR CURETTAGE AND BIOPSY

Once osteotomy or trephination has been completed, curettage needs to be performed at the periradicular area. It comprises the removal of the cyst, granuloma or periradicular inflammatory tissue from its pathological bony crypt. Apart from the lesion, bony sequestrum and debris from the tooth socket are also removed. Special sharp surgical bone curettage instruments of various sizes, shapes and angulation are used, such as the mini curettes, mini Jacquette 34/35, Columbia 13–14, mini endodontic curettes, mini molten curettes, enlarged tips of mini Jacquettes and mini endodontic curettes. The entire pathogenic tissue mass is removed by inserting the bone curette between the lesion and the lateral wall of the bony crypt. The concave surface of the curette should be facing the bone when the lesion is being released from the peripheries and the concave part of the curette should be turned towards the soft tissue and used in a scraping manner to free the tissue completely from the bony crypt (Fig. 20.4A and B). The excised specimen is always sent for histopathological investigation.

ROOT-END RESECTION (APICOECTOMY)

Periradicular curettage only eliminates the effect (periapical lesion) of the leakage, but not the cause/origin of the lesion. Hence, periradicular curettage without root-end resection and root-end filling should never be considered as a terminal treatment in periradicular surgery unless associated with concurrent orthograde root canal treatment (RCT).

Indications and factors determining amount of root resection

They can be classified as:

1. *Biologic factors*
   a. Persistent symptoms and large persistent lesions after RCT
2. *Technical factors*
   a. Failed (RCT/Re-RCT) (Fig. 20.5A)
   b. Intraradicular posts
   c. Crowned teeth without posts
   d. Irretrievable root canal filling materials
   e. Procedural accidents
3. *Anatomic factors*
   a. Calcific metamorphosis (Fig. 20.5F)
   b. Severe root curvatures (Fig. 20.5G)

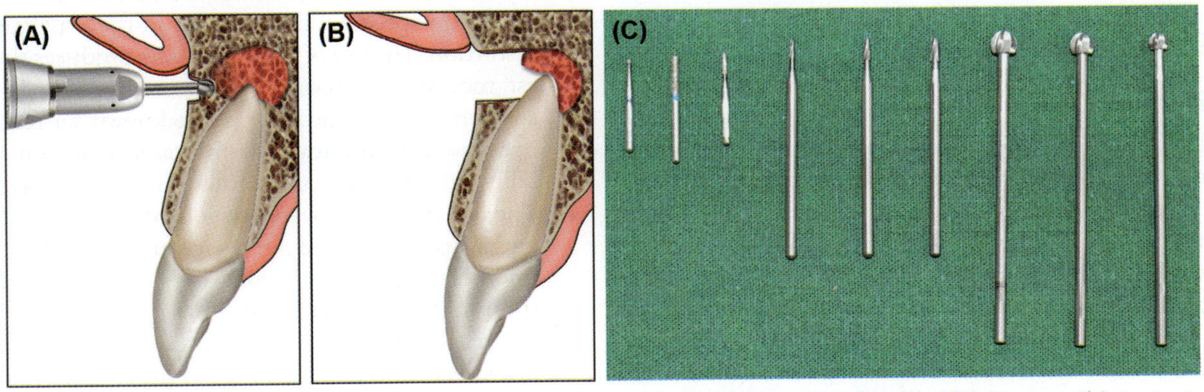

Figure 20.3 Osteotomy. (**A** and **B**) Removal of cortical bone to expose the full extent of lesion. (**C**) Burs used in osteotomy—No. 4 round bur, No. 6 round bur, No. 8 round bur, No. 57 fissure bur, multipurpose bur Endo-Z bur.

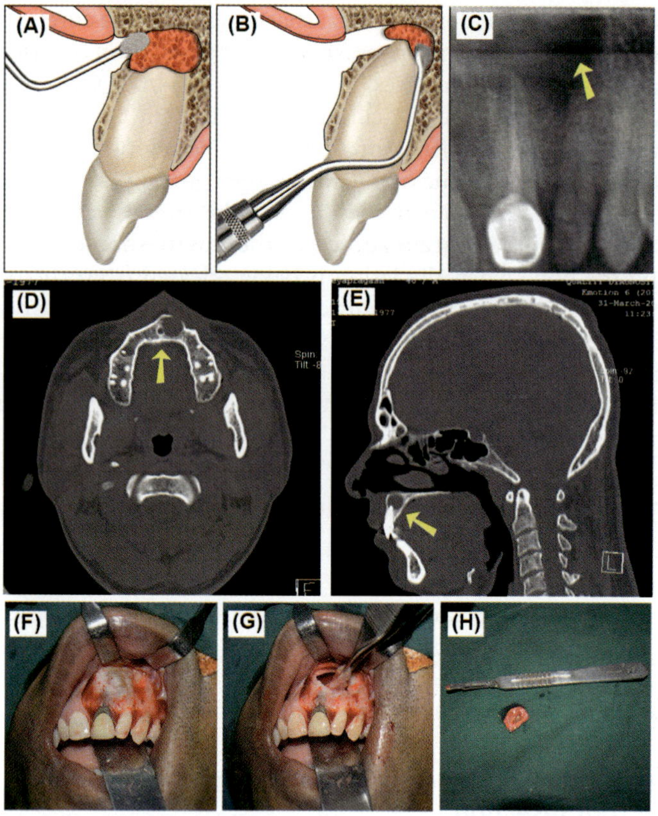

Figure 20.4 (**A**) Periapical curettage—initial release of the lesion from the peripheries. (**B**) Periapical curettage—scraping motion of curettes. (**C–E**) Image showing well-defined unilocular radiolucency involving 21, 22 and 23. (**F** & **G**) Cyst enucleation. (**H**) Excised specimen.

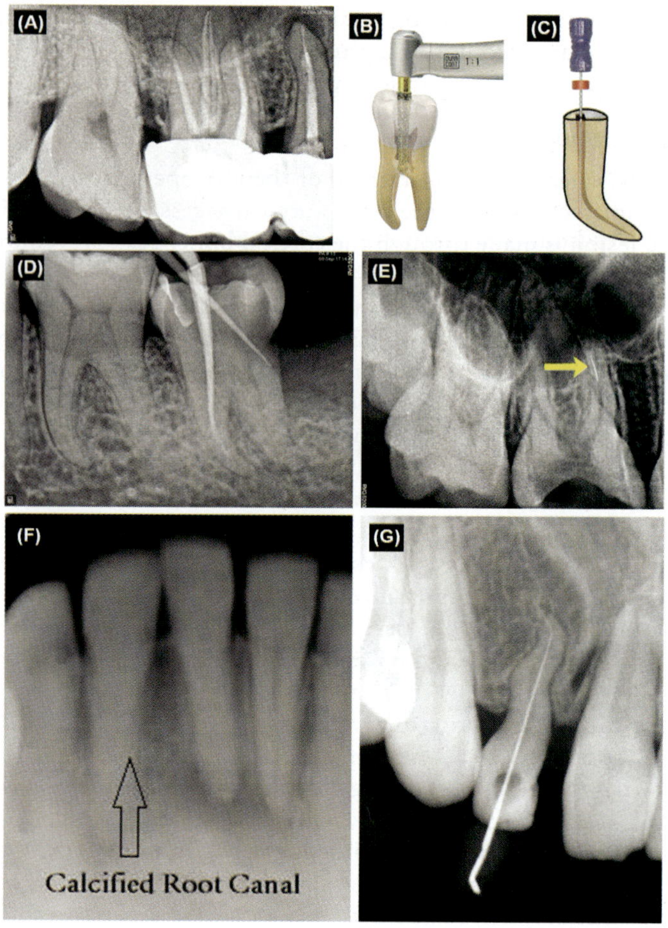

Figure 20.5 (**A**) Failed root canal treatment (RCT) or failed re-RCT. (**B**) Perforation at the furcation. (**C**) Ledging due to curved root and wrong instrumentation. (**D**) IOPA showing distal perforation. (**E**) Broken instrument. (**F**) Calcific metamorphosis. (**G**) Severe root curvature.

4. *Procedural errors*
   a. Perforations (Fig. 20.5B)
   b. Ledging (Fig. 20.5C)
   c. Broken instrument (Fig. 20.5E).

Factors to be considered before performing root-end resection

1. Instrumentation
2. Extent of the root-end resection
3. Apical bevel–angle of the resection.

Instrumentation

The choice of bur type and the use of either a low or high-speed handpiece for root-end resection are considered. Ingle et al., recommended that a tapered fissure bur or a round bur provide the best outcomes for root-end resection when used in a low-speed straight handpiece, but Nedderman et al., found that use of round burs produces ditching due to gouging of the root surface and an uneven and rough surface can result from using crosscut fissure burs. A smooth, flat, resected root surface is preferred clinically and may promote tissue healing. Plain fissure burs, both high-speed and low-speed, produce the smoothest resected root surface.

- High-speed handpiece with straight fissure burs gives the root-ends a satisfactory resection, whereas crosscut fissure burs produce the roughest root surface. The plain fissure bur and a low-speed handpiece result in the least gutta-percha distortion. The use of low-speed burs produces the smoothest root surface, but Er:YAG laser produces a clean and smooth root surface. Laser is also known for reduced post-operative pain, improved haemostasis, reduction of permeability of root surface and sterilisation of the root surface
- The ultrasonic tips were previously preferred. Abedi et al., and Waplington et al., in their study have described that microcracks in root walls after resection were noted though the ultrasonic tips allowed the operator to follow the natural course of the root canal and the cracks did not affect the sealing capacity of the sealer. Ishikawa et al., used stainless steel tips with diamond and zirconium coating, which were compared revealing that tips with a

diamond coating took lesser time for preparing the apical bevel than with the zirconium coating.

Extent of root-end resection

In the past, it was thought that failure to remove all foci of infection would result in a persistent periapical lesion. Hence, it was advised to resect the root surface to the level of healthy bone, but Andreasen and Rud showed no correlation between the presence of microorganisms in dentinal tubules and the degree of periapical inflammation.

Root-end resection improved access and visibility of the surgical site. It also reduced the root-end surface with lateral canals, thus reducing the disease process and increasing access to the location of iatrogenic errors.

According to Cohen et al., the length of root tip for resection depends upon the frequency of lateral canals and apical ramifications at the root-end. They found that when 3 mm of apex is resected, the lateral canals are reduced by 93% and apical ramifications decreased by 98% whereas root resection of 3 mm at a 0-degree bevel angle eliminates most of the anatomic features that are the possible cause of failure (Fig. 20.6E).

The amount of root to be resected depends on various factors. They are as follows:

1. Ability to access and visualise the surgical site (Fig. 20.6G & H)
2. Anatomy of the root
3. Incidence of lateral canals and apical ramifications at the root-end—3 mm root-end resection significantly eliminates the major anatomic entities
4. Number of canals and their position in the root
5. Need to place a retrofilling material surrounded by solid dentine
6. Presence and location of procedural error
7. Presence and extent of periodontal defects
8. Level of remaining crestal bone.

Apical bevel—angle of the resection

The access through the buccal bone to the apex of the affected root can be done with a low-speed handpiece under saline irrigation as high-speed handpieces may cause emphysema. Thesis et al., suggested the use of a fissure bur below 90 degrees with a phase no greater than 10 degrees for complete removal of the apical delta and lateral apical tubules. Histopathological analysis is obtained for the curetted apical tissues. The angle of the cut along with the depth of the cavity also influence microleakage. In the application of the cut angle of 0, 30 and 45 degrees, the least microleakage was found in section of 0 degrees and most at 45 degrees (Fig. 20.6I and J). A *bevel of 0 to 10 degrees* is recommended with resection at the level of 3 mm (Fig. 20.6I).

Short bevel of 0 degrees is almost perpendicular to long axis of the tooth. It has the following advantages:

1. Inclusion of more of lingual anatomy with less reduction
2. Decreases the distance between the canals
3. Short bevels are easier to create
4. Short bevel causes less of tooth destruction
5. Avoids unnecessary removal of radicular dentin
6. Reduces microleakage even after retrofilling.

ROOT-END PREPARATION OR RETROPREPARATION

The purpose of a retropreparation in periradicular surgery is to create a class 1 cavity with a depth of 3 mm into root dentine, to receive a root-end filling. An isthmus or anastomosis is a complete or incomplete narrow connection that can be present between the root canals of the same root, containing pulp tissue. Thus, the isthmus is a significant factor in determining the design and placement of the root-end preparation. *Five* requirements have been identified for retropreparation; they are as follows:

1. Apical 3 mm of the root canal must be freshly cleaned and shaped
2. Preparation must be parallel to the anatomic outline of the pulp space
3. Adequate retention form must be created
4. All isthmus tissue must be removed
5. Remaining dentine walls should not be weakened.

A small round bur or an inverted cone bur with a contra-angle or straight handpiece is dependent on the physical access available around the root apex. These preparations are often

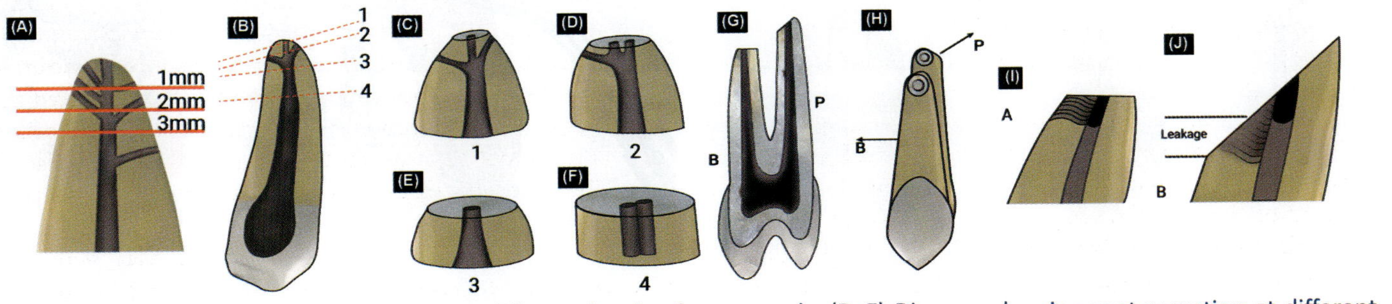

Figure 20.6 (**A**) Frequency of canals found at different levels of root canals. (**B–F**) Diagram showing root resection at different levels. (**G & H**) Resection of buccal root to gain access to the lingual root (access for palatal root is about 0–10 degrees). (**I**) Zero-degree bevel exposes lesser dentinal tubules to oral environment. (**J**) Bevelling results in opening of dentinal tubules on resected tooth surface, which communicate with root canal space and result in apical leakage.

placed obliquely into the root, resulting in a risk of perforation and/or weakening of the dentine walls (Fig. 20.7A–C). Ultrasonic microtips can also be used as they are about a one-tenth diameter smaller than a conventional microhead handpiece. Specially designed tips produce smooth cutting with relatively little chatter. A light touch with a brush type motion with irrigation should be used for maximum cutting efficiency (Fig. 20.7D).

Advantages of ultrasonic preparation are as follows:

- Better access, especially in difficult-to-reach areas (e.g. a lingual apex)
- More thorough debridement of tissue debris
- Conservative preparations tracing the long axis at a precise depth of 3 mm
- Precise isthmus preparations with parallel canal walls for better retention of filling materials.

Root conditioning

Root conditioning removes the smear layer and improves the mechanical adhesion of retrograde fillings as it exposes the dentine tetraacetic acid. The common conditioners used are 15%–24% EDTA with a pH of 7.3, tetracycline HCl 1% and 50% citric acid.

ROOT-END FILLING

The purpose of placing a retrograde filling is to provide a tight, biocompatible apical seal, which prevents the leakage of potential irritants from the root canal into the periradicular tissues (Fig. 20.8D)

Ideal retrograde filling materials should

- be well tolerated by periapical tissues
- adhere (i.e. ideally bond) to the tooth structure
- be dimensionally stable
- be resistant to dissolution
- promote cementogenesis
- be bactericidal or bacteriostatic
- be noncorrosive
- be electrochemically inactive
- not stain tooth or periradicular tissue
- be easy to handle
- provide sufficient working time followed by a quick setting time
- be radiopaque
- insulate periradicular tissues from seepage of bacteria and their by-products
- be nontoxic and noncarcinogenic
- be biocompatible with the host tissues
- be insoluble in tissue fluids
- unaffected by moisture during setting.

Root-end restoration materials

Numerous materials beginning from silver amalgam, zinc oxide eugenol to a more recent mineral trioxide aggregate (MTA) have been used as a retrofilling material. So far, no material appears to be an ideal root-end filling material. Materials that most closely meet the requirements are (1) intermediate restorative material (IRM), (2) super-ethoxy benzoic acid (EBA) and (3) MTA. IRM and super-EBA are modified zinc oxide eugenol cement whereas MTA principally consists of compounds containing calcium and phosphorus ions. MTA is hydrophilic with excellent biocompatibility and has a superior sealing ability of all the available retrofilling materials. The unique advantage is the regeneration of new cementum over MTA. However, difficult manipulation and long setting time are the greatest disadvantages of MTA. Common retrofilling materials are as follows:

- MTA
- IRM
- Super-EBA
- Glass ionomer cement
- Dialect
- Composite resin and resin ionomer hybrids
- Cavit

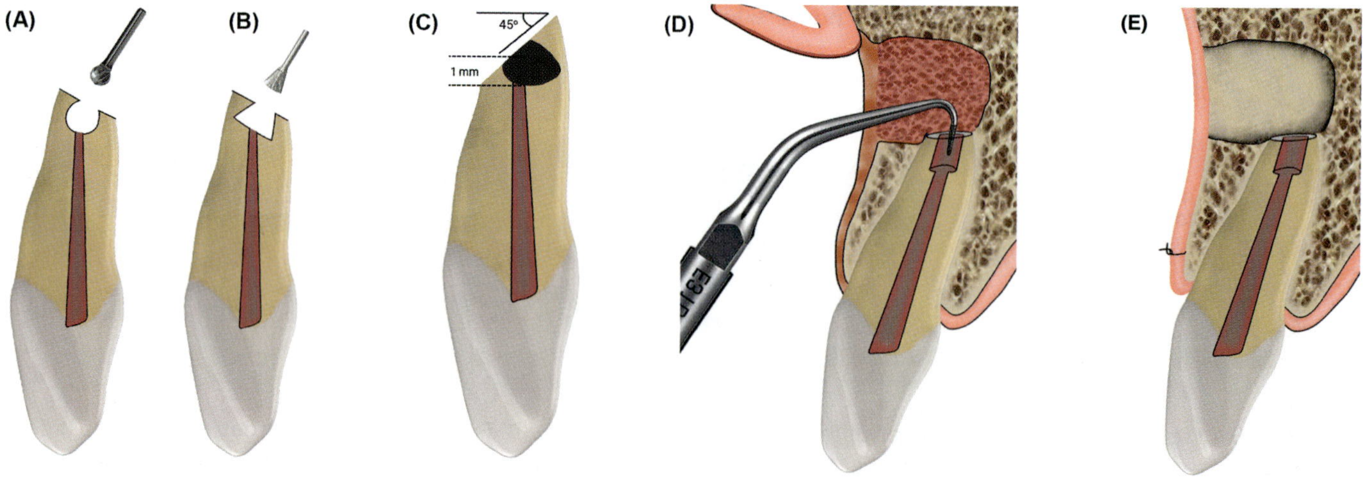

Figure 20.7 (**A** and **B**) Obliquely placed retropreparation with conventional handpiece. (**C**) Perforation and weakening of dentinal walls. (**D**) Ideal retropreparation achieved with ultrasonic. (**E**) Root-end filling.

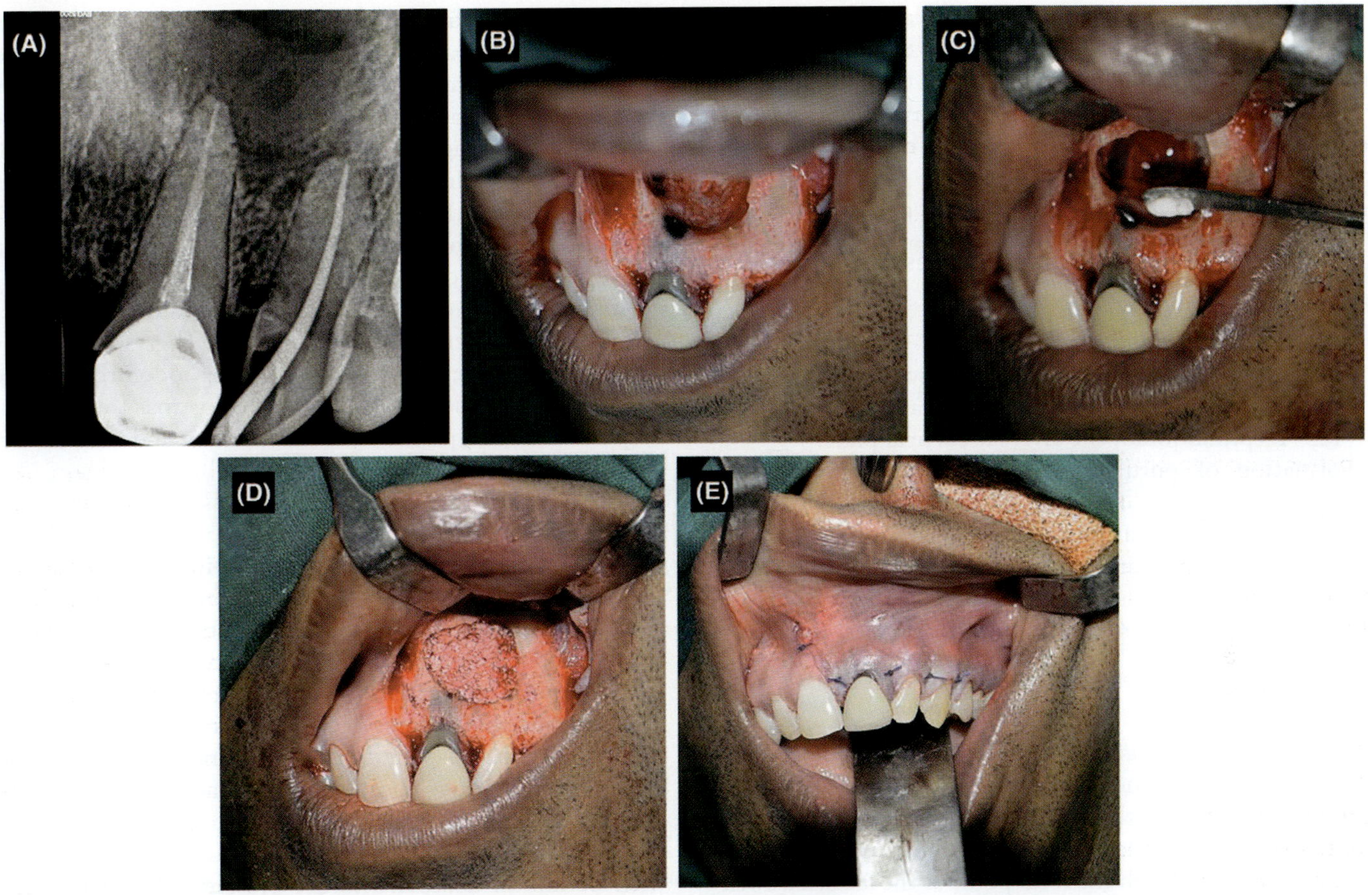

Figure 20.8 (**A–E**) Root-end retropreparation with retrofilling.

- Amalgam
- Carboxylate cement
- Zinc phosphate cement.

Instruments for apical placement of fillings

- Reverse fill carriers—two, one large and one small
- Reverse fill pluggers—two, one large and one small
- Amalgam squeeze clothes (used if amalgam is being employed as reverse filling material)
- Stellate plastic instrument
- Miniature reverse fill mirrors
- Miniature head aspirator tips—to fit on surgical aspirator, but much smaller than normal size; may be fabricated by cutting and bevelling tip from a 16-gauge needle and using an adapter on the usual aspirator tip holder
- Ultrasonic holder and appropriate tips.

SOFT TISSUE REPOSITIONING AND SUTURING

After completion of the root-end filling, a postoperative radiograph is taken to evaluate the placement of the root-end filling and to check for the presence of any root fragments or excess root-end filling material. The surface of the flap is thoroughly examined to remove any debris or foreign material. Then the elevated mucoperiosteal tissue is replaced in its original position with the incision lines approximated as closely as possible. A surgical gauze, slightly moistened with sterile saline is applied gently with firm pressure to the flap tissue for 2–3 min before suturing. Tissue compression, both before and after suturing enhances clotting and also approximates the wound edges. A single interrupted suture or interrupted looped suture is placed depending on the need of approximation (Fig. 20.8E).

POSTOPERATIVE INSTRUCTIONS

1. Patient should be careful and rest the entire day. Refrain drinking any alcohol or using any tobacco (smoke or chew) for the next 3 days
2. To follow a good diet and drink plenty of liquids for the 1st few days of the surgery
3. Avoid disturbing the surgical site as it can loosen the stitches and cause bleeding
4. A mild bleeding from the surgical site is normal for the initial few hours. There may be a mild swelling and bruising of the face
5. Place an ice bag (cold) on the face where the surgery was done. Leave it on for 20 min and remove it for 20 min. Do this for 6–8 h after the procedure

6. After 8 h, the ice bag should not be used. For the next 2–3 days, put a soft, wet hot towel on the face where the surgery was done
7. Rinse the mouth with 1 tablespoon of chlorhexidine mouthwash 2 times a day, once in the morning and once at night for 5 days
8. It is important to remove the stitches after 7 days.

Surgical drainage for periapical abscess

Surgical drainage

1. Incision and drainage of soft tissue
2. Trephination in case of periapical abscess
   a. Apical trephination through the apical foramen
   b. Trephination of the alveolar cortical plate.

Formation of purulent and/or haemorrhagic exudate within the soft tissue or a periradicular abscess within the alveolar bone are indications for surgical drainage. A significant reduction of pain and a decrease in the length of morbidity will follow the release of pressure and evacuation of the by-products of inflammation and infection.

Periapical abscess management—incision and drainage of soft tissue

When a patient presents with a fluctuant soft tissue swelling where inflammatory exudate exits through the medullary bone and cortical plate and the exudates spread into surrounding soft tissues, this is called a soft tissue abscess. An incision should be made through the focal point of the localised swelling on the gingiva to relieve the pressure and eliminate exudates, thus stimulating healing (Fig. 20.9A and B). The exudates should be aspirated and a sample collected for bacteriologic culture. Probing with a curette or haemostat into the incisional wound to release exudates entrapped in tissue compartments will facilitate a more effective result. Incision into a diffuse or indurated swelling before its localisation is often unsuccessful. In this situation, it has been suggested that the patient be placed on appropriate systemic antibiotic therapy and instructed to use hot salt water 'mouth holds' (¼–½ tsp of salt in a 10–12 oz glass of hot water) in the swollen area to assist in localisation of the swelling to a more fluctuant state. The clinical situation should be monitored every 24 h. As soon as the swelling has localised and a fluctuant area has developed, surgical drainage should be performed. Nerve blocks are performed for this procedure instead of local infiltration as local anaesthesia may not work in an acidic environment with pus. Insertion of a drain is only indicated when initial drainage is limited and in cases presenting with moderate to severe cellulitis and other positive signs of an aggressive infective process. The drain may be made of either iodoform gauze or rubber dam material cut in an 'H' or 'Christmas tree' shape. It may be sutured in place for added retention and should be removed after 2–3 days.

Trephination for periapical abscess

Trephination is a perforation made through the buccal cortical plate and through the apical foramen. Steps of trephination techniques are (1) apical trephination and (2) cortical trephination. Trephination allows the release of pressure in the periapical area caused by the accumulation of exudate (pus) within the alveolar bone. Patients who present with moderate to severe pain, but with no intraoral or extraoral swelling may require drainage of periradicular exudates to alleviate the acute symptoms.

Apical trephination is the treatment of choice for patients with periapical abscess who are present with pain but no swelling or drainage. The apical foramen is penetrated with small endodontic files, thus enlarging the apical opening to a 25K-file size (Fig. 20.10A). This cause drainage from the periradicular lesion into the canal space.

Accumulation of infectious exudate within the alveolar bone causes pressure to build up within the bone. Cortical trephination is the procedure that is performed by perforating the buccal cortical bone to drain the exudate and release the pressure. It is performed through a small incision placed over the periapical region. The flap is reflected and bone is exposed. A radiopaque

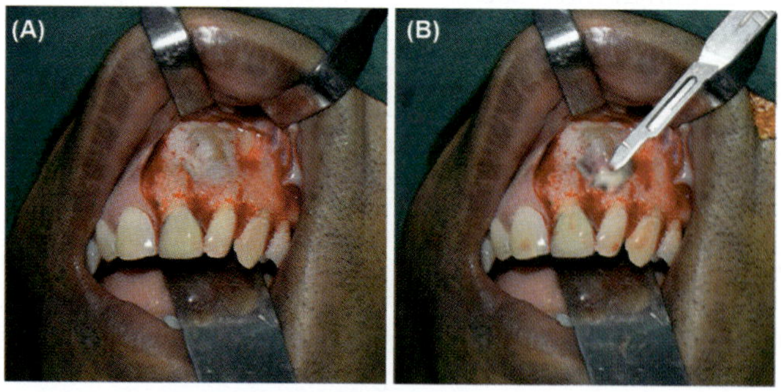

Figure 20.9 **(A)** Soft tissue abscess—a fluctuant swelling in relation to the affected tooth. On administration of the appropriate nerve block, surgical area should be isolated with sterile gauze sponges. **(B)** Incision should be horizontal and placed at dependent base of the fluctuant area. This will allow the greatest release (flow) of exudates.

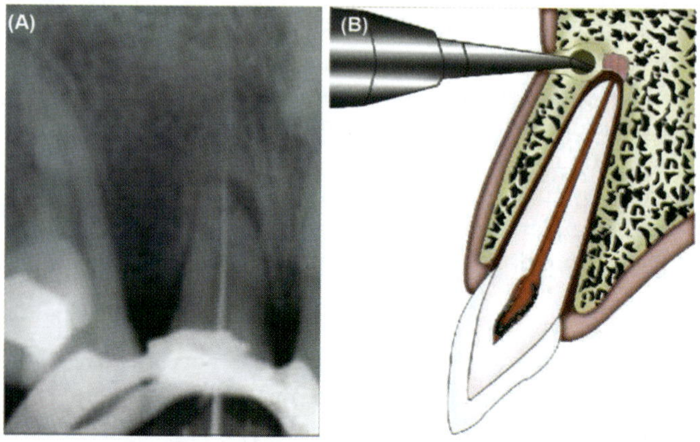

Figure 20.10 **(A)** Apical trephination. **(B)** Site of cortical trephination—perforation of cortical plate.

marker (such as gutta-percha) is placed over the bone and a radiograph is taken. Once the root apex is localised, the buccal cortical trephination is performed. This prevents penetration in the wrong area (Fig. 20.10B). A No. 6 or No. 8 round bur in a high-speed handpiece is used to penetrate the cortical plate. A reamer or K-type file is then passed through the cancellous bone into the vicinity of the periradicular tissues.

CORRECTIVE SURGERY

'Corrective surgery can be defined as the surgical procedure required to repair a defect that occur in the root or furcation area as a result of therapeutic misadventures of pathologic process'.–John I. Ingles. Corrective surgery is performed when procedural accidents, resorption (internal or external), root caries, root fracture and periodontal disease occur.

Reparative defects of the root and associated procedures are classified as follows:

1. Perforation repair
   a. Mechanical
   b. Resorptive and root caries
2. Periodontal repair
   a. Guided tissue regeneration (GTR)
   b. Root resection
   c. Hemisection
   d. Bicuspidisation

PERFORATION REPAIR

MECHANICAL

Perforations are procedural accidents that can occur during root canal or postspace preparation. High potential areas for perforations are pulp chamber, floor of molars, distal aspect of the mesial root of mandibular molars and mesiobuccal root of maxillary molars. Corrective surgery should be reserved for those teeth when internal repair is not a treatment option or when internal repair has failed.

Midroot perforations, such as those resulting from postspace preparations, should be immediately sealed internally if possible or calcium hydroxide should be placed as an intracanal dressing and sealed at the subsequent appointment. If the perforation is excessively large or long standing, a full mucoperiosteal flap should be reflected, the perforation site identified and the repair made with an appropriate repair material. If the perforation is located in the apical 3rd of the root, a root-end resection extending to the point of the perforation and a root-end filling should be considered as a more effective and efficient way of handling this clinical situation.

RESORPTION (EXTERNAL OR INTERNAL) AND ROOT CARIES

Repair of a defect on the root surface depends to a large extent on whether there is communication between the resorptive defect and the oral cavity and/or the pulp space. Corrective surgery is usually indicated when communication between the resorptive defect and the oral cavity exists.

In case of a resorptive defect that opens into the gingival sulcus, the approach depends to a great extent on the location and extent of the defect. If it is approachable from the buccal or facial side, a full mucoperiosteal flap should be raised and extent of the defect visualised. If the resorptive defect has not extended into the pulp space, it is restored with a suitable material. If the defect extends into the pulp space, a temporary internal matrix (large gutta-percha point) is placed in the root canal and the resorptive defect repaired. After that, the flap is repositioned and stabilised with sutures and the endodontic treatment can be completed at the same or subsequent appointment.

PERIODONTAL REPAIR

GUIDED TISSUE (BONE) REGENERATION

Before the advent of guided tissue bone generation and demineralised freeze-dried bone allografts, extensive periodontal defects required extraction or root amputation. The quality and quantity of the alveolar bone regenerated with GTR is found to be superior than without the GTR and an allograft.

ROOT AMPUTATION

Root resection is where one or more diseased or failed roots of a tooth are removed at the level of the furcation. The crown and remaining roots are functional. This is indicated when one root of the multirooted tooth undergoes failure due to periodontal or endodontic failure. It is also indicated in roots that have undergone resorption due to caries or iatrogenic perforation, fractured roots and in roots that undergo treatment, but is impeded by calcifications. The other roots have adequate periodontal support and the remaining crown structure can be restored. Root amputation is most frequently indicated for a maxillary molar, thus allowing preservation of a posterior abutment (Fig. 20.11A–D).

HEMISECTION

Hemisection is the surgical removal of one root and the overlying crown. It is indicated when root removal is required for a mandibular molar due to a vertical root fracture caused by procedural error or pathologic resorptive process (Fig. 20.12).

Indications

- Extensive bone loss in relation to one root and periodontal therapy cannot treat it
- Severely curved canal, which cannot be treated
- Extensive calcifications in root
- Fracture of one root, which does not involve another root
- Resorption
- Caries
- Perforation involving one root.

Contraindications of hemisection and root amputation

1. Lack of bone support for the remaining root
2. Fused root

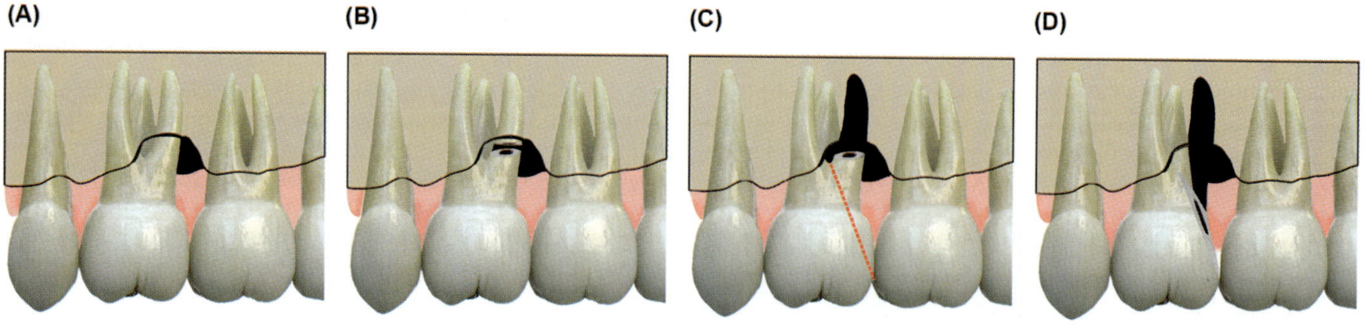

Figure 20.11 Root resection. (**A**) Grade II furcation involvement of the maxillary 1st molar and a crater between the 1st and 2nd molars. (**B**) Oblique cut placed separating the distal root from the mesial and palatal roots of the 1st molar. (**C**) Sectioned root portion removed and oblique section marked to expose less pulp of the tooth. (**D**) Final contours of the resection.

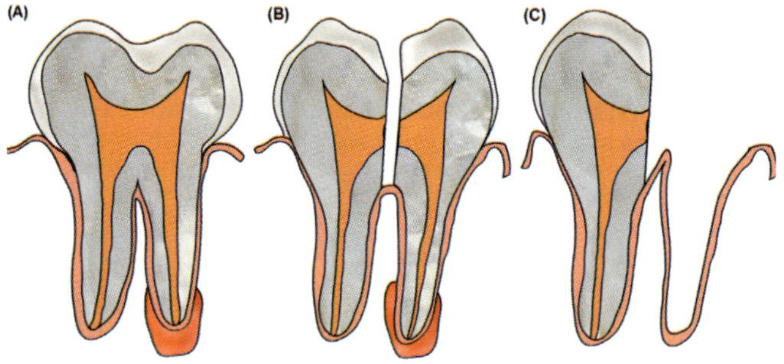

Figure 20.12 Hemisection. (**A**) Endodontic treatment completed prior to hemisection. (**B**) Vertical cuts placed extending from the crown to the furcation of the tooth. (**C**) The affected root segment removed.

3. If remaining roots are endodontically inoperable
4. Roots in close proximity to each other
5. Uncooperative patient.

Technique of root amputation

Before root resection or hemisection, endodontic treatment in roots to be retained should be completed. The entire root canal and the coronal pulp chamber should be filled with MTA. The occlusion of the tooth is checked and adjusted. Once MTA has set completely, the surgical procedure can be performed. The surgical procedure has been briefed in Flowchart 20.1 and Fig. 20.13.

Administration of local anaesthesia
↓
Probe the area to determine the extent and outline of alveolar bone destruction at the root to be removed
↓
Elevate the mucoperiosteal flap
↓
With the contra-angle handpiece and crosscut bur severe the root at the furcation and remove the root
↓
With a stone or diamond point smooth the resected root stump and contour
↓
The flap is repositioned and sutured
↓
The coronal portion and the socket is allowed to heal
↓
Refinement of the contour of the coronal tooth structure and the appropriate final restorative procedure can be completed

Flowchart 20.1 Surgical procedure of root amputation.

BICUSPIDISATION (FIG. 20.14)

Bisection or bicuspidisation refers to a division of the crown that results in two halves and their respective roots. Through bicuspidisation, a single molar tooth can be converted into two bicuspids. Indications for the procedure are **severe bone destruction in the bifurcation**, but excellent support on the nonfurcation sides of each root or severe destruction of tooth structure in the furcation area. If both roots are to be retained, there should be a considerable spread between them for restorative procedures to be successful. If a greater spread is needed and there is room on the distal aspect, orthodontic movement may be employed to spring the distal root distally and give a more desirable interfurcal area that allows for efficient patient home care. If the spread is minimal, it is best to amputate the weaker root and restore accordingly.

The procedure involves making the vertical cut after endodontic therapy. The crowns and furcation areas are trimmed with the diamond stone. The restoration will include two separate post and core crowns with a superstructure that allows for adequate hygiene in the area (Fig. 20.12A–F).

Indications

1. Furcation perforation
2. Furcation pathosis from periodontal disease
3. Buccolingual cervical caries
4. Fracture into furcation.

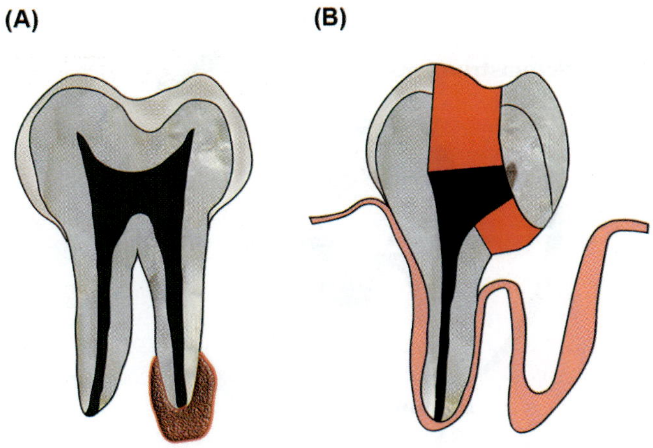

Figure 20.13 Root amputation. (**A**) Periapical lesion noted in relation to the root portion of molar tooth. (**B**) Endodontic treatment completed, intracoronal restorative material placed in coronal one-third of the crown and the affected root portion is amputated.

Contraindications

1. Deep furcation
2. Unrestorable half of the tooth
3. Severe periodontal disease
4. Fused root
5. Able to complete RCT.

REPLACEMENT SURGERY (EXTRACTION/REPLANTATION)

INTENTIONAL REPLANTATION

Grossman defined intentional replantation as the act of deliberately removing a tooth and after examination, diagnosis, endodontic manipulation and repair, returning the tooth to its original socket. The procedure has been briefed in Flowchart 20.2.

Indications

1. Inadequate interocclusal space to perform nonsurgical endodontic treatment caused by the patient's limited range of motion of temporomandibular joint (TMJ) and associated muscles
2. Nonsurgical treatment and retreatment are not feasible because of canal obstructions

Incision of the periodontal fibres

↓

Appropriate forceps are applied
without injury to the buccal, lingual plates and to the interradicular bone the tooth is extracted atraumatically

↓

The tooth is covered with gauze saturated with normal saline, leaving only the apex exposed
The gauze should be frequently saturated during the procedure to keep the roots wet

↓

Resect the apical 3–5 mm with a new, sharp fissure bur under copious irrigation
This will provide an apical space for pooling of fluids in the postoperative phase

↓

Retropreparation of the apex
Using a small round bur, prepare a cavity 3 mm deep into the apical foramina

↓

Seal the root-end cavity with retrofilling material

↓

Periapical Curettage
Remove granulation tissue and the recently accumulated blood at the apical part of the socket

↓

Irrigate thoroughly with 0.9% saline

↓

Gently reinsert the tooth, pushing it back slowly into the socket so that pooled blood will escape from the socket

↓

Stabilise with wire or with composite if the tooth is mobile
If fixation is required, it should be removed after 7 days

↓

Reduce occlusal surface of the opposing maxillary tooth to minimise occlusal trauma

↓

The patient should be advised not to chew on the tooth for up to 2 weeks

Flowchart 20.2 Intentional replantation.

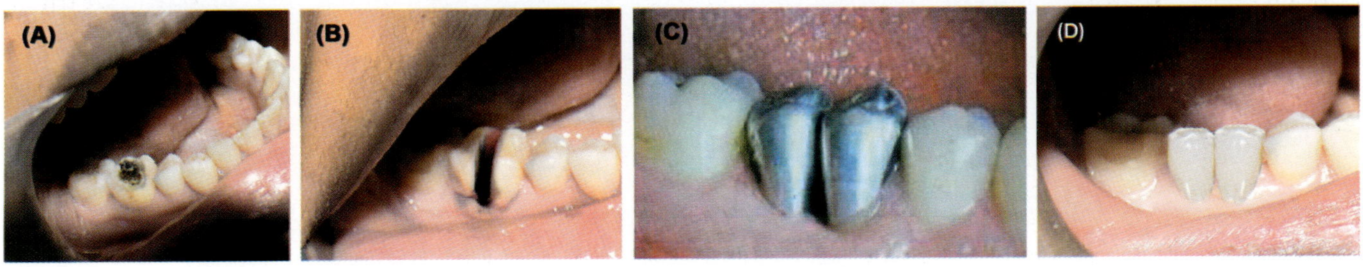

Figure 20.14 (**A–D**) Steps in bicuspidisation.

3. Surgical approach for periradicular surgery is not practical because of limiting anatomic factors
4. Nonsurgical and surgical treatments have failed and symptoms or pathoses persist
5. Visual access is inadequate to perform root-end resection and root-end filling
6. Root defects exist in areas that are not accessible through a periradicular surgical approach without excessive alveolar bone loss
7. To thoroughly examine the root or roots on all surfaces to identify or rule out the presence of a root defect.

Contraindications

- Poor periodontal condition
- Furcation involvement
- Widely divergent or curved roots
- Medically compromised patients.

Prognostic factors

Three factors that determine the outcome of replantation are as follows:

1. Keeping the extraoral time as short as possible
2. Maintaining the periodontal ligament cells on the root surface moist with saline or Hanks' balanced salt solution
3. Minimising the damage to the cementum and periodontal ligament cells by gentle elevation and extraction of the tooth.

ENDODONTIC MICROSURGERY

Microsurgery is limited to a surgical procedure on exceptionally small and complex structures with the aid of an operating microscope. Microscope allows the surgeon to assess pathologic changes more precisely and to remove pathologic lesions with a far greater precision, thus minimising tissue damage during the surgery. Precision is a key element in endodontic microsurgery because of the restricted access to the surgical field. The triad of magnification, illumination and microinstruments provides the greater accuracy required (Fig. 20.15 and Table 20.1).

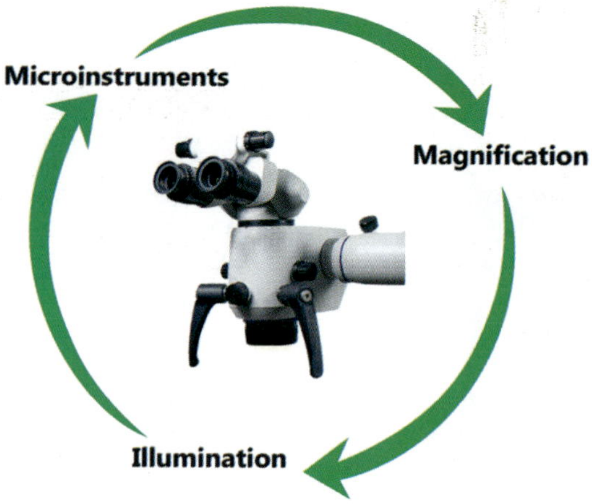

Figure 20.15 Endodontic microsurgery.

ADVANTAGES OF SURGICAL OPERATING MICROSCOPE

1. Visualising the surgical field
2. Evaluating the surgical technique
3. Reducing the number of radiographs needed
4. Increasing patient education through video use
5. Providing reports to referring dentists and insurance companies
6. Creating documentation for legal purposes.

TRADITIONAL ENDODONTIC SURGERY VERSUS MICROSURGERY

TABLE 20.1 Endodontic Microsurgery

	Procedure	Traditional surgery	Microsurgery
1	Identification of the apex	Sometimes difficult	Precise
2	Osteotomy	Large (>10 mm)	Small (<5 mm)
3	Root surface inspection	Imprecise	Precise
4	Bevel angle	Large (45 degrees)	Small (<10 degrees)
5	Isthmus identification	Nearly impossible	Customary
6	Retropreparation	Approximate	Precise
7	Root-end filling	Imprecise	Precise

Chapter 21

Preprosthetic Surgery

OUTLINE

IDEAL EDENTULOUS RIDGE

Goodsell had recommended the following criteria for a healthy and ideal edentulous ridge for dental rehabilitation:

- Adequate bony support for the dentures—the bony ridge should have adequate width and height and U-shape for a denture to be retentive and efficient
- The bone should be covered with adequate soft tissue—the covering oral mucosa should have adequate uniform thickness
- The ridge should not have any undercuts or sharp ridges
- No bony or soft tissue protuberances should be present
- It should have adequate buccal and lingual sulci depth
- It should not have any scar bands that prevent normal seating of the denture
- No muscle fibres or frena should dislodge the prosthesis
- Relation of maxillary and mandibular ridge should be satisfactory in all the planes
- No soft tissue hypertrophies or redundancies should be present on the ridge or the sulci.

RESIDUAL RIDGE RESORPTION (RRR)

The term used for the diminishing quantity and quality of the residual ridge after removal of teeth (Table 21.1). Rate of resorption depends upon the general health status of the patient, the shape, size and density of the residual alveolar ridge and the number of masticatory forces exerted by the patient with or without denture.

PATHOPHYSIOLOGY

- Secondary maxillary/mandibular bone loss is an insidious regressive remodelling of alveolar and basal bone that is a sequela of tooth loss. This secondary process is referred to as edentulous bone loss and is caused by characteristic anatomy, metabolic state, jaw function and prior use of any prosthesis
- Bone requires stimulation referred to as 'the minimum essential strain' to maintain its normal strength, dimension and function
- Both insufficient strain and excessive loads can lead to regressive remodelling of bone
- In long-term edentulism with no rehabilitation, the ridge undergoes extreme ridge resorption. Similarly, ridge underneath poorly fitting, improper denture shows the extreme bone loss
- Anatomic factor—Dolichocephalic faces have greater vertical ridge dimensions than brachycephalic faces
- Metabolic factors—Nutritional and endocrine disorders affecting bone such as osteoporosis, osteomalacia, hyperparathyroidism and Cushing's disorder have significant influence on bone remodelling and resorption. They also affect osseous reconstructive surgery.

CLASSIFICATIONS OF RESIDUAL RIDGE RESORPTION

MERCIER'S CLASSIFICATION (1995)

- Type I—Minor ridge modelling—The ridge is wide enough at its crest to accommodate the recently extracted teeth

TABLE 21.1 Cawood and Howell's Classification of Residual Ridge Resorption

Classification	Radiographic Image	Illustration
Class I—Dentate	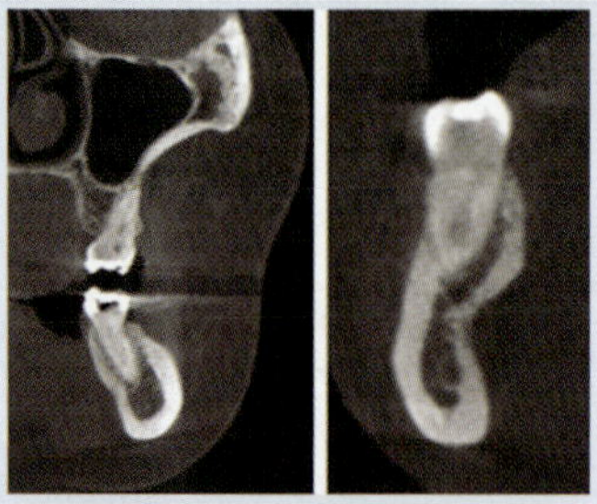	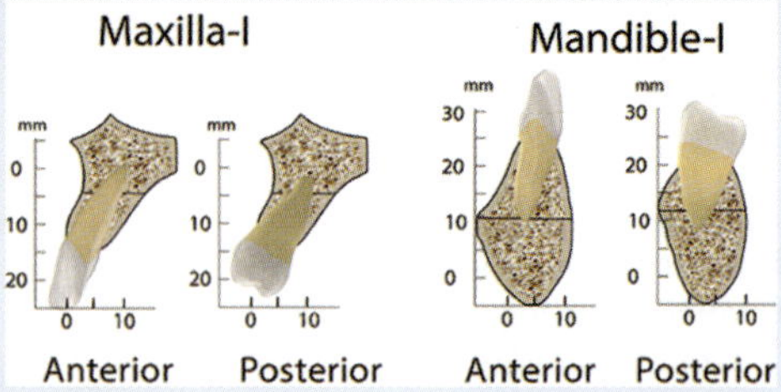
Class II—Immediate postextraction no defect or buccal wall defect/multiwall defect or deficiency	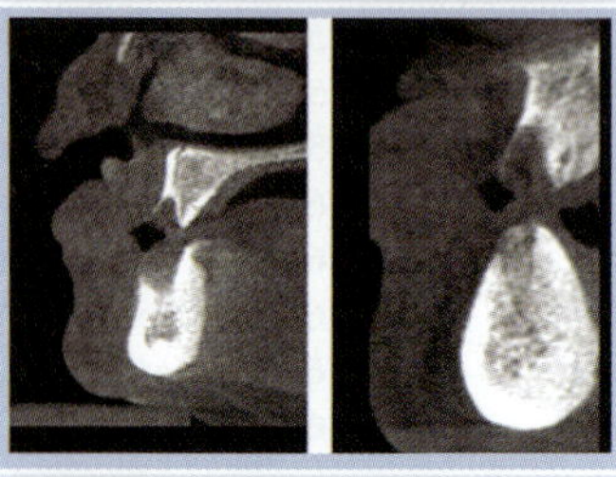	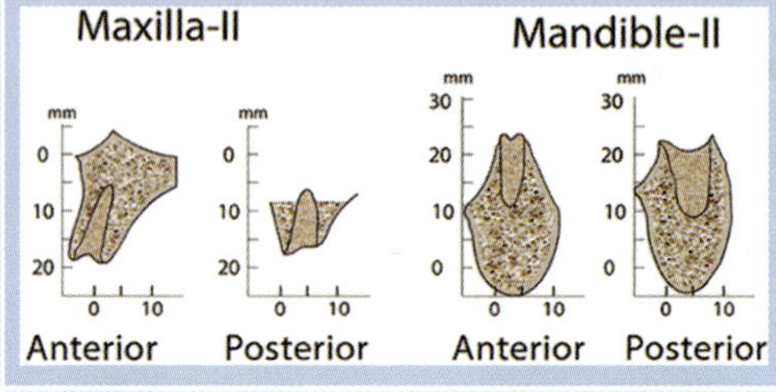
Class III—Convex ridge form, with adequate height and width of alveolar process	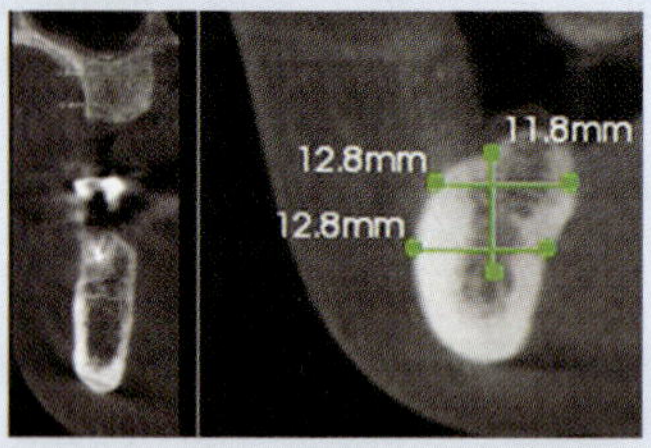	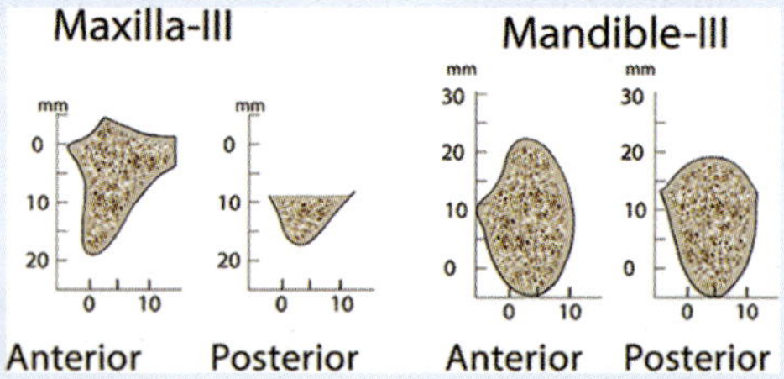
Class IV—Knife-edge form with adequate height but inadequate width of alveolar process	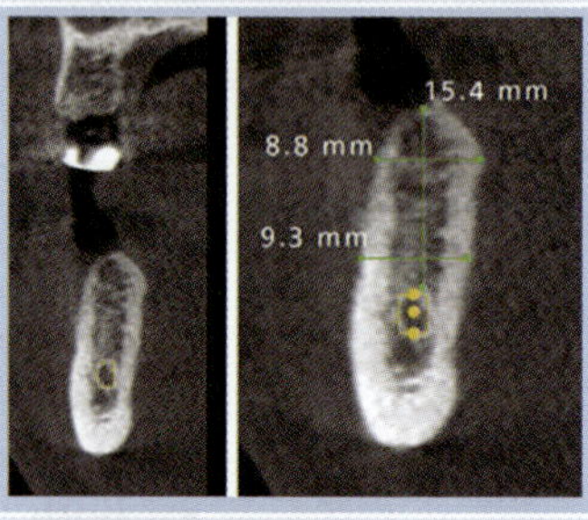	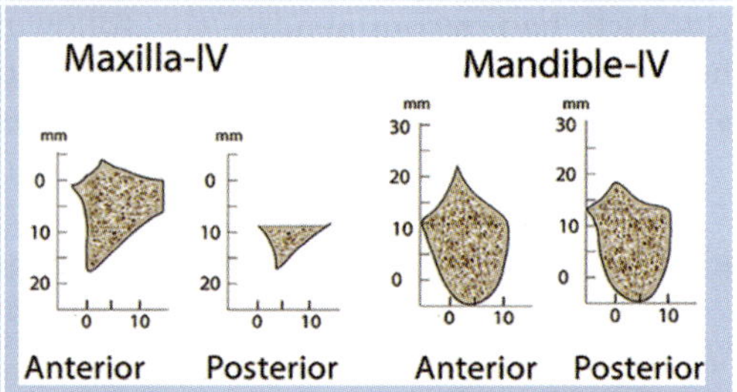
Class V—Flat-ridge form with loss of alveolar process	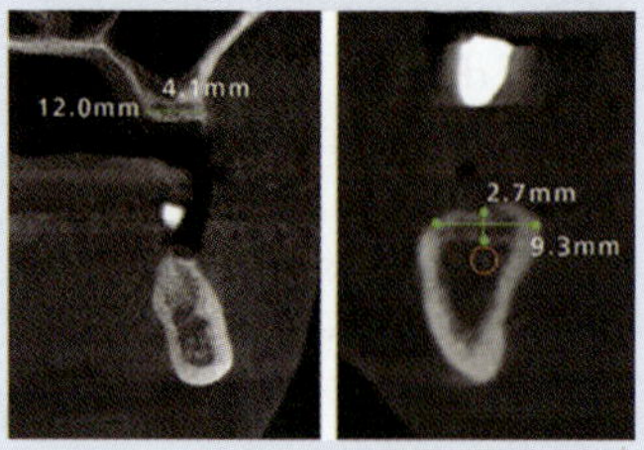	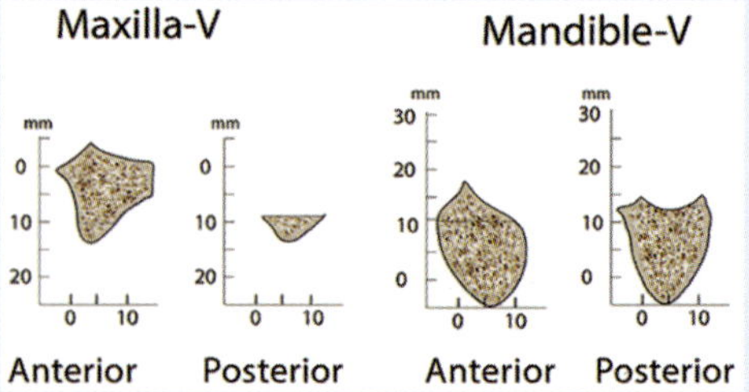
Class VI—Loss of basal bone that may be extensive but follows no predictable pattern. Submarginal resection defect or continuity defect	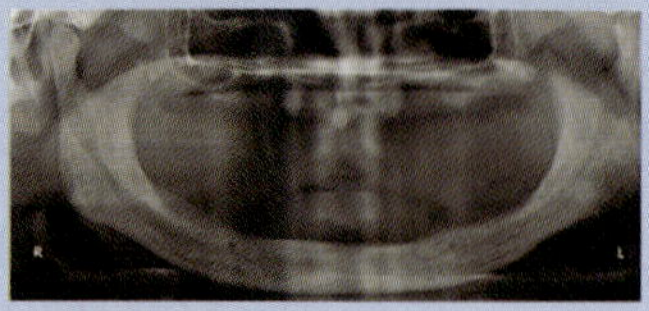	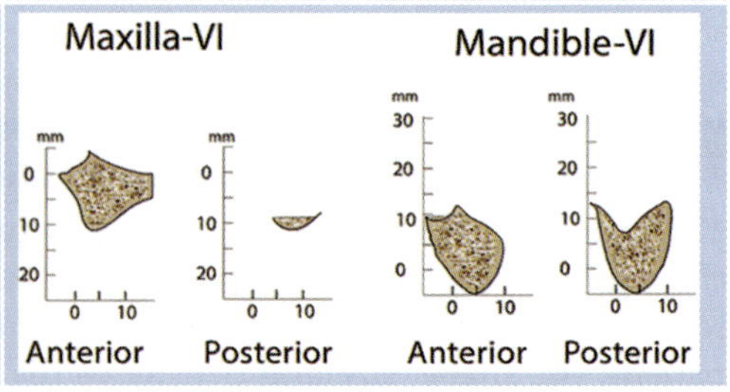

- Type II—Sharp atrophic mandible alveolus—The ridge becomes thin and pointed
- Type III—Basal bone ridge (concave form in posterior mandible and sharp bony form with flabby soft tissue in maxilla)—The pointed ridge flattens to the level of the basal bone
- Type IV—Basal bone resorption (pencil thin flat mandible/maxilla)—Flattened ridge becomes concave.

CAUSES OF ATROPHIC MAXILLA AND MANDIBLE (Fig. 21.1)

- Pathological diseases like ectodermal dysplasia, osteomalacia and osteoporosis
- Nutritional deficiency
- Prolonged usage of denture may exert compression in certain stress bearing areas of the edentulous ridge
- Extraction of single or multiple mandibular or maxillary teeth at different periods of life may lead to differential resorption of the ridge resulting in a 'roller-coaster' or 'hills and valleys' type of ridge
- Improper alveoloplasty techniques at the time of extraction predisposes to increased ridge resorption
- Chronic periodontal diseases result in vertical or horizontal loss of alveolar bone, which becomes evident after extraction
- Presence of sharp buccal plate after extraction, presence of bony exostoses and maxillary or mandibular tori also cause irregularity of the alveolar ridge
- Disuse of the alveolar ridge is also one of the common causes of atrophy of the ridge.

PREPROSTHETIC SURGERY

Preprosthetic surgery is defined as the surgical procedure to prepare the remaining oral tissues to best support a prosthesis. It is concerned with the surgical modification of the alveolar process and its surrounding structures to enable the fabrication of a well-fitting, comfortable and aesthetic dental prosthesis. When the natural dentition is lost due to periodontal disease, trauma, pathologies such as cyst, tumour and extraction, the alveolus and the surrounding soft tissue undergoes variable changes. Some of these changes may be unfavourable for the ridge to undergo dental rehabilitation. There may be:

- Bone loss with irregularities
- Prominences
- Undercuts
- Superficial location of mental nerve and foramen with associated soft tissue changes
- Scarring and changes in insertion of the perioral muscles
- Reduced vestibular depth
- Flabby hypertrophic ridge.

These unfavourable changes mandate correction before attempting for a dental rehabilitation. In addition, certain preexisting conditions such as maxillary and mandibular tori or prominent maxillary tuberosity pose problems in dental rehabilitation with prosthesis.

AIMS OF PREPROSTHETIC SURGERY

- To provide adequate height, length, breadth, width and shape of residual tissue with which the ridge can support and retain the denture and withstand masticatory stress

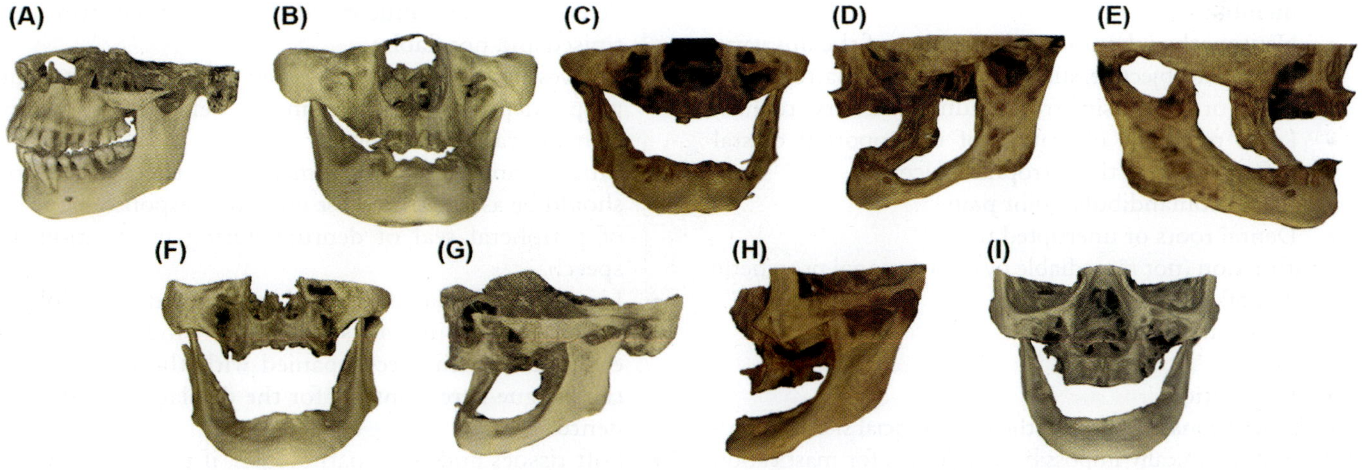

Figure 21.1 Patterns of residual ridge resorption. **(A)** Completely dentulous mandible with normal position of mental foramen 10–12 mm from alveolar crest. **(B)** Completely edentulous mandible after recent loss of teeth (extracted) with unchanged position of mental foramen and no evident ridge resorption. **(C)** Completely edentulous mandible with loss of teeth in different time periods. Left posterior zone of disuse atrophy from long-term absence of stimulation. **(D)** Atrophic left alveolar ridge with superior positioned mental foramen after no dental rehabilitation for many years. **(E)** Right posterior edentulous irregular ridge after recent loss of teeth from extraction. **(F)** Completely edentulous mandible with severe resorption and superiorly positioned mental foramina requiring mental nerve repositioning. **(G)** Mandibular resorption pattern evident by posterior and lingual version of alveolar ridge. **(H)** Mandibular ridge resorption more on buccal and posterior direction while maxillary resorption creates a buccal and anterior shift of ridge resulting in Class III. **(I)** Atrophic mandible with knife-edge meagre alveolar bone with residual basal bone only.

- To help in proper speech and deglutition
- Satisfy the aesthetic concerns of the patient
- Remove all the hard and soft tissue protuberances and undercuts
- Provide adequate vestibular depth
- Provide appropriate frenal attachment
- Achieve proper jaw relationship in anteroposterior, transverse and vertical dimensions
- Relocate the mental nerve and establish correct vestibular depth
- Reduce the pain and discomfort produced by the denture pressure on a narrow alveolar ridge and unsupported (by soft tissue) alveolus due to the presence of a superficial mental nerve or an impacted or buried tooth or root, which was asymptomatic prior to denture placement
- Insert endosseous implant.

INDICATIONS

Specific indications for preprosthetic surgery include:

1. Complete or partial edentulism secondary to early tooth loss (as in anodontia, ectodermal dysplasia)
2. Naturally occurring reduction of the residual bony ridge
   - Jaw atrophy (Class II–VI)
   - Mucosal atrophy
   - Interarch changes (vertical, anterior/posterior, transverse)
   - Reduction of denture bearing area
   - Muscle hypotonia
   - Facial changes
3. Pain (not remedial by conventional prosthetic measures) due to:
   - Mucositis (a burning discomfort of the mucous membrane)
   - Neuropathy (alteration of sensation of the lips varying from objective/subjective paraesthesia to anaesthesia or pain arising from traumatised nerve trunks)
   - Local recurrent ulceration of unsupported crestal soft tissues and thin atrophic mucosa
   - Temporomandibular joint pain
   - Dental roots or unerupted teeth
4. Dysfunction (not remediable by conventional prosthetic means) of:
   - Mastication
   - Speech
   - Deglutition
5. Disproportionate growth of the jaws or facial skeleton produces mechanically impossible conditions for mastication and denture retention. This skeletal deformity may be:
   - Class II or relative mandibular retrusion/maxillary protrusion
   - Class III or relative mandibular protrusion/maxillary retrusion
6. Craniofacial deformity which results from abnormal growth patterns of the skull base and facial skeleton
7. Oligodontia, anodontia: a naturally occurring failure of tooth development
8. Enhanced gag reflex: patients have an excessive sensitivity of the soft palate which if contacted produces 'retching'.

CONTRAINDICATIONS

1. General contraindications to surgery—medically compromised state
2. Generalised bone disorders such as osteoporosis, hyperparathyroidism, etc
3. Patient on bisphosphonate therapy—at risk of osteochemonecrosis (BRONJ)
4. Patient with a recent history of head and neck irradiation.

PATIENT EVALUATION

A thorough patient evaluation is very essential before beginning any surgery to receive prosthesis. A complete history should be taken and physical examination should be carried out:

- Chief complaint of the patient
- The patient's aesthetic and functional goals must be assessed and clinician should determine if these needs can be met
- The patient's psychological adaptability helps in determining the efficient use of dentures by them
- Evaluation of previous experience with the prosthesis further helps in assessing the patient's ability to adapt to the prosthetic treatment
- General health status, any medications being taken and risk values should be evaluated.

EXAMINATION OF INTRAORAL SOFT TISSUES

- Quantity and quality of the overlying tissues should be determined. The mucosa ideally should be firm, keratinised and not flabby
- The vestibule should be palpated manually to determine proper depth for self-cleansing, as well as any inflammation, ulceration, or growth
- Muscles and frenal attachment with the alveolar crest should be assessed as these are often responsible for loss of peripheral seal of denture during mastication and speech
- Lingual vestibular depth and attachment of mylohyoid muscle on the lingual aspect of the mandible should be evaluated as this accompanied with the movement of the tongue is responsible for the displacement of lower denture
- Soft tissues and bony pathologies, if present, should be investigated
- A thorough examination of the palatal vault and soft palate for lesions, papillary hyperplasia or abnormalities interfering with denture placement.

EXAMINATION OF INTRAORAL BONY STRUCTURES

- All the areas of the maxilla and the mandible should be inspected, palpated and radiographically examined (Table 21.2) and models should be assessed

TABLE 21.2 Radiological Evaluation of the Bony Structures

Plain radiographs: Intraoral and Orthopantomogram (OPG), lateral cephalogram for routine assessment ***CBCT scan:*** For assessment of pathologies, impactions	
Radiologic assessment is a useful preoperative assessment aid in:	
• Detecting any embedded root apices and impacted teeth • Presence of cyst and tumour • The position of the mental foramen in relation to ridge crest to assess risk of compression under denture as well as in planning implant placement • The density of the maxillary and mandibular bone to evaluate risk of resorption, suitability for implant placement	Completely edentulous atrophic mandible with severe RRR, mental foramen 4 mm from alveolar crest requiring mental nerve repositioning and bone graft augmentation 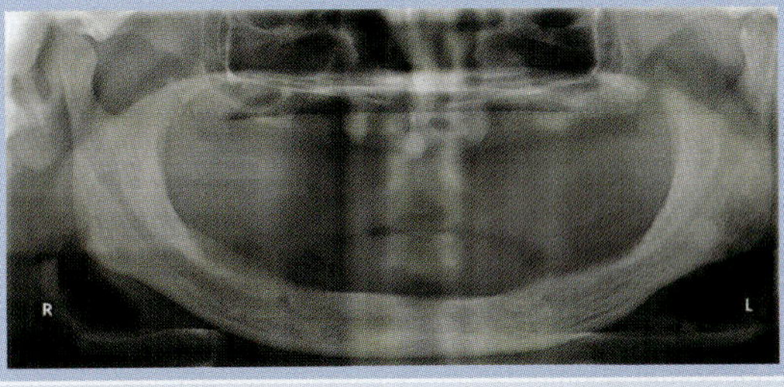
• Position of inferior alveolar canal for implant placement	CBCT used to measure alveolar ridge height width and relation to inferior alveolar canal (IAC) before implant placement. CBCT used to trace IAC course before planning, implant placement in mandible 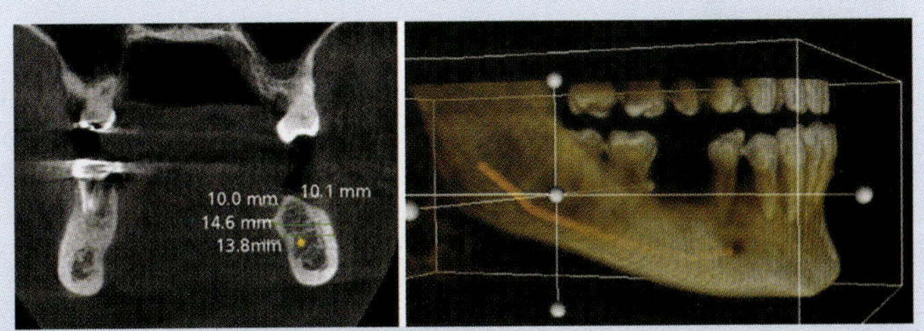
• Height and width of alveolar ridge to plan implant placement or need for augmentation.	CBCT used to assess maxillary alveolar ridge and relation to sinus before implant placement 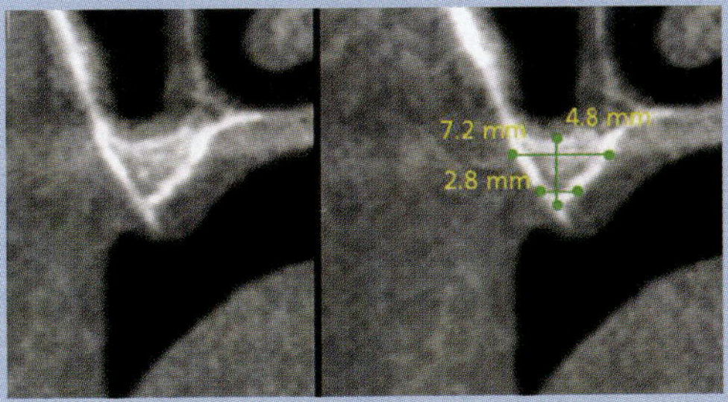
• Relation of maxillary sinus to alveolar crest to assess adequate height of alveolar bone, pneumatisation of alveolar ridge, need for sinus lift, sinus disease if any impacted tooth in sinus, etc.	CBCT coronal section showing pneumatisation of left maxillary ridge even though the alveolar height and width are preserved. CBCT sagittal section sagittal section showing alveolar ridge pneumatisation requiring sinus lift 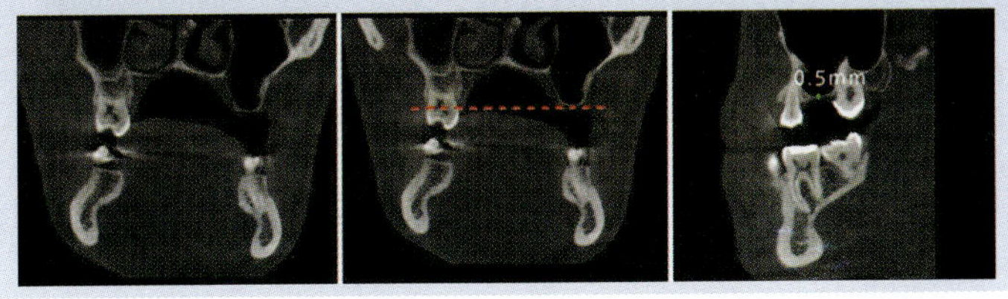

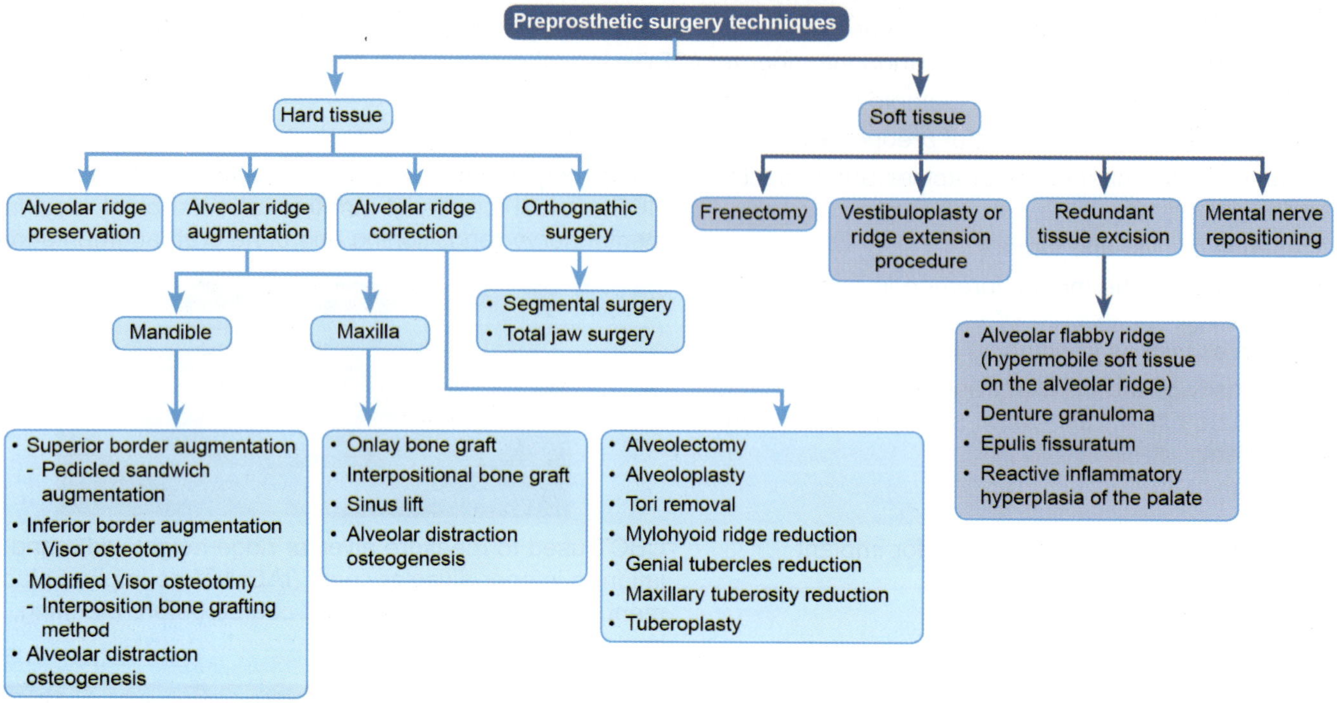

Flowchart 21.1 Preprosthetic surgery—classification.

- The bony ridge of the maxilla and the mandible should be evaluated for the presence of gross irregularities like exostoses, undercuts, prominences, tori, sharp mylohyoid ridges, etc
- Attachment of the frena and the muscles in alveolar crest should be evaluated
- The ridge should have proper contour, height, width and shape
- The interarch relationship between the maxilla and the mandible must be defined in all three planes. For any vertical excess of the tuberosity, the interarch distance should be measured, particularly in the region of maxillary tuberosity
- The interarch resistance is assessed. In case of deficiency from supraerupted opposing tooth onto ridge, it is planned for coronoplasty or extraction.

CLASSIFICATION OF PREPROSTHETIC SURGERY AND TREATMENT PLANNING

A thorough evaluation should be followed with an appropriate treatment plan. The type of surgery, type of anaesthesia and the expected postoperative sequelae should be explained to the patient before surgery. Whenever possible, informed consent should be obtained prior to the surgery. If there is any benign growth or cyst, they should be treated 1st. Small benign pathological entities can be removed at the time of tooth extraction. When planned for total extraction, a dental diagnostic cast aids in treatment plan. When extraction of the teeth is planned in stages, extraction of teeth in one area should be accomplished 1st and ridge preparation done later. This allows the patient to retain at least some dentition for a longer time. Whenever possible, a few occluding teeth should be left until last visit, so that the patient does not bite against a healing ridge. The hard and soft tissues are evaluated and the necessary preprosthetic surgery is performed (classification of procedures shown in Flowchart 21.1).

HARD TISSUE SURGERIES

ALVEOLAR RIDGE CORRECTION

ALVEOLECTOMY

Alveolectomy is the surgical removal of some or all of the alveolar process. In an impacted 3rd molar, an alveolectomy is performed to remove the impacted tooth. The alveolar bone above the impacted tooth is removed as the tooth cannot erupt. This procedure is done to remove retained roots of infected teeth, preparation of the alveolar ridges for denture placement, for removal of impacted teeth and for removing protuberant alveolar bone.

ALVEOLOPLASTY (Fig. 21.2)

Alveoloplasty is the surgical recontouring of the alveolar process. A U-shaped well-contoured smooth ridge is essential for proper construction of a denture. While contouring the ridge, it is highly essential to remember that greater the excision of

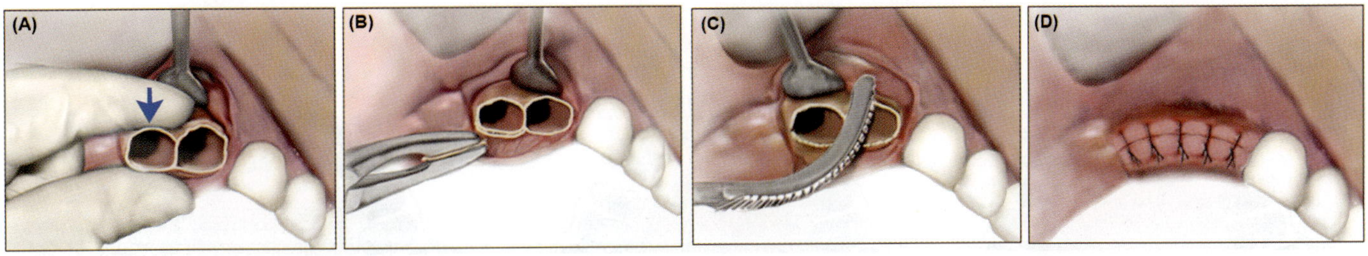

Figure 21.2 (A-D) Alveoloplasty performed immediately after extraction.

bone, greater will be the resultant resorption. Therefore, the procedure of contouring should be limited to the excision of irregular sharp ridges and unfavourable undercuts, which are unsuitable for denture construction. Alveoloplasty should be deferred until all the teeth have been extracted to permit healing of sockets and filling of any periodontal defects with bone and allow some spontaneous resorption of prominent or undercut areas, which give the best possible chance for maintaining the greatest amount of bone.

Goals of alveoloplasty

- To provide optimal ridge contour quickly
- The alveolar ridges should be left as broad as possible for maximum distribution of the masticatory load
- The ridge need not be perfectly smooth but sharp irregularities should be removed and the edges should be rounded
- The mucosa covering the ridge should have uniform thickness, density and compressibility for even transmission of the masticatory forces to the underlying bone
- In younger patients, less amount of bone should be removed as the process of resorption extends for a longer number of years than the older patients.

Primary or simple alveoloplasty

Primary alveoloplasty is the term used to describe the trimming and removal of the labio-buccal alveolar bone along with some interdental and interradicular bone and is carried out at the time of extraction of teeth.

Indications

- Patients with prominent and dense alveolar bone undergoing extraction
- Done as a procedure prior to the construction of an immediate denture.

Technique

- The crevicular incision is placed along the free gingival margin and a full thickness mucoperiosteal envelope flap or a triangular flap is elevated, which extends up to one tooth distance on either side of the sockets
- The alveolar ridge is palpated for sharp bony points or irregularities
- A sharp cutting rongeur forceps is held with one beak beneath the bony rim of the socket and the other on the crest of the ridge
- Small pieces of required amount of bone are removed and bone file is used to smoothen the bone
- The mucous membrane is then held with sutures over the interradicular bony septa
- If any excess flap is present, it is trimmed away and the edges are approximated
- In case of immediate denture, the previously prepared template is fitted on and noted for the presence of any pressure points, indicated by the blanching of the mucosa under the transparent acrylic template. If such pressure points are present, they should be trimmed again
- If there are no bony irregularities, the buccal and lingual plates should be compressed with firm digital pressure
- If the patient presents with severe periodontitis, alveoloplasty should be performed 4–6 weeks after extraction.

Dean's intraseptal alveoloplasty for anterior maxilla (Fig. 21.3)

This procedure helps in eliminating anterior maxillary undercuts, gross maxillary overjet and reducing the large anterior maxilla by removing interseptal bone between the teeth. The procedure involves preparation of six anterior teeth and sometimes the premolars are included. The advantage of this technique is that it reduces bone resorption postoperatively due to the procedure retaining much of the compact labial cortical bone, the reduction in space for formation of cancellous bone and no requirement to raise a mucoperiosteal flap. According to Dean, the most posterior teeth should be removed 1st to preserve the integrity of labial cortical plate and avoid any disturbance to its blood supply. Dean's intraseptal alveoloplasty is based on the following biological principles:

- The prominence of the labial and buccal alveolar margin is reduced to facilitate the reception of dentures
- The muscle attachments are undisturbed
- The periosteum remains intact
- The cortical plate is preserved as a viable onlay bone graft with an intact blood supply
- Since the cortical bone is spared, postoperative resorption is minimised.

Indications

- To decrease gross maxillary overjet
- Adequate bone height
- Multiple extractions.

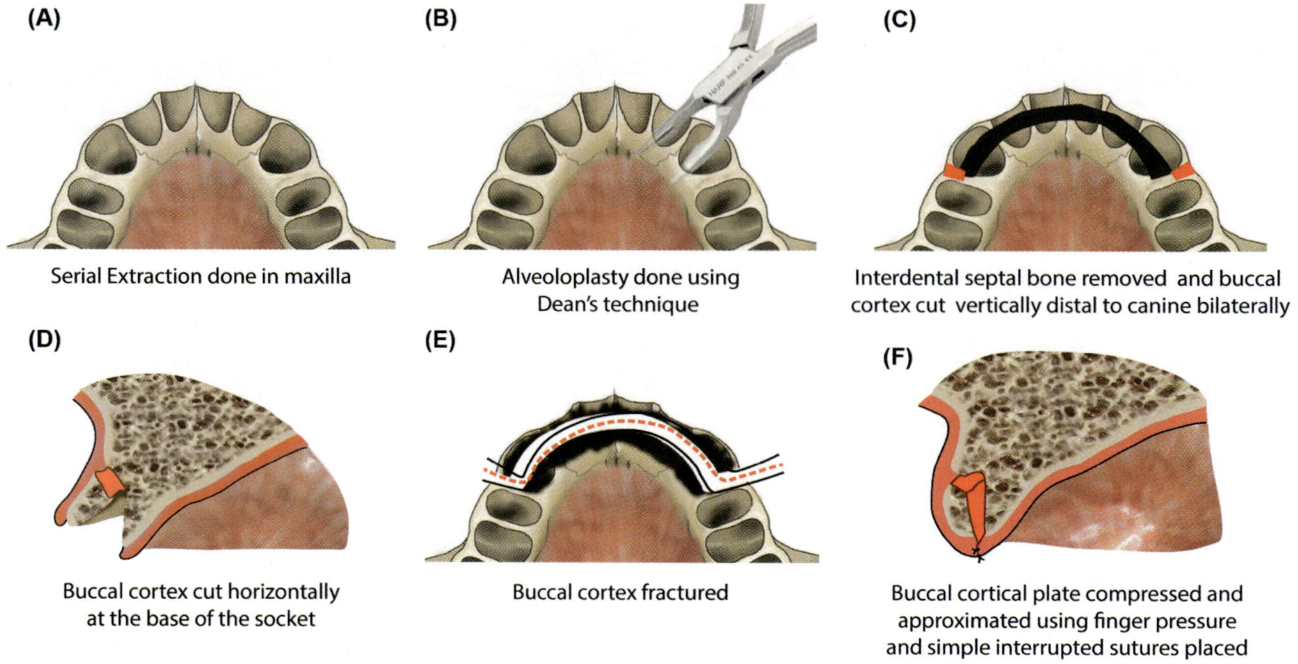

Figure 21.3 (A-F) Dean's intraseptal alveoloplasty.

Technique

- Incision is made along the gingival margin with epithelial attachment (crevicular incision) and interdental papilla attached to the respective teeth. Multiple extraction of the maxillary anterior segment starting from the canine to the incisors are performed
- The interradicular bony septa should be removed with a rongeur forceps or rotatory drill introduced into the socket to separate the labial and palatal cortical plate
- A V-shaped bone excision is performed with a rotatory drill in the labial cortical plate, distal and posterior to the canine eminence, as close to the alveolus as possible. A periosteal elevator or osteotome can also be used to fracture the base of the canine sockets
- Thus, three sides of the labial cortex become free and the labial cortex becomes a freely movable osteoperiosteal graft attached to only the labial mucoperiosteum from which it receives its blood supply like a greenstick fracture
- **Obwegeser's modification:** When inward compression of the labial cortex is not sufficient to correct maxillary overjet, Obwegeser modified the traditional technique to include the palatal cortex also. After extraction, an inverted cone vulcanite bur is used to widen the base of the socket followed by a disc bur at the base of the labial and palatal cortices through the socket to make the horizontal osteotomy cuts. The vertical cuts are made bilaterally with the straight fissure bur on the canine sockets (Fig. 21.4)
- Now finger pressure is applied to the labial cortical plate, which is collapsed towards the socket. Sutures are placed to stabilise the tissues
- Immediate denture in clear acrylic is prepared to identify and relieve the visible pressure points for healing.

Secondary alveoloplasty (Fig. 21.5)

- Secondary alveoloplasty refers to bone corrective surgery performed on the edentulous ridge for irregularities after the commencement of extraction socket healing. A sharp knife-edge like edentulous ridge causes great denture irritation. They are usually found in the anterior part of the mandible. Localised tenderness over such ridge on palpation or on wearing denture is common. The ridge may also show an irregular pattern known as *feather-edged ridge*
- Incision should be made on the crest of the alveolar ridge
- Usually an envelope flap would suffice, but a releasing incision can be made on the labial or buccal side to provide a broad base to the flap
- Bony contouring is accomplished with bone files, rongeurs or burs
- The ridge is made free of sharp irregularities and is not aimed at attaining a perfectly smooth ridge, requiring excessive bone removal. Digital palpation can be used to determine the uniformity of the ridge
- On achieving satisfactory results, the site is irrigated thoroughly with saline to eliminate debris and small avascular bone pieces at risks of necrosis, and the flaps are closed.

TORI REMOVAL

Tori are small developmental anomalies that occur in constant sites on the jaw bones.

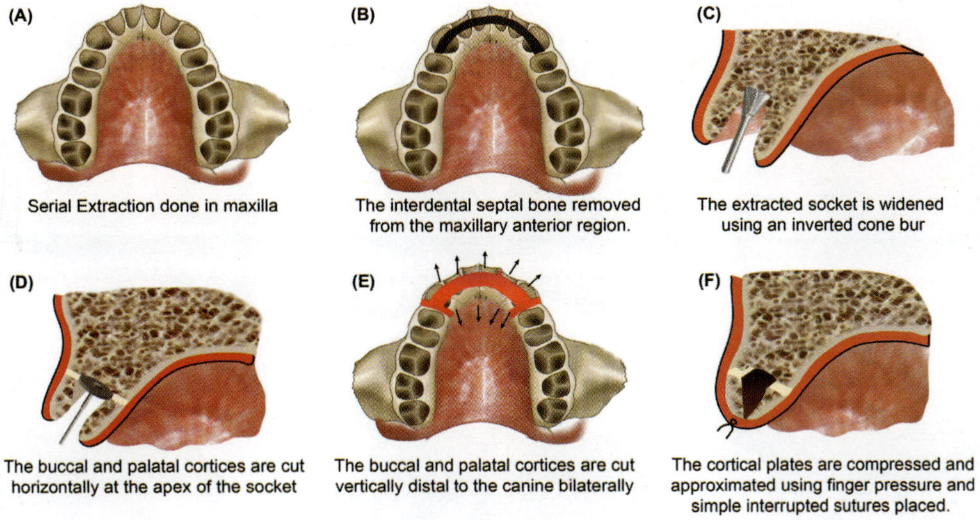

Figure 21.4 (A-F) Obwegeser's modification of Dean's intraseptal alveoloplasty.

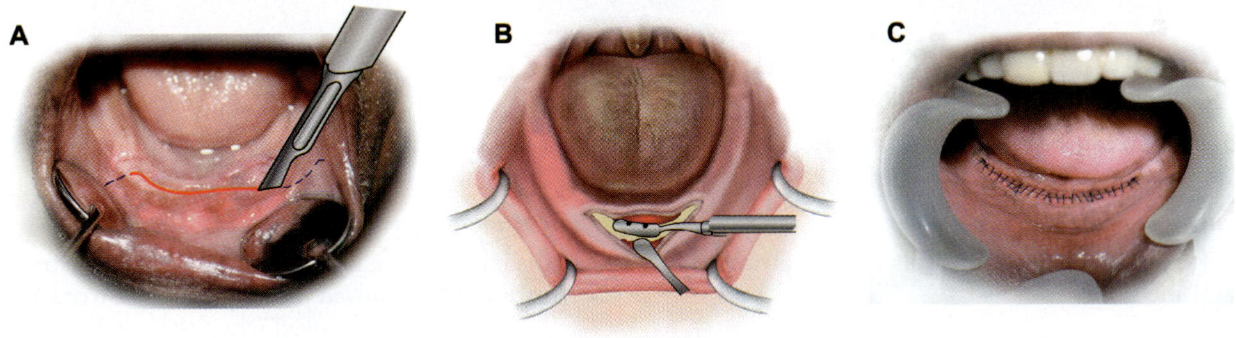

Figure 21.5 (A-C) Alveoloplasty performed on edentulous ridge.

Maxillary torus or Torus palatinus (Fig. 21.6)

A torus palatinus is an exostosis found along the suture line of the hard palate. Not all tori require to be removed as all of them do not cause prosthetic difficulty. Sometimes, the bony exostoses may be present on the buccal buttressing bone.

Indications

- Smooth maxillary torus can be ignored, but when it is extensively irregular, large and extends beyond the junction of the hard and soft palate and interferes with the post-dam seal of the denture, it should be removed
- Sometimes the torus may be subjected to constant trauma during mastication
- When it interferes with normal speech
- When a patient is concerned about malignancy.

Technique

- Before surgical excision of the tori, an impression should be taken and the models should be prepared
- The tori should be removed in this model and an acrylic stent should be made
- A Y-incision for small tori and a double Y-incision for the large tori is made. A full thickness mucoperiosteal flap is elevated carefully to expose the tori entirely
- The tori is divided by transverse and anteroposterior bur cuts to a depth of 1–2 mm above the level of horizontal palatal shelf in order to prevent any fracture of the palate and perforation into the nasal cavity
- These cut sections are removed with the help of a chisel and mallet
- The surface should be finely smoothened using large bone files or vulcanite bur. The torus can also be removed with the help of rotary burs alone without the use of chisels, but this may cause accidental perforation into the nasal cavity or trauma to the soft tissues
- This area should be copiously irrigated and the mucoperiosteal flap is trimmed accordingly and sutured back
- The acrylic stent, which was initially constructed must now be inserted
- This stent supports the flap and prevents any haematoma formation and covers the wound. The stent can be used until wound healing is completed.

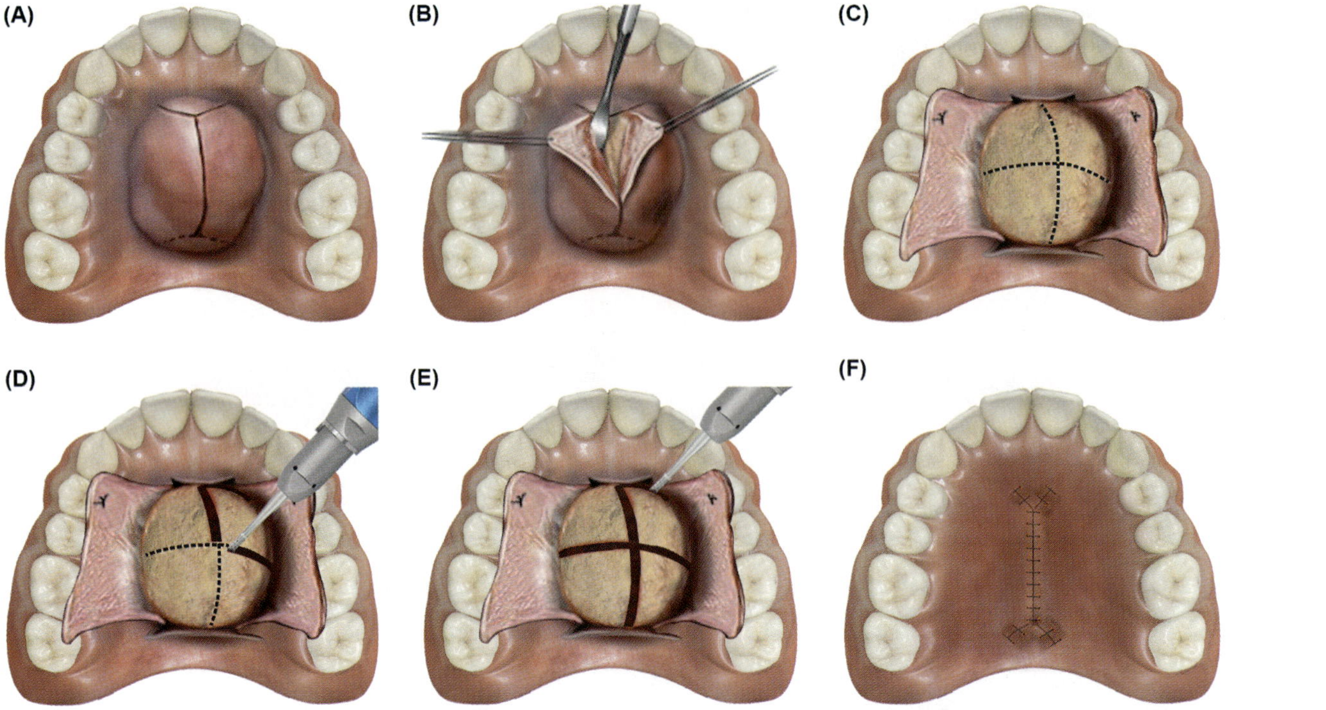

Figure 21.6 Removal of maxillary tori. (**A**) Placement of double-Y incision. (**B**) Elevation of full thickness mucoperiosteal flap. (**C**) Transverse and anteroposterior depth cuts marked. (**D** and **E**) Depth cuts made using rotary bur. (**F**) Mucoperiosteal flap trimmed and sutured.

Complications

The risk of creation of oronasal fistula is more owing to the thin palatal shelf.

Mandibular tori or Torus mandibularis (Fig. 21.7)

It is an exostoses located on the lingual aspect of the mandible in the region of the premolar above the mylohyoid line. They may be unilateral or bilateral.

Indications for removal

- It is removed if a lower denture is to be constructed
- It should be removed if there is chronic irritation
- Very rarely, it is removed when the patient is concerned about malignancy.

Technique

- Inferior alveolar nerve (IAN) and lingual nerve block are given along with local infiltration anaesthesia on the tori

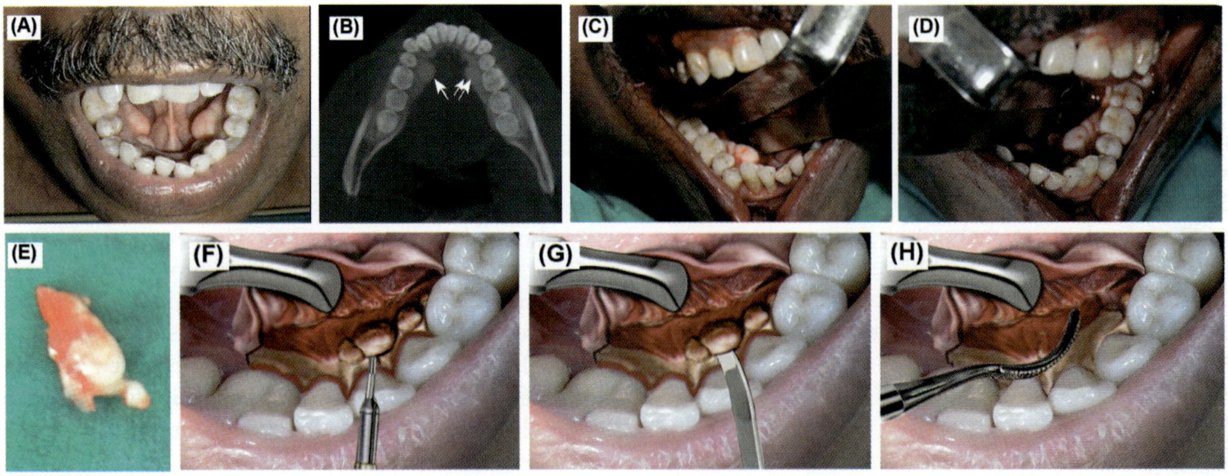

Figure 21.7 (**A**) Mandibular tori in a dentulous arch. (**B**) CBCT showing torus mandibularis on the lingual aspect of the mandible. (**C** and **D**) Surgical excision of mandibular tori—demonstration. (**E**) Excised tori specimen. (**F–H**) Illustration of mandibular tori removal in a dentulous arch.

- Once anaesthetised, an incision is made on the crest of the alveolar ridge for sufficient length to expose the entire tori
- In case of edentulous patients, incision can be placed on the gingival sulcus
- Soft tissues are elevated using a periosteal elevator to expose the tori
- Using a chisel, bur or rongeur, tori is removed and the rough bony surface is smoothened using a bone file
- Excess soft issue is trimmed, wound irrigated and sutured back.

Precaution

- To prevent formation of sublingual haematoma while removing bilateral mandibular tori, the flap should be kept intact in the midline
- A gauze pack is placed below the torus to be removed to prevent the loss of excised bone into the soft tissues since displacement of bone chips may lead to sublingual space infection.

MYLOHYOID RIDGE REDUCTION

Mandibular lingual shelf area contains mylohyoid ridge and houses the 3rd molar tooth. This area is used extensively by the prosthodontists to extend the lingual flanges of the mandibular denture to gain stability and retention.

This shelf, along with the mylohyoid muscle insertion (Fig. 21.8), becomes more prominent and superficial with time due to atrophy of the mandible. A sharp lingual shelf interferes with denture construction and insertion and the mylohyoid muscle attachment here dislodges the denture.

Therefore, this shelf needs to be reduced and the mylohyoid muscle attachment should be released.

Technique

- A linear incision is made on the crest of the ridge, on the posterior aspect of the mandible, laterally and superiorly on the external oblique ridge
- A full thickness mucoperiosteal flap is elevated to expose the lingual shelf area and the mylohyoid muscle

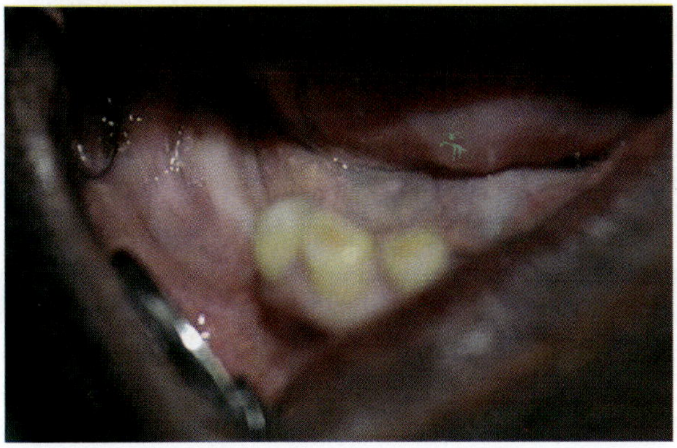

Figure 21.8 Posterior mandibular ridge resorption with prominent mylohyoid ridge and higher muscle attachment.

- Care should be taken to avoid any injury to the lingual nerve in this area
- The mylohyoid muscle is released by sharply incising the muscle attachment at bony origin
- A chisel is then placed parallel to the ramus and in accordance with the direction of the bone grain of the mandible and the shelf is split off
- The bone is trimmed and smoothened with the help of bur and bone files. The wound is closed with sutures after irrigation with saline
- Immediate replacement of the denture helps in repositioning the muscle attachments inferiorly; however, downward repositioning can be best established with the help of a rubber catheter placed in the floor of the mouth and securing it with sutures passed through the skin with an awl. The catheter is retained in position for a period of 5 days.

GENIAL TUBERCLES REDUCTION (Fig. 21.9)

Genial tubercles are the bony projections located on the lingual aspect of the mandible, two on either side of the midline, which gives attachment to the genial muscles. The two genial tubercles located superiorly are more prominent than the inferior due to the gross resorption of the mandibular ridge. This may elevate the ridge lingually giving a shelf-like appearance and making the anterior lingual seal impossible. This is also a frequent site of ulceration when a lower denture is used.

Technique

- An incision is placed in the midline in an anteroposterior direction, and the tubercles are exposed by blunt dissection
- The muscle is secured using catgut before separating the tubercle
- Using bur, chisel or rongeurs, the tubercle is removed and the rough bony margins are smoothened using a file
- The wound is closed using suture.

MAXILLARY TUBEROSITY REDUCTION (Fig. 21.10)

Enlarged maxillary tuberosity may be either fibrous or bony in nature. Unilateral hypertrophic maxillary tuberosity is favourable for construction of denture if sufficient space exists between the tuberosity and the ascending ramus of the mandible for the denture flange to fit in without any difficulty during opening and closing of mouth. However, bilateral hypertrophic tuberosity needs reduction.

Causes of enlarged tuberosity

- Prolonged retention of maxillary 3rd molar with loss of mandibular 3rd molar resulting in supraeruption of the maxillary molar along with alveolar hyperplasia
- Enlargement of the maxillary antrum with the pneumatisation of the tuberosity region
- Gingival fibromatosis.

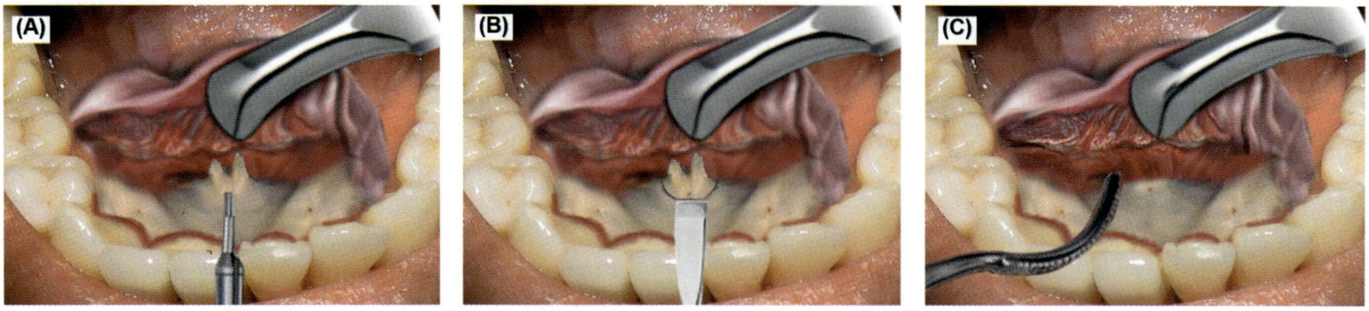

Figure 21.9 Resection of genial tubercle. (**A**) Superior position of the genial tubercle interference in the lingual seal of denture. (B) The tubercle exposed, genioglossus muscle is secured. (**C**) Genial tubercles resected.

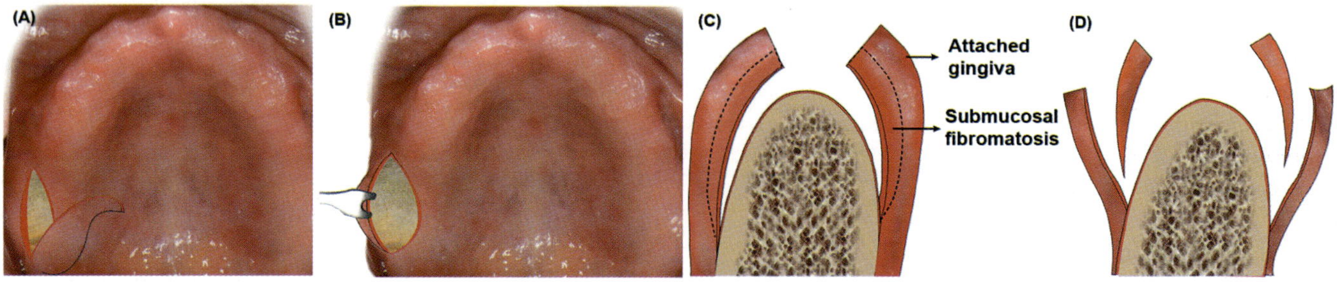

Figure 21.10 (**A**) Elliptical incision made on the crest of the alveolar ridge. (**B**) Reflection of the buccal flap to expose the bony tuberosity. (**C** and **D**) Excision of the submucosal fibrous tissue for reduction.

Techniques

Crestal approach

- An interarch space of at least 1 cm should exist between maxillary and mandibular arches in the posterior region for proper denture construction. A radiograph of the tuberosity region would help in detecting if the enlargement is a fibrous or bony one
- Usually this is a combined procedure, which requires removal of both soft and hard tissue
- A wedge-shaped or elliptical incision is made on the crest of the alveolar ridge to the depth of the bone. This piece of the tissue is then removed
- The buccal and palatal margins of the flap are then thinned by removing the submucosal tissues beneath these flaps
- A rongeurs or a large oval bur is used to remove the bony undercut
- The area is then smoothened with the help of bone files and irrigated with saline
- Before closure, undermined buccal and palatal flaps may need to be trimmed for proper approximation. The wound is closed primarily.

Lateral approach

When the tuberosity is very narrow and overlying keratinised mucosa requires to be preserved for vestibuloplasty in this region, the tuberosity is reduced using a lateral approach instead of a crestal approach.

- An incision is made on the lateral side of the maxillary ridge superior enough to pass below the malar buttress
- Two relaxing incisions are made on either side of the crestal incision anteriorly and posteriorly and the flap is retracted and submucosal excision of the fibrotic tissue is done
- The sulcus is extended superiorly from the lateral incision to deepen the sulcus. The palatally based flap is now advanced to cover the bone such that it lines the newly created sulcus and it is sutured here to the new periosteum
- A maxillary denture splint is used to stabilise the tissue in the new position.

TUBEROPLASTY

The tuberosity, and the hamular notch region help in retention of denture and also aid in peripheral seal of the maxillary denture. This procedure is undertaken to increase the depth between the hamular notch and the distal aspect of the maxilla. In this technique, to deepen the hamular notch, the pterygoid plate and the hamulus are repositioned in the posterior direction (Fig. 21.11).

ALVEOLAR RIDGE PRESERVATION

Most of the measures which are undertaken to prevent or reduce the prosthetic difficulties are related to extraction of teeth. Conservative extraction techniques using periosteotomes to maintain alveolar continuity, orthodontic guided tooth or root extraction, immediate grafting of extraction sites, relief of undercuts using bone grafts or hydroxyapatite (HA) augmentation and guided tissue regeneration are some

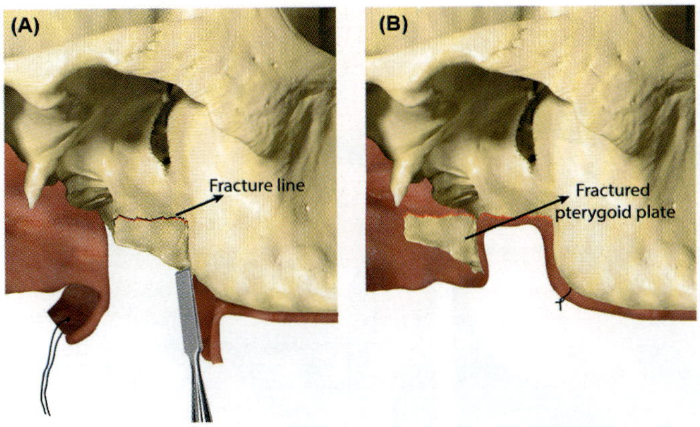

Figure 21.11 (A & B) Maxillary tuberoplasty.

of the current techniques in ridge preservation. Proper radiographs should be taken prior to extraction of any teeth to detect the presence of any abnormality related to the teeth and predict the difficulty in removing the teeth. In edentulous ridge, the radiographs help in viewing any retained root apices, embedded teeth or other bony pathologies.

Technique

- Meticulous extraction technique with appropriate extraction forceps can avoid most of the difficulties of prosthetic rehabilitation
- Avoid improper soft tissue handling, extreme forces in extraction that causes buccal bone fractures and injudicious bone removal for root retrieval
- When multiple teeth are extracted in a quadrant, primary alveoloplasty is required
- In case of multiple maxillary anterior teeth extraction, canine extraction is done prior to premolars to prevent alveolar bone fracture. When premolars and lateral incisors are extracted before canine extraction, the long root of canine fractures the thin buccal cortex along with portions of alveolar bone of adjacent sockets
- After extraction, the socket should be compressed with the thumb and forefinger to reposition the expanded socket
- Any sharp bony spicule or other debris like loose bone, calculus should be removed prior to suturing (intraseptal alveoloplasty)
- When the tooth root is fractured, it should be removed with minimum manipulation (like dividing the roots or removing via apicoectomy window), while preserving the crestal bone, to ensure adequate bony support for the denture construction
- Wherever possible, an osteoplastic flap (i.e., the bone is mobilised with attached mucoperiosteum) should be raised during removal of buried teeth, root apices or cysts
- If the radiograph shows a fractured tooth root with normal surrounding periodontal ligament and vital pulp, it can be left as such as it does not pose any danger, but when it is related to a granuloma or a cyst or otherwise, it should be removed
- Periodontally involved teeth should be extracted early to prevent excessive bone loss
- Ankylosed tooth, hypercementosis or long dilacerated root are extracted by transalveolar method with judicious bone removal since buccal cortex fracture occurs with intraalveolar extraction.

Preservation of uninfected root stumps

In an edentulous ridge, if uninfected root stumps are present without any periodontal disease or periapical pathology, it may be retained to maintain the alveolar ridge height and width. These roots if firmly placed in the ridge can also be used to support the denture with precision attachments such as ball-retained dentures.

MENTAL NERVE TRANSPOSITION

Gross resorption of the alveolar bone may lead to mental foramen becoming superficial until it reaches to the crest of the ridge. When this occurs, mental nerve may be subjected to pressure from dental flange which causes a dull burning sensation or sudden sharp severe pain. The pain can be elicited during mastication or by applying digital pressure. In some cases, pain can be eliminated by simply relieving the denture in that area, provided the denture has enough support for the remaining denture bearing area. Preoperative radiograph is taken to assess the level of mental foramen.

Technique

- The nerve is approached via along incision made in the crest of the alveolar ridge
- If the mental foramen is located on the crest of the ridge, the incision should curve lingually to avoid the foramen
- Mucoperiosteal flap is reflected and the mental foramen and the neurovascular bundle are located
- The nerve should be retracted carefully and held with hook
- A vertical groove is drilled below the mental foramen on the buccal cortex with a dental drill
- The nerve is now repositioned in the inferiorly created cortical groove
- The nerve can be secured to the new position with the help of absorbable haemostatic gauze such as Surgicel, and the mucoperiosteal flap is sutured back
- Postoperative anaesthesia may persist if there happens to be any damage caused to the nerve during surgery.

REPOSITIONING OF INFERIOR ALVEOLAR NERVE

In 1987, Jenson and Nock carried out IAN transposition (IANT) for the placement of dental implants in posterior mandibular regions. Dental implants are often placed in the posterior mandible, but in many cases, the bone has so severely atrophied that sufficiently long fixtures cannot be placed without encroaching on the IAN. IAN lateralisation (IANL) and IANT are surgical procedures that reposition the IAN for the purpose of implant placement without bone augmentation (Fig. 21.12).

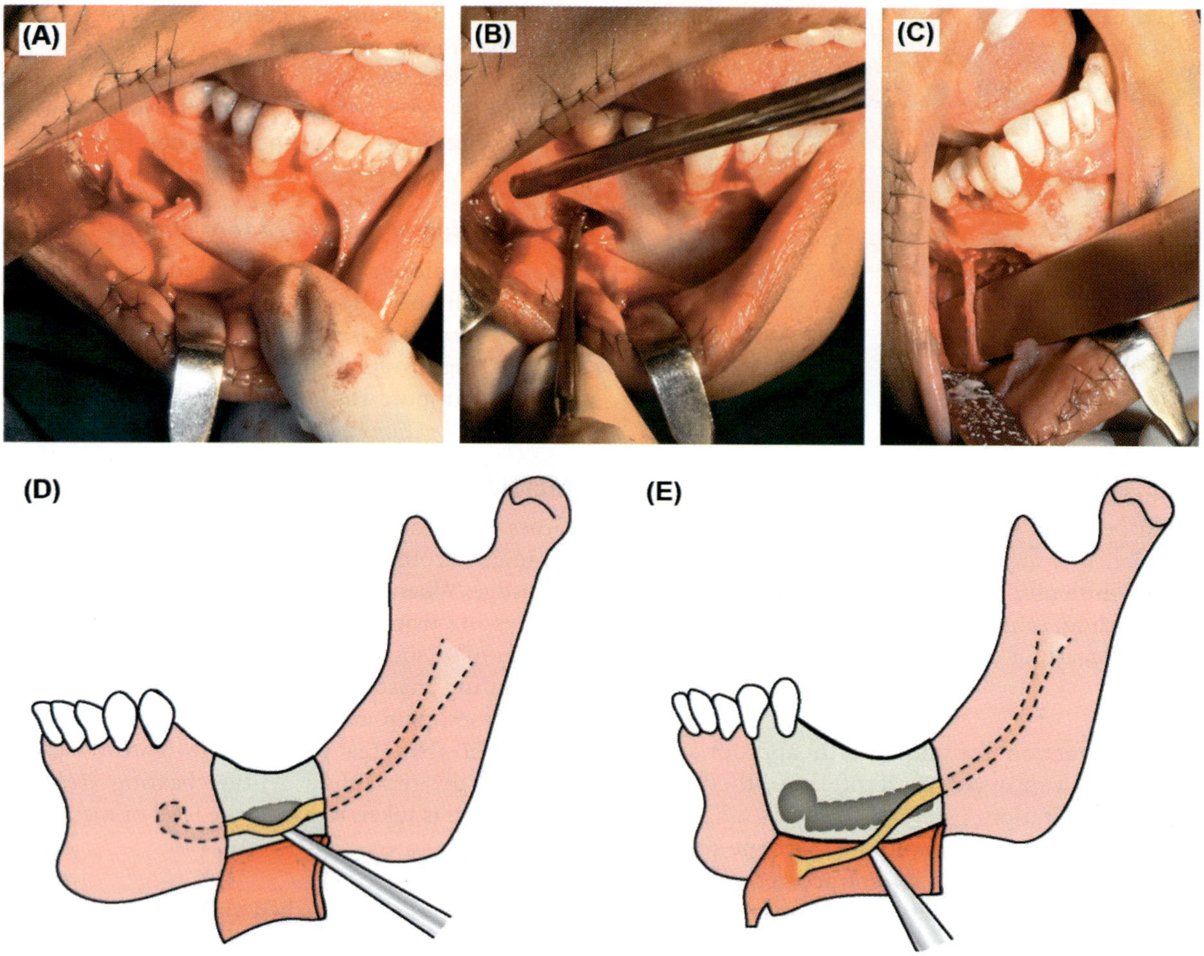

Figure 21.12 **(A-E)** Inferior alveolar nerve repositioning.

IAN LATERALISATION

IANL is the lateral reflection of the IAN without incisive nerve traction. The incisive branch is 5 mm from the mental foramen, a posterior window is created by osteotomy around the IAN. Preservation of the incisive nerve and lateralisation of inferior alveolar neurovascular bundle posterior to the mental foramen is done with a periosteal elevator. The nerve bundle should be protected and the implants are placed under direct visualisation.

IAN TRANSPOSITION

In IANT, a corticotomy is done around the mental foramen and the incisive nerve is transected (incisive neurovascular bundle is sacrificed) to allow transposition of both the mental foramen and the IAN such that the mental foramen is repositioned more posteriorly.

Advantages

- Prevents injury to the IAN and vessels during implant placement in edentulous posterior atrophic mandible
- Eliminates the need for bone grafts
- Greater implant stability.

Indicated during orthognathic surgeries, such as lower border shaving and total mandibular subapical osteotomy.

ALVEOLAR RIDGE AUGMENTATION

The augmentation of the bone is achieved by building up the atrophied jaw bone using autogenous bone—iliac crest, rib grafts, allogenic bone—freeze-dried cadaver bone, alloplastic material—Hydroxyapatite (HA), metal mesh with autogenous corticocancellous bone or metal mesh with HA (Table 21.3).

Criteria for ridge augmentation (*Fig. 21.13*)

- Gross atrophy of the jaws with the risk of mandibular fracture
- Atrophy of the jaws with knife-edge ridge causing prosthetic difficulties
- Insufficient alveolar dimension for implant placement.

Goals of ridge augmentation

- Restoration of the optimum ridge height and width, vestibular depth, ridge form and optimum denture bearing area

TABLE 21.3 Mandibular and Maxillary Augmentation Procedures

Mandibular Augmentation Procedures 1. Superior border augmentation a. Bone graft—Iliac crest b. Bone graft and rhBMP-2/PRP c. Alloplastic graft d. Alveolar transport distraction osteogenesis (DO)
2. Inferior border augmentation a. Bone grafts b. Cartilage graft
3. Interpositional or sandwich bone grafting a. Bone graft b. Cartilage graft c. Hydroxyapatite blocks
4. Visor osteotomy—Vertical osteotomy
5. Onlay grafting
6. Pedicled augmentation—Horizontal osteotomy
7. Ridge split technique for implant placement
Maxillary Augmentation Procedures 1. Onlay bone grafting
2. Onlay grafting of alloplastic material
3. Interpositional or sandwich graft a. Sinus lift procedures b. Ridge split technique for implant placement
4. Bone graft and rhBMP-2
5. Alveolar transport DO
Augmentation in Combination with Orthognathic Surgery 1. Mandibular osteotomy procedures
2. Maxillary osteotomy procedures
3. Combination procedures
4. Segmental jaw surgeries
Distraction osteogenesis—Vertical, Anterior—Posterior Vector

- To increase retention and stability of the denture
- To attain a proper interarch relationship
- To protect and prevent injury to anatomic vital structures such as the neurovascular bundle, maxillary sinus, mental nerve.

MANDIBULAR AUGMENTATION PROCEDURES

Mandibular augmentation is a procedure used to improve the height, strength and contour of an extremely deficient mandible before placement of a denture or an implant (refer to Chapter 22, Table 22.14). Autogenous bone, allogeneic bone or alloplastic material can all be used for this purpose as a source of bone graft material. Recently the use of rhBMP-2 and alveolar distraction osteogenesis has gained immense popularity. The following are different techniques for mandibular augmentation.

SUPERIOR BORDER AUGMENTATION

Superior border augmentation described by Davis (1970) was performed in ridge height less than 10 mm. Two long autogenous grafts (any of 5th to 8th rib grafts) approximately 15 cm are harvested. Kerfing of one of the rib grafts to adapt to the mandibular curvature should be performed by creating vertical cuts on the inner surface of the rib. This is fixed to the superior border of the mandible by transosseous wiring, circummandibular wiring, miniplates or microplates. The other rib is made into corticocancellous particles and packed into the dead spaces around and in between the graft and the mandible. This procedure is indicated when the mental foramen is situated on the superior border. In this procedure, the 2nd rib graft can be used or excluded with addition of rhBMP-2 in absorbable collagen sponge fixed to the superior border of the mandible (Fig. 21.14). Mandibular symphysis graft or external oblique ridge (Refer to Chapter 22, Figs. 22.30 & 22.32) or iliac crest can also be used instead of rib grafts. Precarved HA blocks are also available for mandible as alloplastic grafts.

Disadvantages

- Morbidity of the donor site
- Secondary surgical site

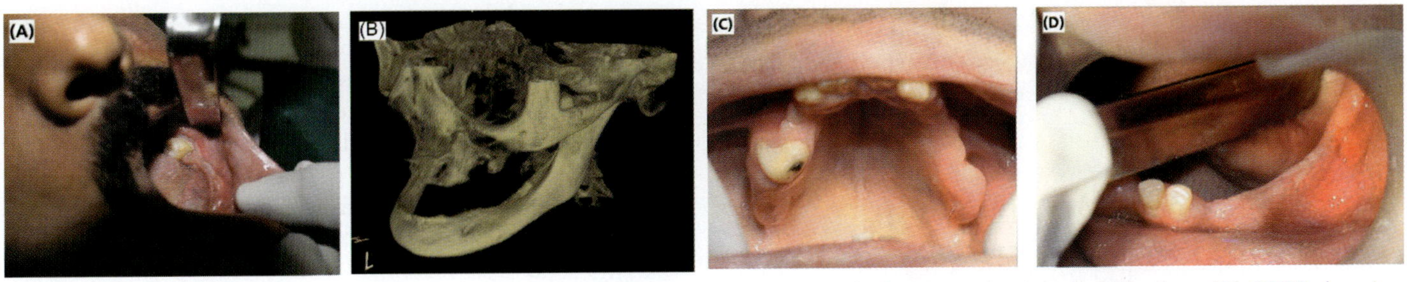

Figure 21.13 (**A**) Knife-edge alveolar ridge indicated for ridge augmentation before prosthetic rehabilitation. (**B**) CBCT showing severe atrophic mandible with knife-edge ridge, insufficient alveolus for implant placement. (**C and D**) Partial anodontia with resorbed maxilla and mandible indicated for augmentation.

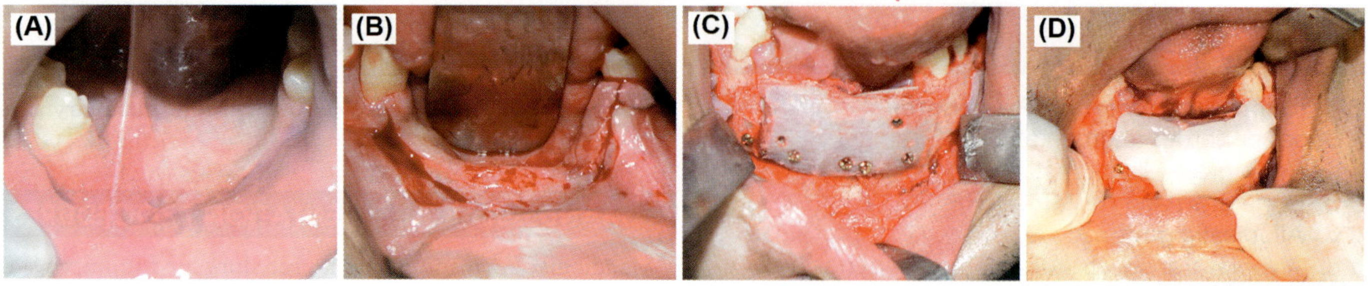

Figure 21.14 **(A-D)** Superior border augmentation for atrophic knife-edge mandibular ridge using rib graft and rhBMP-2.

- Necessity of the patient to withdraw denture till the surgical wound heals for a period of 6–8 months
- Postoperative resorption of the graft is common. This has been overcome well by concurrent use of rhBMP-2.

PEDICLED SANDWICH AUGMENTATION

Pedicled sandwich augmentation was described by Schettler and Holtermann (1977). A cranially pedicled periosteal flap is raised at the depth of the lower labial vestibule. This is achieved by a vestibular incision and soft tissue dissection to the lower border of the chin where the periosteum is incised. The atrophied ridge is sectioned horizontally. It is important to make sure the lingual pedicle containing the attachments of the genioglossus and suprahyoid muscles are not damaged. The osteotomised segment is handled carefully to keep the lingual pedicle intact. The defect of 15–20 mm can be augmented with bone or cartilaginous graft in a sandwich technique. The surgical site is then closed with the periosteal flap. Vestibuloplasty can be performed after 4–12 weeks. The resorption after 2–3 years was about 1 mm in alveolar bone graft (ABG).

INFERIOR BORDER AUGMENTATION (Fig. 21.15)

This technique was 1st described by Sanders and Cox in the year 1986 for reconstruction of a resected mandible. This procedure is indicated to prevent and manage fractures of an atrophic mandible.

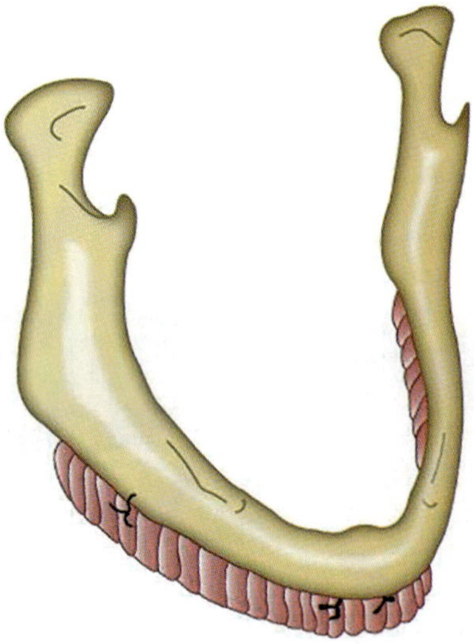

Figure 21.15 Inferior border augmentation with rib graft.

Indications

- Augmentation of severely atrophic edentulous mandible
- Prevention of pathological fracture of atrophic edentulous mandible
- Management of malunion or nonunion of edentulous mandible.

Procedure

A submandibular incision is made from angle-to-angle region and subplatysmal dissection is done to the inferior border of the mandible. An incision through periosteum is made from the angle of mandible of one side to the other. Two ribs obtained are kerfed and abutted against the lingual and buccal aspect of the inferior border. The graft material is fixed to the mandible by means of circummandibular wiring. The flap is closed primarily.

Using freeze-dried cadaveric mandible

A freeze-dried allogenic cadaver mandible can be used as a tray by hollowing it out. Cancellous bone graft harvested from the iliac crest is then filled into it, and multiple perforations are made on the cadaveric mandible to allow for revascularisation of the packed cancellous bone graft.

Advantages

- Does not obliterate the vestibule
- The superior border and alveolar ridge is not altered in this procedure, so patient's old dentures can be used as transitional dentures
- Interim denture can be worn immediately
- Implant placement can also be planned
- No change in vertical dimension
- Graft is not subjected to direct masticatory force
- Extraoral flap gives better tissue coverage postgrafting
- Increasing lower 3rd of the facial height improves aesthetics.

Disadvantages

- It will not correct the abnormalities of denture bearing areas
- It will not protect a highly placed mental nerve

- Donor site morbidity
- Resorption of the graft
- Presence of scar.

VISOR OSTEOTOMY (Fig. 21.16)

This technique was 1st described by Harle to overcome the resorption of free onlay bone graft. This technique is designed wherein the muscle insertion into the mandible and nutrient supply are maintained. The mandible is divided buccolingually by a vertical osteotomy from external oblique ridge of one side of the mandible to the other side. The osteotomised lingual segment is pushed superiorly and fixed with the buccal segment using stainless steel wire in the lower border of the lingual segment and upper border of the buccal segment.

MODIFIED VISOR OSTEOTOMY (Fig. 21.17)

Visor osteotomy was modified by Peterson and Slade in 1977. Here the vertical osteotomy cut is made only in the posterior region to divide the segments buccolingually. A horizontal osteotomy is performed in the anterior mandible to divide the anterior segment superiorly and inferiorly, and bone grafting (usually corticocancellous bone from iliac crest or HA granules) is done into the osteotomised gap and the two osteotomised segments are fixed with wires.

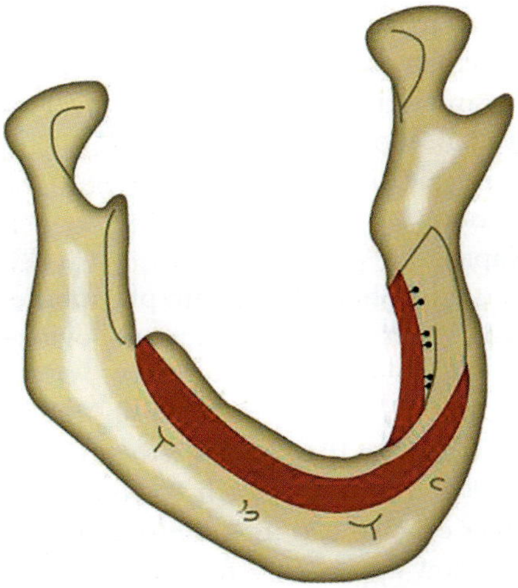

Figure 21.16 Visor osteotomy.

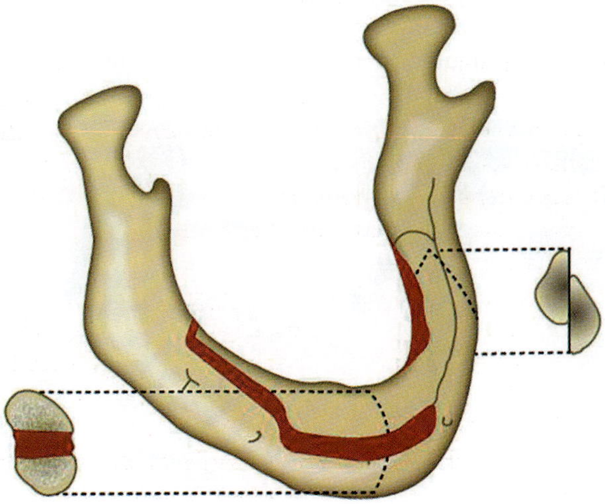

Figure 21.17 Modified visor osteotomy.

Advantages

- The rate of resorption is less when compared to onlay grafts
- Correction of mild to moderate anterior–posterior discrepancies
- Better positioning of superior and posterior segments allows a stable area for augmentation, thus resulting in ridge height of at least 80% after 3–5 years of RRR
- Incidence of nerve paraesthesia is less when compared to visor osteotomy.

Disadvantages

- Chances of nerve damage causing paresthesia and dysesthesia is higher
- Donor site morbidity for autogenous graft
- Inability to wear the dentures for 3–5 months following surgery for healing of the ridge.

INTERPOSITION BONE GRAFTING METHOD

This procedure is also called as sandwich grafting advocated by Danielson and Nemarich. This procedure can be performed in both maxillary and mandibular ridges with a horizontal osteotomy that splits the residual maxilla or mandible creating space for the graft. Autogenous bone/cartilage or allogenic bone is grafted into this osteotomised gap or HA granules can also be packed (Fig. 21.18). In mandible, sandwich technique is used for the augmentation of the anterior mandible, within the bilateral mental foramina. For the posterior mandibular region, a good amount of vertical bone height should be present above mandibular canal to perform this procedure. Prosthetic dentures or implant placement is delayed from 3 to 6 months for complete remodelling of the bone. Secondary vestibuloplasty for better denture retention may be performed.

Advantages

- Sandwich technique has a lesser resorption rate than onlay grafting with predictable long-term results
- Incidence of nerve paresthesia is reduced compared to the technique-sensitive visor osteotomy and modified visor osteotomy
- Implant placement through the superior free segment of the bone and through the interpositional grafted bone can be secured to the inferior segment of the mandible with implant success rate of 98% and with low resorption rate.

MAXILLARY AUGMENTATION PROCEDURE

ONLAY GRAFTING (Fig. 21.18)

Onlay grafting of the edentulous maxilla or mandible is done when there is adequate bone height but inadequate bone width. It is most commonly done for the anterior segment of the maxilla compared to that of the posterior segment where sinus augmentation technique is preferred.

Procedure and grafting techniques

- **Outline Procedure:** With a high vestibular incision, mucoperiosteal flap is reflected and the bony surface is exposed. The defect is analysed and small perforations may or may not be made on the outer cortex. This is performed to facilitate neovascularisation. The choice of graft as discussed below is moulded over the cortex and immobilised as required. A barrier membrane may be placed to preserve the graft from resorption. The flap is mobilised over the graft and a watertight closure is done
- Bone grafting of the maxilla using autogenous bone from the mandible or costochondral rib graft (described by Terry et al.,) is performed to increase the height and width of the maxillary alveolar process. To facilitate good closure and to achieve good undermining of tissues, a high vestibular incision is made and mucoperiosteal flap is reflected to expose the alveolar ridge. The rib graft is harvested and placed over the alveolar defect. The wound is closed with sutures

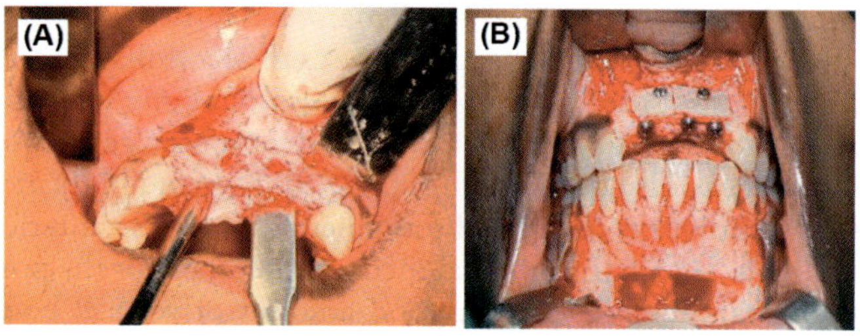

Figure 21.18 Maxillary bone grafting. (**A**) Atrophic edentulous maxillary ridge. (**B**) Bone graft taken from the mandible.

- A split thickness costochondral (rib) graft, which has a uniform structure, can be placed as a whole graft, or iliac crest graft in multiple blocks can be used as only grafting
- HA crystals is the prototype of nonresorbable ceramic bone substitute with chemical and physical structures of calcium phosphate similar to tooth enamel. Grafting can also be done using allograft-like HA as described by Obwegeser, wherein a vertical incision is made in the midline and mucosa is tunnelled on both sides of the midline. HA crystals are mixed either with blood or saline and injected through this incision. A solid or porous HA block can be used as an only graft
- Some literatures also mention mixing of the autogenous bone graft and HA crystals as grafting material.

SINUS AUGMENTATION TECHNIQUE OR SINUS LIFT PROCEDURE (Fig. 21.19)

Due to excessive pneumatisation of the maxillary antrum and atrophy of the maxillary ridge, floor of the sinus almost comes to lie very close to the maxillary alveolar crest. Maxillary sinus lift procedure is carried out to lift the floor of the sinus lining by placing a graft in between the maxillary sinus lining and the floor of the maxillary antrum in the posterior aspect.

The various materials used for this surgical procedure are:

- Iliac crest cancellous graft
- Costochondral (Rib) graft
- Allogenic bone
- Hydroxyapatite
- Tricalcium phosphate or calcium phosphate
- Calcium deficient carbonate apatite—bovine bone.

Technique

In 1977, Tatum was the 1st to perform the sinus lift operation. He introduced a crestal approach to the sinus membrane, which was later on changed in 1986 to a modified Caldwell-Luc lateral window approach. An incision is made on the alveolar crest extending from canine to the tuberosity region with two vertical releasing incisions placed. Full thickness flap is elevated and horizontal bony cut is made inferiorly 2–4 mm above the floor of the sinus. A vertical bony cut is made perpendicular to the horizontal cut in the anterior

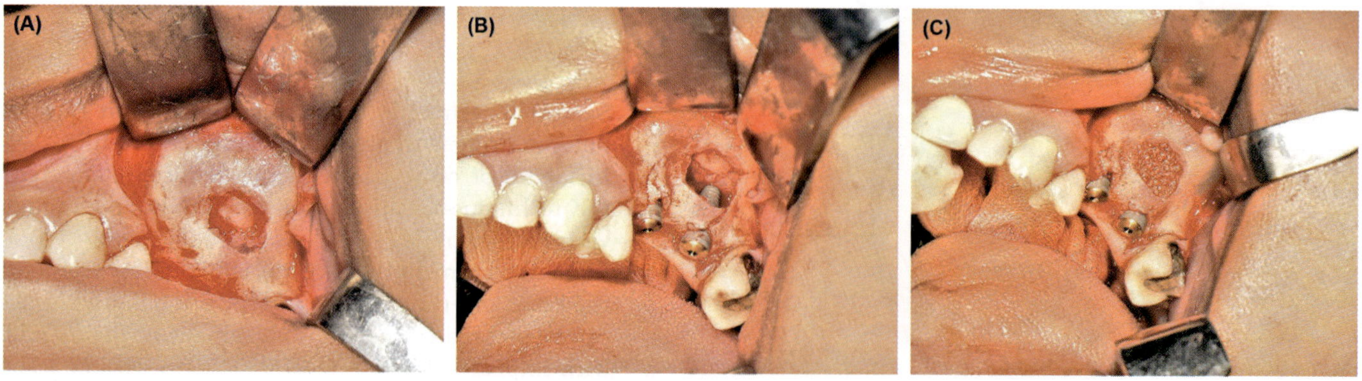

Figure 21.19 **(A-C)** Sinus lift procedure.

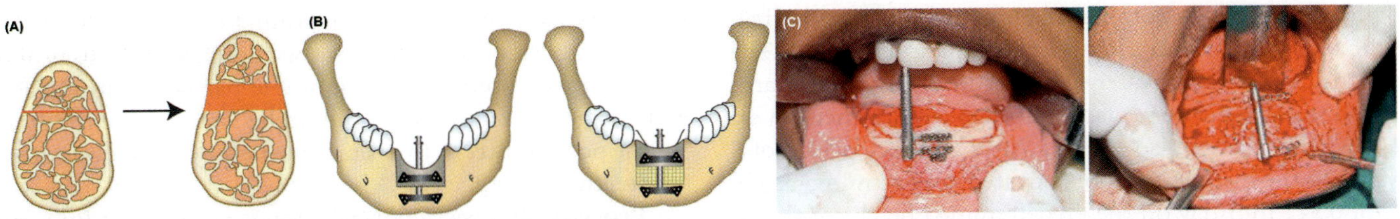

Figure 21.20 **(A)** Illustration of vertical alveolar distraction osteogenesis. **(B)** Technique for intraoral vertical distraction osteogenesis of the mandibular anterior alveolar ridge. **(C)** Vertical distraction osteogenesis.

region parallel to the lateral nasal wall. Another vertical cut is made posteriorly perpendicular to the inferior horizontal cut in the region of the maxillary buttress. Two vertical cuts are joined superiorly by an interrupted osteotomy cut to create a hinged bony window. The bone is feathered till grey colour of the maxillary sinus is seen. A surgical curette is placed between the bone and the antral lining in the inferior osteotomy cut and the bone is gently peeled from inside of the lining of the sinus. The graft is now inserted between the lining and the floor of the sinus. The flap with its intact periosteum is approximated over the graft and closed with interrupted sutures. Instead of bone graft, rhBMP-2 can also be used by the same technique. The waiting period for the healing of the bone graft is 6–9 months (refer Chapter 22, Fig. 22.31).

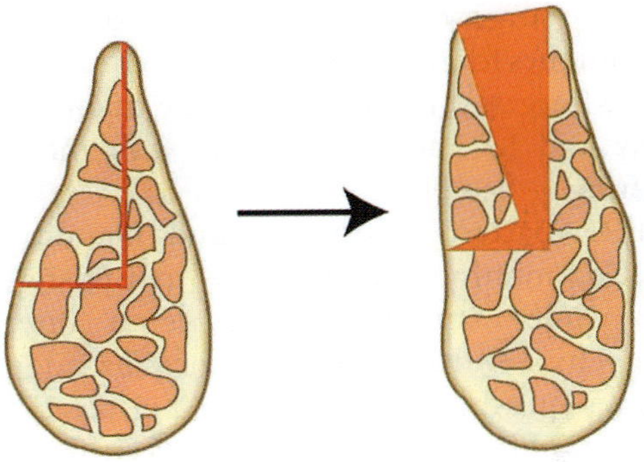

Figure 21.21 Illustration of horizontal alveolar distraction osteogenesis.

MAXILLARY AND MANDIBULAR AUGMENTATION

ALVEOLAR RIDGE DISTRACTION

Alveolar ridge distraction refers to alveolar reconstruction by means of bone transport technique, whereby the transport segment would be moved using a special device called distractor. Alveolar ridge augmentation can be divided into two categories: **Vertical augmentation**, in which the transport alveolar segment is translated vertically and the height of the alveolar ridge is increased (Fig. 21.20). In **horizontal augmentation**, the transport alveolar segment is translated horizontally, thereby increasing the alveolar ridge width (Fig. 21.21).

Indications

- Atrophic alveolus with defects of the vertical height or horizontal width
- Alveolar insufficiency with sufficient basal bone (segmental).

Contraindications

- Cases of inadequate bone volume, especially in severe atrophic mandible with only basal bone with danger of fractures
- Osteoporosis
- Systemic or osseous disorders.

Advantages

- No visible scars
- No bone harvesting required
- Implants can be placed 3 months after surgery
- Shortening of the entire treatment time
- Precise positioning of the device
- Transport of vital alveolar bone, safe blood supply
- Less resorption
- No infection and periodontal problems
- Early vascularisation of new bone
- Teeth vitality remain intact.

Disadvantages

- Temporary nerve disturbance is possible
- A 2nd intervention for removal of the distractor under local anaesthesia is mandatory.

Procedure

A horizontal incision is made buccally at the site where the distractor should be placed. The mucoperiosteal flap is raised similar to the pedicled augmentation flap. The lingual pedicle is maintained intact to the lingual periosteum and alveolar bone. This maintains the viability of the osteotomised segment and allows vascularisation for the bone during distraction. It is important to make sure the lingual pedicle containing the attachments of the genioglossus and suprahyoid muscles are not damaged. The defective alveolar ridge is exposed on the buccal side at the level of the planned horizontal osteotomy. Using a micro-sagittal saw, a segmental osteotomy is created to mobilise the deficient alveolar ridge. The osteotomy cuts made are of two vertical components, which are parallel to the roots of adjacent teeth and one horizontal component connecting the two vertical cuts. The segment is mobilised with an osteotome. The distractor device is then fixed on both the movable and immovable component. The wound is closed with a water-tight closure. The activator arm of the distractor device is placed through a small incision on the mucosa, which is also sutured. After a latency period of 5 days when the distractor is not activated, it is activated at the rate of 0.5–1 mm/day till the predetermined height of the alveolar segment is achieved. The consolidation period for the distracted bone is 3–4 months (Fig. 21.20).

ORTHOGNATHIC SURGERY FOR RIDGE AUGMENTATION

Orthognathic surgery is used in combination with augmentation techniques for reconstruction of edentulous mandible or maxilla. Surgeries normally used are anterior maxillary osteotomy and Le Fort I osteotomy with interpositional bone grafting.

The RRR pattern of maxilla and mandible is very variable. Commonly, maxilla resorbs in a posterosuperior direction while mandible resorbs in an anteroinferior direction. This results in Class III anterior ridge relation, very often requiring jaw correction (Fig. 21.22A and B). Similarly, variable resorption pattern of either jaw in posterior can also mandate segmental jaw surgery for favourable occlusion.

1. Mandibular osteotomy procedures
2. Maxillary osteotomy procedures (Fig. 21.23A–G)
3. Combination procedures
4. Segmental jaw surgeries (Fig. 21.23 (H-M), 21.23 (N & O)).

POSTERIOR SEGMENTAL OSTEOTOMY TO ACHIEVE INTEROCCLUSAL CLEARANCE

Failure to rehabilitate maxillary posterior teeth prosthetically for a long period of time can cause supraeruption of the mandibular posteriors, which decreases the interocclusal clearance. To regain the lost interocclusal clearance, extraction of the offending teeth, intentional root canal therapy, crown shortening or orthodontic intrusion of teeth using cortical implants have been done. Performing a posterior maxillary segmental osteotomy is a versatile alternative for cases of bilateral distal extension of removable partial denture (RPD). The vertical osteotomy cut should be 5 mm above the apices of the posterior teeth to protect the neurovascular bundles of the teeth involved.

Procedure: A vestibular incision is made extending from 1st premolar to 2nd molar followed by raising of a full thickness mucoperiosteal flap. Buccal osteotomy cut 5 mm above the apices of teeth are made with fine surgical burs, with care taken not to damage the roots. The palatal osteotomy cut is completed transantrally. The anterior cut and posterior cut up to the socket of the 3rd molar are made. The osteotomised segment is downfractured, repositioned and fixed with miniplates and screws.

SOFT TISSUE PROCEDURES

FRENECTOMY

A frenum is a fold of tissue or muscle connecting the lips, cheek or tongue to the jawbone (Fig. 21.24). A frenectomy is removal of one of these folds of tissues. Patients receiving dentures may need a frenectomy if the position of a frenum interferes with the proper fit of the denture, thereby frequently ulcerating and reducing the stability of the denture. Indications for frenectomy are high frenal attachment and fibrous bands attached to the alveolar ridge.

Procedures performed on the labial frenum and lingual frenum are termed as labial frenectomy and lingual frenectomy, respectively.

Techniques

1. Simple excision
2. Z-plasty: This technique is used when the base of the frenum is broad and the vestibule is short. The z-plasty can increase the depth of the vestibule. The z-plasty also relieves the tension at the scar postoperatively

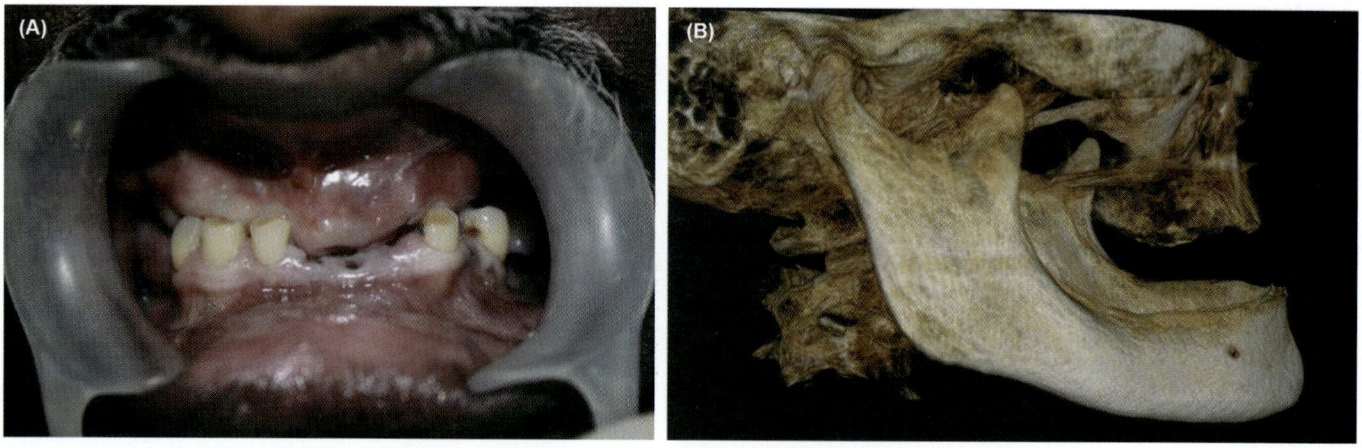

Figure 21.22 **(A)** Class III relation of maxillary edentulous ridge against mandibular teeth requiring corrective orthognathic surgery. **(B)** CBCT showing Class III skeletal relation of completely edentulous maxilla and mandible.

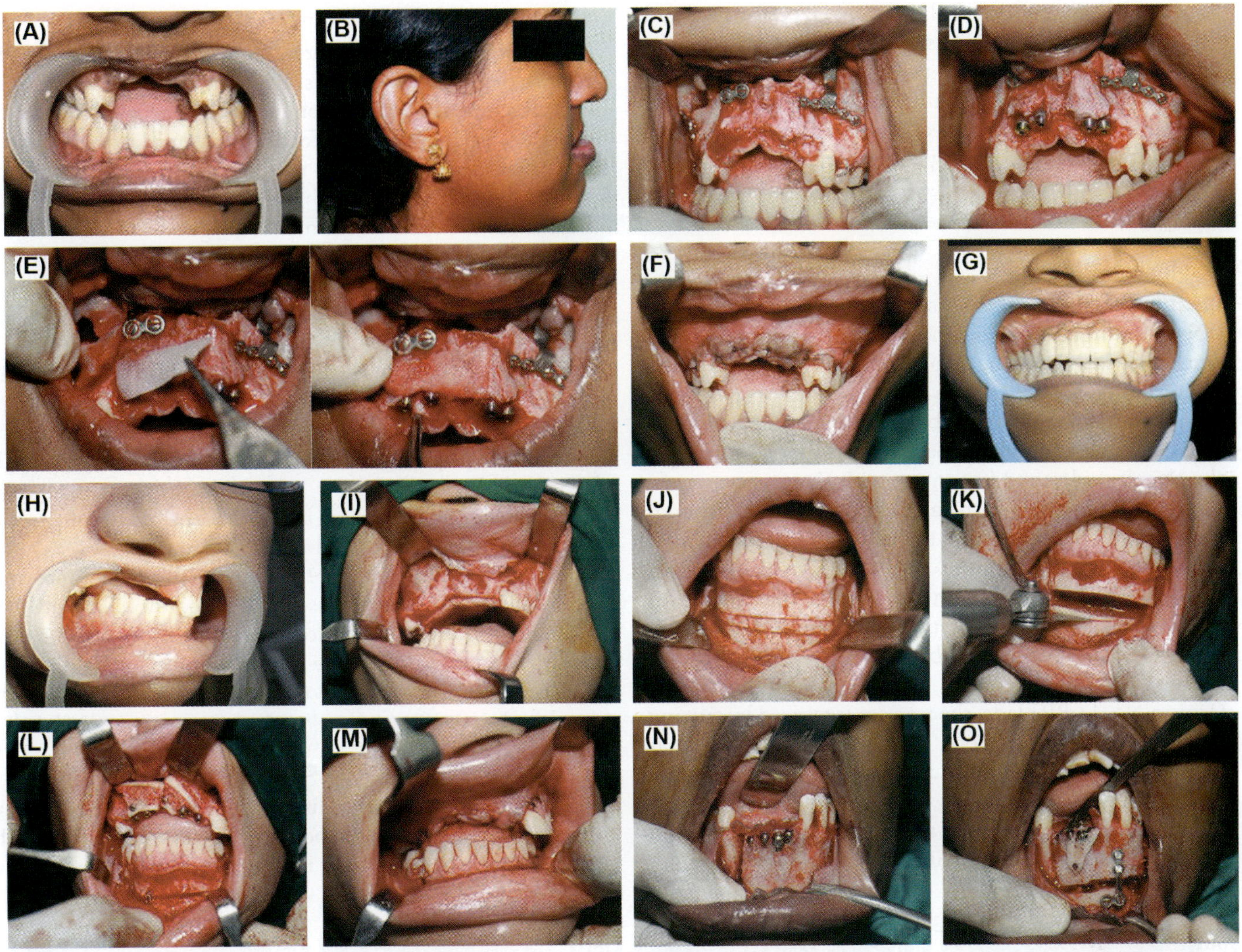

Figure 21.23 Maxillary osteotomy and segmental jaw surgery: **A-G, (A)** Partially edentulous anterior maxilla due to trauma. Skeletal Class III relation. **(B)** Post traumatic deformity with no dental support for upper lip: **(C)** Le Fort I advancement **(D)** Dental implant placed in anterior maxilla. **(E)** Absorbable collagen soaked rhBMP-2 placed for ridge augmentation. **(F)** Primary closure. Note advancement of maxilla with favourable occlusion. **(G)** Prosthetic rehabilitation with incisors in Class I relationship; **H-M, (H)** Partially edentulous resorbed maxilla with reduced interarch space. Note altered mandibular occlusal plane superiorly to right. **(I)** Exposure of the edentulous maxillary alveolus. **(J)** Mandibular segmental subapical osteotomy–planned cuts with excess bone removal on left to correct occlusal cant. **(K)** Osteotomy performed with oscillating saw. **(L)** Implant placement in maxilla with primary onlay bone grafting with bone harvested from mandible. **(M)** Primary closure showing adequate interarch space with mandibular occlusal plane modified; **N&O (N)** Implant placement in mandibular anterior edentulous region. **(O)** Subapical osteotomy–segmental surgery to achieve class I incisor relation, primary bone grafting done in relation to the implant.

3. Cross diamond excision: used when there is a lot of tissue available. The base of the frenum is grasped with a haemostat followed by incisions above and below the haemostat. The fibrous bands are excised and closure done with interrupted sutures
4. V–Y plasty for frenectomy: V–Y incision can lengthen a localised area by creating a localised vestibuloplasty with secondary epithelialisation. When vestibular depth at the premolar and molar area is less, the broad frenum can be excised by a semilunar incision at the mucogingival

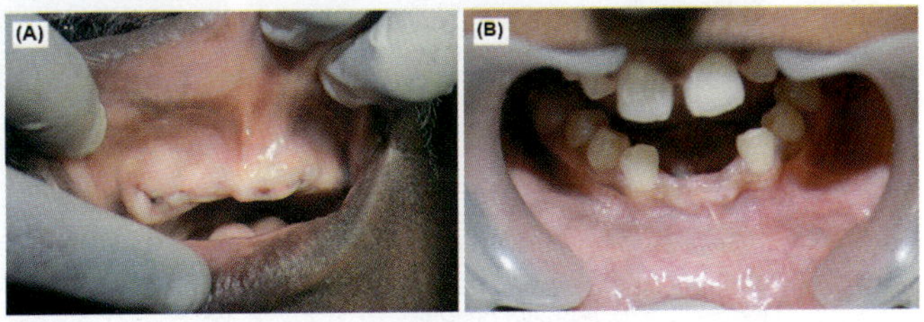

Figure 21.24 **(A)** High frenal attachment in maxilla requiring labial frenectomy. **(B)** Lower labial high frenal attachment requiring frenectomy.

junction. Supraperiosteal dissection is performed and the superior edge of the incision is sutured vertically (the tail of the Y). This increases the depth of the vestibule to the periosteum. The remaining part of the incision is either sutured or left raw to heal by secondary epithelialisation. A prefabricated stent postoperatively is placed for retaining the depth created

5. Laser-assisted frenectomy.

LABIAL FRENECTOMY (FIG. 21.25)

- Local infiltration anaesthesia is used to anaesthetise the labial frenum at its origin and insertion
- Once anaesthetised, the upper lip is everted so that the frenum is kept taut
- Using two haemostats, the fibres of the frenum are locked (the 1st haemostat is placed parallel to the labial surface of the alveolar ridge and in contact with the mucosa covering the labial surface of the mucobuccal fold, and the 2nd haemostat is placed parallel to the lip and perpendicular to the 1st haemostat)
- The haemostats are kept in such a way that their tips touch each other, so that the entire fibrous tissue of the frenum, which has to be removed, lies within the haemostat
- Using a No. 11 BP blade, the frenum is excised by cutting the outer surface of both the haemostats such that the excised tissue comes out separately along with the haemostats
- Now the lateral margins of the wound are undermined and the wound is sutured without tension.

LINGUAL FRENECTOMY (FIGS. 21.26 & 21.27)

This procedure is performed when there is ankyloglossia (tongue-tie) or when there is high lingual frenal attachment. This attachment binds the tongue to the lingual surface of the alveolar ridge. Lingual frenectomy is performed in these patients even when prosthesis is not required as it interferes with the normal speech. Once the teeth are lost, it disturbs the stability of the denture each and every time the tongue is moved.

Technique

- A 3-0 silk suture is passed through the midline of the tongue around 2 cm from the tip (traction suture)
- This is done to hold the tongue up so that the frenum becomes taut
- Using a sharp scissors, a cut is made 1–2 cm midway between the tip of the tongue and the lingual surface of the mandible
- The cut is made in such a way that the blades of the scissors are parallel to the floor of the mouth
- Care should be taken not to injure the submandibular duct, papilla and the blood vessels in the floor of the mouth
- In certain cases, genioglossus muscle should also be dissected in addition to the lingual frenum
- The wound margins are undermined, approximated and closed without tension.

Vestibuloplasty or ridge extension procedures

'Vestibuloplasty is a procedure to increase the depth by uncovering the existing basal bone of the jaws surgically and by repositioning the overlying mucosa, muscle attachments to

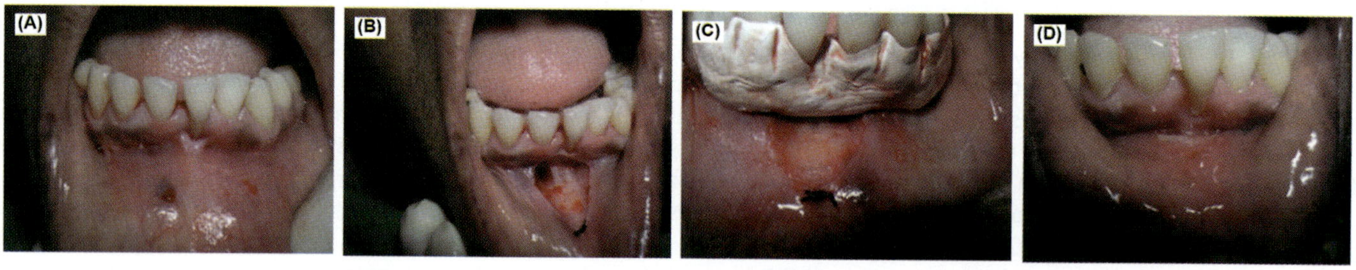

Figure 21.25 (**A–D**) Clinical pictures of labial frenectomy.

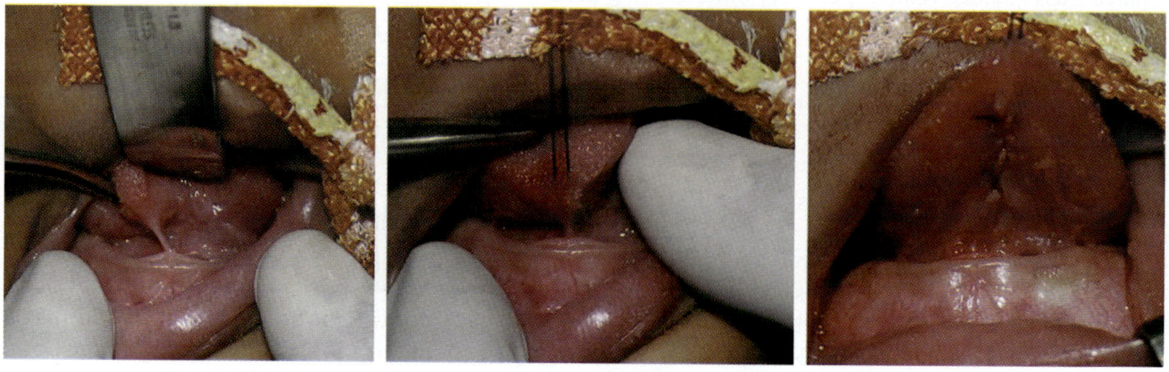

Figure 21.26 Lingual frenectomy—lingual frenal attachment to alveolar ridge.

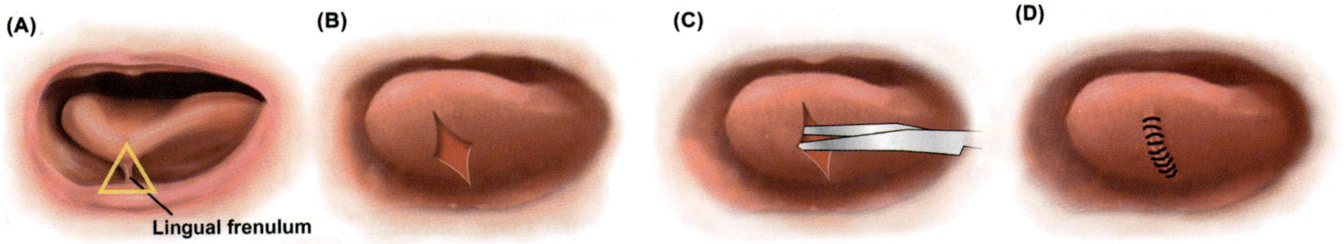

Figure 21.27 (A-D) Illustration of lingual frenectomy.

a lower position in the mandible/superior position in the maxilla'. Vestibuloplasty can be done either on the labial or the lingual side for mandibular atrophy and for high muscle or soft tissue attachments.

Goals of the surgery

- To increase the size of denture bearing area
- Increase the retention and stability of the dentures
- To increase the height of the residual alveolar ridge.

Types of vestibuloplasty

The type of vestibuloplasty technique based on procedures done on the maxilla or mandible either on labial and/or lingual side is as shown in Flowchart 21.2.

Maxilla
- Submucosal Vestibuloplasty - Mucosal advancement vestibuloplasty
- Obwegeser's Maxillary "Pocket Inlay" Vestibuloplasty
- Tissue/ alloplastic grafts - Grafting vestibuloplasty

Mandible
- Submucosal Vestibuloplasty
- Labial Vestibuloplasty - Secondary epithelisation procedure
  - *Lipswitch technique*
  - *Kazanjian's technique*
  - *Godwin's modification*
  - *Clark's technique*
  - *Obwegeser's modification*
- Lingual Vestibuloplasty -Secondary epithelisation procedure
  - *Trauner's technique*
  - *Caldwell's technique*
  - *Obwegeser's technique*
- Tissue/ alloplastic grafts vestibuloplasty

Flowchart 21.2 Types of vestibuloplasty.

LABIOBUCCAL VESTIBULOPLASTY OF MAXILLA

Different techniques:

i. Mucosal advancement vestibuloplasty (submucosal vestibuloplasty)
ii. Obwegeser's maxillary 'Pocket Inlay' vestibuloplasty
iii. Grafting vestibuloplasty.

Mucosal advancement vestibuloplasty

This procedure is also known as submucosal vestibuloplasty, wherein the mucous membrane of the vestibule is undermined and advanced to line both sides of the extended vestibule. The prerequisite for this kind of procedure is that there should be presence of adequate amount of healthy mucosa determined by the mouth mirror test where a mouth mirror is placed in the vestibule and retracted against the bone. If there is no abnormal shortening of the lip, then submucosal vestibuloplasty can be performed. Different types of mucosal advancement vestibuloplasty are:

i. Closed submucosal vestibuloplasty (Obwegeser)
ii. Open view submucosal vestibuloplasty.

Closed submucosal vestibuloplasty (Fig. 21.28)

This procedure is indicated where there is enough bone and healthy tissues but with muscle attached closer to the alveolar crest. It is performed to extend the vestibule for providing additional ridge height and to prevent relapse by excising or transferring submucous tissue and the muscles to a position farther from the crestal ridge.

Technique

A vertical incision is made in the midline of the vestibule extending till the mucogingival junction. Blunt dissection is

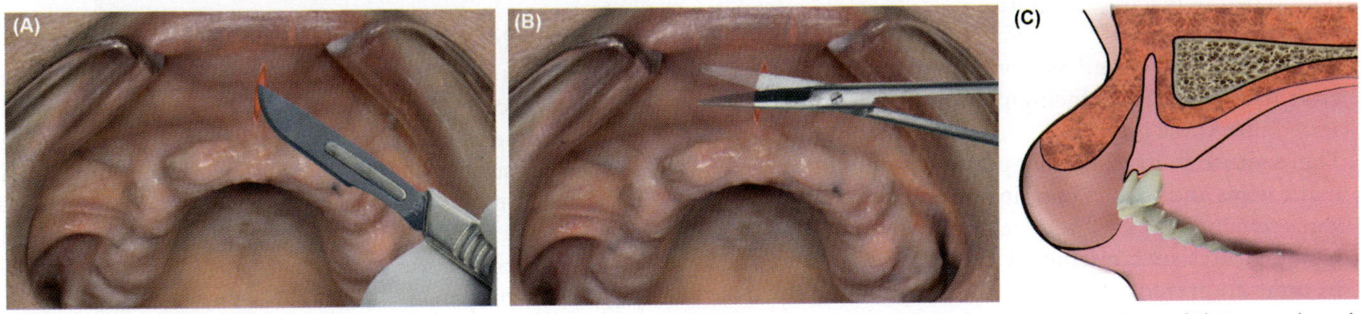

Figure 21.28 Closed submucosal vestibuloplasty of the maxilla. **(A)** Incision made. **(B)** Blunt dissection done. **(C)** Stent placed to maintain the depth of the vestibule.

carried out separating the mucosa from the submucosa to create a submucosal tunnel. The tunnel is extended till the zygomatic buttress on either side. Next supraperiosteal dissection is carried out by freeing the underlying muscles and connective tissue from the periosteum. The vertical incision is closed and a stent is placed for 10–14 days after adapting the mucosa to the deepened vestibule.

Open view submucosal vestibuloplasty (Obwegeser)

Wallenius advocated an open method to overcome the relapse of the closed vestibuloplasty. A horizontal incision is made in the mucogingival junction. A thin mucosal flap is elevated by submucosal dissection followed by supraperiosteal dissection to the desired extent, excising muscle and subcutaneous tissues. Stay sutures are used to fix the flap to the periosteum deep in the vestibule. The free flap is returned to its original position and sutured.

Obwegeser's maxillary 'Pocket Inlay' vestibuloplasty

This procedure is used for extension of ridge (by increasing vestibular area) in the atrophic maxilla for better retention of the dentures and to restore deficiency in the region of nasolabial fold with improved contour. It is indicated for patients with mandibular anterior teeth that cause occlusal trauma to the maxillary anterior ridge. Here pockets are created on either side of the pyriform aperture and denture flanges are extended into these pockets for stability.

Technique

- Preoperatively patient's denture is modified with extended labial flanges
- Incision is made along the vestibule from one zygomatic buttress to the other
- Supraperiosteal dissection is carried out and two pockets are created on either side of the pyriform aperture extending up to the level of levator anguli oris
- In midline, the dissection is performed up to the pyriform aperture
- Care should be taken not to cause any injury to the nasal cavity
- Impression of the pouch is made with impression compound before placing the graft
- Now, labial flanges of the prefabricated denture are lined with gutta percha and is covered with split thickness graft (the raw surface facing pyriform aperture) and inserted into these pouches
- The denture is fixed in this position with circumzygomatic wires and wound margins sutured to the graft. The wires remain in place for a week
- New dentures are constructed after a period of 6 weeks
- In order to prevent contracture of the pouches, the denture must be worn for a period of 1 year throughout the day and night.

Grafting vestibuloplasty

Indications

- When the available bone is inadequate to compensate for relapse of the vestibuloplasty
- When a bone graft has been previously placed in the surgical site
- When a large surgical defect is present.

Grafts used

- Skin graft
- Mucosal graft (palatal and buccal mucosa)
- Xenograft
- Amnion graft.

Advantages

- Relapse caused by contracture of the wound margin is reduced
- Due to early covering of the surgical defect, patient discomfort is reduced
- Healing is faster.

Disadvantage

Depending on the type of the graft, a 2nd wound would be present at the donor site.

Obwegeser's skin graft technique (1959)

The difference is that here the raw surface of the ridge with its periosteal attachment is covered with a split thickness skin graft in order to maintain the depth of the vestibule at the desired level. Mucosal grafts can also be used for this purpose. In all the ridge extension procedures, a new prosthesis is made after 4–5 weeks. The flange of the new denture should be of sufficient length to maintain the new depth of the sulcus. The denture flange should not irritate the periosteal surface. In spite of all the efforts to increase the vestibular depth, 50% relapse can occur. Therefore, overcorrection is done to compensate this relapse. When the residual bony ridge is too small to perform overcorrection, a free epithelial graft should be considered to cover the wound.

MANDIBULAR VESTIBULOPLASTY TECHNIQUES

Mandibular vestibuloplasty is performed to deepen the labial/buccal or lingual sulcus. It also involves muscle repositioning.

Labial approach

An incision is made deep in the sulcus and supraperiosteal dissection is carried out till the predetermined depth. The raw surface heals by secondary epithelialisation. The drawback of this surgery is that during the healing process, the sulcus tends to get obliterated due to scar contracture. In order to prevent scar contracture, techniques have been designed to reposition or 'switch' the mucosa to cover the raw defect of the deepened vestibule. They are:

- Kazanjian's technique
- Godwin's technique

- Clark's technique
- Obwegeser's modification
- Lip switch technique.

Kazanjian's technique (1924) (Fig. 21.29)

An incision is made in the mucosa of the lip and a large flap of labial and vestibular mucosa is retracted. The mentalis muscle is detached from the periosteum to required depth and the vestibule is deepened via supraperiosteal dissection. The periosteum is left intact. A flap of the mucosa from premolar to premolar is turned downwards from the attachment of the alveolar ridge and is placed directly against the periosteum to which it is sutured. A rubber catheter stent can be placed in the deepened sulcus and secured with percutaneous sutures. This catheter helps to hold the flap in its new position and maintain the depth of the vestibule. It is removed after 7 days. The labial donor site is coated with tincture of benzoin compound. The surface heals by granulation and secondary epithelialisation. Contracture of the wound margins takes place. This procedure has a poor prognosis as severe scarring of the lip mucosa occurs, which decreases proper movement of the lower lip.

Godwin's technique (1947) (Fig. 21.30)

It is similar to the Kazanjian's method in which a flap of labial mucosa is raised, but the vestibule is deepened by subperiosteal stripping instead of supraperiosteal dissection. The periosteum and the connective tissue attached to it are pushed downwards and the flap of labial and vestibular mucosa is placed against the bone and sutured to the connective tissue beyond the deepened vestibule with the help of resorbable sutures. Now, a rubber catheter is placed in the deepened sulcus and secured by means of percutaneous sutures. The catheter is left in place for 11 days. Meanwhile, raw tissue on the labial side is packed with zinc oxide eugenol dressing, which heals by secondary epithelialisation and scar contracture. The greatest disadvantage of Kazanjian's and Godwin's technique is that the scar contracture, which takes place on the labial side, leads to reduction in the vestibular depth.

Clark's technique (1953) (Fig. 21.31)

Clark's technique is the reverse technique of the Kazanjian's technique. It is based on the following principles:

1. Raw surface on connective tissue contracts, whereas when covered with epithelium will have minimum contracture

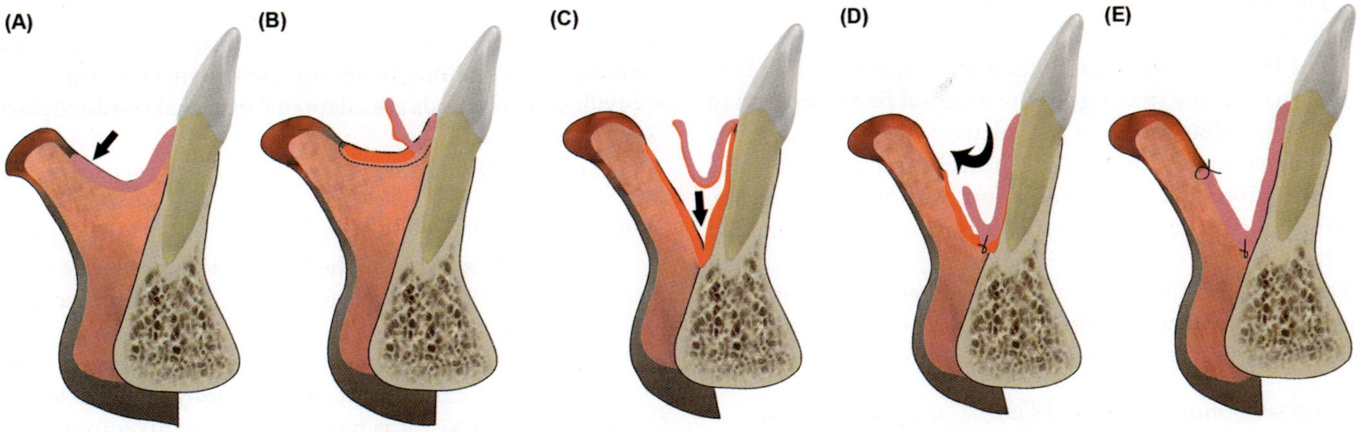

Figure 21.29 **(A–E)** Kazanjian's method of vestibuloplasty.

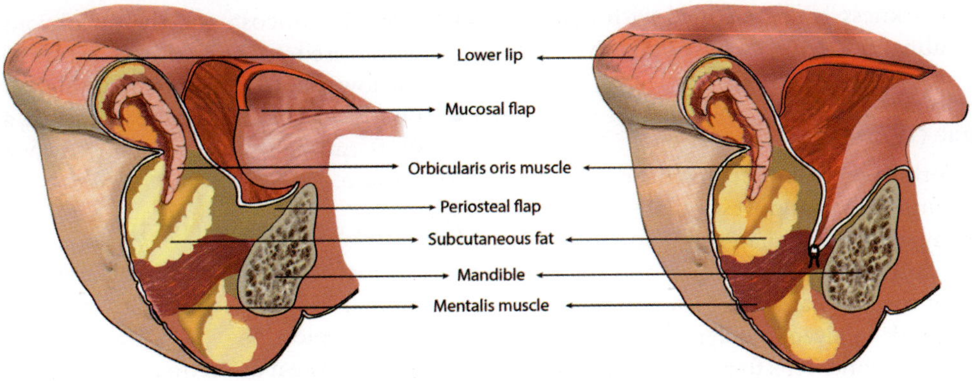

Figure 21.30 Godwin's method of vestibuloplasty.

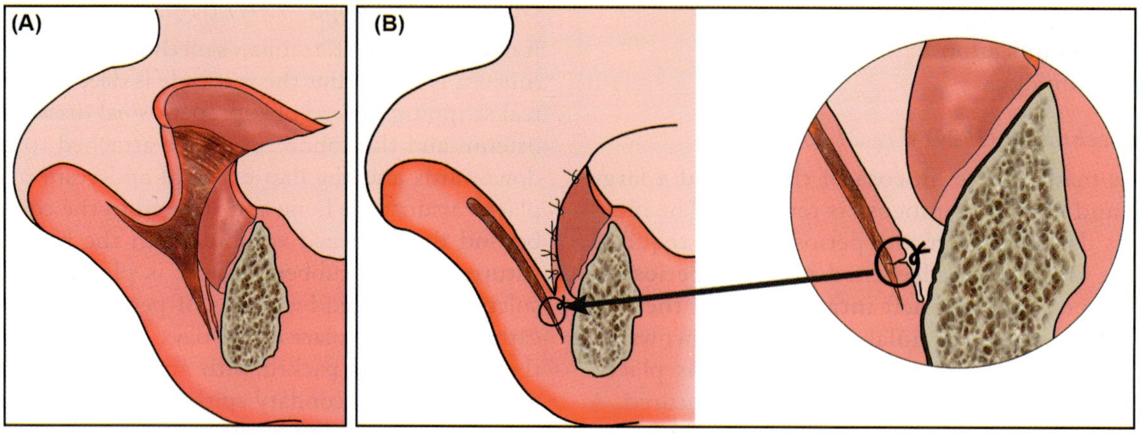

Figure 21.31 (A & B) Clark's method of vestibuloplasty.

2. Raw surface on bone does not undergo contracture
3. For repositioning and fixation, epithelial flap must be undermined adequately
4. Soft tissues which are repositioned tend to return to their normal position, therefore overcorrection is necessary
5. The flap is pedicled off from the lip, the raw surface of the bone is left exposed
6. An incision is made slightly labial to the crest of the alveolar ridge
7. The dissection is carried out supraperiosteally till the desired depth of the sulcus
8. The lip mucosa is undermined up to the vermilion border so that the free edge of the mucosal flap is secured to the periosteum deep in the sulcus
9. The raw surface on the bone heals by granulation tissue formation and epithelialisation without contracture. Initially the depth of the sulcus is maintained for a long time.

Drawback of the technique is that relapse is common since the attachment of the lip musculature to the alveolar bone shifts towards the alveolar crest, obliterating the sulcus.

Obwegeser's modification (1959)

This was a modification of Clark's technique for the mandibular vestibuloplasty. Similar to the maxillary graft vestibuloplasty, the area of periosteum over the alveolar bone is covered with a split thickness graft and held with a stent. This allows faster healing and reduces post-operative scarring and infection.

Lip switch technique (1978)

It was described by Kethley and Gamble. In this procedure, mucosal flap containing labial and vestibular mucosa is raised in a similar way as in Kazanjian's and in Godwin's technique which has its free margin in the lip and the base attached to the crest of the alveolar ridge. However, here the periosteum is incised high in alveolar ridge below the crest and it is reflected from the bone. This flap consisting of periosteum, connective tissue and muscle is turned outwardly and sutured to the margins of the raw labial surface. Now the mucosal flap is turned downwards against the bare bone and sutured to the periosteum deep in the vestibule.

Lingual vestibuloplasty

Lingual vestibuloplasty is used in patients with extensively resorbed mandible. Mylohyoid and genioglossus muscles attached to the lingual aspect of the mandible interfere with the stability of the prosthesis and try to dislodge them. In these patients, extension of the lingual sulcus (or lowering of the floor of the mouth) can help in increasing the denture retention and stability by increasing the surface area.

Following methods are adapted for lingual vestibuloplasty:

- Trauner's technique
- Caldwell's technique.

Trauner's technique (1952)

- An incision is made in the floor of the mouth extending from the 2nd molar of one side to the 2nd molar of the other side
- The mucosa is reflected lingually and supraperiosteal dissection is carried out, once mylohyoid muscle is exposed, a haemostat is passed through this muscle in the canine region and the muscle fibres incised on the haemostat to avoid any injury to the periosteum and the lingual nerve
- Now the mucosa and the mylohyoid muscle are secured with percutaneous sutures extraorally over the skin to the lower border of the mandible
- On the lingual side of the mandible, a split thickness skin graft can be used on a stent to cover the raw periosteal surface.

Caldwell's technique (1955)

- An incision is made in the crest of the posterior mandibular ridge extending from one molar to the other molar region
- Subperiosteal dissection is carried out and a full thickness mucoperiosteal flap is elevated and reflected medially.

The mylohyoid muscle is detached and mylohyoid ridge is removed or reduced

- The subperiosteal stripping is carried out till the desired depth and sometimes even to the inferior border of the mandible. A rubber catheter is placed in the bottom of the lingual sulcus and secured with percutaneous suture. It is left in place for 7–10 days.

Combination of buccal and lingual vestibuloplasty (Fig. 21.32)

Obwegeser's technique (1963)

- The lingual sulcus is 1st deepened as described by Trauner
- Genioglossal fibres are detached leaving the medial and inferior fibres to maintain muscular control of the tongue
- The mylohyoid muscle attachment is detached next
- Now the labiobuccal vestibule is deepened as described by Obwegeser for skin graft vestibuloplasty
- The edges of the buccal and the lingual flaps along with mylohyoid are sutured to each other below the inferior border of the mandible with the help of an awl. Entire alveolar ridge is now covered with skin graft
- Prepared stent is lined with a split thickness skin graft, which is ligated to the mandible using circumferential sutures. The stent can be removed after 7–10 days.

REDUNDANT TISSUE EXCISION

Alveolar flabby ridge (hypermobile soft tissues on the alveolar ridge) (Fig. 21.33)

As a result of resorption of the residual alveolar bone or ill-fitting dentures or both, excessive hypermobile tissue can be seen on the residual alveolar ridge. This is most commonly

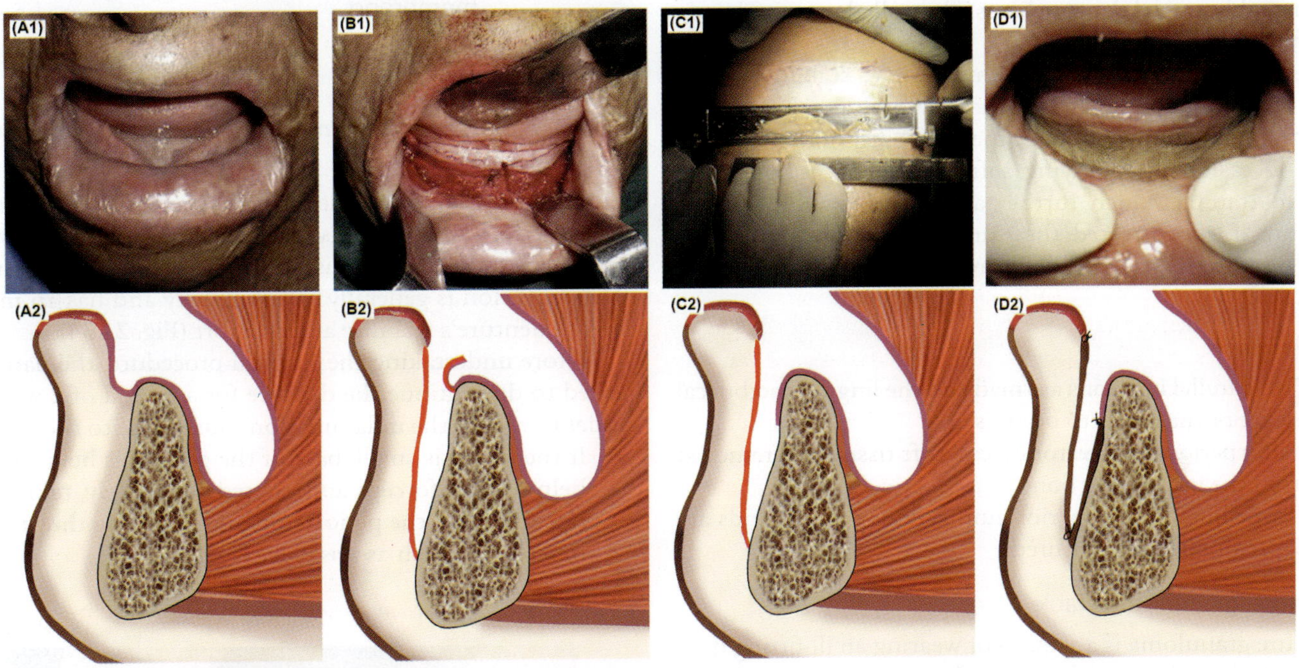

Figure 21.32 (A1-D2) Obwegeser's technique—grafting vestibuloplasty (SSG—split thickness skin graft harvested from thigh region).

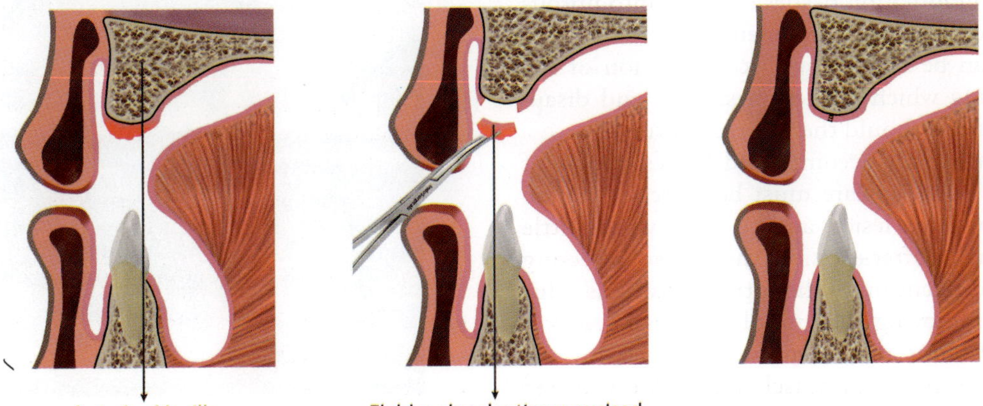

Figure 21.33 Removal of hypermobile tissue from the anterior maxillary alveolar ridge.

seen in maxillary anterior region, most commonly as a part of Kelly's combination syndrome.

Kelly's combination syndrome

In 1972, Kelly collectively called the sequential destructive changes in the hard and soft tissues of the oral cavity seen in patients requiring singular restoration of a completely edentulous arch opposing a natural dentition as combination syndrome.

The characteristic features that occur when an edentulous maxilla is opposed by natural mandibular anterior teeth are:

- Loss of bone from the anterior portion of the maxillary ridge
- Overgrowth of the tuberosity
- Papillary hyperplasia of the hard palatal mucosa
- Extrusion of mandibular anterior teeth
- Loss of alveolar bone and ridge height beneath the removable partial denture bases, also called anterior hyperfunction syndrome.

As these soft tissues are compressible, stability of the denture is jeopardised (the denture will have a rocking movement), which in turn increases the possibility of bone resorption. Occasionally, overlying soft tissue may get ulcerated due to trauma, which further affects the stability of the denture. If left untreated, these unsupported alveolar tissues may increase in size and even prolapse towards the palatal direction.

Technique

- Two parallel incisions are made on the lingual and buccal aspect of the tissue to be excised
- Using periosteal elevator excess, soft tissues are removed from the underlying bone
- Tunnelling of mucoperiosteum is done and the ends are approximated and sutured.

Denture granuloma (Table 21.4)

Denture granuloma is a sequela of wearing an ill-fitting denture. An ill-fitting denture and its flanges compress the adjacent soft tissues, causing formation of ulcers and granulation tissues. These granulation tissues organise into fibrous tissues and the lesion becomes permanent.

- Early lesions can be treated by discontinuation of the denture following which the lesion shrinks and disappears. New dentures should then be reconstructed
- Late lesions are mostly accompanied by resorption of the underlying bone, so care must be exercised not to remove the unwanted lesion and to preserve the little sulcus that remains after excision, thereby not affecting the stability and retention of the future prosthesis. This is achieved by removing the granulation tissue with a combination of blunt and sharp dissection, leaving the underlying periosteum and muscle intact. Care should be taken not to injure the mental nerve while performing the procedure on the mandible.

TABLE 21.4 Howe's Classification of Denture Granuloma

Class	Situation of the Lesion	Treatment protocol
I	Lesions entirely situated upon the mucoperiosteum	Heals well with minimum scarring
II	Lesions entirely attached to the mucous membrane of the cheek, lip or floor of the mouth	The wound should not be closed under tension; heals by primary intention
III	Lesions whose attachments saddle and obliterate the reflection of mucous membrane	Needs epithelial covering

Epulis fissuratum (inflammatory fibrous hyperplasia, denture fibrosis)

Epulis fissuratum is a generalised hyperplastic expansion of the mucosa and fibrous tissue in the vestibular and alveolar area that is frequently caused by chronic denture irritation. The condition is generally inflammatory and has an impact on the denture's stability and comfort (Fig. 21.34).

Before undertaking the surgical procedure, the patient is asked to discontinue the denture for a period of 2 weeks in order to reduce the inflammation caused due to the denture.

- If the lesion is small, base of the growth is held with the help of Allis forceps and excised completely, taking care not to violate the periosteum and retaining the attached mucosa as much as possible (Fig. 21.35)

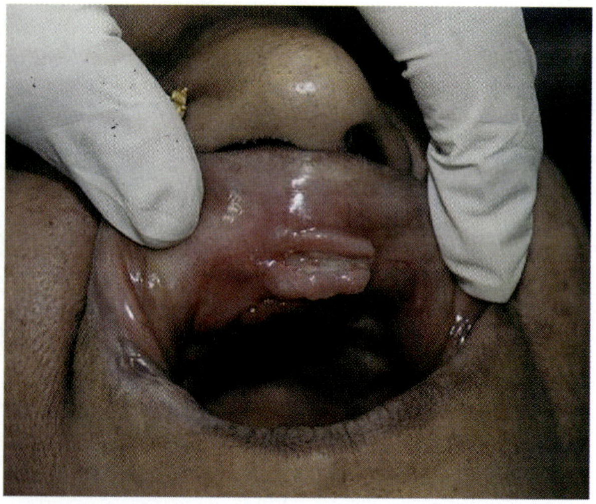

Figure 21.34 Epulis fissuratum in maxillary anterior region following prolonged denture usage.

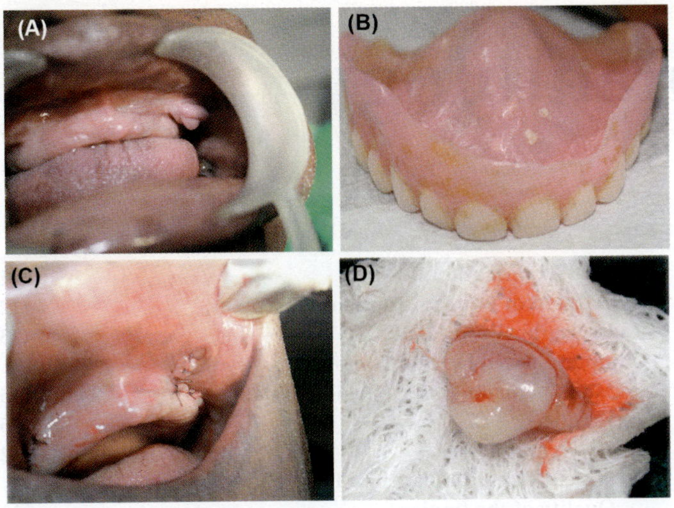

Figure 21.35 **(A)** Epulis fissuratum in left maxillary posterior region in relation to sharp edge of complete denture (inset). **(B-D)** Surgical excision of the growth at the base of the lesion.

- Sometimes, sharp submucosal dissection is done to form a flap followed by sharp submucosal excision of the growth. The flap is then sutured back to the periosteum in order to maintain the vestibular depth
- When severely scarred tissues are present, excision or submucosal dissection of the growth leads to extensive contracture relapse and loss of vestibular depth. Therefore, in these cases, the epulis is 1st excised followed by supraperiosteal placement of free mucosal palatal graft to extend the depth of the vestibule
- Denture splints can be used to protect the graft site.

Reactive inflammatory hyperplasia of the palate (Fig. 21.36)

Reactive inflammatory hyperplasia of the palate is characterised by the presence of red nodules or papillary growth on the palatal mucosa. It is a sequela of chronic use of ill-fitting maxillary complete or partial denture. Sometimes construction of a denture on a preexisting papillomatosis also leads to the situation (Fig. 21.13).

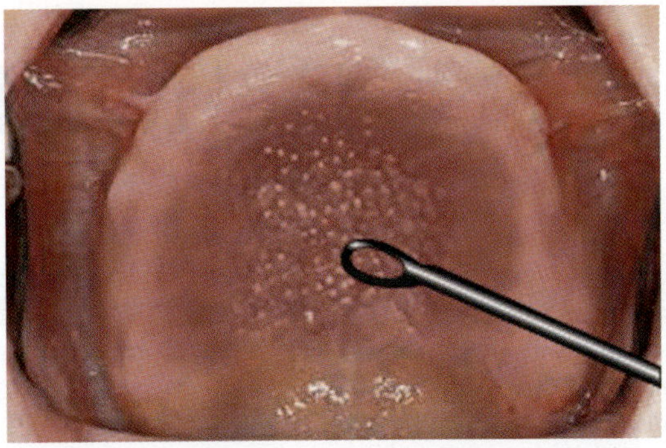

Figure 21.36 Removal of papillary hyperplasia.

- Initial treatments involve discontinuation of the denture or reducing its use
- If candidiasis is present, it should be treated 1st with appropriate antifungal agents and the denture should be relined
- Small masses can be removed with the help of a curette by scraping on the surface of the palate until the corium is reached
- Mucoabrasion can be done with slow-moving, nongouging bur at a slow speed accompanied with copious irrigation
- Electrocautery and loop electrodes can also be used for complete excision. The loop is used slowly in a paintbrush fashion but may require several procedures for complete removal. The proper depth of excision is till the submucosa. Care should be taken not to penetrate the periosteum as this might result in sloughing of the palate resulting in delayed healing
- Once the growths are excised, a relined denture or a prefabricated acrylic stent with soft reline must be used to prevent haemostasis and for wound protection
- Usually healing by epithelialisation is complete within 3–5 weeks.

Chapter 22

Dental Implantology

OUTLINE

INTRODUCTION

DEFINITION

A prosthetic device made of alloplastic material(s) implanted into the oral tissues beneath the mucosal and/or periosteal layer and on or within the bone to provide retention and support for a fixed or removable dental prosthesis; a substance that is placed into and/or on the jaw bone to support a fixed or removable dental prosthesis (GPT—Glossary of Prosthodontic Terms) (Fig. 22.1).

HISTORY/EVOLUTION

Dental implants are surgically fixed substitutes made up of biomaterials for roots of missing teeth. They are embedded in the bone and act as anchors for a replacement of tooth or teeth crown or a full set of dentitions. Dental implantology is the study of the art and science concerned with surgical insertion and restoration of materials and devices restoring the function of the partially or totally edentulous patient. Replacing a single missing tooth with a dental implant has high success rates. It also does not compromise the adjacent natural dentition.

EVOLUTION OF DENTAL IMPLANT MATERIALS (Table 22.1)

CONCEPTS OF OSSEOINTEGRATION

Definition of osseointegration (Fig. 22.2)

The apparent direct attachment or connection of osseous tissue to an inert, alloplastic material without intervening fibrous connective tissue is defined as osseointegration.

BIOLOGICAL PRINCIPLES FOR OSSEOINTEGRATION

Theories on bone to implant interface

1. Weiss' theory of fibro-osseous integration (Linkow 1970, James 1975 and Weiss 1986).
2. Brånemark's theory of osseointegration (supported by Brånemark, Zarb and Albrektsson 1985).

Weiss' theory of fibro-osseous integration

Weiss stated that the presence of collagen fibres at the interface between the implant and bone is a periimplant membrane with an osteogenic effect. He believed that these collagen fibres weave around the implant, originating at the trabeculae of cancellous bone on one side and reinserting into a trabeculae on the other side. He suggested early loading of an implant. However, the collagen fibres around the implant are oriented differently from fibres in the periodontal ligament (PDL) of natural teeth. The implant fibres are usually irregular and parallel to the implant body rather than perpendicular like PDL fibres. Fibro-integration is seen with implant systems that may have a good initial success rate but whose success rates drop off rapidly in the long term.

Brånemark's theory of osseointegration

In 1985, Brånemark, Zarb and Albrektsson defined osseointegration as the direct structural and functional connection between ordered, living bone and the surface of a load-carrying implant. Brånemark proposed that implants integrate such that the bone is laid very close to the implant without any intervening connective tissue. The titanium oxide permanently fuses with the bone, as Brånemark showed at the light microscopic level of magnification in the 1950s. With osseointegration, the root form of dental implant became the most dominant design in implantology. Rigid fixation is denoted by the absence of mobility with 1–5 N force applied in vertical or horizontal direction. There are 14 factors necessary to achieve a successful osseointegrated bone-to-implant interface. These factors are discussed in Table 22.2.

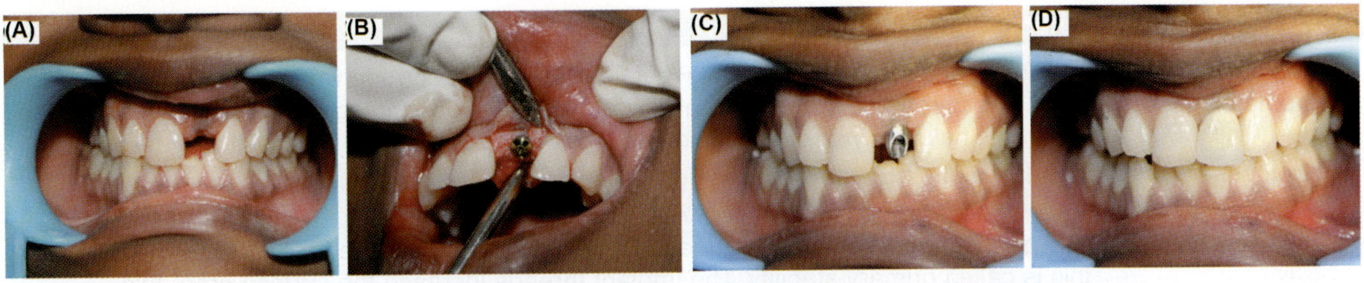

Figure 22.1 (**A-D**) Restoration of partially edentulous space with implants.

TABLE 22.1 Evolution of Dental Implant Materials

2500 BC	Egyptians	Gold wire to stabilise teeth
500 BC	Etruscans	Oxen bones
600 BC	Mayans	Shells
1700	J. Hunter	Teeth transplantation between humans
1809	J. Maggiolo	Gold implant tube as artificial root—failed
1930	A. and M. Strock	Vitallium orthopaedic screws as implants
1938	P. B. Adams	Cylindrical endosseous implants
1940s	M. Formiggini and F. Zepponi G. Dhal	Post-type endosseous implant Subperiosteal implants—Sweden
1952s 1965	Per-Ingvar Brånemark	Discovers osseointegration Treated 1st patient for full mouth rehabilitation with titanium implants
1968	L. Linkow	Blade implants for partially edentulous
1983	M. Anderson	1st CAD/CAM ceramic coping
1986	Lederman	Hand titanium system
1996	Doughlas et al.,	Endopore implant
1996	Per-Ingvar Brånemark	Novum concept—full set mandibular implants in a single day
1998	P. Malo	All-on-four treatment concept
1998	Per-Ingvar Brånemark	Zygomaticus implants
2005	Nobel Biocare	3D treatment planning and guided surgery

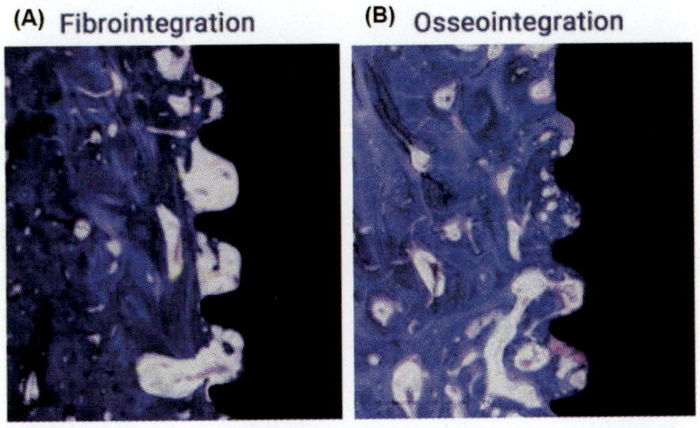

Figure 22.2 (**A**) Fibro-osseous integration can be seen at the pitch of the implant. Fibrous tissue is seen in between the bone and implant surface. (**B**) Bone-implant contact with healthy dense collagenous tissue between the implant and bone showing complete osseointegration.

Bone tissue responses to implants (*Fig. 22.3*)

Healing process may be by primary bone healing or secondary bone healing. Primary bone healing is ideal where well organised bone forms with minimal granulation tissue. Secondary bone healing is undesirable as it has granulation tissue formation; this prolongs the healing period. Fibrocartilage is sometimes formed instead of bone. The implant design consists of two consecutive profiles of the pitch. Pitch is the U-shaped circumferential trough that runs throughout the implant. It engages hard tissue walls. Initially after placement of the implant, the void between the pitches is filled with blood clot. This area is called the wound chamber. Erythrocytes, neutrophils and monocytes are present in the wound chamber, and leukocytes start the cleansing process. Four days into healing, fibroplasia starts where coagulum gets replaced by granulation tissue. Mesenchymal cells are

TABLE 22.2 Factors Determining Osseointegration

1	Implant biomaterial	Titanium is the most biocompatible metal as it does not corrode when in contact with bodily fluids. It is unreactive with biological tissue and allows osseointegration. The protective oxide film forms naturally with oxygen and prevents reactions between the metal and the tissues.
2	Biomechanics	The 1st month after implant insertion is critical for initial healing. If loads are applied to the implants during this stage, primary stability may be destroyed.
3	Implant design	The geometry of the implant influences its initial stability at the time of placement—this is called primary stability. The implant threads increase the surface area, this distributes the forces of occlusion into the bone. Thread design, Thread pitch, Thread shape, Thread depth.
4	Implant taper	The taper should not be greater than 30 degree. The larger the taper, greater the compressive load to the interface.
5	Apical design	Anti-rotational features in the implant like • a vent or hole in the apex of the implant • grooves at the apex
6	Implant width	Cylindrical preparations are made in the correct size and shape with precision instrumentation and a sound surgical procedure. This will minimise the distance between the implant and bone.
7	Crest module design	A smooth crest module design will result in shear stress. Angled crest module of more than 20 degree is beneficial. Crest module should be a little larger than the outer thread diameter.
8	Implant surface topography	Surface texture increases the surface area of the implant and thus the area of bone-implant contact. Research has shown that rougher the surface, faster the osseointegration. However, it also facilitates the growth of bacteria. The neck of the implant is kept polished to reduce plaque retention where the implant is exposed to the oral cavity.
9	Implant surface modifications	The methods of creating a roughened surface are by sandblasting particles of aluminium or titanium oxide or acid etching the surface. Pits of 1.5 μm are created as a result of the sprayed particles.
10	Contamination	The implant should be sterile to produce osseointegration.
11	Heat production	If the gap between the implant and the bone is minimal and surgery is atraumatic to allow minimal mechanical and thermal injury, osseointegration will be rapid. More than 47 degree during drilling can cause cell death.
12	Loading time	Early loading causes fibrous connective tissue encapsulation around the implant. *Minimum integration time:* Anterior mandible—3 months Posterior mandible—4 months Anterior maxilla—6 months Posterior maxilla—6 months Bone graft—6–9 months
13	Surgical factors	Tissue handling Profuse irrigation Sharp drills Drill speed less than 2000 rpm Torque wrench with moderate torque of 45 N/cm is ideal
14	Patient factors	Age Compromised oral hygiene Smoking Anaemia Vitamin C deficiency Periodontal disease Uncontrolled systemic disease Chemotherapy/Radiotherapy Bone density Available bone

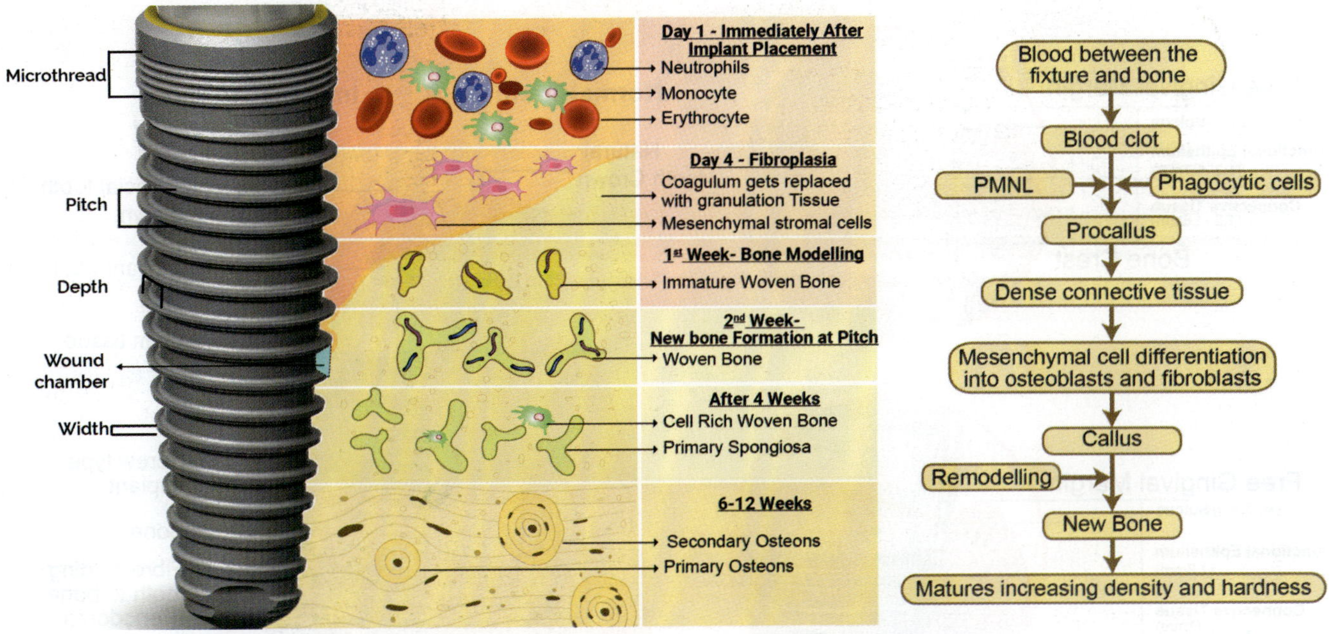

Figure 22.3 Bone tissue response to implant placement, the parts of the implant body have been marked. At day 1, the area between the bone and implant consists of blood clot. The bone response from day 1 to 12 weeks (3 months) have been illustrated. The wound chamber fills up with new bone at the 2nd week. After 12 weeks, remodelling of the callus occurs (PMNL-Neutrophils).

formed with the other components of the matrix. Angiogenesis occurs in the matrix and provisional connective tissue forms. The next stage is bone modelling at 1 week of healing, vascular structures with few inflammatory cells develop cell rich immature (woven) bone. This also occurs at the centre of the wound chamber and at direct contact of implant surface. This is followed by the 1st phase of osseointegration at 2 weeks; in this phase, the woven bone becomes pronounced. Woven bone extends from the parent bone into the connective tissue, making mature osseointegration possible. At the pitch, new bone formation starts. At the recipient site, the site immediate to implant in direct contact with bone, bone resorption occurs with new bone formation. After 4 weeks, cell-rich woven bone covers most of the titanium. The central portion contains primary spongiosa with vascular structures and mesenchymal cells. After 6–12 weeks, mineralised bone forms by the primary and secondary osteons, forming bone marrow with adipocytes and mesenchymal cells.

COMPARISON BETWEEN TOOTH AND IMPLANT SURFACE (Fig. 22.4)

The PDL is a suspension system for the natural tooth to transfer all occlusal loads to the alveolar bone. This micromovement to dissipate limited overloads is seen with natural teeth. Implants transfer occlusal loads directly to the bone due to the absence of PDL. Overload in off-axis directions lead to immediate bone loss. While the teeth start moving with these stresses, implants cannot orthodontically move to dissipate loads. Therefore, stresses easily result in bone loss or other clinical complications like screw loosening, implant fracture and sudden bone necrosis with excessive parafunctional loads.

The implant surface is porous and rough in most implant designs. This can allow bacterial biofilm to exist in numbers more than on the natural tooth's root surface. Detoxification of implant surface can prevent periimplantitis as described in page 434 (Table 22.18).

SOFT TISSUE-IMPLANT INTERFACE

Comparison of normal teeth and implant (Fig. 22.4)

Gingiva and periimplant soft tissues

In the healthy adult, the gingival margin is located on the enamel. A group of gingival connective tissue fibres that form bundles of interdental fibres, dentogingival fibres, are inserted into the root cementoenamel junction, and they depend on the presence of natural teeth. In case of implants, a transmucosal element protrudes through the overlying mucosa, which adapts around the implant. The collagen fibres within the periimplant mucosa run parallel to the abutment with no insertion in the abutment surface. This tight cuff of the fibrous connective tissue, which runs parallel to the implant surface, supports the epithelial seal and forms an effective barrier to periimplant pocket formation and bone loss. This may be supported by collagen fibres attached to the adjacent natural tooth, but in case of implants without any neighbouring natural teeth, formation of soft tissue papilla is less predictable.

Junctional epithelium

In natural healthy teeth, the junctional epithelium is attached to the enamel by hemidesmosomal contacts and a basal lamina-like structure formed by the epithelial cells. A

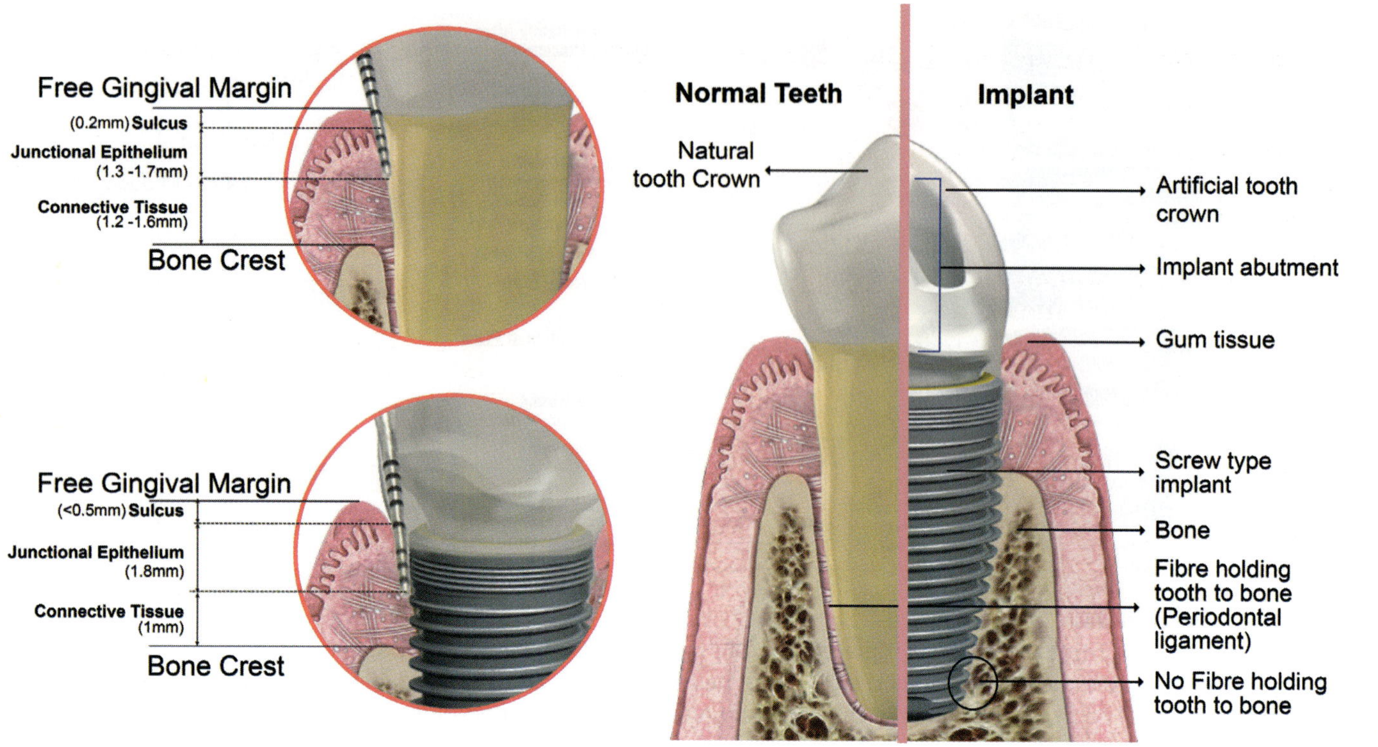

Figure 22.4 Gross difference of implant and tooth has been illustrated. The biological width has also been marked for normal teeth and implant.

similar normal junctional epithelium can be regenerated from the adjacent oral mucosa following excision or damage. This helps in any form of breach in the integrity of the junctional epithelium around the implants.

Biological width

It is the zone of attached connective tissue that separates the underlying alveolar bone from the apical termination of the junctional epithelium. The length of the junctional epithelium is about 1.5 mm and the connective tissue zone is about 2 mm wide. This may vary in various implant systems. Periodontal probing of natural teeth forms an important part of any dental examination. The probe penetrates the junctional epithelium to some degree while examining, and this penetration increases in the presence of inflammation. It usually stops about 2 mm from the bone. In implants, probing depth is generally deeper than around the natural teeth. Hence, clinicians are advised to rely on radiographic assessment of bone level rather than probing.

Periodontal ligament and osseointegration

PDL is a complex structure with a width of 0.1-0.2 mm that supports the natural teeth. Sharpey's fibres are embedded in the root cementum and alveolar bone. On the contrary, precise nature of osseointegration at the molecular level is not yet defined. At the low-power microscopic level, bone is very closely adapted to the implant. However, at a higher magnification, a small gap can be identified, occupied by the intervening collagen rich zone near the bone and an absolute phenomenon. It only represents the proportion of the total implant surface that is in contact with bone. It is similar to ankylosis where absence of mobility and the absence of intervening fibrous tissue are the indications of successful osseointegration.

Components of endosteal implants

A generic language for endosteal implants has been developed by Misch. The components are described in Table 22.3.

TABLE 22.3 Components of Endosteal Implants

Implant body regions	Crest module Body Apex
Surgical accessories	Surgical guide/implant stent Cover screw Transepithelial portion (permucosal extension, healing abutment, gingival former)
Prosthetic accessories	Abutment Superstructure Transfer coping Prosthetic coping Analogue

IMPLANT BODY REGION/IMPLANT FIXTURE

It is the component that is surgically fixed into the bone.

Crest module

Crest module of an implant is that portion designed to retain the prosthetic component. It is the transition zone between the implant fixture and the implant at the crest of the ridge. The abutment connection area often has a platform on which the abutment is set, the platform offers physical resistance to axial occlusal loads. The crest module is often smoother which impairs plaque retention if crestal bone loss occurs.

Body

The body of the implant may be cylindrical or tapered, with a threaded or a smooth surface. It can contain holes or vents to cancel antirotational forces. The most preferred type is those with threads as it increases the surface area for osseointegration. The threads also maximise the contact with bone to dissipate stresses. Threads have different shapes and designs (Fig. 22.5).

Apex

The design of the apex provides antirotational features in the implant like a vent or hole in the apex of the implant or grooves at the apex. A maximum of 30 N/cm rotational force can be applied. The apex design is better flat than sharp to protect soft tissue.

IMPLANT COMPONENTS USED IN SURGICAL STAGE I (Fig. 22.6)

Surgical guide/Implant stent

Surgical template is a guide used to assist in proper surgical placement and angulation of dental implants. The main objective of the surgical template is to direct the implant drilling system into the bone and provide accurate placement of the implant according to the surgical treatment plan (Fig. 22.7A).

In case of a one-stage procedure, after placement of the implant body, the surgeon decides to either place the cover screw or the healing abutment based on the attainment of primary stability and the loading protocol.

Cover screw

It is placed in the stage I surgery and is used to cover the implant to prevent bone, soft tissue or debris from invading the abutment connection area during healing (Fig. 22.7B).

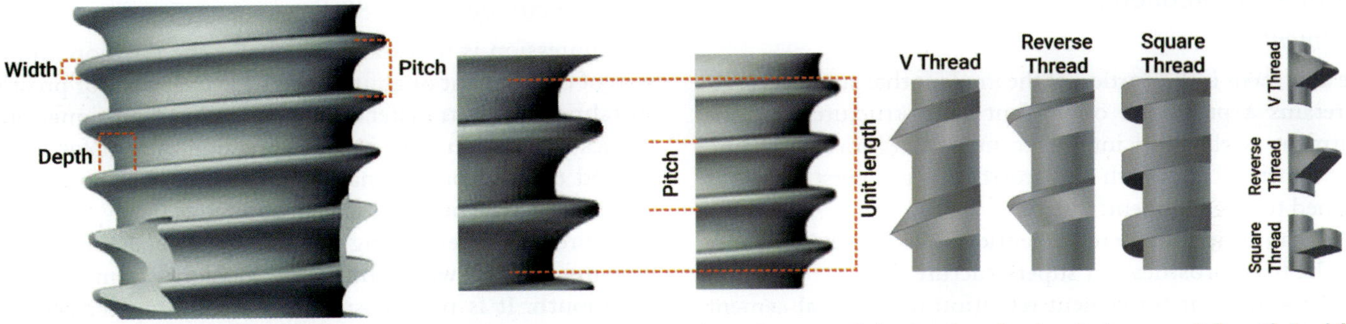

Figure 22.5 Thread design—V thread, square thread and reverse thread, parts of the implant body, pitch per unit length in different implants.

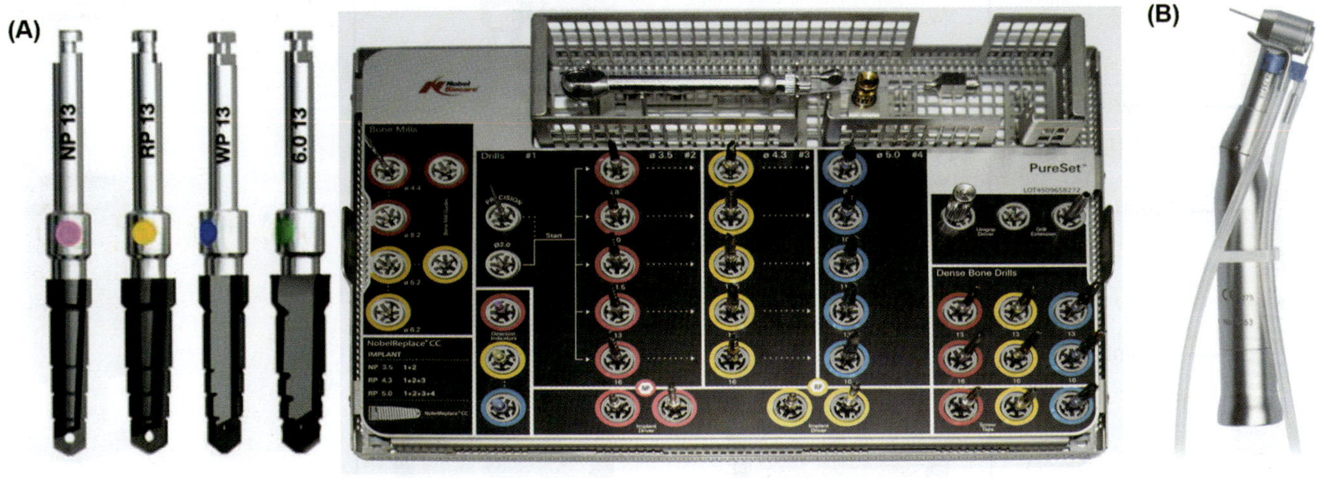

Figure 22.6 (**A**) Dental implant kit with drills of various sizes. (**B**) Handpiece with external and internal irrigators.

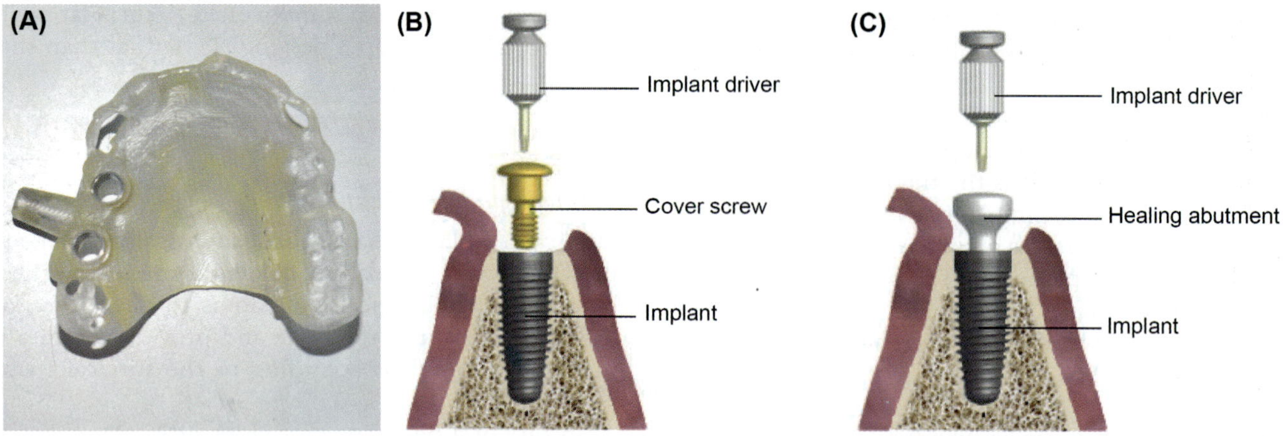

Figure 22.7 (A) Surgical implant guide (B) Cover screw with the implant screwdriver (C) Healing abutment with implant screwdriver.

IMPLANT COMPONENTS USED IN SURGICAL STAGE II

Transepithelial portion (permucosal extension, healing abutment, gingival former)

It is attached to the implant in the stage II surgery after removing the cover screw. This portion extends from the implant above the soft tissues and results in the development of a perimucosal seal around the implant (Fig. 22.7C).

Prosthetic components

Abutment

The abutment is the portion of the implant that supports and/or retains a prosthesis or implant superstructure. Implant abutment is classified into three main categories according to the method by which the prosthesis or superstructure is retained to the abutment:

(1) An abutment for screw retention uses a screw to retain the fixed prosthesis or superstructure

(2) An abutment for cement retention uses dental cement to retain the fixed prosthesis or superstructure

(3) An abutment for overdentures uses an attachment device to retain a removable prosthesis (RP4, RP5).

An abutment for screw retention uses a hygienic cover screw placed over the abutment to prevent debris and calculus from invading the internally threaded portion of the abutment during prosthesis fabrication between prosthetic appointments (Fig. 22.8A).

Transfer coping (Fig. 22.8B)

An impression is necessary to transfer the position and design of the implant or abutment to a master cast for prosthesis fabrication. A transfer coping is used in traditional prosthetics to position a die in an impression. A transfer coping is used to position an analogue in an impression material requiring elastic properties.

Indirect transfer coping is screwed into the abutment. It remains in place when the set impression is removed from the mouth. It is parallel-sided or slightly tapered to allow ease in removal of the impression and often has flat sides or

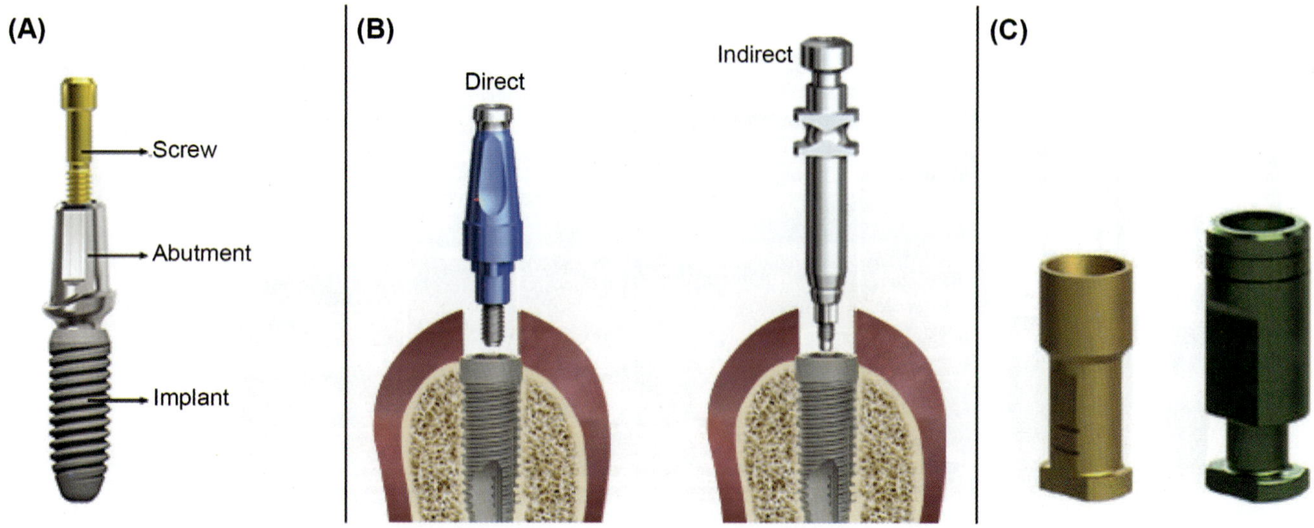

Figure 22.8 **(A)** Titanium abutment with screw **(B)** Transfer coping **(C)** Analogue.

smooth undercuts to facilitate reorientation in the impression after it is removed. A direct transfer coping usually consists of a hollow transfer component and often a square and long central screw to secure it to the abutment of the implant body. After the impression material is set, direct transfer coping remains within the impression until the master model is poured.

Prosthetic coping

A prosthetic coping is a thin covering, usually designed to fit the implant abutment for screw retention and serve as connection between the abutment and the prosthesis for superstructure. A prefabricated coping usually is a metal component machined precisely to fit the abutment. A castable coping usually is a plastic pattern cast in the same prosthesis or suprastructure, secured to the implant body or abutment with a prosthetic screw.

Analogue

An analogue is a replica for the master cast to replicate the abutment. After the master impression is obtained, the corresponding analogue is attached to the transfer coping and assembly is poured in stone to fabricate the master cast (Fig. 22.8C).

CLASSIFICATION/TYPES OF IMPLANTS (FIG. 22.9)

Implants have been classified based on different criteria, but the most easily understood classification is based on the implant-bone relationship, which will be described in detail (endosteal, subperiosteal and transosteal).

Based on the implant-tissue interface

a. Direct bone-implant interface, for example, endosseous implants (osseointegration)
b. Indirect interface, for example, blade and subperiosteal implants.

Based on design and location

a. Submucous
b. Supraperiosteal
c. Subperiosteal
d. Endosseous
e. Transosseous
f. Endodontic.

Based on function

a. Retentive implants: It provides additional retention for the prosthesis with mucosal inserts and magnetic implants
b. Supportive implants: Supportive type provides support to the prosthesis. At the same time, mucous membrane and teeth are relieved from any functional load. They may be intraosseous or extraosseous (subperiosteal).

Based on implant materials

a. Metallic implants
b. Polymer implants
c. Ceramic implants
d. Vitreous carbon implants.

Based on implant design

a. Brånemark implant—Threaded screw
b. Core-vent implant—Open basket with vents combined with threads
c. IMZ implant—Rough plasma sprayed implant surface
d. Stryker implant—Fluted design.

Based on loading protocol

a. Conventional loading/delayed loading/two-stage loading
b. One-stage protocol:
    - Immediate loading
    - Early loading.

Based on bone the implant is placed on

- Alveolar implants
- Pterygoid implants
- Zygoma implants.

Based on implant–bone relationship

- Endosteal implants
- Subperiosteal implants
- Transosteal implants.

ENDOSTEAL IMPLANTS

Endosteal (in the bone) implants are the most commonly used type of implant, which are placed directly into the bone like natural tooth roots and can be used for many purposes. There are various types like root form (screws and cylinders) or blade form, surgically placed into the jaw bone. Each

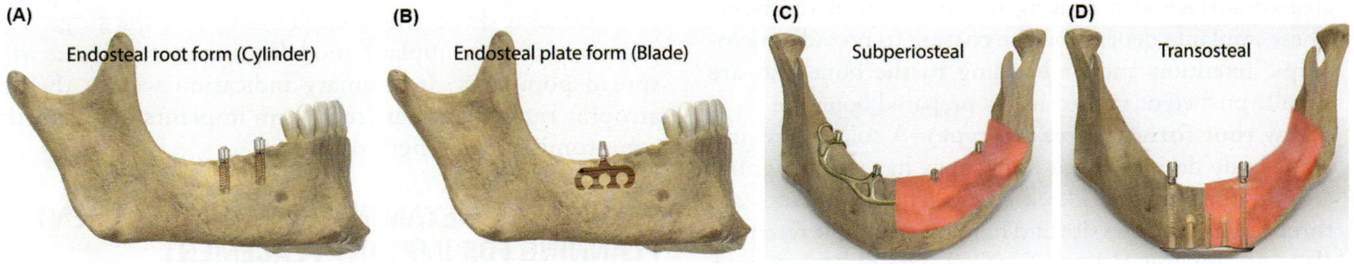

Figure 22.9 **(A)** Endosteal implant—root form. **(B)** Endosteal implant—blade form. **(C)** Subperiosteal implant. **(D)** Transosteal implant.

implant holds one or more prosthetic teeth. Since this implant is placed into the bone, the bone area must be sufficient to support the implant in height, width and length.

ROOT FORM IMPLANTS

- Root form implants mimic the basic shape of the natural root
- Available in a variety of lengths, widths and designs including cylinders (also known as press-fit) and screws (also referred to as threaded) or a combination of the two
- May be used in any area of the mouth
- May replace one or more teeth
- Root forms are further divided based on design into.

Classification of root form endosteal implants

Combination root forms have macroscopic features of both the *cylinder and screw root forms*. The screw or combination root form designs may also benefit from microscopic retention to bone by the addition of coatings. Root forms have also been described by their means of insertion, healing, surgical requirements, surface characteristics and interface.

I. *Their macroscopic body design can be:*
   - Cylindrical
   - Threaded
   - Plateaued
   - Perforated
   - Solid
   - Hollow or vented

II. *Their surface can be:*
   - Smooth—no coating
   - Coated
   - Textured

III. *They are available as:*
   - Submersible
   - Nonsubmersible

IV. *Three basic screw-threaded geometrics:*
   - V-threaded
   - Buttress thread
   - Power (square) thread designs

V. *Surgical stages:*
   - One-stage endosteal implants
   - Two-stage endosteal implants

a. **Cylinder root form implants (press-fit type)**—Most cylinder implants are essentially smooth-sided and bullet-shaped implants and require a bioactive or increased surface area coating for retention in the bone. These implants depend on the coating to provide microscopic retention and/or bonding to the bone and are usually pushed or tapped into a prepared bone site

b. **Screw root forms (threaded type)**—A solid screw implant body design with a blunt apex has threads going around the implant like a screw. These implants are threaded into a bone site and have macroscopic retentive elements for initial bone fixation. The most common thread outer diameter is 3.75 mm, a 0.4 mm depth of thread, with a crest module approximately 2 mm in height and crestal diameter of 4.1 mm. Various lengths range from 7 to 20 mm; lengths from 10 to 16 mm are the most widely used (Fig. 22.5).

Advantages of the screw type of endosteal implant: It permits the preparation and placement of the implant in dense cortical bone as well as in fine trabecular bone. The implant can be removed at the time of surgery if placement is not ideal. If the implant perforates the inferior border of the mandible or maxillary sinus, it avoids complication most of the time if the apex is smooth or blunted. The functional surface area of threaded implant is greater than a cylinder implant depending on the thread geometry. This increase in functional implant surface area decreases the stress imposed on the bone-implant interface. *The choice of whether to use a threaded implant or a press-fit is dependent on the quality of the bone that will support the implant and what will be placed upon the implant when it is healed.*

BLADE FORM IMPLANTS

Blades are wedge-shaped or rectangular in cross-section. They are generally 2.5 mm in width, 8–15 mm in depth and 15–30 mm in length. These implants are flat rectangles of metal with one or two metal prongs on one side. A blade implant is placed in the jaw so that the prongs stick out into the mouth where they will support the crown or bridges.

SUBPERIOSTEAL IMPLANT

To overcome the problem of insufficient bone width to place an endosteal implant, subperiosteal implant can be placed on and around the maxilla and mandible. A subperiosteal implant is a framework specially fabricated to fit on top of supporting areas in the mandible or maxilla under mucoperiosteum with perimucosal extensions for support and attachment of the prosthesis. This is rarely used in practice, especially after the introduction of pterygoid and zygoma implants.

TRANSOSTEAL IMPLANTS

Transosteal implants were inserted through an extraoral incision below the chin with a series of projections that penetrate the mandible from its inferior border and were connected by a bone plate that rests on the inferior border of the mandible. Several of the projections completely transverse the mandible to enter the oral cavity and anchor the lower denture. Transosteal implants can only be used in the anterior mandible due to the complex nature of the surgical approach, and this implant modality has not enjoyed widespread popularity. Its primary indication was in the very atrophic mandible where root form implants might further compromise the strength of the jaw.

PREOPERATIVE EXAMINATION AND TREATMENT PLANNING FOR IMPLANT PLACEMENT

IMPLANT TREATMENT PROTOCOL

Protocol for treatment of implant is depicted in Flowchart 22.1.

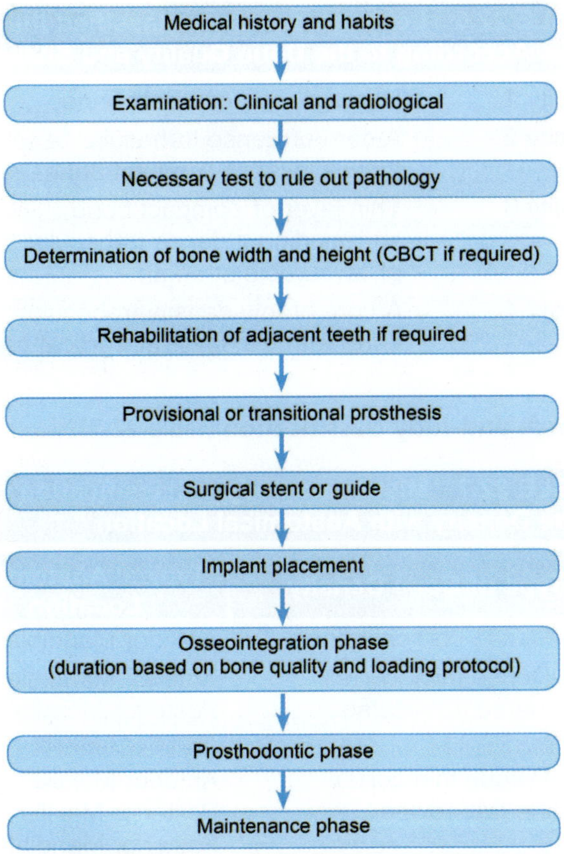

Flowchart 22.1 Implant treatment protocol.

PATIENT SELECTION

The clinician should ensure that the provision of implants will provide better prosthodontic service. The general health conditions and dental status should be evaluated. Availability of sufficient bone should be verified to accommodate the implant. Ridge should be at least 5 mm in width to accommodate any type of implant with a marginal safety of 1 mm on either side; 10 mm in vertical height (in maxilla from alveolar crest to the sinus floor and, in mandible, from the alveolar crest to the mandibular canal). The bony contour below the mylohyoid line is evaluated. If extensive undercuts are present, the implant might perforate the lingual cortex. Study models are necessary to evaluate the occlusion and determine the correct positioning of implants. Radiographic evaluation should be done to aid in the diagnosis.

INDICATIONS & CONTRAINDICATIONS OF IMPLANT TREATMENT (Tables 22.4 and 22.5)

CLINICAL EXAMINATION

Prior to the placement of implants, the patient should be assessed: (1) medical and dental history, (2) clinical examination and (3) radiographic examination.

Medical history: The absolute and relative contraindications have been discussed earlier. Apart from those, the

TABLE 22.4 Indications of Dental Implant

- Patient who does not want removable prosthesis
- Patient with poor oral muscular coordination
- Patient with high gag reflex
- Prolonged edentulous span—multiple implants
- Low tissue tolerance
- To resolve psychological problems associated with edentulism
- When implant achieves superior results in terms of functions and aesthetics

TABLE 22.5 Absolute and Relative Contraindications of Dental Implant

Absolute Contraindications

- Poorly controlled diabetes
- Blood dyscrasias
- Ischaemic heart disease
- Cerebral palsy
- Immunocompromised patients
- Patient on bisphosphonates or other antiangiogenic drugs
- Jaw bone radiation less than 1 year before implant placement
- Acute psychotic disorders
- Acute bone resorption
- Poor patient cooperation
- Underlying bone atrophy due to abnormal stress
- Metabolic disorders
- Musculoskeletal disorders
- Focal and systemic disorders
- Oral submucous fibrosis with limited mouth opening
- Drug or alcohol dependence
- Patient who lacks manual dexterity
- Renal osteodystrophy
- Pregnancy
- Regional malignancy
- Recent myocardial infarction (MI)
- Recent cardiac valve prosthesis

Relative Contraindications

- Patients with uncontrolled diabetes mellitus
- Significant history of smoking
- Cardiac patients with stable condition
- Patient on antidepressant or anticoagulant
- Habits like bruxism or tongue thrusting
- Endocrine disorders
- Trismus
- Chronic maxillary sinusitis (for maxillary implant which may require sinus lift procedures-direct or indirect)
- Erosive diseases
- Hyposalivation
- Osteoporosis
- Uncontrolled hypothyroidism
- History of radiation/chemotherapy

patient should not have any uncontrolled systemic disorders. If the patient is on treatment and the condition is under control, there is no contraindication for placement of implants. History of irradiation should be considered and subsequent hyperbaric oxygen therapy (HBOT) (20 treatments of 90 min each at 2–2.4 atm before surgery) should be advised before implant placement. Emotionally intolerant, perfection-seeking patients may not be willing to wear dentures. All these factors should be considered.

Intraoral assessment: A thorough dental history is taken to rule out any dentofacial disease, which is contraindicated for implant placement. Abnormal jaw relation, atrophic ridge, inadequate and shallow vestibule, abnormal tongue position are some of the structural diseases of the oral cavity, which interfere with denture retention. Periapical and panoramic radiographs provide adequate information with reference to the volume and quality of bone and the location of anatomical limiting factors.

Personal history: Smoking causes vasoconstriction and reduces the blood flow to the healing bone. It compromises polymorphonuclear leukocytes (PMNL) function and increases platelet adhesiveness. Smokers comparatively have more marginal bone loss than a nonsmoker. Smoke cessation is advised. Parafunctional habits like bruxism and clenching produce forces that are greater than 1000 psi that can cause overload on implants. These habits should be corrected before implant placement. If that is not possible, the number of implants should be increased and patients should be given an occlusal splint. Oral hygiene maintenance should also be evaluated and the patient should be advised to maintain good oral hygiene.

ASSESSMENT OF BONE FOR IMPLANT PLACEMENT

CLASSIFICATION OF THE BONE

I. Lekholm and Zarb classification (Fig. 22.10 and Table 22.6)

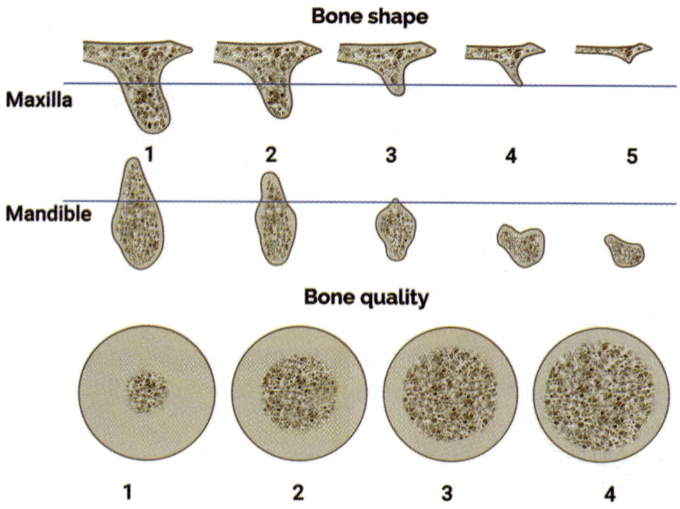

Figure 22.10 Lekholm and Zarb's classification of jaw bone densities.

TABLE 22.6 Lekholm and Zarb Classified the Jaws According to the Bone Quality and Shape

Quality 1	Homogenous compact bone
Quality 2	A core of dense trabecular bone with a thick layer of compact bone
Quality 3	Thin layer of compact bone surrounding a dense trabecular bone of favourable strength
Quality 4	A core of low-density trabecular bone with thin layer of cortical bone

II. Misch and Judy classification (Table 22.7)

TABLE 22.7 Misch and Judy's Classification of Bone Density with Anatomical Location

Type of Bone Density	Typical Anatomical Location
D1—Dense cortical bone	Anterior Mandible
D2—Dense thick cortex and coarse trabeculae	Anterior Mandible Posterior Mandible Anterior Maxilla
D3—Porous thin cortex and fine trabeculae	Anterior Maxilla Posterior Maxilla Posterior Mandible
D4—Fine trabeculae	Posterior Maxilla

BONY CRITERIA FOR IMPLANT PLACEMENT

- *Bone height*
- *Bone width*
- *Bone length*
- *Bone angulation.*

Bone height

The height of available bone is measured from the crest of the edentulous ridge to the opposing landmark such as the maxillary sinus or mandibular canal in the posterior regions. Anterior regions are limited by nasal cavity or inferior border of the mandible. Maxillary canine eminence region offers greater height of available bone than the maxillary anterior or posterior regions. The minimum bone height for predictable long-term endosteal implant survival approaches 10 mm. There should be a minimum of 2 mm height between the apex of the implant and the inferior alveolar canal (Fig. 22.11). In the maxilla due to excessive pneumatisation of the maxillary antrum, atrophy of the maxillary ridge and the floor of the sinus almost comes to lie very close to the maxillary alveolar crest. Maxillary sinus lift procedure is carried out to lift the floor of the sinus lining by placing a graft in between the maxillary sinus lining and the floor of the maxillary antrum in the posterior aspect (Fig. 22.12).

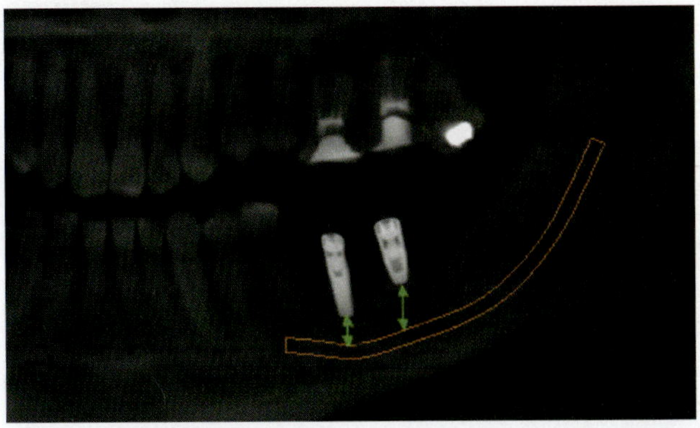

Figure 22.11 Position of implant in relation to inferior alveolar nerve (minimum of 2 mm height between apex of the implant and the inferior alveolar canal).

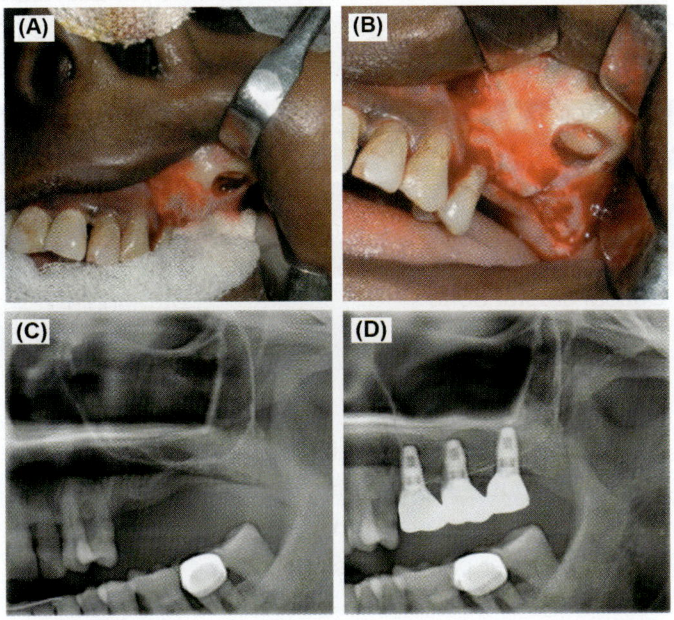

Figure 22.12 Sinus lift procedure. (**A** and **B**) Intraoral view showing infracturing of the bony window and lifting of the left maxillary sinus. (**C**) Preoperative OPG showing reduced bone height in relation to 26, 27 and 28. (**D**) Postoperative OPG showing adequate bone fill favourable for implant placement.

Bone width

The width of available bone is measured between the buccal and lingual plates at the crest of the potential implant site. Crest of the edentulous ridge is supported by a wider base. Root form implants of 4.0 mm crestal diameter usually require more than 5.0 mm of bone width to ensure sufficient bone thickness and blood supply around the implant for predictable survival. These dimensions provide more than 0.5 mm bone on each side of the implant at the crest. Because bone usually widens apically, this minimum dimension rapidly increases. In case of bony defects, local regional bone graft, bone shavings near the implant area and cortico-cancellous graft can be used.

Bone mesiodistal length (Fig. 22.13)

Mesiodistal length is the area of bone that is usually limited by adjacent teeth or implants. For a mesiodistal length of 7 mm, a minimum width of 5 mm implant will be sufficient to bear the load. For mesiodistal length of 14 mm, one implant will have a cantilever of 5 mm of the prosthesis. This will reduce the health of the implant due to the cantilever. In that case, the use of two implants is ideal. For a bone width less than 5 mm, it requires a 3.2 mm implant with compromises such as less surface area and greater crestal concentration of stress.

Bone angulation

Bone angulation is the 4th determinant for available bone. Ideally, it is aligned with the forces of occlusion and is parallel to the long axis of the prosthodontic restoration. The incisal and occlusal surfaces of the teeth follow the curve of Wilson and curve of Spee. This results in roots of the maxillary teeth being angled towards a common point approximately 4 inches away. The 1st premolar cusp tip is usually vertical to its root apex. The mandibular roots flare, so the anatomic crowns are more lingually inclined in the posterior regions and labially inclined in the anterior area compared to the underlying roots. Implants should be placed in the same angulation as the adjacent teeth to bear the occlusal load.

RADIOGRAPHIC EXAMINATION

Preoperative radiographic examination should reveal the following for evaluation of the implant treatment (Table 22.8).

- Position and extent of the normal anatomic boundaries of the site of implant (inferior alveolar nerve canal, mental foramen, incisive foramen, nasal floor, sinus floor) (Table 22.9)
- Quantity of available bone: Shape and size of the alveolar ridge (length, width, height and angulation of the ridge and adjacent teeth)
- Quality of available bone: The bone quality should be provided in a standardised format (in Hounsfield unit or other standardisation protocols)
- Presence of any pathologies that can affect the implant treatment (cyst, bone tumours–fibrous dysplasia, underlying disease–osteosclerosis, presence of any buried teeth/root).

TWO-DIMENSIONAL RADIOGRAPHIC MODALITY

Periapical radiograph

It helps to identify the interradicular space, prognosis of adjacent teeth and location of critical structures. It is useful in case of a single tooth implant. But it has a limited value in determining bone quantity and density.

Cephalometric evaluation

Lateral cephalogram is used to identify anterior alveolus and the relationship of lingual plate to the patient's skeletal anatomy. It can also identify the vertical dimension loss, interarch relation and crown-to-implant relation.

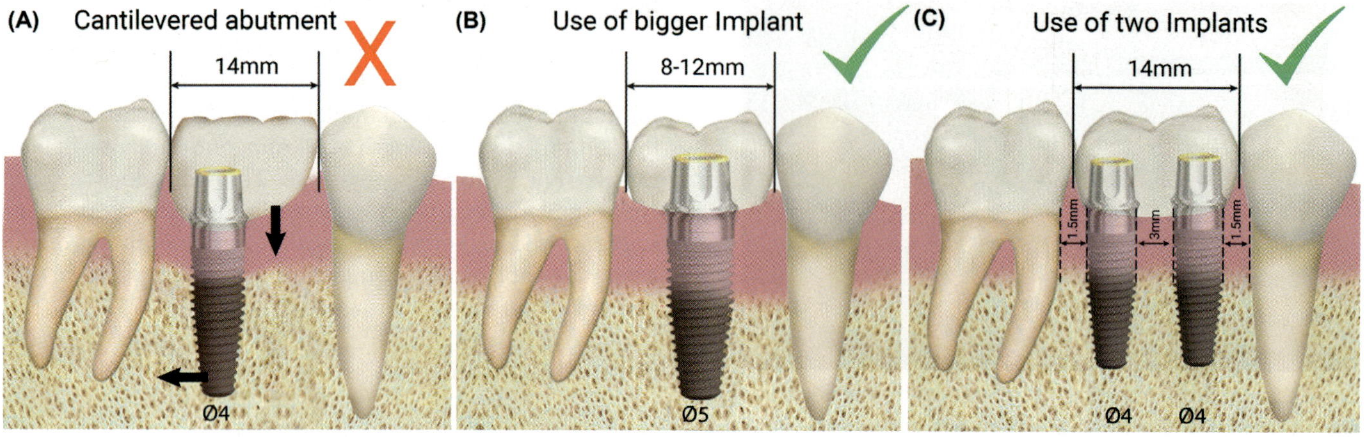

Figure 22.13 Illustration shows the proper use of the mesiodistal length of an edentulous molar region. (**A**) Cantilevered abutment should not be used when the mesiodistal length is more than 12 mm. The black arrows indicate the path of stress and areas where the bone loss will occur when cantilevered abutment is used. (**B**) Use of wider implants is indicated when the length is above 8–12 mm. (**C**) Two implants can be placed at the mesiobuccal and the distolingual sites of the molar region.

TABLE 22.8 Radiographic Bone Density Classification by Kirkos and Misch

Density	Hounsfield Unit
D1	>1250
D2	850–1250
D3	350–850
D4	150–350
D5	<150 (pathology)

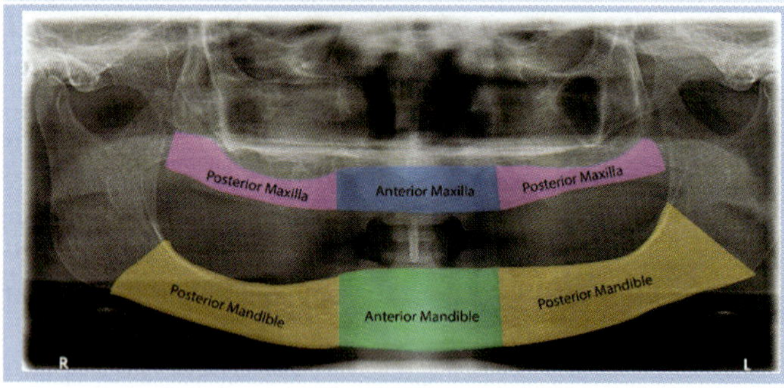

TABLE 22.9 Anatomic Boundaries and Limitations of Implant

Anatomic Boundaries	Anatomic Limitations (mm)
Buccal crestal bone	1
Lingual crestal bone	1
Adjacent implant	3
Adjacent tooth	1.5
Nasal cavity—Anterior maxilla	1
Maxillary sinus—Posterior maxilla	1
Mental foramen—Anterior mandible	5
Inferior alveolar canal—Posterior mandible	2

Orthopantomograph

Orthopantomograph is most commonly used for implant placement and helps to identify vertical bone height and general dental status. It shows the gross anatomy and rules out pathology of the jaws. It can also monitor the prosthetic outcome but does not provide three-dimensional information (bone width, angulation—all these have to be evaluated clinically).

THREE-DIMENSIONAL RADIOGRAPHIC MODALITY

3D scans are better at determining the information needed for implant placement. While CT scan uses more radiation, cone beam computed tomography (CBCT) seem to lean towards being the gold standard due to the advantages it possesses.

Computed tomography (CT) scan

CT scans can analyse bone height, width, density and distance from vital structures. It provides a standardised protocol for bone quality based on Hounsfield units. It can also guide the position and orientation of implants. Acrylic template with barium sulphate film helps to precisely identify position and orientation of proposed implant. The disadvantage is the radiation exposure.

Cone beam computed tomography (CBCT) (Fig. 22.14)

CBCT can trace the mandibular canal, maxillary sinus and other structures. The software can also identify the bone's length, width, height and angulation. Bone quality and measurements of available bone can be determined but it is not

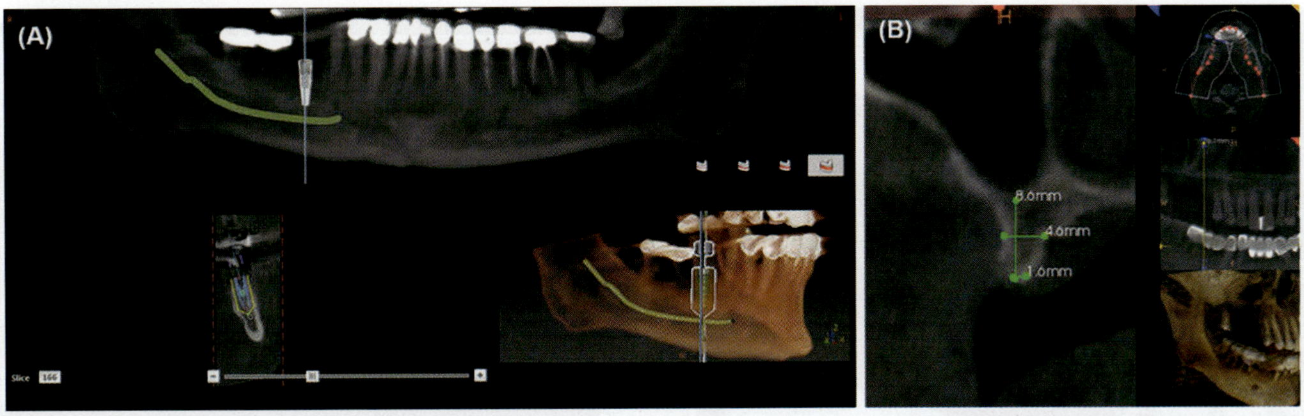

Figure 22.14 (**A** and **B**) CBCT images showing the measurement of bone height and width for implant placement.

calibrated for Hounsfield measurement; this seems to be the disadvantage of CBCT, but the advantages are that with reduced radiation exposure, sectional images can be obtained, reduced cost when compared to CT scan and we can accurately determine the number and size of implants. CBCT is best for preoperative planning and postoperative maintenance or diagnosis of periimplantitis.

Key implant position and implant number

Misch's guidelines for key implant positions:

- Avoid cantilevers as they are force magnifiers.
- No three adjacent pontics (Fig. 22.15).

1. Maxillary bone requires multiple implants in key positions to compensate for its bone density. When multiple maxillary teeth are missing, the following key positions are used based on the maxillary open pentagon:
   a. One central incisor position
   b. Bilateral canine positions
   c. Bilateral 2nd premolar positions
   d. Bilateral sites on the distal half of the 1st molars
2. For the mandibular edentulous arch:
   a. Overdenture option
   b. Fixed prosthesis option: five treatment plans
      i. Branemark approach: Use five to six implants between the mental foramen to support a cantilevered prosthesis
      ii. Modified by Bidez and Misch: five to seven implants; The mandatory key positions are two over mental foramina, two in canine positions, one in midline
      iii. Modified by Misch: five to seven implants; The use of one posterior ridge as cantilever—The key positions are: two canine positions, two premolar positions and one 1st molar site
      iv. Treatment plan 4 is used when the bone density is poor: seven implants—two 1st molar positions, two premolar positions, two canine positions and one incisor position
      v. Treatment plan 5 is used to fabricate three independent prosthesis: one anterior prosthesis (two premolar sites, two canine sites) and two posterior prosthesis (L&R) (one premolar and one 1st molar position)
3. Implant body size: Ideal size—12 mm up to 15 mm for softer bone
   a. Step 1: Consider biomechanics and aesthetics for initial selection of implant body size
   b. Step 2: After radiographic evaluation, consider bone length, width, height and adjacent structures.

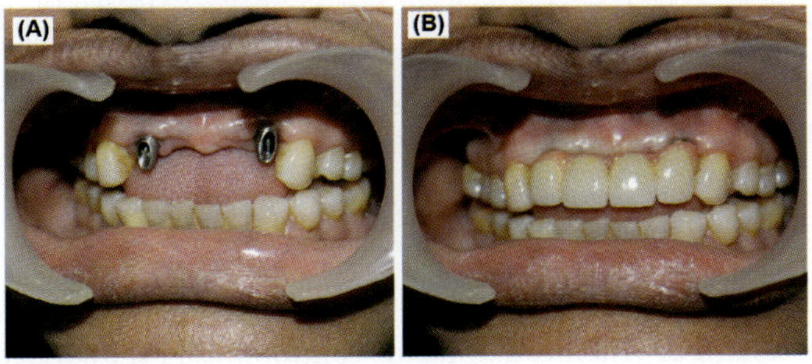

Figure 22.15 (**A** and **B**) A clinical situation where the use of only two pontics has been shown.

Diagnostic casts

Diagnostic casts are the complete representation of the patient's maxillary and mandibular arches. Diagnostic wax up is the ideal representation of the teeth to be replaced (Fig. 22.16). The procedure after making the diagnostic casts to fabrication of the surgical guide has been described in Flowchart 22.2.

Surgical guide template

Computer-guided implant treatment (Fig. 22.17)

COMPUTER-AIDED DESIGN/COMPUTER-ASSISTED MANUFACTURING-BASED SURGICAL GUIDE

Computer-aided design/computer-assisted manufacturing (CAD/CAM) technology uses data from CT scan to plan

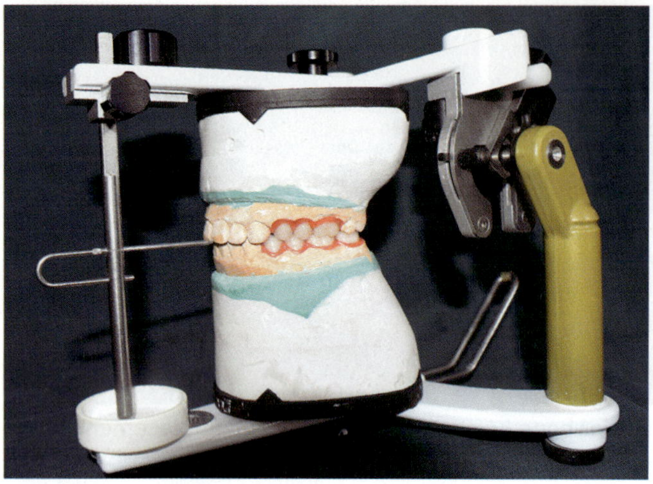

Figure 22.16 Diagnostic casts articulated with diagnostic wax up done for partially edentulous maxillary and mandibular ridge.

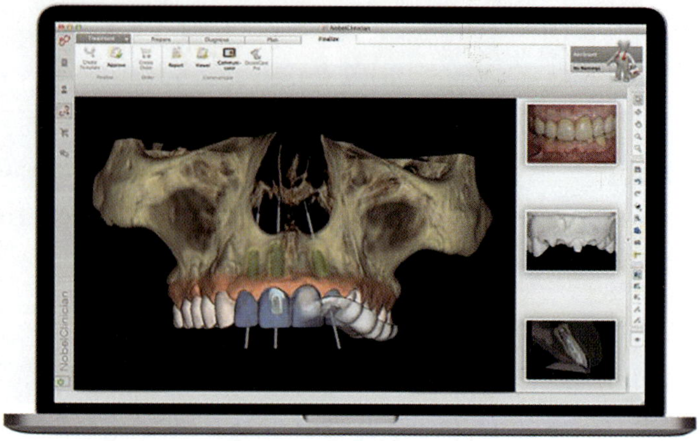

Figure 22.17 Presurgical treatment planning software for surgical guide fabrication with implant angulation, bone width and height taken into consideration. For example, Nobel Clinician Software as shown in the image.

Diagnostic casts are made

↓

Selection of Articulator type
- Choice of articulators depending on the edentulous space
- Requirement of Face bow transfer, Centric jaw relation, Protrusive movement, Bennett movement and intercondylar distance for fully-adjustable articulators – Full mouth rehabilitation

↓

Mounting of diagnostic casts on to the articulator

↓

Diagnostic wax up is done (ideal positioning of the missing tooth)

↓

Implant positioning co-relation with CT imaging considering the following requirements is deviced
- Implant Natural tooth distance
- Implant – Implant distance
- Distance from IAN/Mental foramen
- Distance from Nasal Cavity
- From Maxillary sinus
- Implant angulation and position
- Number and size of implants
- Implant depth

↓

Fabrication of radiographic templates is done

↓

Fabrication of surgical templates is done either by Hand (Laboratory fabricated) or by CAD/CAM using the radiographic template

Flowchart 22.2 The procedure from the making of diagnostic cast to the fabrication of the surgical guides have been described.

implant rehabilitation. CT images are converted into data that is recognised by a CT imaging and planning software. The software transfers the presurgical plan to the surgical site with stereolithographic drill guides. The surgical templates fabricated by this technology are preprogrammed with individual depth, angulations, mesiodistal and labiolingual positioning of the implant.

Advantages

1. Precise placement of implants
2. Conservation of anatomic structures
3. Three-dimensional technology allows precise evaluation of anatomic points such as the size of the maxillary sinus in the upper jaw and location of the alveolar nerve in the lower jaw
4. Precise analysis of osseous topography
5. Provides information about size, direction and bone location for accurate positioning of implants
6. High observed accuracy of 0.1 mm
7. Reduced surgical exposure time
8. Swelling is less likely with minimally invasive flapless surgery
9. Less postoperative strain on dentist and patient
10. Transparency of material, which allows seeing through the model
11. To summarise stereolithography fabrication process
12. A CT scan procedure is performed with a radiographic template fabricated using radio-opaque marker in place.

Disadvantages

1. Lack of visibility and tactile control during the surgical procedure
2. Insufficient mouth opening jeopardises surgical procedure.

TIMING OF IMPLANT PLACEMENT (Flowchart 22.3)

Surgical placement of a conventional implant

Surgical protocol

Anaesthesia

Local anaesthesia versus conscious sedation versus general anaesthesia

Most endosseous implant operations can be performed using local anaesthesia with or without conscious sedation. A thorough review of the patient's medical history may reveal medical problems that limit the amount of local anaesthesia or epinephrine that can be administered or that the patient's condition must be monitored by a clinician trained in anaesthesia, such as an anaesthesiologist or an oral and maxillofacial surgeon.

Routine inferior alveolar nerve blocks and maxillary infiltration anaesthesia provide satisfactory local anaesthesia for the implant patient. Local anaesthesia infiltrated directly into the planned incision line reduces bleeding and simultaneously performs a hydropic dissection. This eases the subperiosteal dissection during development of a full thickness mucoperiosteal flap.

The specific local anaesthetic is chosen by operator preference. Lidocaine 2% (Xylocaine) with 1:100,000 or 1:20,000 epinephrine or a similar anaesthetic is most commonly used.

Conscious sedation may be replaced by general anaesthesia in patients with extreme dental phobia or those requiring bone graft harvesting from multiple intraoral or extraoral sites.

Incision

A scalpel blade no. 15 is used to make the crestal incision. The incision has to be placed carefully enough to allow 2 mm of buccal keratinised gingiva. A distal releasing incision may be given depending on the requirement of exposure (preferably avoided as the blood supply to the bone may get compromised).

Incision design—anterior mandible: The crestal incision is used when the mandible has sufficient height and the mentalis and lip musculature insert below the alveolar crest. For a patient without an adequate band of attached gingival tissue or for a patient whose mentalis muscle inserts close to the crest, a vestibular incision is recommended. High muscle attachment with the mobile tissue against the labial portion of the implant's abutment requires simultaneous vestibuloplasty or presurgical soft tissue grafting.

Type 1
- Implant is placed Immediately after extraction

Type 2
- Implant is placed 4 - 8 weeks after extraction
- Only soft tissue healing

Type 3
- Implant is placed 12 -16 weeks after extraction
- Partial bone healing

Type 4
- Delayed Implant placement
- 6 months after extraction
- Complete bone healing

Flowchart 22.3 International Team for Implantology (ITI) consensus classification on timing for Implant placement.

FLAP DESIGN AND SOFT TISSUE HANDLING

Flap versus Flapless design (Fig. 22.18)

Traditionally, access for implant placement has been achieved by a flap approach. Studies have demonstrated that flap reflection often results in bone resorption around the natural teeth. Postsurgical tissue loss from flap reflection has also been reported.

Principles of flap design for dental implants

Using a periosteal elevator, a clear incision is made to prevent the need for retraction and elevation, with removal of minimal amount of periosteum to retain the maximum vascular supply. Identification of the contours of the adjacent teeth as well as the concavities or protrusions on the surface of the bone is essential and will facilitate implant placement. All wounds should have clean edges, which will facilitate closure and optimise healing by primary intention. Provide for closure away from the submerged implant. In cases of reduced quantity of keratinised tissue, it is beneficial to position the crestal incision towards the palatal aspect, the area of more keratinised tissue as it extends onto the palatal mucosa. Avoid any local or external pressure on the wound during the healing period.

Drilling

Drilling should be done with proper irrigation using saline, cold saline can also be used. The speed of the drill ranges between 800 and 1500 rpm. It is important to maintain the temperature, because bone exposed to a temperature of 47°C for more than 1 min can cause bone necrosis. The speed should not increase by more than 2000 rpm. The steps in drilling are explained in Table 22.10 (Fig. 22.19).

Implant placement (Table 22.11)

Flap closure and postoperative care

Stage I surgery

The operative site is thoroughly irrigated and all sharp bony edges are smoothened. Depending on the type of loading, the stages in the surgical phase are decided. If the procedure is a ***stage I*** surgical phase and has a ***stage II surgery*** planned, then once the implant is firmly placed and seated, cover screws are placed into the implant body. The flap is sutured completely

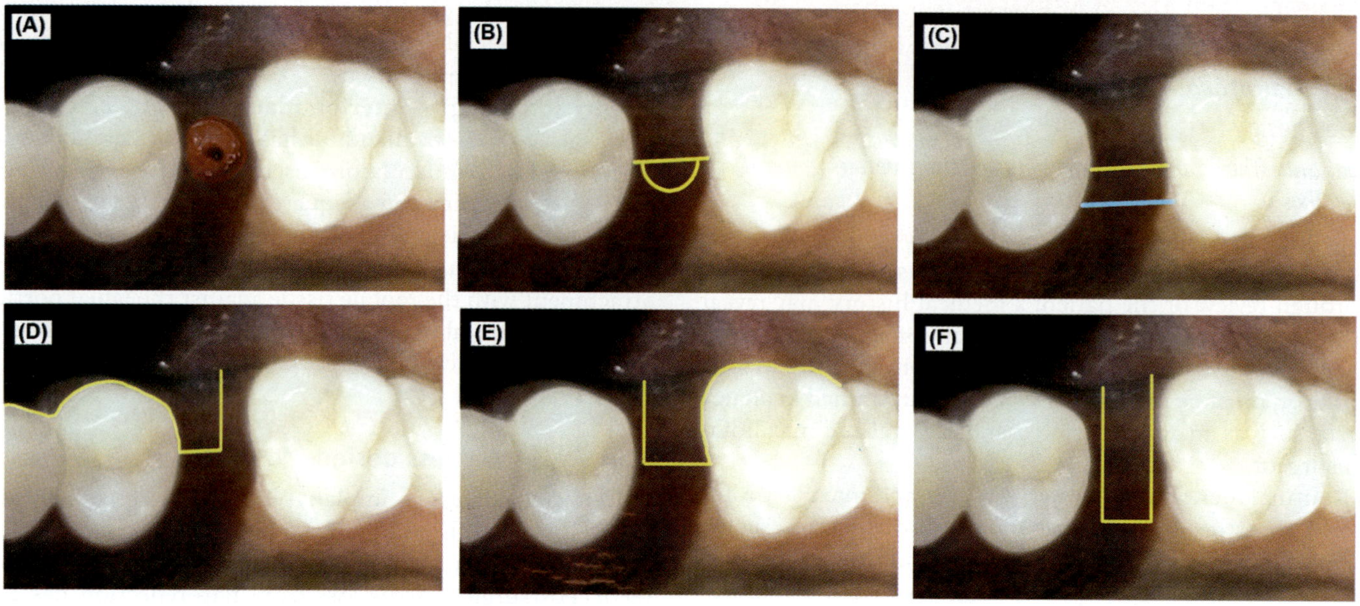

Figure 22.18 (**A**) Punch approach. (**B**) Half punch approach. (**C**) Midcrestal, Palatal/lingual crestal. (**D**) Mesial papilla preservation. (**E**) Distal papilla preservation. (**F**) Double papilla preservation.

TABLE 22.10 Steps in Drilling

Drill	Procedure	Illustration
Pilot drill also called sharp or precision drill	This is a preliminary drill used to mark the site of osteotomy. It has a sharp point at the end that makes it easier to puncture even dense bone. It has a marking at 10 mm. It prevents the next drill from slipping on the bone surface. It is more often used for the flapless technique. Maximum speed: 2000 rpm	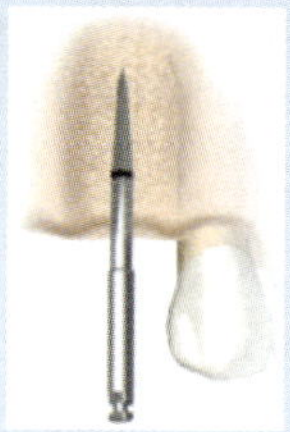
Drill stop	Is a guide for the clinician to know the height marked on the drill. It is fit over the drills at the desired length.	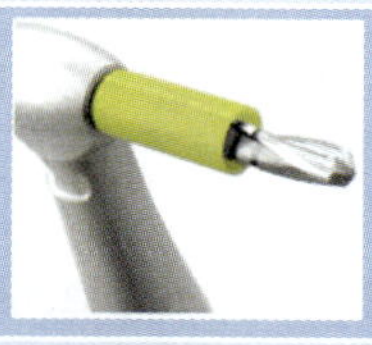
Twist drill 2 mm	**Height determination:** The pilot drill is the 1st drill used to create the osteotomy. It is determined by the length of the implant to be placed. The length of the implant socket is chosen to be 1.5–3 mm more than the implant height for subcrestal placement of the implant. **Flapless design:** This is not followed for the flapless procedure as the implant will be placed at the crest in the flapless technique. But the flap depth is measured with a probe and that is added to the height of the implant. **Emergence profile:** To achieve this, the shoulder of the implant should be 1 mm below the cementoenamel junction of the adjacent teeth. **Drilling angulation:** The correct axis or angulation should be maintained. **Maximum speed:** 2000 rpm	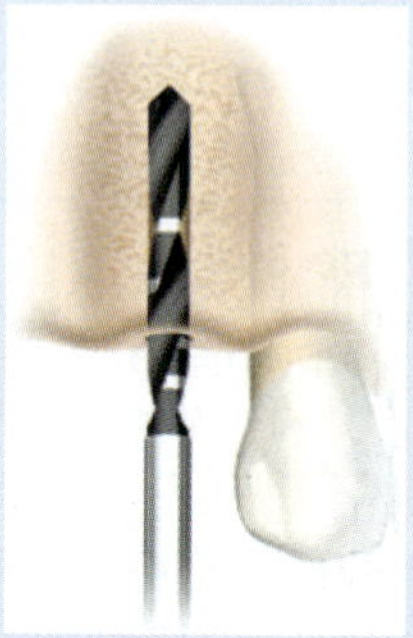
General rule of using the implant drills: The drilling should be done in a pumping in and out manner, this exposes the bone debris, drill and the osteotomised socket to the water coolants for clearing and cooling of the bone.		

Drill	Procedure	Illustration
Guide pin (used when surgical template is not used)	Single implant: Used to check angulation with the adjacent tooth. Multiple implants: When multiple implants are placed before the use of the subsequent drills, a guide pin is inserted into the 1st osteotomised socket. This aligns the 2nd implant's drilling angulation for the clinician. Once all the implant sites are drilled with the Twist drill (2 mm), the next sequence of drills are used. Floss: A floss is tied to the instrument to prevent loss.	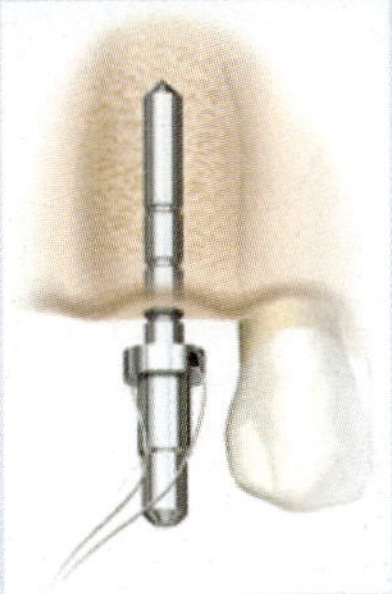
Subsequent drills or twist step drills	The twist step drills are available in diameters 2.4/2.8 and 3.2/3.6. They are used to enlarge the osteotomy socket to the desired width. These drills have cutting edges only at the lateral sides and not for depth. This helps maintain the planned depth of the implant socket. The guide pin is used in between every drill to check angulation. Maximum speed: 2000 rpm	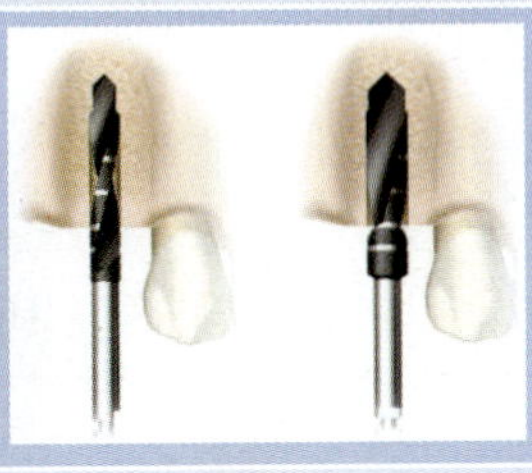
Depth probe	It helps the clinician to verify the depth of the implant socket. It is used in between the subsequent drill and wider twist step drill.	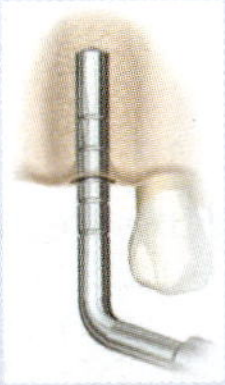
Wider twist step drills or profile drills or cortical drills	Used only when bone is dense. They are used between the sequential drills to widen the crestal part of the implant socket to allow the next drill inside. These drills also flare the preparation for the cover screw over the implant without any bony interference. Maximum speed: 2000 rpm	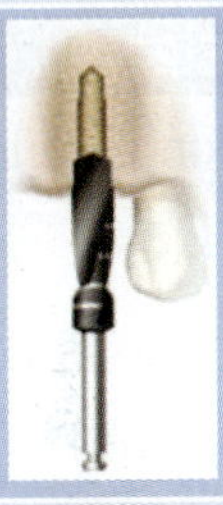
Bone tapping drill/ screw tap	Bone tapping is done only in dense bone. Dense bone can hinder the placement of threaded implants. Screw tap makes a screw shape inside the osteotomised implant socket to allow the threads of the implants to fit inside the implant socket smoothly. This is done at very slow speeds (20–40 rpm) without water irrigation. Maximum speed: 25 rpm	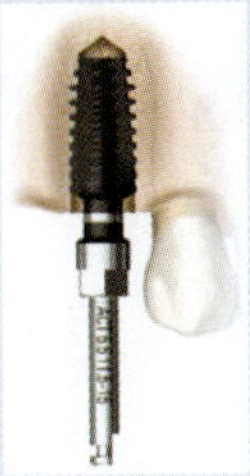

burying the implant and cover screw under the soft tissue. This is called the ***Two-stage delayed function***. If a ***One-stage delayed function*** has been planned, the healing abutment or the gingival former is placed. The surgical site is irrigated, the mucosal flap sutured around the healing abutment and closed with 3-0 black silk or 5-0 resorbable sutures. The healing abutment will be visible in the oral cavity and attached gingiva forms around it. Sutures are removed after 7–10 days. Following implant surgery, the patient is given systemic antibiotics and analgesics (Fig. 22.20).

Stage II surgery

If the cover screw was placed in the stage I surgery, the next stage II surgery is planned. In this stage, the healing abutment is attached to the implant after removing the cover screw. The implant site is identified radiographically and clinically with a probe. The soft tissue is removed from over the cover screw. A curette, piezo, or drill is used to remove any bone overgrowth that has formed over the cover screw. When the implant is subcrestal, the bone collar may hinder the attachment of the abutments. In that case, a

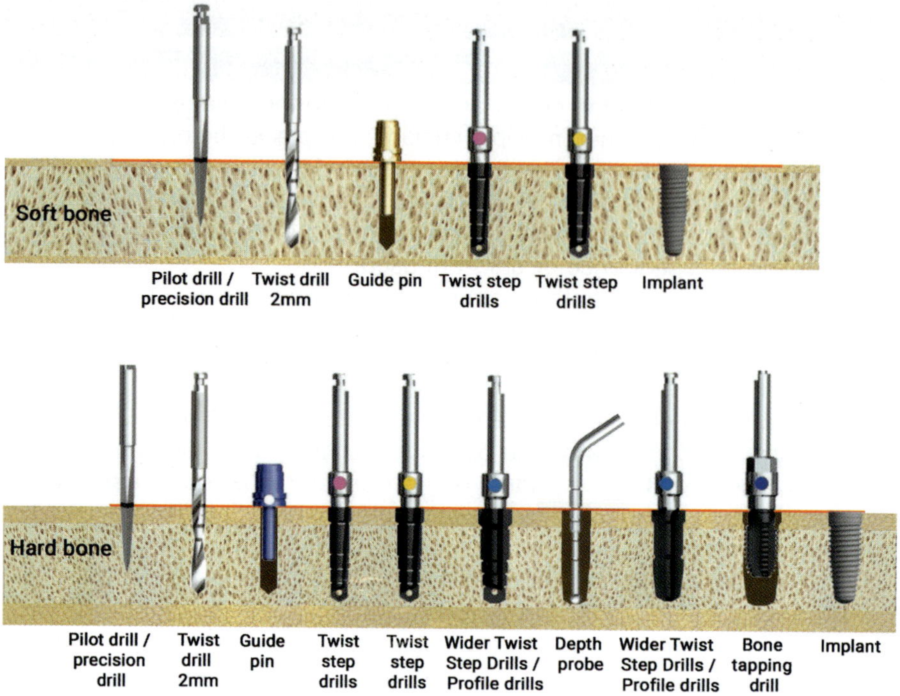

Figure 22.19 Drills used in the sequence depending on the type of bone density. Sequence of drills till implant placement. The height of the crestal bone and other marking in the drills can be noted.

TABLE 22.11 Steps in Implant Placement

Unpacking the implant	The implant will be provided in a metal sterile vial that is packed in a plastic vial. The plastic vial is opened and the sterile metal vial is dropped in the sterile tray. This can now be handled by the surgeon. The surgeon picks up the implant in the desired device. The plastic vial contains two labels which provides all information about the dimensions of the implant. This can be placed in the patient records.	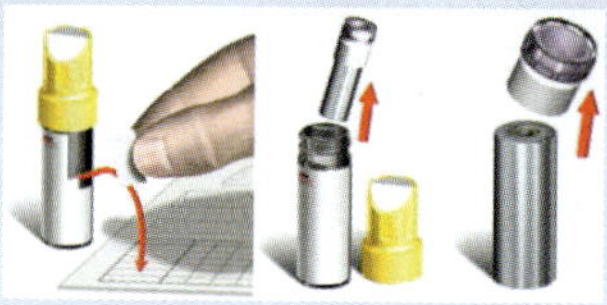
Implant pick up	The implant can be placed by the torque wrench or the surgical driver or the drilling unit itself. The clinician should make sure that the implant is fully seated in the implant driver to prevent it from falling, leading to contamination.	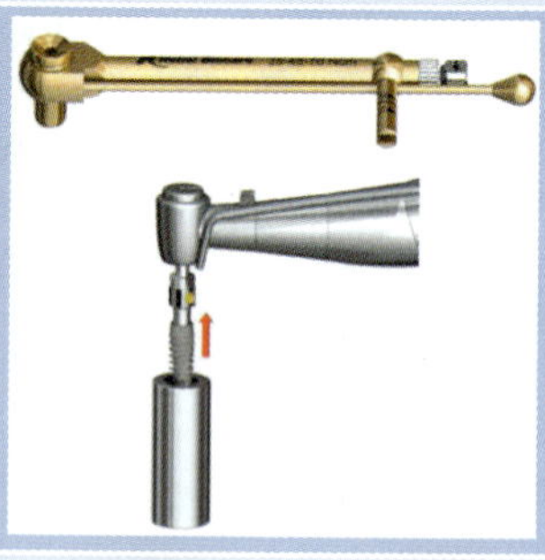
Inserting the implant into the osteotomised implant socket	Maximum speed on drilling unit: 25 rpm Maximum torque: 70 N/cm for smaller diameter implants, less than 3 mm 45 N/cm. Giving torque force more than 70 N/cm can fracture the implant. Chances of implant fracture is higher while using surgical driver as the clinician can give varied forces up to 200 N/cm easily.	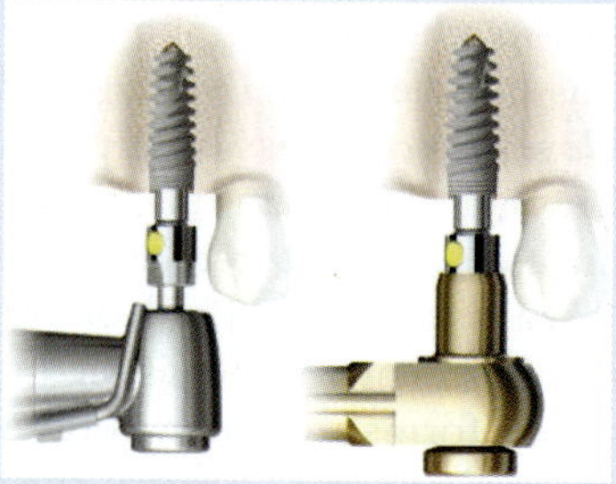

TABLE 22.11 Steps in Implant Placement—cont'd

Check final insertion torque with torque wrench	The torque wrench is inserted and the final insertion torque is measured. Above 35 N/cm can withstand immediate loading.	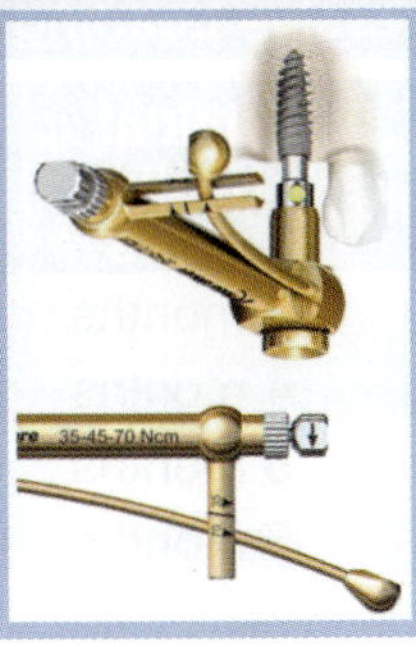

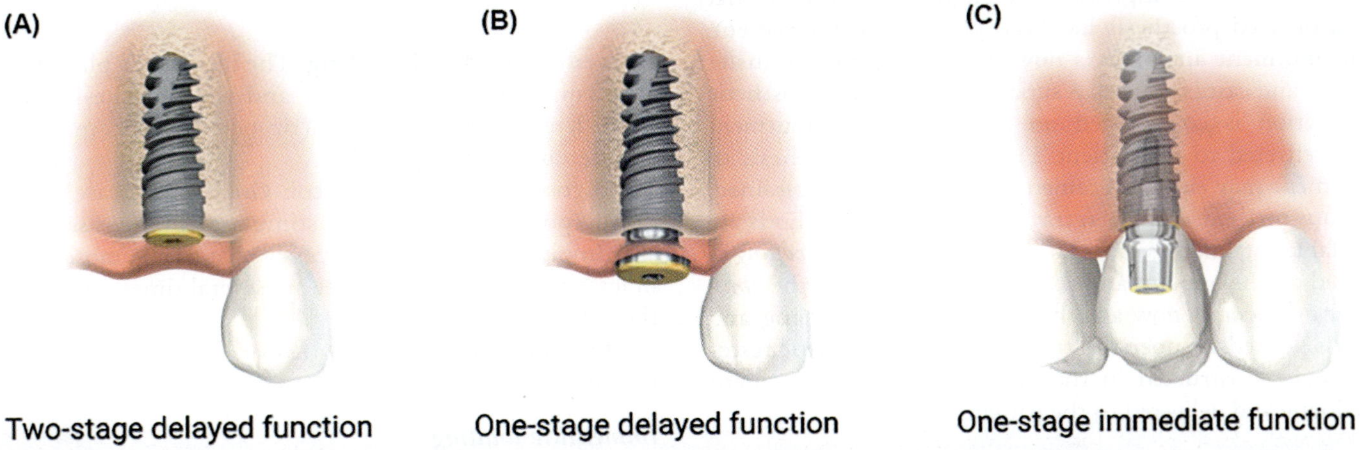

Figure 22.20 (**A**) Two-stage delayed function is also called conventional implant loading system, where the cover screw is placed and completely sutured. (**B**) One-stage delayed function is where only one surgical procedure is done, healing abutment placed and delayed loading of the implant. (**C**) One-stage immediate function is where a single surgical procedure and immediate loading of the implant is done.

bone mill kit may be provided by some implant systems. The respective size bone mill for each implant size can be used manually or with a drill to remove this bone overgrowth.

For early and delayed loading, surgical stage II is done just before the final prosthesis appointments. Till then, the temporary removable prosthesis is made and given for aesthetics.

Abutment connection (Fig. 22.21)

For immediate loading (one-stage immediate function): A temporary single unit or multiple unit restoration (cement retained) can be given in case of a missing tooth/teeth in stage I surgical phase. After attaining primary stability, the premade temporary abutment is fixed into the implant, tightening torque of the abutment is at 35 N/cm for smaller implants (3 mm or lesser) is done. If the implant starts rotating, consider delayed loading after 3–4 months of submerged healing. If tightened correctly and primary stability is intact, adjust abutment height and other clearance. Place the plastic coping, fabricate a temporary crown or bridge and cement with temporary cement.

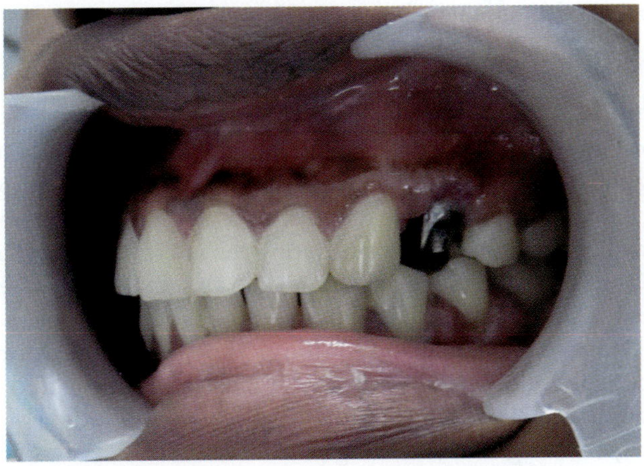

Figure 22.21 Abutment connection shown in a clinical situation.

Final prosthesis

After 2 weeks for early loading and after 3 or 6 months for delayed loading, to achieve the final restoration, the patient undergoes a series of impressions. These appointments can be based on the ***progressive loading protocol*** explained in

TABLE 22.12 Appointment Timings in Progressive Loading Technique

Bone Density	Initial Healing Time	Weeks Between Appointments	Total Time for Progressive Loading
D1	3 months	1 week	4 months
D2	4 months	2 weeks	5.5 months
D3	5 months	3 weeks	7 months
D4	6 months	4 weeks	9 months

Table 22.12. These impression techniques are based on what kind of fixed prosthesis has been planned for the patient. The abutment analogue is now attached into the transfer coping and cast is poured. A superstructure or the prosthetic restoration is constructed on the implant or abutment and delivered to the patient. Fixation of the prosthesis to abutment may either be cement retained or screw retained. Various methods like open tray and closed tray methods are available for impression taking. Once the ***transfer coping*** is placed on the implant and the impression is made, the ***abutment analogue*** is now attached to the transfer coping and cast is poured. A superstructure or the final prosthetic restoration is constructed in the dental lab on the abutment analogue and delivered to the patient.

Prosthetic phase

The clinician must comprehend that the patient's normal dentition has been affected, resulting in a loss of normal contour, comfort in function, aesthetics, speech, and health. The clinician must endeavour to provide the greatest possible outcome to the patient.

Concept of implant loading

Loading concepts

Bone interface is strong on the day of implant placement. During the healing phase, the lamellar bone becomes woven bone for repair. Thus, the bone experiences a phase where the bone is weakest. This period occurs during the interface, which lasts 3–6 weeks. There are many studies showing that this phase is the weakest phase due to the bone remodelling process.

Branemark's original loading: This was the traditional protocol followed in the past. It has been illustrated in Flowchart 22.4.

Early loading: Early loading protocol is when a provisional prosthesis is inserted before osseointegration (within 2 weeks after surgery).

Conventional loading protocol: The original healing periods as suggested by different implant systems are followed (i.e. after 12–24 weeks).

Delayed loading protocol: The healing period is extended due to the compromised site conditions, and prosthesis is provided later than the conventional healing period.

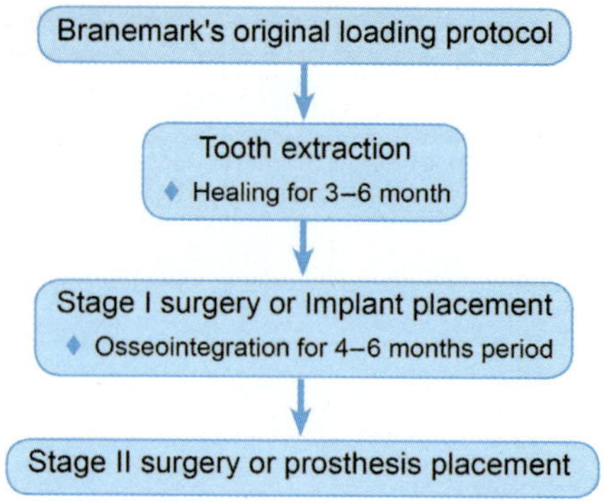

Flowchart 22.4 Brånemark's original loading system or conventional loading system.

Immediate occlusal loading: The implant is placed with adequate primary stability and the prosthesis placed 48 h postsurgery has centric occlusion at maximum intercuspation.

Progressive loading protocol: Gradual increase in load during prosthetic fabrication stimulates an increase in density. Implementation of progressive loading is more critical in lesser bone densities as they are several times weaker than the cortical bone.

Only immediate and progressive loading have been explained in detail.

Immediate loading

Indications:

- Adequate bone quality (type I, II and III)
- Sufficient bone height (i.e. approximately 12 mm)
- Sufficient bone width (i.e. approximately 6 mm)
- Ability to achieve an adequate anteroposterior spread between the implants.

Rationale for implant immediate loading:

- Primary implant stability is the most important determining factor for immediate implant loading. Micromovements of more than 100 μm are enough to jeopardise healing with direct bone-implant contact
- Proper implant placement technique includes copious irrigation both internally and externally to maintain temperatures less than 47 °C for prevention of necrosis of the surrounding bone (47 °C for 1 min can cause bone necrosis)
- Bone microstrain: Loaded bone changes its shape. This change may be measured as strain. At microstrain levels of 20%–40%, bone already starts to form fibrous tissue and is called the pathologic overload zone. To decrease microstrain, the surface area of load may be increased by the implant number (>8 in maxillary arch and >6 in mandibular arch), implant size (wider implants increase surface area), implant design (threaded implants) and implant body surface conditions (hydroxyapatite-coated)

- Torque during implant placement is a good predictor of implant stability (insertion torque greater than 30–35 N cm)
- Force factors: Parafunctional forces, crown height, muscular dynamics
- Implant position and number: For maxilla—bilateral canine position and bilateral molar position are mandatory, and for mandible—at least three implants, one in the anterior and one in each posterior region. If clinician anticipates increases in forces—Increase the implant number
- Occlusal load direction: No posterior cantilevers.

Success criteria of immediate loaded implants:

1) The individual unattached implant should be immobile when tested clinically
2) No periimplant radiolucency
3) Vertical bone loss around the fixtures should be less than 0.2 mm annually after the 1st year of implant loading
4) The implant should not show any signs and symptoms of pain, infection, neuropathies, paraesthesia, violation of mandibular canal and sinus drainage
5) Success rate of 85% at the end of 5 year observation period and 80% at the end of 10 year service
6) Implant design allows the restoration to be satisfactory to patient and dentist.

Progressive loading protocol

The progressive loading protocol gradually increases the load during prosthetic fabrication, this stimulates an increase in bone density. This was initially demonstrated by Pierazzini in animals, where development of dense trabeculae around progressively loaded implants was seen, but implementation of progressive loading is more difficult in lower bone densities as they are weaker. This protocol is followed based on the following factors: procedural interval, diet, occlusal material, occlusion and prosthetic design (Table 22.12).

Time interval: The two surgical appointments between stage I and stage II implant surgery are separated by 4–8 weeks. The prosthetic appointment during which implants are sequentially load are separated by 2–4 weeks.

Role of diet in progressive loading: Apart from these procedures, the patient's diet is initially restricted to soft food. The food habit is controlled to prevent overloading of the implants. Once the final prosthesis function, occlusion and cementation are evaluated, a normal diet is advised.

Role of occlusal material: The load is progressively increased by using acrylic as the occlusal material initially, this is called the transitional prosthesis. Acrylic has lower impact force than metal. Metal or ceramic are used as the occlusal material in the final prosthesis.

Role of occlusion: The occlusal contacts are gradually intensified. While placing the final abutment, no occlusal contact is allowed as this is the healing phase. This is gradually increased when the final prosthesis is given.

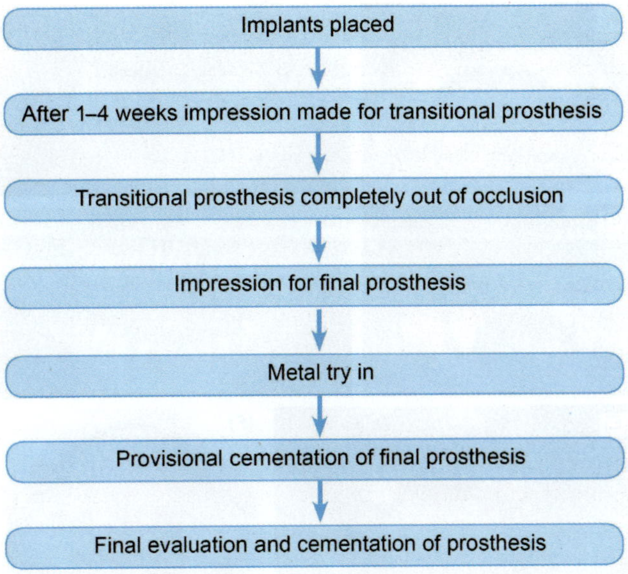

Flowchart 22.5 The flowchart illustrates the procedures after implant placement till final cementation of prosthesis.

Prosthetic design: Avoid load on implants during initial healing. The transitional prosthesis splints the implants together to reduce the stress and bear masticatory load.

Procedure: Given in Flowchart 22.5 for easy understanding.

Advantages: A stage II surgery is eliminated. Removable prosthesis is not required. Soft tissue is allowed to mature. Implant healing is better when splinted together during healing phase.

Disadvantages: Risk of failure. More numbers of implants are placed making treatment expensive.

Implant prosthetic options

The prosthetic options can be classified based on the type of prosthesis or based on the number of missing teeth (Fig. 22.22).

Fixed/removable prosthesis (*Table 22.13*)

Single-tooth implant restorations: FP1 or FP2

When an implant is used to replace a single missing tooth at any position in the arches, the major advantages are not damaging the adjacent teeth for support, less decay risk, decreased sensitivity and many more. It benefits the adjacent teeth health.

CONSIDERATIONS

Anterior teeth replacement with implant:

- Distance from adjacent tooth—1.5 mm
- Do not disturb the incisive foramen
- Buccal bone of 1.5 mm should be present
- Lingual/palatal bone of at least 0.5 mm
- Angulation: under incisal edge of crown
- Depth between 2 and 4 mm from free gingival margin for soft tissue emergence profile

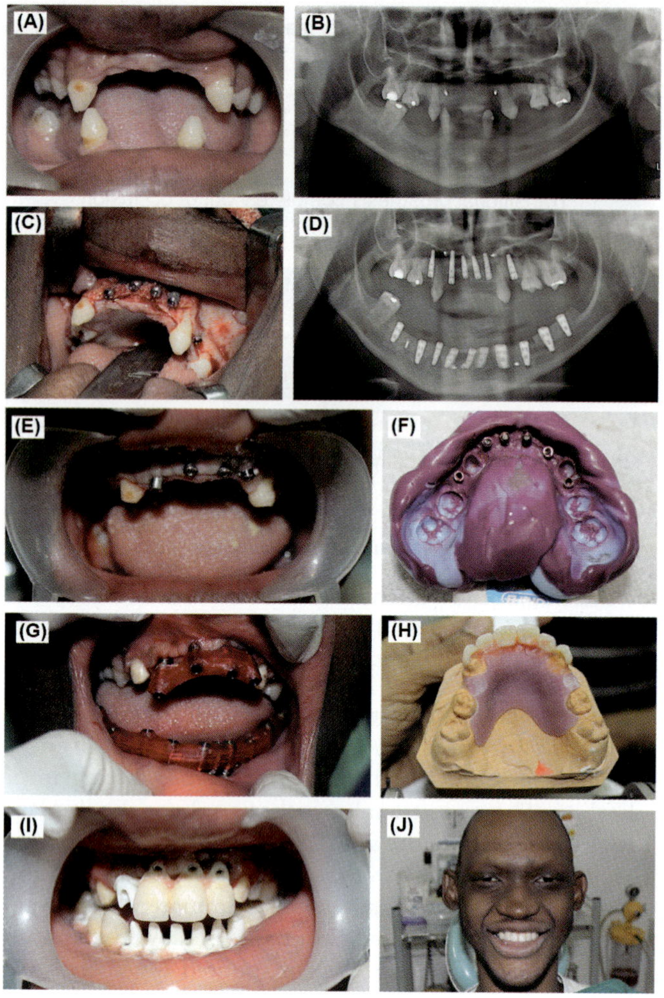

Figure 22.22 **(A–J)** Sequential steps showing rehabilitation of edentulous space with implants.

Molar replacement with implant:

- Mesiodistal space (MD) space—Implant diameter
  a. 7–8 mm—4 mm implant
  b. 8–12 mm—5–6 mm
  c. 12–14 mm—gain space to achieve MD width of 14 mm and place two implants (4 mm each) (Fig. 22.13)
  d. 14–20 mm—two implants. One can be placed on the mesial marginal ridge and the other on the distal marginal ridge. The prosthesis should be splinted
- The prosthesis should not have a cantilever of more than 3.5 mm on one side.

Immediate implant placement after extraction

Important points

The tooth position should be in relation to the free gingival margin. The form of the periodontium should be adequate for proper soft tissue healing. The tooth shape should be adequate and easily replaceable without rotation. The presence of the osseous crest before extraction of the tooth. The type of extraction plays an important role as it should be atraumatic. In the anterior region, the buccal bone should not fracture. Atraumatic extraction with a piezo is indicated. The angulation of the implant should not be hindered. In case of using an implant longer than the socket, the preparation should be done adequately.

Fixed treatment plan for partially and completely edentulous arches FP1, FP2, FP3

Indications

Fixed prosthesis is given for patients with good bone quantity and quality and the patient has other implants already. The crown space plays a vital role in this decision.

TABLE 22.13 Classification of the Bone-prosthesis (Fixed/Removable Relationship)

Type	Fixed/ Removable	Dentition to be Replaced	Description	Illustrations—Lateral View	Profile View
FP1	Fixed	Single tooth, multiple missing teeth	Replaces only the crown, looks like the natural teeth	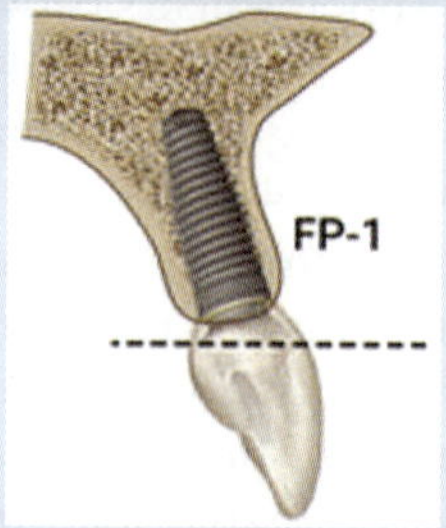	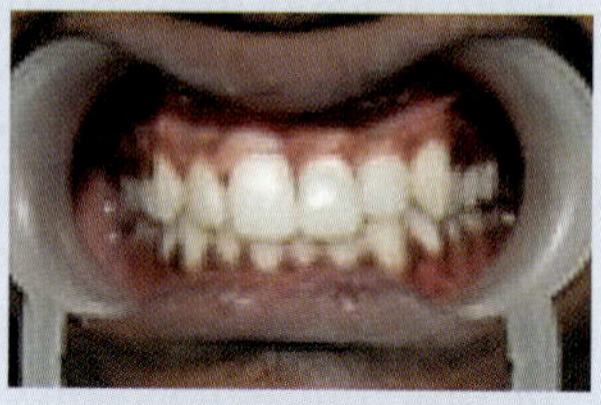
FP2	Fixed	Single tooth and for partially and completely edentulous jaws	Replaces crown and a portion of the root; tooth may look elongated	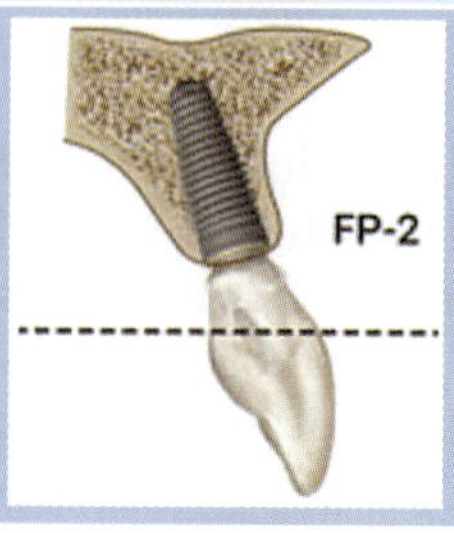	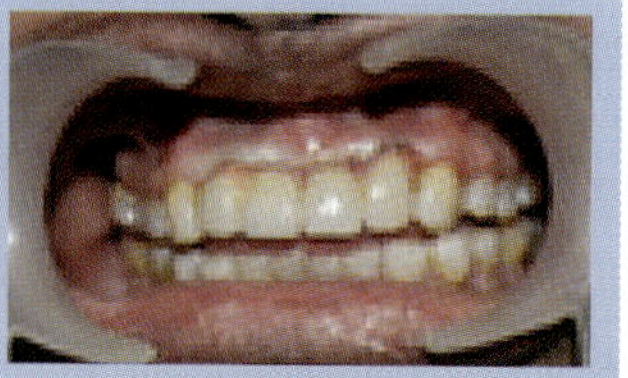

TABLE 22.13 Classification of the Bone-prosthesis (Fixed/Removable Relationship)—cont'd

Type	Fixed/ Removable	Dentition to be Replaced	Description	Illustrations—Lateral View	Profile View
FP3	Fixed	Mostly for partially and completely edentulous jaws	Replaces crown, gingiva and a portion of edentulous site	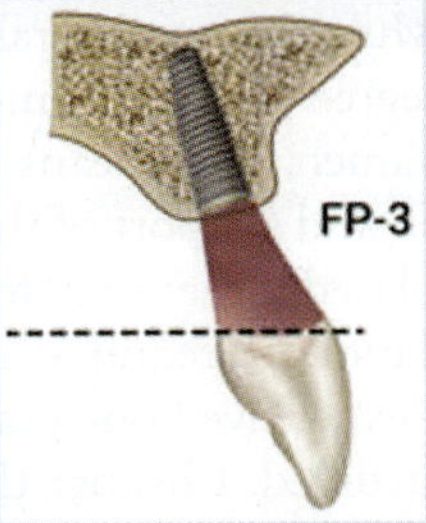	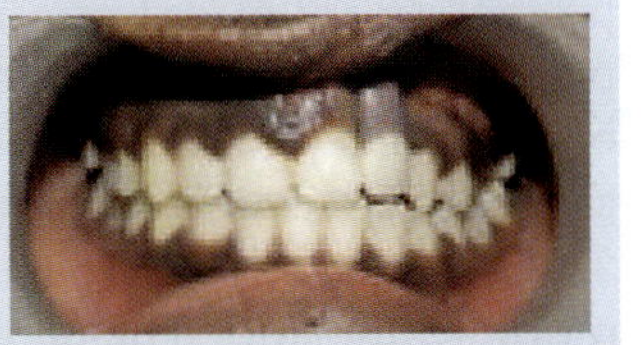
RP4	Removable	Completely edentulous jaws	Overdenture supported by implant	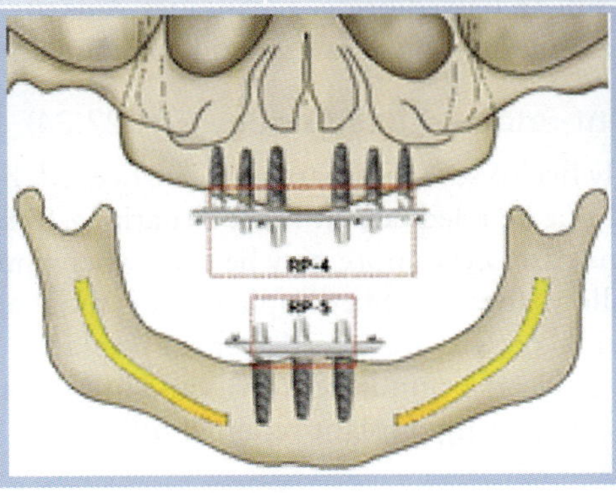	
RP5	Removable	Completely edentulous jaws	Overdenture supported by both oral musculature and implant		

Fixed prosthesis consideration

Crown height space (implant crown ratio)

Crown height space is measured from the alveolar crest to the occlusal plane in the posterior region and incisal edge in the anterior region. Ideal crown length for fixed implants is 8–12 mm and removable prosthesis is >12 mm. Excessive length can cause increased stress accumulation leading to crestal bone loss. It can also produce different stress and is a considerable force magnifier; various methods are adopted to decrease the stress, like shortening the cantilever length, minimising the offset loads to the buccal and lingual, increasing the number of implants, increasing the diameters of implants, fabricating removable restorations, which are less retentive and incorporates soft tissue support, and for >15 mm of crown length—all occlusal contacts in centric relation in most posterior parts are eliminated.

Key positions of maxilla and mandible

The classification and the key positions for partially and completely edentulous arches have been discussed earlier in page 415.

Implant—natural tooth splinting

It is not advisable to attach the pontic from a fixed implant restoration to a natural tooth as an abutment. It will result in the failure of the implant.

Completely edentulous fixed prosthesis design

Patient desire for fixed prosthesis is the primary concern. To make the procedure cost effective, many full mouth rehabilitation (FMR) designs with less number of implants have been described like the all-on-four concept. If bone quantity and quality is compromised, then conventional full-arch implants for each arch have been illustrated and content described in page 415. Patients also have the option of choosing zygoma implants or pterygoid implants if all factors are satisfied.

ALL-ON-FOUR CONCEPT (Fig. 22.23)

All-on-four technique enables a full arch of teeth to be replaced with just four dental implants. This technique eliminates the traditional need of six to eight implants for

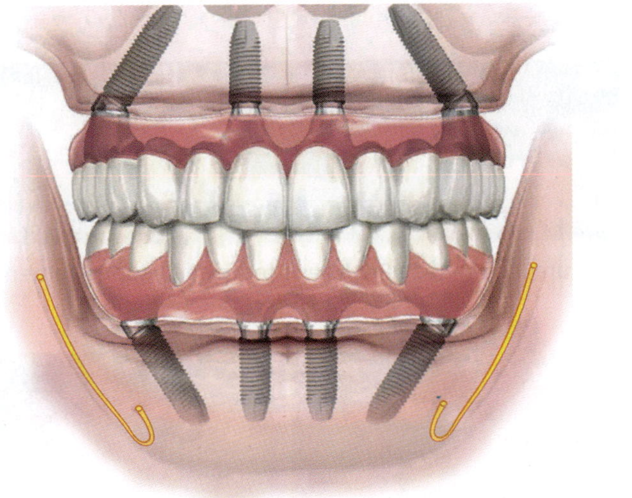

Figure 22.23 Implant placement based on all-on-four concept with fixed denture.

conventional full-arch implant treatment. All-on-four implants are actually similar to the normal screw-like implants, but the implants are positioned at a specific angle in the jaw bone. The two central implants are placed at the conventional angle of 90 degree to the alveolar ridge, while the two lateral implants posteriorly are placed at a 45 degree angle. All implants are placed anterior to the mental foramen. This means that more bone is utilised in the stabilisation and support of the implant allowing full set of teeth to be replaced rather than fewer teeth.

Advantages: Only four implants are required instead of multiple implants. The need for expensive bone grafting and sinus lift in most cases can be avoided. Cheaper than traditional full-arch fixed-bridge techniques. Aids the prevention of further bone loss in the jaw. Requires minimal recovery time.

Cement-retained fixed bridge (Fig. 22.24)

Usually five to seven implants may be needed. Four implants would not be adequate in most situations. Ten implants or in some cases even more may be used when amount of bone only allows for very short implants. It is more aesthetic since individual crowns are placed over the implants. The patient's ability to clean around the crowns and implants is important when considering implant retained full mouth prosthesis.

Screw-retained fixed bridge (Fig. 22.25)

Similar to the cement-retained prosthesis, screw-retained prosthesis needs five to seven implants depending on the amount and quality of the bone present. The teeth are built upon a metal base through which screws are inserted and secured the crown onto the implants. The metal base does not come in contact with the gingiva and sits like a 'platform' above it. This 'high water line' may be inconvenient for some cases, especially for upper teeth replacements.

Zygoma implants (Fig. 22.26)

The zygomaticus system, developed as part of the Brånemark system, allows reconstruction of a severely resorbed maxilla without the need for bone grafting. This approach is especially recommended for cases in which the maxillary sinuses extend anteriorly up to the bicuspid area. These implants were introduced in 1998 by ***Professor Per-Ingvar Brånemark*** and his team. The implant is a titanium endosteal implant. These are self-tapping screw-shaped implants in commercially pure titanium with a well-defined machined surface. They are available in eight different lengths ranging from 30 to 52.5 mm and their diameter tapers from 4 mm superiorly to 5 mm at the fixture level. They present a unique 45 degree angulated head to compensate for the angulation between the zygoma and the maxilla. The path of the zygoma implant lies along the crest of the zygomaticomaxillary buttress, and its external hex fixture head emerges in the 2nd premolar–1st molar area.

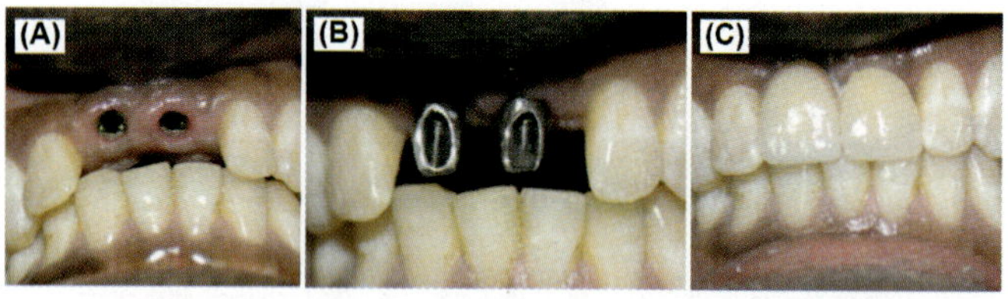

Figure 22.24 (A-C) Prosthesis retained by luting cement.

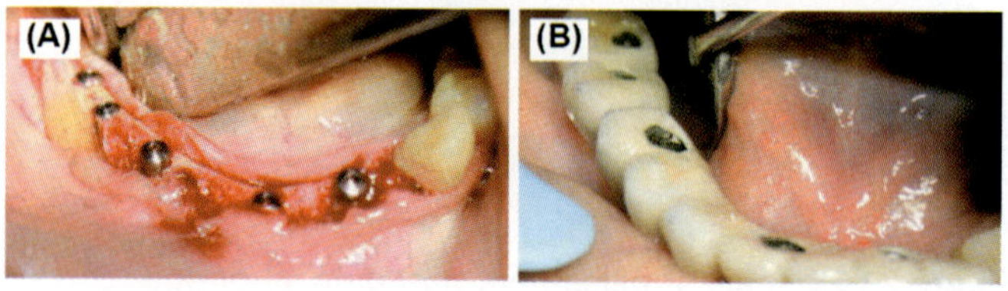

Figure 22.25 (A-B) Screw-retained prosthesis.

Important points

The tooth position should be in relation to the free gingival margin. The form of the periodontium should be adequate for proper soft tissue healing. The tooth shape should be adequate and easily replaceable without rotation. The presence of the osseous crest before extraction of the tooth. The type of extraction plays an important role as it should be atraumatic. In the anterior region, the buccal bone should not fracture. Atraumatic extraction with a piezo is indicated. The angulation of the implant should not be hindered. In case of using an implant longer than the socket, the preparation should be done adequately.

Classification: ***Aparicio's classification consists of*** five basic anatomical groups named as ZAGA 0, ZAGA 1, ZAGA 2, ZAGA 3 and ZAGA 4.

Advantages: It avoids use of grafts in atrophic maxilla. No additional donor site morbidity. Zygomatic implants placed with two to four traditional premaxillary implants can be either immediately loaded or more traditionally, a final fixed prosthesis can be placed after a 6 month healing period. Good anchorage from tough zygomatic bone, which enhances stability of prosthesis. Fewer implants are required to support a prosthesis compared to traditional bone grafting and implant placement.

TECHNIQUE (Fig. 22.26)

Surgical access: The patient may have either general anaesthesia or deep sedation for this surgery. Incision is made slightly palatal to the crest and a full thickness reflection is performed. Dissection up to the infraorbital foramen is done, a sinus window and dissection to the inner aspect of the zygoma is also done. **Osteotomy preparation:** Identify the implant trajectory and starting point for drilling using depth gauge. **Drilling sequence:** A long round bur to make an entrance mark into the maxilla from the palatal aspect of the ridge. Continue with 2.9 mm pilot drill (maximum speed ≤2000 rpm). Determine the implant length using the straight depth indicator. Widen the osteotomy with pilot drill 3.5 mm through the previously made osteotomy. Again, continue the osteotomy with the

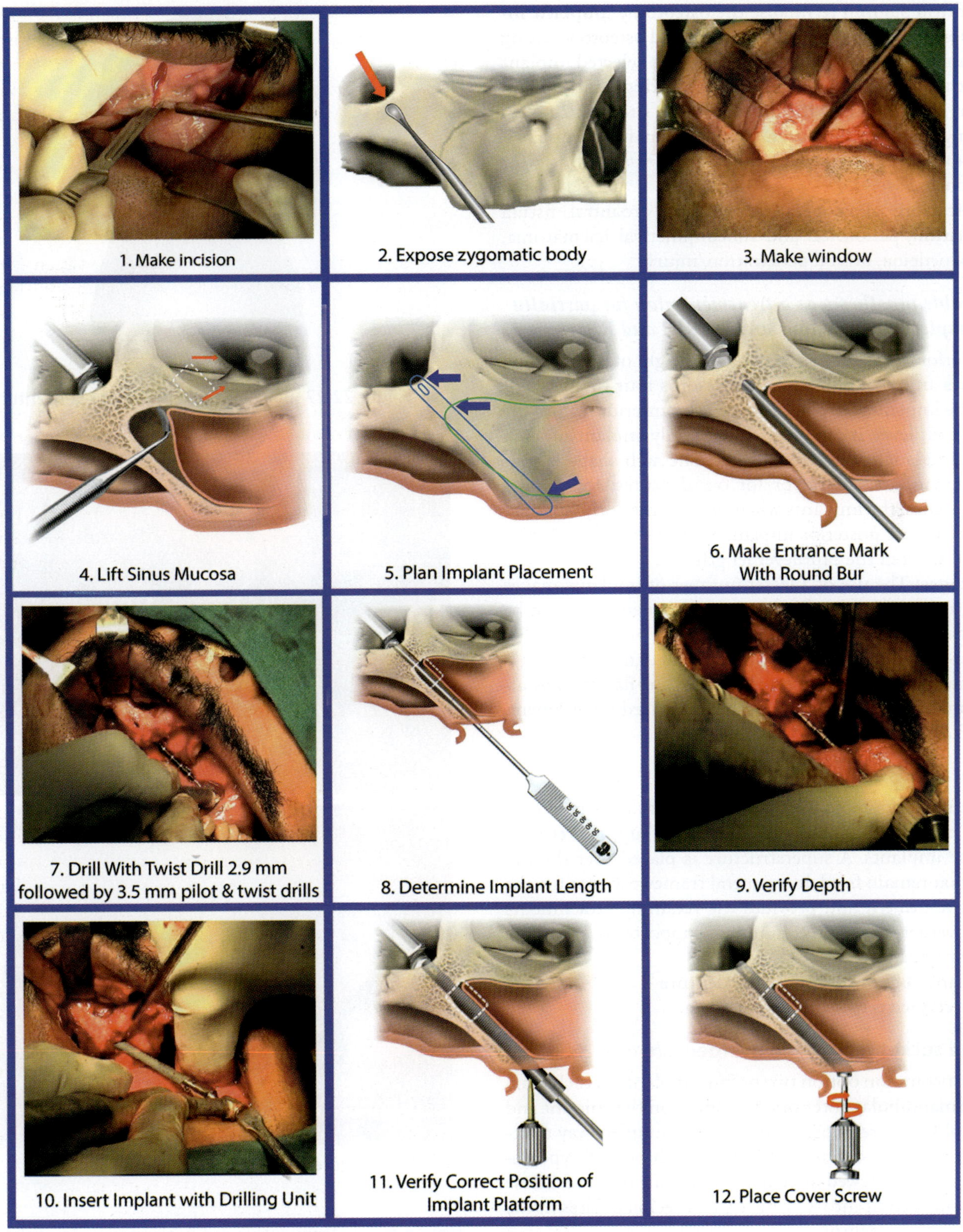

Figure 22.26 Zygomatic implant placement procedure.

twist drill 3.5 mm to finalise the osteotomy. **Implant insertion:** Verify the depth of the prepared osteotomy using the angled depth indicator to ensure the selected implant length. Irrigate the sinus before inserting the implant. Insert the implant in the prepared bone site with 20 Ncm setting on the drilling unit. Place the remaining implants. Close the flap and wait for sufficient healing (for 6 months).

Complications: Postoperative sinusitis, oroantral fistula formation, periorbital and subconjunctival haematoma, facial oedema, orbital penetration/injury.

Removable prosthesis as a treatment plan for partially and completely edentulous arches (RP4 and RP5)

The anterior mandible has the greatest height of bone among all arches and posterior mandible resorbs four times faster. Thus, the implants are placed only in the anterior region; the rest is a cantilever. It can be made with only implant support or with implant and tissue support. The arch shape is considered an important factor for overdentures; for square-shaped arches, the implants when placed anteriorly can have a short anterior posterior implant area (A-P area) ~ 5 mm. This will shorten the cantilever length.

Advantages: The use of a lesser number of implants makes this treatment cost effective. Bone augmentation can be avoided, thus reducing treatment time. Daily home care is easier. Better retention than traditional dentures.

Disadvantages: Food entrapment below the flanges. The attachments may fail over time and will need replacement. Acrylic will wear faster than porcelain.

Implant-supported overdenture—RP4

Overdentures are removable prosthesis that have better retention than a regular denture due to the support received from the implants. A superstructure is placed over the implants that remain fixed. It is a metal framework that fits the implant abutment and provides the retaining attachments for the overdenture. Types of implant supported overdenture for edentulous patients:

- Ball and socket removable overdenture
- Bar-retained removable overdenture.

Ball and socket removable overdenture (Fig. 22.27)

The most common option two or four implants in each maxillary or mandibular anteriors depending on the amount and quality of bone present. This may be the simplest way to replace an ill-fitting denture. The implants have 'ball-type' inserts which are screwed or cemented into the denture. These inserts will then fit into 'O-ring' type of recipient sites in the underside of the denture.

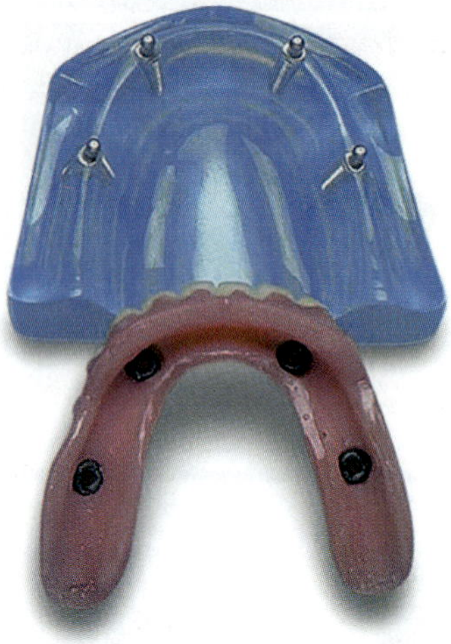

Figure 22.27 Ball and socket type of overdenture.

Bar-retained removable overdenture (Fig. 22.28)

It may require two to six implants depending on the amount and quality of bone, as well as for which jaw (upper or lower) the overdenture is being planned. The bar-retained overdenture is frequently used in the upper jaw if the patient has had a severe gagging problem with a conventional full upper denture. When patients have had severe bone resorption from previously wearing a lower denture, a new denture or a ball and socket supported implant overdenture, which rests on the gums, may compress the underlying mental

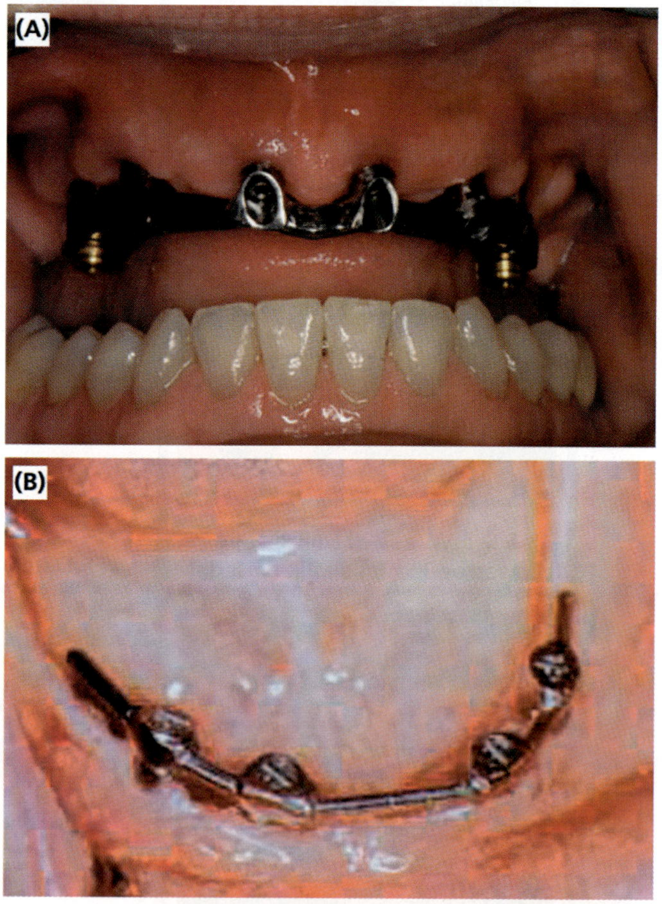

Figure 22.28 Bar type of overdenture.

nerve that lies in close approximation with this severely resorbed residual alveolar ridge. Bar-retained overdenture is recommended in resorbed ridges where the mental foramen lies at the level of the alveolar crest.

Implant and tissue-supported overdenture—RP5

The mandible between the mental foramen is divided into five equal parts (A, B, C, D and E). These sites represent the placement of the implant for RP5. Unlike RP4, where an extension bar completely supports the overdenture, in RP5, the implants only partially support the overdenture. The implants are placed perpendicular to the occlusal plane. The rest of the denture follows traditional dentures with complete flange and other components. The RP5 overdentures have some disadvantages like the need to keep relining them, and the tissue support movements can cause complete failure of the implants.

Treatment of children and adolescents with oral implants

Causes for use of dental implants in children: Ectodermal dysplasia, dental trauma, nonsyndromic agenesis, congenital aplasia, anodontia, oligodontia, missing anterior teeth, special cases of total jaw bone reconstruction.

Placement site: Maxillary and mandibular jaw bone—anterior or posterior alveolus.

Types of prosthesis that can be given for children: Fixed bridge crowns, fixed or removable prosthesis, overdentures, single crowns.

Loading of the implant: The loading of the implant has been done based on the clinical state of the implant. For implants with proper primary stability, studies show that loading it according to the adult protocol has shown success. Most studies show the clinicians allowing the healing phase to extend up to 9–12 months. This allows the clinician to analyse the implant before loading it.

Maxillary growth: Maxilla has a pronounced vertical growth, which can result in infraocclusion of the implants, but in patients younger than 10 years old, sagittal growth of maxilla can change the position of the implant as the patient grows. The midline can get shifted.

Mandibular growth: The mandible has a more pronounced sagittal growth when compared to the maxilla. The transverse growth of the mandible can result in lingual positioning of the implants. When the implant is placed in the interforaminal region, the implant can rotate due to rotational growth of the jaw.

Complications: Infraocclusion of implant supported prosthesis due to vertical growth of bone, rotation of dental implants for lower arch, loosening of implant supported restoration. Implant placed in the posterior maxilla during growth can get exposed into the sinus.

Recommendations according to literature

For the maxilla, it is better to wait till 10 years to place the implants as this avoids structural and growth complications. Placing the implants in a more coronal position prevents infraocclusion of the implants as the patient grows. More studies need to be done to achieve a specific protocol.

Bone augmentation in implantology (Figs. 22.29–22.32)

Bone augmentation is required when a patient has a vertical or horizontal bone loss. The bone dimensions are not enough to place an implant. The various bone augmentation techniques used for implant placement have been described in Table 22.14.

Case report 1: Management of bone loss up to 4 mm. Bone shaving from the nearby site.

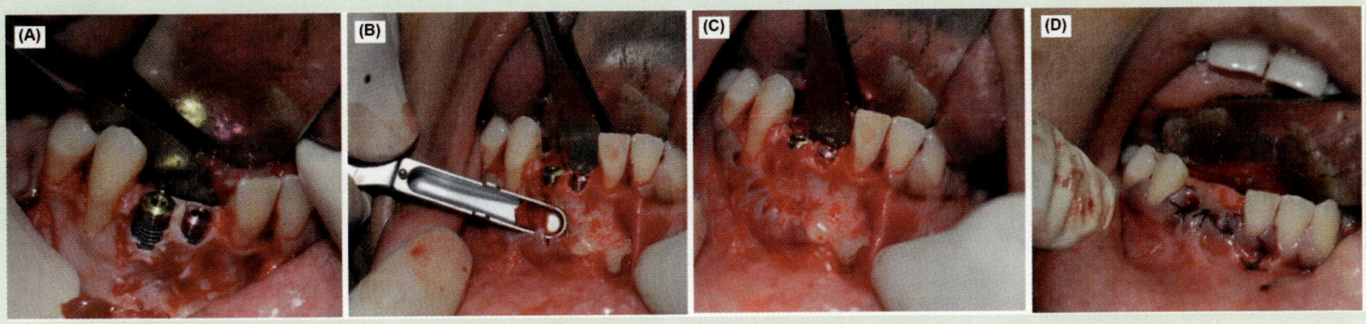

Figure 22.29 (**A–D**) Bone shavings for small bony defects in relation to the implant.

Continued

Case report 2: Management of post-surgical alveolar defect followed by bone grafting and implant fixation.

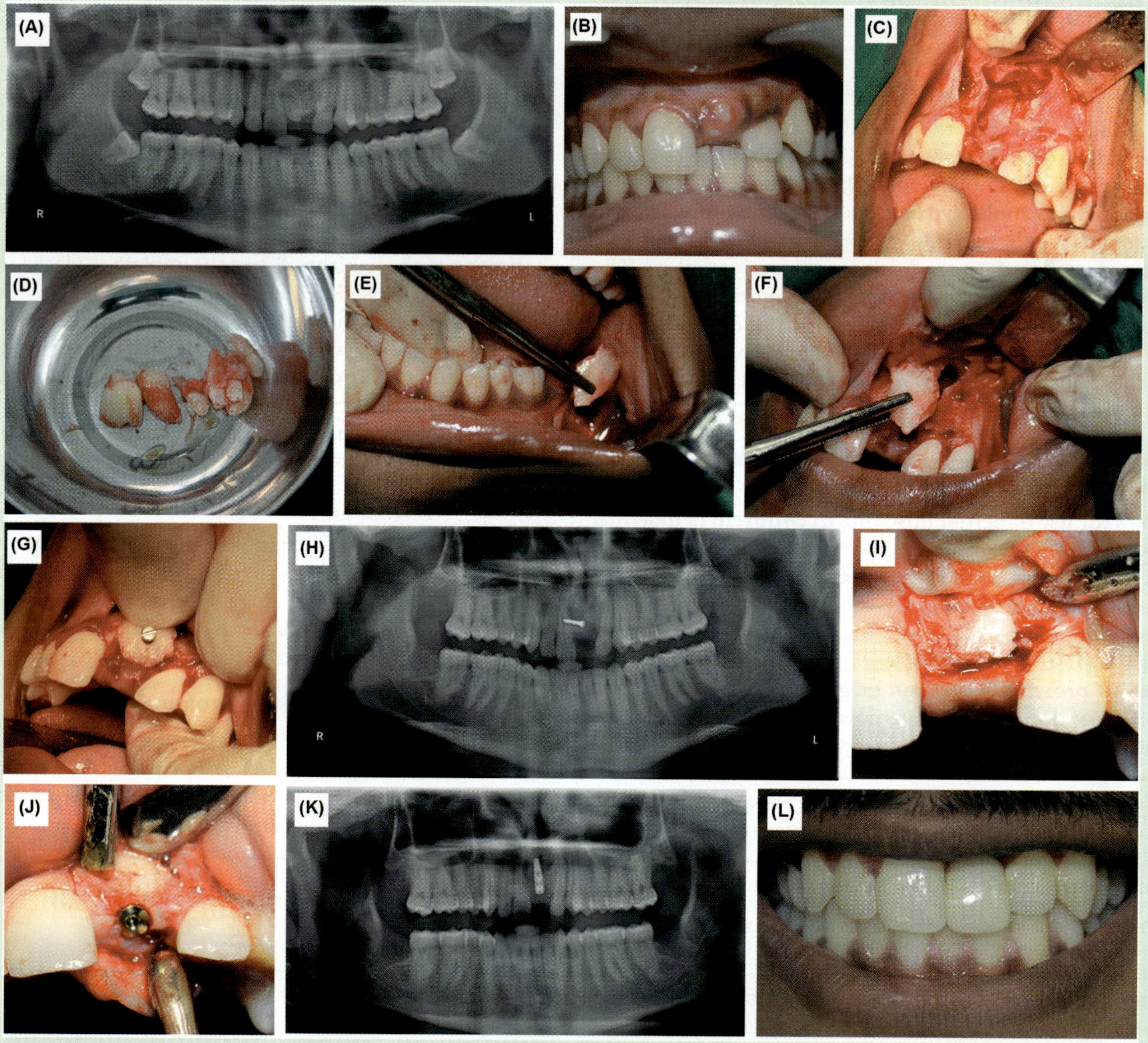

Figure 22.30 (**A**) Preoperative OPG showing odontome in the 21 region. (**B**) Odontome in the anterior maxillary region in relation to 21. (**C**) Bony defect in the excised area. (**D**) Excised odontome. (**E**) Bone graft taken from external oblique ridge region. (**F**) Filling of the bony defect using the graft. (**G**) Graft retained using screw. (**H**) Postoperative OPG showing odontome removed and graft retained with screw. (**I**) Bone fill in the defect area after a period of 3 months. (**J**) Implant fixation in the grafted area. (**K**) OPG showing Implant in relation to 21. (**L**) Postoperative view.

Case report 3: Use of bone mill for autogenous bone chips.

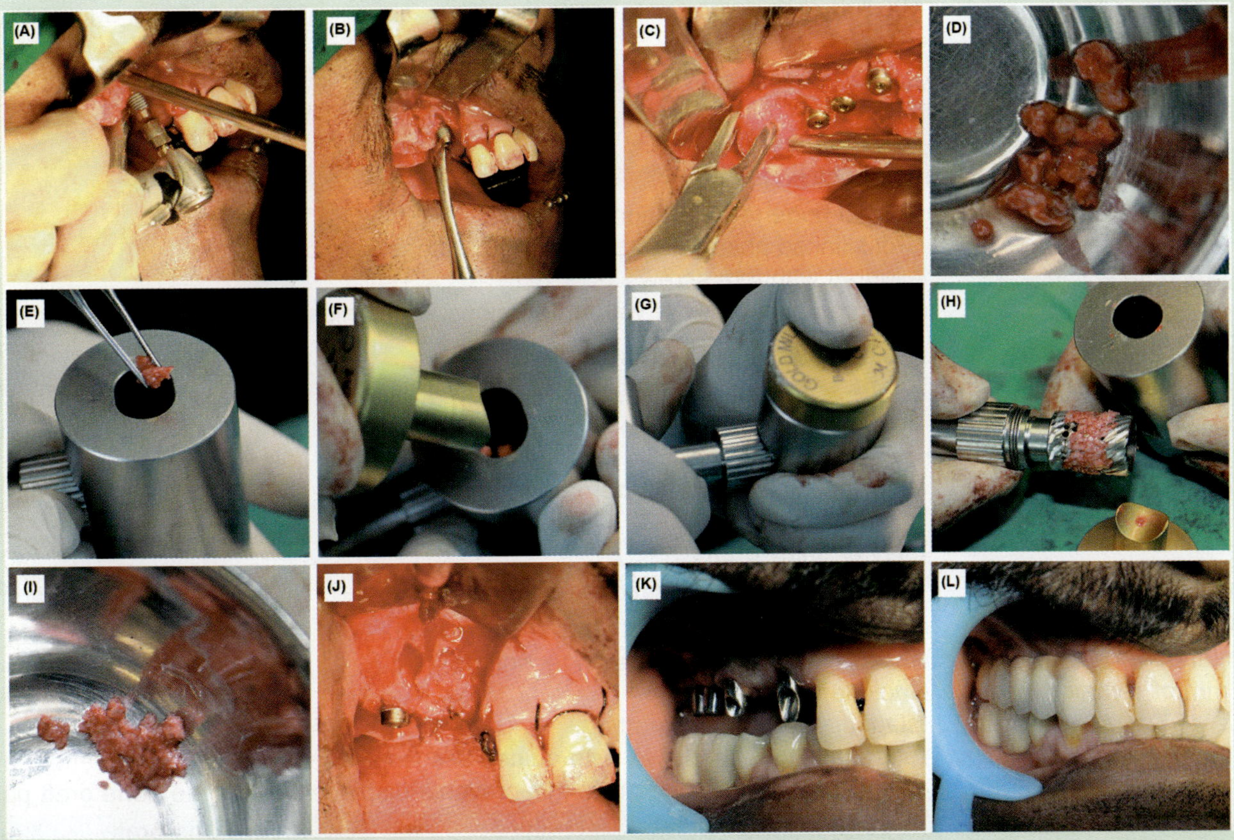

Figure 22.31 (**A**) Implant placement in 13 region. (**B**) Buccal wall defect in relation to implant. (**C**) Cortical graft from the right zygomaticomaxillary buttress region using rongeur (locoregional site of harvesting). (**D**) Cortical graft obtained from the zygomaticomaxillary buttress region. (**E–I**) Use of bone mill for the ease of adaption of the graft in the defect area. (**J**) Cortical bone fill of the defect. (**K**) Abutment placement after 3 months. (**L**) Dental rehabilitation.

Case report 4: Use of block graft from the symphysis.

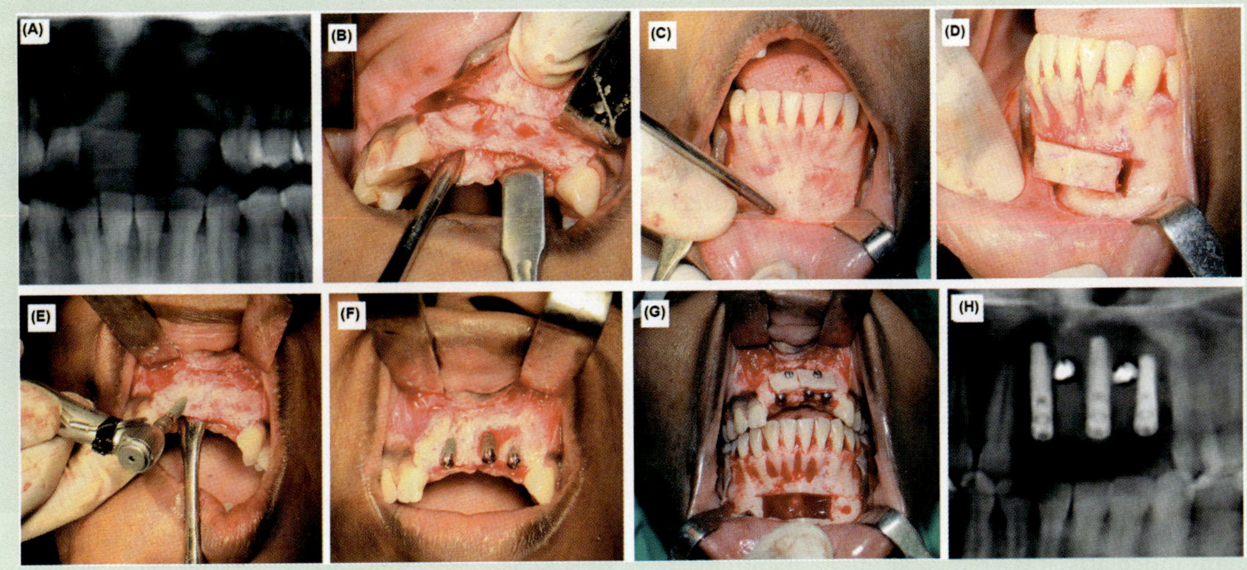

Figure 22.32 (**A**) Preoperative radiograph. (**B–G**) Simultaneous implant placement and ridge augmentation using mandibular symphysis bone graft. (**H**) Postoperative radiograph.

TABLE 22.14 Bone Augmentation Techniques for Vertical and Horizontal Bone Loss

Severity of bone loss—detected prior to extraction	Maxillary bone augmentation techniques	Mandible bone augmentation techniques
Ridge preservation techniques	Socket preservation techniques PRP Hydroxyapatite Bone shavings	Socket preservation techniques PRP Hydroxyapatite Bone shavings
Horizontal bone loss—defect 4 mm or less Vertical bone loss—defect 4 mm or less	Guided bone regeneration: Cross linked absorbable barriers with autogenous bone chips Allograft with tent screws Non-resorbable barrier with autogenous bone chips (Case report 1)	
Vertical bone loss—defect more than 5 mm	Guided bone regeneration: Nonresorbable barrier with autogenous bone chips	
Horizontal bone loss less than 6 mm of remaining width	Bone block augmentation: • Autogenous bone from the iliac crest, calvarium, maxillary tuberosity, mandibular retromolar, symphysis Inlay or onlay grafts	Bone block Augmentation Inlay or onlay grafts
Vertical bone loss—less than 6 mm of remaining bone	Indirect sinus augmentation technique	Bone block Augmentation Inlay or onlay grafts
Horizontal bone loss less than 5 mm of remaining width	Alveolar ridge split expansion technique: Book flap Island flap with bone grafting (both flaps can be closed with guided tissue regeneration membrane after packing the split area with bone graft, this prevents displacement of the bone graft particles)	
Vertical bone loss—less than 4 mm of remaining bone	Direct sinus augmentation technique: • Autogenous bone from the iliac crest or maxillary tuberosity, mandibular retromolar, symphysis • Freeze-dried bone • Xenogeneic bone • Demineralised freeze-dried bone • Hydroxyapatite Onlay bone graft Alveolar distraction osteogenesis	Onlay bone graft Alveolar distraction osteogenesis

Complications of implant therapy

Periimplantitis

The microorganisms responsible for periimplantitis and periodontitis seem to be the same. Periimplantitis affects the entire circumference of the implant resulting in a 'gutter'-like bone loss filled with inflammatory tissue. The destructive inflammatory lesions have rapid stages called 'Burst phenomenon', followed by periods of relative dormancy (Figs. 22.33). Implant failure due to periimplantitis is attributed to the interaction of certain host factors like microbiology, genetic susceptibility and host-modifying factors (Table 22.15).

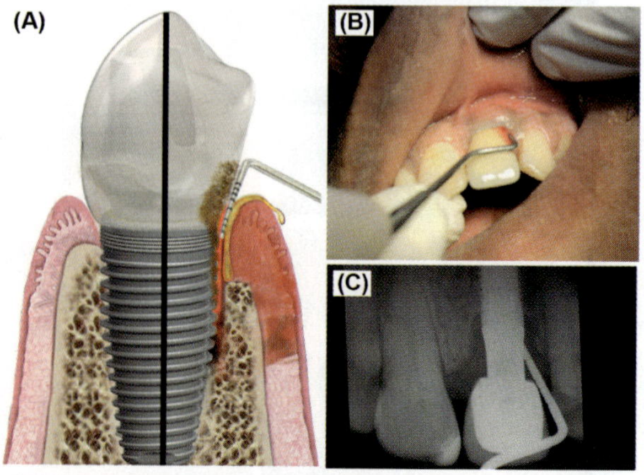

Figure 22.33 (**A**) Healthy implant and periimplantitis illustrated, (**B** & **C**)- Periimplantitis—loss of attachment to the surrounding bone.

OTHER TERMINOLOGIES

Periimplant mucositis: it is a reversible inflammation localised to the soft tissues only.

TABLE 22.15 Periimplantitis Based on Origin

Origin	Caused by
Biofilm	Bacteria induced biofilm, plaque, calculus.
Irritants	Residual cement or other irritants like smoking, food debris.
Iatrogenic factors	Implant malposition, increased functional overload, faulty technique, overheating bone during procedure.
Extrinsic pathology	Other local or systemic diseases like periapical pathology, pathological changes of adjacent tissue (benign or malignant).
Loss of periimplant junctional epithelium or connective tissue	No gingival attachment is formed, maybe due to loss of all adjacent teeth before procedure or loss of attached gingiva during traumatic extraction.

TABLE 22.16 Spiekermann's Classification 1991

Class	Description	Initial Treatment	Surgical Treatment
Class I	Slight horizontal defect from the surface of the alveolus	Conservative treatment—eliminate possible aetiologic factors	Cleaning implant surface Revising osseous topography Apical repositioning for pocket elimination Local and systemic antibiotic treatment
Class II	Moderate bone loss with isolated vertical defect		In addition to the above, systemic antibiotic treatment
Class III	Broad circular defect		Pocket elimination with osseous regeneration and adjunctive antibiotic treatment
Class IV	Broad circumferential defect with loss of buccal/lingual/palatal wall		In addition to the above, autologous bone regeneration techniques can be advised with autologous bone transfer

Periimplant disease: pathological change of periimplant tissue.

Retrograde periimplantitis: clinically, a periapical lesion develops within the 1st few months around the apex of the implant, but the coronal portion sustains normal bone-implant interface (McAllister et al., 1992).

Symptoms: bleeding on probing, increased probing pocket depth, mobility, suppuration and pain.

CLASSIFICATION (Table 22.16)

CAUSES OF PERIIMPLANTITIS

- Several experimental studies suggest that plaque accumulation can cause progressive bone loss around the implant
- It has also been stated that overloading the dental implant may result in loss of marginal bone.

CLINICAL DIAGNOSIS (Table 22.17)

The well-advanced periimplantitis lesion may be clearly identifiable via evidence of radiographic bone loss, mobility and clinical signs of infection. It is the early lesion that poses the greatest challenge to the clinician and is undoubtedly of greatest value in order to avoid further bone resorption and subsequent loss of the implant. Diagnosis of periimplantitis relies on crude parameters commonly used for the diagnosis of periodontal diseases.

TABLE 22.17 Stages of Periimplantitis Based on Periodontal Probing Depth for Diagnosis

Stage	Probing Depth	Characteristics
Early	≥4 mm	Bleeding and/or suppuration on probing is present
Moderate	≥6 mm	
Advanced	≥8 mm	

CLINICAL SIGNS OF PERIIMPLANTITIS (Fig. 22.33)

- Evidence of vertical destruction of the crestal bone, often 'saucer-shaped'
- Formation of a periimplant pocket (>4 mm)
- Bleeding or suppuration after gentle probing
- Tissue redness and swelling
- Mobility (late implant failure).

TREATMENT OF PERIIMPLANTITIS: THE 1st STEP IS ANALYSING THE QUALITY OF THE IMPLANT (Table 22.18)

IMPLANT QUALITY SCALE

The implant quality scale was updated by Misch for better clinical assessment of the patients. Once the patient has

TABLE 22.18 Management of Periimplantitis Based on Implant Quality Scale

Group	Clinical Condition	Management
Success	No pain, no mobility, no exudate <2 mm bone loss <5 mm probing depth	Normal maintenance therapy
Satisfactory health	No pain, no mobility, no exudate 2–4 mm bone loss 5–7 mm probing depth (stable) Radiographic bone level is stable	• **Occlusal therapy:** • Reduction of stress by change in prosthesis design, occlusal adjustment. • Long-span prosthesis: increase implant number and position. • **Antiinfective therapy**: • *Mechanical debridement* • Mechanical cleaning with Prophy jets • Plastic curettes • Titanium brush • Rubber cups • Polishing accessible surface with pumice • *Detoxification:* • Use of subgingival medications like Chlorhexidine chips, Chlorhexidine lavage, local doxycycline or metronidazole gel • Ligosan 260 mg slow release up to 12 days • *Systemic antimicrobial therapy* for 10 days—Metronidazole 400 mg BD • **Laser decontamination without flap**
Compromised health	No pain, no mobility Bleeding on probing is present Suppurative exudate may be present > 4 mm bone loss > 7 mm probing depth Radiograph shows bone loss more than 2 mm	**Occlusal therapy** *(same as above)* **Mechanical debridement** *(same as above)* **Ultrasonic debridement** **Laser decontamination with flap** **Drug therapy** • Metronidazole 350 mg TID • Ornidazole 500 mg BD **Surgical debridement** • Open flap debridement • Open flap debridement with guided bone regeneration (GBR) Post-GBR – Doxycycline + Ornidazole
Clinical failure	Pain, mobility, uncontrolled exudate > 50% bone loss Vertical and/or horizontal mobility of the implant	Removal of implant Allow healing of the bone
Absolute failure	Implant gets exfoliated Vertical mobility of the implant is present It is surgically removed	Allow healing of the bone Bone grafting of the site after assessment

been classified correctly, the treatment plan can be finalised easily.

IMPLANT FAILURE

Implant failure is defined as a total failure of the implant to function or provide aesthetics or phonetics due to loss of mechanical and biological support. Ailing implant is an implant that shows radiographic bone loss without inflammatory signs or mobility. Failing implant has a progressive bone loss with bleeding on probing and may have exudate but no mobility. Failed implant has progressive bone loss with clinical and radiological bone loss and clinical mobility.

CAUSES (Table 22.19)

Indications of implant removal: Fractured implant, malposition, infection, advanced periimplantitis and implant failure.

TABLE 22.19 Factors that Cause Implant Failure

Host Factors	Surgical Placement	Implant Selection Factor	Restorative Factors
Medical status Habits Poor home care Irradiation therapy	Improper angulation of implant Loss of primary stability Improper healing due to bad flap design Overheating bone more than 47°C Immature grafted site Contamination of implant body	Improper implant type Length of implant Width of the implant Number of implants Improper implant design	Excessive cantilever Pier abutment No passive fit Improper fit of abutment Bending moments Connecting implant to natural teeth Improper occlusal scheme

Removal of mobile implant: A mobile implant may easily be removed by rotating it counter-clockwise using a driver or counter-torque ratchet or forceps. Rotating with minimum luxation allows reduced trauma and damage to the surrounding bone and soft tissue.

Removal of fractured implant: These may be partially or fully osseointegrated (Fig. 22.34).

Techniques of implant removal:

- Counter-torque ratchets
- Piezo tips
- High-speed burs
- Elevators
- Forceps
- Trephine burs

Counter-torque ratchet technique: This is the least invasive technique for removing an implant without damaging surrounding structures. It should be used if the implant is able to be engaged and reverse-torqued until mobile. Care must be taken with narrow-diameter implants that are less than 4 mm in dense cortical bone to avoid further implant fracture.

Piezo tips: Piezo tips allow for better intraoperative control than high-speed burs during bone-cutting because they prevent damage to the surrounding soft tissue. It is less efficient for deep cuts into bone. Another disadvantage is when the cutting speed is decreased, the tip's temperature rises.

High-speed burs: The use of high-speed burrs under copious irrigation is an efficient method to remove a failed implant. Air from the high-speed handpiece can be forced into a surgical wound or a laceration in the mouth causing an air embolism. When using high-speed burrs, the residual apical part of the implant should be carefully approached in order to prevent damage to anatomical structures such as the sinus floor, inferior alveolar nerve and mental foramen.

Trephine burs: The smallest effective size trephine should be selected to avoid collateral damage to the neighbouring

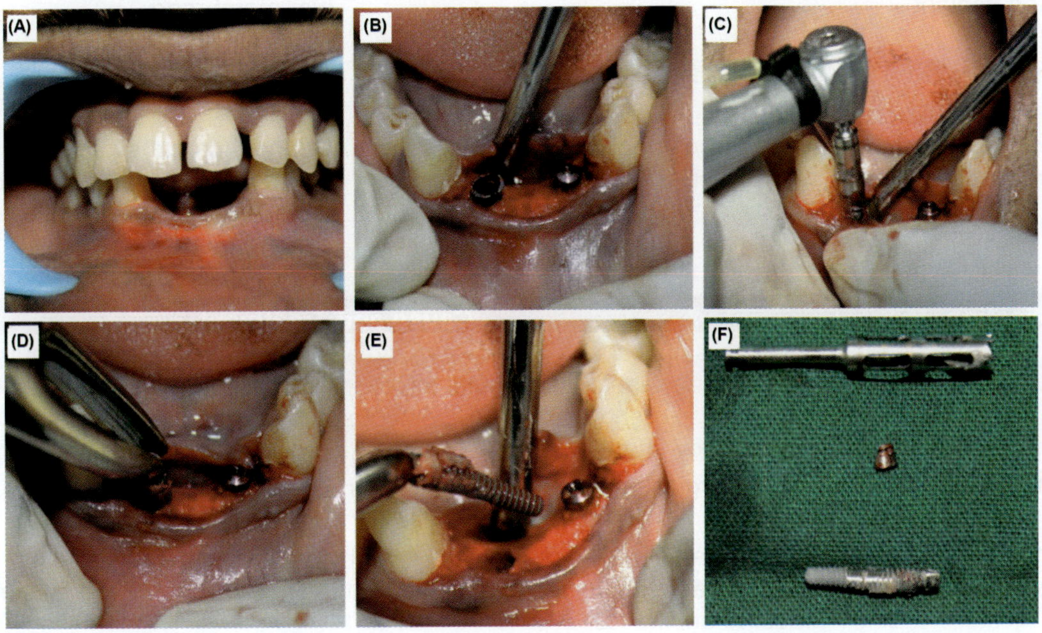

Figure 22.34 **(A–F)**—Sequential steps showing removal of fractured implant using trephine and forceps followed by replacement with another implant.

bone, teeth and/or implants. The internal diameter of the trephine needs to be slightly larger than the implant to avoid engaging the implant body. This technique is one of the most invasive options for implant removal. Osteomyelitis may occur as a complication after using a trephine burr, particularly if bone is overheated. Trephine burrs are only indicated when absolutely necessary and the retrieval procedure should be carefully planned and performed under copious irrigation with cooled saline. The coronal half of the bone around the implant should be removed to loosen the implant at which point elevators, forceps and torque drivers may be used.

Combination technique: If the integrated implant cannot be removed with less-invasive methods, the piezo tips or drill are used to remove sufficient supporting bone around the coronal parts of the implant. The counter-torque ratchet or forceps are then employed to remove the implant to reduce damage to the surrounding bone. If there is no movement, a bur or trephine can be used to cut through the surrounding cortical bone and into the trabecular bone. The reverse-torque technique is then attempted again. The goal is to preserve the remaining bone as much as possible. Alternating between the counter-torque ratchet and the elevator and occasionally drilling with the bur or trephine can then be used in combination to remove the implant.

OTHER IMPLANT COMPLICATION (TABLE 22.20)

TABLE 22.20 Describing the Complications with Cause and Treatment

Complication	Cause and Treatment	
Stage I—Intraoperative Complications		
Haemorrhage during drilling	Injury to artery Risk sites in the posterior mandible include the sublingual fossa and lingual cortex. The posterior superior alveolar and infraorbital arteries are located approximately 19 mm above the maxillary alveolar ridge and the anastomoses of these arteries can pose a risk during sinus lift procedures by lateral window preparation.	Implant placement itself can stop the bleeding or use of bone wax or Gelfoam or Surgicel to stop bleeding.
Implant mobility immediately after placement	Lack of primary stability Soft bone (D3, D4) Improper preparation	Remove the loose implant and place a larger implant. Give implant a longer healing time.
Cortical plate perforation causing exposed implant threads	Narrow crest	The threads can be covered with a coagulum membrane.
Lingual swelling	Injured sublingual artery	Send to the emergency room for vascular surgeon intervention.
Drop feeling while drilling in the posterior mandible	When alveolar ridge height is less and the surgeon is inexperienced.	Change to next size of drill and maintain the required height 2 mm above the nerve canal. Place the implant 2 mm above the nerve canal. Postoperative nerve function evaluation.

Complication	Cause and Treatment
Nerve injury	Other possible causes of nerve injury include poor flap design, traumatic flap reflection, accidental intraneural injection, traction on the mental nerve in an elevated flap, penetration of the osteotomy preparation and compression of the implant body into the canal. It has to be prevented by proper use of implant stent.
Wrong angulation	Use of surgical guides and proper treatment planning can alleviate angulation problems.
Improper implant location	Adjacent teeth should be at least 1.5 mm from the implant body and more than 3–4 mm between adjacent implants to prevent horizontal bone loss as well as to preserve aesthetics.

TABLE 22.20 Describing the Complications with Cause and Treatment—cont'd

Complication	Cause and Treatment	
Sinus or nasal floor perforation	Sinus complications often occurred when the membrane is perforated at the time of surgery. Perforations were more common in areas with minimal amount (<5 mm) of residual alveolar bone. Use of surgical guides and proper treatment planning can prevent this.	
Devitalisation of adjacent teeth	Dilacerated roots and excessive tilting in the mesiodistal direction that invade the implant space and often prevent ideal placement. If a drill and/or implant fixture invades the PDL space, hard tooth structure and/or vital pulp of the adjacent teeth, this will lead to endodontic lesions.	
Mandibular fracture	Proper implant selection and patient selection can prevent this. Immediate open reduction and internal fixation should be done.	
Ingestion and aspiration	Treat as emergency, Heimlich manoeuvre.	
Stage II Surgery and During Abutment Connection		
Sensitivity during removal of cover screw Immobile implant	Osseointegration is incomplete	Allow the healing phase to extend (2–3 months).
Pain and mobile implant	Complete lack of osseointegration	Remove the implant. Allow the socket to heal.
Difficulty in attaching gingival former or abutment screw	Bone may have covered the area where screw should lie	Under local anaesthesia, remove extending bone with a drill, irrigate well. Place the screw.
Postoperative complication	• Postoperative infection • Periimplantitis • Cover screw exposure (healing period) • Bleeding • Swelling • Transient pain or paraesthesia • Neuralgia • Fracture • Implant mobility • Recession Prosthetic complication—combination syndrome	

Section VII

Infections in Oral and Maxillofacial Surgery

Chapter 23

Head and Neck Space Infections

OUTLINE

ODONTOGENIC INFECTION

Odontogenic infection originates from the dental pulp, periodontium and jawbones or in tissues that closely surround it. **Periapical infections** are localised dental infections that spread across the pulp to the area extending beyond the apex of the tooth. When this periapical infection undergoes an acute exacerbation with pus formation within the bony confines, it becomes a **periapical abscess**. When a periapical abscess extends beyond the confines of the dentoalveolar bone into the vestibular space (space between oral vestibular mucosa and buccinator mucosa), it becomes a classic **dentoalveolar abscess**. It remains as a thick-walled cavity containing pus.

When a periapical infection fails to localise as an abscess, it results in **cellulitis** where infection rapidly spreads through fascial tissue planes diffusely.

The introduction of ***antibiotics*** has had a profound influence on the treatment of odontogenic infections. The significance of this type of infection lies in that when untreated or improperly treated, it can cause life-threatening complications by spreading to distant vital structures, for example, intracranial, retropharyngeal, pulmonary or pleural infections. The complications arising from odontogenic infections can have systemic manifestations as well as the potential to develop into life-threatening deep fascial infections. Though incidence, severity, morbidity and mortality of odontogenic infections have declined after the advent of antibiotics, basic knowledge of management of such infections is necessary to prevent morbidity.

FASCIAL SPACES

Shapiro defined fascial spaces as potential spaces between the layers of fascia. These spaces are normally filled with loose connective tissues and various structures like veins, arteries, glands, lymph nodes, etc. *Space is a misnomer as there are no voids in the tissues in actual reality.*

Purulent exudate accumulates in these potential tissue spaces, which are not actual spaces until the purulent exudate is formed. This exudate (pus) destroys the loose connective tissue and separates the anatomical boundaries of the compartment. Some of these potential spaces are compartments, which contain structures like submandibular salivary gland, lymph nodes or buccal pad of fat. Normally these structures are surrounded by deep connective tissue (Fig. 23.1A).

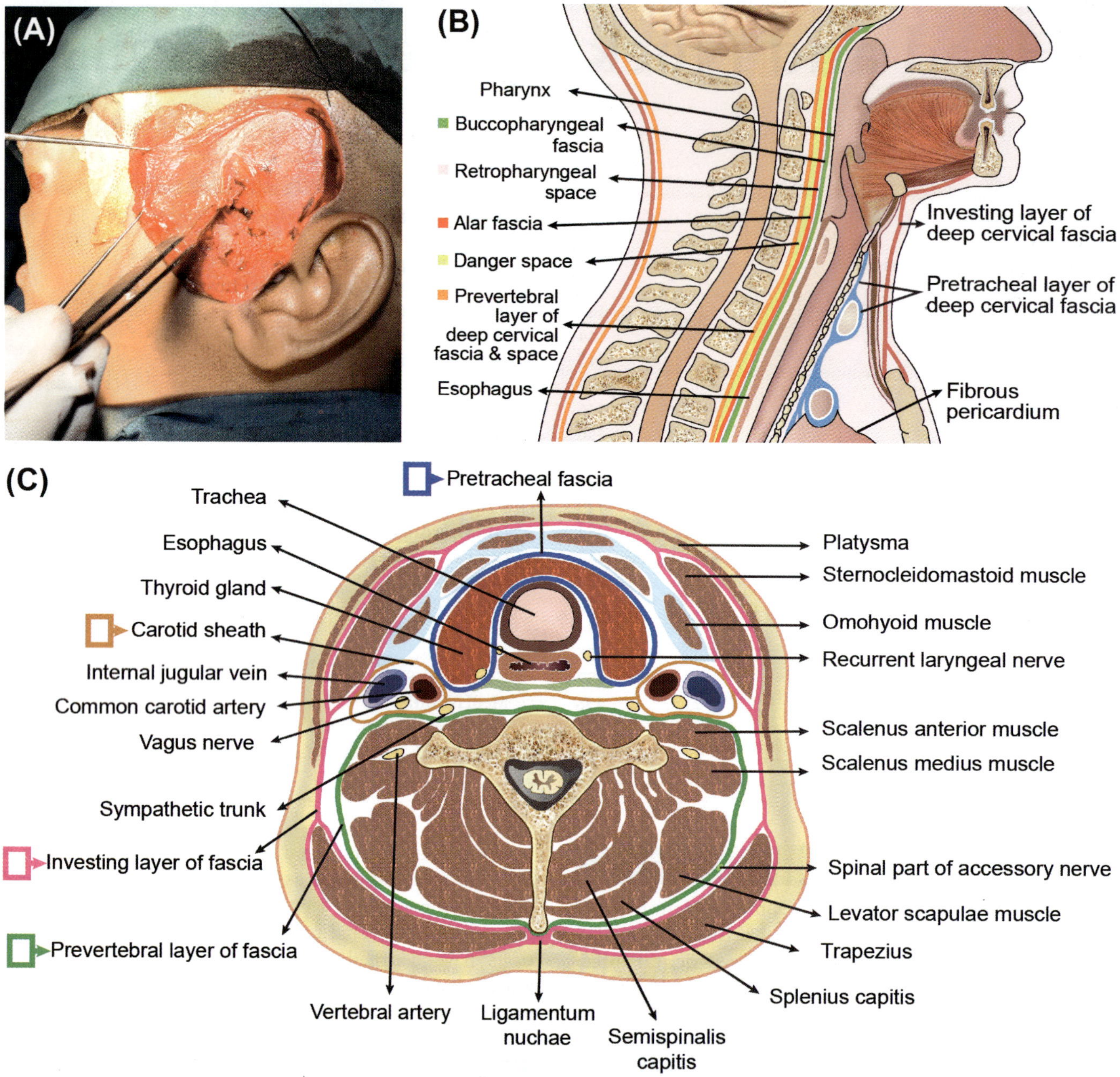

Figure 23.1 (**A**) Fascia—the photograph shows the fascia being elevated during temporomandibular joint (TMJ) surgery; the fascia has been dissected and the plane beneath the fascia accessed in order to reach the TMJ. The temporalis muscle is preserved. The temporal space is the potential space between the fascia and muscle. (**B** and **C**) Colles' fascia—superficial and deep cervical fascia.

The head and neck region has structures separated from each other through specific natural connective tissue barriers called ***fascia***. Fascia is fibrous connective tissue, which binds together various structures of the body. These fascial layers can be anatomically divided into ***superficial*** and ***deep***. The fascial spaces are potential spaces formed by the division and union of various fascial layers at different levels. They are separated by pus, blood, drain or surgical instruments during surgery. Potential spaces are present between the fascial layers. *Fascial planes offer anatomic highways for infection to spread from superficial planes to deep planes.* ***Superficial fascia*** are sheets of fibrous connective tissue, encircling the head and neck with attachments to the fascia of the shoulders, thorax and axilla. It contains the platysma muscle, external jugular vein and the marginal mandibular branch of the facial nerve, which lies just deep to it. ***Deep cervical fascia*** has three layers, the superficial layer—also called enveloping or investing or anterior layer. The middle layer—also called visceral layer or pretracheal layer. The deep layer—prevertebral fascia or carpet fascia. The cervical fascia or ***Colles' fascia*** is divided into superficial cervical fascia and deep cervical fascia (Fig. 23.1B and C).

According to Hollinshead

1. ***Superficial fascia***
2. ***Deep cervical fascia***
   a. *Anterior layer*
      i. Investing fascia
      ii. Parotidomasseteric fascia
      iii. Temporal fascia
   b. *Middle layer*
      i. Sternohyoid–omohyoid division
      ii. Sternothyroid–thyrohyoid division
      iii. Visceral division
         a. Buccopharyngeal
         b. Pretracheal
         c. Retropharyngeal
   c. *Posterior layer*
      i. Alar division
      ii. Prevertebral division.

MECHANISM OF SPREAD OF INFECTION

Depending on the virulence of the organism and host resistance, these bacterial infections have the potential to spread beyond the bony confines of the teeth and jawbones, and into the surrounding potential soft tissue spaces. These potential spaces are created by the fascia. Fascia are sheets of dense connective tissues that separate muscles, nerves, arteries, veins and glands that pass over each other. These fascial planes or spaces between the structures and the fascia are the potential spaces as described by Shapiro et al. They are called potential spaces as they are not physiologically present, but appear when a pathological collection of fluid occurs. Under ***hydrostatic pressure***, the infection follows the ***path of least resistance*** into loose areolar connective tissue of the fascia that surrounds the muscles. This type of tissue is easily destroyed by the ***hyaluronidases and collagenases*** produced by the bacteria, thus opening ***potential spaces*** surrounding the muscles. Most of these infections can be managed by early extraction of the offending tooth, incision and drainage.

The type and virulence of the microorganisms involved and the immunological condition of the patient influences the degree of spread of infection. Some organisms remain localised whereas other organisms tend to spread rapidly through the tissues along the lines of least resistance into the tissue spaces. To a greater degree, muscle attachments determine the route taken by the infection (Fig. 23.2).

Factors influencing spread of infection

Factors influencing the spread of infections are of two types—general factors and local factors. While the local factors are anatomical barriers that remain constant in all patients, the general factors vary depending on the host resistance, host defence and virulence of the microorganism as shown in Flowchart 23.1.

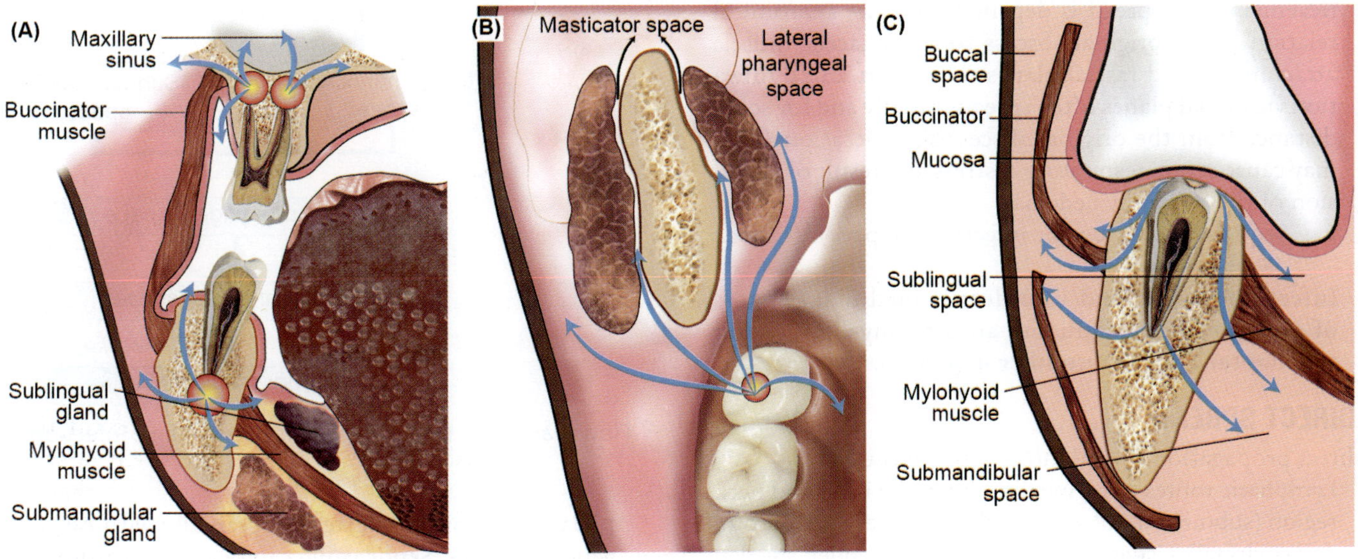

Figure 23.2 (**A**) Pathways of dental infections from maxillary and mandibular teeth. (**B**) Posterior spread of infection from mandibular 3rd molar. (**C**) Lateral spread of infection from mandibular 3rd molar.

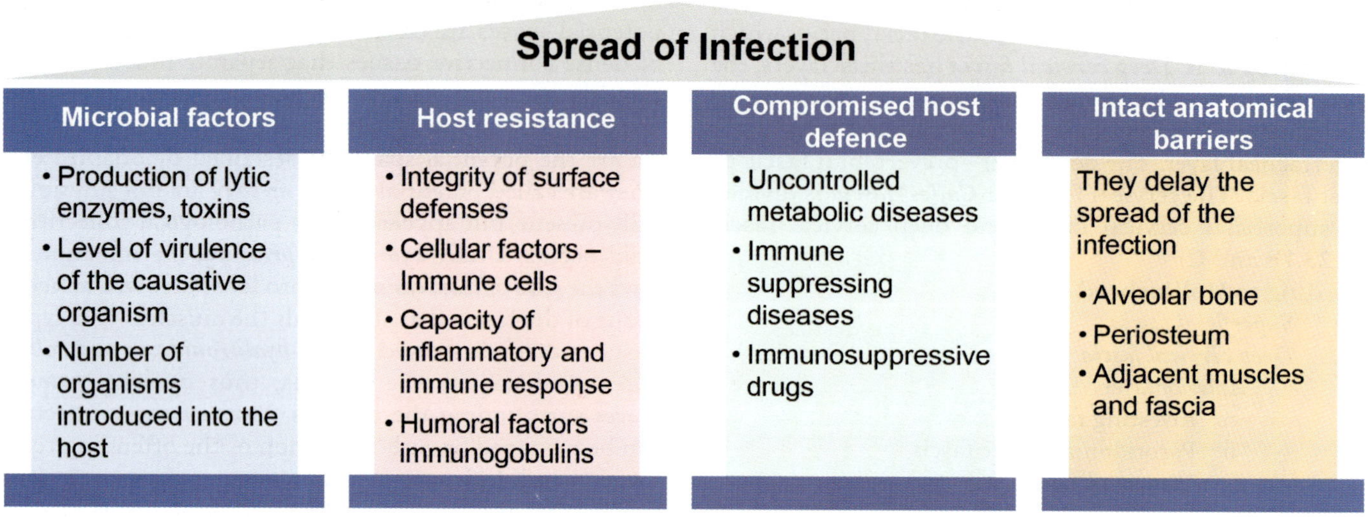

Flowchart 23.1 Systemic and local factors that affect spread of infection.

ROUTES OF SPREAD

DIRECT SPREAD

1. Direct propagation of oral infections is through local spread by direct extension—fascial space infections
   a. Localise as a soft tissue abscess
   b. Extend through the overlying oral mucosa or skin, producing a 'sinus' connecting the main abscess cavity to the exterior
   c. Extend through the soft tissue to produce cellulitis
2. Spread may occur into the adjacent fascial spaces, following the path of least resistance resulting in space infection, which can further lead to life-threatening septicaemia. Such spread is dependent on the anatomical relation of the original abscess to the adjacent muscle attachments and fascial planes (Flowchart 23.2). Infection via fascial planes often spreads rapidly and for some distance from the original abscess site. Occasionally, it may cause severe respiratory distress as a result of occlusion of the airway by oedema
   a. Sequelae: Odontogenic infection → space infections → septicaemia
3. Infection may extend into deeper medullary spaces of alveolar bone producing an osteomyelitis. (Refer to Chapter 24, page number 474–486).

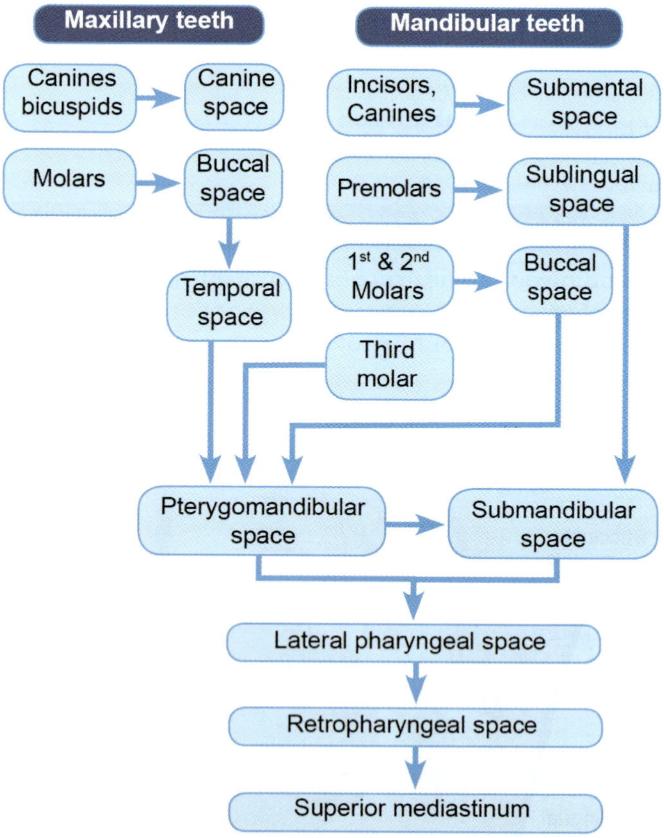

Flowchart 23.2 Direct spread of odontogenic infections.

INDIRECT SPREAD

Indirect propagation of oral infections is through:

1. Lymphatic routes to regional nodes in the head and neck region (submental, submandibular, deep cervical, parotid and occipital). Usually involved nodes are tender, swollen and rarely may suppurate requiring drainage
2. Haematogenous routes to other organs such as brain is possible through deep facial vein and pterygoid venous plexus that communicate intracranially with cavernous venous sinuses. Septicaemia can be caused through haematogenous spread (Flowchart 23.3). Venous spread—cavernous sinus thrombosis—valveless veins of the face—retrograde spread.

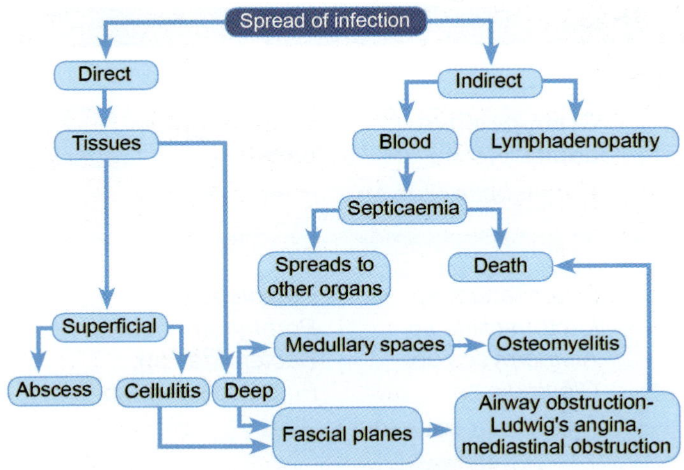

Flowchart 23.3 Routes of spread of infection.

AETIOLOGY OF SPACE INFECTIONS

DENTAL CARIES

Dentoalveolar abscess usually develops by extension of dental caries lesion causing the spread of bacteria to the pulp via the dentinal tubules. When the decay reaches the dental pulp, it will lead to pulpitis. Infection from here may spread to supporting bone resulting in periapical abscess, which in turn may spread subperiosteally. The pulp responds to infection either by rapid acute inflammation involving the whole pulp, which quickly becomes necrosed or by development of a chronic localised abscess with most of the pulp remaining viable (Flowchart 23.4).

1. Traumatic root fracture or pathological exposure due to tooth wear
2. Traumatic pulpal exposure due to dental treatment
3. Through periodontal membrane and accessory root canal
4. Rarely by anachoresis, that is seeding of the organisms directly into the pulp via pulpal blood supply during bacteraemia
5. Periapical abscess may occur in seemingly intact but devitalised teeth (trauma, cracks or decay under fillings)
6. Periapical and periodontal abscess may result from chronic gingivitis and periodontitis.

PERICORONITIS

Partially impacted 3rd molars with a gingival flap serves as a nidus for food accumulation and infection, very often leading to a space infection. The infection from the 3rd molar can spread posteriorly to the lateral pharyngeal space, masticator space and laterally to the buccal space, sublingual space and submandibular space below the mylohyoid (Fig. 23.1B and C).

MICROBIOLOGY OF ODONTOGENIC INFECTIONS

Of all the infections resulting from microorganisms contained in the oral flora, the leading ones are related to odontogenic

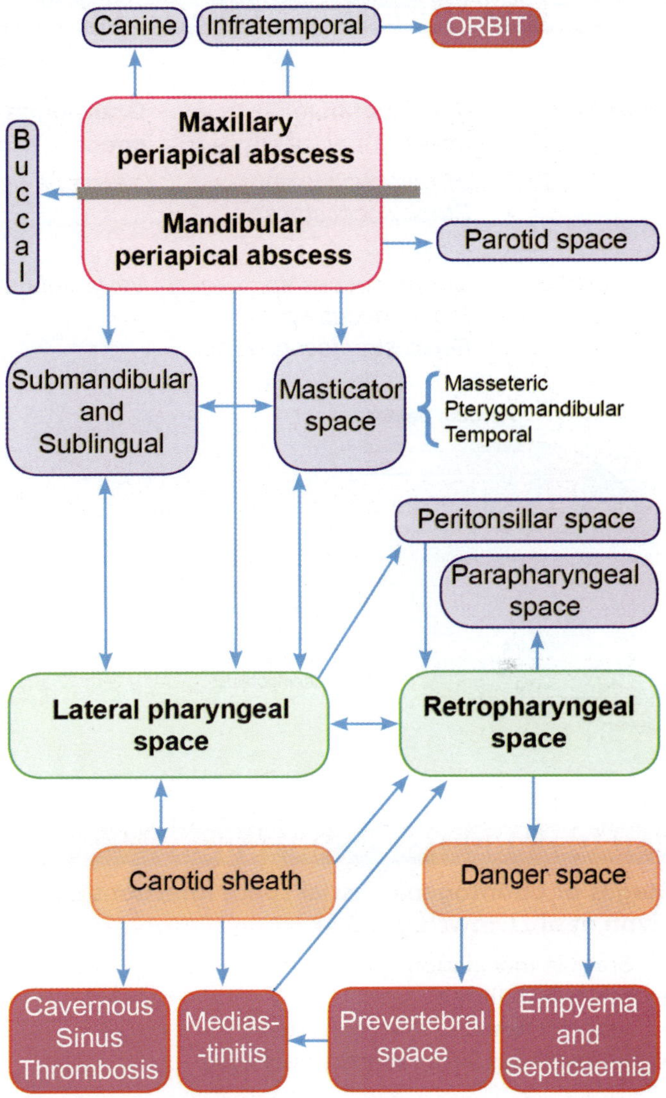

Flowchart 23.4 Spread of maxillary and mandibular dental infection into fascial spaces.

infections. Almost all are polybacterial, caused by five different species on average and by mixed aerobic–anaerobic flora, especially Gram-positive aerobic, anaerobic cocci and Gram-negative anaerobic bacilli in more than 95% of cases. Approximately, 5% of odontogenic infections are caused by aerobic bacteria, 35% are due to anaerobic bacteria and the remaining 60% are jointly caused by aerobes and anaerobes (Table 23.1). The infections caused by these microorganisms follow a well-defined pattern of evolution. Following inoculation in deep tissue, there is a proliferation of aerobic bacteria, such as the more invasive and virulent *Streptococcus* sp., which leads to a decrease in the tissue oxidation–reduction potential, thereby creating the ideal conditions for anaerobic bacteria to proliferate; these anaerobic bacteria will predominate or may be the only ones encountered in suppurative and chronic phases of the infectious process.

TABLE 23.1 Bacterial Causes of Odontogenic Infection

	Microorganism			
Aerobic	**Gram-positive cocci**	**Gram-negative cocci**	**Gram-positive bacilli**	**Gram-negative bacilli**
	Streptococcus sp. *Staphylococcus* sp. *Eikenella* sp.	*Neisseria* sp.	*Corynebacterium* sp.	Haemophilus sp.
Anaerobic	*Streptococcus* sp. *Peptococcus* sp. *Pepto streptococcus* sp.	*Veillonella* sp.	*Eubacterium* sp. *Lactobacillus* sp. *Actinomyces* sp. *Clostridia* sp.	*Prevotella* sp. *Porphyromonas* sp. *Bacteroides* sp. *Fusobacterium* sp.

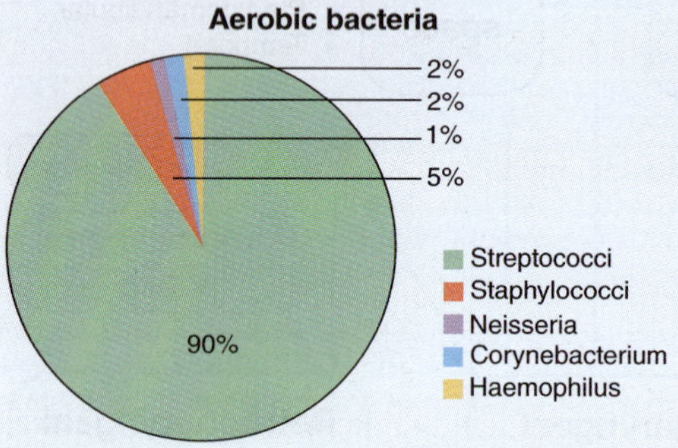

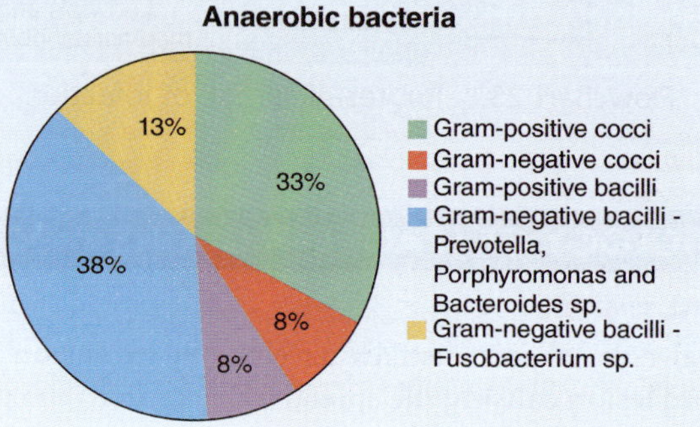

STAGES AND TYPES OF INFECTION

Stages of odontogenic fascial space infections by Flynn et al., (Flowchart 23.5)

- Stage I—inoculation
- Stage II—cellulitis
- Stage III—abscess/space infection
- Stage IV—resolution/septicaemia.

CELLULITIS

Cellulitis is defined as a 'diffuse, nonsuppurative inflammatory reaction of the fascial tissue planes (submucosal or subcutaneous) or loose connective tissues, usually as a result of bacterial odontogenic infections'.

Clinical findings

Cellulitis of head and neck involves the face and orbit commonly. Cellulitis of clinical importance involving bilateral submandibular, sublingual and submental spaces is called ***Ludwig's angina.***

Cellulitis presents with classical clinical findings of diagnostic values:

- Acute onset (short duration of within 3 days)
- Fever and malaise
- Swelling of the involved tissues causing facial asymmetry
- Skin over the swelling appears erythematous, shiny and nonpinchable. It may show secondary changes such as discolouration
- Swelling is painful and tender with firm board like consistency and induration
- Regional lymphadenopathy is common
- *Ludwig's angina*—presents classically as a swelling of the lower face extending to the neck. Involvement of the floor of the mouth causes raising of the tongue, extension to the neck (laryngoedema) may cause airway obstruction—hyperventilation, increased respiratory rate, use of accessory muscles of respiration (sternocleidomastoid), which may further spread to the mediastinum (mediastinitis)
- Cellulitis may involve the orbital tissues resulting in orbital cellulitis.

ORBITAL CELLULITIS

Periorbital and orbital cellulitis may result from maxillary infection. It is an uncommon sequela, usually seen in immunocompromised patients (Fig. 23.3).

Classification of orbital cellulitis

Chandler et al., classification of orbital cellulitis includes five groups (Table 23.2). Difference between cellulitis and abscess are depicted in Table 23.3.

ABSCESS

PERIAPICAL ABSCESS

- An abscess is a thick-walled cavity containing pus
- Periapical abscess refers to an abscess of odontogenic origin that occurs mainly in relation to the root apices. It may be confined to the alveolar bone, perforate through the bone and reaching the surface or invade the soft tissues subperiosteally or supraperiosteally. Abscess formation may be well circumscribed or may be associated with regional cellulitis

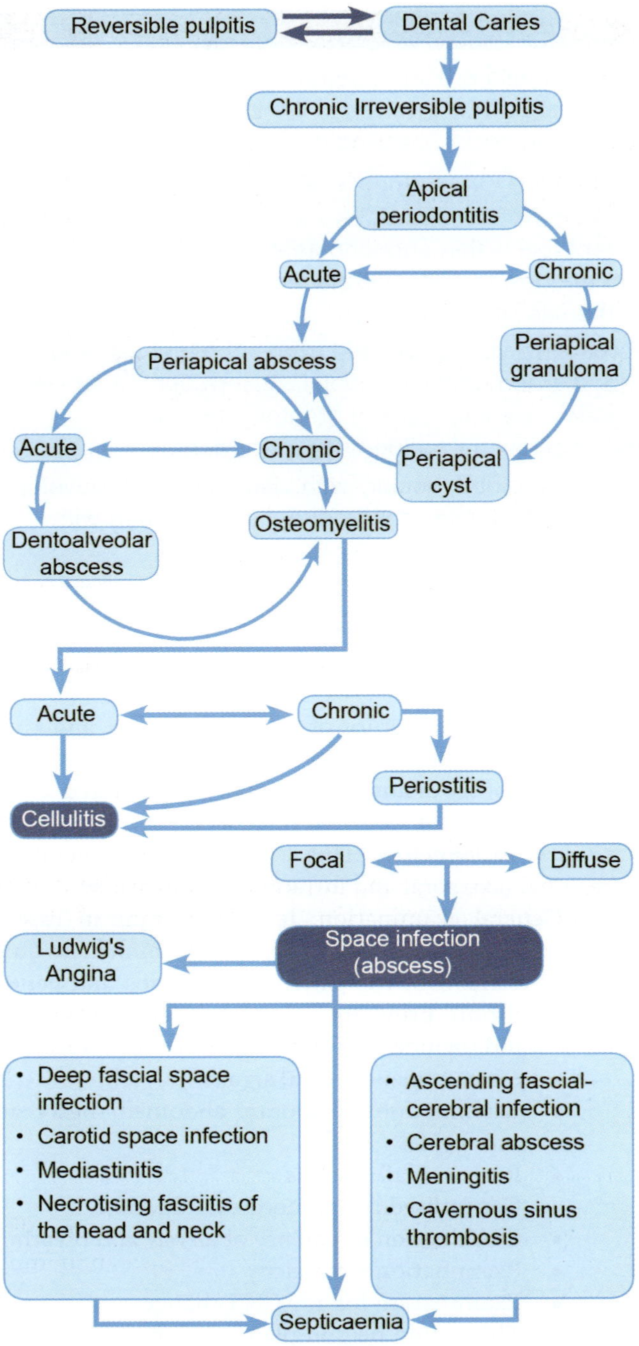

Flowchart 23.5 Sequelae of odontogenic infection.

- *Staphylococcus* is associated with abscess formation that produces coagulase (coagulase-positive staphylococci) in contrast to association of streptococci in cellulitis
- The number, position, shape and curvature of roots and their apices determine the common site of localisation of abscess
- Common sites for the localisation of dental abscess in maxillary and mandibular teeth:
  a. Mandibular incisors—labial/lingual
  b. Mandibular canines—labial

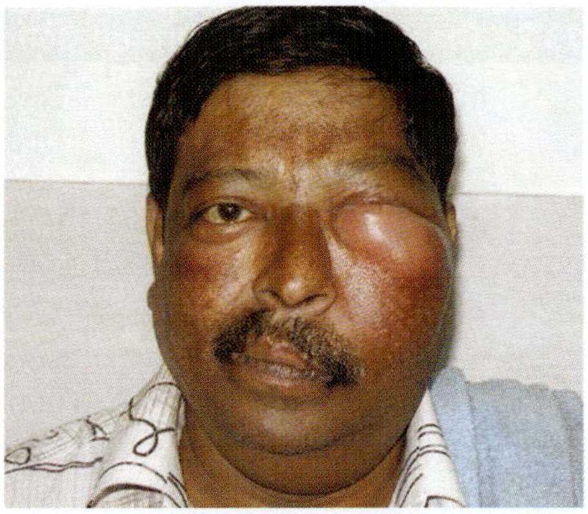

Figure 23.3 Preoperative view of the patient with preseptal cellulitis (canine space infection).

  c. Mandibular premolars—buccal
  d. Mandibular molars—buccal
  e. Maxillary incisors—labial
  f. Maxillary canines—labial
  g. Maxillary 1st premolars—labial and palatal
  h. Maxillary 2nd premolars—buccal
  i. Maxillary molars—buccal and palatal
- Differences between periapical and periodontal abscesses are depicted in Table 23.4.

DENTOALVEOLAR ABSCESS

The infection that has extended beyond the alveolar bone and comes into the adjacent soft tissues as a localised form is known as dentoalveolar abscess.

Abscess pass through three stages before they undergo resolution:

1. During 1–3 days—the swelling is soft, mildly tender and doughy in consistency
2. Between 5 and 7 days—the centre begins to soften and the underlying abscess undermines the skin or mucosa making it compressible. The underlying pus may be seen through the epithelial layers making it fluctuant
3. Finally, there is a resolution of the abscess that may be spontaneous or after surgical drainage. During the resolution phase, the involved region is firm on palpation due to the process of necrotic tissues and bacterial debris removed by the macrophages and alternating repair mechanism.

EVALUATION OF THE PATIENT WITH OROFACIAL INFECTION

Evaluation of a patient with odontogenic infection follows the same basic principles of diagnosis as with any oral disease. The steps include the following:

1. ***History taking:***
   In case of odontogenic infections, this should mainly include:
   - Onset, duration and course of present condition
   - Any associated symptoms such as fever, chills, etc

TABLE 23.2 Classification of Orbital Cellulitis

Group I	Inflammatory Oedema (Preseptal Cellulitis, Periorbital Cellulitis)	Swelling of the eyelids with mild orbital oedema Upper eyelid (usually medial part) is involved in the initial stages. More advanced stage includes 'chemosis' (swelling of the conjunctiva)
Group II	Orbital cellulitis	Infiltration of the orbit, leading to oedema, congestion, proptosis, motor and visual impairment
Group III	Subperiosteal abscess	Accumulation of purulent foci within subperiosteal space leads to nonaxial displacement and tenderness. Displacement of the globe is nonaxial and reflects the site of the abscess
Group IV	Orbital abscess	Progression of intraorbital cellulitis or spread from subperiosteal space leads to intracoronal or extracoronal loculations. Severe ophthalmoplegia, orbital cellulitis, visual loss and marked proptosis produced by localised necrosis and abscess formation within central orbital fat
Group V	Cavernous sinus thrombosis	Proptosis and fixation of the globe, usually with visual loss and development of similar signs in the opposite orbit frequently associated with signs of meningitis

TABLE 23.3 Differences Between Cellulitis and Abscess

Features	Cellulitis	Abscess
Duration	3–7 days	More than 5 days
Size	Large	Small
Localisation	Diffuse	Circumscribed
Palpation	Hard and tender	Fluctuant
Skin	Thickened, board hard	Undermined and shiny
Temperature	Warm	Moderately warm
Loss of function	Severe	Moderately severe
Tissue fluid	Serosanguineous	Pus
Bacteria	Mixed	Anaerobic
Degree of seriousness	Very severe	Moderate to severe

TABLE 23.4 Differences Between Periapical and Periodontal Abscesses

Features	Periapical Abscess	Periodontal Abscess
Site	Usually over the apex of tooth	Usually over gingival 3rd of alveolar process
Aetiology	Necrosis of pulp	Periodontal pockets
Tooth mobility	Only in late stages	In early stages
Age	Young and middle age	Middle to older age

- History of extraction or any other trauma to the site
- Previous history of similar infection and treatment administered
- History of any radiotherapy administered
- History of recurrent infections

2. ***Clinical examination:*** This would include general and regional (extraoral and intraoral) examinations
   a. General examination: It is important in case of odontogenic infections to have an immediate quick assessment of the patient's vital signs and general condition prior to a complete evaluation. This should include the following:
      - Measurement of vital signs
      - Examination of thorax, abdomen, heart and extremities
      - Review of all systems
      - Generalised lymph node examination
      - Examination of patency of airway and breathing
      - Examination for toxicity
      - Examination for any CNS changes
      - This would help in planning for any emergency medical or surgical intervention (e.g. tracheostomy) if needed
   b. Regional examination
      i. Extraoral examination
         1. Skin changes—swelling, redness, ulcers, etc
         2. Bony enlargements
         3. Lymph node swellings
         4. Presence of any sinus openings, fistula, etc
         5. Restrictions in mouth opening—trismus
         6. Ophthalmic examination
      ii. Intraoral examination
         1. Swelling (consistency, fixity), discharge, dental caries, deviation of tissues (tongue, uvula)

3. ***Clinical features of odontogenic infections***
   a. Signs and symptoms of early complications of space infection
      i. A nonvital tooth with or without a carious lesion or with a large restoration
      ii. Pallor
      iii. Rapid breathing or difficulty breathing
      iv. Pounding pulses
      v. Fever and shivering
         1. Fever/pyrexia: normal oral temperature is 97.7°F–99.5°F
         2. Chills—this is typical in bacteraemia and pyogenic abscesses
         These two symptoms are direct consequence of increased levels of systemic inflammatory cytokines such as interleukins and tumour necrosis factors in response to bacterial products such as lipopolysaccharides (i.e. endotoxins)
      vi. Lethargy
      vii. Diaphoresis—heavy perspiration
      viii. The cardinal signs of inflammation are present. If they are absent, then it is an indication that the infection is spreading to the deeper tissues
         1. ***Rubor*** or redness: Present when infection is close to the tissue surface; markedly seen in light-complexioned patients. It is due to vasodilatation
         2. ***Tumour*** or swelling: This is caused by the build-up of inflammatory exudate or pus
         3. ***Calor*** or heat: It is the result of inflow of warm blood from the deeper tissues, increased velocity of blood flow and increased rate of metabolism
         4. ***Dolor*** or pain: It is due to the pressure on sensory nerve endings caused by distention of tissues by oedema or spreading of infection, liberated or activated factors such as kinins, histamine, metabolites or bradykinin-like substances on nerve endings
         5. ***Functio laesa*** or loss of function: Reflected as difficulty in chewing, swallowing and respiratory embarrassment. Also associated with the reflex inhibition of muscle movements associated with pain
      ix. Headache is commonly accompanied with fever and is thought to be caused by straining of sensitive areas surrounding dilated intracranial arteries
      x. Lymphadenopathy: In acute infections, lymph nodes are enlarged, soft and tender. In chronic infections, nodes are less firm, often nontender. Suppuration of the nodes occurs when infecting organism overwhelms the local defence mechanism in the node and produces excessive cellular reaction and collection of pus
      xi. Presence of draining sinuses or fistulae
      xii. Trismus—difficulty opening the mouth
      xiii. Difficulty swallowing
      xiv. Increased salivation
      xv. Changes in phonation
      xvi. Presence of halitosis due to intraoral pus discharge
   b. Clinical symptoms of late (systemic) complications of space infection
      i. Impairment of respiratory system
      ii. Difficulty in swallowing
      iii. Impaired vision or eye movement. Oedema of the upper and lower eyelids, as well as atypical eye signs (CNS symptom)
      iv. Severe headache, stiff neck and vomiting are all symptoms of meningeal inflammation (CNS symptom)
      v. Change in the quality of one's voice
      vi. A reduced level of consciousness (CNS symptom)
      vii. Agitation and restlessness as a result of hypoxia
4. ***Laboratory investigations:*** Other than the usual laboratory investigations, it is imperative to do a bacterial culture and an antibiotic sensitivity test. This will help in directly eliminating the source of infection
5. ***Radiological investigation:***
   i. Intraoral periapical (IOPA) radiograph and Orthopantomogram (OPG): Conventional radiographic methods may be used to determine the underlying cause (carious/impacted teeth, foreign body)
   ii. Lateral view of mandible, lateral view of neck
   iii. Anteroposterior (AP) view
   iv. CT and MRI: It is especially useful in special infections as they clearly show the extent of soft tissue damage. Moreover, with the advent of 3DCT and other advances in imaging, the extent can be studied in all planes. Other than their diagnostic and prognostic uses, these imaging methods can also be used as treatment aids, for example, in CT-guided percutaneous drainage (Table 23.5 and Fig. 23.4)
6. ***Interventional procedures:***
   i. Fine Needle Aspiration Cytology (FNAC)
7. ***Diagnosis and treatment planning*** (Flowchart 23.6).

PRINCIPLES OF MANAGEMENT OF ODONTOGENIC INFECTIONS

TREATMENT OF THE CAUSES

Most infections have a distinct cause and only surgical treatment will prevent worsening and recurrence, though antibiotics play a supportive role. In early cases, surgical treatment may be as simple as root canal treatment of the suspected tooth or alternatively simple tooth extraction followed by oral antibiotics. However, in advanced infections resulting in

TABLE 23.5 CT View of the Suprahyoid Neck Spaces Commonly Seen in Oral and Maxillofacial Surgery

CT View of Various Spaces	Contents
Submandibular space 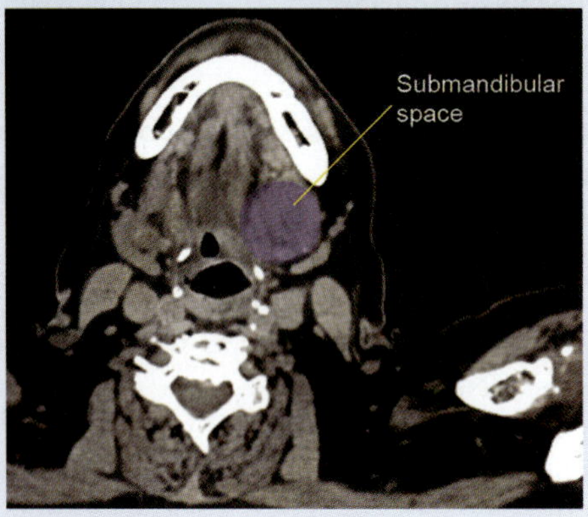 Figure 23.4 (A) CT scan view of Submandibular space.	• The superficial lobe of the submandibular gland appears as a well-defined soft tissue density that is frequently bordered by a fat plane. • The lymph nodes of the submandibular region have a homogeneous, nonenhancing appearance and are 1.5 cm in diameter. • The deep lobe can be seen in the coronal section. • The mylohyoid muscle is a soft tissue band that runs as a coronal sling between the medial aspect of the mandible. • The genioglossus is a muscular band divided by a low-density midline lingual septum. Cellulitis or abscess cause loss of submandibular soft tissue plane.
Sublingual space 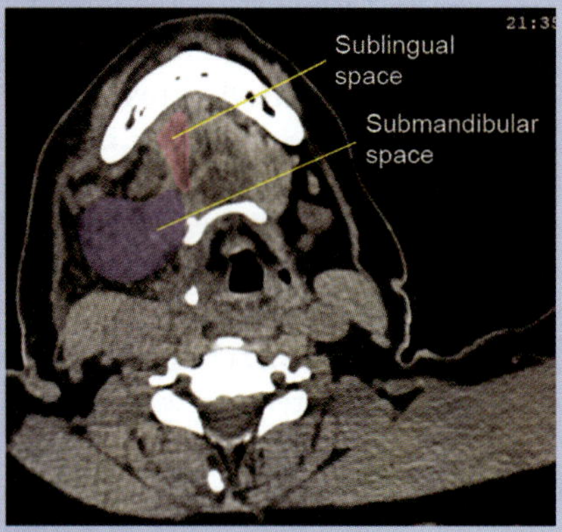 Figure 23.4 (B) CT scan view of Sublingual space.	• Sublingual space is a low-density area located between the paramidline and the genioglossus muscle on the medial side of the mandible and the mylohyoid muscle and the medial surface of the jaw on the lateral side of the mandible. With IV contrast, the lingual blood vessel, which is a very significant landmark, may be seen clearly. The hyoglossus and styloglossus are two muscles that appear as a narrow curvilinear muscle complex in this space. • On axial CT, the anterior belly of the digastric can be seen in the digastric fossa on the undersurface of the anterior jaw. • Below the level of the mandible on an axial CT image, paired anterior bellies of the digastric can be seen stretching between the anterior mandible and the larger cornu of the hyoid bone.
Masticator space 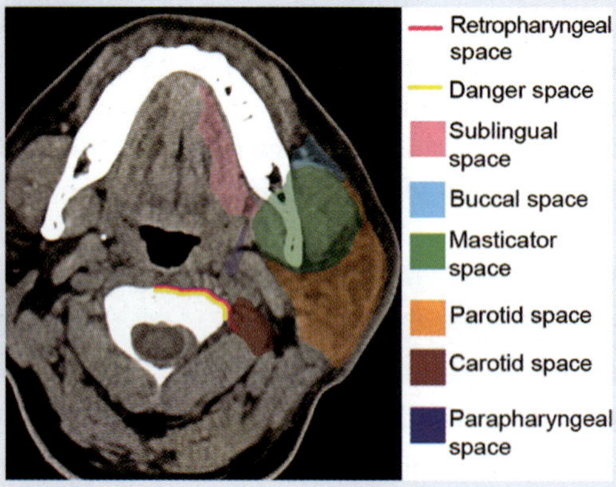 Figure 23.4 (C) CT scan view of Masticator space.	• Masticator space is a separate deep fascial space, surrounded by layers of deep cervical fascia. The deep cervical fascia acts as an early line of defence against transmission of infection. Masticator space infection causes a complicated drainage issue once the fascial limits have been compromised. • Trismus complicates clinical examinations of patients with masticator space infection and so a CT imaging may be advised. The lack of visible pus on CT images indicates cellulitis, which restricts surgical drainage. A subperiosteal drainage is required for osteomyelitis. Spread of infection beyond the masticator space requires an extensive drainage technique. Presence of pus confined to masticator space, facilitates intraoral drainage.

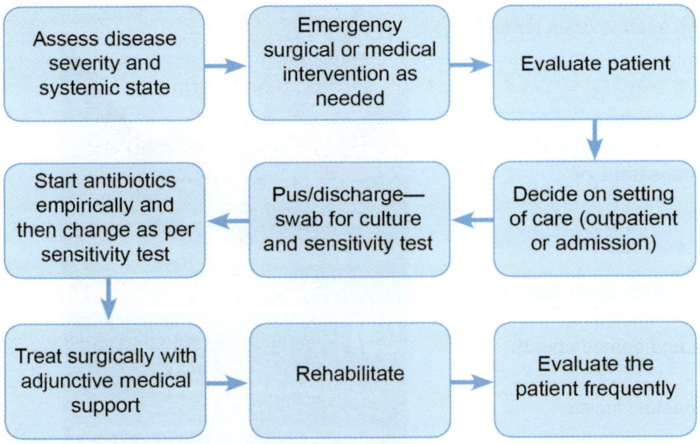

Flowchart 23.6 Algorithm for management of odontogenic infections.

space infection and septicaemia, management strategies shift to medical management. Surgically, most cases can be approached transorally. Removal of the cause (usually tooth) is followed by incision and drainage of the infection. Early diagnosis, prompt empirical antibiotic treatment together with early removal of the cause can prevent most complications and result in early recovery. Therefore, management of acute odontogenic infections involves both surgical and supportive therapies. Depending upon the stage of infection, treatment will vary from tooth extraction to evacuation of pus as in cases of abscesses from extraoral space infections.

EXCISION OF SINUS

In most cases, the abscess escapes the tissue spaces spontaneously through a sinus if left without any treatment for a sufficient period of time. Pus discharge through the skin in a location unfavourable for drainage follows and the resulting scar is always puckered, thickened and depressed. Further, the sinus will become chronic unless the original source of infection is removed, and it is subjected to exacerbations and remissions with attempts at healing during the quiescent phase. To treat this sinus, an elliptical incision is made around its external orifice so that on closure the scar lies in Langer's line without puckering. Using a pair of scissors, the sinus tract is followed to its source, which is usually found on the bony surface of the jaws. Then a deep soluble suture is inserted to eliminate the dead space and the skin wounds are closed with careful eversion of the edges.

INCISION AND DRAINAGE

Incision and drainage (I&D) are the foremost surgical method in treating space infection (Fig. 23.5A–F).

Objectives

- Create an escape route for the necrotic tissues, pus and microbes from the tissue space
- Removal of dead tissue, pus, toxins and infective material, which would facilitate better immune defence mechanism.
- Effectively reduce the surface area of infected tissue, thus minimising the dosage of antibiotic required
- Blunt dissection into the tissue spaces breaks the pus locules and fibrous barrier, thus facilitating reach of the antibiotics into the infective site
- Drainage is used for culture and sensitivity (C&S) based on which empirical antibiotic therapy may be continued or changed.

Indications

1. Space infections (primary) that has localised pus collection with a clinically evident point of fluctuance. Example: buccal space infection with point of fluctuance on the face (Fig. 23.5C)
2. Space infections (secondary) that have pus collection with no clinical sign of fluctuance, but require immediate drainage to prevent progression. Example: masseteric space infection–only clinical sign is trismus
3. Nonsuppurative space infection such as Ludwig's angina, where I&D serves as a method of decompression of the tissue planes, which could be lifesaving.

HILTON'S DRAINAGE METHOD

1. Take the shortest and most direct route to the exudate or pus accumulation, while preserving anatomical structures
2. Performing aesthetic incisions in low-impact places like the face. Infections of the buccal space can be drained intra- or extraorally by placing incisions along the lower border of the mandible
3. Create incisions in healthy mucosa or skin, avoiding atrophic and fluctuant areas
4. Only perform cutaneous or mucosal incisions (with a No. 11 blade)
5. The incision is then pierced with a haemostat or sinus forceps in closed position, then blunt dissection is performed by opening it into the pus locules. It is withdrawn in the same place to prevent damaging anatomical structures like nerves and arteries (Hilton's drainage method, Fig. 23.5D)
6. The choice of the most appropriate drainage material is dictated by the site of the infection. Use of gauze as a drainage material should be avoided since secretions would be trapped and coagulate, resulting in a tamponade that would allow the infection to continue to spread.

PLACING A SURGICAL DRAIN

Insert the drain into the most dependent part of the cavity. In cases of infections such as abscesses and/or osteomyelitis, a noncollapsible drain that would facilitate irrigation should be chosen. Drain should preferably exit the wound through a separate stab incision away from the necrotic unhealthy tissue. Fix it with a suture or any other device to prevent the drain from getting dislodged into or away from the wound. Check regularly for the patency of the drains.

Drain removal: When the discharge ceases, the drain can be removed at 48 h or earlier if drainage becomes minimal.

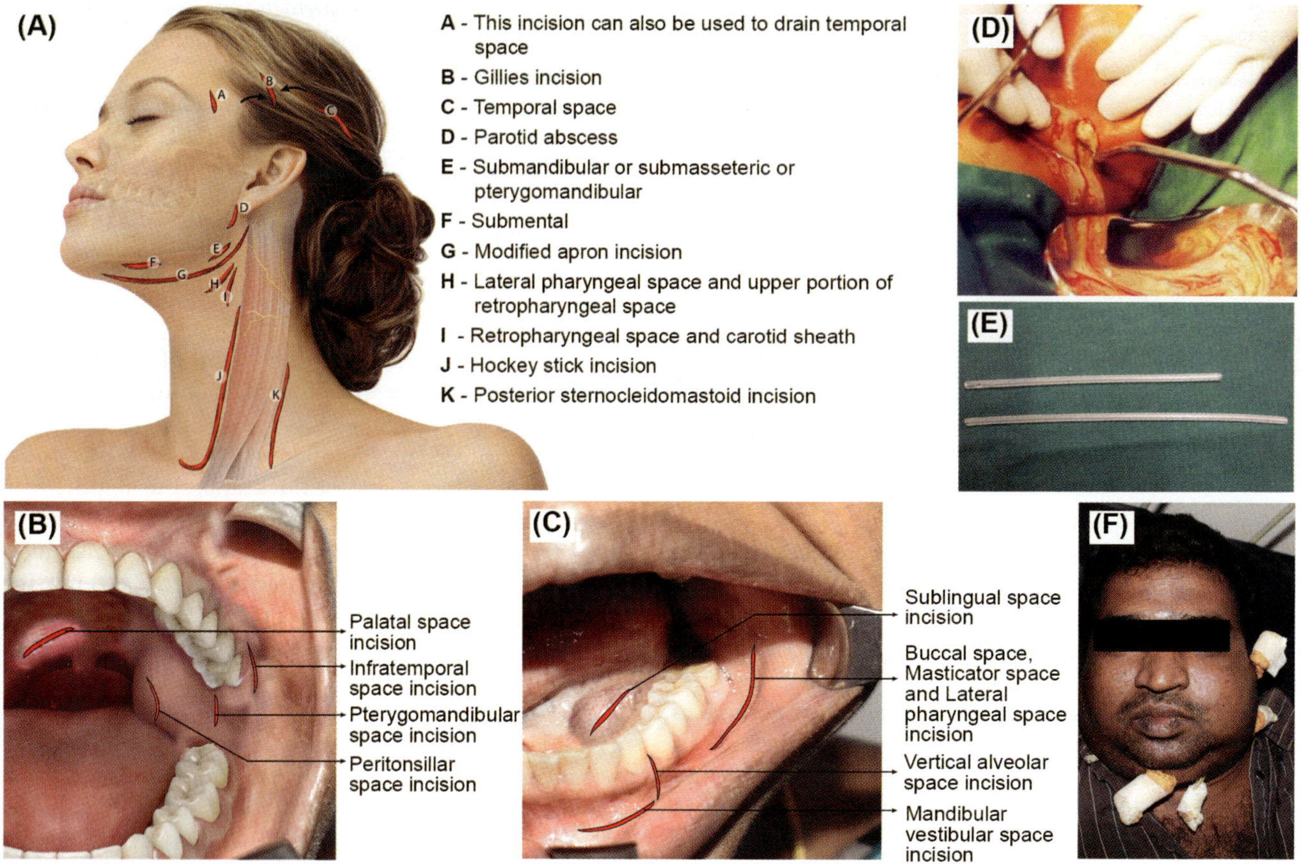

Figure 23.5 **(A)** Extraoral incisions. **(B** and **C)** Intraoral incisions. **(D)** Hilton's method of drainage of abscess. **(E)** Simple drain—perforated and nonperforated. **(F)** Simple drain placed for draining Ludwig's angina.

Simple rubber drains are used for infections (Fig. 23.5E and F):

- Red rubber catheter
- Rubber dam material
- Latex Penrose drain
- Corrugated rubber drain: Rubber sheet with corrugations on the surface. One end is inserted into the dead space containing the fluid and the other end projects out through the incision line. Antiseptic solutions can be instilled through these drains in deep wounds. It is adaptable, soft and inexpensive but it does not prevent clotting and is difficult to irrigate the wound.

ANTIBIOTIC THERAPY

Odontogenic infections are caused by a highly predictable group of bacteria, so choice of the initial antibiotic is empirical. More than 90% of odontogenic infections are caused by aerobic and anaerobic streptococci, peptostreptococci, prevotella, fusobacterium and bacteroides.

AS THE 1st-CHOICE THERAPY

1. Synthetic penicillin and cephalosporin
2. Amoxicillin/clavulanic acid 2 g, 1 h prior to starting the surgical intervention, followed by 2 g every 12 h for 5–7 days. This is the most appropriate option since it offers greater coverage than penicillin against oral streptococci and beta lactamase. Alternatively, 3rd or 4th generation cephalosporins are active against Gram-positive and Gram-negative anaerobic bacteria and have bone penetrating properties
3. Other alternative regimens
4. Clindamycin 300 mg every 6 h (per os), for 5–7 days
5. In all cases, treatment must be initiated approximately 1 h prior to surgery
6. Culture sensitivity test should be routinely performed, using drains, pus cells; this is of clinical significance in:
   a. When the patient fails to respond to empirical antibiotic therapy (Table 23.6) and after treatment of the causes within 48 h
   b. When the infection is disseminated to other fascial spaces despite initial treatment
   c. In an immunosuppressed patient or if he/she has a prior history of bacterial endocarditis and does not respond to the initial antibiotic.

SUPPORTIVE THERAPY

- Patients with facial cellulitis may also need other treatments, such as when the disease spreads to other parts of the body or when they are in a life-threatening situation

TABLE 23.6 Antimicrobial Therapy Based on the Severity of Infection

Severity of the Infection	Empirical Antibiotic of Choice
Mild to moderate—the patient can be treated as an out-patient (only primary space is affected)	• Amoxicillin • Clindamycin (penicillin allergy) • Azithromycin • Moxifloxacin
Moderate to severe—treated as an inpatient; Airway compromise may begin due to multiple spaces affected or secondary space involvement	• Ampicillin + sulbactam • Ampicillin + metronidazole • Clindamycin (penicillin allergy) • Ceftriaxone • Moxifloxacin—*Eikenella corrodens* sp. • Vancomycin + metronidazole with or without moxifloxacin—*MRSA, Pseudomonas—deep neck infections*

MRSA - Methicillin-resistant Staphylococcus aureus

- Analgesics, nonsteroidal antiinflammatory drugs (NSAIDs) and nutritional support must be administered to patients
- People who have an infection and a fever present a considerable loss of body fluids, about 250 mL for every degree (centigrade) temperature rise. It is important for ambulatory patients to drink 8–10 glasses of water or another liquid. Intravenous fluids can be given to people who are hospitalised to help them stay hydrated. For every degree (centigrade) above normal body temperature, the daily calorie needs rise by up to 13%
- An important factor to be noted in these patients is the potential danger of start of respiratory impairment, requiring airway monitoring, maybe even on an emergency basis, by means of endotracheal intubation, cricothyrotomy or tracheotomy
- In the treatment of deep neck infections, intensive care, antibiotic therapy and surgical drainage are all beneficial
  a. Dehydration must be addressed immediately. To maintain serum electrolyte balance, Ringer's lactate (RL) is preferable
  b. Antibiotic coverage via intravenous injection is critical. In small abscesses, antibiotic therapy alone can be tried without causing systemic toxicity
  c. If the general condition worsens or the abscess cavity does not heal, surgery may be required
  d. Since most "pure" parapharyngeal abscesses are difficult to aspirate, empirical antibiotic therapy with amoxicillin and clavulanic acid (150 mg/kg per day) for the 1st 72 hours is required. This is because beta-lactamase-producing bacteria are usually present in deep neck abscesses. For anaerobic coverage, administer 0.5 g of metronidazole every 6 hours.

CLASSIFICATION OF FASCIAL SPACES

1. Topazian classification (Flowchart 23.7)
2. Classification according to involvement of spaces: The spaces have been described based on the classification of clinical significance (Table 23.8)
   - Direct involvement: Primary spaces
     1. Maxillary spaces
     2. Mandibular spaces
   - Indirect involvement: Secondary spaces
3. **Grodinsky and Holyoke classification:** This classification is based upon the data of dissected materials spread of injected masses and infections observed clinically. Grodinsky and Holyoke designated these spaces by numerals (spaces of anterior triangle) and numerals followed by letter 'A' (spaces of posterior triangle) as follows:
   - ***Space 1:*** Superficial fascial compartment
   - ***Space 2:*** Potential space between the superficial layer of deep fascia and the deep layer of the sternothyroid–thyrohyoid sheath
     - ***Space 2A:*** Space between the superficial layer of deep fascia and the sheath of the posterior belly of the omohyoid muscle
   - ***Spaces 3 and 3A:*** Visceral compartment and space within carotid sheath, respectively
   - ***Space 4:*** Space between two laminae of prevertebral fascia
     - ***Space 4A:*** The potential space between the superficial layers of deep fascia and the scalenus fascia
   - ***Space 5:*** This is a potential space between prevertebral fascia and vertebral bodies limited laterally up to transverse processes of vertebrae
     - ***Space 5A:*** This lies in the posterior triangle deep to scalenus fascia. This space, posterior to the scalenus fascia, lies between the deep muscles of the back of the neck
4. **Based on the hyoid:** The structures of the deep cervical fascia are slightly different above and below the hyoid bone, the neck spaces are typically categorised into two: **suprahyoid** (between the base of the skull and the hyoid bone) and **infrahyoid** (between the hyoid bone and the clavicles) (Table 23.7). Some of the spaces traverse the hyoid bone and run through the length of the neck. **Masticator spaces** are suprahyoid spaces but only those that involve the muscles of mastication—consists of ***the***

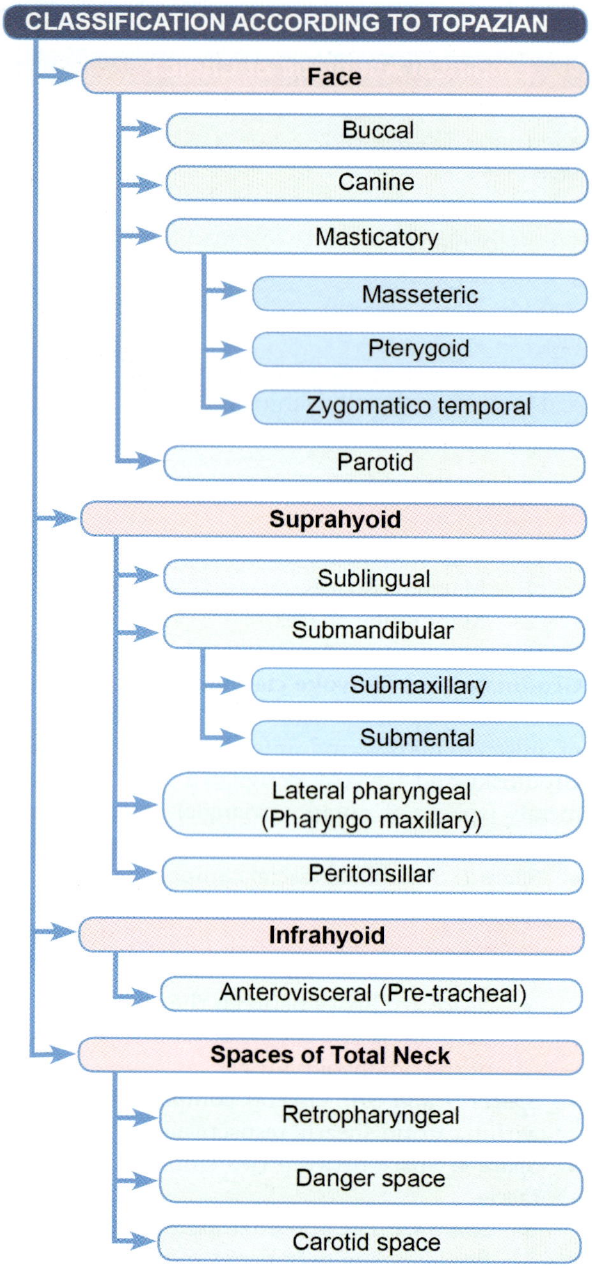

Flowchart 23.7 Topazian classification (based on clinical significance).

TABLE 23.7 Classification of the Head and Neck Spaces Based on the Anatomical Position of the Hyoid Bone

Suprahyoid neck
• Masticator space
• Parotid space
• Sublingual space
• Submandibular space
• Parapharyngeal space
  • Prestyloid space
  • Poststyloid space
• Pharyngeal mucosal space

Infrahyoid neck • Visceral space • Carotid sheath

Suprahyoid and infrahyoid neck
• Superficial compartment and fascia
• Retropharyngeal space
• Danger space
• Perivertebral space
  • Prevertebral space
  • Paraspinal space
• Posterior cervical space

TABLE 23.8 Classification of Head and Neck Spaces Based on Clinical Significance

Primary maxillary spaces	Canine (infraorbital) Buccal Infratemporal
Primary mandibular spaces	Submental Submandibular Sublingual Buccal
Secondary fascial spaces	Masseteric Pterygomandibular Superficial and deep temporal Lateral pharyngeal Retropharyngeal Prevertebral

superficial temporal space, masseteric space, pterygomandibular space, deep temporal space and the infratemporal space (Fig. 23.6 & 23.7).

SUPRASTERNAL SPACE OF BURNS

The **suprasternal space of Burns** is a space of the inferior neck. Superficial fascia splits below the level of the hyoid bone to form two spaces:

1. It forms the lower part of the root of the posterior triangle, the fascia splits into two layers, both of which are attached to the clavicle
2. It forms the lower part of the roof of the anterior triangle and the fascia splits in form the suprasternal space or the space of Burns. The layers pass down to get attached, one to the anterior and the other to the posterior border of the manubrium sterni.

Contents

- Sternal head of the sternocleidomastoid muscle
- Anterior jugular vein anastomoses
- Lymph nodes
- Interclavicular ligament.

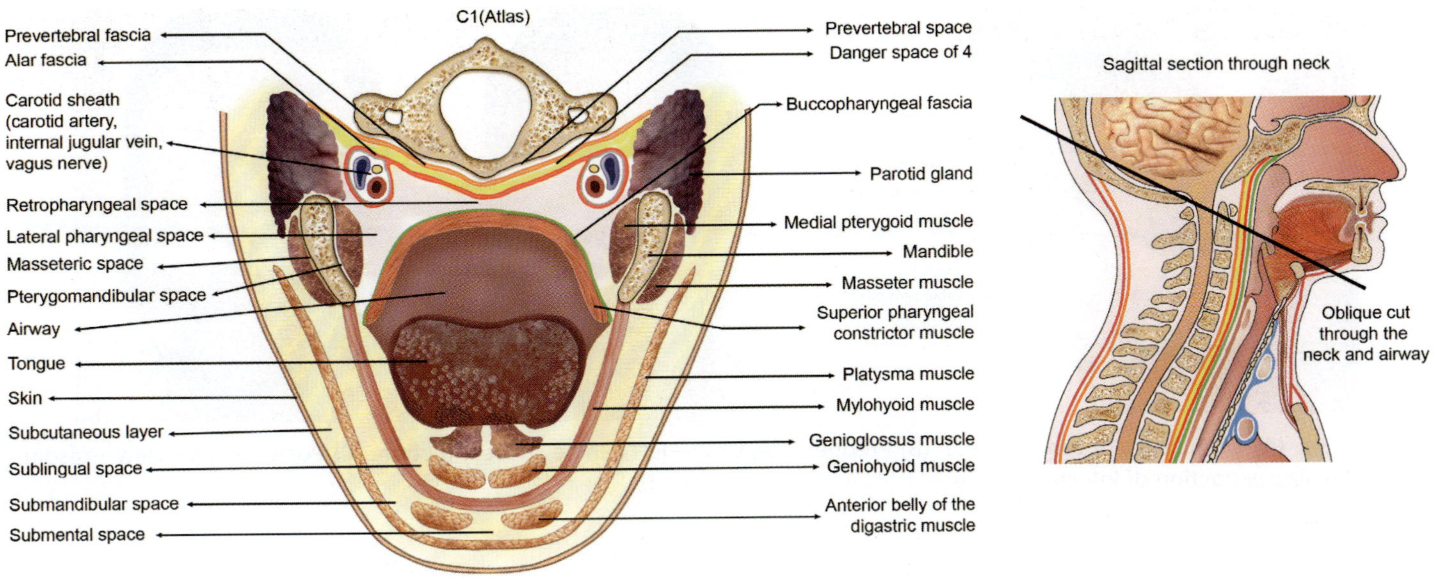

Figure 23.6 Illustration showing all primary and secondary spaces encountered in the head and neck region.

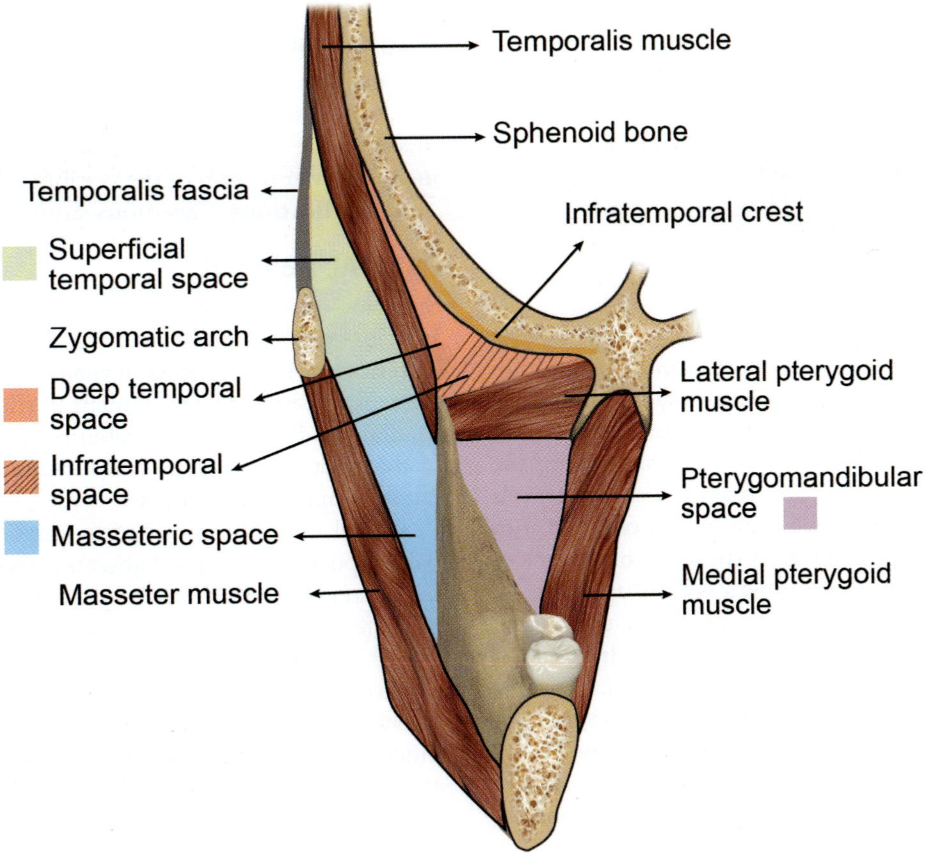

Figure 23.7 Masticatory spaces.

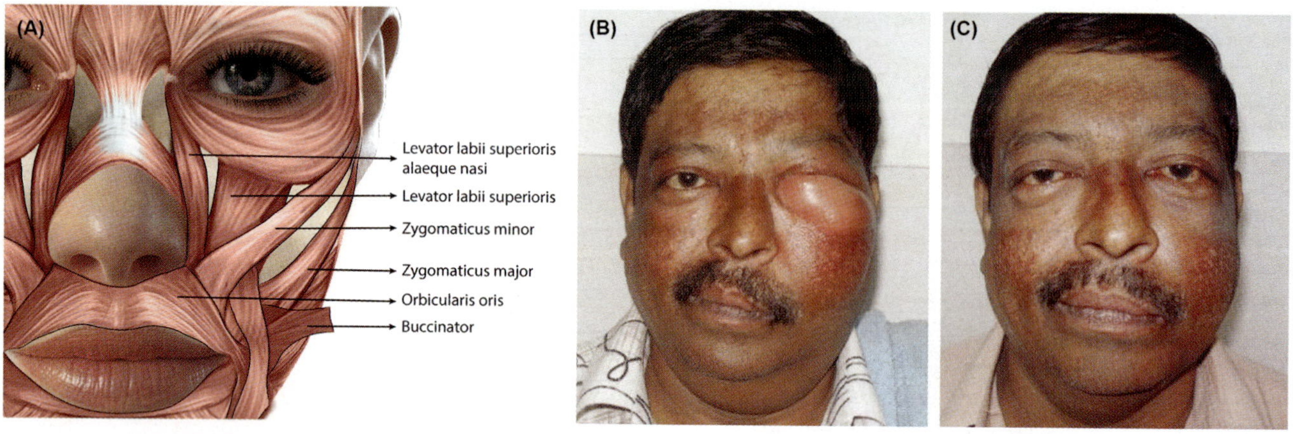

Figure 23.8 (**A**) Boundaries of canine space. (**B**) Preoperative view—left canine space infection. (**C**) Postoperative view—resolution following extraction of infected canine.

PRIMARY FASCIAL SPACES—DIRECT INVOLVEMENT

CANINE SPACE—INFRAORBITAL SPACE

Boundaries of canine space

Superficial and superior—quadratus labii superioris.
Inferior—orbicularis oris.
Deep—levator anguli oris, anterior surface of maxilla.
Medial—levator labii superioris alaeque nasi.
Lateral—zygomaticus major (Fig. 23.8).

Contents

- Angular artery and vein
- Infraorbital nerve.

Quadratus labii superioris originates from above the infraorbital foramen and overlaps the levator anguli oris muscle, which originates below the infraorbital foramen.

When the root of the canine is long and the origin of the levator anguli oris is low, infection from the canine travels along the medial border of the levator anguli oris and into the canine space (the region between the anterior surface of the maxilla and overlying levator muscles of the upper lip). If the swelling is untreated, pus points out below the medial corner of the eye by emerging in between quadratus labii superioris and levator labii superioris alaeque nasi.

Cause

Maxillary canine, 1st premolar infection and sometimes mesiobuccal root of 1st molars; infrequently nasal infections.

Clinical features

1. Periapical abscess of canine usually presents as a labial sulcus swelling and less commonly as a palatal swelling
2. Swelling of the cheek and upper lip (vestibular abscess)
3. Obliteration of the nasolabial fold (pus accumulation in the nasolabial fold)
4. Oedema of the lower eyelid
5. Marked periorbital oedema forcing the eyelids closed
6. Marked tenderness and redness in the facial tissue (Fig. 23.8B and C).

Surgical management

The incision is made intraorally high in the maxillary labial vestibule. Insert a small haemostat through the levator anguli oris into the abscess cavity, place a rubber drain and suture into the lower margin of the vestibular incision (Fig. 23.5B).

Complications: Cavernous sinus thrombosis.

PALATAL ABSCESS

Superior—palatal bone
Inferior—periosteum of the hard palate.
Anterior—alveolar process of the maxilla.
Posterior—periosteal attachment of the hard and soft palate.
Medial—midline; the periosteum attachment is firm and does not typically allow the infection to cross the midline.
Lateral—maxillary alveolus.

Palatal infection is caused by periodontal abscesses from palatal pockets and apical abscesses from the palatal roots of the posterior teeth. When infected lateral incisors are present, the infection can move posteriorly, as far as the soft palate. This is because of the increased palatal inclination of its roots. The palatal space is bounded inferiorly by the cortical plate of the hard palate, superiorly by the overlaying periosteum and mucosa, and laterally by the alveolar process of the maxilla and the teeth. It is possible to drain the abscess cavity by ***making an incision through the palatal mucosa that runs parallel*** to the greater palatine neurovascular bundle (Fig. 23.9).

Clinical features

Intraorally, a well-defined circumscribed fluctuant swelling on one side of the palate is present, close to the offending tooth. There may or may not be any discolouration. Tenderness on percussion of the affected tooth is present.

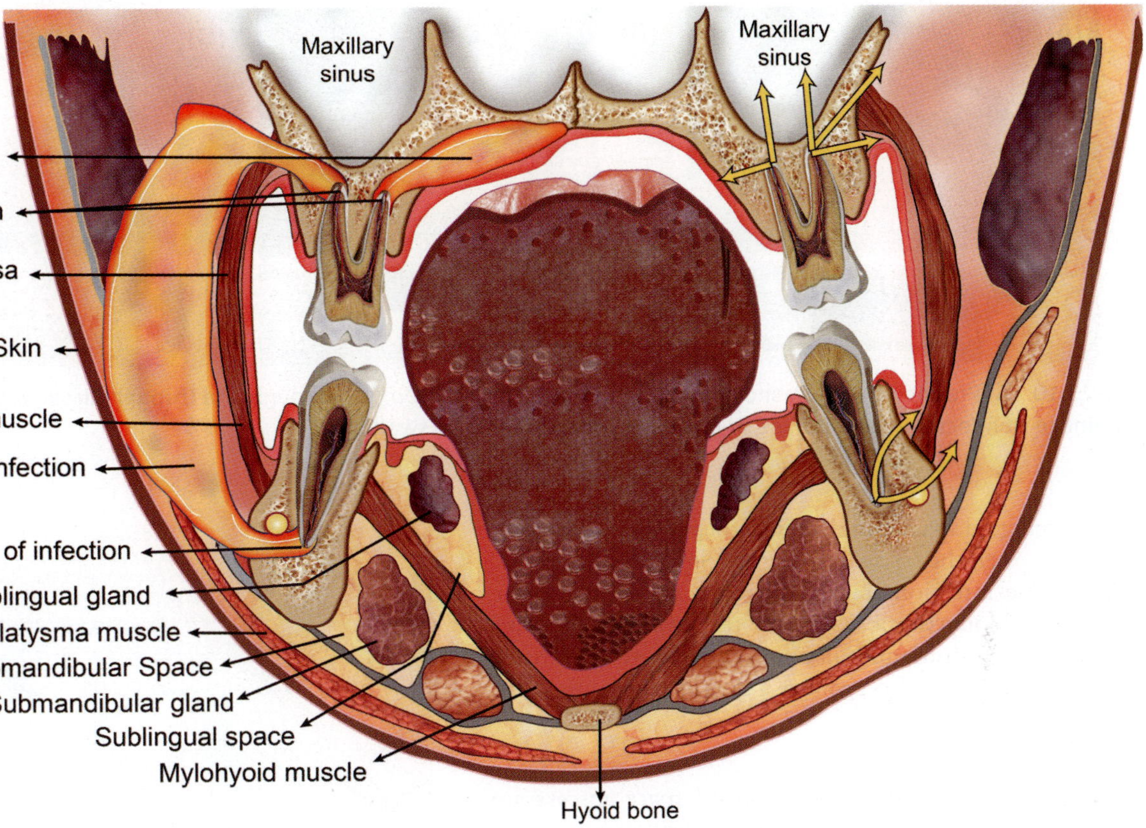

Figure 23.9 Buccal space infection—lateral to buccinator. Plane of spread lateral to buccinator muscle.

BUCCAL SPACE

Boundaries of buccal space

Superior—zygomatic arch.
Inferior—inferior border of the mandible.
Anterior—posterior border of the zygomatic bone above and depressor anguli oris below.
Posterior—anterior border of the masseter muscle.
Medial—buccinator muscle and its fascia.
Lateral—skin and subcutaneous tissue.

Contents

This space between the buccinator and masseter muscle consists of:

- Space filled with buccal pad of fat (adipose tissues)
- Parotid duct—Stensen's duct
- Facial nerve—CN VII
- Anterior and transverse facial artery and vein (Fig. 23.9).

Teeth involved

Maxillary and mandibular premolars and molars.

Clinical features

1. There is an obvious and dome-shaped swelling on the anterior aspect of the cheek beginning at the lower border of the mandible, extending upwards to the level of the zygomatic arch. This can extend to the lower eyelid rarely (Fig. 23.10)
2. Usually, infections from maxillary premolars and molars perforate the buccal aspect of the alveolar process
3. *Relationship of the root apices* to the attachment of the buccinator muscle is the factor that determines whether localisation is intraoral or extraoral or deep into the buccal space
   a. If perforation is below the buccinator attachment on the maxilla, swelling will be located in the oral vestibule
   b. If perforation is above the buccinator attachment, the infection extends laterally to the buccinator muscle forming a buccal space abscess
4. Communications—infection in the buccal space can spread to or from the teeth. Inferiorly, there is no discernible boundary between the buccal space and the submandibular space. Posterior communications are with the pterygomandibular space, infratemporal space and parapharyngeal space
   a. The buccal space is continuous posteromedially, around the buccal pad of fat, and with the ***pterygoid space.*** This is through the interval between the buccinator and anterior border of the coronoid process. In this case, the infection spreads deeper into the

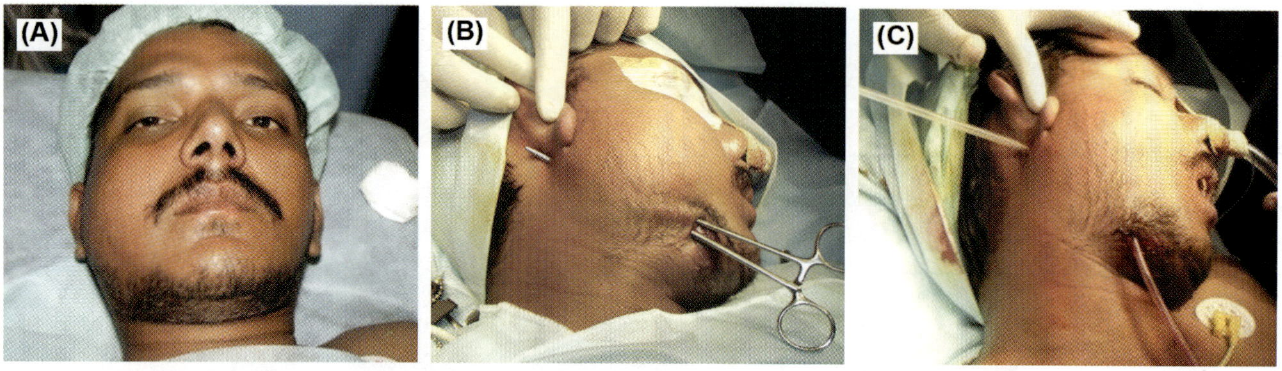

Figure 23.10 (**A**) Preoperative view showing right buccal space infection. (**B**) Through and through dissection into the buccal space for drainage of infection. (**C**) Drainage in most dependent region of swelling.

pterygoid space and then into the ***infratemporal space*** (through the fascia covering the Stenson's duct)

b. If the infection tracks backward, it penetrates the parotidomassetric fascia into the ***submasseteric space***

5. Infections from mandibular molars and pericoronitis of the 3rd molar can also produce a buccal space infection.

Surgical management

Two stab incisions for drainage of buccal space abscess are made extraorally through the skin and subcutaneous tissue with No. 11 scalpel blade, below the lower border of the mandible for a dependent drainage. A curved haemostat is inserted through the anterior incision into the abscess cavity; exited through the posterior incision; the beaks are opened and a strip of rubber drain is grasped; the haemostat is then withdrawn carrying the drain through the tissues. The ends are tied with suture to prevent dislodgement. This incision also hides the scar in the shadow of the mandible. In case of buccal space abscess, intraoral incision (Fig. 23.5D) is not preferred because it is difficult to maintain a patent opening for drainage since the buccinator muscle tends to contract, especially when a vertical incision is made. If an intraoral incision is preferred, horizontal incision should be placed just above the depth of the vestibules. This not only prevents damage to the parotid duct, but also provides dependent drainage.

INFRATEMPORAL SPACE

It is also called as 'retrozygomatic space' as it is partly situated behind the zygomatic bone. It is a masticatory space shown in Fig. 23.7 and the boundaries are shown in Fig. 23.11.

Boundaries

Superior—skull base-sphenoid crest.
Inferior—lateral pterygoid muscle.
Medial—lateral pterygoid plate.
Lateral—temporalis muscle and tendon.
Anterior—maxillary tuberosity.
Posterior—mandibular condyle.

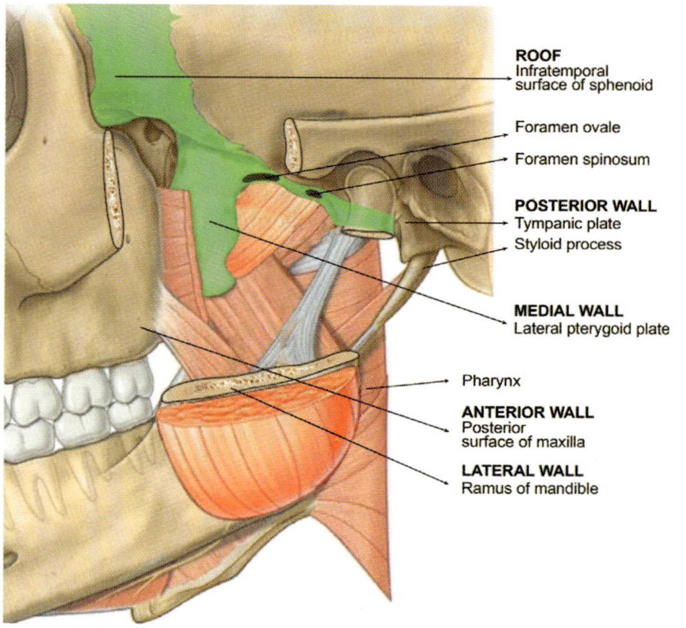

Figure 23.11 Boundaries of infratemporal fossa.

Contents

- Internal maxillary artery (2nd part)
- Pterygoid venous plexus
- Mandibular division of trigeminal nerve
- Origins of medial and lateral pterygoid muscles
- Middle meningeal artery.

Neighbouring spaces

- Buccal space
- Pterygomandibular space—the space is anteriorly connected with the upper section of the pterygomandibular space. However, it is separated from it posteriorly by the lateral pterygoid muscle. As a result, the infratemporal fossa serves as the upper extremity of the pterygomandibular area
- Superficial temporal space
- Inferior petrosal sinus space.

Involvement

Infratemporal fossa may also become secondarily infected from infections of the submasseteric, parotid and lateral pharyngeal spaces.

Clinical features

1. The swelling is characterised by severe trismus and pain
2. If the swelling is present over the tuberosity area, the swelling can then be seen extraorally over the temporomandibular joint and zygomatic arch. From here, it extends to the cheek and if left untreated may involve the whole side of the face
3. Optic neuritis might also occur
4. Occasionally, the swelling may also extend into the neck
5. The presence of the pterygoid plexus of veins makes the infection of the infratemporal space dangerous. Emissary veins connect the pterygoid plexus with the cavernous sinus. Therefore, infections from here can spread to the cavernous sinus and present with symptoms like headache, irritability, photophobia, vomiting and drowsiness.

Surgical management

Infratemporal space can be reached either intraorally or extraorally.

Internal approach **(Kruger)** consists of an incision made in the buccolabial fold lateral to the maxillary 3rd molar. A curved haemostat is introduced carefully behind the tuberosity of the maxilla and directed medially and superiorly within the cavity. A drain is then inserted.

According to **Laskin**, a vertical incision is made medial to the upper extent of the anterior border of the ramus of the mandible. A haemostat is introduced and passed superiorly into the infratemporal region and a drain is inserted. In the presence of severe trismus, intraoral approach may not be possible.

In such cases, external approach consists of a horizontal incision made just above the zygomatic arch—at the upper and posterior edge of the temporalis muscle. A curved haemostat is introduced and directed in an inferior and medial direction into the infratemporal space followed by the insertion of a drain. The main disadvantage of this procedure is that it cannot produce a dependent drainage.

SPACES RELATED TO LOWER JAW

SUBMENTAL SPACE

Boundaries

Superior—mylohyoid muscle.
Inferior—skin and subcutaneous tissue, platysma and investing layer of deep cervical fascia.
Medial—submental space is a single midline space with no medial wall.
Lateral—anterior belly of digastric (bilateral).
Anterior—inferior border of mandible.
Posterior—hyoid bone (Fig. 23.12A and B).

Contents

- This space has no vital structures
- Lymph nodes and anterior jugular veins.

Involvement

Infection from lower incisors, lower lip, chin, tip of the tongue and anterior part of floor of the mouth can spread to the submental lymph nodes and subsequently cause infection of the submental space (Fig. 23.12C).

Neighbouring space

Submandibular space—the infection can spread posteriorly to involve the submandibular space or it may discharge on the face to the submental region.

Clinical features

Distinct and firm swelling in the midline, in the region of the chin and the region just beneath it. The skin is taut and board-like.

Surgical management

The incision for drainage is made bilaterally through the skin, subcutaneous tissue and platysma muscle at the most inferior aspect of the swelling (Fig. 23.12A). Unsuccessful drainage requires a horizontal midline incision just anterior to the hyoid bone. The hyoid bone is the inferior boundary of the submental space, therefore incisions near it offer gravity-dependent drainage. Blunt dissection enters the

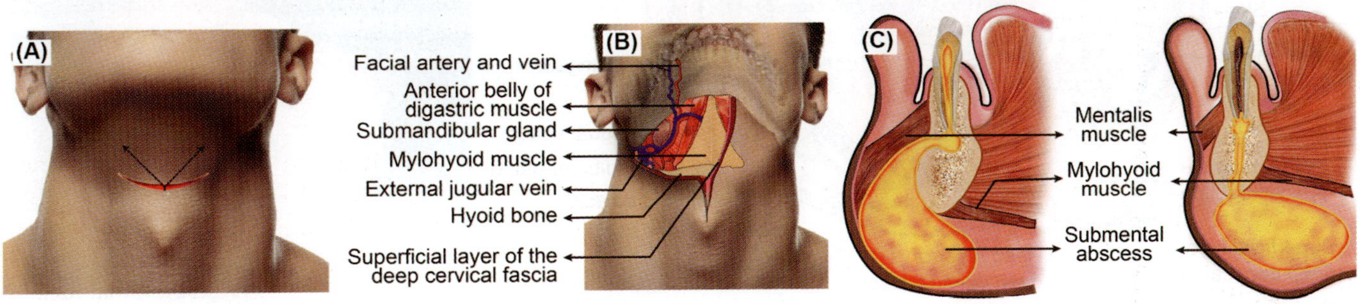

Figure 23.12 Submental space infection. (**A**) Submental incision. (**B**) Boundaries of submental space. (**C**) Pathway of infection from lower incisors.

submental space superiorly through the skin, subcutaneous tissue, and platysma avoiding the anterior jugular veins. A vestibular incision through the mentalis muscle can potentially drain the submental space intraorally. The intraoral method lacks dependent drainage. Rubber drain is inserted through one incision, exited through the other and secured with the help of sutures and dressing is applied.

SUBMANDIBULAR SPACE

Also called submaxillary space, submylohyoid space.

Boundaries

Lateral—skin, superficial fascia, investing fascia, platysma.

Medial—mylohyoid, hyoglossus, superior constrictor, styloglossus muscles.

Superior—inferior and medial surface of the mandible and attachment of mylohyoid muscle.

Inferior—anterior and posterior bellies of the digastric muscle (Fig. 23.13A).

Contents

- Submandibular salivary gland and lymph nodes
- Facial artery
- Lingual nerve
- Lymph nodes.

Submandibular space is enclosed by the investing layer of deep cervical fascia and lies lateral to the submental space.

Involvement

Infection from the mandibular molars, most commonly 2nd and 3rd molars, penetrates the thin lingual plate to pass directly into the submandibular space (inferior to the attachment of mylohyoid muscle).

Infection from submental and sublingual spaces can pass backwards via lymphatics.

Infection from the submandibular salivary gland may pass via lymphatics to the submandibular lymph node.

Infection from the middle 3rd of the tongue, posterior part of the floor of the mouth, maxillary teeth, cheek, maxillary sinus and palate.

Neighbouring spaces

- Sublingual space
- Submental space
- Lateral pharyngeal space
- Buccal space.

Clinical features

Extraoral manifestations include a firm swelling in the submandibular region at the point where the facial artery crosses it. It extends till the level of hyoid bone in a shape of inverted cone, below the lower border of the mandibular jawbone with widespread physiological symptoms including tenderness and redness of the skin covering the affected area.

Intraoral findings include infected teeth that are tender to percussion and may or may not be mobile. The swelling may cause dysphagia and significant trismus (Fig. 23.13B).

Spread

There are no anatomical barriers between the bilateral submandibular and submental spaces, hence the infection can easily spread across the midline and involve the submandibular space on the contralateral side.

The submandibular space communicates with the sublingual space around the posterior border of mylohyoid muscle.

Submandibular space infection may extend backwards to involve the parapharyngeal spaces.

Surgical management

An extraoral submandibular technique is used for drainage, in which a 1.5–2 cm long incision is made in the skin creases, 2 cm caudal to the inferior border of the mandible. The incision is made at the plane of the hyoid bone, parallel to the resting skin tension lines (Fig. 23.5A). Thus, a gravity-dependent

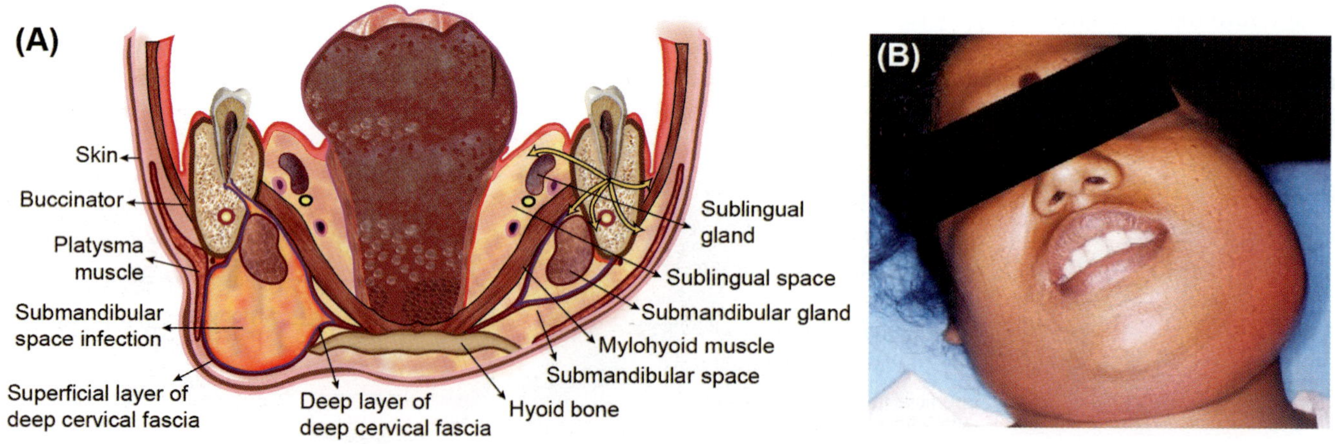

Figure 23.13 (**A**) Infection of submandibular space and routes of spread. (**B**) Left submandibular space infection.

drainage can be accomplished to its fullest extent. A sinus forceps is introduced through the incision and directed towards the inferior border of the mandible from both the superior and posterior sides. Once this has been accomplished, it is guided to lingual side of the jaw, superiorly towards the mylohyoid, in order to discharge pus from the submandibular region. A corrugated rubber drain is placed into the abscess cavity and fixed with a suture, after which a dressing is administered to the wound.

SUBLINGUAL SPACE

Boundaries

Superior—mucosa of the floor of the mouth.
Inferior—superior surface of mylohyoid muscle.
Medial—midline raphae.
Lateral—medial surface of mandible (Fig. 23.14).

Contents

- Deep part of submandibular gland, sublingual gland and their draining ducts (Wharton's duct and ducts of Rivinus)
- Lingual nerve.

Infections, which take a route on the lingual aspect of the mandible at a point above the origin of the mylohyoid muscle and below the mucosa of floor of the mouth, end up in sublingual space. These infections usually arise from mandibular premolars or molars or from any direct trauma to the region.

Neighbouring spaces

- Submandibular space
- Lateral pharyngeal space.

Clinical features

- Swelling is seen on the anterior part of floor of the mouth, interferes with swallowing and has severe tenderness.
- Difficulty in speaking.
- Floor of the mouth is raised and the tongue may be pushed superiorly causing airway obstruction.
- Source: Chronic decayed mandibular anterior teeth, infected ranula, infected lymph node with purulent discharge—lymphadenitis or an extension of infections of the submandibular space.

Surgical management

Surgical approaches to the sublingual space for incision and drainage of the abscess is obtained through the following:

1. Extraoral approach—an external transverse skin incision between the hyoid bone and the inferior border of the mandible (Fig. 23.5A)
2. Intraoral approach—drainage can be obtained transorally by incising the mucosa in the anterior part of the floor of the mouth, the incision should be placed parallel to the submandibular duct. Blunt dissection is indicated so as to not injure the lingual nerve or the submandibular ducts (Fig. 23.5C)

   When the submandibular space is affected, both spaces can be simultaneously reached via a submandibular approach (extraoral).

SECONDARY FASCIAL SPACES—INDIRECT INVOLVEMENT

PAROTID SPACE INFECTION

Parotid space is enclosed by the superficial layer of the deep cervical fascia surrounding the parotid gland.

Extension of odontogenic infections into the parotid space is difficult since the fascial covering is firmly attached to the gland. Parotid space can be invaded by infections from the pterygomandibular, submasseteric or lateral pharyngeal spaces (Fig. 23.5A).

Clinical features

Swelling extends from the zygomatic arch to the lower border of the mandible anteriorly and from the anterior border of the mandible to retromandibular region posteriorly.

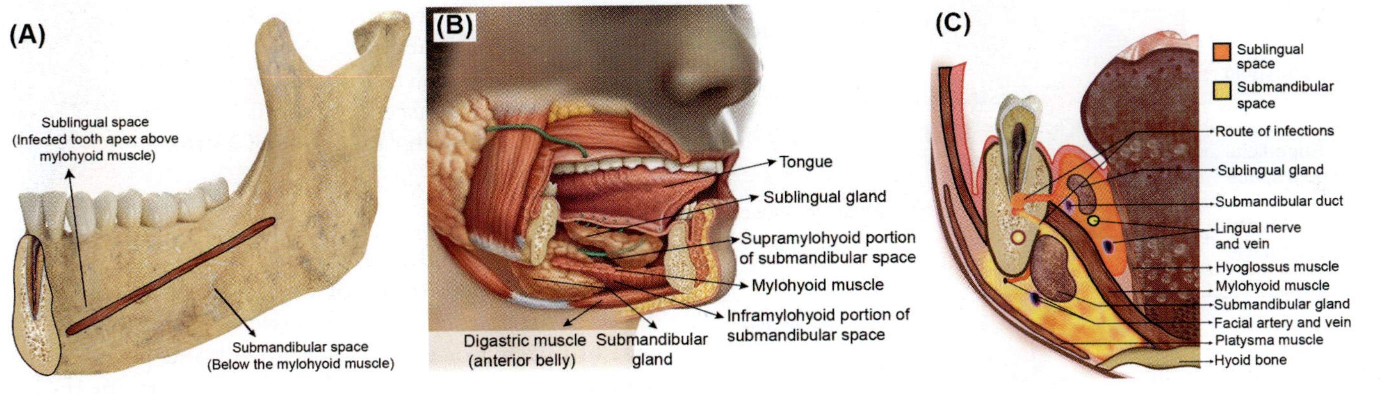

Figure 23.14 (**A**) Boundaries of sublingual space. (**B**) Mylohyoid muscle separating both spaces. (**C**) Infection of submandibular and sublingual space.

Swelling everts the lobule of the ear and presents with severe pain especially while eating. Intraorally, pus may be milked from the parotid duct. Trismus is not a sign of this space infection.

Differential diagnosis

Submasseteric space infection

Trismus will be present.

Management

The pus within the parotid space is present in different loculations, which necessitates an approach that covers a wide area. A large incision is made in the ***retromandibular area*** from the lower aspect of the lobule of the ear to the angle of the mandible. Blunt dissection with a haemostat is done, avoiding injury to the branches of the facial nerve. Multiple drains are used for drainage of the pus. A curved incision at the angle of the mandible can also be made; blunt dissection is done with a haemostat and a drain is placed.

TEMPORAL SPACE

Temporal space has two compartments: superficial and deep.

Boundaries

Superficial compartment

Laterally—temporal fascia.
Medially—lateral surface of the temporalis muscle (Fig. 23.15).

Deep compartment

Laterally—medial surface of the temporalis muscle.
Medially—temporal bone.

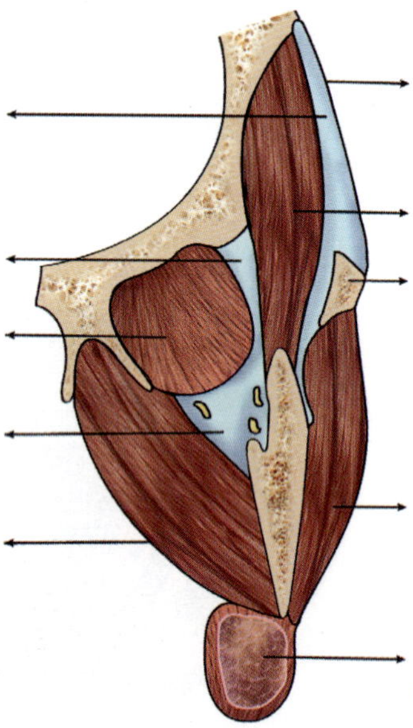

Figure 23.15 Boundaries of superficial and deep temporal spaces.

Contents

Superficial temporal vessels, auriculotemporal nerve and temporal fat pad.

Clinical features

Patient complains of severe pain and trismus. Swelling is more obvious in the superficial temporal space infection and will be restricted by the outline of the temporal fascia superiorly and laterally and by the zygomatic arch inferiorly. In case of associated buccal space infection, swelling has a characteristic dumbbell shape due to absence of swelling over the zygomatic arch. A deep temporal space infection produces less swelling and there will also be pain and trismus.

Surgical management

Intraoral incision for drainage of the temporal abscess is the same as that of infratemporal space. The haemostat is passed superiorly along the lateral aspect of the coronoid process to enter the superficial compartment. ***If the haemostat is passed superiorly along the medial aspect of the coronoid process, it will enter the deep temporal compartment.***

In case of severe trismus, an extraoral approach can be used to gain access into the temporal space. This incision is also the same as that used for extraoral incision of infratemporal space. At 1st, the haemostat is passed medially to enter the superficial space followed by blunt dissection through the temporalis muscle to enter into the deep temporal space. An intraoral approach is preferred over an extraoral since *intraoral approach provides more dependent drainage* over the entire area whereas the extraoral approach does not enter the inferior aspect of the temporal space. Moreover, intraoral approach prevents the fibres of the temporalis muscle from contracting against the drain and affecting the flow of pus from the deep temporal space.

SUBMASSETERIC SPACE

Boundaries

Anterior—buccal space, parotidomasseteric fascia.
Posterior—parotid gland and its fascia.
Superior—zygomatic arch.
Inferior—inferior border of mandible.
Superficial or medial—ascending ramus.
Deep or lateral—masseter muscle (Fig. 23.16).

Contents

Masseteric artery and vein.

Especially pericoronitis of vertical or distoangular mandibular 3rd molars leads to submasseteric space abscess. Presence of buccinator muscle attachment and position of the mandibular 3rd molar in relation to that determine the backward extension of pericoronal pus. This space communicates freely with the temporal space superiorly.

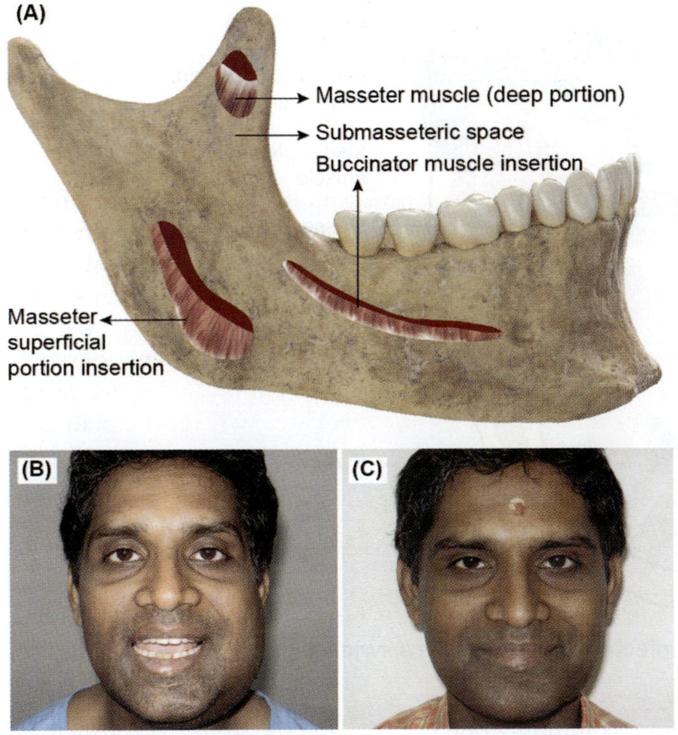

Figure 23.16 **(A)** Illustration showing submasseteric space. **(B)** Submasseteric space infection. **(C)** Postoperative view.

Neighbouring spaces

- Buccal space
- Pterygomandibular space
- Superficial temporal space
- Parotid space
- Infratemporal space

Clinical features

Extraorally, the swelling is seen mainly over the angle of the mandible. It is restricted to the masseter muscle as the forward spread is confined by the tendon of temporalis, which is inserted into the anterior border of the ramus (Fig. 23.16B and C). The lower border of the ramus controls inferior spread. Sometimes, the posterior mandibular sulcus may be obliterated. The infection is characterised by severe trismus and throbbing pain. Chronic submasseteric space infection can be punctuated by recurrent exacerbation, which can be controlled through drainage and antibiotics, but without complete resolution. The masseter muscle supplies more blood to the ramus of the mandible than to the body, which is mainly supplied by the mandibular artery. Because of this, ischaemia results in that part of the bone denuded of periosteum by the abscess, which leads to osteomyelitis with sequestrum formation. Extent of bone destruction depends upon the area of bone in contact with the pus. Often, submasseteric infection leads to subperiosteal new bone deposition beneath the periosteum, an important clue to the diagnosis.

Surgical management

A vertical incision is made intraorally along the external oblique line of the mandible. A haemostat is inserted through this incision and passed posteriorly along the lateral aspect of the ramus beneath the masseter muscle and the beaks are opened for free escape of the pus. A rubber drain is inserted and sutured to the incision margin. Extraoral approach involves a small incision beneath the angle of the mandible and blunt dissection is done with the help of the haemostat. A rubber catheter is inserted into the wound for drainage.

Differential diagnosis

Peritonsillar abscess

However, there is no trismus or dental involvement in this condition (refer page 466).

PTERYGOMANDIBULAR SPACE

Boundaries

Anterior—buccal space.
Posterior—parotid gland with lateral pharyngeal space.
Superior—lateral pterygoid muscle.
Inferior—inferior border of mandible.
Superficial or medial—lateral surface of medial pterygoid muscle.
Deep or lateral—medial surface of ascending ramus of mandible (Fig. 23.17).

Contents

Mandibular division of trigeminal nerve, inferior alveolar artery and vein.

Infection can spread to pterygomandibular space from mandibular 3rd molar region, especially from pericoronitis involving the 3rd molar. Infection can also be caused by contaminated needle and maxillary 3rd molar. Infection can also spread into the parapharyngeal space by extending medial to the medial pterygoid space.

Neighbouring spaces

- Buccal space
- Lateral pharyngeal space
- Submasseteric space
- Deep temporal space
- Parotid space
- Peritonsillar space

Clinical features

Extraorally, the swelling is not very obvious. Intraorally, there is visible swelling of the soft palate on the same side, swelling of the anterior tonsillar pillar and deviation of the uvula to the opposite side. The patient has severe trismus and dysphagia. Therefore, in cases of pterygomandibular space infection, we have to carefully examine intraorally using anaesthetic spray to arrive at a proper diagnosis.

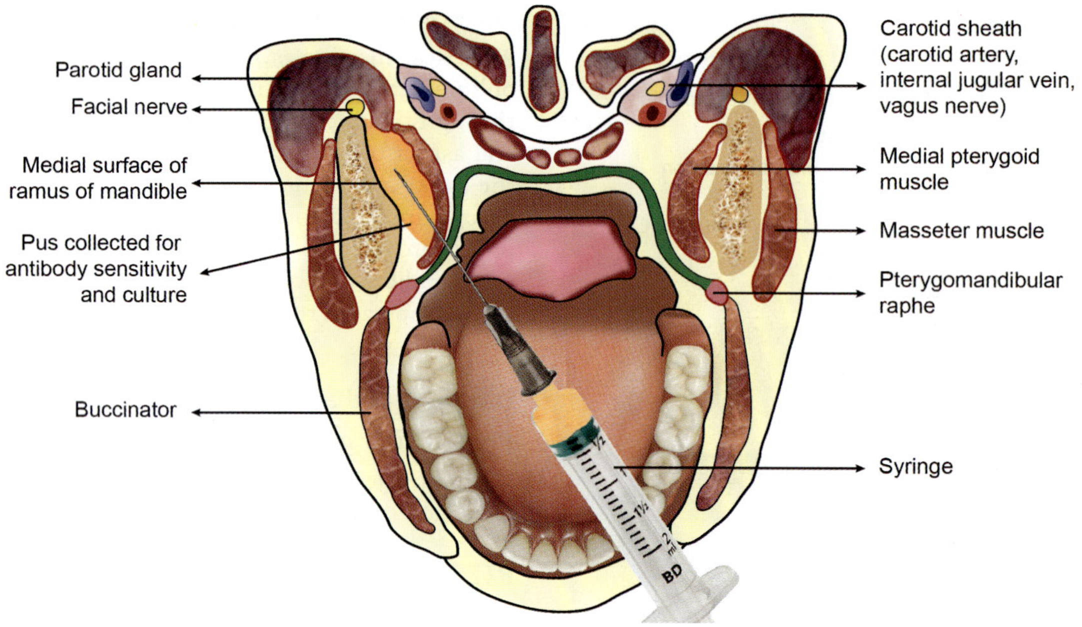

Figure 23.17 Pterygomandibular space infection accessed with a syringe.

Surgical management

Because of the severe trismus, either general anaesthesia is used or the mandibular nerve is blocked extraorally with local anaesthetic. The incision for drainage is made between medial aspect of the ramus of mandible and the pterygomandibular raphae, and the abscess cavity is opened by blunt dissection using a haemostat. Rubber drain is placed and sutured to one of the margins of the incision to prevent dislodgement. This would help in sufficient drainage.

PARAPHARYNGEAL SPACE INFECTIONS

LATERAL PHARYNGEAL SPACE

Lateral pharyngeal space is a part of the suprahyoid spaces and is also called pharyngomaxillary space.

Boundaries

Anterior—superior and middle pharyngeal constrictor.
Posterior—carotid sheath, stylohyoid, styloglossus and stylopharyngeus.
Superior—skull base.
Inferior—hyoid bone.
Superficial or medial—superior pharyngeal constrictors and retropharyngeal space.
Deep or lateral—medial pterygoid muscle and capsule of parotid gland.

Contents

Carotid artery, internal jugular vein, vagus nerve and cervical sympathetic chain.

Lateral pharyngeal space may be infected from abscess extending backwards from the mandibular 3rd molar area or more commonly one passing laterally from the tonsillar abscess. Infection can also spread backwards from a sublingual, submandibular and pterygomandibular space infection.

Neighbouring spaces

- Pterygomandibular
- Submandibular
- Peritonsillar
- Sublingual
- Retropharyngeal

Clinical features

Severe pain on the affected side of the throat and dysphagia are present. The tonsil, tonsillar pillar and uvula are seen to be displaced to the medial side. The four cardinal signs of lateral pharyngeal abscess are trismus, induration and swelling of angle of the jaw, fever and pharyngeal bulging. Rotation of the neck away from the side of the swelling causes severe pain from tension on the ipsilateral sternocleidomastoid muscle. Complications of lateral pharyngeal abscess include septic jugular thrombophlebitis and carotid artery erosion. Inequality of the pupils due to involvement of the cervical sympathetic and bleeding from nose, mouth or ear can be a warning of such disastrous sequelae. These infections have a potential to spread upwards causing cavernous sinus thrombosis, meningitis and brain abscess. They can also spread into the retropharyngeal space.

Surgical management

There are multiple approaches to the lateral pharyngeal space: intraoral, extraoral and a combination of both.

Intraoral incision can be either ***transpharyngeal or lateral***. The transpharyngeal approach is made through the tonsillar fossa, but this approach is not recommended since adequate drainage is very difficult to obtain.

Intraoral approach is more easily performed by making an incision between the ramus and medial pterygoid and dissecting bluntly with a haemostat medial and posterior to the medial pterygoid muscle into the parapharyngeal space. All peroral incisions are contraindicated when there has been prior haemorrhage no matter how minimal.

Extraoral submandibular incision is the safest approach and should be used if there is any involvement of the posterior compartments. In extraoral approach, an incision is made anterior and inferior to angle of the mandible and blunt dissection with haemostat is carried superficially and medially along the medial pterygoid muscle into the pharyngeal space.

In the combined intraoral and extraoral approach, the lateral mucosal incision is made and a large curved haemostat is passed lateral to the superior constrictor and medial to the medial pterygoid muscle. A blunt dissection is carried out posteroinferiorly below the angle of the mandible. The tip of the instrument is palpated extraorally anterior to the sternocleidomastoid and a cutaneous incision is made over the tip. This technique offers direct access into the lateral pharyngeal space and aids in correct placement of the external incision in a swollen face. To enable drainage, a drain is placed and sutured to the wound margin. Other extraoral incisions are the modified apron and hockey stick incisions on the side of the neck (Fig. 23.5A).

RETROPHARYNGEAL SPACE

Boundaries

Anterior—superior and middle constrictors.
Posterior—alar fascia.
Superior—skull base.
Inferior—fusion of alar and prevertebral fascia at T4.
Superficial or medial—common space, no wall.
Deep or lateral—carotid sheath and lateral pharyngeal space (Figs. 23.6 and 23.18).

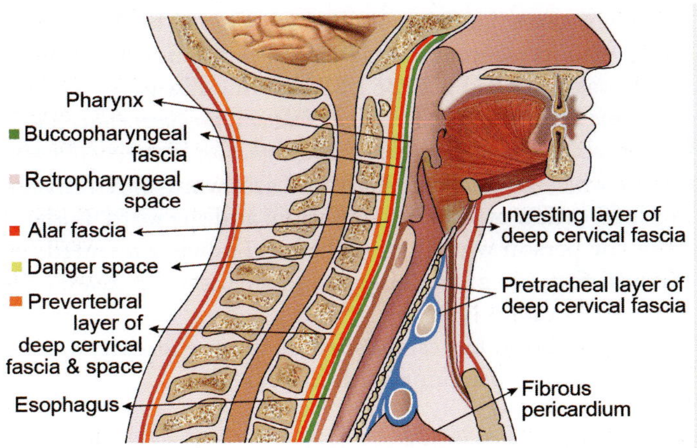

Figure 23.18 Retropharyngeal space (sagittal view of the fascia and space).

Contents

Lymph node, no major structures.

Clinical features

Clinical symptoms include **pain, fever, stiffness of the neck, dyspnoea, drooling** and **dysphagia**. ***Bulging of the posterior pharyngeal wall*** is often more prominent on one side because of adherence of the median raphae of the prevertebral fascia, but this is difficult to appreciate. Retropharyngeal abscess should be considered the most dangerous deep neck space abscess because complications include **supraglottic oedema with airway obstruction and aspiration pneumonia** due to rupture of the abscess and **acute mediastinitis**. It represents the main avenue for spread of infections into the mediastinum. Mediastinitis is the most feared complication that may result in **empyema or pericardial effusion**. If the infection perforates the alar layer posteriorly, it enters the **danger space** (between the alar and prevertebral layers), which extends down the entire mediastinum to the level of diaphragm (Box 23.1). This condition is characterised by **dyspnoea and chest pain**.

Surgical management

In most of the cases, the retropharyngeal space abscess will result from an extension of lateral pharyngeal space infection and therefore will not be drained independently.

In conditions where independent drainage is necessary, an intraoral approach is made. A vertical incision is made on the pharyngeal wall lateral to the midline. Using a haemostat, abscess cavity is opened by blunt dissection while the patient is in Trendelenburg's position to avoid aspiration of the pus.

In case of concerns about the rupture of the abscess, an extraoral approach is used for drainage. The muscle and carotid sheath are retracted laterally after an incision is made along the anterior border of the sternocleidomastoid inferior to the hyoid bone. Dissection between the carotid sheath and the inferior constrictor helps in drainage of the retropharyngeal space (Fig. 23.19).

BOX 23.1 Danger Space

It is the potential space between the alar and prevertebral division of the deep layer of the deep cervical fascia.

Why is it called danger space?

The danger space at its inferior border is continuous with the posterior mediastinum containing vena cava, arch of aorta, thoracic duct, trachea and oesophagus. Erosion of the major blood vessels, lower airways and upper digestive tract leads to death of the patient.

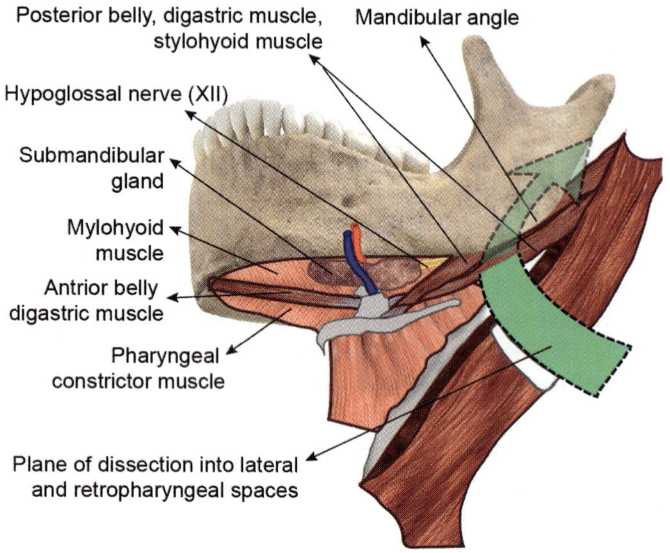

Figure 23.19 Extraoral approach for the drainage of retropharyngeal abscess.

FACTORS AFFECTING THE TREATMENT AND POSTOPERATIVE PHASE OF PARAPHARYNGEAL INFECTIONS (LATERAL AND RETROPHARYNGEAL SPACE)

1. When an abscess is large and has complicating conditions like diabetes mellitus (DM), it is likely to recur following drainage. This may need revisiting. In such instances, ***corrugated drains*** are preferred
2. ***Closed vacuum drains*** can be used for minor cavity abscesses without Diabetes mellitus (DM). This gives superior cosmetic results
3. Antibiotics normally last 3–6 weeks
4. Septicaemia, internal jugular vein thrombophlebitis and septic emboli are all symptoms of **Lemierre's syndrome**, which develops as a result of severe oropharyngeal infections
5. **Metastatic emboli** are common. Hence, anticoagulation is indicated to prevent infection spread and septic emboli catastrophe
6. Antibiotics and anticoagulants are given until **leukocytosis and erythrocyte sedimentation rate (ESR)** return to normal
7. The nasogastric tube is recommended for proper nutrition.

PERITONSILLAR ABSCESS (QUINSY)

Peritonsillar abscess or quinsy is a deep neck infection that is usually secondary to contiguous spread from the local sites or as a complication of acute tonsillitis that is rarely life threatening in itself. It can spread to involve the lateral pharyngeal space. The peritonsillar space is a potential space of loose areolar tissue that surrounds the tonsil and is bounded laterally by superior constrictors.

Clinical features

The infection is characterised by **swelling of the tonsils**, deviation of the **uvula** towards the unaffected side, **trismus** and a **muffled voice**. The infection generally starts in the intratonsillar fossa, which is situated between the upper pole and body of the tonsil and eventually extends around the tonsil. Quinsy is **usually unilateral**, but can rarely occur bilaterally. Most abscesses occur in younger patients who present with **fever**, **sore throat** and **dysphagia**.

Complications

Spontaneous rupture and aspiration, contiguous spread to pterygomaxillary space.

Surgical management

If the patient is not treated until the pus is formed or if antibiotic therapy fails, the abscess must be drained through an incision on the affected tonsillar swelling (Fig. 23.5B), but since peritonsillar abscess often tends to recur, tonsillectomy should be performed 6–8 weeks after formation of the abscess.

LIFE-THREATENING COMPLICATION OF OROFACIAL INFECTIONS

Related to lower jaw:

1. Ludwig's angina
2. Mediastinitis
3. Involvement of carotid sheath

Related to upper jaw:

1. Intracranial complications like cavernous sinus thrombosis, brain abscess, dural meningitis and osteomyelitis of skull
2. Retrobulbar cellulitis leading to blindness.

LUDWIG'S ANGINA

Ludwig's angina is a form of a firm, acute, toxic and severe diffuse cellulitis/induration that spreads rapidly, bilaterally affecting the submandibular, sublingual and submental spaces. It was 1st described by Wilhelm Friedreich Von Ludwig in 1836. The term 'Ludwig's angina' was coined by Camerer in 1837, who presented the classic case of Ludwig's angina, which was described in 1836 by Wilhelm Ludwig.

Classic Ludwig's angina—definite bilateral involvement of all the three spaces, that is submandibular, sublingual and submental spaces.

The word 'angina' derived from Latin word '*angere*' meaning suffocation or choking sensation; and the word 'Ludwig' from the person who 1st described it. Ludwig presented the classical features of the disease and successfully treated the same for Franklin NN.

The condition has established its unique identity among general medical personnel with three 'F'.

It was to be *feared*.
It rarely become *fluctuant*.
And it was often *fatal*.

Other names:
- *Marbus strangulatorius*: Chocking effect of the disease
- *Angina maligna*
- *Garrotillo*: Spanish term for Hangman's noose.

Aetiology

Ludwig's angina is a disease primarily of dental origin although various causes can also be related.

1. **Odontogenic infection:**
   a. Dental aetiology has been reported as the causative factor in 90% of cases, either as primary dental infection or as postextraction phenomena
   b. It is generally of dental origin, following infection of the 2nd and 3rd mandibular molars (70%–80%). The roots of these teeth often spread below the crest of the mylohyoid muscle, leading to periapical infection that reaches the submandibular space and from here, bilaterally to the contralateral submandibular, submental and sublingual spaces
   c. Acute dentoalveolar abscess (commonly from mandibular 2nd and 3rd molars)
   d. Acute periodontal abscess
   e. Acute pericoronal abscess (in relation to the erupting 3rd molar)
   f. Infection from these causes may spread to submandibular spaces, buccal space, sublingual space and pterygomandibular space. Mostly originate in association with mandibular 2nd and 3rd molars due to the anatomical relationship of the teeth and the involved spaces. The buccal bone around the teeth is thicker than the lingual bone
2. Traumatic injuries of orofacial region:
   a. Compound/comminuted mandibular fractures
   b. Oral soft tissue lacerations
   c. Puncture wounds of the floor of the mouth
   d. Osteomyelitis secondary to compound mandibular fractures
3. Submandibular and sublingual sialadenitis
4. Secondary infections of oral malignancies
5. Pharyngeal infection or tonsillitis
6. Iatrogenic: Use of contaminated needle for giving local anaesthesia
7. Cervical lymphoid tissues
8. Miscellaneous: Foreign bodies such as fish bone.

Pseudo-Ludwig's angina/pseudo-Ludwig's phenomena

This term is applied to cases of nondental origin.

Microbiology

- As Ludwig's angina is commonly of dental origin, streptococci or mixed oral flora are the most commonly reported organisms
- Presence of staphylococci, *Escherichia coli*, *Pseudomonas* and anaerobes including *Bacteroides*, *Pepto streptococcus*, *Prevotella* species and fusospirochetes have also been isolated
- The role of anaerobes as primary or synergistic organisms should not be omitted in culture.

CLINICAL FEATURES

General examination

General constitutional symptoms: Patient looks toxic, very ill, dehydrated, chills and malaise.
Marked pyrexia.
Difficulty in swallowing (dysphagia).
Impaired speech and hoarseness of voice.

Regional examination

Extraoral examination:
- Bilateral suprahyoid swelling is observed with a hard, cardboard-like consistency
- Swelling is firm/hard brawny involving bilateral submandibular and submental regions, which soon extends down the anterior part of the neck of the clavicles, swelling present with ill-defined borders. It is nonpitting, not fluctuating and tender on palpation
- Airway obstruction and cyanosis may occur due to progressive hypoxia
- *Difficulty in swallowing and breathing, chills, fever, increased salivation, restricted tongue movements and inability to close the mouth are the most salient presenting clinical features of the illness*
- Early presentation has no suppuration, but occurs late in the course of the disease. Further, this phenomenon appears very rapidly and does not respect any anatomic barrier.

Mouth remains open due to oedema of the sublingual tissues and there is a resultant raised tongue with restricted movements.

- Shallow breathing with accessory muscles of respiration being used and respiratory rate may be raised
- Severe muscle spasm leading to trismus with restricted mouth opening and also jaw movement
- Fatal death may occur in untreated cases of Ludwig's angina within 10–24 h due to asphyxia

Intraoral examination:
- Swelling develops rapidly and involves sublingual spaces causing elevation of tooth against the palate
- Increased salivation, stiffness of tongue, difficulty in swallowing with hot potato speech is noted
- Drooling of saliva due to reduced control of muscles and jaw posture
- Backward spread of infection leading to oedema of the glottis, which leads to obstruction of airway

- Development of stridor being the alarming sign for fatal extension necessitating emergency intervention to keep airway patent.

Potential complications

It is a potentially serious infection that can lead to septicaemia, upper respiratory airway obstruction and provoke oedema of the epiglottis.

On the other hand, it can also spread to the submassetric, pterygopalatine spaces, parapharyngeal and paratonsillar spaces and proceed onwards to the mediastinum, producing thoracic empyema.

Aspiration pneumonia and vascular erosion have been cited as possible complications. The most common cause of mortality is acute obstruction of the airways.

Rarely the infection may spread below and reach close to the carotid sheath and pterygopalatine fossa, leading to cavernous sinus thrombosis with subsequent meningitis.

If untreated, Ludwig's angina can be fatal within 12–24 h due to asphyxia.

Diagnosis

Diagnosis is made on the basis of clinical findings although CT studies can help to determine the extent of the infection, especially when there is abscess formation.

Treatment

Ludwig's angina should be considered as the life-threatening emergency. Treatment must be vigorous and initiated early with administration of antibiotics as for any odontogenic infections and prophylactic incision and drainage of the spaces involved, without waiting for fluctuation to appear. The airway must also be controlled, often requiring tracheostomy (Flowcharts 23.8).

Surgical management

Surgical management is necessary in case of rise of tissue tension and as a provision for drainage. In a classic case of Ludwig's angina, a little amount of pus is evacuated. Bilateral drainage of submandibular spaces along with drainage of

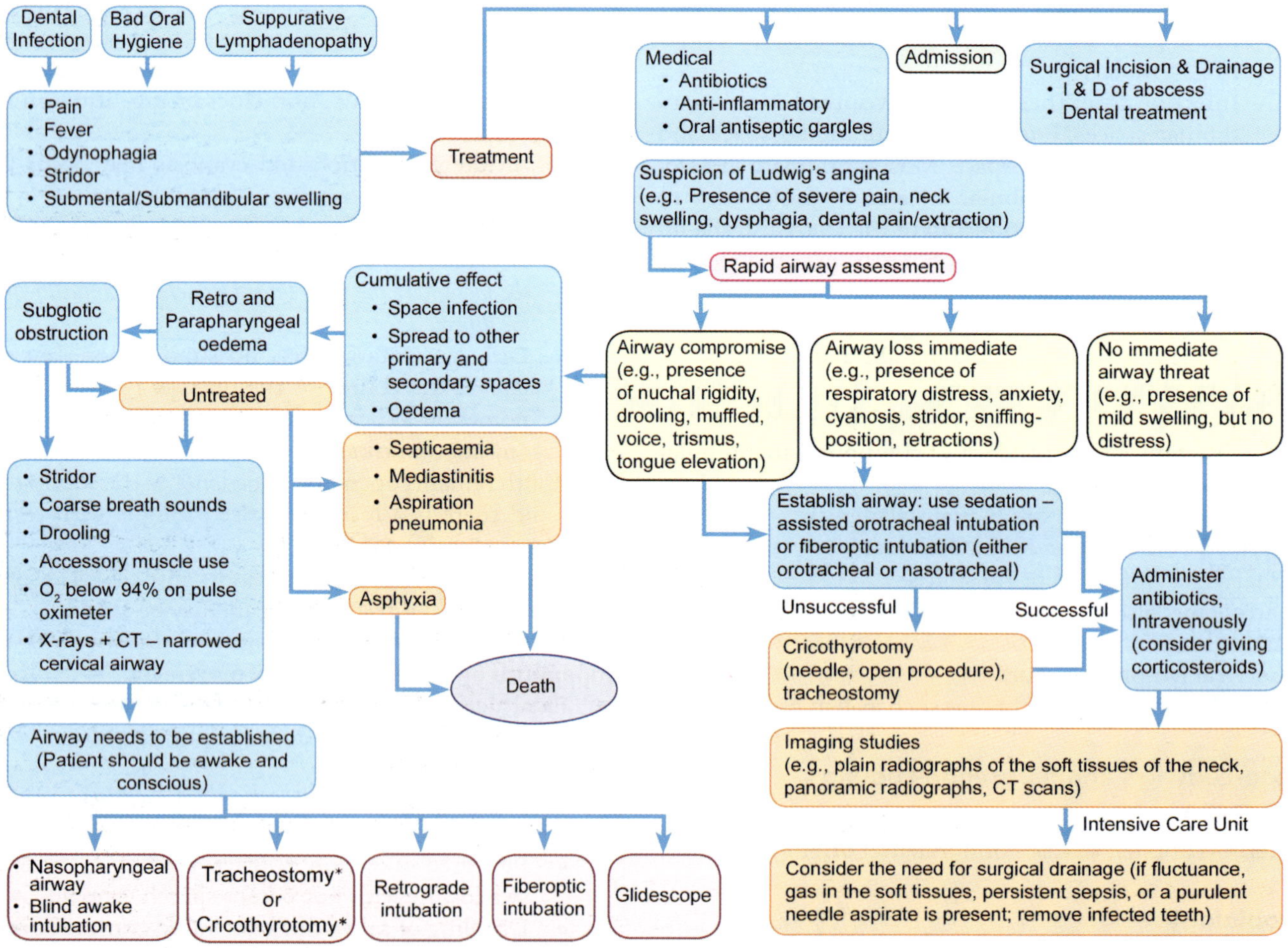

*Sometimes pharyngeal wall may have a soft point on the mucosa where the pus may rupture out and lead to aspiration of pus when traumatised by endotracheal tube. Hence, tracheostomy and cricothyrotomy are consider safer.

Flowchart 23.8 Management of Ludwig's angina with various severity of airway compromise along with timing of surgical management.

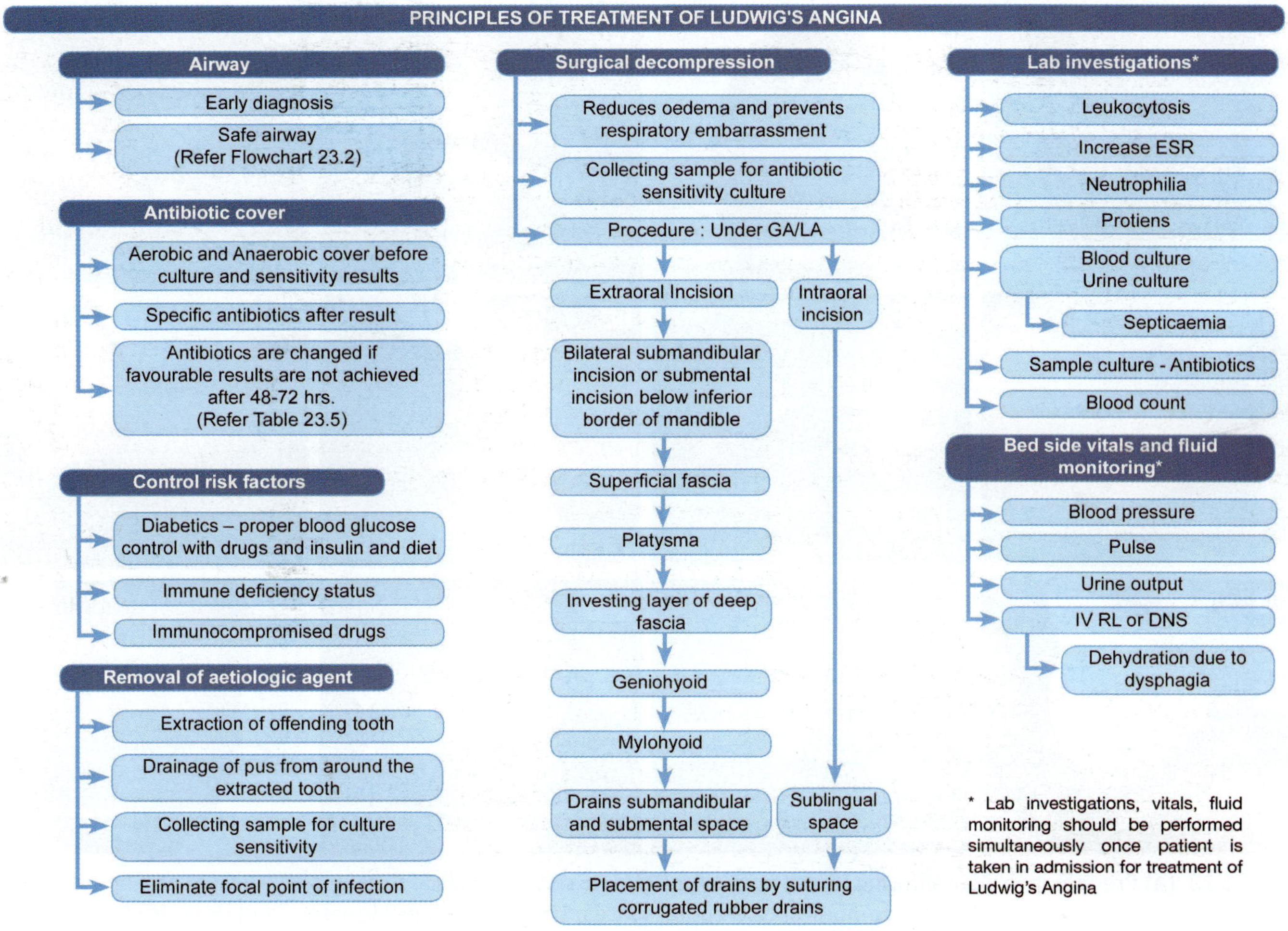

Flowchart 23.9 Principles of treatment of Ludwig's angina.

sublingual and submental spaces is the recommended therapy. It is preferable to drain sublingual and submental spaces separately to avoid perforation of the mylohyoid muscle (Flowchart 23.9 and Fig. 23.20A–J).

DISTANT SPREAD

Distant spread can occur by means of the bloodstream, essentially via the internal jugular vein in the same direction as the blood flow. Cardiac colonisation can result, leading to bacterial endocarditis, although the disease may be seeded practically in any organ. It can also follow a retrograde pathway towards cavernous sinus of the skull, establishing thrombophlebitis at some point in the facial venous system. Aseptic thrombus is formed, replete with microorganisms, which can then spread to distant areas, causing the much-feared neurological complications, such as thrombosis of the cavernous sinus, encephalic abscesses and meningitis.

CAROTID SPACE INFECTION

Carotid space infection produces a tender swelling in the lateral aspect of the neck under the sternocleidomastoid muscle. Patients will experience pain on palpation while rotating the head laterally. Usually there will be torticollis towards the unaffected side. The carotid sheath is made up of the superficial, middle and deep layers of the deep cervical fascia.

An incision is made along the middle 3rd of the anterior border of the sternocleidomastoid muscle. Through a vertical incision, carotid sheath is exposed carefully after retracting the muscle posteriorly. Internal jugular vein should be ligated to prevent infection if it is thrombosed (Fig. 23.21).

Lincoln's highway: It is a potential space within the carotid sheath, which extends from jugular foramen and carotid canal to the mediastinum.

CEREBRAL ABSCESS

Cerebral abscess may be the consequence of cavernous sinus thrombophlebitis, but can also be due to septic metastasis and bacteraemia accompanying odontogenic infections. Organisms on reaching the brain produce inflammation, localised oedema and septic thrombosis.

Brain abscesses have been associated with oral manipulations such as dental extractions, dental and periodontal

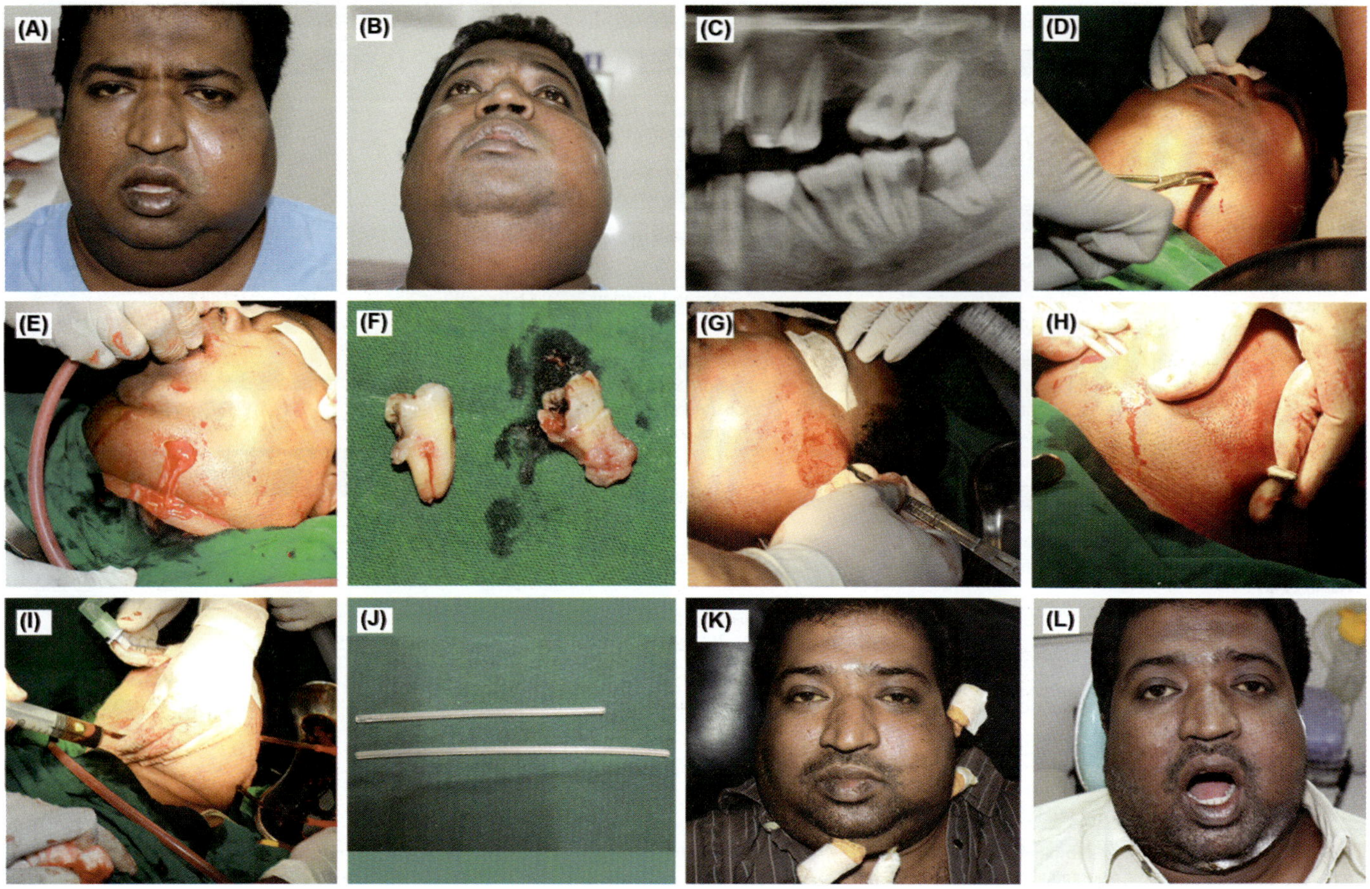

Figure 23.20 (**A**) Preoperative view showing raised tongue position, trismus and facial distress. (**B**) Swelling of bilateral submandibular, submental, left masseteric, infratemporal and temporal spaces. Skin appears erythematous and shiny. (**C**) Orthopantomogram showing grossly decayed left mandibular 2nd and 3rd molars. (**D**) Blunt dissection done into both submandibular and submental spaces breaking the pus locules. (**E**) Active pus discharge. (**F**) Removal of the source of infection—extracted mandibular left 2nd and 3rd molars. (**G**) Through and through drain placement connecting both submandibular and the submental spaces. (**H**) Stab incision made for drainage of left temporal space. (**I**) Irrigation using two-way drain. (**J**) Simple drain—perforated and non-perforated. (**K**) Simple drain placed for draining Ludwig's angina. (**L**) Postoperative view after 1 week.

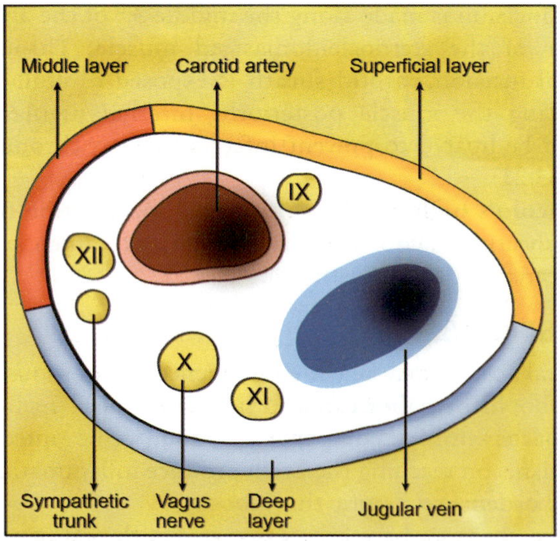

Figure 23.21 The carotid space contents and boundaries.

surgery and injection of local anaesthetics or dental prophylaxis, which suggests that the mechanism responsible for producing septicaemia is not as critical as the host response. There has been an increase in the incidence of brain abscesses in immunocompromised patients in both transplant recipients as well as in AIDS patients. Brain abscesses are rare with a prevalence of 1 per 100,000 inhabitants and a mortality rate of 0%–24%.

Cerebral abscesses consist of localised suppurative areas inside the cerebral parenchyma, preferentially located in the temporal lobe, followed by the cerebellum. They can occur following brain trauma, after surgery or they may be secondary to septic infection located anywhere in the body that can disseminate by means of direct spread or via the bloodstream, as seen in odontogenic infections.

The agents that are isolated from samples of brain abscess contents depend on the source of infection; when the cause is dental, *Streptococcus viridans, Bacteroides, Actinobacillus actinomycetemcomitans* have all been isolated.

Clinical presentation

Clinical signs necessarily depend on location of the infection site in the brain, but common symptoms result from elevated intracranial pressure, with intense headache, nausea and projectile vomiting. Cerebral irritation may present as convulsions, asphyxia, changes in character and behaviour, when the frontal lobe is involved. The patient may also present with temporal-spatial disorientation, etc. Diagnosis is confirmed by means of a CT scan and papillary stasis evident with ophthalmoscope. Other signs and symptoms are hemiplegia, papilloedema, hemisensory deficit and abducent nerve palsy.

Management

The main line of management is the use of antibiotics, anti-inflammatory drugs, steroids and mannitol to reduce cerebral oedema as well as surgical drainage.

MENINGITIS

Meningitis is the most commonly occurring neurological complication though rare. It may develop from metastatic spread or it may be due to nearby thrombophlebitis.

Clinical features

Clinically, it debuts with an intense headache, mental confusion, irritability, stupor, high fever with chills, vomiting and stiff neck (Brudzinski's sign). Convulsions may occur.

Kernig's sign: Flexing the patient's hip 90 degrees, then extending the patient's knee causes pain.

Brudzinski's sign: Flexing the patient's neck causes flexion of the patient's hip and knees.

Diagnosis

It is based on cerebrospinal fluid (CSF) analysis of cloudy or purulent opalescent fluid obtained on spinal tap. Upon examination of the CSF, polymorphonuclear leucocytes as well as elevated protein levels and decreased glucose levels are detected.

Management

Neurological complications require hospital care. Initiating treatment with chloramphenicol 4 g/day i.v. because of its broad-spectrum activity, associated with penicillin G at a dose of 24 million units/day i.v., while the microorganism is being identified through culture and sensitivity and its sensitivity profile is being determined. The maintenance of hydro electrolytic balance is also recommended in addition to controlling cerebral oedema and preventing collapse and shock.

CAVERNOUS SINUS THROMBOSIS

When a thrombus is formed at some point in the facial venous system, it can undergo retrograde spread towards the cavernous sinus, giving rise to thrombosis. It has been estimated that 7% of all cases of thrombosis of the cavernous sinus are of dental origin. The infection begins with unilateral involvement, but can develop bilaterally through the intercavernous sinuses.

Route:

1. Danger area of face (external route): Infection of the face and lip is carried by facial and angular veins and nasofrontal veins (danger area of face) to the superior ophthalmic veins, which enter through the superior orbital fissure to the cavernous sinus. External route-facial route is a very rapid short fulminating course because of large open system of veins leading directly to cavernous sinus. Infection from one side will involve the opposite side through circular veins
2. Pterygoid plexus of veins (internal route): Infection of dental origin enters the pterygoid plexus from posterior maxillary region, from here through inferior orbital fissure into the terminal part of the inferior ophthalmic vein and then through the superior orbital fissure into the cavernous sinus
3. Emissary vein: Pterygoid plexus is connected to cavernous sinus through emissary vein.

Clinical features

The 1st symptoms to appear are **eye pain, sensitivity of the eyeball** to pressure and signs of **severe toxic infection, high fever, chills, tachycardia and sweating. Pulsatile exophthalmos** is seen where the carotid pulse is transmitted through retrobulbar oedema. Subsequently, venous obstruction produces **palpebral oedema, ptosis, tearing of the eye, chemosis and retinal bleeding**. When the process progresses further, cranial nerves are also affected, producing **ophthalmoplegia** and **palpebral ptosis**; **corneal reflexes** are decreased or absent leading to **mydriasis**. The involvement of cranial nerves III, IV, VI and the carotid sympathetic plexus also occurs. The organisms that have been identified as causal agents are *Streptococcus, Staphylococcus* and Gram-negative bacteria.

Late complications like **thrombophlebitis, loss of vision, retroorbital bleeding** are seen in untreated cases.

Advanced stage presents with **toxaemia, meningitis, stiffness of neck with positive Kernig's and Brudzinski's sign and Biot's respiration.**

Eagleton criteria: Diagnostic criteria were suggested by Eagleton prior to the introduction of modern investigative procedures and comprise of:

1. A known site of infection or septicaemia
2. Early destructive signs (such as full retinal veins, proptosis, exophthalmos, collateral venous circulation)
3. Oculomotor paresis and trigeminal nerve involvement
4. Neighbourhood abscesses from the thrombophlebitis situated in the orbit, nasopharynx, occiput or neck
5. Symptoms of complications such as headache, papilloedema and meningeal signs.

Treatment

1. Early diagnosis is necessary for prompt treatment and favourable prognosis

2. Treatment involves therapy with antibiotics and steroids
3. Surgical treatment includes exploration of the cavernous sinus, which is not regularly performed. Removal of the septic focus, extraction of odontogenic focus and surgical drainage of paranasal sinuses
4. Antibiotics for empiric coverage of gram positive, negative and anaerobic bacteria is administered with 3rd generation cephalosporins, vancomycin and metronidazole
5. If fungal in origin, debridement of fungal paranasal sinusitis and Amphotericin-B (liposomal) 10 mg/kg/day is given
6. Administering steroids is controversial
7. Heparinisation—to prevent the extension of thrombosis. Intravenous heparin 24,000–30,000 units/day in 1.5 L of 5% dextrose or dicumarol 200 mg may be given orally for 1st day and 100 mg daily
8. Mannitol—to reduce oedema.

MEDIASTINITIS

Odontogenic infections and Ludwig's angina are uncommon, but when they occur, they are life threatening due to airway obstruction or mediastinitis. The spaces that are mainly involved are lateral pharyngeal space and the retropharyngeal space. In the neck, the muscles and aponeurosis are oriented in the vertical plane, creating a space that joins the posterior part of the mouth with the mediastinum in a chimney-like manner. This is where the major structures, the carotid artery, vagus nerve and internal jugular vein covered by perivascular fascia pass through. When this area becomes infected, it can lead to mediastinitis, also known as descending necrotising mediastinitis. It is an uncommon and serious complication. The rapid spread of cellulitis is caused by both aerobic and anaerobic bacteria acting in synergistic fashion.

Clinical features

The clinical signs are classically presented by these abscesses in the parapharyngeal and retropharyngeal spaces include dysphagia, dyspnoea, stiff neck and oesophageal regurgitation. Swelling appears on the side of the neck underneath the sternocleidomastoid muscle. It is painful on palpation and, on a functional level, causes stiff neck. When infection reaches the mediastinum, the patient experiences retrosternal pain, severe dyspnoea and nonproductive cough. It may also present as oedema and crepitation in the upper thorax. The patient's general health status deteriorates with fever and chills.

Diagnosis

The anteroposterior chest X-ray reveals broadening of the mediastinal space and presence of air at this level. Lateral X-ray of the neck reveals displacement of posterior wall of the pharynx together with the presence of free gas. Mortality rate associated with this form of mediastinitis is high, often due to difficulty in making an early diagnosis, since dysphagia, dyspnoea, swelling of the neck and crepitation are all late signs of the condition.

Potential complications

Mediastinitis can course with severe complications such as septicaemia, abscess formation, pleural effusion, empyema, compression of the local blood vessels, pericarditis and death. When there is vascular involvement, there will be septicaemia with an abrupt rise in temperature, chills, sweats and shock.

Medical management

In these patients, intravenous administration of antibiotics at maximum doses and support measures that can only be given in intensive care units (ICU) are mandatory. The association of penicillin G and metronidazole or chloramphenicol against the anaerobes is often considered shock therapy; when the Gram-negative microorganisms are also involved, gentamicin or tobramycin is added.

Surgical intervention

Surgical intervention is aimed at incision and drainage. A transcervical approach has been recommended, performing a wide incision in the area of the anterior edge of the sternocleidomastoid muscle and reaching all the way to the mediastinum by means of blunt finger dissection through the pretracheal space. This procedure reduces the risk of injuring vascular structures. After abundant irrigation of the affected spaces, continuous suction drains are placed. During the postoperative period, the patient must be placed in the Trendelenburg's position to facilitate drainage of the mediastinum.

NECROTISING FASCIITIS OF THE HEAD AND NECK

Necrotising fasciitis of the head and neck is a multimicrobial, uncommon soft tissue infection that spreads fast. It is characterised by formation of large necrotic lesions and gas formation, located in the subcutaneous tissue and in the superficial fascia. As the disease progresses, muscle and skin involvement develops, giving rise to myonecrosis and spots in the area, as a consequence of the feeder vessels that pass through the infected fasciae.

If the necrotising fasciitis does not receive surgical care, generalised toxicity occurs with multisystem organ failure. Necrotising fasciitis is a rare, but potentially fatal disease that occurs predominantly in the limbs and abdominal wall following trauma or surgery and less commonly in the head and neck. Dental infections comprise the most frequent cause in the head and neck although it can also be due to pharyngeal infections. Immunosuppressed states of peripheral vascular disease and diabetes mellitus have also been reported to be predisposing factors, although the illness has also been detected in healthy patients (Fig. 23.22).

Causative organism

Aerobic microorganisms, particularly Group A-haemolytic *Streptococcus* and *Staphylococcus,* were initially considered to be the causal agents in necrotising fasciitis. It was later demonstrated that the strict anaerobes played a very important role, representing a mixed or synergistic infection.

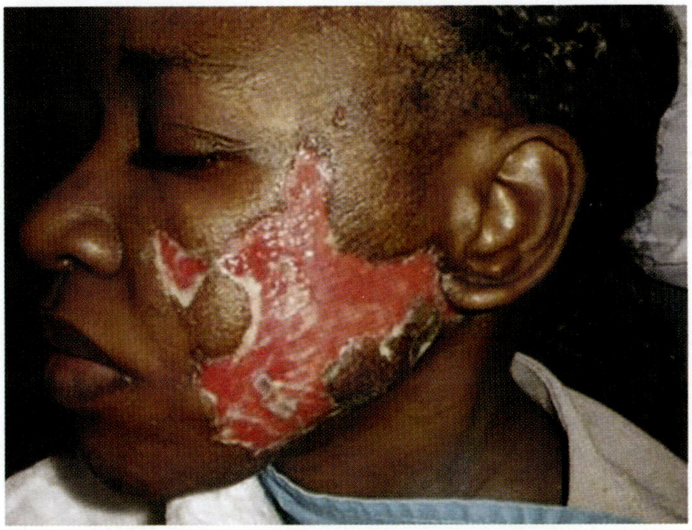

Figure 23.22 Necrotising fasciitis of face.

Microorganisms of the *Bacteroides* genus, *Proteus*, coliforms and *Pepto streptococcus* as well as *Enterobacter* and Pseudomonas have been isolated. The fulminating nature of the necrotic process is the result of a symbiotic relationship between both types of bacteria, with alteration of the oxygen reduction potential and a microenvironment that fosters the growth of anaerobic bacteria. Bacterial enzymes and cell wall components play an essential role in local tissue destruction, dissemination of the infection and systemic toxicity.

Clinical features

- The initial clinical signs and symptoms are nonspecific soft tissue involvement, which then progresses, producing gangrene of the subcutaneous cell tissue and muscular aponeurosis
- There may be intense pain at the onset of the disease, whereas during the course of illness, paraesthesia or even anaesthesia may develop in the affected area as a result of nerve involvement
- As the necrotising fasciitis evolves, the skin is affected; it turns purple or dark with poorly defined edges
- Vesicles later appear with a foul-smelling, purulent exudate
- Cutaneous necrosis is detected on the 4th or 5th day. Over time, necrotic tissue begins to separate with suppuration (approximately on the eighth day)
- If the necrotising process continues to spread, it involves the neighbouring tissues and provokes local or systemic complications such as neck organ involvement, pneumonia, pulmonary abscess, vascular erosion, venous thrombosis and cranial neuropathies
- The classical triad of symptoms include local pain, swelling and erythema.
- The most common vital sign abnormalities are tachycardia (>100 beats/min), fever followed by hypotension (< 100 mmHg) and tachypnoea (>20/min), which along with skin erythema helps in diagnosis of necrotising fasciitis from other soft tissue infections.
- It is not hard to confuse necrotising fasciitis with cellulitis of dental origin, erysipelas and gangrenous necrosis due to *Clostridium*.

Investigations

- CBC- Complete blood count (Leukocytosis, Band cells, and Toxic granules in Leukocytes)
- USG- Ultrasonography of the neck helps to visualize the fluid collection in the superficial planes as well as the extent of infection.
- CT scans are helpful in detecting the necrosis, extent of tissue infection, and gas formation.

Treatment

1. Necrotizing infections often cause significant fluid loss and a marked hemodynamic response. Severe septic shock may occur. There is always a risk for cardiovascular, respiratory or renal failure. Therefore, an ICU monitoring with continuous pulse oximetry, hourly monitoring of urine output and frequent recording of the haemodynamic values and respiratory rate are required.
2. Broad spectrum antibiotic therapy.
   - i.v. Benzyl penicillin 2.4 g, 4 hourly + flucloxacillin 1 g, 6 hourly + metronidazole 500 mg, 8 hourly)
   - i.v. Cefotaxim 2 gm + Metronidazole 500 mg or Clindamycin 900 mg, 8 hourly
   - i.v. Imipenem/Cilastatin 500 mg, 6 hourly or add penicillin 20 million units

   Antibiotics should be administered for 5 days to 6 weeks, until the local signs and symptoms have resolved. These antibiotics can be subsequently modified once the culture results are obtained.
3. If necessary, tracheostomy to maintain the airway.
4. Surgical debridement includes excision of the necrotic tissue, up to the point of fresh bleeding or healthy tissue appears. The procedure is repeated every day and the wounds are left open. Drains can be inserted into the deeper fascial planes. Irrigation of the wound can be done with NaCl 0.9% and H_2O_2.
5. Hyperbaric oxygen therapy can also be used as an adjunct.
6. Once the wound granulates healthily, a skin graft can be placed or primary closure can be attempted.

Chapter 24

Osteomyelitis, Osteoradionecrosis and Osteochemonecrosis

OUTLINE

OSTEOMYELITIS

The term osteomyelitis was 1st coined by Nelaton in 1934. It is primarily an inflammation of the medullary portion of the bone. The process is rarely confined to the ***endosteum*** and usually affects the ***cortical bone*** and the ***periosteum*** as well. Therefore, osteomyelitis may be considered as an inflammatory condition of the bone that begins as an infection of the ***medullary cavity***, rapidly involves the ***Haversian system*** and quickly extends to the periosteum of the area. When infection becomes established in the calcified portion of the bone, the pus in the medullary cavity and subperiosteal compartment compromises or obstructs the blood supply. Following ischaemia, the infected bone becomes necrotic.

Microcirculation failure in the cancellous bone is a significant element in the development of osteomyelitis. The illness spreads in the direction of least resistance. Because normal blood-borne defences do not reach the tissue when the affected area becomes ischaemic and bone becomes necrotic, allowing bacteria to proliferate and osteomyelitis to spread unless medical and surgical treatment is administered. The predisposing factors for the formation of osteomyelitis are:

Conditions that alter host defences: Diabetes mellitus, malnutrition, autoimmune disorders, agranulocytosis, anaemia especially sickle cell, leukaemia, drug abuse, AIDS, syphilis, chemotherapy for cancer, steroid use, alcohol and tobacco abuse are frequently associated with osteomyelitis.

Conditions that alter vascularity of bone: Radiation, osteoporosis, osteopetrosis, Paget's disease, fibrous dysplasia, bone malignancy, bone necrosis caused by mercury, bismuth and arsenic.

The aetiologic factors are described in Flowchart 24.1.

PATHOGENESIS (Fig. 24.1)

The extensive blood supply to the maxilla makes it less susceptible to osteomyelitis than the mandible. There is a medullary cavity, dense cortical plates and a distinct periosteum in the mandible. The thin cortical plates and porosity of the medullary part allow oedema and purulent discharge to spread into neighbouring tissues. Insufficiency of blood flow is a crucial element in the development of osteomyelitis. The inferior alveolar artery supplies the mandible with blood, while the periosteum receives blood from a secondary source.

Increased capillary permeability and granulocyte infiltration due to infection trigger osteomyelitis. This occurs when proteolytic enzymes are released along with bacterial breakdown. Osteomyelitis occurs when the infection escapes from the medullary bone into neighbouring soft tissues. The accumulation of necrotic tissue and pus (dead bacteria in white blood cells) causes an increase in intramedullary pressure. Pus flows through the Haversian system and the nutrient canals, accumulating beneath the periosteum, which elevates from the cortex and reduces blood supply. When the inferior alveolar neurovascular

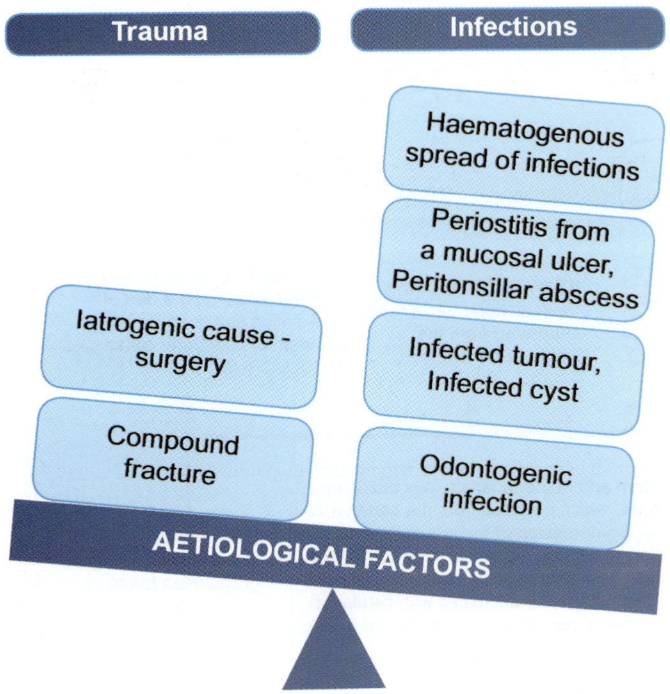

Flowchart 24.1 Aetiological factors for the formation of osteomyelitis.

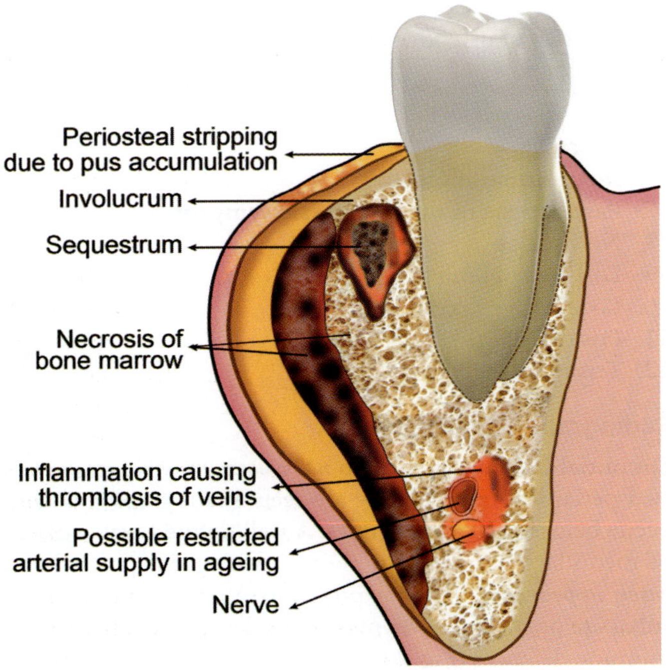

Figure 24.1 Pathogenesis of mandibular osteomyelitis.

bundle is compressed, thrombosis and ischaemia progress more quickly.

In **osteomyelitis-induced inferior alveolar nerve dysfunction**, if the pus persists, the periosteum is penetrated, resulting in mucosal and cutaneous abscesses with fistulae. In children, the periosteum is less bound to the cortical bone, allowing for more extensive elevation.

With a good host defence system, chronic inflammation subsides and granulation tissue forms. The necrotic bone separates from the viable bone and is called the **sequestrum**. Small sections of bone may be completely lysed, while larger sections may be isolated by a bed of granulation tissue encased in a sheath of new bone called the **involucrum**. Sequestrum may be revascularised, remain dormant, resorb, or become chronically infected, necessitating surgical removal for complete infection cure. When the involucrum is punctured by channels known as **cloacae**, pus escapes and forms fistulae on the epithelial surface (Flowchart 24.2).

CLASSIFICATION

Osteomyelitis is classified as either acute or chronic or suppurative or nonsuppurative (presence or absence of pus). Acute or subacute osteomyelitis is always accompanied with pus discharge due to the rapid progression of the illness. Osteomyelitis without pus development is predominantly chronic in nature. There are additional causes of osteomyelitis, such as syndromes associated—SAPHO (Synovitis, acne, pustulosis, hyperostosis, osteitis), juvenile and infantile osteomyelitis (Flowchart 24.3). Three common classifications of osteomyelitis are presented in Table 24.1.

TYPES OF OSTEOMYELITIS

ACUTE/SUBACUTE SUPPURATIVE OSTEOMYELITIS

Acute suppurative osteomyelitis is a serious sequela of a periapical infection that results in a diffuse spread of the infection throughout the medullary spaces with subsequent necrosis of a variable amount of bone. **History may reveal any one of the following: recent extraction, infection or debilitating disease.** The causative organisms are *Staphylococcus aureus* and *Staphylococcus albus*. The osteoblasts surrounding the trabeculae of bone are eliminated. The trabeculae lose their viability and undergo a slow resorption process. As the condition progresses, the bone loses its vitality and begins to detach from the living bone. Each separated dead bone piece is known as a ***sequestrum***. Each sequestrum is gradually exfoliated through the mucosa; when a large sequestrum forms, it can be surgically removed. When the sequestrum becomes encircled by new living bone, this is known as the ***involucrum***.

Clinical features

1. Either the maxilla or the mandible might be affected by acute or subacute osteomyelitis
2. In the maxilla, lesions are typically localised to a small area, whereas in the mandible, they are more widespread and diffuse
3. It can affect people of any age
4. Deep and intense jaw pain

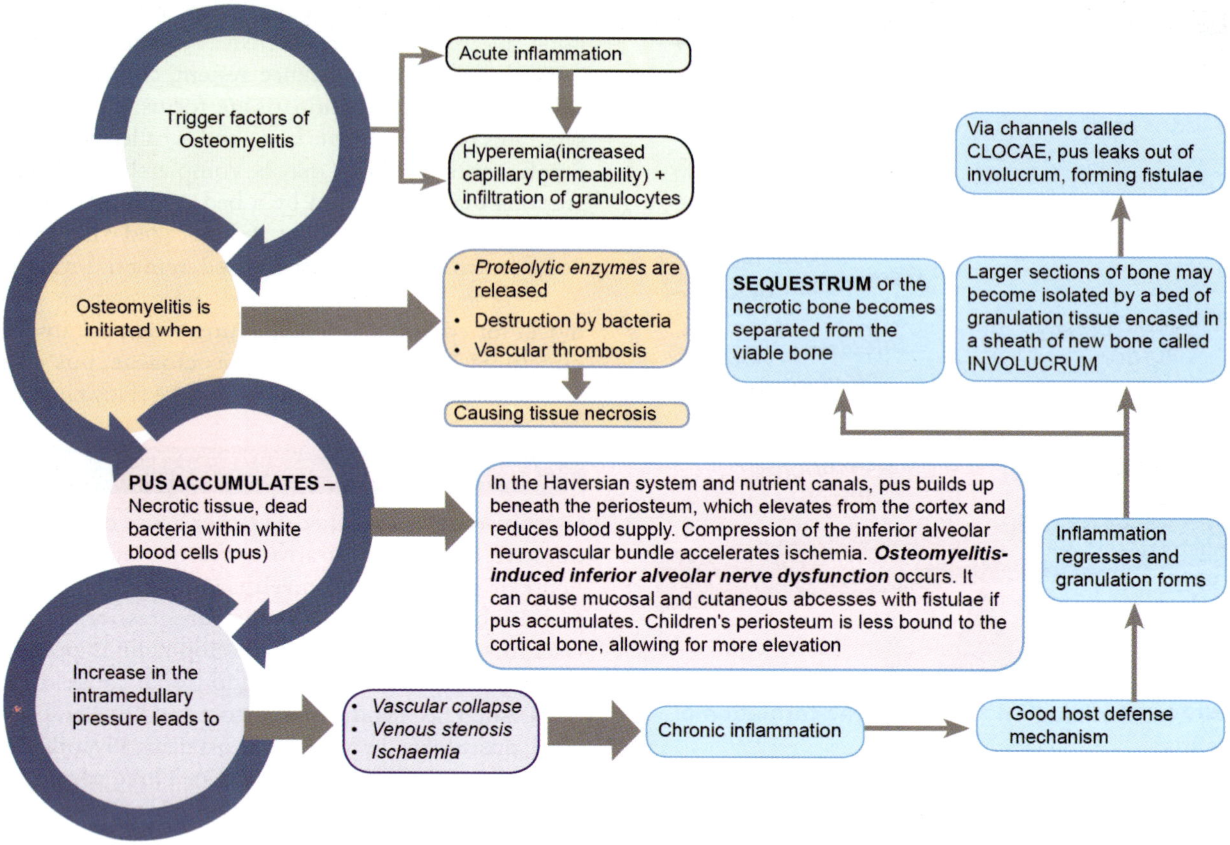

Flowchart 24.2 Pathogenesis for the formation of osteomyelitis.

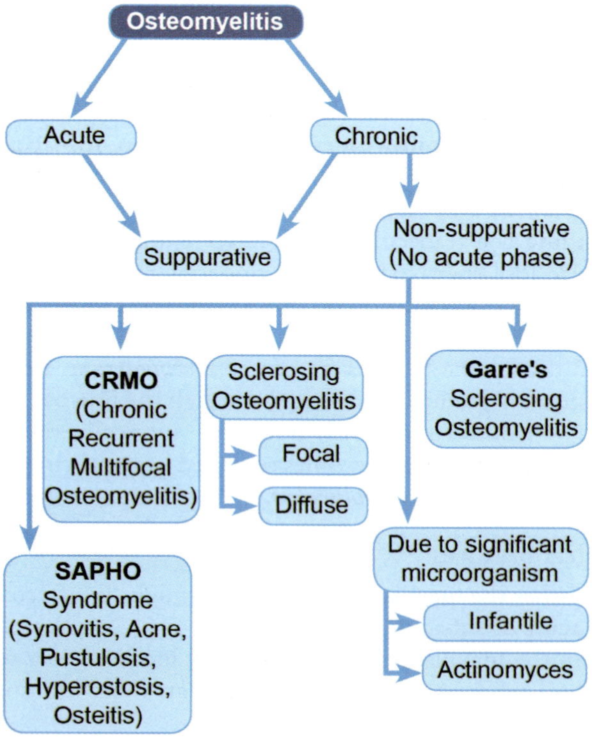

Flowchart 24.3 Types of osteomyelitis.

5. Abscess
6. Intermittent high fever
7. Paraesthesia of the lip (**classic symptom**)
8. No fistulae
9. Diffuse swelling
10. Loosening of teeth
11. Pus discharge
12. Trismus.

Radiographic features

On initial examination, often *no radiographic findings* or localised periapical radiolucency are seen. Radiographic changes occur between 10 and 20 days. A well-defined trabeculation of medullary bone is lost, giving an irregular patchy ***moth-eaten appearance***. If inadequately treated, progression to a subacute or chronic form may occur depending on the host's immune defences (Fig. 24.2).

CHRONIC SUPPURATIVE OSTEOMYELITIS

It may develop after the acute phase of the disease has subsided (secondary), or it may arise from a dental infection without a preceding acute stage (primary). History of previous episodes of acute suppurative osteomyelitis or odontogenic infection may be seen (Fig. 24.3).

TABLE 24.1 Classifications of Osteomyelitis

Marx and Mercuri's classification based on clinical picture, radiology, aetiology and pathophysiology	I. Acute osteomyelitis: 1. Associated with haematogenous spread 2. Associated with intrinsic bone pathology or peripheral vascular disease 3. Associated with odontogenic and nonodontogenic local processes II. Chronic osteomyelitis: 1. Chronic recurrent multifocal osteomyelitis of children 2. Garre's osteomyelitis 3. Chronic suppurative osteomyelitis: – Foreign body related – Systemic disease related – Related to persistent or resistant organisms 4. True chronic diffuse sclerosing osteomyelitis
Hudson's dual classification based on pathological anatomy and pathophysiology	I. Anatomic types: Stage I: medullar osteomyelitis—involved medullar bone without cortical involvement; usually haematogenous Stage II: superficial osteomyelitis—less than 2 cm bony defect without cancellous bone Stage III: localised osteomyelitis—less than 2 cm bony defect on radiograph, defect does not appear to involve both cortices Stage IV: diffuse osteomyelitis—defect greater than 2 cm. Pathologic fracture, infection, nonunion II. Physiological class: A: normal host B: systemic compromised host, local compromised host C: treatment worse than disease
Topazian's classification based on clinical picture, radiology and aetiology	I. Suppurative osteomyelitis: 1. Acute suppurative osteomyelitis 2. Chronic suppurative osteomyelitis: – Primary chronic suppurative osteomyelitis – Secondary chronic suppurative osteomyelitis 3. Infantile osteomyelitis II. Nonsuppurative osteomyelitis: 1. Chronic sclerosing osteomyelitis: – Focal sclerosing osteomyelitis – Diffuse sclerosing osteomyelitis 2. Garre's sclerosing osteomyelitis 3. Actinomycotic osteomyelitis 4. Radiation osteomyelitis and necrosis

Clinical features

1. Clinical features of chronic suppurative osteomyelitis are similar to that of acute osteomyelitis in a milder form
2. Acute exacerbations of the chronic stage may occur periodically
3. Paraesthesia of the lip may be seen, though not classically seen in chronic suppurative osteomyelitis
4. The pain is less severe
5. The temperature is still elevated
6. Leukocytes count is elevated
7. The teeth may not be mobile.

Radiographic features

Irregular radiolucent areas are superimposed on more sclerotic and nontrabeculated zones (Fig. 24.3B).

INFANTILE OSTEOMYELITIS

Although it is an uncommon disease for the jaws, it merits special attention since it involves risks of ocular, intracranial spread and subsequent facial deformities. Infantile osteomyelitis is believed to occur ***by haematogenous route or from perinatal trauma*** that occurs few weeks after birth and usually involves the maxilla (Fig. 24.4).

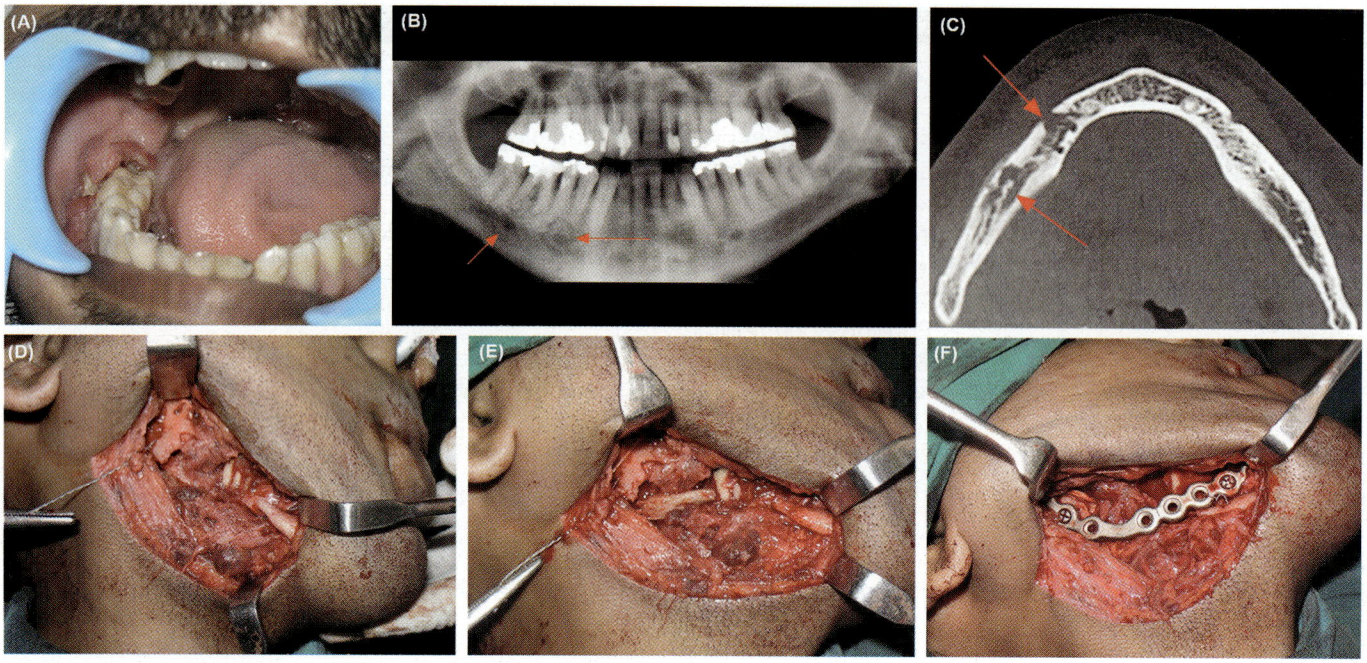

Figure 24.2 Acute suppurative osteomyelitis. (**A**) Intraoral view showing induration and pus discharge. (**B**) OPG showing bone destruction in the molar area with moth-eaten appearance of the bone in relation to the lower right molars. (**C**) CT scan showing bone destruction in the molar region and sequestrum in the premolar region. (**D**) Through an extraoral incision, the affected bone is exposed, the sequestrum can be seen. (**E**) Bony excision of the sequestrum performed and the normal bone is exposed. (**F**) The bony segments are stabilised with a reconstruction plate.

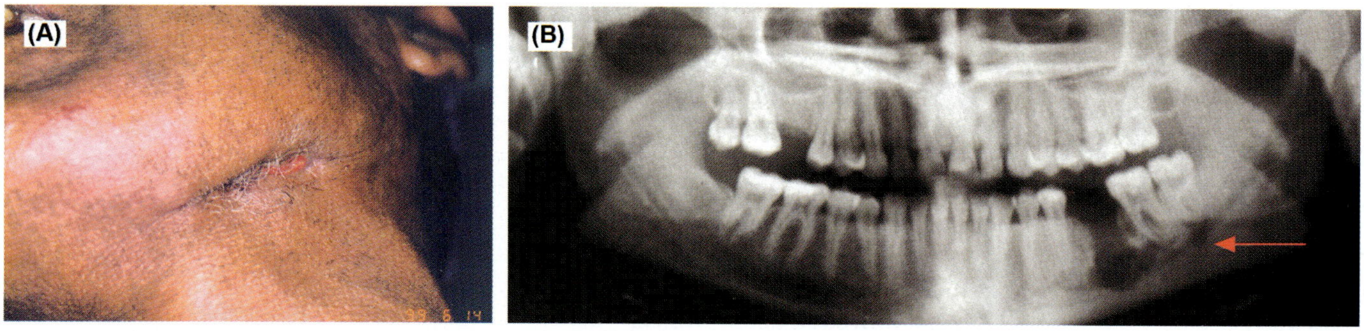

Figure 24.3 Chronic suppurative osteomyelitis. (**A**) Extraoral sinus tract. (**B**) Irregular radiolucent areas superimposed on more sclerotic and nontrabeculated zones.

Clinical features

1. Facial cellulitis centred about the orbit
2. Inner and outer canthal swelling
3. Palpebral oedema
4. Closure of the eye and proptosis
5. Purulent discharge from the nose and medial canthus.

Generalised symptoms include fever, irritability, malaise, anorexia, dehydration and even convulsions and vomiting. Intraoral buccal or palatal fistulae may be occasionally present. Osteomyelitis of the ribs and femur is also an important finding in infantile osteomyelitis, with ill-defined lytic lesion, found in the lateral distal femoral metadiaphysis, there is a thick periosteal response that is accompanied with soft tissue oedema. Rib osteomyelitis is presented with chest wall swelling, fever, leukocytosis and elevated C-reactive protein.

Investigations

Radiographic change is noted early. CT scans may be used to investigate extension of orbital abscess, possible dural extension or involvement of the sinus. Leucocytosis is usually present and the usual offending microorganism is *S. aureus.*

DIFFUSE SCLEROSING OSTEOMYELITIS

Diffuse sclerosing osteomyelitis is a chronic condition and represents a proliferative reaction of the bone to a low-grade

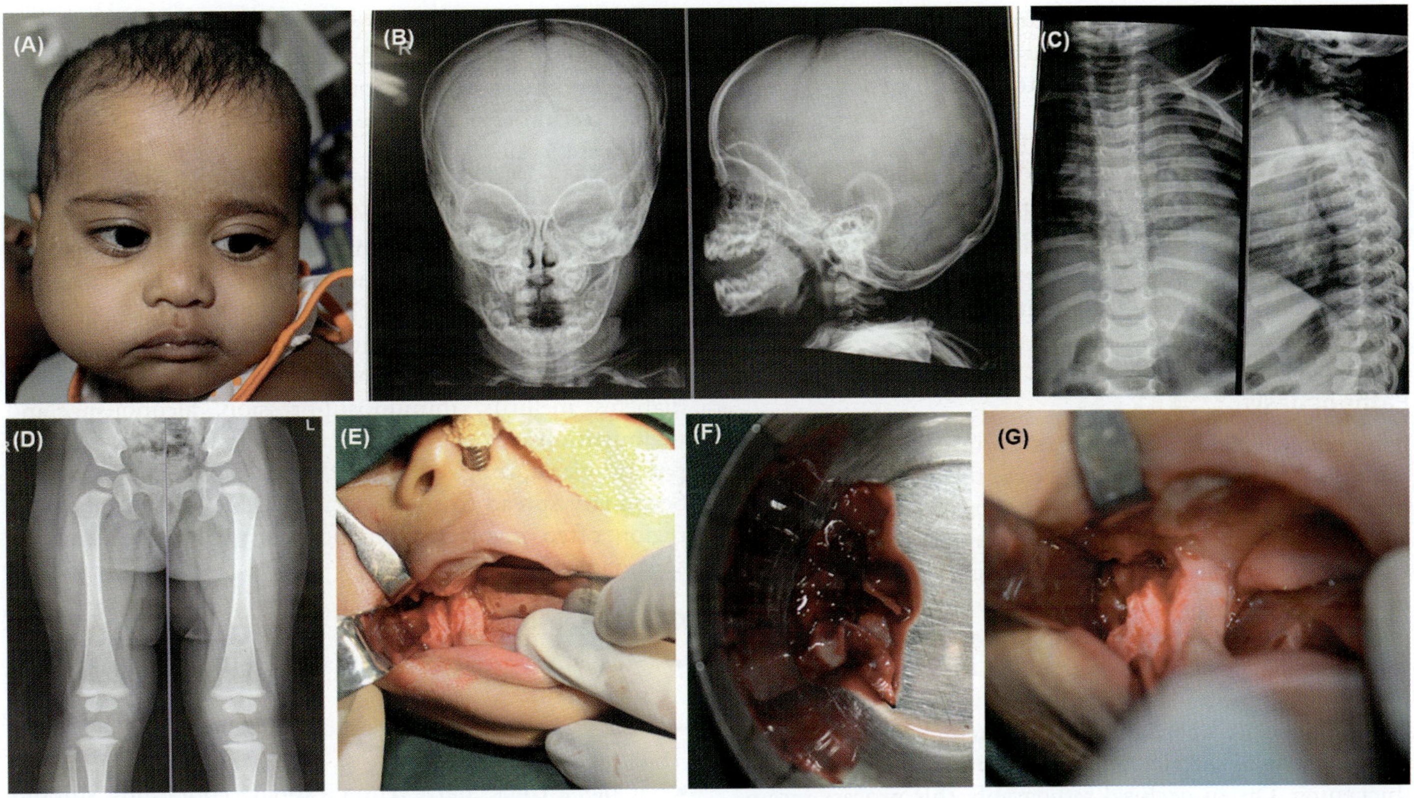

Figure 24.4 Infantile osteomyelitis. (**A**) Preoperative photograph of infant with infantile osteomyelitis. (**B**) Skull views showing osteomyelitis lesion in the right condylar region. (**C** and **D**) Osteomyelitis of the ribs and femur are also an important finding in infantile osteomyelitis, with ill-defined lytic lesion, found in the lateral distal femoral metadiaphysis, there is a thick periosteal response that is accompanied with soft tissue oedema. Rib osteomyelitis is presented with chest wall swelling, fever, leukocytosis and elevated C-reactive protein. (**E–G**) Intraoperative photographs showing resection of the affected bone.

infection. The portal of entry for the infection is diffuse periodontal disease.

Clinical features

It can occur at any age. Often the disease shows no clinical sign of its presence. In some cases, the 1st symptom may be a fistula on the mucosal surface. The patient may complain of vague pain and a bad taste.

Radiographic findings

Extensive radiopaque lesion, at times bilateral. Mimics Paget's disease of the bone by having a ***cotton wool appearance***.

SAPHO SYNDROME—CHRONIC RECURRENT MULTIFOCAL OSTEOMYELITIS

- The SAPHO syndrome, 1st described by Chamot et al. consists of symptoms–synovitis, acne, pustulosis, hyperostosis and osteitis, associated with the syndrome
- Several case studies concluded that there may be a link between SAPHO syndrome and diffuse sclerosing osteomyelitis (DSO) of the mandible
- Chronic recurrent multifocal osteomyelitis (CRMO) and SAPHO are linked, due to the likelihood that it is related to other dermatoskeletal associated illnesses
- CRMO is a type of osteomyelitis that lasts for many years and is characterised by intervals of exacerbation and remission
- Despite the fact that it is more common in youngsters, this highly rare illness can afflict both adults and children
- A number of research published in recent years have discussed the possibility of a categorical link between DSO and CRMO.

FOCAL SCLEROSING OSTEOMYELITIS—CONDENSING OSTEITIS

It is another chronic condition which occurs in cases of extremely high host tissue resistance, or in cases of low-grade medullary infection which causes endosteal or periosteal reactions.

Clinical features

Most common in younger individuals in the mandibular 1st molar region with mild pain and decreased sensitivity in the tooth related to the radiopacity with no specific clinical findings.

Radiographic findings

The Intraoral periapical (IOPA) radiograph demonstrates pathognomonic well-circumscribed radiopaque mass of sclerotic bone surrounding and extending below the apex of one or both roots. The border of the lesion may be smooth and distinct or may appear to blend into the surrounding bone.

GARRE'S OSTEOMYELITIS—CHRONIC NONSUPPURATIVE SCLEROSING OSTEITIS

In 1983, Carl Garre described a distinctive type of chronic osteomyelitis as a '*focal gross thickening of the periosteum*' of the long bones with peripheral reactive bone formation resulting from mild irritation or infection. It is essentially a periosteal osteosclerosis.

Pathogenesis

It is prevalent among children and young adults. The mandible is more frequently afflicted than the maxilla. The aetiological agents may include a carious tooth, a low-grade chronic infection, or an infection of the overlying soft tissue. In cases where the causal agent persists, radiographic evidence of bone thickening might be observed. The infectious process caused by a tooth infection travels to the periosteum. It localises in the periosteum or under the periosteal layer of the cortical bone and spreads slightly within the bone. New bone is deposited beneath the periosteum. This peripheral development of reactive bone results in localised periosteal thickening. On an occlusal radiograph, this process resembles the appearance of an ***onion peel***.

Clinical features

1. The patient usually presents with a complaint of toothache or pain in the jaw
2. Acute caries in a young patient
3. The characteristic feature of Garre's osteomyelitis is the presence of a localised hard and nontender bony swelling, most commonly at the lateral and inferior areas of the mandible–also called the peripheries of the jaw.

Radiographic features

1. An IOPA radiograph often reveals a carious tooth opposite the hard bony mass. This mass of bone is smooth, may calcify and itself shows a thin but definite cortical layer
   a. Plain radiography of the mandible depicts areas of local decalcification or sclerosis
   b. Occlusal radiograph–***onion peel appearance***
   c. CT scanning or MRI allows early diagnosis and extent of the disease. Single photon emission computed tomography (SPECT) imaging is gaining importance in the recent times.

Management

Conservative management includes hyperbaric oxygen therapy and endodontic treatment along with antibiotics and tooth extraction. Studies have shown improved bone contours in the sixth month post extraction reviews. Surgical bone recontouring in Garre's osteomyelitis by bone excision and secondary reconstruction with distraction osteogenesis after infection resolution are indicated when bone contours remain stagnant.

LUMPY JAW—ACTINOMYCOSIS

Actinomycosis is a rare chronic disease caused by *Actinomyces israelii*. A granulomatous and suppurative lesion affecting soft tissues and occasionally bone.

Oral mucosa trauma (dental extraction, gingival trauma), and cervicofacial surgery are risk causing procedures and diabetes mellitus, immunosuppression, alcoholism, and malnutrition are risk factors. It affects the maxillary sinuses, parotid gland, tongue and soft tissues above the mandible. Secondary spread to the skull is possible. The cervicofacial region often involves submandibular, submental and nasogenian soft tissues.

Clinical features

- Slowly progressing, fluctuant, painless, firm swelling with fistulae
- It is a widespread infection that affects the submandibular area
- It has a thick, hard yellow exudate containing sulphur particles
- Sulphur granules are actinomycetes colonies that resemble sulphur grains. They are visible to the naked eye and are firm, yellowish macroscopic formations
- It can cause trismus and pain due to masticatory muscle infiltrations
- Osteomyelitis can develop if the infection extends to the facial and maxillary bones.

Diagnosis

For the detection of sulphur granules and filamentous Gram-positive fungi-like infections, a microscopic inspection is required. The bacteria must be detected by histological investigation and bacterial culture. Occasionally, a misleading negative culture result can occur due to the frequent prescription of oral antimicrobials, especially in patients with odontogenic cervicofacial actinomycosis, this occurs primarily prior to surgery. CT and MRI imaging techniques are beneficial for demonstrating bone involvement.

Management

- The most effective treatment is an antimicrobial regimen consisting of a high dose of amoxicillin
- In severe situations, the patient must initially receive large doses of either ***amoxicillin*** (up to 200 mg/kg/day) or ***penicillin G*** (up to 24 million units/day) by intravenous administration
- Patients allergic to penicillin have the option of using an alternative medication, such as ***erythromycin, clarithromycin, azithromycin, doxycycline or clindamycin***

- Although the addition of a companion medicine like ***metronidazole or a beta-lactamase inhibitor*** is contentious, it might be helpful in treating infections caused by multiple microorganisms at the same time
- If an optimal surgical resection of infected tissues has been performed, in the absence of bone involvement, and if a satisfactory patient response to treatment is rapidly observed, then it is likely that the traditional prolonged course of treatment, which can last anywhere from 6 to 12 months, can be shortened. In point of fact, numerous observations have indicated acceptable cure rates with antimicrobial treatment lasting between 4 and 6 weeks
- The purulent material must be drained and then the sinus tracts must be surgically excised. This is all covered in the surgical management
- If patients with deep infections do not have surgical therapy, they may be forced to undergo treatment for a period of up to a year.

CLINICAL FEATURES OF OSTEOMYELITIS

Early signs and symptoms

1. *Generalised symptoms of infection*: High intermittent fever, malaise, nausea, vomiting, decreased food intake and anorexia in chronic cases
2. Deep seated gnawing, continuous intense pain in the affected area
3. Intermittent paraesthesia of the lower lip
4. Facial cellulitis, or indurated swelling of moderate size, which is more confined to the periosteal envelop and its contents
5. Thrombosis of inferior alveolar vasa nervorum
6. Rise in pressure from oedema in inferior alveolar canal
7. Affected teeth are tender to percussion and are mobile
8. Trismus
9. *In children*: It develops suddenly and severely occurring in both the maxilla and mandible. Osteomyelitis is worsened by the existence of unerupted teeth buds that become necrotic, act as foreign bodies and prolong the progression of the disease
10. Ankylosis of the temporomandibular joint (TMJ) can result from long-term TMJ involvement, which can impact face growth and development
11. Mild leucocytosis and albuminuria are present in laboratory tests.

Established cases are characterised by:

1. General symptoms: Deep gnawing pain, fatigue, fever, dehydration and anorexia
2. Local symptoms: Teeth in the affected region become loosened and tender to percussion
3. Sinus discharge containing pus: (a) Intraorally—surrounding gingival sulcus, through buccal vestibule and (b) extraorally on the face, via cutaneous fistulae. Often a foetid odour is present
4. Clinical signs:
   a. Exposed bone
   b. Persistent sinus tract
   c. Tissue necrosis overlying bone
   d. Chronic soft tissue wound overlying fracture or surgical hardware
5. Trismus could cause dehydration. Typically, regional lymphadenopathy is present
6. Lab investigations:
   i. Moderate polymorphonuclear leukocytes (PMNL)
   ii. Slightly raised erythrocyte sedimentation rate (ESR)
   iii. Anaemia
   iv. Albuminuria
   v. Elevated C-reactive protein
   vi. Blood cultures, wound culture and sensitivity, are important diagnostic tools for monitoring risk of septicaemia.

MANAGEMENT OF OSTEOMYELITIS

Marx's guidelines for the treatment of osteomyelitis

The main goals of treating osteomyelitis were described in Marx's guidelines as follows:

1. To disrupt the foci of infection by eradicating the causing bacterium
2. Meticulous debridement with removal of dead bone, foreign bodies, necrotic tissue and sequestrum
3. Antibiotic therapy: antibiotic therapy by culture sensitivity. The treatment depends on the type of osteomyelitis. Antibiotic therapy remains constant in acute and chronic osteomyelitis. Once the culture specimen is obtained, start the i.v. antibiotic treatment. Treatment should be changed based on culture and sensitivity results. The antibiotic regimen should be continued if clinical symptoms improve (decrease in pain, swelling, erythema and fever) (Flowchart 24.4)

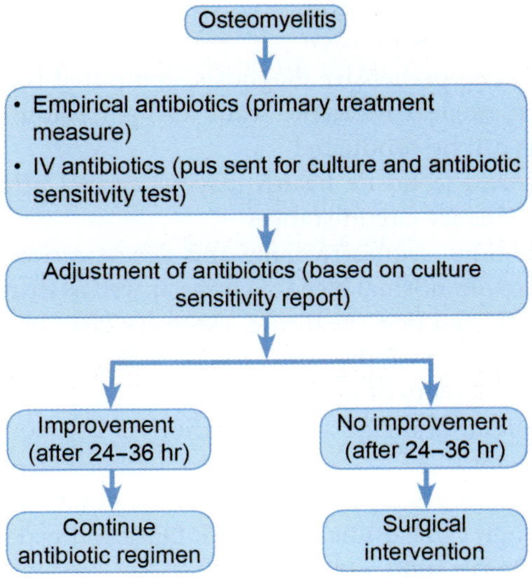

Flowchart 24.4 Management of osteomyelitis.

4. Drain fixation and irrigation of the affected area
5. Adjunctive treatment:
   a. Trephination
   b. Decortication
   c. Hyperbaric oxygen therapy (HBO)
   d. Vascular flaps
6. The bone may be disrupted by sequestrum or involucrum. Once they are removed and modified, the remaining bone may be structurally weak. This may require reinforcement with plates and screws until healthy bone formation occurs
7. Reconstruction of the defect.

Hudson's treatment plan for osteomyelitis

Acute osteomyelitis in a healthy host

1. Conservative decompression and debridement of infection in conjunction with extraction of all offending teeth
2. Drainage and irrigation of the suppuration; if pus exists
3. Culture and sensitivity testing is done with a sample from the infected foci
4. Antibiotic treatment for 3 to 4 weeks, depending on the Gram's stain, culture and sensitivity, blood culture and ESR
5. Regional bony stabilisation, if pathology itself or the surgical debridement and decompression causes regional instability.

Acute osteomyelitis compromised host

1. Stabilise the host's medical condition, including nutritional status
2. Aggressive debridement and decompression with periosteal rind disruption to encourage healing
3. Sensitivity and culture of infected foci
4. Persistent antibiotic therapy for 6–12 weeks, according to a culture sensitivity test
5. Regional skeletal stabilisation, if required.

Chronic osteomyelitis

Chronic infection present more than 1 month.

1. The host is always compromised, even if it is only due to the infectious process
2. For a comprehensive diagnosis, computed tomography scans, nuclear medicine scans and perfusion investigations can be conducted
3. Restore the host's health, paying special attention to their dietary circumstances
4. Wide bony sequestrectomy and decortication to reveal and retain normal bleeding bone as well as disruption of the affected periosteal rind, extensive layer by layer core out excision of the sinus tracts with extended culture and sensitivity of sequestrum
5. Consider drainage and irrigation if the condition is purulent
6. Antibiotic therapy for 3-6 months, potentially longer, through central line as needed. Duration is determined by Gram's stain and culture
7. Consider nonsteroidals against steroids
8. Use of plates and screws for regional bone stabilisation
9. Hyperbaric oxygen treatment before surgery 20–40 dives bid on 100% O_2 for 90 minutes at 2.5 ATA
10. Reconstruction is performed as needed. When immediate reconstruction is not preferred due to risk of infection, delayed reconstruction is performed based on the defect (refer Chapter 34).

ANTIBIOTIC THERAPY

1. The most frequent microorganisms associated with osteomyelitis are the *Streptococcus viridans*, *Peptostreptococcus*, *Eikenella corodens*, *Fusobacterium* sp. and *Actinomyces* sp. The 1st line of management should be the prompt diagnosis of the type of osteomyelitis by both clinical history and radiological examination. The treatment is based on the type of osteomyelitis
2. Recovery of the patient's clinical condition is the most important factor in determining the shift of the i.v. antibiotics to the oral antibiotics (PO)
3. The positive findings which denotes good response to antibiotic treatment are absence of fever, improvement in symptoms like malaise, tenderness, anorexia, night pain and reduction in C-reactive protein (CRP).
4. Slow clinical response indicates virulent or resistant organisms. In such cases, the i.v. antibiotic should be continued instead of shifting to oral therapy
5. If there is no clinical response within 48 h of medical management, the possibility of the presence of bone abscess should be suspected. Re-evaluation by additional CT or MRI and surgical management should be considered
6. The most frequently employed broad-spectrum antibiotics are included in Table 24.2. Utilised empiric antibiotics are arranged in order of choice. In the case of a penicillin allergy, the alternative to the 1st-choice treatment becomes the remaining option.

SURGICAL TREATMENT (Flowchart 24.5)

Antibiotic therapy is considered to be the primary form of treatment for acute osteomyelitis, as opposed to surgical treatment (minor debridement may be needed in some cases). On the other hand, surgical intervention is required in cases of chronic osteomyelitis that have resulted in bone necrosis or dead space. In addition to sequestrectomy, hyperbaric oxygen therapy and decortications are secondary measures. If the clinical symptoms do not improve, surgery is required. Surgical treatment is indicated in cases of TMJ involvement, bone or subperiosteal abscess, and failure to recover after 48 h of i.v. antibiotic therapy. Surgical treatment is not necessary in acute cases if antibiotics work. Chronic cases require surgery owing to bone alterations.

The following surgical procedures should be considered for the management of osteomyelitis:

- Trephination or fenestration
- Sequestrectomy
- Saucerisation

TABLE 24.2 Spectrum of Antibiotic Routine followed for Osteomyelitis

Broad Spectrum Antibiotics for Osteomyelitis		Dosage	Duration	Organism
1st choice	Aqueous Penicillin	2 million units i.v.	Every 4 h	*Streptococcus* sp.
	Oxacillin	1 g i.v.	Every 4 h	*S. aureus*, Methicillin-sensitive
	If patient is asymptomatic for 48–72 h, then switch to – Penicillin V or Penicillin V + dicloxacillin	500 mg Oral 500 mg + 250 mg Oral	Every 4 h for 2–4 weeks	Anaerobes
2nd choice	Clindamycin	600 mg i.v. 300–600 mg Oral	Every 6 h	Anaerobes, bacteroides, penicillinase secreting staph. cocci, streptococci
3rd choice	Cephalosporin a. Cefazolin b. Cephalexin	250–500 mg Oral 500 mg 500 mg	Every 6 h 8 h 6 h	Penicillinase secreting staph. cocci, *Escherichia coli*, Moderately against anaerobes
4th choice	Erythromycin	2 g i.v. Then, 500 mg Oral	Every 6 h Every 6 h	

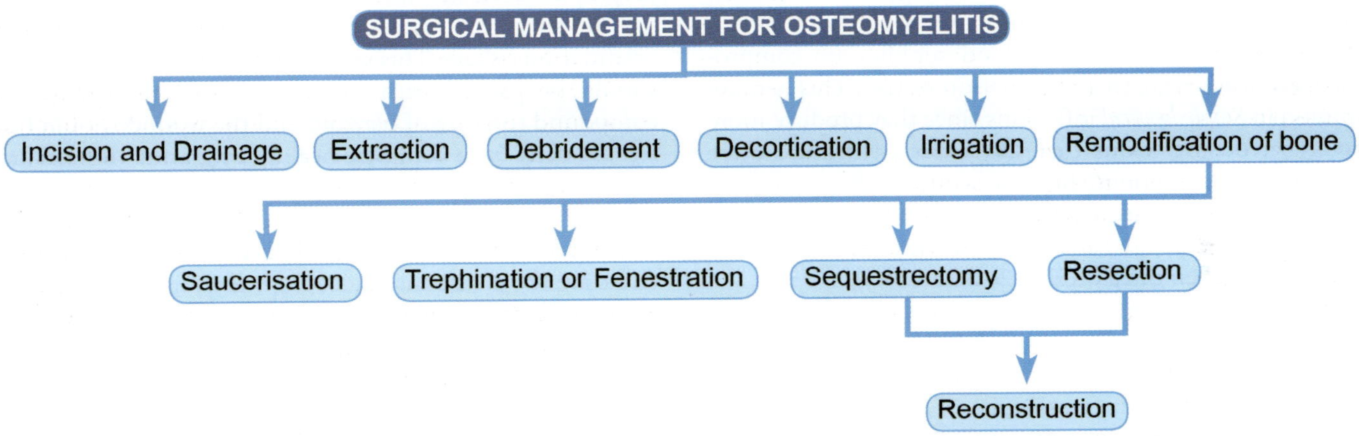

Flowchart 24.5 Surgical management for osteomyelitis.

- Decortication
- Resection.

The primary indication of surgical management is the presence of abscess within the bone (chronic). Lack of response to high dose parenteral antibiotic therapy is another important indication for the surgical management (acute). The reason for antibiotic therapy failure should be carefully analysed before proceeding to the surgical treatment. Re-examination of the culture sensitivity, antibiotic dose and identification of any other possible reason like bone or soft tissue abscess should be undertaken. If no possible reason can be correlated, then CT or MRI should be performed to locate the possible abscess. Incision and drainage is performed followed by irrigation.

IRRIGATION TECHNIQUES

In addition to utilising closed suction, it is important that irrigation tubes be inserted through their own distinct stab incisions.

Continuous or intermittent indwelling closed catheter irrigation: Following intraoral sequestrectomy and saucerisation or decortication, two small paediatric suction tubes, nasogastric feeding tubes, catheters or polythelene drain tubes, measuring 4 mm in diameter and 8 inches in length, are positioned against the bony bed through separate skin incisions at some distance and are then secured with sutures. One tube is attached to the low-pressure suction to allow drainage of pus and serum, and another one is kept patent to provide a route via which local antibiotics may be infused in very high concentrations. Both of these tubes are kept open so that the patient may get treatment.

It is recommended that on a daily basis, 1st saline irrigation and then antibiotic instillation be performed until negative culture results are achieved. It is also recommended to keep taking systemic antibiotics for at least 2 to 3 months after the last sign of infection has disappeared clinically.

TREPHINATION OR FENESTRATION

Trephination is the process of creating bony holes or windows in the overlying cortical bone that are adjacent to the infectious process. This allows for tissue approximation and decompression of the medullary compartment. Trephination can also be referred to as fenestration. When holes are drilled into the cortex and continued to the medulla, several surgical transcortical ports are created. These ports enable for vascular communication to take place between the periosteum and the medullary cavity.

SEQUESTRECTOMY

The process by which necrotic bone is separated from the living bone is called *sequestration* and the dead bone thus formed is called *sequestrum*. The resorption of living bone around the dead bone results in the formation of the sequestrum. When both endosteal and periosteal blood supplies are compromised, extensive sequestrum formation results. This is more common in *Staphylococcal* infections since they produce more potent necrotising toxins than *Streptococci*, which are more likely to cause resorption. The bone is often radiopaque since dead bone including sequestrum attracts calcium. Periosteal bone is usually deposited and an involucrum (new bone) may form to strengthen the jaw (Figs. 24.5 and 24.6).

Procedure

Using the preoperative radiograph, which shows the exact location of the sequestrum, the site of incision is decided. The approach may be either intraoral or extraoral. To expose entire sequestrum, intraoral incision is made over the alveolar ridge, but in many instances, entry can be gained by excising the fistulous tract. Following this, soft tissue is detached

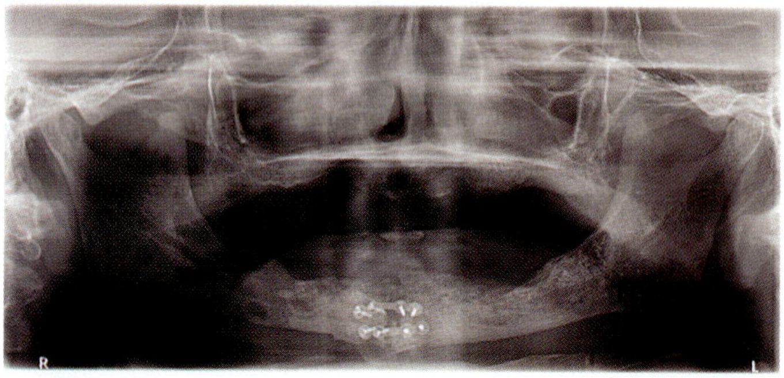

Figure 24.5 OPG showing osteomyelitis on the right side of the mandible.

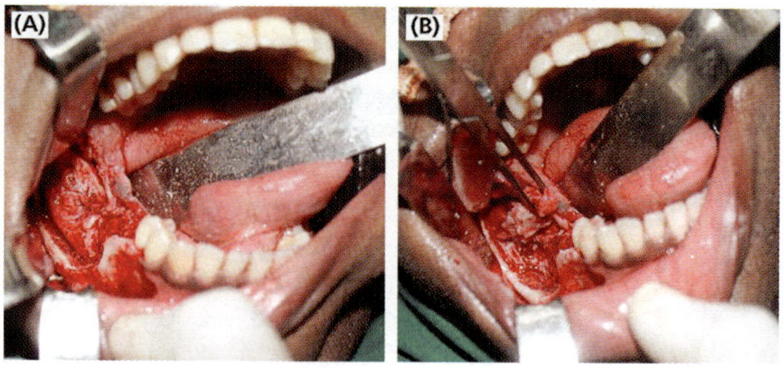

Figure 24.6 (**A** and **B**) Sequestrectomy.

from the bone by blunt dissection and the sequestrum is lifted and removed. In case of partial attachment of the sequestrum to the bone beneath, it is separated by using an air drill or sharp osteotome. Rongeurs are used to remove any remaining necrotic bone. If the sequestrum is encased by involucrum, a window must be cut to allow it to be taken out.

This is also done using an air drill or a sharp curette. The border of the necrotic bone is identified by the initiation of bleeding during drilling. The excision of bone should be made at least 1.5 cm in front of or behind the area of the radiographic bone necrosis.

The cavity is thus exposed and almost always contains granulation tissues. This should not be disturbed. The defect should be packed with iodoform gauze, moistened with compound tincture of benzoin and the wound should be irrigated daily until complete healing by granulation occurs.

SAUCERISATION

When saucerisation is performed in combination with sequestrectomy, the incision is made longer than usual to expose the entire infected portion of the bone and extended through the periosteum. Whenever possible the sinus tract should be included. The periosteum is stripped off the part of the cortex, which is to be removed. The walls of the bone overhanging the cavity resulting from the removal of the sequestrum are chipped off with the use of rongeurs or sharp osteotomes. This exposes extension of the disease. The additional sequestrum and granulation tissue present should be cleaned out and more of the cortex should be removed if necessary to saucerise the cavity completely, so that the overlying tissue can be pressed into it to eliminate the dead space. The bone is made smooth with the help of bone files or round burs. The wound is packed tightly with gauze covered with antibiotic ointment and the flap is loosely sutured over it. The packing is removed after 3–7 days and replaced several times until the exposed raw surface of the bone is epithelialised. There is minimal or no risk of fracture of jaws with this type of procedure. In case complete primary suture is not feasible because the infected bone cannot be removed completely or because there is active suppuration, the wound may be open, packed loosely with gauze and closed later. This procedure is done mainly in the mandible. Saucerisation of the maxilla is rarely required (Fig. 24.7).

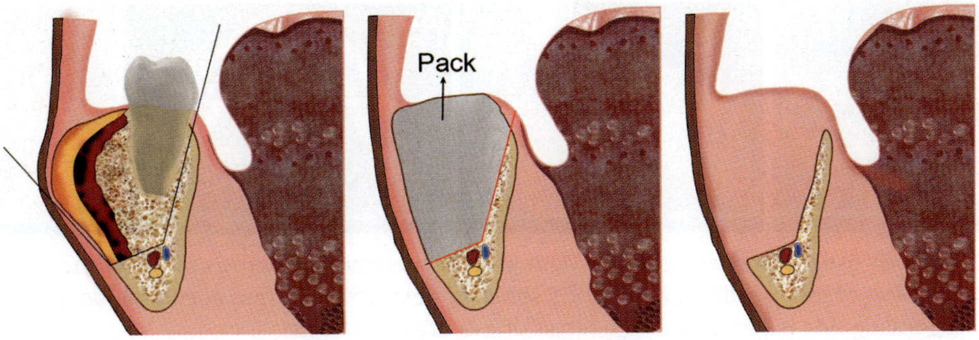

Figure 24.7 Saucerisation.

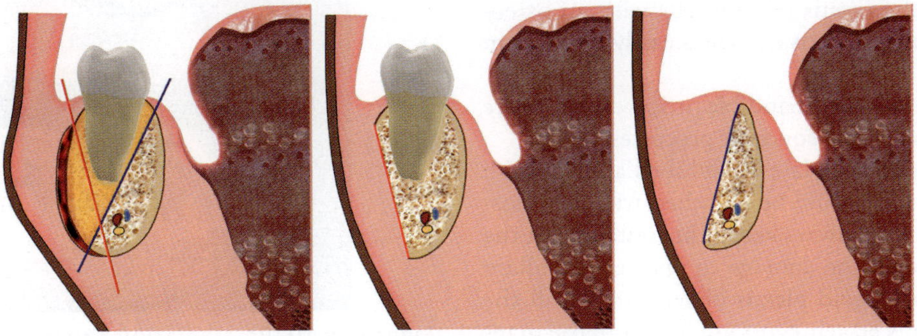

Figure 24.8 Decortication.

DECORTICATION

1st introduced in 1917 by Mowlem. Decortication involves removal of the chronically infected cortex; usually the buccal and the inferior border are removed 1 to 2 cm beyond the affected area. It can be used as initial treatment of primary or secondary chronic osteomyelitis or more commonly when initial conservative treatment has failed (Fig. 24.8).

Procedure

1. Full thickness mucoperiosteal flap is reflected buccally and extended to the inferior border
2. Involved teeth are removed
3. The buccal cortex and inferior borders are removed until bleeding bone is encountered
4. Primary closure is achieved and pressure dressing is applied to provide better support of the bone bed with its related vascular soft tissue. Drain or antibiotics are used *in situ*.

In case of excessive debridement, adequate stabilisation and reconstruction to support the remaining bone is necessary.

Complications

1. Undue bleeding which may occur in the bone
2. Injury to the mandibular nerve results in anaesthesia of the lip
3. Fracture of the weakened bone.

Postoperative treatment

Antibiotic treatment should be continued for 10 days to 2 weeks postoperatively or longer if signs of infection persist. Intravenous infusion of distilled water with 5%–10% glucose is required to counteract dehydration. Diet should be rich in protein and vitamins and complete bed rest is essential.

RESECTION

Indications for resection

Excision of a part of the mandible is seldom necessary. Most patients with osteomyelitis can be cured by antibiotic treatment combined with sequestrectomy and saucerisation. However, if the patient has constant recurrences for many years or months and is suffering from disability and pain, the disease may have to be treated by resection. After resection is done, continuity of the mandible can be restored with the help of bone grafts or other reconstruction techniques.

Procedure

The patient is properly prepared to increase his/her general resistance to infection at an optimal level. Antibiotic therapy is started 24 h before surgery. IMF is done, reconstruction plate contoured and screws drilled before resection in order to maintain preoperative occlusion.

Mandibular resection can either be partial or total. *Partial resection* involves preservation of the condylar and coronoid

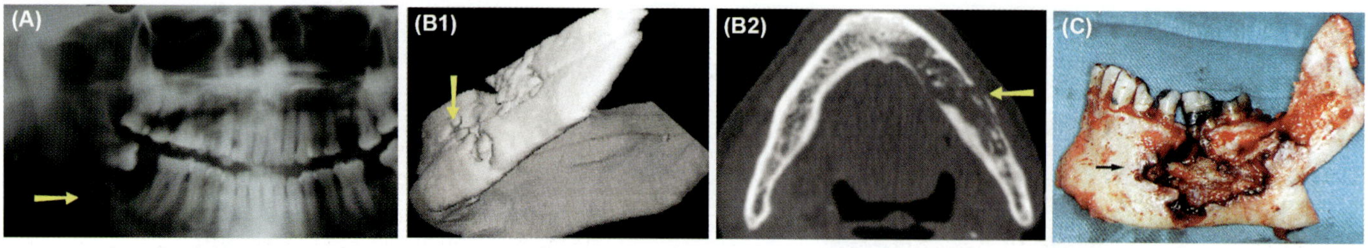

Figure 24.9 (**A**) OPG showing osteoradionecrosis of the right jaw. (**B1**) Osteoradionecrosis of the left mandible in an 80-year-old man, CT showing destruction of left mandible, (**B2**) 3D CT showing destruction of buccal cortical bone. (**C**) Hemisection of the mandible of the corresponding side is carried out as a result of osteoradionecrosis.

processes. Condylar and coronoid processes may be preserved by sectioning the ramus horizontally with an osteotome. Segment of mandible thus excised is easily lifted from its soft tissue bed.

Total disarticulation of the mandible involves complete stripping of the coronoid and condylar processes.

Therefore, insertions of the lateral and medial pterygoid, temporalis and masseter should be detached with a periosteal elevator taking care to always keep it in contact with the underlying bone to avoid the damage to internal maxillary artery and vein and pterygoid plexus of veins. After all the muscle and ligamentous attachments are free from the mandible, it may be removed by grasping it with a large bone-holding forceps and literally rolling it out of the glenoid fossa. The wound is closed in layers to eliminate the dead space. A rubber drain may be placed if any infection or haematoma formation is suspected. A temporary condyle prosthesis or an intraoral splint is used to reduce the postoperative scar contracture. However, usage of such appliances is discouraged as these may cause the mucosal closure to take place under tension, leading to dehiscence of the wound. When the anterior part of the jaw is to be removed, the insertion of the geniohyoid and genioglossus muscles have to be stripped, which results in falling back of the tongue and interference with breathing. A silk suture placed through the anterior aspect of the tongue in such cases pulls the tongue forward and prevents any difficulty with breathing. Prophylactic tracheotomies should be considered if the airway is severely compromised.

OSTEORADIONECROSIS

Osteonecrosis is a term derived from the Greek words *osteon* = *bone, nekros* = *dead, osis* = *condition*, meaning the destruction and death of bone tissue, such as from ischaemia, infection, malignant neoplastic disease or trauma.

In the maxillofacial bones, osteonecrosis is common and significant because of two main sources:

- Radiation, that is osteoradionecrosis (ORN)
- Bisphosphonate-related osteonecrosis of the jaw (BRONJ), that is osteochemonecrosis.

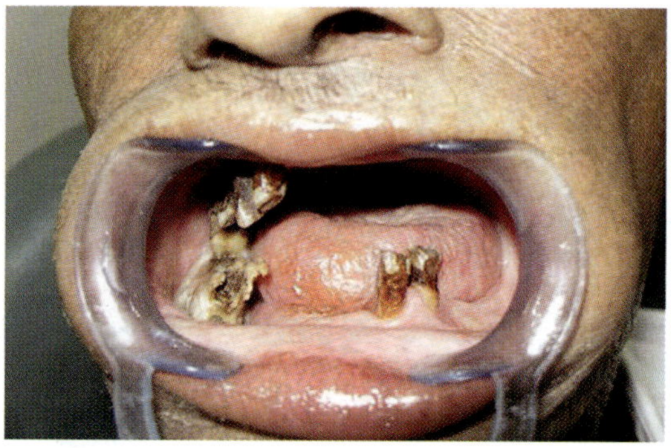

Figure 24.10 Postradiation exposed necrotic bone in right mandible.

Osteoradionecrosis or postradiation osteonecrosis

It was 1st described by Regaud in 1920. ORN is an exposure of a nonviable, nonhealing, nonseptic lesion in the irradiated bone, which fails to heal without intervention. It is a radiation-induced wound healing defect (Figs. 24.9 and 24.10).

Definition:

Exposed irradiated bone that has failed to heal over a period of 3 months in absence of local tumours (Harris, 1992). It may be chronic or progressive.

In the past, the radiation therapist used orthovoltage therapy and there was a high incidence of ORN. However, the modern radiation therapists use megavoltage, which is felt to be less harmful to the bones and soft tissues.

Aetiology:

Doses above 50 Gy usually are required to cause this irreversible damage. Dental extraction and denture trauma after radiation therapy.

Types of ORN:

1. Spontaneous ORN (39%)—degradative function exceeds new bone production
2. Trauma-induced ORN (61%)—reparative capacity of bone is insufficient to overcome an insult

Bone injury can occur through direct trauma:

1. Tooth extraction (84%)
2. Related cancer surgery or biopsy (12%)

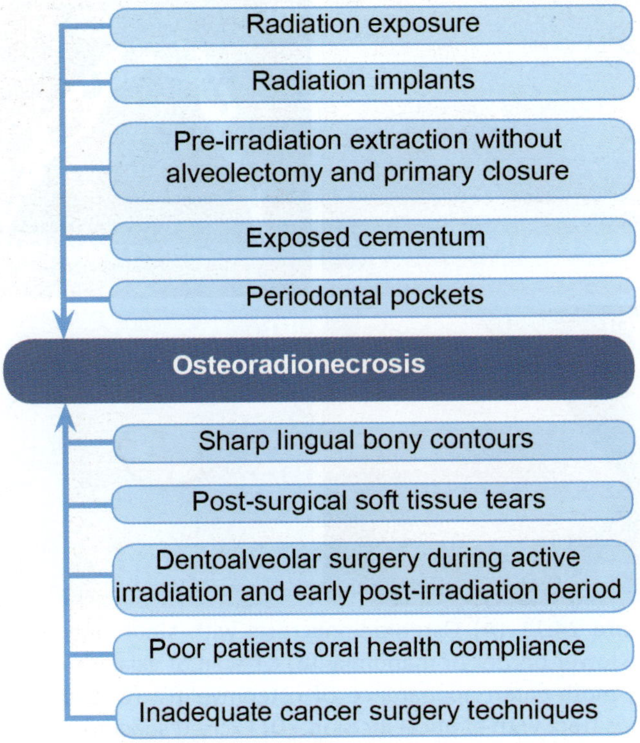

Flowchart 24.6 Risk factors of osteoradionecrosis.

3. Denture irritation (1%)
4. By exposure of the oral cavity to the environment secondary to overlying soft tissue necrosis.

RISK FACTORS (Flowchart 24.6)

The risk of developing ORN depends on the following:

1. Primary site
2. *T stage* of the malignancy
3. **Proximity of the tumour to bone**—bone is 1.8 times as dense as soft tissue and thereby absorbs a proportionately larger dose of incident radiation than does soft tissue.
4. **Dentition**—dentate patients have 2.6-fold higher risk
5. **Type of treatment** (external beam radiotherapy, brachytherapy, surgery and chemotherapy)
6. **Time of radiation dose delivery:** Radiotherapy results in continuous damage to the tissues at both the cellular and humoral levels. If the stipulated dose is given in a rapid phase, the recovery of remaining normal viable cells is prevented thus causing more loss of normal cells than anticipated. There are different schemes of fractionated delivery of irradiation which are aimed at reducing the complications of radiotherapy
7. **Radiotherapy dose:** Patients who receive a total of 80 Gy have 2.9-fold higher risk of developing osteomyelitis
8. **Mode of delivery, location and volume of irradiated tissue:** The conventional external beam irradiation causes more complications due to exposure of the lesion as a whole, especially areas of less blood supply such as the posterior part or surgically manipulated parts are at risk of ORN. This is overcome by more localised delivery such as brachytherapy. In brachytherapy, the delivery of radiation is localised, thus limiting the radiation damage to adjacent tissues
9. **Status of oral hygiene—inadequate oral hygiene:** The cell damaged during irradiation is not compensated by cell multiplication over time, resulting in mucositis and xerostomia. This is accelerated further with poor oral hygiene, ill-fitting tissue-borne prosthesis leading to odontogenic and periodontal infections which in turn lead to osteoradionecrosis
10. **Surgery:** The chances of developing ORN increases with jaw surgery after radiotherapy. This is due to the reduction in blood supply to the tissues. The potential risk of ORN in jaw surgery prior to radiotherapy has also been suggested. This may be due to reduction in periosteal blood supply in a marginal mandibular resection, unstable fixation of the mandibular split osteotomy leading to malunion or nonunion, and inadequate tissue coverage of the bone after resection of a tumour

    External radiotherapy has shown more detrimental effects than brachytherapy. The risk of developing ORN is decreased if hyperfractionation techniques and intensity-modulated radiotherapy (IMRT) are used. The prevalence of ORN was 20.1% and 6.6% in conventional fractionation and hyperfractionation groups, respectively. In studies using IMRT, researchers found that postradiation osteonecrosis (PRON) developed in up to 0.01% of patients

    Risk factors for developing ORN include old age, poor nutritional status of the patient and prolonged tobacco or alcohol abuse.

PATHOGENESIS

ORN was 1st described by Marx in 1983 as hypovascularity, hypocellularity and local tissue hypoxia.

MARX'S THEORY: THREE 'H' CONCEPT—HYPOCELLULARITY, HYPOXIA AND HYPOVASCULARITY

- Following radiotherapy, hyperaemia, inflammation and endarteritis occur in the mandible, periosteum and the related soft tissues. This eventually results in thrombosis, cellular death, progressive hypovascularity and fibrosis
- The irradiated block becomes less cellular and lacks fibroblasts, osteoblasts and undifferentiated osteocompetent cells
- The irradiated tissues become hypovascular, hypocellular and hypoxic. This is mainly due to the damage of DNA, RNA and other cellular units by the free radicals released from water molecules
- The free radicals such as hydrogen ions and hydroxyl ions react with the nucleotide or amino acid sequences resulting in cell death, or total reversible repair or repairs with some impaired function

- Mandible is more prone to ORN (it occurs in 5%–15% of cases) than maxilla. This is because the mandible is supplied mainly by the inferior alveolar artery, whereas the maxilla is supplied by the anterior, middle and posterior superior alveolar arteries and collateral blood vessels.

Marx proposed three types of osteoradionecrosis

Type I

ORN that is seen soon after radiotherapy due to devascularisation resulting from combined side effect of surgery and radiation.

Type II

ORN that occurs many years after radiotherapy following a known traumatic episode. These results from vascular endarteritis of nutrient vessels of the jaw bone combined with poor wound healing of surrounding soft tissues.

Type III

ORN occurring between 6 months and 3 years post radiotherapy with no specific preceding traumatic episode.

CLINICAL FINDINGS

Mandible is commonly affected than maxilla due to microanatomy and less vasculature.

Posterior mandible is more commonly affected than the anterior portion because of radiation treatment for tumours in this region.

The patient complains mainly of pain, bad breath and food lodgement in the affected area. On examination, the bone is exposed and the associated soft tissues are ulcerated and necrosed. Additional findings such as intraoral or extraoral fistula, mandibular discontinuity, or evidence of secondary local or systemic infection may also be present.

Loss of mucosal covering and exposed bone are hallmarks of ORN.

Why mandible is at an increased risk?

Generally, a bone—with more tenuous blood supply and more mechanical stress—more susceptible to the development of ORN.

The craniofacial skeleton receives its blood supply in three distinct manners:

Vessels that enter the bone via direct muscular attachments, periosteal perforators and intramedullary vessels.

In a study by Bras et al., radiation-induced obliteration of the inferior alveolar artery was consistently found in ORN of the mandible and was felt to be a dominant factor in the onset of the disease.

TREATMENT

Treatment of ORN of the mandible is aimed at:

1. Removal of the necrotic bone and soft tissue (Fig. 24.11)
2. Enhancement of vascularity of the remaining radiation-damaged tissues (Flowchart 24.7).

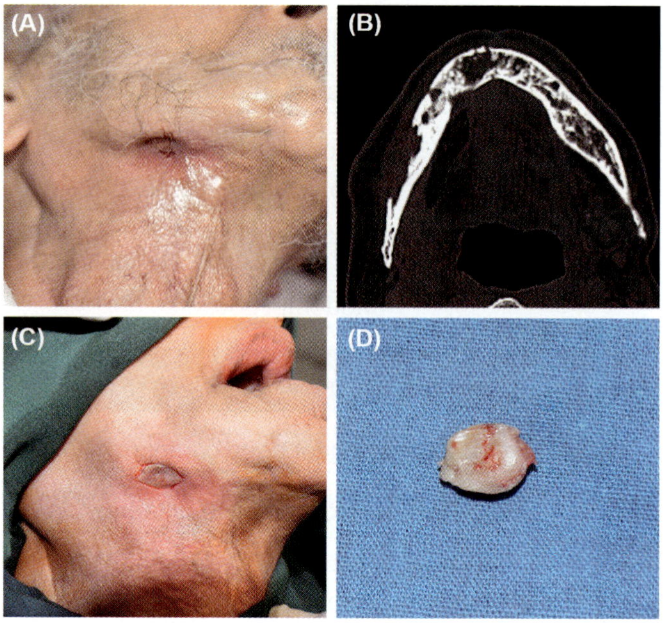

Figure 24.11 (**A**) Osteoradionecrosis with sinus opening on the lower border of mandible. (**B**) CT scan of axial view showing moth-eaten appearance of osteomyelitis. (**C**) Excision of sinus tract with eliptical incision. (**D**) Excised specimen.

Marx protocol

- **Stage I**—a total of 30 hyperbaric oxygen exposures at 2.4 atmospheres absolute pressure (ATA) for 90 min in a multiplace chamber or 2.0 ATA for 120 min in a monoplace chamber is needed. The wound is examined for signs of improvement such as mucosal cover, resorption of nonviable bone, or a decrease in the size of the exposure. Patients with improvement are labelled stage I responders and additional dives up to 60 is given until full mucosal covering is achieved. The stage I nonresponders are treated by stage II protocol.
- **Stage II**—undergo a transoral debridement/sequestrectomy which attempts at primary mucosal closure. For postoperative healing, an additional 10 sessions of hyperbaric oxygen exposure is given. If there is wound dehiscence with bone exposure, stage III protocol is adhered. Patients excluded from entering stage I because of fistula formation, fracture, or inferior border of the mandible osteolysis undergo initial hyperbaric oxygen therapy consisting of 30 dives.
- **Stage III**—undergo mandibular resection of the necrotic segment until the bone margins yield viable bone, that is till bleeding is encountered. In those with orocutaneous fistula, the involved skin and fistulous tract are excised followed by closure.

  Stabilisation of the segments of the mandible is done with an external fixator or maxillomandibular fixation, and the patient undergoes additional hyperbaric oxygen therapy postoperatively.

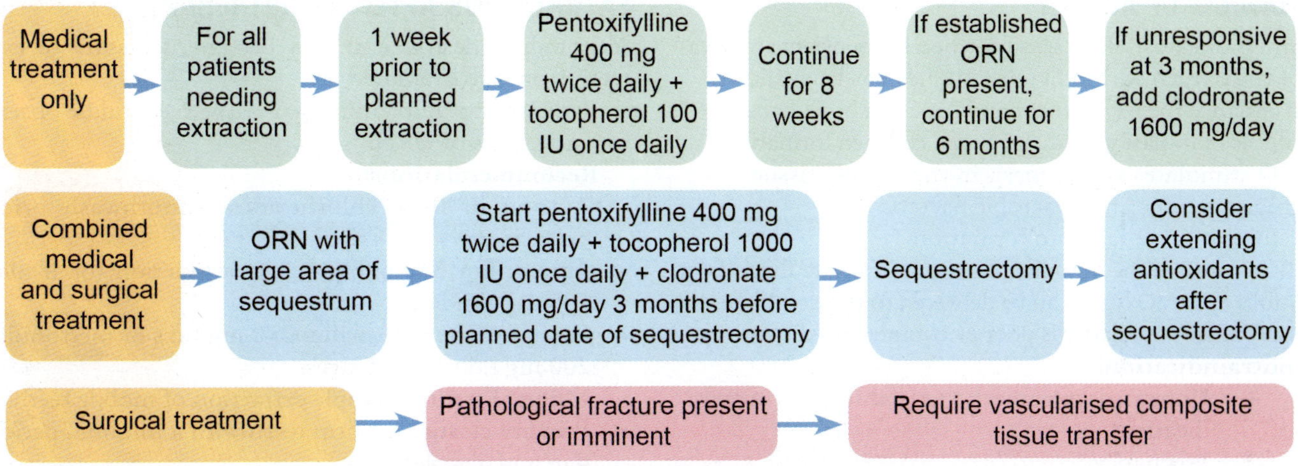

Flowchart 24.7 Treatment of osteoradionecrosis.

- **Stage III R:** Marx proposes that the reconstructive surgery should be done 10 weeks after resection thus enabling the graft to be placed, into a sufficiently vascular and cellular bed with intact mucosa. Before reconstruction, an additional 20 dives were planned with 10 dives postoperatively. Mostly, autogenous particulate bone and marrow within a custom-made stainless steel metal crib or autogenous particulate bone and marrow within a freeze-dried allogenic bone framework is used for reconstruction of mandible in such patients.

Management (Fig. 24.9):
Initial treatment—control of infection, if present.
Gentle irrigation of the soft tissue margins—removes debris and reduces inflammation.
Supportive treatment with fluids and a liquid or semi-liquid diet high in proteins and vitamins.
Pain may be controlled with:

- Narcotic analgesics
- Bupivacaine
- Alcohol nerve blocks
- Nerve avulsion
- Rhizotomy

Hyperbaric oxygen therapy
Pentoxifylline
Clodronate
Antioxidant (vitamin E).

HYPERBARIC OXYGEN THERAPY (FIG. 24.12)

Hyperbaric oxygen (HBO) therapy for radiation-damaged tissue was introduced in 1973 by Greenwood, Gilchrist and Mainous.

Since there is a decrease in vascularity and cellularity of both the hard and soft tissues following irradiation of the bone, the hypoxic compromised tissues when challenged by a traumatic episode fail to heal. Delayed fibroblastic activity in neocollagen formation results in chronic nonhealing wound. These wounds commonly get infected secondarily. The goal of treating ORN is to overcome the hypoxia and increase vascularity of tissues. In order to increase tissue oxygenation, the patient is subjected to increased oxygen concentration and pressure. HBO therapy consists of **100% oxygen administered at more than one absolute atmospheric pressure**. This 100% oxygen is a means of increasing the oxygen dissolved in plasma and tissues that in turn induces angiogenesis in the compromised tissues.

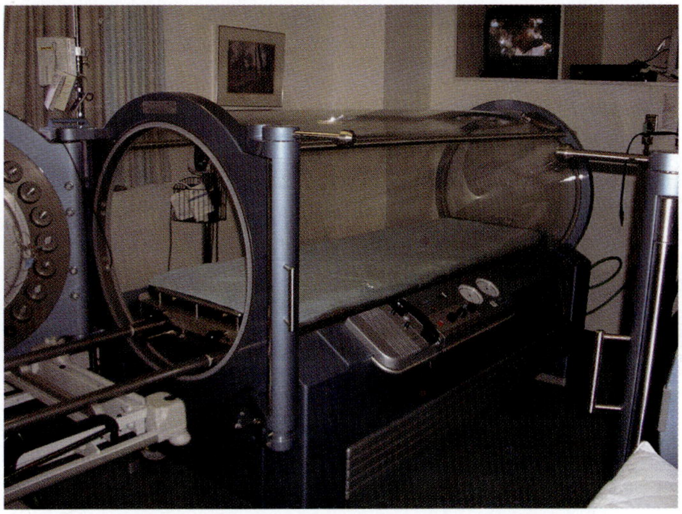

Figure 24.12 Hyperbaric oxygen chamber.

METHODS OF DELIVERY

HBO therapy is administered in a chamber called the hyperbaric chamber which may be **monoplace (single patient) or multiplace (multiple patients)**. Each session ranges from 90 to 120 min where patient breathes 100% oxygen at 2 to 2.4 ATA. Each session is termed a dive. A total of 20–30 dives spanning 5 days a week is planned preoperatively.

MECHANISM OF ACTION

The timeframe post HBO session when there exists an elevation of the oxygen within hypoxic tissues has been shown:

- To enhance the recruitment and function of leukocytes
- Induces fibroblast growth, increased collagen formation
- HBO stimulates angiogenesis in the healing tissue
- Inhibits aerobic and anaerobic bacteria
- To inhibit bacterial toxin formation
- HBO increases the amount of oxygen in tissue fluids by a 10-fold factor. Oxygen can be delivered to the depths of the tissue where vascularity is poor or compromised

Contraindication:

1. Untreated pneumothorax—(absolute contraindication)
2. Pregnancy
3. Emphysema
4. Upper respiratory tract infection
5. Uncontrollable fever
6. Optic neuritis
7. Ear problems.

PENTOXIFYLLINE AND VITAMIN E

Pentoxifylline lowers blood viscosity, increases tissue oxygen level, reduces fibroblast proliferation and increases collagenase activity; it is used to treat intermittent claudication.

Vitamin E is an antioxidant. These drugs have been used to treat advanced cases of ORN, with promising results. These drugs are believed to promote healing (Refer Chapter 57).

Recent guidelines:

Prevention of ORN:

- Every patient should have a dental assessment prior to radiotherapy for the best outcome following cancer treatment
- Extraction of all teeth before radiotherapy has been recommended
- Removal of all teeth with poor prognosis, generally considered less than 5 years is recommended
- Extractions are planned with the view to avoiding extractions in the future
- Removal of all mandibular molars in fields over 60 Gray, unless the patient has excellent oral hygiene.

PREVENTIVE REGIME

- If the mouth becomes too sore during radiotherapy, a soft brush may be necessary for a time, supplemented with chlorhexidine mouth wash, which may be diluted with an equal volume of water if too sore on the mucosa
- In addition, a fluoride regime, either high fluoride toothpaste, fluoride gel in splints for 10 min each day or alcohol-free fluoride mouth rinse
- Saliva substitutes should be pH neutral
- Dentures should be regularly checked for pressure areas and adjusted, but it may be preferable to avoid dentures.

EXTRACTIONS AFTER RADIOTHERAPY

Although undesirable, it may become necessary to extract teeth from the irradiated jaw.

Patients should be informed of the risk and be observant for early signs of ORN.

Recommendations:

- A total of 0.2% chlorhexidine mouthwash prior to extractions.
- Amoxicillin 3 g orally 1 h preextraction (or if allergic 600 mg clindamycin).
- Postoperative amoxicillin 250 mg t.d.s or metronidazole 200 mg t.d.s for 3–5 days.
- Minimal trauma, simple extraction of mobile teeth.
- Primary closure for firm teeth with a minimal periosteal flap and alveolectomy.
- An experienced operator.
- Possibly preoperative HBO for mandibular molars in areas of high radiation.
- Review after 5 days, weekly review until healing is complete.

OSTEOCHEMONECROSIS (OCN) - MEDICATIONS ASSOCIATED OSTEONECROSIS OF JAWS

Osteochemonecrosis (OCN) can be defined as necrosis of bone resulting from oncologic chemotherapy or medications. The drugs implicated can be VEGF inhibitors, bisphosphonates, RANKL antibodies, tyrosine kinase inhibitors, cathepsin K inhibitors, or immune modulators such as sirolimus.

Terminologies

- Bisphosphonate osteonecrosis (BON)
- Bisphosphonate associated osteonecrosis of the jaws (BONJ)
- Bisphosphonate related osteonecrosis of the jaws (BRONJ)
- Antiresorptive osteonecrosis of the jaw (ARONJ)
- Medication related osteonecrosis of the jaw (MRONJ)

The term **BRONJ** was given by American Association of Oral and Maxillofacial Surgeons (AAOMS) and was widely accepted till 2014. BRONJ is a condition where necrosis of the jaw bone occurs in patients under treatment with bisphosphonates. In 2014, AAOMS changed the nomenclature from BRONJ to MRONJ, which is "medication-related osteonecrosis of the jaw" to accommodate the growing number of osteonecrosis cases associated with other antiresorptive and antiangiogenic therapies.

MRONJ DRUGS

1. Antiresorptive (bold format):
   a. Bisphosphonates (BPs):
      - Aminobisphosphonates
      - Nonaminobisphosphonates
   b. Receptor activator of nuclear factor kappa-B ligand (RANKL) inhibitors:
      - Denosumab

2. Antiangiogenic (bold format):
   a. Bevacizumab
   b. Tyrosine kinase inhibitor (sunitinib, sorafenib)
   c. mTOR inhibitor (sirolimus).

MRONJ is defined by SICMF (Italian Society for Maxillofacial Surgery) and SIPMO (Italian Society of Oral Pathology and Medicine) as "A severe adverse drug reaction, consisting of progressive bone destruction and death of bone in the maxillofacial region of patients exposed to the treatment with nitrogen-containing BPs, in the absence of a previous radiation treatment". Clinically, it is characterized by the following manifestations:

- The presence of exposed bone in the maxillofacial region that has not healing for more than 8 weeks
- History of ongoing or antecedent treatment with an antiresorptive or antiangiogenic drugs
- There is no documented history of radiation exposure to the head and neck region.

CLINICAL SIGNS AND SYMPTOMS OF OCN

1. None/ asymptomatic
2. Pain
3. Soft tissue infection that causes inflammation, ulceration, and suppuration
4. Intra and/or extraoral formation of sinus tracts and fistulas
5. Paresthesia of the associated nerve
6. Pathological Fracture of jaw
7. Chronic maxillary sinusitis
8. In 2006, Ruggiero et al. designed the **MRONJ staging system** and subsequently updated by AAOMS in 2014. It facilitates the creation of treatment guidelines for MRONJ patients (Table 24.3).

TABLE 24. 3 MRONJ Staging and Treatment Strategies

Stages	Clinical findings	Treatment
At risk category	No apparent necrotic bone in patients	No treatment. Patient education about the possible signs and symptoms of the condition and regular dental follow-up.
Stage 0	• Patients with no clinical evidence of necrotic bone *Non-specific signs and symptoms include,* • Odontalgia without any odontogenic cause • Dull, aching bone pain in the jaw • Loosening of teeth • Swelling (intra or extra oral) *Radiographically,* • Alveolar bone loss • Trabecular pattern sclerotic bone without any new bone in extraction socket • Thickening of lamina dura with decrease in periodontal ligament space	Symptomatic treatment to control pain and infections (antiseptic, analgesic, antibiotic, and antiphlogistic therapy) Low-level laser therapy
Stage 1	• Exposed and necrotic bone or fistula that probes to the bone • Patients are asymptomatic with no evidence of infection • Radiographic findings as mentioned in stage 0, but localised to the alveolar bone region	Chlorhexidine mouthwash 0.12% and regular follow-up appointments.
Stage 2	• Exposed and necrotic bone, or fistula that probes to the bone, with evidence of infection • Patients are symptomatic (pain, erythema of the exposed bone, with or without discharge) • Radiographic findings as mentioned in stage 0, and localised to the alveolar bone region	Antibiotic regimen with an antimicrobial mouthwash Surgical debridement
Stage 3	• Exposed and necrotic bone extending beyond the region of alveolar bone • Pathologic fracture, extraoral fistula, oro-antral communication • Osteolysis extending to the sinus floor or inferior border of the mandible	Surgical management (marginal to segmental resection) is indicated in combination with an antibiotic regimen

Blood Test

The amount of octapeptide fragment is measured by the C-terminal telopeptide (CTX) value, which is released during osteoclastic bone resorption.

- CTX < 100 pg/ml indicates high risk
- CTX 100 to 150 pg/ml indicates moderate risk
- CTX > 150 pg/ml indicates minimal or no risk.

RADIOGRAPHIC APPEARANCE OF MRONJ

Although imaging modalities (CT Scan, OPG) are useful for assessing the area involved and identifying the extent of bone and soft tissue involvement, they cannot provide any definitive differentiation of osteonecrosis of the jaw.

The radiographic manifestations include altered bone morphology, increase in bone density, periosteal bone formation, or formation of sequestrum. The severity and extent of a lesion can be assessed by the presence of diffuse osteosclerosis, degenerated cortical bone, bone resorption, periosteal reaction, and bone fistulas.

In the early stages, it manifests as diffuse sclerotic bone, ill-defined radiolucency, or a mix of a radiopaque and radiolucent lesion in addition to a non-healing extraction socket.

In advanced stages, the MRONJ can resemble chronic osteomyelitis, resulting in formation of sequestrum, thickening of lamina dura, and pathological fractures.

PATHOGENESIS OF MRONJ

Antiresorptive drugs (bisphosphonate and denosumab).

Bisphosphonates are used in the treatment of patients with osteoporosis, metastatic bone cancers, multiple myeloma, Paget disease, osteosclerosis, and fibrous dysplasia. They act by directly inhibiting the osteoclastic activity and accumulating the bone minerals. As a consequence of this, bone resorption is unable to take place, which allows the older bone to persist beyond its lifespan. The lack of maintenance of its capillary networks ultimately results in avascular necrosis of the jaw. Bisphosphonates can also lead to necrosis of the soft tissues and bone cells. Alterations in wound healing and delay in the epithelial closure of a mucosal opening in the mouth, causes chronic infection and bone necrosis. Various bisphosphonates used are alendronate, pamidronate, zoledronate, ibandronate, etc.

Antiangiogenic drugs (bevacizumab or sunitinib).

These drugs are used in the treatment of cancer patients to prevent metastasis through the blood and lymph nodes. These medications obstruct the development of new blood vessels, leading to ischemia and ultimately, osteonecrosis.

RISK FACTORS THAT CONTRIBUTE TO MRONJ FORMATION

A. **Local risk factor**
   - Pre-existing dental or periodontal infection, Micro-trauma, Inflammatory diseases, removable prosthesis, implant placement

B. **Systemic factors**
   - Medical illness (Diabetes, anemia, hypocalcemia, rheumatoid arthritis, immunosuppression, renal dialysis)
   - Age, sex
   - Obesity, Alcohol
   - Genetic predisposition: polymorphism in farnesyl pyrophosphate synthase or CYP2C8 coding for a cytochrome P450 enzyme

C. **Type of medications (bisphosphonate and denosumab)**
   - Concomitant medications: corticosteroids and H2 blocking drugs, erythropoietin and cyclophosphamide therapy
   - Total amount of drug administered
   - Length of therapy
   - Way of administration

HISTOPATHOLOGY

Resected necrotic bone from MRONJ patients does not demonstrate any unique features of the disease. The most frequently found microorganisms in the exposed bone sites are *Actinomyces*, *Eikenella*, *Veillonella*, and *Moraxella* species - penicillin-sensitive organisms.

MANAGEMENT OF MRONJ

Each patient will have a unique treatment plan developed based on their specific condition's stage and symptoms.

- Conservative treatment
- Surgical debridement
- Resection of the lesions
- Adjunctive treatments such as oxygen therapy
- Mesenchymal cell therapy to regenerate the damaged bone

CONSERVATIVE MANAGEMENT

Conservative management is indicated for patient's at-risk and early asymptomatic stages. Conservative treatment includes antibiotic therapy, maintenance of good oral hygiene, periodic dental visits, and chlorhexidine mouthwash. A combination of conservative treatment with adjunctive treatments such as hyperbaric oxygen, ozone therapy, or low-intensity laser therapy can be preferred for higher success rate (Box 24.1)

SURGICAL MANAGEMENT

MRONJ Stages II and III often requires surgical intervention. The surgical approach involves debridement of the superficial necrotic bone (sequestrectomy) and antibiotics and antiseptic mouth rinses. Surgical procedures can sometimes be combined with alternative treatments such as ozone therapy and leukocyte-platelet rich fibrin (L-PRF). When conservative debridement and other less invasive treatments have failed, Segmental resection may be necessary. Debridement and marginal resection is characterized by the removal of all necrotic material, leaving only healthy bone at the inferior border

BOX 24.1 Conservative management of MRONJ

Medical Management

1. Antimicrobials
   - Topical antimicrobials
   - Oral antimicrobials
   - Intravenous antimicrobials
2. Pentoxifylline and vitamin E therapy
3. Teriparatide
4. Hyperbaric oxygen therapy

Topical Antimicrobials

Patients with MRONJ have exhibited improvement while using the chlorhexidine gluconate 0.12%, which is a topical bactericidal and bacteriostatic agent. The use of topical antimicrobials disrupts the oral flora, and biofilms, that contributes to the disease process. Chlorhexidine is suggested as a standalone therapy for stage 1 disease and in combination with other medical and surgical treatments for more advanced stages.

Oral Antimicrobials

The mainstay in the management of MRONJ are oral antimicrobials. Infections typically involve are polymicrobial, such as Actinobacteria, Fusobacteria and Bacteroides. Since penicillin is effective against these organisms, it remains the first choice of antibiotic. Antibiotics that can be used as alternative to penicillin are clindamycin, fluoroquinolones and/or metronidazole.

For stage 1 disease, a 2-week course is prescribed and for more severe cases a 4–6-week course of antibiotic is recommended.

Intravenous Antimicrobials

When oral antibiotics no longer work against these pathogenic organisms, Intravenous antimicrobials are effective, as they have greater tissue penetration. Long-term i.v. antibiotic treatment (6-week) is recommended.

Pentoxifylline and Vitamin E

The osteoradionecrosis and MRONJ of jaw are effectively treated by combination of pentoxifylline and vitamin E. A xanthine derivative, pentoxifylline (Trental), is largely used to treat the vascular diseases. Vitamin E acts as a scavenger of free radicals that can cause cellular injury and reduce tissue fibrosis and inflammation.

Dose: Pentoxifylline (400 mg sustained release twice daily) and vitamin E (1000 IU daily) for 36 months.

Teriparatide

Teriparatide (Forteo) is primarily used in the treatment of osteoporosis. It stimulates new bone formation and activate osteoclasts. Dose: 20 mcg SC daily for up to 2 years.

Hyperbaric Oxygen Therapy

It can be used for the management of ORN and MRONJ. It provides greater oxygen to the tissues with impaired vascularisation.

of mandible. The term "segmental resection" describes an en bloc removal of affected bone, including the inferior border of the mandible, leaving a defect in the bone's continuity.

The following surgical principles should be applied for the removal of necrotic bone:

- A full-thickness mucoperiosteal flap should be adequate to reveal the entire area of exposed bone and beyond the disease-free margin
- Resection of the affected bone to achieve healthy, bleeding bone
- Sharp edges and spicules should be smoothed
- Primary soft tissue closure to facilitate tension-free mucosal healing
- Postoperative antibiotic therapy

ADJUVANT TREATMENT OPTIONS

Adjuvant treatments for MRONJ includes laser-assisted surgical debridement/ low-level laser therapy and the application of ozone oil or platelet-rich plasma/ platelet-derived growth factor to the surgical wound.

Chapter 25

Maxillary Sinus and Its Disorders

OUTLINE

INTRODUCTION

Paranasal air sinuses are air-filled, mucosa-lined cavities which develop in facial and cranial bones and the spaces communicate with the nasal airway. There are total of four paired sinuses and are named in relation to the bone in which they are located—maxillary, frontal, sphenoid and ethmoid (Fig. 25.1 and Flowchart 25.1). The four paranasal sinuses develop as outpouchings of the nasal mucosa. The lining of each sinus is made up of ciliated pseudostratified epithelium, interspersed with mucus-secreting goblet cells.

FUNCTIONS OF PARANASAL SINUSES

The functions of the sinuses are to help in reducing the weight of the skull (pneumatisation of sinus) and moreover, to act as shock absorber of face or skull. Sinuses provide humidification of inspired air and their production of mucus aids in moistening the nasal chambers and inspired air. Their mucus secretion assists in air filtration and mechanical rigidity. They help in increasing the olfactory area, vocal resonance and diminution of auditory feedback. They also provide thermal insulation for intracranial structures. The sticky mucus absorbs pollutants and entraps the bacteria. Small, hair-like projections called cilia must move in unison to propel mucous outward, expelling bacteria and other particles. The mucus also contains adequate amount of bacteria-fighting substances, as well as immune factors called antibodies.

OPENINGS

The ostia of the frontal, maxillary and anterior ethmoid sinuses open into the ostiomeatal complex, which lies in the middle meatus lateral to the middle turbinate. The sphenoid sinuses and posterior ethmoid opens into the superior meatus and sphenoethmoid recess. The ostiomeatal complex is important because the frontal, ethmoidal and maxillary sinuses drain through this area.

MAXILLARY SINUS

Maxillary sinus (sinus maxillaris or antrum of Highmore), the largest of the paranasal sinuses is a pyramidal cavity in the body of the maxilla. In 1651, Highmore described maxillary sinus, but its existence was known before his description. The possible relation between dental pathology and the spread of infection to the maxillary antrum was later on described by John Hunter.

EMBRYOLOGY

The paranasal sinuses develop as a diverticula of the lateral nasal wall and extend into the frontal, ethmoid, sphenoid and maxillary bones. Maxillary sinus is the 1st of the sinuses to develop at around 10th week. It begins as a mucosal invagination that grows laterally from the middle meatus of the nasal cavity. The enlargement of this outgrowth is restricted by the perichondrium of nasal capsule, limiting its extension into the maxillary process (maxilla). Only after the resorption of capsule, the maxillary sinus enters the developing maxilla.

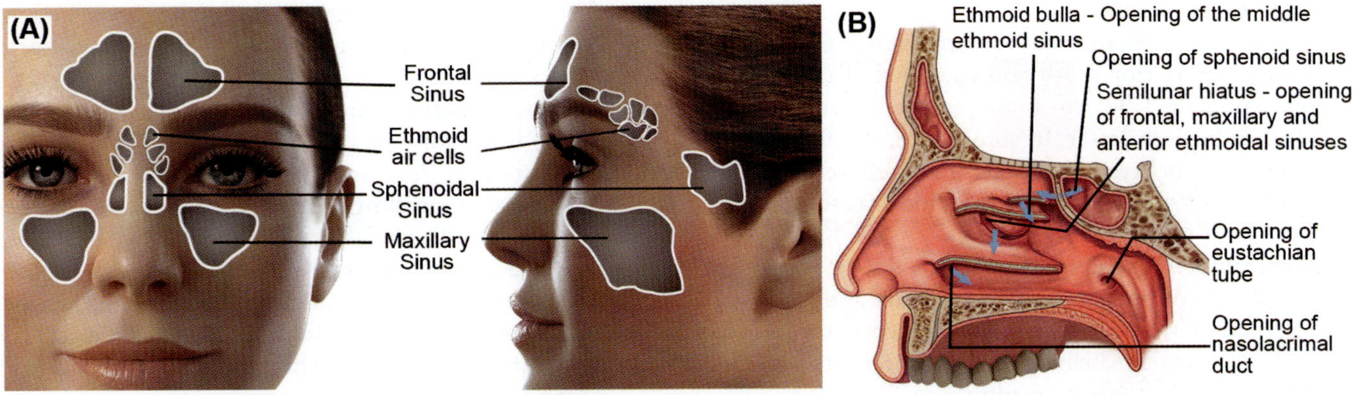

Figure 25.1 **(A)** Paranasal air sinuses **(B)** Lateral wall of the nose showing openings of the sinuses.

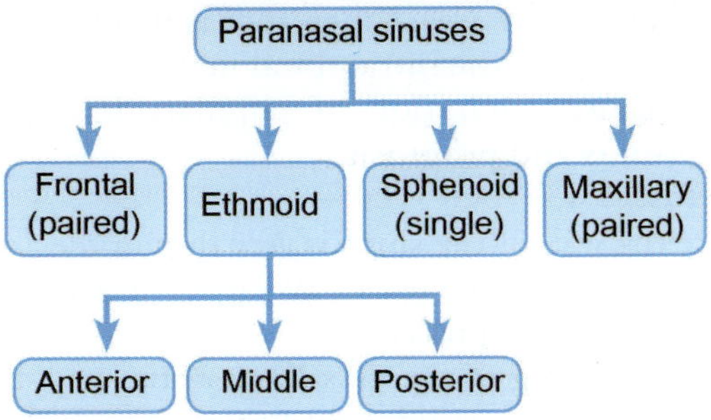

Flowchart 25.1 Group of paranasal air sinuses.

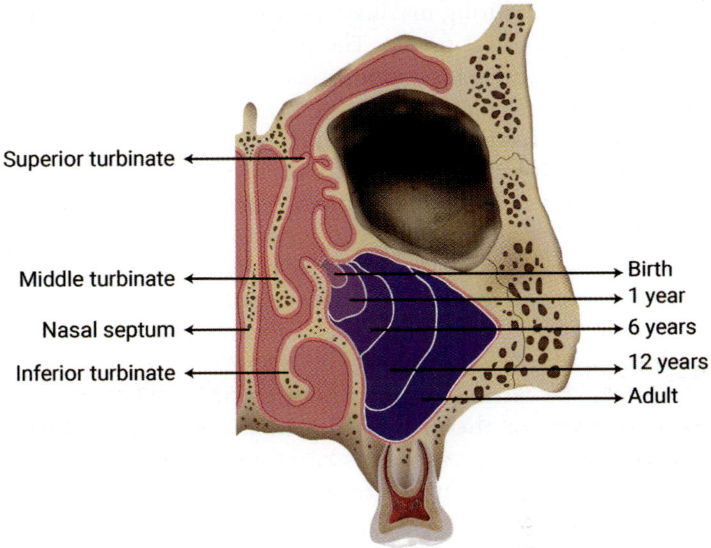

Figure 25.2 Developmental pattern of the maxillary sinus.

The maxillary sinus expands by pneumatisation and extends anteriorly and inferiorly from the base of the skull closely matching the growth rate of maxilla and development of dentition. In the neonates, the lower border of the sinus lies above that of the nasal floor whereas along with the developing midface and the eruption of permanent dentition, the floor of the sinus migrates to a lower level than that of the nasal cavity (0.5–10 mm).The expansion of the sinus normally stops around eruption of the permanent teeth (Fig. 25.2). Sometimes it may pneumatise further after removal of one or more of the maxillary posteriors, which extends into the residual alveolar process.

ANATOMY

The maxillary sinus is the largest of the paranasal sinuses, located within the body of the maxillary bone. It is pyramidal in shape having an apex, a base and four walls.

- **The base:** Directed medially and is formed by the lateral wall of the nasal cavity
- **The apex:** Directed laterally, is formed by the zygomatic process of the maxilla
- **Anterior wall:** The facial surface of the maxilla
- **Posterior wall:** The infratemporal surface of the maxilla
- **Roof:** Floor of the orbit
- **Floor:** Alveolar process of the maxilla.

The size of the sinus varies in different skulls and even on the two sides of the same skull. The average dimensions of the sinus are approximately 3.75 cm (vertical height) × 2.5 cm (transverse breadth) × 3 cm (anteroposterior depth). The adult average capacity of maxillary sinus varies from 9.5 to 20 cc, average about 14.75 cc. The blood supply to the mucous membrane of the sinus is derived from facial, infraorbital and greater palatine arteries. The veins accompany the arteries and drain into facial veins and the pterygoid plexus of veins. The lymphatic drainage is through the infraorbital foramen or through the ostium and then to submandibular nodes and upper deep cervical lymph nodes. Nerve supply is derived from all the branches of V2 (maxillary division of trigeminal nerve)—infraorbital, anterior, middle and posterior superior alveolar nerves.

APPLIED ANATOMY

Root anatomy:

The most common teeth whose roots are in close approximation to the maxillary sinus are 2nd maxillary molar followed by 1st and 3rd molars, 2nd premolar, 1st premolar and canine.

Maxillary sinus in adult:

In adults, the distance between the apical ends of the maxillary posterior tooth and the floor of the sinus is approximately 1–1.2 cm but in some individuals, this gap may be even lesser. In some cases, the floor of the sinus lies in between the roots of the adjacent teeth or adjacent roots of the same tooth, which causes elevation of the floor of the sinus.

Maxillary sinus in children:

Completion of pneumatisation occurs at about 15 years of age, hence the chances of creating an oroantral fistula (OAF) in a patient below the age of 15 years are comparatively lesser than in an adult.

Oroantral fistula and maxillary sinus:

Large sinuses may pose a risk of sinus wall fracture if the force used during maxillary posterior extraction results in an oroantral fistula. The presence of an unerupted tooth in the maxillary tuberosity is a potential line of weakness (Fig. 25.3).

Periapical infection and maxillary sinus:

Periapical infection of the tooth, which is in relation to maxillary antrum, might cause an oroantral fistula. Acute or chronic periapical infection may secondarily involve the maxillary sinus. The pus may discharge into the sinus increasing the fluid level, and the extraction of such tooth might result in oroantral fistula.

Antral puncture—intranasal antrostomy:

It can be carried out by puncturing into the sinus cavity through the middle meatus in children and the inferior meatus in adults creating a point of dependent drainage. In the case of acute sinusitis, pus is formed inside the antrum which in turn increases the intra-antral pressure because of occlusion of the lining mucosa.

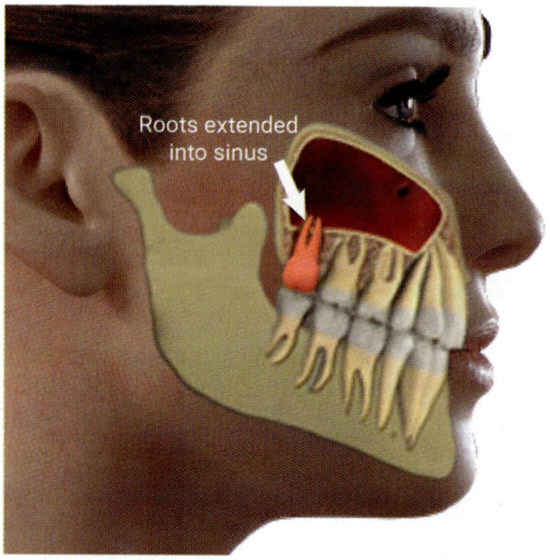

Figure 25.3 The root tips of the maxillary molar tooth commonly protrude the antrum. Extraction of those teeth often results in the formation of oroantral communication.

Tumours in maxillary sinus:

Since walls of the maxillary sinus are thin, any tumours that develop here may erode these walls and present as a swelling on the cheek, palate or buccal mucosa. Swelling of the cheek is noted, when the anterior and infratemporal walls are involved. Swelling in the palate or buccal sulcus is presented, when the tumours penetrate the floor of the sinus. Obstruction of nostrils is seen when the medial wall (nasal side) is involved. When a tumour involves the posterior wall, the posterior superior alveolar nerves are destroyed, resulting in paresthesia of the gingiva or teeth in the maxillary molar area. When roof is involved, it causes paraesthesia of the infraorbital nerve. Orbital involvement causes alteration of pupillary level, diplopia, strabismus and proptosis.

Canine fossa:

Since the wall of the sinus is very thin in the area of canine fossa, it can be used for diagnostic aspiration; site for Caldwell-Luc procedure.

The mucous lining of the maxillary sinus:

Sinus is lined by pseudostratified columnar ciliated epithelium which might regenerate once the infection is treated. But in cases where the lining is stripped, nasal mucosa extends through the ostium.

Fractures in the middle 3rd of face:

Fractures of the middle 3rd of the face might cause fracture of the sinus walls since these are very thin. Le Fort I, II and III show disturbances in the wall of the maxillary sinus. Zygomatic buttress may be pushed into the maxillary sinus during the fracture of the zygomatic bone.

Developmental anomalies:

The hypoplastic or underdeveloped maxillary sinus is presented in

- Crouzon syndrome
- Treacher Collins syndrome
- Binder syndrome.

CLINICAL EXAMINATION OF MAXILLARY SINUS PATHOLOGY

- **Extraoral examination:** Pain and tenderness, swelling over the prominence of cheekbones
- **Intraoral examination:** Pain and tenderness, swelling if present may be seen in the canine fossa and zygomatic buttress
- **Transillumination test:** Affected sinus shows reduced transmission of light due to accumulation of fluid, debris, pus and thickening of the sinus mucosa.

RADIOLOGICAL INVESTIGATION AND ASSESSMENT FOR MAXILLARY SINUS PATHOLOGY (Fig. 25.4)

The radiologic assessment of the maxillary sinus is usually done along with all other paranasal sinuses. Various radiographs used for assessment include following:

Intraoral views: Periapical radiographs help in locating and retrieving the foreign bodies like teeth, root tips, osseous fragments and also for planning. It also helps to differentiate the root apices which are intra-antral but extramucosal to visualise maxilla from the palatal aspect. **Anterior and lateral maxillary occlusal** projection provides excellent visualisation.

Extraoral views: The bony perimeter of the frontal, maxillary and sphenoid sinuses are visualised in the **lateral view**. The bony perimeter of the frontal sinus is best seen in **Caldwell's view**, which is helpful in cases of pansinusitis. The **submentovertex view** evaluates the sphenoid sinus and the anterior and posterior walls of the frontal sinuses. A good display of the lower aspects of the antrum is seen in **panoramic view** (orthopantomography) and also useful for routine detection of lesions of odontogenic origin. Detailed demonstration of mucosal abnormalities of sinuses and nose is given by CT scan or MRI. **CT scan** clearly shows the fine bony anatomy of the ostiomeatal channels in the coronal plane and also, the relationship of the brain and ethmoid roof as well as the relationship of the orbits to the paranasal sinuses (Fig. 25.4F). Whereas, the frontal recess is best visualised on the sagittal images. **MRI** is helpful in diagnosing fungal concretions, mucoceles and cephaloceles.

CLASSIFICATION OF DISEASES AFFECTING MAXILLARY SINUS

Diseases affecting the maxillary sinus are classified as depicted in Table 25.1.

ODONTOGENIC MAXILLARY SINUSITIS

Intimate anatomical relation of the upper teeth to the maxillary sinus promotes the development of periapical or periodontal odontogenic infection into maxillary sinusitis.

Aetiology: (1) Infections (periapical abscess, common cold, upper respiratory infection), (2) trauma (fracture of antral floor and walls), (3) allergy, (4) neoplasm or cyst of odontogenic origin, (5) oroantral fistula and (6) displaced tooth or root. The most common cause of maxillary sinus by oral infection is due to periapical abscess, as the roots

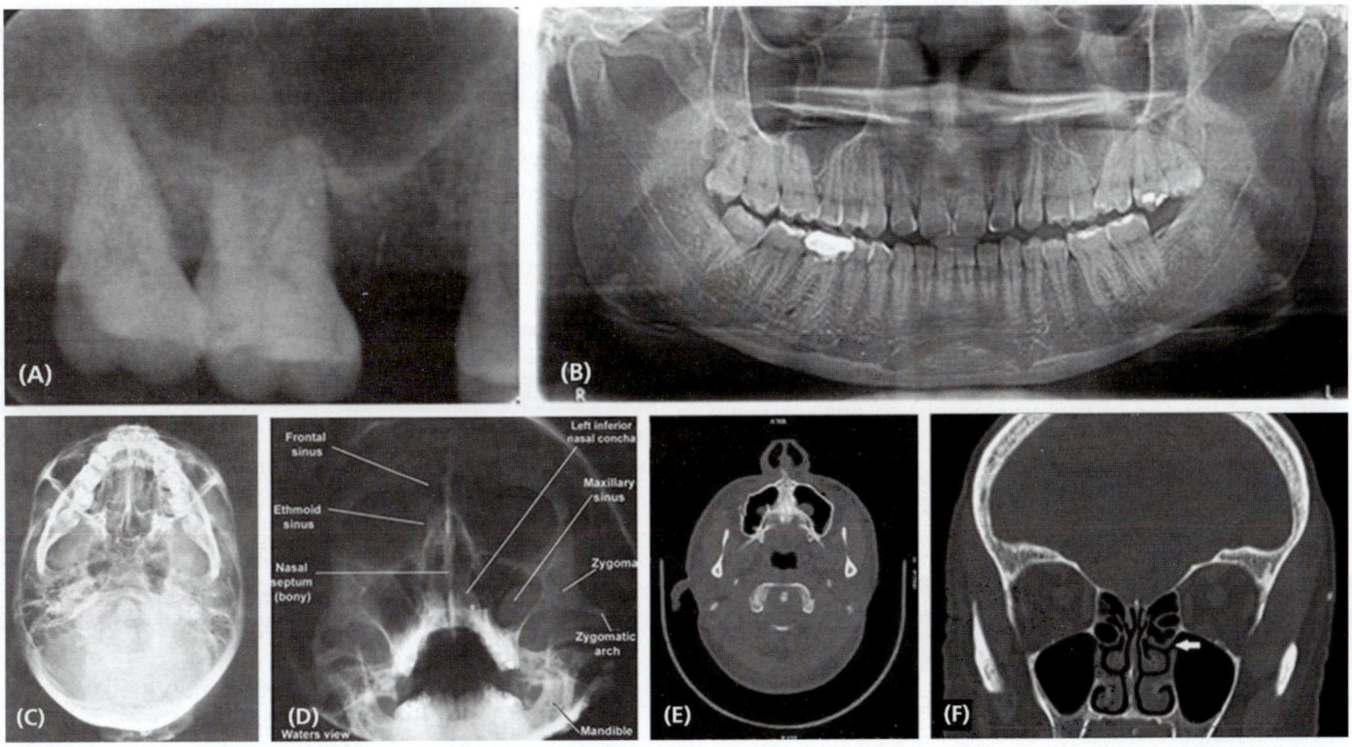

Figure 25.4 (**A**) Intraoral periapical radiograph showing the posterior teeth in connection with maxillary sinus. (**B**) Orthopantomogram (OPG) (**C**) Submentovertex view. (**D**) Waters view (occipitomental view) for evaluation of sinus pathology. (**E**) Axial CT section showing nasal polyp in left maxillary sinus. (**F**) Coronal view maxillary sinus showing ostium, maxillary sinus opening through the middle meatus.

TABLE 25.1 Classification of Diseases Affecting the Maxillary Sinus

1. Maxillary sinusitis
   a. Odontogenic
   b. Inflammatory
      - Acute
      - Subacute
      - Chronic
2. Oroantral fistula
   a. Acute
   b. Chronic
3. Traumatic
   a. Haematoma in the sinus
4. Iatrogenic
   a. Tooth or root displaced into the sinus
5. Tumour—carcinoma of maxillary sinus
6. Antral rhinoliths

of molars (1st and 2nd molars) are in close proximity to the sinus.

Clinical features:

Sinonasal symptoms include unilateral nasal obstruction, rhinorrhoea and/or foul odour and taste. Headaches, unilateral anterior maxillary tenderness and postnasal drip. Mild swelling in the cheek is seen. Dental symptoms include severe throbbing pain due to collection of pus in the apical region within the bone. Unpleasant smell or taste in mouth. Mobility of teeth (depending on the periodontal involvement).

Diagnosis: The accurate diagnosis of odontogenic maxillary sinusitis is important. Radiologic imaging can provide useful adjunct information in the diagnosis of sinusitis and particularly whether an odontogenic source may be responsible for the infection.

Management:

Elimination of the source of the infection (e.g. removal of an external dental root from the sinus cavity, extraction or root canal therapy of causative tooth) to prevent recurrence of the sinusitis.

Adequate care must be taken during extraction to avoid oroantral fistula. Antibiotic prophylaxis and nasal decongestant should be used.

INFLAMMATORY MAXILLARY SINUSITIS (Fig. 25.5)

Maxillary sinusitis is classified according to the duration of its course into: (1) acute, (2) subacute and (3) chronic maxillary sinusitis.

- **Acute maxillary sinusitis (AMS)** has a sudden onset and duration of 4 weeks or less
- **Subacute maxillary sinusitis** has a duration of 4–12 weeks

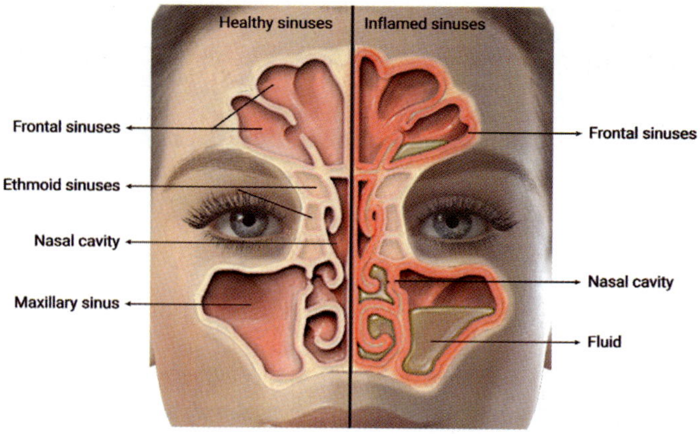

Figure 25.5 Illustration of healthy sinus (right) versus inflamed sinus (left); note the sinuses are swollen due to inflammation, blocking the passage and leading to mucus build-up.

- **Recurrent subacute maxillary sinusitis** occurs at least four times per year with each episode lasting 7–10 days. The symptoms are completely absent in between the episodes
- **Chronic maxillary sinusitis** has duration of at least 12 weeks.

ACUTE MAXILLARY SINUSITIS

AMS may be clinically defined as an inflammatory response involving mucous membranes of the nasal cavity and paranasal sinuses. Most cases of AMS involve inflammation of more than one of the paranasal sinuses, most commonly maxillary and ethmoid sinuses. When all the paranasal sinuses are either acutely or chronically infected, the condition is called pansinusitis, which may be either unilateral or bilateral.

AETIOLOGY OF MAXILLARY SINUSITIS (Table 25.2)

TABLE 25.2 Aetiology of Maxillary Sinusitis

Dental Cause	Others
• Dental infection • Oroantral communication	• Allergy • Anatomic abnormality of the ostiomeatal complex • Nasal anatomic variations • Cystic fibrosis • Immune deficiency (common variable, IgA, IgG subclass, specific antibody) • Acquired immunodeficiency syndrome (AIDS) Wegener's granulomatosis • Swimming/diving • Topical nasal medications • Cocaine abuse • Injury

PATHOPHYSIOLOGY

Maxillary sinusitis is a disease of multifactorial aetiology. The ostia are the most important foci for development of disease. Inflammatory changes of the ostiomeatal complex result in decreased mucociliary clearance, retention of secretions and decreased sinus ventilation. Swelling of the mucosa impedes drainage and creates an environment predisposed to the development of infection.

MICROBIOLOGY

Bacteria: The bacteria most often isolated from patients with acute sinusitis are *Streptococcus pneumoniae, Haemophilus influenzae* and *Moraxella catarrhalis*. However, *Staphylococcus aureus*, other streptococci and anaerobes may also be isolated from patients with bacterial AMS.

CLINICAL FINDINGS

Extraoral

- Headache
- Facial pain/pressure/swelling
- Mild fever, chills
- Nasal obstruction/blockage
- Nasal or postnasal discharge/purulence (by history or physical examination)
- Fatigue
- Hyposmia/anosmia
- Cough
- Ear pain

Intraoral

- Halitosis
- Presence of fistula
- Discharge of pus from fistula into the mouth
- Teeth in the area of the sinus may be painful and mobile.

INVESTIGATIONS

Transillumination: This is a method of examination performed in a darkened room. A light is placed in the mouth. It transilluminates normal sinus but fails to do so in presence of pus, polyps or thickening of antral membrane due to acute or chronic infection.

Rhinoscopy: Anterior rhinoscopy reveals pus draining downwards with oedema and erythema of mucosa.

Radiographic findings

Waters view is the screening tool for all paranasal sinuses. It also gives a clue regarding involvement of other sinuses. The level of fluid and any deviation of the septum that is obstructing the ostium can be detected.

MANAGEMENT

Symptomatic therapy: Primary aim for patients with AMS is to facilitate drainage of the sinuses and nasal passages. Patients should be hydrated, and analgesics and decongestant should be administered to relieve pain and malaise associated with AMS.

Nonsteroidal anti-inflammatory drugs (NSAIDs): Paracetamol, aspirin, ibuprofen.

Antimicrobial therapy–erythromycin: 250–500 mg 4/day for 5 days, **amoxicillin** 250–500 mg 3/day for 5 days. If there is no response within 72 h, culture sensitivity test must be carried out.

Decongestant–nasal drops or sprays: Ephedrine sulphate 0.5%–1% in normal saline, six hourly. Xylometazoline hydrochloride 0.1% shrinks the mucosa and eliminate the mucosal discharge.

Mucolytic agents: They reduce the viscosity of the mucus and increase drainage by the ciliary complex. Ordinary steam inhalation, camphor, menthol, tincture benzoin, etc. are used.

Topical corticosteroids: To reduce inflammation in patients with chronic rhinitis or recurrent infections.

CHRONIC MAXILLARY SINUSITIS

Chronic maxillary sinusitis refers to inflammation of the sinus membrane for duration of at least 12 weeks. Either a sudden worsening of baseline chronic maxillary sinusitis symptoms or appearance of new symptoms characterises acute exacerbation of chronic maxillary sinusitis. During an acute exacerbation, prominent symptoms include pain and tenderness in the area of antrum and unilateral foul discharge through posterior nares.

MICROBIOLOGY

Staphylococci, streptococci and Gram-positive organisms may be found.

AETIOLOGY

- Periapical abscess gaining access into the maxillary sinus due to close proximity of the involved tooth with the floor of the sinus
- Infections of neoplasm or cysts of odontogenic origin
- Fracture of the maxillary floor
- Displaced tooth into the maxillary sinus.

PATHOPHYSIOLOGY

Chronic inflammation may cause hyperplasia or atrophy of the lining epithelium. Multiple polyp formation or degeneration of epithelium, where the cilia are lost can be seen. The ostium may be blocked completely due to oedema thus affecting drainage of the sinus.

CLINICAL FINDINGS

- The predominant symptom is severe pain of constant and localised character. This pain may be referred to the cheek and frontal region above the eye
- Discharge into the nose may at 1st be profuse, but soon it assumes a mucopurulent form, dripping into the nasopharynx from where it is expectorated or swallowed
- If the head is bent forward, it may run out of the nostril

- In maxillary sinusitis that originates from diseased teeth, the secretion has a foul, saprophytic odour
- General toxaemia accompanies the disease, with chills, sweats and a rise in temperature, often nausea and dizziness
- Breathing may be obstructed or impaired on the side affected by the antral infection.

INVESTIGATIONS

Radiographic findings

Waters view: The sinus reveals thickening of lining membrane and radiopacity on the affected side due to the presence of fluid. In case of presence of tooth or root, the characteristic outline is seen within the sinus.

Diagnosis

- Anterior rhinoscopy shows nasal congestion and mucopurulent material in middle meatus
- History of repeated attacks of acute mucopurulent rhinitis and long-standing nasal or postnasal discharge
- Inspection of oropharynx may reveal pharyngeal exudates
- Prolapse of polypoidal mass into the mouth forming a lump may be seen
- Transillumination—negative
- Presence of chronic oroantral fistula may be an associated finding.

MANAGEMENT

Goals of management

General goals for treatment of the patient with odontogenic sinusitis that is bacterial are as follows:

- To control infection
- Diminish tissue oedema
- Reverse sinusoidal obstruction so that the mucus can drain.

Medical and surgical management

- Appropriate antibiotic therapy
- Nasal drops or inhalations of decongestants
    1. If the chronic sinusitis is caused by chronic periapical infection, then the affected tooth must be extracted and the socket should be surgically closed completely as there is a risk of oroantral fistula formation
    2. In case, the cause is a foreign body, such as tooth or root in the sinus, it is necessary to retrieve these foreign bodies prior to considering any other form of treatment
    3. The presence of a chronic pyogenic sinusitis subsequent to an oroantral fistula requires surgical closure of fistula. The polyps found at operation should also be removed
        a. The antrum should be irrigated with warm saline or Betadine daily
        b. Once the antral washouts appear to be clear, the fistula should be repaired surgically
    4. In cases, where there is no oroantral fistula present, but there is chronic maxillary sinusitis nonresponsive to other conservative regime, then a surgical drainage should be considered.

Surgical drainage

The thin medial wall of the antrum is punctured by introducing the sharp trocar and cannula along the floor of the nasal cavity inferior to inferior turbinate. The trocar is withdrawn and the pus is drained under pressure through suction tip. Warm saline irrigation should be done till symptoms resolves.

COMPLICATIONS OF UNTREATED MAXILLARY SINUSITIS

Due to the proximity of paranasal sinus to the eyes and brain, complications of sinusitis can be divided into two broad categories: *orbital and intracranial*. These infections usually originate from ethmoid sinus and extend into the orbit and associated soft tissues through any of the following mechanisms:

- Direct extension to the orbital wall
- Retrograde spread through veins between the sinuses and the orbit.

It is very rare for the infection to spread through lymphatics because they are absent in the orbit. If not effectively treated, the following serious complications may occur rarely:

- Cellulitis
- Abscess
- Meningitis
- Cavernous sinus thrombosis
- Osteomyelitis
- Oroantral fistula.

PERIORBITAL CELLULITIS

This is also known as preseptal cellulitis, which is oedema and inflammation of the skin and muscle anterior to the orbital septum. This results due to impairment of venous drainage from these tissues. There are no visual symptoms. Depending on the size of the abscess, associated mass effect and degree of inflammation, ocular muscles and visual acuity are variably affected.

CAVERNOUS SINUS THROMBOSIS

This occurs as a sequelae of direct extension or retrograde thrombophlebitis of ethmoid or sphenoid sinuses. Clinical features include proptosis, chemosis, restriction of extraocular mobility, visual loss and signs of meningitis, intracranial complications occur less frequently than orbital complications.

OROANTRAL FISTULA

Oroantral fistula is a pathological communication between the oral cavity and the maxillary sinus. Immediate oroantral fistulae usually do not have any epithelial lining but chronic oroantral fistulae are epithelialised.

AETIOLOGY

EXTRACTION OF TEETH

- The sinus attains its maximum size by the age of 15; therefore, perforation is more common in adults than in children. Sometimes, the roots of the posterior teeth are in close proximity with the sinus floor. There might be only a thin lamina of bone or sometimes only the antral mucosa may be present in between the root apices and the maxillary antrum. This is due to greater degree of pneumatisation of the maxillary sinus. In such cases, chances of creation of oroantral fistula are greater during extraction of teeth (Fig. 25.6)
- The shape of the tooth might be such that when extraction forceps are applied, the tooth slips into the antrum like the popping of the 'orange seed' held between the fingers
- The most common reason of oroantral fistula is the iatrogenic, which occurs while extracting the maxillary tooth. Most commonly, the 1st maxillary molar tooth's palatal root which breaks during extraction might create an oroantral communication (OAC). Attempt to retrieve retained apices in posterior teeth by 'blind instrumentation' might result in displacement of root into the maxillary sinus through perforation
- Surgical removal of impacted teeth (maxillary 3rd molar, supernumerary), submerged, hypercementosis, geminated, diverged root teeth carries the risk of inadvertent breech in continuity of antrum.

PERIAPICAL LESIONS OF TEETH

The periapical lesions which are in close proximity with the sinus floor and necrotic lesion of the maxilla such as noma may erode the sinus floor. Apicoectomy of root, which is adjoining with the sinus lining, will create OAF.

IMPLANT

Implant dentures can cause considerable destruction of the antral floor creating OAF and also the use of contaminated or diseased maxillary implant dentures forms the fistula.

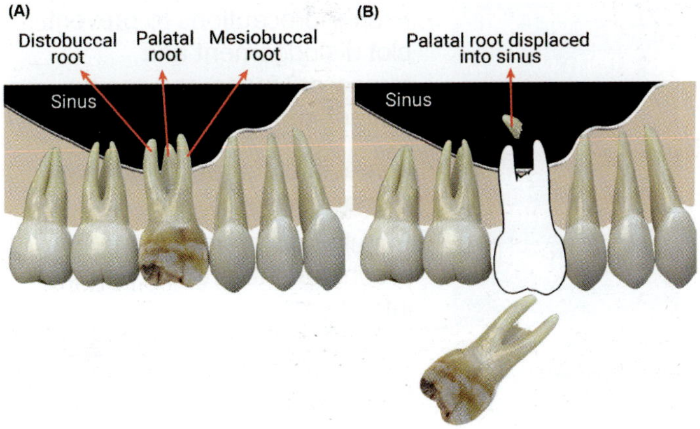

Figure 25.6 Schematic diagram showing distobuccal root in close proximity to maxillary sinus. (**A**) Decayed tooth. (**B**) Broken root after extraction.

SURGERIES

Surgical procedures such as maxillary sinus surgeries, marsupialisation, orbital floor fracture treated by antral pack support by Caldwell-Luc incision, partial maxillectomy (malignancy or antral neoplasm).

Maxillary sinus surgery performed to remove a large abscess or cystic lesion may lead to fistula formation.

- Marsupialisation performed on defective alveolar antral wall may also result in the fistula
- Orbital floor fracture treated by antral pack support by Caldwell-Luc incision. Usually the end of the pack is sutured to the buccal vestibule, and the pack is removed through the buccal vestibule creating the orifice. If the orifice fails to heal, it might lead to OAF
- Partial maxillectomy (malignancy or antral neoplasm) involves the removal of alveolus, part of palate and antral walls creating OAF.

EXTENSIVE FACIAL TRAUMA

- Multiple and extensive midfacial trauma, particularly, because of sharp objects or missiles inserted into the sinus via mouth will lead to oroantral fistula. Even gunshot injuries/penetrating type of injuries affecting the sinus walls create huge defect resulting in OAF.

NEOPLASMS

Malignant granuloma and other malignant disorders of the maxillary sinus may erode the oral cavity. Tumours of the upper jaw may reach into the sinus, forming the fistula.

SYPHILIS

Gummatous lesion of palate results in extensive OAF due to destruction of bone. Secondary and tertiary forms of syphilis involving nose may create OAF.

OSTEOMYELITIS

Osteomyelitis is commonly seen in mandible, but the maxillary osteomyelitis might occur rarely in some systemic conditions such as diabetes, leukaemia, uraemia and irradiation.

INVESTIGATIONS TO CONFIRM THE PRESENCE OF FISTULA

In case of large fistula, assessment can be done from inspection. Whereas, if the opening is small, other test must be done.

- **Nose blowing test:** A cotton wisp is kept near the fistulous opening and the patient is asked to blow the nose with closed nostrils and open mouth. In the presence of oroantral communication, air will pass through the defect and will displace the cotton wisp, whereas any blood present will be seen to bubble
- **Mouth mirror test:** The patient is made to perform Valsalva manoeuvre, with a mouth mirror placed facing the oral opening of fistula. If the mirror gets fogged, it indicates the presence of oroantral communication
- **Sinus probing:** To diagnose an oroantral fistula, a sinus probe can be safely used. However, in case of suspicion of

an acute oroantral communication, the use of probe for assessment is contraindicated. Instrumentation of the site will lead to breakdown of blood clot and leads to fistula

- **Water holding test:** When the patient is asked to hold fluid within the mouth, fluid can be seen escaping through the nose. Betadine can be mixed with the fluid to differentiate between the nasal secretion and the rinsing fluid
- **Radiological examination:** Best way to detect OAC.

SYMPTOMS OF RECENTLY CREATED OROANTRAL COMMUNICATION (REMEMBER 5 E'S)

1. **Escape of fluids:** Fluid regurgitation and escape of air through the nose from the site of extraction
2. **Epistaxis:** Unilateral epistaxis is seen due to escape of blood from the sinus into the nose through the ostium
3. **Escape of air:** Air escapes into the nose from the mouth during sucking, inhaling. Due to escape of air patient has inability to blow their cheeks
4. **Enhanced column of air**: Which causes a change in the vocal resonance and consequently change in the voice
5. **Excruciating pain**: Severe pain in and around the region of affected sinus.

SIGNS OF RECENTLY CREATED OROANTRAL COMMUNICATION

1. Disappearance of the root piece of the extracted tooth.
2. Positive nasal blow test.

SYMPTOMS ESTABLISHED OROANTRAL FISTULA (REMEMBER 5 P'S)

1. **Pain:** As the fistula is established by epithelisation, it allows free escape of fluids, so the pain is a less dominant feature than seen in early stage
2. **Purulent nasal discharge:** When the head is lowered, there is persistent, purulent unilateral discharge from the affected side of nostril
3. **Postnasal drip:** There is unilateral nasal discharge from the posterior nares, down the pharynx. The discharge is associated with foul smell and thus leads to unpleasant taste
4. **Possible sequelae of general systemic toxaemic condition:** Fever, anorexia, malaise, parietal and frontal headaches and in extreme cases, anosmia
5. **Popping out of an antral polyp:** The opening of long-standing OAF is occluded by an antral polyp, which is seen as bluish red bulge extruding through the fistula.

SIGNS OF ESTABLISHED OROANTRAL FISTULA

1. **Early signs:** Disintegration of blood clot as a result of forceful nose blowing, excessive mouth rinsing and infection. Therefore, the breach in the antral lining remains patent
2. **Late signs:** Signs and symptoms of sinusitis and rhinitis, escape of fluids or air through nose, development of polyp.

DECISION-MAKING IN TREATMENT OF OAC AND OAF (FLOWCHART 25.2)

SIZE OF COMMUNICATION

The closure of the defect and prevention of oral bacteria and food debris penetrating the sinus is the main objective in the management of OAC/OAF. If the OAC is ***less than 2 mm*** in diameter, without epithelialisation and in the absence of sinus infection, there can be spontaneous healing if proper precautions are taken. Inadvertent probing into sinus through socket must be avoided. Proper high-quality blood clot within the socket must be ensured and sinus precautions are advised to the patient. However, if the defects are **larger than 5–6 mm**, spontaneous healing rarely takes place and will require surgical intervention.

PREOPERATIVE CONDITIONS OF MAXILLARY SINUS

Even small communications fail to heal if the maxillary sinus is infected. If the patient has maxillary sinusitis, healing of OAC is impaired leading to the formation of chronic oroantral fistula, which requires surgical intervention

MANAGEMENT OF ACUTE OROANTRAL FISTULA

TEMPORARY MEASURE

1. **Whitehead's varnish pack**
   The pack is used over the socket and secured with sutures
   Whitehead's varnish:
   - Benzoin 10 parts 44 g
   - Storax 7.5 parts 33 g
   - Balsam of Tolu 5 parts 22 g
   - Iodoform 10 parts 55 g
   - Solvent ether to 1 fl oz or 100 parts

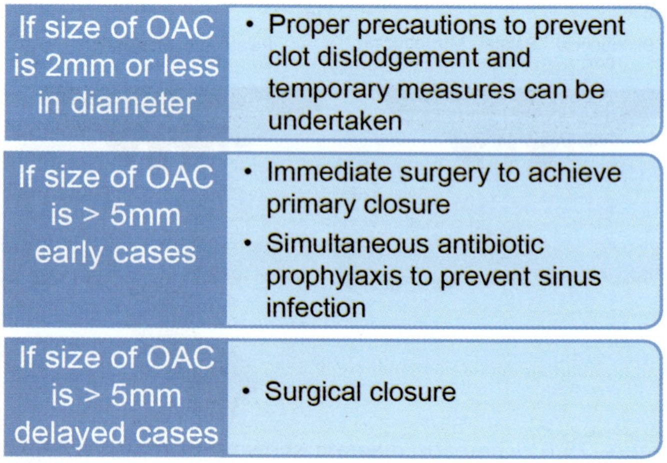

Flowchart 25.2 Decision-making in treatment of OAC based on size.

2. **Denture plate**
Indicated when there is delay in surgical repair of fistula. Denture plate acts as barrier to prevent entry of food particles into the antrum.

IMMEDIATE CLOSURE

The simplest method is primary closure of the socket by mucoperiosteal flaps, obtained by reducing the height of the bony socket. The flaps are approximated and are loosely sutured over the defect. Antibiotics are prescribed to prevent sinus infection. This requires minimum time, surgical skill and facilities and can be done in all cases at risk of oroantral fistula (Figs. 25.7 and 25.8).

SUPPORTIVE MEASURE

- **Antibiotics:** Antibiotics are prescribed to prevent secondary infection at the site, to prevent pre-existing infection of antrum. Based on culture and sensitivity testing, the selection of antibiotic must be done. Penicillin and its derivatives—initially i.v. route and later switched to oral route. Dose—Penicillin V 250–500 mg six hourly

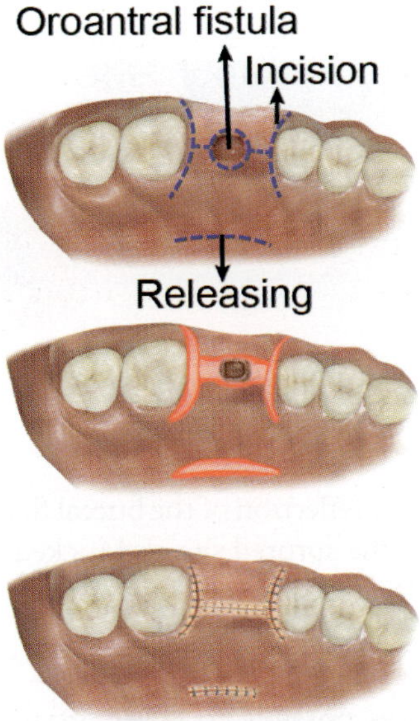

Figure 25.7 Immediate closure of Oroantral fistula.

- **Nasal decongestants**: They facilitate the drainage of pus and secretions. For example, Ephedrine (0.5%) or Otrivin nasal drops 3 drops three times a day for 7 days
- **Analgesics:** NSAIDs: (1) Tablet Aspirin 500 mg four times daily, (2) tablet Paracetamol 500 mg three times daily and (3) tablet Ibuprofen 400 mg three times daily.

SURGICAL OPTIONS FOR CLOSURE OF OROANTRAL FISTULA

Surgical management for closure of OAF is briefed in Flowchart 25.3.

SURGICAL PROCEDURES FOR CLOSURE OF OROANTRAL FISTULA

The success of closure of oroantral fistula depends upon the complete elimination of sinus pathology, fistulous tract and infected bone. Numerous surgical techniques can be used for the closure of defect depending on the requirement. Various flap techniques can be used to close OAF and all these flaps should follow the basic requirements of an ideal flap.

BUCCAL FLAP (VON REHRMANN FLAP) (Fig. 25.9)

- Local anaesthesia: Adequate local anaesthesia is given to reduce the bleeding and risk of formation of postoperative haematoma
- The fistulous tract is excised by placing an incision 2–3 mm around the orifice. The entire epithelium of the fistula along with any nasal polyp (as in chronic fistula) should be removed
- Incisions are made on either side of the orifice and extended into the buccal sulcus. Buccal vestibular height may be affected through this procedure
- A broad-based trapezoidal buccal flap is raised by means of subperiosteal dissection, which is carried out well above the reflection of the mucous membrane. A horizontal cut is then made through the periosteum alone above the reflection and inherent elasticity of the mucous membrane then permits the mucosa to be advanced and sutured to the palatal mucoperiosteum without tension.
- Bleeding should be completely controlled to prevent any haematoma formation inside the sinus

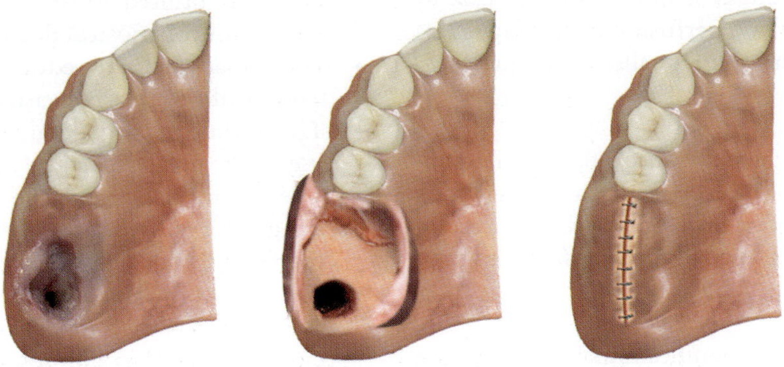

Figure 25.8 Immediate closure of large sinus opening in the tuberosity region after extraction.

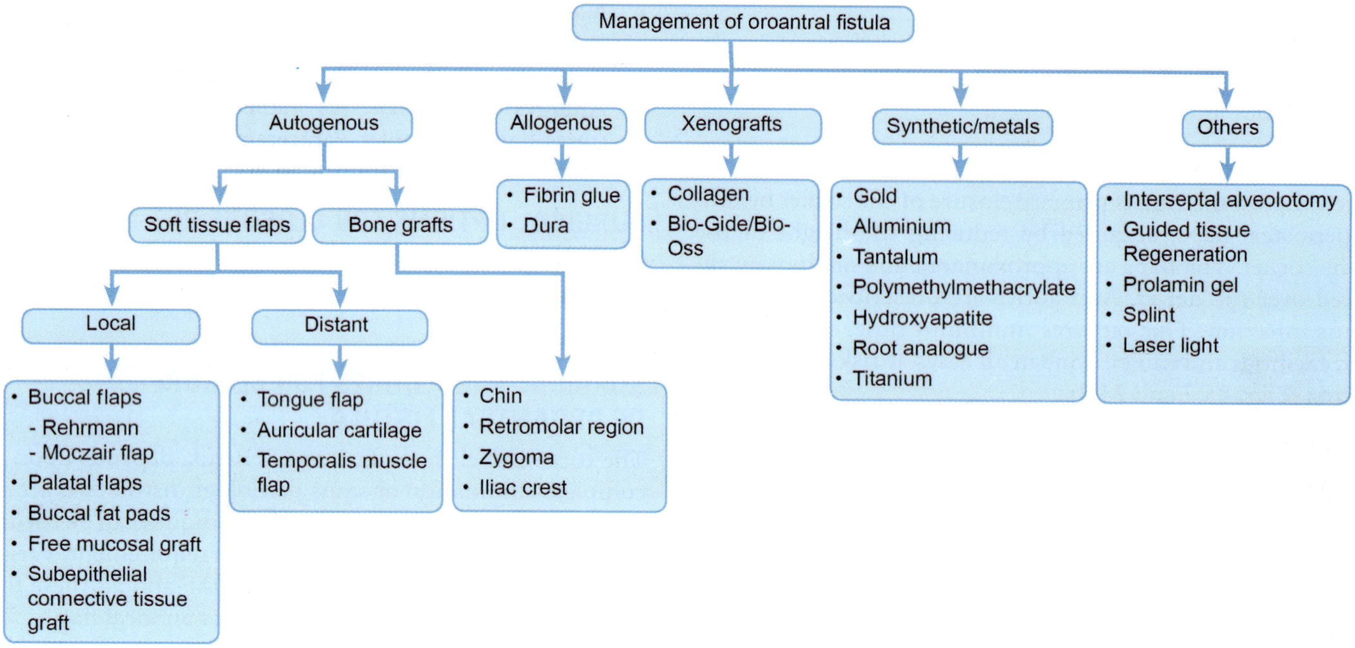

Flowchart 25.3 Various surgical options for the management of oroantral fistula.

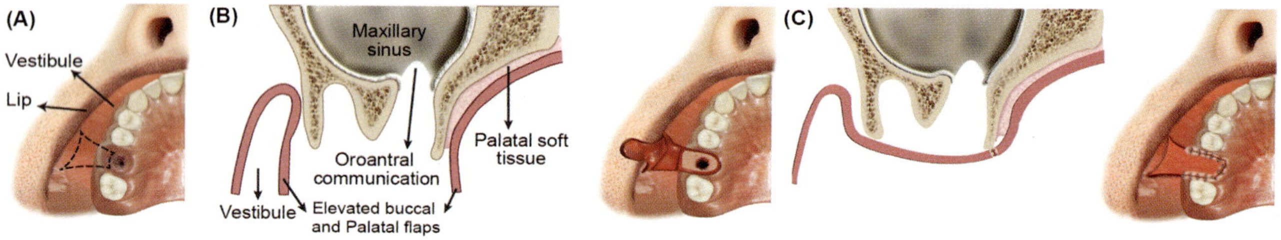

Figure 25.9 (**A–C**) Closure of oroantral fistula using buccal flap.

- Horizontal mattress sutures should be employed for this purpose and left in situ for 2 weeks

  Advantages: This is a simple and safe technique with excellent method of repair which, however, requires more operating time and surgical skill. It is often accompanied by some postoperative haematoma formation and loss of depth in the buccal sulcus and in edentulous patients, a secondary vestibuloplasty may be required. This technique is not a choice in case of larger defects as the blood perfusion of the flap is less and is only recommended for smaller techniques.

MOCZAIR FLAP

A modification of this flap where the buccal flap is raised anterior to the defect, buccal of healthy teeth, following which the flap is slided into the defect horizontally (buccal sliding flap). Advantages include less vestibular sulcus flattening.

FALCI ET AL.,

Falci et al., has described another modification of this technique in which the mucosal margins of the fistula are sutured together prior to the reflection of the buccal flap. Later the buccal flap is pulled over the sutured site and tucked inside the palatal flap, which was elevated simultaneously with the buccal flap.

PALATAL FLAP (ASHLEY'S FLAP) (FIG. 25.10)

- It is not always possible to cover oroantral communications situated high up in the sulcus with a buccal flap, even when the soft tissues lying either behind or in front of the defect are utilised. In such cases, it is often better to use a palatal mucoperiosteal flap based upon its blood supply
- Local anaesthesia to reduce the bleeding
- The fistulous tract is excised as previously mentioned
- The outline of the palatal flap should be marked according to the greater palatine artery and incised
- The palatal flap should be elevated carefully preserving the greater palatine artery. It is then rotated and approximated with the buccal margin
- The bare bony base of the resultant palatal defect may be covered by a pack, composed of Whitehead's varnish on ribbon gauze, held in position by means of mattress sutures inserted into the margins of the attached mucoperiosteum

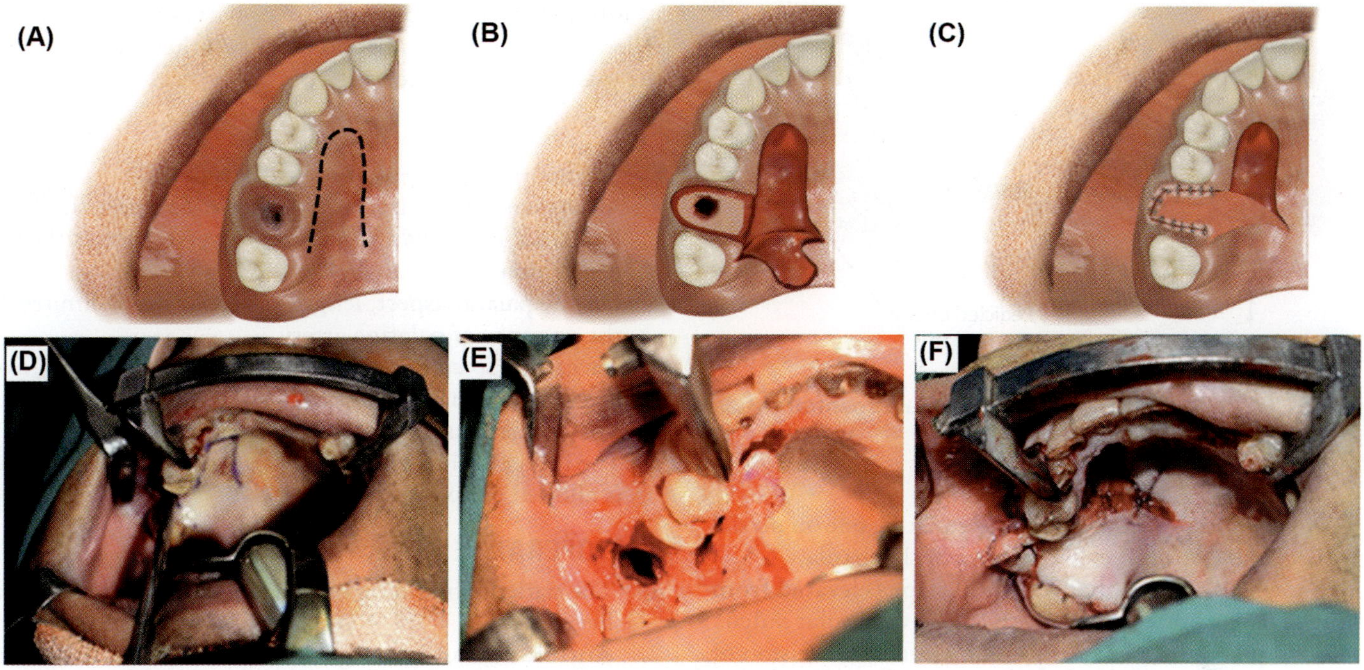

Figure 25.10 (**A–C**) Illustrations showing closure of oroantral fistula using palatal flap. (**D–F**) Intraoperative view showing the closure of oroantral fistula using palatal flap. (Scan to play oroantral fistula closure by palatal flap).

- **Kruger's modification**: A back cut at the posterior end of the flap for ease of rotation and to avoid kinking.

Advantages

- The rich blood supply of the palatal flap provides satisfactory healing
- Buccal vestibular height is unaffected. Hence, prosthetic rehabilitation is unimpaired.

Disadvantages

- Limitation in the rotation of thick keratinised palatal flap, if the OAF is located at the maxillary tuberosity
- Kinking or 'dog-ear' formation can occur during rotation of the flap which compromises the vascular blood supply predisposing to vascular congestion and also adaptation of distal part of flap is impaired
- Palatal flaps tend to shrink when elevated from the bone and their thickness and consistency make them more difficult to reposition than buccal flaps
- In systemically compromised patients, risk of necrosis of the exposed bone at the donor site.

COMBINATION METHOD (Fig. 25.11)

In combination method, both buccal and palatal flaps are used to cover the defect.

- Usually used when re-repair is required
- Two layered closure is obtained using buccal and palatal flaps
- The thick covering gives more strength and reduces shrinkage and risk of infection

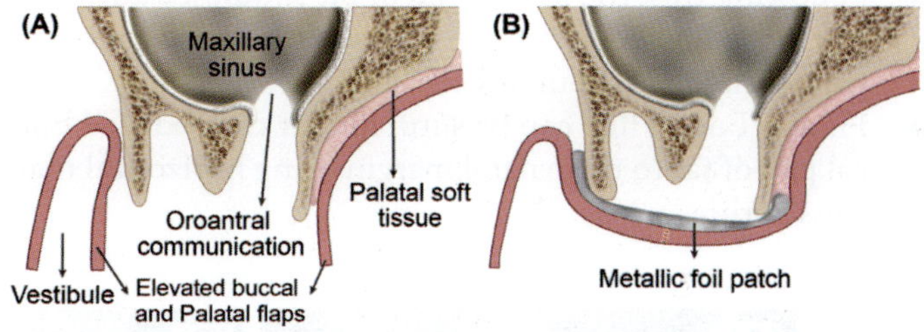

Figure 25.11 (**A** and **B**) Illustrations showing closure of oroantral fistula using both buccal and palatal flaps along with metal foil covering the defect.

- Metallic foil can also be used. Following reflection of buccal and palatal mucoperiosteal flaps, metallic foil 'patch' (usually gold foil) is adapted over the defect. The flaps are repositioned and sutured over the foil.

PEDICLED BUCCAL PAD OF FAT (Fig. 25.12)

The technique was 1st described by Egyedi in the late 1970s, following a study by Tideman et al., its use became more common. This technique is indicated in case of larger defects (>7 mm) associated with inflammatory conditions. This procedure can be employed when all other methods have failed to yield desired result.

- Buccal pad of fat is a simple lobulated mass, situated deeply along the posterior maxilla and superior fibres of buccinators muscles. Its blood supply is derived from the maxillary artery, superficial temporal and facial arteries
- Under local anaesthesia, a circular incision is placed around the fistula and the epithelial lining is removed

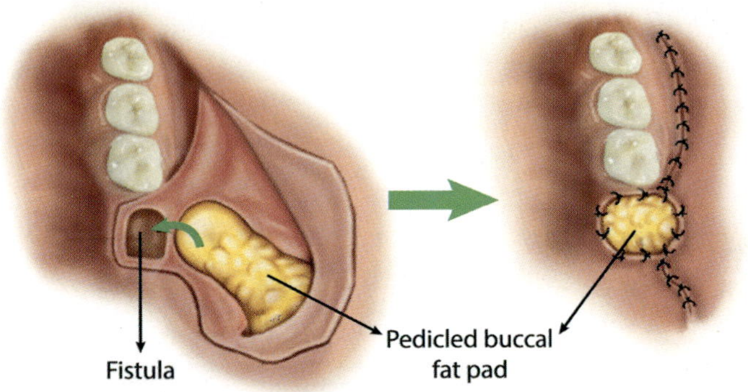

Figure 25.12 Illustrations showing closure of oroantral fistula using pedicled buccal pad of fat.

- Two diverging vertical incisions are placed, one on mesial aspect and one on the distal aspect of the fistula
- Now, the trapezoid-shaped buccal flap is elevated from the alveolar bone to the depth of the vestibular sulcus
- Buccal pad of fat can be exposed by a vertical incision of 1 cm long on the posterior aspect of the zygomatic buttress region and periosteum is teased open upwards until the lobulated mass is seen popping out
- Following this, the buccal pad of fat should be advanced along the bony defect to be sutured in the margin of the palatal tissue without any tension
- Finally, buccal flap can be sutured over the pedicled buccal pad of fat to the palatal margin using horizontal mattress suture.

Advantages: Location and ease of harvesting the flap. Excellent blood supply and good rate of epithelisation without the loss of vestibular depth.

BRIDGE FLAP (Fig. 25.13)

- Commonly employed in edentulous maxilla
- After excising the lining epithelium covering the fistulous tract, incisions are placed transversely across the line of the arch
- On the palatal aspect, length of the bridge is limited by the presence of palatine artery
- Buccally, flap can be elevated sufficiently and lifted over the fistula without tension
- The bridge must be wider than the bony defect
- The bridge is shifted to cover the fistula and the raw area is allowed to epithelialise.

POSTOPERATIVE CARE

1. The patient should be instructed to avoid blowing his/her nose
2. **Antibiotics and analgesics:** Antibiotics are used to eliminate any infection and prevent any further infection of the sinus. Culture and sensitivity test can be done to determine the appropriate antibiotic. Analgesics are used to control postoperative pain
3. **Nasal drops and inhalations:** Ostium of the maxillary antrum is situated high up on the wall of the sinus and decongestant nasal drops and inhalations (e.g. ephedrine, benzoin) should be prescribed to the patient whenever it is essential to ensure the patency of this natural

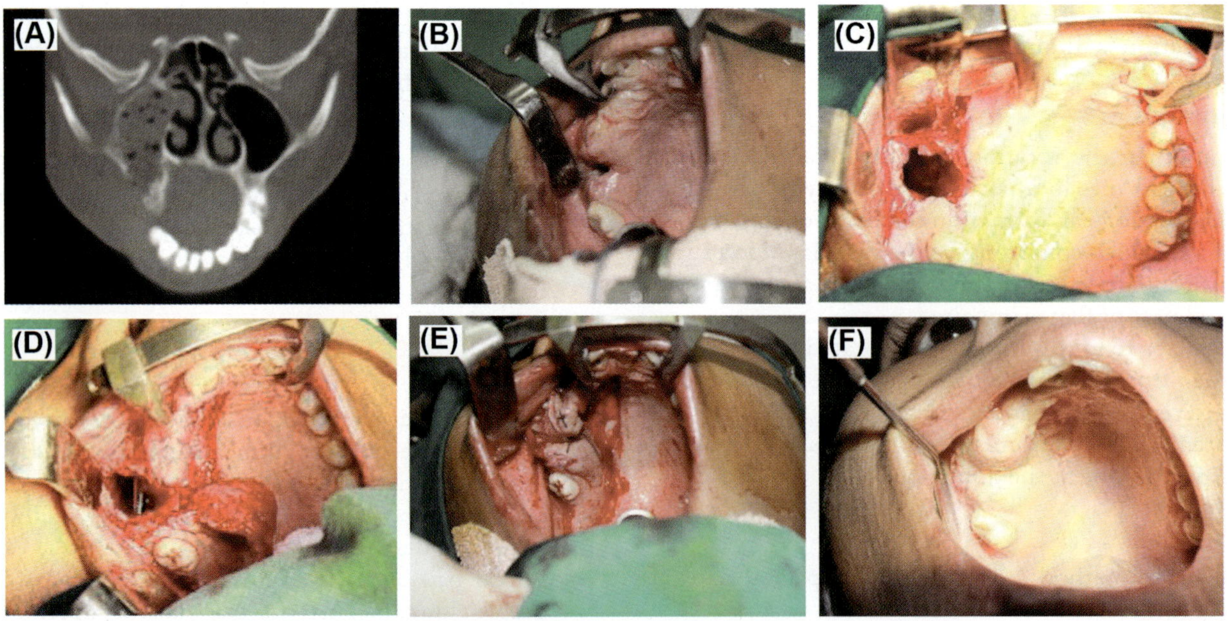

Figure 25.13 Bridge flap in partially edentulous maxilla. (**A**) CT showing infected right maxillary sinus in relation to the edentulous region. Note the complete obliteration of the sinus by the infection. (**B**) Oroantral fistula in relation to the right maxillary edentulous region. (**C**) Excision of the fistulous tract done and buccal flap is raised. (**D**) Raising of the palatal flap based on greater palatine artery. (**E**) Sinus cavity packed with betadine gauze and communication is primarily closed using buccal and palatal flaps. Note the raw area in the palate which will heal by secondary epithelialisation. (**F**) Postoperative view showing complete secondary healing.

opening. Nasal drops should be instituted whenever a freshly created oroantral opening has been repaired and should be continued until healing is complete

4. **Mechanical support for the flap:** Whichever method is utilised to cover the bony defect, additional support for the flap should be provided by covering the area with either an acrylic extension to a denture or a shellac base plate. The cover may be either ligated to adjacent teeth if any are present or sutured to the soft tissue overlying edentulous regions
5. **Nasal antrostomy:** It is performed by introducing a nasal rasp through the nostril below the inferior turbinate bone. It enters the sinus when force is applied. By moving the rasp back and forth, an oblong aperture can be created for drainage of the cavity. Alternatively, nasoantral bone may be removed with an osteotome and the nasal mucosa cut on three sides, leaving it attached only at the floor of the nose so that it can be folded into the antral cavity
   - Along strip of plain or iodoform tape saturated with petrolatum (a uterine pack may be employed) is inserted. End of the tape is pulled through the created stoma and hence the nostril. Since it is to be taken out through the nose, it should be carefully folded into the antral cavity to facilitate the removal. Finally, the mucoperiosteal flap is replaced and primary closure is done.

COMPLICATIONS

The flap might breakdown, either due to poor blood supply owing to improper design or by excessive suture tension. Condition of the antrum should be reviewed carefully, especially if the antrum was not drained by means of a nasoantral perforation. A new closure may be attempted after the infection in the sinus has been cleared up.

CHRONIC OROANTRAL FISTULA

A persistent acute OAC may lead to a chronic oroantral fistula. Any OAF present for more than a period of 15 days is known as chronic oroantral fistula. Due to persistence of the communication, the sinus gets infected by the oral microorganisms. Hence, goal of the treatment should be eradication of the infection and closure of the fistula.

CLINICAL FEATURES

- Continuous unilateral foul smelling nasal discharge
- Unpleasant taste may result due to discharge of postnasal drip down the pharynx from the posterior nares
- Systemic complication includes pyrexia, malaise, headache and anosmia
- Healing of fistulous tract will be delayed by projection of the polyp from the antrum into the oral cavity.

MANAGEMENT

- The 1st aim of treatment is to eliminate any coexisting antral infection. Oroantral reflux can be prevented by insertion of a well-fitting acrylic base plate, which covers the defect without entering it
- The antrum is washed out with warm normal saline, usually via the fistula, twice weekly until a clean return is obtained. Decongestant nasal drops and inhalations are prescribed for use by the patient and antibiotic therapy is sometimes required
- When treatment of this nature is employed most oroantral fistulae shrink in size and may even heal spontaneously, especially if there is any epithelium lining the track is removed either by cauterising the track with a silver nitrate solution or trichloroacetic acid or by freshening the edges of the fistulous tract with a barbed broach
- Antral lining is sometimes said to prolapse through any defect in the bony wall of the maxillary air sinus. It has been proved that these soft tissue projections are usually polypoid in nature. In vast majority of instances, careful examination will reveal presence of an oroantral fistula and a chronically infected antrum. It is imperative that such lesions should be biopsied and sent for histologic examination at the earliest opportunity.

CALDWELL-LUC PROCEDURE

George Caldwell (1893) and Henri Luc (1897) described a new method of entering into the maxillary sinus where two separate openings are made, one in the canine fossa to gain access to the antrum and the other in the nasoantral wall for drainage. Therefore, this procedure has been known as Caldwell-Luc procedure.

Two radical antrum operations have been devised; one is Caldwell-Luc and the other is Denker operation. In Denker operation, perforation in the canine fossa is extended medially to include the piriform aperture and join the window cut under the inferior turbinate bone. Caldwell-Luc operation is preferred, since Denker operation frequently interferes with innervation of the teeth.

INDICATIONS

The Caldwell-Luc procedure is used for:

- Removal of teeth and fragments of roots or impacted teeth in the antrum
- Treatment of chronic maxillary sinusitis with polyps and cystic degeneration of the mucosa
- Excision of cysts and benign tumours of the maxillary sinus
- For management of haematoma or haemorrhage in the maxillary sinus
- To treat fractures involving floor of the orbit or anterior maxillary sinus wall (transantral repair).

SURGICAL PROCEDURE (Fig. 25.14)

- Under anaesthesia (general anaesthesia preferred), incision is placed extending from apex of the canine down to near the gingival margin and posteriorly to the 2nd molar. In edentulous cases, it is carried to and along the alveolar ridge

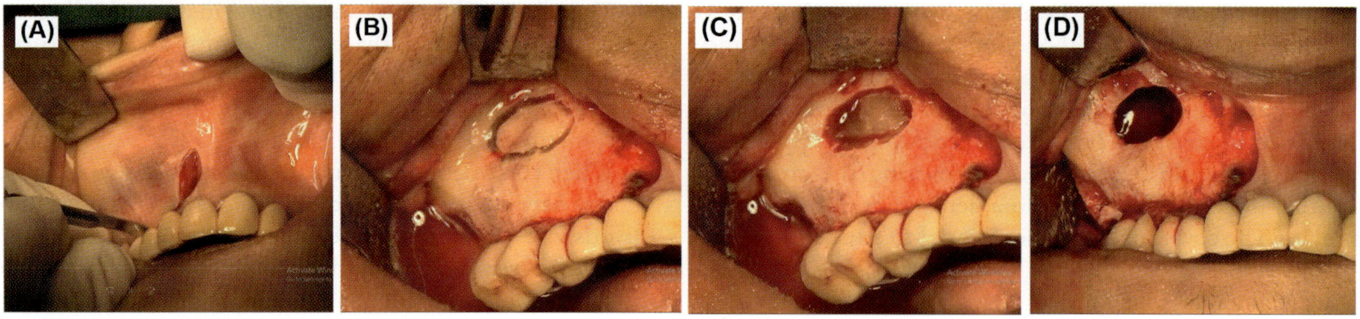

Figure 25.14 Caldwell-Luc surgical procedure. (**A**) Intraoral incision placed in the buccal vestibule. (**B**) Elevation of mucoperiosteal flap and creation of bony window with drill. (**C**) Antral walls showing thickened, hyperplastic tissue. (**D**) Diseased tissue is removed and cavity is allowed to fill with healthy blood clot.

- The incision should be larger than the window to be cut in the bone
- The mucoperiosteum is then detached and retracted till the infraorbital ridge taking care to preserve integrity of the infraorbital nerve
- Bony window is created in canine fossa with the help of drills or gouges or chisels and enlarged to allow introduction of at least the index fingers
- Blood and pus contained in the sinus are removed by means of the aspirator. Bleeding may be arrested by inserting small sponges saturated with adrenaline and antral wall is inspected
- If the entire antral membrane is thickened, hyperplastic or altered by cystic degeneration and filled with polyps, all the diseased tissue should be removed
- Granulomatous tissue may be found on the floor of the sinus if an abscessed tooth has been the cause of the infection or if a perforation has been made while extracting a tooth tissue. A curette may be useful for removing the inflammatory granulation
- Irrigation is done using normal saline and ribbon gauze impregnated with antibiotic solution or paste is placed and removed later (within 5 days) to assist in healing
- The socket should be allowed to fill with a healthy blood clot and finally gingival margins may be approximated by a suture.

POSTOPERATIVE CARE

Advised postoperative antibiotics, analgesics and nasal decongestants. Postoperative sinus instructions (head end up position, avoiding nose blow for 2 weeks). Advised removal of nasal pack after 48 h.

COMPLICATIONS

Complications associated with Caldwell-Luc procedure include facial oedema and pain, bleeding and haematoma, creation of oroantral fistulae, injury to the tooth root (devitalisation), paraesthesia due to involvement of infraorbital and anterior superior alveolar nerves, dacryocystitis (inflammation of the nasolacrimal sac) and persistent epiphora.

TRAUMATIC DISEASE

HAEMATOMA IN MAXILLARY SINUS

A fracture involving infraorbital artery or posterior superior alveolar vessels injury frequently results in a haematoma formation in the maxillary sinus. Usually the blood, which accumulates in the maxillary sinus, is eliminated by the activity of the ciliated epithelium of the antral membrane promoting normal drainage through the ostium. If the haematoma is not removed, infection might occur. Radiologically this is evident by air–fluid demarcation in the CT scan, in contrast to chronic sinusitis where the sinus lining appears as thickened hyperdense mass with central hypodensity of air (Fig. 25.15).

Treatment: Uncontrolled bleeding into sinus with epistaxis may require surgical haemostasis. Surgery consists of a Caldwell-Luc procedure by which the bleeding vessel in the sinus is located. Oxidified cellulose is applied and held in place by an iodoform pack, which is allowed to protrude from the nostril. It may be withdrawn gradually or completely.

IATROGENIC DISEASE

TEETH DISPLACED INTO SINUS

Foreign body, which is usually displaced into the maxillary sinus, is a tooth or a fragment of a tooth root.

AETIOLOGY

1. Absence of intervening bone in between the tooth root and the antrum

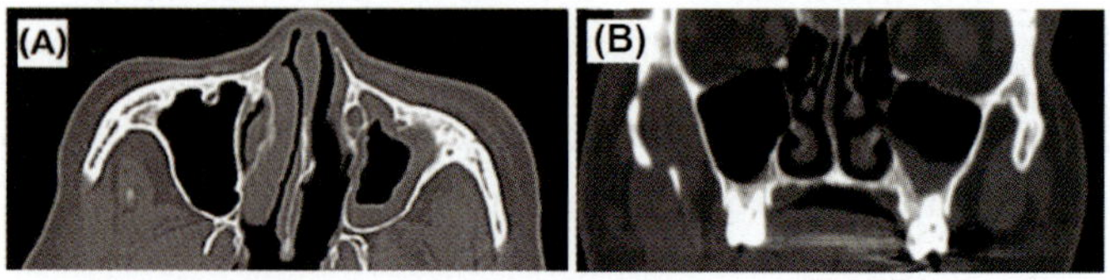

Figure 25.15 (**A**) CT section showing chronic sinusitis (left). Note the thickened hyperdense sinus lining with central hypodensity of air. (**B**) Haematoma in left maxillary sinus due to trauma. Note the air–fluid demarcation.

2. Aggressive instrumentation to retrieve fractured maxillary molar root
3. Solitary maxillary molar around which the bone is dense and cortical, extraction of which may lead to fracture of the alveolus
4. The tooth may displace into the maxillary antrum during extraction just like an orange seed if there is no intervening bone and the instrument slips of the tooth.

DIAGNOSIS

The root fragments do not always penetrate the membrane of the antrum. Frequently they can be found between the membrane and the bony wall. Sometimes a radiograph shows the root in the sinus when it is actually outside between the bone and the mucoperiosteum. Apart from intraoral periapical radiograph (IOPA), upper occlusal posterior nasal spine (PNS) view can also be used.

MANAGEMENT

1. Powerful suction is kept at the entrance of the fistula and the root recovered
2. If the tooth is lying loose in the antrum, it can be removed by packing roller gauze and withdrawing in a jerky motion
3. Surgical approach (Caldwell-Luc operation). Saline is continuously irrigated into the sinus through the window created by the Caldwell-Luc procedure.

Formation of whirlpool inside the sinus is observed, which can displace the root from its position and then it can be retrieved.

FUNGAL DISEASE IN THE MAXILLARY SINUS

Paranasal mycoses is caused by different variety of organisms, the most common being Aspergillus and Mucor. Fungal infections of maxillary sinus manifest as two different entities noninvasive or a benign infection and more serious invasive infection which occurs commonly in immunocompromised individuals (Table 25.3). Symptoms of fungal sinusitis include severe headache, nasal obstruction, rhinorrhoea, severe facial pain and opthalmoplegia at a later stage. Proper and early diagnosis is crucial. Delay in the treatment initiation is life-threatening as the affinity of the fungi to invade the surrounding connective tissue and the blood vessels causes thrombosis and finally leads to necrosis of hard and soft tissue structures.

The organism involved in the most of the fungal disease of the maxillary sinus is aspergillus, which enters the body through inhalation by respiratory system. This organism is confined to maxillary sinus and the foci of infection result in dystrophic calcification and leads to the formation of rhinoliths. These larger rhinoliths are identified as fungal balls. Treatment includes surgical removal of the cause to restore normal ciliary function. Fungal infections in immunocompromised patients such as poorly controlled diabetes mellitus, HIV infections and chemotherapy are more invasive. The extensive nature of the aspergillosis or mucormycosis involves orbit, temporal fossa or oral cavity extending from the maxillary sinus fabricating symptoms and signs suggestive of malignant disease.

TABLE 25.3 Classifications of Fungal Sinusitis

Noninvasive	Invasive
• Saprophytic fungal infestation • Sinus fungal ball (mycetoma) • Allergic fungal sinusitis	• Acute fulminant invasive fungal sinusitis • Chronic invasive fungal sinusitis • Granulomatous invasive fungal sinusitis

FUNCTIONAL ENDOSCOPIC SINUS SURGERY

Functional endoscopic sinus surgery (FESS) (Fig. 25.16) is a minimally invasive technique used to restore sinus ventilation and one of the primary approach used today for the surgical treatment of recurrent acute or chronic infective sinusitis. It is called functional because it aims to return the functioning of the sinuses to normal. This procedure is usually reserved for use in patients in whom medical treatment has failed. To return the mucociliary drainage of the sinuses to normal function.

INDICATIONS

Endoscopic sinus surgery is most commonly performed for inflammatory and infectious sinus diseases. Most common indications for endoscopic sinus surgery are as follows:

- Chronic sinusitis refractory to medical treatment
- Recurrent sinusitis
- Nasal polyposis
- Antrochoanal polyps

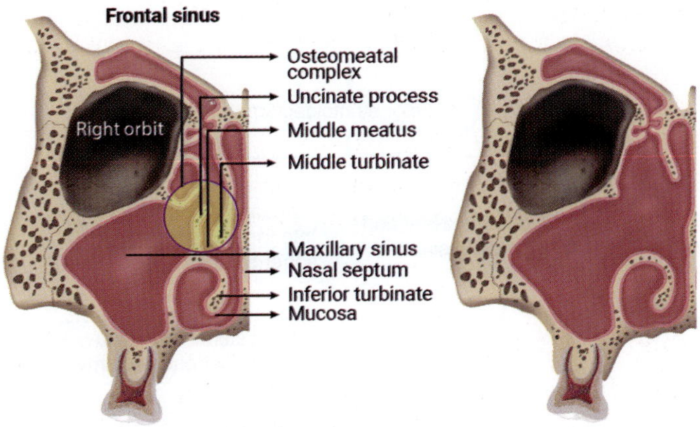

Figure 25.16 Illustration of functional endoscopic sinus surgery (FESS). (Left) Narrowing in the circled region (middle meatus, middle turbinate, uncinate process) may precipitate sinusitis. (Right) After FESS, the osteomeatal area is open.

- Sinus mucoceles
- Excision of selected tumours
- Cerebrospinal fluid (CSF) leak closure
- Orbital decompression (e.g. Graves' ophthalmopathy)
- Optic nerve decompression
- Dacryocystorhinostomy (DCR)
- Choanal atresia repair
- Foreign body removal
- Epistaxis control.

CONTRAINDICATIONS

- Orbital abscess
- Frontal osteomyelitis with Pott's puffy tumour
- Previously failed endoscopic procedures associated with CSF rhinorrhoea and frontal sinus disease
- Nasal and sinus malignancies.

PROCEDURE (Flowchart 25.4)

- After suitable vasoconstriction using cocaine or ephedrine, middle turbinate is identified. This is the most important landmark for the procedure. **Uncinectomy (infundibulotomy):** FESS may begin with uncinectomy either by direct visualisation of the uncinate process or by medialisation of the middle turbinate. On the lateral wall of the nose at the level of the anterior end of the middle turbinate lies the uncinate process. **Maxillary antrostomy:** Now the maxillary sinus ostium, which can be easily identified and visualised following uncinectomy, is enlarged to a diameter of 1 cm so that it allows adequate outflow. **Anterior ethmoidectomy**: Next, the ethmoid bulla should be identified and opened at its interior and medial aspect. This minimal surgery will often be sufficient to greatly improve the function of the ostiomeatal complex and therefore provide better ventilation of the maxillary, ethmoidal and frontal sinuses. If radiographic interpretation shows disease spread to the posterior ethmoidal and sphenoidal cells, then dissection should further continue with **posterior ethmoido-frontosphenoidectomy.** Once the procedure is complete and haemostasis is achieved, an antibiotic gauze pack is placed into the nostril.

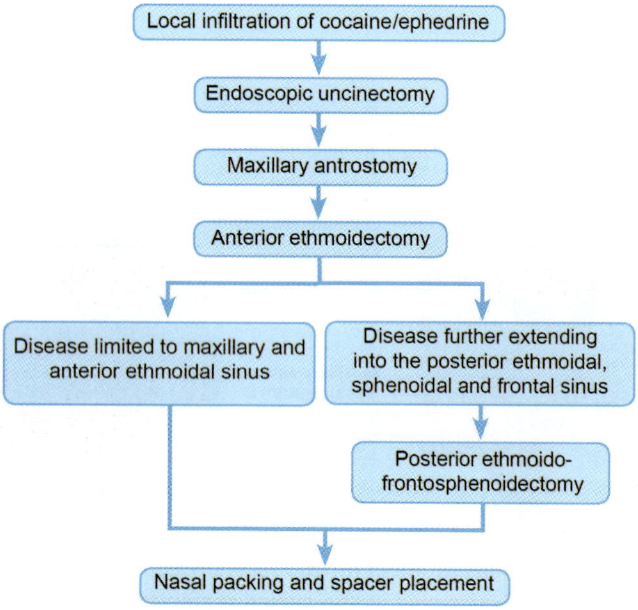

Flowchart 25.4 Functional endoscopic sinus surgery (FESS).

POSTOPERATIVE CARE

Nose should be kept free from build-up of crusts as much as possible. In patients with gross inflammation or polyps, a short course of systemic steroids combined with antibiotics will hasten postoperative recovery. Nasal packing is removed prior to discharge of the patient. The patient is to be discharged with nasal spray and antibiotics, as well as instructions for a follow-up visit in 1 week.

Postoperative complications include bleeding, synechiae formation, orbital injury, diplopia, orbital haematoma, blindness, CS leak, direct brain injury, nasolacrimal duct injury/epiphora, orbital haematoma/postoperative proptosis requires immediate removal of nasal packing, urgent ophthalmologic consultation and emergency lateral canthotomy.

EXTENDED USES OF FESS

- Endoscopic dacryocystorhinostomy
- Endoscopic orbital decompression.

EPISTAXIS

Epistaxis or nosebleed is a common problem seen in children and elderly patients. Failure to control the bleeding might result in life-threatening problems. While trauma is the most common cause, epistaxis can be associated with an underlying conditions such as bleeding disorders, anatomic disorders, telangiectasia and intranasal tumours. The most common site of epistaxis is from the anterior nasal septum (Little's area or Kiesselbach's plexus), which is an area of vascular anastomosis of five arteries that supply the nasal septum. Bleeding during surgical procedures can lead to the formation of haematoma within the sinus, which might get infected secondarily. Therefore, it is important to control bleeding. Minor bleeding at this site can be controlled simply by pinching of nose or by cauterisation. Whereas major bleeding from the posterior region of nasal cavity (spheno-ethmoidal recess) and epistaxis associated with midface trauma necessitate more aggressive treatment. Management of the cases that are refractory to medical measures and cauterisation requires nasal packing (anterior or posterior nasal packs) under antibiotic coverage. Foley catheter can be used for posterior nasal packing. If these above measures fail, surgical management by arterial embolisation is considered to control bleeding.

Section VIII

Maxillofacial Pathologies

Chapter 26

Cysts of the Oral Cavity

OUTLINE

DEFINITION

Killey and Key (1966): Cyst is defined as an epithelium-lined sac filled with fluid or semifluid material.

Kramer (1974): 'Cyst is defined as a pathological cavity having fluid, semifluid or gaseous contents and which is not created by the accumulation of pus'. Most cysts, but not all, are lined by epithelium.

True cysts: Cysts which are lined by epithelium, for example, dentigerous cyst, radicular cyst.

Pseudocysts: Cysts which are not lined by epithelium, for example, solitary bone cysts, aneurysmal bone cysts, traumatic bone cysts and mucous extravasation cysts. Few authors describe pseudocysts as the pathological cavities not lined by epithelium.

CLASSIFICATION

According to **Shear**, the cysts were classified under three main categories:

A. Cysts of jaws.
B. Cysts associated with the maxillary antrum.
C. Cysts of the soft tissues of the mouth, face, neck and salivary glands.

SHEAR'S CLASSIFICATION (Flowchart 26.1)

Odontogenic cysts refer to the cysts arising from tooth-forming tissues. Nonodontogenic cysts refer to the cysts arising from ectoderm involved in the development of the facial tissues or fissures.

JOSEPH REGEZI'S CLASSIFICATION BASED ON THE TISSUE OF ORIGIN (Table 26.1)

In the WHO classification (2005), the odontogenic keratocysts (OKC) were considered as benign tumours, as they closely correspond to neoplastic lesions, and are classified as keratocystic odontogenic tumour. Both Regezi and Shafer considered OKC as cyst and not a tumour. Reclassification of OKC and calcifying odontogenic cyst (COC) (calcifying cystic odontogenic tumour) remains a controversy and has not been fully accepted.

PATHOGENESIS AND DEVELOPMENT OF CYST

The pathogenesis of cysts basically originates from the remnants of the embryonic tissue responsible for the teeth and jaw development. The formation of a cyst involves various steps:

- Attraction of fluid into the cystic cavity
- Retention of fluid inside the cavity
- Increase in internal hydrostatic pressure
- Increase in size of the cavity by resorption of the surrounding bone.

Cyst formation requires three elements: A source of epithelium, a stimulus for epithelial proliferation, and bone resorption with cyst growth. Thus, the development of a cyst has been explained under three phases: (1) *cyst initiation,* (2) *cyst formation* and (3) *cyst enlargement or expansion* (Fig. 26.1).

CYST INITIATION (SOURCE OF EPITHELIUM)

Odontogenic cysts arise from the remnants of dental lamina, reduced enamel epithelium, cell rests of Malassez within the jaw

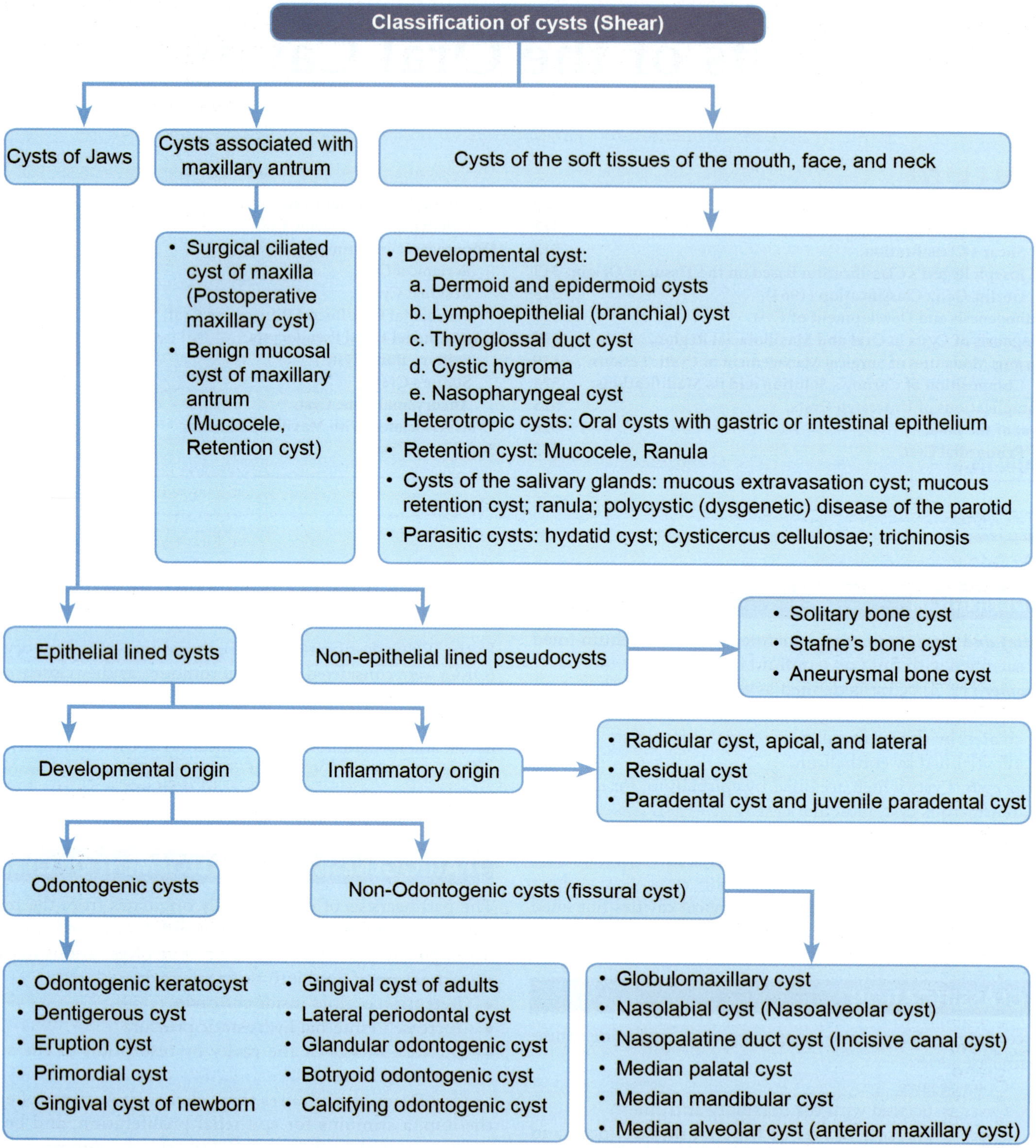

Flowchart 26.1 Classification of cysts according to Shear.

TABLE 26.1 Joseph Regezi's Classification Based on the Tissue of Origin

Type	Source	Origin of Rests	Example
Odontogenic rests	Rest of Malassez	Epithelial root sheath	• Periapical (radicular) cyst • Residual cyst
	Reduced enamel epithelium	Enamel organ	• Dentigerous cyst • Eruption cyst • Calcifying odontogenic cyst
	Rests of dental lamina (rest of Serres)	Epithelial connection between mucosa and enamel organ	• Odontogenic keratocyst (OKC) • Gingival cyst of newborn • Gingival cyst of adult • Lateral periodontal cyst • Glandular odontogenic cyst
Nonodontogenic rests	Remnants of nasopalatine duct	Paired nasopalatine duct (vestigial)	• Nasopalatine canal cyst • Thyroglossal tract cyst • Nasolabial cyst

GORLIN-GOLTZ CLASSIFICATION (1964) (Table 26.2)

TABLE 26.2 Gorlin-Goltz Classification (1964)

A. Odontogenic cysts
- Dentigerous cyst
- Eruption cyst
- Gingival cyst of newborn infants
- Lateral periodontal and gingival cyst of adults
- Keratinising and calcifying cyst (OKC)
- Radicular cyst
- Primordial cyst
- Multiple cysts of jaws and multiple cutaneous nevoid basal cell carcinoma and skeletal anomalies

B. Nonodontogenic and fissural cysts
- Globulomaxillary cyst (premaxilla maxillary cyst)
- Nasoalveolar (nasolabial Klestadt's) cyst
- Nasopalatine (median anterior maxillary) cyst
- Median mandibular cyst
- Anterior lingual cyst
- Dermoid and epidermoid cyst
- Palatal cyst of newborn infants

C. Cysts of neck and floor of mouth and salivary gland
- Thyroglossal duct cyst
- Lymphoepithelial (branchial cleft) cyst
- Oral cysts with gastric or intestinal epithelium
- Salivary gland cyst
- Mucocoele and ranula

D. Pseudocyst
- Aneurysmal bone cyst
- Static (developmental latent) bone cyst
- Traumatic (haemorrhagic solitary) bone cyst

or gingiva, or from the accumulation of fluid between the reduced enamel epithelium and the crown of an erupted tooth. The *cyst of infective* origin arises from the bacterial invasion and inflammatory components. The factors/stimulus that may be responsible for cyst initiation include genetics, immunological compromise, inflammatory mediators or local factors such as decreased oxygen tension and increased carbon dioxide tension.

CYST FORMATION (EPITHELIAL PROLIFERATION)

After initiation, the *epithelial cells proliferate to form a mass*. The innermost cells become deprived of nutrients and blood supply, resulting in liquefactive necrosis in the centre and leading to cyst formation. Release of proteolytic enzymes and high levels of acid phosphate activity in the central cells results in central degeneration along with proliferation of surrounding epithelium, leading to the formation of several microcysts (central cavity surrounded by viable epithelium). These microcysts increase in size and coalesce to form a single large cyst.

CYST ENLARGEMENT OR EXPANSION

Once the cysts are formed, it continue to grow and enlarge slowly for over months. The process of cyst enlargement is similar for all epithelium-lined cysts, with some variations. Breakdown of cellular debris within the cyst lumen increases the *osmotic pressure*, resulting in fluid transport into the lumen and this fluid ingress produces outward growth of the cyst. Many theories have been put forth to explain the mechanism of cyst enlargement.

THEORIES OF CYST ENLARGEMENT OR EXPANSION

Malcolm Harris (1975) proposed various theories of cyst expansion in the following manner:

1. Mural growth theory
2. Osmotic theory/hydrostatic enlargement
3. Bone resorption theory.

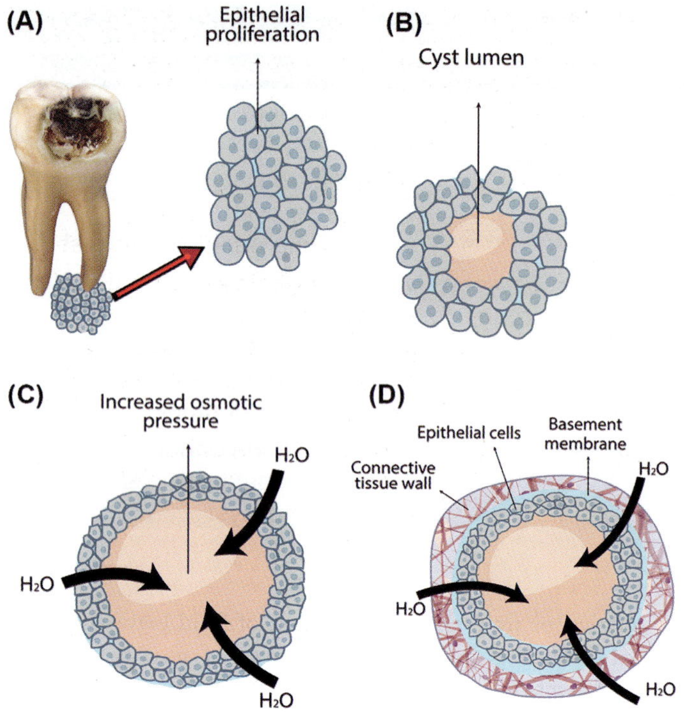

Figure 26.1 Mechanism of cyst development. (**A**) Proliferation of epithelium to form a mass. (**B**) Liquefactive necrosis of cells in the centre forming lumen. (**C**) Expansion of the cyst due to increase in osmotic pressure. (**D**) Cyst maturation and expansion with resorption of bone.

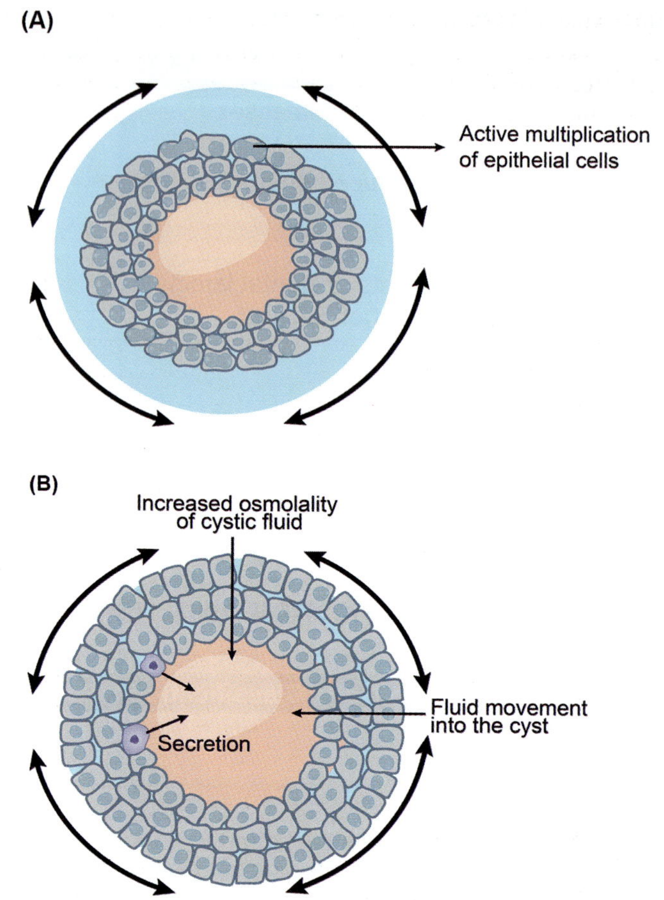

Figure 26.2 Theories of cyst expansion. (**A**) Mural theory. Cyst enlargement by active division of the peripheral lining epithelial cells. (**B**) Hydrostatic pressure. Cyst enlargement by osmolarity.

MURAL GROWTH THEORY (Fig. 26.2A)

Cyst expansion by this theory is explained by two proportions.

a. ***Peripheral cell division:***
   The surface area of the cystic sac increases due to *active division of the peripheral lining epithelial cells*, in response to any irritating stimulus. The contents of a cyst support the cystic lining and also cause rapid resorption of surrounding bone to accommodate the enlarging cyst. Cyst regression takes place following the removal of the stimulus.
b. ***Accumulation of cellular contents:***
   Kramer (1974) explained that as the *mural squamous cells are shed off the lining epithelium, they accumulate* and increase the keratocyst volume. The sites of expansion and growth are represented by finger-like projections which are zones of active cell division or proliferation.

The growth of OKC, although persistent, is a poor bone resorber and extends preferentially along the less dense cancellous bone with little resorption and expansion of dense cortex.

This explains why keratocyst very rarely causes expansion or resorption of the cortical plates.

Kubota et al., (2002) showed in his study that interleukin **(IL)-1α** stimulates enzymatic degradation of extracellular matrices of the bone around the cyst causing expansion of OKC.

Oka et al., (2005) proposed that the positive intracystic fluid pressure in OKCs stimulates the expression of IL-1α in epithelial cells.

OSMOTIC THEORY/HYDROSTATIC ENLARGEMENT (Fig. 26.2B)

The *pressure difference and increased intraluminal concentration* inside the cystic cavity than the peripheral surroundings, influences the fluid movement into the cyst, resulting in increase in the size of cyst. The fluid moves into the cyst from the surrounding area and the cysts start to expand and grow in size.

James and Tratman proposed the osmotic theory or dialysis to explain the hydrostatic enlargement of the cyst. The mean *osmolality of cystic fluid is 10 millimoles higher than the serum*. This gradient causes the accumulation of all the shed degenerated cells from the cyst lining. In addition, the *inadequate lymphatic drainage* further favours the accumulation of the fluid from the capsular capillaries thereby aiding the cyst enlargement. Accumulation of fluid within the cyst wall causes secondary proliferation of epithelial cells and expansion of the cyst wall. Thus, plasma protein exudate, hyaluronic acid, products of epithelial cell breakdown together contribute to the high osmotic pressure of the cystic fluid, causing bone resorption and cyst enlargement.

BONE RESORPTION THEORY

Harris et al., proposed that the cystic capsule contains very potent *bone resorbing factors like prostaglandin PGE2, PGE3 and leukotrines* (Keratocysts are found to secrete very less amount of bone resorbing factors per unit surface area compared to other cysts. This explains the burrowing nature or intramedullary growth of the keratocyst). *Increased internal pressure* also causes bone resorption and enlargement of cyst cavity. This bony expansion causes *egg shell crackling* on palpation due to microcracks on the thinned out cortical bone. Complete resorption and perforation of cortical bone occurs on further expansion.

CYST REGRESSION

Any process that leads to the involution of cyst epithelium, for example, extraction of tooth or reduction of intracystic pressure as with marsupialisation, may cause connective tissue capsule to regress and the cavity to be filled by bone or scar tissue.

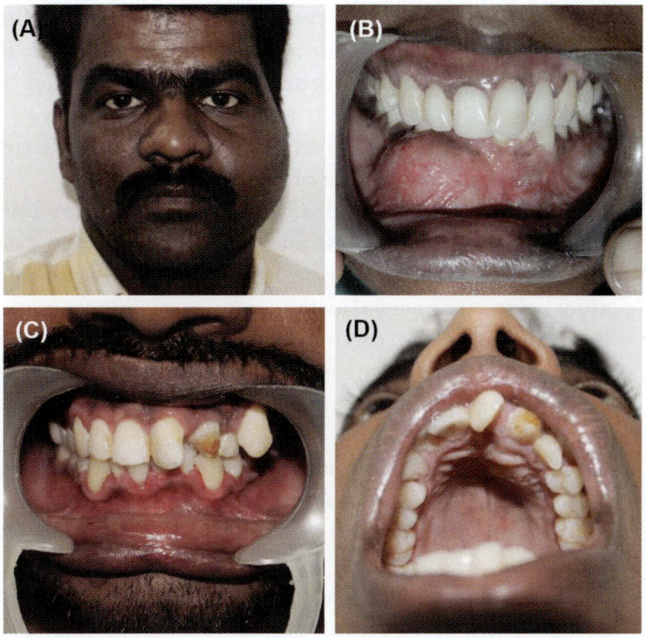

Figure 26.3 Clinical presentation of cysts. **(A)** Extraoral expansion of the cyst causing facial deformity. **(B)** Intraoral expansion of cyst seen as swelling in the lower vestibular region. **(C)** Supernumerary teeth in relation to maxillary left lateral incisor area associated with the periapical cyst. **(D)** Note the cystic expansion of the palatal area.

DIAGNOSIS OF CYSTS IN ORAL AND MAXILLOFACIAL REGION

In jaws, the odontogenic cysts are more prevalent than the nonodontogenic cyst. Odontogenic cysts are the 2nd most common oral lesions in adults. The commonest being periapical cyst, dentigerous cyst and OKC.

The peak incidence of jaw cyst is between 21 and 30 years, and are more prevalent in males than females.

CLINICAL PRESENTATION (Fig. 26.3)

The patient often presents with complaints of pain, swelling, discharge, sinus tract, deranged occlusion and delayed eruption of teeth.

1. *Expansion of the jaw*—The cysts can be small or large. A small cyst can be detected only as an incidental finding, as they do not produce any signs and symptoms. As the cyst grows larger, the expansion of the bone usually occurs on the buccal aspect of the jaw (*buccal cortical expansion*). Expansion in the lingual aspect of the jaw are usually seen in the cysts of ramus and 3rd molar area.
   - This expansion of the cyst stimulates the periosteum to form a *new layer of bone* (subperiosteal bone), which later forms the outline of the affected portion of the jaw
   - In the early stage, the bony expansion will be smooth, hard and painless, and can obliterate the buccal vestibule intraorally. As the cyst expands, the bone covering the centre of the convexity of the cyst becomes thinned and can be *indented with pressure*. This consistency is described as elastic
   - The cyst with an outer-thinned cortex can be described as *'Ping Pong/Table Tennis Ball'* with spring consistency
   - In few cases, when the periosteum is not able to maintain the new bone formation, it results in area of summit of convexity or *'window' formation*. This window presents as round and smooth margins
   - Later on, the fragile outer shell of the bone becomes fragmented and cracks, producing a sensation of *'egg shell cracking'* on palpation
   - In advanced cases, the bone pieces might disappear and the cyst lining lies immediately beneath the mucosa, eliciting *fluctuation on palpation*. A cyst that has encroached on the soft tissues appears as a compressible and fluctuant swelling
   - Very rarely, the larger cysts can cause pathological fracture of the jaw bone
   - Progressive enlargement of the cyst leads to eventual *discharge of the fluid* into the mouth. In some cases, the discharge of fluid from the cyst can be detected as a *sinus* tract, either intraorally or extraorally and the patient may complain of salty taste
2. Cysts are generally *painless*, unless they get secondarily infected

3. Large expansion of the cyst can cause *loosening of the adjacent teeth*. In edentulous patients, *a change in the fitting of denture* may occur due to the presence of swelling
4. *Missing* one or more *teeth* without history of extraction may indicate the presence of dentigerous or OKC
5. The teeth adjoining an OKC, fissural cyst, solitary bone cyst, nonodontogenic cyst and lateral periodontal cysts are *vital*, whereas those associated with radicular or periapical cysts are *nonvital tooth*
6. Percussion of the teeth overlying the solitary bone cyst produces a *dull or hollow sound* in contrast with the high-pitched note produced by percussing normal teeth
7. Large and infected cyst exerts pressure on the neurovascular bundle resulting in *neuroparaxia* of the nerve. Surgical drainage of the infection returns the sensation back to normal
8. *Site of occurrence*—Dentigerous cysts are usually associated with impacted canines, premolars and molars. OKC are often associated with the lower 3rd molar region extending into the ramus. Fissural cysts like nasopalatine cysts are usually confined to the upper jaw, whereas Stafne's bone cyst exclusively occurs beneath the mandibular canal. Solitary bone cyst usually occurs in the mandible, whereas periodontal cyst can occur anywhere in the alveolar process
9. If infected cyst is present inside the maxillary antrum, signs of *sinusitis* can occur. A large cyst under the nasal floor can cause distortion of the nostril.

RADIOGRAPHIC EXAMINATION (Fig. 26.4)

Periapical and occlusal views give essential information as far as small cysts are concerned. For large cysts, extraoral radiographs like lateral oblique and PA view of the mandible along with the intraoral radiographs. Occlusal radiographs are especially used for viewing the extent of palatal bone destruction in the cysts of the maxilla. Waters view is used for cysts in maxillary sinus. Orthopantomogram helps in viewing the entire jaw.

- A typical odontogenic cyst appears as a *well-defined round or oval radiolucency* circumscribed by a sharp radiopaque margin. Intrabony cysts can present as unilocular or multilocular radiolucency with or without cortication
- The shape of the cyst varies depending on the type of cyst: Oval or round for dentigerous cyst, scalloped margins in OKC, heart shape in nasopalatine cyst
- Cortical expansions, perforations, displacement of the adjacent structures or pathological fracture can also be seen.

ASPIRATION (Fig. 26.5)

The fluid inside the cystic cavity varies in colour, consistency and protein content that helps in differentiating the various

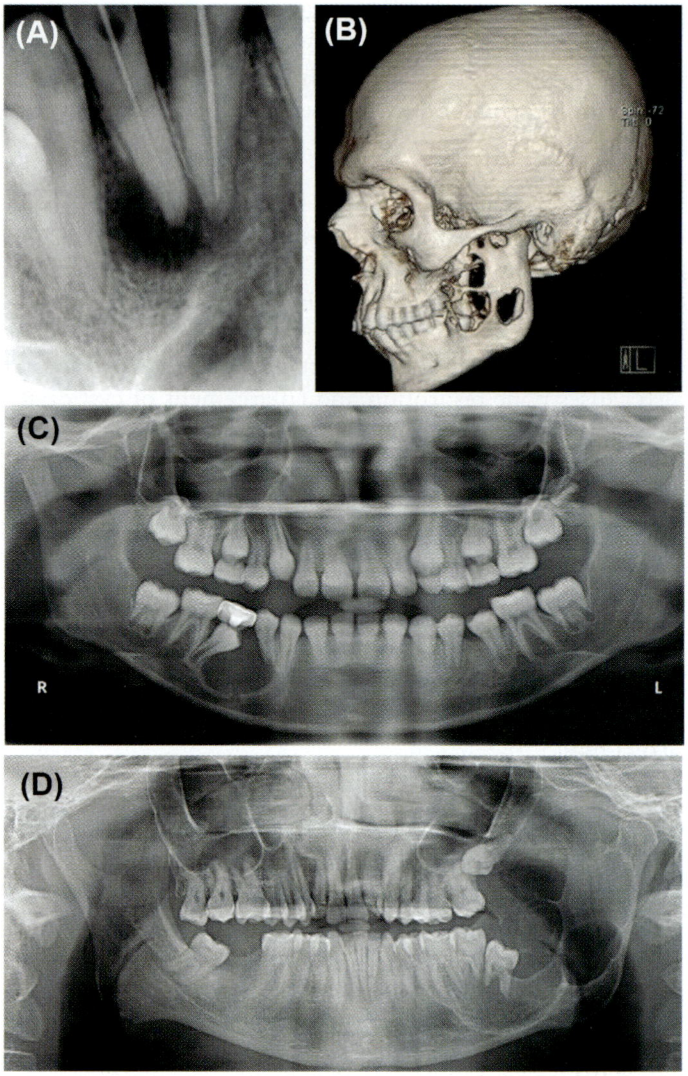

Figure 26.4 Radiographic presentation of cysts. (**A**) IOPA showing well-defined radiolucency in the periapical region of 42. (**B**) 3D CT scan showing multilocular radiolucency in the left side of mandible. (**C**) OPG showing well-defined unilocular radiolucency with sclerotic margin in the right mandibular premolar region. (**D**) OPG showing multilocular radiolucency in the left side of mandibular ramus, angle and body region.

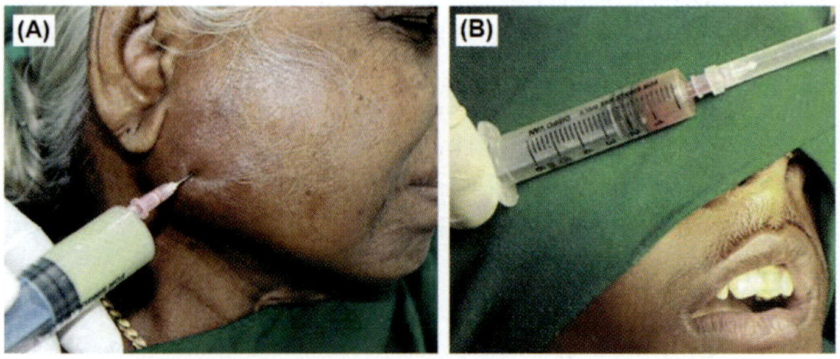

Figure 26.5 (**A**) Aspiration of pus from an infected cyst of mandible. (**B**) Blood tinged straw-coloured fluid.

TABLE 26.3 Cystic Lesions and their Aspirates

Type of Cysts	Aspirate Colour	Other Features
Dentigerous cyst	Clear, pale straw colour fluid	Contains cholesterol crystals Purulent material if infected Total protein >4.0 g/100 mL
OKC	Dirty, creamy white, viscous fluid	Parakeratinised or orthokeratinised epithelium keratin flakes Total protein <4.0 g/100 mL (majority of content is albumin)
Periodontal cyst	Serous caseous content	Contains cholesterol crystals Total protein content between 5 and 11 g/100 mL
Infected radicular cyst	Contains pus or brownish fluid	Contains inflammatory cells like polymorphonuclear leukocytes, foam cells, cholesterol crystals
Gingival cyst	Clear fluid	
Mucocoele/ranula	Viscous and thick mucous	
Solitary bone cyst	Serous or serosanguinous fluid, sometimes with blood or empty cavity	
Stafne's bone cyst	Empty cavity filled with air	
Dermoid cyst	Thick sebaceous material	
Fissural cyst	Mucoid material	
Haemangioma/arteriovenous (AV) malformation	Dark venous blood/bright red blood, pulsatile	
Unicystic ameloblastoma	Chocolate brown fluid	

cysts. Aspiration biopsy indicates the nature of the cystic lesion and hence used for initial diagnosis of cysts.

Aspiration of the intralesional fluid is done under local anaesthesia (LA) with the help of a *wide bore needle of 18 gauge and 5 mL syringe*. The needle is introduced at the thinner area of the cyst and aspirated. The aspirated cystic fluids can range from clear yellow to cheesy material (Table 26.3).

Analysis of the cystic fluid's protein content (albumin, globulin, keratin flecks and total protein) can be done using biochemical techniques. When the air is aspirated, it is an indication that the needle has entered the antrum. When aspiration yields no contents, it is a sign that there is a tumour growing.

BIOPSY

Biopsy is the gold standard for determining the type of cysts and arriving at a final diagnosis. Refer to chapter 6 for incisional biopsy and for larger lesions and excisional biopsy for small lesions.

VARIOUS MODALITIES OF SURGICAL MANAGEMENT OF CYSTIC LESIONS (Flowchart 26.2)

Goals of surgery

- Complete elimination of the pathologic lesion
- Minimal destruction and damage to the adjacent structures
- Decrease the recurrence rate and morbidity of the patient
- Restore normal function and aesthetics

Factors to be considered before surgical treatment

- Patient's age and their general health
- Number of cystic lesions (solitary/multiple)
- Location of the lesion
- Cortical perforation
- Involvement into the adjacent structures
- Presence or absence of infection
- History of recurrence
- Size of the lesion
- Histological variant of the lesion
- Pulp vitality of the related teeth
- Risk of pathological fracture
- Requirement of bone graft and reconstruction plate.

Surgical treatment

The principle treatment of the cyst involve complete removal of the cyst lining with preservation of the adjacent vital structures like the neurovascular bundle, nasal or antral lining mucosa. The surgical procedures in the treatment of jaw cysts are placed under two categories: Conservative and aggressive surgical management.

1. CONSERVATIVE SURGICAL TREATMENT

i. Decompression

Decompression of cysts is a less invasive surgical procedure than enucleation and marsupialisation, to *create a small bony*

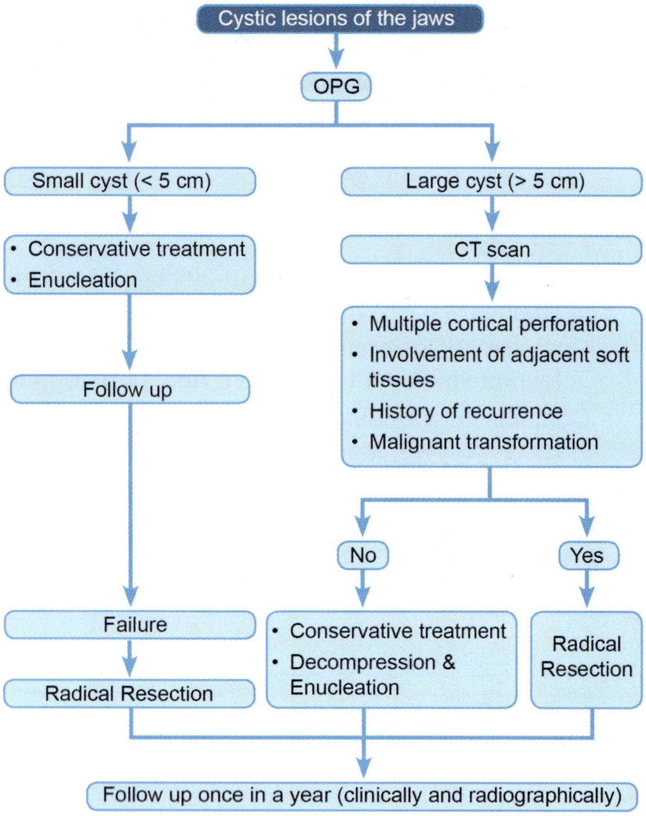

Flowchart 26.2 Algorithm for the management of cystic lesions of jaw.

window and decrease the intracystic pressure by constant drainage. The aim of decompression is to decrease the intracystic hydrostatic pressure, and encourage the formation of new bone from the bony cystic walls with minimal complications (Fig. 26.6).

Procedure

Decompression can be achieved under LA, by creating a small opening in the cystic wall and keeping the opening patent by suturing a drain to the peripheral overlying mucosa. The patency of the opening can be maintained by suturing devices such as drains, acrylic tubes, polyethylene tubes, Luer's syringes, nasal cannulas, intravenous tubes or gauze to its periphery. Through the opening, the cystic lumen can be irrigated with saline or antiseptic wash twice or thrice a day. This reduces the intramural pressure and encourages new bone formation.

Advantage

It spares the tissue, minimises the damage to the adjacent structures, and avoids hospitalisation.

Disadvantages

The duration of treatment, discomfort, patient compliance and chance of recurrence of the cyst from the remaining remnants of epithelium.

Decompression are more successful for patients under 30 years of age and are mainly performed to avoid morbidity. It can be performed as a single, complete procedure or combined with subsequent enucleation, depending on the type of the cyst.

ii. Marsupialisation/cystotomy/Partsch I operation (Figs. 26.7 and 26.8)

Principle

It was 1st described by Partsch in 1892. It is a surgical procedure, where a cystic sac is transformed into an open pouch, through a *wide opening* in the superficial aspect of the cyst. It aims at releasing the intraluminal pressure with progressive reduction of the volume and size of the lesion, and promotes a gradual growth of a new bone. It is basically a surgical externalisation of the cystic cavity.

It involves surgical resection/ostectomy of the cortical bone and partial removal of the external cystic wall. The removed cystic wall is sent for biopsy and the remaining borders of the cystic wall are sutured to the surrounding oral

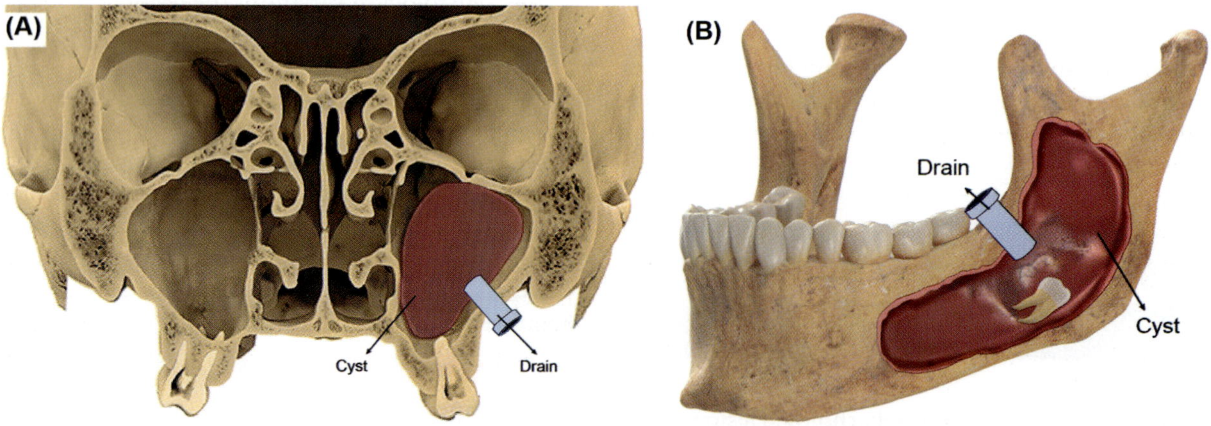

Figure 26.6 Decompression of a cyst with a drain sutured to the oral mucosa. (**A**) Cyst in the left maxilla. (**B**) Cyst involving the body, angle and ramus of mandible.

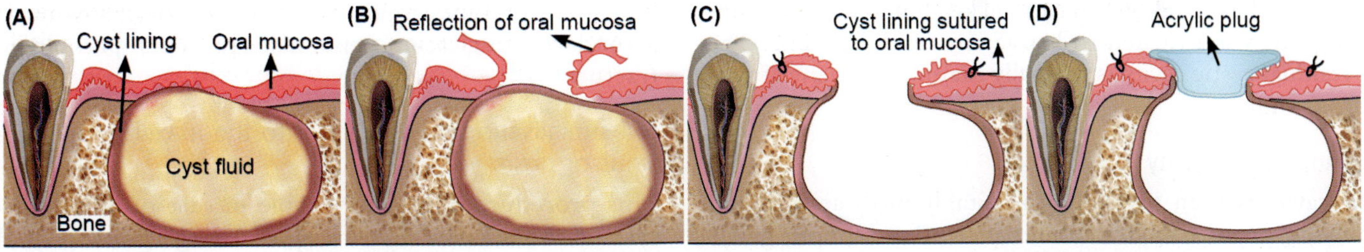

Figure 26.7 Marsupialisation procedure. (**A**) Cyst covered by oral mucosa. (**B**) Incision and reflection of mucosa. Creation of a window by removing the bone and epithelial lining. (**C**) The lining at the cystic boundaries are turned outwards and sutured to the adjacent oral mucosa. The cystic contents are irrigated and packed with gauze. (**D**) An acrylic plug is placed to cover the defect.

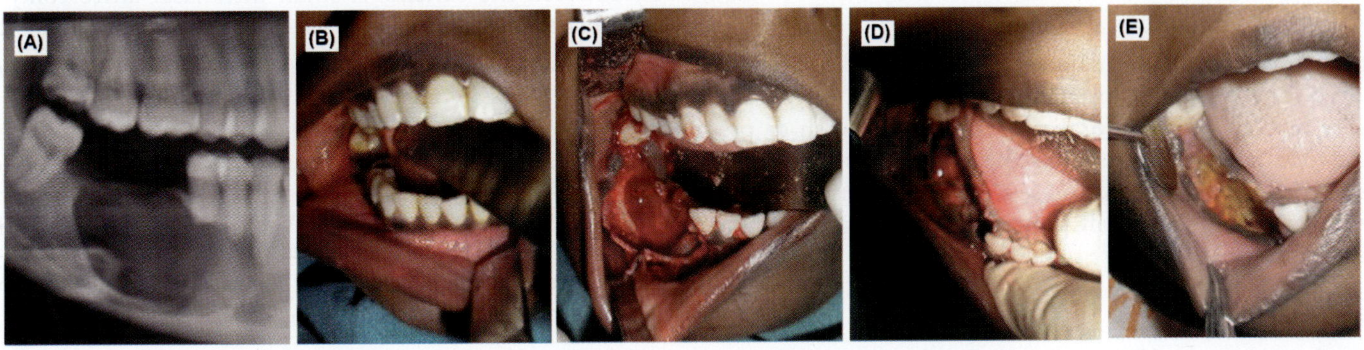

Figure 26.8 Marsupialisation. (**A**) OPG showing well-defined radiolucency involving the right side body of mandible. (**B**) Transoral approach to the cyst. (**C**) Creation of window on the roof of the cyst. (**D**) The patency of the cystic cavity is maintained by suturing the cyst lining to the oral mucosa. (**E**) Healing cystic cavity after 2 weeks.

mucosa. Thus converting an enclosed cystic sac into an open pouch. It generally requires frequent gauze packing or obturators to prevent food impaction and infection. Marsupialisation can be used as a solo regime or combined with secondary enucleation.

Indications

- Very large cyst
- Large cyst with difficult surgical access
- Cysts lying in close proximity to the vital structures
- Young children with developing tooth buds (to preserve the tooth germ and guide the eruption of developing teeth)
- When the root apices of many adjacent teeth are involved in a cyst (to maintain the vitality of these teeth)
- Possibility of pathological fracture of the jaw bone during enucleation
- Medically compromised patients.

Advantages

- It is a relatively simple procedure and can be done under LA
- Prevents injury to the adjacent vital structures
- Avoids pathological fracture of the jaw bone
- Maintains the vitality of teeth and avoid extraction
- Gradually decreases the size of cystic cavity and reduces the intracystic pressure
- It induces endosteal bone formation
- The fragile cystic lining may become thick, favouring secondary enucleation.

Disadvantages

- Leaving a pathological lining behind, might pose a risk of recurrence or neoplastic changes in the future
- Longer healing time in older patients
- Needs patient cooperation to maintain hygiene
- Requires repeated irrigations and long follow-up
- Need for secondary surgical intervention
- Formation of tissue pockets may lodge food material.

Surgical technique (Partsch I operation)

Marsupialisation can be performed either under general or local anaesthesia.

Elevation of flap: An elliptical, oval, circular or inverted U-shaped incision are made in the buccal sulcus with a broad base and a mucoperiosteal flap is reflected.

Removal of bone: A bony window of 1 cm is created by using burs or rongeurs.

Removal of cystic lining: The cystic lining in the window created can be sent for biopsy. The thinned out bony cortex and the oral mucosa covering the surgical window is removed.

Suturing: The lining at the cystic boundaries are turned outwards and sutured to the adjacent oral mucosa.

Irrigation: The cystic contents are sucked out and the remaining cavity is irrigated to lavage any residual debris. The residual cystic cavity is carefully examined for any abnormal findings.

Packing of the cavity

The cavity is then packed with suitably medicated ribbon gauze to prevent food contamination. For example, gauze soaked in Whitehead's varnish (Box 26.1) or tincture of benzoin or liquid paraffin, or an antibiotic ointment, or bismuth iodine paraffin paste (BIPP paste), with the gauze end protruding through the cyst opening.

Maintenance of cavity

Approximately after 10 days of operation, the pack is removed. The patient is instructed to clean and irrigate the cavity regularly with an oral antiseptic mouthwash to prevent food accumulation. After the wound has completely healed, it is recommended to use a durable material that can be plugged in it. This will preserve the healing cavity and ensure that the cyst orifice remains patent.

Healing and follow-up

The slow process of bone regeneration begins and the patient is reviewed at monthly intervals for progressive reduction in the depth of the plug, but the diameter at the opening must be fully maintained. For large cysts, the patient is usually under surveillance for 18–20 months before he/she is able to discard the plug. Although there is often extensive bone regeneration, the alveolar contour usually has a degree of depression and distortion.

Modifications of marsupialisation

Waldron's method—two-stage procedure—marsupialisation followed by enucleation

Once the large cyst is marsupialised, the cystic lesion regresses in size and bone healing progresses. The smaller size cystic cavity is then removed completely by enucleation as a secondary surgery. This two-stage procedure is known as Waldron's method.

The 2nd surgery (enucleation) is done when the adequate bone is formed around the adjacent vital structures. This new bone prevents injury to the vital structures during secondary enucleation, and also prevents pathological fracture.

BOX 26.1 Composition of Whitehead's Varnish

- Benzoin: 10 grams
- Iodoform: 10 grams
- Storax: 7.5 grams
- Balsam of Tolu: 5 grams
- Solvent ether upto 100 mL.

Marsupialisation by opening into the maxillary sinus or nose

This procedure can be applicable in case of an extensive cyst of the maxilla that occupies a large portion of the antrum.

The entire cystic lining is removed unless there is concern about the damage to adjacent vital structures. The partition between the cyst and antrum is removed to provide continuity between the cavities. A small intranasal antrostomy is established by packing the cyst cavity with any one of the following:

- Iodoform gauze coated with tincture benzoin
- Antral balloon
- Foley's catheter with balloon
- Sterile polyethylene tube.

A curved hemostat is passed via the nostrils into the antrostomy made in inferior meatus and the end of the drain is pulled outwards and secured by means of a suture or tape. The wound is closed without tension.

iii. Enucleation/cystectomy/Partsch II

Enucleation is 'complete removal or excision of the cyst and its contents in toto without rupture'. Surgical enucleation of a cyst in one piece helps in reducing the rate of recurrence. Enucleation can be done with or without adjunct procedures and has been the most recommended surgical modality for all the orofacial cysts.

Complete excision of the cyst is possible because of the presence of a fibrous connective tissue layer between the cystic lining and bony wall. This layer acts as cleavage point and helps in separating the cyst from the bone. A mucoperiosteal flap covers the cyst cavity, and blood clots fill it up, which eventually transforms into a new bone.

Indications

- Small cysts
- Small or large cysts not endangering vital structures, tooth vitality or risk of pathologic fracture
- Cysts as OKC that have a high recurrence rate
- Medically fit patients with larger lesions
- As a 2nd stage procedure after decompression or marsupialisation.

Advantages

- Primary closure and rapid healing of the wound
- Entire cystic lining is removed making the pathologic tissue available for microscopic study
- Chances of recurrence of cyst are reduced when used along with adjunct procedures
- Easy oral hygiene maintenance

- Postoperative treatment is reduced
- Comfortable for the patient.

Disadvantages

- Direct observation of wound healing is not possible due to primary closure
- In young people, tooth germ or unerupted teeth involved with the cyst are extracted or removed along with the lesion
- Removal of large cyst can make the jaw more prone to pathological fracture
- Possibility of damage to the adjacent vital structures
- Damage to the adjacent teeth or pulp necrosis.

Surgical procedure (enucleation with primary closure)

Enucleation of smaller cysts are done under LA, whereas the larger cysts can be treated under general anaesthesia (GA). The approach (intra or extraoral) and the mucoperiosteal flap are designed based on the location and size of the lesion.

If the overlying bone is thin, access to the cyst is achieved by removing the cortical bone using rongeurs. But if the overlying bone is thick and hard, then the bony window is created by using rotary burs.

The cyst should be removed entirely without tearing or puncturing. When separating the cyst lining from inferior alveolar neurovascular bundle, antral floor or apices of teeth, atraumatic enucleation should be carried out. In places where the lining of the cyst is adherent to the cavity, blunt instruments or a piece of rolled gauze held in a hemostat can be used to separate the cystic lining from the bone (Fig. 26.9).

After complete removal of the cyst, thorough irrigation and cleaning of the entire cavity is done with saline. Any roughened bony margins are smoothened with bur. The cavity and its margins are inspected for any irregularities and remnants.

It is followed by tight closure of the flap with sutures over a sound bone. Few cases might require mobilisation of soft tissue flaps for watertight closure. If complete closure is not possible, the defect can be packed with gauze soaked in Whitehead's varnish, bismuth iodoform paraffin paste (BIPP) or antibiotic ointment. Frequent change of this packing is required until complete epithelisation of the wound has taken place.

Enucleation along with adjunctive procedures

Enucleation with open packing

This technique is preferred in cases of infected large cyst, where primary closure of the cyst might lead to breakdown of the wound and interfere with healing.

Mucoperiosteal flap is raised and the cyst is enucleated as described above, but instead of primary closure, the flap is turned into the bone cavity. It is fixed with a medicated gauze pack for 10 days. A change of pack is followed by the construction of an acrylic plug as used in marsupialisation. In case of extremely large defects where pathological fractures are suspected, bone graft can be used to obliterate the cavity (Fig. 26.10).

Enucleation and peripheral ostectomy

It involves enucleation of the cyst along with a peripheral bone trimming with powered rotary instruments. It is basically an additional adjunctive step to avoid resection of the jaw. It is indicated for cyst with high recurrence rate or large cyst with scalloped border or cysts with difficult access, where there is a possibility of leaving residual pathological fragments.

A peripheral ostectomy is the removal of 2–5 mm of bony margin using a rotary bur with sterile irrigation. This procedure helps in removing the lesion in one piece along with an enveloping border of bone, which helps to remove all the microscopic residual pathological tissue. Thus, the recurrence of the cyst is prevented by this procedure (Fig. 26.11).

Enucleation and chemical cauterisation

Few cysts may present with thin, friable wall and many satellite cysts, making it difficult to enucleate the cyst in one piece. Hence, chemical cauterisation is applied after cyst enucleation to eliminate all the residual epithelial fragments. Most commonly used cauterising agent is Carnoy's solution.

- It was 1st described by *Cutler and Zollinger (1933)*
- Carnoy's solution acts as a potent haemostatic, cauterising and fixative substance. It works by penetrating the

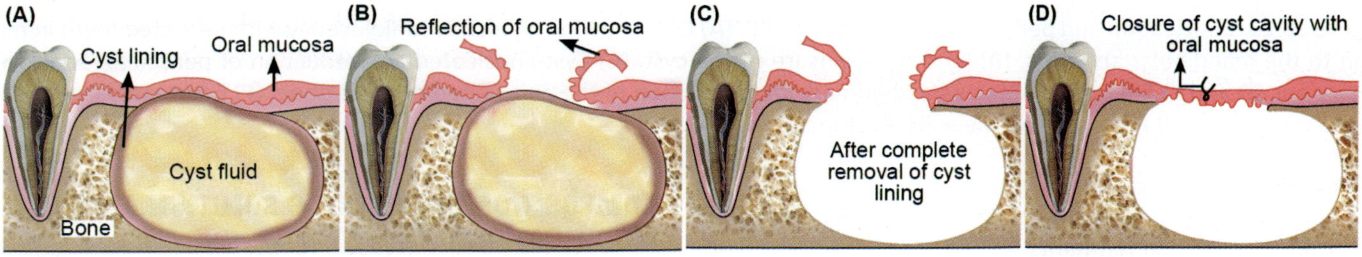

Figure 26.9 Enucleation of cyst. (**A**) Cyst covered by oral mucosa. (**B**) Incision and reflection of the oral mucosa. (**C**) Creation of a window by removing the bone. The cyst lining is separated from the surrounding bone and is completely removed. The cystic cavity is irrigated and packed with gauze. (**D**) Closure of the defect using flaps or oral mucosa.

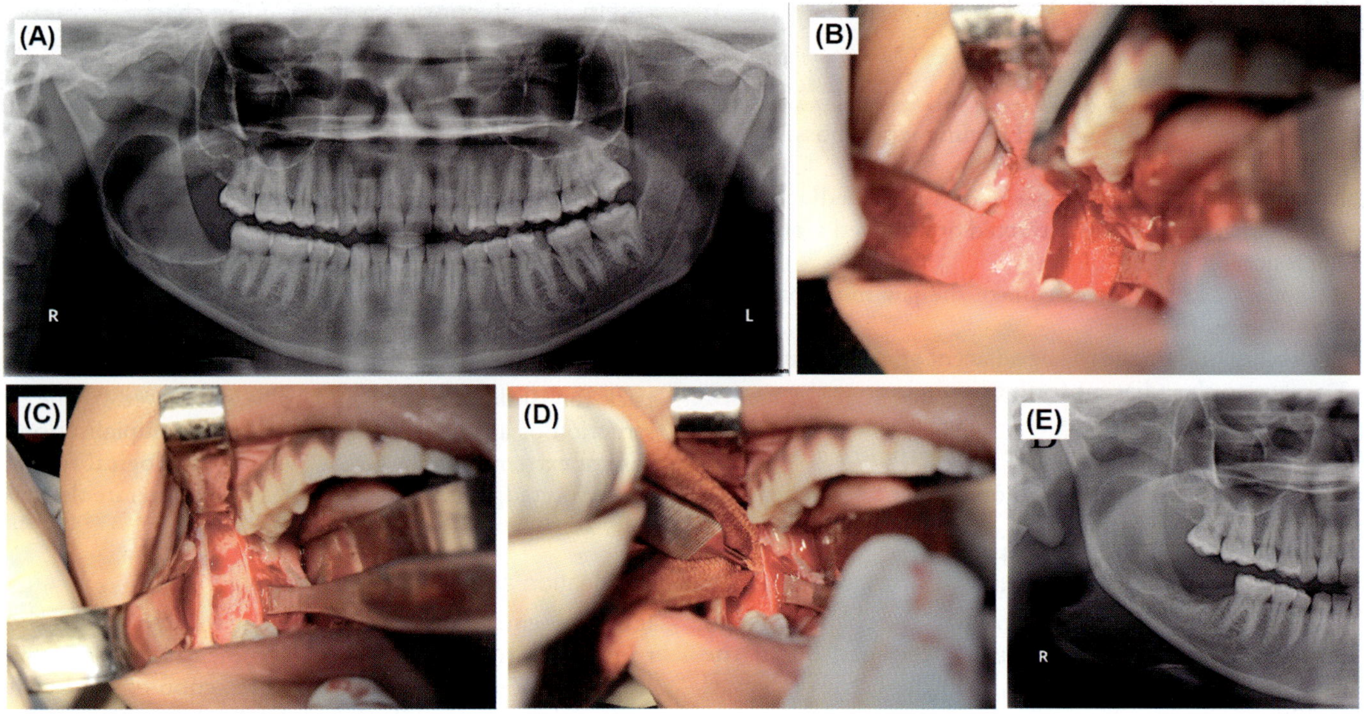

Figure 26.10 Enucleation with open packing. (**A**) Preoperative OPG showing a well-defined large unicystic radiolucency involving the right side angle and ramus of mandible. (**B** and **C**) Intraoperative picture showing enucleation of the cyst. (**D**) Packing of the cystic cavity with iodine gauze. (**E**) Postoperative OPG showing spontaneous bone fill reducing the cavity size.

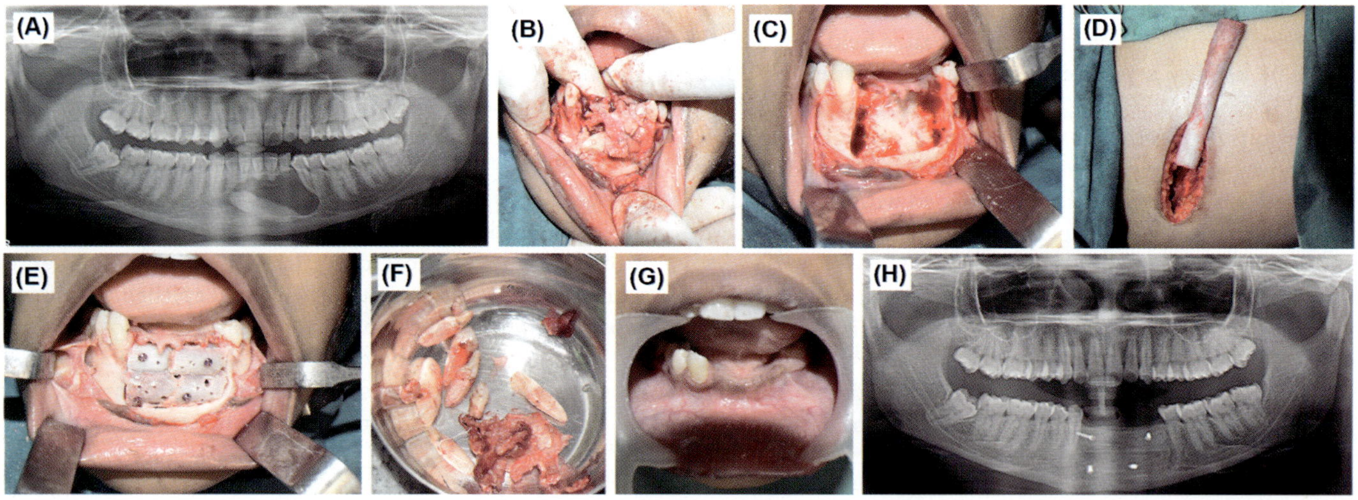

Figure 26.11 Enucleation and peripheral ostectomy of OKC. (**A**) OPG showing unilocular radiolucency with impacted teeth in relation to the mandibular anteriors. (**B**) Intraoral exposure of the cyst. (**C**) Cyst enucleated and reduction of peripheral bone with rotary bur. (**D** and **E**) Rib graft is obtained and primary reconstruction of the enucleated cavity is done. (**F**) Enucleated cyst and its associated teeth. (**G**) Postoperative view. (**H**) Postoperative OPG.

cancellous bone, where it devitalises and then fixes the residual epithelial remnants
- The average depth of penetration in bone is 1.54 mm, after 5 min of application
- It is always recommended to use a freshly prepared solution
- It is applied on the cystic cavity following enucleation.

COMPOSITION OF CARNOY'S SOLUTION AND ITS MODIFICATIONS (Table 26.4)

As chloroform is considered to be very hazardous and can trigger malignant transformation, many surgeons do not recommend its use. Recent literature recommends the use of modified Carnoy's solution without chloroform.

TABLE 26.4 Composition of Carnoy's Solution and its Modifications

Cutler and Zollinger Composition	Composition II	Composition III	Composition IV
Ferric chloride: 1 g Glacial acetic acid: 1 mL Chloroform: 3 mL Absolute alcohol: 6 mL	Ethyl alcohol 96%: 3 mL Glacial acetic acid: 1 mL	Ethyl alcohol 96%: 6 mL Glacial acetic acid: 1 mL Chloroform: 3 mL	Ethyl alcohol 96%: 6 mL Ferric chloride: 1 g Glacial acetic acid: 1 mL

SIDE EFFECTS OF CARNOY'S SOLUTION

- Prolonged application of Carnoy's solution on the blood vessels can result in damage to the vascular walls, such as vascular wall clots and fibrosis
- Neurotoxic–it can result in irreversible damage to the nerve. Hence, nerve should be protected using bone wax, wooden spatula or paraffin gauze and its use should not exceed 2–3 min for safe application
- It may cause necrosis of the maxillary sinus.

Enucleation followed by liquid nitrogen cryotherapy

It is commonly recommended for aggressive cysts like OKC and ameloblastoma. These cysts are treated by enucleation followed by cryotherapy using liquid nitrogen (which boils at–196°C). Cryotherapy destroys the epithelial lining cells and leaves behind an intact inorganic bone matrix, which acts as a scaffold for osteoconduction. Liquid nitrogen has the ability to devitalise the bone from ice crystal formation and subsequent osmotic and electrolytes disturbance. The adjoining tissues are shielded by wooden spatula or gauze strip. The cystic cavity is sprayed with liquid nitrogen twice for 1 min, with 5 min thaw between freezes.

Advantages

- Bony matrix is left behind, which acts as a scaffold for new bone formation
- Bone grafts can be placed immediately to promote healing and decrease the risk of pathological fracture
- Acts as haemostatic agent and reduces scarring.

Disadvantages

- Bone necrosis and postoperative swelling from uncontrolled spray of liquid nitrogen
- Contact with nerve can result in altered sensation of nerve.

Enucleation followed by bone grafting

After enucleation, the dead space in a large cyst can be eliminated by packing the defect with bone grafts. Bone grafts can also be used to avoid pathological fracture and long-term functional problems of the jaw. Autogenous cancellous bone grafts are the gold standard, as it possess both the osteoconductive and osteoinductive qualities. Synthetic substitutes such as calcium phosphates, calcium sulphate, bioactive glasses, glass ionomers and hydroxyapatite (HA) can also be used to fill the defect. The synthetic defects are osteoconductive in nature. (Refer to Chapter 34)

2. AGGRESSIVE SURGICAL TREATMENT/RESECTION OF JAW (FIG. 26.12)

Resection modalities of the jaw:

Marginal resection–It is the surgical removal of a lesion in toto along with a small area of uninvolved bone, thus maintaining the continuity of the bone.

Segmental resection–It is the surgical removal of a segment or portion of maxilla or mandible without maintaining the continuity of the bone. In maxilla, the resections can be classified as partial maxillectomy (alveolectomy) or subtotal or total maxillectomies (Fig. 26.13).

Indications

For recurrent cystic lesions, large multilocular cysts with severely thinned out bone or multiple perforations, malignant transformation within the cysts, and patients with poor compliance for follow-up.

Advantages

Resections have the lowest recurrence rate as compared to other conservative measures.

Disadvantages

- The highest morbidity rate, which frequently requires reconstructive treatments to restore jaw function and aesthetics
- The patient's quality of life seems to be poor
- Restoration of the continuity of defects and functions remains a challenge.

COMPLICATIONS OF UNTREATED CYSTS

Cysts that are not treated develop potential complications such as:

- The cystic content being a rich source of bacterial nutrition could lead to secondary infection. This could spread into tissue spaces causing cellulitis or osteomyelitis
- On expansion, the cyst can cause damage to the surrounding tissues and vital structures. Fast growing cysts exert a pressure on the surrounding bone leading to resorption. Further it could cause 'pressure effects' on

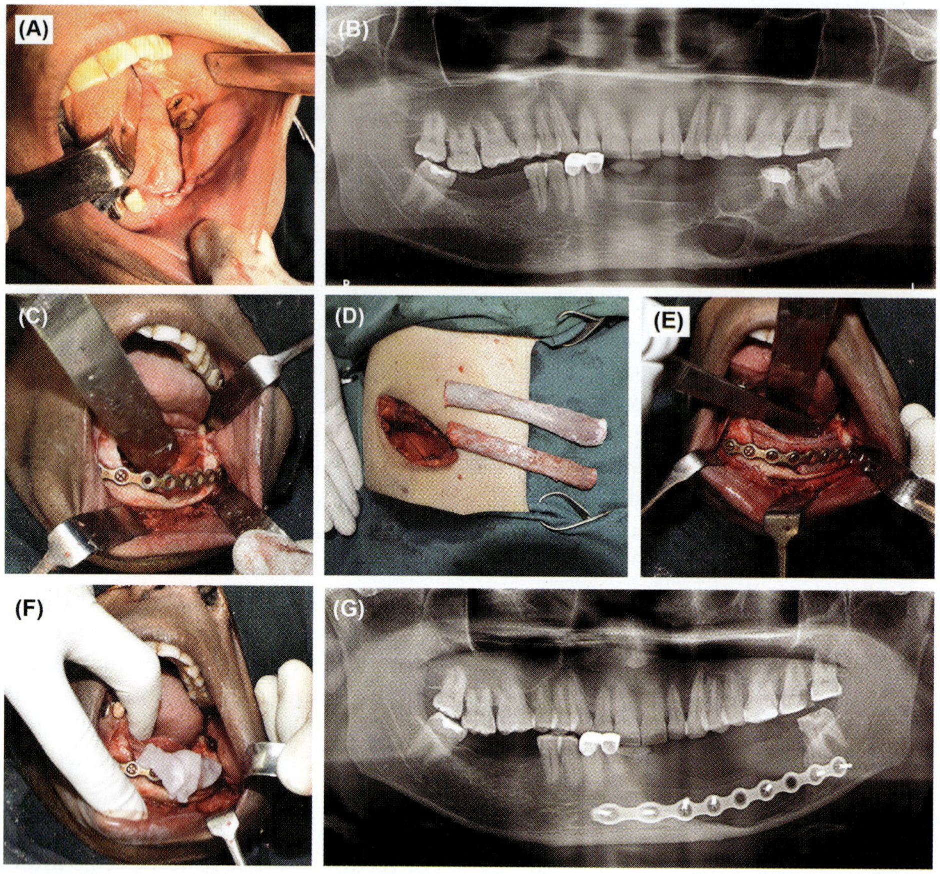

Figure 26.12 Marginal resection of mandible. (**A**) Intraoral view showing cyst expansion in the left side lower jaw in relation to premolar and molar region. (**B**) OPG showing multiple radiolucencies in the left lower jaw. (**C**) The lesion is resected completely along with a small area of uninvolved bone, maintaining the continuity of the bone (marginal resection). (**D**) Rib graft. (**E** and **F**) Reconstruction of the defect with rib graft and rhBMP-2. (**G**) Postoperative OPG showing reconstructed defect.

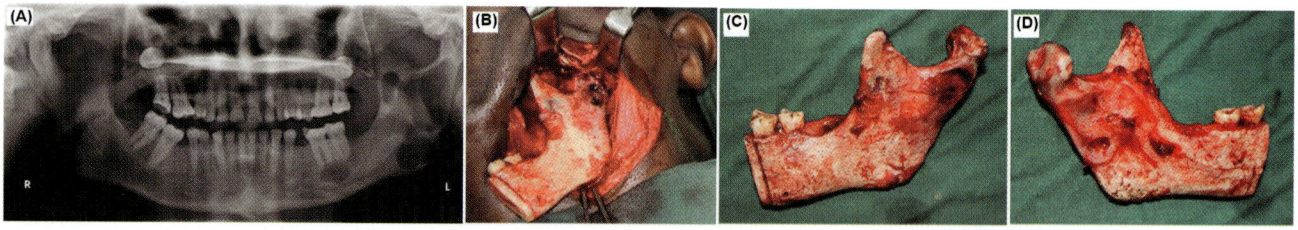

Figure 26.13 Segmental resection of jaw. (**A**) OPG showing multilocular radiolucency in the left mandibular ramus, diagnosed as OKC. (**B**) Segmental resection done as a curative surgery for OKC. (**C** and **D**) Resected mandibular specimen showing bicortical expansion.

nerves and vessels that may cause symptoms of paraesthesia, neuropraxia or decreased blood flow
- The cystic lining may act as precursor to odontogenic tumours or primary intraosseous carcinoma. Untreated dentigerous cysts have been reported to give rise to ameloblastomas and primary intraosseous carcinoma
- Resorption of surrounding bone may lead to thinning down of the bone that predisposes the jaw bones to pathologic fractures or oroantral fistula
- Loss of vitality of teeth
- Gross facial deformation.

CYST OF THE JAWS

EPITHELIAL CYSTS

Odontogenic Developmental Cysts

DENTIGEROUS CYST

Other names

Follicular cyst or Periodontal cyst

It is a developmental odontogenic cyst of epithelial origin. The term dentigerous cyst was coined by Paget in 1863, meaning 'tooth bearing or producing'.

It encloses the crown of an unerupted or impacted tooth by enlargement of the follicular space and is attached to the cementoenamel junction. It is always associated with the crown of a fully or partially impacted tooth. This is the most common type of developmental odontogenic cyst, making about 20% of all epithelium-lined cyst of the jaws.

Origin

A dentigerous cyst develops from the *remnants of enamel organ or reduced enamel epithelium*. In normal tooth development, enamel is produced by the enamel organ, an ectodermally derived epithelium. After enamel formation is complete, the enamel organ epithelium atrophies. This reduced enamel epithelium eventually merges with the overlying mucosal epithelium to form the initial gingival crevicular epithelium of the newly erupted tooth.

Pathogenesis

Dentigerous cysts form when fluid accumulates between the reduced enamel epithelium and the crown of the unerupted tooth. This fluid accumulation or expansion of the cyst can be intrafollicular or extrafollicular.

Intrafollicular theory

Fluid accumulation occurs:

- Between the layers of reduced enamel epithelium (inner and outer enamel epithelium) after formation of the crown
- Cyst formation occurs within the enamel organ by degeneration of the stellate reticulum at an early stage of tooth development
- The pressure from the fluid provokes a proliferation of the outer enamel epithelium and presses the inner enamel epithelium onto the crown surface (Fig. 26.14A)

Extrafollicular theory

- Fluid accumulation occurs between the unerupted tooth and the reduced enamel epithelium
- Increased osmolality (hydrostatic pressure) of the cystic fluid causes expansion of the cyst wall (Fig. 26.14B).

Clinical features

Age and gender: It is usually found in 1st, 2nd and 3rd decades of life, between 1 and 30 years of age. It appears to have an equal incidence on both sexes with a slight predilection for male.

Site

By definition, a dentigerous cyst occurs in association with an unerupted tooth. More frequently in the *mandible* than the maxilla. The most frequently involved teeth in descending order are *mandibular 3rd molars, maxillary canines, maxillary 3rd molars and mandibular 2nd premolars*. Occasionally, they may also be found enclosing a supernumerary teeth or odontomas. Distinctly rare to occur around an unerupted primary teeth.

Signs and symptoms

- Generally asymptomatic, but pain may occur on secondary infection

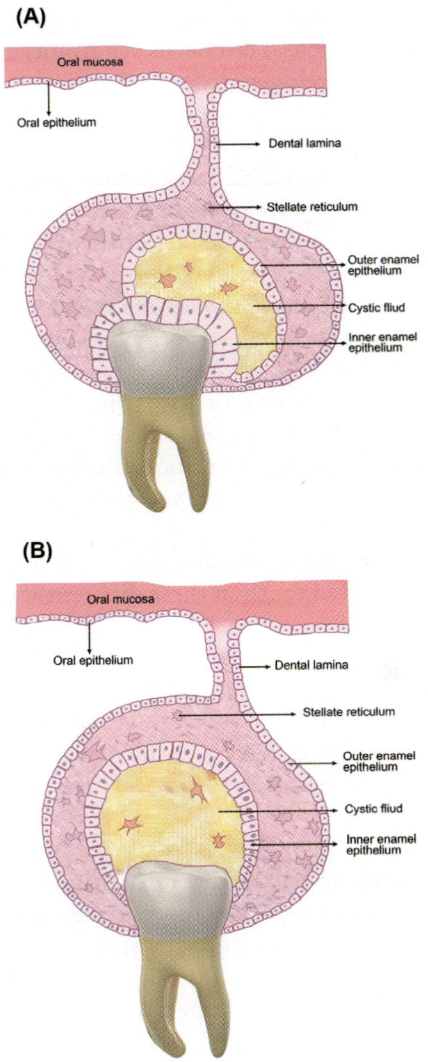

Figure 26.14 **(A)** Intrafollicular formation of cyst between the layers of reduced enamel epithelium. **(B)** Extrafollicular origin of cyst between the unerupted tooth and reduced enamel epithelium.

- Identified on routine radiographs or on investigating a delayed eruption of tooth
- Clinically, the most common indication is missing tooth, tilted or malaligned tooth
- An important feature of the dentigerous cyst is its potential for lateral/cortical expansion of bone. The lateral expansion produces a painless and hard prominence of the bone. Extensive lesions may result in facial asymmetry, extreme displacement and resorption of teeth
- Dentigerous cyst involving an unerupted 3rd molar may result in; expansion of the cortical plate, displacement of the 3rd molar towards the lower border of the mandible, compression on the inferior alveolar nerve, hollowing out of the entire ramus up to the coronoid process
- Dentigerous cyst involving an unerupted maxillary canine may result in anterior maxillary expansion and may resemble sinusitis

- Bilateral or multiple dentigerous cysts may be found in association with basal cell nevus syndrome, cleidocranial dysplasia and amelogenesis imperfecta.

Radiographic features

Most commonly it occurs as a *well-defined, unilocular radiolucency associated with the crowns of an unerupted impacted teeth*. Sometimes, it may present as a multilocular lesion with irregular shape due to the persistence of bony trabeculations. The margins are *well-defined and sclerotic*. In an enlarging cyst, the *unerupted tooth can be pushed away* from its direction of eruption. The lower molar can be pushed to the lower border of mandible or into the ascending ramus, whereas the maxillary canine can be displaced into the maxillary sinus, nasal floor or floor of orbit. The dentigerous cyst presents with *resorption of the roots of the adjacent teeth*.

According to ***Thoma***, the dentigerous cyst may expand around an unerupted tooth in three different ways:

Central or coronal type

The crown is enveloped by the cyst symmetrically surrounding the entire crown of tooth. In this type, pressure is applied to the tooth crown and can be pushed away from its direction of eruption (Fig. 26.15A).

Lateral type

The radiographic appearance results from dilation of the follicle on one aspect of the crown. It develops at lateral side of the tooth and only partially surrounds crown. It is commonly seen in a partially erupting mandibular 3rd molar, where the superior aspect is exposed intraorally (Fig. 26.15B).

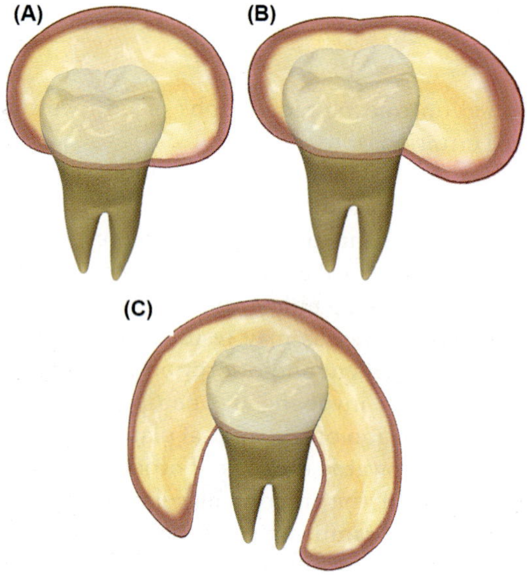

Figure 26.15 Variants of dentigerous cysts: (**A**) central, (**B**) lateral and (**C**) circumferential.

Circumferential type

In this type, the entire tooth appears to be enveloped by cyst. The entire enamel organ around the tooth becomes cystic often allowing the tooth to erupt through the cyst. This variety should be differentiated from OKC (Fig. 26.15C).

According to ***Mourshed***:

Class I:

- Cyst associated with a completely unerupted teeth
- Cyst associated with an unerupted tooth, which has failed to erupt due to the lack of space in dental arch
- Dentigerous cyst associated with unerupted teeth, which has failed to erupt due to malpositioning of the tooth germ
- Dentigerous cyst associated with unerupted supernumerary teeth

Class II:

Dentigerous cyst associated with a partially erupted teeth.

Histologic features

In a noninflamed dentigerous cyst:

- It is made of a thin cystic wall with nonkeratinising stratified squamous epithelium
- The lining epithelium is two to four cell layers thick
- Rete ridges formation is absent
- The cells are cuboidal or low columnar
- The connective tissue wall shows bundles of collagen fibres. Sometimes, odontogenic epithelial islands can be seen
- The cystic lumen contains thin, watery and yellowish straw-coloured fluid

In an inflamed dentigerous cyst:

- The epithelial lining may show varying thickness/ hyperplasia due to inflammation
- Formation of rete ridges and a more definite squamous features
- The connective tissue wall is more thickened and is composed of organised fibrous connective tissue
- Juxtaepithelial inflammatory cells infiltrate the connective tissue
- *Rushton's bodies* can be seen within the epithelium lining. These are linear or hairpin-shaped curved bodies that appear as a result of inflammation.

In case of metaplasia, mucous or ciliated epithelial lining with hyaline bodies within the epithelium can be seen. Cholesterol crystals may be found in the connective tissue.

Aspiration: The cystic fluid is usually thin, watery, yellow straw-coloured fluid.

Differential diagnosis

- Ameloblastoma and ameloblastic fibroma—they are usually not associated with the crown of an unerupted tooth and grow laterally away from the tooth unlike dentigerous cyst which envelops the tooth
- OKC—presence of keratin pearls

- Adenomatoid odontogenic tumour—they occur in the maxillary anterior region
- COC—it contains calcifications
- Primordial (developmental and follicular) cyst—the cystic lining surrounds the crown, whereas in dentigerous cyst it is attached to the neck of tooth.

Treatment

The treatment method for a dentigerous cyst depends on various factors such as patient age, site and size of the cyst and involvement of vital structures. The definite treatment for a dentigerous cyst is *enucleation of the entire cyst together with removal of the unerupted tooth*. A large cyst in young children is treated by *marsupialisation or decompression* to relieve the pressure and allow for gradual shrinking of the cyst. The tooth may erupt into occlusion as the cyst heals (Fig. 26.16).

Potential complications of dentigerous cyst

Dentigerous cysts have the potential for *neoplastic proliferation* besides the possibility of recurrence. The development of ameloblastoma from the lining of dentigerous cyst or rests of odontogenic epithelium in the wall of the cyst is called as *mural ameloblastoma*.

The dentigerous cyst may contain cells with the potential of mucus secreting ability, which may transform into *mucoepidermoid carcinoma*. The cyst lining with long standing keratin metaplasia can initiate neoplastic changes to form *squamous cell carcinoma*.

ODONTOGENIC KERATOCYST (OKC) (Fig. 26.17)

OKC is an epithelial odontogenic developmental cyst of the oral and maxillofacial region. It is a benign locally aggressive developmental cyst with specific characteristics such as high recurrence rate, rapid infiltrative growth, locally aggressive nature and defined histopathological features.

It was 1st described by ***Philipsen*** in 1956 as 'odontogenic keratocyst'. *Pindborg and Hansen* (1963) designated the term 'keratocyst' and it was used to describe the jaw cyst in which keratin is formed to a large extent.

Odontogenic keratocyst as benign neoplasm

Many terminologies have been under discussion in the past.

- Shear used the term *'keratocystoma'*
- Philipsen (2005) has suggested the term *'keratocystic odontogenic tumour'*
- Reichart and Philipsen (2004) redesigned OKC as 'keratinising cystic odontogenic tumour—KCOT'

OKC is classified under odontogenic neoplasm than cyst due to the following reasons:

- Aggressive behaviour
- High recurrence rate
- Asymptomatic until it grows larger
- Extends through the medullary cavities resulting in hollowing of the mandible
- High mitotic count of the basal and parabasal layers of epithelium
- Increased proliferative rate of the epithelium.

This consideration of OKC as tumour suggested a change in the management protocol, which was not widely accepted. As the researchers proposed that marsupialisation can revert the fragile cystic lining epithelium to normal mucosa. So, WHO in 2017, moved the KCOT back into the cyst category as the evidence supporting OKC as neoplasia is considered insufficient.

Shear had emphasised *the association of OKC with the Gorlin–Goltz syndrome*/nevoid basal cell carcinoma syndrome. Histochemical studies have proved the expression of the following proteins in OKC, which are not present in normal epithelium.

- Altered gene expression of the epithelial cells
- Increased expression of cell proliferation markers, such as p53 protein, Ki-67 and PCNA
- Mutation of PTCH.

Aetiology and pathogenesis

Origin

It originates from the odontogenic epithelium. Most OKCs (60%) arise from *remnants of dental lamina or from the basal cells of oral epithelium*, and are therefore known as primordial origin OKCs and the remaining 40% arise from the reduced enamel epithelium of the dental follicle and are therefore considered as of dentigerous origin OKCs.

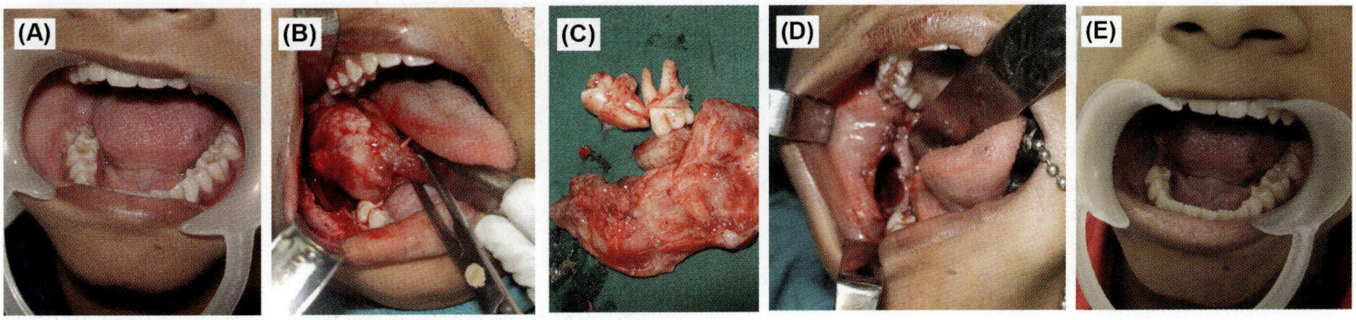

Figure 26.16 Dentigerous cyst. (**A**) Intraoral view. (**B**) The cyst is completely enucleated through an intraoral approach. (**C**) Excised specimen along with the involved tooth. (**D**) Primary closure of the wound. (**E**) Postoperative view.

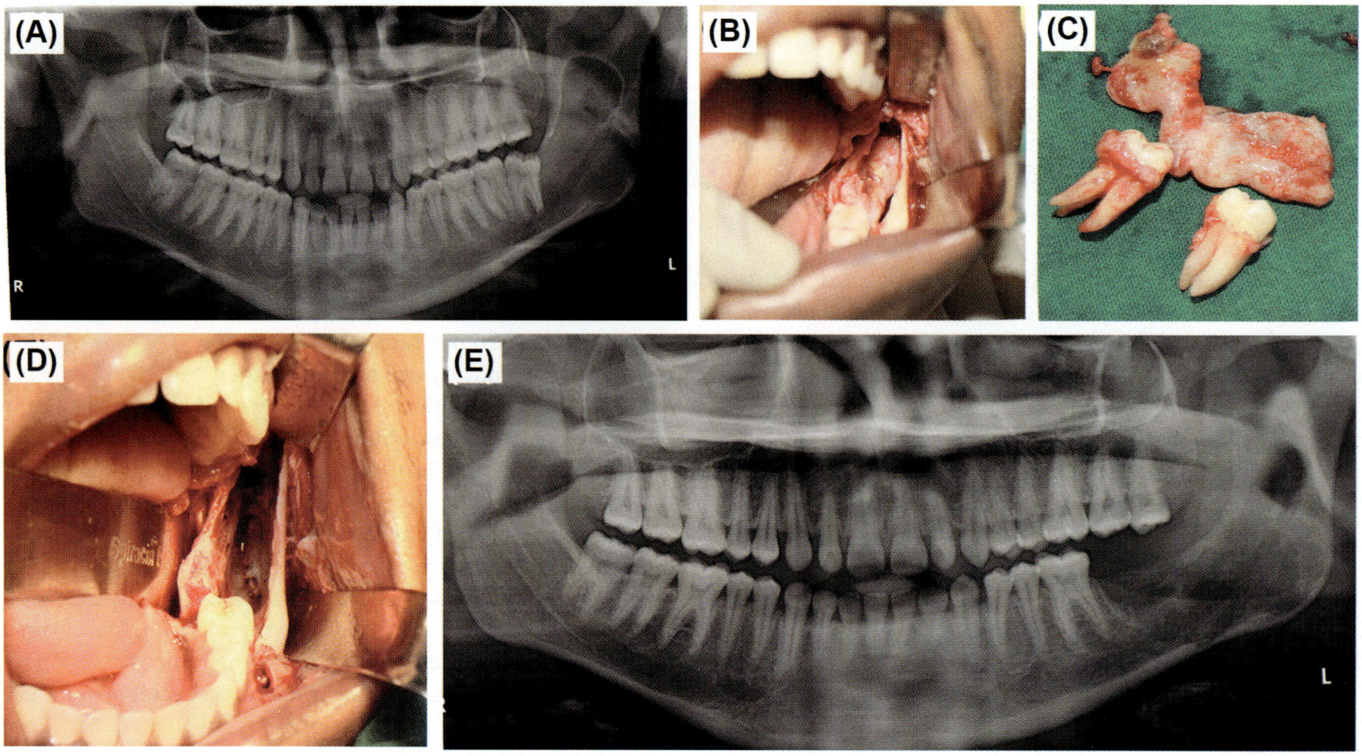

Figure 26.17 Odontogenic keratocyst. (**A**) Preoperative OPG showing unilocular radiolucency in the left mandibular ramus and angle region. (**B**) Exposure of the cyst through intraoral approach and creation of bony window. (**C**) Enucleated cyst with associated teeth. (**D**) Bone cavity after enucleation of the cyst. (**E**) Postoperative OPG.

Pathogenesis of odontogenic keratocyst

The factors that contribute to the pathogenesis of OKC includes high proliferation rate, overexpression of the antiapoptotic protein Bcl-2, overexpression of interface proteins (MMPs 2 and 9, TGF, IL-1α, IL-6) and mutations in PTCH tumour suppressor gene.

Clinical presentation

Age and gender:

It occurs at all ages with peak incidence in 2nd and 3rd decades of life, with male:female ratio of 1.6:1.

Site:

Central intraosseous lesion:

- It occurs more frequently in mandible than in maxilla
- In mandible, it usually occurs at the angle region—extending from the ascending ramus region (69%–83%) it moves forward into the body
- Maxillary cyst may involve the maxillary sinus, nasal floor, premaxilla and maxillary 3rd molar region. OKC may also arise from Temporomandibular joint (TMJ)

Peripheral OKC:

- It occurs in the buccal gingiva with female predominance

Number of cyst:

- Usually solitary in nonsyndromic lesions
- In syndromic patients, multiple OKCs can be seen at a time (Box 26.2)

Signs and symptoms:

- Mostly asymptomatic, swelling appears late as the cyst initially extends in the *medullary cavity along the path of least resistance*, rather than expanding the cortex (early stage)
- Pain and swelling with discharge only when they get secondarily infected
- The expansion of the cyst is very minimal in the initial stage and it is due to the classical characteristic of the cyst to *grow in anteroposterior direction* in the medullary space of the bone

BOX 26.2 Syndromes Associated with Multiple OKC

- Nevoid basal cell carcinoma syndrome (NBCCS) or Gorlin–Goltz syndrome.
- Marfan's syndrome.
- Ehlers–Danlos syndrome.
- Noonan's syndrome.
- Orofacial digital syndrome.
- Simpson–Golabi–Behmel syndrome.

- Buccal expansion is more common than the palatal or lingual expansion
- Perforation of the bony cortex in expanded lesions
- Displacement of teeth
- Percussion of teeth produces dull hollow sound
- Paraesthesia of the lower lip and teeth in expanded lesions
- Maxillary lesions get infected in the initial phase and are hence detected earlier than the mandibular cyst
- Enlarging maxillary lesion may produce displacement and destruction of the floor of orbit and proptosis of eye
- Associated with missing tooth (not always)
- Displacement of inferior alveolar canal in large lesions.

Recurrences (Box 26.3)**:**

It has a high rate of recurrence of about 25%–60%. The mean time of recurrence for males was found to be 4 years and for females it came out to be 7 years.

Radiological features (Box 26.4)**:**

- Most commonly involve the mandible molar ramus area
- OKC presents as well-defined unilocular or multilocular (25%–40%) radiolucent lesion with smooth margin (corticated margin in secondarily infected cases)
- Radiolucency is usually hazy due to the presence of keratin and is surrounded by a thin sclerotic rim
- Size may be 5 cm or more in diameter
- Shape of the cyst is usually oval extending along the body of mandible
- **Borders:** Smooth or scalloped suggesting unequal growth activity

  Effect on bone:
  - Expansion and perforation of the buccal and lingual cortex
  - Downward displacement of the inferior alveolar canal with resorption of the lower cortical plate
  - Pathological fracture of bone
  - Extensive involvement of the ascending ramus and body of mandible with no bony expansion

  Effect on teeth:
  - Tooth displacement
  - Deflection of the unerupted tooth
  - Resorption of adjacent tooth root
  - Associated with teeth either in pericoronal, interradicular or periapical or in association with missing teeth.

BOX 26.3 Contributing Factors for and Mechanism of Recurrence of OKC

These Factors Contribute to the Recurrence of OKC

- Thin and friable nature of epithelial lining, which may be left behind.
- Higher level of proliferative activity in the epithelium.
- Presence of satellite cyst.
- Presence of intrinsic growth potential in the epithelial lining.
- Cyst can arise from the proliferation of the basal layer.
- Firm adherence of the cyst to the overlying soft tissue.
- Perforation of the cortex, cyst lining adheres to the adjoining bone or soft tissue.
- Enucleation in one piece is difficult for cysts with scalloped margins and those present in areas with difficult access.

Mechanism of Recurrence by Brannon (1976)

- Incomplete removal of the cystic lining.
- Growth of new OKC from satellite cyst/daughter cyst/dental lamina remnants or odontogenic rests left behind during surgery.
- Development of new OKC in the adjacent areas such as the bone or overlying mucosa from the dental lamina remnants.

BOX 26.4 Radiological Types of Keratocyst (Main 1970)

- **Replacement type:** Cyst which forms in the place of normal teeth.
- **Envelopmental type:** Cyst which embraces an adjacent unerupted tooth.
- **Extraneous type:** Cyst which occur in ascending ramus away from the teeth.
- **Collateral type:** Cyst which occurs adjacent to the root of teeth which are indistinguishable radiologically from lateral periodontal cyst.

Histological features of odontogenic keratocyst by WHO (Phillipsen 2005) (Box 26.5)

- Regular *parakeratinised stratified squamous epithelium without rete ridges* (80%–90%)
- The pathognomic feature is the *corrugated* epithelium with a thickness of five to eight cell layers
- The basal layer is well defined with columnar or cuboidal epithelium frequently containing basophilic nuclei in a palisaded fashion described as '*picket fence or tombstone appearance*'. The nuclei is placed away from the basement membrane (reversed polarity)
- Weak epithelial-connective tissue attachment
- Presence of *satellite cysts/daughter cysts*

BOX 26.5 Histopathological Groups of OKC

Based on the occurrence of satellite cysts and squamous islands in the cystic wall:

- **Group I:** Unicystic, without any satellites (63%).
- **Group II:** With few satellites and squamous islands in the cystic lining less than 10%–27%.
- **Group III:** Abundant presence of satellite cyst and squamous islands 6%–10%.

- Basal cell hyperplasia
- The cystic wall is thin and composed of fibrous connective tissue (mucopolysaccharide)
- Fibrous connective tissue wall may get mineralised and may include cholesterol crystals and Rushton's bodies

Malignant transformation:

Rarely, OKCs may undergo malignant transformation into *primary intraosseous squamous cell carcinoma* (PIOSCC). Patients persisting with unresolved disease after treatment should be investigated for malignant transformation. Detailed histopathological examination of OKC specimens is recommended to detect small foci of SCC which may be present in the epithelium

Aspiration:

- Odourless, thick, creamy, dirty white, caseous, viscoid suspension of keratin (shimmering keratin crystals)
- Total protein less than 4 g/100 mL, mostly albumin
- Other contents: Cholesterol crystals, hyaluronic acid, keratin, Rushton's bodies, heparin and chondroitin sulphate
- Protein-53 is positive in Gorlin-Goltz syndrome
- Immunofluorescent studies demonstrate 'keratocyst antigen—KCA' in the cystic fluid, which is not present in other cystic lesions

Differential diagnosis:

Histologically: Myxoma, ameloblastoma, central giant cell granuloma, odontogenic cysts

Radiographically: Dentigerous cyst (40%), residual cysts, radicular cyst, lateral periodontal cysts (25%), primordial cyst (25%), globulomaxillary cyst (10%), unicystic ameloblastoma, A-V malformation, fibroosseous lesion at initial stages.

Treatment modalities for odontogenic keratocyst

A wide range of treatment modalities have been tried in the past for successful treatment of OKC, which includes the following:

i. Decompression alone
ii. Marsupialisation alone
iii. Enucleation alone
iv. Enucleation with adjuvant therapy (mechanical curettage, chemical curettage, cryotherapy)
v. Marsupialisation followed by enucleation
vi. Resection without continuity defect—peripheral ostectomy.
vii. Resection with continuity defect—segmental resection.

Definitive treatment of OKC depends on various factors such as the patient age, size, extent and location of cyst, bony perforation, soft tissue involvement, radiographic appearance and histological variant of lesion.

Bramley's (1974) approach to surgical management of odontogenic keratocyst

- Single, small cystic lesion with a regular spherical outline and good surgical access are treated with *enucleation from an intraoral approach*
- Single, large, less accessible lesions with regular spherical outline are *enucleated through extraoral approach*
- Unilocular lesions with scalloped margins and small multilocular lesions are treated by *marginal excision*, maintaining the continuity of the posterior and inferior borders in the ascending ramus, angle and body of mandible. The defect cavity can be left to heal secondarily or filled with *bone grafts* and closed primarily. Access may be gained through extraoral approach
- Large multilocular or multicystic lesions (with or without bone perforation) are treated with *resection and primary or secondary reconstruction* with bone grafts and reconstruction plates.

According to *Stoelinga and Van Hoelst (2003)*, larger lesions are treated by enucleation with excision of the overlying muscle or mucosa, if attachment of the cyst existed. The bony defect was cauterised with Carnoy's solution to prevent recurrence.

To summarise, both conservative and aggressive approach have been advocated in the treatment of OKC. Conservative methods have not been recommended because of thin, friable lining making it difficult to remove the cyst completely and its potential for recurrence. The most commonly accepted and followed treatment modalities for OKC are as follows:

- Large expanding lesions and younger age group—marsupialisation followed by enucleation
- Smaller and easily accessible lesions—enucleation with chemical cauterisation with Carnoy's solution or enucleation with cryosurgery
- Multiple recurrent lesions or lesions with extensive soft tissue invasion and large bony perforations—resection of the jaw bone followed by extensive rehabilitation. Resections should be used as a last alternative method
- Follow-up—the patient should be followed yearly, at least for 5 years postoperatively.

Features of nevoid basal cell carcinoma (Gorlin-Goltz syndrome) is discussed in Table 26.5.

ERUPTION CYST

It is a dentigerous cyst occurring in the soft tissues. Eruption cyst develops when a tooth is impeded during its eruption, *within the soft tissues* overlying the bone. Whereas, the dentigerous

TABLE 26.5 Features of Gorlin-Goltz Syndrome

Cutaneous • Basal cell epitheliomas • Milia • Palmar pits • Plantar pits • Epidermal cysts of skin • Subcutaneous calcifications • Cleft lip or palate • Polydactyly
Skeletal • Odontogenic keratocysts • Bifid ribs • Scoliosis • Mandibular prognathism • Increased calvarial diameter • Well-developed supraorbital rims • Spina bifida of cervical or thoracic spine • Hyperpneumatisation of paranasal sinuses • Short 4th metacarpals • Marfanoid build
Ocular • Glaucoma • Cataracts • Coloboma of the iris • Hypertelorism • Strabismus • Nystagmus
Neurologic • Calcified falx cerebri • Mental retardation • Cerebral tumours • Agenesis of corpus callosum • Calcified tentorium cerebelli
Sexual • Undescended testes • Ovarian tumours • Hypogonadism

cyst develops around the crown of an unerupted tooth lying in the bone. It results from accumulation of fluid within the follicular space of an erupting tooth. Accumulation of blood within the follicular space has often been termed as 'eruption haematoma'. It appears as a well-circumscribed purple or deep blue swelling.

Pathogenesis

It is similar to dentigerous cyst. Browne and Smith (1991) proposed that as the crown of the tooth associated with an eruption cyst usually projects into the cyst lumen, the epithelium is derived from reduced enamel epithelium.

Clinical features

- It appears as a soft, circumscribed, translucent swelling in the gingival mucosa or alveolar ridge of an erupting deciduous or permanent tooth
- Common in children below the age of 10 years
- More commonly seen in erupting 1st permanent molars and maxillary incisors.

Radiographic features

It presents as an expansion of the normal follicular space of an erupting tooth crown. In some cases, the cyst may show a soft tissue shadow without bone involvement.

Histologic features

The superficial aspect of the cyst wall is covered by the stratified, squamous, keratinised epithelium of the overlying gingiva (oral epithelium) of two to three layers thick. The gingival connective tissue is acellular and densely collagenous. As the cysts are frequently exposed to masticatory trauma, there is an increase in the inflammatory infiltrate towards the cyst lining.

Treatment

No treatment is required because the tooth erupts through the cyst causing spontaneous rupture of the cyst. Few cases might require excision of the cyst exposing the crown and allowing the tooth to erupt.

Differential diagnosis

Gingival cysts.

PRIMORDIAL CYST

Robinson defined a primordial cyst as '*a cyst which arises from the breakdown of stellate reticulum of the enamel organ before any hard tissue is formed*'. It is an uncommon odontogenic cyst. The term primordial cyst indicates that the cyst arises from the primordial odontogenic epithelium (remnants of dental lamina, basal cells, enamel organ), prior to the formation of tooth structures. Thus, this cyst is found in place of a tooth rather than being associated with it.

Pathogenesis

It may originate from the remnants of dental lamina, enamel organ or the basal cells of the odontogenic epithelium in place of a tooth.

Clinical features

It is less common and comprises of about 5% to 6% of odontogenic cysts. It is predominantly seen in children and young adults between 10 and 30 years of age, although it may occur at any age group. It occurs in both the sexes with a slight predilection for males than females. The primordial cyst occurs more commonly in the mandible than the maxilla. It can arise from any portion of the jaw, but mostly seen in the region posterior to the bicuspids (ascending ramus of the mandible and 3rd molar area).

- The cyst develops and *slowly enlarges along the medullary cavity* before the expansion of the cortical plate. A small cyst is usually diagnosed only on routine radiographic examination, whereas a large cyst appears as a painless, bony expansion
- Large cyst may present with tooth displacement, dull or hollow sound on percussion of the overlying tooth or associated with a missing tooth
- The vitality of the associated tooth is usually not affected
- When a large cyst is infected, it may present with pain, perforation of the cortical plate or paraesthesia of the nerve.

On aspiration, it may yield a thick granular yellowish material.

Radiographic features

It appears as a unilocular, well-circumscribed radiolucency with hyperostotic borders. It may or may not have a scalloped outline. The involved tooth is usually missing and the adjacent tooth may be deflected or its roots resorbed.

Histologic features

The primordial cyst are lined by a keratinised stratified squamous epithelium of 6–10 layers thick, devoid of rete pegs. These cells are arranged in a *'picket fence' or 'tombstone pattern'*. Few cases may exhibit a surface layer of orthokeratin. The basal cell layer is not prominent and sometimes with an atypical corrugated appearance. The connective tissue capsule is usually thin, and may contain strands of odontogenic epithelium resembling daughter cysts.

Treatment

Primordial cysts are treated with surgical enucleation. Due to its tendency for recurrence, the patients should be under regular follow-up.

Differential diagnosis

Odontogenic keratocyst

GINGIVAL CYST OF NEWBORN

Other names

Dental lamina cyst

They appear as multiple, solitary, superficial raised nodules on the edentulous alveolar ridges of the infants.

Pathogenesis

They are derived from the epithelial remnants of dental lamina (glands of Serres) and keratin-producing epithelial lining.

Clinical features

In infants, the dental lamina cysts appear as asymptomatic, isolated, small discrete white papules of 2–3 mm on the crest of the alveolar ridge of newborns. They are more commonly found on the maxilla.

Radiographic features

No imaging is required as they are extraosseous and do not involve the bone. Few may show faint shadow indicative of superficial erosion of bone. They are usually diagnosed based on their clinical appearance.

Histologic features

These are true cysts with a thin stratified squamous epithelium, parakeratotic, flat basal cells and with no rete pegs. The lumen of the cyst is filled with desquamated keratin and inflammatory cells. Sometimes, *dystrophic calcification and hyaline bodies of Rushton* are also found in this cyst.

Treatment

No treatment is required as these lesions invariable disappears, either by involution or rupture through the surface epithelium or by disruption of the cyst from the erupting teeth. They regress spontaneously within a few weeks or months. They can be rarely seen after 3 months of age.

PALATAL CYSTS OF THE NEWBORN

Other names

Epstein's pearl, Bohn's nodule

These cysts are similar to gingival cyst, but their location and aetiology of the lesions are different.

Pathogenesis

- Epstein's pearls arise from the epithelial inclusions entrapped along the line of fusion of palatine shelves and the nasal processes
- Bohn's nodules are derived from the minor salivary gland structures (palatal).

Clinical features

Epstein's pearls appear as cystic, keratin-filled nodules *along the midpalatine raphe*.

Keratin-filled cysts known as Bohn's nodules can be seen dispersed all over the palate. But they are most abundant along junction between the hard and soft palates. They are also found on the buccal or lingual aspects of the alveolar ridges.

These cysts are small, 1–3 mm in size, firm and white or greyish white nodules. Sometimes, a cluster of two to six cysts may be observed. Epstein's pearls are white and quite large when compared to small Bohn's nodules.

Radiographic features

No imaging is required as they are extraosseous and do not involve the bone.

Histopathological features

Microscopic examination reveals keratin-filled cysts that are lined by parakeratinised stratified squamous epithelium.

Treatment

They resolve spontaneously.

Differential diagnosis

Natal or neonatal teeth and congenital epulis.

GINGIVAL CYST OF ADULTS

It is an uncommon cyst of gingiva, occurring in the *free or attached gingiva*. The gingival cyst of adults and the lateral periodontal cyst are similar both clinically and histologically (Fig. 26.18).

Pathogenesis

According to Ritchey and Orban, the possible sources of cystic formation are as follows:

- Cystic transformation of the dental lamina or rests of Serres
- Traumatic implantation of surface epithelium.

The gingival cyst of adults and the lateral periodontal cyst may arise from the same source. The lateral periodontal cyst develops from reduced enamel epithelium before eruption of the tooth, whereas the gingival cyst of adults may also arise from the reduced enamel epithelium but after the eruption of tooth.

Clinical features

- The gingival cyst may occur at any age, most commonly in adults over 40 years
- Common sites are mandibular canine and premolar area.
- They appear as a painless, small, well-circumscribed swelling of the gingiva
- The lesion is usually less than 1 cm in diameter and the colour appears similar to that of the adjacent normal mucosa
- It is soft and fluctuant and the adjacent teeth are usually vital
- They occur in the free or attached gingiva, some may occur in the gingival papilla.

Radiographic features

As it is a soft tissue lesion, it does not manifest on the radiographs. If the lesion is large, it may show faint shadow indicative of superficial erosion of the cortical bone.

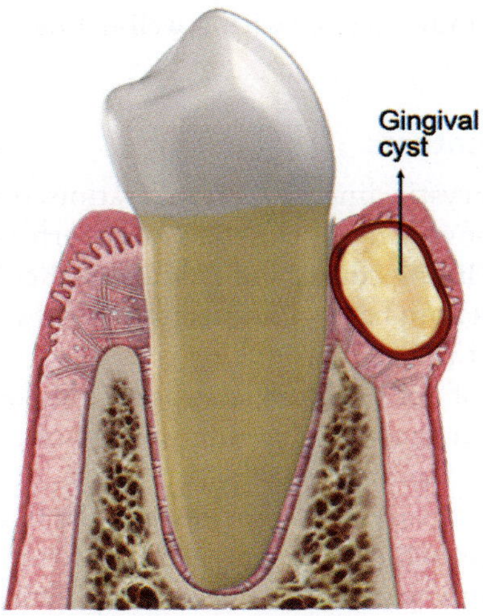

Figure 26.18 The gingival cyst of adults after eruption of the tooth.

Histologic features

- It is a true cyst with a thin stratified squamous epithelium, without rete ridges of varying thickness. The lining epithelium is similar to that of lateral periodontal cyst
- The focal thickenings or plaques of the lining may contain glycogen-rich clear cells. The connective tissue wall may also contain remnants of dental lamina
- This lesion can be unicystic or polycystic
- The connective tissue may or may not exhibit an inflammatory reaction, as the cyst lies in the gingiva
- In implantation type of gingival cyst, calcification or ectopic ossification may be associated with the cyst.

Treatment

Local surgical excision of the lesion and generally this lesion does not tend to recur.

Differential diagnosis

Lateral periodontal cyst.

LATERAL PERIODONTAL CYST

The lateral periodontal cyst occurs adjacent or *lateral to the roots of a vital teeth*. It is an uncommon, slow growing, nonexpansile odontogenic cyst. It is histogenetically similar to gingival cyst of adults.

Pathogenesis

The possibilities of development of a lateral periodontal cyst include the following:

- It may originate initially as a dentigerous cyst along the lateral surface of the crown, as the tooth erupts, the cyst assumes a position lateral to the root surface
- It can arise from the proliferation of rests of Malassez in the periodontal ligament
- It may form as a primordial cyst of a supernumerary tooth germ, in the mandibular premolar area
- It may origin from proliferation and cystic transformation of the rests of dental lamina.

Clinical features

- It occurs more commonly in adults of age 22–85 years with a distinct male predilection
- Most common location of the lesion are *mandibular premolar and canine*, and occasionally incisor area. In maxilla, lesions are found more commonly in the lateral incisor region
- It is an uncommon, slow growing, nonexpansile odontogenic cyst
- The majority of the lesions are asymptomatic and have been diagnosed during radiographic examination of the teeth
- The *associated tooth is vital*
- It may appear clinically as a slight mass, with a normal overlying mucosa.

Radiographic features

It discloses as a well-delineated, *round or teardrop-shaped unilocular radiolucency* with an opaque margin along the lateral surface of a tooth root. The lesion is usually small and less than 1 cm in diameter. In most cases, it presents with definitive border surrounded by a thin layer of sclerotic bone. A polycystic variant of lateral periodontal cyst is termed as *'botryoid odontogenic cysts'*.

Histologic features

- It is characterised by a thin, nonkeratinised epithelium of around one to five layers thick, resembling the reduced enamel epithelium
- The lining cells may be cuboidal or columnar in shape and have a *clear, vacuolated, glycogen-rich cytoplasm*. Sometimes, rests of dental lamina can be found in the connective tissue wall
- Few may show *focal thickened plaques* of proliferating lining cells projecting into the lumen. These epithelial plaque protrusions in the cyst wall may be 'pinched off' and develop into daughter cysts, leading to the formation of botryoid variant
- Inflammatory cells may occur as a secondary reaction
- The connective tissue exhibits a zone of hyalinisation, with a thick fibrous cyst wall.

Treatment

The lateral periodontal cyst is treated by local surgical enucleation with or without preserving the associated tooth. Recurrence is rare, but reported in botryoid variant.

Differential diagnosis

OKC, traumatic cysts, lateral radicular cyst.

BOTRYOID ODONTOGENIC CYST

It refers to a *multilocular lateral periodontal cyst* or botryoid variety of the lateral periodontal cyst. The term 'botryoid odontogenic cyst' was proposed by Waldron, as their specimen resembled *a cluster of grapes*.

Pathogenesis

It is similar to lateral periodontal cyst developing from the multiple islands of dental lamina rests.

Clinical features

It is commonly found in adults of age between 5th to 7th decades. It is most often seen as an asymptomatic swelling in the mandible, predominantly the premolar region.

Radiographic features

It appears as multilocular radiolucency on the lateral surface of a tooth.

Histologic features

- The lesion is multilocular with thin fibrous connective tissue septa
- The cyst cavities are lined by a thin, nonkeratinised epithelium of about one to two layers of flat cells
- There are many foci of plaque-like thickenings, consisting of flat fusiform cells
- The cystic cavities are grossly similar to that of a cluster of grapes.

Treatment

The lesion can be excised by surgical enucleation. This cyst has an increased tendency for recurrence and the patients treated for a botryoid cyst should be followed periodically.

GLANDULAR ODONTOGENIC CYST

Other names

Sialo-odontogenic cyst or Mucoepidermoid cyst

It is described as an unusually large solitary or multilocular odontogenic cyst. It is a rare and recently recognised developmental odontogenic cyst with a *remarkable aggressive behaviour*. As it is similar to lateral periodontal cyst, it is considered a variant of it by some authors. The name 'glandular odontogenic cyst (GOC)' was favoured by Gardner et al., based on its histological features and biological behaviour.

Pathogenesis

It arises from the epithelial rests of the dental lamina.

Clinical features

- Most commonly in middle-aged adults with a mean age of 49 years and a slight male predilection
- It is more commonly seen in the mandible, with a strong predilection for *anterior region* of the jaws (incisor and canine areas). Many mandibular lesions can cross the midline
- Root resorption or divergence of adjacent teeth can be seen in some cases
- The lesions shows painless, slow progressive growth, and locally aggressive.

Radiographic features

Multilocular radiolucency with a well-defined margin and a sclerotic rim.

Histologic features

- It is multicystic, lined by a nonkeratinised stratified epithelium of varying thickness. The superficial layer of the epithelial lining consists of columnar or cuboidal cells
- The epithelium has a glandular structure with microcysts and goblet mucous producing cells
- Presence of focal epithelial thickenings or plaques are identical to those in the gingival cyst of adults and the lateral periodontal cyst
- The connective tissue may present with islands of odontogenic epithelium and irregular calcifications
- Mucous and cylindrical cells in the epithelium and mucinous material within the cystic spaces are all characteristics of *a gland-like structure*.

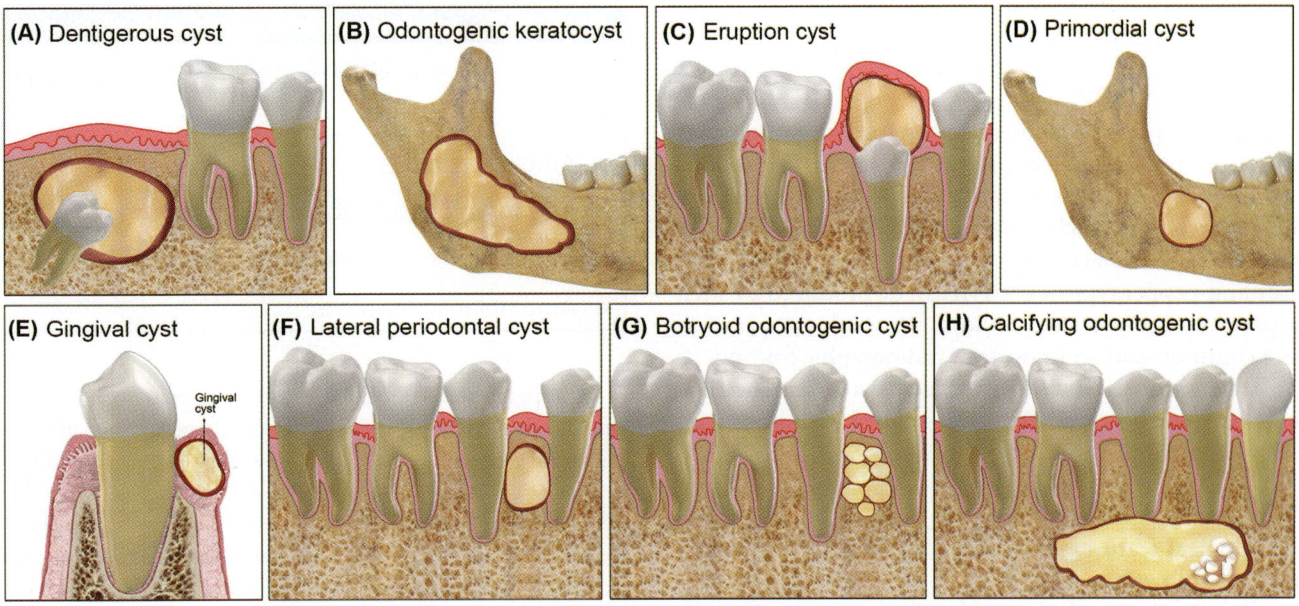

Figure 26.19 Various cysts of odontogenic origin and their development.

Treatment

The lesion is locally aggressive, therefore surgical management involves enucleation with peripheral curettage or marginal excision. Long-term follow-up is essential to avoid recurrences.

CALCIFYING ODONTOGENIC CYST (Fig. 26.19)

Other names

Keratinising or Calcifying epithelial odontogenic cyst, Gorlin-Goltz cyst, Cystic keratinising tumour

The COC is composed of two entities: cyst and a true neoplasm. In **WHO classification (2005)**, it was classified as a benign odontogenic tumour and renamed as calcifying cystic odontogenic tumour (CCOT). Li and Yu (2003) proposed the name 'ghost cell lesions' as cysts, neoplasms and even malignancies.

Praetorius classification of the odontogenic ghost cell lesions is described in Box 26.6.

The COC was 1st described by Gorlin *et al.* because of the presence of **'ghost cells'** and its histological resemblance to the cutaneous calcifying epithelioma of Malherbe.

Classification of COC:

1. Cystic:
   a. Simple unicystic
   b. Unicystic odontome associated type
   c. Ameloblastomatous proliferating type
2. Neoplastic.

Pathogenesis

COC is developed from reduced enamel epithelium or remnants of odontogenic epithelium in the gingiva of the maxilla or mandible.

BOX 26.6 Classification of the Odontogenic Ghost Cell Lesions by Praetorius 2006

Group 1: Simple cysts

Calcifying odontogenic cyst (COC)

Group 2: Cysts associated with odontogenic hamartomas or benign neoplasms

Calcifying cystic odontogenic tumours (CCOT)

Group 3: Solid benign odontogenic neoplasms with similar cell morphology to that in the COC, and with dentinoid formation

Dentinogenic ghost cell tumour

Group 4: Malignant odontogenic neoplasms with features similar to those of the dentinogenic ghost cell tumour

Ghost cell odontogenic carcinoma

Clinical features

- A wide age range has been reported, with a peak incidence in the 2nd and 3rd decades of life. The mean age is 40 years, with a slight predilection for females
- The majority of the lesions are found within the bone (intraosseous), though extraosseous forms also occur in the gingiva. The frequency of lesion is equal in both the maxilla and mandible with a predilection for the canine–premolar region of the maxilla
- Painless swelling or bony expansion can be observed
- Displacement of the adjacent teeth are seen in some cases

- Extraosseous lesions may appear as a pink to red, circumscribed elevated masses.

Radiographic features

The intraosseous lesions present as unilocular radiolucent area with a discrete and well-demarcated margins. Few lesions may occasionally occur as multilocular. Within the lesion, radiopaque structures such as *irregular calcifications or tooth-like densities* may be seen scattered.

A salt-and-pepper type of pattern can be produced by such radioopacities. The presence of adjacent tooth root resorption is a common and an important radiographic finding.

The extraosseous lesions may present with localised superficial bone resorption, or saucer-shaped radiolucencies with displacement of the adjacent tooth.

Histologic features

The histological features of a COC are characteristic which includes the following:

- A well-defined cystic lesion with a fibrous connective tissue wall lined by an odontogenic epithelium of 6–10 cells thick
- The prominent basal layer consists of *palisaded cuboidal or columnar cells* with a *hyperchromatic nuclei which are polarised* away from the basement membrane
- The overlying layer of loosely arranged epithelium may resemble the stellate reticulum
- Occasionally, intraluminal epithelial proliferation may occur obscuring the cyst lumen, which produces the impression of a solid tumour
- The most prominent microscopic feature of the COC is the presence of *'ghost cells' in the epithelial component* or in the fibrous capsule. The ghost cells are enlarged, ovoid or elongated elliptoid epithelial cells
- Ghost cells are altered epithelial cells that are characterised by the loss of nuclei (anucleate) with preservation of the basic cell outline
- These ghost cell may undergo dystrophic mineralisation resulting in large sheets of calcified material
- In some cases, dysplastic dentine or an area of more extensive dental hard tissue formation resembling an odontoma may be laid down adjacent to the basal layer of the epithelium. About 20% of *COC are associated with odontomas*
- Neoplastic (solid) calcifying odontogenic cysts are uncommon, accounting for 2%.

Treatment

The treatment is usually aggressive because of the unpredictable biological behaviour of this lesion. It is treated by surgical enucleation unless it is associated with another odontogenic tumour, in which wider excision may be required. When associated with ameloblastoma or other tumours, the treatment and prognosis are likely to be the same as for the associated tumour.

BOX 26.7 Lesions with Ghost Cells

- Calcifying odontogenic cysts.
- Odontomas.
- Ameloblastomas.
- Adenomatoid odontogenic tumours.
- Ameloblastic fibroodontomas.
- Ameloblastic fibromas.

The peripheral neoplastic COCs appear to have the good prognosis, with a minimal chance of recurrence after simple surgical excision.

Differential diagnosis (Box. 26.7)

Dentigerous cyst, OKC, ameloblastoma, adenomatoid odontogenic tumour, a partially mineralised odontoma, calcifying epithelial odontogenic tumour, and ameloblastic fibroodontoma.

Nonodontogenic Epithelial Cysts (Developmental Fissural Cyst)

Fissural or inclusion cysts are jaw cysts caused by epithelial inclusions along the lines of fusion of the various bones or embryonic processes.The epithelium for these cysts are derived from the cells that are entrapped between the embryonic or facial processes. Hence, each cyst is correlated to its actual anatomical location. (Fig. 26.20).

GLOBULOMAXILLARY CYST

Pathogenesis

The globulomaxillary cyst was 1st described by Thoma (1937) as fissural cyst arising from the nonodontogenic epithelium at the site of fusion of the globular process of the medial (frontonasal) process and the maxillary process. The

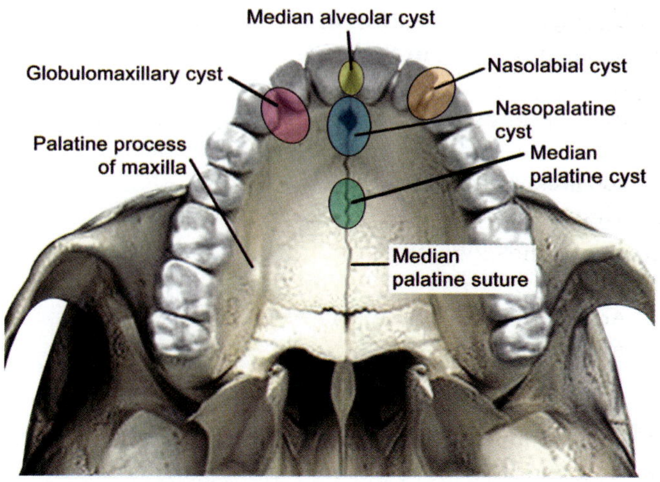

Figure 26.20 Fissural cyst of maxilla.

globular process is now embryologically referred to as premaxillary process.

Ferenczy (1958) proposed that the cysts actually forms in the suture, at the junction of premaxilla and maxilla and that they should be called as '*premaxillary–maxillary*' cysts.

Clinical features

- It is uncommon and can be seen in adults of varying age
- It develops between *the maxillary lateral incisor and cuspid teeth*
- It is asymptomatic and usually found during routine radiological examination. When the cyst becomes infected, pain may develop
- Expansion of the buccal cortex between maxillary lateral incisors and canines in large cysts
- Rotation of the crown and divergence of the roots between the maxillary lateral incisors and canines
- The involved teeth are usually vital
- Mucosa over the swelling retains the normal colour
- On aspiration, typical amber-coloured cystic fluid is encountered.

Radiographic features

- It characteristically appears as an *inverted, pear or tear-shaped radiolucency* between the roots of maxillary lateral incisors and canines. Inverted pear shape—the small end of the pear is directed towards the alveolar crest
- It causes divergence of the roots of adjacent teeth
- The lamina dura of the involved teeth are usually intact.

Histologic features

It is lined by stratified squamous epithelium or ciliated columnar epithelium. The connective tissue is fibrous with inflammatory cell infiltrates.

Treatment

Surgical enucleation of the cyst preserving the adjacent teeth is the treatment recommended for globulomaxillary cyst.

NASOLABIAL CYST

Other names

Nasoalveolar cyst, Kledstadt's cyst

Nasolabial cysts are *soft tissue cyst of the upper lip*. It is a rare fissural cyst and is not found within the bone but may involve the bone secondarily.

Pathogenesis

It arises as a proliferation of entrapped epithelium along the fusion of the globular process, the lateral nasal process and the maxillary process.

According to Roed-Petersen, this cyst probably originates from the lower part of the nasolacrimal duct rather than from the epithelium entrapped in the furrow.

Clinical features

- It is a rare lesion with an incidence ranging from 12 to 75 years of age, and a mean age between 41 and 46 years
- It occurs in both sexes with a slight predilection for women
- It is usually unilateral but can occur bilaterally also
- It is a painless swelling unless infected secondarily
- It appears as a soft tissue swelling in the mucolabial fold over the canine region
- Larger swelling can be seen as a bulge in the floor of the nose, obstructing the nasal cavity. They can be associated with flaring of the ala of nose, distortion of the nostril and fullness of the upper lip.

Radiographic features

The cyst can cause erosion of the underlying bone.

Histologic features

The nasoalveolar cyst is commonly lined by pseudostratified columnar epithelium, sometimes ciliated with goblet cells, or by stratified squamous epithelium.

Aspiration shows straw—coloured or whitish mucous fluid.

Treatment

The cyst should be removed intraorally through surgical excision.

NASOPALATINE DUCT CYST

Other names

Nasopalatine canal cyst, incisive canal cyst, median anterior maxillary cyst or vestigial cyst

The nasopalatine duct cyst is the *most common nonodontogenic cyst* of the oral cavity, occurring in about 1% of the population. It is formed within the incisive canal, located in the palatine bone or in the soft tissues of the palate overlying the foramen (incisive papilla).

Pathogenesis

The *nasopalatine ducts* undergo progressive degeneration, however, the persistence of epithelial *remnants* can become the source of epithelium in the development of nasopalatine duct cyst. It arises from spontaneous proliferation or proliferation of epithelium following trauma, bacterial infection or mucous retention.

Clinical features

- It can occur over a wide age range, with a mean age of 40–60 years
- Most commonly affects the males
- Smaller cysts are frequently asymptomatic
- Larger cysts presents as a swelling of the anterior palate with pain and discharge
- Larger cysts with perforation of the labial and palatal bony plates may present as an expansile, fluctuant swellings of the anterior palate
- The associated teeth are usually nonvital
- Few patients may complain of salty taste in mouth, which is produced by small sinus or remnant of nasopalatine duct that permits the cystic fluid to drain into the oral cavity

- The soft tissues cysts at the incisive papilla presents as a translucent or bluish coloured, dome-shaped swelling. This discolouration is due to the accumulation of fluid contents within the cyst
- Displacement of tooth is a common finding.

Radiographic features

It appears as a *radiolucency superimposed on the apices of the central incisors*. The anterior nasal spine may superimpose the cystic cavity giving it a *heart shape or inverted tear drop shape*. The size of the nasopalatine duct cysts is variable, but usually *from 6 mm* to several centimetres. Displacement of the adjacent teeth and divergence of central incisor roots are common features. Hence a radiolucency of less than 6 mm at the incisive canal fossa should be considered as normal.

Histologic features

The cavity is usually lined by stratified squamous epithelium or ciliated columnar epithelium with a relatively dense fibrous connective tissue band. A chronic inflammatory reaction consisting of lymphocytes and plasma cells can be observed in the cyst wall. Collections of mucous glands, goblet cells and cilia can also be often seen, which are highly indicative of their origin. The characteristic feature of this cyst is the *presence of structural elements in the cyst wall* that are native to the nasopalatine canal (neurovascular bundles in the wall). Aspiration shows a clear or straw-coloured fluid.

Treatment

Excision of the cyst by surgical enucleation through a palatal flap extending from canine to canine. Care should be taken to preserve the neurovascular bundle. A palatal acrylic splint can help in healing of the wound.

MEDIAN PALATAL (PALATINE) CYST

It is a rare cyst. This cyst may be difficult to differentiate from a nasopalatine duct cyst. In fact, most 'median palatal cyst' may represent as posteriorly positioned nasopalatine duct cysts.

Pathogenesis

It develops from the epithelium entrapped along the line of fusion of the palatal processes of the maxilla.

Clinical features

The median palatal cyst presents as a firm or fluctuant swelling in the midline of the hard palate, between the lateral palatal processes and posterior to the palatine papilla. The lesion is seen frequently in young adults. It must be stressed that a true median palatal cyst exhibits clinical enlargement of the palate.

Radiographic features

It appears as a well-circumscribed radiolucent area opposite to the bicuspid and molar region, with a sclerotic layer.

Histologic features

The cyst is lined by stratified squamous epithelium with a dense fibrous connective tissue band. Occasionally, it may be lined by pseudostratified ciliated columnar epithelium or a modified squamous epithelium.

Treatment

Surgical enucleation of the cyst through palatal approach.

MEDIAN MANDIBULAR CYST

It is an extremely rare lesion occurring in the midline of the mandible. It is a controversial lesion of questionable existence.

Pathogenesis

It develops from the epithelial remnants entrapped in the median mandibular fissure during fusion of the bilateral mandibular arches.

In reality, the mandible actually develops as a single bilobed proliferation of mesenchyme with a central isthmus in the midline. As the mandible develops, this isthmus is eliminated. Hence, fusion of epithelium is not possible.

Clinical features

Most of them are clinically asymptomatic and are discovered only on routine radiographic examination. They rarely cause obvious expansion of the cortical plates of bone. The associated teeth are usually vital.

Radiographic features

It appears as a well-circumscribed, unilocular radiolucency in the mandibular midline, between or apical to the mandibular central incisor teeth.

Histologic features

It is composed of stratified squamous epithelium with many folds and projections lining a central lumen.

Treatment

Surgical enucleation of the cyst with preservation of associated teeth. Recurrence is not expected in most cases.

MEDIAN ALVEOLAR CYST

Other names

Anterior maxillary cyst

Median alveolar cyst arises in the intermaxillary suture anterior to the anterior palatine cyst.

Clinical feature

It arises as a painless swelling on the labial surface of the premaxilla between the two incisors.

Radiographic features

An area of radiolucency in the midline, *close to the shadow of the incisor crowns* rather than the root. The periphery of the cavity may or may not be a lined with a thin layer of cortical bone.

Some cases might present with symmetrical resorption of the roots of teeth.

Treatment

Surgical excision of the cyst.

ODONTOGENIC INFLAMMATORY CYSTS

Inflammatory cysts are a group of lesions that arises from the epithelial proliferation within an inflammatory focus.

PERIAPICAL CYST

Other names

Radicular cyst/Apical periodontal cyst/Dental root end cyst

It is the most common odontogenic inflammatory cyst. It arises from the epithelial remnants in the periodontal ligament following necrosis of the pulp of an infected tooth.

The radicular cyst is classified as inflammatory cyst because the cyst develops *from periapical inflammatory response*. It can be considered as odontogenic cyst as it originates from the cell rests of Malassez, from the odontogenic epithelial layer (Fig. 26.21).

Pathogenesis

Arises from the epithelial residues (rests of Malassez) within the periodontal ligament as a result of inflammation (Flowchart 26.3).

Islands of squamous epithelium developed from odontogenic rests of Malassez can be found in a periapical granuloma without cystic transformation, which is referred to as '*bay cyst*'.

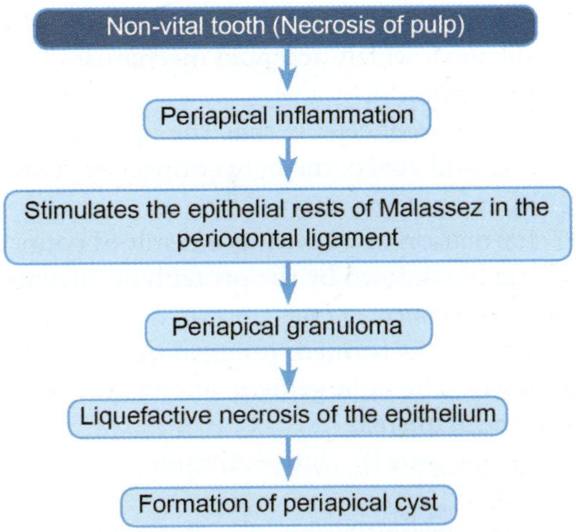

Flowchart 26.3 Pathogenesis of periapical cyst for non-vital tooth.

Development of a radicular cyst occurs in three phases:

1. *Phase of initiation:*
   Inflammation and bacterial antigens from the necrotic pulp, initiates the epithelial cell rests for cyst formation. It has been found that the bacterial endotoxins (from the necrotic pulp) and the inflammatory cytokines are the key initiating factor in the pathogenesis of radicular cysts
2. *Phase of cyst formation:*
   It is the process in which a cavity is lined by the proliferating epithelium (stratified squamous epithelium)
   The mechanism of cyst formation are as follows:
   - In a proliferating epithelial mass degeneration and death of cells occur in the centre, due to

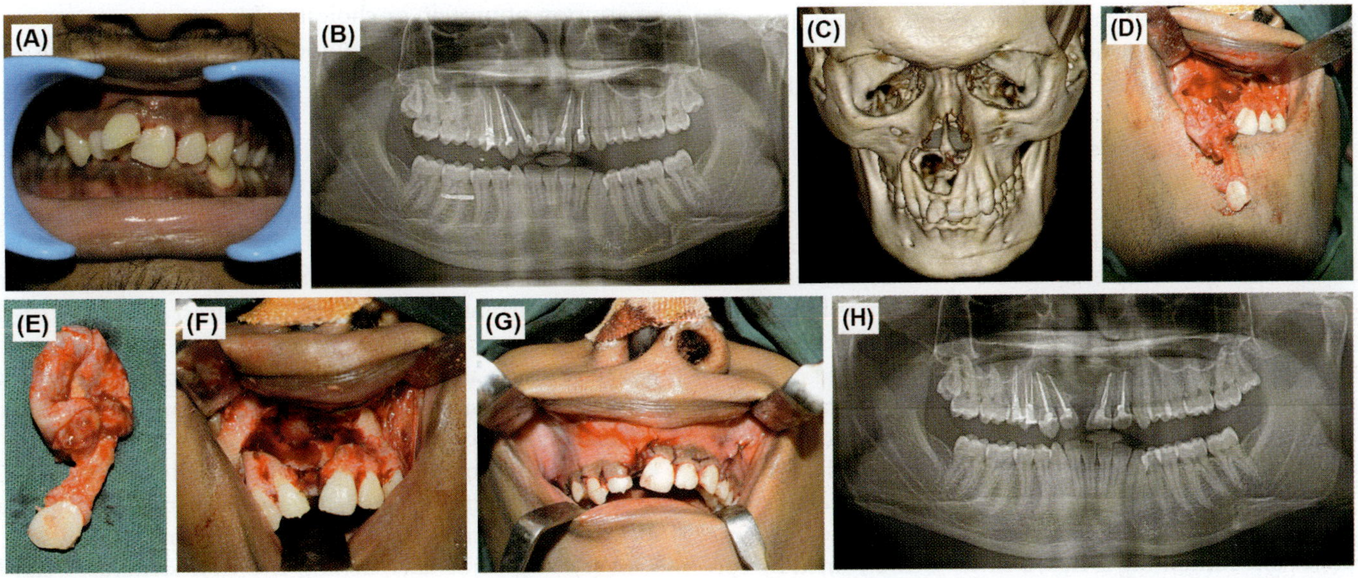

Figure 26.21 Periapical cyst. (**A**) Preoperative view. (**B**) OPG showing unilocular radiolucency in the periapical region of 11, 13 and 21. (**C**) CT scan showing bone resorption in the periapical region of 11 and also involving the nasal floor. (**D**) Mucoperiosteal flap raised and the cyst is enucleated along with the involved teeth. (**E**) Enucleated cyst with 11. (**F and G**) The cavity is irrigated and primary closure of the defect is done using vicryl. (**H**) Postoperative OPG.

increase in the size of the cells and hypoxia. It is the most widely accepted mechanism for cyst cavity formation
  - Another concept is that the epithelium proliferates and covers the bare connective tissue surface of an abscess cavity
  - Formation of a cavity as a result of connective tissue breakdown by the proteolytic enzymes

3. *Phases of enlargement of cyst:*
   Once the cysts is formed, it continues to grow and enlarge slowly. The enlargement of the cyst can occur by various mechanisms:
   - Mural growth–active division of the peripheral cells
   - Fluid accumulation–the cystic contents and the absence of lymphatic drainage creates an osmotic imbalance with the surrounding tissues of the cyst and supports the accumulation of fluid inside the cyst
   - Bone resorption–the growth of the cyst is accompanied by bone resorption and degradation of adjacent connective tissues.

Clinical features

It is the most common type of odontogenic cyst for about 60% of all the jaw cysts. It occurs from 2nd to 6th decades of age with a peak incidence in the 3rd decade. More commonly affects the males than the females.

The anterior region of maxilla has the highest incidence of the cyst, followed by the posterior region of maxilla, mandible and the anterior region of mandible.

- These cysts are usually asymptomatic and are often discovered on routine radiographic examination
- The periapical cyst cause bone resorption and does not produce bone expansion
- Often, the presence of a *nonvital tooth* assist us in the diagnosis of periapical cyst
- Sometimes, it presents as a slowly enlarging swelling. The enlargement is bony hard initially, but as the cyst increases in size, the covering becomes very thin and the swelling exhibits 'springiness' or 'egg shell crackling'
- When the cyst completely erodes the bone, the lesion becomes fluctuant. In the maxilla, it presents as buccal and palatal enlargement, whereas in the mandible it involves the buccal plate and rarely the lingual plate
- Pain may become significant on infection. Occasionally, a sinus tract may develop from the cyst to the oral mucosa
- *Cysts* that are retained even after the removal of the involved nonvital tooth are called as *residual radicular cysts.*

Simon (1980) showed two types of radicular cyst. (1) *True radicular cyst* containing a closed cavity entirely lined by epithelium, and (2) *periapical pocket cyst*/bay cyst where the epithelium is attached to the margins of the apical foramen and the cyst lumen opens into the affected root canal.

Radiographic features

It generally presents as a round to ovoid radiolucency surrounded by a narrow radiopaque margin, which is contiguous with the lamina dura of the involved tooth. Periapical cysts usually ranges from 1.5 to 3 cm, with a *well-defined outline with hyperostotic borders.* In long-standing cases, root resorption of the involved tooth may be seen.

Histologic features

- The radicular cyst is lined by stratified squamous epithelium of 6–20 cell layers thick. Occasionally, it is lined by pseudostratified, columnar or respiratory type of epithelium
- The epithelial lining may present with inflammatory cell infiltrates, predominantly of polymorphonuclear leucocytes and few lymphocytes
- The characteristic feature of radicular cyst is the presence of '*hyaline body or Rushton's body*' in the epithelial lining. It is rarely seen in connective tissue. The hyaline bodies are arc-shaped or tiny linear bodies, amorphous, eosinophilic and brittle in nature. They are believed to be the secretory product of odontogenic epithelium
- Foci of dystrophic calcification, cholesterol clefts and multinucleated foreign body-type giant cells may also be seen
- The connective tissue wall is more collagenous with abundant fibroblasts. The wall may presents with an inflammatory infiltrate, predominantly with lymphocytes. Lymphocytes appear as darkly stained nucleus occupying most of the cytoplasm. Plasma cells are also seen as eccentric nucleus with a cartwheel arrangement of the nuclear chromatin
- The cyst lumen usually contains fluid with a low concentration of protein or cholesterol
- Aspiration shows a shimmering gold or straw-coloured fluid.

Treatment

The various treatment options are as follows:

- Extraction of the associated nonvital tooth and curettage of the periapical region
- Endodontic treatment (root canal filling) of the nonvital tooth with an apicoectomy and direct curettage of the lesion
- Performing a root canal filling only, because most of the periapical lesions resolve after the removal of the inflammatory stimulus
- The commonly used procedure for radicular cyst is RCT of the nonvital tooth, enucleation of the cyst, apicoectomy and retrograde filling of the tooth
- Very large cyst encroaching the vital structures can be treated by marsupialisation
- If the cyst lining is incompletely removed, a residual cyst may develop later.

Differential diagnosis

Periapical granuloma, periapical cementoma, traumatic bone cyst, periodontal abscess.

RESIDUAL CYST

These are actually retained periapical cysts from the teeth they have been removed.

Pathogenesis

The possible causes are as follows:

- Incompletely removed periapical granuloma after an extraction
- Unrecognised cystic lesion after removal of an impacted tooth, associated with a lateral dentigerous cyst
- A cystic lesion develops on either a deciduous tooth or a retained tooth which either exfoliates or is extracted without the knowledge of the underlying pathologic process.

Clinical features

The residual cyst is more commonly seen in the middle-aged and elderly people. It is found in *any of the tooth bearing areas* of the mandible or maxilla or in edentulous sites, with a greater incidence in maxilla.

In most of the cases, the cyst is asymptomatic and are usually found on routine radiographic examination. They become symptomatic upon secondary infection. The residual cysts usually do not produce expansion of the bone.

Radiographic features

It appears as a well-defined round or ovoid radiolucency that can vary in size from a few mm to several cm.

Treatment

The commonly employed surgical procedure is enucleation with primary closure.

PARADENTAL CYST/BUCCAL BIFURCATION CYST

A paradental cyst is defined as *'a cyst originating near the cervical margin of the lateral aspect of a root as a consequence of an inflammatory process'* in the periodontal pocket of a vital tooth. Paradental cyst has been used synonymously for the buccal bifurcation cyst (BBC).

Paradental cyst is a rare inflammatory cyst that is most commonly seen in the buccal side of permanent mandibular 1st molars. The exact cause of paradental cyst is unknown.

WHO have included the BBC under the category 'paradental cysts' and suggested the term 'mandibular infected buccal cyst'. Thus BBC is defined as an inflammatory cyst arising on the *buccal side of a vital tooth.*

PATHOGENESIS

The aetiology of the BBC remains unclear, and various theories have been proposed.

During eruption of the permanent mandibular 1st molar, as cusps of the tooth penetrate the oral epithelium, an area of inflammation may occur in the connective tissue, which stimulates the epithelial proliferation and cyst formation. It may also develop from the junctional or crevicular epithelium, cell rests of Malassez, or the reduced enamel epithelium.

Clinical features

It commonly occurs in the age group of *4 and 14* years, with an equal sex predilection. It characteristically develops on the *buccal aspect of the mandibular 1st permanent molar* and occasionally with the mandibular 2nd molar.

It appears as a swelling over the gingiva of the affected molar or as bluish appearance on the alveolar ridge. Some cases may present with pain, tilting of the tooth, and suppuration from the pericoronal sulcus. It may also be associated with foul-tasting discharge and pocket formation in the buccal side.

Radiographic features

It presents as a *U-shaped well-defined radiolucency on the buccal aspect of a tooth* with a normal periodontal ligament space and lamina dura. Few cases may present with a periosteal reaction on the buccal surface and tilting of the apices of the affected roots towards the lingual cortex.

Histologic features

The histopathology is nonspecific for BBC. It is lined by nonkeratinised stratified squamous epithelium with areas of hyperplasia and chronic inflammatory cell infiltrate in the fibrous connective tissue capsule.

Treatment

Many methods of treatment have been proposed including tooth extraction and curettage of the lesion, curettage of the lesion without tooth extraction, endodontic treatment of the tooth and curettage of the lesion or enucleation of the cyst without tooth extraction.

NONEPITHELIAL LINED PSEUDOCYSTS

Pseudocystic lesions have a radiographic appearance similar to that of a cyst, but on microscopic examination, they lack an epithelial lining. These bone benign lesions are completely harmless and can develop in the maxilla, mandible or any other bones in the body.

SOLITARY BONE CYST

Other names

Traumatic or haemorrhagic cyst/extravasation cyst/unicameral bone cyst/idiopathic cyst/simple bone cyst

It is an uncommon pseudocyst comprising of about 1% of all jaw cysts. Solitary bone cysts are either *fluid-filled or empty intraosseous lesions*, found most commonly *in the long bones* of children and adolescents. In craniomaxillofacial region, it is more common in the mandible than the maxilla.

Pathogenesis

The aetiology is unclear, and a number of theories have been proposed of which, the most accepted theory is the ***trauma-haemorrhage theory***. According to the traumatic theory, in normal bone, trauma causes haemorrhage within the medullary spaces, which heals by organisation of the clot and eventual formation of new bone. In solitary bone cysts, the blood clot breaks down and leaves an empty cavity within the bone. Any obstruction in the lymphatic or venous drainage produces expansion of the lesion along the medullary spaces. On reaching the buccal cortex, this expansion tends to cease.

Other theories of origin by Whinery are as follows:

- Cystic degeneration of the primary bone tumours
- As a result of faulty calcium metabolism (e.g. parathyroid disease)
- Necrosis of the fatty marrow due to ischaemia
- End result of a low-grade chronic infection
- A result of osteoclasis. Trauma causes disturbed circulation from an unequal balance of osteoclasis and repair of bone
- Implantation type of cyst. The epithelium of the maxillary sinus becomes entrapped along the line of surgical entry into the sinus and subsequently proliferates to form a true cystic cavity.

Clinical features

- It is more frequent in the 2nd decade of life (young persons) with a mean age of 18 years
- Males are affected more commonly than females
- Mandible is more commonly involved than the maxilla. Majority of them are seen in the posterior portion of the mandible above the inferior dental canal
- It presents as an asymptomatic swelling mostly on the buccal side
- The involved teeth are usually vital.

Radiographic features

It appears as a unilocular radiolucency of variable size with a smooth outline and a thin sclerotic border. It may range from a centimetre to large lesions involving most of the molar area as well as part of the ramus. When the lesion involves the roots of the teeth, the margins may have a lobulated or scalloped appearance extending between the roots of these teeth. The lamina dura of the teeth appears intact. It rarely causes cortical expansion and pathological fracture.

Care must be taken to differentiate the small solitary traumatic cyst from the lingual salivary gland depression, which has a similar radiographic appearance.

Histologic features

It consists of a thin fibrous connective tissue membrane without any other significant features. There can be fragments of fibrin with *few red blood cells, haemorrhage and haemosiderin* fragments, or giant cells adhering to the bone surface.

Cystic contents

On surgical opening of the cyst, the cavity contains a deep yellow-coloured serosanguinous fluid, necrotic blood clots, and fragments of fibrous connective tissue. Some cysts may be empty.

Treatment

The cyst has to be opened to determine the nature of the lesion. It is usually treated by *surgical exploration* of the cavity. Curettage of the cystic wall stimulates haemorrhage and eventual healing by the formation of new bone.

STAFNE'S CYST

Other names

Static bone cavity, static bone cyst, latent bone cyst, defect of the mandible, lingual mandibular bone cavity, developmental lingual mandibular salivary gland depression

Stafne's cyst *is not a cyst*. It is an *anatomic indentation* of the posterior lingual mandible that has a cystic appearance on radiographs. It may be a form of slightly aberrant salivary gland tissue adjacent to the lingual surface of the body of the mandible. Hence, it is considered as a developmental entity rather than a pathologic defect.

Pathogenesis

The lesion is due to the entrapment of the salivary gland tissue or other soft tissues during development of the mandible.

Clinical features

The lesion is rare. The lesion is asymptomatic and is discovered during radiographic examination. It presents as a deep well-circumscribed depression adjacent to the lingual surface of the body of mandible, with an indentation on the lingual surface of mandible, within which lies a portion of the submandibular gland.

Radiographic features

The lesion appears as an *ovoid radiolucency generally situated between the inferior alveolar canal and the inferior border of mandible* in the 2nd or 3rd molar regions. Anteriorly, it presents as a round or ovoid radiolucency in between the central incisors and 1st premolars.

Histologic features

These are cavities and does not require diagnostic tissue. They may have sublingual salivary gland tissue or lymph nodes. Sialography can be done to confirm the presence of salivary gland tissue.

Treatment

As these are cavities, no treatment is required.

ANEURYSMAL BONE CYST

Aneurysmal bone cyst was 1st described by *Jaffe and Lichtenstein in 1942*. It is a rare haemorrhagic lesion of the bone. It does not contain vascular aneurysms and hence it is not considered as a true bony cyst. It can be considered as a *tumour like reactive lesion of bone* with exaggerated proliferative response of the vascular tissue similar to the peripheral and central giant cell granuloma (Fig. 26.22).

The lesion is characteristically *a blood-filled cyst*. The term 'aneurysmal bone cyst' was suggested by Jaffe to describe the characteristic 'blown-out' contour of the affected bone in the radiographs.

Pathogenesis

Lichtenstein put forth that aneurysmal bone cyst arises from a *local alteration in the haemodynamics,* which results in increased venous pressure and subsequent development of an engorged vascular bed. It is followed by resorption of bone, which is replaced by connective tissue, osteoid and new bone.

The aetiology is controversial and numbers of possibilities have been proposed, which includes the following:

- Cyst formation as the end result of a common pathophysiological process with a variety of causes
- It may result from a *vascular disturbance* in the form of sudden venous occlusion or the development of an arteriovenous shunt
- As a secondary phenomenon arising from the breakdown of a part of preexisting bone lesion
- Arises as a modification of some other lesion of bone, most of which may be destroyed by haemorrhage
- Few lesions showed evidence of an associated lesion of bone with the cyst. They hypothesised that the primary lesion initiated an arteriovenous malformation in the bone and that *its haemodynamic forces* is responsible for the formation of aneurysmal bone cyst. The most frequently associated lesions were solitary bone cysts, giant cell tumours and osteosarcomas.

Clinical features

It is commonly seen in long bones and vertebral column (50%), the pelvis and vertebrae (20%) and also frequently seen in clavicle, rib, innominate bone, skull and bones of the hands and feet. The lesion is commonly encountered in adults, predominantly young persons of 18 years, with a slight female predilection. It is more commonly seen in mandible than the maxilla.

On surgical exploration of the cyst, excessive bleeding and the *blood 'welling up'* from the tissue is encountered, which is an important characteristics of aneurysmal cyst. The tissue inside the cyst resembles a blood-soaked sponge with large pores which represents the cavernous spaces of the lesion. Few cysts have elevated vascular pressures as high as arteriolar levels.

The pathogenesis of aneurysmal cyst undergoes four phases:

- **Initial osteolytic phase**
- **Active growth phase**—rapid destruction of bone and a subperiosteal blow out pattern

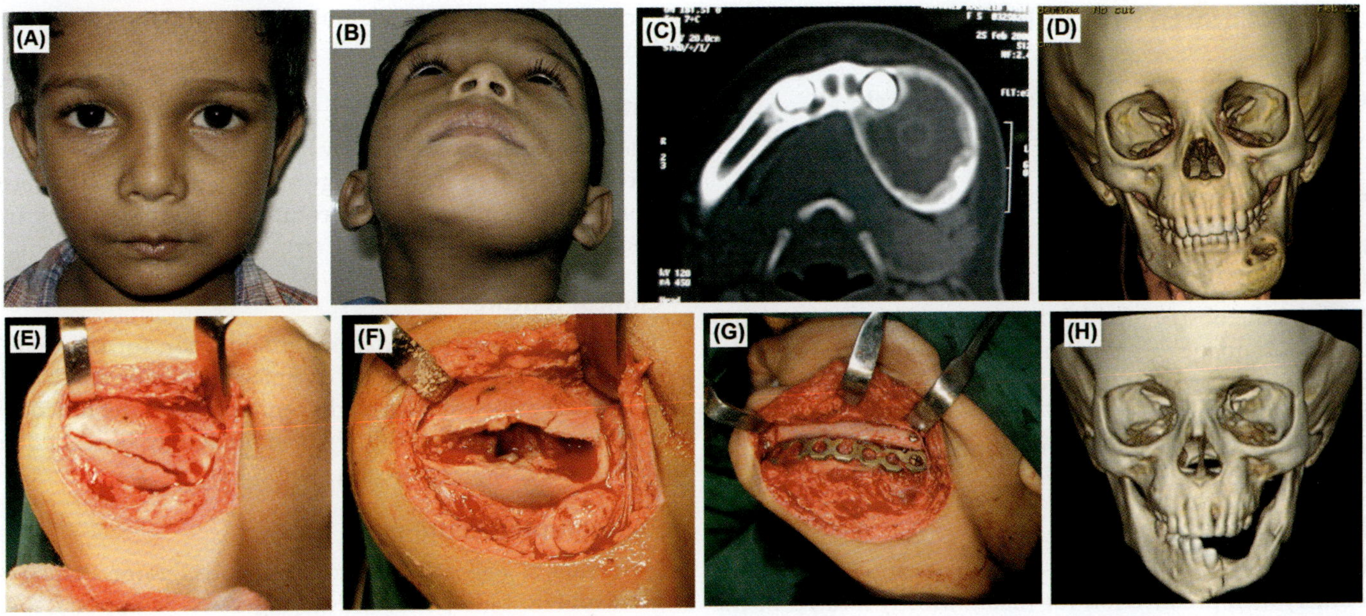

Figure 26.22 Aneurysmal bone cyst. (**A** and **B**) Preoperative view with swelling on the left side of mandibular body. (**C** and **D**) Axial section and 3D CT scan showing bucco-lingual expansion of the left side of mandible with perforation of the buccal cortex. (**E**) Through submandibular approach, the cyst is exposed. (**F**) On surgical exploration, the tissue inside the cyst resembled a blood-soaked sponge and the cyst was excised. (**G**) Reconstruction of the defect with bone graft and reconstruction plate. (**H**) Postoperative OPG and CT scan.

- **Mature phase (stage of stabilisation)**–formation of peripheral bony shell and internal bony septa and trabeculae, which is responsible for the classic soap-bubble appearance
- **Healing phase**–progression of calcification and ossification of the cyst and its eventual transformation into a dense bony mass.

Radiographic features

Its radiographic picture is distinctive. It presents with cortical expansion of bone that appears cystic with a *honeycomb or soap-bubble appearance* and is eccentrically ballooned. The cortical bone appears destroyed with periosteal reaction.

Histologic features

It consists of fibrous connective tissue stroma containing many cavernous or sinusoidal blood-filled spaces, with or without thrombosis. The connective tissue stroma shows numerous young fibroblasts and multinucleated giant cell. Traces of haemosiderin, new osteoid and bone formation are also encountered.

Treatment

Surgical curettage or excision is the treatment of choice as it has a relatively high recurrence rate. It can be supplemented with cryotherapy.

Differential diagnosis

OKC, central giant cell granuloma and ameloblastic fibroma.

CYSTS ASSOCIATED WITH MAXILLARY ANTRUM

SURGICAL CILIATED CYST OF MAXILLA

Other names

Postoperative maxillary cyst, sinus mucocele

It was originally reported by Gregory and Shafer. It is termed as postoperative maxillary cyst as it arises as a delayed complication of surgery involving the maxillary sinus, after many years.

Pathogenesis

The cyst develops either after trauma or *surgery to the sinuses* or due to the obstruction of the ostium. The cyst most frequently originates after a Caldwell-Luc procedure in the floor of maxillary sinus. It develops as an implantation type of cyst, in which a portion of the sinus lining becomes entrapped and subsequently forms a true cyst, which gets anatomically separated from the sinus.

Clinical features

The majority of the cases are in 4th to 5th decades (middle-aged or older) with predilection for males. Mostly located in the premolar and molar regions of maxilla.

The patient often gives history of surgical procedure involving the maxilla, frequently of 10–20 years back.

It presents as an extraoral in the cheek or intraoral swelling of the palate or alveolus. The patient may complain poorly localised pain, tenderness or discomfort in the maxilla, associated with pus. When the lesion with mucocoele is infected, it is called as mucopyocele.

Radiographic features

It reveals a well-defined unilocular radiolucency closely related to the maxillary sinus. The postoperative maxillary cyst appears to encroach the sinus but remains anatomically separate from it (without any communication).

Histologic features

The cysts are lined by respiratory epithelium–pseudostratified ciliated columnar epithelium. In case of infection, squamous metaplasia may be found. The connective tissue wall of the cyst may be fibrous or cellular.

On aspiration, the fluid shows presence of hyaluronic acid and chondroitin-4-sulphate.

Treatment

The treatment for this lesion is surgical enucleation of the cyst and in case of thin wall and extensive bony perforation marsupialisation is appropriate.

BENIGN MUCOSAL CYST OF MAXILLARY ANTRUM

RETENTION CYST OF MAXILLARY SINUS

Other names

Secretory cyst of maxillary antrum, mucocoele of maxillary sinus, mucosal cyst of maxillary sinus

It represents a retention phenomenon of the mucous glands associated with the lining of maxillary sinus. It is commonly encountered as an accidental finding in the radiographs (Fig. 26.23).

Pathogenesis

The cause of development may be traumatic injury associated with extraction of tooth, allergy or sinus infection. They arise from blockage of an antral seromucous gland, resulting in a ductal epithelium-lined cystic structure filled with mucin.

Clinical features

There is no clear-cut age or sex predilection for this cyst. A majority of the patients are completely asymptomatic. Few cases might present with slight tenderness on the mucobuccal fold and numbness of the upper lip. Rarely, buccal expansion of the maxillary antrum can be seen.

Radiographic features

It reveals a well-defined, homogeneous, dome-shaped or hemispheric radiopacity of varying sizes. It appears to be arising from the floor of the antrum and superimposed on it. As the sinus mucocoeles arise from the sinus lining, there is no bone on the surface. The radiopacity appears as a soft tissue mass rather than as a calcified area and other landmarks can be visualised through the lesion.

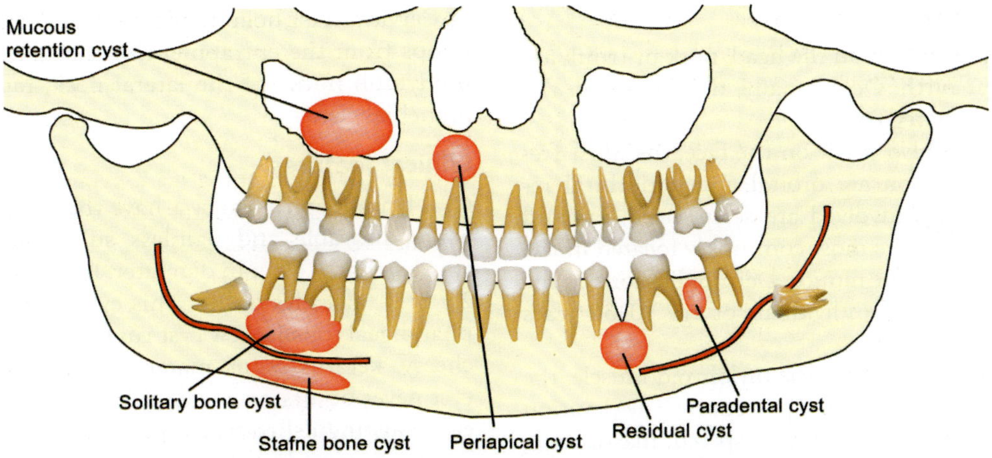

Figure 26.23 Locations of inflammatory cyst, pseudocysts and maxillary antral cyst.

Histologic features

Two forms:

Nonsecretory cyst—no definite lining. But have fluid (mucoid material) surrounded by a compressed connective tissue.

Secretory type of antral cyst—the lesion may be lined by a respiratory type of epithelium (pseudostratified columnar epithelium) with occasional interspersed mucous cells.

Inflammatory cell infiltrates are present in the connective tissue wall of both forms of cyst.

Treatment

They show limited growth and are not destructive, hence left untreated. They either remain unchanged or disappear spontaneously within a relative period of time.

MUCOCOELE OF THE MAXILLARY ANTRUM

It is a true cyst lined by the mucoperiosteum of the involved sinus and filled with mucus.

Pathogenesis

It is caused by blockage of the ostium from inflammatory changes associated with chronic sinusitis. The obstruction results in accumulation of mucus and cystic growth by an osmotic mechanism.

Clinical features

Commonly seen in middle age with no sex predilection. It presents as a gradually enlarging swelling of the cheek and lateral nasal region with obliteration of the buccal sulcus or nasolabial fold intraorally. It causes ballooning expansion of the surrounding bone and displacement of adjacent structures, resulting in nasal blockage and proptosis.

Radiographic features

It reveals a well-defined radiolucency with expansion and perforation of the bone margins. The lesion is spherical with medial expansion. The characteristic feature is *complete opacification of the maxillary sinus* with evidence of bony expansion, anteriorly and superiorly resulting in elevation of the orbital floor.

Histologic features

The cyst is lined by normal antral mucosa (ciliated respiratory type epithelium or flattened simple cuboidal or squamous epithelium) filled with mucus or mucoid material. Chronic inflammatory cells may be present in the wall.

Treatment

This cyst may be managed by decompression or complete removal by curettage through a Caldwell-Luc approach, or by an endoscopic approach through the middle meatus with marsupialisation of the cyst.

SOFT TISSUE CYSTS

DEVELOPMENTAL CYST

DERMOID AND EPIDERMOID CYSTS

Other names

Dermoid cystic tumour, cystic teratoma, ovarian cystic tera-toma, congenital cyst of spine

It is considered as a hamartomatous tumour containing multiple sebaceous glands and almost all skin adnexa (nails and dental, cartilage-like and bone-like structures). When it occurs on the skin, these are thin-walled tumours containing different amounts of fatty masses.

Pathogenesis

The development of dermoid cyst may be due to the entrapment of multipotential cells or implantation of epithelium. It arises from sequestration of skin and subsequent implantation of it along the lines of embryonic closure. Seward (1965) suggested that the origin of dermoid cysts on the floor of the mouth is contributions from the mandibular arches to the tongue.

Clinical features

- Congenital dermoid cysts on the head, neck or trunk are usually visible at birth. Occasionally, they occur on the neck or in a midline region
- Dermoid cysts may also occur on the face, the most frequently involved region are orbital and periorbital region. The other sites involved are scalp, neck, ear and nose. The oral lesions are most commonly located in the midline of the floor of the mouth. Dermoid lesions of the floor of mouth occur in individuals of age 10–30 years with no gender predilection
- When the cyst is present above the mylohyoid muscle, the tongue is displaced superiorly and posteriorly. The elevation of the tongue results in difficulty of speech, mastication, breathing and closure of the mouth
- When the cyst is present below the mylohyoid muscle, it appears as a midline swelling of the neck
- When the lesions are deeper between the geniohyoid and mylohyoid muscles, it produces a submental swelling in the neck giving the patient a '*double-chin*' appearance
- The dermoid cysts occur as painless and slow growing swelling of size 1–4 cm. These cysts may be soft and doughy or fluctuant because of the presence of keratin and sebum in the lumen
- The congenital mouth cysts are subdivided into: *epidermoid (simple) cysts, dermoid (complex) cysts and teratoid (complex) cysts.*

Histologic features

Dermoid cysts are lined by stratified squamous epithelium supported by a fibrous connective tissue wall. The presence of skin appendages (hair follicles, sebaceous glands and sweat glands) are characteristic features of dermoid cyst.

Epidermoid cysts also have an epithelial lining but the skin appendages are absent.

Sometimes, the lining epithelial may proliferate as papillary boundaries, which may superficially resemble epidermal carcinoma, and may be misdiagnosed as a cancer.

Treatment

Intraoral lesions are removed by surgical excision through a midline incision in the free edge of the lingual frenum. If the cyst is located below the mylohyoid muscle, it is approached extraorally by a horizontal submandibular incision.

LYMPHOEPITHELIAL CYST

Other name

Branchial cleft cyst

Cervical lymphoepithelial cysts or branchial cleft cyst are usually located in the lateral portion of the neck, anterior to the sternomastoid muscle. Oral lymphoepithelial cysts appear most commonly in the floor of the mouth.

Pathogenesis

Oral lymphoepithelial cyst develops within a benign lymphoid aggregate or accessory tonsil of the oral or pharyngeal mucosa.

Cervical lymphoepithelial cyst or branchial cleft cyst develops from the entrapment of salivary duct epithelium in the lymph nodes of the lateral neck, rather than from the branchial cleft.

Clinical features

Oral lymphoepithelial cyst have the appearance of a yellow-white, movable and painless submucosal nodule that is smaller than 0.6 cm in diameter. It is usually seen during the 2nd or 3rd decades of life. This cyst usually occur within the pharyngeal tonsils. Few cyst rupture to release a foul-tasting, cheesy, keratinaceous material. The oral lymphoepithelial cyst never occurs on the alveolar mucosa, hence they can be easily distinguished from other cyst.

The cervical lymphoepithelial cysts appear in late childhood or young adulthood. It is most commonly found in the lateral aspect of the neck anterior to the sternocleidomastoid muscle at the level of angle of the mandible. It appears as a soft and fluctuant mass which may form a fistulous tract and drain externally.

Histologic features

The intraoral cysts are usually lined by atrophic stratified squamous epithelium, lacking rete pegs and with a minimal granular cell layer. The cyst is entangled within an aggregate of mature lymphocytes. This combination *of epithelium-lined cyst with lymphoid aggregates* is a characteristic feature of oral lymphoepithelial cyst.

The cervical lymphoepithelial cysts are lined by stratified squamous epithelium, pseudostratified columnar epithelium or both. The connective tissue may show lymphoid aggregates. The lumen contains mucus and desquamated parakeratotic cells.

Treatment

The oral lymphoepithelial cyst does not require any treatment unless it is being constantly traumatised. The cervical lymphoepithelial cysts are best treated by complete surgical excision either by cervical or intraoral approach.

THYROGLOSSAL DUCT CYST

It is a rare cyst occurring in the midline of neck. It arises from the epithelial remnants of the thyroid gland development.

Pathogenesis

The pathogenesis is related to the *thyroid gland development*. During the formation of the posterior portion of the tongue in the region of foramen caecum, the thyroid anlage grows downwards from the foramen caecum to its permanent position in the neck. Any residual epithelial elements along this pathway which has not completely atrophied may give rise to cysts in the later life.

Clinical features

- It is often seen before 20 years, but can also be seen in the older population

- These cyst are most commonly located in the midline below the level of the hyoid bone or within the tongue (2%). Intraoral lesions arise at the foramen caecum or in the floor of mouth
- The cyst appears as an asymptomatic, soft, movable and sometimes tender swellings in the midline of the neck, at or below the level of the hyoid bone. When the patient swallows or protrudes the tongue, the swelling also moves
- If the mass is located high in the tract, they may cause dyspnoea or dysphonia.

Histologic features

It may be lined with stratified squamous epithelium, ciliated columnar or an intermediate transitional type of epithelium depending upon the level of the cyst in relation to the hyoid bone. The fibrous connective tissue wall frequently contains thyroid tissue, lymphoid tissue and mucous glands. The cysts present in the lingual area might have mucous cells in the cyst lining and seromucous glands in the fibrous wall.

Treatment

Complete surgical excision along with its tract and branches is essential to avoid recurrence. Because of the intimate association of the tract with hyoid bone, simultaneous removal of the central portion of the hyoid bone is necessary to ensure the complete removal of tract.

As a result, the Sistrunk's treatment requires the removal of approximately 1 cm of tissue that surrounds the duct in addition to 1–2 cm of the central part of the hyoid bone.

CYSTIC HYGROMA

It is a developmental abnormality arising as a progressive dilatation of the lymphatic channels. It is a type of lymphangioma. Lymphangiomas of the neck are commonly called as cystic lymphangioma or cystic hygroma.

Pathogenesis

Cystic hygromas occur embryologically as a result of the sequestration of lymphatic tissue from lymphatic sacs during the development of lymphaticovenous sacs. These sequestered tissues fail to communicate with remainder of the lymphatic or venous system. Dilatation of these sequestered lymphatic tissues results in the development of cystic hygroma.

Clinical features

- It is often present at birth and most commonly diagnosed before the age of 2 years
- It can occur anywhere in the body, but frequently presents as a swelling in the neck or face
- The lesion usually appears unilateral but may involve the entire side of the neck and lower face
- It presents as a painless, soft, compressible and nontender swelling with a bluish colour skin overlying the swelling. The patient may give a history of gradual or sudden enlargement of the swelling
- The transillumination of the swelling is positive.

Histologic features

It consists of dilated cystic spaces lined by endothelial cells. Aspiration of these cysts may show milky, serous, serosanguinous or straw-coloured fluid.

Treatment

Complete surgical excision of the mass is the definitive treatment for cystic hygroma. As it lacks encapsulation, recurrences are common. Sclerosing solutions can be injected into cystic areas to produce scarring of the lesion and avoid recurrence.

NASOPHARYNGEAL CYST

Other name

Tornwald's cyst

It is a rare, benign, developmental lesion in the midline of the nasopharynx. It may be classified as congenital or acquired.

Pathogenesis

It arises as a result of abnormal embryological development at the posterior wall of nasopharynx. Congenital nasopharyngeal cyst may arise from the *'pharyngeal bursa or Rathke's pouch'*.

Clinical features

The most common age of presentation is in the 2nd and 3rd decade of life, around 15–30 years.

Based on the drainage, the nasopharyngeal cyst is classified into two categories: crusting and cystic. The cystic type has an obstruction in their drainage pathway and therefore resulting in cyst formation, whereas the crusting type without any obstruction drains spontaneously into the nasopharynx.

It appears as a pendulous polyp or a generalised bursa like swelling in the midline, of the posterior wall of the nasopharynx. It can be diagnosed by nasoendoscopic examination.

Patients may present with nonspecific nose or ear symptoms such as snoring, nasal obstruction, postnasal drip, ear block, conductive hearing loss and neck stiffness. On infection of the cyst, it may lead to foul odour, sore throat or headache in the occipital region.

Histopathological features

They are lined by stratified squamous epithelium, with chronic inflammatory cells and congested vessels.

Treatment

The cyst can be managed surgically by means of simple excision of the pendulous polyp or a marsupialisation of a cyst appearing as a bursa.

HETEROTOPIC CYSTS

Other names

Oral cysts with gastric intestinal epithelium, oral alimentary tract cyst, anterior median lingual cyst, intralingual cyst of foregut origin

Developmental anomalies of the foregut form a group of disorders, referred to as foregut duplications. Foregut anomalies in the head and neck are rare. In the neck and oral cavity, lesions have been described under a number of terms based on the histological nature of their lining. The lingual cyst is used to describe cysts of foregut origin that arise within the tongue.

Pathogenesis

It arises from the embryonal rests of foregut that becomes entrapped between the parts of the developing tongue.

Clinical features

It is a rare lesion and in most cases occur in infants and young children, between the ages of 2 and 11 years, with a predilection for males.

It appears as an asymptomatic, fluctuant swelling in the anterior part of the tongue or floor of mouth, covered by normal mucosa. These cyst may be entirely enclosed or may communicate with the surface. Patient may often complain difficulty in feeding.

Histopathological features

The lingual cyst may be lined partly by stratified squamous epithelium and partly by the intestinal mucosa.

Treatment

Treatment involves complete surgical excision of the lesion.

PARASITIC CYSTS

Other names

Hydatid cyst, Cysticercus cellulosae, trichinosis

Parasitic cysts in mouth are rare. Parasitic cysts are caused by *Echinococcus* and *Taenia.*

Hydatid disease is caused by the larvae of *Echinococcus granulosus*, the dog tapeworm.

Pathogenesis

The humans may accidentally ingest the ova, which gets hatched to the upper gastrointestinal (GI) tract. From the GI tract, small embryos permeate through the intestinal mucosa and are dispersed by the blood vessels and lymphatics to all parts of the body.

Clinical features

It is most commonly seen in the salivary glands and the pterygopalatine or infratemporal fossa. Other sites that are reported includes the tongue, maxillary sinus, buccal mucosa and the subcutaneous tissues of the neck.

Histopathological features

The mature hydatid cyst is comprised of three layers: an outer layer of host origin and two inner layers of parasitic origin. The outer host layer contains fibrous tissue with chronic inflammatory cells, eosinophils and giant cells. The intermediate layer has white, nonnucleated and delicate laminations. The inner layer is made of nucleated germinal layer.

The cystic fluid is relatively clear, albumin-free and contains the 'hydatid sand'. Hydatid sand consists of brood capsules and scolices (daughter cysts).

Cysticercosis is caused by the larval form, *Cysticercus cellulosae*, of the pork tapeworm *Taenia solium.* Trichinosis is caused by *Trichinella spiralis*, a roundworm parasite of rats and pigs.

Cysts of the salivary glands–(mucocoele, ranula, mucous extravasation cyst, mucous retention cyst, polycystic disease of the parotid) Refer to Chapter 31.

Chapter
27

Odontogenic Tumours

OUTLINE

INTRODUCTION

According to Sir Rupert Willis, ***a tumour or neoplasm*** is defined as 'an abnormal mass of tissue, the growth of which is uncontrolled and uncoordinated with that of the normal tissue and persists in the same excessive manner even after the cessation of the stimulus that evoked the change'.

The term '*odontogenic*' signifies all the primordial tissues—epithelium, mesenchyme and ectomesenchyme of the *tooth-forming apparatus*. Any aberrance or abnormal proliferation of such tissue at any stage of differentiation gives rise to an odontogenic tumour. The oral tissues retain some remnants of these embryonic tissues, postnatally. These tissues have inherent potential for replication and growth, the stimulus for which has been controversial. These dormant cells and tissues that give rise to the odontogenic tumour histologically resemble the native embryonic tissue of origin and are unique to the jawbones.

The possible source of cells that give rise to odontogenic tumours are:

- *Cell rests of Serres*
- *Cell rests of Malassez*
- *Oral epithelium*
- *Ectomesenchyme/mesenchyme.*

The jaw tumours that arise from tissues other than the tooth-forming tissues are referred to as nonodontogenic and is not exclusive to the jawbone. As with all *tumours, odontogenic tumours are classified as benign and malignant*, based on their biological behaviour.

Benign tumour

These are a mass of cells or tissues which proliferate and divide in their primary location without invading the surrounding tissues or other parts of the body. They tend to grow slowly with distinct borders and enlarge by peripheral expansion. The benign tumours are not life threatening and their clinical course is predictable.

Malignant tumour

These are composed of embryonic, primitive or poorly differentiated cells that grow uncontrollably and rapidly, invading the surrounding tissues or distant sites. The spread to the distant sites is through the bloodstream or the lymphatic system and this process of rapid spread is called as metastasis. They grow quickly with irregular borders, and their clinical course is destructive.

Odontogenic tumours

Odontogenic tumours are a heterogeneous group of lesions arising from the cells of odontogenic origin (teeth). They present with diverse clinical behaviour, ranging from hamartomatous lesions to malignancy. They are found exclusively in the jaws as they are derived from the tooth-forming apparatus.

Clinically, they are asymptomatic, with jaw expansion, displacement of teeth, root resorption and bone loss. Microscopically, they mimic the cell or tissue of origin. Histologically, they resemble enamel organ or may contain hard tissue elements of enamel, dentin or cementum.

CLASSIFICATION OF ODONTOGENIC TUMOURS

Several classifications have been proposed based on the histological pattern or the cell of origin. The odontogenic tumours are commonly divided into three broad groups:

- The lesions comprising odontogenic epithelial elements
- Those originating from odontogenic mesenchyme
- Lesions with a mix of both epithelium and mesenchyme.

The WHO's 1st classification of neoplasms in 1971 was titled as 'Histological typing of odontogenic tumours, jaw cysts and allied lesions', with the inclusion of all neoplasms and cysts of odontogenic origin. The latest WHO (2017) Classification on 'Odontogenic and Maxillofacial Bone Tumours' proposed various modifications based on the evidence and molecular studies. In this, the odontogenic tumour is primarily divided into benign and malignant tumours (Boxes 27.1 and 27.2).

According to WHO classification (2017), the odontogenic and maxillofacial bone tumours include 'a heterogeneous group of lesions ranging from cysts, benign neoplasms, hamartomas to malignant neoplasms, with metastatic potential'. The

BOX 27.1 WHO Classification of Odontogenic and Maxillofacial Bone Tumours (2017)

A. Benign Odontogenic Tumours

i. Epithelial origin/Odontogenic epithelium without odontogenic ectomesenchyme
1. Ameloblastoma
2. Ameloblastoma, unicystic type
3. Ameloblastoma, extraosseous/peripheral type
4. Metastasising (malignant) ameloblastoma
5. Squamous odontogenic tumour
6. Calcifying epithelial odontogenic tumour (CEOT)
7. Adenomatoid odontogenic tumour (AOT)

ii. Mixed origin/Odontogenic epithelium with odontogenic ectomesenchyme, with or without dental hard tissue formation
1. Ameloblastic fibroma
2. Primordial odontogenic tumour
3. Compound odontoma
4. Complex odontoma
5. Dentinogenic ghost cell tumour (calcifying odontogenic cyst)

iii. Mesenchymal origin/Odontogenic ectomesenchyme with or without included odontogenic epithelium
1. Odontogenic fibroma
2. Odontogenic myxoma (myxofibroma)
3. Cementoblastoma
4. Cemento-ossifying fibroma

B. Malignant Odontogenic Tumours

i. Odontogenic carcinomas
1. Ameloblastic carcinoma
2. Primary intraosseous carcinoma, Not otherwise specified (NOS)
3. Sclerosing odontogenic carcinoma
4. Clear cell odontogenic carcinoma
5. Ghost cell odontogenic carcinoma

ii. Odontogenic sarcomas

iii. Odontogenic carcinosarcoma

BOX 27.2 Biological Classification of Odontogenic Tumours

A. Benign, No Recurrence Potential
- Adenomatoid odontogenic tumour
- Squamous odontogenic tumour
- Cementoblastoma
- Periapical cemento-osseous dysplasia
- Odontoma

B. Benign, Some Recurrence Potential
- Cystic ameloblastoma
- Calcifying epithelial odontogenic tumour
- Central odontogenic fibroma
- Florid cemento-osseous dysplasia
- Ameloblastic fibroma and fibro-odontoma

C. Benign Aggressive
- Ameloblastoma
- Clear cell odontogenic tumour
- Odontogenic ghost cell tumour
- Odontogenic myxoma
- Odontoameloblastoma

D. Malignant
- Malignant ameloblastoma
- Ameloblastic carcinoma
- Primary intraosseous carcinoma
- Odontogenic ghost cell carcinoma
- Ameloblastic fibrosarcoma

metastatic ameloblastoma was shifted to the benign category, as the metastatic ameloblastoma is histopathologically identical to the benign ameloblastoma. Three new lesions were included namely *sclerosing odontogenic carcinoma, primordial odontogenic tumour and odontogenic carcinosarcoma.*

BENIGN ODONTOGENIC TUMOURS

EPITHELIAL ORIGIN

AMELOBLASTOMA

(Adamantinoma, adamantoblastoma, multilocular cyst)

It is the 2nd most common odontogenic tumour of enamel organ-type tissue, which does not undergo differentiation to the point of enamel formation.

Definition

The term 'adamantinoma' was created by *Malassez* (1885), which refers to the development of hard tissues. In 1934, *Churchill* replaced the term adamantinoma with the now accepted term *'ameloblastoma'*. Ameloblastoma has been defined by *Robinson* as 'usually unicentric, nonfunctional, intermittent in growth, anatomically benign and clinically persistent'.

WHO (1991) defined ameloblastoma as a benign but locally aggressive tumour with a high tendency for recurrence, composed of odontogenic epithelium proliferating within a fibrous stroma.

It is a low-grade, malignant, basaloid tumour with a variable range of histopathologic patterns, clinical forms and behaviour.

Pathogenesis

Ameloblastoma is believed to be derived from

- Remnants of dental lamina, cell rests of the enamel organ, epithelial rests of Malassez or remnants of Hertwig's sheath in the periodontal ligament of the erupted teeth
- *Epithelium of odontogenic cysts*—17% are associated with impacted teeth and dentigerous cysts
- *Disturbance of developing enamel organ, dental lamina or tooth buds*, which may result from trauma or chemical insult in utero
- *Basal cells of surface epithelium*—thought to result from invagination of the basal cell of epithelium into the developing jawbone
- Heterotopic epithelium—epithelium from other areas of the body (e.g. pituitary gland) that migrates to the jaw.

Classification of ameloblastoma (Flowchart 27.1)

Ameloblastoma was simply classified into three types: conventional, peripheral and unicystic. The term multicystic or solid type was discarded, as it led to confusions.

Clinical classification of ameloblastoma

a. Conventional or multicystic or solid ameloblastoma
b. Unicystic ameloblastoma
c. Peripheral (extraosseous) ameloblastoma
d. Malignant ameloblastoma

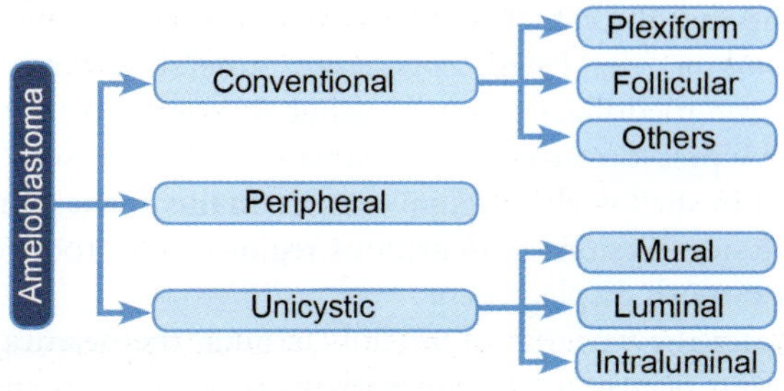

Flowchart 27.1 New classification for ameloblastoma by WHO, 2017.

e. Pituitary ameloblastoma (craniopharyngioma or Rathke's pouch tumour).

CONVENTIONAL AMELOBLASTOMA/MULTICYSTIC/ SOLID AMELOBLASTOMA

Clinical features

Ameloblastoma represents approximately 1% of all oral tumours and 18% of all odontogenic tumours. The most common type is conventional ameloblastoma, which accounts for about 85% of all ameloblastomas. It occurs in people of all ages, with a peak incidence in the 3rd to 4th decades (33–39 years). Males and females have the same rate of occurrence.

It occurs most commonly in the mandible (>80% of all cases), with 75% of these in the mandibular molar-ramus region and 20% in the maxilla. It is often associated with an impacted mandibular 3rd molar. In the maxilla, it is more common in the molar area.

- The lesions are asymptomatic and present as a *slow-growing, hard and nontender* swelling
- Ameloblastoma usually starts to grow along the *medullary spaces of the mandible* and may attain a substantial size before the outer contour of the bone is appreciably altered. Later on, both the buccal and lingual aspects of the mandible expand, presenting as an intra- or extraoral swelling and facial disfigurement
- The lesion enlarges and invades the neighbouring tissues by replacing them. As a result, it is regarded as a *benign but locally aggressive, invasive and persistent tumour*
- As the surrounding bone is thinned in large tumours, they produce 'fluctuation and egg-shell cracking'. The vital structures can be compressed by the larger lesions. The lesions involving the maxillary sinus and nasal cavity may lead to *nasal obstruction* and proptosis of eye
- Occasionally, they may present with displaced, mobile or exfoliated teeth, ill-fitting dentures or malocclusion
- Pain, *paraesthesia* or sensory nerve damage may occur with infection of the lesion.

Radiographic features

Conventional ameloblastoma presents as a *multilocular radiolucency with a well-defined and sclerotic margins.* The lesion exhibits a compartmented appearance with septa of bone extending into the radiolucent tumour mass, which is described as *a honeycomb or soap bubble appearance*. Ameloblastoma grows within the medullary cavity, causing scalloping of the inner cortex by pressure erosion. The erosion may be so severe that only a thin shell of the original cortex remains at the periphery of the lesion. Lesions in dentulous regions cause root resorption and tooth displacement.

Among the variants of ameloblastoma, the desmoplastic type often occurs in the anterior maxilla and presents as a relatively radiopaque lesion because of its dense connective tissue content.

Histological features

The histological subtypes of ameloblastoma are: *follicular, acanthomatous, granular cell, basal cell, desmoplastic and plexiform*. Most ameloblastomas fall into two major morphologic configurations—follicular and plexiform types. It may present purely as one histopathologic subtype or with predominance of one pattern or mixture of different patterns. The follicular type has the highest rate of recurrence with the acanthomatous type having only a 4.5% recurrence rate.

Common histological presentations of ameloblastoma are:

- Proliferating odontogenic epithelium in the form of islands, strands or cords within a densely collagenised connective tissue stroma
- The tall columnar cells in the peripheral layer presents typically with hyperchromatic nuclei, nuclei with reverse polarity and subnuclear vacuole. The nuclei of adjacent cells are at roughly in the same place within the cytoplasm, producing the *characteristic palisading pattern*
- Budding of the tumour cells as small, rounded extensions of epithelium emerging from larger islands, representing the various stages of tooth development can be seen.

Follicular type (most common type)

It is composed *of small, discrete islands of tumour cells that mimic the normal dental follicle*. It is made of a peripheral layer of cuboidal or columnar cells with a well-polarised nuclei. These cells look similar to preameloblasts or ameloblasts and surround a central mass of loosely arranged cells that resemble the stellate reticulum. The tiny cysts are formed by the complete breakdown of the stellate reticulum-like cells. Thus, *cyst formation* is a regular occurrence in the follicular type.

Plexiform type

The tumour cells are arranged in *irregular masses* or as a network of *interconnecting strands*. The strands are lined by a layer of columnar cells, and stellate reticulum-like cells between them. Cystic degeneration of the stroma can also be seen.

Acanthomatous type

The stellate reticulum undergoes *squamous metaplasia, and keratin* is formed in the central portion of the tumour islands. Keratin pearls may be seen occasionally.

Basal cell type

It is a rare type of ameloblastoma. The tumour cells are less columnar and are arranged in sheets with a considerable resemblance to the basal cell carcinoma of the skin.

Granular cell type

The cytoplasm transforms into a coarse, granular appearance. These cytoplasmic granules are lysosomal aggregates with no cellular components. The peripheral cells may be cuboidal, columnar or rounded. The granular type appears to be *aggressive with a marked tendency for recurrence.*

Desmoplastic type

It is composed of a *densely collagenised stroma with a hypocellular and hyalinised (Desmoplasia) appearance*. The presence of desmoplasia in the stromal connective tissue can be considered as the maturation stage of a tumour. In this type, the epithelium tends to grow in long, thin strands or cords rather than islands of epithelium. The periphery of the strands and cords are flattened or cuboidal cells with scant central cells. Occasionally, classic islands of follicular ameloblastoma among the strands and cords can be seen in desmoplastic type.

Surgical management of conventional/multicystic ameloblastoma

Treatment of ameloblastoma is dependent on the individual status of the patient as well as the surgeon's judgement. The surgical plan is greatly impacted by the presence of lesion in either the mandible or the maxilla. Ameloblastoma tends to spread more easily through the maxilla's cancellous bone than through the mandible's dense cortical plates.

The goals of the treatment are to completely remove the tumour, rebuild the defect with the least amount of deformity possible and continue monitoring the patient over the long term.

The treatment for multicystic ameloblastoma includes both conservative and radical methods (Box 27.3).

BOX 27.3 Multicystic Ameloblastoma

Conservative Methods

- Curettage
- Enucleation
- Surgical excision with peripheral ostectomy
- Surgical excision with other adjuvant therapies such as cryotherapy, carnoy's solution or liquid nitrogen therapy
- Marsupialisation

Radical Methods

- Resection with continuity defect
- Resection without continuity defect

Enucleation and curettage

As the tumour spreads to the adjacent cancellous bone (locally invasive), enucleation and curettage are considered to be ineffective. Among all conservative techniques, performing enucleation alone showed the highest recurrence rate. As a consequence, it is recommended to do adjunctive procedures, in addition to enucleation, which includes chemical cauterisation or peripheral ostectomy. Enucleation is performed in some cases, such as when the patient is either too young or too old for segmental resection or when the patient is medically compromised.

Surgical excision

Regarding the surgical treatment of multicystic ameloblastoma, there is a significant amount of controversy. According to some authors, *the initial treatment should be conservative, as the tumour has a minimal metastatic potential, and radical treatment should be reserved for situations of recurrence.* Small multicystic, solid lesions can be successfully treated with marsupialisation (Fig. 27.1).

- The most effective treatment for ameloblastomas is surgical excision of the lesion with a marginal clearance of 1.5–2 cm of normal bone
- The integrity of the inferior cortex determines whether the lesion can be removed as a block and with or without a continuity defect
- Postoperatively, there must be at least a minimum of 1 cm of residual bone at the inferior border of mandible to prevent the pathologic fracture
- Inferior alveolar nerve should be sacrificed if it lies within the lesion
- The greatest concern with mandibular ameloblastomas is that they spread into the soft tissues, making it difficult to determine the tumour boundaries and endangering vital structures

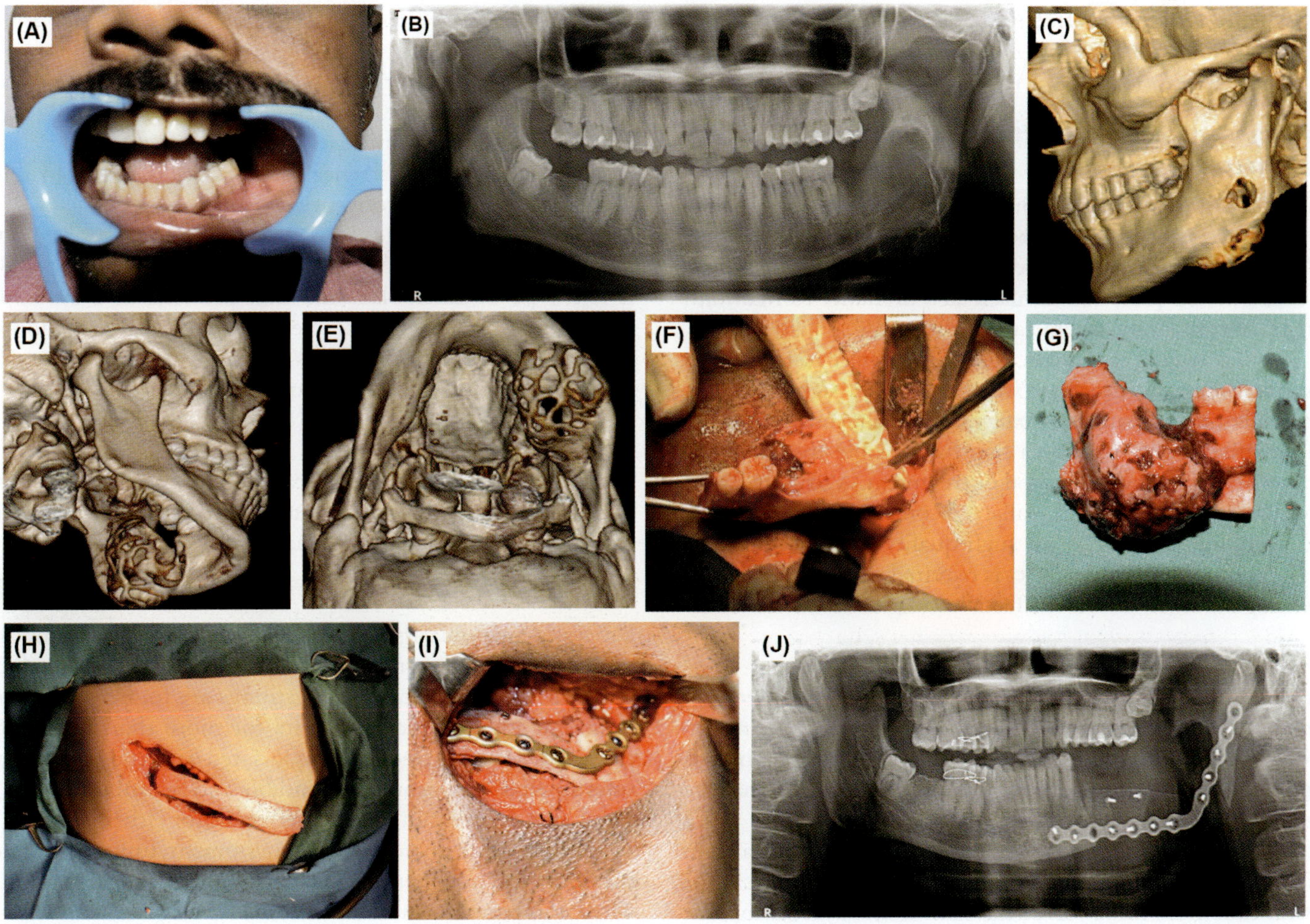

Figure 27.1 Multicystic ameloblastoma. (**A**) Preoperative intraoral view. (**B**) OPG showing multilocular radiolucency in the left mandibular body, angle and ramus. (**C–E**) CT scan in various views showing expansion of the bone in the angle and ramus region of left mandible. The lesion shows penetration of the buccal cortex and expansile multilocular appearance on the lingual side. (**F**)Through submandibular incision, segmental resection of the mandible was done. (**G**) Resected specimen with the lesion. (**H**) Rib graft. (**I**) Reconstruction of the mandible using rib graft and reconstruction plate. (**J**) Postoperative OPG.

TABLE 27.1 Surgical Treatment on the Basis of Anatomical Locations of Ameloblastoma

Mandibular anterior region (canine to canine)	• In smaller lesions, conservative management with preservation of the inferior border of mandible (marsupialisation, enucleation or curettage, peripheral oste ctomy or en bloc resection) • In large lesions with cortical perforation, marginal mandibulectomy followed by reconstruction of the segment with plate and long-term follow up
Posterior mandible (bicuspid to condyle)	• Marginal mandibulectomy while maintaining the inferior and posterior border whenever possible • A reconstruction plate to maintain the normal anatomic relationship
Anterior maxilla (canine to canine)	• Less aggressive treatment • Conservative methods (marsupialisation into oral cavity, enucleation or curettage)
Posterior maxilla (bicuspid to pterygoid plates)	• Resection of the tumour (low level or high level maxillectomy) • Reconstruction of the defect, after maxillectomy local flap by temporalis muscle or free-flap reconstruction

- Ameloblastomas in the maxillary region are considered to be more dangerous because of the thinner bones, which provide less effective support than those of mandible. Therefore, radical excision is essential, preferably maxillectomy (Table 27.1).

Reconstructive options after surgical resection of the maxilla/mandible

In order to restore the anatomical form and function of the maxilla and mandible, it is required to reconstruct the jaw. When immediate reconstruction is not possible, titanium reconstruction plate can be used as a modality to maintain the bone continuity and facial contours.

The immediate reconstruction of the defect restores both the aesthetics and function, which results in significant improvement in the patient's quality of life. In reconstruction of the mandible, the free fibula flap has become the most frequently recommended method of treatment. A scapula flap is an effective method for maxillary reconstruction due to the length of its pedicle and the high quality of its bone. When restoration of soft tissue defect is required, the radial forearm-free flap becomes the most effective and preferred treatment.

Bone graft substitutes

The calcium phosphate cement is the most widely used material because of its effectiveness in osteointegration and osteoconductive properties. High-density porous polyethylene implants are one of the other implantable materials that are available.

For reconstructing the mandibular defect, a titanium mesh tray filled with autologous cancellous bone blocks, or a titanium mesh filled with fresh bone marrow, recombinant human bone morphogenic protein (rhBMP) or xenogenic bone mineral can be utilised. The BMP is the most important stimulator for bone formation.

Tissue engineering, transport distraction osteogenesis and modular endoprosthesis are three recent advancements in the reconstruction of mandible. Dental implants are frequently used to restore the patient's masticatory function.

Prognosis

Ameloblastoma is a persistent, locally invasive lesion and has a high recurrence rate. Recurrence rates of 10%–20% have been reported after enucleation and curettage of unicystic ameloblastoma. A recurrence rate of 15% is reported after marginal resection of conventional ameloblastomas.

UNICYSTIC AMELOBLASTOMA

It is a type of ameloblastoma that presents as a cyst with clinical and radiologic characteristics similar to an odontogenic cyst. It is the 2nd and less common pattern to develop in the intraosseous ameloblastoma.

Pathogenesis

The unicystic ameloblastoma can development from the reduced enamel epithelium, dentigerous cyst or cystic degeneration of multicystic ameloblastoma.

Clinical features

Unicystic ameloblastomas are most often seen in young patients with 50% diagnosed in the 2nd decade of life (16–35 years). Most unicystic ameloblastomas are found in the posterior mandible, which accounts for more than 90% of all cases. The lesion is frequently associated with the crown of an unerupted 3rd molar in the mandible and resembles a dentigerous cyst. It does not have a preference for either gender.

Because of its cystic type of development, unicystic ameloblastoma has a higher prognosis and a lower recurrence rate when compared to the conventional ameloblastoma.

- The lesion is usually asymptomatic
- Facial asymmetry from expansion of the buccal or lingual cortices
- Occasionally associated with dental mobility, malocclusion and nasal block.

Radiographic features

It presents as a unilocular radiolucent lesion with a well-circumscribed radiopaque border.

Histological features

It is characterised by a solitary cystic cavity with ameloblastomatous differentiation in the epithelial lining. The basal epithelial layer is composed of columnar cells with hyperchromatic, palisaded nuclei, reverse polarity and a subnuclear vacuole.

The characteristic features of unicystic ameloblastoma are:

- Projection of tumour nodules intraluminally
- Proliferation of ameloblastomatous lining epithelium into the connective tissue wall
- Formation of ameloblastoma islands are in the connective tissue wall as solitary clusters.

Ackermann's histopathological classification of unicystic ameloblastoma

Group 1—Luminal

The tumour is confined to the cyst's luminal surface.

Group 2—Intraluminal

It presents with an extension of ameloblastic epithelium projecting from the cyst lining into the lumen, without invasion of tumour cells in the connective tissue wall.

Group 3—Mural

Islands of ameloblastomatous epithelium in the connective tissue wall without involving the entire epithelium. The fibrous wall may be infiltrated by typical follicular or plexiform ameloblastoma. This is the only variant with high recurrence rate.

Treatment

Before surgery, an incisional biopsy can be performed to establish an accurate diagnosis as well as a comprehensive representation of the tumour. Both *conservative and radical excision* may be performed as a part of the treatment (Fig. 27.2).

The most widely recommended and implemented procedures for treating unicystic ameloblastoma include:

- Enucleation as the 1st line of therapy because they manifest clinically as cysts. Depending on the histologic type, the patient should be followed up for 5–10 years
- Mural unicystic ameloblastoma, as well as lesions with root resorption and cortical bone perforation, have a high recurrence rate requiring long-term follow-up
- Following the early procedures of enucleation and curettage, marginal resection is regarded as the treatment of choice for infiltrating and mural type of ameloblastomas
- Few authors recommended curettage, peripheral ostectomy and adjuvant procedures such as Carnoy's solution and Liquid Nitrogen
- For large benign aggressive lesions, conservative management has been advocated. Marsupialisation has been proved to be a successful treatment option.

PERIPHERAL (EXTRAOSSEOUS) AMELOBLASTOMA

Ameloblastomas that are found in the *gingival or alveolar mucosa* is called as peripheral ameloblastoma. It is characterised by infiltration into the surrounding tissues, mostly the gingival tissues, without affecting the underlying bone.

Pathogenesis

It appears to develop from the remnants of dental lamina, surface epithelium or pluripotent cells of minor salivary glands.

Clinical features

The average age of occurrence is between 30 and 50 years, with a slight predilection for males. The mandible has an incidence ratio of 2:1 over the maxilla. The mandibular premolar is the common site of occurrence.

The peripheral ameloblastoma presents as an *exophytic growth on the gingiva*, varying in size from 3 mm to 2 cm in diameter, overlying the alveolar bone. It is considered as a soft tissue counterpart of the central intraosseous ameloblastoma. It is a slow-growing lesion with little or no bone erosion.

It is relatively innocuous and lacks the invasive nature of the intraosseous lesion, hence it has a low recurrence rate.

Radiographic features

In majority of the patients, there is no radiological evidence of bone involvement, but rather a superficial erosion of bone described as cupping or saucerisation can be seen.

Histological features

Histologically, the peripheral ameloblastoma exhibits the same pattern as the central ameloblastoma (multicystic). The majority of the lesions are acanthomatous, with only a few appearing to be follicular. The characteristics of tumour resemble the site of origin, surface epithelium (gingiva) or odontogenic remnants.

Treatment

The peripheral ameloblastoma is often treated by a wide local excision. Although malignant transformation is rare, recurrence after treatment has been recorded. If prior biopsy indicates involvement of bone, block resection with continuity defect is the choice of treatment.

PITUITARY AMELOBLASTOMA

Other names

Craniopharyngioma/Rathke's pouch

It is a neoplasm of the CNS, which grows as a pseudoencapsulated mass in the suprasellar or intrasellar area with tendency to encroach the frontal, temporal lobe or brain stem.

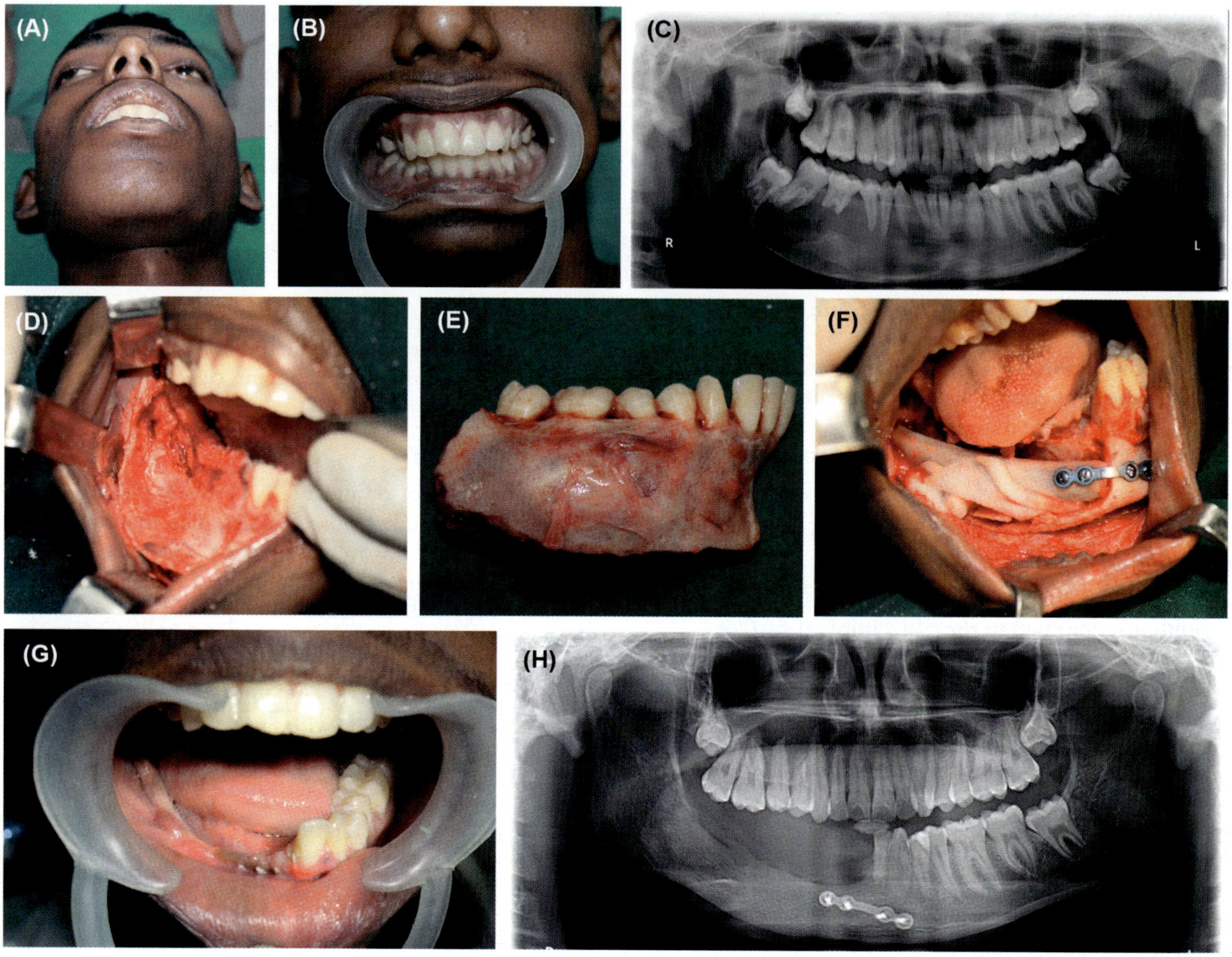

Figure 27.2 Unicystic ameloblastoma. (**A** and **B**) Preoperative view. (**C**) Preoperative OPG showing unilocular radiolucency with sclerotic margins at the right side of mandible extending from midline to 48 region. Root resorption seen in 46 and 47. (**D**)The lesion was excised by marginal resection of mandible, retaining the continuity of lower border of mandible. (**E**) Excised specimen showing the buccal and lingual side. (**F**) The resected area is reconstructed using bone grafts. (**G**) Postoperative view. (**H**) Postoperative OPG.

It often destroys the pituitary gland. It consists of 25% of all CNS tumours regardless of the age. It is the most common tumour of childhood and adolescents with an average age of 3–23 years.

Pathogenesis

Derived from unobliterated portions of the *foetal craniopharyngeal duct* formed by the Rathke's pouch (oral ectoderm). This craniopharyngeal duct epithelial remnants are extremely common in adults and has the potential to develop into tumours that are histologically comparable to those of the jaw.

Histological features of craniopharyngioma that are not commonly seen in central ameloblastoma are irregular calcified masses and foci of metaplastic bone or cartilage. Some cases present with islands and nests of 'ghost' cells, calcifications and sometimes tooth materials.

The pituitary ameloblastoma grows at a variable rate. Clinical symptoms can vary depending on the exact location of the tumour, such as endocrine imbalance, sleepiness or even toxic symptoms. The neoplasm requires neurosurgical intervention.

ADAMANTINOMA OF LONG BONES

Adamantinoma is a rare, low-grade malignant bone tumour that most commonly affects the diaphyses and metaphyses of long bones, between 20 and 40 years of age. The term adamantinoma was given to this tumour because of its histological resemblance to ameloblastoma of mandible.

There are two kinds of adamantinoma: *classical and differentiated*, which resembles osteofibrous dysplasia. The characteristics of this lesion are still unknown, although they are proven to be aggressive and capable of metastasising locally.

Though the **aetiology** of this lesion is not clear, it may be due to the early displacement of the basal epithelial cells of the skin during embryological development. It frequently occurs in young adults of age 20–40 years with slight male predominance. It most commonly affects the anterior metaphysis or diaphysis of the tibia. Other locations include the fibula, femur, humerus, ulna and radius.

Clinically, it appears as a well-defined, yellowish-grey tumour with a firm to bony consistency. It is characterised by a slow-growing swelling with or without pain, as well as with bone deformities and pathological fractures.

The tumour appears **radiographically** as a cortical, well-circumscribed, multilocular opacities with peripheral sclerosis producing the characteristic 'soap-bubble' appearance.

Histiologically, it is characterised by epithelial and osteofibrous components mixed in various proportions. Classic adamantinoma is distinguished by four distinct patterns: basaloid, tubular, spindle cell and squamous.

The most successful treatment for adamantinoma is wide resection with clear margins.

METASTASISING (MALIGNANT) AMELOBLASTOMA

Traditionally, ameloblastoma has always been thought to be a benign tumour that can be locally aggressive but can occasionally metastasis and kill the patient. The term 'metastasising ameloblastoma' refers to a tumour that possesses the histologic characteristics of a classic ameloblastoma but has *metastatic deposits in other parts of the body*.

Clinical features

The primary ameloblastoma occurs more commonly in the mandible of a young adult, with an average age of 30 years. The *lung* accounts for 80% of all metastatic nodule development, while cervical lymph nodes and extragnathic bones each account for 15%.

The pulmonary metastases are typically *multifocal and involve both the lungs*. The median survival time following the identification of a metastatic lesion is roughly 2 years. Innocuous lung 'granulomas' found on routine chest images of an ameloblastoma patient can be silent metastases.

Kunze et al., (1985) reported that the majority of patients with ameloblastoma had several recurrences. Multiple recurrences may be the result of an inherently more aggressive tumour, surgery-associated tumour 'spillover' into neighbouring tissue or tumour embolisation of lymphatic or blood arteries.

Histological features

Ameloblastomas with metastatic potential are histologically identical to normal ameloblastoma. In most cases, the metastatic form of ameloblastoma does not display a higher level of cytologic atypia or mitotic activity than the main form. Metastasising ameloblastoma exhibits the biologic characteristics of a *well-differentiated low-grade carcinoma*.

Treatment

The best method to treat the metastatic ameloblastoma is surgical excision of the lesion, although the evidence for increase survival rate is minimal. The metastatic cervical lymph node is treated by neck dissection. Metastases to the lungs are managed by lobectomy that helps to preserve the pulmonary function. Chemotherapy has often been ineffective; however, a short-term partial response is possible.

SQUAMOUS ODONTOGENIC TUMOUR

Other names

Benign epithelial odontogenic tumour

Squamous odontogenic tumour (SOT) is a relatively uncommon odontogenic neoplasm that was initially identified and described as a distinct entity in 1975.

Pathogenesis

These tumours originate from:

- *Rests of dental lamina* associated with the crowns of unerupted or impacted teeth
- *Epithelial rests of Malassez* associated with the alveolar process of the lateral root surface of teeth.

Clinical features

SOTs have been seen in patients at an average age of 38 years with no site predilection. It most commonly occurs in the mandible's premolar-molar area, whereas in the maxilla, the lesions are centred in the incisor-canine area. The tumours present as an asymptomatic lesion, occasionally with mobility of involved teeth, tenderness on percussion and abnormal sensations.

Radiographic features

It presents as a roughly triangular radiolucent defect, with or without a sclerotic border, typically associated with the cervical part of the tooth root.

Histological features

The tumour is unique and consists of *islands of mature squamous epithelium in a fibrous connective tissue stroma*, without a peripheral palisaded or polarised columnar layer.

This peripheral layer is typically flattened or cuboidal. There is *no pleomorphism, nuclear hyperchromatism or mitotic activity in the squamous cells*. Individual cell keratinisation occurs on occasion, but no epithelial pearls are visible. Other findings that can be seen are microcyst formation, laminar calcifications in the epithelium and globular, hyaline structures inside the island which are not amyloid.

Treatment

The SOT is effectively treated with conservative local excision. Because of the nature of the maxillary bone, the maxillary

SOT is found to be more aggressive, with a greater potential to invade the surrounding structures.

CALCIFYING EPITHELIAL ODONTOGENIC TUMOUR

Other names: Pindborg's tumour

Pindborg was the 1st person to describe this extremely rare tumour as a distinct entity (1956). It is an extremely uncommon form of benign odontogenic tumour that originates entirely from epithelial cells.

Pathogenesis

The tumour is thought to arise from:
- The epithelial elements of the enamel organ
- Remnants of the primitive dental lamina found at the early stage of odontogenesis.

Clinical features

- The tumour occurs at any age, most frequently in middle-age with equal sex distribution
- Occurs mainly in the premolar and molar regions
- Affects the mandible twice as frequently as the maxilla
- It presents usually as an expansile, painless, slow-growing swelling
- Most commonly associated with impacted or embedded teeth.

Radiographic features

- It has a variable radiographic appearance
- May appear as a diffuse or a well-circumscribed unilocular radiolucent area, mimicking an odontogenic cyst
- As it progresses, it tends to become multilocular or honeycomb as a result of destruction of bone and deposition of calcium. It is a mix of radiolucency and radiopacity pattern with many tiny, irregular bony trabeculae traversing the radiolucent area in many directions
- The *'driven snow' appearance* is due to the scattered flecks of calcification throughout the radiolucency. It may present as diffuse radiopacities within the lesion.

Histological features

Tightly packed huge sheets of *polyhedral epithelial cells* or as scattered islands dispersed in a plain fibrous connective tissue stroma. The intercellular bridges are found to be prominent.

Pleomorphic with giant nuclei and multinucleation are common. Binuclear and even trinuclear cells may be present.

A well-known type of this tumour is the *clear-cell variant*. The tumour cells have a distinct clear vacuolated cytoplasm, with a circular or oval nucleus in the centre of the cell or flattened towards the cell membrane.

One of the tumour's distinguishing microscopic features is the presence of a *homogeneous, eosinophilic material* that has been variously interpreted as amyloid. According to ultrastructural studies, this amyloid-like material is composed of at least three different types of fibrils; nevertheless, they are smaller in size compared to the 'normal' amyloid fibres.

Another distinguishing feature of Pindborg's tumour is the presence of calcifications within the amyloid-like area, in significant amounts as concentric rings or crenate-like shapes known as *Liesegang rings*, which accounts for the radiopacities.

Treatment

Surgical treatment of this tumour should be case specific and based on anatomic location, size and perforation of the bone. Enucleation or curettage can be used to treat the intrabony tumours that are small and well-defined, which is accompanied by removal of a thin layer of bone located near the tumour.

Marginal or segmental resection is the treatment of choice for recurrent or persistent tumours. As with other odontogenic tumours, radical excision of the affected jaw and accompanying soft tissues with not less than 1 cm in every direction is recommended. Immediate or delayed reconstruction can be performed. The tumour recurs after inadequate treatment.

ADENOMATOID ODONTOGENIC TUMOUR (Fig. 27.3)

Other names

Adenoameloblastoma, ameloblastic adenomatoid tumour

Adenomatoid odontogenic tumours (AOTs) are benign lesions that were originally known as adenomatoid ameloblastoma. They are distinct from ameloblastomas in that they lack a glandular component and do not behave like ameloblastomas. Some researchers classify it as a benign tumour, while others classify it as a hamartomatous malformation due to its *small size and the lack of recurrence* in most cases.

Pathogenesis

The tumour is thought to arise from epithelium of the dental lamina complex or its remnants.

Clinical features

- This is a rare tumour that usually arises in conjunction with an unerupted maxillary canine. It occurs as a slow-growing, painless swelling, usually in the anterior maxilla
- It occurs in people between 10 and 21 years of age
- Females are more commonly affected
- Most of the lesions occur anterior to the canine tooth and are frequently associated with impacted or unerupted teeth
- The great majority of lesions are measured between 1.5 and 3.0 cm, although massive lesions of over 7.0 cm have been documented
- It can develop in the jaw bones or gingiva. Peripheral lesions appear as a painless, gingival-coloured lump of 1–1.5 cm in diameter, more frequently in the maxillary gingiva.

Radiographic features

It appears as a well-defined unilocular radiolucency with margins showing definite sclerosis. There have been a few

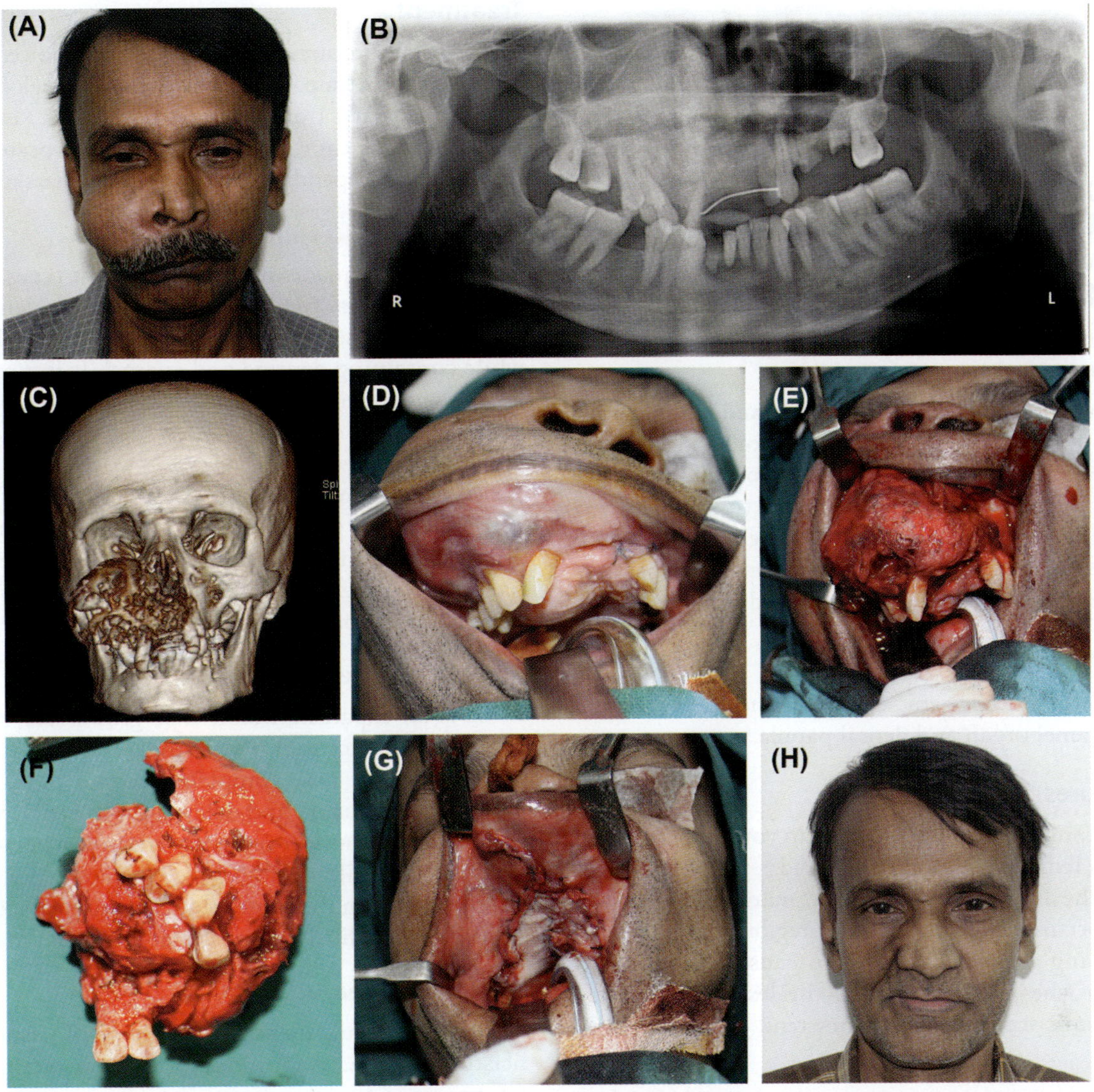

Figure 27.3 Adenomatoid odontogenic tumours (AOT). (**A**) Preoperative view showing swelling over the right side of cheek, with obliteration of the maxillary vestibule. (**B**) OPG reveals radiopacity on the right maxilla obliterating the maxillary sinus. (**C**) Preoperative CT scan showing the lesion. (**D**) Preoperative intraoral view showing the lesion. (**E**) Through intraoral incision, the lesion is exposed and segmental resection of the maxilla is done. (**F**) Resected specimen. (**G**) Intraoperative view showing primary closure of the palate. (**H**) Postoperative view.

reports of multilocular radiolucency, with a scalloped border occasionally. It may enclose a part of the root usually on the lateral aspect. Root divergence and tooth displacement occur more commonly than root resorption.

Histological features

Central AOTs appear as a *soft, spherical mass with a prominent fibrous capsule*. On gross sectioning, white, solid to crumbly tissue or cystic cavities with yellowish brown fluid or semi-solid material; *hard 'gritty' granular material; and large calcified masses* may be present in the tumour.

The AOT has a variety of histomorphologic traits. The tumour is composed of a proliferation of spindle, cuboidal and columnar cells in various patterns, as well as dispersed duct-like structures, eosinophilic material and calcifications in various forms, all surrounded by a fibrous capsule of varying thickness. Cytologic atypia is never noticeable.

The characteristic microscopic features of AOT are:

- Presence of duct-like structures with varied lumina
- Bordered by a single layer of cuboidal to columnar epithelial cells
- Polarised nuclei
- These duct-like structures or microcyst lumina are typically lined with an eosinophilic rim of varied thickness called as *hyaline ring*.

Treatment

The tumour is encapsulated and the marrow space around the lesions is free of tumour, so the lesions may be removed by the simple curettage or enucleation.

MIXED ORIGIN/TUMOURS OF ODONTOGENIC EPITHELIUM WITH ODONTOGENIC ECTOMESENCHYME WITH OR WITHOUT DENTAL HARD TISSUE

AMELOBLASTIC FIBROMA

Other names

Soft mixed odontogenic tumour, soft mixed odontoma
Ameloblastic fibroma is a benign mixed odontogenic tumour that is histologically similar to ameloblastomas. The ameloblastic fibroma is a rare odontogenic tumour defined by the simultaneous development of epithelial and mesenchymal tissue without the formation of enamel or dentin. As a result, this may be considered a true mixed tumour.

Pathogenesis

It arises from the odontogenic epithelial and mesenchymal cells of the enamel organ and dental papilla.

Clinical features

- Typically found in the 1st 2 decades in younger people
- Males and females are equally affected
- Most of the lesions appear in the mandible, with the majority occurring in the posterior region
- Slow-growing asymptomatic lesion causing gradual expansion of the jaw. As a result, the lesion's periphery often remains smooth. It does not tend to infiltrate the bone.

Radiographic features

Appears as a unilocular or multilocular radiolucency with smooth, sclerotic margins and bulging of the bone. It ranges from 1 to 8 cm in diameter.

Histological features

The *ectodermal component* is made up of dispersed islands of epithelial cells that organise themselves into rosettes, nests, cords and long finger-like strands. The epithelium consists of columnar or cuboidal cells resembling the primitive odontogenic epithelium.

The *mesenchymal component* is composed of primitive connective tissue with densely intertwining fibrils interspersed by large connective tissue cells similar to those found in the dental papilla. There may be a lack of blood vessels and juxtaepithelial hyalinisation of connective tissue.

This tumour has a dense fibrous capsule enclosing epithelial and connective tissue components. The connective tissue collagen production resembles that of the immature dental papilla.

Treatment

Conservative excision is the treatment of choice. As it does not appear to penetrate bone as actively as ameloblastoma does and also separates from the bone more easily. Resection including 0.5–1 cm of clinically sound bone is advocated. Recurrence in these cases depends upon the completeness of excision.

AMELOBLASTIC FIBRO-ODONTOMA

This tumour is made up of two different types of growth: an *ameloblastic fibroma and an odontoma*. It was defined as a neoplasm having the general features of an ameloblastic fibroma while containing dentine and enamel. It is a more common and less-aggressive lesion.

Pathogenesis

It develops from an abnormal proliferation of odontogenic epithelium of a permanent tooth germ. It contains proliferating epithelium as well as calcified tooth tissues. The epithelial cells differentiate into functional ameloblasts before enamel matrix production.

Clinical features

- It is an expansile lesion that grows very slowly, with a little tendency to infiltrate the bone
- The patient may complain of mild pain, swelling, deranged occlusion and delayed tooth eruption
- Occurs in younger patients—mean age being 8 years
- No sex predilection
- Appears with the same frequency in the maxilla and mandible, most likely in the molar–premolar area.

Histological features

The lesion is made up of the same type of tissue as in ameloblastic fibroma. Additionally, a characteristic composite odontoma is discovered.

Radiographic features

It appears as a well-circumscribed radiolucent area with opaque odontomatous tissue. The odontoma part of the lesion is represented by a single radiopaque mass or multiple small opacities.

Treatment

Conservative excision with a margin of sound bone is the treatment of choice.

AMELOBLASTIC ODONTOMA

Other names

Odontoameloblastoma
Ameloblastic odontoma is classified as a rare neoplasm characterised by the presence of enamel, dentine and odontogenic epithelium resembling that of an ameloblastoma, both in structure and behaviour. It is a tumour in which odontogenic cells give rise to both an ameloblastoma and a composite odontoma. It is more aggressive than the ameloblastic fibro-odontoma.

Clinical features

- Occurs in any age group, particularly during childhood
- Males and females are equally affected
- The mandible is more frequently involved than the maxilla
- The site of predilection is the molar–premolar region
- Patient gives a history of slow expansion of the jaw, dull pain and disturbance of occlusion.

Radiographic features

- Either as a well-defined unilocular radiolucency or multilocular radiolucency with numerous dense opacities, which can be solid masses or small particles
- These opacities may or may not resemble miniature teeth
- Infiltration by the lesion results in disruption of the bone.

Histological features

The tumour shows a variety of cells and tissues, which include ameloblasts, enamel, dentine, stellate reticulum-like tissue, dental papilla and cementum. The characteristic feature is the presence of cells resembling typical ameloblastoma.

Treatment

Surgical management is same as that of ameloblastomas because of its resemblance and behaviour to it, namely, progressive infiltration and local destruction of surrounding tissues.

PRIMORDIAL ODONTOGENIC TUMOUR

The primordial odontogenic tumour (POT) is a recently described entity by WHO in 2017 classification of Head and Neck Tumours. It is benign tumour that is believed to develop during the early stages of odontogenic process (late cap and early bell).

Clinical features

This tumour develops in the 1st and 2nd decades of life and affects the posterior area of the jaw, specifically the mandible.

Radiographic features

It manifests as a well-defined unilocular radiolucent lesion associated with the crown of an unerupted tooth. It is responsible for the varying degrees of bone expansion, root resorption and tooth displacement.

Histological features

POT is characterised by a firm, multilobulated whitish, glossy mass that is devoid of cystic spaces and is encircled by a capsule that differentiates it clearly from the surrounding structures. POT is composed of mesenchymal fibromyxoid tissue with varied cellularity that mimics the dental papilla and is bordered at the periphery by a cuboidal to columnar epithelium similar to the inner epithelium of the enamel organ.

The surrounding epithelium can invaginate the mesenchymal component, resulting in ameloblastic fibroma-like islands.

The tumour lacks dental hard tissues; no evidence of odontoblastic differentiation or dental hard tissue deposition has been described.

Treatment

Simple excision or enucleation, followed by extraction of the involved teeth.

ODONTOMAS

The term 'odontoma' refers to any tumour of odontogenic origin. The odontomas are considered as hamartomatous malformation and not a neoplasm. It is one of the most common odontogenic tumour.

- They are the result of anomalous completion or incomplete tooth formation by odontogenic epithelium and ectomesenchyme
- They tend to form during the period of odontogenesis approximately up to 20 years
- All the four types of dental tissues are found within them—enamel, dentine, pulp and cementum
- They are slow growing and asymptomatic, occurring particularly in the incisor–canine region and 3rd molar region
- They are identified on routine radiographic examination
- They can also be found during investigation of retained deciduous tooth or delayed eruption of the permanent tooth.

When a lesion is composed of more than one type of tissue, it is known as a *composite odontoma*. Some composite odontomas have enamel and dentin put down in such a way that the structures resemble the normal teeth anatomically, except that they are often smaller. The term *compound composite odontomas* are used to describe the abnormal growths that have anatomical similarity to the normal teeth. The term *complex composite odontoma* is used to describe the calcified dental tissues that appear as an irregular mass with no morphologic similarity to the teeth.

Odontomas have been divided into two types radiologically and histologically: (1) Complex odontoma and (2) Compound odontoma.

COMPLEX ODONTOMA

Complex odontoma consists of an irregular calcified mass of hard and soft dental tissues, displaying a disorderly and haphazardly arranged calcified dental structures.

Structural differentiation is poor, having little resemblance to the normal form of teeth. Frequently, it forms a cauliflower-like mass of hard dental tissues which is surrounded by a fibrous follicle.

Pathogenesis

Complex odontomas develop in the place of a normal tooth, either from the dental lamina or enamel organ. It is believed that odontomas can be caused by any local injury or infection that occurs in the area of tooth formation.

Clinical features

- It occurs in 2nd and 3rd decades of life
- It shows a slight preference for males over females
- The majority of the complex odontomas are found in the mandible, with a predilection for the *posterior jaws*
- Both forms of odontomas are more common on the right side of the jaw than on the left side
- Complex odontoma is less common than the compound odontoma
- Odontomas are typically asymptomatic small hard masses, associated with unerupted or impacted teeth as well as retained deciduous teeth
- Occasionally, it may get larger and cause expansion of the bone, along with swelling and evidence of infection.

Radiographic features

Complex odontoma appears as an irregular dense radiopaque mass, surrounded by a thin radiolucent area, associated with or overlying the crown of an unerupted tooth or impacted tooth (Fig. 27.4).

Histological features

Presence of *mature dental tissues* such as enamel, dentine, pulp tissue and cementum *arranged as unstructured sheets*. These tissues are frequently surrounded by a thin connective tissue capsule. Occasionally, *ghost cells* can be seen in the enamel forming cells.

Treatment

Odontomas have a limited capacity to grow larger and do not recur. When the odontoma causes obstruction to the erupting teeth or acts as a possible source of infection, they are treated by surgical excision of the tumour. Large complex odontomas should be cut in segments for removal in order to conserve normal bone and prevent jaw fracture.

COMPOUND ODONTOMA (Fig. 27.5)

Compound odontoma consists of calcified tooth-like structures or miniature teeth.

Pathogenesis

Compound odontoma may be produced by repeated divisions of a tooth germ or by multiple budding off from the dental lamina with formation of many tooth germs. They begin as lesions within the bone over the period of tooth formation.

Clinical features

- Seen in the 2nd and 3rd decades of life
- Males and females are equally affected
- Occurs most commonly in the maxilla, especially in *the anterior jaw* (incisor–canine region)
- It presents as a slow-growing, noninfiltrative lesion
- Failure of eruption of permanent teeth is seen due to interference from the compound odontoma.

Radiographic features

Compound odontoma is seen as a packet *of malformed or dwarfed teeth or tooth-like forms* surrounded by a thin radiolucent zone.

Histological features

Histologically, the lesion is composed of *anatomically distinct, small, well-formed or numerous dwarfed teeth* with enamel, dentine, pulp and cementum surrounded by a connective tissue capsule which represents the follicle.

Treatment

The most effective treatment for compound odontoma is *enucleation or surgical removal*. The presence of compound odontoma can increase the risk of cystic change and cause significant bone destruction. The tumour can be accessed through intraoral incision and removal of sufficient overlying bone is necessary to expose the lesion. When fully calcified, the odontomas do not recur. Recurrence is more

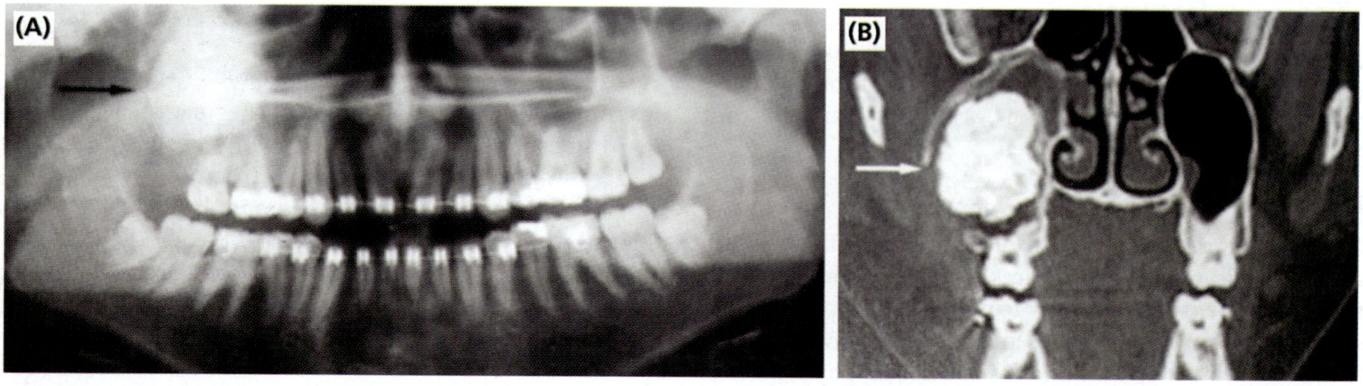

Figure 27.4 Complex odontoma. **(A)** OPG showing a large radiopaque mass in the right maxillary sinus. **(B)** Coronal CT showing a large mass in the right maxillary sinus, which is surrounded by fibrous capsule with resorbed lateral wall of maxillary sinus.

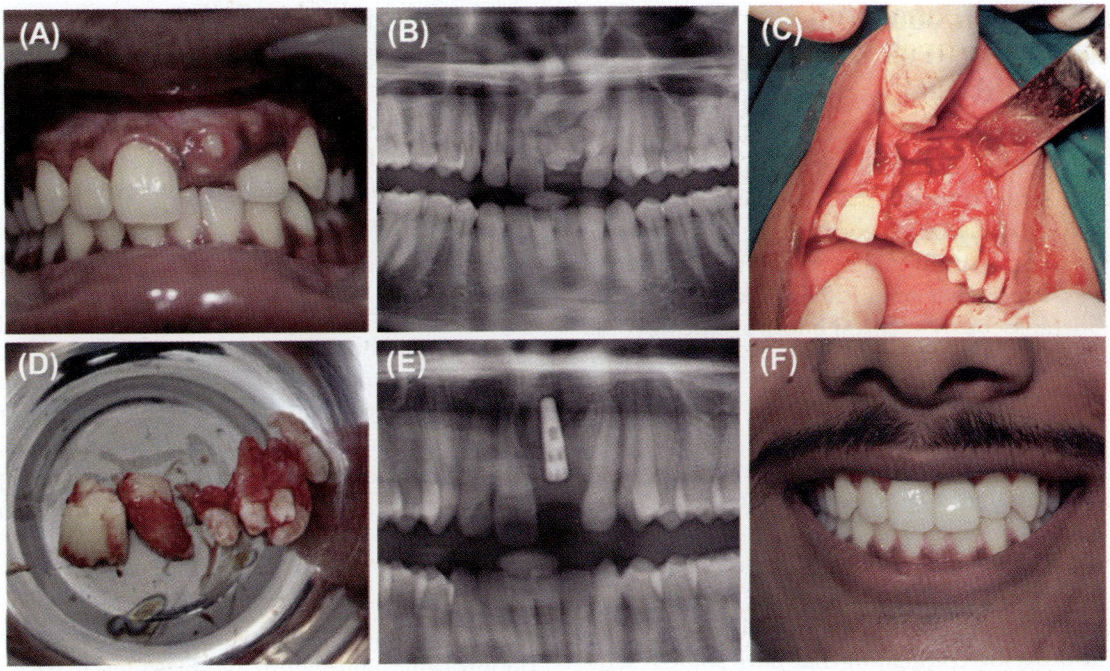

Figure 27.5 Compound odontoma. (**A**) Clinically missing 21, replaced by an irregular hard swelling. (**B**) OPG showing multiple small tooth-like structures in the region of 21, 22. (**C**) The bone cavity after excision of the odontoma. (**D**) Excised specimen. (**E**) After 6 months, OPG revealing dental rehabilitation with implant. (**F**) Postoperative photograph.

common after inadequate removal of the early soft stage of the lesion. Removal of the entire soft tissue portion is recommended to prevent recurrence.

DENTINOGENIC GHOST CELL TUMOUR

Other names

Calcifying odontogenic cyst

Gorlin and colleagues were the 1st to define the calcifying odontogenic cyst (COC) as a unique clinicopathologic entity in 1962. Gold (1963) used the phrase 'keratinising and calcifying odontogenic cyst' to describe the lesion. The term 'Calcifying ghost cell odontogenic tumour' was proposed by Fejerskov and Krogh, while 'cystic calcifying odontogenic tumour' was proposed by Freedman and his colleagues. Neither of these terms were accepted.

The two main types of COCs are (1) *cystic lesions and (2) solid neoplastic* lesions. It is possible to add a 3rd malignant counterpart to the neoplastic lesion.

Clinical features

It is an uncommon lesion with same incidence rate for both genders, in adults in their 2nd and 3rd decades. It arises centrally from within the jaws and appears either as a painless expansile lesion or as an abnormality during routine radiographic evaluation.

Radiographic features

Lesions may show as radiolucencies or *radiolucencies with foci of opacification*, particularly when coupled with odontomas. The dentinogenic ghost cell variety presents with expansile radiopacity.

Histological features

The epithelium lining of the cyst proliferates to the point that it resembles ameloblastoma. Within this epithelium, the cells undergo *distinctive 'ghost cell' keratinisation*. The COC is frequently found in conjunction with an odontoma, which can be identified next to the proliferative lining epithelium or mixed with the ghost cells, referred to as '*dentinoid*'.

The term 'dentinogenic ghost cell tumour' is used when there is abundance of '*dentinoid*' material and the lesion appears 'solid' rather than 'cystic'. *The most important part of the diagnosis is the presence of ghost cells within the proliferating odontogenic epithelium.*

The ghost cells have nuclear remnants, cytoplasmic organelles and numerous tonofilaments within it. Ghost cells are larger, often vacuolated with prominent remnants of nuclear membranes. This could be because of oedema inside the cell and the presence of swollen, degenerated membrane organelles.

Treatment

Enucleation or complete curettage can be used to successfully treat the COC. The central dentinogenic ghost cell tumour is treated by surgical excision. Depending on the tumour's size and anatomic extent, it may require block excision or segmental resection for removal.

MESENCHYMAL ORIGIN/ODONTOGENIC ECTOMESENCHYME WITH OR WITHOUT INCLUDED ODONTOGENIC EPITHELIUM

ODONTOGENIC FIBROMA

Odontogenic fibroma is classified as a benign, relatively rare connective tissue tumour that contains a variable amount of inactive odontogenic epithelium. Odontogenic origin of this tumour is confirmed by its formation only in the jaws and by the presence of epithelial rests. The lesion is found both intraosseously—central odontogenic fibroma and extraosseously on the gingiva known as peripheral odontogenic fibroma.

Central odontogenic fibroma

It is a rare central tumour of jaws. Concerning this tumour, there are three basic concepts, which include:

- It is a lesion around the crown of an unerupted tooth that looks like a little dentigerous cyst
- It is a fibrous connective tissue lesion with dispersed islands of odontogenic epithelium that have some resemblance to the dental follicle
- It is a fibroblastic neoplasm containing varying amounts of odontogenic epithelium and calcified material resembling dysplastic dentin or cementum-like material. Thus, except for the location, it is histologically identical to the peripheral odontogenic fibroma.

Pathogenesis

It is thought to be derived from the mesenchymal portion of the tooth germ, either from the dental follicle, papilla or periodontal ligament.

Clinical features

- Wide range of age distribution with a mean of 23–37 years.
- Females are more frequently affected
- Has a predilection for occurrence in the mandible
- Appears as an asymptomatic, progressive enlargement of the jaw
- Swellings or routine radiographic examinations are the only means of identifying this tumour
- Displacement of adjacent teeth and mobility of teeth may become apparent.

Radiographic features

- Appears as a sharply defined radiolucency in a tooth-bearing area
- Small lesions are unilocular while large ones tend to show multiloculation
- May cause root resorption and root divergence
- Most of these lesions are associated with unerupted or displaced teeth
- Occasionally a '*ground-glass appearance*' is noted, due to the calcifications present in the form of flecks, resulting in patchy radiopacity.

Histological features

The lesion's histology displays mature collagen interspersed with fibroblasts. The collagenous tissue is moderately to densely packed with nests of inactive odontogenic epithelium in strands possible. Gardner (1980) separated the central odontogenic fibroma into two types based on the histological presentation.

Epithelial-poor type or simple type

The simple fibroma differs from the WHO type in that its stroma resembles that of a tooth follicle, from which it is most likely generated. It is acellular and comprises delicate fibres interspersed with considerable amount of ground substance. A variable feature is the presence of small strands of inactive epithelium. Islands of odontogenic epithelium resembling dental follicle can be seen scattered throughout the lesion.

Epithelial rich type or WHO type or complex

It exhibits high cellularity or densely packed with cells. The odontogenic epithelium is an essential part of the WHO type. It also presents with foci of calcifications of the collagenous materials such as cementoid, osteoi, and dysplastic dentin.

To put it another way, odontogenic fibromas have more cells and collagen in them when compared to odontogenic myxomas.

Treatment

Odontogenic fibromas separate out from the bone easily and thus, can be treated by enucleation and curettage. Recurrence is not common with these lesions.

PERIPHERAL ODONTOGENIC FIBROMA (Fig. 27.6)

Clinically, this tumour is mistaken for a fibrous epulis. It can only be differentiated histologically by the presence of odontogenic epithelial rests.

Clinical features

- The lesion appears as a slow growing, pink, firm, sessile or pedunculated mass on the attached gingiva, particularly on the anterior teeth
- Found more frequently in the mandible
- No specific sex predilection
- Occurs from 1st to 8th decade
- The lesions measure around 1–3 cm and are found anterior to the 2nd premolar.

Radiographic features

Calcifications are seen more commonly in these lesions than the central lesions.

Histological features

The tumour consists of cellular and collagenous fibrous tissue and small discrete strands or rests of epithelial content.

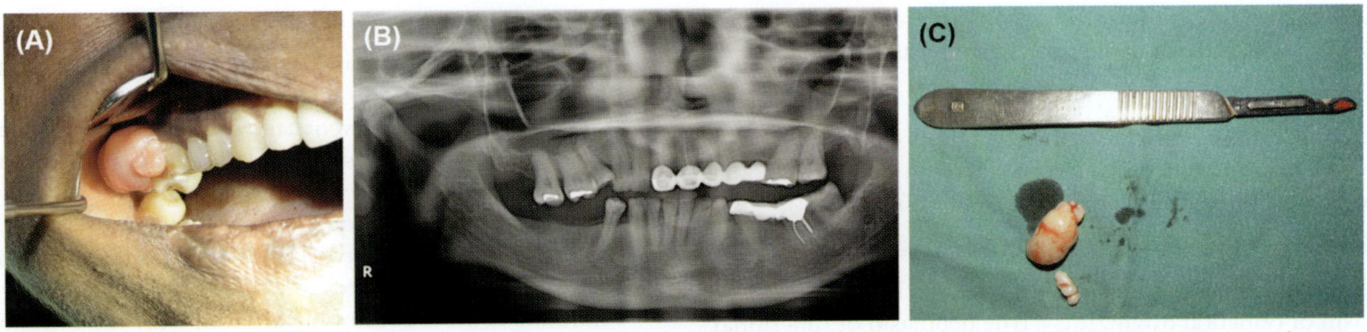

Figure 27.6 Peripheral odontogenic fibroma. (**A**) A small, sessile pink mass is seen attached to the gingiva in relation to the 15, 16 region. (**B**) OPG reveals radiolucency in relation to 15-17 region. (**C**) Excised specimen.

Calcifications may be present. A stroma of mature fibrous connective tissue is present and can be extensively vascularised, especially in the less-cellular portions.

Treatment

Excision is the preferred treatment for extraosseous odontogenic fibroma.

ODONTOGENIC MYXOMA (Fig. 27.7)

Other names

Odontogenic fibromyxoma or myxofibroma

Odontogenic myxoma is an odontogenic tumour, based on the evidence that it is distributed in the jaws and facial skeleton. It is a benign, nonencapsulated, slow-growing, infiltrative tumour of mesenchymal tissue.

Pathogenesis

It is thought to arise from the *mesenchymal portion* of the tooth germ, dental papilla or the dental follicle.

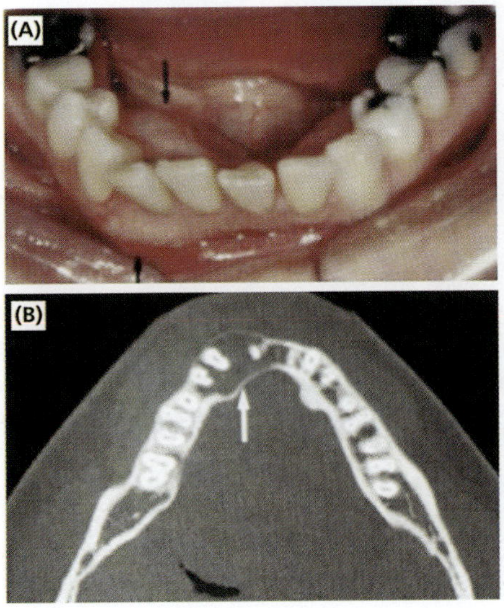

Figure 27.7 (**A**) Odontogenic myxoma in a 40-year-old female showing expansion of buccal and lingual cortical plate. (**B**) Corresponding CT image showing expanded buccal and lingual cortical bone.

Clinical features

- Has a wide age range, but occurs mostly in the 2nd and 3rd decades of life, with a mean age of 28–30 years.
- No particular gender predilection
- Both jaws are affected with a slight preponderance in the mandible
- Usually unilateral but may extend beyond the midline
- It appears as an asymptomatic, slow-growing swelling of the jaw with the overlying mucosa uninvolved
- The myxoma starts as a central mass and tends to spread slowly through the marrow spaces, followed by the expansion of bone.

Radiographic features

Appears as a unilocular or multilocular radiolucency with well-defined or *moth-eaten margins*. The most common appearance is as a radiolucent area with scalloped margins and trabeculations, giving a *honeycomb or mottled appearance*. May cause displacement of teeth in involved dental areas.

Histological features

The mesenchymal cells are spindle shaped or angular with long, fine protoplasmic processes in a loose mucoid intercellular material. The tumour margins are ill-defined and peripheral bone is progressively invaded and resorbed.

In the odontogenic myxoma, Hodson and Prout found two acid mucopolysaccharides: relatively significant levels of hyaluronic acid and smaller amounts of chondroitin sulphate. They believe that the high hyaluronic acid content of the tumour is a crucial determinant for its neoplastic activity.

Treatment

Myxomas are benign but can infiltrate widely. Enucleation and curettage are restricted to unilocular lesions of 1–2 cm in diameter. Teeth within the limit of the lesion should also be removed. Chemical cauterisation of the tumour bed may be of value.

Enucleation or curettage of large lesions is associated with high recurrence. Large lesions should be treated by wide excision or en bloc resection including a perimeter margin of tumour free bone, followed by reconstruction. Radical treatment should be considered for recurrent cases.

CEMENTOMAS

Cementoma is the term given to a group of lesions of the jaws producing cementum-like calcifications. These tumours contain either acellular or cellular cementum.

Cementoblastoma (true cementoma) (Fig. 27.8)

Benign cementoblastoma is considered as the only true neoplasm of cemental origin. It is a true neoplasm of functional cementoblasts that forms a mass of cementum or cementum-like tissue fused to the root of a tooth. It is defined by the WHO as a neoplasm characterised by the formation of sheets of cementum-like tissue, which may contain a very large number of reversal lines and may be unmineralised at the periphery of the mass or in the more active growth areas.

Pathogenesis

Though the exact pathogenesis of cementoblastoma is not known, connective tissue of the periodontal ligament and dental follicle are thought to give rise to the lesion.

Clinical features

- Clinically, it is characterised as a painless bony expansion of the jaw
- It is slow-growing but eventually produces a large lesion that may expand and resorb the lateral and medial cortical bone
- Males and females are equally affected
- Occurs in the age range of 15–30 years but most commonly seen in the 2nd decade
- Mandible is more commonly affected with the 1st molar and premolar being the most frequently affected tooth. The associated tooth is usually vital
- Often detected during routine examination.

Radiographic features

The lesion usually appears as a *solitary, well-defined radiopacity* with a peripheral radiolucent rim *attached to the root of a tooth*. Centre of the lesion appears mottled and at the periphery, radiating trabeculae of calcified tissue may be seen. Root resorption and fusion of the mass to the tooth is common.

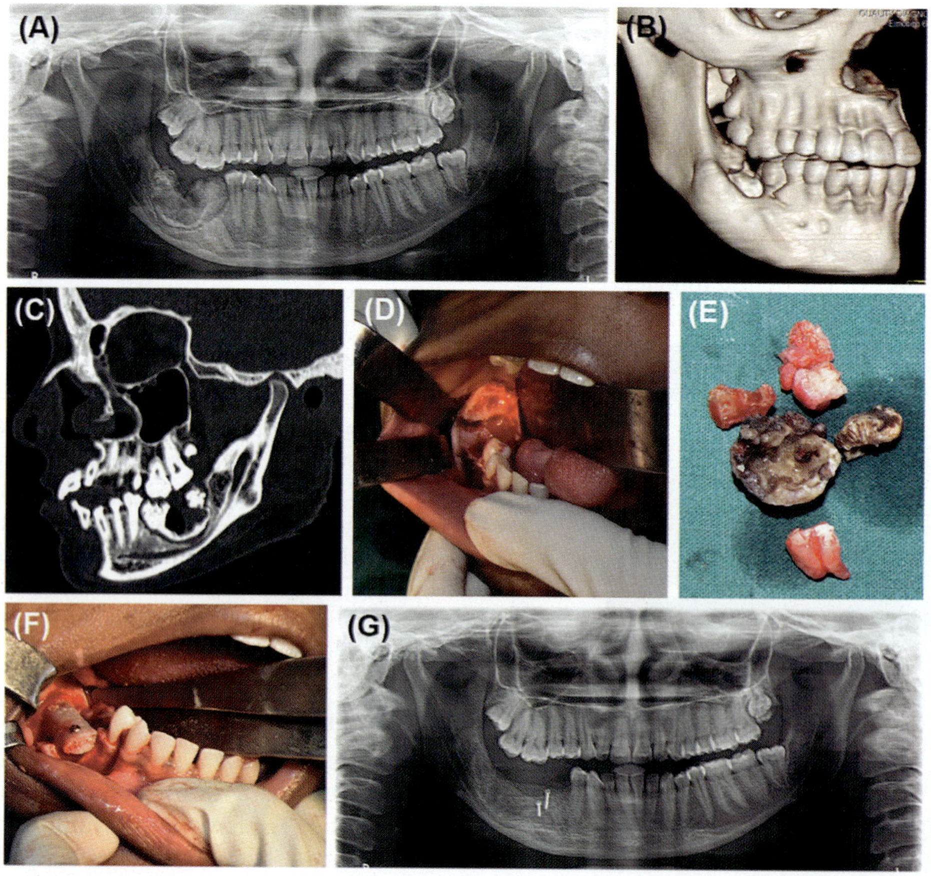

Figure 27.8 Cementoma. (**A**) Preoperative OPG showing well-defined radiopacity with a peripheral radiolucent rim in relation to 46, 47 and 48 region. The lesion appears to be fused with the roots of an impacted molar. (**B** and **C**) CT scan showing bone loss and buccal expansion at the right lower jaw in 47 and 48 region. (**D**) The lesion is removed surgically by enucleation along with the removal of involved teeth. (**E**) Excised specimen. (**F**) Reconstruction of the defect with bone grafts. (**G**) Postoperative OPG.

Histological features

Central part of the lesion consists of a cementum-like tissue deposited in a globular pattern resembling giant cementicles. Throughout the calcified tissue, scattered reversal lines can be seen frequently and has a pagetoid appearance. The trabeculae radiating from the centre of the tumour have prominent cementoblasts. At the periphery, there is a broad zone of unmineralised tissue and the mass has a soft tissue cellular layer resembling capsule.

Treatment

Extraction of the related tooth and complete enucleation of the mass have been suggested. Recurrence is highly unlikely.

CEMENTO-OSSIFYING FIBROMA (CEMENTIFYING FIBROMAS)

WHO defined central ossifying fibroma as a demarcated or rarely encapsulated neoplasm, composed of fibrous tissue with varying amounts of mineralised material (bone and/or cementum). The term 'cemento-ossifying fibroma' (COF) is commonly used because both the osseous and cemental tissues are present in a single lesion.

The COF is a controversial central tumour of bone and periodontium. The COF originates from the odontogenic tissue, whereas the ossifying fibroma originates in the bone.

Pathogenesis

COF is a disorder with no identified cause. According to Bernier, COF can be caused by an irritant stimulus (such as tooth extraction) that could initiate the formation of new tissue from the retained periodontal membranes. The cells in the periodontal membrane are multipotent and are capable of forming cementum, lamellar bone and fibrous tissue.

Clinical features

- Commonly appears between 20 and 40 years of age
- Females are more frequently affected than males
- Occurs more commonly in the mandibular premolar or molar region
- It is a slow-growing, painless expansile lesion that replaces normal bone as it enlarges
- The 1st presenting symptom is displacement of the teeth and facial asymmetry
- It is confined to the periapical region of the jaws in contrast to the more diffuse distribution of fibrous dysplasia
- Juvenile presentation of this lesion are extremely aggressive and may involve both the jaws.

Radiographic features

It can be divided into three stages: the initial or early stage, the mixed stage and the mature stage.

The COF presents initially as a well-defined radiolucent lesion with no signs of internal radiopacities. As the tumour develops, the radiolucent area gradually gets flecked with opacities. Eventually, the lesion will appear as a highly radiopaque mass after reaching the mature stage.

The diagnostic characteristics of COF is that the lesion appears as a round mass and its growth pattern is centrifugal. That is the lesions expand uniformly in all directions.

The *margins of the lesion are well-defined* and is separated from the surrounding bone by a thin radiolucent line depicting a fibrous capsule. The outer cortical plate, despite being shifted and weakened, remains intact. Large mandibular lesions may result in *the thinning and 'bowing' of the inferior border*. Teeth affected by the lesion may be displaced; however, resorption of the tooth is not commonly seen.

Histological features

- It is a well-defined lesion, made of fibrous tissue with varied levels of mineralised material resembling bone (ossifying fibroma), cementum (cementifying fibroma) or both
- Discrete bundles of collagen fibres are interspersed with significant numbers of proliferating fibroblasts and cementoblasts
- As the lesion progresses, the cementum islands increase in number and size, and ultimately coalesce
- Spherical cementicle-like calcifications are also found
- Spicules of bone which can be recognised radiographically as well as microscopically are of diagnostic importance
- A COF can be differentiated from a fibrous dysplasia, based on the presence of osteoblasts along the surface of bone deposits.

Treatment

Due to the fact that COFs have a definite capsule and can be well-demarcated from the bone, they can be removed in a conservative manner through an intraoral approach. When larger lesions that destroys the jaws are present, they require local resection and if necessary bone grafting. Prognosis is good.

MALIGNANT ODONTOGENIC TUMOURS

ODONTOGENIC CARCINOMAS

AMELOBLASTIC CARCINOMA

Ameloblastic carcinoma is either a malignant transformation of an ameloblastoma or has a histological resemblance to ameloblastoma. Ameloblastic carcinoma is an aggressive tumour that is locally invasive and can spread to regional lymph nodes or distant locations such as the lungs and bones.

- **Clinically,** it presents as a swelling of the jaw, which grows rapidly than conventional ameloblastoma. Mandible is most frequently involved
- **Radiographic features** show an ill-defined area of radiolucency with focal radiopacities within the radiolucency. Root resorption, perforation of the buccal and lingual plate of the jaw can also be seen
- **Histologically,** it seems to exhibit a greater cytologic atypia as well as mitotic activity than ameloblastoma

- **Treatment** for ameloblastic carcinoma consists of a complete surgical excision, neck dissection and postoperative radiation due to its aggressive nature.

CARCINOMA EX AMELOBLASTOMA

A carcinoma that is directly adjoining to an ameloblastoma is referred to as a 'carcinoma arising from an ameloblastoma' or carcinoma in ameloblastoma.

DE NOVO AMELOBLASTIC CARCINOMA

If a carcinoma lacks a component of traditional ameloblastoma, and its clear identification it is considered as de novo ameloblastic carcinoma. The tumour should have nonspecific ameloblastomatous characteristics, including a plexiform pattern that demonstrates budding and anastomosing epithelial processes, peripheral palisaded cuboidal to columnar cells and centre polygonal to angular cells.

PRIMARY INTRAOSSEOUS CARCINOMA

Primary intraosseous carcinoma (PIOC) is a form of squamous cell carcinoma that develops within the jaw bone. It is referred to as 'primary' because it does not occur as a secondary deposit or metastases from a distant site. It is called as 'intraosseous' because it grows centrally from the bone.

PIOC originates either from the central odontogenic epithelium, or occasionally, from incisive canal epithelium.

It appears as a diffuse enlargement of the jaw, confluent with the gingival surface after erosion of bone. Radiographically, it appears to have an intraosseous origin, as well as destruction of the buccal and lingual cortices.

Solid primary intraosseous carcinoma

It appears as a painful swelling in the posterior mandible. It demonstrates a cup-shaped radiolucency or poorly-circumscribed 'moth eaten' radiolucency.

Cystic primary intraosseous carcinoma

It is a type of squamous cell carcinoma having a cystic component and a lumen containing fluid or keratin, as well as a lining of stratified squamous epithelium with cytologic atypia.

Treatment of PIOC involves surgical excision, neck dissection and/or postoperative radiotherapy.

SCLEROSING ODONTOGENIC CARCINOMA

It is a PIOC of the jaws that has a bland cytology, a *sclerotic stroma*, and a locally aggressive and infiltrative development pattern. Sclerosing odontogenic carcinoma (SOC) has been introduced by WHO (2017) as an independent entity. It is considered as a low-grade malignant tumour.

The patient presents with nonspecific features ranging from completely asymptomatic to swelling with pain. It occurs most commonly in the mandible.

Radiographically, it appears to be lytic with thinning of the cortical bone or perforation of bone.

Histologically, SOC is composed of a single thin cords, nests or strands of epithelium in a *heavily sclerosed stroma.* Epithelial cells appear bland or slightly hyperchromatic with infrequent mitoses and vacuolated cytoplasm. *Perineural or intraneural infiltration and soft tissue or vascular infiltration* are described as a striking features of SOC.

Treatment involves surgical resection of the tumour with a 5 mm margin followed by a close follow-up. Neck dissection is not necessary as metastasis has not been reported so far.

CLEAR CELL ODONTOGENIC CARCINOMA

It is a type of low-grade carcinoma composed of homogenous nuclei and clear cytoplasm. It is a potentially aggressive tumour, capable of frequent recurrences as well as metastases to the local and distant areas.

It arises most commonly in the mandible with slight female predilection and an age range of 17–89 years. It presents as a painless swelling in the mandible or maxilla, occasionally associated with teeth mobility and paraesthesia.

The **radiographic** appearance of the tumour varies. It most commonly appears as an expansile, unilocular radiolucent lesion with an unclear periphery; nevertheless, few cases are multiloculated and well-circumscribed.

Histologically, it shows budding and branching cords, islands and sheets of neoplastic polygonal epithelial cells. They have small dark uniform nuclei, little nuclear pleomorphism, abundant pale cytoplasm, 'clear cells' and distinct cell borders. The clear cells have diastase-sensitive, Periodic Acid Schiff–positive glycogen, but are negative for mucicarmine.

Treatment is primary resection with a wide margin. Patients with significant soft tissue or perineural invasion may benefit from adjuvant radiation therapy.

GHOST CELL ODONTOGENIC CARCINOMA

Other names

Odontogenic ghost cell carcinoma, malignant epithelial odontogenic ghost cell tumour

An ameloblastic carcinoma with evidence of ghost cell keratinisation is called as ghost cell odontogenic carcinoma (GCOC). As a result, it is classified as a variant of ameloblastic carcinoma.

Pathogenesis

It can arise from malignant transformation of preexisting CCOT or other odontogenic tumours.

Clinical presentation

The age of presentation ranges from 13 to 72 years, with male predominance. They are more common in maxilla. They present as a painful swelling associated with paraesthesia, root resorption or tooth displacements. It may result in the expansion of the maxilla or mandible.

Radiographic features

It is usually a mix of radiolucent and radiopaque pattern, with varying degrees of bone destruction and ill-defined borders.

Histological features

GCOC presents with atypical histological features such as groups of *ghost cells*, prominent mitoses, necrosis, aggressive behaviour, infiltrative growth pattern and elevated Ki-67 and p53 expression.

Because ghost cells are immunoreactive for amelogenin (a protein found exclusively in the enamel matrix), the existence of ghost cells in jaw malignancies indicates ameloblastic differentiation. The epithelial cells have lost nuclei, leaving just a faint outline of the original nuclei.

Treatment

The recommended treatment is wide surgical excision with adjuvant radiotherapy, with or without chemotherapy.

ODONTOGENIC SARCOMA

Other names

Ameloblastic fibrosarcoma

It is a malignant odontogenic tumour characterised by having both a benign epithelium and a malignant mesenchymal component in its typical structure. WHO defines ameloblastic fibrosarcoma as a 'neoplasm similar to ameloblastic fibroma, but the ectomesenchymal component presents the characteristics of a sarcoma'.

Odontogenic sarcoma is divided into two types: primary (arising de novo) and secondary (as a result of malignant transformation of ameloblastic fibroma).

Pathology

It can develop spontaneously without any prior lesion or as a result of the malignant transformation of ameloblastic fibroma.

Clinical features

- It is the malignant counterpart of ameloblastic fibroma
- It is a very rare tumour
- It occurs mostly in young adults with an age ranging from 3 to 89 years
- The mandible is the most common site with slight predilection for posterior mandible. No sex predilection
- It is locally aggressive tumour that grows rapidly and causes destruction of the jaw bone and loosening of teeth. At times, pain may be present
- Very rarely, ulceration and bleeding of the overlying mucosa can be seen.

Radiographic features

It appears as a large multilocular radiolucencies. Extensive areas of bone destruction with irregular and indistinct margins from expansion or thinning of cortical bone are seen.

Histological features

Mostly shows malignant transformation of a benign ameloblastic fibroma.

- Benign ameloblastic columnar or cuboidal epithelial cells are found grouped in budding and branching cords, admixed with islands and knots. All of these components are seen in a highly cellular malignant connective stromal component with varying degrees of anaplasia
- Malignant cells exhibit a considerable mitotic activity and resemble immature fibroblasts. They appear as elongated cells containing hyperchromatic nuclei with varying degree of pleomorphism.

Treatment and prognosis

This condition is treated by radical surgery and resection of the affected jaw. It can be combined with chemotherapy or radiotherapy. Recurrence is common, hence prognosis is poor.

ODONTOGENIC CARCINOSARCOMA

Odontogenic carcinosarcoma is an exceptionally rare malignant tumour composed of odontogenic carcinoma and sarcoma, with both epithelial and mesenchymal components exhibiting malignant activity.

WHO's definition of odontogenic carcinosarcoma is 'a very rare neoplasm, similar in pattern to ameloblastic fibrosarcoma, but with cytological hallmarks of malignancy in both the epithelium and ectomesenchymal components'.

Pathogenesis

It is thought to develop from preexisting tumours including ameloblastoma, ameloblastic fibroma or ameloblastic fibrosarcoma or de novo. De novo odontogenic tumours develop from the remnants of embryologic process of odontogenesis.

Clinical features

It occurs more commonly in the posterior region of the mandible. It affects mainly the middle-aged patients, without any gender predilection. Clinically, it presents as a highly aggressive lesion with high rates of recurrence and metastasis.

Radiographic features

It shows an irregularly shaped radiolucency with ill-defined margins.

Histological features

It is a heterogeneous neoplasm consisting of biphasic malignant cells. It shows mixed features of both carcinomatous and sarcomatous elements.

Proliferation of cords and nests of odontogenic epithelium in a hypercellular odontogenic mesenchyme, both with cellular pleomorphism, hyperchromatism and mitotic figures, are the predominant histological features of this tumour.

Treatment

The majority of the patients have been treated with radical resection. Few cases may require adjuvant therapy such as chemotherapy and/or radiotherapy.

Chapter 28

Nonodontogenic Tumours

OUTLINE

INTRODUCTION

Nonodontogenic tumours are defined as tumours that originate from the tissues other than the tooth or tooth-forming tissues. They can occur in the jaw, with or without the involvement of other bones of the skeleton. These tumours can be the oral manifestations of a generalised disorder like polyostotic fibrous dysplasia, Paget's disease, Brown's tumour.

Nonodontogenic tumours of the jaws comprise tumours which are solely made up of bone or cartilage and fibrosseous lesions which may contain bone, fibrous tissue, osteoid, cartilage and cementum (Box 28.1).

Osseous tumours are slow-growing and cause bony expansion and facial deformity. A few of the most common nonodontogenic tumours are elaborated in this chapter.

CLASSIFICATION OF NONODONTOGENIC TUMOURS

BOX 28.1 WHO Classification of Maxillofacial Bone Tumours (2017)

A. Benign maxillofacial bone and cartilage tumours
- Chondroma
- Osteoma
- Melanotic neuroectodermal tumour of infancy
- Chondroblastoma
- Chondromyxoid fibroma
- Osteoid osteoma
- Osteoblastoma
- Desmoplastic fibroma

B. Malignant maxillofacial bone and cartilage tumours
- Chondrosarcoma
- Osteosarcoma

C. Haematolymphoid tumours
- Solitary plasmacytoma of bone

D. Fibro-osseous and osteochondromatous lesions
- Ossifying fibroma
- Familial gigantiform cementoma
- Fibrous dysplasia
- Osseous dysplasia
  - i) Periapical osseous dysplasia
  - ii) Focal osseous dysplasia
  - iii) Florid osseous dysplasia
  - iv) Familial gigantiform cementoma
- Cemento-osseous dysplasia
- Osteochondroma

E. Giant cell lesions and simple bone cyst
- Giant cell granuloma
- Cherubism
- Aneurysmal bone cyst
- Simple bone cyst

BENIGN MAXILLOFACIAL BONE AND CARTILAGE TUMOURS

OSTEOMA

Osteomas are benign tumours that are composed of *mature, compact and cancellous bone*. They are distinguished by the proliferation of compact or cancellous bone in an endosteal or periosteal position.

Osteomas are classified into two types:

(1) ***Central (endosteal) osteomas***
(2) ***Peripheral (periosteal) osteomas.***

Osteomas that originate centrally within the bone are referred to as *endosteal* or *central osteomas*. Endosteal osteomas within medullary bone may be detected as dense, well-circumscribed radiopacities during routine radiographic evaluation because significant growth must occur before cortical expansion is visible (Fig. 28.1).

Osteomas that arise on the surface of bone from the periosteum or from the bone itself are called *peripheral osteomas*. Periosteal osteomas appear as asymptomatic, slow-growing, bony, hard lumps. When lesions enlarge to a substantial proportion, asymmetry may be observed.

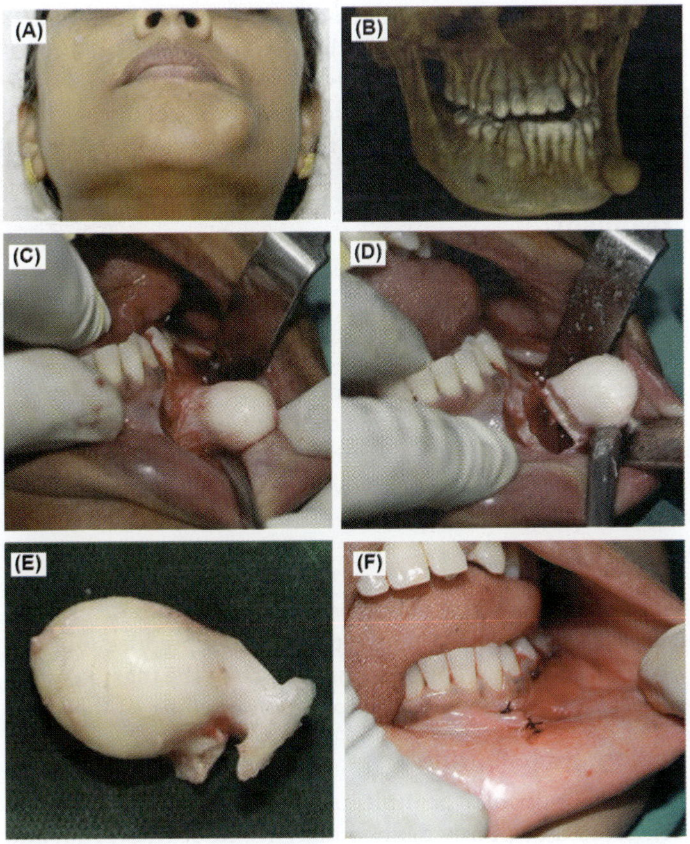

Figure 28.1 Osteoma. **(A)** Bony hard swelling in left mandible. **(B)** CBCT (Cone Beam CT) showing an osseous tumour (osteoma) in relation to mandible left canine/premolar region. **(C–E)** Intraoperative picture showing resection of the osteoma and the excised specimen. **(F)** Closure of the wound.

Clinical features

- Osteomas are most commonly seen in young adults and anywhere between 2nd and 5th decades. These occur both in males and females, with a greater proclivity for males
- It occurs anywhere on the maxilla (hard palate and maxillary sinus) and are most frequently found in the mandible (angle more common)
- It presents as slow growing, asymptomatic, bony hard masses causing asymmetry of the affected bone
- Lesion in the maxillary sinus may cause sinusitis, headache and ophthalmic symptoms depending on the site of the lesion.

GARDNER'S SYNDROME

Gardner's syndrome is an important marker of internal malignancy. Multiple peripheral osteomas of the jaws or sino-orbital region should give rise to suspicion of the possibility of Gardner's syndrome. It is inherited as an autosomal dominant trait.

The syndrome comprises:

1. Adenomatous polyps of the large intestine with a high malignant potential
2. Multiple osteomas of the jaws, skull or long bones
3. Multiple desmoid tumours
4. Epidermal and trichilemmal cysts of the skin
5. Compound odontomas
6. Impacted supernumerary and permanent teeth.

Radiographic features

Endosteal lesion appears as well-circumscribed radiopaque mass surrounded by a radiolucent line. Periosteal form manifests as a sclerotic mass.

Histological features

There are two different histologic forms of osteoma. One type is composed of dense, mature, lamellar, compact bone with sparse marrow tissues, and another type is composed of lamellar trabeculae of cancellous bone with abundant marrow tissue between them.

Osteons and haversian canals are seen in the compact type. Compact osteomas consist of dense lamellar bone arranged like *layers of onion* with occasional blood vessels. No haversian system is seen.

Spongy osteomas consist of cancellous bone with intertrabeculae bone marrow or fat in between and are surrounded by a lamellated cortex.

Treatment

- Conservative excision is the appropriate treatment. Small, asymptomatic, nonprogressive deep lesions need not be removed and can be observed periodically

- Osteomas causing functional and aesthetic problems are removed surgically. Endosteal osteomas are usually approached intraorally and enucleated. Periosteal osteomas require surgical excision as they cause swelling and facial symmetry
- Osteomas attached to the lingual surface of the mandibular alveolar process, the buccal surface of the alveolar portion of the mandible, and the coronoid process can be approached intraorally. Osteomas present on the inferior border, angle, and external surface of the ramus of the mandible can be approached via an extraoral incision
- Maxillary sinus osteomas are removed through a Caldwell-Luc approach. Once the osteoma is exposed, it is removed by means of burs and osteotomes.

OSTEOID OSTEOMA/OSTEOBLASTOMA

It is a rare benign osseous tumour and is seldom seen in the jaws. It has been confused with chronic sclerosing osteomyelitis in some cases, and the osteoid osteoma may be a manifestation of a form of osteomyelitis. They are clinically and histologically similar to osteosarcoma.

Clinical features

It is seen in young people of age group less than 30 years. Males are more frequently affected than females. The mandible is affected twice as frequently as the maxilla. One of the classical presenting symptom is pain, which is characteristically worse at night. It may present as a tender localised soft tissue swelling over the involved bone. Pain is relieved by antiinflammatories.

Radiographic features

It appears as a small ovoid or round *radiolucency surrounded by a rim of sclerotic bone*. Some *calcification* may be present in the radiolucency. It is more frequently cortical than medullary in site. The lesion is usually less than 1 cm in size but the overlying cortex thickens due to subperiosteal new bone production.

Histological features

It has a characteristic appearance of a *central nidus consisting of compact osteoid tissue*, calcifications to varying degrees, interspersed by vascular connective tissue. Definite trabeculae are formed, which are outlined by active osteoblasts. Osteoclasts and bone resorption are also seen. The overlying periosteum shows new bone formation, and lymphocyte collections can be seen in this interstitial tissue.

Treatment

Treatment is complete surgical removal of the lesion. Recurrence is usually not expected.

BENIGN OSTEOBLASTOMA (GIANT OSTEOID OSTEOMA)

The difference between the benign osteoblastoma and the osteoid osteoma is that benign osteoblastoma has a *far greater growth potential.*

Further, the benign osteoblastoma *lacks the characteristic pain* and sclerotic bone associated with osteoid osteoma. When an ambiguous lesion was *larger than 1.5 cm* in its largest dimension, McLeod and colleagues arbitrarily classified it as an osteoblastoma.

Benign osteoblastoma has pathological resemblance to osteoid osteoma, while demonstrating a difference in the average size of the tumour.

Clinical features

It occurs most frequently in young persons of age range 20–30 years. It has a predilection for males. Pain and swelling at the tumour site characterise the lesion, which can last anywhere from a few weeks to a year or more. The most prevalent site is vertebral column followed by sacrum, long tubular bones and calvarium. It occurs in both the maxilla and mandible.

Radiographic features

It appears as a well-circumscribed radiolucent lesion. Few tumours present with only bone degeneration, while others show sufficient bone formation producing a mottled or mixed radiolucent-radiopaque appearance.

Histological features

The benign osteoblastoma has the following characteristics:

- The lesion's vascularity includes numerous dilated capillaries spread throughout the tissue
- Multinucleated *giant cells* scattered throughout the tissue
- *Proliferating osteoblasts* that form the irregular trabeculae of new bone.

Treatment

Treatment is complete surgical removal of the lesion. Recurrence is rare.

DESMOPLASTIC FIBROMA

Desmoplastic fibroma is a benign, *locally aggressive* bone lesion that might be considered as the gnathic and extragnathic counterpart of fibromatosis. Typically, the lesion demonstrates locally aggressive clinical behaviour, indicating a neoplastic development.

Clinical features

It occurs frequently in young people of age less than 30 years, with a mean age of 14 years, with no gender predilection. The mandible is affected more commonly than the maxilla. It appears as a slow growing, asymptomatic swelling of the jaw.

Radiographic features

It shows unilocular or multilocular radiolucency with well-demarcated or poorly defined margins. Root resorption and cortical perforation may also be seen.

Histological features

Interlacing bundles and aggregates of extremely collagenous tissue along with homogeneous spindled and elongated fibroblasts are seen in this lesion. *Hypercellularity with plumper fibroblast nuclei* may be present in some locations. However, no cytologic atypia or mitotic figures are observed.

Treatment

Surgical excision of the lesion is the treatment of choice.

CHONDROMA

Chondroma is a benign cartilaginous tumour of unclear origin. Chondromas are uncommon in the jaws, especially when compared to other bone regions.

Clinical features

A chondroma typically manifests as a painless, gradually increasing swelling. Mucosal ulceration is uncommon when the lesion grows gradually.

The nasal septum and ethmoid sinuses are the sites of the majority of craniofacial complex lesions. The majority of maxillary chondromas are seen in the anterior area. Mandibular chondromas have been seen in the body and symphysis areas, as well as the coronoid process and the condyle.

Chondromas occur equally in both genders, with the majority of tumours appearing before the age of 50.

Radiographic features

It presents as an irregular radiolucent area with foci of calcification within the radiolucency.

Histological features

The lesion is made up of distinct lobules of mature hyaline cartilage. Chondrocytes are tiny, solitary with regular nuclei. Within the chondroma, the degree of cellularity varies greatly.

Treatment

Surgical excision of the chondroma is the treatment of choice. The recurrence is unusual.

MALIGNANT MAXILLOFACIAL BONE AND CARTILAGE TUMOURS

CHONDROSARCOMA

The malignant analogue of the chondroma is chondrosarcoma and is the 3rd most prevalent bone malignancy after myeloma and osteosarcoma.

Pathogenesis

The actual cause of chondrosarcoma is unknown; however, the most important primary growing tissue is cartilage throughout. Chondrosarcoma usually develops from de novo, although secondary chondrosarcoma can develop in preexisting benign cartilaginous tumours such as osteochondroma or enchondroma.

Clinical features

The majority occur between the ages of 30 and 60 years, with men accounting for 75% of all cases. The maxillofacial area is more commonly affected than the mandible. The anterior portions (lateral incisor–canine region) and the palate are commonly involved in maxillary lesions. Whereas in mandible, the most common sites are premolar and molar regions, symphysis, coronoid process, as well as the condylar process.

The appearance of chondrosarcoma is determined by the tumour's grade. A *high-grade*, rapidly developing tumour can cause excruciating pain. An elderly patient complaining of discomfort and swelling is likely to have a *low-grade*, more indolent tumour.

It presents as a painless swelling and expansion of the affected bones, which leads to the loosening of teeth or ill-fitting denture. Chondrosarcoma that has spread from the jaw to adjacent structures might cause pain, vision abnormalities, nasal symptoms and headache.

Radiographic appearance

It has a wide range of presentation from solitary or multilocular moth-eaten radiolucencies to diffusely opaque tumours. Numerous chondrosarcomas have zones of calcification and ossification that correspond to areas of mottled densities.

Histological features

Grade I (well differentiated)—They have a lobular structure with proliferations similar to benign cartilage and an increase in the number of chondrocytes present in a chondroid or myxomatous stroma (hypercellular compared and have moderate cytologic atypia).

Grade II (intermediate)—They have an enlarged chondrocyte nuclei with occasional mitotic patterns in a myxoid stroma. At the periphery of the cartilaginous lobules, an increased cellularity can be frequently observed (more cellular than grade 1 and cytologic atypia is more pronounced).

Grade III (poorly differentiated)—They are distinctly cellular with a spindle cell component and numerous mitotic figures (extreme cellularity with large bizarre nuclei, and tiny spindle-shaped foci at the periphery of the lobule).

Treatment

The treatment of choice is wide local or radical surgical excision. Metastasis is more frequent in high-grade chondrosarcoma, typically occurs in the lung or the bone. Since chondrosarcoma is radioresistant, the treatment with radiotherapy is of little value. Even chemotherapy does not offer any significant advantages.

OSTEOSARCOMA (OSTEOGENIC SARCOMA)

It is the 2nd most common bone malignancy after plasma cell neoplasm (myeloma).

Pathogenesis

It originates from a primitive mesenchymal bone-forming cell and is distinguished by the production of osteoid. Osteosarcomas can develop either spontaneously (de novo) or as a result of other bone abnormalities such as Paget's disease, fibrous dysplasia, multiple osteochondromas, chronic osteomyelitis and osteogenesis imperfecta.

Hereditary retinoblastoma (Rb) and Li-Fraumeni syndrome are two cancer susceptibility syndromes that can lead to osteosarcoma.

Clinical features

- It is a bone tumour that can develop in any bones in the body, especially common in the *extremities of long bones,* near the metaphyseal growth plates. The most common sites being femur, tibia, humerus, pelvis and skull or jaw
- It is frequently seen in young people of age range 10–25 years, with slightly higher incidence in male. It is very rare in children. The mandible is more commonly affected than the maxilla
- It often presents with swelling and localised pain. Patients could complain of sprains, arthritis or the so-called growing discomfort associated with this condition. Teeth loosening and displacement may occur in some circumstances
- Paraesthesia, a cardinal sign of malignancy, is produced by tumour compression or invasion of adjacent nerves
- Maxillary tumours also produce similar symptoms but can also produce epistaxis, nasal obstruction, proptosis or diplopia
- In most cases, mucosal ulceration appears at the late stage of disease
- Variants of osteosarcoma are:
  a. Conventional
  b. Multifocal
  c. Telangiectatic
  d. Small cell
  e. Intraosseous well-differentiated
  f. Intracortical
  g. Periosteal & Paraosteal
  h. High-grade surface
  i. Extraosseous.

Radiographic appearance

- The lesion is destructive and shows an irregular margin with cortical disruption, variable mineralisation and no marginal sclerosis
- The early stages of osteosarcoma, that involve the alveolar process, are characterised by the widening of the periodontal ligament space. In advanced tumours, the radiolucencies are irregular with poorly marginated radiopacities that produce a *'moth-eaten' appearance*
- The majority of these neoplasms exhibit mixed radiographic characteristics. A characteristic *'sunray' or 'sunburst' radiopaque appearance* caused by periosteal response may be noticed in jaw lesions but is not indicative of osteosarcoma.

Histological features

All osteosarcomas share a common sarcomatous stroma, which directly creates *osteoid*. Histological subtypes are:

- **Chondroblastic**–Predominantly with malignant cartilage
- **Osteoblastic**–Predominantly with malignant bone and osteoid
- **Fibroblastic**–Predominantly with spindle cells
- **Telangiectatic**–It shows multiple aneurysmal gaps that are filled with blood and lined by malignant cells. In certain types of osteosarcomas, multinucleated giant cells can be found in the tumour.

All histologic types of conventional osteosarcoma show the *multipotentiality of neoplastic mesenchymal cells* in forming osteoid, cartilage and fibrous tissue.

Treatment

- Osteosarcomas are treated with a combination of surgery, chemotherapy and radiotherapy. However, surgery is the mainstay of treatment for mandibular osteosarcoma
- Physical examination or specific imaging techniques can be used to assess the invasion of anatomic barriers surrounding any head and neck malignancy
- The fundamental difference between the resection of carcinoma and sarcoma is the recommended bony marginal clearance. Carcinomas are recommended to have a 2 cm marginal clearance in bone, whereas sarcoma resections require a 3 cm marginal clearance
- Chemotherapy can be given either before or after surgery (neoadjuvant or adjuvant chemotherapy).

HAEMATOLYMPHOID TUMOURS

SOLITARY PLASMOCYTOMA OF BONE

It is an uncommon malignant tumour of plasma cell without any systemic involvement. Plasma cell neoplasms are characterised as neoplastic transformation of B lymphoid cells.

The solitary plasmacytoma (SP) has two kinds:

EXTRAMEDULLARY SOLITARY PLASMACYTOMA

Extramedullary solitary plasmacytoma (ESP) arises from the soft tissues and is more common in the head and neck region. ESP is produced by the cells in the mucosal surface.

SOLITARY BONE PLASMACYTOMA

Solitary bone plasmacytoma (SBP) originates as an intramedullary bone lesion in the axial skeleton and develops as an isolated disease or as the 1st manifestation of a subsequent multiple myeloma. SBP is produced by the plasma cells in bone marrow. The prognosis for patients with the solitary form appears to be more favourable.

Pathogenesis

The origin of SP is unknown; however, it has been hypothesised that persistent stimulation, excessive exposure to radiation, viral infections and genetic interaction in the reticuloendothelial system may all have had a role in the development of the lesion.

Clinical features

Although the SP is most common in males in their 60s and 70s, it can strike people at any age. In general, patients present with the primary symptom of swelling in conjunction with minimal pain.

In cases of larger lesions infiltrating the neurovascular bundle, a pathologic migration of teeth along with swelling and paraesthesia may be noticed.

The current diagnostic criteria for SP are as follows:

- Isolated area of bone destruction caused by clonal plasma cells
- Plasma cell infiltration in the bone marrow not exceeding 5% of all nucleated cells
- Absence of other tissue involvement
- Absence of anaemia, hypercalcemia or renal impairment attributable to myeloma
- Low concentrations of serum or urine monoclonal protein
- Preserved levels of immunoglobulins.

Radiographic features

SBP can present itself as any of the following two patterns. The 1st radiographic pattern can be a circumscribed radiolucent area, while the 2nd can be a destructive lytic mass in the mandible.

Histological features

A monoclonal proliferation of plasmacytoid cells that have eccentric nuclei and basophilic cytoplasm can be seen under the microscope.

Treatment

Radiotherapy is generally considered to be the most effective treatment for SBP. The combination of chemotherapy and surgical surgery is typically reserved for specific cases. Due to the fact that the patient may eventually develop Multiple Myeloma, they will need to be monitored on a regular basis for at least 3 years after they have been diagnosed.

FIBRO-OSSEOUS AND OSTEOCHONDROMATOUS LESIONS

OSSIFYING FIBROMA

Ossifying fibroma is considered as a benign fibro-osseous neoplasm arising from undifferentiated cells of the periodontal ligament tissue. It consists of bone, cementum and fibrous tissue in varying proportion. Cementifying and ossifying fibromas are now considered as the same and are categorised together as cemento-ossifying fibroma.

Clinical features

It is a slow-growing, painless expansile lesion that replaces normal bone as it enlarges. The 1st presenting symptom of the patient is facial asymmetry.

Commonly appears between 20 and 40 years of age. Females are more frequently affected than males in a ratio of 5:1. It occurs more commonly in the mandibular premolar or molar region.

It is confined to the *periapical region of the jaws* in contrast to the more diffuse distribution of fibrous dysplasia. Juvenile presentation of this lesion are extremely aggressive and may involve both the jaws (Fig. 28.2).

Radiographic features

It is a well-circumscribed radiolucency with a sharply defined border between the lesion and adjacent normal bone. The appearance is variable. The radiolucent stage progresses to a radiopaque stage as the matrix is mineralised. A fully mature lesion appears as radiopaque mass surrounded by a thin radiolucent rim.

Histological features

- The lesions have well-defined capsules. They consist of numerous stellate or spindle-shaped fibroblasts
- Collagen fibres are arranged in whorled or stori-form pattern
- Trabeculae of woven bone with osteoblastic rimming and also lamellar bone are seen
- Spherical cementicle-like calcifications are also found
- Focal presence of osteoblasts along the surface of bone deposits distinguishes a cemento-ossifying fibroma from a fibrous dysplasia
- *Spicules of bone* which can be recognised radiographically as well as microscopically are of diagnostic importance.

Treatment

Cemento-ossifying fibromas have a definable capsule and can be readily enucleated by intraoral approach. Large lesions which distort the jaws require local resection and bone grafting if necessary. Prognosis is good.

FIBROUS DYSPLASIA

Fibrous dysplasia is a condition characterised *by the replacement of normal bone by an excessive proliferation of fibrous connective tissue intermixed with irregular bony trabeculae.* There is arrest of bone development in the woven bone stage with failure to mature to lamellar bone. It is a congenital dysplastic disease of the bone that may occur in a single bone or multiple bones.

It was 1st described by Von Recklinghausen in 1891. In 1937, Albright described a syndrome of polyostotic fibrous dysplasia. Lichtenstein in 1938 delineated the clinical spectrum and pathological anatomy, which he named fibrous dysplasia. It is a benign but, at times, destructive disease.

Pathogenesis

The exact aetiology of this condition is not known. Lichtenstein and Jaffe indicated an aberrant activity in the bone-forming mesenchymal tissues as the cause.

Patients with a mutation in the gene which codes for 'Gs' alpha membrane associated protein can induce altered proliferation of osteoblastic cells. It is also thought to develop as a result of postzygotic mutation in the GNAS I (guanine

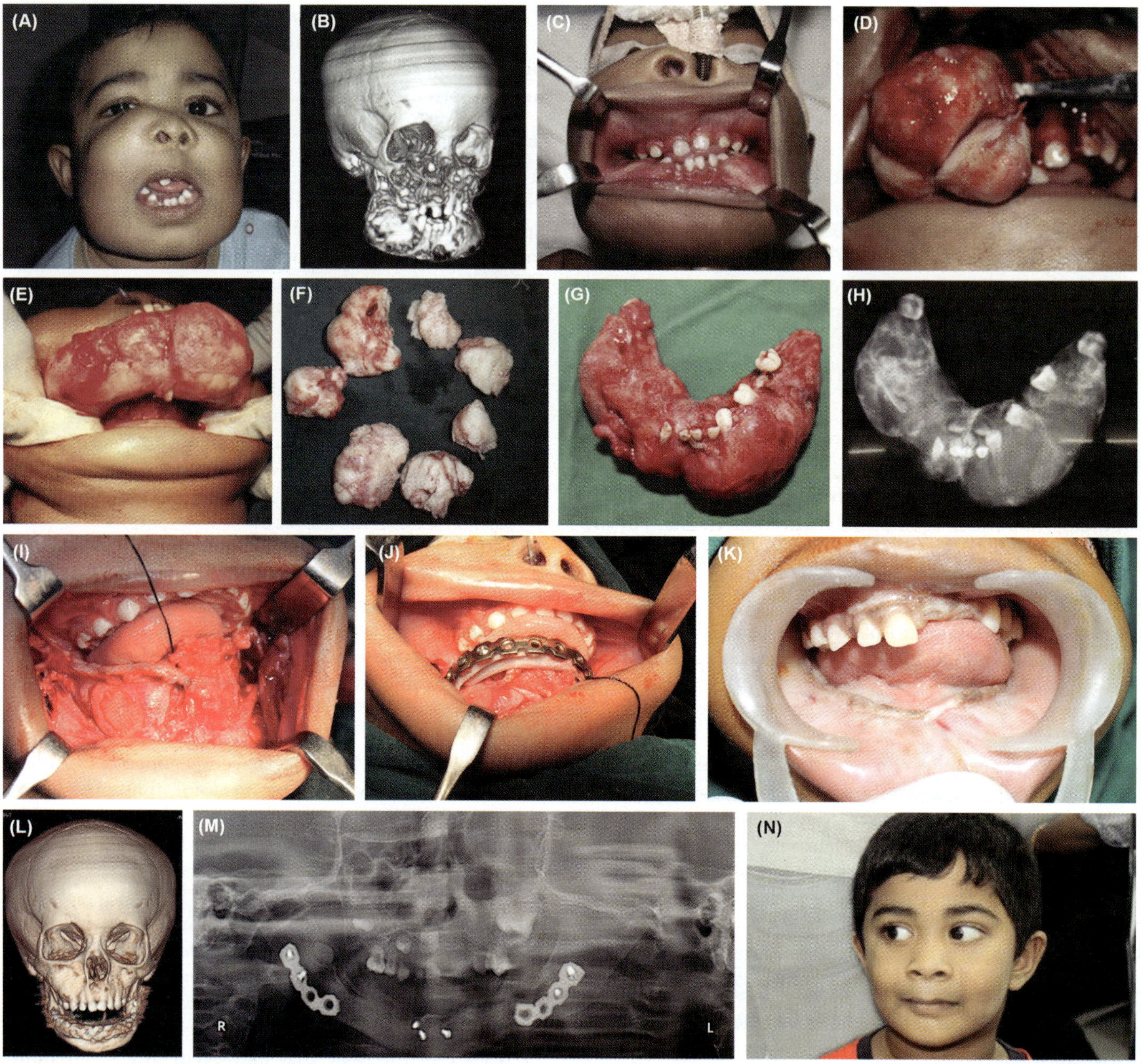

Figure 28.2 A rare juvenile aggressive cemento-ossifying fibroma of both jaws. **(A)** Swelling of midface and lower face in a 1½-year-old boy. **(B)** CT scan showing a variable multilocular expansile mass in maxilla and mandible. **(C)** Preoperative intraoral view showing obliteration of the vestibular sulcus and prominent bony hard swellings in the maxilla and mandible. **(D)** Resection of the fibroma on the right and left side of the maxilla. **(E)** Transoral exposure of the mandibular lesion. **(F)** Excised maxillary lesion. **(G)** Resected mandibular specimen. **(H)** Digital X-ray image of the resected mandible. **(I** and **J)** Reconstruction of the mandible using bone grafts and reconstruction plate. **(K)** Postoperative intraoral view. **(L** and **M)** Postoperative CT scan and OPG. **(N)** Postoperative view.

nucleotide-binding protein, alpha-stimulating activity polypeptide I) gene.

Clinical features

Fibrous dysplasia presents as a painless, slow enlargement of the involved bone. Normal appearance of a bone is altered, causing expansion in various directions, presents as *facial asymmetry or pathological fracture of an extremity*. The lesions are recognised in early childhood, grow slowly and stabilise in early adult life. There is a tendency for the disease to arrest with skeletal maturation or by puberty. But this is unpredictable and may not happen by puberty.

Two forms of fibrous dysplasia have been described:

- Monostotic—where one bone is involved
- Polyostotic—where several bones are involved along with cutaneous and endocrine abnormalities.

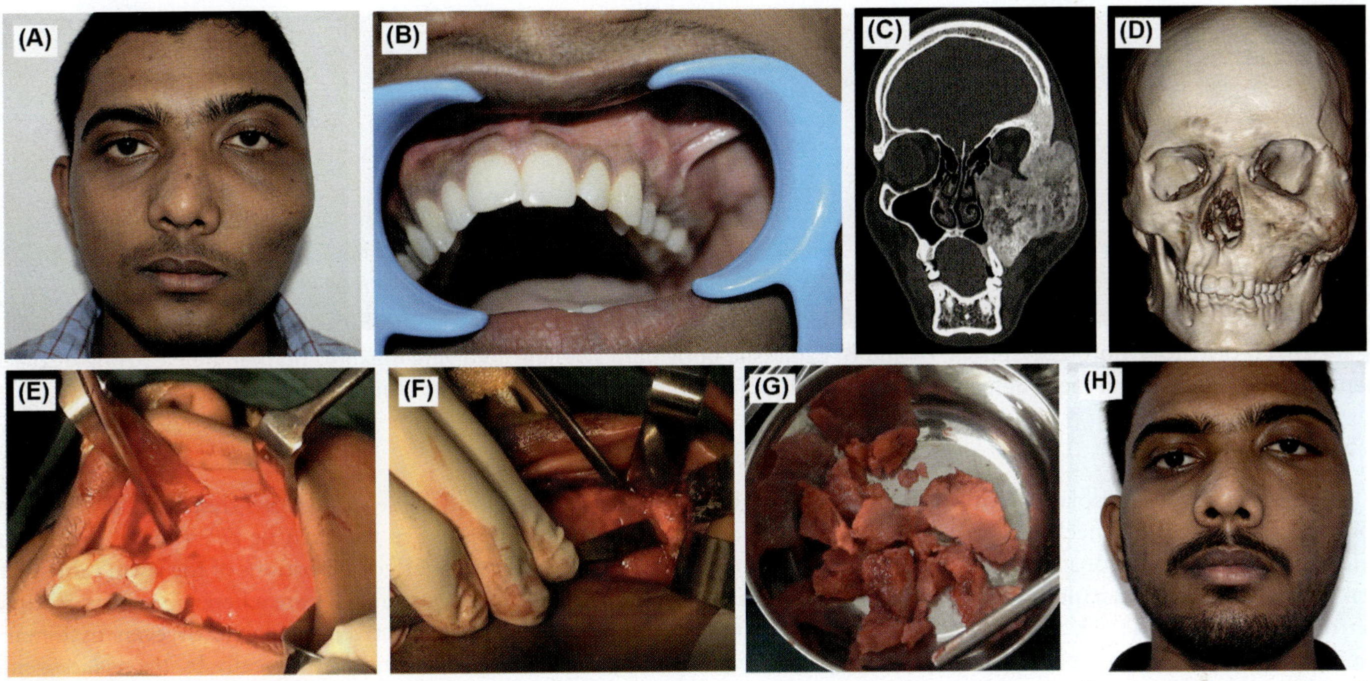

Figure 28.3 Monostotic fibrous dysplasia. (**A** and **B**) Expansile bony hard swelling in the left maxilla causing facial deformity. (**C–D**) CT showing expansile radiopaque mass in the left maxilla, encroaching the maxillary sinus almost obliterating the sinus. Note the ground glass appearance of the mass. (**E** & **F**) Intraoperative view showing the paring down procedure (excision of the lesion and sculpting of the bone). (**G**) Excised specimen. (**H**) Postoperative picture after excision of the lesion.

MONOSTOTIC FIBROUS DYSPLASIA

It is more common than the polyostotic form and accounts for 80% of cases (Fig. 28.3).

It is characterised by focal but poorly circumscribed fibro-osseous replacement of an area of bone. The jaws, particularly the maxilla, is the most frequently affected site.

Frontal bone is the other bone in the craniofacial skeleton that is commonly involved. Other frequently involved bones include the ribs, femur, long bones and skull.

Clinical features

- Onset of the disease usually occurs during the 1st or 2nd decade of life
- Males and females are equally affected
- The lesion forms a diffuse painless, smooth rounded swelling
- It is usually but not always unilateral
- As the lesion grows and expands, facial asymmetry develops
- Buccal cortical plate expansion is common.
- Displacement of teeth can cause malocclusion
- Interference with normal eruption of teeth may occur
- Normal occlusion is often seen, as normal teeth erupt
- While the disease develops in the maxilla, outer surface of the alveolar process is extremely enlarged
- Maxillary lesions frequently involve adjacent bones such as zygoma, sphenoid, maxillary sinus and floor of orbit. In the mandible, the mandibular body area is most frequently affected.

Radiographic features

Typical appearance is a homogeneous radiopacity with the numerous trabeculae of woven bone giving a *ground glass or orange peel appearance*.

An important feature is that the lesion merges imperceptibly with surrounding normal bone without a circumscribed border. The lesion may also present as a radiolucent area with patchy irregular opacities.

Histological features

It consists of areas of loose cellular fibrous tissue interwoven with irregular trabeculae and newly formed bone. The trabeculae are discrete, slender and accurate or branched. Some are slender and *C-shaped called 'Chinese characters' trabeculae*. Osteoblasts are scattered throughout the substance of the trabeculae. Lamellar bone formation is not seen in the classic microscopic picture of fibrous dysplasia.

POLYOSTOTIC FIBROUS DYSPLASIA (Fig. 28.4)

Polyostotic fibrous dysplasia is uncommon. Several or many bones may be involved. Females are more often affected than males in a ratio of 3:1. When seen with cutaneous pigmentation (café-au-lait macules), the disease is termed ***Jaffe-Lichtenstein syndrome***.

McCune-Albright syndrome comprises polyostotic fibrous dysplasia, skin pigmentation and endocrine abnormalities. Precocious sexual development and onset of puberty in females is the common endocrine disorder.

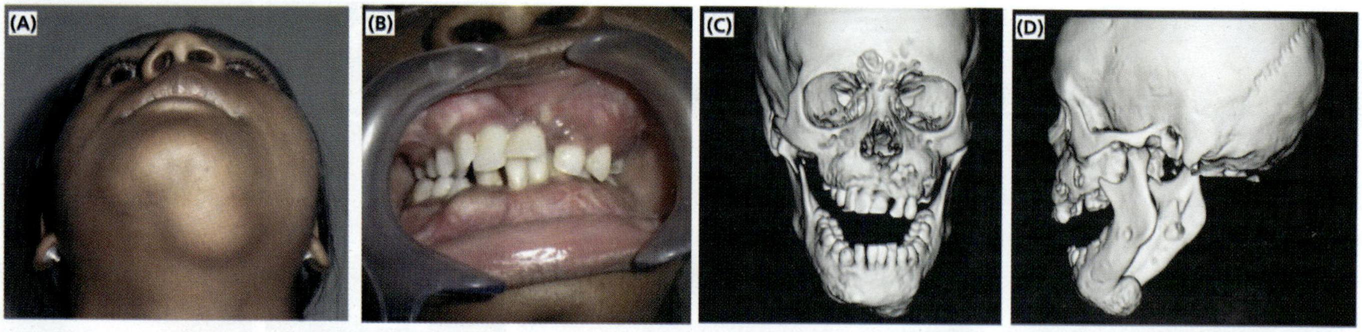

Figure 28.4 Polyostotic fibrous dysplasia. (**A** and **B**) Expansile bony hard swelling involving maxilla and mandible causing displacement, tipping of teeth and facial deformity. (**C** and **D**) 3D CT showing osseous expansion of maxilla and mandible.

Polyostotic fibrous dysplasia is more frequent in childhood. Involves head and neck region in 50% of cases. A jaw lesion may be the most conspicuous feature. Skin pigmentation consists of brown macules measuring 1 cm or more with an irregular outline. The risk of sarcomatous change is greater in polyostotic disease and typically develops in early adult life.

Treatment

- Radiotherapy is contraindicated because of its potential for malignant transformation as it may lead to postradiation bone sarcoma
- Small lesions may only require biopsy for confirmation and periodic follow-up. Lesions that cause functional disability or cosmetic deformity are treated by osseous recontouring
- Surgical intervention is generally done following active growth stage and during the period of stabilisation of the disease process. Entire disease cannot be eradicated by surgery, it is only a sculpting manoeuvre to improve the patient's appearance and provide a better functional masticatory apparatus
- Complete excision of the lesion is not possible because of the diffuse nature of the lesion and poorly defined borders
- In many cases, disease tends to stabilise and essentially stops enlarging when skeletal maturation is reached. As long as possible, therapy is postponed in adolescents since the dysplastic process can continue to proceed after surgery
- Lesions involving the anterior wall of the maxilla and the zygoma can be approached intraorally. An extraoral approach—Weber-Ferguson flap is required for lesions extending into the nasal or posterior maxillary regions. Lesions of the mandible connected to the alveolar ridges or inner aspect of the mandible are approached intraorally, whereas lesions in the posterior mandible are best accessed through a submandibular incision. Periodic follow-up is necessary because of the possibility of spontaneous malignant transformation.

CEMENTO-OSSEOUS DYSPLASIA

Cemento-osseous dysplasia is a group of disorders that includes periapical cemento-osseous dysplasia, focal cemento-osseous dysplasia and florid cemento-osseous dysplasia. These are all similar disease processes that can be *differentiated based on the extent of involvement* of affected portions of the jaws (Table 28.1).

These fibro-osseous diseases are a heterogeneous group of lesions that can be reactive, dysplastic or even malignant. They are distinguished microscopically by *the replacement of normal bone with a collagenous matrix* that contains trabeculae of immature bone or cementum-like material.

Pathogenesis

It is believed to originate from cells of the periodontal ligament or due to a defect in the remodelling of the extraligamentary bone.

Clinical features

The vast majority of these lesions are symptom-free and are typically discovered by chance during the radiographic examination. When these lesions become secondarily infected, as a result of poor endodontic therapy, tooth extraction or any other cause, they become symptomatic, at which point they need to be surgically removed.

GIANT CELL LESIONS AND SIMPLE BONE CYST

GIANT CELL GRANULOMA

Giant cell granuloma is considered widely to be a nonneoplastic lesion. Although formerly designated as 'giant cell reparative granuloma', there is little evidence that the lesion represents a reparative response.

A benign proliferation of fibroblasts and multinucleated giant cells within a well-vascularised stroma that occurs nearly exclusively within the jaws is known as a *central giant cell lesion.*

Clinical features

Giant cell granuloma may be encountered in patients ranging from 2 to 80 years of age, although more than 60% of all cases occur before the age of 30. A majority of giant cell granulomas are noted in females and approximately 70% arise in the mandible. Lesions are more common in the

TABLE 28.1 Characteristics of Types of Cemento-Osseous Dysplasia

Periapical Cemento-Osseous Dysplasia	Florid Cemento-Osseous Dysplasia	Focal Cemento-Osseous Dysplasia
• Most frequently in women above 40 years • Asymptomatic • Common sites are the apices of the anterior mandible • Vital teeth Radiographically, Progresses from radiolucent to opaque lesion (osteolytic, cementoblastic and mature phase) Histologically, Heterogeneous pattern-numerous cementum-like substances characterised by islands of calcified deposits in loose fibrocollagenous stroma • Mature and immature bone • Few inflammatory cells Treatment • No treatment • Endodontic treatment of teeth • Extraction is usually not recommended • On extensive lesions, surgical resection and saucerisation of the lesion	• Exuberant variant of periapical cemento-osseous dysplasia • Middle-aged woman • Predominantly multiquadrant involvement in both maxilla and mandible • Commonly posterior mandible • Bilateral and symmetrical distribution • Asymptomatic unless secondarily infected • Teeth are vital • Radiographically-Large radiolucency with opaque zones in the tooth-bearing regions • Histologically-Cementum-like calcifications embedded in a fibroblastic stroma • No treatment unless secondarily infected	• Incidence is from 3rd to 5th decade • More commonly in females • Asymptomatic, with an average size of 1.5 cm • Occurs at the apices of mandibular posterior teeth • Local jaw expansion and mild discomfort • Three developmental stages • Early or osteolytic stage is characterised by a well-defined radiolucent region together with the loss of periodontal ligament and lamina dura • Intermediate or cementoblastic stage is characterised by tiny opacities inside the radiolucent area • Mature, osteosclerotic or 'inactive' stage shows radiopacity throughout the lesion

anterior portions of the jaws and mandibular lesions frequently cross the midline.

1. ***Nonaggressive lesions*** make up most cases, exhibit few or no symptoms, demonstrate slow growth and do not show cortical perforation or root resorption of teeth involved in the lesion
2. ***Aggressive lesions*** are characterised by pain, rapid growth, cortical perforation and root resorption. They show a marked tendency to recur after treatment, compared to the nonaggressive types.

Radiographic features

Radiographically, central giant cell lesions appear as radiolucent defects, which may be unilocular or multilocular with well-demarcated margins (Fig. 28.5).

Histological features

Presence of abundant *multinucleated giant cells* in a background of mononuclear stromal cells in fibrous connective tissue. These giant cells represent osteoclasts and may be aligned more closely with macrophages.

Treatment

Central giant cell lesions of the jaws are usually treated by thorough curettage. Excision of aggressive lesion is required.

In patients with aggressive tumours, three alternatives to surgery, namely *(1) intralesional corticosteriods, (2) exogenous calcitonin, (3) interferon alpha-2* are being investigated.

Bisphosphonates have been proposed as an adjuvant to surgery due to their inhibitory effects on osteoclasts.

Similarly, targeting osteoclast-like large cells in this lesion with RANK ligand antibodies (denosumab) may be beneficial. In spite of the reported recurrence rate, long-term prognosis of giant cell granulomas is good and metastasis does not develop.

CHERUBISM

(Familial fibrous dysplasia of jaws, disseminated juvenile fibrous dysplasia, familial multilocular cystic disease of jaws)

Cherubism is a rare developmental jaw condition that is generally inherited as an autosomal dominant trait with high penetrance but variable expressivity.

Clinical features

Onset is typically between the ages of 6 months and 7 years. Severely affected cases are manifested before 1 year of age, whereas mild forms are not evident until 10–12 years of age. Most cases are identified between the age of 2 and 7 years. Males are more commonly affected than females.

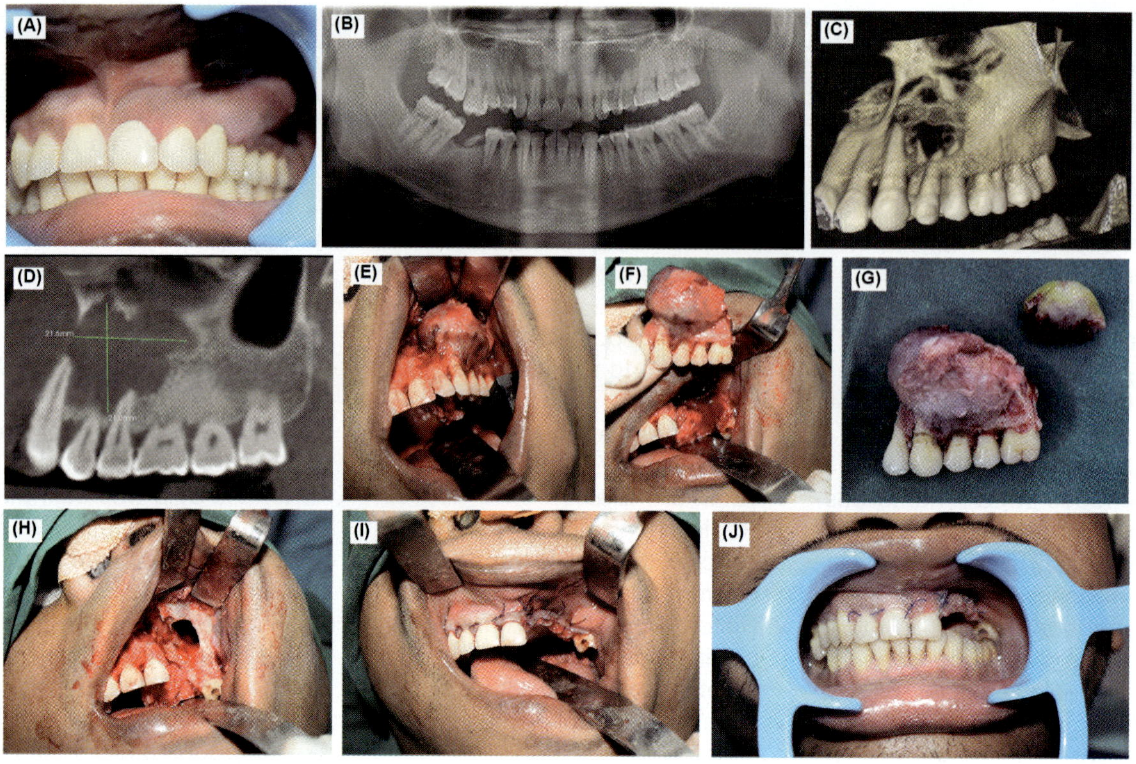

Figure 28.5 Giant cell granuloma. (**A**) Preoperative view showing a mild swelling in the upper left anterior maxilla. (**B**) OPG showing unilocular radiolucency in relation to apical region of 23–26. (**C** and **D**) CBCT showing bone loss and radiolucency with well-defined margins of about 2 × 2 cm in the left anterior maxilla. (**E** and **F**) Exposure and segmental resection of the lesion through intraoral approach. (**G**) Excised specimen. (**H**) After excision of the lesion, the bone cavity showing communication to the maxillary sinus. (**I**) Primary closure of the defect. (**J**) Postoperative view.

The lesion presents as a painless, slow expansion of affected areas of the jaw. Mandible, particularly the region of the angle is frequently involved. Maxilla is less commonly affected, though its involvement is usually associated with widespread mandibular diseases.

Involvement of the anterior maxillary segment produces the most characteristic deformity. Expansion of the anterior maxilla causes stretching of the skin and retraction of the lower lid exposing the sclera. As a result, the patient's eyes appear to be turned upwards ('eye to heaven' appearance). Inverted 'V' shape of the palate is due to maxillary expansion.

Premature exfoliation of primary teeth and absence or displacement of permanent teeth. Regional lymphadenopathy is seen as a result of reactive hyperplasia and fibrosis.

GRADING OF VARIABLE CLINICAL PRESENTATIONS OF CHERUBISM

Grade I: Bilateral involvement of ascending rami of mandible.

Grade II: Bilateral maxillary tuberosity involvement along with ascending rami of the mandible.

Grade III: Extensive involvement of anterior and posterior regions of the maxilla and mandible.

Grade IV: Extensive involvement of anterior and posterior region of the maxilla and mandible along with involvement of coronoid and condylar process.

Radiographic features

Produces well-defined multilocular radiolucency of the affected portions of the jaws with expansion and thinning of cortical bone (Fig. 28.6). Displaced or malformed teeth may be evident within the radiolucency. This existence of a large number of unerupted teeth and alveolar bone destruction can cause displacement of teeth, producing a radiographic appearance

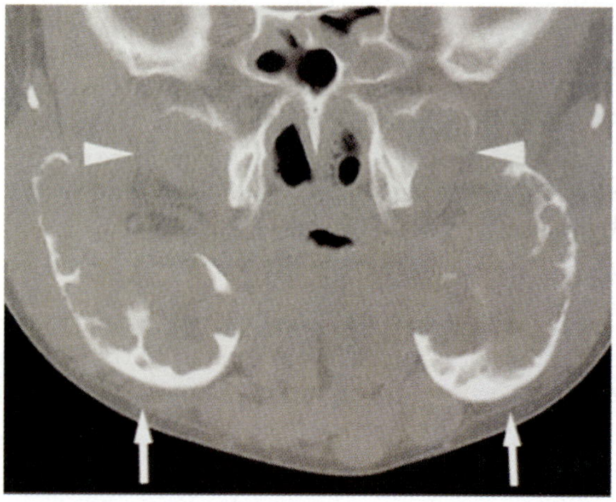

Figure 28.6 Coronal CT of a 6-year-old child with cherubism showing bilateral jaw expansion.

known as '*floating tooth syndrome*'. As the child develops, these cystic areas tend to re-ossify resulting in uneven patchy sclerosis and producing the typical '*ground glass appearance*'.

Histological features

It is characterised by the presence of cellular and vascular fibrous tissue containing many *multinucleated giant cells*. The collagenous stroma with large number of spindle-shaped fibroblasts are considered as unique. A resolving cherubism shows signs of an increase in fibrous tissue, a decrease in giant cells and formation of new bone.

Treatment

The treatment of cherubism should be based on the disease's natural course as well as the clinical behaviour of each case. Surgical intervention is usually done after puberty, consisting of curettage or debulking of lesion with recontouring is the treatment of choice.

Patients were observed until the postpubertal stage to assess lesion regression and any remaining deformity. Extensive lesions interfering with function may be treated surgically. Repeated procedures may be necessary to provide the desired result.

VASCULAR ANOMALIES OF OROFACIAL REGION

Vascular anomalies are a broad category of pathologies that affect the vascular structures of the human body. Vascular tumours are typically benign, show neoplastic features and represent disorganised angiogenesis. Vascular anomalies have been classified into ***haemangiomas and vascular malformations*** based on the clinical behaviour and endothelial cell characteristics (Table 28.2).

Haemangiomas are a *benign blood vessel tumour* composed of arterioles with proliferative and hyperplastic endothelial cells. They clinically appear as a soft, pink to red or purple, smooth or lobulated mass of any size ranging from few millimetres to several centimetres. The lesion blanches on pressure and bleeding can occur either spontaneously or as a result of minor trauma. There are two subtypes of haemangioma, which are infantile and congenital (Fig. 28.7).

Infantile haemangiomas are the most prevalent type and are found in children under the age of 1 year. Congenital haemangiomas are completely formed at birth and does not show any signs of rapid growth after birth.

Lesions arising from arterial, venous and lymphatic circulation are referred to as ***vascular abnormalities*** (AV malformations, venous malformations, capillary malformations, Lymphatic malformations).

Radiological assessment

To effectively diagnose and manage the vascular abnormalities, clinical and radiological assessments must be combined. Commonly used imaging modalities for assessment of vascular anomalies are:

- Ultrasound (US)
- Doppler ultrasound
- Computed tomography (CT) with contrast
- Digital subtraction angiography (DSA)
- Magnetic resonance imaging (MRI)
- MRI angiogram.

Treatment

The mode of treatment is determined by the type of vascular abnormality and its flow parameters. These are typically divided into three categories: *medical management, interventional therapy and surgical management.*

The primary goal of nonsurgical therapies is to limit the proliferation of cells, the extension of the lesion as well as its effect on the surrounding tissues.

TABLE 28.2 Features of Vascular Lesions

Haemangiomas	Vascular Malformations
Present at birth, mostly diagnosed within 1 year old	Although present at birth, it is frequently not detected until the 2nd decade
Rapid growth occurs until the age of 6–8 months, after which it slows and involutes during the next 5–9 years	Slow development throughout life, with increases in reaction to infection, trauma or hormonal changes
Endothelial cell turnover increases with neoplastic progression	Growth as a result of flow dynamics through the lesion and collateral supply
Reddish discolouration of skin	Red, pink or bluish swelling
Depth-skin, subcutaneous tissue	Superficial or deep
Rare osseous involvement	35% Osseous involvement
Female-to-male ratio (5:1)	Female-to-male ratio (2:1)
Low flow	May be low flow or high flow
Functionally—Ulceration/vision, hearing or airway problems	Pain, airway problems, dysphagia, difficulty in mastication, cosmetic disfigurement
Does not necessitate treatment	Treatment is frequently required

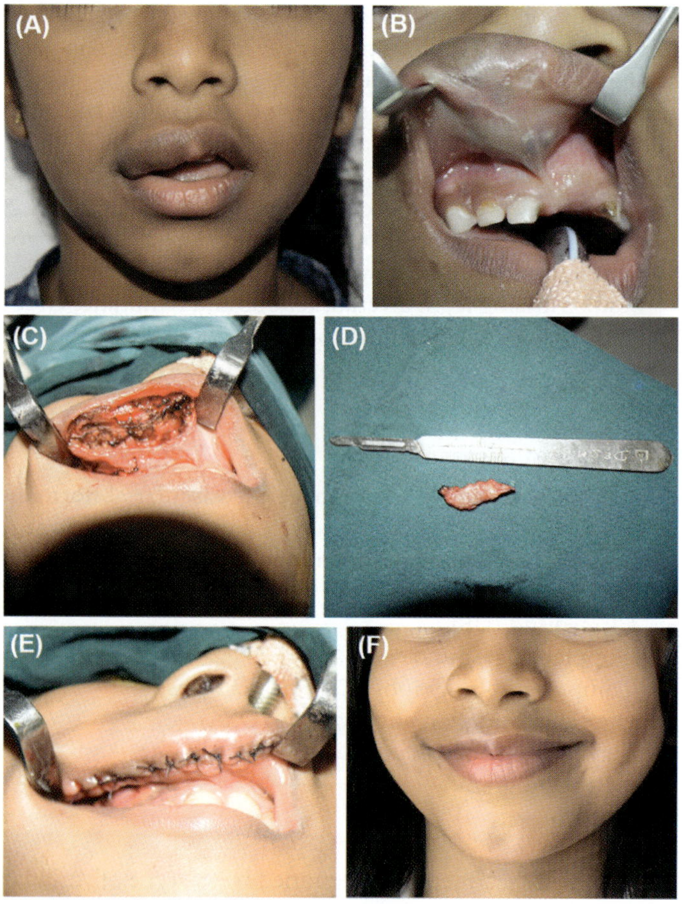

Figure 28.7 Haemangioma. (**A** and **B**) Preoperative view showing soft purple swelling in the upper lip. (**C**) Surgical excision of the lesion using electrocautery. (**D**) Excised haemangioma. (**E**) Primary closure of the defect. (**F**) Postoperative view.

MANAGEMENT OF HAEMANGIOMAS

More than 85% of patients show signs of involution and a strategy of '*wait and observe*' is recommended. The treatment options available for haemangioma include:

1. Propranolol
2. Systemic steroids
3. Embolisation
4. Surgery
5. Sclerotherapy
6. Pulsed dye laser.

Propranolol produces vasoconstriction and also reduces the expression of pro-angiogenic factors responsible for the growth of haemangioma. It is given in a dose of 1 mg/kg/day for 12 months or longer. It helps to prevent the complications that could arise from haematomas near the vital regions.

Systemic steroids are used extensively, for the purpose of early involution of large and rapidly growing haematomas, particularly during the initial period of life. *Prednisone* of dose 2 mg/kg/day for 2 weeks to 4 months is the recommended regimen. Systemic steroids have been linked to a variety of adverse effects, including growth retardation, personality changes, gastric irritation and opportunistic infections. Additionally, it is common for the lesion to experience rebound growth after the treatment has been discontinued.

BOX 28.2 Intralesional Sclerosing Agents
• Bleomycin
• 5% Sodium morrhuate
• Absolute ethanol
• OK-432 (Picibanil)
• Ethanolamine oleate
• Doxycyclin

Trans-arterial embolisation can be used to supplement or even increase the natural process of involution. Embolisation entails the installation of coils or glue, and it can be performed by accessing the malformation through a proximal artery or retrograde venous approach, or by directly puncturing the bone through the osseous tissue.

Sclerotherapy includes injection of foreign agents into one of the primary vessels of haemangioma. It results in endothelial damage and obliteration of the lumen. Studies have shown that sclerotherapy produces favourable results, with minimal adverse responses; nonetheless, there is still a possibility of thrombosis associated with embolisation. Commonly used sclerosing agents are shown inBox 28.2.

Pulsed dye laser are effective for the treatment of ulcerated haemangiomas. They are not recommended for growing haemangiomas due to their inability to penetrate adequately into the tumour.

Surgery—The therapy of choice for majority of haemangiomas is excision of the lesion surgically, *with or without ligation of the vessels and embolisation*. The surgical management should be carried out with extreme caution, taking into consideration the likelihood of bleeding both during and after the surgery. Surgical management is also recommended for patients who does not respond to medications or have compromised function.

Surgical resection is considered as a definitive treatment for haemangiomas and is often preferred for smaller lesions. Large lesions are not preferred for surgical resection because it may require a significant amount of tissue removal.

In the treatment of haemangiomas, there are two different types of surgical excisions: *lenticular and circular*. Lenticular excision increases the scar length, while circular excision with purse-string closure reduces the dimensions and turns a large circular lesion into a small ellipsoid scar.

Popescu (1985) presented a new technique known as intratumoural ligation. This technique blocked the intratumoural blood flow and results in endothelial atrophy, formation of blood clot, obstruction of vascular lumina and subsequent fibrous hyperplasia. It is followed by splitting of the haemangioma mass into segments and eliminates the blood flow.

MANAGEMENT OF VASCULAR MALFORMATIONS

Management of vascular malformations are challenging because of their aggressive nature and significant life-threatening complications such as massive haemorrhage. The various treatment options available for vascular malformations include:

- Sclerotherapy
- Embolisation
- Pulsed dye laser
- Surgery
- Reconstruction with flaps.

The type of treatment is determined by the severity, depth, extent and the anatomical location of the lesion. The treatment options available for various vascular anomalies include:

Capillary malformations—Pulsed dye laser.

Venous malformation—Lasers, surgical excision, sclerotherapy and combinations.

Arteriovenous malformations (AVMs)—Embolisation, surgical resection and combinations.

Lymphatic malformations—Laser/photo ablation, surgery and sclerotherapy (Fig. 28.8).

Sclerotherapy

It is still a viable alternative in the treatment of venous abnormalities in the head and neck. Sclerosing agents such as ethanol and sotradecol remain the mainstay with a long-term efficacy. The technique of sclerotherapy involves percutaneous injection of a substance to induce fibrosis and limit the expansion of the lesion.

Embolisation and surgery

Surgery to remove an AVM may result in significant blood loss, but if the tumour is not completely removed, it may regrow and becomes more difficult to treat. A proximal ligation of the parent artery is unsuccessful and ought to be avoided because it can make subsequent therapy difficult or impossible. Hence, management of AVMs requires multimodal treatment, which includes *preoperative embolisation and complete surgical resection*.

Preoperative embolisation of the feeding arteries helps in reducing the blood flow within the tumour, decreases the blood loss during surgery, thereby making it possible to remove the entire tumour. The current treatment method in AVMs are *arterial embolisation to obstruct the nidus followed by surgical excision after 24–72 h*. The surgical treatment is aimed in removing the AVM nidus and the surrounding tissues.

Commonly used embolic agents (Box 28.3)

Embolisation rarely results in complications; however, necrosis of the neighbouring tissues is a possibility.

- Vascular abnormalities can be diagnosed by using noninvasive imaging techniques such as *ultrasonography and MRI*. In most cases, a high-flow AVM is diagnosed based on the findings of an MRI, which indicates the presence of rapid flow within the lesion
- An *angiography* is essential to completely see the vascular architecture of the lesion, identify all the arteries and veins that are feeding the lesion and create a 'plan of attack'
- *Selective arterial embolisation* is performed by an interventional radiologist, by injecting polyvinyl alcohol or Cyanoacrylate into the external carotid artery. Selective embolisation blocks the high-flow shunt between the arterial and venous system.
    a. Under direct fluoroscopy, a 16-gauge needle trocar is inserted straight through the bone or alveolus intraorally

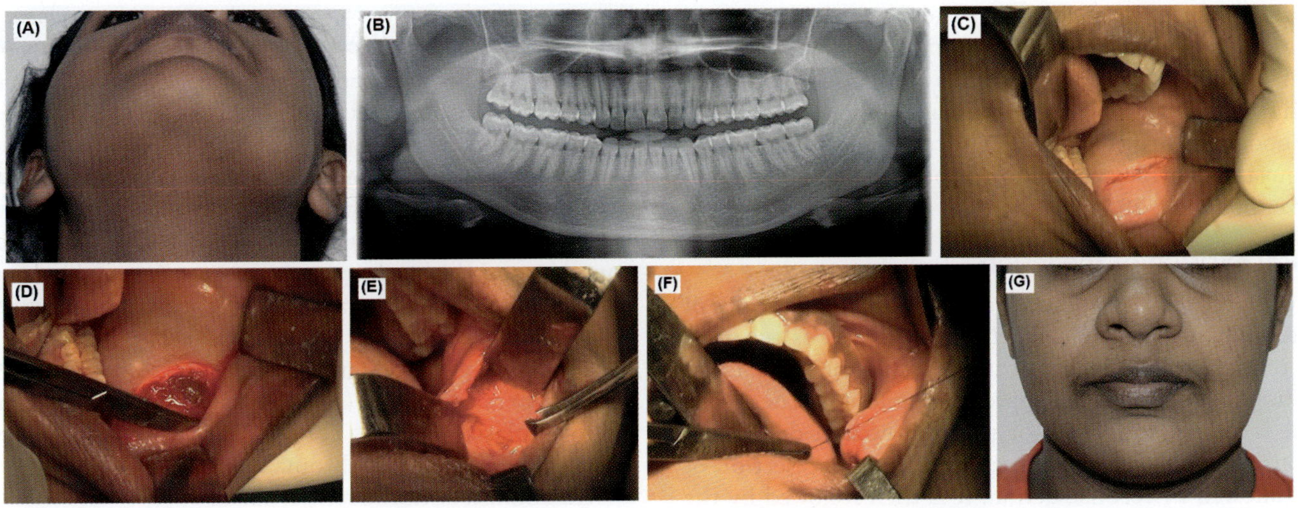

Figure 28.8 Lymphangioma. **(A)** Preoperative view with soft swelling in the mandibular left ramus and angle region. **(B)** OPG shows no evidence of bone and tooth involvement. **(C)** Surgical exposure through an incision over the lesion. **(D)** Dissection of the mucosa exposing the purplish lesion. **(E)** Surgical excision of the lesion. **(F)** Primary closure of the wound. **(G)** Postoperative view.

BOX 28.3 Commonly Used Embolic Agents

A. Temporary (resorbable)
- Gelfoam
- Collagen
- Iodine oil

B. Permanent
- Polyvinyl alcohol particles
- Cyanoacrylate (acrylic glue)
- Platinum coils
- Silky thread
- Stainless steel

b. The position of the trocar into the AVM is verified by arteriogram
c. An 18-gauge catheter is inserted through the trocar, with the assistance of a guide wire
d. Through the catheter, the embolisation substance is delivered directly into the AVM nidus
f. This procedure is carried out several times to treat the different varices of AVMs.

- Both before and after the selective embolisation, a *diagnostic angiogram* needs to be performed to assess the flow and location of arterio-venous shunting.

One to three days after the embolisation procedure, a surgical excision of the lesion and the surrounding tissues may be performed, either partially or completely. Except for the major and proximal arteries, it is necessary to ligate all of the smaller arteries that supply the AVM.

EXTERNAL CAROTID ARTERY (ECA) CONTROL

A cervical incision is placed, and the sternocleidomastoid muscle is retracted at the hyoid cornu to expose the carotid sheath. The distal external carotid is recognised and is encircled by a vascular sling. This vascular compression reduces the blood supply to the lesion. ECA control is often used as an adjuvant to achieve haemostasis because of its collateral blood supply (Fig. 28.9).

Surgical excision of the lesion

Incisions over the face and neck are placed along the lines of skin tension to avoid unaesthetic results. Care is taken to avoid thinning of the skin flap and avascular necrosis. Layer wise dissection is done to approach the lesion. The lesion (AVM) is either completely or partially excised depending upon its size. Few cases may require segmental resection of bone followed by reconstruction. It is then followed by the closure of the defect.

The management of vascular lesions involves a wide range of considerations. However, surgery is usually an essential component in the vast majority of cases, and it plays a significant role in achieving faster and more stable outcomes.

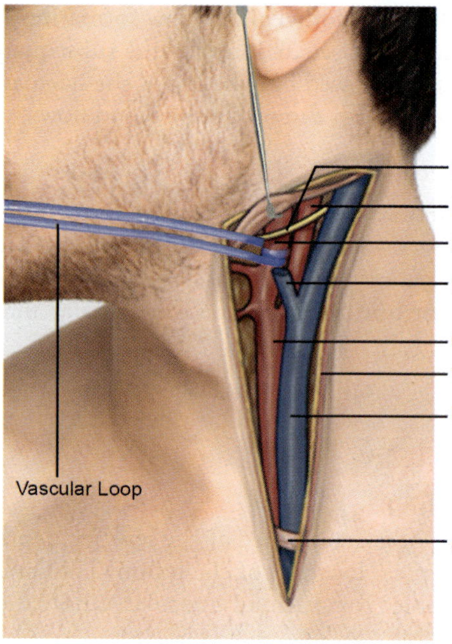

Figure 28.9 ECA control.

Complications

- Massive blood loss during surgery
- Recurrence of the lesion
- Development of collaterals after embolisation
- Embolisation can cause ischaemic stroke
- Extrusion of embolisation materials.

Conclusion

Vascular anomalies are a diverse group of lesions that require a multidisciplinary approach involving oral and maxillofacial surgeon, radiologist, vascular surgeon, anaesthetist and blood bank.

REACTIVE LESIONS OF ORAL CAVITY

Reactive lesions are benign, reactive, isolated swellings, caused by persistent and recurring tissue damage. They are usually caused by chronic inflammation from oral mucosa irritations such as broken teeth, overhanging restorations, food impaction, etc. In spite of the fact that the lesion is not malignant, it has a propensity to recur, if the excision is incomplete and the local irritants are not eliminated.

The common peripheral reactive lesions of oral cavity are:
- Pyogenic granuloma
- Peripheral giant cell granuloma
- Peripheral fibroma (fibrous epulis and focal fibrous hyperplasia)
- Peripheral ossifying fibroma
- Inflammatory fibrous hyperplasia.

Reactive lesions are more likely to appear in the gingiva than in other parts of the oral cavity including the tongue, palate, cheeks and floor of the mouth.

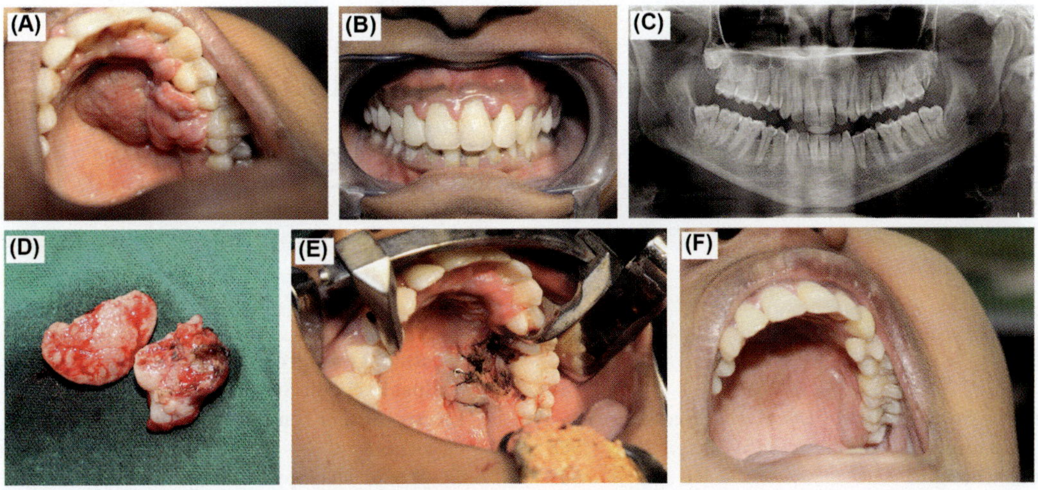

Figure 28.10 Pyogenic granuloma. (**A** and **B**) Preoperative view of the lesion that presents as a soft sessile mass in relation to the palatal aspect of 24–26 region. (**C**) OPG shows resorption of the alveolar bone and increased periodontal ligament space in between 25 and 26. (**D**) Excised specimen. (**E**) Primary closure of the defect. (**F**) Postoperative view.

Clinically, they manifest as:

- Sessile or pedunculated masses with smooth or injured surfaces
- Different colours from bright pink to red
- Similar to neoplastic lesions
- Striking predilection for gingiva.

Based on their histopathological features, these lesions can be divided into fibrous and inflammatory type.

PYOGENIC GRANULOMA (Fig. 28.10)

It is also known as pregnancy tumour, benign vascular tumour, lobular capillary haemangioma or vascular epulis.

Aetiology

It appears as a reparative response to different stimuli such as chronic irritation, hormonal changes, trauma, and bone marrow transplants. Daley et al., found a significant link between the blood levels of oestrogen and progesterone hormone, as well as prostoglandins. These hormones make the gingival tissues more susceptible to inflammation.

Clinical features

The most common site of appearance is gingiva, even though it can occur in the lips, mucosa, and the tongue. It can affect people of any age and of either gender, although there is a female predominance in their 2nd decade of life. This is due to higher levels of circulating hormones like oestrogen and progesterone during this time. Both the jaws have been found to have an equal incidence, with a slight predilection for the anterior maxilla.

It manifest as a painless, pedunculated or sessile, soft mass that is prone to bleeding with occasional ulcerations on the surface.

Radiographic features

In most cases, pyogenic granuloma does not show any appreciable radiological alterations; nevertheless, in some cases, a cup-like resorption of the underlying alveolar bone can be detected on an IOPA or OPG.

Histological features

Pyogenic granulomas can be divided into two subtypes based on their histological appearance: the nonlobular capillary haemangioma (non-LCH) type, and the lobular capillary haemangioma (LCH) type.

Non-LCH type—It is characterised by high vascular proliferation with foci of fibrous tissue.

LCH type—It is characterised by lobular aggregates of proliferating blood vessels without any signs of inflammation.

Treatment

The therapy consists of surgical removal of the lesion, followed by the elimination of any local irritants, which may include calculus, a foreign body, etc. The excision of the lesion is made up to the periosteum, followed by primary closure or healing by secondary intention using (Coe-Pak/Peripac/Ward's Wondrpak). It is common to encounter bleeding during removal of the lesion that necessitates electrocoagulation. Electrocautery, cryosurgery, sclerotherapy and laser are some of the further treatment possibilities.

Chapter 29

Premalignant Lesions and Conditions

OUTLINE

INTRODUCTION

For individuals exposed to carcinogens premalignant lesions, particularly erythroplakia and leukoplakia may be a potential finding. The risk of these premalignant lesions for malignant change is exceedingly high, especially if the carcinogenic assault is not ceased. Practitioners must be able to recognise these lesions before malignant transformation. Learning about these conditions and lesions become fundamental for diagnosis and treatment planning.

DYSPLASIA

Chronic irritation to tissues can cause a series of changes at the cellular level. The cell's response to a noxious stimulus is adaptation followed by reversible damage, but when the stimulus is not removed, it can lead to irreversible damage. Dysplasia can be graded as mild, moderate and severe dysplasia. Cellular level atypia with marked aberrant and uncontrolled cellular proliferation leads to tissue level dysplasia. Krammer et al. described the features of dysplasia as cells showing the following features (Table 29.1). The criteria and grading of dysplasia is shown in Fig. 29.1.

TABLE 29.1 Cellular Features of Epithelial Dysplasia Seen in Oral Mucosa Described by Krammer et al.

1. Loss of basal cell polarity
2. Increased layers of basaloid cells
3. Increased nuclear cytoplasmic ratio
4. Rete process shape changes to drop shape
5. Epithelial stratification becomes irregular
6. Abnormal mitosis
7. Mitosis in superficial cells of epithelium
8. Cellular pleomorphism
9. Nuclear hyperchromatism
10. Enlarged nucleoli
11. Decreased cellular cohesion
12. Keratinisation

CLINICAL METHODS FOR INVESTIGATION OF DYSPLASIA, PRECANCEROUS LESIONS AND SQUAMOUS CELL CARCINOMA (SCC)

1. Vital staining:
   a. **Toluidine blue staining:** It is performed for diagnosis of the dysplastic areas in the oral cavity (Fig. 29.2A & B)

Procedure: The patient is asked to rinse the mouth twice with water (20 s each time), followed by a rinse with 1% acetic acid (20 s). The suspicious area is dried with gauze. Toluidine blue solution 1% is applied over the dry mucosa. The patient is asked to rinse with 150 mL of acetic acid for 1 min, followed by a rinse with water. The positive stained mucosa is recorded. This procedure is repeated in 1 week. All areas that stained positive in both visits are subjected to biopsy.

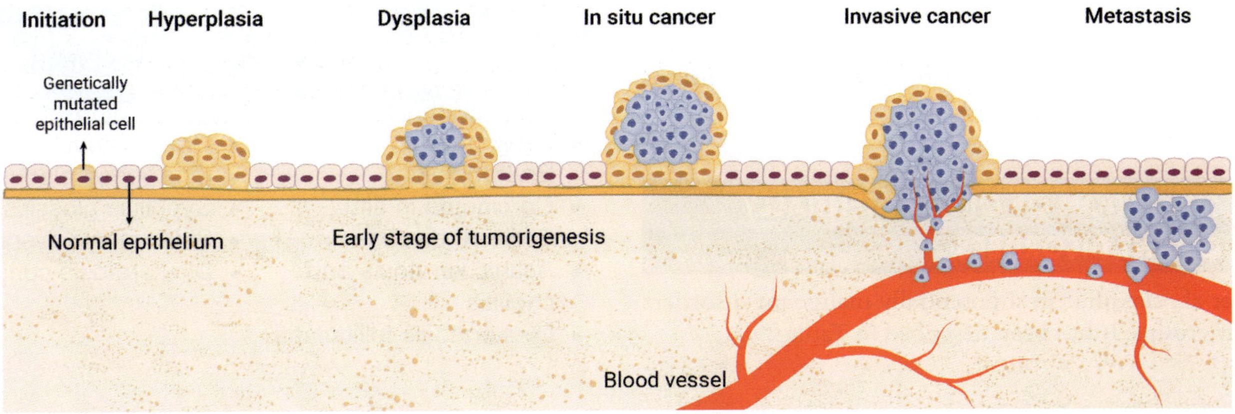

Figure 29.1 The illustration shows the changes of a normal tissue on continuous stimulation by noxious stimuli. Normal cells 1st show reversible changes like hyperplasia followed by mild, moderate or severe dysplasia. The next stage is carcinoma in situ followed by invasive cancer and metastasis.

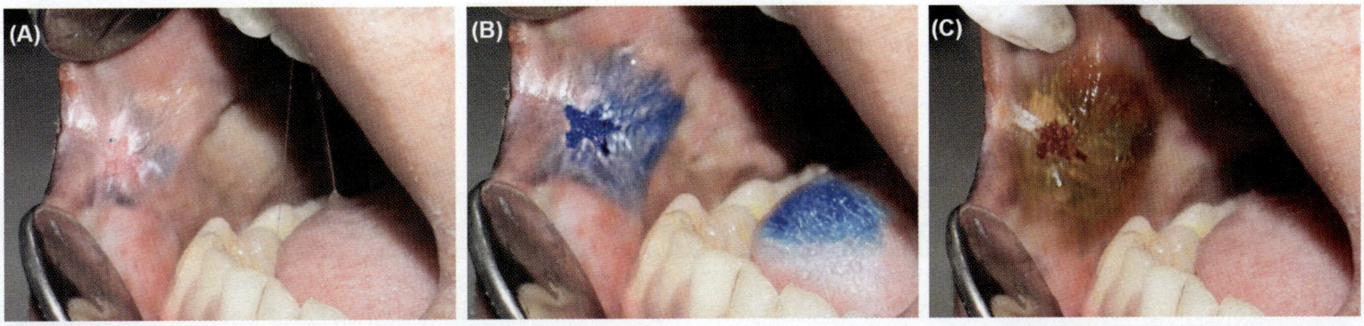

Figure 29.2 (**A**) Area of suspicion in the oral cavity. (**B**) Use of Toluidine blue staining. (**C**) Use of Lugol's iodine staining.

   b. **Lugol's iodine staining:** Lugol's iodine staining has greater specificity for the detection of oral squamous cell carcinoma (Fig. 29.2A & C).
2. ViziLite: It is a chemiluminescent (CL) light shined over areas in the oral cavity after an acetic acid rinse. The acetic acid changes the refractile properties of lesions like leukoplakia. When ViziLite is shown on the mucosa, the abnormal tissue shines brighter than the normal tissues.
3. Acridine binding.

CLINICAL PRECANCEROUS CHANGES

Types of alteration of dysplasia in the oral cavity after continuous irritation to normal mucosa are depicted by four types of cellular changes. These changes are the clinical formation of precancerous lesions.

Type I—when only genetic changes occur in the normal epithelium, the changes are detected at molecular levels.

Type II—genetic changes with dysplasia can be detected at molecular and histological levels.

Type III—genetic changes, dysplasia with hyperplasia and clinical leukoplakia can be detected clinically.

Type IV—genetic changes, dysplasia with atrophy and clinical erythroplakia can be detected clinically.

POTENTIALLY MALIGNANT DISORDERS OF THE ORAL CAVITY

PREMALIGNANT LESION

A premalignant lesion is 'a morphologically altered tissue in which oral cancer is more likely to occur than in its apparently normal counterpart'—WHO workshop 1978. The important premalignant lesions discussed in this chapter are leukoplakia, erythroplakia and carcinoma in situ.

PREMALIGNANT CONDITION

Premalignant condition is 'a generalised state associated with a significantly increased risk of cancer'—WHO workshop 1978.

Premalignant condition is a group of disorders of varying aetiologies, usually tobacco; characterised by mutagen associated, spontaneous or hereditary alterations or mutations in the genetic material of oral epithelial cells with or without clinical and histomorphological alterations that may lead to oral squamous cell carcinoma transformation'—WHO workshop 2005.

The most common premalignant lesions and conditions have been listed out in Table 29.2.

TABLE 29.2 List of Premalignant Lesions and Conditions	
Premalignant Lesions	**Premalignant Conditions**
• Leukoplakia • Erythroplakia • Carcinoma in situ • Bowen's disease • Actinic keratosis and cheilitis • Dyskeratosis follicularis	• Oral submucous fibrosis • Oral lichen planus • Syphilitic glossitis • Sideropenic dysphagia • Dyskeratosis congenita

CLASSIFICATION OF ORAL POTENTIALLY MALIGNANT DISORDERS

Sarode et al., classified oral potentially malignant disorders into four groups. It has been described in Table 29.3.

TABLE 29.3 Classification of Oral Potentially Malignant Disorders

GROUP I: Morphological alteration due to external factor	**Group IA—Habit Related** 1. Tobacco associated lesions: a. **Leukoplakia** b. Tobacco pouch keratosis c. Stomatitis palatine nicotine 2. Betel nut associated: a. Oral submucous fibrosis 3. *Sanguinaria*-associated keratosis	**Group IB—Nonhabit Related** • Actinic cheilosis • Chronic candidiasis
GROUP II: Morphologically alteration due to chronic inflammation	**Group II A: Chronic inflammation caused by internal derangement** 1. Lichen planus 2. Discoid lupus erythematosus	**Group II B: Chronic inflammation caused by external factors** 1. Chronic mucosal trauma 2. Lichenoid reactions 3. Poor oral hygiene 4. Chronic infections: • Chronic bacterial infections • Chronic viral infections • Chronic fungal infections 5. Prolonged untreated chronic inflammation
GROUP III: Inherited disorders with risk of malignant transformation	1. Inherited cancer syndromes: a. Xeroderma pigmentosum b. Ataxia telangiectasia c. Fanconi's anaemia d. Li–Fraumeni syndrome 2. Dyskeratosis congenita 3. Epidermolysis bullosa 4. White sponge nevus 5. Darier's disease 6. Hailey–Hailey disease	
GROUP IV: Premalignant conditions	1. Immunosuppression: a. AIDS b. Immunosuppression therapy (for malignancy or organ transplant) 2. Alcohol consumption and abuse 3. Nutritional deficiency: a. Sideropenic dysphagia b. Deficiency of micronutrients	

DIAGNOSIS AND TREATMENT PLAN OF POTENTIALLY MALIGNANT LESIONS AND CONDITIONS (FLOWCHART 29.1)

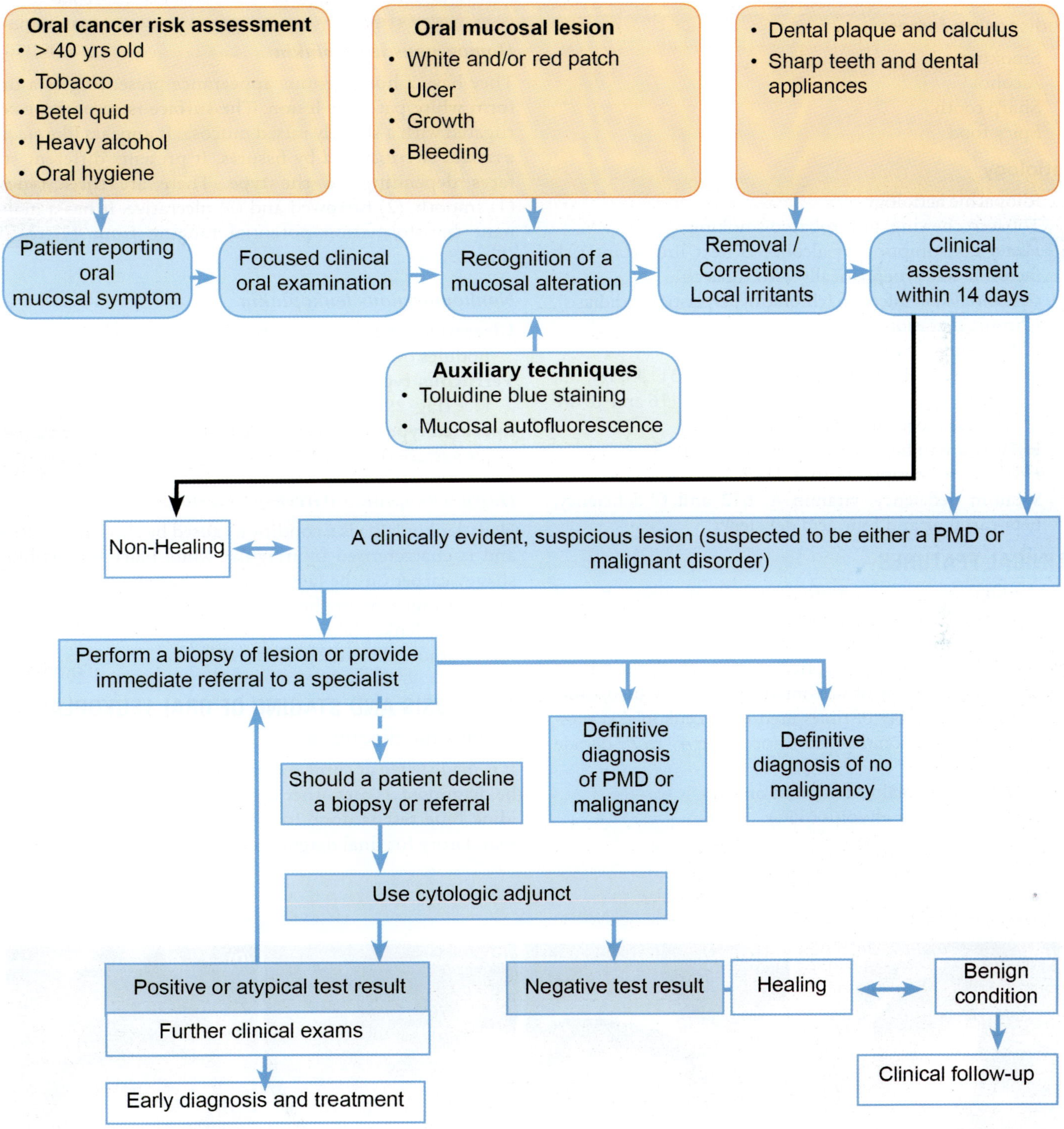

Flowchart 29.1 Steps in clinical risk assessment, removal of causative agent of lesions, biopsy, diagnosis and treatment plan of potentially malignant lesions and conditions.

LEUKOPLAKIA (LEUKO—WHITE; PLAKIA—PLAQUE)

Leukoplakia WHO definition

'A white patch or plaque that cannot be characterised clinically or pathologically as any other disease'.

Predisposing factors

1. Smoking
2. Alcohol
3. Sharp tooth
4. Spicy food

Aetiology

1. Idiopathic aetiology
2. Tobacco chewing, bidi/tobacco smoking
3. Heavy consumption of alcohol is next important risk factor, it acts synergistically with tobacco
4. *Candida albicans* infection (chronic hyperplastic candidiasis).
5. Chronic irritation
6. HPV–human papilloma viruses
   - High-risk HPV include types 16, 18, 31, 33, 34, 35, 39, 45, 51, 52, 56, 58, 59, 66, 68 and 70 (16 and 18 are the most common causes)
7. HHV–human herpesviruses, HHV-6, HHV-8
8. HSV–herpes simplex viruses, HSV-1
9. Vitamin deficiency–vitamin A, B12 and C deficiency, beta-carotene and folic acid deficiency.

CLINICAL FEATURES

Oral leukoplakia carries a fivefold risk of mutating into oral cancer. Tobacco produces a specific clinical feature of leukoplakia on the oral mucosa, a characteristic pumice stone appearance. Clinical appearance often correlates with the type of tobacco used, duration of use, intensity (amount used/time) and frequency (number of times used/day). Leukoplakia presents a male predilection that mostly occurs in 4th to 7th decade of life.

Site: Oral leukoplakia are found on the:

1. Upper and lower alveolus (36%)
2. Buccal mucosa (22%)
3. Lips
4. Palate
5. Floor of mouth
6. Gingiva
7. Tongue
8. Retromolar trigone.

CLINICAL TYPES

Homogenous leukoplakia

They have a homogenous appearance presenting as a uniform white patch or lesion. The surface is smooth or corrugated with a slightly raised mucosa. It appears like *plaque, wrinkled or crisscrossed* by fissures. It presents different surfaces depending on the type. There are three types—(1) smooth, (2) furrowed and (3) ulcerative. It has a malignant transformation potential ranging from 1% to 7%. (Fig. 29.3A).

Nonhomogenous leukoplakia

Ulcerative type–red ulcerative lesion with white specks or nodules over it.

Verrucous type–white lesion with hyperplastic warty surface (Fig. 29.3B).

Speckled type–mixed red and white patches with an irregular surface (Fig. 29.3D).

Hairy leukoplakia (Greenspan lesion)

Hairy leukoplakia is a condition caused by chronic irritation, and is characterised by irregular white hairy lesions like a shaggy carpet on the lateral side of the tongue and dorsum of the tongue or in the oral cavity. The viruses associated with hairy leukoplakia are Epstein–Barr virus (EBV) and human immunodeficiency virus (HIV).

DIAGNOSIS AND STAGING OF ORAL LEUKOPLAKIA

Provisional diagnosis

It is made when at clinical examination a white lesion cannot be diagnosed as any other disease of the oral mucosa. Toluidine blue test is done for dysplastic changes. A biopsy is mandatory for final diagnosis (Flowchart 29.2).

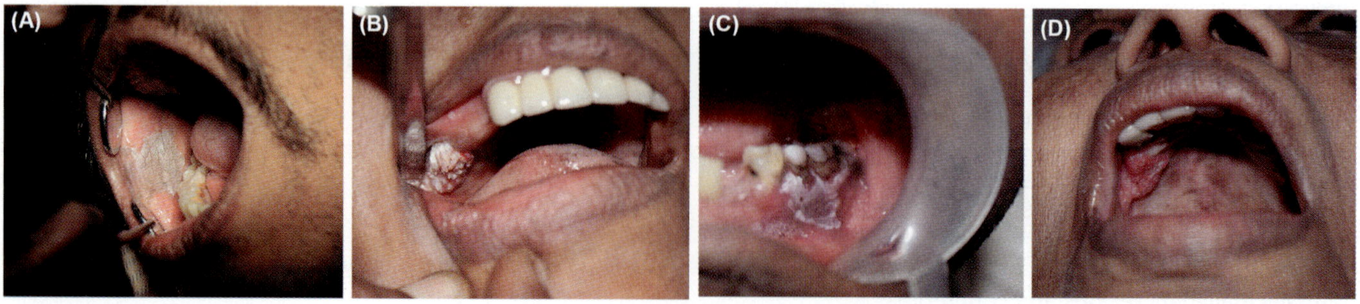

Figure 29.3 (**A**) Homogenous leukoplakia. (**B**) Verrucous leukoplakia. (**C**) Candidal leukoplakia. (**D**) Speckled leukoplakia.

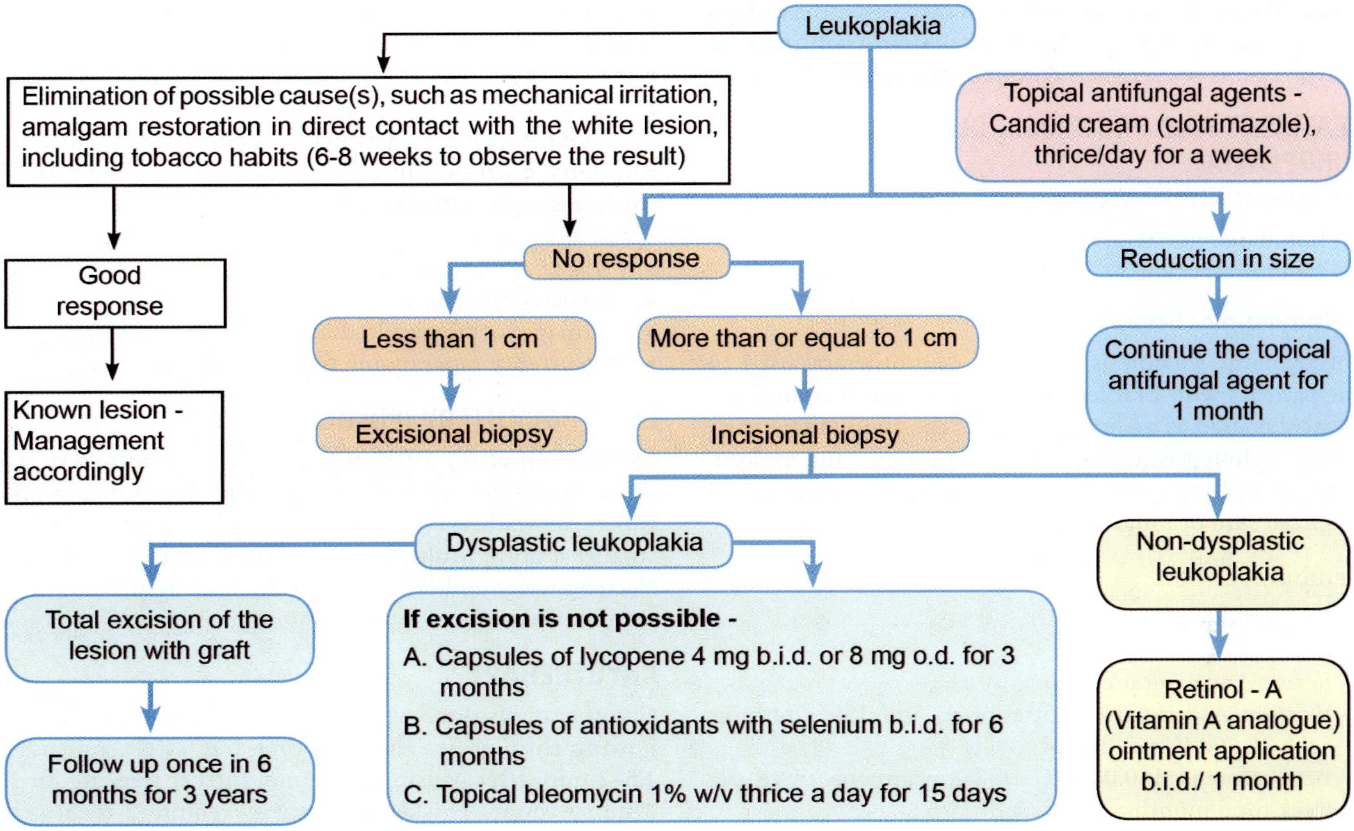

Flowchart 29.2 Diagnosis and management of oral leukoplakic lesions.

Differential diagnosis

White sponge nevus, acute pseudomembranous candidiasis, chronic hyperplastic candidiasis, leukoedema and lichen planus (plaque type).

Histopathology

Epithelial dysplasia is noted in the histopathological examination. This can be graded based on the system shown in the Table 29.4. This grading helps in the treatment of leukoplakia as the treatment varies for high risk and low risk leukoplakia.

Final diagnosis

A biopsy is mandatory for all lesions provisionally diagnosed as leukoplakia as this will guide the course of treatment. The site of biopsy should be from the clinically most 'severe' areas of involvement, multiple sites for biopsy can be taken in

TABLE 29.4 Clinical Grading, Histopathological Grading and Staging of Oral Leukoplakia has been Described

Clinical Grading of Oral Leukoplakia	Histological Grading of Leukoplakia	Staging of Oral Leukoplakia
Clinical lesion size and number	1. Squamous hyperplasia	Stage I: L1 P0
Lx: Size not specified L1: Single or multiple lesions together <2 cm L2: Single or multiple lesions together 2–4 cm L3: Single or multiple lesions together >4 cm	2. Mild dysplasia—better prognosis	Stage II: L2 P0
Histopathological presence of dysplasia	3. Moderate dysplasia	Stage III: L3 P0 or L1/L2 P1
Px: Epithelial dysplasia not specified P0: No epithelial dysplasia P1: Mild to moderate epithelial dysplasia P2: Severe epithelial dysplasia	4. Severe dysplasia 5. Carcinoma in situ—poor prognosis	Stage IV: L3 P1 or Lx P2

Clinical grading includes histopathological grading.

larger lesions. A definitive diagnosis is made after the clinical and histopathological grading of the lesion. High risk and low risk lesions are staged accordingly for better treatment.

TREATMENT AND PROGNOSIS OF ORAL LEUKOPLAKIA

NONSURGICAL TREATMENT

- Photodynamic therapy
- Chemoprevention.

Photodynamic therapy

Photodynamic therapy is a type of phototherapy used to treat patients with oral leukoplakia in which 5-aminolevulinic acid is used as a photosensitiser. The simultaneous use of light, a photosensitising chemical substance and molecular oxygen will cause cell death. It is used in the treatment of superficial skin or mucosal lesions.

Chemoprevention

1. L-ascorbic acid (vitamin C)
2. α-Tocoferol (vitamin E)
3. Retinoic acid (vitamin A)
4. Vitamin A derivative, isotretinoin, and 13-cis retinoic acid: 28,500 IU per day
5. Beta-carotene 150,000 IU of beta-carotene twice per week for 6 months
6. Isotretinoin alone or in combination with beta-carotene
7. Bleomycin—0.5%/day for 15 days or 1%/day for 14 days.

SURGICAL TREATMENT

1. Scalpel excision/stripping
2. Electrocautery
3. Cryotherapy
4. CO_2 laser therapy.

SCALPEL EXCISION/STRIPPING

The traditional surgical method of excision of oral leukoplakia is by using a blade or electrocautery. After local anaesthetic solution is deposited to attain anaesthesia of the surgical site, the area is outlined with a mucosal marker. This should include a few millimetres of normal tissue for further investigation on field cancerisation. Before incision, a suture can be used to take a bite without affecting the lesion. The borders are incised with a scalpel and the lesion is undermined by blunt dissection to a depth of 2–4 mm. This allows the lesion to be removed as a whole with the borders. The mucosal defect is closed primarily if possible or is closed by a rotational mucosal flap. Larger defects are covered with split thickness skin graft (Fig. 29.4).

Complications

- Persistent bleeding
- Damage to submandibular duct or lingual artery
- Recurrence rate ranging from 20%–35%.

ELECTROCAUTERY (FULGURATION)

Destruction of the affected tissue with electrocautery is another treatment of leukoplakia. This procedure requires general anaesthesia (GA) and is done for a greater number of smaller lesions. Multiple areas of the lesion are subjected to electrocautery and left to heal. The healing process is slow and painful.

CRYOTHERAPY

Cryotherapy is done with a probe that has liquid nitrogen flowing through it. The cryoprobe freezes the mucosa for 1.5–2 min, after pausing for 2 min, further freezing for 1.5–2 min is done. Thicker lesions may require 2 to 3 min of freezing. Though cryotherapy is simple, painless and well tolerated by patients, there is no surgical specimen for histopathological examination. The healing phase is better without infection and pain as the wound is cleaner but the margins are inaccurate and cannot be as controlled as in traditional surgical excision. General anaesthesia is not required and scar formation is minimal. Postoperatively there is marked oedema. Sometimes, there is delayed necrosis, which separates as a slough and it might stimulate epithelial changes. Literature shows 20% recurrence rate, and for the verruciform or granular types, 83% may recur and will require additional removal or destruction.

CO_2 LASER THERAPY

CO_2 lasers can be used either to excise the lesion or destroy the affected tissues. CO_2 laser beam wavelength is about

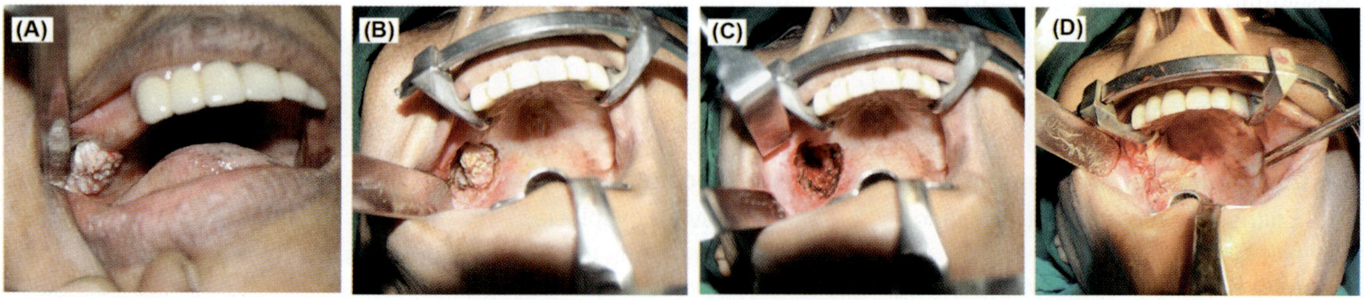

Figure 29.4 **(A)** A verrucous leukoplakic lesion. **(B)** Incision placed with electrocautery forceps. **(C)** The site has been completely cleared with submucosal tissue. **(D)** Buccal advancement flap to close the defect.

10.6 μm. CO_2 lasers are well absorbed by water and hence by soft tissues. It causes vaporisation of the intracellular and extracellular fluid leading to the destruction of cell membrane and depositing a carbonised layer on the tissue surfaces. There are two techniques which can be used to remove oral leukoplakia lesions using CO_2 lasers.

1. ***Excision:*** The laser beam is used to incise around the margins. The lesion can be held with tissue forceps while the laser undermines the leukoplakic lesion.
2. ***Vaporisation:*** Vaporisation can be done by moving the laser beam back and forth across the surface of the lesion. This technique risks leaving small areas of abnormal tissue.

Advantages

- Excellent visibility
- Excellent precision while dissecting through the tissue planes
- Less contraction or scarring
- Patients usually feel less pain.

Disadvantages

- High cost of equipment
- Requires eye protection for both patient and surgeon
- Delayed wound healing
- 20% recurrence rate.

MALIGNANT POTENTIAL OF LEUKOPLAKIA

INCIDENCE OF MALIGNANT TRANSFORMATION OF LEUKOPLAKIA

While most studies predict that 7%–13% of lesions have potential for malignant transformation, some studies show the potential risk to be up to 39.2%. Certain characteristics may predict an increase in the risk of transformation. These features are dependent on clinical appearance, aetiology, duration of existence and site, and have been briefed as follows:

- Longer the duration of existence at the site
- Idiopathic leukoplakia
- Lesion located at sites of higher risk like the floor of mouth, retromolar area and tongue
- Nonhomogenous type of leukoplakia
- Candidal leukoplakia (Fig. 29.3C)
- Speckled leukoplakia (Fig. 29.3D)
- Syphilitic leukoplakia
- Dysplastic leukoplakia.

RISK OF MALIGNANT POTENTIAL BASED ON TYPE OF LEUKOPLAKIC LESION

The phases of leukoplakia have been described based on clinical appearance and type. Phase I may or may not have malignant transformation potential. The other three phases have malignant transformation potential in increasing order.

- **Phase I**—thin homogenous leukoplakia or preleukoplakia
- **Phase II**—fissured, thick and smooth homogenous leukoplakia
- **Phase III**—granular, verrucous candidal homogenous leukoplakia
- **Phase IV**—speckled, candidal nonhomogenous leukoplakia

GUIDELINES FOR FOLLOW-UP AFTER DIAGNOSIS OF LEUKOPLAKIA

Periodic follow-up is mandatory for all leukoplakic lesions with photographs. If any change in the clinical appearance is noted, malignant transformation potential should be considered. These changes include the following:

- Change in colour to red
- Fissuring or ulceration, which fails to heal after removal of the cause like a sharp tooth
- Induration of the area
- Fixation of the lesion to the structures below.

To identify these, the clinician should be well versed in clinical investigation and palpation during follow-up.

CRITERIA FOR COMPLETE EXCISION OF LEUKOPLAKIC LESIONS

- If lesion fails to regress after conservative treatment
- Faster growth of the lesion
- Development on healing/nonhealing ulcers
- Change in colour—erythroplakia/speckled leukoplakia
- Induration of the lesion
- Any kind of dysplasia noted in the histological investigation
- Leukoplakia due to smokeless tobacco
- Risky dysplasia in the histopathological investigation.

ERYTHROPLAKIA

Erythroplakia is a potentially malignant lesion that is rare but more likely to show dysplasia or carcinoma. Literature reveals that every erythroplakia lesions show some degree of epithelial dysplasia; majorly as invasive squamous cell carcinoma, carcinoma in situ or severe epithelial dysplasia, and to a lesser extent as mild-to-moderate dysplasia. Erythroplakia is a riskier lesion compared to leukoplakia (Fig. 29.5).

Erythroplakia WHO definition

'A fiery red patch that cannot be characterised clinically or pathologically as any other definable disease'.

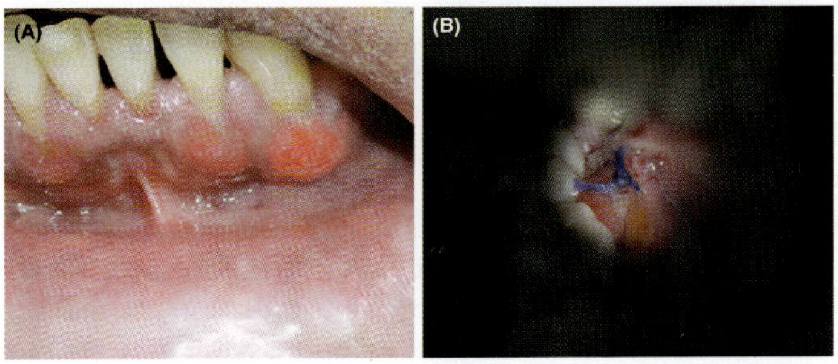

Figure 29.5 (**A**) Erythroplakia lesion on the attached gingiva. (**B**) Erythroplakia on the posterior buccal mucosa.

Aetiology

- Idiopathic
- Alcohol and smoking
- *Candida* infection.

Clinical presentation

- Red, often velvety, nonelevated and well-defined patches
- Most commonly present on floor of mouth, retromolar trigone area, and lateral border of tongue
- Usually asymptomatic
- May be smooth to nodular
- It is clinically similar to candidiasis, tuberculosis, histoplasmosis and nonspecific conditions such as denture irritation.

Clinical types

1. Homogenous form of erythroplakia, which appears as a red, velvety lesion with straight or scalloped well-defined margins. It usually involves an extensive area, which is commonly found on the buccal mucosa, sometimes on the soft palate, and more rarely on the tongue and floor of the mouth
2. Speckled leukoplakia/erythroplakia are soft, red lesions that are slightly elevated with an irregular border and a nodular surface speckled with tiny white plaques
3. Smooth erythroplakia–soft and velvety, may feel pebbled
4. Erythroleukoplakia–mostly seen on tongue or floor of mouth.

Diagnosis

- Clinical appearance helps in diagnosis
- 1% Toluidine blue staining test (Fig. 29.2)
- History of tobacco/alcohol use
- Histopathological investigation with a biopsy is mandatory for diagnosis and treatment planning.

Differential diagnosis

- Erythematous (atrophic) candidiasis
- Kaposi's sarcoma
- Ecchymosis
- Contact stomatitis
- Vascular malformation
- Squamous cell carcinoma
- Geographic tongue/erythema migrans.

Treatment

Step 1: Removal of the cause.

Step 2: Incisional biopsy for final diagnosis as the treatment is similar to invasive carcinoma or carcinoma in situ with planned complete surgical excision, radiation and cauterisation of the lesion. Surgical stripping is not indicated for these lesions.

Step 3: Clinical follow-up is mandatory at 3 months, 6 months and every year.

CARCINOMA IN SITU

It is also called intraepithelial carcinoma (Ca in situ). It occurs less commonly on the mucous membrane of the oral cavity. Severe dysplasia can be classified as Ca in situ, but the dysplastic epithelial cells do not invade into the connective tissue. Histologically, all features of dysplasia are present but there is no break in the epithelium. It has combined features of leukoplakia and erythroplakia, and clinically appears as a white plaque or ulcer and reddened areas with well-defined borders. The absence of induration is the key point in differentiating carcinoma in situ from invasive carcinoma. Common sites of carcinoma in situ are the floor of the mouth, tongue and lips. Many studies show the presence of multiple sites of carcinoma in situ in asymptomatic oral SCCs and in erythroplakia lesions.

Treatment

Wide local excision is the treatment of choice for lesions of oral carcinoma in situ.

ORAL SUBMUCOUS FIBROSIS

INTRODUCTION

Oral submucous fibrosis (OSMF) is a potentially malignant disorder that was 1st described by Joshi and Schwatz among East Indian women. OSMF is a chronic insidious disease affecting all parts of the mucosa of the oral cavity and oropharynx (Fig. 29.6).

DEFINITION (J.J. PINDBORG AND SIRSAT, 1966)

'It is a chronic insidious disease affecting any part of the oral cavity and sometimes the pharynx, occasionally preceded by or associated with vesicle formation. It is always associated with juxta-epithelial inflammatory reaction followed by fibro-elastic changes of the lamina propria with epithelial atrophy leading to stiffness of the oral mucosa, causing trismus and inability to eat'.

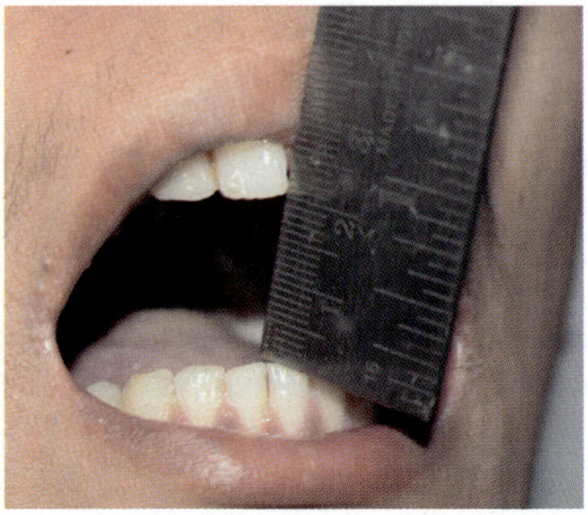

Figure 29.6 Oral submucous fibrosis with limited mouth opening.

EPIDEMIOLOGY

OSMF is an oral fibrotic disorder causing a decrease in the functioning of the oral cavity, commonly seen in India. Sporadic cases are seen in Malaysia, Nepal, Thailand, and South Vietnam. Incidence of OSMF in India is 0.2%–0.5% of the population.

AETIOLOGY

1. Chronic irritation—chillies, lime, areca nut, tobacco
   a. The continuous action of mild irritants like capsaicin found in chillies, *Capsicum annuum* and *Capsicum frutescens*
   b. Arecoline and arecaidine found in areca nut—fibroblast proliferation—stimulate collagen synthesis tannin, catechin—makes collagen fibrils resistant to collagenase
2. Defective iron metabolism
3. Bacterial infections
4. Collagen disorders
5. Immunological disorders
6. Genetic disorders.

CLINICAL FEATURES AND STAGING

Prodromal symptoms

- Burning sensation of oral mucosa when consuming spicy food
- Appearance of blisters especially in the palate
- Ulcerations
- Recurrent generalised inflammation of the oral mucosa
- Excessive salivation
- Defective gustatory sensation
- Dryness of the mouth
- Appearance of small vesicles in the cheek and palate
- Focal vascular dilatations manifest clinically as petechiae
- Trismus
- Palpable bands.

Sites involved

Buccal mucosa: The fibrous bands in the buccal mucosa run in a vertical direction, sometimes so marked that the cheeks are almost immovable.

Faucial pillars, uvula, hard palate and soft palate: The fibrous bands in the soft palate radiate from the pterygomandibular raphae and the faucial pillars bilaterally. It has a scar-like appearance on clinical inspection. The uvula has a hockey stick appearance or a bud-shaped appearance, as it shrinks and appears like a small fibrous bud. The bilateral faucial pillars become thick, short and extremely hard with the tonsils placed in between them.

Lips: Circular bands can be felt around the entire upper and lower lip mucosa.

Tongue: The tongue becomes pale and bald.

Clinical classification (Table 29.5)

Staging of functional mouth opening (refer Chapter 3—Fig. 3.3)

M1: Interincisal mouth opening more than 35 mm.
M2: Interincisal mouth opening between 25 and 35 mm.
M3: Interincisal mouth opening between 15 and 25 mm.
M4: Interincisal mouth opening less than 15 mm.

Pindborg's clinical staging of OSMF (Table 29.6)

Stage I: Stage of stomatitis and vesiculation.
Stage II: Stage of fibrosis.
Stage III: Stage of sequelae and complication.

Histopathological features

- Atrophic oral epithelium
- Loss of rete pegs
- Epithelial atypia may be observed
- Hyalinisation of collagen bundles.

MANAGEMENT OF ORAL SUBMUCOUS FIBROSIS

The treatment modalities available for OSMF are conservative treatment, medical treatment, and surgical treatment. The patient is usually subjected to a combined therapy protocol as described in Table 29.7.

FIBROTOMY

Simple excision of the fibrous bands with a scalpel, laser or electrocautery was done in the past. However, fibrotomy or excision of the fibrous bands without proper reconstruction can result in contracture of the tissue, which may worsen the condition by decreasing the mouth opening.

BILATERAL NASOLABIAL FLAP

In a nasolabial flap, the donor site is in close proximity to the defect. The procedure is performed under general anaesthesia with nasal intubation. The incisions on the affected buccal mucosa can be made with a scalpel or an electrosurgical knife at the level of the occlusal plane away from the Stensen's duct. The incision should extend to the pterygomandibular raphae, faucial pillars and anteriorly till the fibrotic bands are present, restricting mouth opening. This may extend up to the corner of the mouth in advanced stages. This incision frees and allows manipulation to allow mouth opening of at least 35 mm. A wide spindle-shaped flap is raised superior to the nasolabial fold, pedicled to the facial artery. The length of the flap is 5 cm and the width is measured based on the lesion intraorally. The incision is made on the medial margin of the nasolabial fold (Fig. 29.7). The flap is raised in a subcutaneous fat plane preserving the pedicle. The flap is rotated at 90 degrees and tunnelled intraorally with the pedicle. The skin flap is placed over the raw excised area of the buccal mucosa where fibrotomy was done. Suturing the margins of the mucosa to the skin flap closes the defect in the mucosa and the donor site is closed in layers. Nasolabial region has an excellent dual blood supply, which assures successful uptake of the flap. The mouth opening has minimal relapse. This flap has less chances of partial or complete flap failure. Bilateral inferiorly based nasolabial flaps can be used for the treatment of advanced OSMF.

TABLE 29.5 Clinical Gradings Based on Clinical Features and the Subsequent Treatment Modalities

Grade	Clinical Features	Treatment Modalities
I	• Stomatitis • Burning sensation in the buccal mucosa • No detection of fibres	• Antioxidants and multivitamins • Iron supplements • Lycopene
II	• Stomatitis • Burning sensation • Fibrous bands • Fibrosis of soft palate • Mouth opening reduces to 26–35 mm	• Antioxidants and multivitamins • Iron supplements • Lycopene • Inj. Dexamethasone
III	• Symptoms of Grade II OSMF • Blanched mucosa • Fibrosis of tongue starts in this stage • Mouth opening reduces to 6–25 mm	• Antioxidants and multivitamins • Iron supplements • Lycopene • Inj. Dexamethasone • Inj. Placentrix • Inj. Hyaluronidase
IV	• Symptoms of Grade III OSMF • Fibrosis of lips • Mouth opening less than 5 mm	• Antioxidants and multivitamins • Iron supplements • Lycopene • Inj. Dexamethasone • Inj. Placentrix • Inj. Hyaluronidase • Surgery • Lasers
V	• Symptoms of Grade IV • Histopathological carcinomatous changes	Surgical excision, radical neck dissection, etc., depending on the tumour, nodes and metastases (TNM) staging and reconstruction

TABLE 29.6 Pindborg's Clinical Staging of OSMF

Stage I	Stage of stomatitis and vesiculation	Includes erythmatous mucosa, vesicles, mucosal ulcers, melanotic mucosal pigmentation
Stage II	Stage of fibrosis	There is inability to open mouth completely and stiffness in mastication. As disease advances, there is difficulty in blowing out cheek and protruding tongue. Sometimes pain in ear and speech is affected. On examination, there is an increasing amount of fibrosis in the submucosa. This causes blanching of mucosa. Lips and cheeks become stiff and lose their normal resistance. Shortening and disappearance of uvula in advanced cases. Mucosa of floor of mouth shows blanching and stiffness
Stage III	Stage of sequelae and complication	Patient presents with all the complaints as in stage II. Also there may be evidence of leukoplakia. Changes in mucosa are whitish or brownish black. Pindborg et al. (1967) found that OSMF was found in 40% cases of oral cancer than in general population (1.2%)

TONGUE FLAP

An anteriorly based tongue flap can be designed on the dorsal surface of the tongue or on the lateral border, dimensions approximately 4×1.5 cm in size. The flap is dissected with the lingual artery pedicle and sutured to the created cheek defect after sectioning of fibrous bands. After 21 days, the flap is sectioned from the pedicle and donor site is sutured, once the graft has been vascularly taken up in the recipient site. The disadvantages of tongue flaps are that they are bulky when used bilaterally. This can cause disarticulation of the flaps, dysphagia, and increased chances of aspiration, which can be life threatening. In addition, the tongue itself is involved in all cases of advanced OSMF after grade III involvement, compromising the vascular supply.

TABLE 29.7 Treatment Modalities Including Conservative, Medical and Surgical Management of OSMF

Conservative treatment	Restriction of habits/behavioural therapy: • The consumption of pan, betel nut, chillies, spices, pan masala and gutka with or without tobacco should be restricted • Affected patients should be counselled about the disease and malignant potential of OSMF • Removal of all irritants Nutritional or supportive therapy: • Vitamin A, B, C, D and E • Fe, Cu, Ca, Zn, Mg, Se Oral physiotherapy Microwave diathermy		
Medical treatment	Steroids Collagenase Hyaluronidase Placental extracts Chymotrypsin INF—gamma—intralesional inj. (0.01–10 μ/mL) Pentoxifylline therapy—400 mg three times a day (TDS) for 7 months Turmeric	• Intralesional injections of hyaluronidase • Hydrocortisone • Placentrix 2 ml solution intralesional injection every 3 days.	Systemic administration of immunomodulators • Levamisole 150 mg for 3 weeks • Dapsone 75 mg O.D. for 90 days
		• Topical application • 4% Acetic acid TDS • 5-Fluorouracil	Antioxidants and multivitamins Lycopene 8 mg BD Iron supplements
Surgical management	Nasolabial flap Buccal fat graft Lingual pedicle flap ErCr: YSGG lasers	Fibrotomy (scalpel, electrocautery, laser) Coronoidectomy and temporalis myotomy Extraction of 3rd molars Reconstruction: • Bilateral nasolabial flaps • Pedicled tongue flaps • Buccal fat pad • Split thickness skin grafting • Collagen membrane • Temporalis fascia • Tongue flap • Palatal flap • Free flap (radial forearm)	
Combined therapy	A combination of steroids and topical hyaluronidase is 1st given Nutritional and iron supplements with intralesional injection of: • Hyaluronidase • Dexamethasone • Topical triamcinolone acetonide 0.1% Bilateral nasolabial flap technique can be performed for buccal vertical bands causing reduced mouth opening		

BUCCAL FAT PAD GRAFT (BFPG)

The BFPG is a flexible and lobulated mass which can be easily mobilised. Many studies conclude that BFPG gives best results for early stages of OSMF. It may be used to cover the defects after excision of the fibrous bands. Harvesting of buccal pad fat (BPF) is easy, but the anterior reach of the flap is often inadequate and cannot be used for larger defects as in advanced OSMF.

The procedure is performed under general anaesthesia (GA) with nasal intubation. The incisions on the affected buccal mucosa can be made with a scalpel or an electrosurgical knife at the level of the occlusal plane away from the Stenson's duct. The incision should extend to the pterygomandibular raphae, faucial pillars and anteriorly till the fibrotic bands are present, restricting mouth opening. This may extend up to the corner of the mouth in advanced stages. This incision frees and allows manipulation to allow mouth opening of at least 35 mm. Coronoidectomy is done if the temporalis muscle is also affected as this can allow for more manipulation and better mouth opening (refer Chapter 25, Fig. 25.12).

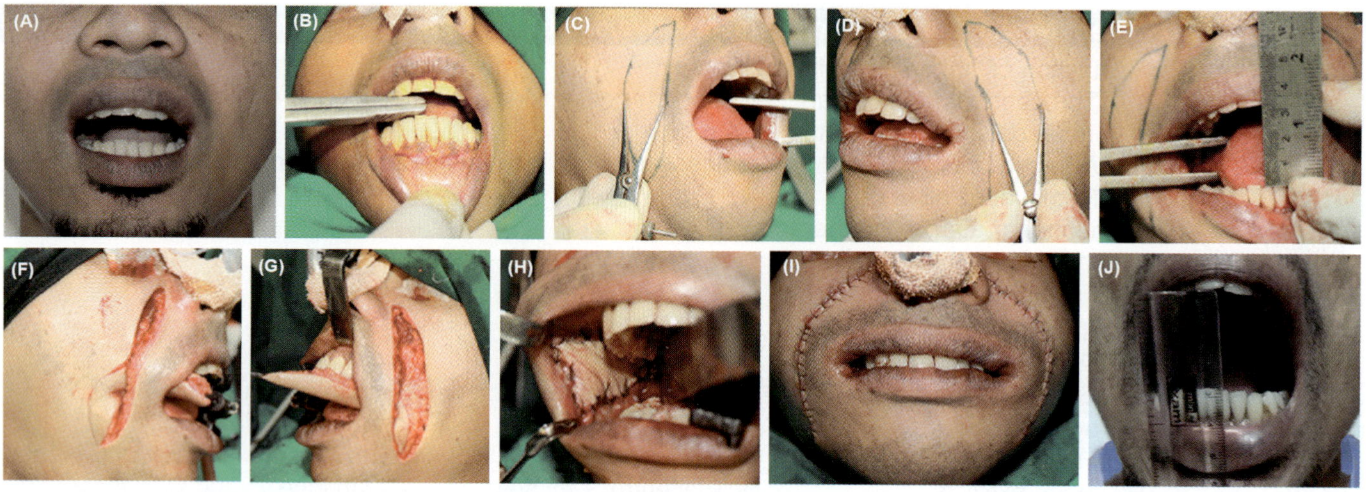

Figure 29.7 **(A)** Preoperative mouth opening. **(B)** Intraoperative mouth opening before surgery. **(C and D)** Marking of bilateral nasolabial flap. **(E)** Increase in mouth opening after lease of fibrotic bands. **(F and G)** Nasolabial flap transfer bilaterally. **(H)** Intra-oral suturing of flap. **(I)** Primary closure. **(J)** Postoperative increase in significant mouth opening.

The buccal fat pad is approached through the posterior-superior margin of the created buccal incision. Blunt dissection with an index finger is done. The fat pad is teased out gently until a sufficient amount is obtained to cover the defect without tension. It is then secured in place with a horizontal mattress suture.

SPLIT THICKNESS SKIN GRAFT

Split thickness graft—0.014 to 0.018-inch thick can be harvested from the lateral aspect of the thigh, using a dermatome or a skin knife (refer Chapter 34, Fig. 34.14). The donor site is covered with antibiotic-impregnated gauze and pressure dressing. Puncture holes are created on the harvested graft and sutured to the mucosal margins using vicryl sutures. A quilt suturing is done to minimise dead space. A mucosal graft is the best treatment for OSMF, but is usually unavailable in oral mucosa affected by advanced OSMF. Split-skin grafting has a high failure rate as the fibrotic areas have less vascular supply.

ORAL LICHEN PLANUS

Oral lichen planus (OLP) is an immune-mediated chronic disorder that can affect the oral mucosa. The most common aetiology is T cell-mediated disease targeting the basal keratinocytes. Other causes are lichenoid changes associated with galvanism, graft versus host disease (GvHD), certain drugs, contact allergens and idiopathic causes. Up to 3% to 4% of the Indian population presents with OLP. Clinical variants are the reticular type which is the most common oral form, the erosive type which is the most painful, the atrophic type, the papular or plaque type and the bullous type (Fig. 29.8). Clinically, it appears bilaterally and is often symmetric in distribution. The lesion most frequently appears on the buccal mucosa, followed by the tongue, the gingiva and the lips.

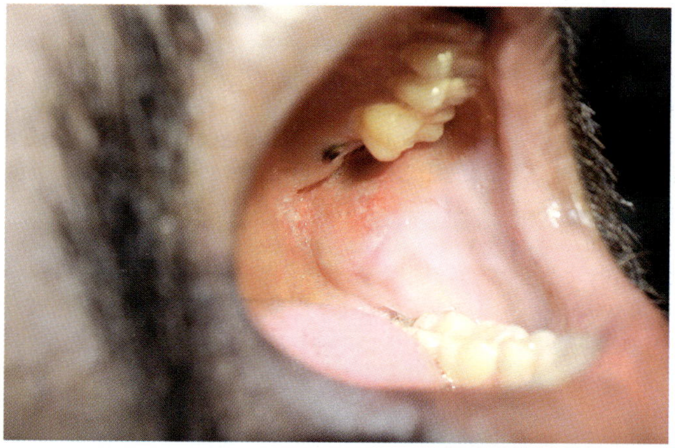

Figure 29.8 Oral lichen planus. A network of connecting and overlapping thin white lines can be observed.

Diagnosis

- Examination of oral mucosa, skin
- H/o galvanism
- Graft-versus-host disease (GvHD)
- Biopsy—confirmatory
- Direct immunofluorescence—presence of fibrinogen and cytoid bodies at interface.

Management of oral lichen planus

For mild to moderate OLP lesions, topical corticosteroids are the line of treatment. Intralesional triamcinolone can also be

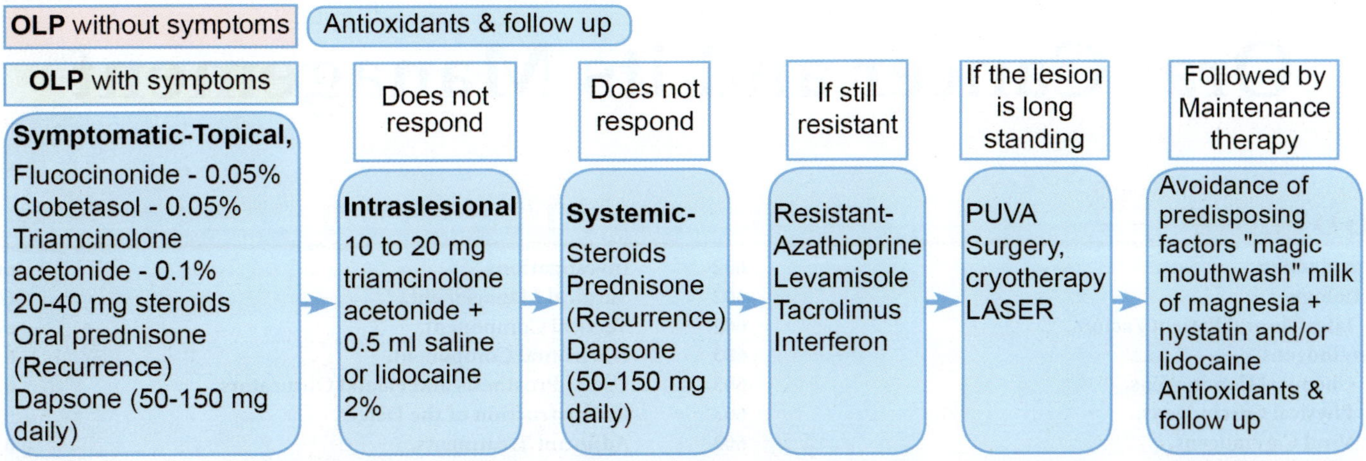

Flowchart 29.3 Medical, surgical and maintenance therapy for oral lichen planus. The treatment is given from conservative to aggressive approach. Aggressive approach is given for lesions that fail to respond or are resistant (erosive or atrophic types of OLP).

injected into the lesion. For severe OLP lesions, systemic immunosuppression with prednisone and topical tacrolimus ointment is given. Complete management of OLP is illustrated in Flowchart 29.3. Malignant transformation can be seen in the erosive and atrophic forms of OLP, for which the treatment plan changes completely. Erosive and atrophic forms need to be surgically excised and field cancerisation should be considered before excision. Surgical management of the lesion is dependent on the size of the lesion and the degree of dysplasia. For small lesions without any dysplasia clinically or histologically, a simple excision and closure is done with scalpel or with laser. For larger lesions with dysplasia, wide local excision with proper follow-up and maintenance therapy is performed (Flowchart 29.3).

ACTINIC (SOLAR) KERATOSIS, ELASTOSIS AND CHEILITIS

Actinic keratosis is a potentially malignant disorder. It is associated with long-term exposure to radiation. The lesions are found on the vermilion border of the lips on the face. Clinical features are crusted, keratotic lesions on the vermilion border of the lip. If the labial mucosa has been exposed, a white area of atrophic epithelium with underlying scarring of the lamina propria referred to as elastosis is seen. When this atrophic tissue ulcerates, it is called *actinic cheilitis*. Treatment with 5-flurouracil is found to be effective, but if dysplastic changes in the epithelium still remain, then surgical removal is performed.

Chapter 30

Oral Cancer and its Management

OUTLINE

INTRODUCTION

A tumour growth is an abnormal mass of tissue, the expansion of that exceeds normal tissue and is uncoordinated with normal tissue. This growth persists in the same excessive manner even after the stimuli that induced the change has been removed. Tumours of the head and neck comprise an important group of neoplasia, the incidence of which is increasing in many parts of the world. More than 95% of the carcinomas of the oral cavity are of squamous cell type in nature. Since the oral cavity is more accessible to complete examination, ***early detection*** of precancerous and cancerous lesions is possible.

Tumour progression in epithelium has been classified as normal, hyperplastic (nondysplastic), dysplastic, carcinoma in situ and invasive carcinoma. The majority of the alterations of premalignant lesions and malignant neoplasms are not readily recognisable during clinical or histopathological examination.

AETIOLOGY

The major aetiology of cancer can be classified as chemical carcinogens, physical carcinogens and viral carcinogens. Tobacco and alcohol are the two most important known risk factors for the development of oral cancer. The higher incidence of carcinoma of the head-neck in relation to other malignancies in India may be due to use of tobacco in various forms, consumption of alcohol, low socioeconomic status associated with poor hygiene, poor diet and viral infectious agents. Dietary factors, immune deficient conditions and human papilloma virus (HPV)-16/18 are well-known cofactors in oral squamous cell carcinoma (OSCC).

LIFESTYLE AND PATIENT FACTORS

DIET

Fruits and vegetables (high in vitamins A and C) are described as protective in oral neoplasia, whereas meat and red chili are thought to be risk factors.

FAMILY HISTORY OF HEAD AND NECK SQUAMOUS CELL CARCINOMA

The ability to repair DNA damaged by tobacco carcinogens, such as benzo[a]pyrene diol epoxide is defective in some patients with head and neck cancer. These patients show an increased susceptibility to chromosome damage by mutagens.

IMMUNE DEFICIENCY

Human immunodeficiency virus (HIV)-infected individuals, due to a compromise in immunity, may be predisposed to cancer. The most common oral malignancy in HIV-infected patients is Kaposi's sarcoma and the human herpes virus type 8 (HHV-8) has been implicated as the aetiological agent. Lymphoma, mostly non-Hodgkin B cell lymphoma in HIV-infected individuals or other immunosuppressed states, is commonly associated with Epstein–Barr virus (EBV) and may occur in the head and neck region. Squamous cell carcinoma of the lip is more common in transplant recipients receiving immunosuppressive therapy, but HIV infection does not predispose to intraoral squamous cell carcinoma.

CARCINOGENS

There are various carcinogens for cancer. The carcinogens in oral cancer can be classified as follows:

CHEMICAL CARCINOGENS

TOBACCO AND ALCOHOL

Chewing of tobacco with betel quid, smoking and heavy alcohol consumption are the main risk factors.

BETEL QUID AND ARECA NUT

Betel quid chewing produces reactive oxygen species (ROS), which are detrimental to oral mucosa and can be directly involved in tumour initiation process by inducing mutation or by making the mucosa susceptible to betel quid ingredients and environmental toxicants.

ALCOHOL

Alcohol may act as a solvent and enhance the penetration of carcinogens into target tissues. Acetaldehyde, which is an alcohol metabolite, has been identified recently as a tumour promoter.

PHYSICAL CARCINOGENS

CHRONIC TRAUMA

Sunlight

Broad spectrum UV radiation is a known carcinogen.

VIRAL CARCINOGENS

Most common viral carcinogens are DNA viruses:

- Human papilloma virus (HPV) (cervical cancer)
- Hepatitis B (liver cancer)
- Epstein-Barr virus (EBV) (a type of lymphoma).

HPV has been found to be associated with several types of cancers, most commonly of cervical, vulvar, vaginal, penile, anal and head & neck cancers.

HPV-16/18 has been detected in condylomas, squamous cell papilloma and malignant oral lesions.

HUMAN PAPILLOMA VIRUS IN ORAL CANCER

The association of HPV with oral cavity and oropharyngeal cancer was 1st reported by Loning et al., and de Villiers et al., in 1985 (Flowchart 30.1) HPV types detected were classified into:

1. Nononcogenic (low-risk, such as HPV6, 11, 26)
2. Oncogenic (high-risk, such as HPV16, 18, 31).

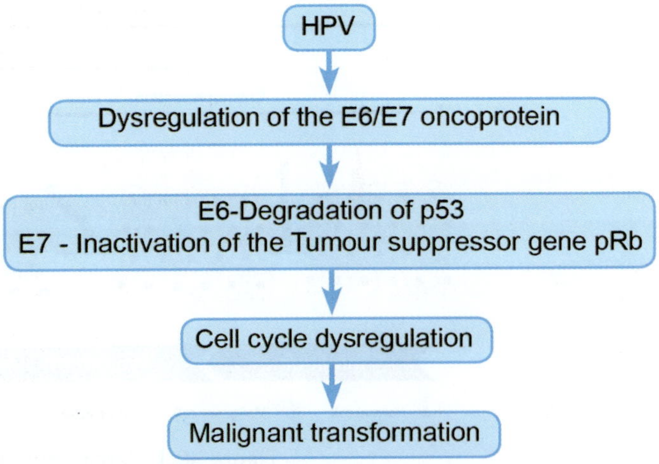

Flowchart 30.1 p53, pRb–tumour suppressor gene.

CARCINOGENESIS

INITIATION

The beginning of mutation of the gene that controls the cell proliferation is called initiation. This occurs after at least one round of mutation has occurred. Initiation is an irreversible process (Fig. 30.1).

PROMOTION

Proliferation of the mutated cells without change in DNA mitogenicity is called promotion. Promotion is reversible. It causes both normal and mutated cells to proliferate. The promoters cause promotion, these promoters are ROS, metals, phorbol esters, tissue plasminogen activator (TPA), dioxin, oxidised fats and endocrine disruptors like estradiol and diethylstilbestrol (Fig. 30.1).

PROGRESSION

Progression causes the dysplastic cells to metastasise. This occurs when there is chromosomal instability, presence of inflammatory immune cells at the tumour site, secretion of angiogenesis factors, proteases and presence of progressor agents like inflammation, asbestos, benzene, peroxides, oxidative stress and inflammation (Fig. 30.1).

CONCEPT OF FIELD CANCERISATION

Field cancerisation is also termed field change, field change cancerisation, field carcinogenesis, cancer field effect or premalignant field defect. **Field cancerisation** is a biological process in which carcinogenic changes affect vast areas of cells on a tissue surface or inside an organ (Fig. 30.2A). The

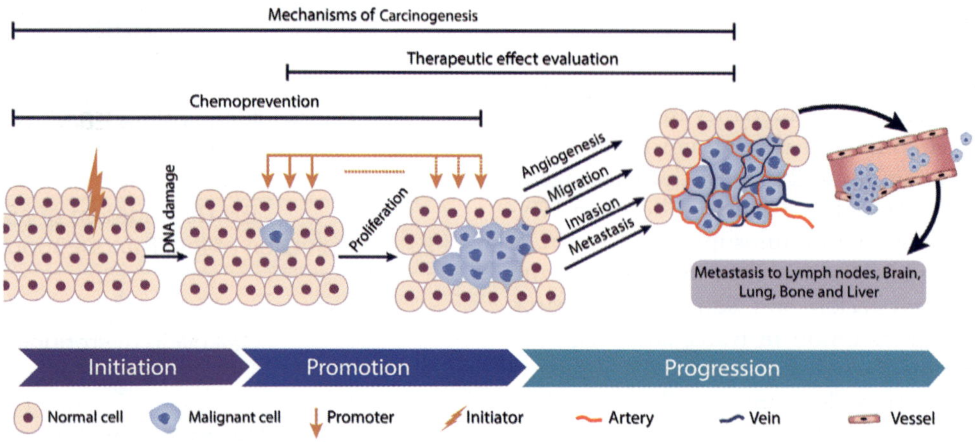

Figure 30.1 Carcinogenesis process has been illustrated.

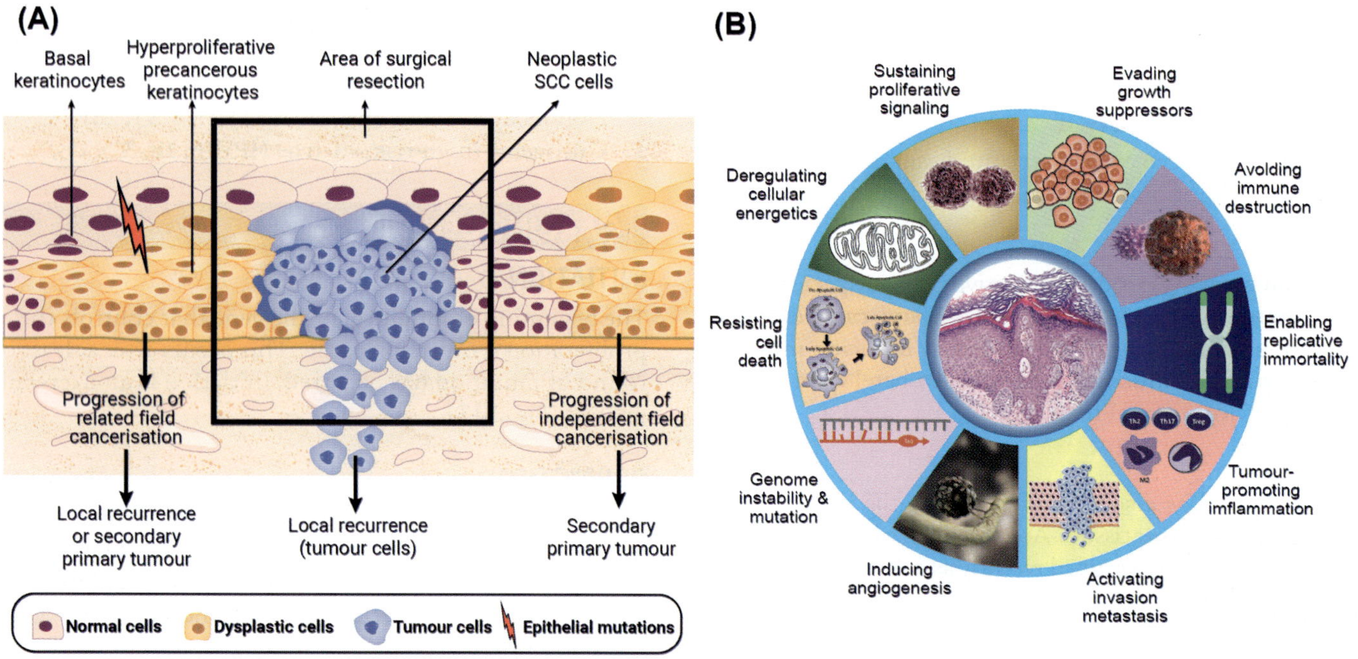

Figure 30.2 (**A**) Field cancerisation. (**B**) Hallmarks of oral cancer.

normal tissues surrounding the cancerous cells have changes or atypia; this is called the field of cells that have the capacity to form mutant clones (TP53). This can cause a subsequent tumour growth if left without treatment. This is important in oral squamous cell cancers. Fields greater than 7 cm have been detected in the mucosa of the head and neck. Patients with field cancerisation will require more aggressive treatment approach. The phenomenon of field cancerisation explains the following:

1. A multifocal precancerous lesion or area in the oral cavity transitioning into a malignant lesion
2. Abnormal tissues surrounding the tumour
3. Oral cancer often consists of multiple independent lesions that may coalesce
4. Persistence of abnormal tissue even after surgery may explain secondary primary tumour and recurrences.

HALLMARKS OF CANCER

The hallmarks of cancer comprise of 10 biological capabilities acquired by a normal cell mutating into a cancer cell (Fig. 30.2B). The hallmarks constitute of the following:

1. Sustaining proliferative signalling
2. Evading growth suppressors
3. Avoiding immune destruction
4. Resisting cell death
5. Enabling replicative immortality
6. Inducing angiogenesis
7. Tumour promoting inflammation
8. Genome instability
9. Activating invasion
10. Invasion and metastasis.

Recognition of the cellular hallmarks of cancer will help in the treatment of the disease. These cellular changes represent the the transition from a precancerous lesion and condition to carcinoma. These cellular hallmarks also play an important role in field cancerisation.

SPREAD OF ORAL CANCER FROM ORAL CAVITY

1. Local infiltration:
   Spreads in centrifugal manner in soft tissue, but altered when bone is encountered
2. Various modes of spread in bone:
   - Via periosteal or subperiosteal layer, particularly on lingual alveolar aspect of mandible
   - Through periodontal membrane when teeth are present
   - Diffuse spread within marrow cavity
3. Perineural spread: Perineural spread, especially along inferior alveolar nerve, most often proximally in direction of pterygoid fossa and skull base and then towards trigeminal ganglion
4. Lymphatic spread: OSCC, unlike other types of cancers, has a characteristic cervical lymph node metastasises through the draining lymphatics in the early stages
5. Haematological spread: Metastasis through blood vessels occurs rarely in oral cancers, during early stages and visceral spread occurs in later stages of the disease.

STAGING AND GRADING OF ORAL CANCER

Oral cancer has been conventionally graded and staged according to the Tumour-Node-Metastasis (TNM) classification by American Joint Committee on Carcinoma (AJCC) for ease of communication and prognosis prediction (Tables 30.1 and 30.2).

TABLE 30.1 TNM Classification by AJCC

T—Primary Tumour	
TX	Primary tumour cannot be assessed
T0	No evidence of primary tumour
Tis	Carcinoma in situ
T1	Tumour 2 cm or less in greatest dimension
T2	Tumour more than 2 cm but not more than 4 cm in greatest dimension
T3	Tumour more than 4 cm in greatest dimension
T4a (lip)	Invasion of tumour through cortical bone, inferior alveolar nerve, floor of mouth or skin of chin or nose
T4a (oral cavity)	Invasion of tumour through cortical bone, into deep/extrinsic muscle of tongue (genioglossus, hyoglossus, palatoglossus and styloglossus), maxillary sinus or facial skin
T4b (lip and oral cavity)	Tumour invades masticator space, pterygoid plates or skull base, or encases internal carotid artery
N—Regional Lymph Nodes	
NX	Regional lymph nodes cannot be assessed
N0	No regional lymph node metastasis
N1	Metastasis in a single ipsilateral lymph node of greatest dimension not exceeding 3 cm
N2a	Metastasis in a single ipsilateral lymph node of greatest dimension between 3 and 6 cm
N2b	Metastasis in multiple ipsilateral lymph nodes of greatest dimension not exceeding 6 cm
N2c	Metastasis in bilateral or contralateral lymph nodes, not more than 6 cm in greatest dimension
N3	Metastasis in a lymph node more than 6 cm in greatest dimension
M—Distant Metastasis	
MX	Distant metastasis cannot be assessed
M0	No distant metastasis
M1	Distant metastasis

TYPES OF CANCER IN THE HEAD AND NECK

HISTOLOGICAL TYPES OF MALIGNANT CANCERS OF HEAD AND NECK

1. Epithelial tissue:
   a. Squamous cell carcinoma
   b. Basal cell carcinoma (Table 30.3)
   c. Verrucous carcinoma
2. Bone:
   a. Osteosarcoma (Table 30.4)
   b. Ewing's sarcoma
3. Salivary gland tumour:
   a. Adenocarcinoma
4. Plasma cells of blood:
   a. Multiple myeloma.

SITE BASED MALIGNANT CANCERS IN THE HEAD AND NECK

1. Carcinoma of the oral cavity—subsites:
   a. Lip mucosa
   b. Buccal mucosa
   c. Upper or lower alveolar ridge
   d. Retromolar trigone
   e. Floor of mouth
   f. Hard palate
   g. Anterior two-thirds of the tongue

TABLE 30.2 TNM Staging and Illustration of Staging

Stage	Tumour	Node	Metastasis
Stage I	Tis, T1	N0	M0
Stage II	T2	N0	M0
Stage III	T3	N0	M0
	T1	N1	M0
	T2	N1	M0
	T3	N1	M0
Stage IVa	T4a	N0	M0
	T4a	N1	M0
	T1	N2	M0
	T2	N2	M0
	T3	N2	M0
	T4a	N2	M0
Stage IVb	T4b	Any N	M0
	Any T	N3	M0
Stage IVc	Any T	Any N	M1

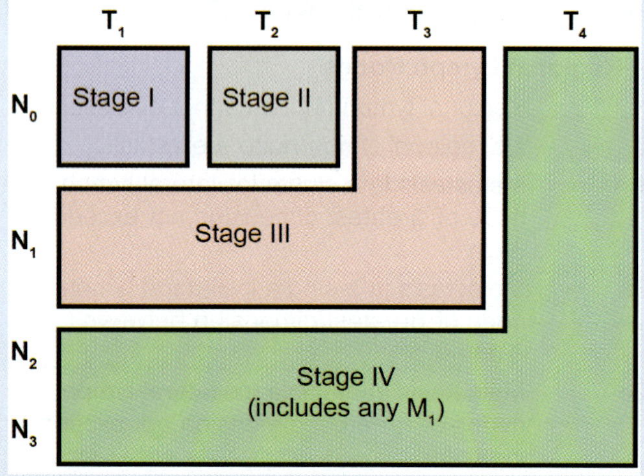

2. Cervical lymph node metastasis
3. Salivary glands
4. Nasal cavity and paranasal sinuses:
   a. Maxillary sinus
   b. Nasal cavity and ethmoid sinus
5. Larynx:
   a. Supraglottis
   b. Glottis
   c. Subglottis
6. Pharynx:
   a. Nasopharynx
   b. Oropharynx
   c. Hypopharynx
7. Thyroid gland
8. Nonmelanoma skin cancer
9. Melanoma of skin.

CARCINOMA OF THE NASAL CAVITY, MAXILLARY SINUS AND OTHER PARANASAL SINUSES

Malignancies of the nasal cavity and paranasal sinuses are relatively less in occurrence. These malignancies are predominantly of epithelial origin (SCC). More common are carcinomas of the maxillary sinus than the other regions. The other malignant carcinomas that can occur in this area are adenocarcinoma, adenoid cystic carcinoma, mucoepidermoid carcinoma and melanoma. The carcinoma of maxillary sinus may extend into the nasal cavity and sinus in the later part of the disease. Exposure to wood dust and chemicals for leather manufacturing are risk factors for maxillary adenocarcinoma.

SITE AND ROUTE OF SPREAD

- Most commonly:
  a. Maxillary antrum
  b. Lateral wall of nasal cavity
  c. Septum
  d. Ethmoidal air cells

TABLE 30.3 Clinical and Histopathological Features of Basal Cell and Verrucous Carcinoma

Basal Cell Carcinoma	
Basal cell carcinoma (BCC) is a slow-growing tumour, which infiltrates locally; pattern of spread lateral rather than deep. It does not metastasise. Treatment is dependent on the size and depth of the lesion (Fig. 30.3A & B). Rotational flaps are planned based on the post-resection defect. Refer Chapter 33 for other flaps.	
Clinical Features	**Histopathological Features**
• Common in the older age group. • Rolled out edges. • Early stage - a nodule with a pearly appearance. • In larger lesions, presence of telangiectatic vessels - diagnostic feature.	• Clumps of cells lying in a connective tissue stroma. • In infiltrative BCC, the presence of morphemic and sclerosing patterns.

TABLE 30.3 Clinical and Histopathological Features of Basal Cell and Verrucous Carcinoma—cont'd

Verrucous Carcinoma or Ackerman's Tumour	
Characterised by an extension of lesion into underlying connective tissue, deep to adjacent normal epithelium. It has more favourable prognosis.	
Clinical Features	**Histopathological Features**
• Low-grade variant • Found in elderly (>60 years) who chew tobacco or consume snuff • Predilection for buccal mucosa • Characterised by their whitish, warty, bulky, cauliflower-like growth with a broad base • Pebbly lesion with multiple small protuberances, piled up folds and cleft-like spaces between them.	• Thickened epithelium, prominent surface keratin, down growth of club-shaped fingers of hyperplastic epithelium that push rather than infiltrate deeply towards an intact basement membrane • Prominent inflammatory reaction in the underlying connective tissue.

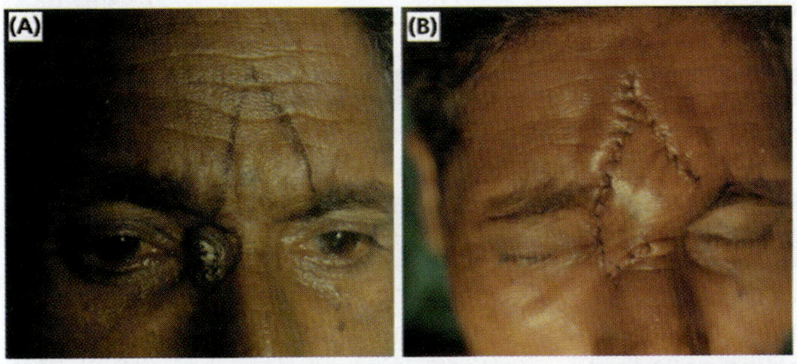

Figure 30.3 (A) Basal cell carcinoma of the medial canthus. Limberg's rotational flap planned. (B) Postoperative photograph.

- Maxillary sinus carcinoma route of spread to other sites can be understood by drawing a line from the medial canthus to the angle of mandible. Area above this line is called superstructure and below is called infrastructure
- Tumour of superstructure can spread to base of skull:
  a. Through posterior wall of antrum:
     - To pterygomaxillary space
     - To infratemporal fossa
     - Middle cranial fossa
  b. Through roof of antrum to orbit
  c. Through ethmoid sinus to anterior cranial fossa

TABLE 30.4 Clinical, Radiographic, Histopathological Features, Treatment & Prognosis of Osteosarcoma, Ewing's Sarcoma & Multiple Myeloma

Osteosarcoma			
Osteosarcoma is commonly understood as malignancy of the bone. It is common in the long bones and is an aggressive type of malignant neoplasm. The mesenchymal cells like the osteoblasts under mutation produce osteoid or immature bone. It is the primary neoplasm originating within bone. About 6%–8% accounts for jaw osteosarcomas.			
Clinical Features	**Radiographic Features**	**Histopathological Features**	**Treatment and Prognosis**
• Common in the 3rd and 4th decades of life. • Can occur in maxilla and mandible. • More frequent in the posterior body of mandible. • Swelling and pain are the most common symptoms. • Metastasis to lungs develops early. • Osteosarcoma of the jaws is rapidly invasive.	• Varying sclerosis from dense to a mixed, somewhat radiolucent lesion to complete radiolucency of the anatomical site. • The classic 'sunburst' or 'sunray' appearance caused by osteophytic bone production.	• Osteoid formation by malignant mesenchymal cells. The tumour cells may vary from relatively uniform round or spindle-shaped cells to highly pleomorphic cells with bizarre nuclear and cytoplasmic shapes.	• Early radical excision is the 1st requirement. This may be combined with pre- or postoperative radiotherapy and adjuvant chemotherapy. Recurrence of tumour in excised margin is the major problem.

Continued

TABLE 30.4 Clinical, Radiographic, Histopathological Features, Treatment & Prognosis of Osteosarcoma, Ewing's Sarcoma & Multiple Myeloma—cont'd

Ewing's Sarcoma

Ewing's sarcoma is an uncommon malignant neoplasm, which occurs as a primary destructive lesion of bone that most commonly involves the pelvis and lower extremities. Origin of the cells might be derived from marrow endothelium or from undifferentiated cells of the reticuloendothelial system (Fig. 30.4).

Clinical Features	Radiographic Features	Histopathological Features	Treatment and Prognosis
• Occurs in children and young adults, rarely in older patients. • An episode of trauma often precedes development of the tumour. • Intermittent pain. • Swelling of the involved bone. • Low-grade fever. • Elevated WBC count due to infection. • Metastatic foci appear in other bones and organs.	• Layers of new subperiosteal bone producing 'onion skin' appearance. • Osteophyte formation similar to the 'sunray' appearance of osteosarcoma.	• Solid sheets of small round cells with large nuclei and minimal stroma. • Necrosis is also a common microscopic feature.	• Surgery, chemotherapy and radiotherapy

Multiple Myeloma

Origin - cells of the bone marrow. Multiple myeloma has a multicentric origin at approximately the same time and each independent of the other lesions.

Clinical Features	Radiographic Features	Histopathological Features	Treatment and Prognosis
• Occurs mostly in adults • Anaemia is a common finding in multiple myeloma • Signs and symptoms of jaw involvement include • Pain • Swelling • Expansion of the jaw • Numbness • Abnormal healing. • Mandibular fracture. • Mobility of teeth.	• It reveals numerous sharply punched-out areas in numerous bones of active haematopoiesis like vertebrae, ribs, skull, jaws and ends of long bones. • Diffuse destructive lesions of bone may be seen.	• Consists of sheets of closely packed cells that resemble plasma cells. These cells exhibiting chromatin clumping in a 'cartwheel' or 'checkerboard' pattern.	• Chemotherapy is presently the treatment of choice for multiple myeloma using alkylating agents such as melphalan or cyclophosphamide in combination with prednisone. • Bone marrow transplant. • Radiation therapy is also used, often in combination with chemotherapy.

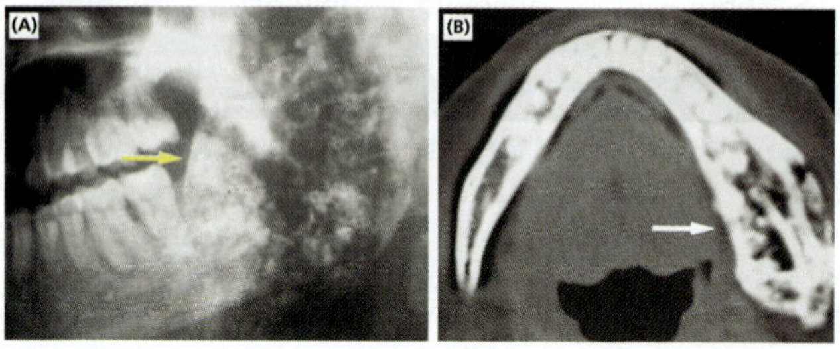

Figure 30.4 **(A)** Panoramic radiograph of a 26-year-old female with Ewing's sarcoma showing bone formation. **(B)** CT image showing bone formation both buccally and lingually.

- Infrastructure:
  a. Through floor of antrum to oral cavity
  b. Through medial wall to nasal cavity
  c. Through anterior wall to the cheek and skin of the face.

CLINICAL FEATURES

The carcinoma of nasal cavity and sinus does not present with symptoms in the early stages. The clinician should carefully evaluate older patients with unilateral symptoms.

- Early-stage symptoms—rare
- Late-stage symptoms:
  a. Nasal obstruction
  b. Epistaxis
  c. Epiphora
  d. Headache
  e. Symptoms of obstructive sinusitis
  f. Facial pain
  g. Congestion
  h. Swelling on hard palate
  i. Mass on maxillary alveolus or buccal sulcus
  j. Mobile teeth on the upper arch around the swelling

k. Paraesthesia of the skin of cheek or lip and buccal or labial mucosa
l. Diplopia
m. Proptosis
n. More advanced stages can present with trismus—masticatory muscle involvement
o. Posterior extension of the lesion:
   - Paraesthesia of distribution of trigeminal nerve
   - Paralysis of oculomotor nerve, trochlear nerve and abducent nerve
p. Anosmia is a rare symptom when olfactory nerve is involved.

INVESTIGATIONS

- Anterior rhinoscopy or nasal endoscopy: For intranasal lesions, endoscopy can provide very less information related to the extent of the lesion. It can only confirm the presence of the lesion. Care should be taken to prevent excessive manipulation to prevent bleeding from the tumour
- Radiographic investigation:
  a. CT scan is the 1st line of investigation
     - Better delineation of bone matrix with regard to:
       - Expansion
       - Remodelling
       - Erosion or destruction
     - Delineation of the cartilaginous matrix
     - Malignant calcification
  b. Contrast—enhanced CT scan
  c. MRI—T1/T2 weighted MRI and contrast enhanced MRI (CEMRI):
     - Better delineation of tumour to adjacent tissues
     - Tumour changes
     - Orbital extension
     - Intracranial extension
     - Perineural extensions
- Positron emission tomography (PET) scan is important for postoperative evaluation
- Biopsy:
  a. If the lesion is visible through the nasal or oral cavity, a punch biopsy is performed
  b. If the lesion is not approachable directly:
     - Transnasal endoscopic biopsy
     - CT-guided needle biopsy
  c. Avoid surgical biopsy with Caldwell–Luc antrostomy or other surgical approaches to access site for biopsy. This will violate the surgical planes for the surgical excision of the lesion.

SURGICAL MANAGEMENT

MAXILLECTOMY

In case of tumours involving the maxilla, a partial or total maxillectomy is done depending on the extent of involvement of the tumour.

Brown et al., in 2000 presented the Liverpool classification of maxillectomy defects (Fig. 30.5).

VERTICAL COMPONENT

CLASS I - MAXILLECTOMY WITH NO OROANTRAL COMMUNICATION

Surgical excision of the alveolar bone without causing oronasal or oroantral fistula. Surgical excision of ethmoidal sinus or frontal sinus or lateral wall of nose are included in this class.

CLASS II - LOW MAXILLECTOMY

Surgical excision of alveolus, antral wall. This excision will cause oroantral or oronasal fistula.

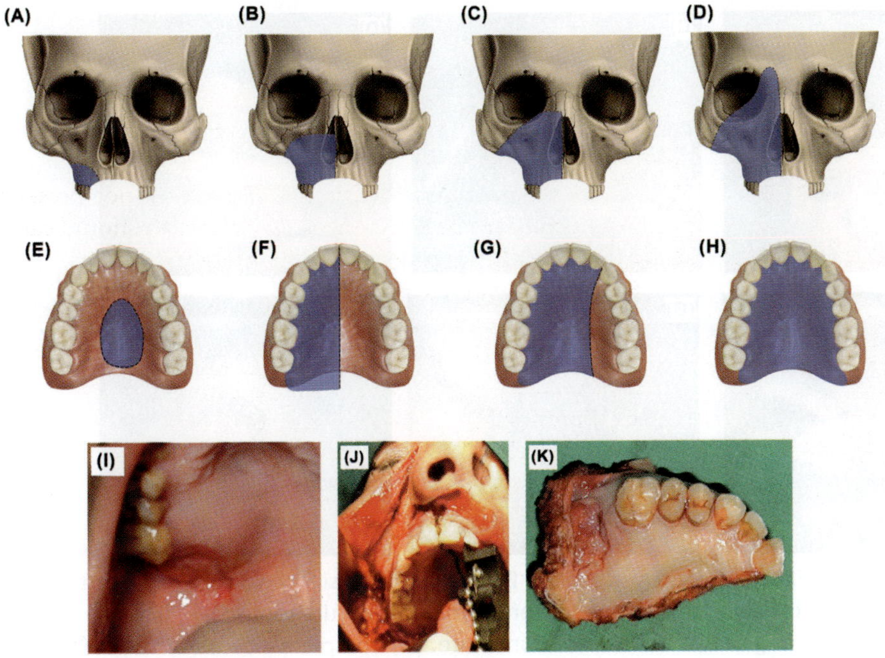

Figure 30.5 (**A–H**) Liverpool classification of maxillectomy. (**A–D**) Vertical component. (**E–H**) Horizontal component. (**A** and **E**) Class I. (**B** and **F**) Class II. (**C** and **G**) Class III. (**D** and **H**) Class IV. (**I–K**) Maxillectomy through a Weber–Ferguson approach. Class II Liverpool classification.

CLASS III - HIGH MAXILLECTOMY

Entire maxilla with floor of orbit with or without periorbital tissues are resected. Skull base resection may be done.

CLASS IV - RADICAL MAXILLECTOMY

Maxillectomy with orbital exenteration is performed. Anterior skull base resection is done based on the extent of the lesion.

HORIZONTAL COMPONENT

a. Unilateral maxillary alveolus and hard palate are resected
b. Resection extends partially to the contralateral maxilla
c. Maxillary alveolus and hard palate are completely resected.

SURGICAL APPROACHES FOR MAXILLARY CARCINOMA

1. Lateral rhinotomy—Moore's incision for medial maxillectomy
2. Lateral rhinotomy with:
   a. Lip split (Weber–Ferguson) (Fig. 30.12)
   b. Subciliary
   c. Supraciliary
   d. Lateral canthotomy
   e. Dieffenbach's extension
   f. Lynch extension
   g. Nasal rotation—for bilateral access
3. Midfacial degloving—Denker and Kahler approach
4. Classic Weber–Ferguson approach.

Maxillectomy via Weber–Ferguson approach

- An incision is made to split the lip along the philtrum up to and around the alar base, continuing along the lateral surface of the nose up to the medial canthus of the eye. The incision can also be extended beneath the lower eyelid up to the lateral canthal region
- The lip incision is made from the skin to the mucous membrane, continuing intraorally to the buccal sulcus incision extending posteriorly to the tuberosity
- The soft tissue incision is carried down till the bone of the lateral wall of maxilla
- A subperiosteal flap is elevated extending superiorly till the infraorbital rim, thus exploring the lateral surface of the maxilla and the zygoma
- Depending on the planned level of osteotomy like limited (alveolar) Class I, subtotal (low or Class II) or total maxillectomy (high or radical—Class III/IV), the osteotomy cuts are made
- The cut is next extended on to the hard palate, which is sectioned along the floor of the nose
- The pterygoid plates are then separated using a curved osteotome to separate the maxilla
- The sectioned maxilla is then removed and haemostasis achieved
- A skin graft can be used to cover the raw wound
- The defect is packed with a tincture benzoin gauze and maintained with a maxillary splint or obturator
- The skin incisions are closed in layers.

USE OF PROSTHESIS AND PALATAL OBTURATORS

For patients who did not undergo surgical reconstruction, prosthesis for aesthetics and palatal obturators for the palatal defect can been fabricated. Palatal obturators assist in closure of the oronasal fistula. It will need support from the remaining dentition.

RECONSTRUCTION OF THE DEFECT

Some of the reconstructive procedures for closure and reconstruction of the defect include palatal flap, pectoralis major myocutaneous (PMMC) flap (Fig. 30.6), forehead flap (Fig. 30.7),

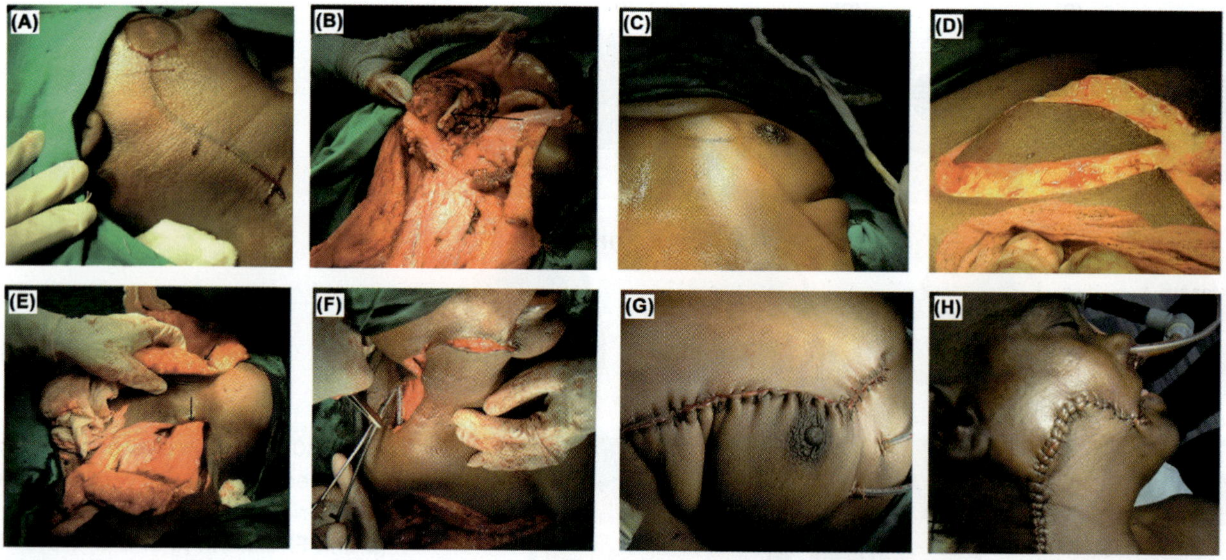

Figure 30.6 Pectoralis major myocutaneous flap. **(A)** Carcinoma-buccal mucosa. **(B)** Excision of the lesion with external skin, tumour excision, hemimandibulectomy and neck dissection. **(C)** Incision marked for pectoralis major myocutaneous flap. **(D)** Flap raised. **(E)** Flap tunnelled to buccal defect site. **(F)** Closure of oral region. **(G)** Closure of donor site. **(H)** Complete closure of the defect.

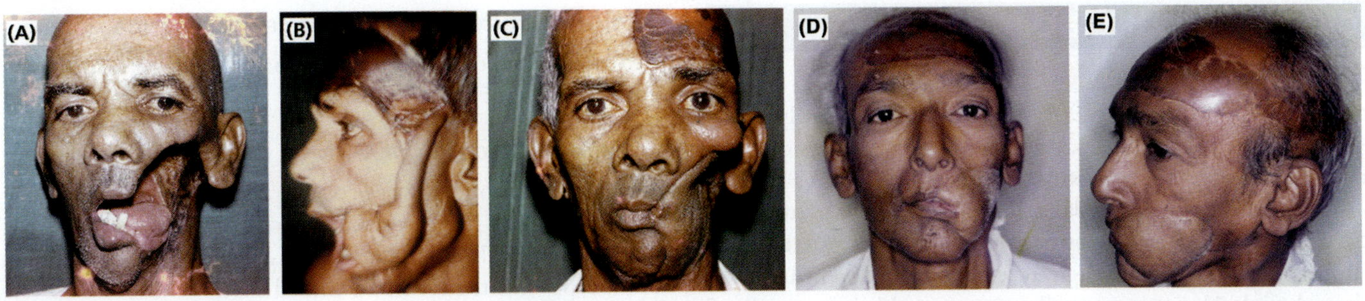

Figure 30.7 (**A**) Defect caused by resection of carcinoma of buccal mucosa. (**B**) Forehead flap used for soft tissue reconstruction, the pedicle is still intact. (**C**) Postoperative photograph after division of the flap. (**D** and **E**) Six months postoperative view of the patient.

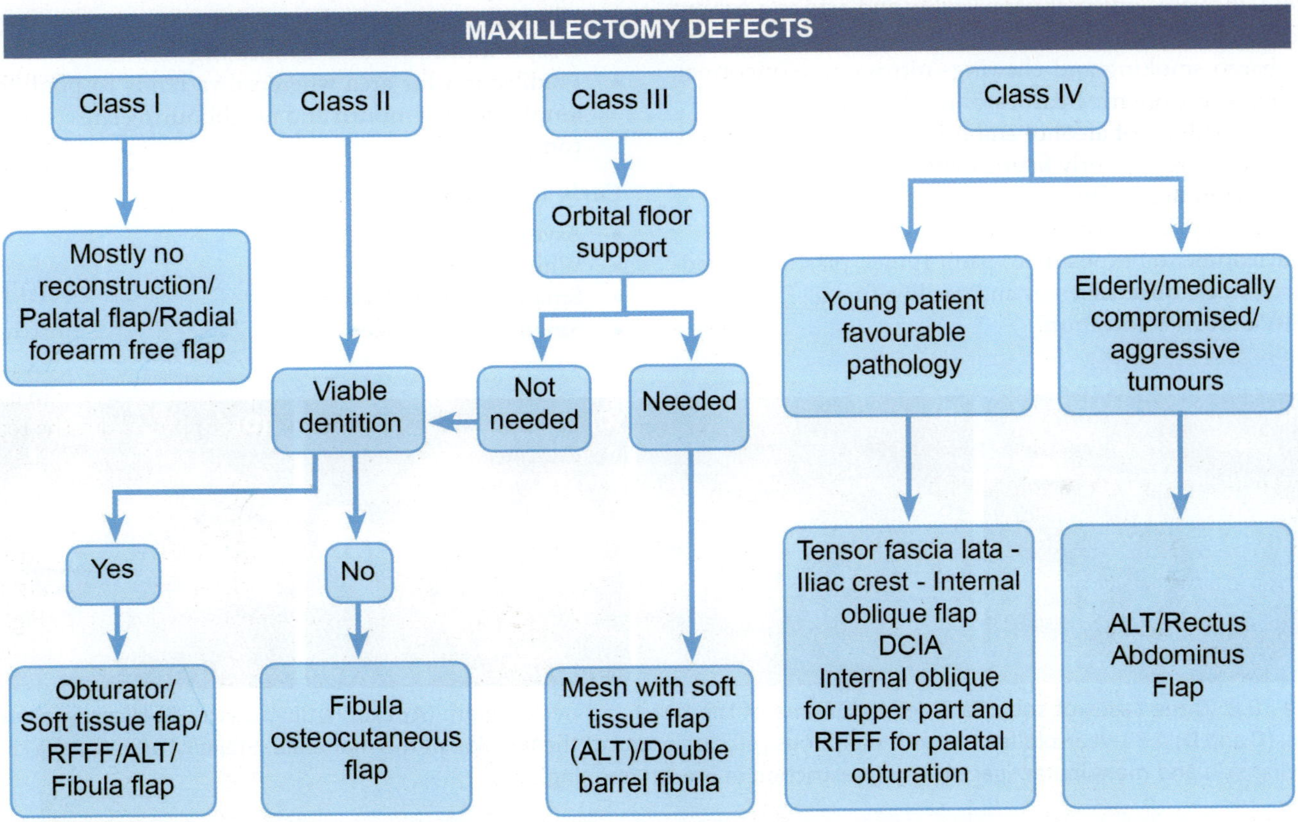

Flowchart 30.2 Reconstructive options and management of maxillary defects based on the Brown's classification of maxillectomy. DCIA - deep circumflex iliac artery.

radial forearm free flap (RFFF), anterolateral thigh flap (ALT), fibula osteocutaneous flap, double barrel fibula flap, rectus abdominus flap, etc. can be used. For young patients with favourable pathology, tensor fascia lata-iliac crest-internal oblique free flap for composite orbitomaxillary defect with orbital exenteration can be done. Another option would be to use deep circumflex iliac artery flap or internal oblique for upper part and RFFF for palatal obturation (Flowchart 30.2). Refer Chapter 33.

ADJUVANT TREATMENTS

- Systemic chemotherapy followed by intensity modulated radiotherapy (RT)
- Chemotherapy drugs:
  a. Cisplatin or carboplatin
  b. 5-Fluorouracil (5-FU)
  c. Taxotere

COMPLICATIONS

- Haemorrhage
- Infection
- Epiphora—treatment is dacryocystorhinostomy (DCR)
- Paraesthesia—infraorbital nerve is resected
- Atrophic rhinitis
- Breakdown of split thickness skin graft.

CARCINOMA OF THE ORAL CAVITY

SQUAMOUS CELL CARCINOMA

Carcinoma of oral cavity is 90% of times pathologically squamous cell carcinoma (SCC), the other malignant lesions are from the minor salivary glands. According to the WHO histological publication of oral and oropharyngeal tumours, OSCC is described as tumours consisting of irregular nests, columns or strands of malignant epithelial cells, infiltrating subepithelial. The tumour cells may resemble any or all of the layers of stratified squamous epithelium (Fig. 30.8).

Aetiology

- Unknown
- Alcohol consumption–irritation and dehydration of mucosa, increases mucosal permeability and acts as a solvent for carcinogens
- Tobacco smoking and chewing–nitrosamine (nicotine), polycyclic aromatic hydrocarbons (3,4-benzopyrene)
- Combined use of alcohol and tobacco–synergistic effect
- Irritation from poorly fitting dentures
- Oral submucous fibrosis
- Plummer–Vinson syndrome
- Environmental exposure to paint fumes, plastic by-products, wood dust, asbestos and gas line fumes
- EBV and HPV infection.

Clinical features—squamous cell carcinoma

SCC is most often characterised as *exophytic or ulcerative* or a combination of both.

Exophytic lesions of SCC

- Less common, slower growing and less infiltrative
- Cauliflower-like irregular growth
- Pinkish proliferative lesion (Fig. 30.9)
- Deeply infiltrative in advanced cases.

Ulcerative lesions of SCC

- More common
- The lesion bleeds easily
- Ulcers are reddish or greyish
- Ulcer edges are everted
- Deeply infiltrative and nonhealing
- Predilection for area where saliva tends to pool, for example, floor of mouth and neighbouring sites (side of the tongue).

Early lesions of SCC

- Asymptomatic
- White or red patches
- Small exophytic growth
- Small indolent ulcer.

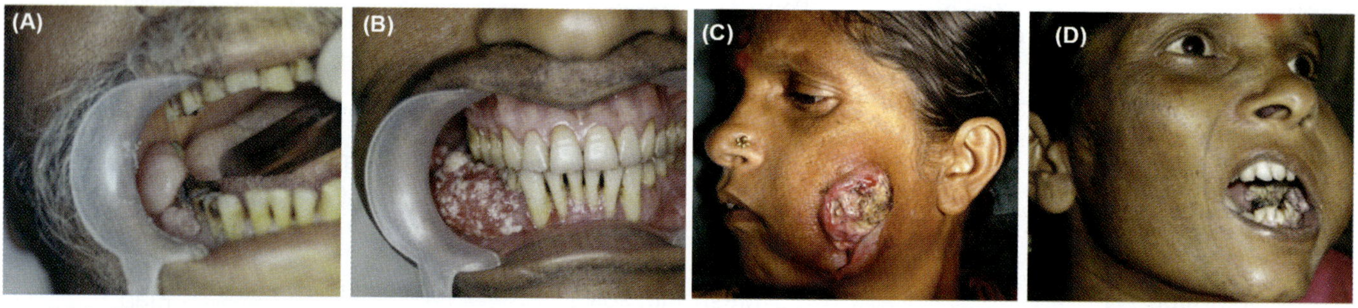

Figure 30.8 Three cases of squamous cell carcinoma of the head and neck region. (**A**) Exophytic growth. (**B**) Ulceroproliferative lesion. (**C** and **D**) A 32-year-old female with squamous cell carcinoma of the left side of the mandible. Stage IV or end stage disease involving skin and mandibular space causing restriction in mouth opening.

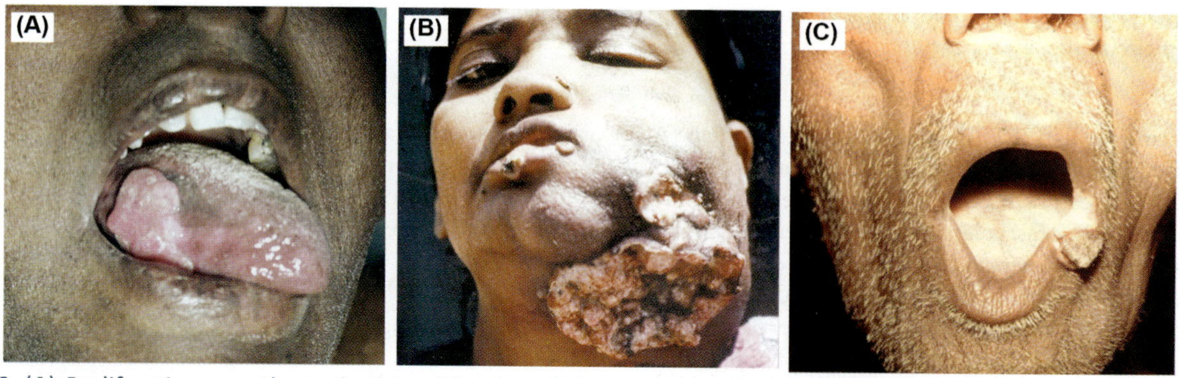

Figure 30.9 (**A**) Proliferative growth on the lateral border of the tongue—squamous cell carcinoma. (**B**). Squamous cell carcinoma—ulceroproliferative lesion with secondary changes on the skin. Necrosis of the exophytic mass can be noted in the centre of the lesion. (**C**) Verrucous carcinoma.

Intermediate lesions of SCC

- Persistent ulceration
- Induration
- Fixation to underlying structures
- Lymph node enlargement.

Advanced lesions of SCC

- Haemorrhage or necrosis of exophytic mass (Fig. 30.9B)
- Destructive crater-like ulcer with raised or rolled edges
- Pain, paraesthesia
- Bone destruction, invasion, fracture
- Mobility of teeth.

Clinical features—verrucous carcinoma

- White proliferative growth (Fig. 30.9C and D)
- Keratin heaped up over the lesion
- Papillary projections
- Bleeding from surface.

Pathway of oral cancer

The dysplastic cells of SCC from the oral mucosa spreads to the bone. This is through the attached gingiva (Flowchart 30.3). The cells cannot cross the periosteum as it acts as a protective barrier.

INVESTIGATION

Radiographic screening

- Orthopantomogram (OPG):
  a. Best for routine screening
  b. To assess general architecture of bone
- PET scan:
  a. Neoplastic screening
  b. Shows inflammatory lesions also should be differentiated
  c. Best for postoperative screening during follow-up.

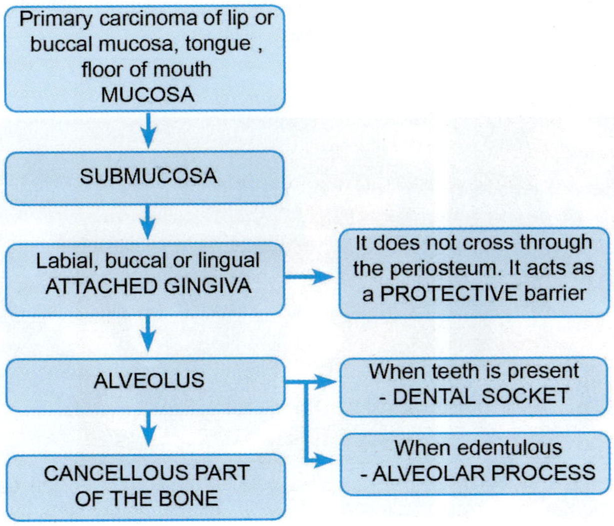

Flowchart 30.3 Pathway of oral cancer.

Radiographic investigation for surgical planning

- Occlusal radiographs and intraoral radiographs:
  a. Best for bone—early lesions
- OPG:
  a. To assess invasion of tumour
  b. To assess the tumour relation with dentoalveolar structures
- Bone scintigraphy
- Contrast enhanced CT scan
- CT scan:
  a. For tumour invasion into bone
  b. Bone destruction
  c. Relation of tumour to bone
- 3DCT scan
- Cone-beam computed tomography (CBCT)
- Magnetic resonance imaging (MRI)

Biopsy

- Wedge biopsy or punch biopsy
- Adequate volume of tissue
- Vascularised, viable tumour specimen
- Avoid superficial biopsy
- Biopsy site should be chosen on the adjacent invasive zone with complete depth of lesion
- Lesions thicker than 4 mm have increased risk of lymph node metastasis (Fig. 30.10)
- **Low-grade tumours:**
  a. More extensive keratinisation, infrequent mitoses and little nuclear pleomorphism
  b. Maintain orientation from basal to keratinised layers
- **High-grade tumours:**
  a. Little keratin, increased mitosis and extreme nuclear pleomorphism
- **Well differentiated:**
  a. Presence of keratin pearls
  b. Basement membrane is absent

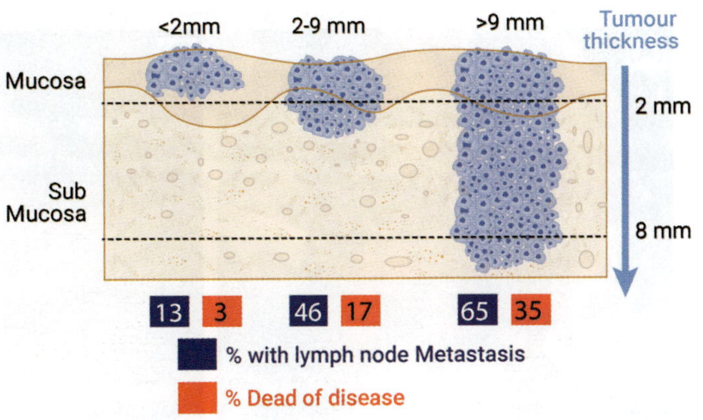

Figure 30.10 Impact of tumour thickness on lymphatic spread and survival rate.

- **Moderately differentiated:**
  a. Keratin pearls are sparse or absent
  b. Prickle cells are more pleomorphic
  c. A typical mitotic figure
- **Poorly differentiated (anaplastic):**
  a. No keratin
  b. Extreme pleomorphism and hyperchromatism
  c. Cells cannot be recognised as keratinocytes
- ***Histologic variants of squamous cell carcinoma:***
  a. Basaloid SCC—aggressive variant:
    - Basaloid cells that are arranged in nests
    - High mitotic rate
    - Worse prognosis
    - Develop distant metastasis more frequently
  b. Verrucous SCC
- ***Recurrence:***
  a. After postoperative excision, the margin of lesions less than 5 mm from resected margin should be pathologically investigated for carcinoma in situ and severe dysplasia. This predicts future probability of recurrence.

SURGICAL MANAGEMENT OF ORAL CANCER

Surgical management remains the primary modality of management of oral cancer. The principle of treating oral cancer is eradication of the disease.

Preoperative dental evaluation and treatment before cancer treatment

- Mobile teeth involved with the tumour are not extracted. Extraction of these teeth can cause implantation of the cancer cells in to the mandibular canal, or can cause further invasion into the bone
- Complete removal of calculus and sharp cusps have to be done
- Planning for fixed prosthesis, removable dentures or palatal obturators can be done prior to the surgery
- Dental treatment before radiation therapy becomes mandatory to prevent osteoradionecrosis (refer Chapter 24—page 486).

SURGICAL APPROACHES TO ORAL CARCINOMA

Factors affecting choice of approach

1. Size and site of tumour
2. Depth of infiltration
3. Proximity of tumour to maxillary or mandibular bone
4. Dentition
5. Size of oral aperture
6. Mouth opening length
7. Trismus
8. Size and mobility of tongue.

Various surgical approaches

1. Per-oral approach
2. Lower cheek flap (lip-split) with or without mandibulectomy
3. Upper cheek flap (Weber–Ferguson approach)
4. Visor flap.

PER-ORAL APPROACH

This approach is when the lesion is accessed for surgical excision through the mouth (Fig. 30.11). Per-oral approach does not give adequate access for larger posterior lesions. If the patient presents with malignancy due to oral submucous fibrosis (OSMF), per-oral approach will not be possible. If cervical node metastasis is present, a separate incision is made on the neck to access the lymph nodes. Per-oral approach is used for carcinoma of tongue, floor of the mouth, gingiva, buccal mucosa, and hard or soft palate when the lesion is:

- Small
- Anteriorly located
- Easily accessible
- Superficial
- Not too close to the bone
- No bone invasion of tumour.

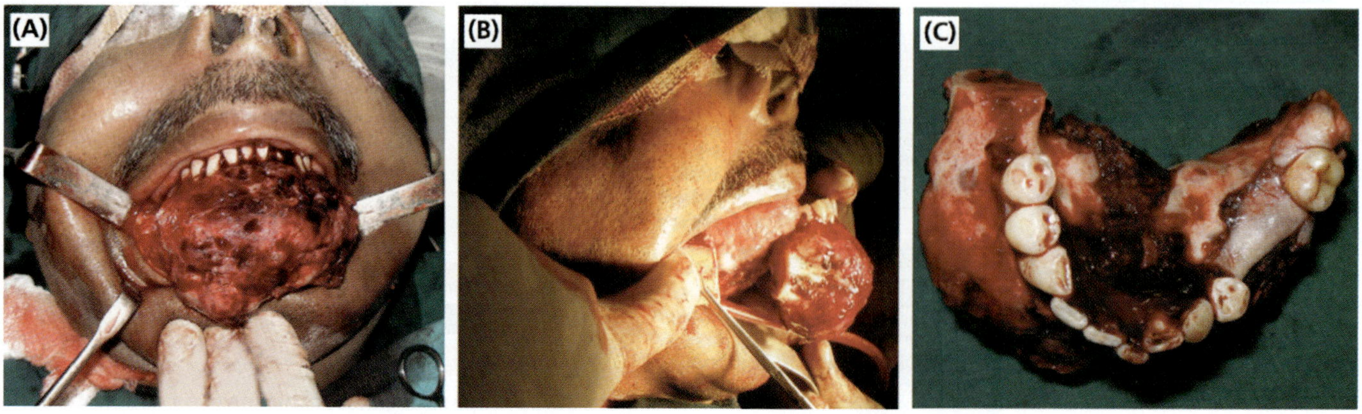

Figure 30.11 (**A–C**) Mandibular segmental resection through a per-oral approach.

LOWER CHEEK FLAP (LIP-SPLIT)

The lower cheek flap is used when the lesion cannot be accessed by the per-oral approach. This flap gives better access to the pathological region for surgical excision. When a mandibulotomy is also done, this approach can access the larger tumours of the base of the tongue, oral cavity, oropharynx, pharynx and up to the upper cervical spine. A type of mentolabial incision called lip-split incision is used for this flap. In the classic lip-split, the incision involves splitting of the lower lip on the midline, this results in notching of the lip at the incision's scar. The most common complications of this incision are as follows:

- Scar contracture causes notching at the scar
- Functional defect of the depressor muscles causing lip incontinence
- Loss of function of the mandibular branch of CN VII
- Loss of function of buccinator muscle fibres involved with the incision.

There are many modifications to the lower lip-split incisions to overcome these complications (Fig. 30.12). These modifications are based on the relaxed skin tension lines (RSTL). When the incision lies on these RSTL, it produces better aesthetic results.

The lower lip-split incision and its modifications

1. *Roux–Trotter incision*—classic lower lip-split incision (Fig. 30.12):
   a. Best to avoid damage of nerves, vessels and muscle fibres
   b. Produces an unaesthetic scar and scar contracture
2. *McGregor's incision* (Fig. 30.12):
   a. This incision breaks up the straight line to conceal scar in the skin crease
   b. More noticeable scar
3. *Robson's incision* (Fig. 30.12):
   a. Lateral approach
   b. This can damage the terminal branches of facial nerve, mental nerve
   c. It causes paraesthesia, incompetence and incontinence of lower lip
4. *Bhatt's incision* (Fig. 30.12):
   a. The incision goes along the vermilion border with the skin, goes downward and goes back to the midline to create a vermilion flap
5. *Hayter's incision* (Fig. 30.12):
   a. This is a modification of the McGregor's incision, but with V-shaped lines on the vermilion and skin.
6. *Rassekh's incision* (Fig. 30.12):
   a. Similar to Hayter's incision but extends as a high cervical incision for neck dissection.

Mandibulotomy

Mandibulotomy is a procedure of splitting the mandibular bone to access the tissues behind the mandible for resection. After tumour excision, the mandible with no lesions is fixed back in place by rigid or semi-rigid fixation. The mandible is split into two segments allowing for surgical access to locations like the base of the tongue, posterior areas of the oropharynx, and up to the cervical spine. Once the tumour has been completely excised, the mandible is fixed with plates and screws.

Types (Table 30.5):

1. Posterior lateral mandibulotomy—not recommended (Fig. 30.13)
2. Anterior midline mandibulotomy:
   a. Midline osteotomy (Fig. 30.14A)
   b. Stepped mandibulotomy (Fig. 30.14B)
3. Paramedian mandibulotomy (Fig. 30.15).

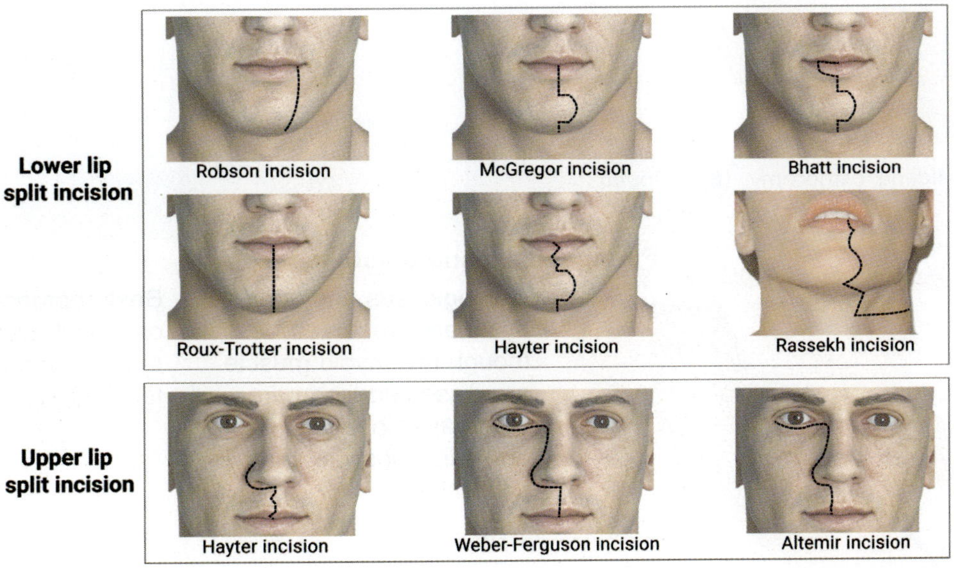

Figure 30.12 Types of upper and lower lip-split incisions.

TABLE 30.5 Types of Mandibulotomy

	Advantages	Disadvantages
Posterior Lateral Mandibulotomy		
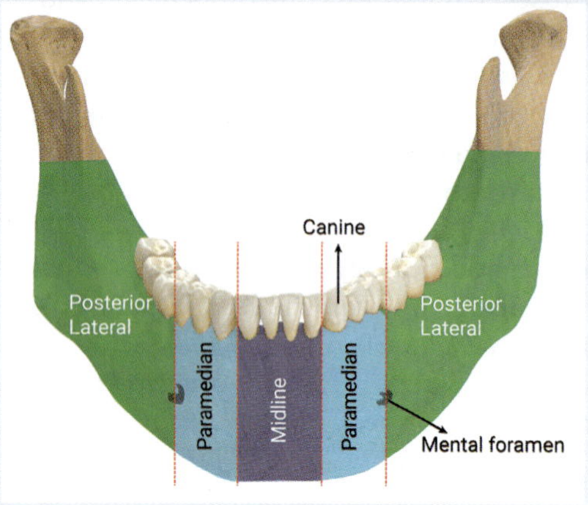 Figure 30.13 Posterior lateral mandibulotomy.	• The cut is made in the posterior lateral area of the mandible as seen in the figure. • This technique of mandibulectomy is not recommended due to the disadvantages.	• Muscle pull for the mandibular segments are different causing an unbalanced stress during healing. • This will require IMF to overcome the forces. IMF can cause sepsis at suture line due to poor oral hygiene. • Denervation of teeth. • Devascularisation of teeth. • Exposure is limited. • The area of osteotomy lies at the line of radiation therapy. This can cause delayed healing of the bone.
Anterior Midline Mandibulotomy		
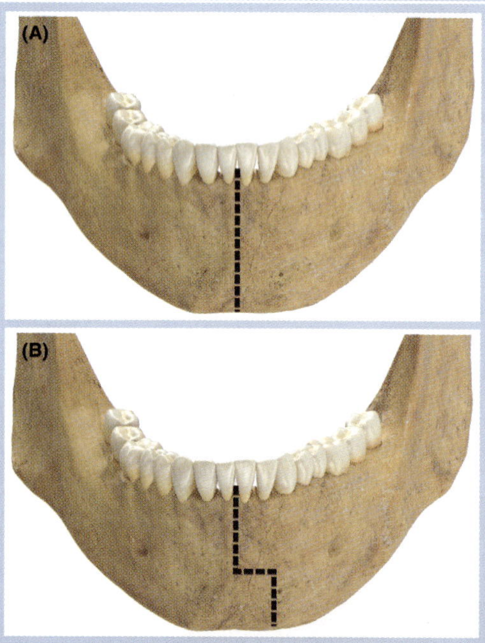 Figure 30.14 **(A)** Midline osteotomy. **(B)** Stepped mandibulotomy.	• Easier technique to follow for edentulous arches. • Better healing for patients undergoing radiation therapy as the osteotomy cut is completely out of line of radiation.	• Requires extraction of one lower central incisor to provide space to make the osteotomy cut. • The genioglossus and geniohyoid have to be elevated from the genial tubercle. This causes delayed recovery of swallowing.
Paramedian Mandibulotomy		
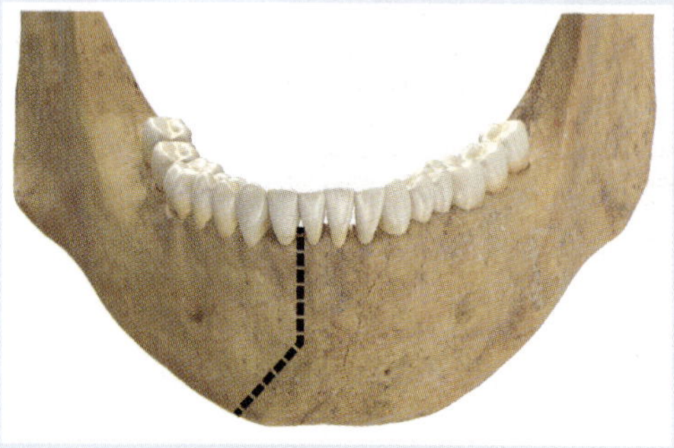 Figure 30.15 Paramedian mandibulotomy.	• Genioglossus and geniohyoid are preserved though mylohyoid muscle are dissected, comparatively faster healing and minimal swallowing difficulties.	• Best approach for mandibulotomy as it avoids the disadvantages of the other two techniques.

UPPER CHEEK FLAP (WEBER–FERGUSON APPROACH)

Upper lip-split is used when per-oral approach cannot be used and when carcinoma of the hard palate and upper alveolus presents with tumour invasion that is deeper, larger and located at a more posterior site.

Upper lip-split incisions and modifications

1. *Weber–Ferguson* approach (Fig. 30.12):
   a. A midline split of the upper lip to the base of the columella is made, which then proceeds towards the lateral nasal contour and up to the medial canthus
   b. From here, the incision can extend as a subciliary incision or a lateral canthotomy incision or above the upper eyelid as an eyelid crease incision. For further approach into the orbit, it can extend as an incision onto the temporal area
2. *Altemir's incision* (Fig. 30.12):
   a. In this modification, the lip-split starts at the philtral crest
3. *Hayter's incision* (Fig. 30.12):
   a. Similar to the lower lip-split Hayter's modification, V-shaped cuts are given at the vermillion of the lip and at the upper lip.

VISOR FLAP

This flap is used for large anterior lesions like carcinoma of the floor of the mouth, anterior tongue, anterior gingiva, and carcinoma extending into the mandibular bone where segmental osteotomy of the mandible is indicated. This approach avoids lower lip-split incision. It is indicated when per-oral approach is not possible. The disadvantages of this approach are paraesthesia of the chin as the mental nerve is transected, sagging of the lower lip, lip incontinence and incompetence (Fig. 30.16).

PER ORAL EXCISION OF ORAL CARCINOMA

Resection of early oral cancer using conventional surgical techniques

- Margins: In situations where achievable, all lesions should be resected with a margin of at least 1 cm in every direction(mucosa and soft tissue). It is considered a compromised margin if it is smaller than 0.5 cm.
- Technique of excision: Excisions can be performed using a cautery, laser (CO_2), or scalpel. As far as cancer control is concerned, the outcomes are the same regardless of the technique.
- Neck dissection as well as the resection of the jaw's maxilla or mandible portion

Guidelines for the management of locally advanced oral cavity malignant tumours

Stage III and IV malignancies are tumours that have spread locally. They need a multimodal approach to treatment. This leads to the most important development: deciding which lesions are operable and which of those are inoperable.

Stage III and IVa oral cancers are those that can be removed via surgical procedure (operable). Once the surgical excision is performed, radiotherapy, with or without chemotherapy, is performed.

Oral cancers that have passed stages IVb and IVc are inoperable.

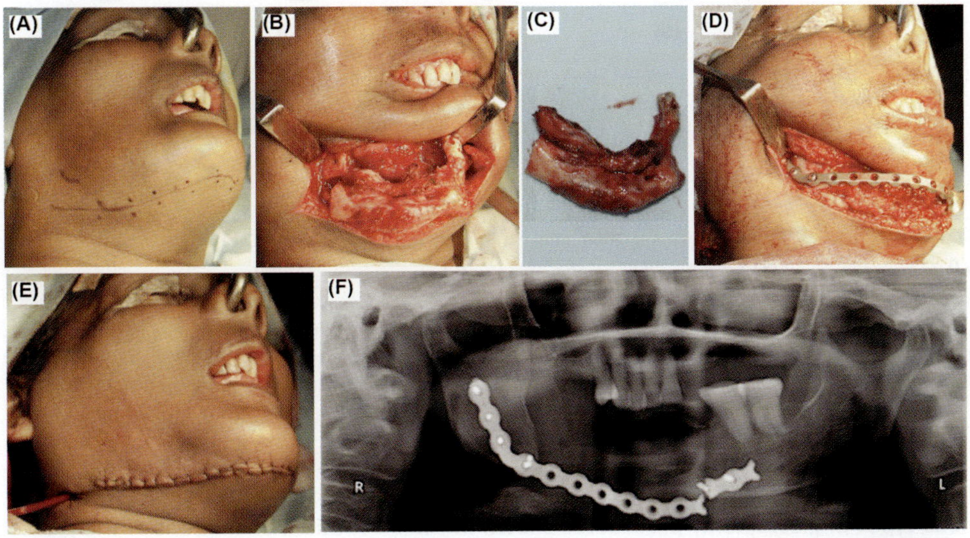

Figure 30.16 Least favoured form of reconstruction—reconstruction plate. (**A**) Preoperative view of the patient showing a mild lower facial asymmetry with marking for right submandibular incision. (**B**) Exposure of the lesion via submandibular approach. (**C**) Resected specimen. (**D**) Placement and fixation of the reconstruction plate according to the planned position of the template. (**E**) Primary closure of the surgical wound. (**F**) OPG showing fractured reconstruction plate.

Criteria that indicate oral cancer is inoperable include: fixed neck nodes on clinical palpation; recent onset of trismus due to gross infratemporal fossa invasion; extensive involvement of the base of the skull; extensive involvement of soft tissues up to the zygoma or hyoid bone; and distant metastasis or blood vessel infiltration. Inoperable lesions culminate in palliative CT/RT and symptomatic care.

Surgical treatment for locally advanced cancer

The majority of patients with locally advanced oral cavity malignancies undergo composite resections. All lesions should be removed, with a margin of at least 1 cm on all sides. For the mucosa, soft tissue, and bone, a sufficiently wide margin must be attained. Any margin that is compromised is one that is less than 0.5 cm. Removal of the entire lesions, including any affected lymph nodes, mucosa, skin, or bone, is required for composite resections, usually done in continuity.

GLOSSECTOMY

The type of glossectomy procedure is selected depending on the TNM staging. The types of glossectomy are as follows:

1. Partial glossectomy (Fig. 30.17A and B) and (Fig. 30.30)
2. Hemiglossectomy (Fig. 30.17C and D)
3. Base of tongue resection with or without hemiglossectomy:
   a. Unilateral base of tongue resection without hemiglossectomy (Fig. 30.17F)
   b. Unilateral base of tongue resection with hemiglossectomy (Fig. 30.17G)
   c. Bilateral base of tongue resection without hemiglossectomy (Fig. 30.17H)
   d. Bilateral base of tongue resection with hemiglossectomy (Fig. 30.17I)
4. Subtotal glossectomy (Fig. 30.17J and K)
5. Anterior tongue total glossectomy (Fig. 30.17E)
6. Anterior and posterior tongue total glossectomy (Fig. 30.17L and M).

MEDIAN LABIOMANDIBULAR GLOSSECTOMY PROCEDURE (TROTTER'S OPERATION)

It is a procedure that is similar to mandibulotomy procedure. Trotter's operation is done to access the posterior tumour site. The tongue is split in the centre to access the tumour site. It is used in conjugation with mandibulotomy for access. This procedure is done for tumours of:

- The base of the tongue
- Posterior pharyngeal wall
- Cranio-cervical junction
- Midline oropharynx.

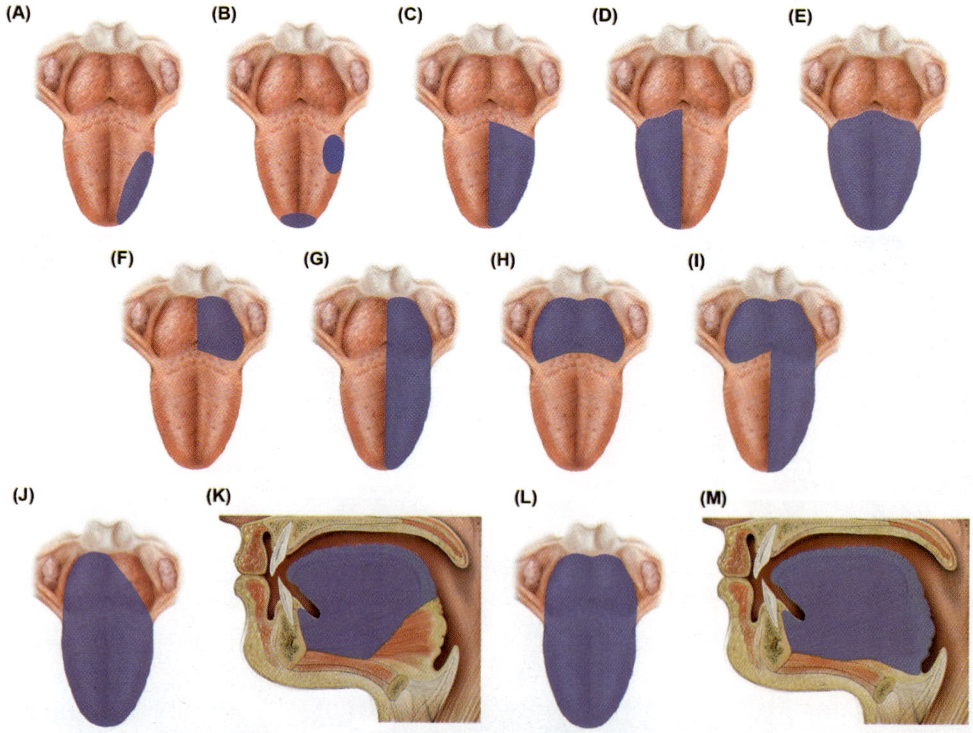

Figure 30.17 The various types of glossectomy procedures shown in the illustration. The extent of the glossectomy is dependent on the extent and type of malignancy. (**A** and **B**) Partial glossectomy. (**C** and **D**) Hemiglossectomy. (**E**) Anterior tongue total glossectomy. (**F**) Unilateral base of tongue resection without hemiglossectomy. (**G**) Unilateral base of tongue resection with hemiglossectomy. (**H**) Bilateral base of tongue resection without hemiglossectomy. (**I**) Bilateral base of tongue resection with hemiglossectomy. (**J** and **K**) Subtotal glossectomy. (**L** and **M**) Anterior and posterior tongue total glossectomy.

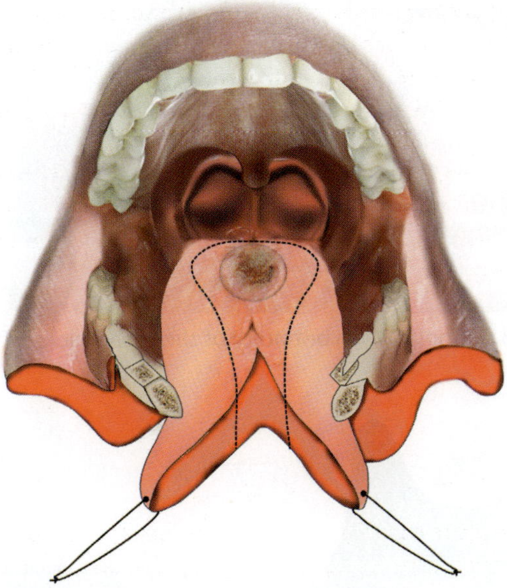

Figure 30.18 Trotter's operation to reach the base of the tongue lesions.

Splitting the tongue in the midline prevents damage to the nerves and vessels of the tongue, thus preventing functional defect like movement of the tongue (Fig. 30.18).

MANDIBULECTOMY

Types of mandibular resection:
1. Composite or commando resection
2. Marginal mandibulectomy
3. Segmental or rim mandibulectomy
4. Hemimandibulectomy.

Composite or commando resection

- COMMANDO procedure—combined mandibulectomy and neck dissection operation
- Wide local excision with hemimandibular resection, total glossectomy (if the lesion extends to the tongue), resection of the floor of the mouth and block dissection of the neck to remove the entire lymphatic drainage with sternocleidomastoid (SCM) muscle and internal jugular vein (IJV)
- This is a procedure of the past when recent advances in cancer were not available.

Marginal mandibulectomy

- It was termed mandibular en-bloc resection in the past
- In this procedure, the tumour is removed along with a rim of uninvolved bone, while maintaining the continuity of the jaw
- This is the treatment of choice for small malignant lesions of the gingiva with minimal bony invasion or suspected field cancerisation of the alveolar process
- Postresection, a minimum of 1 cm height of normal bone must be present to avoid pathologic fracture
- Types of marginal mandibulectomy (Fig. 30.19):
  a. Horizontal or classical alveolar rim resection
  b. Vertical or sagittal alveolar rim resection
  c. Oblique alveolar rim resection
- Reverse marginal mandibulectomy (Fig. 30.20):
  a. Resection of the inferior border of mandible for fixed submandibular lymph nodes to the inferior border of mandible
  b. For advanced cervical secondaries infiltrating into the mandible
- Indications:
  a. Minimal or no bony erosion
  b. Carcinoma of lip with mandibular invasion

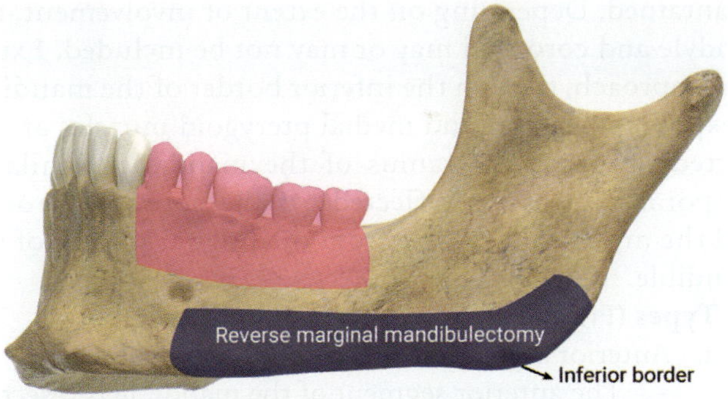

Figure 30.20 Regular marginal mandibulectomy (pink) and reverse marginal mandibulectomy (purple) on the inferior border of the mandible.

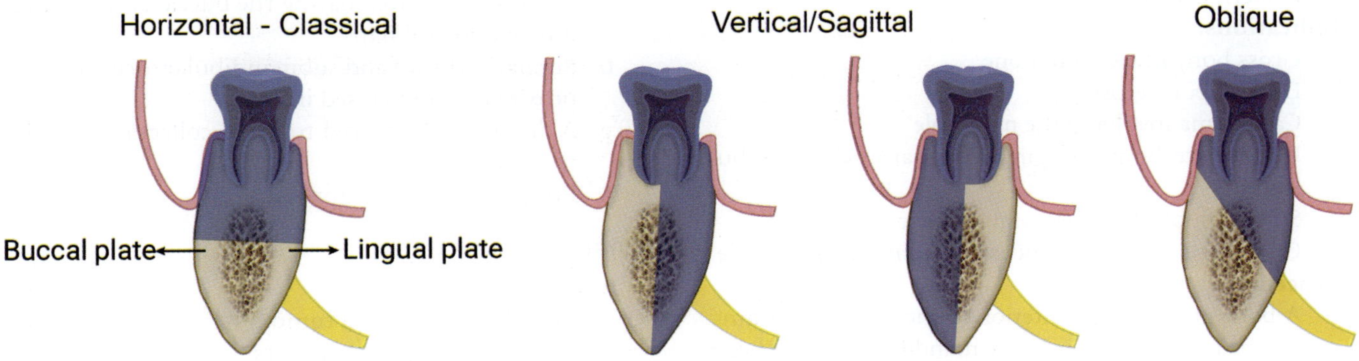

Figure 30.19 Types of marginal mandibulectomy based on the cortical involvement.

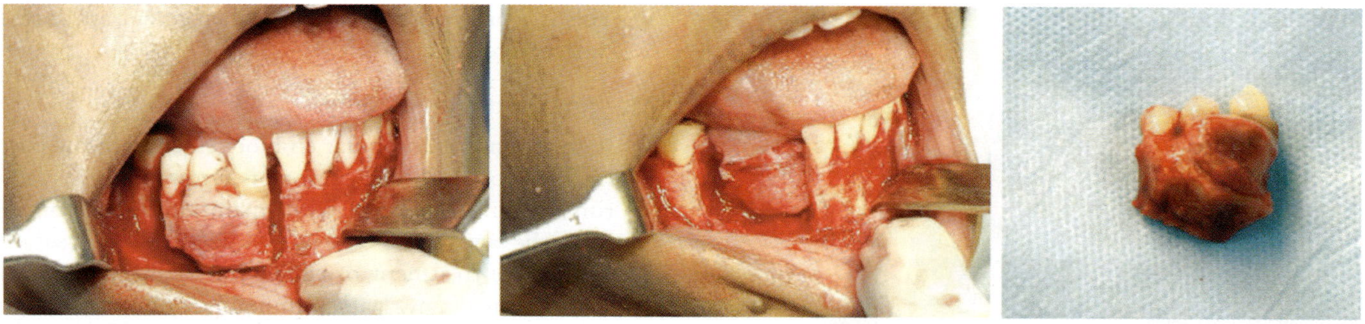

Figure 30.21 Marginal mandibulectomy of a lesion in relation to the canine and premolar. The continuity of the mandible is left intact.

  c. Carcinoma of mandibular alveolus
  d. Carcinoma of buccal mucosa invading the mandible
  e. Carcinoma of floor of the mouth
  f. Retromolar trigone carcinoma—posterior alveolus extending up to coronoid process is resected
- Contraindications:
  a. Irradiated mandible
  b. Edentulous mandible—segmental resection is indicated
  c. Gross erosion of the bone
  d. Carcinoma involving both cortices of the mandible (Fig. 30.21).

Segmental mandibulectomy

In this technique, continuity of the inferior border is not maintained. Depending on the extent of involvement, the condyle and coronoid may or may not be included. Extraoral approach, though the inferior border of the mandible is exposed, masseter and medial pterygoid muscles are reflected off from the ramus of the mandible. Similarly, temporalis muscle is reflected off the coronoid process and the mylohyoid muscle from the lingual surface of the mandible.

- **Types** (Fig. 30.22):
  a. Anterior segmental:
    - The anterior segment of the mandible is resected
    - The primary tumour can originate from the gingivolabial sulcus, invasive lip carcinoma, mucosa of anterior floor of mouth
  b. Lateral segmental
  c. Posterior segmental
- **Indications:**
  a. Gross bony invasion of bone
  b. Evident bony erosion
  c. Carcinoma involving the mandible
  d. Inadequate bony margin after marginal mandibulectomy
  e. SCC of floor of mouth, oral cavity, oropharynx
  f. Carcinoma of buccal mucosa invading the mandible
- **Procedure:**
  a. A bone cut is made anterior to the lesion extending till the inferior border of the mandible, using either a Gigli's saw or bur

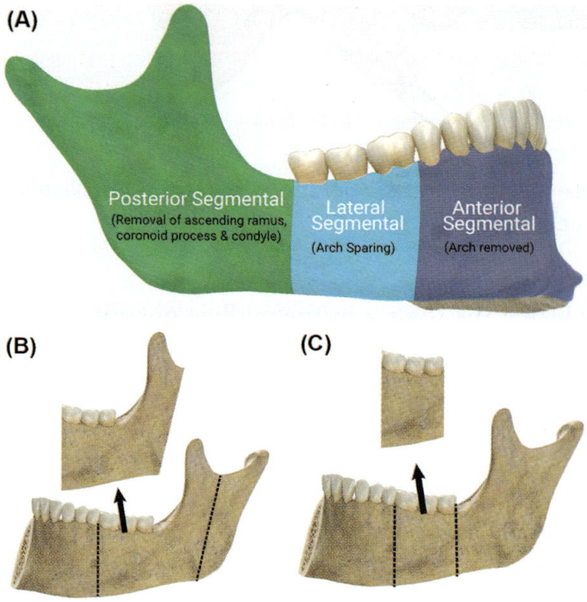

Figure 30.22 (**A**) Types of segmental mandibulectomy. (**B** and **C**) Variation in lateral segmental mandibulectomy depending on the extent of the malignant lesion.

  b. Once the cut is made, the segment is rotated laterally, on entering the mandibular foramen, the inferior alveolar bundle is identified and ligated
  c. The condyle is then freed from the lateral pterygoid muscle and the mandible disarticulated
  d. Haemostasis is achieved
  e. Closure by approximating the buccal and the lingual mucoperiosteal flaps
  f. Similarly, the lip and submandibular incisions are approximated and closed in layers
  g A drain may be placed to avoid collection of fluid in the dead space
  h. Pressure dressing is applied.

Hemimandibulectomy

- **Indications:**
  a. More laterally placed tumours
  b. Retromolar trigone tumours
  c. Advanced stage tumours

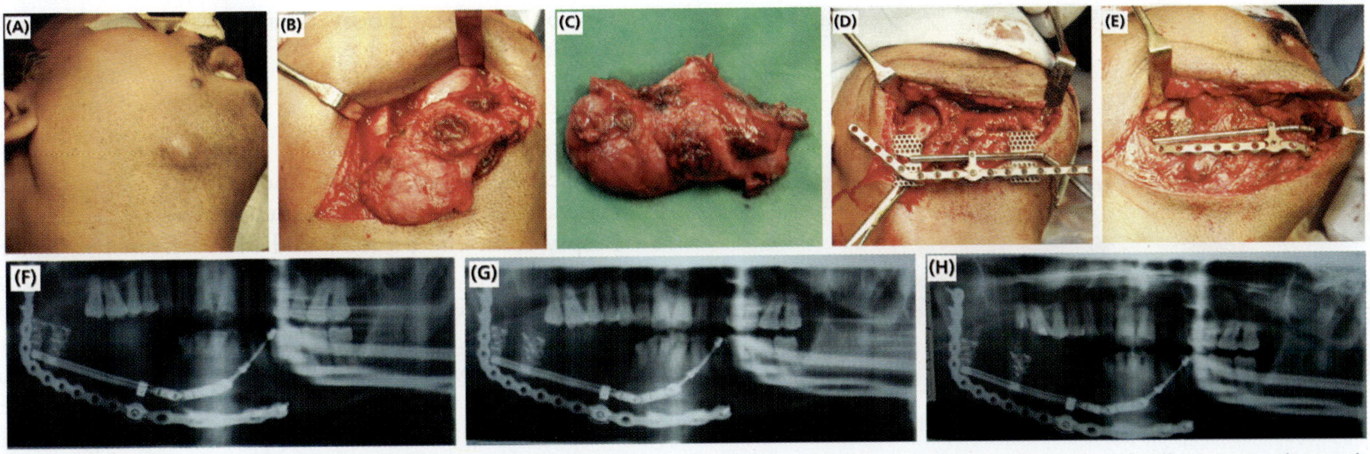

Figure 30.23 Transport distraction osteogenesis. (**A** and **B**) Note the skin over the swelling is inflamed and adherent to the underlying bone lesion. (**C**) Resected specimen. (**D**) Plate guided univector unidirectional straight mandibular distractor. (**E**) Fixation of the mesh footplates and completion of planned osteotomy. (**F–H**) Sequential OPG showing the movement of transport disc with daily activation.

- The mandible is resected from the symphysis to the condyle on one side
- This procedure produces a major functional loss
- Reconstruction can be done with composite fibula osteocutaneous flap with microvascular surgery.

Mandible reconstruction

The reconstruction of the resulting defect may be treated primarily or secondarily depending on the diagnosis of the lesion. Defect from aggressive lesions with high recurrence rate are reconstructed secondarily. Mandible reconstruction ranges from simple reconstruction plate, free bone grafts, microvascular vascularised graft to distraction osteogenesis or use of rhBMP-2 with free grafts (Fig. 30.23). Refer to Chapters 33, 34 and 44.

CERVICAL LYMPH NODE METASTASIS

Metastasis in the cervical lymph nodes are of three types:

1. Metastasis in the neck with clinically unidentified primary
2. Metastasis in the neck with an occult primary
3. Metastasis in the neck with known primary.

METASTASIS IN THE NECK WITH CLINICALLY UNIDENTIFIED PRIMARY

- Hard neck lymph nodes are metastases from the primary tumour. They can be palpated clinically, but primary tumour has not yet been identified
- **Differential diagnosis:**
  a. Lymphomas
  b. Tuberculous lymphadenitis
  c. Nonspecific lymphadenitis
  d. HIV
  e. Chronic lymphatic leukaemia
- **Investigations:**
  a. Fine needle aspiration cytology (FNAC) from the positive cervical nodes
  b. Search for the primary tumour should be performed through:
     1. PET scan
     2. CT scan
     3. Pan-endoscopy:
        - Nasopharyngoscopy, laryngoscopy, oesophagoscopy and bronchoscopy
     4. Surveillance biopsy:
        - Blind biopsies are taken from tonsillar bed, base of tongue, fossa of Rosen Muller, lateral wall of pharynx, pyriform fossa and subglottic region (larynx)
     5. FNAC of thyroid and other suspected areas.

METASTASIS IN THE NECK WITH AN OCCULT PRIMARY (OCCULT HIDING FROM VIEW)

- Metastasis in the neck lymph nodes revealed by FNAC, but primary site of tumour is still not found clinically
- Occult primary cervical metastasis: No evidence of primary tumour
- **Causes**
  1. Too small a primary to detect
  2. Immunological spontaneous regression of primary
  3. Inability of the diagnostic tools to detect the primary
- **Histological causes**
  1. SCC
  2. Adenocarcinoma
  3. Poorly differentiated tumours like lymphoma, sarcoma, melanoma (Fig. 30.24)
- **Investigations for occult primary**
  1. PET scan
  2. FNAC

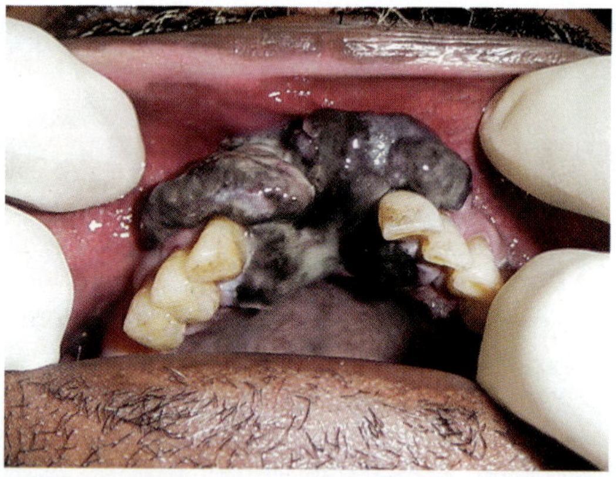

Figure 30.24 Malignant melanoma of the soft palate.

3. Open biopsy (if FNAC is inconclusive) after open biopsy with frozen section confirmation, immediate neck dissection has to be done
4. CT with contrast
5. MRI
6. Triple endoscopy
7. Surveillance biopsy
8. FNAC of thyroid
9. Ipsilateral tonsillectomy if surveillance biopsy and other methods are negative

- **Treatment**
  1. Neck dissection
  2. Regular follow-up (at 3 monthly intervals) until the primary reveals
  3. After detection of primary tumour
  4. Confirmed by biopsy treated by curative RT or by wide excision.

METASTASIS IN THE NECK WITH KNOWN PRIMARY TUMOUR

- Cervical nodes are present and primary tumour in the oral cavity has been identified clinically
- Biopsy from the primary and FNAC from the cervical node
- Neck dissection with surgical excision of primary tumour.

This is the most common kind of cervical metastasis in oral cancer. Oral cancer is commonly associated with regional metastasis to neck nodes, which has been graded according to the site of involvement based on the lymph node classification (Table 30.6). Early-stage localised cancers have an 80% 5-year survival rate, but presence of lymph node metastases decreases survival by 50%. Thus, early detection is important for survival of oral cancer patients.

Anatomical path of lymphatic drainage

In the head and neck, the lymph nodes are arranged into different levels. The path of lymphatic drainage can be easily understood as two rings. The outer and bigger ring is called the 'outer circle' consisting primarily of the superficial nodes of the head, the ***submental nodes, submandibular nodes, parotid nodes, mastoid nodes and the occipital nodes***. The inner ring is called the 'inner circle' and contains the lymph nodes primarily in the neck region, the ***pretracheal nodes, paratracheal nodes and the retropharyngeal nodes***. The lymphatic

TABLE 30.6 Classification of Superficial Cervical Lymph Nodes by the AJCC

Levels	Region	Landmarks
IA	Submental triangle	Triangle bounded by anterior belly of the digastric and the mylohyoid
IB	Submandibular triangle	Triangle bounded by the anterior and posterior belly of the digastric and body of mandible
II	Upper jugular/jugulodigastric nodes	Nodes around the middle 3rd of internal jugular vein
IIA	Anterior to the spinal accessory nerve	Digastric muscle superiorly and the hyoid bone or the carotid bifurcation inferiorly
IIB	Posterior to the spinal accessory nerve	Digastric muscle superiorly and the hyoid bone or the carotid bifurcation inferiorly
III	Middle jugular nodes/juguloomohyoid	Carotid bifurcation superiorly to the cricothyroid notch inferiorly
IV	Lower jugular nodes	Omohyoid muscle superiorly to the clavicle inferiorly
V	Posterior triangle—spinal accessory nerve and the transverse cervical artery	Nodes are present along the lower half of the spinal accessory nerve and the transverse cervical artery. Level V includes supraclavicular nodes
VI	Anterior triangle—anterior jugular chain, juxtavisceral chain—prelaryngeal, pretracheal and paratracheal	Hyoid bone superiorly to the suprasternal notch inferiorly
VII	Superior mediastinal nodes	Lymph nodes in the tracheoesophageal groove

system is interconnected starting from the organ or the tissues or from the Waldeyer's ring to the superficial nodes of the outer circle or to the deeper nodes of the inner circle. All of the nodes in the outer circle and the inner circle drain into the deep cervical nodes around the Internal jugular vein (IJV) (Fig. 30.25A).

The lymph nodes of the head and neck drain directly or indirectly into the deep cervical group of nodes. They are all interconnected and collected by the jugular lymph trunk. The left jugular lymph trunk joins the thoracic lymph trunk. The right jugular lymph trunk empties independently at the junction of the IJV and subclavian vein (Fig. 30.25B).

Patterns of neck metastasis

The lymph nodes that are affected can show a sequential pattern, as only a selective group of nodes will be affected when a particular site is affected with cancer. For **oral cavity** as the primary site of cancer, for **submandibular and sublingual gland** primary tumours, the 1st ranks of lymph nodes affected will be **levels I, II and III**. For tongue cancers, the commonly metastasised lymph nodes are levels IIA and III, and tumours on the buccal mucosa usually metastasise to levels IB and IIA. Anatomically these levels of lymph nodes are contained in the supraomohyoid triangle. For tumours with primary site as **larynx and pharynx**, the 1st rank of affected nodes will be **levels II, III and IV**. For **primary parotid tumours**, the 1st rank lymph nodes are the **preauricular, parotid, levels II and III** lymph nodes are affected.

To understand the lymphatic spread of oral cancer, it is important for the clinician to have a sound knowledge of the lymph nodes draining the head and neck region (Flowchart 30.4).

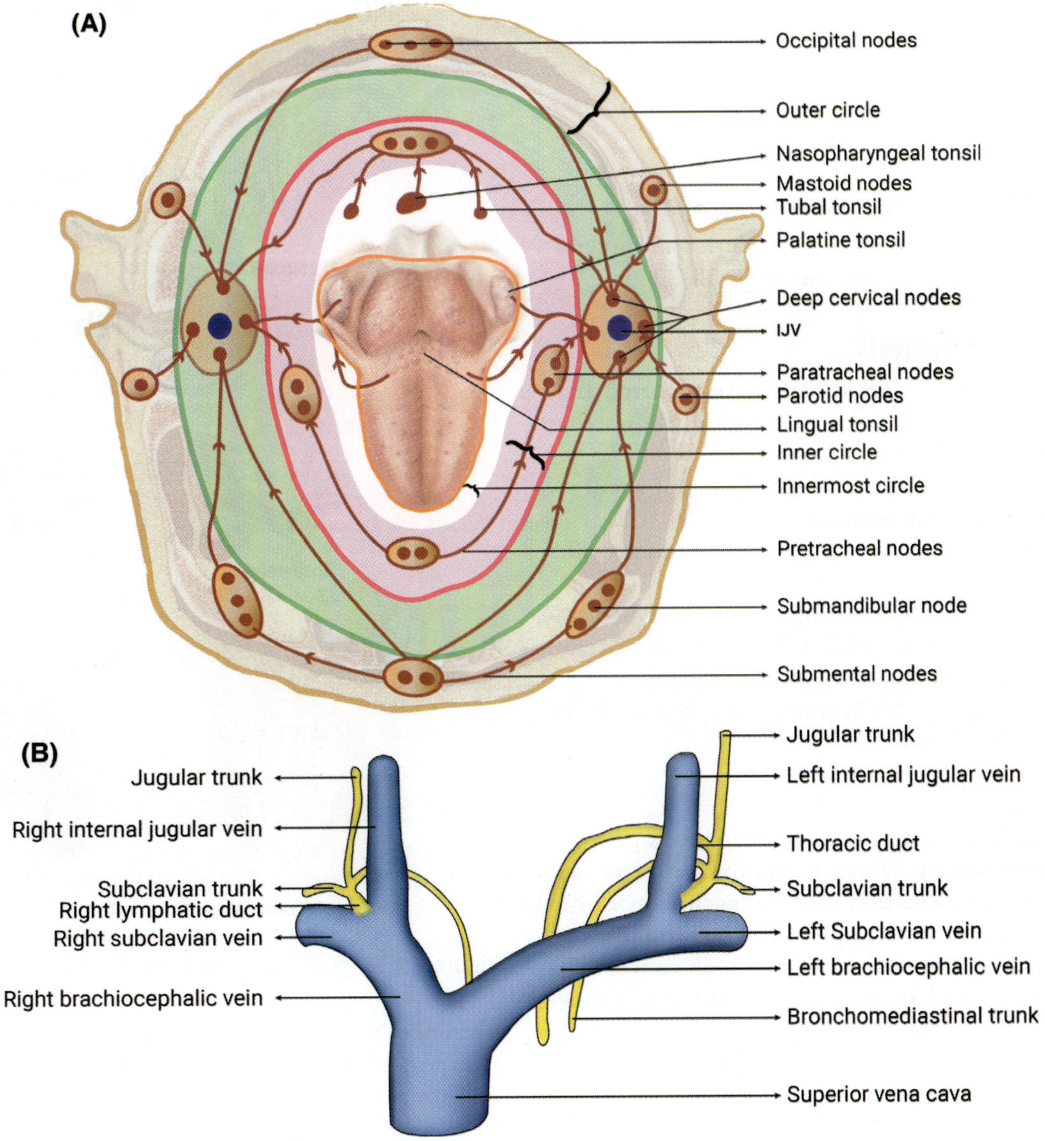

Figure 30.25 (**A**) Illustration showing path of lymphatic drainage of the lymph nodes of the head and neck. (**B**) Lymph drainage.

Skin of the Scalp	Occipital, Mastoid and Parotid Nodes
Lower Eye Lid and Malar Areas	Buccal Nodes which Drain into the Submandibular Lymph Nodes
Posterior Cheek Area	Parotid, Buccal and Submandibular Nodes
Upper Lip and Area Lateral to the Lower Lip	Submandibular Nodes
Medial Middle Third of the Lower Lip Crossover	Submental Nodes
Upper and Lower Gingivae	Submandibular, Submental and Upper Deep Cervical Lymph Nodes
Palatal Lymph Vessels	Submandibular and then into the Superior Deep Cervical Nodes
All Teeth	Submandibular and Deep Cervical Lymph Nodes
Anterior Floor of Mouth	Submental and Upper Deep Cervical Nodes
Posterior Floor of Mouth	Submandibular and Upper Deep Cervical Nodes

Flowchart 30.4 Showing lymphatic drainage of the areas of the head and oral cavity.

Factors that predict neck node metastasis

- Tumour thickness—above 5 mm—30% chance of neck node metastasis
- Depth of invasion more than 8 mm—presence of neck nodes.

Nodal staging in cervical metastasis (Fig. 30.26)

Staging for metastatic carcinoma or secondaries in the cervical lymph nodes by the AJCC 7th edition (Table 30.7):

Detection of neck metastasis

1. Clinical examination—many studies have reported that clinical examination is inferior to imaging studies that are available for the clinician
2. CT scan—investigation of choice due to better accuracy compared to clinical examination
3. USG-guided FNAC—has a better sensitivity and specificity for detection of nodal metastasis
4. PET-CT scan—is best for detecting occult node metastasis of neck for N0 patients. PET-CT has a higher overall cost and is not recommended as 1st line imaging
5. Sentinel node biopsy (SNB)—most accepted tool for management of neck nodes.

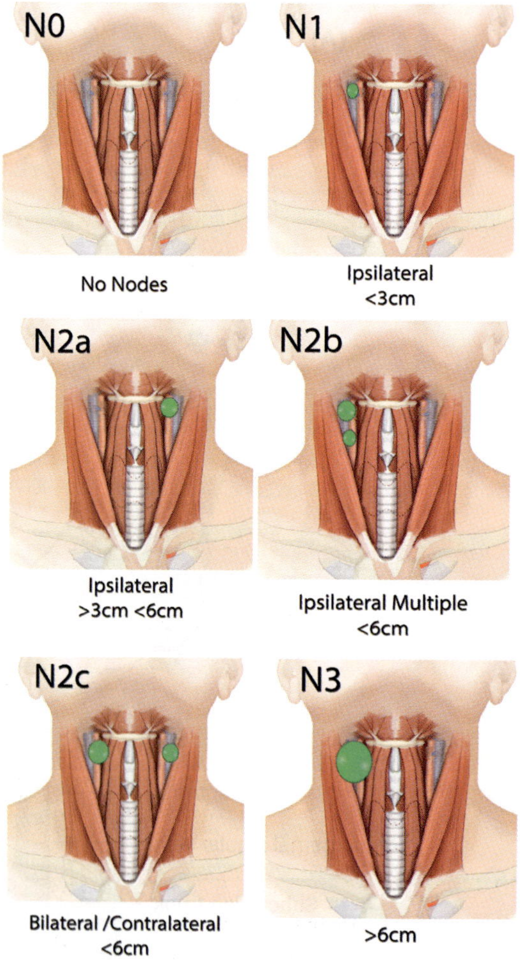

Figure 30.26 Nodal staging in cervical secondary metastasis.

SENTINEL NODE BIOPSY

SNB is a minimally invasive tool, used for intraoperative identification of metastatic lymph nodes for complete surgical excision. The identification rate and accuracy of SNB for head and neck tumours are up to 96%. A ***sentinel lymph node*** is defined as 'the 1st lymph node to which cancer cells are most likely to spread from a primary tumour. Sometimes, there can be more than one sentinel lymph node' (Fig. 30.27).

Sentinel lymph node biopsy is a procedure by which the sentinel lymph node is identified with a gamma probe, excised, and histologically examined to determine the presence of metastatic cancer cells from the primary tumour. A positive sentinel lymph node indicates the presence of metastases in nearby regional lymph nodes. Thus, SNB allows to determine the stage of the cancer for a better treatment plan.

TABLE 30.7 AJCC Staging for Metastasis of the Cervical Lymph Nodes

Nodal Staging	ECS Clinical/ Radiological	ECS—Histopathological	Description
NX			Regional lymph nodes cannot be assessed
N0			No regional lymph node metastasis
N1	E−: ECS is absent E+: ECS present	Eg: ECS is gross Em: ECS is microscopic En: ECS is not present	Metastasis in a single ipsilateral lymph node, 3 cm or less in greatest dimension
N2			Metastasis in a single ipsilateral lymph node, more than 3 cm but not more than 6 cm in greatest dimension; or in multiple ipsilateral lymph nodes, none more than 6 cm in greatest dimension; or in bilateral or contralateral lymph nodes, none more than 6 cm in greatest dimension
N2a			Metastasis in single ipsilateral lymph node more than 3 cm but not more 6 cm in greatest dimension
N2b			Metastasis in multiple ipsilateral lymph nodes, none more than 6 cm in greatest dimension
N2c			Metastasis in bilateral or contralateral lymph nodes, none more than 6 cm in greatest dimension
N3			Metastasis in a lymph node more than 6 cm in greatest dimension

ECS, extracapsular spread.

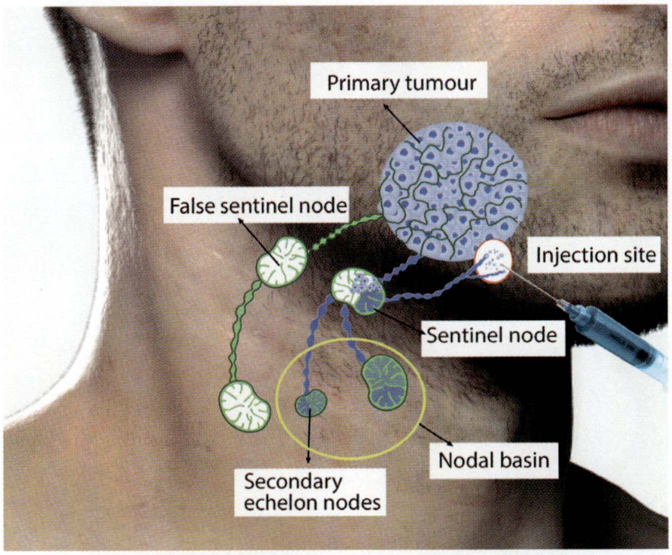

Figure 30.27 Sentinel lymph nodes are the 1st nodes that show metastasis due to a primary tumour.

Procedure

The primary tumour site is injected with a radiolabelled colloid and its flow from the primary tumour can be recorded on a gamma camera. The most commonly used radiolabelled colloid is 99mTc attached to sulphur colloid. The transit time of 99mTc sulphur colloid for mucosal head and neck cancer is less than 30 min and radioactivity can be detected 3–6 h after injection. The sentinel lymph nodes are those that show localisation of radioactivity after injection. The entire nodal basin is scanned by dynamic lymphoscintigraphy preoperatively. Intraoperatively, static lymphoscintigraphy is done with a handheld gamma probe. The nodal basin is exposed by surgery for neck dissection and the lymph nodes with higher radioactivity are termed as 'hot' lymph nodes. All nodes that are more than 10% hot are removed (Fig. 30.28).

TREATMENT OF CERVICAL LYMPH NODE METASTASIS

Cancer of the head and neck occurs in a region, which is highly vascular with rich lymphatic drainage; this facilitates early metastasis to regional lymph nodes. Neck dissection is the major part of surgical management of metastatic/secondary neck nodes.

Approaches to different neck dissections (Fig. 30.29)

The most commonly used incisions for neck dissections are as follows:

- Apron incision
- Half-apron
- Conley's incision
- Double Y incision

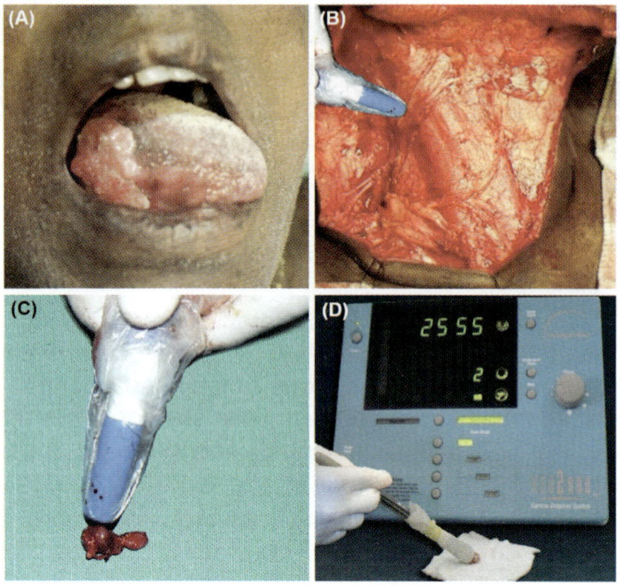

Figure 30.28 Procedure of sentinel lymph node biopsy with dynamic and static lymphoscintigraphy.

- McFee's incision
- H incision
- Schobinger's incision
- Modified Schobinger's incision
- Supraomohyoid neck dissection (SOHND) incision
- Extended SOHND incision for parotidectomy
- Extended SOHND incision for submental dissection
- Jugular node dissection incision.

TYPES OF NECK DISSECTION

Classical radical neck dissection (Crile's neck dissection)

The classic procedure involves en-bloc removal of the cervical lymphatics, IJV, spinal accessory nerve, submandibular gland, SCM muscle and the primary tumour. This usually causes disadvantages such as shoulder drop due to loss of accessory nerve supplying the trapezius muscle, neck deformity, facial swelling, numbness, neuromas and may also cause severe postirradiation complications such as carotid rupture.

- Lymph nodes excised are the levels I–V
- Structures excised are the:
  a. Spinal accessory nerve
  b. SCM muscle
  c. IJV
  d. Submandibular salivary gland.

Modified radical neck dissection

This type of neck dissection involves preserving undoubtful nonlymphatic structures in the neck, while removing all nodal groups (IV). The spinal accessory nerve is preserved at

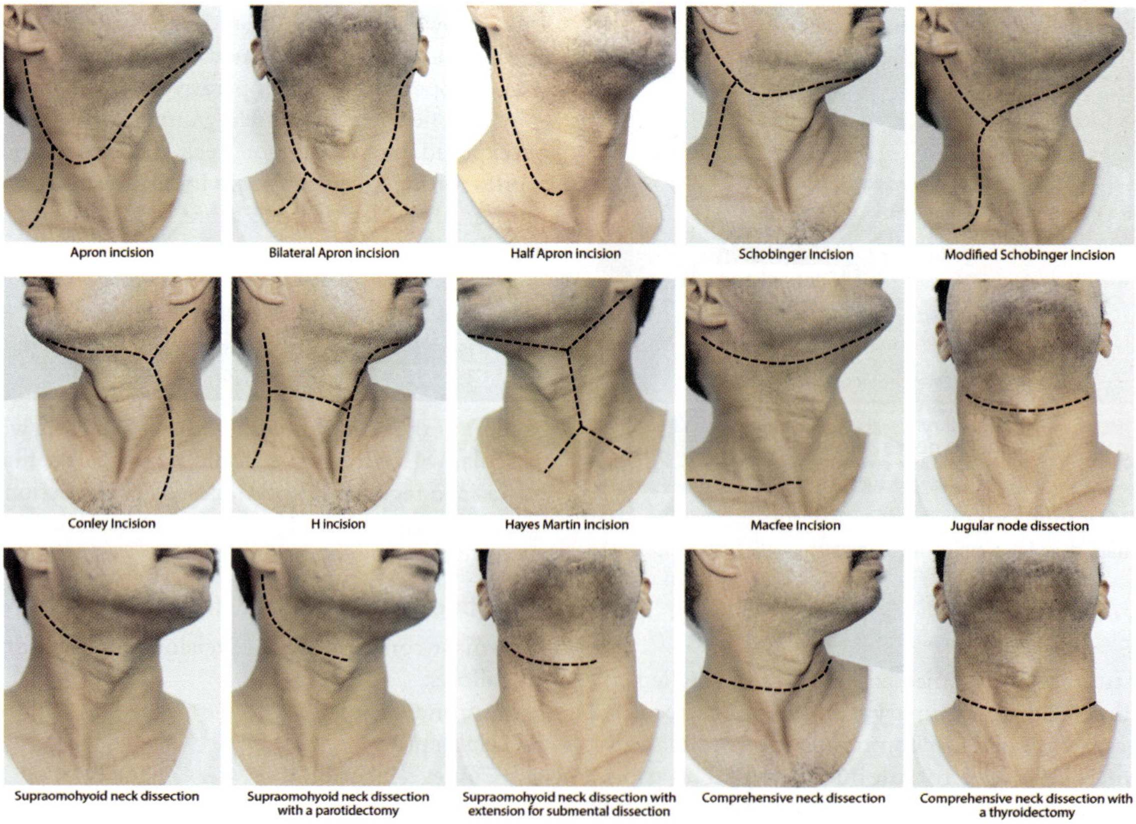

Figure 30.29 The most commonly used incisions for various types of neck dissections.

TABLE 30.8 Modified Radical Neck Dissection (MRND)

Types	Lymph Nodes Excised	Structures Excised	Structures Preserved
MRND I	Levels I–V	Sternocleidomastoid muscle Internal jugular vein Submandibular salivary gland	Spinal accessory nerve
MRND II	Levels I–V	Internal jugular vein Submandibular salivary gland	Spinal accessory nerve Sternocleidomastoid muscle
MRND III	Levels I–V	Submandibular salivary gland	Spinal accessory nerve Sternocleidomastoid muscle Internal jugular vein

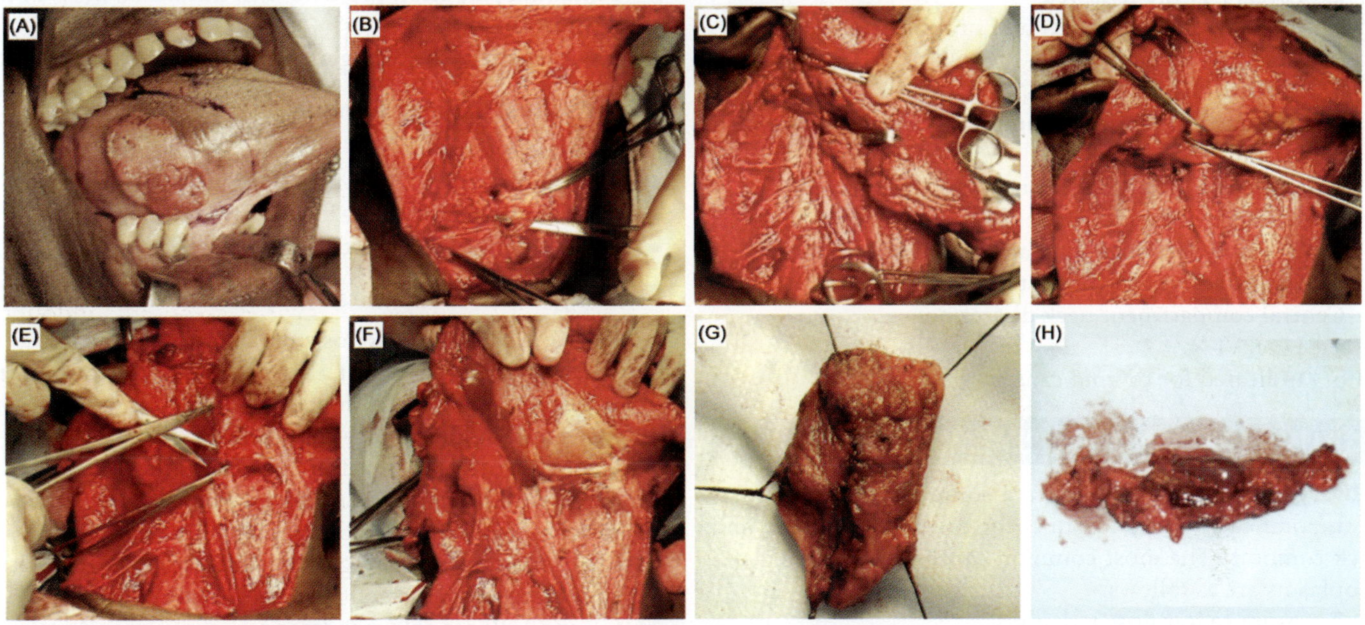

Figure 30.30 **(A)** Squamous cell carcinoma of the right lateral border of tongue. Incision marking for performing a wide excision of the primary tumour. **(B)** Subplatysmal dissection exposing right anterior and posterior triangles, the lower border of the sternocleidomastoid (SCM), the internal jugular vein (IJV) are identified and ligated. **(C)** Neck dissection—IJV ligation and clearance of levels I–V lymph nodes, followed by ligation of the branches of the external carotid artery. Dissection is continued in the posterior aspect of the anterior triangle of the neck to remove the fibrofatty tissue along with the radical neck dissection specimen. **(D)** Dissection performed to identify the posterior belly of the digastric muscle. **(E)** Ligation of the upper part of the IJV. **(F)** After completion of the radical neck dissection prior to excising the radical neck dissection specimen, viewing the clearance of the levels IV, III, II and I lymph nodes along with the SCM, IJV and fibrofatty tissue. **(G)** Excised tumour of tongue. **(H)** Cleared lymph nodes of lymphatic chain.

Erb's point, with the nerve exiting the posterior SCM and the greater auricular nerve arising from under it (Table 30.8).

- Type I modified radical neck dissection (MRND) preserves only the spinal accessory nerve (Fig. 30.30)
- Type II preserves the accessory nerve and the IJV
- Type III preserves these structures as well as the SCM muscle
- MRND III is also called the functional neck dissection. MRND should be performed when there is an evidence of nodal disease or there is a risk of probable nodal metastasis and surgery is being performed for the primary cancer.

Advantages include improved shoulder function, lower morbidity and mortality for bilateral neck dissections, protection for the carotid artery, staging for prognosis and/or use of adjuvant therapy, less cosmetic deformity and less facial oedema. Disadvantages include possibility of leaving positive nodes behind or cutting into positive nodes and seeding cancer.

Selective neck dissection

Selective neck dissection (SND) is done to remove a group of lymph nodes that are at risk of having secondaries due to micro metastasis. Clinically, the patient presents with a N0 neck. This is a modification of the RND in which one or more lymph node groups are removed. The SND is divided into subtypes:

1. Supraomohyoid neck dissection (SOHND)
   a. Levels I–III are removed
   b. Indicated for primary tumours of the oral cavity
2. Extended SOHND:
   a. Levels I–IV are removed
   b. Indicated for primary tumours of the lateral border of tongue
3. Anterolateral neck dissection:
   a. Levels I–IV are removed
   b. Indicated for oral cavity and oropharynx
4. Jugular node dissection:
   a. Levels II–IV are removed
   b. Indicated for primary tumours of hypopharynx and larynx
5. Posterolateral neck dissection:
   a. Suboccipital nodes, nodes of posterior triangle, levels II–V and deep jugular chain of nodes are removed
   b. Indicated for SCC of posterior scalp
6. Central compartment neck dissection:
   a. Level VI
   b. Indicated for thyroid cancer.

SALIVARY GLAND NEOPLASMS

Salivary gland neoplasms are rare compared to carcinomas of the oral cavity as it accounts for 3%–6% of all head and neck tumours. The most common causes for salivary gland neoplasms are as follows:

- Exposure to low dose radiation
- Exposure to wood dust
- Exposure to chemicals from leather tanning—adenocarcinoma of minor salivary glands of nasal cavity.

Majority of the malignant neoplasms of the salivary gland occur in the minor salivary glands. Pleomorphic adenomas are slow growing benign tumours of the parotid gland, but clinicians should be cautious if there is a sudden quickening of the growth as it may indicate malignant transformation. Mucoepidermoid carcinoma is most commonly seen in parotid and adenoid cystic carcinoma in the submandibular gland (Refer to chapter 31).

CLINICAL FEATURES

Parotid gland superficial lobe

- Asymptomatic mass in the superficial lobe anterior to the lobule of ear
- Enlarged ipsilateral cervical lymph node
- Facial nerve paralysis
- Invasion of overlying skin—surface ulceration
- Involvement of facial nerve.

Parotid gland deep lobe

- Diffuse enlargement
- Fullness of area posterior to the ramus
- Medial displacement of:
  a. Soft palate
  b. Tonsil
  c. Lateral pharyngeal wall
- Palpable parotid mass
- Trismus
  a. Dysphagia.

Submandibular gland tumour

- Painless swelling in the submandibular triangle
- Pain can occur with obstruction of the ducts
- Bimanual palpation presents with indurated mass in the floor of the mouth
- Involvement of the hypoglossal nerve or mandibular nerve.

Minor salivary gland tumour

- Submucosal mass
- Ulceration
- It may mimic mucocoele, but is firm on palpation
- Involvement of the greater palatine nerve.

Investigations used for salivary gland tumours

- FNAC: Gives 95% diagnosis of the malignancy status of salivary gland tumour. It also differentiates lymphomas, epithelial origin of tumour, metastatic or primary tumour and inflammatory conditions
- USG-guided FNAC for deep lobe tumours
- Large core biopsy and incisional biopsy are contraindicated as it can cause seeding of tumour cells
- Plain radiograph, sialography, nuclear scan and ultrasound are not indicated for final diagnosis
- CT and MRI are gold standards for salivary gland tumours
- CT scan and CECT: Differentiates cystic lesion and solid lesion, differentiates from normal surrounding tissue, show bony erosion and invasion. Allows better treatment planning
- MRI scan and contrast enhanced MRI: MRI differentiates deep lobe of parotid tumour from that of minor salivary gland tumour. It also shows enlargement or bony erosion of skull base neural foramina. Contrast enhanced MRI shows perineural tumour extension and invasion along cranial nerves
- PET scan: Useful to diagnose unknown primary or subclinical lesions. CT/PET combination can be used for determining exact extension of tumour.

Tumour staging (Table 30.9)

Treatment

1. Surgery
2. RT
3. Chemotherapy
4. Targeted therapy

TABLE 30.9 AJCC Staging of Salivary Gland Tumour

Tumour staging	Description
TX	Primary tumour cannot be assessed
T0	No evidence of primary tumour
T1	Tumour 2 cm or less in greatest dimension without clinical extra parenchymal extension
T2	Tumour more than 2 cm but not more than 4 cm in greatest dimension without clinical extra parenchymal extension
T3	Tumour more than 4 cm and/or tumour having clinical extra parenchymal extension
T4a	Moderately advanced local disease Tumour invades skin, mandible, ear canal and/or facial nerve
T4b	Very advanced local disease Tumour invades skull base and/or pterygoid plates and/or encases carotid artery

5. Immunotherapy
6. Combination therapy.

Surgery

- Surgery is the primary treatment modality for salivary gland neoplasms.
- The steps followed are:
  a. Resection of tumour
  b. Comprehensive neck dissection
  c. Reconstruction of defect (when skin or bone is involved)—local flap, distant flap or free flap are used
  d. Functional, aesthetic and psychological rehabilitation
  e. Follow-up
- Stages I and II can be cured by surgery alone
- Adjuvant therapy is required for Stages III and IV. Radiation therapy and chemotherapy are added along with the surgical excision
- Factors that influence surgery:
  a. Age
  b. Metastatic spread
  c. Skin, nerve and bone involvement
  d. Size, extent, grade, stage and site of tumour
- Parotid mass:
  a. Near-total parotidectomy:
     - Complete excision of lateral and deep lobes of the salivary gland and complete dissection of the facial nerve
     - Some salivary gland tissue may be left over
  b. Total radical parotidectomy/total conservative parotidectomy:
     i. Complete excision of the salivary gland and complete dissection of the facial nerve
  c. Extended radical parotidectomy:
     i. Complete resection of all salivary gland tissue with complete or partial resection of the facial nerve
- Submandibular mass:
  a. Complete resection of the gland and nerves with suprahyoid lymph node dissection

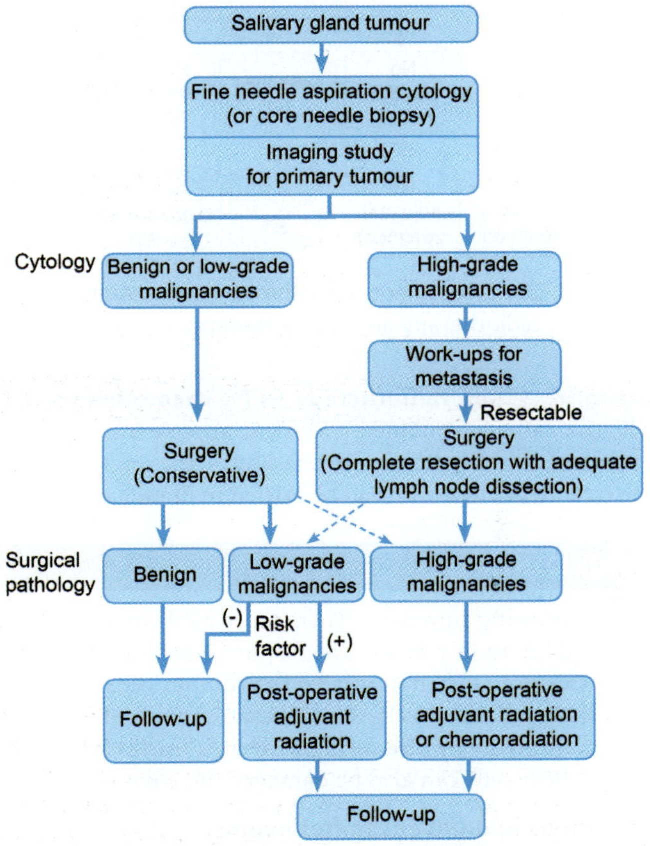

Flowchart 30.5 Treatment algorithm of salivary gland tumours.

- Minor salivary glands:
  a. Maxillectomy depending on involvement
- Treatment algorithm has been briefed in Flowchart 30.5.

ADJUVANT TREATMENTS FOR ORAL CANCER

General principles and management guidelines in oral cancer

The treatment for oral cancer depends on the diagnostic staging of the patient. The management of oral cancers include

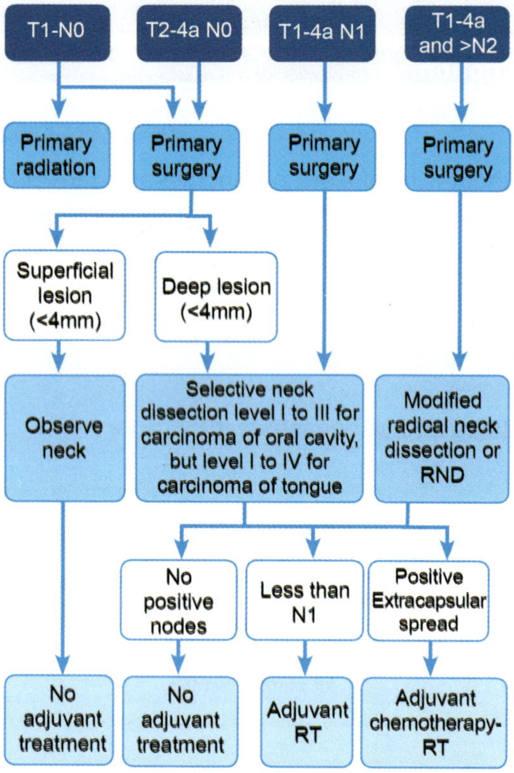

Flowchart 30.6 Treatment algorithm including surgery, neck dissection, radiotherapy and chemotherapy.

surgical resection, **radiotherapy (RT), chemotherapy** and palliative care. A combined treatment approach is indicated for patients with this disease depending on the stage of cancer. The treatment algorithm can be briefed in Flowchart 30.6.

RADIOTHERAPY

Actively growing tumour cells are more liable to ionising radiation than adult tissues. The faster the cells are multiplying or the more undifferentiated the tumour cells, the more likely that radiation is effective. Radiation prevents the cells from multiplying by interfering with their nuclear materials. Normal host cells can also be damaged by radiation.

Indications of adjuvant radiotherapy

1. T1–T2 lesions
2. Advanced T-stage (T3/T4)—locally advanced lesion
3. Presence of lymphovascular invasion
4. Presence of perineural invasion
5. Positive surgical resection margins
6. Multiple lymph node involvement (level IV/V)
7. Extracapsular nodal extension.

Radiation for oral cavity

- External beam radiation
- Interstitial implants (brachytherapy)
- Intraoral cone therapy.

Types of radiotherapy

The principal methods employed are as follows:

- X-ray therapy:
  a. Superficial X-ray therapy 45–100 kV
  b. Kilovoltage X-ray therapy 300 kV
- Electron therapy
- Surface applicator (radium mould)
- Brachytherapy—interstitial implantation—radium or equivalent source
  a. Placement of radioactive source on or in the tumour site.

Most commonly radiation is delivered externally by the use of large X-ray generators. The normal amount of tolerable radiation for a person should not be exceeded and adjacent uninvolved areas are spared by the use of protective shielding.

The patient's host tissues are protected from radiation by two mechanisms of delivery: (1) fractionation and (2) multiple ports.

FRACTIONATION

Fractionation of the delivery of radiation means that instead of giving the maximal amount of radiation a person can withstand at one time, smaller increments of radiation (fraction) are given over several weeks, which gives a time period for the normal tissues to recover between doses. The tumour cells, however, are less liable to recover between doses.

MULTIPLE PORTS

The 2nd method employs multiple ports for radiation exposure. Instead of delivering the entire dosage through one beam (port), multiple beams are used. All beams are focused on the tumour but from different angles. Thus, the tumour is exposed to the entire dosage of radiation. In this method, normal tissue exposure is reduced more as compared to fractionation method.

Radiation therapy is generally delivered on a 5-day-a-week basis in any of the several delivery schemes. The general therapeutic dose for head and neck cancer falls between 60 and 72 Gy, most commonly delivered on a once-a-day schedule. Fractionated regimens that deliver the radiation on a twice-a-day basis have shown greater efficacy in tumour elimination and even hyper-fractionated plans have been designed. The intensity of side effects, most notably mucositis, with the later approaches, however, has all but disallowed their use (Table 30.10).

Radiosensitisers

Radiosensitisers are compounds that sensitise the tumour cells to radiation during RT (Box 30.1).

Radioprotectors

Radioprotectors are chemical compounds that protect the non-tumour (normal) cells from radiation during RT (Box 30.1).

TABLE 30.10 Effects of Radiation

Mucositis and Candidiasis

- Usual treatment schedule 200 rad/day for 6 to 7 weeks
- Skin reaction prominent in 2–4 weeks; peak in 5 to 6 weeks; resolving by 6–8 weeks
- Mucositis becomes prominent in 1 to 2 weeks and peak in 4 to 5 weeks
- Clears shortly after or at completion of therapy (Fig. 30.31, Flowchart 30.7)

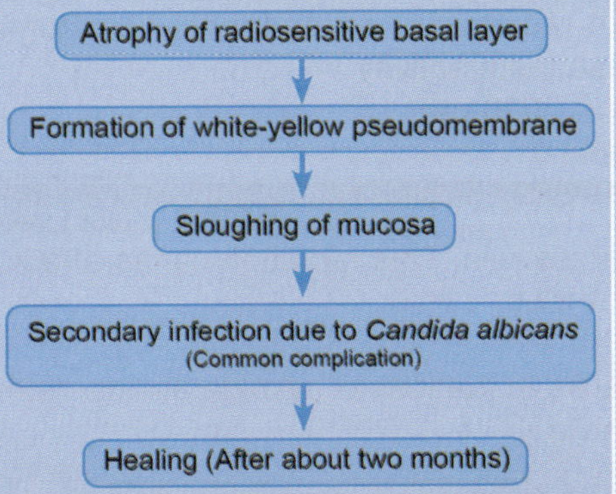

Flowchart 30.7 Pathway of mucositis and candidiasis for patients under radiotherapies.

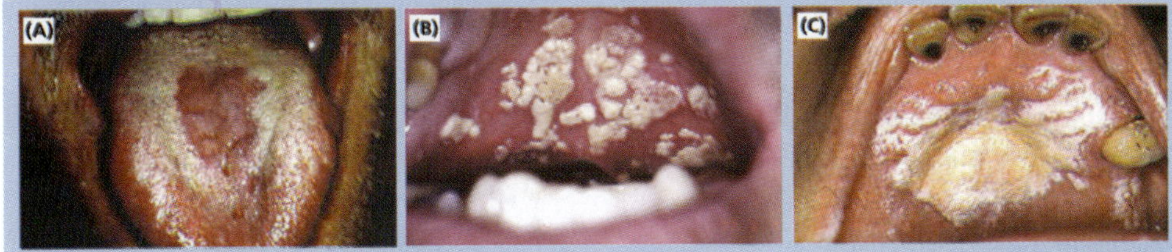

Figure 30.31 **(A)** Erythematous candidiasis on the dorsum of the tongue. **(B)** Candidiasis seen on the palate. **(C)** Pseudomembranous candidiasis.

Management

1. Diluting agents: Saline bicarbonate rinses, frequent rinses with water, dilute H_2O_2 rinses
2. Coating agents: Kaolin/pectin, aluminium chloride, aluminium hydroxide, magnesium hydroxide, hydroxypropyl cellulose, sucralfate
3. Lip lubrication: Water-based lubricants, lanolin
4. Topical anaesthetics: Xylocaine HCl, benzocaine HCl
5. Analgesic agents: Benzydamine HCl
6. β-Carotene

Xerostomia

- Results from direct effect on major salivary glands
- Salivary glands are affected when upper limit of field is at chin to mastoid
- Doses more than a total dose of 3000 Gy poses a risk if all major glands are in the field of radiation
- Irreversible effects occur with a total dose of 6000 Gy for 5 weeks
- Decrease in the rate of salivary flow occurs in the 1st week of treatment due to atrophy and necrosis of acinar cells, changes in the vascular connective tissues and altered neurologic function
- Serous acini are affected earlier. This results in thick and viscous secretions
- Changes in composition of saliva results due to decrease in secretory IgA and buffering capacity and acidity. This affects microbial flora and remineralising potential of teeth (Fig. 30.32).

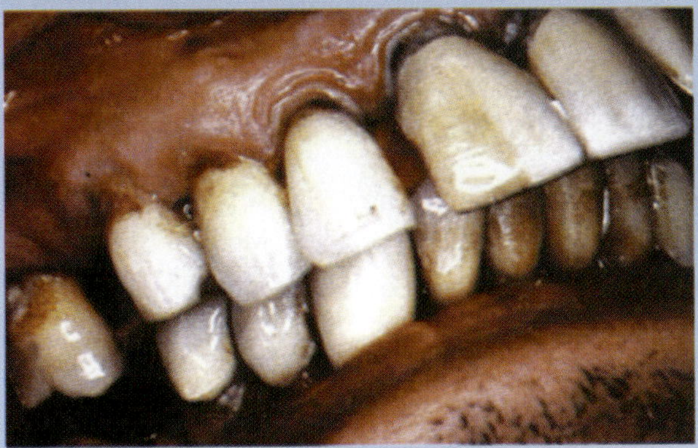

Figure 30.32 Xerostomia. Note the dry gingival mucosa and cervical caries.

Management

1. Stimulation of remaining salivary gland function:
   - Use of sialogogues Pilocarpine 15 mg/day
   - Anetholetrithione
   - Bethanechol and bromhexine
2. Radiobiologic approach to protect salivary glands from radiation:
   - Isoproterenol
   - Prophylactic use of pilocarpine (5 mg q.i.d.) stimulates salivary glands during radiotherapy
3. Palliation of xerostomia:
   - Mouth-wetting agents or saliva substitutes can be used
   - Frequent sipping of water and moist diet may be helpful
   - Carboxymethyl cellulose

Continued

TABLE 30.10 Effects of Radiation—cont'd

Loss of Taste	Management
• It may occur as a primary effect of radiation or secondary to xerostomia • Doses less than 2000 rad decrease taste activity • Complete subjective loss is seen at 3000 rad Patient notices this at 2nd or 3rd week	Taste loss is reversible, recovery happens in 60–120 days
Radiation Caries	**Management**
Usually, caries is associated with xerostomia. This radiation caries affects the gingival 3rd and incisal cusp tips of teeth *Aetiology of caries:* • Lack of production of saliva results in the loss of remineralising potential • Loss of buffering capacity of salvia • Increased acidity of saliva • Change in bacterial flora of saliva	• Oral hygiene maintenance • Manage xerostomia • Use of fluorides to harden tooth structures • Chlorhexidine rinses to reduce levels of *Streptococcus mutans* • Extract the teeth with doubtful prognosis 7–10 days before radiotherapy or within 7–10 days after commencement of radiotherapy with antibiotic coverage • Avoid surgical extractions
Osteoradionecrosis	**Management**
Inflammatory condition of the bone in line of fire, that occurs after radiation therapy for malignant neoplasms (Flowchart 30.8) 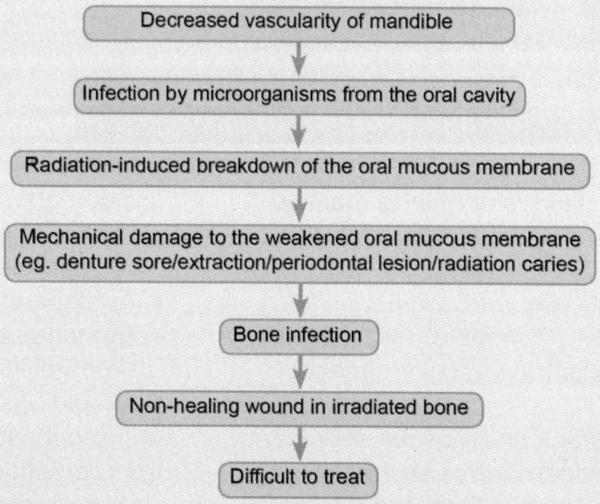 Flowchart 30.8 Pathogenesis of osteoradionecrosis.	• Debridement • Antibiotics • Supportive therapy • Analgesics • Good oral hygiene • Bone resection • Hyperbaric oxygen therapy (Refer chapter 24)
Muscular Fibrosis	**Management**
• Causes mandibular dysfunction • It occurs due to fibrosis of muscles • Inflammation and fibrosis of muscles due to radiation • Mandibular discontinuity • Restriction in mouth opening occurs 2 months after completion of radiotherapy • Masseter and pterygoid are involved	• Physiotherapy • Occlusal stabilisation appliances • Mandibular stretching exercises • Trigger point injection • Analgesics • Muscle relaxants • Tricyclic medication

BOX 30.1 The different radiosensitisers, radioprotectors and radiation mitigators are listed in the box

Radiosensitisers
- Hyperbaric oxygen
- Carbogen
- Nicotinamide
- Metronidazole and its analogues (Misonidazole, etanidazole, nimorazole)
- Hypoxic cell cytotoxic agents (mitomycin-C, tirapazamine)
- Membrane active agents (procaine, lidocaine, chlorpromazine)
- Radiosensitising nucleosides (5-fluorouracil, fluorodeoxyuridine, bromodeoxyuridine, Iododeoxyuridine, hydroxyurea, gemcitabine, fludarabine)
- Texaphyrins (Motexafin gadolinium)
- Suppressors of sulphydryl groups (N-ethylmalemide, diamide and diethyl maleate)
- Hyperthermia
- Novel radiosensitisers (paclitaxel, docetaxel, irinotecan)

Radioprotectors
- Amifostine
- Nitroxides (tempol)
- Other antioxidants (glutathione; lipoic acid; vitamins A, C and E; superoxide dismutase)
- Cysteine and cysteamine
- Melatonin
- Novel radioprotectors (tetracyclines and fluoroquinolones)

Radiation Mitigator
- Palifermin
- Halofuginone
- TGF-13
- Keratinocyte growth factor
- ACE inhibitors (captopril, enalapril, ramipril)
- COX-2 inhibitors/NSAIDs (celecoxib, aspirin, ibuprofen)

Radiation mitigator

Radiation-induced late normal tissue toxicity includes ongoing mitotic cell death and perpetually active cytokine cascades that can lead to vascular damage, tissue hypoxia and excessive extracellular matrix deposition. Radiation mitigators aim to interrupt these cascades or intervene to prevent the perpetuation of damage and thus reduce the expression of toxicity (Box 30.1).

CHEMOTHERAPY

Chemotherapy approaches

Chemotherapeutic agents are used in several therapeutic regimens and approaches. They are as follows:

1. Combination therapy
2. Induction chemotherapy
3. Concomitant chemotherapy
4. Adjuvant chemotherapy
5. Palliative chemotherapy
6. Chemoprevention.

These approaches are described in relation to head and neck squamous cell carcinomas (HNSCC), which are the primary focus of head and neck oncology.

Chemotherapeutic agents

- Cisplatin
- Carboplatin
- Taxanes
- 5-fluorouracil (5-FU)
- Methotrexate
- Ifosphamide
  a. Vincristine, bleomycin and methotrexate in various combinations have been used, but more recent protocols include platinum compounds most commonly in combination with 5-FU
  b. In cases of sarcoma, most regimens are combinations of vincristine, actinomycin D, cyclophosphamide and doxorubicin (adriamycin)
  c. Chemotherapy finds its main role as a support for radiation and/or surgical care. It is most effective for lesions confined strictly to the soft tissues.

Mechanism

- Drugs that interfere with the rapid growth of tumour cells are used for treating malignancies
- Chemotherapy is not as selective to the cells as RT, as it affects normal cells also during treatment
  a. Chemotherapy in combination with radiation is used as a radiation sensitiser.

Routes of administration

Intravenous and intraarterial

- The drugs are predominantly injected intravenously
- Recently intraarterial route for certain drugs have been introduced
- This systemic delivery of the drug produces adverse effects especially in the hematopoietic system, due to the rapid rate of cellular turnover of the blood cells
  a. Thus, patients under chemotherapy present with anaemia, neutropaenia and thrombocytopaenia

   b. Infections and bleeding are common complications in these patients
- To reduce the toxicity of a single agent given in large quantities, multiple-agent therapy is preferred
- Patients are subjected to three to five chemotherapy agents at the same time
   a. Each agent works at a different point in the life cycle of the tumour cell, thus increasing effectiveness with less toxicity to the host
- Intraarterial therapy is reserved for T3 and T4 lesions due to:
   a. Difficulties in performing and maintaining an intra-arterial catheter
   b. Excessive local tissue toxicity
   c. Difficulties in repeated therapy
- The drugs are introduced through branches of the external carotid artery
   a. In the superficial temporal branch, the drugs are injected in a retrograde manner.

Intralesional chemotherapy

- Intralesional injection of vinblastine, vincristine or interferon has been shown to be effective in the local control of epidemic Kaposi's sarcoma
- It can be used in combination with systemic chemotherapy or RT
- Lesions are reinjected at 3–6 week intervals
- In a study, 40% of Kaposi's sarcoma lesions require done injection for initial control, 31% required two injections and 29% required three injections. No lesions required more than three injections for initial control. This is followed by protocolled treatments.

Topical chemotherapy

- Actinic keratosis lesions have been effectively treated with the application of 5% fluorouracil (5-FU) cream
- 5-FU cream is applied twice daily for 3 to 4 weeks, by then the area shows an expected inflammatory reaction and ulceration
- Similar topical application of 5-FU in selected cases of multiple superficial BCC, basal cell naevus syndrome, has been effective
- Topical therapy is not effective for invasive lesions
- Surgical excision is still the treatment of choice for most cases of BCC.

Induction chemotherapy

- Initial chemotherapy before definitive local therapy
- Improves locoregional control by reducing size of primary tumour and reduces risk of metastatic recurrence
- Drugs used: Docetaxel, cisplatin, 5-FU.

Adjuvant chemotherapy

- It is the standard intervention after primary surgery for Stages III and IV
- Postoperative cisplatin and 5-FU
- Administered with adjuvant radiation therapy.

Chemoprevention

- Chemo preventive agents are used to prevent or to reverse carcinogenesis before an invasive cancer develops
- They also prevent a 2nd primary cancer in patients who have had a previous cancer cured
- The most effective preventive strategy for upper aerodigestive tract cancer is the cessation of smoking or any other carcinogenic habit
- ***Retinoids:***
   a. Retinoids regulate gene expression
   b. Synthetic retinoids have been produced by advances in molecular biology
      - This is less toxic and more effective in the prevention of cancer.

Chapter 31

Salivary Gland Pathologies

OUTLINE

SURGICAL ANATOMY

PAROTID GLAND

Parotid gland is the largest of the salivary glands and is a predominantly serous gland. In adults, it occupies a position from the zygomatic arch downward about 6 cm to just below the angle of the mandible and from just in front of the ear extending forward 3 or 4 cm on the surface of the masseter muscle. It is inverted pyramidal in shape with the apex towards the angle of the mandible and the base at the external acoustic meatus.

The capsule of the parotid gland is extensive and is derived from the investing layer of deep cervical fascia (Table 31.1).

Structures within the gland (Fig. 31.1)

- Arteries—external carotid artery, posterior auricular, superficial temporal and maxillary artery
- Veins—retromandibular vein forms from superficial temporal and maxillary vein
- Nerves—facial nerve
- Parotid duct (Stensen's duct)—It extends from anterolateral surface of the masseter muscle parallel to zygomatic branch 1.5 cm below it. It is 35–50 mm in length and 3 mm in diameter
- At the anterior border, it bends and pierces the buccal fat of pad and buccinator muscle and opens into the oral cavity opposite the crown of the maxillary 2nd molar
- Faciovenous plane of Patey.

TABLE 31.1 Relations of Parotid Gland

Borders	Structures
Anterior	• Masseter muscle • Ramus of mandible
Anteromedial	• Medial pterygoid muscle • Stylomandibular fascia
Medial	• Styloid process superomedially • Transverse process of the atlas inferomedially
Posteromedial	• Stylohyoid muscle • Posterior belly of the digastric muscle
Posterior	• Mastoid process of the temporal bone • Sternocleidomastoid muscle
Lateral	• Investing layer of deep cervical fascia, helping form the capsule
Superior	• External acoustic meatus • Condylar head of the mandible articulating in the glenoid fossa
Inferior	• *Angular tract of Eisler* between the angle of the mandible and the sternocleidomastoid muscle

Blood supply

External carotid artery supplies the parotid gland. The venous drainage from the gland is to the posterior facial vein and then to the internal jugular vein through the common facial vein.

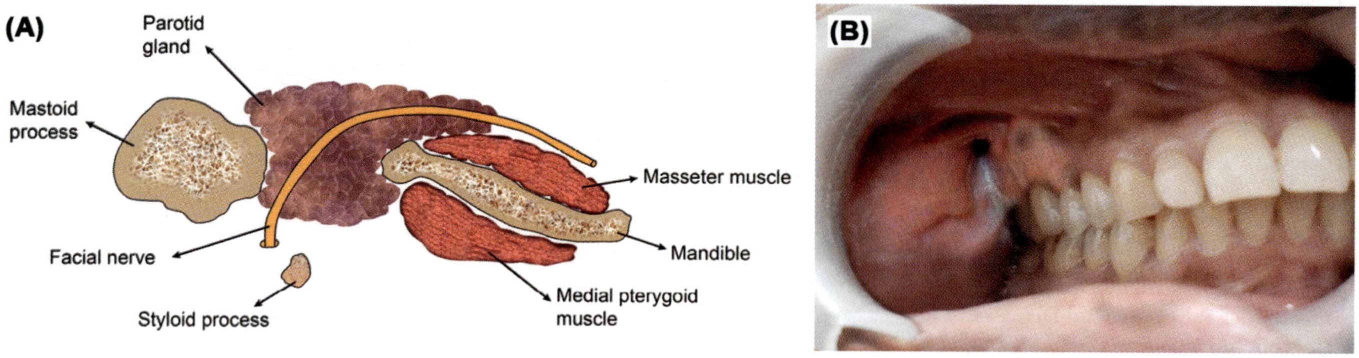

Figure 31.1 (A) Faciovenous plane of Patey. (B) Stensen's duct opening seen intraorally.

Nerve supply

The auriculotemporal nerve carries secretomotor fibres to the parotid gland and frequently anastomoses with the temporal branch of the facial nerve.

Lymphatic system

The parotid gland contains two layers of lymph nodes: superficial and deep. These two lymph nodes ultimately drain into the superior deep cervical nodes.

CLINICAL CONSIDERATIONS AND APPLIED ANATOMY OF THE PAROTID GLAND

- Due to the tight lateral (outside) fascial capsule, parotid gland enlargement is frequently excruciatingly painful
- Due to the loose medial capsule, gland enlargement is typically visible externally in the late stages of illness
- Before its exit, the parotid duct widens, and the right-angle bend of the parotid duct causes saliva to stagnate. Here, epithelial cells and other organic materials can become entrapped, producing blockages, stone formation, etc
- In Frey's syndrome/auriculotemporal syndrome, the injury to the salivary gland's autonomic innervations and the inappropriate regeneration of parasympathetic fibres are responsible. The auriculotemporal nerve's secretomotor fibres unite with the greater auricular nerve. Stimulation of the salivary glands stimulates sweat glands on the skin's surface
- Mumps or viral parotitis seldom suppurates
- Deep parotid tumours can spread into the lateral pharyngeal space and bulge the lateral pharyngeal wall
- Mixed parotid tumour is slow-growing, lobulated, painless tumour without facial nerve involvement. Pain, fast development, hardness, facial nerve involvement and enlarged cervical lymph nodes suggest malignant transformation
- The facial nerve is near to the parotid gland and should be considered during surgery. In parotid abscess, the skin incision for drainage can be vertical, but the deeper incision must be horizontal to prevent branch damage. During parotidectomy, the facial nerve is protected by removing the gland superficially and deeply
- During surgery, the plane of cleavage is determined by following the nerve from its origin in the back to its ending point in the front of the body
- The facial nerve is located in the superficial zone of Patey's fasciovenous plane. The retromandibular vein is one of the most essential markers in identifying the facial nerve, especially when a retrograde dissection is used. Typically, the retromandibular vein resides deep and medial to either the main facial nerve trunk or its branches. Any alteration in this nerve–vein interaction might make it more difficult to identify the nerve, increasing the risk of damage.

SUBMANDIBULAR GLAND

Submandibular gland is the 2nd largest of the salivary gland weighing 10–15 g. It contains both serous and mucous secreting glandular elements. This gland lies in the submandibular triangle or digastric triangle. It is J-shaped. The largest portion of the gland lies below the mylohyoid muscle. It extends as far anteriorly to the anterior belly of digastric and posteriorly to the stylomandibular ligament, which keeps it separate from the parotid gland.

At the posterior border of the mylohyoid muscle, a process of the gland curves upwards around the muscle and extends medially towards the genioglossus muscle to lie in the lateral sublingual space. It is divided into superficial and deep parts by mylohyoid muscle (Table 31.2).

TABLE 31.2 Relations of Submandibular Gland

Borders	Structures
Anterior	Sublingual gland
Posterior	Posterior belly of digastric, stylohyoid and parotid gland
Medial	Hyoglossus and styloglossus
Lateral	Mylohyoid muscle and superficial part of the gland
Superior	Lingual nerve and submandibular ganglion
Inferior	Hypoglossal nerve

Submandibular duct (Wharton's duct)

Submandibular duct emerges at anterior end of deep part. It is 5 cm long and runs forward between the mylohyoid and hyoglossus muscles and then onto the genioglossus muscle opening in the floor of mouth on the summit of lingual papilla at the side of frenulum of the tongue.

Nerve supply

The parasympathetic nerve supply is via the chorda tympani nerve, which carries preganglionic fibres to the submandibular ganglia. Postganglionic fibres originate in this ganglion and pass to the gland. The sympathetic nerve fibres are carried along the lingual artery to the gland.

Lymphatic drainage

The lymphatic drainage is into the submaxillary nodes and then to the jugular chain.

CLINICAL CONSIDERATIONS AND APPLIED ANATOMY OF SUBMANDIBULAR GLAND

The tortuous path of the submandibular duct causes saliva to stagnate, resulting in the production of ***sialolithiasis***. The Wharton's duct, like the parotid duct, is broader before reaching the papilla. Saliva and organic debris may get stagnant as a result of this. The duct's lengthy and winding path also causes saliva to get stagnant. The Wharton's duct's steep bend at the posterior border of the mylohyoid muscle allows for salivary stasis, which promotes the production of salivary stones. The most common reason for submandibular gland excision is sialolithiasis

Sialadenitis: The gland and duct of the submandibular gland are located below the level of the oral cavity. It makes the gland vulnerable to retrograde infection. The gland's punctum, on the other hand, is narrowed to prevent bacteria-laden oral secretions from flowing backwards

Submandibular gland removal: To avoid injury to the marginal mandibular branch of the facial nerve, the incision for the submandibular gland removal is made 5 cm below the angle of the jaw. The ability to distinguish between an enlarged submandibular gland and a mass of submandibular lymph nodes requires bimanual palpation. The submandibular glands are responsible for the generation of nearly 60% of resting saliva; hence, their preservation, if feasible, will lessen xerostomia after radiation therapy. The submandibular gland is regularly removed during neck dissection, despite the fact that it contains no nodes. According to the most recent research, unless there is an obvious malignancy, it is typically possible to remove all of the nodes in the area without sacrificing the gland, as occult tumours are uncommon.

SUBLINGUAL GLAND

Sublingual gland is the smallest of the salivary gland and usually weighs 2 g. It is mucous in nature. It is almond-shaped and lies in the sublingual depression on the inner surface of the mandible, near the symphysis under the mucosa of the floor of the mouth. It is located above the mylohyoid line of the mandible and rests on the mylohyoid muscle. There is no discrete capsule for the sublingual gland. There are around 20 small sublingual ducts known as *ducts of Rivinus* opening into floor of mouth. Main duct known as Bartholin's duct opens into the submandibular duct.

Nerve supply

The nerves of the glands are the parasympathetic secretory nerves from the chorda tympani nerve, the sympathetic nerves are from the plexus on the facial artery and the sensory nerves are from the lingual nerve.

Lymphatic drainage

Lymphatic drainage is into the submental and submandibular lymph node groups.

CLINICAL CONSIDERATIONS AND APPLIED ANATOMY OF SUBLINGUAL GLAND

The sublingual gland is not amenable to sialography. If the gland is involved in a ranula, the gland is completely removed. The submandibular duct and lingual nerve, as well as the sublingual artery and vein, are among the tissues at risk during sublingual gland dissection.

MINOR SALIVARY GLANDS

Minor salivary glands have been estimated to number between 600 and 1000. They are small, independent, predominately mucous glands except *Von Ebner's glands*, which is a serous gland. Though these glands are found in almost every part of the oral cavity, they are predominant in the posterior palate. The rest are found in the mucosa of the oral cavity—lips, cheeks, the floor of the mouth, the retromolar region, etc. They can also be found in the tongue, oropharynx, larynx, trachea and paranasal sinuses, as well as other parts of the upper aerodigestive tract. This is of significance due to the high occurrence of malignant tumours in the posterior palate.

CONSIDERATIONS IN CLINICAL PRACTICE AND APPLIED ANATOMY OF MINOR SALIVARY GLANDS

The ducts of the sublingual gland and the minor salivary glands are short, reducing the risks of stasis. As a result, these glands do not develop obstructive lesions. Because minor salivary glands are placed so close to the surface, they are more susceptible to traumatic lesions like ***mucocoeles***.

DIAGNOSIS OF SALIVARY GLAND DISEASES

CLINICAL EXAMINATION

Parotid gland

- Normal parotid gland is not evident clinically unless enlarged

- Parotid swelling classically causes ear lobule elevation (superficial lobe), lateral pharyngeal or retromandibular angle swelling (deep lobe)
- Parotid gland can be palpated in the preauricular, inferior auricular and postauricular regions
- Palpate the gland and nodes bilaterally
- Gently dry the opening of Stensen's duct with gauze, milk the gland by external compression to observe salivary flow.

Submandibular gland

- The submandibular gland is checked by *bimanual palpation*, by placing a finger of one hand in the submandibular region and another intraorally in the floor of the mouth
- The submandibular nodes are palpated by tipping the patient's head slightly down and forward to relax the tissues. 'Cup' the mandible with thumb and fingers and palpate bilaterally. Draw tissue against the lateral border of the mandible. Use bidigital and circular compressions
- The gland is palpable by bimanual palpation (intraoral–extraoral), whereas the node is not evident by this manoeuvre (palpable only extraorally).

SALIVARY GLAND INVESTIGATIONS

Salivary gland imaging

Imaging techniques help to diagnose and differentiate the salivary gland diseases from other diseases. Imaging plays an important role in the diagnosis of many salivary gland diseases and disorders. The various imaging techniques include:

Plain radiographs, sialography, computed tomography (CT), ultrasonography (USG), magnetic resonance imaging (MRI), and radioisotope scanning.

PLAIN-FILM RADIOGRAPHS

Plain radiographs have been used widely to visualise calcification within the salivary glands. They have been used to demonstrate bony changes adjacent to those structures and to show distant effects of salivary disease such as metastases but has been effectively replaced by advanced imaging modalities.

It has the potential to identify unrelated pathoses in the area of the salivary glands that may be mistakenly identified as salivary gland disease, such as resorptive or osteoblastic changes in adjacent bone causing periauricular swelling mimicking a parotid tumour.

Panoramic and conventional posteroanterior (PA) skull radiographs may demonstrate bony lesions, thus eliminating salivary pathosis from the differential diagnosis.

A plain film radiograph may demonstrate a deep antegonial notch, overdeveloped mandibular angle and exostosis on the outer surface of the angle in cases of masseter hypertrophy.

1. ***Intraoral radiographs***
   a. **Periapical radiograph**
   b. **Occlusal radiograph**
2. ***Extraoral radiographs***
   a. **Panoramic projection**
   b. **Lateral projection**
   c. **PA skull projection (with puffed cheek).**

Calcification within the glands

- Calculi present in Wharton's duct are best demonstrated by the use of the intraoral occlusal films, and those situated in the submandibular gland by occlusal or extraoral films
- Calculi in the parotid duct canals can be demonstrated on an extraoral film that is placed at a right angle to the surface of the face, with the direction of the tube parallel to the cheek, the exposure is made when the cheek is blown outwardly or laterally by the patient (puffed cheek view). This provides less superimposition of the osseous structures. Other projection used for parotid gland is the frontal view
- Intraoral views are most easily achieved using a dental radiography set. The value of intraoral views in identifying stones in the submandibular and parotid ducts is well known. The periapical film is placed between the teeth and the cheek and is an extremely sensitive method of demonstrating radiopaque calculi in the parotid duct.

Disadvantages

- Limited soft tissue in formation
- Low sensitivity for involvement of adjacent bony structures
- Exposure to radiation doses.

SIALOGRAPHY

It is a specialised procedure for radiographic demonstration of major salivary glands by introducing radiopaque contrast medium into the ductal system and is termed as sialography (Figs. 31.2 and 31.3).

The various contrast agents and sialographic appearances have been enumerated in Tables 31.3–31.4.

Indications

To determine the following:

- Presence and/or position of calculi or other ductal obstruction
- Extent of ductal and glandular destruction secondary to an obstruction
- Extent of glandular breakdown.

Contraindications

- Allergy to the contrast agent (especially iodine)
- Acute infection/inflammation (discharge of pus from the duct opening)
- Radiographs showing calculus close to the duct opening—risk of dislodgement into the gland.

Different sialographic techniques

- Simple injection technique
- Continuous infusion pressure-monitored technique.

Phases of the procedure

The sialographic procedure is divided into three phases:
- Preoperative phase
- Filling phase
- Emptying phase.

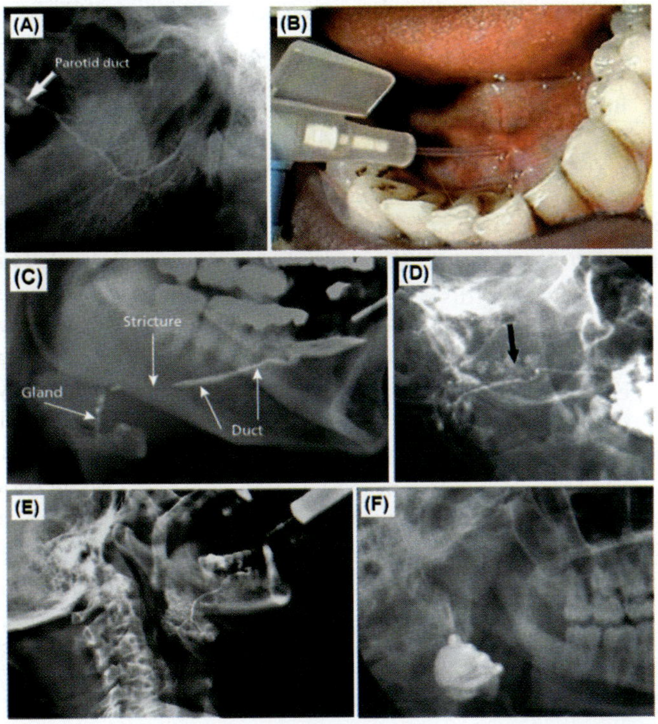

Figure 31.2 **(A)** Normal sialographic view of parotid gland. **(B)** Cannulation at the ductal orifice. **(C)** Sialograph showing submandibular stricture. **(D)** Sialograph of parotid gland demonstrating narrowing and strictures of Stensen's duct. **(E)** Sialography performed in submandibular gland showing normal sialograph. **(F)** Sialography showing salivary fistula as a complication after retromandibular approach to condylar fracture.

Step 1: preoperative phase

This involves taking preoperative (scout) radiographs to assess the following:
- Position and/or presence of any radiopaque obstruction
- Position of shadows of normal anatomical structures that may overlie the gland such as the hyoid bone.

Step 2: filling phase

- A lacrimal or periodontal probe is used to dilate the sphincter at the ductal orifice before the passage of a cannula, which is a blunt needle or catheter connected by extension tubing to a syringe containing contrast agent
- Contrast solution is then slowly infused until the patient feels discomfort (usually between 0.2 and 1.5 mL, depending on the gland being studied). These iodine-containing agents render the ductal system radiopaque
- The filling phase can be monitored by fluoroscopy or with static films. The radiographs are taken, ideally at least two different views at right angles to one another.

Step 3: emptying phase

The gland is allowed to empty for 5 min without stimulation.

The use of lemon juice at this stage to aid excretion of the contrast medium is often advocated.

COMPUTED TOMOGRAPHY

Magnetic resonance imaging (MRI) has become the diagnostic tool of choice in assessing most masses in the head, while computed tomography (CT) is still the most useful imaging modality in the neck. The advantage of MRI over CT is in its superior soft tissue resolution, while CT retains the advantage in defining cortical bone. MRI, however, is much more sensitive to the soft tissue component of bone, that is the marrow space. Therefore, MRI provides the best definition of tumour margins and better localises the extent of regional spread, particularly along nerves.

TABLE 31.3 Contrast Agents Used for Sialography

Aqueous-Based Solutions	Oil-Based Solutions
Contrasts Agents 1. Ionic aqueous solutions Diatrizoate (Urografin), Metrizoate (Triosil) 2. Nonionic aqueous solutions Iohexol (Omnipaque)	**Contrasts Agents** • Iodised oil, e.g. lipiodol (iodised poppy seed oil)
Advantages • Easily introduced because of low viscosity • Easily and rapidly removed from the gland • Easily absorbed and excreted if extravasated	**Advantages** • Densely radiopaque, and thus good contrast
Disadvantages • Less radiopaque, and thus less contrast • Low viscosity, and thus fast excretion	**Disadvantages** • High viscosity, thus slow excretion. High pressure is needed to introduce the contrast agent • Risk of calculi dislodgement into the main duct • Foreign body reaction from remnants of contrast materials

TABLE 31.4 Sialographic Appearances

Normal and Pathological Conditions	Sialographic Appearance
Parotid Gland • Main duct diameter (1–2 mm wide), filled completely and uniformly. • The duct structure within the gland branches regularly and tapers gradually towards the periphery of the gland, the so-called tree in winter appearance	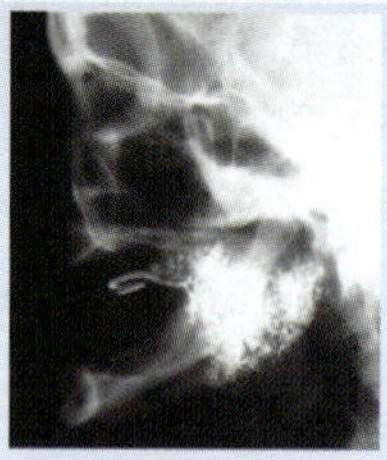 Figure 31.3 (A) Sialograph showing tree in winter appearance
Submandibular Gland • Main duct diameter (3-4 mm wide), filled completely and uniformly • Branching duct structure tapering gradually towards the periphery- the so-called bush in winter appearance	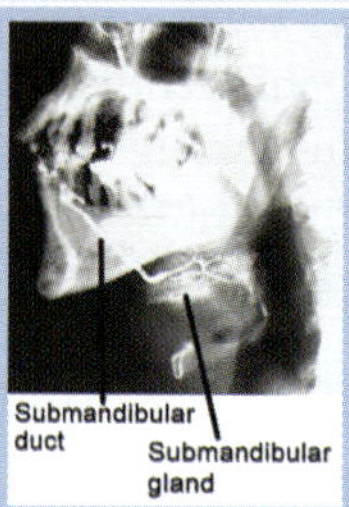 Figure 31.3 (B) Sialographic view of submandibular gland
Nonopaque sialolith • Filling defect(s) in the main duct • Ductal dilatation proximal to the calculus • The emptying phase usually shows contrast medium retained behind the stone	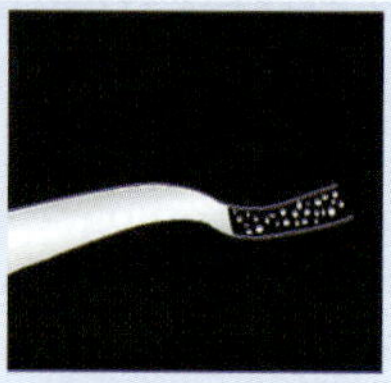 Figure 31.3 (C) Filling defect of stricture
Sialadenitis Dots or blobs of contrast medium within the gland. an appearance known as sialectasis This is due to inflammation of the glandular tissue and saccular acinar dilatation	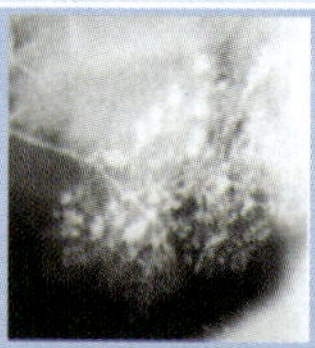 Figure 31.3 (D) Dots or blobs like appearance within the gland
Sjogren's syndrome Snowstorm appearance or punctate sialectasis or cherrv blossom appearance or branchless fruit laden tree appearance	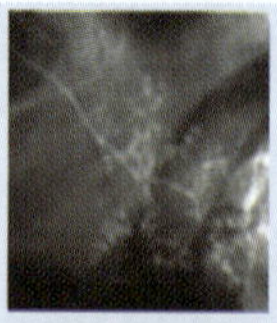 Figure 31.3 (E) Snowstorm appearance
Intraglandular neoplasm This finding is the result of duct displacement and pressure induced b a benign tumour with a capsule or oseudocapsule.	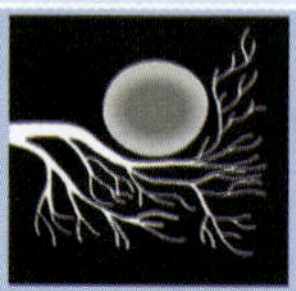 Figure 31.3 (F) Ball in hand appearance

Uses

- CT is remarkably sensitive to the presence of calcification and may demonstrate intraductal or intraglandular calculi, which have escaped detection on good quality plain radiographs
- CT scans helps to define the cystic wall better and thus helps to differentiate between the fluid containing masses like cyst, abscess, etc
- The unexpected involvement of adjacent bony structures in a malignant or inflammatory process is sometimes revealed by CT, which is excellent in demonstrating periosteal reaction and early cortical destruction.

Disadvantages of computed tomography scan for salivary gland imaging

- Parenchymal disease is not well displayed by CT
- In almost all cases, the appearances given by the autoimmune diseases, sialadenitis and sialosis are similar, showing enlarged glands with increased attenuation. Fatty changes may also be apparent as areas of lower attenuation
- CT cannot image the facial nerve and its ability to identify lesions as being in the superficial or deep lobes relies on indirect markers
- Masses within the salivary glands are usually well shown, although the limited soft tissue contrast inherent to this technique may require administration of intravenous contrast medium to render some lesions apparent.

COMPUTED TOMOGRAPHY SIALOGRAPHY

Tumours would be better delineated from the surrounding parenchyma if the parenchyma were opacified with intraductal contrast media. Although majority of salivary tumours are distinguishable by conventional CT, a minority has defied detection, even when intravenous contrast has been administered. CT sialography has also been used to predict the tumour as being superficial or deep to the plane of the facial nerve, the rationale being that the course of the parotid duct and the facial nerve lie in similar planes.

Intravenous contrast media are used in the CT of salivary glands for two reasons:

- To obtain information about the nature and extent of a tumour
- To help delineate blood vessels from lymphadenopathy.

Advantages

- Wide field of view
- Very sensitive for soft tissue calcification and bone involvement
- Usually good soft tissue discrimination
- Not operator dependent.

Disadvantages

- Difficult to scan in planes other than axial plane
- May require intravenous contrast for best results
- Radiation dose received is high.

MAGNETIC RESONANCE IMAGING

MRI relies on the electromagnetic properties of protons and particularly in relation to the energy released when such particles decay from high to a relatively low energy state within an externally applied magnetic field. MRI differs markedly from CT in its apparent sensitivity to calcification. Heavily calcified tissue such as cortical bone or calculi produces no significant signal on MRI and is thus distinguished as a 'signal void'. This means that neither calculi nor dystrophic calcification within a tumour are visible.

Uses

- Sjogren's disease
- Neoplasms: Tumour delineation is assisted in many cases by gadolinium administration. The edge of a lesion may be better evaluated following contrast and the internal structure of tumours can be seen in the images. Unsuspected infiltration of a malignant process beyond the confines of the gland may be seen after gadolinium administration
- Magnetic resonance angiography (MRA) is used in vascular lesions to demonstrate the intraglandular and extraglandular blood vessels in case of any lesions involving or related to the gland. Additionally, the extent of vascular malformations in the region of the salivary glands can be well appreciated.

Advantages

- Nonionising radiation
- Excellent soft tissue (including bone marrow) discrimination
- Ability to reconstruct images in any scan plane
- Not operator dependent.

Disadvantages

- Not widely available
- Poor cortical bone detail
- Long scanning time
- Restricted field of view in some circumstances
- Not tolerated by all patients.

ULTRASONOGRAPHY

Ultrasonography imaging relies upon the transmission of high-frequency sound, which is attenuated as it passes through tissue, at a rate dependent upon the acoustic properties of that tissue and upon the frequency of the incoming waveform (Fig. 31.4).

Uses

- Presence of solid or cystic masses can be detected
- Calculi of the salivary glands can be detected
- Can detect masses present within the gland and outside the gland
- It aids in distinguishing between intraparotid neoplasms and a superficially located lesion extrinsic to the gland.

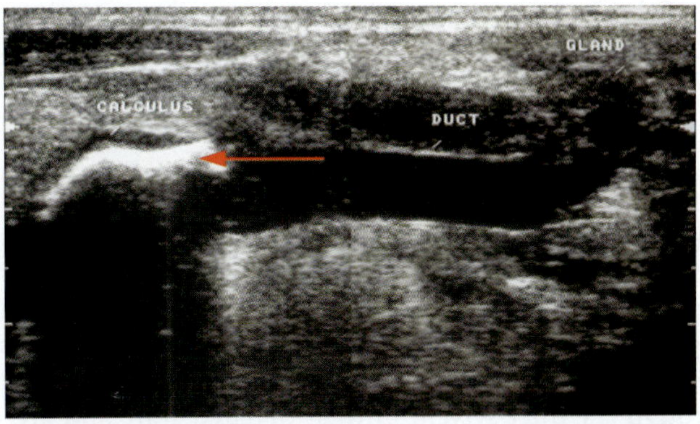

Figure 31.4 Ultrasonograph showing the presence of calculus in the Wharton's duct.

RADIOISOTOPE SCANNING OR SCINTIGRAPHY

The functional basis is a gamma ray-emitting radionuclide, which is directed to a particular area of interest through ingestion, inhalation or intravenous injection. The emitted radiation is detected by a gamma camera consisting of a scintillation crystal and photomultipliers (hence the term scintigraphy)—following computer processing, the activity is displayed in either static or dynamic modes. The radioisotope commonly used is Technetium-99m (^{99m}Tc).

The principal limitation of the radioisotope scan is resolution. Tumours less than 1 cm in diameter cannot be evaluated.

Uses

- It is particularly used in the diagnosis of obstructive sialadenitis. They help to differentiate between acute obstructive and nonobstructive sialadenitis
- Helps in the detection of certain tumours.

Advantage

Pathophysiological information is good for assessment of metastatic spread.

Disadvantages

- Poor anatomical discrimination
- Risk of allergic reaction/anaphylaxis from the radioisotope.

INTERVENTIONAL RADIOLOGY

Interventional radiological techniques are used for minimally invasive procedures with imaging control.

GUIDED BIOPSY TECHNIQUES

Guided biopsy is used widely in many areas of the body, primarily as a method of obtaining material for histological or microbiological examination that would otherwise only be available by open operation.

- CT-guided techniques enable a two-dimensional image using skin markers as a guide, from which the entry point, angulation and depth of insertion of the biopsy device may be electronically planned

- Ultrasonically guided biopsy is particularly suited to relatively superficial regions and not only gives a real-time image of the process but also has the ability to image the needle tip as it is guided into the target lesion.

DILATATION OF DUCT STRICTURES

The high viscosity of the oil-based sialographic contrast media has encouraged attempts to dilate minor duct strictures by hydrostatic pressure transmitted via these agents. High-pressure angioplasty balloon catheters may be used for dilating stenosed ducts. Such balloons are advanced through the duct system in their deflated state and are inflated once accurately positioned across the stricture. A minimal papillotomy may be required for initial passage. The balloons are accurately sized for maximal working dimension and can therefore be used with negligible risk of duct rupture.

USE OF SALIVA AS A DIAGNOSTIC FLUID

1. Changes in salivary composition and flow rate in salivary gland disease.
   a. *Sialadenitis:* Sodium and chloride secretions increased
   b. *Sjogren's syndrome:* Increased sodium and chloride concentration and decreased phosphate concentration. IgA is increased. Rate of salivary flow is reduced. In addition, there are changes in the relative concentrations of some minor salivary proteins
   c. *Cirrhosis of liver:* Calcium, potassium, protein and amylase concentrations are increased. Rate of salivary flow is also increased
   d. *Xerostomia:* Salivary flow rate decreased
   e. *Sialorrhoea:* Salivary flow rate increased
2. The relationship of saliva flow rate and composition to oral disease
   a. There is no association between salivary ionic composition with dental caries or periodontal disease
   b. Salivary IgA concentration is higher in subjects with more dental caries
3. Salivary changes in systemic disease
   a. Generalised immunological reactions as seen in transplant rejection, which may affect major salivary glands, reducing the rate of secretion and raising sodium and chloride concentrations
   b. Cystic fibrosis causes decreased secretion from submandibular, sublingual and minor salivary glands with marked increase in salivary calcium from these glands
   c. Aldosterone increases reabsorption of sodium in the striated ducts, reducing the salivary sodium concentrations and may increase potassium levels. The sodium–potassium ratio in saliva can therefore indicate normal, excessive or deficient aldosterone secretion
   d. Calcium and phosphate concentrations in saliva are thought to be raised in hyperparathyroidism.

BIOPSY

1. Biopsy of salivary glands is mainly used to aid in the diagnosis of Sjogren's syndrome, sarcoidosis and benign lymphoepithelial lesion
2. The most promoted biopsy technique is the extraoral incisional parotid biopsy. It is uncommon for facial nerve damage, salivary fistula, excessive bleeding or difficulty in identifying the parotid gland to occur
3. Submandibular gland biopsy is also done through an extraoral approach; mostly an excisional biopsy
4. *Fine-needle aspiration biopsy (FNAB)* is widely recognised as a practical and useful technique in the diagnosis of masses of the head and neck. It has a high accuracy rate in the diagnosis of lesions of the salivary glands. It is also a valuable adjunct to physical examination in patients with masses in the salivary glands. A palpable enlargement or tumour may be accessible to FNAB for cytology
5. *Fine-needle aspiration cytology (FNAC)* results in accurate diagnosis in 90%–100% of mixed tumours and Warthin's tumour, the most common salivary gland tumour.

CLASSIFICATION OF SALIVARY GLAND DISEASES

Salivary gland diseases are classified as depicted in Box 31.1.

SIALORRHOEA OR PTYALISM

Sialorrhoea or excessive salivation is an uncommon condition and has various causes.

Causes

- Aphthous ulcers or ill-fitting dentures
- Individuals with gastroesophageal reflux disease (GERD) have episodic hypersecretion of saliva, or 'water brash', as a protective buffering system to neutralise stomach acid
- It is a well-known clinical feature of rabies and heavy-metal poisoning
- Medications used to treat dementia such as antipsychotic agents and cholinergic agonists in Alzheimer's type and myasthenia gravis
- Neurological diseases such as cerebral palsy, Parkinson's disease or amyotrophic lateral sclerosis result in drooling due to poor neuromuscular control
- Mentally challenged patients and patients who have undergone surgical resection of the mandible.

Clinical features

- Excessive saliva production produces drooling and choking, causing social embarrassment
- Uncontrolled salivary flow in children with mental retardation or cerebral palsy can cause macerated sores around the mouth, chin and neck that can become secondarily infected

BOX 31.1 Classification of Salivary Gland Diseases

1. **Developmental/congenital disorders**
   a. Agenesis
   b. Aberrancy (ectopic gland)
   c. Aplasia (absence of glands) and hypoplasia
   d. Hyperplasia
   e. Atresia (absence of ducts)
   f. Accessory ducts and lobes
   g. Haemangiomas
   h. Polycystic disease of parotid glands
   i. Heterotrophic salivary glands
   j. Adenomatoid hyperplasia of mucous glands
   k. Oncocytosis
   l. Diverticuli
   m. Congenital fistula
2. **Functional disorders**
   a. Sialorrhea
   b. Xerostomia
3. **Obstructive disorders**
   a. Sialolithiasis/calculi
   b. Mucous plug
   c. Foreign bodies
   d. Stricture and stenosis
   e. Extraductal causes
4. **Cysts**
   a. Mucous extravasation cysts
   b. Mucous retention cysts/mucocele
   c. Ranula
5. **Infection-sialadenitis: Acquired inflammatory enlargement of the gland**
   a. Viral sialadenitis
      - Mumps
      - Coxsackie A
      - AIDS-associated sialadenitis
      - Cytomegalovirus
   b. Bacterial infection:
      - Nonspecific pyogenic infections (aerobic and anaerobic bacterial infection)
        i. Acute bacterial suppurative sialadenitis
        ii. Chronic bacterial sialadenitis
      - Specific bacterial infection
        i. Tuberculosis
        ii. Cat scratch disease
        iii. Syphillis
   c. Mycotic/fungal infection
6. **Noninflammatory asymptomatic enlargement**
   a. Sialosis/sialadenosis-recurrent/persistent benign enlargement due to acinar hypertrophy
   b. Allergic
   c. Associated with nutritional deficiency/malnutrition and alcoholism
7. **Autoimmune/immunologic disorders**
   a. Sjogren's syndrome
   b. Mikulicz's disease
   c. Sarcoidosis-rare
   d. Recurrent nonspecific parotitis
8. **Idiopathic disorder**
   a. Necrotising sialometaplasia
   b. Benign ulcerative lesion located at the back of hard palate due to lack of blood supply
   c. Sarcoidosis
9. **Neoplasms**
   a. Benign but seldom recurrent
      - Warthin's tumour
      - Oncocytoma
      - Monomorphic salivary adenoma
   b. Benign but often recurrent
      - Pleomorphic adenoma
      - Mucoepidermoid tumour (low grade)
      - Acinic cell tumour
   c. Malignant
      - Carcinoma in pleomorphic adenoma
      - Adenoid cystic carcinoma
      - Mucoepidermoid tumour (high grade)
      - Acinic cell carcinoma
      - Squamous cell carcinoma
      - Adenocarcinoma
      - Undifferentiated carcinoma

- Constant soiling of bed linens and clothes can pose a significant problem for the parents and caretakers of these patients
- An interesting type of super-salivation of unknown aetiology has been termed ***idiopathic paroxysmal sialorrhoea***, a condition where an individual experiences short episodes of excessive salivation lasting from 2 to 5 min and are associated with a prodrome of nausea or epigastric pain.

Treatment and prognosis

- Some causes of sialorrhoea are transitory or mild and no treatment is needed
- For GERD patients, medical management for their reflux can be beneficial
- Anticholinergic medications decrease saliva production but also produce unacceptable side effects
- Transdermal scopolamine has been tried with some success, but it should not be used in children younger than age 10. Intraglandular botulinum toxin injection has shown to be successful in reducing salivary secretions with duration of action that varies from 6 weeks to 6 months
- Several surgical techniques have also been used successfully to control severe drooling in individuals with poor neuromuscular control such as:
    a. Relocation of the submandibular ducts (the ducts are repositioned posteriorly to the tonsillar fossa, thereby redirecting salivary flow and minimising drooling)
    b. Relocation of the parotid ducts
    c. Submandibular gland excision plus parotid duct ligation
    d. Ligation of the parotid and submandibular ducts
    e. Bilateral tympanic neurectomy with sectioning of the chorda tympani.

XEROSTOMIA

Xerostomia refers to dry mouth and it is frequently, but not always, associated with salivary gland hypofunction.

Causes

1. Local factors
    a. Decreased mastication
    b. Smoking
    c. Mouth breathing
2. Developmental origin
    a. Salivary gland aplasia
3. Iatrogenic origin
    a. Medications
    b. Radiation therapy to the head and neck
    c. Chemotherapy
4. Water metabolite loss
    a. Impaired fluid intake
    b. Haemorrhage
    c. Vomiting/diarrhoea
5. Systemic diseases
    a. Sjogren's syndrome
    b. Diabetes mellitus
    c. Diabetes insipidus
    d. Sarcoidosis
    e. Human immunodeficiency virus (HIV) infection
    f. Hepatitis C infection
    g. Graft versus host disease (GVHD)
    h. Psychogenic disorders.

Clinical features

- Reduction in salivary secretion and the residual saliva appears either foamy or thick and 'ropey'
- Patient complains of difficulty in mastication and swallowing
- Dental caries seen especially at the cervical region and tooth roots
- Mucosa appears dry
- Often the tongue appears to be fissured along with atrophy of the filiform papillae
- The clinician may encounter examining gloves sticking to the mucosal surfaces
- Due to the reduction in the salivary flow, the cleansing and antimicrobial activities are compromised resulting in oral candidiasis.

Treatment and prognosis

- Maintenance of good oral hygiene and use of oral hygiene products that contain lacto-peroxidase, lysozyme and lactoferrin is advised
- Artificial saliva is available and aids in patient comfort, as may continuous sips of water throughout the day
- Sugarless candy can be used to stimulate salivary flow
- Discontinuation or dose modification can be done if the dryness is secondary to the patient's medication
- Systemic pilocarpine, a parasympathomimetic agonist can be used as a sialagogue at doses of 5–10 mg, 3–4 times daily, it can be an effective promoter of salivary secretion
- Frequent dental visits are recommended due to the increased susceptibility to dental caries
- Fluoride applications can be used to help prevent decay, and chlorhexidine mouth rinses minimise plaque build-up.

OBSTRUCTIVE DISORDERS

SIALOLITHIASIS (SALIVARY CALCULI; SALIVARY STONES)

Sialolithiasis is the mechanical restriction of salivary flow caused by the growth of salivary calculi or stones in the salivary gland or duct. ***Sialoliths*** are calcified formations that form inside the ductal system of a salivary gland, either major or minor. They are often produced with layers of inorganic material around the ***central nidus***. It begins as an organic nidus, which eventually expands in size due to the deposition of layers of inorganic and organic components. The formation rate is around 1 mm/year. They come in single or multiples, round, oval or long shapes, and are yellowish white in colour. They are around 1–10 mm length.

Composition

- *Inorganic salts* of calcium and phosphate like hydroxyapatite, octa calcium phosphate
- *Organic nidus* like desquamated epithelial cells, bacteria, bacterial decomposition, glycoprotein, mucopolysaccharides, etc
- *Foreign bodies* like tooth brush bristles, finger nails, wood splinters, hair, blades of grass, fish bones.

Sialolithiasis is both a cause and a consequence of chronic recurring sialadenitis, and it is frequently a cause of acute suppurative sialadenitis (Fig. 31.5).

Aetiology

The exact cause of sialolith formation is not known, but three prerequisites stand out as primary aetiologic factors:

i. A neurohumoral condition, leading to salivary stagnation
ii. A nidus or matrix for stone formation
iii. A metabolic mechanism favouring precipitation of salivary salts into the matrix in the presence of coexisting inflammation.

Risk factors:

- Dehydration—increase in viscosity and concentration of saliva
- Anorexia/Fasting—decreases the demand for saliva
- Drugs and medications—antihistamines, antipsychotics, antidepressants, antihypertensives, anticholinergics, diuretics, etc
- Irradiation/Radiotherapy
- Tobacco smoking
- Sjogren's syndrome
- Hypercalcaemia
- Gout (uric acid accumulation).

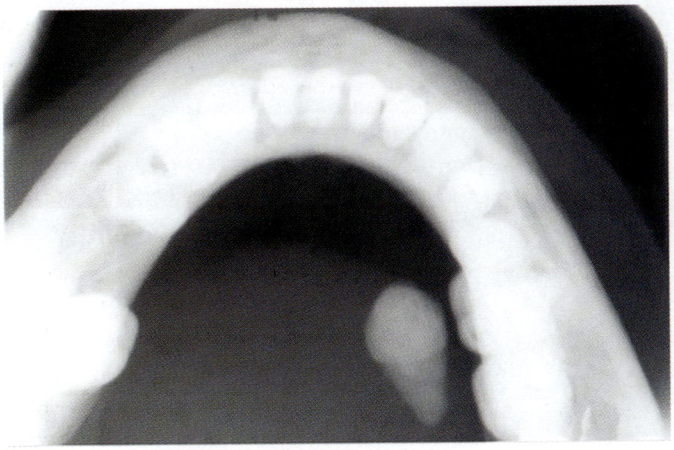

Figure 31.5 Occlusal radiograph of the mandible showing a radiopaque mass in the floor of the mouth on the right side denoting a submandibular gland calculus.

Increased incidence for formation of sialoliths in the ***submandibular gland*** is due to the following factors:

- The pH of saliva from the submandibular gland is about 6.8–7.1 (alkaline), as opposed to the more acidic product of parotid gland (6.3–7.4)
- In addition, the submandibular gland contains a greater concentration of calcium and phosphate salts, mainly in the form of apatites
- The relative alkalinity, in conjunction with alteration in the salivary *calcium–phosphorus ratio*, causes the salivary apatite to exceed its solubility product, resulting in precipitation of these salts
- The mucous content of the submandibular gland and its secretions may become more viscous than those of the parotid gland
- The duct of the submandibular gland is longer, tortuous and situated at a lower level than its orifice (nondependent), leading to increased salivary stagnation in the duct, which can lead to increased calculus formation.

Clinical features

Sialolithiasis occurs in men twice as often as in women. There is a peak incidence between 30 and 50 years of age, and submandibular gland is the most common site of involvement accounting to 80%.

Signs and symptoms

Clinical presentation of sialolithiasis varies. On occasion, there may be a total absence of subjective symptoms; in such cases, the sialoliths are identified accidentally during radiographic examination.

MEAL TIME SYNDROME

Patients complain of moderate to severe pain associated with swelling during and after eating the food (especially when the production of saliva is at peak). The swelling may be diffuse and sometimes resemble cellulitis. Gradual reduction of pain and swelling is noted during the rest period. History of recurrent swelling is seen when the flow is stimulated and is continued till there is complete obstruction. Pain is mainly due to increased pressure in the duct due to obstruction.

- Occasionally, patients report spontaneous extrusion of small calculi from the ducts
- The most common finding on examination is point tenderness in the region of the hilum or near Wharton's duct of the submandibular gland
- Fever occurs due to secondary infection associated with tenseness, tenderness, trismus, decreased or absent salivary flow
- A gelatinous, cloudy, mucopurulent material is seen in basically clear and adequate saliva. This mucopurulent material is derived from the inflammatory ductal changes caused by calculus blockage and salivary stagnation
- If treatment is not instituted early, pronounced exacerbations are seen, characterised by an acute suppurative

process with attendant systemic manifestations. Pus may exude from the duct orifice
- The mucosa around the duct is inflamed, particularly in the floor of the mouth where swelling, redness and tenderness are present along the course of the Wharton's duct
- The glands are enlarged, tender and tense. Palpation of the gland and the duct causes pain and a flow of pus.

Diagnosis

Diagnosis is mainly done by careful bimanual palpation and digital manipulation. Palpation in the floor of the mouth along the duct may reveal the presence of the stone if it is present in the duct. The inability to milk saliva from the duct orifice indicates the presence of calculi/obstructions in the salivary flow path.

Radiographic features

- Occlusal radiograph, lateral view, lateral oblique mandibular view, and AP views (intraoral and extraoral)
- Sialography plays an important role in identifying the location of the calculus
- USG is an inexpensive and noninvasive method used to detect stones more than 2 mm
- CT—to detect gland enlargement, especially in chronic cases
- Scintigraphy and MRI.

Complications

- Acute and chronic suppurative sialadenitis due to bacterial infection of the gland
- **Sialoangiectasis** (dilatation of salivary duct) due to salivary stasis by sialolith, stricture, chronic infection
- **Mucocoele**—due to salivary retention phenomenon
- Atrophy of gland due to complete obstruction of the duct.

TREATMENT OF SIALOLITHIASIS

Conservative treatment

1. Local heat, massage and sialogogues
2. Enhanced use of sialogogues, sour food intake, salivary gland massage, hyperhydration for facilitating spontaneous removal of stones
3. If the stones are located within the duct, intraoral approach is indicated (Fig. 31.6)
4. If the stone is present within the gland and if there are irreversible ductal and glandular changes within the gland, removal of involved gland through an extraoral approach is indicated
5. In the acute phase, standard care includes antibiotics, analgesics and good oral hygiene
6. Surgical intervention for drainage of pus is sometimes necessary. Once the acute stage subsides, definitive surgical treatment can be instituted.

Sialodochoplasty

- Sialodochoplasty refers to salivary duct repair by widening the orifice and shortening of the salivary duct
- It is usually performed during sialolithotomy to prevent re-stenosis or re-narrowing of the ductal system
- The duct may simply be stitched open or may require a stent to be left in place for 7–10 days in order to heal properly.

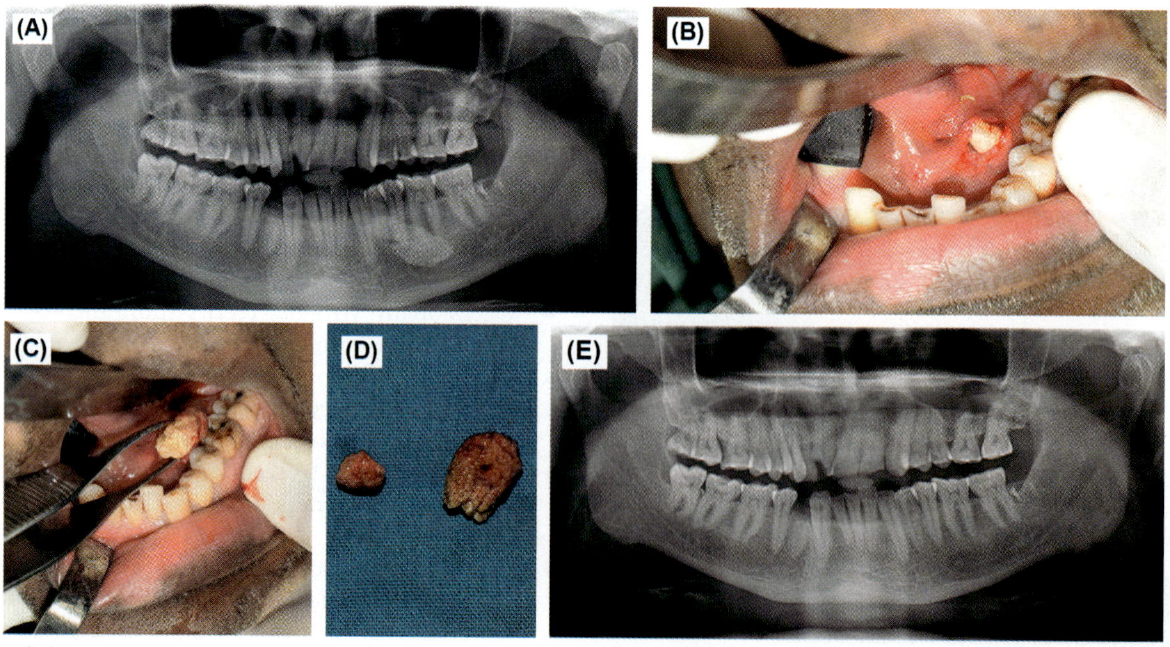

Figure 31.6 (**A**) Preoperative OPG showing the presence of submandibular salivary gland calculus in relation to 34,35,36. (**B**) Submandibular salivary gland calculus present at the entrance of the duct. (**C**) Removal of calculus. (**D**) Excised calculus. (**E**) Postoperative OPG.

Removal of parotid gland calculi

Parotid gland duct is the location of 6%–10% of salivary calculi. The calculi may be located at four basic sites:

- Impacted at the papilla
- In the submucous part of the duct
- In the extraglandular part of the duct external to the buccinator muscle
- In the intraglandular part of the duct.

The technique of removal depends on the site of location of calculi.

Papilla and submucous part of the duct

- Calculi in this region can be released by slitting of the papilla
- Using sharp scissors, a short cut is made in the anterior portion of the way into the duct from the orifice
- If the calculus is not dislodged, as soon as the scissors is removed, gentle pressure on the gland will force a quantity of saliva along the duct, washing out the calculus.

Extraglandular part of duct external to buccinator muscle

Calculi in this part of the duct can be removed through an incision in the intraoral aspect of the check.

- A traction suture is then placed just anterior to the papilla. A Y-incision is made through the mucosa around the papilla with the tail of the Y directed forwards
- Blunt dissection is carried out to separate the mucosa and submucosa from the buccinator muscle
- The tip of the triangle containing the papilla and duct is freed from the undersurface
- The upper and lower flaps are mobilised and stay sutures are placed to hold the flaps out of the way
- Dissection is then carried out laterally into the cheek and posterior to the point where the Stensen's duct pierces the buccinator muscle and turns posteriorly. A suture is then looped around the duct and is retracted medially into the mouth
- Once the site of calculus is located, an incision is made parallel to the long axis of the duct and the stone is removed
- The tissues around the duct are closed with absorbable sutures, leaving the incision in duct open.

Intraglandular portion of the duct

If the calculus is located posterior to the accessory portion of parotid gland, it is generally in the intraglandular course of the parotid duct. These calculi can be removed by an extraoral approach similar to the one used for a parotidectomy (Fig. 31.7).

Removal of submandibular gland calculi

The most frequent location of submandibular gland calculi is extraglandular. They can be present in the anterior or posterior portions of the submandibular duct and also in the intraglandular portion of the duct.

Anterior portion of submandibular duct

- Anterior calculi are those that lie anterior to the mandibular 2nd molars. A suture is then passed into the floor of the mouth around the duct, posterior to the stone to prevent its posterior dislodgement
- A suture is placed across the duct anterior and posterior to the site of calculus
- Traction on these two sutures will steady the tissue in the surgical site by making it taut
- An incision is now made along the line of the duct (along a line that bisects the angle between the root of the tongue and the sublingual plica) and over the stone
- The duct is about 3–4 mm in diameter, pale greyish in colour and identified by the network of fine capillaries that course its surface
- Once the duct is identified, it is mobilised and a suture is passed under it so that it may be pulled anteriorly. The calculus is identified and a longitudinal incision is placed over the duct and the sialolith released.

The incision in the duct is not sutured to prevent stricture formation. The patient is encouraged to drink fluids and use lemon drops to encourage salivary flow and maintain patency of the duct (Fig. 31.8).

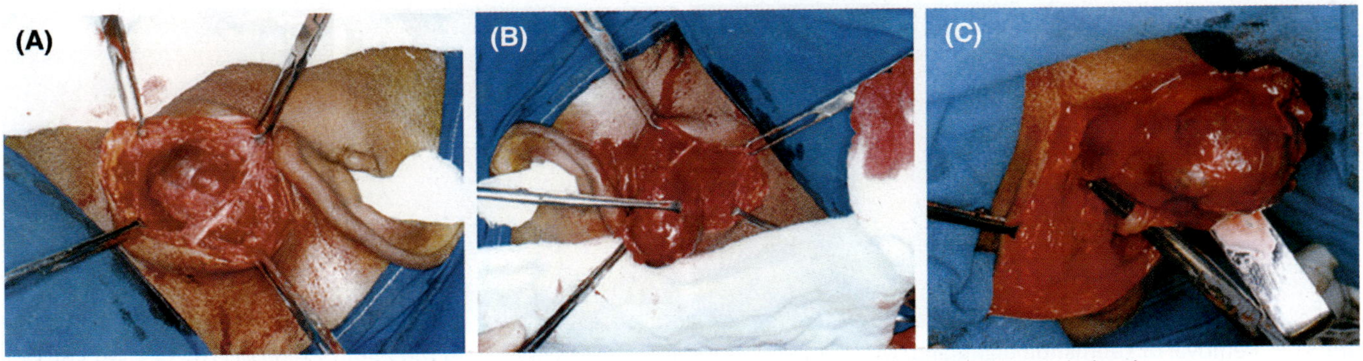

Figure 31.7 Parotidectomy. **(A)** Gland is identified. **(B–C)** Removal of parotid gland.

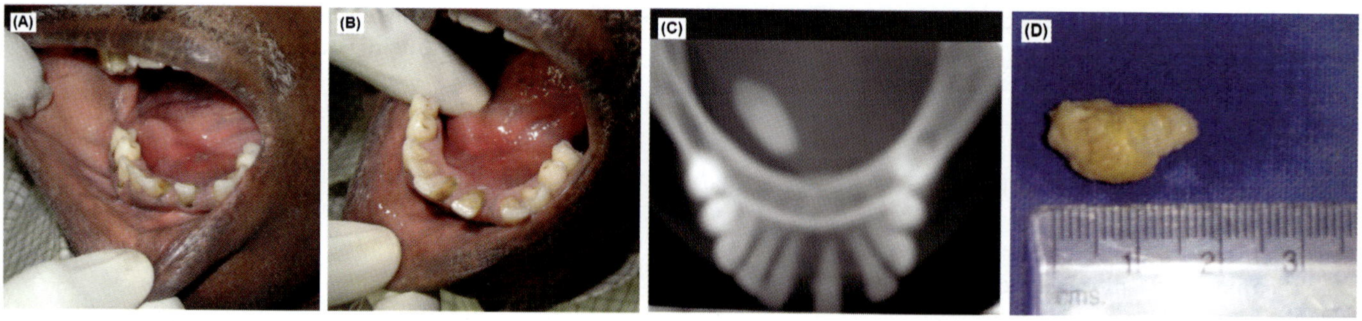

Figure 31.8 (**A** and **B**) A bulge on the right side of the floor of the mouth indicating the presence of submandibular gland calculus. (**C**) Occlusal radiograph of the same person showing an oblong radiopacity of the calculus in the right side of the mandible. (**D**) Excised calculus.

Posterior portion of submandibular duct

- A lacrimal probe can be inserted into the ductal orifice and through the anterior portion of the duct tracing the duct
- An incision is then made in the mucosa opposite the premolar teeth. The duct is traced posteriorly, identifying lingual nerve as it crosses where it is retracted and protected
- Pressure is placed against the lower pole of the gland to raise the upper pole superiorly (since the submandibular duct emerges from the upper and anterior part of the upper pole of the submandibular gland) into the surgical field. The duct is then incised parallel to the long axis of the duct and the calculus removed
- The mucosal tissues closed with interrupted sutures leaving the incised duct open.

Intraglandular portion of submandibular duct

Presence of calculus in the intraglandular portion of the duct affecting the functioning of the gland or infection is an indication for removal of the gland. If the stone is small and the gland is asymptomatic and sialographically normal, it can be left in place and observed for any change in position or function of parenchyma of the gland. If it is symptomatic with abnormal glandular structure, sialadenectomy is done (Fig. 31.9).

INFECTIONS AND SYSTEMIC DISEASES

SIALADENITIS

Sialadenitis is the inflammation of the salivary glands that can arise from various infectious and noninfectious causes.

1. This can be caused by bacteria in the oral cavity contaminating the duct and parenchymal tissues retrograde
2. A restriction of salivary flow, which favours acute suppurative infection
3. Other common causes of sialadenitis include viral infections, bacterial infections, allergic responses and systemic disorders. It might be either acute or persistent.

Causes

- The most common viral infection is mumps, although a number of other viruses can also affect the salivary glands including coxsackie A, parainfluenza and cytomegalovirus (in neonates)
- Most bacterial infections arise as a result of ductal obstruction or decreased salivary flow, allowing retrograde spread of bacteria throughout the ductal system. Blockage of the duct can be caused by sialolithiasis, congenital strictures or compression by an adjacent tumour. Decreased flow can result from dehydration, debilitation or medications that inhibit secretions

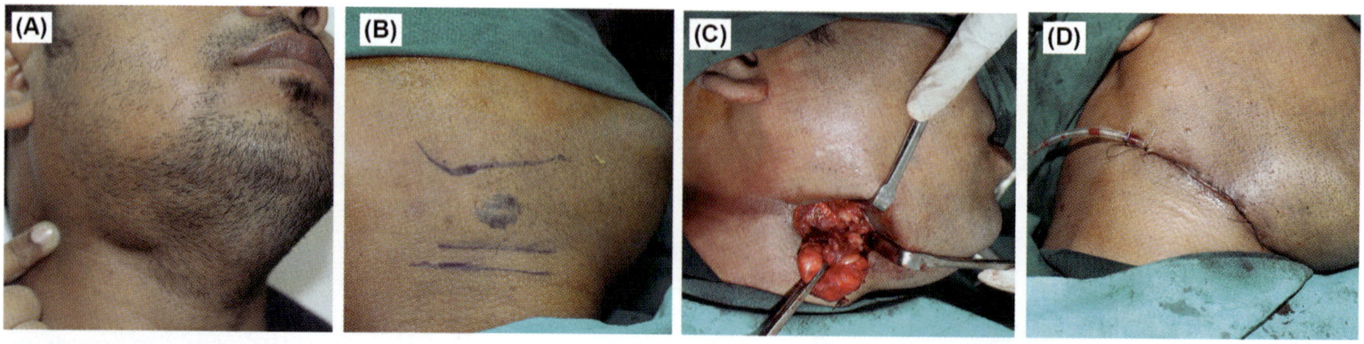

Figure 31.9 Removal of submandibular gland. (**A**) Preoperative view showing swelling on the right side below the jaw. (**B**) Markings placed for incision. (**C**) Submandibular gland is exposed and excised. (**D**) Wound sutured.

- One of the most common causes of sialadenitis is recent surgery after which an acute parotitis (surgical mumps) may arise
- Medications that produce xerostomia as a side effect also can predispose patients to such an infection
- Most cases of acute bacterial sialadenitis are due to *Staphylococcus aureus*, but they also may arise from Streptococci or other organisms
- Noninfectious causes of salivary inflammation include Sjogren's syndrome, sarcoidosis, radiation therapy and numerous allergens.

ACUTE BACTERIAL SIALADENITIS

Clinical features

- Acute bacterial sialadenitis is most common in the parotid gland and is bilateral in 10%–25% of cases
- The affected gland is swollen and painful and the overlying skin may be erythematous in colour. An associated low grade fever may be present along with trismus. A purulent discharge is often observed from the duct orifice when the gland is massaged
- Recurrent or persistent ductal obstruction most commonly caused by sialoliths can lead to a chronic sialadenitis. Periodic swelling and pain occur within the affected gland, usually developing at meal time when salivary flow is stimulated. Sialography often demonstrates sialectasis (ductal dilatation) proximal to the area of obstruction
- Subacute necrotising sialadenitis is a form of salivary inflammation that occurs most commonly in young adults. The lesion usually involves the minor salivary glands of palate, presenting as a painful nodule that is covered by intact, erythematous mucosa. Unlike necrotising sialometaplasia, the lesion does not ulcerate.

Histopathologic features

In patients with acute sialadenitis, accumulation of neutrophils is observed within the ductal system and acini. Chronic sialadenitis is characterised by scattered or patchy infiltration of the salivary parenchyma by lymphocytes and plasma cells.

Treatment and prognosis

Initial treatment of acute sialadenitis includes:

- Appropriate antibiotic therapy
- Rehydration of the patient to stimulate salivary flow
- Surgical drainage may be needed if there is abscess formation.

Although this regimen is usually sufficient, high mortality rate has been reported in debilitated patients because of the spread of infection and sepsis.

Surgical management of chronic sialadenitis depends on the severity and duration of the condition. Early cases that develop secondary to ductal blockage may respond to removal of the sialoliths or other obstruction.

If ***sialectasia*** is present, dilated ducts can lead to stasis of secretions and predispose the gland to further sialolith formation. Surgical removal of the affected gland may be necessary, in case of extensive inflammatory destruction of the salivary tissue.

Subacute necrotising sialadenitis is a self-limiting condition that usually resolves within 2 weeks of diagnosis without treatment.

MUMPS

Mumps sialadenitis is the most common of all salivary gland diseases. It is a nonsuppurative, acute sialadenitis of viral origin. It is a contagious, generalised disease that presents as a painful enlargement of the salivary glands. The live attenuated measles vaccine was introduced in 1967 as a preventative measure. It is usually provided alongside the measles and rubella vaccinations.

- The virus mumps causes an acute febrile illness with a prodromal period of 2–3 weeks
- Mumps primarily infects young adults and children, classically 6–8 years of age. Mumps virus has an incubation period of 2–3 weeks and is transmitted by direct contact or in droplets of saliva
- The onset is sudden with fever, headache and painful swelling of the parotids. Usually one gland is infected 1st and then the other. In 70% of cases, there is bilateral involvement
- Painful swelling occurs rapidly, reaches a maximum size within 1–3 days
- Trismus may be present, with some difficulty in chewing
- Stensen's duct orifice is swollen and erythematous, but there is no purulent material in the saliva. The symptoms subside in 3–7 days
- Orchitis (testicular swelling)
- Oophoritis (Inflammation of ovary)
- Rash
- Chipmunk cheeks.

Diagnosis

Diagnosis is usually made on a clinical basis during epidemics. Serum antibodies to the mumps *S and V antigens* with a titre of greater than 1:192 indicate recent infection. The viruses usually affect the epithelium, although the 1st changes on histologic study are perivascular oedema and white blood cell infiltrates. A diffuse infiltration of the glandular parenchyma by mononuclear cells with acinar degeneration is observed.

Complications

The most important complication of mumps includes parotid gland sialectasia with recurrent chronic and even acute suppuration. Complications of mumps result from generalised viraemia and include pancreatitis (diabetes secondary to pancreatic fibrosis), orchitis (sterility secondary to gonadal involvement), oophoritis, myocarditis, aseptic meningitis, nephritis, and sensorineural hearing loss (frequently unilateral).

The condition resolves spontaneously in 5–10 days. Symptomatic relief of pain and fever is necessary and prevention of dehydration is essential.

Management

This is a self-limiting disease. Antipyretics are able to alleviate symptoms of fever. The subsequent infection can be prevented with antibiotics.

CYSTS OF THE SALIVARY GLANDS

MUCOCOELE

Oral mucocoele is produced by mucus extravasation or mucous retention cyst. Mucous extravasation causes connective tissue hypertrophy. This is due to a damaged salivary gland duct, usually caused by local trauma (injury) in mucous extravasation phenomenon or a blocked or burst salivary duct in mucous retention cysts. The lesion has a blue, translucent appearance and is more common in children and adolescents. Mucocoeles are often called cysts; however, they are actually polyps since they lack an epithelial lining.

Types

There are two types of mucocoeles:

1. Extravasation type
2. Retention type.

Pathogenesis

Mucous extravasation cyst

Mucous extravasation cysts are induced by trauma that lacerates the duct of the minor salivary glands, releasing mucin into the connective tissue. The trauma may be induced by the patient biting the lip and cheek or by iatrogenic trauma via extraction forceps, etc. Mucin that extravasates into connective tissue causes inflammation, attracting neutrophils and macrophages, which leads to the development of granulation tissue, which forms the wall of extravasation cysts. Thus, no epithelial lining is seen. Scarring eventually forms in and around the gland.

Mucous retention cyst

Mucous retention cyst is the collection of saliva within the salivary duct, which is often caused by a sialolith but may also be caused by periductal scarring or an impinging tumour. This causes the duct to dilate, resulting in a cyst-like lesion. Histological examination of these cysts may reveal the presence of ductal epithelium.

Clinical features

- Mucocoeles are nonpainful, potentially recurring swellings. Some individuals report an increase in the size of their mucocoele during meals
- Extravasation-type mucocoeles are most often found on the lower lip and tongue, which are the most common places for injuries to the minor salivary glands
- Retention-type mucocoeles are uncommon and occur rarely on the lower lip. Instead, it manifests in the palate, cheek, gingiva and maxillary sinus
- Mucocoele typically appears as dome-shaped mucosal swellings ranging from one to several centimetres in size
- They are most common in children and young adults
- The spilled mucin below the mucosal surface often imparts a bluish translucent hue to the swelling; however, deeper mucocoeles may be normal in colour
- The lesions are characteristically fluctuant, but some long-standing mucocoeles are firm on palpation (Fig. 31.10)
- Lower lip is the most common site for the mucocoeles, accounting for more than 60% of all the cases
- Mucocoeles are usually found lateral to the midline. Less common sites include the buccal mucosa, anterior, ventral surface of tongue and the floor of the mouth, where it is known as ranula.

Treatment and prognosis

Some mucocoeles are short-lived lesions that rupture and heal by themselves. However, many lesions are chronic in nature and local surgical excisions are necessary.

To minimise the risk of recurrence, when the area is excised, adjacent minor salivary glands should be removed as it may be the source of the lesion. The excised tissue should be submitted for histopathological examination to confirm the diagnosis and rule out the possibility of a salivary gland tumour. The prognosis is excellent, although occasional mucocoeles will recur; prompting re-excision, especially if the other surrounding minor glands are not removed (Fig. 31.11).

RANULA

'Ranula' is a term used for retention cysts of salivary gland origin occurring in the floor of the mouth. The name is derived from the Latin word rana, which means frog, because of the resemblance of the bulging cyst wall to a frog's translucent underbelly. **Formation of ranula occurs by two mechanisms:**

1. Partial obstruction of the distal end of the duct with dilation results in an epithelial lined cyst (*mucous retention cyst*)
2. Disruption of the duct with formation of a connective tissue line space (*mucous extravasation or pseudocyst*). The source of the cystic fluid is believed to be the sublingual glands in the most common form of ranula.

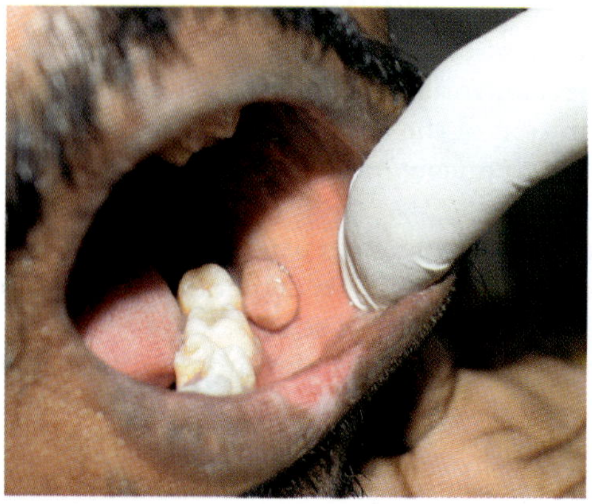

Figure 31.10 Picture showing mucocoele in the region of the left cheek.

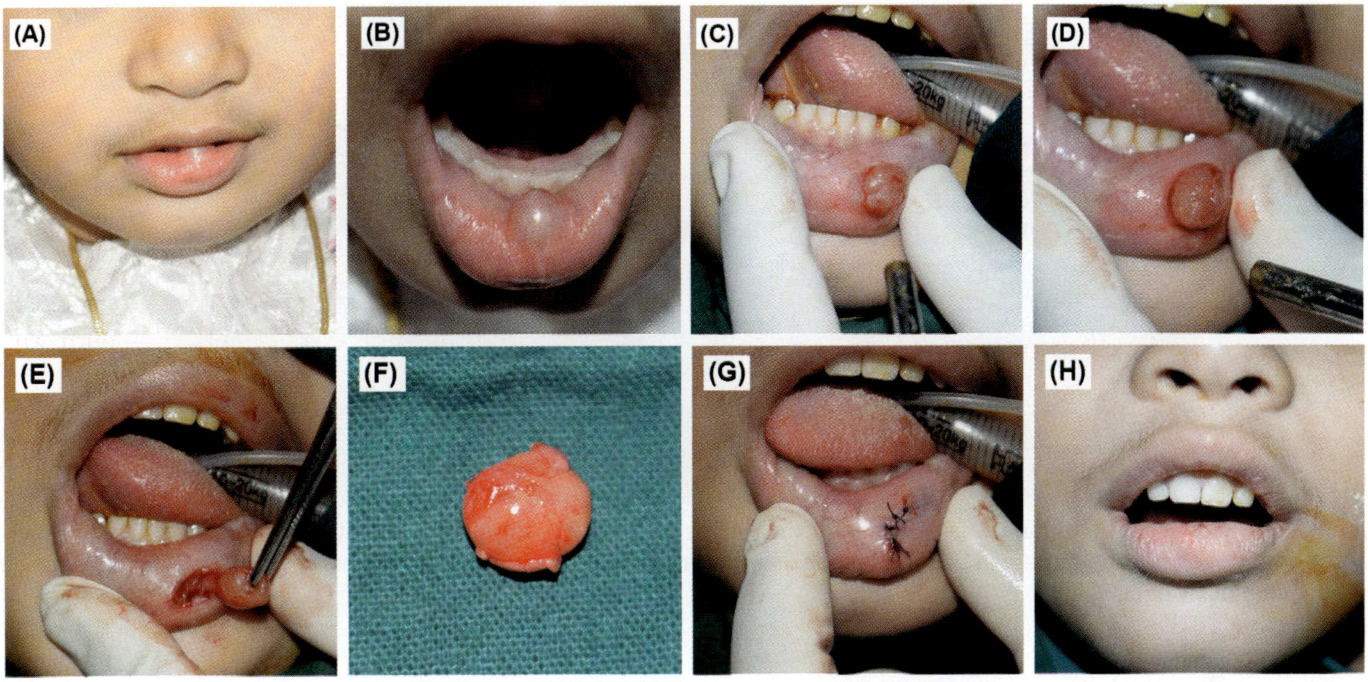

Figure 31.11 **(A–H)** Surgical removal of a mucocoele.

Clinical features

Two varieties of cysts are seen (simple ranula and plunging ranula) that have different clinical behaviour, appearance and they require different methods of treatment.

- Simple ranulas are true retention cysts
- An unusual clinical variant, the plunging or cervical ranula is a cyst that occurs beyond the mucous membranes of the oral cavity into the floor of the mouth, through a hiatus of the mylohyoid muscle and into the fascial planes of the neck. This occurs when the spilled mucin dissects through the mylohyoid muscle and produces swelling within the neck
- Ranula appears as a blue, dome-shaped translucent fluctuant swelling in the floor of the mouth
- They are usually painless and unilateral with increasing size
- They can cause deviation of the tongue
- They can cross the midline submucosally at times
- They may rupture spontaneously with extrusion of a thick, translucent fluid into the mouth. The wall then rapidly heals and the cyst subsequently reforms (Fig. 31.12).

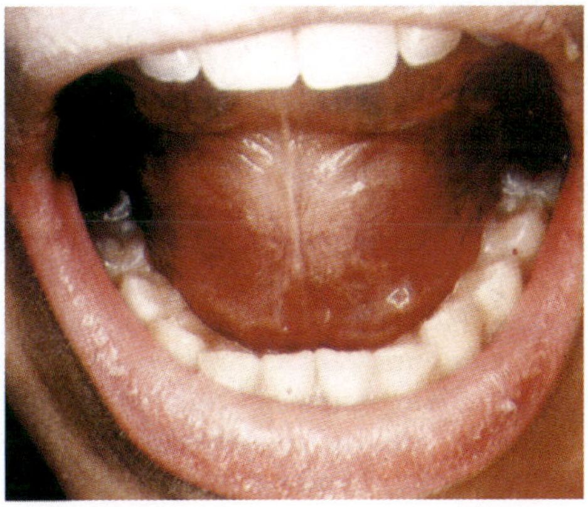

Figure 31.12 Simple ranula.

Treatment

Ranulas do not recede on their own and must be treated surgically. The preferred therapy is marsupialisation. The superior wall of the lesion is excised, and the inner wall is sutured to the mucosa of the floor of the mouth. If recurrence is seen, excision is performed in continuity with the caustic sublingual gland.

Large ranulas are likely to be marsupialised. Because of the great size of the ranulas, the mucosa, which is eventually thinned down, ruptures when injured. Mucoid fluid leaks into the connective tissue. As the region heals, fluid re-collects and the ranula may subside and return.

For simple ranula, the sublingual gland is removed by an intraoral technique. To avoid recurrence of a long-standing plunging ranula, both the sublingual and submandibular glands must be excised simultaneously with the lesion (Fig. 31.13).

NEOPLASMS OF SALIVARY GLANDS

Due to the diversity of salivary gland tumours, various terminologies and categorisation methods are employed. The most generally used method defines salivary neoplasms as primary or secondary, benign or malignant, and by tissue of origin. This system specifies five salivary gland neoplasms as shown in Table 31.5.

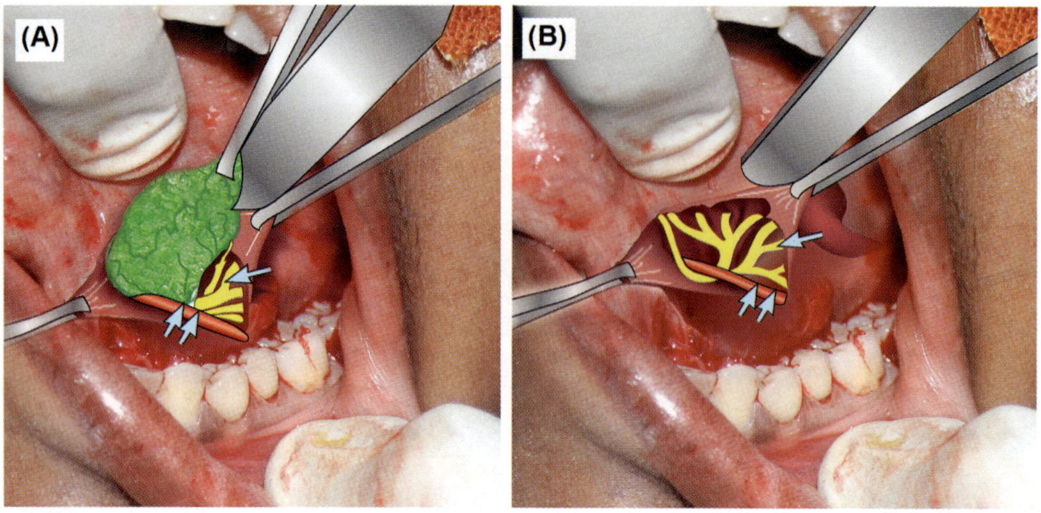

Figure 31.13 Total excision of ranula. (**A**) Excision of the entire mucus-filled capsule and the sublingual gland of origin. (**B**) The single arrow represents the preserved branches of the lingual nerve posterior to the ranula, whereas the double arrow represents the submandibular duct.

AETIOLOGY OF SALIVARY GLAND NEOPLASMS

Viruses

- Epstein–Barr virus
- Polyomavirus
- Cytomegalovirus
- Human papilloma virus type 16 and 18.

Radiation

There is a high correlation between radiation exposure and the growth of tumours in the salivary glands. Studies have shown that the relative risk of both benign and cancerous salivary gland tumours went up in Japan after the atomic bombs went off in Hiroshima and Nagasaki. The risk of salivary gland tumours goes up when therapeutic doses of radiation are used in the head and neck area. Even a dose of only 140 rad is enough to raise the risk. A diagnostic dental X-ray could also lead to the growth of a tumour.

Occupations

- Asbestos mining
- Shoe manufacturing
- Manufacturing of rubber products
- Wood working
- Automobile industry.

Hormones

Endogenous hormones stimulate salivary gland tumours. In 80% of normal salivary gland samples, oestrogen receptors were detected. Same study found increased oestrogen receptors in salivary gland tumours.

TREATMENT

The treatment options for salivary gland tumours ranges from transoral minor salivary gland tumour excision surgery to total excision of the major salivary glands, based on the type and severity of the disease and the involvement of the adjacent structures as follows.

1. **Transoral minor salivary gland tumour surgery**
   a. ***Soft tissue palatal excision*** for benign and low-grade malignant tumours of the palatal mucosa, for example, Pleomorphic adenoma and low-grade mucoepidermoid carcinoma
   b. ***Soft tissue excision of salivary gland tumours in the oral mucosa*** indicated for benign tumours and mucous retention phenomena, for example–Pleomorphic adenomas, canalicular adenomas
   c. ***Palatectomy*** is indicated for low grade and intermediate grade malignant tumours, for example, Polymorphous low-grade adenocarcinoma
2. **Maxillectomies** either partial maxillectomy or total maxillectomy for malignant tumours of the palatal mucosa, for example, intermediate and high grade mucoepidermoid carcinoma, adenoid cystic carcinoma (ACC), squamous cell carcinoma (refer Chapter 30, Flowchart 30.2)
3. **Parotid gland surgeries**
   a) FNAC for diagnostic cytology
      i. Solitary parotid gland masses
      ii. To assess the effect of treatment
      iii. To obtain tissue for special studies
   b) Incisional parotid biopsy to confirm or rule out autoimmune or systemic diseases of the salivary gland tissues
   c) Superficial parotidectomy
      i. Benign tumours in the superficial lobe and some low-grade malignant tumours
      ii. Also indicated in cases of Sjogren's syndrome, HIV parotitis, symptomatic sialosis, parotid

TABLE 31.5 WHO Histologic Classification of Tumours of the Salivary Glands, 2005

Categories	Subcategories
1. Benign epithelial tumours	• **Pleomorphic adenoma** • Basal cell adenoma • Canalicular adenoma • Sebaceous adenoma • Lymphadenoma • Myoepithelioma • Ductal papilloma • **Warthin's tumour** • **Oncocytoma** • Cystadenoma
2. Malignant epithelial tumours	• Acinic cell carcinoma • Mucoepidermoid carcinoma • Adenoid cystic carcinoma • Carcinoma ex pleomorphic adenoma • Metastasising pleomorphic adenoma • Polymorphous low-grade adenocarcinoma • Mucinous adenocarcinoma • Basal cell adenocarcinoma • Sebaceous lymph-adenocarcinoma • Cystadenocarcinoma • Low-grade cribriform cystadenocarcinomas • Epithelial-myoepithelial carcinoma • Clear cell carcinoma • Oncocytic carcinoma • Salivary duct carcinoma • Squamous cell carcinoma • Small cell carcinoma • Large cell carcinoma • Lymphoepithelial carcinoma • Sialoblastoma • Carcinosarcoma
3. Based on tissue origin	Soft tissue tumours—haemangiomas, haematolymphoid tumours, intraosseous central salivary gland tumours
4. Secondary tumours	Metastasised tumours
5. Hybrid tumours	

injuries, refractory sialocoele or salivary cutaneous fistulae

d) Total parotidectomy with nerve preservation
   i. Benign and low-grade malignant tumours that encroach upon or extend into the deep lobe

e) Total parotidectomy with nerve transection and nerve grafting
   i. Malignant tumours of the superficial lobe that require aggressive resection and diffuse benign tumours of both lobes

f) Excision of the deep lobe of the parotid gland
   i. Benign and low-grade malignant tumours located and limited to the deep lobe of the parotid gland.

BENIGN TUMOURS

The salivary glands may be affected by a variety of **benign** tumours, including Warthin's tumour, oxyphilic adenoma, oxyphilic canalicular adenoma, basal cell adenoma, canalicular adenoma, myoepithelioma, ductal papilloma and pleomorphic adenoma.

PLEOMORPHIC ADENOMA

Over 50% of all tumours and 90% of benign salivary gland tumours are pleomorphic adenomas. Most experts assume the tumour originates in salivary gland myoepithelial cells. It has both epithelial and connective tissue components, thus the term 'mixed tumour'. It occurs predominantly in the parotid glands, followed by submandibular glands and minor salivary glands. They are rarely seen in the sublingual gland. It can occur at any age, but the peak incidence is in the 4th and 5th decades of life. There is a slight female preponderance.

Clinical features

- Pleomorphic adenoma is the classic benign tumour, but it is also a true neoplasm, meaning that it will continue to develop or regrow. Even if not totally eliminated, the tumour cannot metastasise
- Pleomorphic adenomas of the parotid gland are painless, hard masses located in the superficial lobe of the parotid gland and in the posterior palate mucosa
- The nodule gradually grows in size, with sporadic development being common. The tumour is well-circumscribed, encapsulated, hard and may have regions of cystic degeneration. The tumour is easily moveable and has no attachment to the underlying tissues or the overlying skin. The tumour may grow to be rather big, yet it does not ulcerate. There is no evidence of tissue loss, discomfort or facial paralysis
- Superficial lobe:
  a. Pleomorphic adenomas in the parotid gland form in the superficial lobe, which accounts for 80% of the gland's surface area
  b. Tumour cannot be transferred over the zygomatic arch, as represented by the curtain sign
  c. When the parotid glands in this benign tumour begin to expand, the ear lobules begin to rise
- Deep lobe:
  a. When the deep lobe of the parotid is damaged, it is a dumb-bell shaped parotid tumour

b. Swelling of the deep lobes goes via Patey's tube
c. Pleomorphic adenomas in the deep lobe frequently go undiagnosed for years, until they grow large enough to cause symptoms such as dysphagia or gagging

- Minor salivary gland: The palate is the most frequent intraoral location of occurrence; however, it may also occur in the buccal mucosa, lips or tongue. They appear as a slow-growing swelling with an entirely intact surface. They are detected early due to difficulty with mastication, speech and so forth. The palatal pleomorphic adenoma is attached to the underlying bone but does not invade it.

Differential diagnosis

- Benign: Warthin's tumour, basal cell adenoma
- Malignant: Mucoepidermoid, adenoid cystic and acinic cell carcinomas
- Nonsalivary gland neoplasms: Haemangiomas, lymphangiomas, lipomas and lymphomas within parotid lymph nodes.

Histopathological investigation

Capsule and epithelial cells organised as sheets and ducts. These duct-like regions are surrounded by myoepithelial cells, giving them a 'swarm of bees' look. Myxoid, chondroid and osteoid regions are present. Plasmacytoid cells are also seen. Depending on their histological appearance, pleomorphic adenomas may be myxoid, cellular or cellular with myxoid regions.

Treatment and prognosis

Although benign, pleomorphic adenoma is capable of malignant change but expand and grow in localised areas of proliferation to form irregular nodular masses. These tumours have good prognosis with superficial or total parotidectomy or sialoadenectomy as required (Figs. 31.14–31.16). The treatment for pleomorphic adenomas is surgical removal. The parotid tumours are excised with appropriate margins while intraoral lesions may be handled with a little more restraint. In cases of submandibular cancers, the gland containing the tumour is removed. During a parotidectomy, the tragal

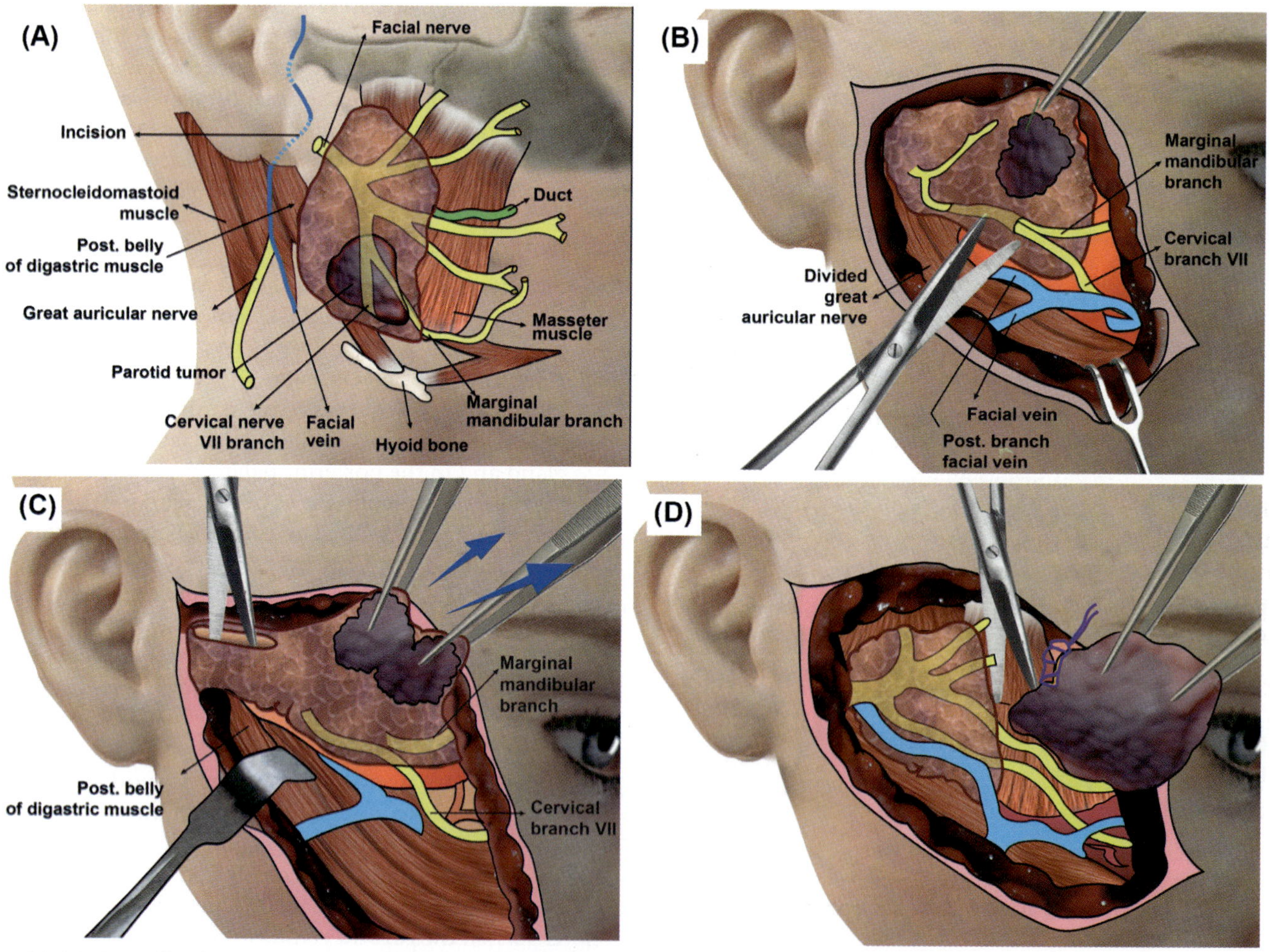

Figure 31.14 Superficial parotidectomy procedure. (**A**) Note the tumour in the superficial lobe at the tail of the parotid gland and the vital structures within the gland. (**B** and **C**) Blunt dissection starts at the inferior pole of the gland and proceeds upwards, separating the main trunk of the facial nerve from the superficial lobe. (**D**) All the facial nerve branches were identified and successively dissected and the superficial lobe of the gland removed in a single block.

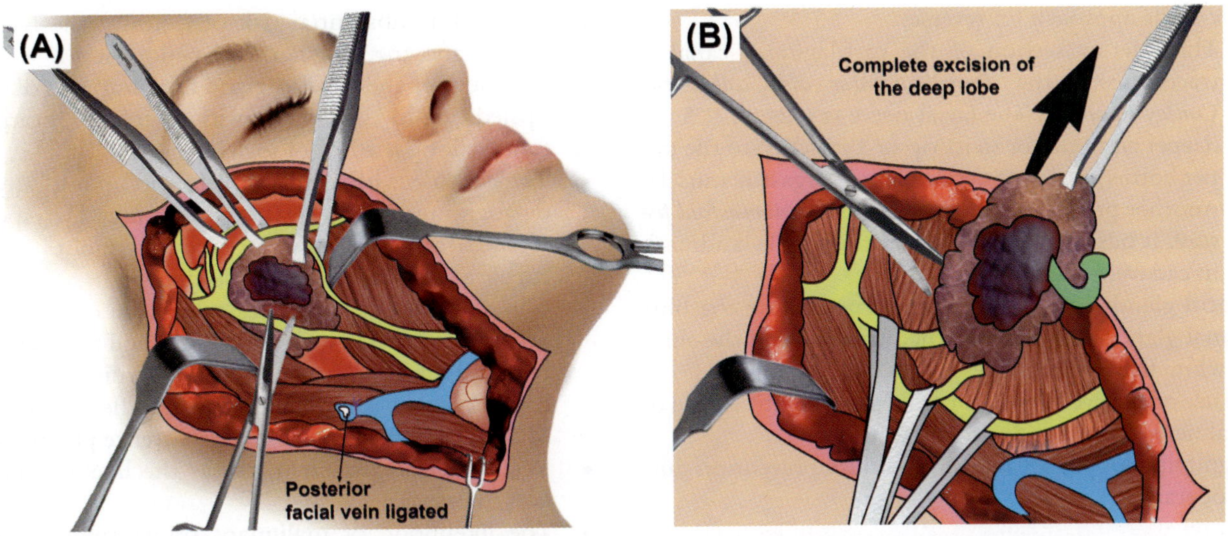

Figure 31.15 Total parotidectomy procedure. (**A**) Tumour present in the deep lobe also. Initial procedure starts with superficial parotidectomy followed by deep lobe parotidectomy. (**B**) Complete parotid gland is removed preserving the facial nerve and its branches.

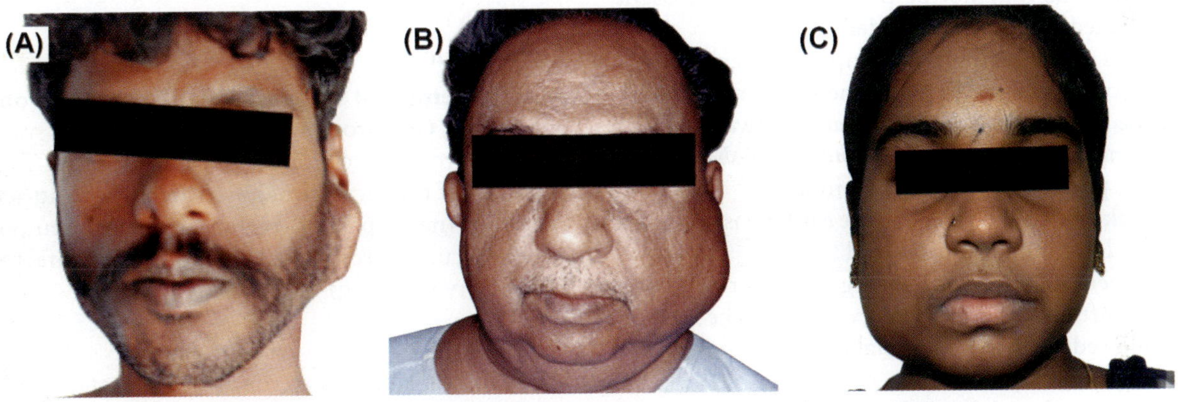

Figure 31.16 Pleomorphic adenoma of the left and right parotid gland.

pointer, the tympanomastoid suture line, the digastric muscle attachment to the digastric groove, retrograde dissection from the distal nerve branch and the nerve in the temporal bone are used to find the facial nerve. Pleomorphic adenoma is radio-resistant.

SUPERFICIAL PAROTIDECTOMY

Indications

1. Pleomorphic adenoma is the most frequent cause of tumour for a parotidectomy
2. Sjögren's syndrome precipitating enlargement
3. Enlargement of the gland owing to chronic sialadenitis
4. Salivary calculus causing enlargement.

Preauricular approach

This is useful for large sialoliths in the posterior portion of the parotid duct. An incision is made on the skin. Dissection of the platysma and superficial fascia is performed. The duct is located on the gland's anterior edge. The duct is traced backwards through the gland's material until the calculus is found and removed. The preservation of facial nerve branches, notably the lower zygomatic branch, which rests on the surface of the duct right below the accessory parotid, should be approached with extreme caution. The fascial sheath that encases the gland is completely sealed preventing salivary seepage into the tissue. A piece of corrugated rubber drain is inserted in the wound. Extraorally, a Y-shaped incision is used for superficial parotidectomy.

Preventing facial nerve injuries

The main stem is identified by following the sternocleidomastoid muscle superiorly. If this approach fails, a peripheral branch, generally the marginal mandibular, can be identified and followed proximally.

One of the following three procedures can be used to identify the facial nerve:

1. Direct detection of the main trunk as it leaves the stylomastoid foramen

2. Retrograde approach (in reverse):
   a. The inferior section of the cartilaginous canal is traced using the ***Tragal pointer also called the Conley's pointer***. The facial nerve is either 1–1.5 cm deeper and inferior to its tip or 1 cm deep to the upper border of the posterior belly of digastric muscle
   b. Another proximal marker is the ***tympanomastoid fissure.*** It has been a reliable and repeatable landmark in cadaveric dissections
3. Parotid gland supravital staining, contrasting the blue normal gland with the unstained tumour and the shining white facial nerve fibres
4. The use of a nerve stimulator aids in the identification of facial nerve branches during dissection
5. Magnifying loops can also aid in injury prevention during operation.

COMPLETE PAROTID GLAND EXCISION

The main goal of total parotid gland excision is to preserve the facial nerve and its branches. However, in the case of malignant tumours, this may not be possible and the patient should be informed of the resulting deformity.

- An incision is made starting at the superior attachment of the pinna downwards, one arm of the incision anteriorly towards the angle of the jaw continuing forward till the hyoid bone and another arm of the ***inverted Y-shaped incision*** is made posteriorly behind the pinna
- On the cheek side of the incision, the ear lobe is retracted upwards and a skin flap is produced
- The facial nerve is identified using an electrical nerve stimulator. After locating the nerve trunk, the nerve's path is followed and the superficial lobe is released from its attachments
- Stensen's duct is found, ligated and severed
- The deep lobe is then addressed by retracting the ear lobe farther posterosuperiorly
- The external carotid artery and the posterior facial vein are both ligated after which the facial nerve is gently lifted from the deep section. The inferior and superior branches of the retromandibular vein are likewise separated and are ligated
- The deep portion of the gland is dissected out. The styloid process, as well as the stylohyoid, styloglossus and digastric muscles, accommodate this deep portion
- The ascending ramus may be split and retracted to ease the excision of the bulky deep lobe tumour following which the mandible is rewired into place. A drain is inserted and the wound is closed in layers.

COMPLICATIONS

- Incomplete excision of the tumour may result in recurrence
- Long-standing benign pleomorphic adenomas that have not been treated may develop malignant transformation
- A tumour that is hard, ulcerates and produces facial paralysis or lymph node involvement may have become malignant
- There is a substantial risk of injuring the facial nerve while removing irregularly formed tumours
- Tumours of the parotid gland are incapable of being biopsied due to their propensity to create repeated recurrences along the line of incision
- The capsule is often incomplete and its integrity cannot be guaranteed if enucleation is attempted irresponsibly
- If enucleation is tried, mucinous tumours may easily rupture and generate many seedlings
- The removal of recurrences, which are often multifocal, gets more difficult with each effort, and the ultimate outcome might be numerous nodules of tumour throughout the neck that extend well beyond the initial location. MUC1/DF3 markers serve as recurrence predictors
- Recurrence treatment increases the likelihood of facial nerve resection
- The likelihood of malignant transformation increases with recurrent recurrences and may rise further if radiation is used
- Frey's syndrome.

FREY'S SYNDROME

Other names

Auriculotemporal syndrome, Baillarger syndrome, Dupuy syndrome, Gustatory sweating syndrome

Frey syndrome is characterised by unilateral flushing and sweating of the facial skin innervated by the auriculotemporal nerve (neck, parotid region and frontotemporal scalp), which occurs in response to gustatory or olfactory stimuli (Gustatory sweating).

Aetiology

- In infants, trauma to the auriculotemporal nerve during forceps-assisted delivery
- Congenital aberration of the auriculotemporal nerve fibres, between the parasympathetic and sympathetic pathways
- Parotid surgery, especially after excision of the superficial lobe or drainage of a parotid abscess
- TMJ surgery
- Rare causes include mandibular condylar fractures, blunt trauma, herpes zoster, associated CNS disorders such as syringomyelia, epilepsy and meningioma of the cerebellopontine angle tumour.

Pathophysiology

Auriculotemporal nerve is a sensory branch of the posterior division of the mandibular division of the trigeminal nerve. It receives the postganglionic parasympathetic secretomotor fibres from the otic ganglion, for parotid glands. Damage to these autonomic fibres causes misdirection of regenerating parasympathetic fibres to join with the sympathetic fibres of the ***great auricular nerve (7th nerve)***, which supplies sweat glands and blood vessels during the process of healing. Because of this, any gustatory stimulus produces erythema and sweating instead of salivation (Fig. 31.17).

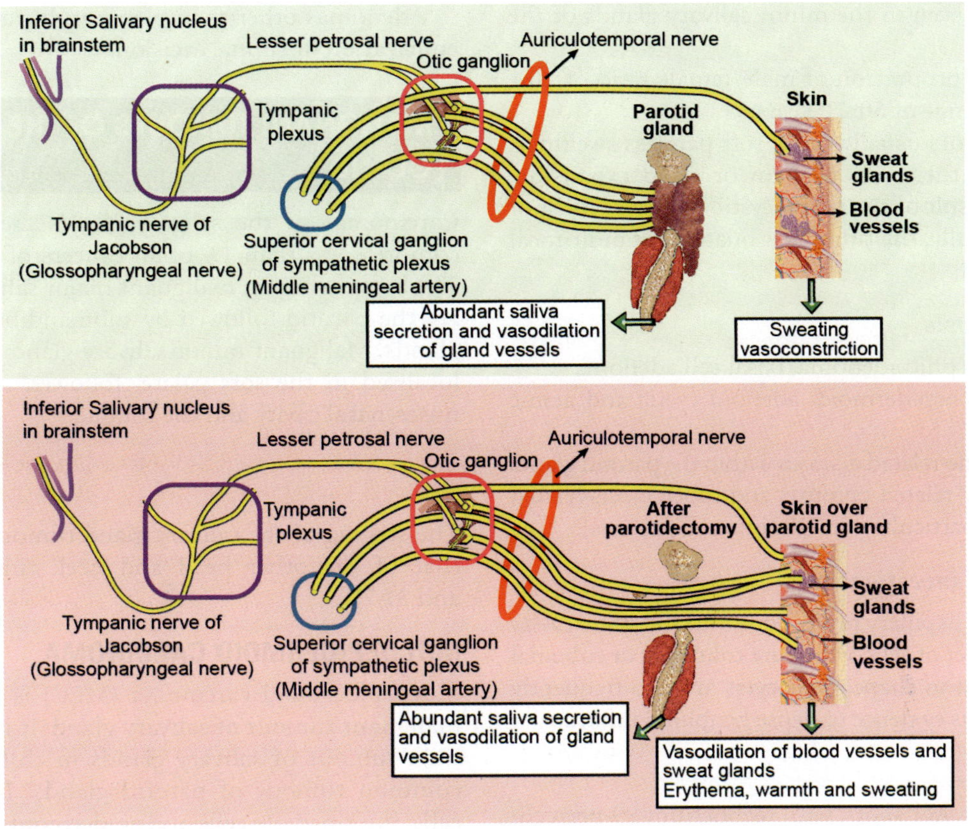

Figure 31.17 Pathophysiology of Frey's syndrome.

Diagnosis

Suspicious areas are painted with iodine and allowed to dry and then dusted with corn starch or potato flour. Sweating is then encouraged via sialogogue (lemon). If positive, the reaction causes change in colour from yellow to black.

Treatment

Topical:

- Antiperspirant—for mild symptoms
- 20% aluminium chloride for a period of 1–2 months
- Anticholinergic—topical glycopyrrolate.

Intradermal:

Intradermal injection of Botulinum Toxin A. Response may last for a period of 6 months. If the treatment is unsuccessful, then surgery is considered.

Radiation:

Radiation of 50 Gy indicated for symptomatic patients.

Surgery:

- Auriculotemporal nerve resection
- Tympanic neurectomy.

WARTHIN'S TUMOUR

Other names

Papillary cystadenoma lymphomatosum

Papillary cystadenoma lymphomatosum is a benign hamartomatous or reactive proliferation of salivary gland ductal cells and lymphoid elements commonly referred to as a *Warthin's tumour*. It is caused by various aetiologies such as smoking (irritates ductal epithelium), autoimmune causes, heterotrophic lymphoid tissue, delayed hypersensitivity reactions and viruses—Epstein–Barr virus.

Pathophysiology

Warthin's tumour is believed to arise from the incorporation of salivary gland cells into lymph nodes during their development; these later become reactive and induce a proliferation of both salivary and lymph node elements.

Clinical features

- Warthin's tumours are common tumours of the parotid glands exclusively in the superficial lobe and periparotid lymph nodes. They are painless and firm to doughy masses
- It is said to occur most frequently in the *'tail' of the parotid gland*, which is the most inferior and posterior portion of the gland below the ear and the angle of the mandible
- They occur as synchronous and metachronous tumours, which mean that they appear bilaterally and two or more tumours occur simultaneously at the same time or years later in the same or opposite gland or may even recur as a new tumour in residual elements of a treated gland

- They can occur even in the minor salivary glands of the oral cavity
- It affects in the proportion of male/female ratio of 10:1 within an age range of 50–70 years
- Warthin's tumours usually cause soft painless swellings, but sometimes there can be pain or rapid expansion, probably as a result of the partly cystic nature of most of them. Occasionally, the tumour is bilateral or multifocal in a single gland.

Differential diagnosis

- Benign: Pleomorphic adenoma, basal cell adenoma
- Malignant: Mucoepidermoid, adenoid cystic and acinic cell carcinomas
- Other lymph node-related diseases within the parotid gland: Lymphoma, HIV-related parotitis and tuberculosis-related lymphadenitis (particularly in HIV infected patients).

Histopathological investigation

There is presence of papillary projections into the cystic cavity lined by a double layer of cells, which are columnar or cuboidal and rarely polygonal in shape. Oncocytes are also frequently encountered. There is evidence of dense lymphoid infiltrate.

Investigation

Tumour presents as 'hot spots' with technetium-99-pertechnetate, other neoplasms show either normal uptake or 'cold nodule'.

Treatment and prognosis

Warthin's tumour must be excised with a superficial parotidectomy which aids in both, a diagnostic biopsy as well as the definitive treatment for this tumour, and the cut specimens often reveal the characteristic finding of a soft, sponge-like, multicystic lesion containing a thin, brown fluid. Prognosis is good and has rare incidence of recurrences, unless incomplete excision and multicentricity become a concern.

ONCOCYTOMA

Oncocytoma is a rare benign tumour that almost exclusively affects the parotids, particularly in the elderly. It consists of large, *eosinophilic cells with small compact nuclei* and is typically arranged in solid cords. There is presence of characteristic granules that represent altered mitochondria and are visible with *phosphotungstic acid haematoxylin (PTAH) stain*.

OTHER ADENOMAS

- Canalicular adenomas particularly affect the upper lip and consist of small darkly staining cells in a tubular or trabecular pattern but sometimes resembling an ACC
- Basal cell adenomas are of different types, namely, solid, membranous, etc. and are mostly encountered in the major salivary glands especially the parotid glands
- Ductal papillomas may also be rarely encountered.

Adenomas other than pleomorphic adenoma respond to enucleation or simple excision.

MALIGNANT TUMOURS OF THE SALIVARY GLAND

Carcinomas of the salivary glands are uncommon. They comprise less than 1% of all cancers of the head and neck. The most common malignant major salivary gland tumours are the parotid followed by submandibular and sublingual glands. Malignant minor salivary gland tumours are mostly localised in the soft palate, followed by the paranasal sinuses/nasal cavity and the tongue.

TNM CLASSIFICATION AND STAGING OF MALIGNANT NEOPLASMS OF THE SALIVARY GLAND

The staging of the salivary gland tumours is different from that of the other head and neck tumours (Tables 31.6 and 31.7).

MUCOEPIDERMOID CARCINOMA

Mucoepidermoid carcinoma (MEC) is the most common malignant tumour of salivary gland. It is the 2nd most common tumour of salivary glands in children and the most common tumour of parotid glands. It contains mucous cells, intermediate cells and epidermoid cells. The low-grade tumour resembles a benign tumour with an extremely favourable prognosis, but the high-grade tumour is very aggressive. The clinical manifestations vary depending on the tumour's grade. Consequently, it may develop slowly or fast; often manifesting as a painless enlargement of the parotid or other major salivary glands, or the minor salivary glands.

A biopsy should be used to confirm the diagnosis.

Variants

- Sclerosing MEC
- Intraosseous MEC.

Clinical features

- Shows wide age predilection from 2nd to 7th decades
- Most common malignant tumour in children
- Shows slight female predilection (3:2)
- Some tumours are associated with previous history of radiation therapy
- It can occur in both major and minor glands, being predominant in major glands
- Features for major glands:
  a. Most common in parotid gland (50%)
  b. Appears as an asymptomatic swelling with duration of less than 1 year
  c. Pain, trismus, discharge from ear, dysphagia. Facial palsy develops in high grade tumours
- Features for minor glands:
  a. Common in palate (20%); Other sites—lower lip, floor of mouth, tongue and retromolar area

TABLE 31.6 TNM Classification by AJCC—American Joint Committee on Cancer

Primary tumour (T)	TX	Primary tumour cannot be assessed
	T0	No evidence of primary tumour
	T1	Tumour 2 cm or less in greatest dimension without extraparenchymal extension
	T2	Tumour more than 2 cm but not more than 4 cm in greatest dimension without extraparenchymal extension
	T3	Tumour having extraparenchymal extension without 7th nerve involvement and/or more than 4 cm but not more than 6 cm in greatest dimension
	T4a	Tumour invades skin, ear canal, mandible and/or facial nerve
	T4b	Tumour invades skull base and/or, pterygoid plates and/or encases carotid artery
Regional lymph nodes (N)	NX	Regional lymph nodes cannot be assessed
	N0	No regional lymph node metastasis
	N1	Metastasis in a single ipsilateral lymph node, 3 cm or less in greatest dimension
	N2	Metastasis in a single ipsilateral lymph node, more than 3 cm but not more than 6 cm in greatest dimension or in bilateral or contralateral lymph nodes, none more than 6 cm in greatest dimension
	N2a	Metastasis in a single ipsilateral lymph node, more than 3 cm but not more than 6 cm in greatest dimension
	N2b	Metastasis in multiple ipsilateral lymph nodes, not more than 6 cm in greatest dimension
	N2c	Metastasis in bilateral or contralateral lymph nodes, not more than 6 cm in greatest dimension
	N3	Metastasis in a lymph node more than 6 cm in greatest dimension
Distant metastases (M)	MX	Distant metastasis cannot be assessed
	M0	No distant metastasis
	M1	Distant metastasis

   b. It is typical for intraoral mucoepidermoid cancer to develop cystic degeneration, clinically imitating the appearance of a mucocoele, as a symptomatic swelling which are sometimes fluctuant and have blue or red colour appearance
- Lesion with ulceration has aggressive clinical course
   a. In its later phases, the high-grade tumour may cause discomfort, ulceration, facial paralysis, local destruction and spread to regional lymph nodes, as well as distant metastases to the lung, bone and brain.

Gross findings

- Appear relatively well circumscribed
- Appear as partially encapsulated
- Difficult to determine the accurate border
- Cut surface shows cystic spaces and contain mucoid material
- Focal haemorrhage sometimes present if biopsy or FNAC has been performed.

Histopathological investigation

- Characterised by the presence of a variety of cells and growth patterns
- The tumour's biologic behaviour of extremely low grade to highly aggressive nature depends primarily on the histology
- Based on this histologic grading, the treatment decisions are made
- These cells form the basis for recognition and grading
- These cells include:
   a. Mucous cells
   b. Epidermoid cells
   c. Intermediate cells
   d. Clear cells.

Differential diagnosis

- Pleomorphic adenoma
- Squamous cell carcinoma
- Retention cysts
- Adenosquamous carcinoma.

Treatment and prognosis

- Treatment depends on:
   a. Location
   b. Histological grade
   c. Clinical stage

TABLE 31.7 AJCC Staging of Salivary Gland Tumour

Stage	Tumour	Node	Metastasis
Stage I	T1	N0	M0
Stage II	T2	N0	M0
Stage III	T3	N0	M0
	T1	N1	M0
	T2	N1	M0
	T3	N1	M0
Stage IVa	T4a	N0	M0
	T4a	N1	M0
	T1	N2	M0
	T2	N2	M0
	T3	N2	M0
	T4a	N2	M0
Stage IVb	T4b	Any N	M0
	Any T	N3	M0
Stage IVc	Any T	Any N	M1

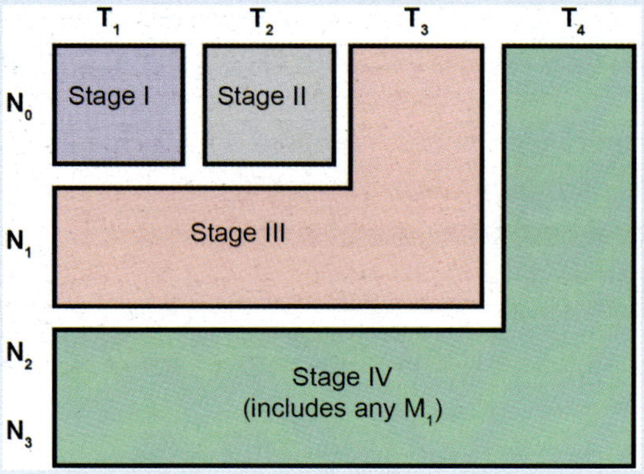

- Early-stage tumours of parotid gland are treated by subtotal parotidectomy with preservation of facial nerve
- Submandibular gland tumours are treated by total sialadenectomy
- For low-grade tumours, modest marginal clearance of 5 mm may be needed, but for high grade tumours, wider excision is required
- If the underlying bone is destroyed, that should be excised
- Regional node dissection is indicated for patient with evidence of metastasis (refer neck dissections in Chapter 30, Page number 625-628)
- Postoperative radiotherapy is needed for some aggressive lesions.

Prognosis depends on grade and stage

- Low grade—good prognosis (cystic)
- Intermediate grade
- High grade—poor prognosis—(perineural invasion)
- Submandibular gland involvement—poor prognosis
- Minor glands—good prognosis
- Recurrence rate—25%.

INTRAOSSEOUS MUCOEPIDERMOID CARCINOMA

Rarely salivary gland tumours arise centrally within the jaws. Entrapped ectopic salivary gland tissue may be responsible for intraosseous salivary gland tumours. When it occurs in the maxilla, the sinus lining may be the source.

Clinical features

- Common in middle age
- Shows light female predilection
- More common in mandible than maxilla
- Most frequent presenting symptom is cortical swelling
- Radiograph reveals—unilocular or multilocular radiolucency
- Some associated with unerupted teeth—misdiagnosed clinically as an odontogenic cyst.

Histopathology

- Same as soft tissue MEC
- Most are low grade in nature.

Treatment

Surgery is the 1st line of treatment (refer Chapter 30, Page 629). Prognosis is fairly good, and there are cases reported with local recurrence and metastasis.

ADENOID CYSTIC CARCINOMA/CYLINDROMA

ACC is a clinically and pathologically well-defined entity that occurs primarily in the major salivary glands (submandibular gland) and relatively frequent in the oral accessory salivary glands, particularly the palate (Fig. 31.18).

Clinical features

- Occur in older individual
- Show equal sex predilection
- Slow-growing tumour
- Pain and tenderness occur during tumour growth
- Fixation to skin and surrounding structures develop in later stages
- Perineural and perivascular spread
- Cause paralysis of facial nerve
- In minor salivary glands, it presents as a swelling or mass.
- Symptoms of facial pain and swelling characterise the ACC of maxillary antrum
- Radiograph is necessary for assessing the extent of osseous destruction
- In major salivary gland—mostly occur in parotid and submandibular gland, rarely in sublingual gland
- In minor salivary gland—palate is most common followed by tongue, cheek, upper lip, floor of mouth, oropharynx, lower lip and orbit
- The characteristic feature of ACC is perineural invasion, which accounts for high incidence of recurrence despite aggressive therapy.

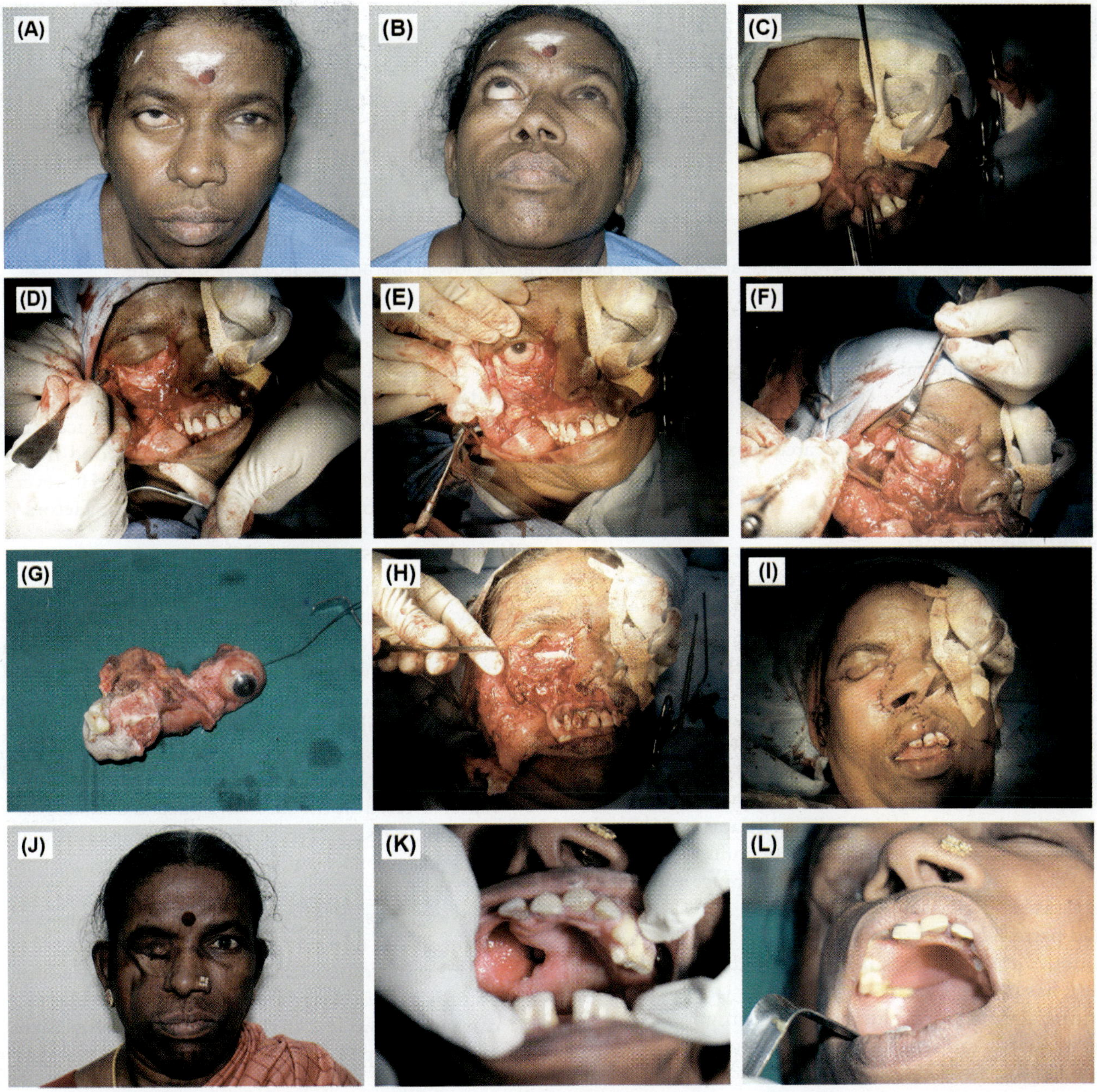

Figure 31.18 **(A–L)** Adenoid cystic carcinoma (ACC) of the right maxilla involving the orbit—Total right maxillectomy with orbital exenteration.

Gross findings

- Present as a fairly well-defined mass within the substance of involved gland
- Oncut section—tumour lacks encapsulation but can be demarcated from surrounding salivary gland tissue.

Microscopic findings

- ACC has a variety of microscopic patterns
- The cells that form various patterns and are uniform in size, shape and staining qualities are called isomorphic cells
- Various microscopic patterns:
  a. Cribriform
  b. Tubular
  c. Solid.

Investigations

1. *FNAC*
   a. Aspiration biopsy consist of round or ovoid basophilic cells arranged in branching structures
   b. Amorphous, hyaline globoid structures with tumour cells is the characteristic feature of ACC

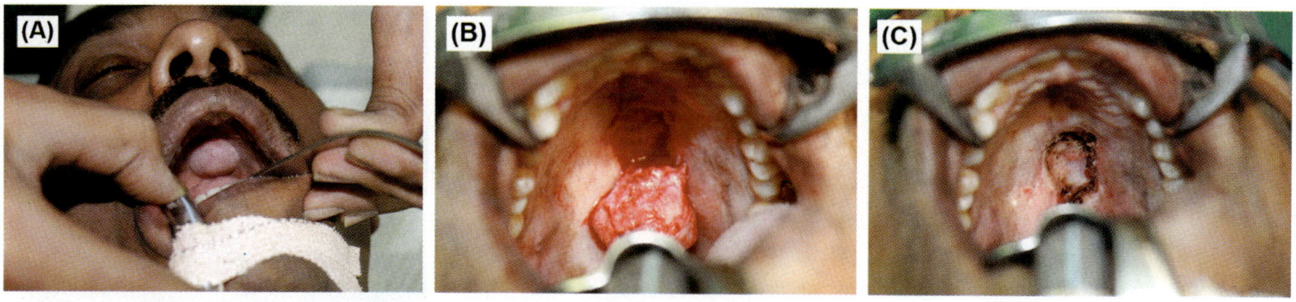

Figure 31.19 (**A–C**) Surgical excision of polymorphous low grade adenocarcinoma of palate.

2. *Immunohistochemistry* reveals the presence of two cell population: (1) ductal cells and (2) myoepithelial cells.

Differential diagnosis

- Polymorphous low grade adenocarcinoma (Fig. 31.19A–C)
- Salivary duct carcinoma
- Pleomorphic adenoma.

Treatment and prognosis

- The treatment of choice for ACC is **radical excision**
- Irradiation is not considered a primary treatment option because the tumour is resistant to being treated by radiation. Radiotherapy is often given after surgery because it is highly susceptible to local recurrence and distant metastasis, adjunct radiotherapy will improve patient survival. Fast neutron therapy is the most effective treatment for inoperable, recurrent or grossly residual salivary gland tumours
- Metastatic disease requires chemotherapy. Chemotherapy is considered situational due to limited data on its benefits
- Regional lymph node metastasis is uncommon
- Prognosis is poor because of local recurrence and distant metastasis
- Solid pattern has worst prognosis
- Tumours arising in maxillary sinus and submandibular gland has poor prognosis
- Perineural invasion has little effect on prognosis
- Metastatic spread most commonly occurs to lungs and bones
- Lesions in the palate and maxillary sinus may invade upward to the brain.

OTHER MALIGNANT TUMOURS

Malignant tumours of salivary glands include basal cell carcinoma, papillary cystadenocarcinoma, serous cell adenocarcinoma, malignant oncocytoma, etc.

They should be treated aggressively and then irradiated because they are biologically aggressive.

IDIOPATHIC DISEASES

NECROTISING SIALOMETAPLASIA

Necrotising sialometaplasia is a rare salivary gland disorder. It may be caused by ischaemia of salivary tissue leading to a localised infarction. Clinically and histopathologically, this lesion mimics a malignant process. Predisposing factors include traumatic injuries, intraoral injections, ill-fitting dentures, upper respiratory infections and adjacent or previous tumours. These factors may reduce blood flow to the affected glands, causing ischaemic necrosis. However, many cases occur without any known predisposing factors.

Clinical features

- Necrotising sialometaplasia usually affects palatal minor salivary glands
- The retromolar pad or minor salivary glands of the lips may be affected. Hard palate is more often affected than the soft palate. Two-thirds of palatal cases are unilateral, the rest are bilateral or midline
- Necrotising sialometaplasia has also been reported in minor salivary glands and the parotid
- Rarely affected are the submandibular and sublingual glands
- Necrotising sialometaplasia can occur at any age, but the average onset age is 46. Nearly twice as many men are affected
- The lesion is a large ulcer or ulcerated nodule well-defined from normal tissue
- Initial symptoms include a nonulcerated swelling with pain or paraesthesia, followed by a crater-like ulcer that can range from less than 1 cm to more than 5 cm in diameter and appear within 2–3 weeks.

Histopathologic features

Early lesions of necrotising sialometaplasia are marked by acinar necrosis, which is followed by squamous metaplasia of the salivary ducts. Although mucous acinar cells are necrotic, the overall lobular architecture of the affected glands is preserved. Mucin liberation could occur, resulting in an inflammatory response. Squamous metaplasia of the salivary ducts can be visually striking, resulting in a pattern that is easily mistaken for squamous cell carcinoma.

Treatment

To confirm the diagnosis, a biopsy should be performed. Because this lesion could be mistaken for malignancy histologically, a sufficient amount of tissue should be included in the biopsy. In most cases, the lesion is self-limiting and heals in 8 weeks without complications. Hydrogen peroxide or saline irrigation for debridement. In the past, clinicians recommended applying gentian violet 2–3 times a day with cotton as a topical antifungal. Since the introduction of nystatin and azole antifungals, this is contraindicated.

SIALADENOSIS

Sialadenosis is an unusual noninflammatory, nonneoplastic disorder characterised by salivary gland enlargement, particularly involving the parotid glands.

Clinical features

Sialadenosis usually appears as a slowly growing swelling of the parotid glands, which may or may not be painful. The condition is usually bilateral, but it can also be unilateral. In some patients, submandibular glands can be involved. Decreased salivary secretion may occur. Sialography demonstrates a ***'leafless tree' pattern***, which is thought to be caused by compression of the finer ducts by hypertrophic acinar cells.

Conditions associated with sialadenosis

A. Endocrine
   a. Diabetes mellitus
   b. Diabetes insipidus
   c. Acromegaly
   d. Hypothyroidism
   e. Pregnancy
B. Nutritional
   a. General malnutrition
   b. Alcoholism
   c. Anorexia nervosa
   d. Bulimia
C. Neurogenic medications
   a. Antihypertensive drugs
   b. Psychotropic drugs
   c. Sympathomimetic drugs used for treating asthma.

Histopathologic features

Microscopic examination reveals hypertrophy of the acinar cells, sometimes 2–3 times greater than normal size.

Treatment and prognosis

Clinical management of sialadenosis is often unsatisfactory because it is closely related to the control of the underlying cause. Pilocarpine has recently been reported to be beneficial in the treatment of bulimic patients with sialadenosis.

SJÖGREN'S SYNDROME

Sjogren's syndrome is a chronic, systemic autoimmune condition characterised by xerostomia and xerophthalmia, which mostly affect the salivary and lacrimal glands. Dry eyes, xerostomia and rheumatoid arthritis were initially grouped together as a triad. There are two types of the disease:

1. Sjogren's syndrome with dry eyes and xerostomia, often known as sicca syndrome; no other autoimmune illness is present
2. Secondary Sjogren's syndrome occurs when a patient has Sicca syndrome and another autoimmune illness such as rheumatoid arthritis, systemic lupus erythematosus or polyarteritis nodosa.

Aetiology

The cause of Sjogren's syndrome is unknown. Although it is not a hereditary disease, there is evidence that it has a genetic susceptibility. It has also been proposed that viruses, such as Epstein–Barr virus (EBV) or human T-cell lymphotrophic virus (HTLV), may have a pathogenic role in Sjogren's disease; however, evidence for this is currently speculative.

Sjögren's syndrome and lymphomas

Patients with Sjögren's syndrome have a greater risk of lymphoma than the general population. These tumours can begin in the salivary glands or in the lymph nodes. Many salivary gland infiltrates that were previously assumed to be benign lymphoepithelial lesions are now recognised as lymphomas. These are mostly low-grade non-Hodgkin's lymphoma of the **mucosa-associated lymphoid tissue** (MALT lymphomas).

Clinical features

- Predominantly women above 40 years of age are affected. However, it may occur in men and young adults. The female to male ratio is 10:1
- Parotid gland is more frequently involved
- Typical features of the disease are the dryness of the mouth and eyes (xerostomia and xerophthalmia), which often results in painful burning sensation and ulcerations on the oral and conjunctival mucosa
- Apart from this, various secretory glands of the nose, larynx, pharynx and vagina are involved with this dryness
- Primary Sjögren's syndrome is characterised by parotid gland enlargement, purpura, lymphadenopathy and other symptoms.

Laboratory findings

- The erythrocyte sedimentation rate is high in individuals with Sjogren's syndrome
- Serum immunoglobulin levels are highly diagnostic
- Whether or not the patient has rheumatoid arthritis, a positive rheumatoid factor is observed in 75% of instances
- In most cases, antinuclear antibodies may also be positive
  a. Anti-SS A (anti-Ro) and anti-SS B (anti-La) are two nuclear autoantibodies that are often identified, particularly in individuals with primary Sjogren's disease
  b. Immunofluorescence: Anti-Ro and anti-La antibodies cause a speckled appearance
- In the Schirmer test, a strip of filter paper is placed in the lower conjunctival sac
  a. In 5 min, normal patients will moisten 15 mm of filter paper
  b. Sjögren's syndrome patients will moisten less than 5 mm of filter paper

- **The Rose-Bengal dye test** is used to identify corneal injury and denudation
- A **slit-lamp** is used to measure the duration between a full blink and the emergence of a dry area on the cornea, which is known as the break up time
- The patient is deemed to have dry eyes if two of the three tests are abnormal
- Salivary gland function may be assessed by parotid flow rate, biopsy and **salivary scintigraphy** in suspected instances. In these cases, **sialochemistry** investigations have shown higher levels of IgA, K, Na and other substances
- Sialography reveals cavitary defects filled with radiopaque contrast media, giving the appearance of a 'branchless fruit laden tree' or 'cherry blossom'.

Criteria for Sjogren's syndrome

1. Ocular symptoms (at least one of the following):
   a. Use of a tear substitute more than three times daily
   b. Persistent, troublesome dry eyes for longer than 3 months
   c. Recurrent sensation of sand or gravel in the eye
2. Ocular signs (at least one of the following):
   a. Positive Rose-Bengal stain
   b. Positive Schirmer's test
3. Oral symptoms (at least one of the following):
   a. Feeling of dry mouth every day for at least 3 months
   b. Need to drink liquids in order to swallow dry food
   c. Recurrent feeling of swollen salivary glands as an adult
4. Oral signs (at least one of the following):
   a. Parotid sialography
   b. Salivary gland scintigraphy
   c. Unstimulated whole saliva (less than 1.5 mL/15 min)
5. Histopathology: Focal lymphocytic sialadenitis of major or minor salivary gland
6. Laboratory abnormalities (at least one of the following):
   a. ANA (antinuclear antibody)
   b. IgM rheumatoid factor (anti-IgG Fc)
   c. Anti-SS-A or anti-SS-B.

Histopathologic features

Basic microscopic finding in Sjogren's syndrome is a lymphocytic infiltration of the salivary glands with destruction of the acinar units. If the major glands are enlarged, microscopic examination usually shows progression to a lymphoepithelial lesion.

Treatment and prognosis

- Treatment of the patient with Sjogren's syndrome is mostly supportive
- The dry eyes are best managed by periodic use of artificial tears with a slowly dissolving methylcellulose preparation, such as Lacrisert (*Merck*) or Restasis (*Allergan*), on a daily basis
- In addition, attempts can be made to conserve the tear film through the use of sealed glasses to prevent evaporation
- The eyes also often require topical antibiotics such as *sulphacetamide* or ophthalmologic gentamycin
- Sealing the lacrimal punctum pack in the inner margin of the eyelids also can be helpful by blocking of the normal drainage of any lacrimal secretions into the nose
- Artificial saliva is available for the treatment of xerostomia: sugarless candy or gum can help to keep the mouth moist
- Symptoms often can be relieved by the use of oral hygiene products that contain lactoperoxidase, lysozyme and lactoferrin. Sialagogues such as *pilocarpine and cevimeline* can be useful to stimulate salivary flow if enough functional salivary tissue still remains
- Because of the increased risk of dental caries, daily fluoride applications may be indicated in dentulous patients
- Antifungal therapy is often needed to treat secondary candidiasis.

Section IX

Reconstructive Surgery

Chapter 32

Introduction to Reconstructive Surgery

OUTLINE

INTRODUCTION

The need for reconstructive surgery arises when the patient experiences a loss of tissue. This may be due to benign and malignant tumours, secondary defects due to trauma, congenital defects and growth disturbances like temporomandibular Joint (TMJ) ankylosis. The hard and soft tissues can be replaced by using flaps and grafts from different parts of the body. In this section, a brief note on the various flaps and grafts used in oral and maxillofacial surgery will be discussed.

RATIONALE OF RECONSTRUCTION

The planning of reconstruction should consider the functional and aesthetic components. For the oral cavity, the functional components include speech, mastication and swallowing. The aesthetic components include contour, expression and competence.

RECONSTRUCTION LADDER

The reconstruction ladder is a guideline for better understanding of the treatment plan for wound closure. Various factors play a role in choosing or surpassing the treatment options in the reconstructive ladder. More complex defects will require treatments mentioned in the higher rung of the ladder. The components of the reconstruction ladder will be discussed in the next two chapters 33 & 34 (Fig. 32.1).

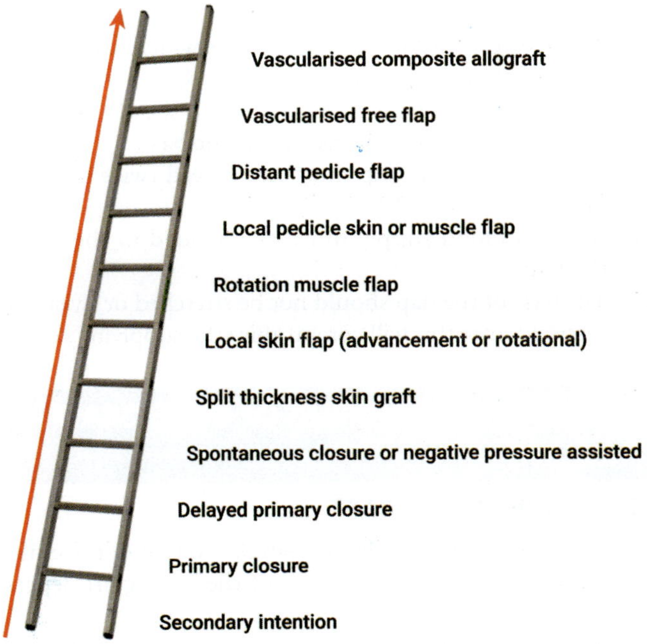

Figure 32.1 Reconstruction ladder.

PRINCIPLES AND GUIDELINES FOR FLAP DESIGNS

1. Replace like with like
2. Reconstruction should be done in terms of the anatomical units
3. Once a surgical plan has been determined, use a template pattern to fit the defect and trace on the donor site
4. Do not advance tissue to the deficient area unless it can be accomplished completely without tension. This will compromise the blood supply of the flap resulting in flap failure
5. The donor site should not result in deformity in terms of function
6. Goals:
   a. Adequate colour match
   b. Adequate thickness—avoid protrusions or deficiencies
   c. Preservation of clinically perceivable sensory innervation
   d. Sufficient laxity—avoid retraction or deranged function

e. Resultant suture lines of either primary or secondary defects are restricted to anatomic units and fall within natural skin lines
7. All surgical instruments used for cutting or incising should be sharp and of appropriate size
8. While incising the tissues, firm continuous strokes should be used
9. Avoid cutting the vital structures like nerves and vessels
10. Instruments should be perpendicular to the epithelial tissue. This angle creates sharp wound edges that heal with minimal scar tissue formation
11. Long incisions not only give better access and ease in tissue separation, but they also heal faster
12. Avoid incisions across major muscle attachments: Difficult repositioning of the flap and healing by secondary intention will result in scar tissue formation if incisions are made across major muscle attachments. This is avoided by including the muscle attachment within the flap
13. Provide adequate visual and operative access with minimal tissue trauma
14. The apex of the flap should never be wider than the base (Fig. 32.2). Exception can be made when a major artery is present in the base. Sides of the flap should be parallel to each other or convergent from the base
15. The length of the flap must not exceed twice the width of the base (Fig. 32.3)
16. An axial blood supply must be included in the base of the flap
17. The base of the flap should not be stretched or twisted excessively since this will compromise the supplying vessels.

BIOLOGICAL PRINCIPLES OF BONE GRAFT HEALING

HEALING OF BONE GRAFT

Bone healing is a unique process similar to that of the embryonic bone formation. The healing of the bone graft depends

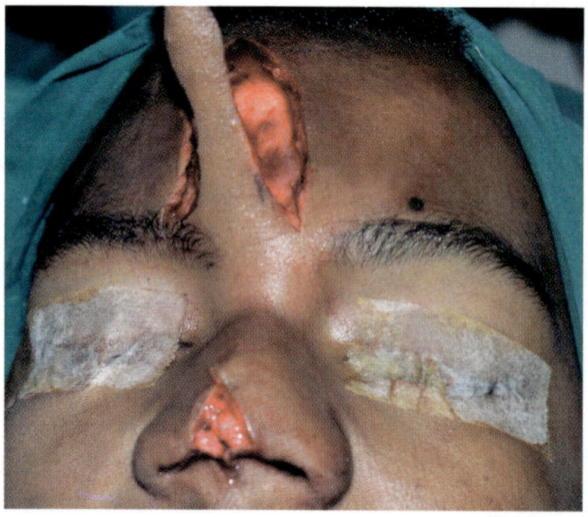

Figure 32.2 The forehead flap for the reconstruction of the nasal deformity. The flap base is wider than the apex.

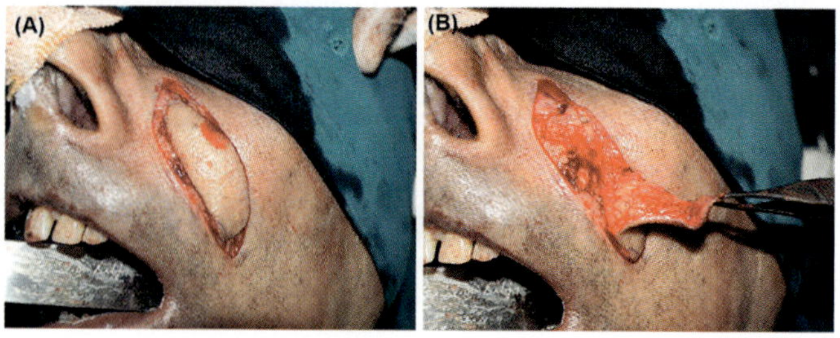

Figure 32.3 The nasolabial flap for intraoral reconstruction of the buccal mucosa in an oral submucous fibrosis patient. This is an axial flap, an islanded pedicle flap raised from the angular artery's pedicle. Note that it follows all principles of flap design.

upon the recipient site's blood supply, oxygen tension and stability of bone segments. Healing of the bone graft may be by primary bone healing or by secondary bone healing (intermediate cartilaginous phase).

Primary bone healing implies direct contact or a gap of less than 1 mm between bone fragments. This healing process occurs by osteoclasts working in groups to create a cutting cone. Following this cutting cone of osteoclasts are osteoblasts secreting osteoid for future mineralisation (Fig. 32.4).

Secondary bone healing occurs after the formation of a callus. Once the primary osteoid and secondary osteoid are formed, mineralisation occurs. This type of bone healing can be divided into the following three major phases (Fig. 32.5):
1. Inflammatory phase (haematoma formation)
2. Reparative phase (soft and hard callus formation)
3. Remodelling phase.

These principles of primary and secondary bone healing can be applied to bone graft healing. The type of graft material used, block versus particulate, dictates which healing process occurs.

Creeping substitution: It is a process by which the cortical bone graft healing occurs and is similar to that of primary

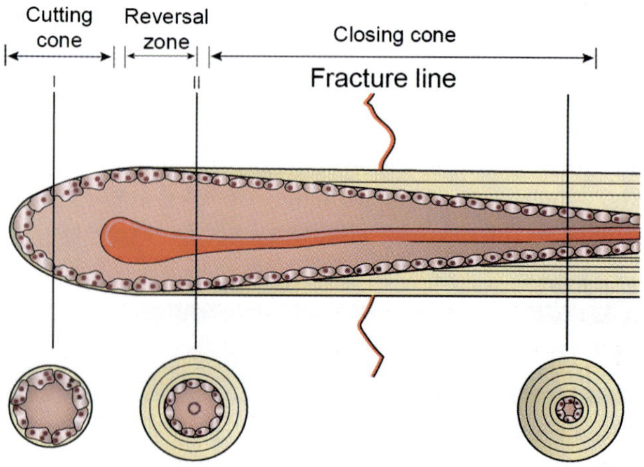

Figure 32.4 Primary bone healing. (I) Osteoclastic cutting cone crossing the fracture gap. (II and III) Bone reconstitution by the trailing osteoblasts.

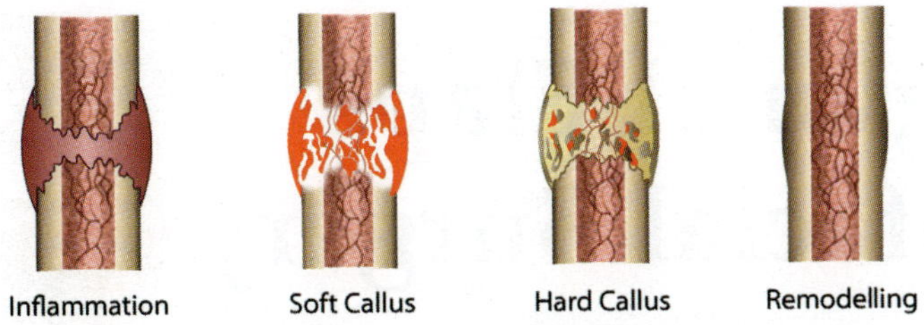

Figure 32.5 Secondary bone healing.

bone healing. Once the nonvascularised graft material is transferred to the defect, osteoclasts create voids in the graft material that are filled with osteoid from osteoblasts. This osteoid then becomes mineralised, undergoes remodelling and maturation. Ideally, the grafted bone would be completely resorbed and new bone would be formed. The grafted bone remains as necrotic centres mixed with the newly formed bone.

Bone apposition: It is a process of bone healing that occurs in particulated cortical or cancellous bone grafts. This bone apposition is followed by the resorption of the graft material. Ideally, there is complete resorption of the graft material which is replaced by mature bone. Cancellous grafts revascularise faster than cortical block grafts as they do not have to 1st undergo resorption before apposition. When particulate bone grafts are used, the newly formed bone undergoes greater resorption.

Reconstruction of craniomaxillofacial region may be achieved with bone grafting or endosseous implant. The basic difference between the bone grafts and the implants must be appreciated to understand the complex healing process of both. By definition, the bone grafting procedure refers to the surgical removal of the living tissue, along with or without its blood supply, from the harvested donor site to the host bed. The implant refers to the surgical placement of the nonviable biocompatible material. Autogenous bone grafts have cells with bone forming ability, platelets and fibrin. The survival of osteoblasts in the endosteum and haematopoietic cells may be around 5 days after transplantation, owing to their capability to absorb nutrients from the adjacent tissues (Flowchart 32.1). Initial regeneration begins within hours of placement of grafts. After revascularisation of the graft, the bone forming units are formed from the circulating stem cells, which are attracted to the wound followed by the remodelling process, which is the end phase of bone healing.

Graft placement

↓

Degranulation of entrapped platelets

↓

Release of growth factors like platelet-derived growth factor (PDGF) from alpha granules and transforming growth factor beta-1 (TGF- β1)

↓

Initiation of capillary Ingrowth by endothelial cells after binding with PDGF

↓

Stimulation of the endosteal osteoblasts and haematopoietic stem cells for initiating mitosis (Increasing numbers)

↓

Osteoid formation (because of the bond between TGF - β1 and cell receptors)

↓

After three days, locally induced macrophages replace the influence of the growth factors

↓

Regulation of bone healing by the synthesis of growth factors by macrophages

↓

By 14th day, the graft will be completely revascularised

↓

Endosteal osteoblasts of the surgically transferred bone graft begin to lay down osteoid and stem cells differentiate into osteoblasts

↓

Small masses of bone formation develop in the transplanted bone graft

Flowchart 32.1 Healing of the bone graft.

CLASSIFICATION OF RECONSTRUCTION

SOFT TISSUE RECONSTRUCTION

Regional soft tissue flaps:

- Submental island flap
- Temporalis flap
- Pectoralis major myocutaneous flap
- Latissimus dorsi myocutaneous pedicled flap
- Forehead flap

Microvascular soft tissue flaps:

- Radial artery fasciocutaneous flap
- Anterolateral thigh flap
- Rectus abdominis myocutaneous flap
- Latissimus myocutaneous free flap

HARD TISSUE RECONSTRUCTION

Nonvascularised bone grafts:

- Iliac crest (anterior and posterior)
- Tibial bone graft
- Cranial bone graft

Vascularised flaps:

- Osteocutaneous radial forearm flap
- Osteocutaneous fibula flap
- Scapula free flap
- Iliac crest free flap

Chapter 33

Local and Regional Flaps Used in Maxillofacial Surgery

OUTLINE

DEFINITION

A flap is defined as a unit or a tongue of tissue consisting of the entire thickness of skin/mucosa, and variable amount of subcutaneous/submucous tissue that is transferred from the donor site to recipient site with its own blood supply.

CLASSIFICATIONS

ACCORDING TO BLOOD SUPPLY

Random flaps are supplied by the dermal and subdermal plexus. The blood supply is not a named artery or vein. It is used for smaller flaps for which the capillaries can maintain the blood supply.

Axial pattern flaps are supplied by a dominant superficial vessel that is oriented along the long axis of the flap.

Pedicle flaps are supplied by vascular units that are larger named arteries. These vascular units that are elevated are called the vascular pedicle, which supplies the skin paddle.

Free tissue transfer are harvested from remote regions and the vascular connection is re-established at the recipient site by microvascular surgery.

ACCORDING TO LOCATION

Local flaps are raised from the tissue adjacent to the defect.

Regional flaps are located near the defect, but are not in immediate proximity. They are usually pedicle flaps. The pedicle needs to be extended to reach certain defects.

Distant flaps are harvested from a different part of the body or different anatomical unit that is not in immediate proximity. These flaps are completely disconnected from the vascular supply of the donor site and microvascularly connected to the recipient site.

ACCORDING TO CONFIGURATION

Bilobed
Rhombic
Z-plasty

ACCORDING TO TISSUE CONTENT

Cutaneous flap: Contains skin only
Myocutaneous flap: Contains skin and muscles
Fasciocutaneous flap: Contains skin and fascia.

ACCORDING TO METHOD OF TRANSFER

Advancement flaps are mobilised along a linear axis in the same plane towards the defect

Rotation flaps are pivoted around a point at the base of the flap, then they are used to cover the complete defect

Transposition flaps are raised from a normal area that is immediate to the defect. It is mobilised to an adjacent defect from an area that is not a part of the defect. Examples of these flaps include rhombic flaps and bilobed flaps

Interposition flaps are mobilised to an adjacent defect over an incomplete bridge of skin, which is also elevated and mobilised. For example, Z-plasty

Interpolated flaps are mobilised over or beneath a part of intact skin through a pedicle of flap containing vascular and tissue pedicle.

LOCAL FLAPS (RANDOM FLAPS AND AXIAL FLAPS)

ROTATIONAL FLAP

Rotational flaps have a curvilinear configuration and a large base. They have a random or an axial blood supply (Fig. 33.1). This type of flap is used majorly to reconstruct scalp defects, for oroantral fistula closure (palatal flaps—Fig. 33.2) and for closure of nasal defects.

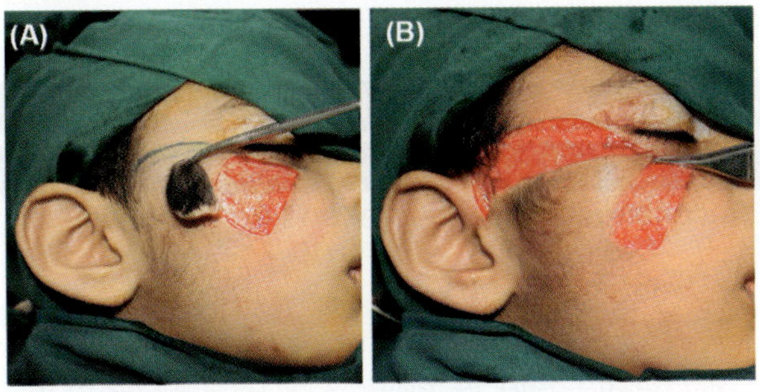

Figure 33.1 (**A**) The photograph shows a case of hairy nevus on the right cheek, the defect is excised. A rotational flap is planned to cover the defect. (**B**) Rotational flap has been raised; the flap movement is in an arc on a fixed plane. The flap gives more movement of tissues for better closure.

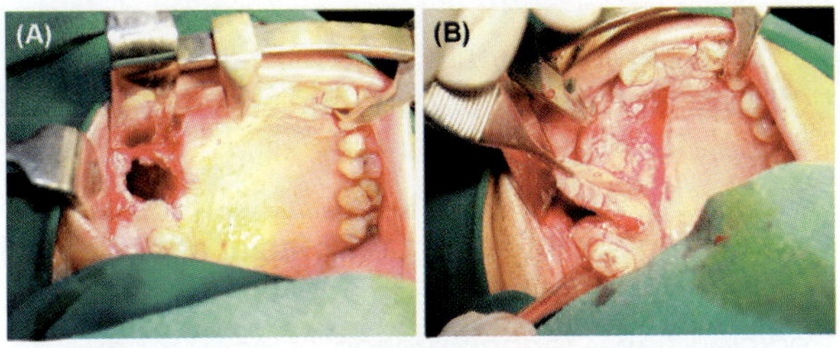

Figure 33.2 (**A** and **B**) Palatal rotational flap.

- The axial frontonasal flap is a pedicled graft from the angular artery and supraorbital artery and are used for closing nasal defects
- The palatal island flap is a pedicled graft on the greater palatine artery for closure of oroantral or oronasal defect
- The buccinator myomucosal flap is an island flap with pedicle on facial artery.

PIVOT FLAPS OR TRANSPOSITIONAL FLAPS FOR TRIANGULAR DEFECTS (Fig. 33.3)

The transposition flaps are designed such that one border of the flap becomes the border of the defect as the flaps are rotated and advanced over the adjacent defect. These transfer tension away from closure of the primary defect. In the head and neck region, it is most commonly used over the nasal tip, the nasal ala, the inferior eyelid and the lips.

There are many types of transposition or pivot flaps like the following:

1. Limberg rhomboid flap, 1963
2. Dufourmentel flap, 1962
3. Bilobed flap (Fig. 33.4)
4. Z-plasty (for lengthening and shortening).

ADVANCEMENT FLAPS

Advancement flaps have a linear configuration, which limits wound tension to a single vector (direction). It is a simple flap used in the defects of the forehead, the helical rim, lips and cheeks. Advancement flaps are also used intraorally for covering oroantral fistulas, but this can decrease the vestibular sulcus depth. If the tissue surrounding the flap has good laxity, scars can be hidden within the skin crease. The most common advancement flaps are described in the Table 33.1.

Extraoral:

1. Single—pedicle advancement flap
2. Bilateral advancement flap (H-plasty)

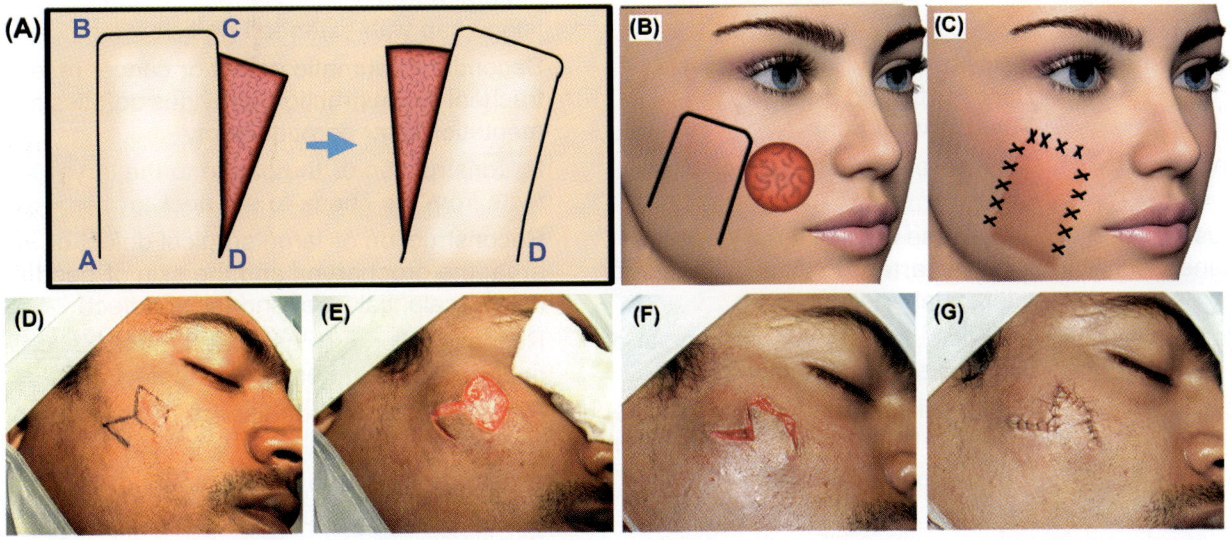

Figure 33.3 (**A**) Transposition flap; a pivot flap, D is the pivot point. (**B**) Defect is shown and the planned transposition flap has been marked. (**C**) Transposition flap sutured. (**D–G**) Limberg's flap—a type of transposition flap.

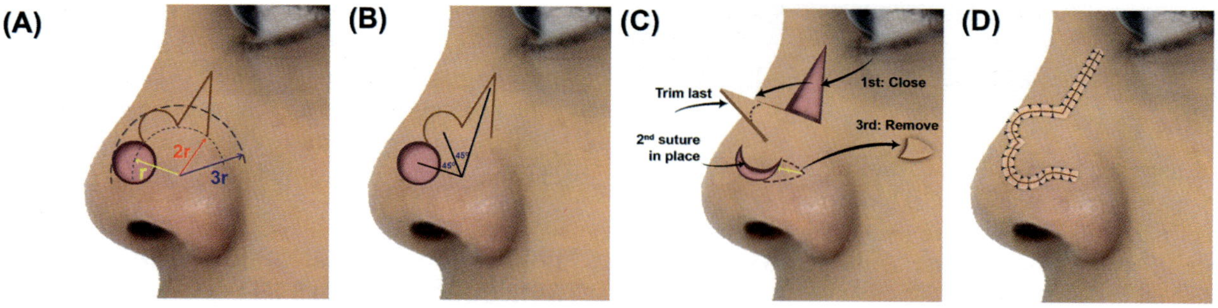

Figure 33.4 (**A–D**) Bilobed flap for small spherical defect on the nose.

TABLE 33.1 Major Composite Flaps used in Oral Surgery with Blood Supply and Reconstructive Uses

Composite Flap	Blood Supply	Used for
Facial artery perforator flap	Based on facial artery perforators—lateral nasal artery or superior alar artery or angular artery or superior labial artery or paramandibular artery—Mitz et al.	Reconstruction of perioral and perinasal defects
Bipedicle advancement flap	Greater palatine artery	Cleft palate defects, defects of palate due to tumour or trauma. Other intraoral defects like alveolar defects (Fig. 33.10A and B).
Glabellar flap	Random flap or pedicled flap based on supratrochlear artery	Reconstruction of defects of the upper 3rd of the nose and periorbital areas Medial canthus reconstruction
Temporalis flap	The anterior and posterior deep temporal arteries	Reconstruction of skull base and orbital defects To close cerebrospinal fluid (CSF) leaks, traumatic defect of soft tissue of zygomatico-orbital complex, soft palate, mandibular and maxillary defects (Fig. 33.10F-I)
Narayanan's bilobed flap	Superficial temporal artery	Obliterating skull base, maxillofacial and orbital defects, cranialisation and facial reanimation.
Submental flap	Superficial and deep submental artery branches	Pedicled flap—reconstruction of chin, tongue defects, buccal defects, floor of the mouth defects, perioral areas Island flap with extended pedicle—temporal region
Sternocleidomastoid flap	Occipital artery Superior thyroid artery Thyrocervical trunk	Secondary traumatic defect or cancer resection, tracheal reconstruction, provides soft tissues augmentation after parotidectomy
Platysma flap	Submental branch of facial artery	Reconstruction of the palate to the larynx and defects from the cheek to the neck
Trapezius myocutaneous flap	Transverse cervical artery Occipital artery, Perforating posterior intercostal artery	Reconstruction of large surgical defect of intraoral area, the oropharynx and the skin of head and neck (scalp, calvarial and facial defect)
Scapular free flap	The scapular artery, parascapular artery and dorsal thoracic artery	Reconstruction of maxilla and mandible, orbital floor defects and hemipalatal defects
Supraclavicular artery flap	Supraclavicular artery, a direct cutaneous branch of the transverse cervical artery	Reconstruction of soft tissues of neck and orofacial regions
Deltopectoral flap	Internal mammary artery	Defects that require large amount of skin Alternative to PMMC flap Soft tissue reconstruction of the mandible and maxilla (Fig. 33.10C-E)

TABLE 33.1 Major Composite Flaps used in Oral Surgery with Blood Supply and Reconstructive Uses—cont'd

Composite Flap	Blood Supply	Used for
Pectoralis major myocutaneous flap	Pectoral branch of thoracoacromial artery Internal mammary artery	Reconstruction of base of the tongue, anterior skull base, total nose and orbital defect
Radial forearm free flap	Branches of radial artery	Reconstruction of soft palate, tongue and floor of the mouth
Latissimus dorsi myocutaneous flap	Thoracodorsal artery——four to six perforators from the posterior intercostal and lumbar vessels	Reconstruction of the entire cheek, hemiface, lower face mandible and maxilla used in large defects of head and neck
Rectus abdominus free flap	Deep epigastric artery	Reconstruction of posterior part of mandible, large tongue defects, orbit and cheek defect

3. Triangular design advancement flap
4. Counter incision advancement flap
5. Curvilinear design advancement flap
6. Z-plasty base advancement flap (Fig. 33.5A–C)
7. O–T plasty or A–T plasty
8. W-plasty or zigzag plasty (hairline transfer) (Fig. 33.6E and F)
9. V–Y advancement flap (Fig. 33.6H and I)
10. M-plasty for dog ear
11. Elliptical flap.

Intraoral:

1. Moczair's buccal sliding flap
2. Rehrmann's buccal advancement flap. (Chapter 25, Fig. 25.9)
3. Buccal advancement flaps (Fig. 33.7).

INTERPOLATION FLAPS

Interpolation flaps have a pedicle that passes either over the skin or under a bridge of intact skin. This pedicle is sutured to form a tube of tissue to prevent infection during flap healing phase. In this technique, the pedicle (tube-like flap) that passes over or under bridging skin must be detached as a 2nd stage surgical procedure. This technique produces excellent vascularity and success of the flap with a flawless skin colour and texture match (Fig. 33.8). The most common interpolation flaps are as follow:

1. *The forehead flap* for large nasal defects with the vascular pedicle of the supratrochlear vessels and angular artery
2. *The melolabial flap,* a type of nasolabial flap based on the pedicle of the angular artery, infraorbital artery and infratrochlear artery (Fig. 33.9). It is used in the reconstruction of the maxillary alveolus, the lip commissure, the lower 3rd of the nose, the chin and the columella
3. *The lip-switch flap,* commonly known as the Abbe's flap based on the labial artery, is ideal in the reconstruction of the columella in bilateral cleft lip defects
4. *Tongue flap* in cleft palate correction, the flap is based on the lingual artery.

REGIONAL FLAPS FOR HEAD AND NECK DEFECTS

Regional flaps are located near a defect, but are not in the immediate proximity like a local flap. While local flaps have a random blood supply, regional flaps have a named blood supply. They are needed when the defects become too large

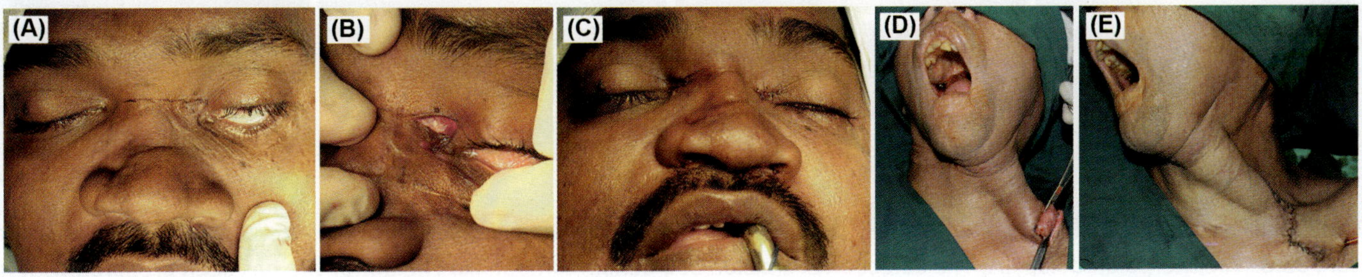

Figure 33.5 **(A–C)** Patient presented with a displaced medial canthus after trauma. Z-plasty done to transport the medial canthus defect to the correct level. **(D and E)** Z-plasty done to the pedicle of the pectoralis major myocutaneous (PMMC) flap to elongate the area to allow better movement. This is done only after the flap has completely healed with good vascularisation.

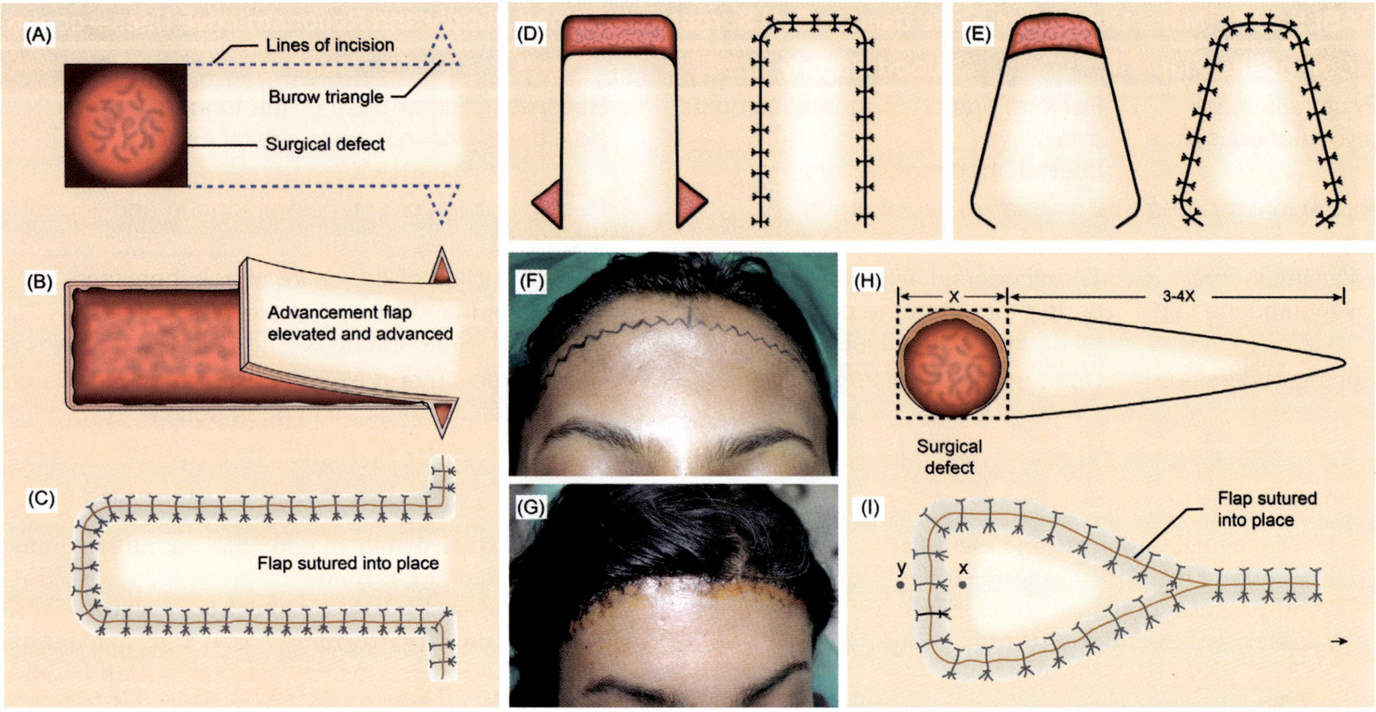

Figure 33.6 Extraoral advancement flaps. (**A–C**) Advancement flap; the flap moves in a single direction. The Burow's triangles are seen bilaterally at the bases of the flap. (**D** and **E**) Burow's triangle can be avoided with a curvilinear pattern advancement flap. (**F** and **G**) Advancement flap by W-plasty or zigzag plasty for hairline transfer. (**H** and **I**) V–Y advancement flap.

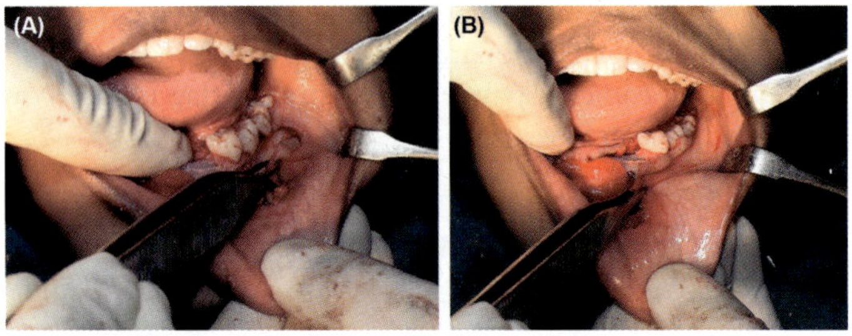

Figure 33.7 (**A** and **B**) Buccal advancement flap.

that a local flap cannot provide sufficient tissue to restore the missing tissue. The regional flaps are raised from the surrounding anatomical units like the neck, chest, temporal region, shoulders, forehead, arm or back.

ISLANDED FLAPS

The islanded flap is a regional flap that does not have a cutaneous attachment to the pedicle. The flap is incised in all sides containing skin and subcutaneous tissue, but the vascular pedicle remains intact. This allows the flap to have its

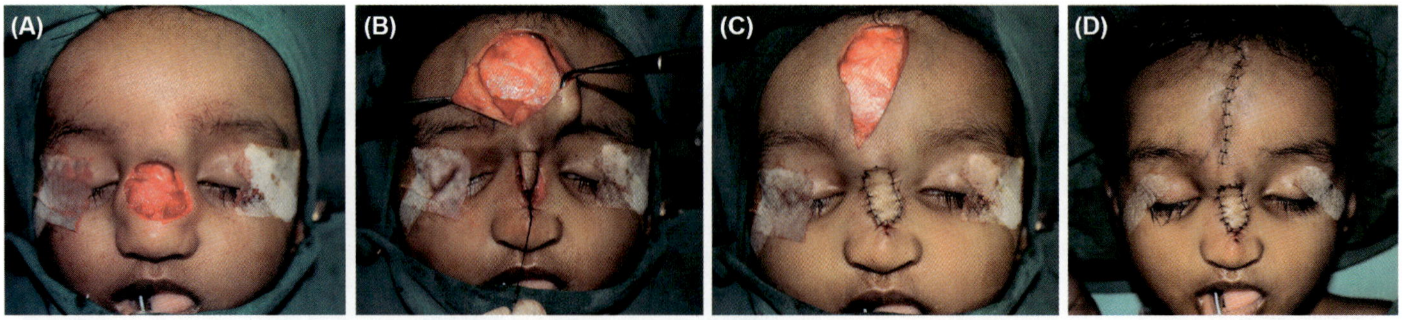

Figure 33.8. An Interpolated flap. (**A**) The defect after excision of a benign tumour. (**B**) The donor site has been prepared with the pedicle and skin island. The pedicle is made to be intact and is tunnelled beneath the bridge of skin to the recipient site as shown in this image. (**C**) The donor tissue is attached to the margins of the defect. The donor skin is being vascularised by the pedicle that has been tunnelled beneath the bridge of skin. (**D**) The donor site has been sutured.

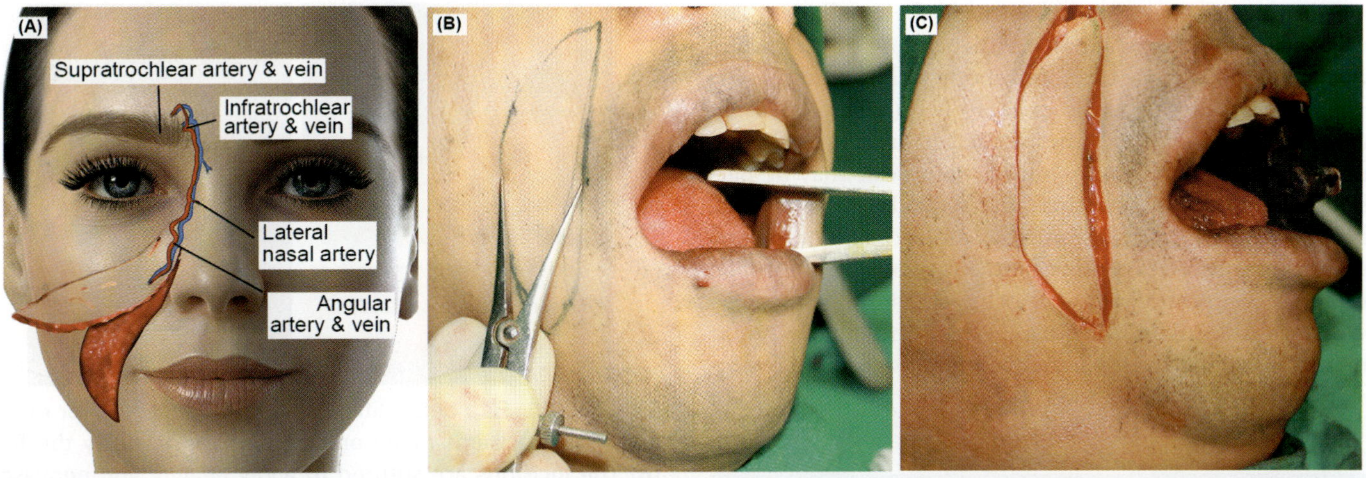

Figure 33.9 (**A**) Superiorly based nasolabial flap. (**B** and **C**) Nasolabial flap (axial pattern); inferiorly based nasolabial flap—angular artery.

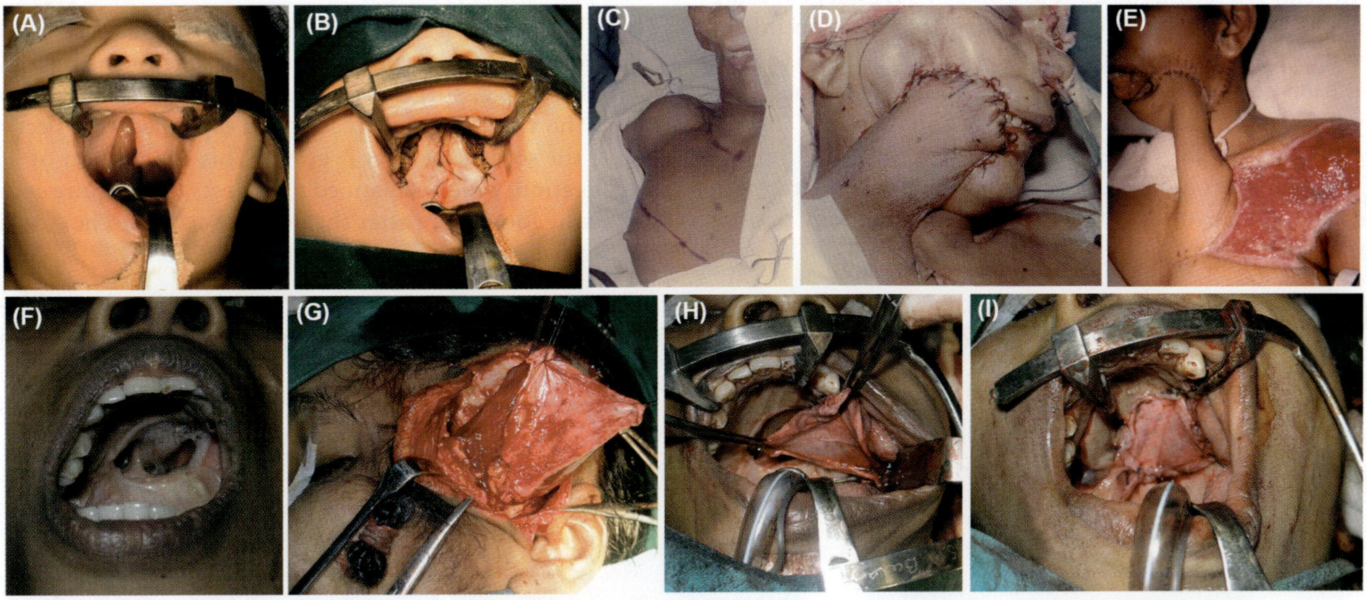

Figure 33.10 Composite flaps. (**A&B**) Bilateral palatal flap raised to close a cleft palate defect. (**C**) Design of the deltopectoral flap on the right side. (**D**) The regional flap has been rotated on to the defect for a right-side buccal defect. (**E**) Another case showing deltopectoral flap on the left side for a defect on the lower half of the face, the chin and submental area. (**F**) Palatal defect caused by a gunshot wound (**G-I**) Temporalis flap raised and rotated into the oral cavity to close the defect.

blood supply at the donor site until healing and neovascularisation of the donor site occurs.

PEDICLED FLAPS

These regional flaps are based on one or more vascular pedicle. Vascular pedicle is the blood supply to the flap. It is based on a named blood vessel. Mathes and Nahai classified pedicled flap as Type 1—flaps with one vascular pedicle. Type 2—flaps with dominant pedicles and minor pedicles. Type 3—flaps with two dominant pedicles. Type 4—flaps with segmental vascular pedicles and Type 5—flaps with dominant pedicle and secondary segmental pedicles.

Major composite flaps used in oral surgery with blood supply and reconstructive purposes are explained in Table 33.1.

DISTANT FREE FLAPS

Free tissue transfer means the transport of donor tissue from one site of the body to the recipient site with its blood supply. The blood supply is maintained in the new donor site by microvascular attachment of the donor vessels with the recipient vessels (both artery and vein). Thus, immediate blood supply to the graft is achieved. Blood thinners like heparin are given to the patient before and after the grafting procedure to prevent blood clot inside the capillaries. The composition of the graft may vary depending on the defective donor site. In some cases, only bone will be required, for example, free vascular fibula graft (FVFG) (page 681). Only the bone, periosteum and the vascular pedicle is harvested. In some defects, periosteum, muscle and bone may be harvested; these are the osteomuscular flaps. In some defects, bone, periosteum, attached muscles and skin island is harvested; this is called osteomyocutaneous flaps, for example, free fibula composite graft. The other types of distant flaps are direct distant flaps, tube distant flaps and microvascular (free) distant flaps. Examples of distant flaps are thoracodorsal artery perforator flap, medial sural artery perforator flap and toe web flap for commissure reconstruction.

FLAP MODIFICATIONS

FLAP DELAY

Flap delay is a technique done as a stage 1 surgical procedure before the actual elevation of the flap. A surgical outline of the flap, the incision is placed 7–14 days before the actual elevation of the flap. This allows the new nutrient blood supply to form on the either sides of the flap incision. This increases the flap tolerance to survive when the actual raising is done. This procedure also increases the tissue tolerance to ischaemia. Flap delay is usually done for random pattern flaps (Fig. 33.11).

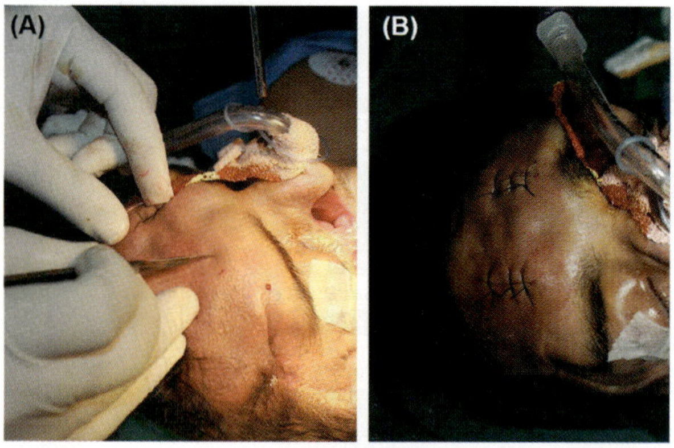

Figure 33.11 Flap delay; Stage 1 surgical procedure for raising a flap. (**A**) Incisions made on the forehead to delay the flap. (**B**) The incisions are sutured to allow healing and neovascularisation for up to 14 days.

TISSUE EXPANSION

Tissue expansion is a procedure where the soft tissue—the cutaneous and subcutaneous layer, is grown by using a balloon-like device, surgically placed below the subcutaneous layer. The tissue expander device is expanded by injecting saline, the soft tissue over it grows. This is a pattern of flap modification, which is planned for defects that require excess soft tissue for closure after the defect is excised. The soft tissue is grown according to the defect (Fig. 33.12).

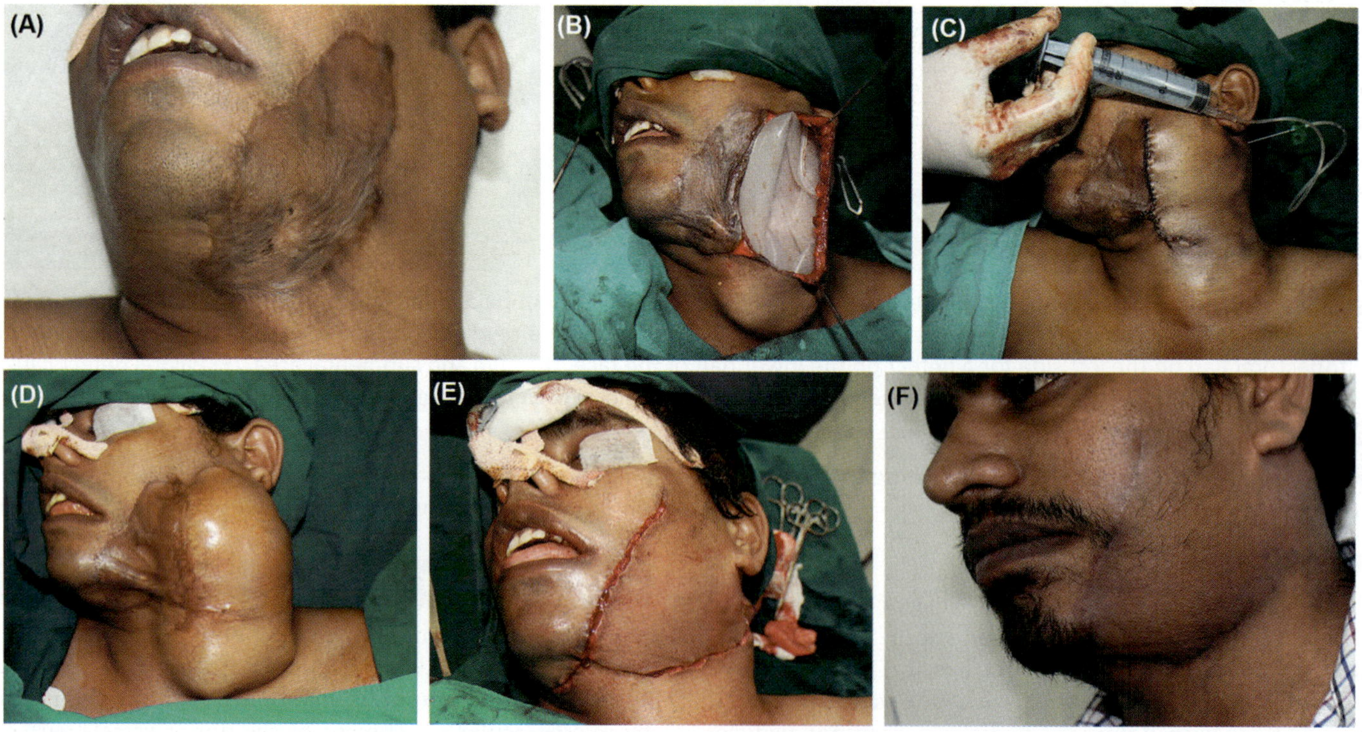

Figure 33.12 (**A**) A case of history of burns on the left side with an unaesthetic scar on his left lower facial region. (**B**) The skin behind the scar was raised and the tissue expander device was inserted and sutured. (**C**) Saline was injected into the device and the tissue expansion has been achieved. (**D**) Result after completion of tissue expansion. (**E**) The scar and the expander have been removed and sutured. (**F**) Postoperative photograph.

Chapter 34

Hard and Soft Tissue Reconstruction Using Vascularised and Nonvascularised Grafts

OUTLINE

INTRODUCTION TO HARD TISSUE RECONSTRUCTION

A defect in the bone is the main component of hard tissue reconstruction. There is no soft tissue defect and it usually involves pathologies pertaining only to the bone. There is no involvement of the soft tissue, as there is in benign tumours. Some malignant tumours do not have margins involving the soft tissues or can be closed by primary intention. In these cases also, only hard tissue reconstruction is done. The gold standard in bone grafts in oral and maxillofacial surgery is autografts. The two types of grafts are vascularised and nonvascularised. The nonvascularised bone grafts are more commonly used as reconstruction options for smaller defects. After complete fusion with the recipient site, the graft receives its blood supply from the recipient site and hence the name nonvascularised grafts. The bone graft healing process has been described in detail in the Chapter 32 (page no. 668–669). With vascular grafting, the bone graft is harvested with its vascular components, for example, free vascularised fibular grafts (FVFG)—the fibula bone is harvested along with the peroneal artery and two peroneal veins. These arteries and veins are joined to the recipient site by microvascular surgery. The recipient vascular structure is either the branches of the facial artery or mandibular artery, if it is viable after surgical excision of the defect/tumour. The major differences between nonvascularised and vascularised bone grafts are explained in Table 34.1.

TABLE 34.1 Differences Between Nonvascularised and Vascularised Bone Grafts

Feature	Nonvascularised Bone Grafts	Vascularised Bone Grafts
Blood supply	Healing of the nonvascularised bone graft is by osteoconductive and osteoinductive properties. They do not have osteogenic properties	The blood supply is immediately provided once the recipient artery is microsurgically attached to the donor artery
Viability	The viability of this graft depends on the time taken for revascularisation by slow resorption of the cortex	The graft viability is better than nonvascularised grafts as the osteocytes survive better due to immediate vascularisation
Remodelling time	Up to 2 years	Remodelling is minimal. Only the bone docking site remodelling may occur
Defect size	Used in defects less than 6 cm	Can be used in defects up to 12 cm

AUTOGENOUS BONE GRAFT PROPERTIES (Table 34.2)

TABLE 34.2 Autogenous Bone Graft Properties

Auto-graft	Structural Strength	Osteo-conduction	Osteo-induction	Osteo-genesis
Can-cellous	No	+++	+++	+++
Cortical	+++	++	++	++

FORMS OF AUTOGENOUS BONE GRAFTS

The autogenous bone grafts (ABGs) can be harvested in two major forms as bone blocks or particulate bone. Bone blocks can be taken from all major sites of bone harvests, for example, mandibular symphysis and ramus. The particulate bone can be obtained in different ways. The most common ways are bone particles scrapped off from the surface of the cortex using an Ebner's knife or milling the block graft to produce particulate bone or by scooping out bone marrow from the iliac crest. Bone blocks can be harvested from all the sites mentioned below. Piezo drills can be used to harvest bone blocks from the intraoral sites. Block bone is grafted into the recipient site with the help of screws or pins to provide an immovable site for bone healing. The other forms used are cortical bone chips and osseous coagulum.

NONVASCULARISED GRAFTS OR FREE GRAFTS

INTRAORAL ACCESSED FREE GRAFTS

The most often used intraoral sites for bone harvesting are the maxillary tuberosity, mandibular symphysis and the mandibular ramus. The other intraoral sites of bone harvesting are the coronoid process, residual alveolar ridge, canine eminence and the area lateral to the anterior nasal spine. The site of bone harvesting is determined based on the volume of the defect (recipient site) (Fig. 34.1).

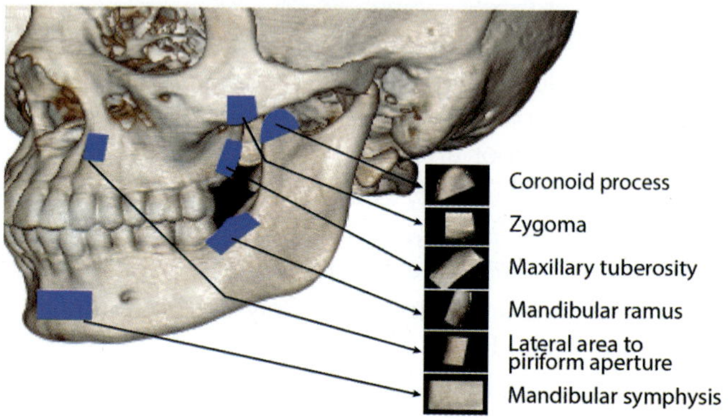

Figure 34.1 Illustration showing various intraoral sites of harvesting autogenous bone grafts.

MAXILLARY TUBEROSITY

The maxillary tuberosity is an easy intraoral site of bone harvest for particulate bone and for block bone grafts. The anatomical limits of this area are the maxillary sinus, the pterygoid plates, the molar teeth and the greater palatine foramen. The tuberosity gives a bone volume of at least 2 mL and dimensions of 10 × 10 mm size grafts. The bone can be harvested by using a drill or by piezo surgery. The use of a bone ronguer and bone scraper like Ebner's knife is indicated for particulate bone harvest. Maxillary tuberosity bone harvesting technique is used mostly in dental implantology or in small defects of the maxilla and mandible (Fig. 34.2).

MANDIBULAR SYMPHYSIS

The bone volume that it provides is approximately 5 mL of particulate bone and up to 2 cm in length of bone. The bone can be used in particulate or block form. The graft is more cortical in nature considering the bone density in the mandibular symphysis. This allows minimal graft resorption. It can be used in both vertical and horizontal bone defects of the alveolus. It is frequently employed in the anterior maxilla when buccal bone loss is present. The particulate bone from this area can be used in direct sinus augmentation technique. The anatomical considerations in this technique are the lower anterior teeth roots, the mental nerve (during flap elevation) and the mental foramen. The osteotomies should be performed at least 5 mm below the root apices and 3 mm away from the mental foramen. The clinician should be aware of the complications of this technique, which include damage to the mental nerve, mental foramen, submental and sublingual arteries (Fig. 34.3).

MANDIBULAR RAMUS

Ramus grafts are used when longer grafts are required. The block bone graft length yield is around 4 mm to 3 cm in length with up to 1 cm of height of bone and yields up to 10 mL of particulate bone. Ramus grafts are used in bone augmentation before dental implants, especially in the posterior maxillary region in orthognathic surgery and for immediate reconstruction of smaller tumour defects. The graft is accessed intraorally and the bone is removed with a chisel following the osteotomy cuts. The anatomical considerations are the lingual

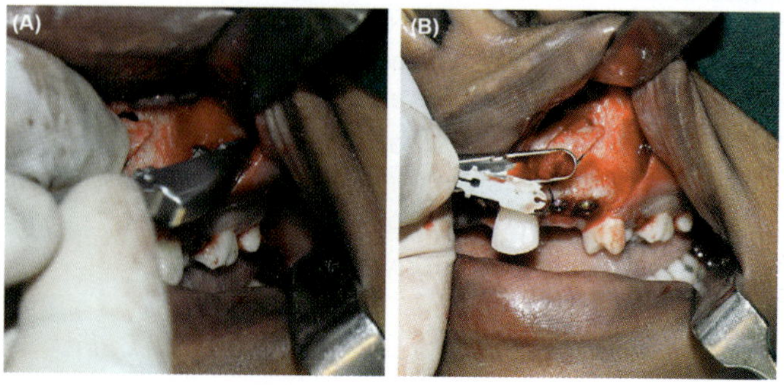

Figure 34.2 (**A** and **B**) A case showing particulate graft harvested from the maxillary tuberosity using Ebner's knife.

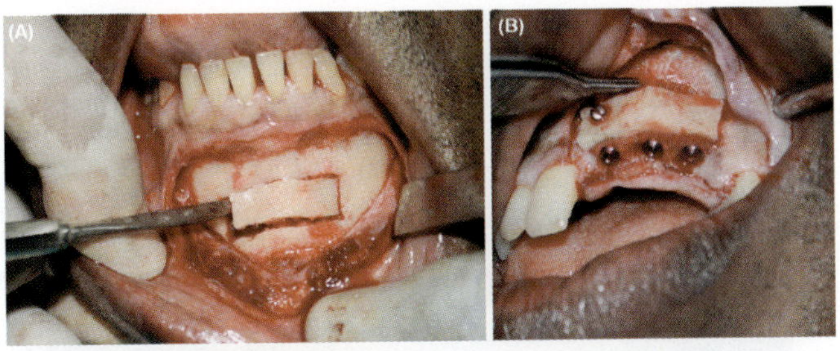

Figure 34.3 (**A** and **B**) Harvesting of block graft from the mandibular symphysis used as an onlay graft for dental implants.

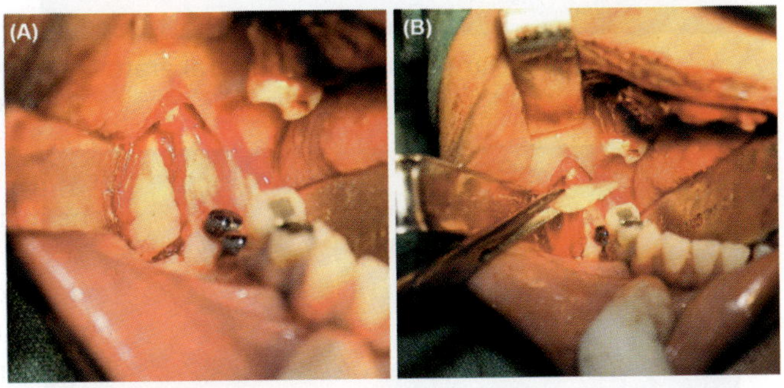

Figure 34.4 (**A** and **B**) Harvesting of block graft from the mandibular ramus at the retromolar area.

nerve while raising the mucoperiosteal flap and the inferior alveolar nerve. Due to the elevation of the temporalis muscle, the patient may experience postoperative trismus (Fig. 34.4).

ZYGOMA

Bone harvesting from the zygoma can provide more volume of graft and has an intraoral approach for access to the site of harvest. A mucoperiosteal flap is raised to the inferior aspect of the zygoma. Block bone graft or small bundles of bone can be harvested with a drill. The drill should be placed parallel to the maxilla and drilled to a depth of 12–14 mm. The graft's dimensions vary depending on the patient, but is usually about 12 × 12 mm. The bone volume yield is up to 5 mL of particulate bone. Before closing, it is critical to accomplish haemostasis with bone wax (Fig. 34.5).

CORONOID PROCESS

The coronoid process can be harvested for alveolar ridge augmentation and orthognathic surgery. The coronoid process can be accessed through an intraoral incision and the temporalis that gets inserted at the coronoid process is stripped off after the osteotomy cut to harvest the coronoid process (Fig. 34.6).

RESIDUAL ALVEOLAR RIDGE

Bone harvesting from the residual alveolar ridge is based on each patient and clinical situation. The graft can be procured using bone trap, trephine bur, bone shaving devices and suction trap. Bone in the form of osseous coagulum can be harvested from the lingual ridge, distal bone to the terminal tooth and any other edentulous areas.

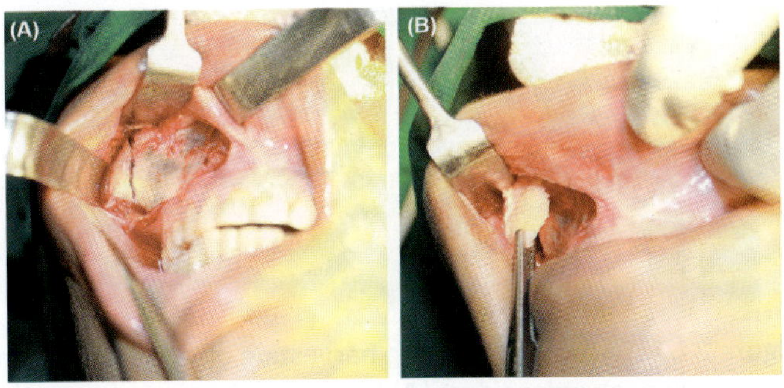

Figure 34.5 (**A** and **B**) Harvesting of block graft from the zygoma.

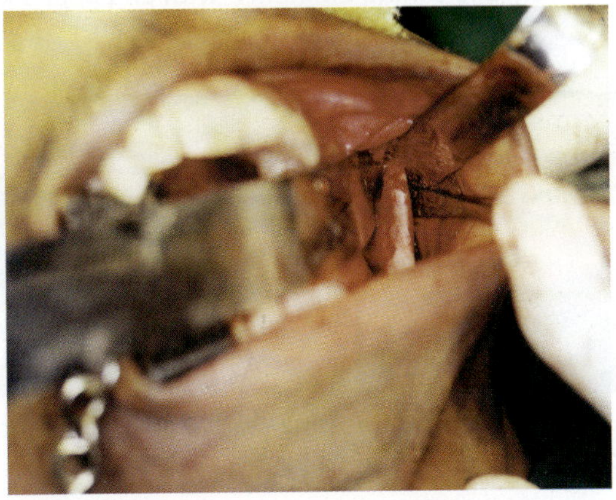

Figure 34.6 Harvesting of block graft from the coronoid process.

CANINE EMINENCE, LATERAL AREA TO THE ANTERIOR NASAL SPINE AND LATERAL AREA TO PIRIFORM APERTURE

The prominence of the bone in the canine area can be used as a site for bone harvest. The area lateral to the anterior nasal spine (ANS) and the piriform aperture are areas that can be accessed easily for small bone defects. Ultrasonic or mechanical bone shaving techniques are the most commonly used methods of bone harvesting. The bone harvested is minimal and can be used for one walled defects or for sinus augmentation techniques (Fig. 34.7).

EXTRAORAL FREE GRAFTS

CRANIUM

The cranial grafts have a characteristic early revascularisation. This allows the graft to survive without much change in dimension. They are used when there is a need of at least 40 mL of bone. The paramedian portion of the parietal bone has thick bone and is away from the superior sagittal sinus. It is approached through a hemicoronal or bicoronal incision. The grafts can be harvested as split thickness or full thickness grafts. Split thickness is only the superficial cortex and is most commonly used in maxillofacial surgery. Bone haemostasis should be achieved with bone wax before closure. The complications faced are haemorrhage due to trauma to the sagittal sinuses or vascular supply. Cranial

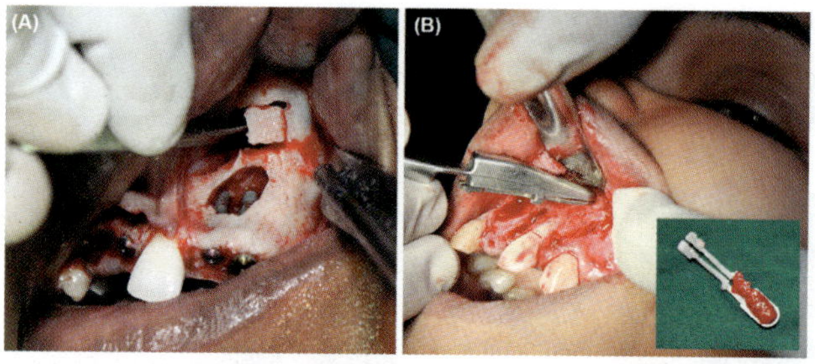

Figure 34.7 Two cases showing harvesting of bone graft from the maxillary alveolar ridge. (**A**) Block graft harvested from the area lateral to the piriform aperture. The graft was used to fill the bony defect caused by the cyst. (**B**) Particulate bone graft harvested from the canine eminence with an Ebner's knife.

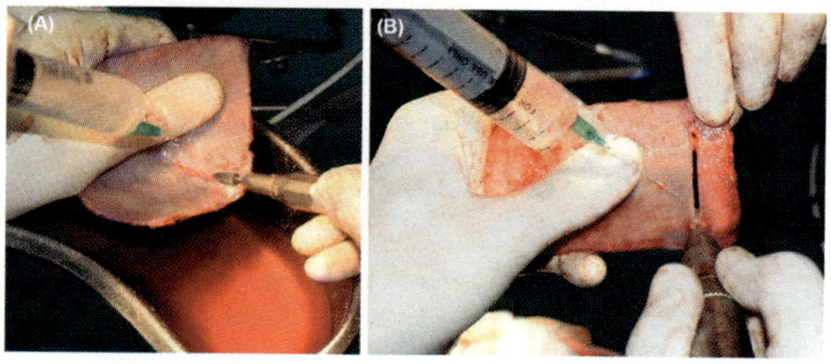

Figure 34.8 (**A** and **B**) Harvesting cranial bone graft through a bicortical incision.

grafts can be used in secondary trauma correction, orbital dystopia correction, etc. (Fig. 34.8).

RIB GRAFT

The ribs that are most commonly harvested as grafts are the 4th, 5th and 6th ribs. The 7th and 8th ribs are harvested when needed for ear reconstruction as they are thinner and more cartilaginous. The 4th rib is more corticocancellous compared to the others, which are costochondral. Rib grafts are also used in children with temporomandibular Joint (TMJ) ankylosis for joint reconstruction (refer to chapter 38 page 734). The most common complications are risk of pleural damage during harvesting and graft overgrowth. If pleural damage is evident, intercostal chest drain (ICD) is done (Fig. 34.9).

ILIAC CREST BONE GRAFT

Trap door technique of particulate bone harvest: In this technique, the corticocancellous bone marrow is scooped out from the iliac bone. The osteotomy cuts are made on the iliac bone and the cortex is partially osteotomised with a chisel. This creates a bony window through which the bone marrow can be harvested. The iliac bone marrow is used in cleft defects and alveolar bone grafting (Fig. 34.10).

Block bone harvest: Block bone can also be harvested from the iliac region. Instead of a trapdoor, the osteotomy cut is made through both the cortex and block bone is harvested for major defects in the maxillary or mandibular bone.

The volume of bone harvested is more in the iliac region than from the tibia (Fig. 34.11).

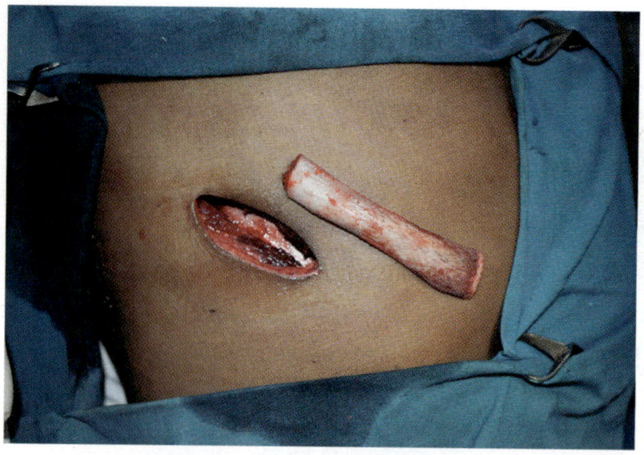

Figure 34.9 Harvested costochondral graft.

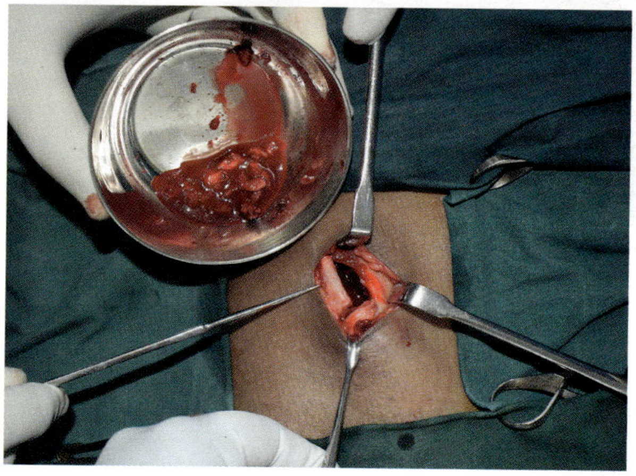

Figure 34.10 Particulate bone graft harvested for autogenous bone grafting of a cleft alveolus, through a trapdoor technique from the iliac crest.

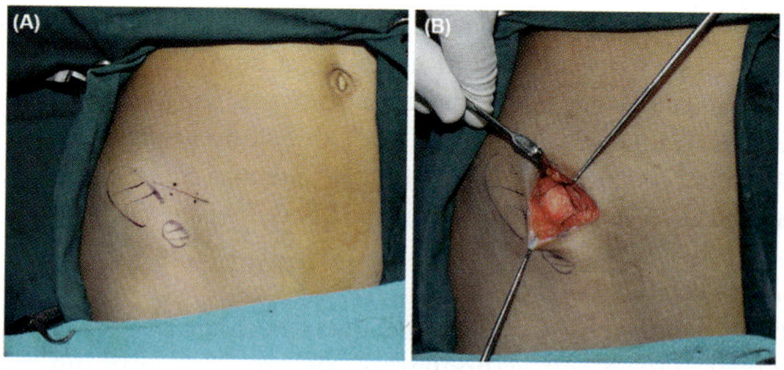

Figure 34.11 (**A** and **B**) Block bone graft harvested from the iliac region.

TIBIAL GRAFT

Particulate bone graft from the tibia contains osteoblasts and osteocytes, mineralised cancellous bone, fibrin and

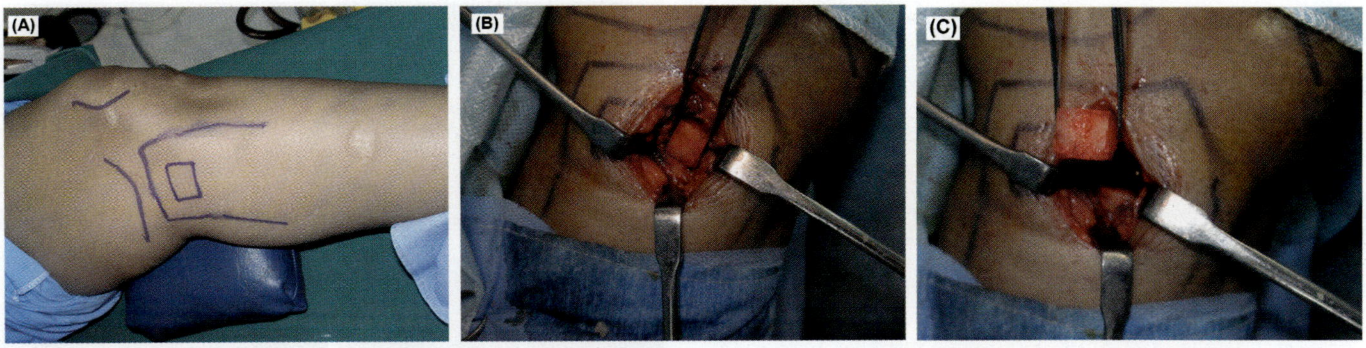

Figure 34.12 **(A–C)** Block graft harvested from the tibia.

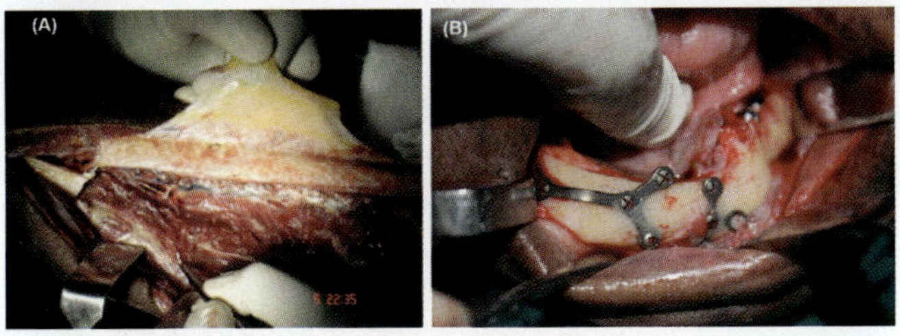

Figure 34.13 **(A** and **B)** Harvesting free vascularised fibular graft for mandibular reconstruction.

platelets from the clot. The platelets degranulate to release platelet derived growth factors and transforming growth factors (TGFs). These are the initial steps for bone regeneration. The bone yield is up to 20 mL of particulate osseous coagulum. Block grafts are also harvested from the tibia according to the bone defect (Fig. 34.12).

FREE VASCULARISED FIBULAR GRAFTS

The fibula bone is present on the lateral surface of the limb. It is connected to the tibia by an intraosseous membrane and laterally by peroneal muscles. The peroneal nerve must be protected while harvesting the graft. The free vascularised fibular grafts (FVFG) are extremely effective in managing larger defects more than 6 cm. It has an endosteal and periosteal blood supply, the endosteal peroneal artery and a nutrient artery are the dominant vascular pedicle. The vascular pedicle is dissected, harvested and attached to the donor vascular segment by microvascular surgery. The ankle joint and the lower quarter of the fibula should be protected. The middle 3rd of the fibula is harvested (Fig. 34.13).

SOFT TISSUE RECONSTRUCTION WITH GRAFTS

The most commonly used soft tissue graft is the skin graft. They are used for closure of wounds that cannot be closed primarily and for wounds that would produce disability due to scarring (Fig. 34.14). The other soft tissue grafts most commonly used in the head and neck region are as follows:

- Composite full thickness skin and cartilage graft harvested from the pinna of ear for small nasal defects
- Fat grafts from the abdominal or gluteal region for facial contours, for example, Parry–Romberg syndrome, hemifacial atrophy
- Fascia as grafts for aesthetic contouring of the face, lips, etc. It is also used for facial reanimation.

FREE SKIN GRAFTS FOR CLOSURE

SPLIT THICKNESS SKIN GRAFT

Split thickness skin grafts are usually taken with skin knives or powered dermatomes. The most commonly used sites are the thighs and buttocks. The split thickness graft is then meshed to improve the 'take' of the graft by allowing the exudate to escape.

Types:

- Thin: 0.2−0.3 mm
- Thick: 0.45−0.75 mm.

FULL THICKNESS SKIN GRAFT

Full thickness (Wolfe) skin graft is prepared from the donor site by cutting the skin without the underlying fat. The commonly used sites are the groin crease and neck where a small defect can allow primary closure of the donor site (Fig. 34.15).

COMPOSITE RECONSTRUCTION WITH OR WITHOUT MICROVASCULAR SURGERY FOR HARD AND SOFT TISSUES OF MAXILLARY AND MANDIBULAR DEFECTS

WITH RECONSTRUCTION PLATE AND PECTORALIS MYOCUTANEOUS FLAP

A reconstruction plate can be used for partial or hemimandibular resection. This is done when the posterior segment of the mandible is salvaged due to pathology. The plate provides the necessary support instead of the

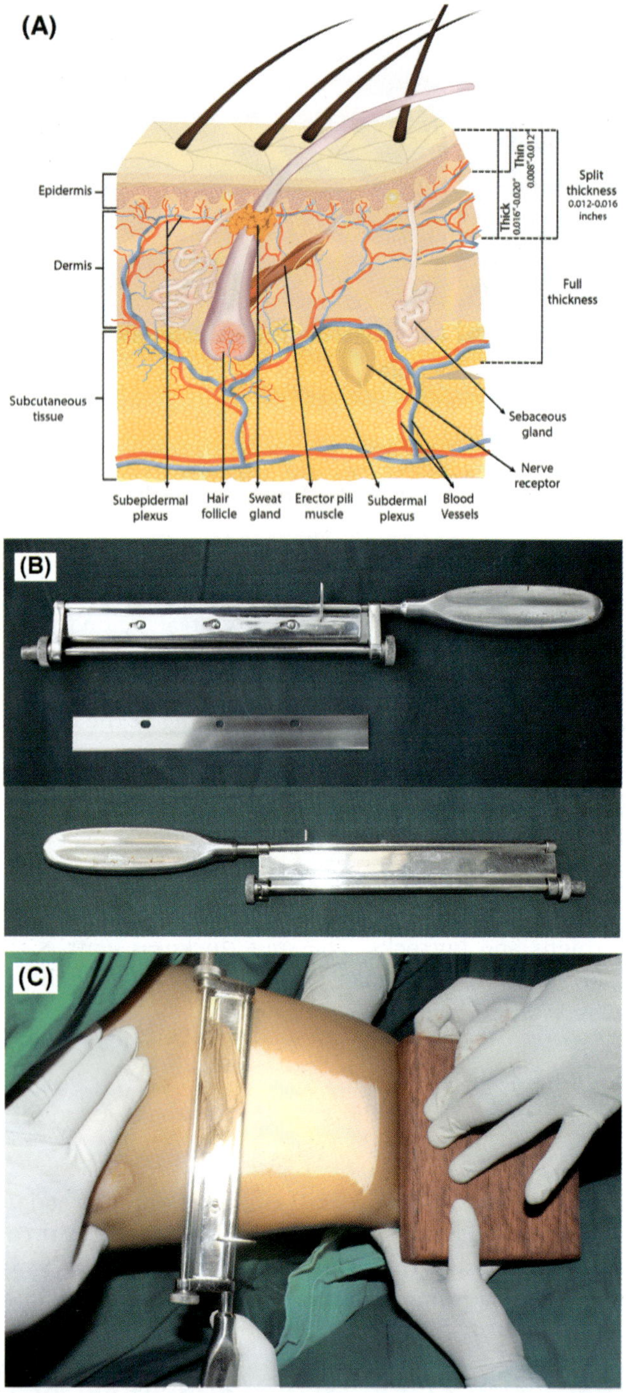

Figure 34.14 (**A**) Illustration showing free skin grafts at different layers. Thin and thick split thickness skin graft contain the epidermis and a part of the dermis. Full thickness skin graft consists of the epidermis, dermis and a part of subcutaneous tissue. (**B**) Skin knife used to harvest split thickness skin grafts. (**C**) Harvesting of a split thickness skin graft with a skin knife.

bone. Pectoralis Major Myocutaneous (PMMC) flap is raised and grafted medial to the plate in case of mucosal loss. The skin from the PMMC flap replaces the lost mucosa at the recipient site. Complication faced is stress fracture of the reconstruction plate (Fig. 34.16).

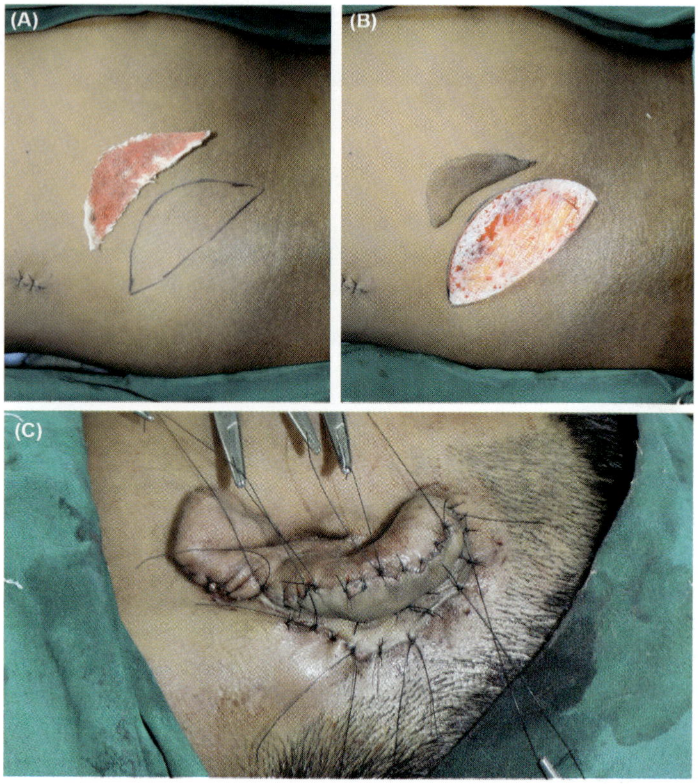

Figure 34.15 Harvesting of a full thickness skin for ear reconstruction. (**A**) The template is taken from the recipient site. The skin to be harvested is planned by marking the incision on the donor site. (**B**) The skin incision made on the donor site and harvested full thickness skin graft is seen in the photograph. (**C**) Suturing of the skin graft to the borders of the recipient site (behind the reconstructed ear).

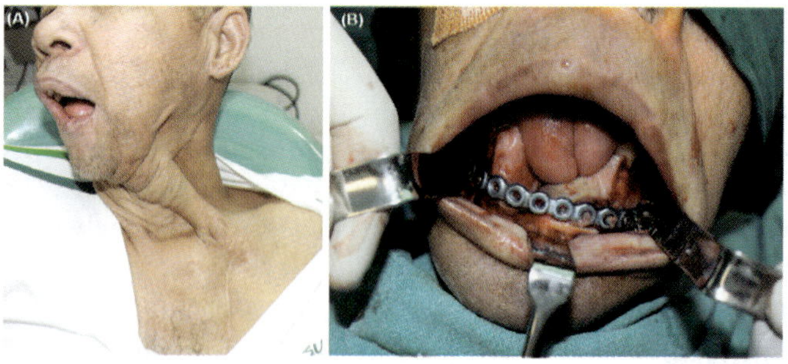

Figure 34.16 (**A** and **B**) Postoperative image of a patient with reconstruction plate and pectoralis myocutaneous flap for mandibular reconstruction.

RADIAL FOREARM OSTEOCUTANEOUS FREE FLAP

The donor flap consists of the skin paddle from the forearm, the vascular paddle that consists of the radial artery, the cephalic vein and other perforators. The osseous component comprises of the radius bone of approximately 10 cm. The major advantage of the radial forearm flap is the thickness of the flap. It is ideal and pliable for reconstruction pertaining to the skin of the head and neck

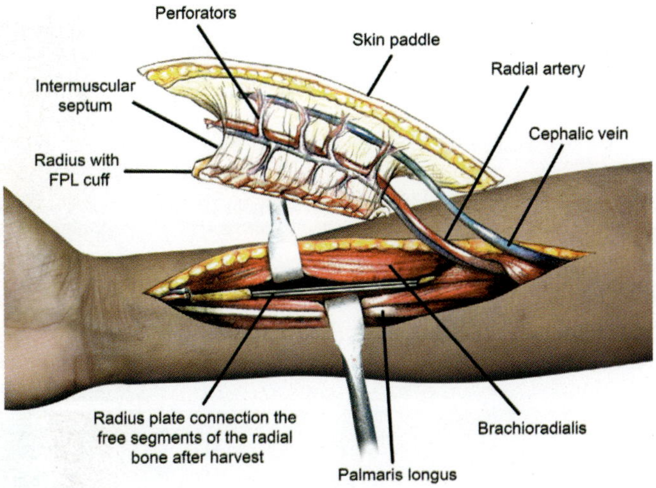

Figure 34.17 Illustration of radial forearm osteocutaneous free flap.

region. The bone available is limited and can be used only for mandibular body defects with large mucosal or cutaneous defects, unicortical defects and for exclusive ramus defects with cutaneous/mucosal loss. Complications are donor site morbidity, hand ischaemia, stricture formation, radial nerve injury and variable paraesthesia over the dorsum of hand (Fig. 34.17).

OSTEOCUTANEOUS FIBULA FREE FLAP

This composite flap consists of an osseous component; the fibula of approximately 22–25 cm and a soft tissue component of a cuff of flexor longus, soleus muscles and skin paddle. The vascular pedicle consists of septocutaneous perforators that is a part of the harvested soleus cuff, the skin perforators from the posterior intermuscular septum and the peroneal artery and vein (Fig. 34.18). Perforators and the vascular pedicle are marked using a Doppler before the grafts are harvested. The vascular pedicle is attached to the recipient site by microvascular surgery (Fig. 34.19). The osseous component is ideal for osseointegration of dental implants. This, with the amount of bone harvested, makes this ideal for mandibular and maxillary reconstructions with mucosal or cutaneous loss. The donor site may need split thickness skin graft for closure.

ILIAC CREST FREE FLAP BASED ON DEEP CIRCUMFLEX ILIAC ARTERY

Iliac crest free flap is used for the reconstruction of lateral and hemimandibular defects. These composite flaps consist

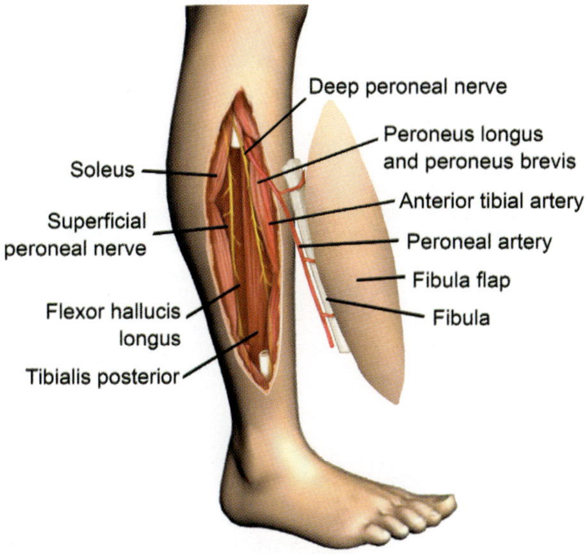

Figure 34.18 Illustration of osteocutaneous fibula free flap.

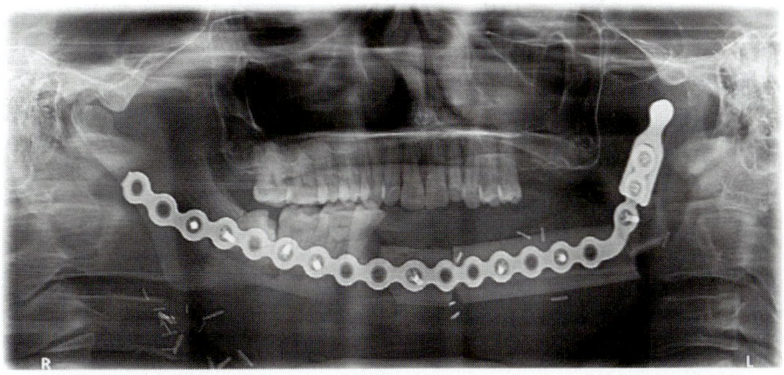

Figure 34.19 Fibula graft used to reconstruct the mandible by microvascular surgery.

of either osteocutaneous or osteomuscular bone flaps from the iliac region. The components are the iliac bone, periosteum, small strip of iliac muscle or larger islands from the internal oblique muscle. The bone harvested can be up to 16 cm and is ideal for osseointegration of dental implants. The vascular pedicle consists of the deep circumflex iliac artery (DCIA) from the lateral aspect of the external iliac artery, which is present 1 to 2 cm cephalic to the inguinal ligament and the deep circumflex iliac vein. Complications seen in this technique are hernia, skin loss due to perforator sheer injury and poor colour match to recipient site.

Section X

Temporomandibular Joint

Chapter 35

Introduction to Temporomandibular Joint

OUTLINE

INTRODUCTION

The temporomandibular joint (TMJ) is a complex craniomandibular articulation where the mandible articulates with the temporal bone of the cranium. It involves two separate synovial joints (right and left) that function in unison. TMJ is considered as an *arthrodial* joint, as it provides sliding or translatory movements, at the same time it also provides hinge or rotatory movements, hence considered as *ginglymoid* joint. Thus TMJ is technically considered as a *ginglymoarthrodial* joint. It is classified as a compound joint with two articulating surfaces: (1) temporal surface (mandibular fossa or glenoid fossa) and (2) condylar surface (mandibular condyle) and an articular disc as a 3rd bone (Fig. 35.1A-D).

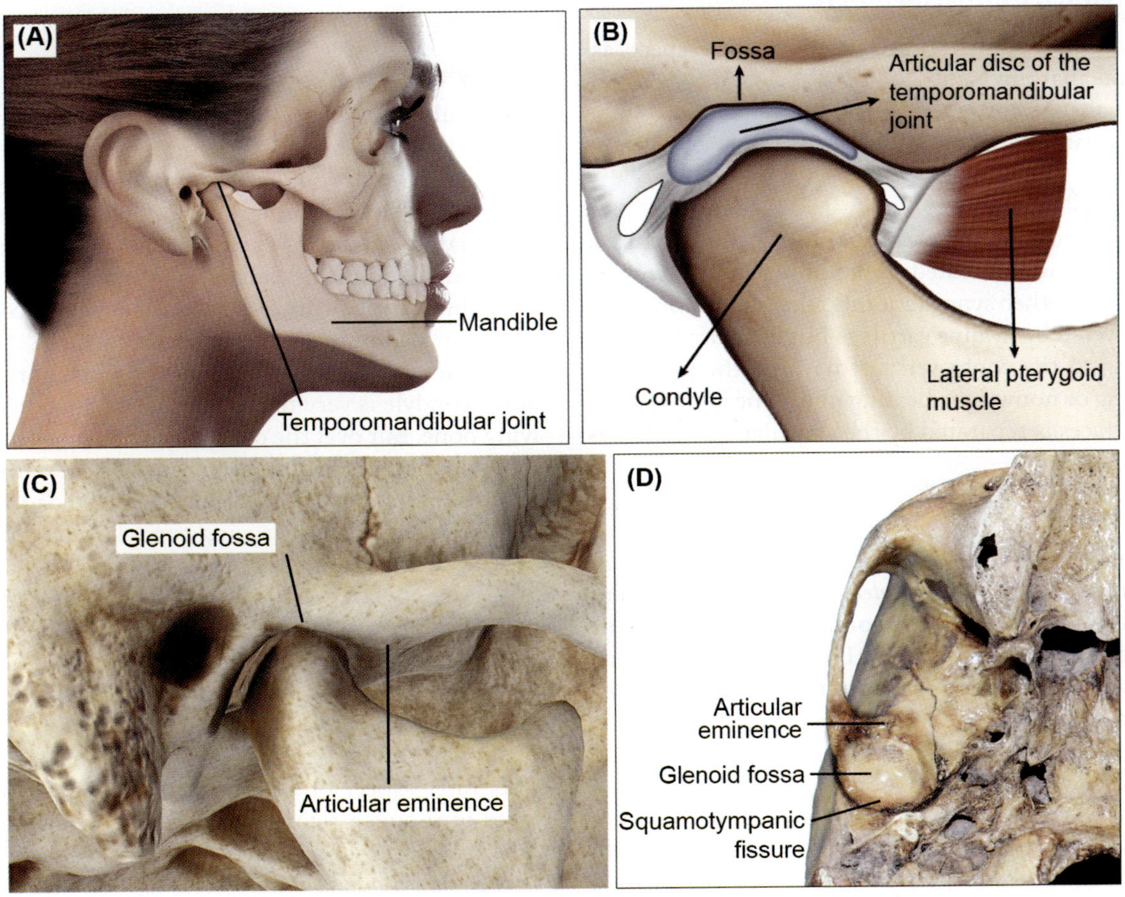

Figure 35.1 (**A and B**) Components of TMJ. (**C and D**) Bony structures of the TMJ.

EMBRYOLOGY

The TMJ begins development in the 10th week of gestation. *Meckel's cartilage*, the skeletal component of the 1st brachial arch, forms the template for the development of inferior bony part of TMJ (mandibular head). The cartilage of the squamous temporal bone forms the superior part of the TMJ, the mandibular fossa. The gap between the mandibular head and the mandibular fossa is filled with ectomesenchyme. These ectomesenchymes differentiate into fibroblasts and produce fibrocartilaginous articular surfaces of the mandibular fossa, mandibular head and articular disc.

The superior and inferior TMJ cavities are formed by apoptosis. The articular capsule is formed by both the joint cavities and is composed of a fibrous stratum and an inner synovial stratum. The centre of the condylar component develops into white fibrocartilage that facilitates subchondral bone formation (endochondral mechanism), thus contributing for condylar growth till adulthood. The meniscus develops into a highly cellular vascular disc that continues anteriorly into the lateral pterygoid muscle and posteriorly as the discomalleolar ligament (Pinto's ligament).

TEMPOROMANDIBULAR JOINT ANATOMY

The joint anatomy can be described based on three aspects as:

a. Structural anatomy
b. Functional anatomy
c. Surgical anatomy.

STRUCTURAL ANATOMY

The TMJ is a synovial joint with a joint capsule lined by a synovial membrane lubricated and nourished by synovial fluid. But unlike other synovial joints, the articulating surface is not covered by hyaline cartilage but by white fibrocartilage, leading to the controversy of terming the joint as a weight-bearing or nonweight-bearing joint. The joint with its two bony surfaces is separated by the articular disc called as meniscus.

BONY STRUCTURES

The articular surface is composed of three portions: *articular eminence, mandibular fossa and preglenoid plane.* The articular surfaces of the joint are the temporal component and the condylar component (Fig. 35.1C & D). The temporal bone surface consists of the articular eminence (convex) and the glenoid fossa (concave).

Articular eminence

Articular eminence is a thick, transverse bony prominence which serves as a major functional component of the TMJ. The articular eminence is present anterior to the glenoid fossa, consisting of a descending slope, a transverse ridge and an ascending slope. The eminence is covered by dense, compact, fibrous connective tissue that consists primarily of collagen with a few fine elastic fibres. The fibrous covering is thickest at the descending slope of the eminence. Underlying the fibrous tissue covering is the chondroid bone. Unlike the glenoid fossa, the articular eminence is subjected to loading during function.

Glenoid fossa

The glenoid fossa, also known as the mandibular fossa, is a concave depression on the petrous part of the temporal bone at its inferior surface. It is bounded posteriorly by the petrotympanic fissure and anteriorly by the articular eminence (Fig. 35.1D). The fossa has medial and lateral rims. The lateral rim proceeds into the zygomatic tubercle anteriorly and into the postglenoid tubercle posteriorly. The medial rim is lateral to the spine of the sphenoid bone and the foramen spinosum along with its middle meningeal artery. A thin fibrous layer covers the fossa.

The chorda tympani nerve appears at the medial end of the petrotympanic fissure close to the spine of sphenoid. The roof of the fossa is thin and separates the brain from the joint cavity; therefore, during surgical manipulation, extreme precaution should be taken to prevent perforation of the roof of the glenoid fossa.

The *preglenoid plane* is a flattened area located anterior to the articular eminence of the temporal bone.

Condyle

The adult condyle is elliptical in shape, the long axis being angled backwards at 15–33 degrees to the frontal plane. The long axis of each condyle is approximately at right angles to the body of the mandible. The condyle has a medial tubercle and a lateral tubercle. The tubercles provide attachments to the medial and lateral collateral ligaments.

A thick layer of fibroelastic tissue which contains fibroblasts and chondrocytes, covers the condyle's articular surface. The fibrous layer covering the posterior aspect of the adult condyle is very thin and adheres directly to the underlying bone. But over the convexity, it becomes thicker with an intervening layer of fibrocartilage. The presence of cartilage facilitates the condyle to adapt to excess loading by becoming hyperplastic. In the ageing condyle, only remnants of the cartilage remain and it becomes calcified.

The condylar head is elliptical in shape and converges medially. The horizontal axis when extended intersects at 145–160 degrees at the foramen magnum. This degree signifies the presence of condylar disease (Fig. 35.2).

CARTILAGE AND SYNOVIUM

The inner aspect of all the synovial joints is lined by two types of tissue: articular cartilage and synovium (Fig. 35.3). The space bounded by articular cartilage and synovium is termed as synovial cavity, which is filled with synovial fluid. The articular surfaces are cored with fibrous connective

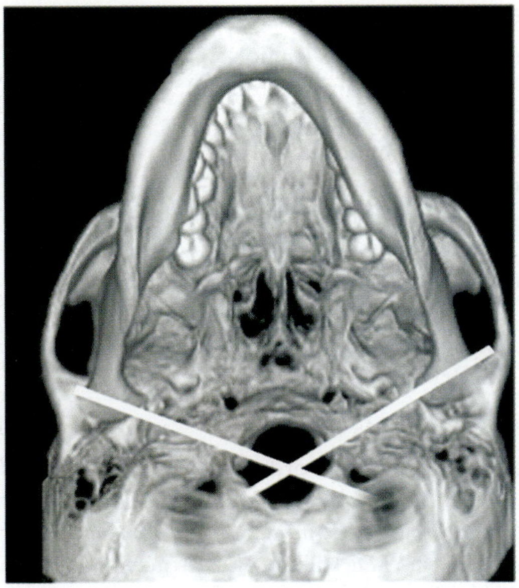

Figure 35.2 Intersection of horizontal axis at foramen magnum.

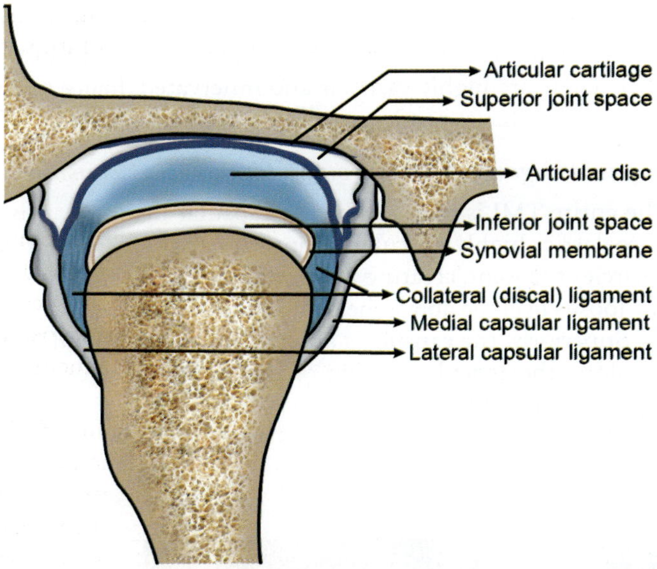

Figure 35.3 TMJ articular cartilage and synovial membrane.

tissue. This fibrocartilage layer has the capacity to regenerate and remodel when placed under functional stress. The articular cartilage is composed of chondrocytes and ground substance (collagen fibres, water and a filler material).

Synovial membrane

The inner surface of the TMJ capsule and the articular disc are lined with a synovial membrane. Various synovial villous projections are present in the anterior, posterior, medial and lateral recesses of the joint cavities.

There are two sources for the synovial fluid: one is from *plasma* by dialysis and the other is by secretion from types A and B synoviocytes. This volume was assessed by Toller in 1961 using contrast radiography studies, and he estimated that the upper compartment can accommodate volume of about 1.2 mL of fluid without undue pressure, whereas the lower compartment had a capacity of about 0.9 mL.

The fluid exists under negative intraarticular pressure. The surface tension of the synovial fluid helps in the spread of the fluid over the articular surfaces as a capillary film, thus helping *lubrication of the joint* during movement of the condyle. It contains *glycoprotein known as lubricin*, which helps in lubrication and reduces the friction between the articular surfaces of synovial joints.

ARTICULAR DISC/MENISCUS (Fig. 35.4)

The disc or the meniscus which is present between the condyle and the temporal bone is semilunar, avascular, noninnervated, fibrocartilaginous structure.

It acts as a shock absorber and provides protection to the bony components of the joint. Sagittal section of the disc reveals a *thick anterior* fibrous band (anterior disc ligament), *thin* intermediate zone and posterior fibrous band (posterior disc ligament). The anterior fibrous band has a superior stratum which inserts itself on the ascending slope of the articular eminence and an inferior stratum which inserts inferiorly at the condyle's anterior aspect.

The anterior fibrous band of meniscus, the capsule and the condyle fix with the superior head of tendons of lateral pterygoid muscle.

In addition to the blood vessels, parotid tissue is usually found between the posterior capsule and the postglenoid tubercle. The parotid gland extends from this location medially until it reaches the lateral wall of the pharynx. Therefore, enlargement of the parotid could impinge on the posterior capsule of the TMJ and cause pain during closure of the mouth or during chewing movements.

The posterior fibrous band (posterior ligament) of the meniscus is a bilaminar structure. The superior lamella of the posterior fibrous band (ligament) is attached to the

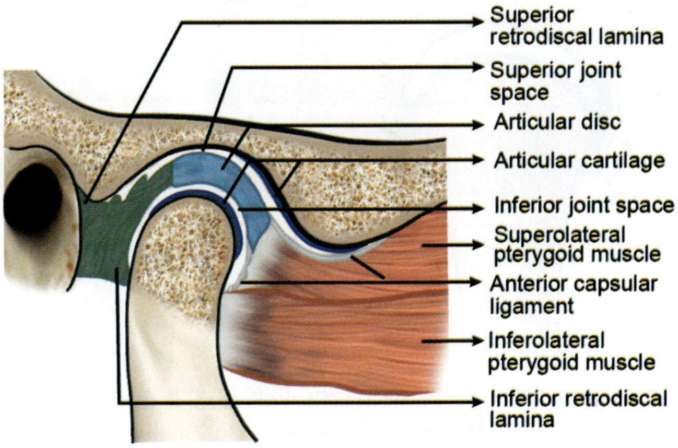

Figure 35.4 Articular disc with attachment of retrodiscal tissue.

posterior margin of the glenoid fossa at the squamotympanic fissure. The inferior lamella of the posterior fibrous band (ligament) attaches with the condyle in the posterior aspect. The area between the lamellae is filled with highly vascular and innervated loose areolar fibrofatty tissue.

Medially and laterally, the meniscus is firmly attached to the periosteum of the condyle's medial and lateral poles through the medial and lateral collateral ligaments. The most medial portion of the disc is connected posteriorly to a ligament referred to as the *discomalleolar or Pinto's ligament*.

The attachments of the disc to the condyle are of significance since the shape of the joint compartment changes during translatory movements according to the position of the condyle. The superior head of the lateral pterygoid muscle is attached to the anteromedial aspect of the disc, and helps in stabilising the mandibular condyle during function.

RETRODISCAL TISSUE

It is a highly vascular and highly innervated structure that blends with the posterior aspect of the articular disc. It is also known as the *bilaminar zone* (superior and inferior retrodiscal laminae), and is involved in the production of synovial fluid. The *superior retrodiscal lamina* contains the elastic fibres, which are attached to the tympanic plate. It functions as a restraint to disc displacement in extreme translatory movements. The *inferior retrodiscal lamina* contains collagen fibres without elastic tissue and functions to connect the articular disc to the posterior margin of the condyle. It also acts as a check ligament in rotational movements, preventing severe rotation of the disc on the condylar head.

LIGAMENTS

Ligaments are composed of collagen and function as restraints to the movements of condyle and disc. The ligaments associated with the joint include functional and accessory ligaments.

Ligaments of temporomandibular joint (Fig. 35.5)

- Functional ligaments (major):
  1. Collateral ligaments (discal)
  2. Capsular ligament
  3. Temporomandibular ligament
- Accessory ligaments (minor):
  4. Sphenomandibular ligament
  5. Stylomandibular ligament
- Other ligaments:
  6. Anterior malleolar ligament (AML)
  7. Discomalleolar ligament (DML)/Pinto's ligament
  8. Mallelomandibular ligament.

Collateral ligaments (discal)

The medial and lateral borders of the articular disc is attached to the condyle by the collateral ligaments. There are two collateral ligaments: *medial discal ligament (MDL) and lateral discal ligament (LDL)*. The MDL attaches the medial edge of the disc to the medial surface of the condyle. Similarly, the LDL attaches the lateral edge of the disc to the lateral surface of the condyle. These ligaments are responsible for dividing the joint into superior and inferior joint cavities. Their function is to restrict the movement of the disc away from the condyle and are responsible for the hinge movement of the TMJ. These are highly vascular and innervated, hence strain on these ligaments produce pain.

Capsular ligament/temporomandibular joint capsule

The entire TMJ is enclosed by the capsular ligament. It is a fibroelastic, highly vascular connective tissue capsule that encircles the joint, creating a closed joint cavity. The capsule is a loose envelope above the disc and taut below it.

- Superiorly, the capsule is attached to the temporal bone along the articular surface of the mandibular fossa and articular eminence
- Inferiorly, the capsule encircles the neck of the condyle

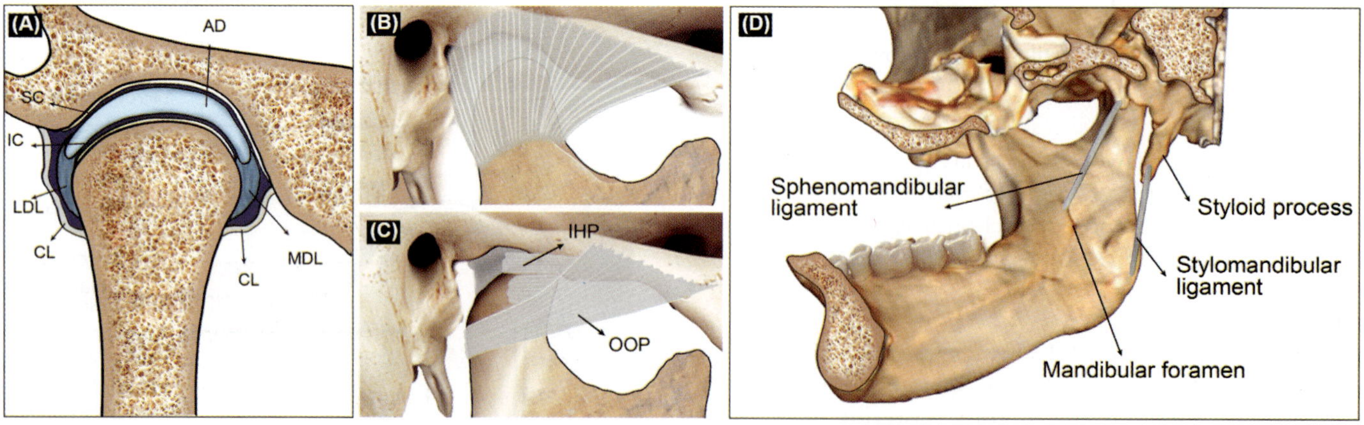

Figure 35.5 **(A)** TMJ ligaments (CL, collateral ligament; AD, articular disc; MDL, medial discal ligament; LDL, lateral discal ligament; IC, inferior joint cavity; SC, superior joint cavity). **(B)** Capsular ligament. **(C)** Temporomandibular ligament (OOP, outer oblique portion; IHP, inner horizontal portion). **(D)** Stylomandibular and sphenomandibular ligament (medial view of mandible).

TABLE 35.1 Muscles Closely Related to the TMJ

Muscles	Origin	Insertion	Nerve Supply	Action
Temporalis	Superior temporal line, Temporal fossa and temporalis fascia	Coronoid process	Trigeminal nerve, mandibular branch	Elevates mandible for biting and chewing; retracts mandible
Masseter	Zygomatic arch	Lateral surface of mandibular ramus and angle	Trigeminal nerve, mandibular branch	Elevates mandible; produces forceful bite and some lateral excursion
Medial pterygoid	Pterygoid process of sphenoid	Medial aspect of mandibular angle	Trigeminal nerve, mandibular branch	Elevates mandible; produces lateral excursion
Lateral pterygoid	Pterygoid process of sphenoid	Slightly anterior to mandibular condyle	Trigeminal nerve mandibular branch	Depresses mandible; produces lateral excursion

- Laterally, the capsule thickens to form the lateral TMJ ligament
- Medially, it is attached to the medial rim of glenoid fossa, spine of sphenoid and sphenomandibular ligament.

The function of the capsular ligament is to resist any medial, lateral or inferior movement of the condyle. It also encompasses the joint and retains the synovial fluid. The ligament is well innervated.

Temporomandibular ligament/lateral ligament

It is a strong tight fibre on the lateral aspect of the capsular ligament. The TM ligament is composed of an *outer oblique portion and an inner horizontal portion*.

The outer portion is attached to the articular tubercle and zygomatic process above, and posteroinferiorly to the outer surface of the condylar neck below. The inner horizontal portion extends from the outer surface of the articular tubercle and zygomatic process, horizontally to the posterior part of articular disc and lateral pole of the condyle.

The lateral ligament supports the mandibular condyle and limits external lateral movement. It limits the rotational movement and also limits the posterior movement of the condyle and disc.

Stylomandibular ligament

The stylomandibular ligament is a specialised band of the deep cervical fascia extending from the apex of the styloid process to the posterior surface and angle of the mandibular ramus. This accessory ligament of the joint limits extreme anterior movement of the condyle in relation to the fossa.

Sphenomandibular ligament

This flat thin band which is extending from the spine of sphenoid to the lingula of the mandible is considered as remnant of Meckel's cartilage. This ligament does not have any significant effects on the mandibular movement.

VASCULAR SUPPLY AND INNERVATION

The TMJ is primarily supplied by the *maxillary artery and superficial temporal artery*. The branches of the maxillary artery that supplies the joint are the deep auricular artery, the anterior tympanic artery and the ascending pharyngeal artery. These vessels converge into the canal of the joint creating a vascular return supplying the joint and the disc.

The venous drainage of the joint is through superficial temporal vein, maxillary plexus and posterior venous plexus.

The joint is innervated by auriculotemporal, maxillary and temporal nerve.

Hilton's law states that nerves which supply a joint also innervate the muscle that moves it. This is well demonstrated by the TMJ which is supplied principally by the auriculotemporal and also by the branches of masseteric and posterior deep temporal nerves.

MUSCLES OF MASTICATION

Muscles that are closely related to the joint (Table 35.1) and influence the joint movements include lateral pterygoid, temporalis and masseter muscles. Among the three muscles, the lateral pterygoid is explained in Table 35.2.

The lateral pterygoid muscle consists of two heads—upper and lower. The lower head of the lateral pterygoid muscle arises from the outer surface of the lateral pterygoid plate, the pyramidal process of the palatine bone and the adjacent portion of the maxillary tuberosity. The superior head originates from the upper 3rd of the lateral pterygoid plate and the infratemporal surface of the greater wing of the sphenoid lateral to the foramen ovale. The fibres from the two heads get closer and almost unite before their insertion sites. The

TABLE 35.2 Actions of TMJ Muscles

Depression of mandible: • Lateral pterygoid • Digastric • Geniohyoid • Mylohyoid	Elevation of mandible: • Temporalis • Masseter • Medial pterygoid
Protrusion of mandible: • Lateral pterygoid • Medial pterygoid	Retraction of mandible: • Posterior fibres of temporalis

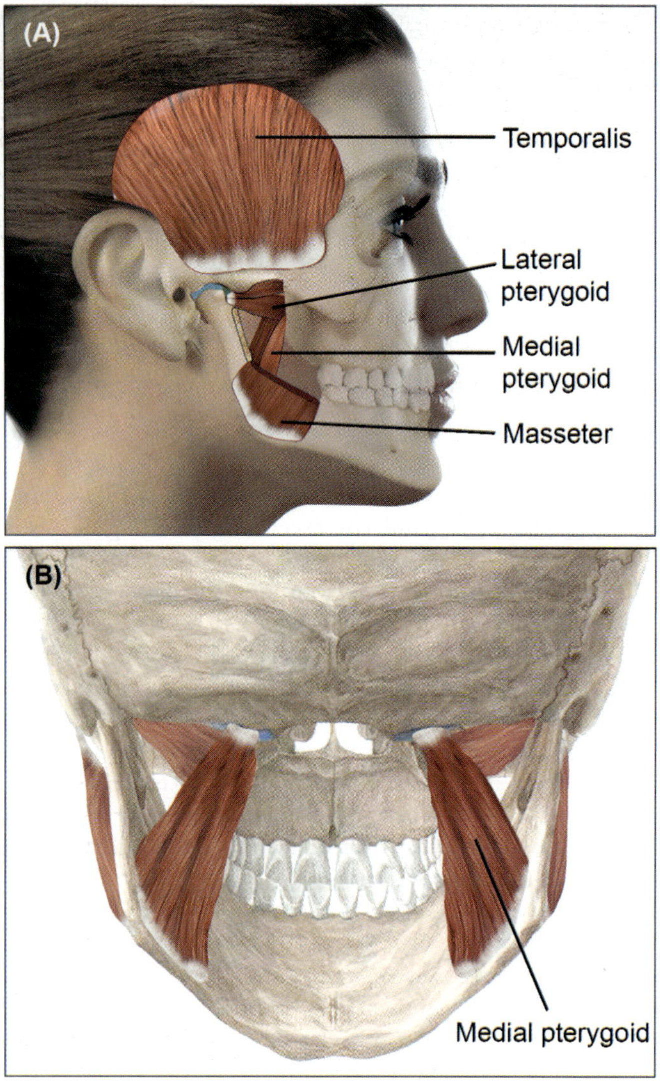

Figure 35.6 (**A** and **B**) Muscles of mastications.

medial half of the condylar fovea receives most of the fibres of both heads of the lateral pterygoid muscles. The upper head inserts some of its fibres (~15%) into the medial portion of the anterior band of the disc.

Spasm of the inferior head of the lateral pterygoid could lead to medial disc displacement. Also, such an anatomic relationship may be important during normal medial rotation of the condyle-disc complex during chewing (Fig. 35.6).

FUNCTIONAL ANATOMY

Functionally, the joint has two components and four articulating surfaces.

Two components: Meniscotemporal (upper) and meniscomandibular (lower).

Four articulating surfaces

1. Articulating facets of temporal bone
2. Articulating facets of condyle
3. Superior surface of disc
4. Inferior surface of disc.

The mandible may be depressed, elevated, protruded or retracted. These mandibular movements are possible as a result of the synchronous and alternating movements of the condyle-meniscus unit in both TMJ. The TMJ exhibits *rotational (hinge) movement in the lower compartment and sliding (translational) in the upper compartment.*

- When the mouth is *opened*, the condyles rotate around a common horizontal axis, resulting in the 1st 10 mm of mouth opening. This initial movement occurs exclusively in the lower joint cavity by *pure hinge or rotation*. At the same time, the disc slides forwards and downwards on the temporal bones
- With further mouth opening (beyond 10 mm), the condyle further rotates and then *translates or glides forwards* and downwards in contact with the lower surface of the articular disc. This movement results from the attachments of each disc to the medial and lateral poles of the head of the mandible and also from the contraction of the lateral pterygoid
- The forward sliding of a disc stops when the fibroelastic tissue of the disc is stretched to its limit. The condylar hinging and gliding forwards occurs until it articulates with the most anterior part of the disc and the mouth is opened fully
- When the mouth is closed, the movements are reversed. Initially, each condylar head glides backwards and then hinges on the disc which is held forward by the lateral pterygoid muscle. The muscle relaxes gradually allowing the articular disc to glide backwards and upwards on the temporal bone
- In the rotatory movements of grinding or chewing, the head of one side with its disc glides forwards, rotating around a vertical axis which passes immediately behind the head as the contralateral head translates forward. These alternating movements swing the mandible from side to side. The medial and lateral pterygoid muscles of each side act alternately to facilitate this action (Fig. 35.7).

SURGICAL ANATOMY (Table 35.3)

- The main trunk of the facial nerve exits the skull through the stylomastoid foramen. The suture line, which lies between the tympanic and mastoid portions of the mastoid bone, is a reliable anatomic landmark because the main trunk of the facial nerve lies 6–8 mm inferior and anterior to the tympanomastoid suture. Approximately 1.3 cm of the facial nerve is visible until it divides into temporofacial and cervicofacial branches (Fig. 35.8)
- Al Kayat and Bramley (1979) observed that the distance from the lowest point of the external bony auditory canal to the bifurcation was about 1.5–2.8 cm and distance from the postglenoid tubercle to the bifurcation was around 2.4–3.5 cm

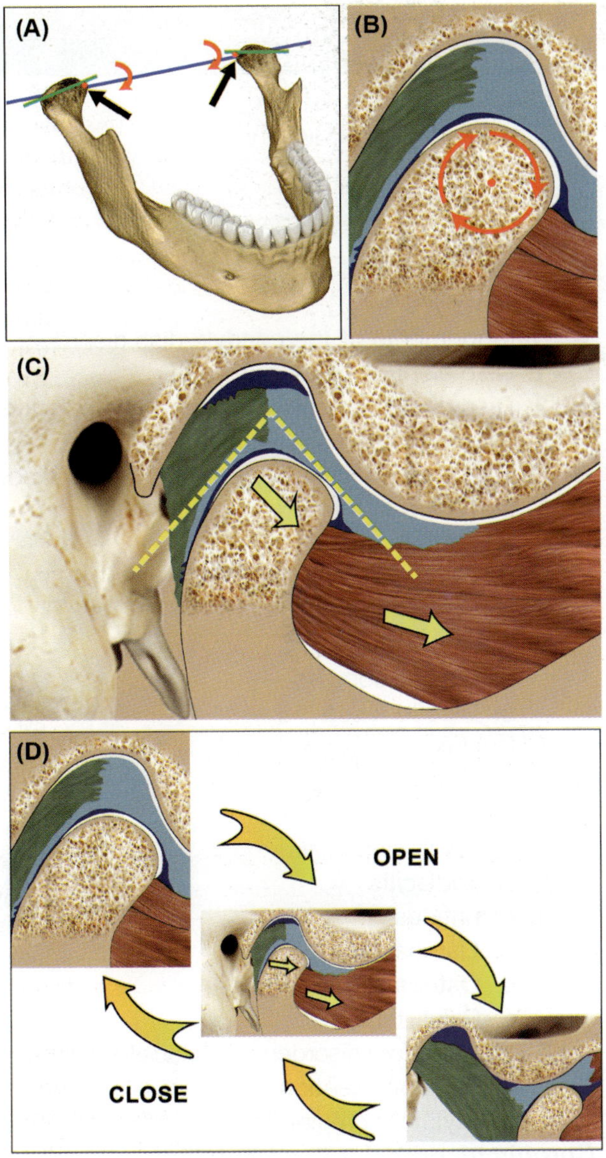

Figure 35.7 (**A** and **B**) Rotation of the mandible around medial pole. (**C**) Translatory movement of the condyle. (**D**) The position of the condyle and disc during normal open and close movements.

TABLE 35.3 Anatomical Relations of TMJ

Anteriorly	Mandibular notch, lateral pterygoid, masseteric artery and vein
Posteriorly	Parotid gland, superficial temporal vessels, auriculotemporal nerve
Laterally	Skin and fascia, parotid gland, temporal branches of facial nerve
Medially	Tympanic plate, spine of sphenoid, auriculotemporal and chorda tympani nerve, middle meningeal artery, maxillary artery
Superiorly	Middle cranial fossa, middle meningeal vessels
Inferiorly	Maxillary artery and vein

- The most variable measurement was the point at which the upper trunk crosses the zygomatic arch, which ranged from 0.8 to 3.5 cm anterior to the most anterior portion of the bony external auditory canal
- The temporal branch of the 7th nerve (facial nerve) emerges from the parotid gland and crosses the zygoma under the temporoparietal fascia to innervate the frontalis muscle
- The auriculotemporal nerve provides most of the innervation to the capsule of the TMJ itself. The anterior portion of the joint also receives innervation from the masseteric nerve and the posterior deep temporal nerve. The articular cartilage on the surface of the condyle, glenoid fossa and the avascular meniscus itself has no innervations.

BIOMECHANICS OF TEMPOROMANDIBULAR JOINT

The TMJ is a compound joint and the free movements of mandible are possible by two distinct systems: *inferior joint and superior joint.*

1. The inferior joint/inferior synovial cavity/condyle-disc complex. As the articular disc is tightly bound to the

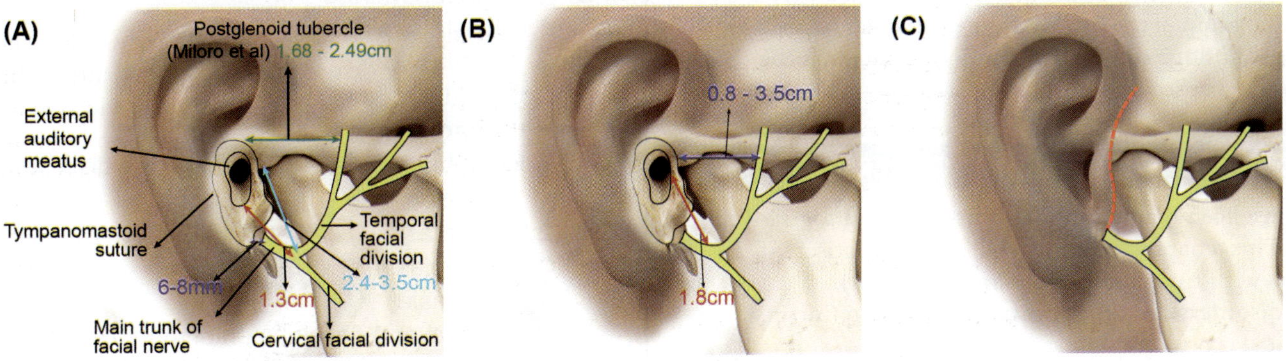

Figure 35.8 (**A**) Surgical landmarks for identifying location of main trunk of facial nerve. (**B**) The facial nerve crosses the zygomatic arch at 0.8–3.5 cm anterior to the bony auditory canal. (**C**) Note that the inferior extent of the incision is the soft tissue attachment of the lobule of the ear.

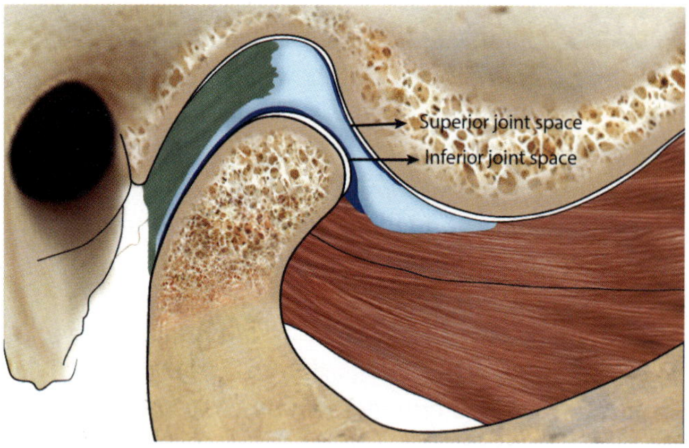

Figure 35.9 Superior and inferior synovial cavity.

condyle by the medial and lateral discal ligaments, the only movement that can occur at these surfaces is rotation. Thus, the *condyle-disc complex is responsible for rotational movement* in the TMJ

2. Superior joint/superior synovial cavity. It is the space between the disc and temporal fossa. *Translatory movements*, involving a gliding motion between the *disc and temporal fossa* occur at the superior joints (Fig. 35.9).

All movements of the mandible involve close contact of the condyle, disc and articular eminence. The position of the condyle and disc within the fossa, as well as the constant contact between the condyle, articular eminence and disc are maintained by the muscles of mastication. Ligaments do not actively participate in the normal TMJ movements. They act as guide wires and restrict joint movements at the extreme range of motion.

The morphology of the disc and the interarticular pressure maintain the condyle in the intermediate zone (ideal position). During translation, the disc moves forward along with the condyle. Thus, *proper morphology of the disc, interarticular pressure and the lateral pterygoid muscle (superior) are important in maintaining the position of disc*. When the morphology of the disc is altered, the ligaments attached to the disc alters the biomechanics of the joint and dysfunction begins.

Centric relation (CR) is defined as the most superior and anterior position of the condyles in the articular fossa against the posterior slope of the articular eminence, with the discs properly interposed.

CLASSIFICATION OF TMJ DISORDERS

There have been many classifications proposed for TMJ disorders. This chapter presents Bell's classification of TMJ disorders with similar characteristics (Box 35.1).

TMJ disorders can be of intraarticular origin (intrinsic) or extraarticular origin (extrinsic) (Box 35.2).

Each broad category has been discussed in Chapters 36–39, according to the aetiology, history, examination, diagnosis and treatment.

BOX 35.1 Bell's Classification of Temporomandibular Disorders

I. Masticatory muscle disorders
- **A.** Protective co-contraction
- **B.** Local myalgia
- **C.** Myospasm
- **D.** Myofascial pain
- **E.** Central mediated myalgia

II. TMJ disorders
- **A.** Derangements of the condyle-disc disorders
  - **1.** Disc displacement
  - **2.** Disc displacement with intermediate locking
  - **3.** Disc displacement without reduction
- **B.** Structural incompatibility of the articular surfaces
  - **1.** Deviation in form
    - **a.** Disc
    - **b.** Condyle
    - **c.** Fossa
  - **2.** Adhesions
    - **a.** Disc to condyle
    - **b.** Disc to fossa
  - **3.** Subluxation (hypermobility)
  - **4.** Luxation
- **C.** Inflammatory disorders of the TMJ
  - **1.** Synovitis/capsulitis
  - **2.** Retrodiscitis
  - **3.** Arthritides
    - **a.** Osteoarthritis
    - **b.** Osteoarthrosis
    - **c.** Polyarthritides
  - **4.** Inflammatory disorders of associated structures
    - **a.** Temporal tendonitis
    - **b.** Stylomandibular ligament inflammation

III. Chronic mandibular hypomobility
- **A.** Ankylosis
  - **1.** Fibrous
  - **2.** Bony
- **B.** Muscle contracture
  - **1.** Myostatic
  - **2.** Myofibrotic
- **C.** Coronoid impedance

IV. Growth disorders
- **A.** Congenital and developmental bone disorders
  - **1.** Agenesis
  - **2.** Hypoplasia
  - **3.** Hyperplasia
  - **4.** Neoplasia
- **B.** Congenital and developmental muscle disorders
  - **1.** Hypotrophy
  - **2.** Hypertrophy
  - **3.** Neoplasia

BOX 35.2 Intrinsic and Extrinsic Disorders of TMJ

I. Intrinsic Disorder

1. Trauma
   - Dislocation, subluxation
   - Haemarthrosis
   - Intra and Extracapsular fracture
2. Internal disc displacement
   - Anterior disc displacement with reduction
   - Anterior disc displacement without reduction
3. Arthritis
   - Osteoarthritis
   - Rheumatoid arthritis
   - Juvenile rheumatoid arthritis
   - Infectious arthritis
4. Developmental defects
   - Condylar agenesis or aplasia-unilateral/bilateral
   - Bifid condyle
   - Condylar hypoplasia
   - Condylar hyperplasia
5. Ankylosis
6. Neoplasm
   - Benign tumours (osteoma, osteochondroma, chondroma)
   - Malignant tumours (osteosarcoma, chondrosarcoma, fibrosarcoma, synovial sarcoma)

II. Extrinsic Disorder

1. Masticatory muscle disorder
   - Protective muscle splinting
   - Masticatory muscle inflammation
   - Masticatory muscle spasm
2. Problems that result from extrinsic trauma
   - Traumatic arthritis
   - Fracture
   - Internal disc derangement
   - Tendonitis
   - Contracture of elevator muscle

Chapter 36

Masticatory Muscle Disorder

OUTLINE

INTRODUCTION

Myalgia is pain felt in muscle tissue and is often associated with a feeling of muscle tightness and fatigue. The severity of pain depends on the functional activity of the muscles involved.

Normal muscle function can be interrupted by an event, which can be either local or systemic factors. The first and immediate response on the masticatory muscle to injury is called *protective co-contraction* or *protective muscle splinting*. It is considered as a normal protective mechanism. If the protective co-contraction continues for several hours or days, the muscle can become compromised and a *local myalgia* can develop. Local myalgia is a noninflammatory, myogenous pain disorder, characterised by deep pain. The muscles present with tender on palpation and increased pain with function. If the local myalgia is resolved, the muscle returns to normal, or else the central nervous system (CNS) is activated resulting in acute myospasm, myofascial pain and fibromyalgia (Flowchart 36.1).

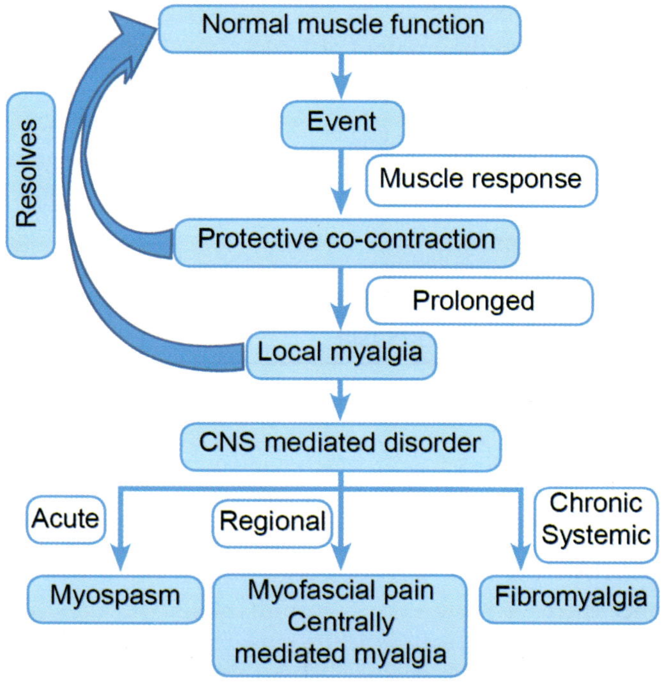

Flowchart 36.1 Relation between the various muscle pain disorders.

Myospasm is a muscle in spasm induced by the CNS. Myospasms are characterised by very firm muscle on palpation and structural dysfunction. They usually lasts only for few minutes.

When the myogenous pain persists, chronicity develops and becomes influenced by the CNS, resulting in a more regional pain condition. The *chronic centrally mediated myalgia* clinically presents as a constant, aching myogenous pain. This pain is constant at rest, with no relief and increases with function. The muscles are very tender on palpation and with structural dysfunction.

MYOFASCIAL PAIN DYSFUNCTION SYNDROME (MPDS)

Myofascial pain (MFP) is a chronic condition with regional myogenous pain associated with ***trigger points*** (TrPs). The TrPs are characterised by local areas of firm, taut bands or hypersensitive areas of muscle tissue, tendons or ligaments (Fig. 36.1). The TrPs are a constant source of deep pain that can produce central excitatory effects, resulting in referred pain, secondary hyperalgesia or autonomic response.

HISTORY

- Costen (1934)—occlusal aetiology in temporomandibular joint (TMJ) pain (bite raising era)
- MFP was first demonstrated by **Travell and Rinzler (1952)**
- Schwartz (1956)—coined the term 'TMJ pain dysfunction syndrome' and reported that the spasm of masticatory and perimasticatory musculature leading towards the symptoms

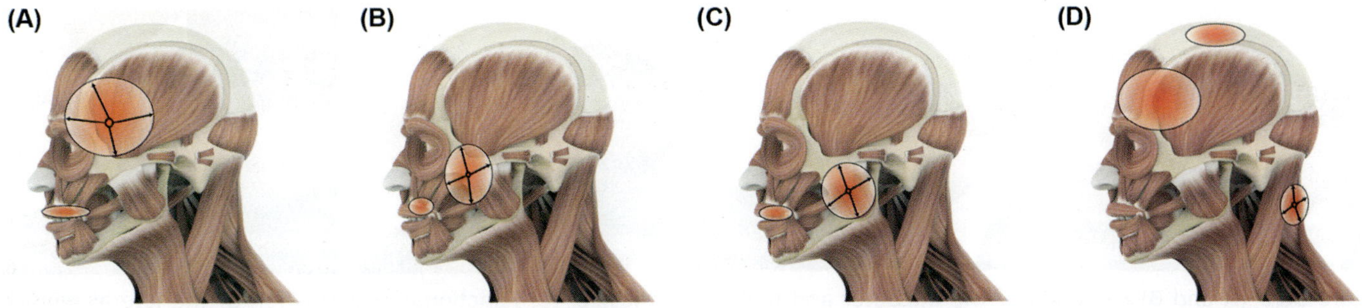

Figure 36.1 Trigger points and associated pattern of referred pain. (**A**) Trigger point—the anterior temporalis. Pain occurs as temporal, frontal and retroorbital headaches and pain in the maxillary anterior teeth. (**B**) Trigger point—the deep masseter trigger point. Pain occurs as preauricular pain, ear aches and pain in the maxillary posterior teeth. (**C**) Trigger point—the middle masseter trigger point. Pain occurs as temple, frontal and retroorbital headaches and as pain in the maxillary anterior teeth. (**D**) Trigger point—the splenius capitus in the posterior cervical area. Pain occurs as posterior cervical pain, vertex headache and frontal headache.

- Laskin in 1969 implicated psychophysiological theory for myofascial pain dysfunction syndrome (MPDS). He suggested that *mechanical factors* (malocclusion) along with the psychophysiological stress motivated oral habits lead to muscle fatigue and painful spasms. To stress the role played by the muscles, *Laskin suggested that the term 'myofascia pain dysfunction syndrome' be more accurate to describe.*

AETIOLOGY

The aetiology of MFP is complex, and several processes have been proposed to explain it.

Continuous source of pain input, sleep disturbance, prosthetic problems, malocclusion, trauma, local factors (habits, muscle strain and posture) & systemic factors (nutritional deficiency, chronic fatigue and poor physical condition, viral infections, emotional stress)

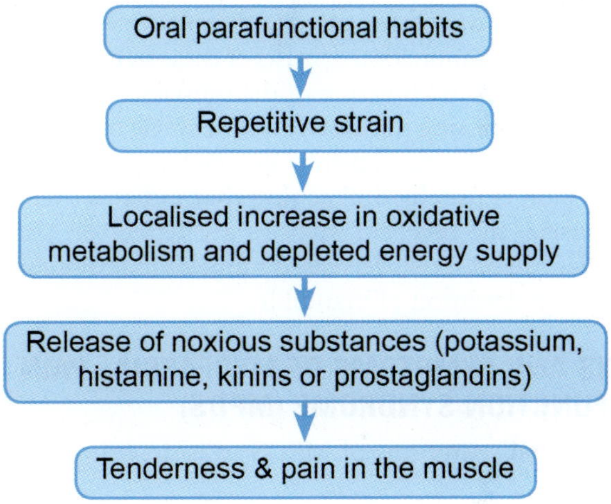

Flowchart 36.2 Development of masticatory myogenous pain.

MECHANISMS OF MASTICATORY MYOFASCIAL PAIN

Since there are no specific anatomic changes in the myogenous pain, there are no conclusive mechanisms identified in nontrauma cases. Therefore, there are several processes that may explain the development and persistence of masticatory myogenous pain.

1. **Repetitive strain hypothesis (**Flowchart 36.2**)**
2. **Neurophysiologic hypothesis:**
   Tonic muscular hyperactivity may be a normal protective adaptation to pain instead of its cause. Phasic modulation of excitatory and inhibitory interneurons supplied by high threshold sensory afferents may be involved
3. **Central hypothesis:**
   Multiple afferent inputs from muscles and other visceral and somatic structures converge in the lamina I or V of the dorsal horn on their way to the cortex, resulting in the perception of local and referred pain
4. **Central biasing mechanism:**
   Multiple peripheral and central factors may inhibit or facilitate central input through the modulatory influence of the brainstem. This may explain the diverse factors that can either exacerbate or alleviate the pain such as stress, repetitive strain, poor posture, relaxation, medications, temperature change, massage, local anaesthetic injections and electrical stimulation.

HISTORY AND CLINICAL EXAMINATION

History should include the following questions to help the clinician identify the TMJ disorders.

Difficulty or pain in opening the mouth, difficulty or pain on using the jaw (chewing, talking), location, onset, characteristics, aggravating and alleviating factors of pain, any noises at the joints, tenderness over individual masticatory muscles, frequent headaches and neck pain, recent injury, and medications.

The patient often complains about the site of referred pain and not the actual source of pain in MFP dysfunction. This will mislead the clinician to treat the referred pain, resulting in unsuccessful treatment. Hence, the clinician must possess adequate skills to identify the primary source of pain and proper treatment.

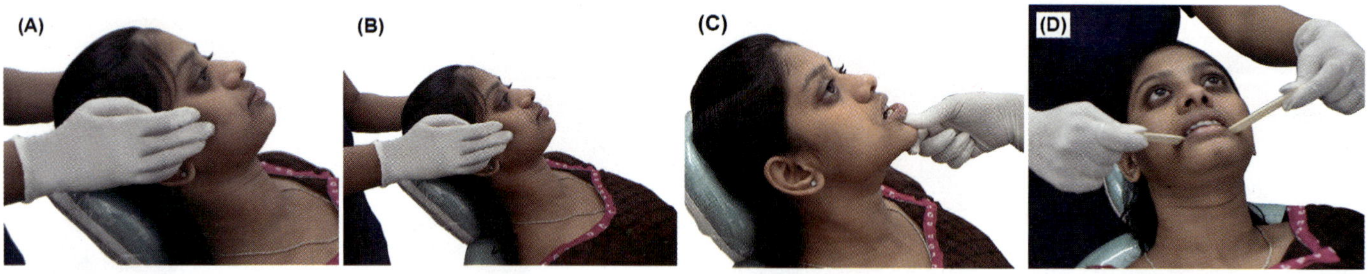

Figure 36.2 (**A** and **B**) Palpation of the masseter and temporalis muscle. (**C**) Functional manipulation of the lateral pterygoid muscle. The patient is protruding the jaw against resistance. (**D**) Functional manipulation of the medial pterygoid muscle. The patient is biting on a tongue blade (clenching of teeth).

CLINICAL EXAMINATION

The source of masticatory pain arises from the masticatory structures: (1) the teeth, (2) supporting structures of the teeth, (3) TMJ, (4) the muscles involved in the movement of mandible. Hence clinical examination consists of these structures in evaluating the health and function of the muscles. The palpation is done by compressing the muscle with a single firm thrust. The degree of discomfort and pain is recorded (Fig. 36.2).

The pain is usually dull aching that radiates over the entire muscle, the involved muscles are tender on palpation with identifiable TrPs, decreased range of mandibular movements, and deviation of mandible.

SIGNS AND SYMPTOMS OF MYOFASCIAL PAIN DYSFUNCTION SYNDROME (MPDS)

The cardinal symptoms of MPDS was described by Laskin (Box 36.1)

Pain in TMJ region, dull aching pain, increased pain on function, referred pain, muscle tenderness and weakness, presence of tight muscle bands with TrPs, limitation of mandibular movement, restricted lateral jaw movement to the contralateral side, unrestricted lateral jaw movement to the affected side, and emotional factors.

TrPs: TrPs are sources of constant deep pain, which produces referred pain, in a predictable area/pattern depending upon the region involved. Palpation of TrPs gives rise to 'Jump sign'

Trigger zone: A circumscribed region near a nerve, often in the head and neck region, which when stimulated, may elicit marked neuralgia accompanied by lightning pain

BOX 36.1 Laskin's Cardinal Symptoms of MPDS

1. Radiating pain or discomfort around head and neck.
2. Restriction of jaw movement.
3. On palpation, TMJ produces grating, clicking, snapping joint noises.
4. On palpation, tenderness of the muscles of mastication felt.

Tender points: Circumscribed regions in muscle, which on palpation produce intense pain in the same region of palpation. No referred pain is present.

DIAGNOSIS

A provisional diagnosis of a pain/dysfunction syndrome is made when no clinically detectable organic lesion can be found.

- Therapeutic anaesthetic block
- Trigger point injections
- Radiographs and other imaging techniques:

Orthopantomogram (OPG), Cone-beam computed tomography, magnetic resonance imaging (MRI) are useful for imaging soft tissues, and arthrography to assess the function of joints.

These imaging techniques are useful only to rule out other contributing factors of pain. Only a thorough clinical examination can provide a reliable diagnosis of MPDS.

TREATMENT

The treatment is focused on eliminating or reducing the aetiological factors (Flowchart 36.3 and Fig. 36.3).

SPRAY AND STRETCH

It consists of spraying of vapocoolant spray on the muscle with a trigger point and then stretching of the muscle, for example, fluoromethane spray.

REASSURANCE

The quality of the doctor–patient relationship is extremely important for the success of treatment as it may help to reduce the emotional problems of the patient, and they must be reassured that there is no serious disease.

OCCLUSAL CORRECTION

Patient should perform bilateral mastication. Any dental pain, substandard restoration or missing teeth should be treated. Habits can be corrected by exercises.

SOFT DIET

To reduce loading forces on joint and reduce muscle activity.

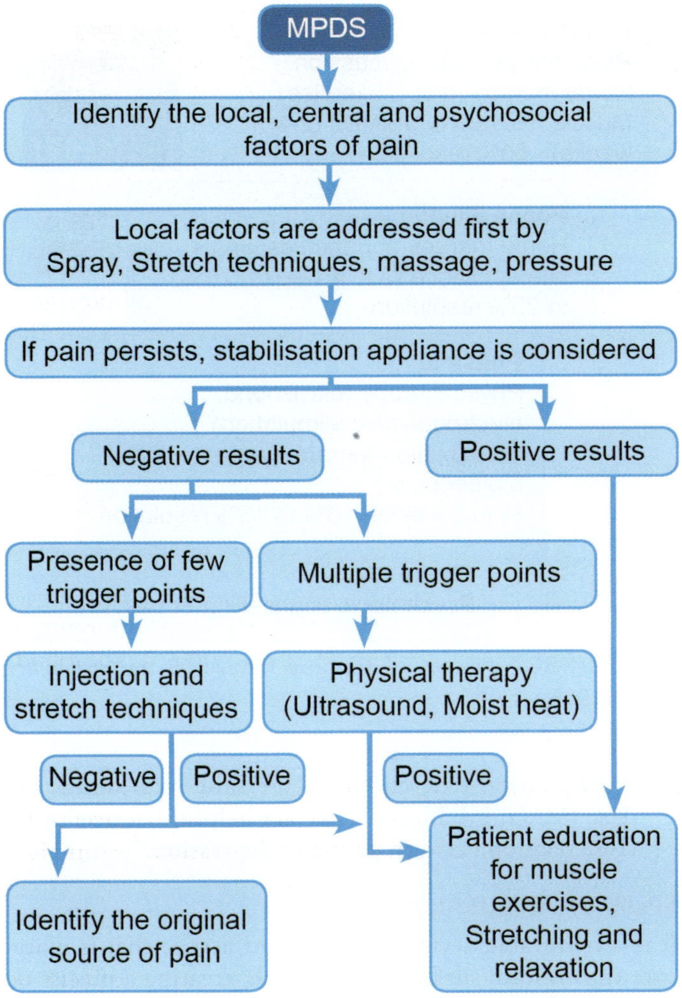

Flowchart 36.3 Management of MPDS.

THERMAL AGENTS

They help in decreasing pain, increasing muscle relaxation and increasing the range of motions.

a. *Superficial moist/dry heat:* Superficial heat produces a therapeutic effect by elevating the pain threshold, altering nerve conduction velocity and decreasing the muscle tension. Muscle relaxation may also result from analgesic effects of heating
b. *Ultrasonography-deep:* They help to increase the elasticity of soft tissues by producing deep heat. It has an antiinflammatory effect
c. *Phonophoresis (electrogalvanic stimulation):* Delivery of topically applied medicines using ultrasonography.

For TMJ inflammation, pulsed ultrasonography is applied at a frequency of 3 MHz and low intensity of 0.5–0.8 w/cm^2 per 5–8 mins. Exercise combined with ultrasonography reported a higher percentage of pain relief.

COLD

Cold can be used to control inflammation by application of ice packs, ice cubes or ice-soaked towels to the TMJ. Cold elevates the pain threshold by decreasing nerve conduction velocity.

IONTOPHORESIS

It is a battery-powered system used to deliver water-soluble ionising drugs through the skin. Common drugs used are dexamethasone sodium phosphate, methyl prednisolone and lidocaine hydrochloride.

TRANSCUTANEOUS ELECTRIC NERVE STIMULATION

Transcutaneous electric nerve stimulation (TENS) is a method of electrical stimulation which provides symptomatic pain relief by exciting sensory nerves. TENS employs a small,

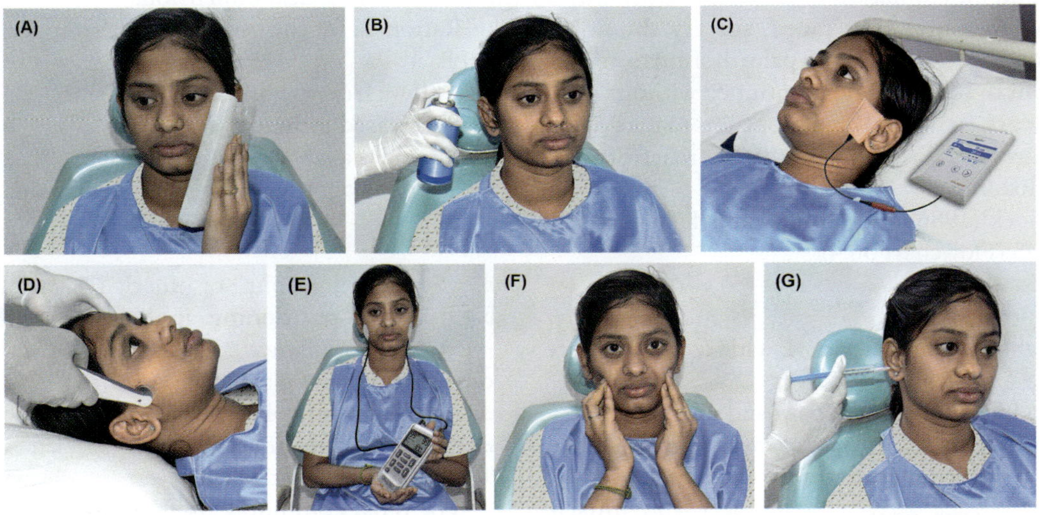

Figure 36.3 Various modalities of physical therapy. (**A**) Cold application. (**B**) Coolant spray. (**C**) Iontophoresis. (**D**) Ultrasound. (**E**) TENS. (**F**) Massage over muscle. (**G**) Injection over trigger points.

portable, battery-operated unit. Frequency, pulse width and amplitude of an alternating current that is to be administered to the patient by electrodes are adjustable. It works on the principle of the '*gate control theory*' of Melzack and Wall. It sends a painless electric current to the specific nerves, which relieves stiffness, improves mobility and relieves pain. It also enhances the healing process by reducing the effects of inflammation. It is a safe, noninvasive and effective method of pain control.

PHYSICAL EXERCISE

Patients with limited mouth opening and associated inflammation should be instructed to open and close their mouth with the tongue against the palate. This should be repeated several times during the day. This aids in increasing joint range of motion and muscular relaxation.

PRESSURE-POINT TECHNIQUES

Extraoral, intraoral massage or pressure-point techniques may be offered to the muscles of mastication. Therapeutic exercises for muscles of mastication can be performed by having the patient place one fist under the chin to resist mouth opening.

INTRAMUSCULAR INJECTION

It is administered to inactivate TrPs, alleviate muscle pain and improve muscle relaxation. Trigger point injection reduces muscle pain and contracture. It is useful when thermal agents and stretching exercises have failed to alleviate muscle dysfunction. 0.5 cc of local anaesthesia (without epinephrine) is injected into each site. The muscle is then passively or actively stretched.

INTRAARTICULAR (IA) INJECTION

Intraarticular injection of steroids has a place in some cases with acute pain and inflammation in relation to the joint.

If conservative measures have failed, surgery should be contemplated for the treatment of pain/dysfunction syndrome. When joint dysfunction has continued without relief over a period of years, structural damage begins to take place. Surgical procedures are directed towards the relief of joint pain due to overloading.

Laskin and Block (1986) suggested phases I–IV for management of MPDS (Flowchart 36.4).

DRUGS

- *Muscle relaxants*—methocarbamol, chlorzoxazone are effective
- *NSAIDs* are helpful in reducing pain and inflammation
- Antiinflammatory action of *corticosteroids* is greater than NSAIDs. Can be given intraarticular or orally
- *Anxiolytics* to reduce anxiety, as anxiety and muscle tension appear to be related. For example, diazepam 5–10 mg

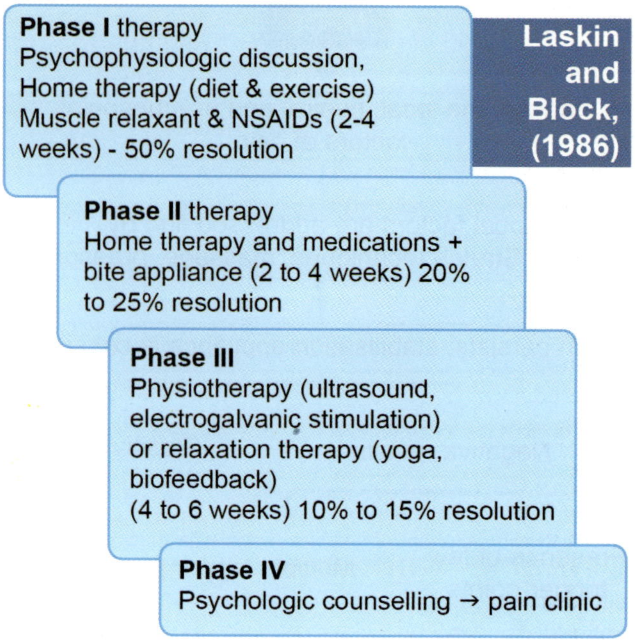

Flowchart 36.4 Phases of therapy for MPDS by Laskin and Block (1986).

- *Antidepressants*—tricyclic antidepressant, monoamino oxidase (MAO) inhibitors. They are helpful because of the close relation between pain and depression.

SPLINTS/OCCLUSAL APPLIANCE

It is a removable device made of hard acrylic that is placed over the occlusal surfaces of the teeth, creating a precise occlusion. It introduces a temporary stable occlusal condition that can improve the muscle pain. A splint inactivates facial muscles, decompresses intracapsular tissue, establishes a balanced occlusal plane, repositions the jaw, stabilises the disc and restores vertical dimension.

Rationale for the use of splint therapy in the treatment of MFP.

- Allows free mandibular movement
- Decreased muscular activity
- Provides a stable dental occlusion
- Aids in cognitive awareness of bruxism.

Types of splints

a. Stabilisation splint or muscle relaxation splint
b. Anterior positioning appliance or orthopaedic repositioning appliance
c. Anterior bite plane
d. Posterior bite plane
e. Pivoting appliance
f. Soft or resilient splint.

The most commonly used appliance in the treatment of TMJ disorders are stabilisation splint and anterior positioning appliance.

a. Stabilisation appliance or splint

The most commonly used splint in the treatment of MFP is the stabilisation splint. It can be used for both the arches but the maxillary arch splint is more stable and has some advantages. It provides an optimal occlusal relationship. The teeth are placed in even contact and at the same time the condyles are in most musculoskeletally stable position. The splint usually has anterior disocclusion in protrusive as well as canine guidance or group function in lateral excursions.

Indications: Muscle pain disorders and retrodiscitis due to trauma.

The advantage of mandibular splint is its less visibility and it is easier for the patient to speak.

b. Anterior positioning appliance

It is an interocclusal device that positions the mandible in a more anterior to intercuspal position. It is primarily used to treat disc derangement disorders with clicking sounds. It provides a better condyle–disc relationship and allows for the repair of retrodiscal tissue.

Indications: Disc displacement with reduction, disc displacement with intermittent locking and some of the inflammatory disorders of the joint.

It can be fabricated on both the arches, but the maxillary arch is preferred. The appliance is similar to a stabilisation splint with an anterior stop/guiding ramp added to it.

Bite plane splint

Bite plane splint, also known as the *Hawley's bite plane*, are used to reduce muscle activity and treat patients with MFP.

c. Anterior bite plane

It is a hard acrylic appliance that provides contact with the mandibular anterior teeth and disengages the posterior teeth, thus eliminating the influence on the masticatory system.

Indications: Muscle disorders due to orthopaedic instability, acute changes in occlusion and parafunctional activity. It consists of an upper acrylic plate without an occlusal cover. Relief from symptoms occurs within a few days of its use. It should be worn only for shorter periods (3 weeks).

d. Posterior bite plane

It is a hard acrylic fabricated on the mandibular posterior teeth and connected by a cast metal lingual bar.

Indications: When there is a need for anterior positioning of the mandible and it requires alterations in vertical dimensions.

e. Pivoting appliance

It is a hard acrylic device fabricated on one arch that provides a single posterior contact in each quadrant. It is indicated for the treatment of TMJ osteoarthritis.

f. Resilient splint (soft splint)

They are soft vinyl plastic occlusal splints (resilient material) made by vacuum-cupping techniques. It is usually fabricated on the maxillary teeth. It aims at achieving even and simultaneous contact with the opposing teeth. Usually this is a full-coverage 'mouth guard'.

Indications: Protective athletic splints, parafunctional habits such as clenching and bruxism. The advantage of a resilient splint is that it can be fabricated in the dental office and more affordable (Fig. 36.4).

INTERMAXILLARY FIXATION

When pain is severe, application of intermaxillary fixation relieves symptoms by inducing absolute rest.

RECENT ADVANCES

Newer methods of management in the treatment of MPDS is Botulinum injection and cold & soft laser.

BOTULINUM INJECTION

Botulinum injection into the TrPs releases endorphins and also increases vascularity to the affected muscles. This releases the tautness of the muscle fibres in MPDS.

COLD & SOFT LASERS (LOW-LEVEL LASER THERAPY)

It reduces pain by elevating the pain threshold and releasing encephalin and endorphin which have analgesic and antiinflammatory effect. They also reduce oedema, inflammation and pain by inhibiting inflammatory components.

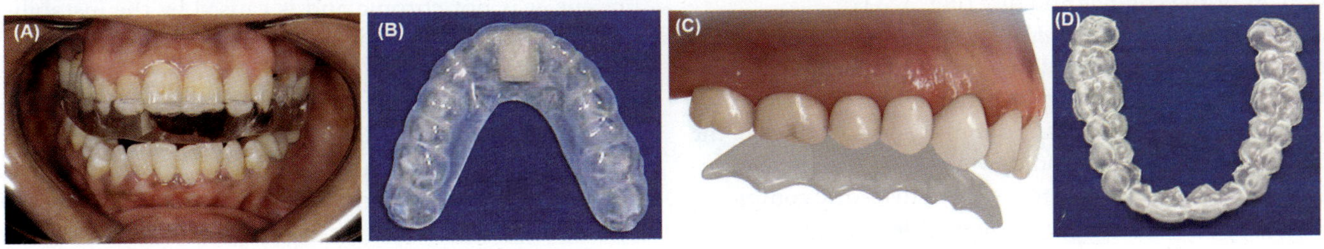

Figure 36.4 Types of splint. (**A**) Stabilisation appliance. (**B**) Anterior positioning appliance. (**C**) Anterior bite plane. (**D**) Soft splint.

Chapter 37

Temporomandibular Joint Disorders

OUTLINE

DERANGEMENTS OF THE CONDYLE–DISC COMPLEX/INTERNAL DERANGEMENT

Internal derangement is defined as a loss or disturbance in the normal structural integrity of the joint. There is disturbance in the normal anatomical relationship of the disc and condyle, which interferes with the smooth movement of the joint and causes momentary catching, clicking, popping or locking. This condition was 1st described by *Hey and Davies (1814)* as a localised mechanical fault interfering with the smooth action of a joint. Temporomandibular joint (TMJ) internal derangement can be defined as a joint dysfunction accompanied with an abnormal disc position.

NORMAL PHYSIOLOGIC MOVEMENTS OF THE TEMPOROMANDIBULAR JOINT

The movements of the condyle–disc complex are extremely intricate and occur in three planes: horizontal, sagittal and frontal. *Translation, sliding or gliding movements occur in the upper cavity, whereas hinge or rotation movements occur in the lower cavity.* A healthy joint allows a smooth, easy and frictionless movement of the condyle and disc (Fig. 37.1).

When the *mouth is opened*, the mandibular heads ***rotate around a common horizontal axis initially, followed by a forward and downward gliding movement*** (rotation or hinge movement followed by translation). Simultaneously, the discs also moves forward and downward on the slope of articular eminence. This movement of condyle–disc complex is maintained by the lateral pterygoid muscle, retrodiscal tissue and interarticular pressure. Further hinging and anterior gliding movement of each condyle continues until they articulate with the most anterior part of the disc and the mouth is open fully (Fig. 37.1).

While *closing the mouth*, the movements are reversed. In the 1st phase, the condyle glides backwards and then hinges on its disc, which is controlled by the lateral pterygoid muscle. Finally, the inferior lateral pterygoid relaxes allowing the disc to glide backwards and upwards along the condyle.

CLASSIFICATION OF TEMPOROMANDIBULAR JOINT INTERNAL DERANGEMENT

TEMPOROMANDIBULAR JOINT DISC DERANGEMENTS CAN BE CLASSIFIED INTO FOUR CLINICAL STAGES

i. Disc incoordination
ii. Disc displacement with reduction
iii. Disc displacement without reduction
iv. Anchored disc phenomenon.

Disc incoordination

Disc incoordination represents the earliest indication of an increase in the frictional properties of the joint. The patients often describe the need to perform a special manoeuvre to achieve a normal opening of the mouth, or they may complain of an annoying terminal jolting sensation associated with mandibular closing. Usually there is no pain, but if present, it is not chronic and is caused by the instability of the condyle–disc relationship.

Disc displacement with reduction

The most frequent TMJ disorder is disc displacement, in which the disc is displaced anteriorly. It could be with or without reduction depending on the circumstances. A *'joint sound or click'* is usually created when the condyle skids across a displaced disc during normal translation of the mandible.

Disc displacement with reduction is a condition in which the articular disc is displaced into an anteromedial position under the influence of lateral pterygoid muscle. The disc can

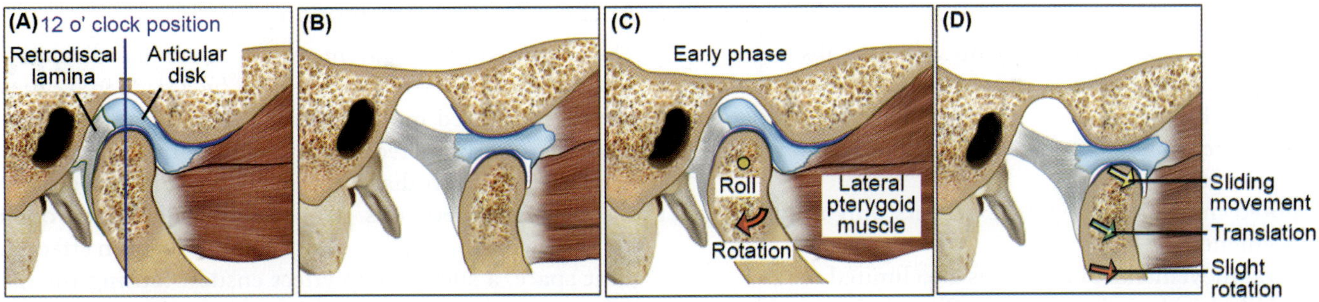

Figure 37.1 Normal relationship of condyle and disc in (**A**) closed mouth—note, the mandibular condyle is located within the glenoid fossa, and the junction of the posterior band of articular disc and the bilaminar zone lies directly above the head of the condyle, at the 12 o'clock position. Also, the thin intermediate zone is between the condyle and the articular eminence, where the two bones are joined intimately. On the other hand, the confluence of the posterior band and the bilaminar zone is within 10 degrees of vertical. (**B**) Open mouth—in the full open mouth position, the condyle is located either exactly under the articular eminence or slightly anterior to it. The intermediate zone maintains its position between the condyle and the articular eminence. (**C**) Early phase of mouth opening with rotation. (**D**) Late phase of mouth opening with translatory or gliding movements.

also be displaced medially or laterally. Reduction refers to the ability of the condyle to transact around the disc, and the disc's ability to resume a normal position relative to the condyle and glenoid fossa. Normally in these patients, *mouth opening is accompanied by a clicking or popping sound.* Clicks are typically reciprocal, occurring during both mouth opening and closing movements and are usually not associated with pain.

In disc displacement with reduction, the *disc is displaced anterior to the condylar head* and remains in this position as long as the mouth is closed (Fig. 37.2A). When the mouth is opened, the condyle passes over the posterior portion of the disc producing a click or popping sound. At maximum mouth opening, *the disc is able to translate/return to its normal position on the condyle* (Fig. 37.2B). As the disc reduces itself, the mandibular movements are not limited. However, the movements may not be as smooth as of normal TMJ.

The **diagnostic criteria** for disc displacement with reduction are as follows:

- When it is associated with pain, any movement of the affected joint significantly increases the pain
- Recurrent clicking or popping sounds are heard upon opening and closing the mouth
- MRI will show the anteriorly displaced disc. The junction of the posterior band and the bilaminar zone will be present at the anterior border of the condyle. It is also important to observe that the intermediate zone will not be situated in between the articular surfaces of the condyle and of the eminence.

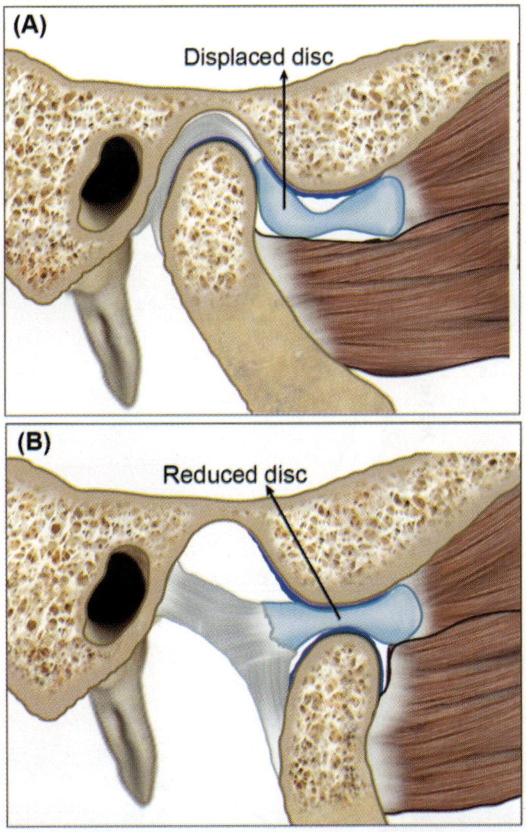

Figure 37.2 Disc displacement with reduction in closed and open mouth position. (**A**) Anteriorly displaced disc in closed mouth. (**B**) On mouth opening the disc returns to its normal position.

Disc displacement without reduction

In disc displacement without reduction, the patient is *unable to return the disc to its normal position* on the condyle during translatory movements. The condition is also referred to as **closed lock**, where the jaw is locked and will not open further. It appears that the disc is impacted in front of the condyle. The mouth opening becomes limited (10–15 mm) as the disc does not get reduced over the condyle or the condyle fails to pass over the posterior band of the articular disc. The only form of movement that can occur in the condyle and disc is rotational or hinge movement.

Diagnostic criteria (acute)

- Joint noises (clicking or popping sound) is absent
- In symptomatic patients, the overloading and stretching of the highly innervated retrodiscal tissue elicits pain at the affected joint. On forceful mandibular movements, the pain gets aggravated
- Limited mouth opening as it permits only initial hinge movement
- Lateral movements of the jaw is also limited
- Mandibular deviation to the affected side can be observed in unilateral cases
- The MRI of the soft tissue demonstrates nonreducing disc displacement or more anteriorly displaced articular disc. The entire disc will be found anterior to the condylar head and inferior to the articular eminence (Fig. 37.3).

Chronic

- Pain may be present but the intensity is much less than that of the acute type
- A history of joint noises (clicking) followed by limitation in mouth opening
- Restricted lateral movements of mandible.

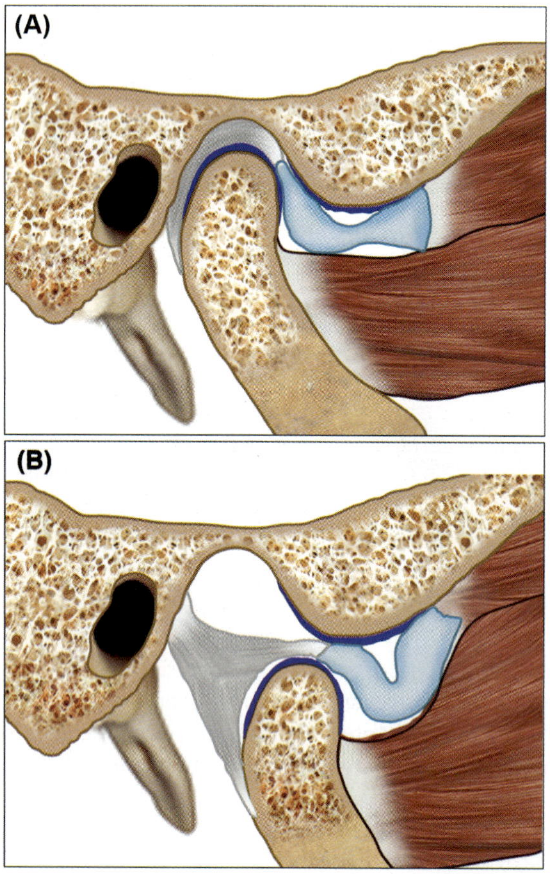

Figure 37.3 Disc displacement without reduction in closed and open mouth position. (**A**) Anteriorly displaced disc in closed mouth. (**B**) On mouth opening the disc has not returned to its normal position.

Anchored disc phenomenon

The anchored disc phenomenon or acute disc displacement without reduction, is characterised by a sudden, severe and persistent limited mouth opening that is less than disc displacement without reduction (10–30 mm). The disc is not displaced, the retrodiscal tissue is also not compressed, but the patient experiences pain on forceful mouth opening. Due to increased joint viscosity and the vacuum effect in the joint space, a suction-cup effect ensues, causing the disc to adhere to the articular eminence.

WILKES CLINICAL STAGING OF INTERNAL DERANGEMENT (1989)

Clinical staging of Internal derangement by Wilkes is depicted in Table 37.1

AETIOLOGY OF INTERNAL DERANGEMENT

The aetiology of TMJ disorders are complex and multifactorial. However, the internal derangement is three to five times more common in females and the symptoms often begin to manifest themselves during the 4th decade of life. The major factors associated with TMJ disorders are as follows:

a. Trauma
b. Unstable occlusion
c. Emotional stress
d. Excessive overloading of the joint
e. Parafunctional activities (bruxism)
f. Local/systemic inflammatory arthropathies
g. Deep pain input (teeth pain).

These factors ultimately results in overloading of the joint as well as degenerative changes in the articular surfaces, increased friction and progressive disc displacement.

TRAUMA

Trauma to the TMJ is one of the most common factor leading to thinning of the disc or elongation of the discal ligaments causing condyle-disc complex disorders. This trauma can be classified as either *macrotrauma or microtrauma* based on the magnitude of the traumatic force.

Macrotrauma

It is a sudden force to the joint, resulting in structural alterations. It can be subdivided into direct or indirect trauma.

Direct trauma

The condyle is suddenly displaced from the fossa if the trauma occurs in an open mouth position, resulting in elongation of the ligaments and condyle-disc derangement.

If the trauma occurs in closed mouth position, that is at maximum intercuspation, the displacement of the condyle is prevented, resulting in reduction of injury to the condyle-disc complex. This is seen in

- Sports injuries
- Assaults
- Intubation procedures

TABLE 37.1 Wilkes Classification of TMJ Internal Derangement

Stage	Characteristics	Imaging
I. Early	• Painless clicking • No restricted motion	• Slight disc displacement with early reduction • Normal disc morphology and osseous contours
II. Early/intermediate	• Increased clicking • Intermittent locking • Headaches	• Moderate disc displacement with late reduction • Early disc deformity • Normal osseous contours
III. Intermediate	• Frequent pain • Joint tenderness, headaches • Locking • Restricted motion • Painful chewing	• Disc displacement without reduction • Deformity in disc • Normal osseous contours
IV. Intermediate/late	• Chronic pain, headache • Restricted motion	• Severe disc displacement without reduction • Severe disc deformity • Abnormal bone contours
V. Late	• Variable pain, joint crepitus • Chronic restriction of motion	• Disc displacement with perforation and gross deformity of disc • Degenerative osseous changes

- 3rd molar extractions
- Long dental appointments
- Overextension of jaw as yawning.

Indirect trauma

The TMJ injury is the result of a sudden force being applied to the mandible. For example, cervical flexion-extension injury (whiplash injury).

Microtrauma

It refers to any small force that is applied to the TMJ repeatedly for over a long period, for example, bruxism or clenching, malocclusion.

EXCESSIVE OVERLOADING OF THE JOINT

The most prevalent cause of internal derangement is the overload on the joint. The overload is commonly produced by stress, unstable occlusion, acute or chronic trauma and joint friction that deteriorates the cartilage metabolism. This process ultimately results in inhibition of the smooth movements of the articular surfaces. Clinically, this is the stage at which joint sounds (clicking) can be observed.

SYSTEMIC ARTHROPATHY

Patients who suffer from systemic arthropathy may experience internal derangement (ID) due to the fact that systemic illnesses influence both the structure and function of the articular tissues. The systemic disorders that can cause ID include rheumatoid arthritis, ankylosing spondylitis, Ehler-Danlos syndrome, Lyme disease, lupus erythematosus, and other connective tissue disorders.

LOCALISED ARTHROPATHY

It is not caused by joint overloading or systemic disease and usually affects one joint only. It can arise from osteochondroma, synovial chondromatosis or synovial cyst.

PATIENT EXAMINATION

Clinical examination should include the following:

TMJ examination:

- *Pain or tenderness* of the TMJ by digital manipulation of the joints, when the mandible is in rest or functional movements. Questions pertaining to pain should include its location, severity, duration, and frequency of episodes, radiation to the surrounding structures; factors that aggravate and relieve the condition; and its associated symptoms
- *Joint sounds* such as click or crepitation can be felt by placing the finger over the lateral surface of joint and making the patient open and close the jaw. A stethoscope or joint recording device can also be used to hear the clicking sounds. It is important to note the sound occur during opening or closing or both. The presence or absence of the sounds gives insight about the disc position
- *Joint restrictions*—restricted or unusual pathways of the mandibular movement should be observed for any irregularities or restrictions in the joint
- Symmetry of motion

Range of mandibular movement:

- The distance between the incisal edges of the upper and lower teeth is the total range of mouth opening. The normal maximal interincisal distance ranges from 35 to 50 mm

- The lateral deviation of mandible or abnormal movements are noted. Normal lateral movements are between 5 and 10 mm. Normal protrusive movement ranges from 7 to 10 mm
- The presence of subluxation or recurrent dislocation of one or both condyles can be determined by abnormal palpation during movement
- The movement of the mandible can be limited by a tightening of one or more muscles, a nonreducible anterior displacement of the articular disc, interference from the coronoid process, a haematoma, an infection, or other conditions like fibrous ankylosis or scleroderma

Dental examination:

Occlusal condition, overjet, overbite, prosthesis, tooth mobility, pulpitis, missing teeth, loss of posterior occlusal contact and tooth wear

Muscular examination:

Each muscle should be examined for tenderness, muscle tone, muscle mass and trigger points (Fig. 37.4).

CLINICAL PRESENTATION OF INTERNAL DERANGEMENT

The most frequent signs and symptoms are as follows:

- Pain over the preauricular area
- Decreased mouth opening
- *TMJ noise—clicking sound, crepitation or popping joint* on mouth opening and closure
- Joint tenderness especially with function
- *Deviation of mandible to the affected side*
- Intermittent lock jaw
- *Trismus:* Present only in disc displacement without reduction
  Disc displacement with reduction: After the initial 10 mm of mouth opening (rotation or hinge), the jaw deviates to the affected side and a *click or pop is heard* or a catch can be felt as the disc pops over the condylar head. A reciprocal click is heard during the mouth closure, when the condyle slips over the posterior rim of the disc
  Disc displacement without reduction: Jaw deviation begins at the commencement of mouth opening and progresses till the end of mouth opening. The mouth can be opened to about <30 mm on exertion of gentle pressure.

RADIOGRAPHIC EVALUATION

- Plain radiographs
- Orthopantomogram (OPG)
- Cone beam computed tomography (CBCT) (Fig. 37.5)
- Magnetic resonance image (MRI)
- Bone scintigraphy (bone scan)
- Electromyography (EMG)
- Ultrasonography (USG)
- Mandibular tracking device
- Arthrography.

Plain radiographs and CT scans show TMJ's bony changes and the condyle-fossa functional relationship. CBCT can evaluate TMJ ankylosis, osteoarthritis, growth anomalies, TMJ fractures, and tumors.

MRIs are more effective for disc positioning and displacement. It may also evaluate the condyle, fossa, eminence (sclerosis, flattening, erosions, and cortical continuity) and disc (position, shape, size, density, and perforation). EMG demonstrates muscle function.

The USG may evaluate masticatory muscle thickness and be used as an image guide for upper and lower joint space injections.

ARTHROGRAPHY

It is injection of a radiopaque material into the joint compartments, followed by evaluation of the intracapsular soft tissues. Assessment of the dynamic and functional movements of the disc and condyle can be done with high precision. It is the method of choice in identifying the disc perforations, adhesions and disc dislocations.

MANAGEMENT OF INTERNAL DERANGEMENT

The treatment of internal derangement should follow the following principles:

- Reduce pain
- Decrease the joint load
- Reduce inflammation
- Identify and remove the cause
- Improvement in the range of movements
- Restore function.

The treatment of internal derangement can be basically divided into two groups: conservative and surgical. According

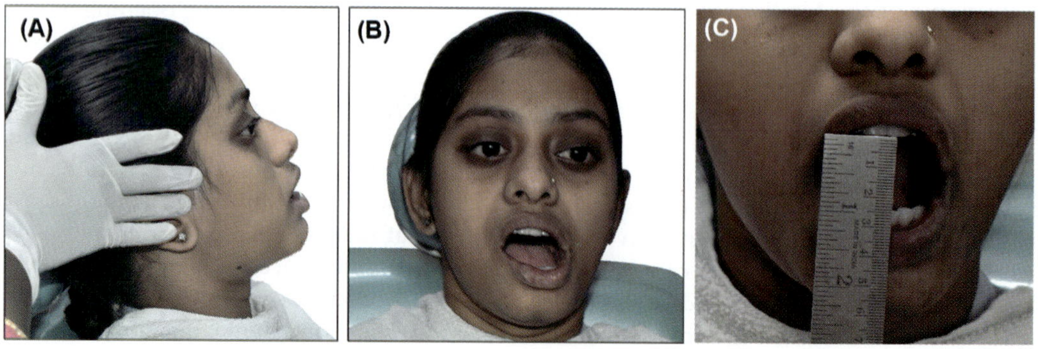

Figure 37.4 **(A)** TMJ examination. (**B** and **C**) Examination of the range of jaw motion (deviation of jaw) and mouth opening.

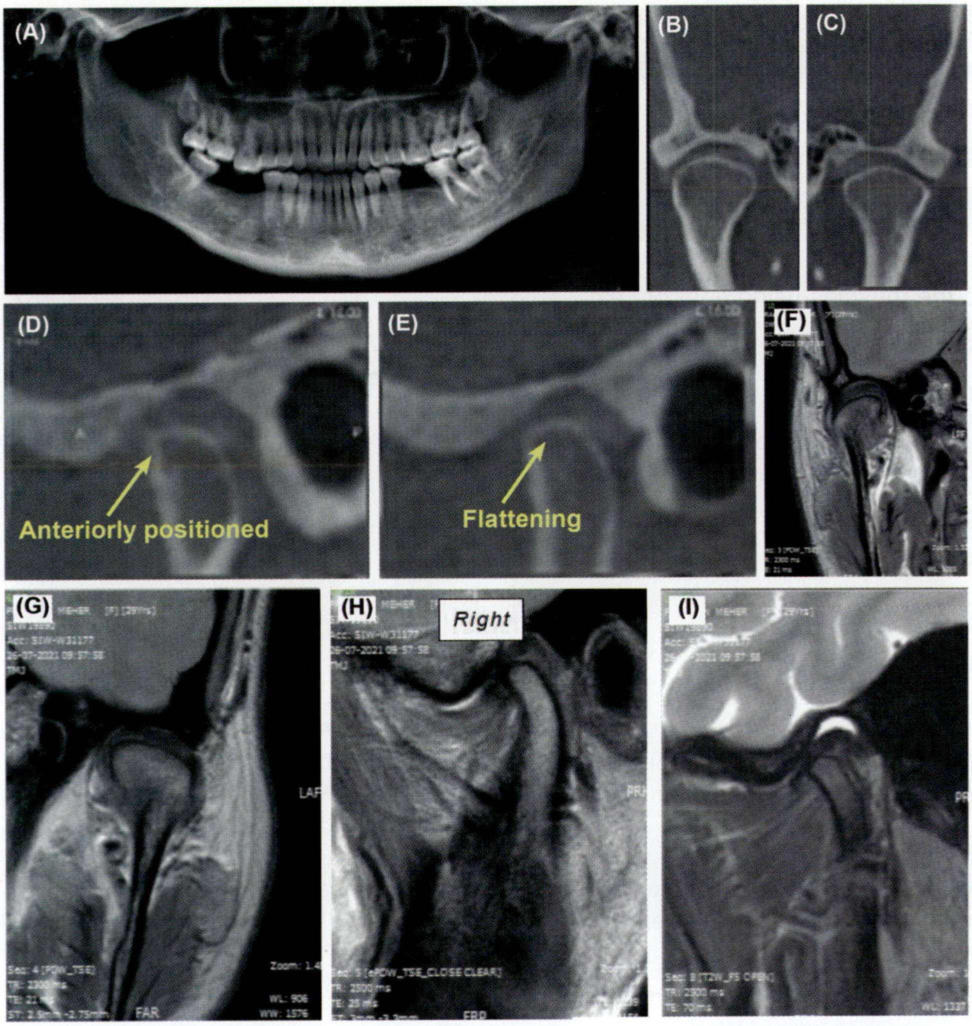

Figure 37.5 **(A)** OPG showing reduced size of the condyle. **(B** and **C)** CBCT image of the right and left condyle. **(D** and **E)** CBCT showing anteriorly positioned condyle, reduced and flattened condylar head. **(F** and **G)** MRI images of right and left condyle. **(H** and **I)** MRI images of right condyle showing focal contour abnormalities in the condyle and deformed disc.

to the Wilkes classification, early stages (I to III) of internal derangement can be managed with conservative or minimally invasive methods; however, advanced stages (IV or V) might require open joint surgery.

NONSURGICAL/CONSERVATIVE MANAGEMENT

It becomes the 1st line of treatment aimed at reducing the joint pain, joint loading, decrease the inflammation, improve healing and restore the function. The conservative therapy includes a number of different methods (Box 37.1).

Patient education and homecare

A successful treatment includes patient awareness, motivation, as well as patient compliance. The patient should be informed about the natural course and aetiology of the disease. Patient education should focus on modifying the patient's diet, helping them sleep better and increasing their awareness of mandibular parafunction. The instructions to the patient should include the following:

- Relaxation of muscles by voluntarily limiting the mandibular function
- Modifying the parafunctional habits
- Physiotherapy sessions in patient's home.

Home physiotherapy includes application of heat (moist towels) over the sensitive areas, which relaxes the muscles, reduces the pain and increase the range of mandibular movements. Patient's stress and parafunctional habits are treated by medications, behavioural modifications and physiotherapy.

Pharmacotherapy

Pharmacotherapy along with other supporting therapies treat ID effectively. No drug treats temporomandibular disorder (TMD) completely. Analgesics, NSAIDs, corticosteroids,

BOX 37.1 Nonsurgical/Conservative Management of Internal Derangement

A. Patient education.

B. Home care instructions:

- Soft diet.
- Avoid clenching habits.
- Massage to the muscles using heat or cold.
- Physical exercises.

C. Pharmacotherapy:

- NSAIDs, antispasmodic and muscle relaxants, tricyclic antidepressants, antibiotics.

D. Occlusal appliance:

- Stabilisation appliance.
- Anterior positioning appliance.

E. Physical therapy:

- Relaxation exercises.
- Physiotherapy to strengthen the muscle and mobilise the joint.
- Physical agents.
- TENS, ultrasound, iontophoresis, phonophoresis, electrogalvanic stimulation, thermotherapy.

F. Stress reduction.

muscle relaxants, and antianxiety medicines perform well for TMD.

NSAIDs–ibuprofen 600-800 mg three times daily or aspirin
Muscle ralaxants–benzodiazepines
Antidepressant drugs–amitriptyline 10 mg before sleep
Antianxiety drugs–diazepam 2.5 to 5 mg
Antibiotics–infectious diseases of joint.

Occlusal splints

An occlusal splint should be symmetrical, strong with smooth edges and have good retention. It should cover only the teeth and should not restrict any functional movement.

The use of occlusal splints in ***disc displacements with reduction*** is to reduce the intracapsular pain and prevent degenerative forces on the TMJ, articular disc and dentition. A *stabilisation appliance* may be considered initially. When this appliance is ineffective, one should consider an *anterior repositioning appliance*, which helps restore the normal condyle-disc relationship. The patient is instructed to wear the device day and night until the symptoms subside. Typically, it takes 8-10 weeks or even longer (Fig. 37.6).

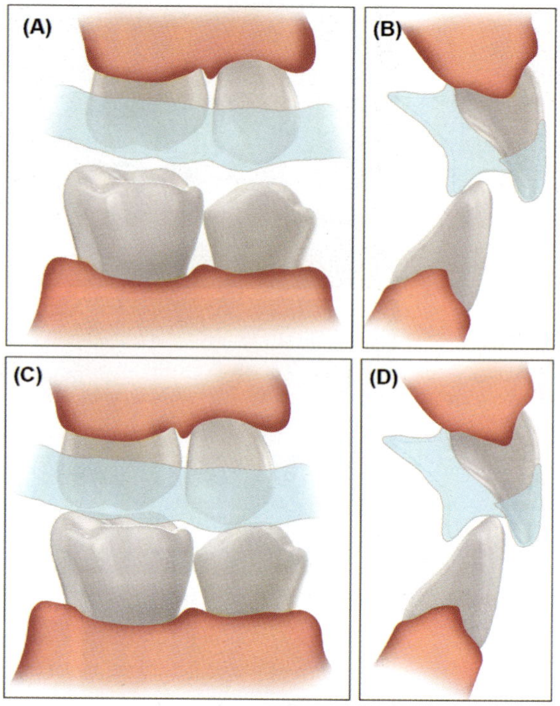

Figure 37.6 Anterior positioning appliance. (**A** and **B**) During normal closure the mandibular anterior teeth is in contact with the anterior guiding ramp. (**C** and **D**) The ramp shifts the jaw forward into a desired position as the mouth closes into occlusion.

For patients with *disc displacement without reduction*, use of an *anterior positioning appliance is contraindicated* as it will aggravate the condition by forcing the disc even more forward.

Management of disc displacement without reduction

The goal of the initial treatment is to reduce the disc through manual manipulation. By grasping the mandibular molars with the thumbs on both sides and pressing the affected side inferiorly, manual reduction is performed. This procedure returns the disc to its normal position over the condyle. It is then followed by an anterior positioning appliance that aids in restoring the disc's normal shape.

Similar to disc displacement with reduction, supportive therapy includes patient education, jaw exercises, avoiding hard biting, NSAIDs, transcutaneous electrical nerve stimulation (TENS).

Intense conservative therapy for 2-3 weeks is advised for patients with internal derangement and signs of joint overload after all other possible causes have been ruled out. If the symptoms begin to resolve, then conservative treatment should be continued. However, if the symptoms persist, surgical interventions should be considered.

SURGICAL MANAGEMENT

Indications for surgery:

- Failure of conservative therapy
- Progression of the disorder

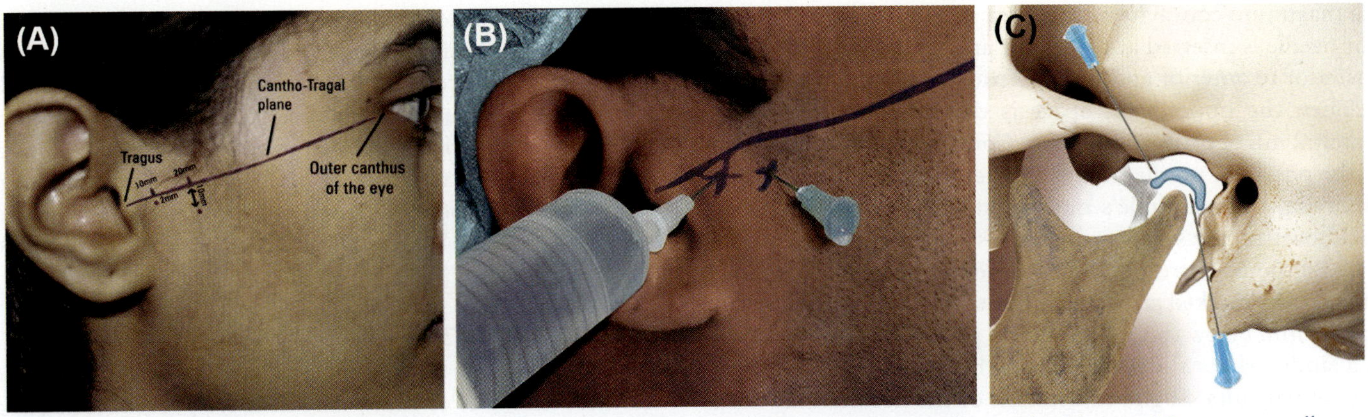

Figure 37.7 (**A**) Landmarks for TMJ arthrocentesis. (**B** and **C**) The upper joint space was lavaged with two 18 gauge needles and irrigation with Ringer's lactate solution.

- Source of pain is intracapsular
- Disc displacement without reduction.

The aim of surgery is to return the disc to a normal functional relationship with the condyle.

Surgical procedures for internal derangement

1. Arthrocentesis
2. Arthroscopy
3. Open joint surgery/arthrotomy:
   - Disc repair or plication
   - Discectomy/meniscectomy
   - Discoplasty
   - Discopexy
4. TMJ replacement.

TMJ arthrocentesis

Arthrocentesis is a safe and rapid procedure used to treat a multitude of disorders affecting the TMJ, 1st described by *Nitzan and colleagues* in 1991 to treat acute closed lock jaw. It is the least invasive of the surgical techniques. Patients with TMJ internal derangements without reduction who do not respond to nonsurgical management benefit from arthrocentesis and/or arthroscopic lysis and lavage (Fig. 37.7).

Indications

- Acute and chronic limitation of opening because of anteriorly displaced disc without reduction
- Chronic pain with good range of motion
- Degenerative osteoarthritis
- Possible sources of pain that include impingement, compression and inflammatory changes in the retrodiscal tissues
- Inflammatory changes in the synovial membrane with joint effusion and capsulitis.

Contraindications

- Patients who have not undergone appropriate conservative/nonsurgical and pharmacologic treatment
- Bony or fibrous ankylosis
- Extracapsular sources of pain
- Pathology involving bony degeneration, osteophytes and bone spicules
- Disc perforation.

Mechanism of arthrocentesis

The concept is based on the observation that simple lysis and lavage of the upper joint space via arthroscopy removes the inflammatory mediators, as well as alters the intraarticular pressure through the addition of more fluid and is highly successful in reestablishing normal range of mouth opening in patients with symptomatic TMJ disease (Table 37.2).

Technique

The procedure is usually performed under intravenous conscious sedation and local anaesthesia (LA) or under local anaesthesia alone. Technique involves the insertion of two 18-gauge needles into the superior joint space of the TMJ.

The patient is seated inclined at a 45-degree angle with the head turned to the opposite side to provide an easy approach to the affected joint. After preparation of the preauricular area, the external auditory meatus is blocked with cotton and a local anaesthetic is infiltrated. The *Holmlund–Hellsing line* is drawn with a marker between the lateral canthus and the apex of tragus (cantho-tragal line). A marking point is made at the midportion of the external tragus. From this point, approximately 10 mm anterior and 2 mm inferior to the line,

TABLE 37.2 Mechanism of Arthrocentesis

Lysis	Lavage
• Adhesions in the space • The lubrication and the flow of synovial fluid is restored • Range of motion is improved	• Inflammatory mediators • Debris • Matrix metalloproteinases (MMPs), cytokines and proteolytic enzymes

the maximum concavity of the fossa is located and the posterior needle is inserted at this point at a 45-degree angle from posterior to anterior and from inferior to superior.

Then the upper joint space is distended with approximately 2 mL of Ringer's solution. Confirmation of placement of the posterior needle into the upper joint space is made by observing the mandible's movement during injection or by backflow into the syringe when pressure is released.

A 2nd point corresponding to the height of the articular eminence is marked at 20 mm anterior to the midtragal point and 10 mm below the cantho-tragal plane. This can function as a landmark for the placement of the 2nd portal for the outflow of irrigants. Slight adjustment of the needles may need to be made if the outflow is sluggish. The upper joint space is then irrigated with 100–300 mL of Ringer's solution.

The outflow is intermittently occluded during the irrigation to distend the joint space. After completion of the irrigation, medication (steroid or hyaluronic acid) may be placed in the upper joint space. Once the procedure is completed, the mandible is moved through opening, excursive and protrusive movements. The range of motion and presence of any mechanical interference to movement are noted. After the procedure, the patient is given a mild analgesic and instructed to perform range-of-motion exercises. This is continued for about a week.

Complications

- Temporary facial nerve weakness or paralysis
- Preauricular swelling
- Haematoma
- Occlusal changes from distention of the upper joint space.

These complications are temporary and generally resolve within 24 h.

Arthroscopy

In this technique, an arthroscope is placed into the joint space and the intracapsular structures are visualised on a monitor. It can be considered as a visually assisted lysis and lavage of the TMJ. In addition, it also helps in identifying intraarticular pathology. This procedure identifies and eliminates joint adhesions, thereby increasing the mobility of joint. It does not correct the disc position but increases the disc mobility. Arthroscopy has been found to be effective and a reliable alternative for many patients undergoing open joint surgery. At the end of the arthroscopic procedure, medications can be *injected intraarticularly* including *steroids, hyaluronic acid (HA) and platelet-rich plasma (PRP)* for improving disc mobility.

Open joint surgery/arthrotomy

Open surgery or arthrotomy is indicated only when the conservative methods or minimally invasive procedures such as arthrocentesis or arthroscopy does not produce adequate success in correcting the disc problems. The open joint surgery can be performed both on the soft and hard tissues of the joint. There are a variety of procedures performed under General anaesthesia, which includes *disc repair or plication, discectomy, discoplasty, discopexy and condyloplasty.*

- *Disc repair or plication*—in this open procedure, a portion of the retrodiscal tissue and inferior lamina is removed and the disc is retracted posteriorly and secured with sutures
- *Discectomy/meniscectomy*—it is a complete removal of the disc and allow the natural mechanism to restore the joint. The removed disc can be replaced with substitutes such as silastic, Proplast-Teflon discal implants, dermal, temporal fascial flaps, fat tissues and auricular cartilage grafts
- *Discoplasty*—it is reparation of small perforations in the disc using sutures. It is indicated in young patients with disc perforation and associated degenerative changes
- *Discopexy*—it is open repositioning of the dislocated disc and its fixation in a suitable position to the condyle using sutures, screw, pin or anchor (Fig. 37.8).

Open surgery often presents with complications such as scarring, postsurgical adhesion, haemarthrosis, risk of damage to the facial nerve. Hence, surgery should be reserved only for patients who do not respond adequately to the conservative methods.

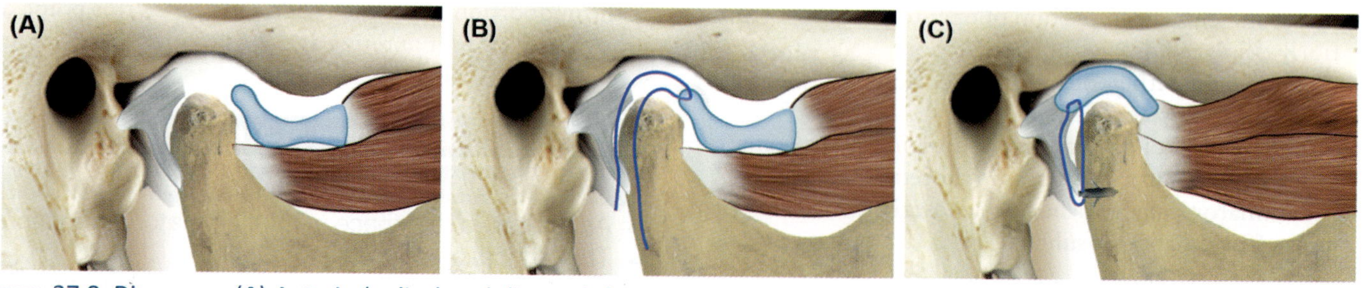

Figure 37.8 Discopexy. (**A**) Anteriorly displaced disc and the excessive bilaminar tissue is excised. (**B**) Anchor sutures are placed through the disc. (**C**) The disc is repositioned over the condyle and stabilised using Mitek anchor suture inserted into the posterior part of condyle.

STRUCTURAL INCOMPATIBILITY OF THE ARTICULAR SURFACES/DISLOCATION

Dislocation—it refers to a situation in which the condyle is displaced out of the glenoid fossa and in front of the articular eminence. The patient cannot reduce it by himself and requires expert assistance for reduction. Dislocation can be unilateral or bilateral

Subluxation/hypermobility—it is a condition in which the dislocated condyle can be reduced back into the normal position by the patient himself without any assistance

Habitual or recurrent dislocation—it refers to frequent and repeated episodes of recurrent dislocation that can be manipulated back into position.

> **Subluxation**—incomplete dislocation.
>
> **Luxation**—dislocation.
>
> **Recurrent dislocation**—repeated dislocation with no strong psychological components.

CONDYLAR DISLOCATION

Dislocation of the TMJ occurs when the mandibular condyle is displaced anteriorly beyond the articular eminence and its inability to descend back to its normal position. In 1832, *Sir Astley Cooper* proposed principles for diagnosis and treatment of dislocation and introduced the terms 'complete dislocation and imperfect dislocation (subluxation)' (Fig. 37.9).

CLASSIFICATION OF DISLOCATION

1. Rowe and Killey classification based on the duration of dislocation:
   - Acute
   - Habitual dislocation/subluxation
   - Chronic recurrent dislocation
   - Long-standing/chronic protracted dislocation

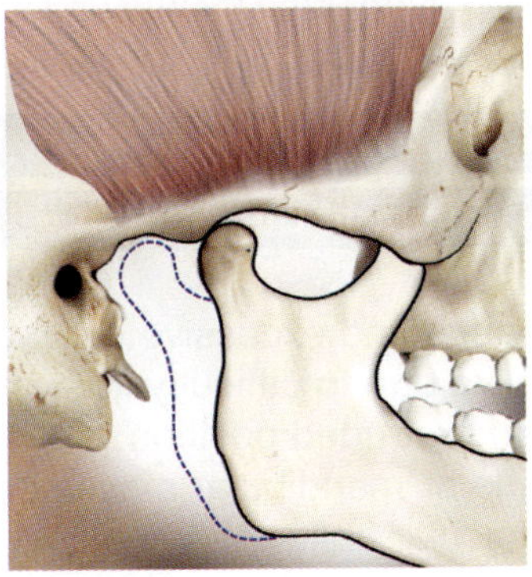

Figure 37.9 Dislocation of condyle out of glenoid fossa.

2. Based on the direction of displacement:
   - Anterior
   - Posterior
   - Medial
   - Lateral
   - Superior
3. Based on the side of displacement:
   - Unilateral
   - Bilateral
4. Based on number of occurrences:
   - Recurrent
   - Nonrecurrent
5. Based on aetiology:
   - Traumatic
   - Nontraumatic (spontaneous).

Anterior dislocation is more common due to the relative weakness of the capsule in the anterior region. Superior dislocation occurs when condyle is pushed into the middle cranial fossa.

Pathogenesis of temporomandibular joint dislocation

The stability of any joint depends on three factors:

1. *The integrity of ligaments associated with the joint:* Laxity of the temporomandibular ligament and joint capsule predisposes the joint to dislocation
2. *Dyssynchronous muscle function:* Abnormalities of neuromuscular mechanisms which control the muscles of mastication may be associated with dislocation
3. *Bony architecture of the joint surfaces:* Myrhaug observed that a deep overbite was frequently associated with a deep glenoid fossa and a steep articular eminence, which may be conducive to dislocation.

The disc–condyle relationship also plays a role in TMJ dislocation, principally in patients with anterior disc dislocation with reduction.

AETIOLOGY OF DISLOCATION

Dislocation can occur either by intrinsic or extrinsic cause.

Aetiology of dislocation has been briefed in Table 37.3.

CLINICAL PRESENTATION

The common clinical features for acute/chronic dislocation as well as unilateral/bilateral dislocation (Table 37.4) are as follows:

- Inability to close the mouth
- Preauricular depression evident on the skin
- Excessive salivation
- Tense, spasmodic muscles of mastication
- Severe pain in the TMJ region
- Protruding chin
- Inability to speak, swallow or masticate
- Condyle palpable anterior to articular eminence
- A 'thud' sound is heard as the condyle quickly jumps forward at maximal mouth opening. This is not same as a subtle clicking sensation.

TABLE 37.3 Aetiology of Dislocation

Trauma	Flexion-Extension Injury to the Mandible
Medical and surgical procedures	Intubation, endoscopy, bronchoscopy, ENT procedures, dental procedures with mouth wide open for prolonged time
Occlusal factors	• Excessive tooth abrasion • Severe malocclusion • Loss of dentition (loss of vertical dimension)
Connective tissue disorders	• Hypermobility syndrome • Ehlers–Danlos syndrome • Marfan's syndrome • Multiple sclerosis • Parkinson's disease
Psychogenic	• Habitual dislocation
Drugs	• Antipsychiatric drugs • Phenothiazines produce extrapyramidal effects resulting in spasm • Antiemetic
Spontaneous	Laughing, yawning, singing, vomiting, biting and seizures
Anatomical aberrations	• Small condyle • Shallow/steep articular eminence • Laxity of ligaments and capsule
Miscellaneous causes	• Internal derangement • Dyssynchronous muscle function • Contralateral intraarticular obstruction

RADIOGRAPHIC EVALUATION

OPG, TMJ tomogram, computed tomography (CT scan) (Fig. 37.10), CBCT, MRI, EMG, and USG.

OPG is the most commonly used modality for screening. It shows the position of the condyle out of the glenoid fossa. TMJ tomogram provides TMJ images in open and closed mouth position. EMG evaluates the activity of the muscles.

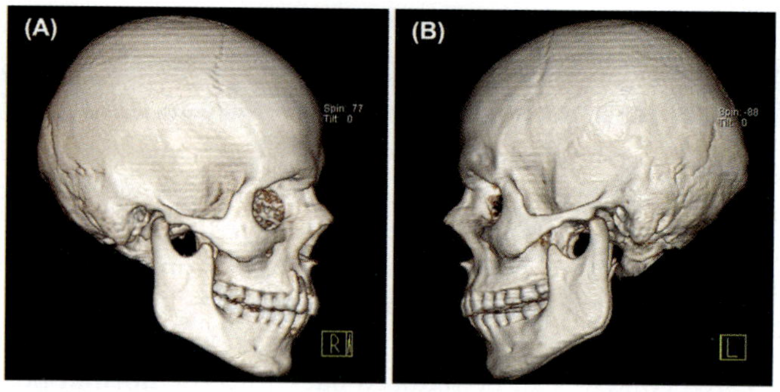

Figure 37.10 CT images showing anteriorly displaced condyle.

USG provides the length and thickness of the muscles at rest and clenching.

MANAGEMENT OF DISLOCATION

Prior to treatment, it is vital to relieve tension, anxiety or muscle spasms by reassuring the patient and prescribing sedatives or tranquillisers.

Management of acute dislocation

Acute dislocation necessitates immediate treatment. *Manual reduction* can be done with or without the *use of local anaesthesia* immediately or within 72 h. Beyond that, reduction may be done *under sedation/LA or general anaesthesia*. Several reduction techniques have been advocated.

Management of Acute Dislocation

1. Nelaton's/hippocratic method
2. Wrist pivot technique
3. Dingman and Natwig
4. Extraoral technique
5. Gag reflex

Nelaton's/hippocratic technique

The patient is made to sit upright in a chair with the clinician standing in front or sometimes behind based on convenience.

TABLE 37.4 Clinical Features of Unilateral and Bilateral Dislocation

Unilateral Dislocation	Bilateral Dislocation
• Mouth is open and the mandible deviated to the opposite side • Deviation produces lateral cross and open bite • Teeth cannot be closed into occlusion • Difficulty in mastication and swallowing • Affected condyle is impalpable • Drooling of saliva with speech difficulty	• Pain • Difficulty in speech and excessive salivation • Drooling of saliva due to difficulty in swallowing • Mouth opens in protruded position • Restricted range of mandibular movements • Bilateral preauricular hollow • Gagging of occlusion (molar teeth) • Anterior open bite

The thumbs of the clinician are covered with gauze or a protective covering and positioned over the lower molar teeth bilaterally. The index fingers are placed under the inferior border of the mandible. The posterior aspect of the mandible is *depressed inferiorly to depress the condyle, while the chin is elevated anteriorly and the entire mandible is pushed backwards with the palm. The mandible is moved downward backwards and then upwards, thus manipulating the condyle back into position.* After reduction, the mandible should be immobilised using *Barton's bandage* for several days to allow for capsular repair, muscle rest and prevention of recurrence (Fig. 37.11).

Wrist pivot method

The thumb is placed under the chin, whereas the other fingers are placed over the occlusal surface. An upward force is given by the thumb, while inferior force is given by other fingers. It utilises the force created by the muscles of mastication than overcoming it.

Dingman and Natwig

They recommended the use of LA based on the theory that dislocation is maintained by muscle spasm secondary to painful stimuli arising from the capsule. When lignocaine is injected into the glenoid fossa or the muscles of mastication, sensory reflex mechanism of the joint is blocked and the muscle spasm is overcome, respectively.

Extraoral technique

Mandibular dislocation can be reduced by pulling one end of the mandible while simultaneously pushing the other end. Hence, reducing the dislocation on one side 1st and then subsequently on the other side. This technique is applicable in unilateral dislocation as one side is reduced 1st, followed by the other.

Gag reflex

The soft palate is probed using mouth mirror and a gag reflex is induced. This reflex relaxes the lateral pterygoid muscle through neuromuscular activities and reduces dislocation.

Following reduction, a Barton's bandage, chin strap, or Intermaxillary fixation (IMF) is advised for 3–6 weeks to prevent redislocation and to allow inflammation and oedema to subside.

Management of chronic recurrent dislocation/subluxation

Encountered mainly in elderly people. Chronic dislocation over time develops *fibrous adhesions* between the disc, condyle and articular eminence. Jaw muscles and ligaments also undergo fibrous change, preventing nonsurgical reduction (Table 37.5).

Following reduction of dislocation, conservative methods are used to prevent further dislocation.

Minimally invasive procedures

Injection of sclerosing solution

Injection of a sclerosing agent into the TMJ capsule results in fibrosis and subsequent capsule tightening, which could

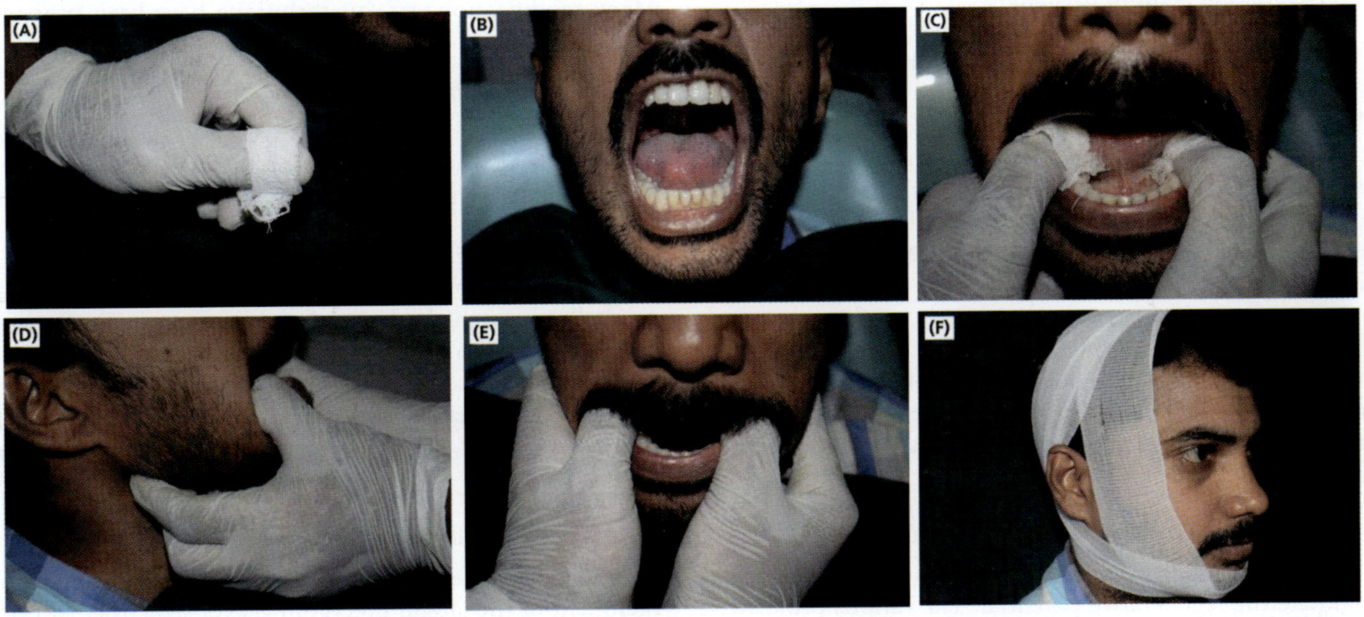

Figure 37.11 Nilaton's technique of reduction. (**A**) Padding of the operator's finger (thumb) before reduction using gauze. (**B**) Bilaterally dislocated condyle. (**C**) Padded thumbs placed over the occlusal surface of the mandibular molars. (**D** and **E**) Other fingers of the hand grasp the lower border of mandible and reduction is done by downward, backwards and upwards movements of the dislocated mandible. (**F**) Bartons's bandage.

TABLE 37.5 Miller and Murphy Management of Chronic Dislocation/Subluxation

Conservative Methods	Surgical Procedures
1. Physiotherapy 2. Intermaxillary fixation 3. Chin straps 4. Barton's bandage 5. Kinesio taping **Minimally invasive:** 1. Injection of sclerosing agents 2. Autologous blood injection 3. Prolotherapy 4. Botulinum toxin injection	1. Capsular tightening procedure: (a) Capsulorrhaphy 2. Creation of mechanical obstacle: (a) Dautrey's procedure (b) Glenotemporal osteotomy (c) Mayer (d) Findley 3. Removal of mechanical obstacle: (a) Eminectomy (b) Condylectomy 4. Creation of new muscular balance: (a) Temporalis scarification (b) Lateral pterygoid myotomy (c) Pterygoid dysjunction

prevent or limit mouth opening. The commonly used solutions are as follows:
- Tincture of iodine
- Five per cent sodium psylliate
- Sodium morrhuate
- Three per cent sodium tetradecyl sulphate
- Ethanolamine oleate
- Picibanil.

The sclerosing injections are given intraarticularly for every 2 to 3 weeks till fibrosis occurs. This procedure might be associated with side effects like pain, muscle tenderness, temporary nerve paresis, TMJ ankylosis and excessive salivation.

Autologous blood injection

It involves injection of the patient's own blood into the pericapsular region and superior joint space. It produces fibrosis, which restricts the mouth opening. PRP can also be injected instead of the patient's own blood.

Prolotherapy/regenerative injection therapy

It involves injection of various solutions into the joint to stimulate the regenerative potential. The various prolotherapy solutions are glycerin, phenol, psyllium oil and dextrose.

Botulinum toxin injection

Botox injection into any muscle weakens the skeletal muscle by preventing the release of acetylcholine at the neuromuscular junction. Injection into the lateral pterygoid muscle prevents forward movement of the condyle.

Surgical methods

Surgical procedures for treating TMJ dislocations has been classified by **MILLER and MURPHY** in 1976:

I. **Capsule tightening procedure:** Capsulorrhaphy
II. **Creation of new muscle balance or direct restraining of condyle:**
   a. Lateral pterygoid myotomy
   b. Temporalis scarification
   c. Pterygoid dysjunction
III. **Removal of mechanical obstruction:**
   a. Eminectomy
   b. Condylectomy
IV. **Creation of mechanical obstruction:**
   a. Linderman/glenotemporal osteotomy
   b. Mayer
   c. Dautrey's procedure
   d. Findley.

Capsule tightening procedure

Capsulorrhaphy

The TMJ is completely covered by capsule which holds the joint components in position. The laxity of the capsule is one of the major reasons for TMJ dislocation. Hence, capsular tightening procedures help in preventing dislocation. Capsulorrhaphy was 1st implemented by Perthes, in which a portion of the lateral capsule is excised and sutured to increase the tautness of the capsule and thus restrain the condyle. Many modifications to this technique have been proposed (Fig. 37.12).

Ligamentorrhaphy

This technique involves anchoring the lateral ligaments of the capsule to the periosteum of the zygomatic arch, followed by IMF for a week.

Capsular plication

This involves exposure of the capsule, followed by an incision vertically through the body of the ligaments. The incision margins are then overlapped and sutured. This technique violates the joint cavity. Several sutures are placed along the inferior aspect of the capsule, to tighten the capsular ligaments (Fig. 37.13).

Creation of new muscle balance

Lateral pterygoid myotomy

It was 1st described by Bowman. In this technique, the attachment of the lateral pterygoid is exposed either through intraoral or extraoral approach and the attachment is severed. Silastic sheet is fixed to the anterior surface of the condyle. It results in restriction of the mouth opening. The disadvantage is loss of translatory movement in the joint (Fig. 37.14).

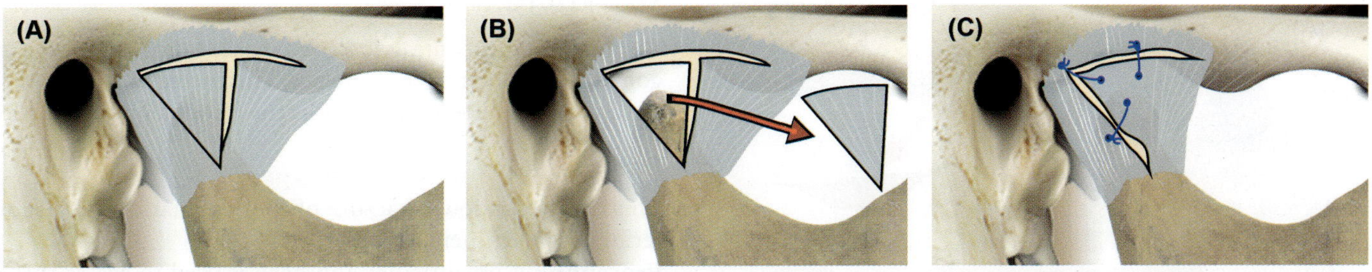

Figure 37.12 Capsulorrhaphy. (**A**) Incision placed over the capsule. (**B**) A portion of the capsule is excised. (**C**) The remaining portion of the capsule is tightened using sutures and its tautness is increased.

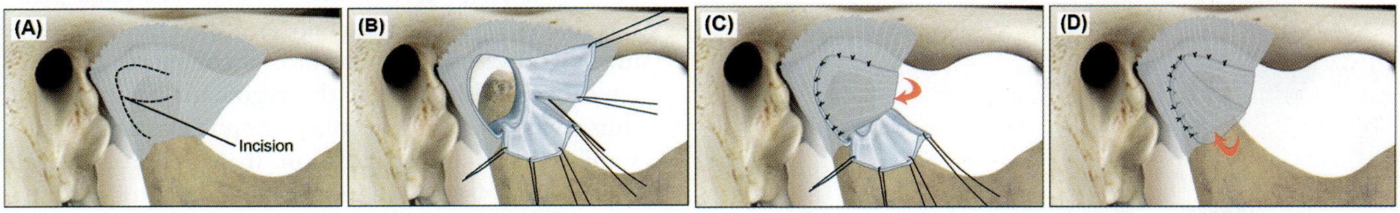

Figure 37.13 Capsular plication. (**A**) Marking of incision over the TMJ capsule. (**B**) Reflection of the flaps. (**C** and **D**) The flaps are overlapped and sutured.

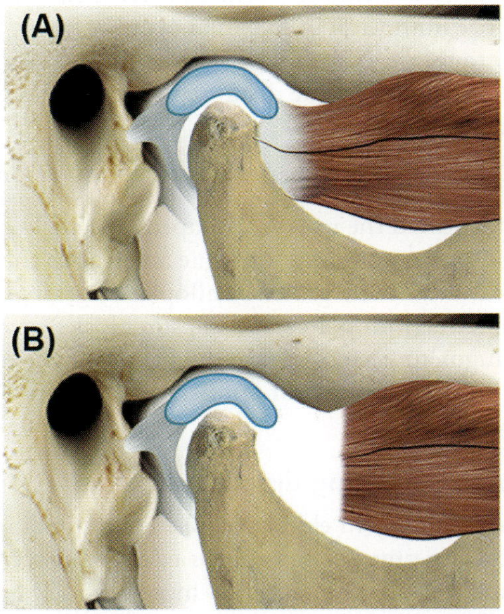

Figure 37.14 Lateral pterygoid myotomy. (**A**) Lateral pterygoid muscle in its normal position. (**B**) A part of lateral pterygoid muscle is excised.

Temporalis scarification

This technique involves removal of a portion of temporalis muscle so that the resultant scar and fibrosis restrict the mouth opening.

Pterygoid dysjunction

Intraoral incision is made to expose the posterolateral wall of maxilla and pterygomaxillary suture. The pterygoid plate is separated from maxilla using pterygoid chisel and the lateral pterygoid muscle is detached along with pterygoid plate. This reduces the activity of lateral pterygoid and forward movement of the condyle.

Removal of mechanical bony obstruction

Eminectomy

1st introduced by Myrhaug (1951). This involves reduction of the height of articular eminence to allow free forward and backward movements of the condyle. The joint can be approached through any of the incisions for TMJ surgery. Following exposure, total eminectomy or partial eminectomy can be done using an osteotome, chisel or piezo. Any irregular bony surfaces are smoothed. Segami described *arthroscopic eminectomy*. Eminectomy allows free movement of the condyle over the articular eminence, thereby preventing locking of the condyle (Fig. 37.15).

Complications: Pneumatisation of eminence and dural tear during its removal, excessive forward movement of the condyle beyond what is required, and excessive stretching of the muscles and ligaments which are injurious to the joint structures.

Condylectomy

Reidel in 1883 performed the 1st condylectomy for treatment of dislocation. Later, Henny and Baldridge (1957) advocated this procedure. It is an intracapsular procedure and involves removal of the entire articular surface of the condyle, above the attachment of the lateral pterygoid. The resulting pseudoarthrosis may limit the range of mandibular motion. Use of chewing gum in early postoperative period is recommended. Modification of this involves condylectomy along with lateral pterygoid myotomy. Occlusion will return to

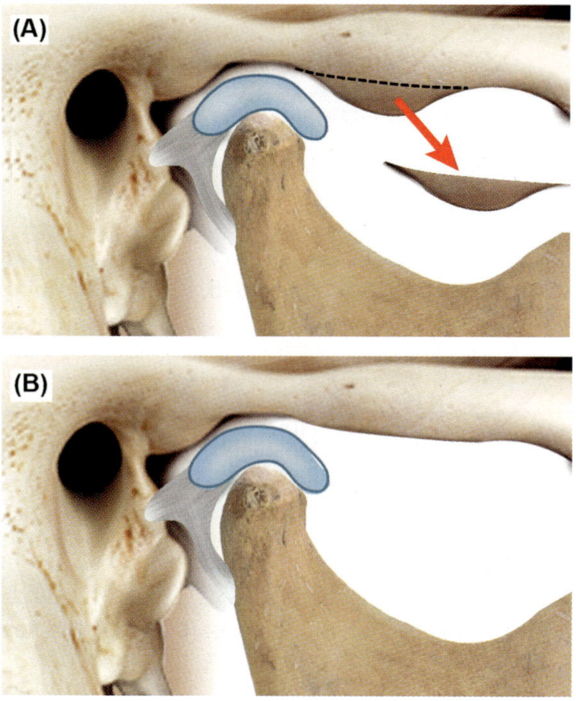

Figure 37.15 Eminectomy. (**A**) Articular eminence is surgically removed. (**B**) After removal.

normal after 4 weeks of surgery; if not, selective grinding is done to eliminate premature contact (Fig. 37.16).

Creating mechanical obstruction

Dislocation of the condyle is prevented by creating an impediment in the path of condyle.

Glenotemporal osteotomy

Norman described glenotemporal osteotomy as a technique to augment the height of articular eminence with interpositional bone grafts. The TMJ is exposed by any of the incisions and an oblique osteotomy is made on the articular eminence and the fragment is gently moved down to create a wedge-shaped defect. The defect can be grafted with bones from the iliac, symphysis and calvarium.

Mayer (1933)

He created a mechanical obstacle by dislocating a part of a zygomatic arch anterior to eminence. This increases the height of the articular eminence and blocks the movement of condyle.

Dautry (1967)

This involves a down fracture of the zygomatic arch just anterior to the eminence.

Procedure: A preauricular approach is used to access the zygomatic arch. Subperiosteal dissection is done over the arch. An oblique cut is made through the arch, running in a downward and forward direction, to divide the lower border just anterior to eminence. Using controlled pressure, the arch is 1st sprung laterally and then downwards to fit into a groove on under surface of eminence. A greenstick fracture should occur at the zygomatic temporal suture, thus giving the segment some rebound elasticity to provide stability in its altered position. It is preferred in younger individuals (<40) to reduce the likelihood of sutural fracture because of increasing brittleness with age (Fig. 37.17)

Advantages:

- Does not violate the joint space
- Allows immediate normal anterior movement with little limitation in maximal opening

Disadvantages:

Risk of fracture of the distal segment and resorption of the distal segment.

Findlay

Findlay advocated the use of 'L'-shaped pins anchored to the zygomatic process of temporal bone anterior to the condyle.

Iliac, calvarial bone grafts or alloplastic grafts (vitallium mesh implants, miniplates and silastic blocks) may also be used to augment or to increase the height of the eminence. Distraction osteogenesis for eminence augmentation is under study (Fig. 37.18).

Chronic/long standing dislocation

Encountered mainly in elderly people. Long standing/chronic dislocation over time develops *fibrous adhesions* between the disc, condyle and articular eminence. Jaw muscles and ligaments also undergo fibrous change, preventing nonsurgical reduction.

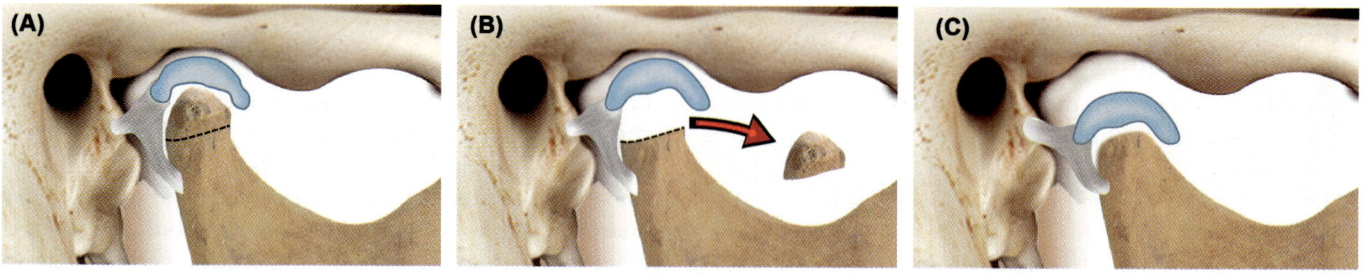

Figure 37.16 High condylectomy and repositioning of the disc. (**A**) Marking of the condyle. (**B**) A portion of the high condyle is surgically removed. (**C**) The sharpened edges on the ramus are smoothed and the condyle is repositioned.

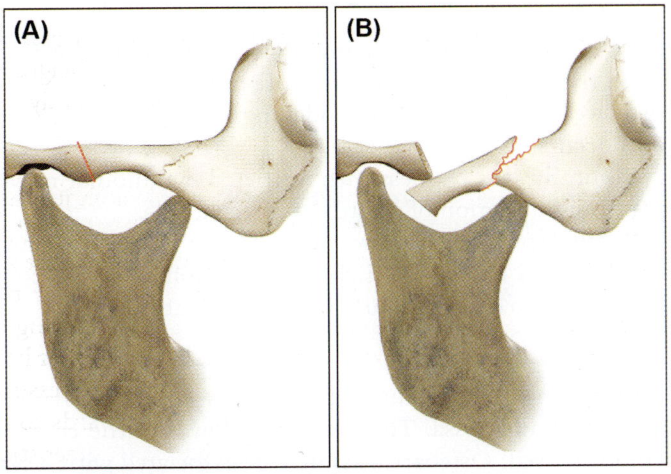

Figure 37.17 (**A** and **B**) Dautry's down fracture of zygomatic arch.

Management of chronic long standing dislocation

Conservative

1. Manual reduction assisted by *use of GA* and a muscle relaxant is helpful
2. Continuous elastic traction using bite block
3. Indirect reduction:
   a. Using a wire passing in the mandibular angle region. A hole is drilled and a traction wire is passed through the inferior border of the ramus to aid in distracting the condyle inferiorly and repositioning the condyle into the fossa
   b. Using a hook in the sigmoid notch *(Finck's technique)*: If this fails, then an *open reduction* should be considered.

Surgical procedures

1. Joint procedures:
   Condylotomy, condylectomy, myotomy or joint prostheses
2. Procedures not involving the joint:
   a. Sagittal split osteotomy
   b. Inverted L osteotomy
   c. Vertical ramus osteotomy
   d. Midline mandibulotomy.

Older techniques include use of *Astley Cooper's basculation and Stromeyer's forceps*. Bilateral ramus osteotomy can be done to restore the occlusion, leaving the condyles in dislocated position.

INFLAMMATORY DISORDERS OF THE TEMPOROMANDIBULAR JOINT

Inflammatory disorders of TMJ are generally characterised by continuous joint pain, which gets accentuated on function. The pain can also present as cyclic muscle pain, hyperalgesia and referred pain. The common inflammatory disorders include: (1) synovitis, (2) capsulitis, (3) retrodiscitis and (4) arthritis.

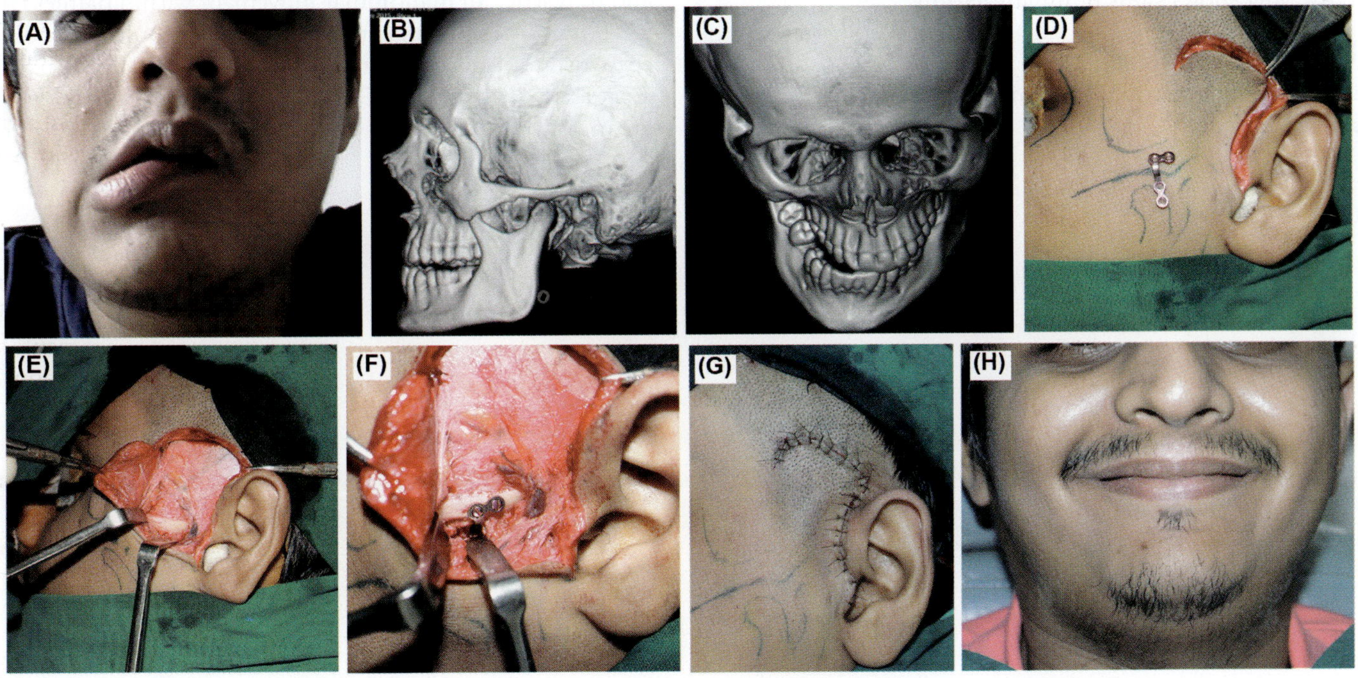

Figure 37.18 Findlay's technique. (**A**) Preoperative view showing deviation of lower jaw to the right side. (**B–C**) CT scan images confirming the anteriorly displaced condyle. (**D**) Intraoperative planning to reduce the condyle. (**E**) Exposure of the zygomatic arch through preauricular incision. (**F**) The dislocated condyle is reduced and L-shaped plate is fixed over the zygomatic arch. (**G**) Closure of the surgical wound. (**H**) Postoperative view.

SYNOVITIS

Any trauma, intracapsular irritation or unusual function of TMJ can result in wearing of the synovial tissue. Synovitis can manifest clinically as local pain that becomes worse with mandibular movements. Pain and fluctuant swelling caused by synovitis are the two most common factors that prevent the posterior teeth from occluding.

CAPSULITIS

It may result from distraction of the capsular ligaments. It can be challenging to distinguish between capsulitis and synovitis clinically. Capsulitis is more painful and is tender on palpation. It is caused by macrotrauma to the joint.

RETRODISCITIS

The application of excessive force to retrodiscal tissues, which are rich in nerves and blood vessels, can lead to inflammation and degeneration of the tissue. It presents with dull pain on clenching of the teeth. It can be caused by both micro and macrotrauma. Any sudden impact to the chin causes the condyle to exert pressure on the retrodiscal tissues, which can ultimately lead to inflammation and degeneration in the long run.

Clinical manifestations

- Localised pain when the patient is at rest, but increases in intensity with function and clenching
- Restriction in mandibular movement's due to pain
- On swallowing, the affected side posterior teeth does not occlude
- An MRI shows signs of inflammation.

ARTHRITIS

The joint inflammations may manifest as osteoarthrosis or osteoarthritis.

OSTEOARTHROSIS

It is a degenerative noninflammatory condition of the TMJ. When the functional forces are more than the adaptive ability as well as the condyle remodelling, osteoarthrosis of the joint occurs.

Clinically, it is painless with restricted mandibular movements and deviation of jaw to the affected side.

Radiographically, it shows signs of bone remodelling, and alterations in the size and shape of the joint. Arthroscopy can be used to diagnose early joint deterioration.

OSTEOARTHRITIS

It is a degenerative condition that results in surface changes of condyle and fossa. The process is slow and the condyle remodels itself. Osteoarthritis may be associated with a systemic disorder.

Aetiology—when articular surfaces cannot withstand the stresses, functional adaptation fails and degeneration occurs.

Clinically there is limitation of mouth opening and tenderness on palpation. It is most commonly associated with crepitus.

Radiographically, it is associated with extensive condyle degeneration. Other bony changes include sclerosis, subarticular cysts, osteophytes and roughness.

MANAGEMENT OF INFLAMMATORY DISORDERS

The inflammatory condition has no definitive treatment. The patient is advised to follow a soft diet with slow movements and to restrict all mandibular movement within painless limits. Physical treatments such as moist heat, ultrasound and corticosteroid injections may be used to alleviate pain. Mild analgesics, such as NSAIDs, should be given to patients who are in constant pain.

Chapter 38

Temporomandibular Joint Ankylosis and Chronic Mandibular Hypomobility

OUTLINE

INTRODUCTION

Temporomandibular joint (TMJ) ankylosis is defined as a fibrous or bony union of the anatomic joint components (condylar head, glenoid fossa and disc), resulting in progressive decrease of the joint mobility and function. Ankylosis is also known as a *'fused joint' or 'stiff joint'* in common parlance. The patient's quality of life is significantly decreased due to the deformed face and decreased jaw function. This has a negative impact on the patient's ability to speak, chew and swallow, which in turn has an adverse effect on the patient's overall health.

AETIOLOGY OF ANKYLOSIS

Trauma—trauma to the joint in childhood has been the foremost and more commonly accepted aetiology of TMJ ankylosis. Key variables that determines the outcome include the presence or absence of mobility during the healing phase, as well as the patient's age at the time of injury

Infection and inflammation of the TMJ—tuberculosis, *Staphylococcus aureus*, *Neisseria gonorrhoeae* and *Haemophilus influenzae* are the most prevalent infections in the joint, but it can also spread from mastoiditis or otitis media

Primary inflammation of the joint may either be of infective origin or autoimmune in nature. Secondary inflammation arises from a local process (e.g. mastoiditis and otitis media)

Systemic aetiology—it includes rheumatoid arthritis, ankylosing spondylitis and psoriatic arthritis. Rheumatoid arthritis is a chronic inflammatory systemic disease that mostly affects the synovial joints, although it can also affect the TMJ. Severe limited motion occurs as the bone is destroyed and the joint space is filled with scar tissue, leading to fibrous ankylosis

Ankylosing spondylitis *(Marie–Strumpell disease, rheumatoid spondylitis)* is a chronic progressive inflammatory disease primarily involving the articulations of the spine and adjacent soft tissues. The sacroiliac joint is always involved with fewer cases affecting peripheral joints such as the hip, shoulder and TMJ leading to ankylosis

Psoriatic arthritis is characterised by the triad of: (1) psoriasis, (2) erosive polyarthritis, (3) negative result of a serologic test for rheumatoid factor. Psoriatic arthritis has been considered to be a predisposing factor for ankylosis.

PATHOPHYSIOLOGY OF TEMPOROMANDIBULAR JOINT ANKYLOSIS

Interfragmentary strain theory or Perren's strain theory

It states that there is a correlation between the TMJ ankylosis and the strain tolerance of bone, cartilage and fibrous tissue. When a condyle is fractured, the stress that is created in the area surrounding the joint space causes tissue deformation, but to varying degree. Even minimal strain or limited jaw movement can cause endochondral ossification, which in turn causes bone development, particularly in the areas of the lateral side of the joint.

Haemarthrosis

Haematoma resulting from trauma to the periosteum and capsular ligament is considered as the main reason for the development of ankylosis. Intracapsular haemorrhage develops fibrosis and ultimately organises to form excessive localised bone/hypertrophic bone. This may lead to hypomobility or bony ankylosis. The right and left joints are dependent on each other and the degree of ankylosis on one side affects the opposite side (Flowchart 38.1).

When compared to fractures of an adult condyle, those of a child's condyle are more likely to develop ankylosis due to the peculiar anatomy of the condyle, which includes a broad neck and a highly vascularised head with abundant osteogenic potential. Thus increasing the risk of ankylosis in paediatric condyle fractures.

It is theorised that haemarthrosis, in conjunction with the loss of fibro-cartilage integrity, makes the development of fibrous connective tissue into the joint, which ultimately leads to ossification. Due to the fact that fusion takes place in the juxtaarticular area, *Ferretti et al.* came to the conclusion that extraarticular haematomas may also contribute to the development of ankylosis.

Yan et al., have suggested a hypothesis that provides support for *hypertrophic nonunion* following TMJ trauma. This hypothesis includes two conditions for the formation of the ankylosis, which are as follows:

- Trauma to the TMJ creates a suitable environment for the bone healing of the two articular surfaces, causing bony ankylosis
- The opening movement of the jaw inhibits bone repair of the injured articular surfaces.

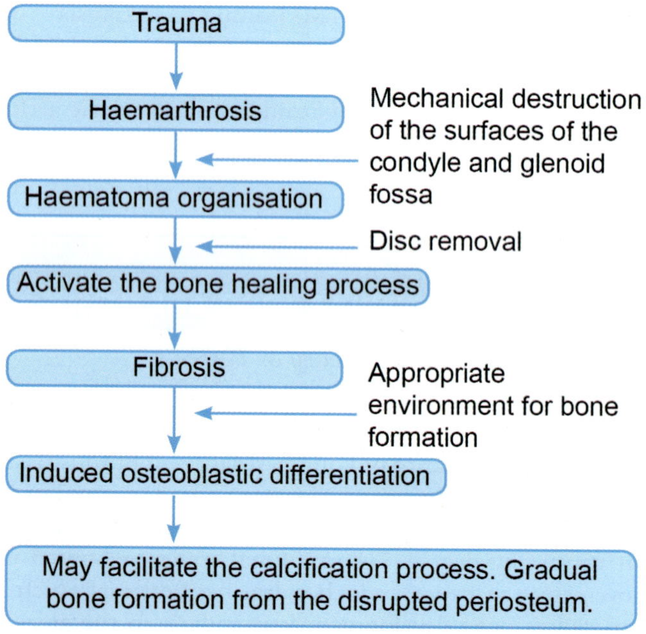

Flowchart 38.1 Process of ankylosis following trauma.

CLASSIFICATION OF ANKYLOSIS

KAZANJIAN'S CLASSIFICATION

TMJ ankylosis was subdivided into extraarticular and intraarticular ankylosis.

- ***Extraarticular* or false ankylosis** is due to the pathological changes in the structures surrounding the TMJ causing limitations in mouth opening. It can be due to enlargement of the coronoid process, infection, irradiation, inferiorly depressed fracture of the zygomatic arch, and scarring after injury. Radiographic findings illustrate normal appearing TMJ and joint spaces
- ***Intraarticular* or true ankylosis** is caused by the fibrous or bony adhesions between the articular surfaces of the mandibular condyle and glenoid fossa. Radiographic evidence of condylar distortion, loss of joint space, and abnormal bone development in and around the TMJ is used to diagnose genuine ankylosis in a patient with limited mouth opening.

Based on the type of tissue formed

- Osseous ankylosis
- Fibrous ankylosis
- Fibro-osseous ankylosis.

Based on the side involved

- Unilateral
- Bilateral.

Topazian (1964)—based on the extension of bone formation

Stage 1: Ankylotic bone limited to the condylar process
Stage 2: Ankylotic bone extending to the sigmoid notch
Stage 3: Ankylotic bone extending to the coronoid process.

MILLER ET AL., (1975)

- False ankylosis: Myogenic, neurogenic, psychogenic, bone impingement, fibrous adhesion
- Tumours.

SAWHNEY'S CLASSIFICATION (1986)—BASED ON THE RADIOGRAPHIC AND OPERATIVE FINDINGS

Type 1: The condyle is medially angulated and associated with a deformed articular fossa together with a mild-to-moderate amount of new bone formation (Fig. 38.1A)
Type 2: There is no recognisable condyle or fossa but instead a large mass of new bone extending from the ramus to the base of the skull (Fig. 38.1B)
Type 3: Medially displaced fracture dislocation with bone bridging the mandibular ramus to the zygomatic arch (Fig. 38.1C)
Type 4: The joint architecture is completely replaced by bone with fusion of the condyle, sigmoid notch and coronoid process to the zygomatic arch and glenoid fossa (Fig. 38.1D)
Type 5: The joint architecture is replaced completely by bone with fusion of the condyle, sigmoid notch, coronoid process to the zygomatic arch, glenoid fossa and maxilla (Fig. 38.1E).

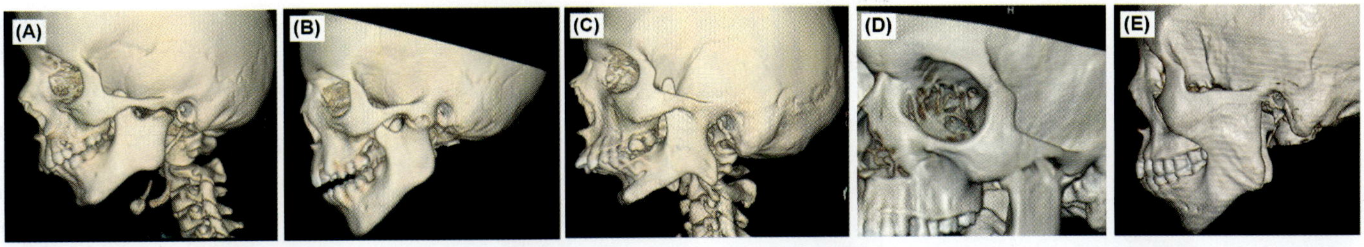

Figure 38.1 Types of ankylosis. (**A**) Type I ankylosis. Condylar head is flattened or deformed with dense fibrous adhesion. (**B**) Type II ankylosis. Bony fusion of the condylar head in the outer aspect of the articular surface and limited to a small area. (**C**) Type III ankylosis. A bony block bridging the mandibular ramus and zygomatic arch. (**D**) Type IV ankylosis. A wider bony block bridges the mandibular ramus and zygomatic arch, extending and obliterating the upper joint space and completely replacing the architecture of the joint. (**E**) Type V ankylosis. A broad bony block bridging the mandibular ramus with the zygomatic arch and maxilla.

TURLINGTON AND DURR (1993)

Classification is based on heterotopic bone formation within the ankylotic mass:

Grade 0: No bone islands visible
Grade 1: Islands of bone visible within the soft tissue around the joint
Grade 2: Periarticular bone formation is visible
Grade 3: Apparent bony ankylosis
Grades 1, 2 and 3 are further classified as symptomatic (S) and asymptomatic (A).

JORAM RAVEH, THIERRY VUILLEMIN CLASSIFICATION (Table 38.1)

DONGMEI HE AND COLLEAGUES CLASSIFICATION (2011) (Table 38.2)

Yan and colleagues (2014)

Based on its development, ankylosis can be classified into three phases:

- *Fibrous-chondral phase* demonstrating fibrous tissue and chondrocytes occupying the gap in the joint
- *Chondral-calcified cartilage phase* manifesting abundant chondrocytes, cartilage matrix, and neoformative endochondral ossification in the joint space
- *Bone-cartilage phase* showing compacted bone in the lateral joint gap and cartilage in the medial joint gap.

TABLE 38.1 Joram Raveh, Thierry Vuillemin Classification

Class 1	Ankylotic bony tissue limited to the condylar process and articulate fossa
Class 2	The bone mass extends out of the fossa involving the medial aspect of the skull base up to the carotid-jugular vessels
Class 3	Extension and penetration into the middle cranial fossa
Class 4	Combination of class 2 and class 3

TABLE 38.2 Dongmei He and Colleagues Classification (2011)

Type A1	Fibrous ankylosis without bony fusion of joint
Type A2	Bony fusion on lateral side of joint while the residual condyle fragment is bigger than half of condylar head on medial side
Type A3	Similar to A2 but the residual condylar fragment is smaller than half of the condylar head
Type A4	Ankylosis with complete bony fusion of the joint

Long Xia, Jingang et al. classification (2019)

Type I—nonbony ankylosis of the joint, with the fossa and condyle clearly seen but with scattered callus (Fig. 38.2)
Type II—lateral bony ankylosis of the joint, with bony fusion on the lateral side of the joint. The medially displaced condyle, residual disc and fossa form a pseudarthrosis
Type III—complete bony ankylosis of the entire joint with a radiolucent line inside the fusion area but no recognisable condyle and fossa
Type IV—extensive bony ankylosis, with complete disappearance of the joint and with no radiolucent line.

Classification of re-ankylosis (Table 38.3)

El-Hakim and Metwalli classification (2002)—based on radiographic presentation (Table 38.4)

CDA classification (2020)

According to the anatomical features of the condyle (C), severity of the dentofacial bone deformity (D) and skeletal age (A).

C—condition of the joint that can be preserved:

C_0—ankylosis of the lateral bone surfaces of both joints, with preservation of the medially displaced condyle heads

C_1—ankylosis of the entire joint with bone fusion and absence of identifiable condyles or fossa on one or both sides of the joint

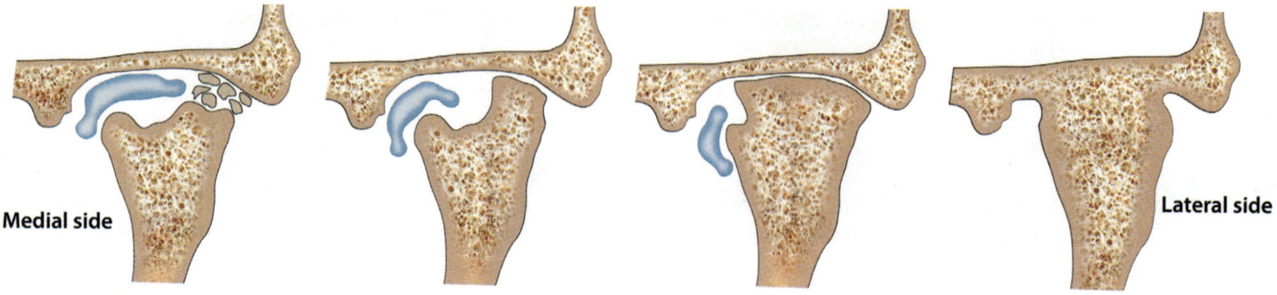

Figure 38.2 Long Xia's classification of ankylosis.

TABLE 38.3 Classification of Re-Ankylosis

Type 1	Fibrous ankylosis, reduction in joint space with clear demarcation of the borders of the temporal and condylar components
Type 2	Bony ankylosis between the condylar region and temporal bone, without involving the coronoid process or the sigmoid notch
Type 3a	Ankylosis between condyle and temporal bone with hyperplasia of the coronoid process without ankylosis
Type 3b	Ankylosis involving the coronoid and the condylar region without obliteration of the sigmoid notch
Type 4	Complete bony union of the condyle and coronoid process to the temporal component, in which sigmoid notch could not be delineated
Type 5	Ankylosis involving the zygomatic arch

D—presence of dentofacial deformity:

D_0—no significant dentofacial deformities

D_1—presence of dentofacial deformities affecting the facial appearance

A—skeletal age of the patient:

A_C—immature skeleton—a young patient with active dentofacial growth

A_a—mature skeleton—an adult patient with a fully developed dentofacial structure.

CLINICAL PRESENTATION

The clinical presentation of TMJ ankylosis is dependent on the age of onset, duration of the disease process and the type of ankylosis. The ankylosed TMJ may present with partial or complete restriction of function. The joint movements are palpable in fibrous ankylosis than bony ankylosis. The *common clinical presentations* of TMJ ankylosis are as follows:

- Significantly *shortened lower face* as the vertical growth of ramus is restricted

TABLE 38.4 El-Hakim and Metwalli Classification (2002)—Based on Radiographic Presentation

	Class I	Class II	Class III	Class IV
Ankylosis	Unilateral and bilateral fibrous ankylosis	Unilateral and bilateral bony fusion between the condyle and the temporal bone	Same as class II	Same as class II
Shape of TMJ on CT scan	The condyle and the glenoid fossa retain their original shape	Bony fusion between the condyle and the temporal bone	Same as class II	Ankylosis extending up to skull base No TMJ anatomy Bony mass of the medial condyle are closed by pterygoid plates, carotid, jugular and spinosum foramina
Relationship with maxillary artery and ankylosed mass	Normal anatomical relationship	Normal anatomical relationship	Maxillary artery and the mandibular condyle's medial pole are more closed on the ankylosed side than the normal side	Same as class III

- *Marked antegonial notching*–the digastric and mylohyoid muscles produce notching at the inferior part of mandible just anterior to the insertion of masseter
- Failure in growth of the condyle impedes the forward and downward movement of the mandible, resulting in *localised thickening of the bone at the angle*
- This warping of the mandible results in *obtuse angle* between the inferior border of the mandible and the base of the skull
- It can give rise to *elongation and thickening of the coronoid process*, ramal shortening and chin recession.

The classical findings described below are of true bony ankylosis in patients afflicted of the disease early in childhood. TMJ ankylosis that occurs after cessation of condylar growth (adult onset) presents only with restricted mouth opening with no other facial deformities.

UNILATERAL TEMPOROMANDIBULAR JOINT ANKYLOSIS

Extraoral findings

1. Gross facial asymmetry
2. Convex profile
3. Restricted mandibular growth on the affected side
4. The ramus and lower facial height is shorter on the ipsilateral side
5. Affected side shows roundening/fullness of the lower face and contralateral normal side shows a flattened elongated appearance
6. Prominent antegonial notch and ill-defined gonium on the affected side
7. Restricted mouth opening
8. Mandible deviates to affected side on opening mouth (Fig. 38.3)
9. On palpating preauricular region, the joint movements will be less or not palpable on the affected side
10. Elongated coronoid on the affected side.

Intraoral findings

1. Decreased maximal interincisal distance
2. Occlusal cant
3. Class II malocclusion with unilateral cross bite on the affected side
4. Dental caries and periodontal disease from poor oral hygiene, inaccessibility for maintaining good oral hygiene
5. Multiple teeth–impacted or submerged.

BILATERAL TEMPOROMANDIBULAR JOINT ANKYLOSIS (Fig. 38.4)

Extraoral findings

1. Gross facial deformity–Andy Gump appearance or ***bird face deformity***. 'Vogelgesicht' (Andy Gump was a cartoon character from the early 20th century in an extremely popular comic strip, *The Gumps*)
2. Highly convex profile
3. Retrognathism and micrognathia
4. Double chin
5. Reduced lower facial height
6. Bilateral reduced mandible height with steep mandibular plane angle

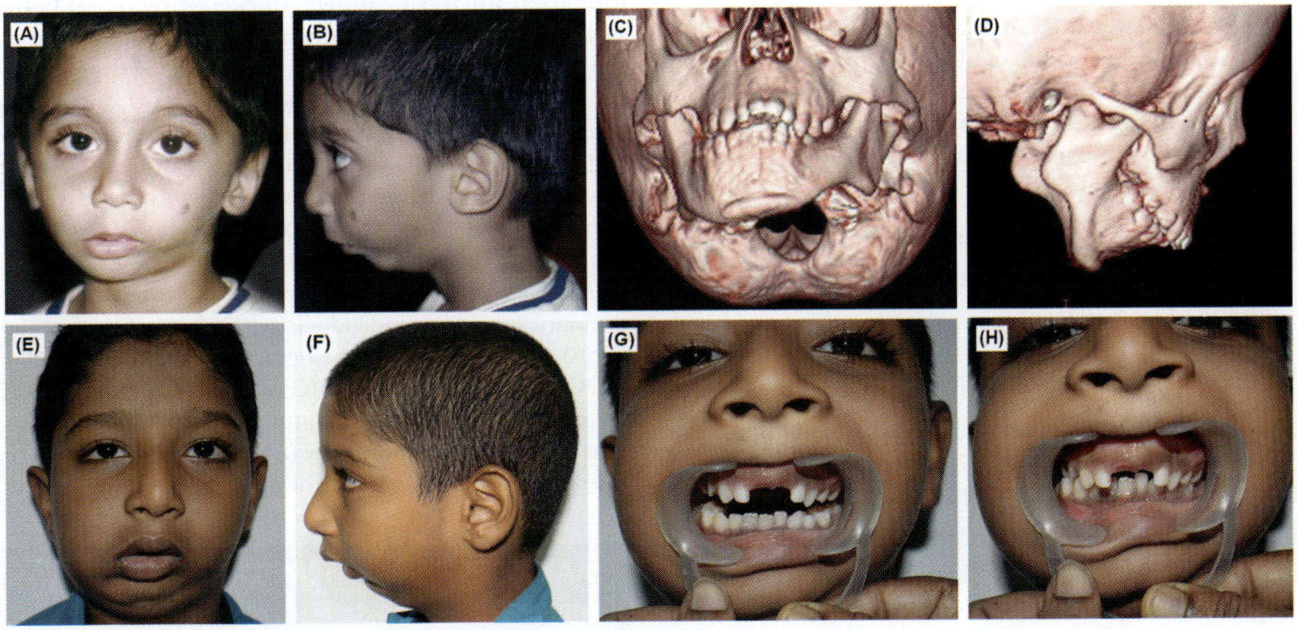

Figure 38.3 Unilateral ankylosis. (**A**) Preoperative view with flattened left side of face with deviation of chin to right side. (**B**) Retruded chin. (**C** and **D**) Preoperative CT scan showing right side TMJ ankylosis with deviation of mandible towards the affected side. (**E** and **F**) Preoperative view of a patient with unilateral ankylosis on the right side. (**G** and **H**) Preoperative intraoral view showing limited mouth opening.

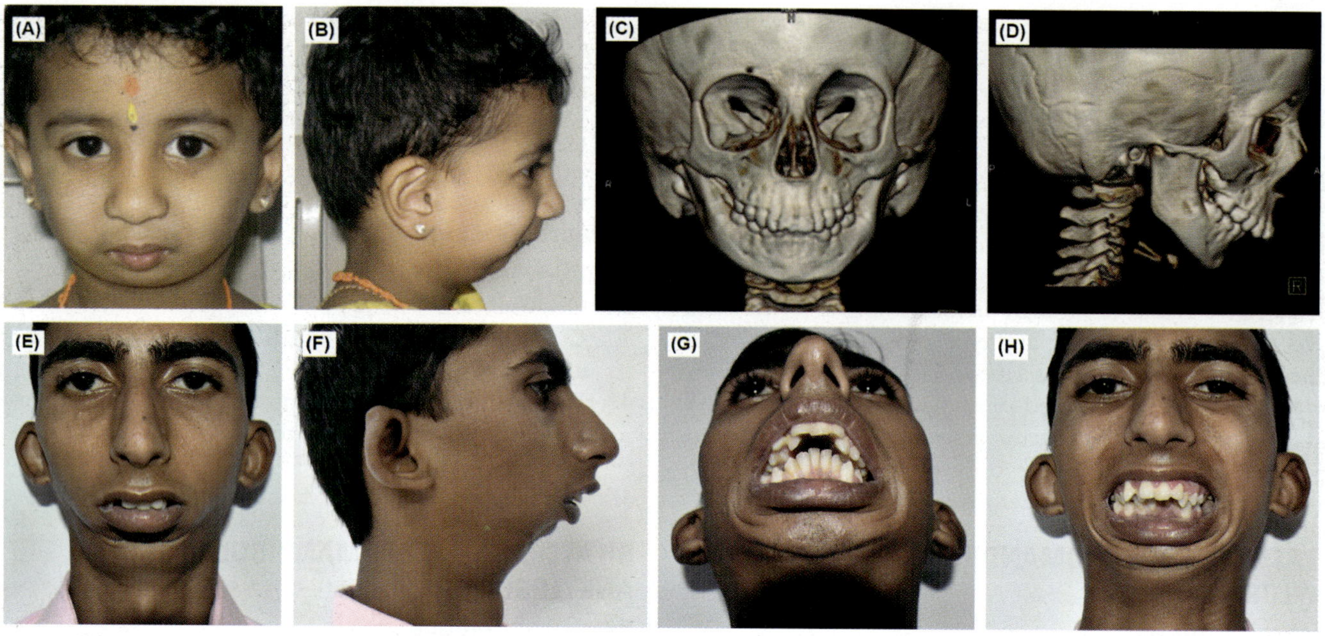

Figure 38.4 Bilateral TMJ ankylosis. (**A** and **B**) Preoperative view showing retruded chin with reduced lower facial height. (**C** and **D**) Preoperative CT scan showing retrognathia with shortened ramus height. (**E** and **F**) Preoperative view of a bilateral ankylosis patient showing bird facies with convex profile. (**G** and **H**) Intraoral view with almost nil mouth opening and Class II malocclusion.

7. Obtuse cervicomental angle
8. Prominent antegonial notch on both the sides
9. Bilateral preauricular palpation reveals no joint movements in true bony ankylosis, whereas in fibrous ankylosis minimal jaw movement may be felt without deviation
10. Elongated coronoids on radiographs.

Intraoral findings

1. Reduced or nil maximal interincisal mouth opening
2. Class II malocclusion bilaterally, with protrusive upper incisors and anterior open bite
3. Dental caries or periodontal disease from poor oral hygiene
4. Multiple teeth—impacted or submerged
5. Presence of occlusal cant.

Sequelae of untreated ankylosis

- The normal growth and development of the face is affected
- Respiratory problems
- Impediment in speaking
- Nutritional deficiency
- Malocclusion
- Poor oral hygiene.

RADIOLOGICAL ASSESSMENT (Figs. 38.5 and 38.6)

Radiological investigation helps in the following:

1. Differentiating fibrous ankylosis from bony ankylosis
2. Extraarticular ankylosis if any (involvement of zygoma, coronoid process)
3. Degree and extent of involvement (e.g. mediolateral width of the ankylotic mass)
4. Relation of the vital structures to the ankylotic mass (e.g. mandibular nerve, internal carotid artery [ICA]).
5. Preoperative surgical planning.

The suggested radiologic films are orthopantomogram (OPG) for initial screening and CT scan with 3D reconstruction for assessing the extent of ankylosis and presurgical planning.

The deformed TMJ is characterised by an excessive bone formation, enlarged condyle, thickened temporal bone, and a radiolucent line in the bony fusion area. The lateral part of the joint shows bony fusion with decreased bone marrow cavity, whereas the medial nonbony fused area shows an atrophic condyle with rudimentary joint space.

In fibrous ankylosis, fibrous tissue can be seen intruding into the bone marrow of the condyle with degeneration. In bony ankylosis, new bone formation can be seen on the rough ankylotic surface of the condyle.

Polysomnography is widely regarded as the diagnostic gold standard for use in individuals with obstructive sleep apnoea (OSA). The electroencephalogram (EEG), electrooculogram (EOG), electromyogram (EMG) and electrocardiogram (ECG) are the four conventional components of a polysomnogram. The apnoea–hypopnoea index (AHI) is used to evaluate the frequency of recurrent episodes of pharyngeal airway obstruction.

MANAGEMENT OF TEMPOROMANDIBULAR JOINT ANKYLOSIS

AIRWAY IMPLICATIONS OF TEMPOROMANDIBULAR JOINT ANKYLOSIS

Anaesthetic administration during ankylotic surgery presents a challenge due to its difficult airway and severely limited

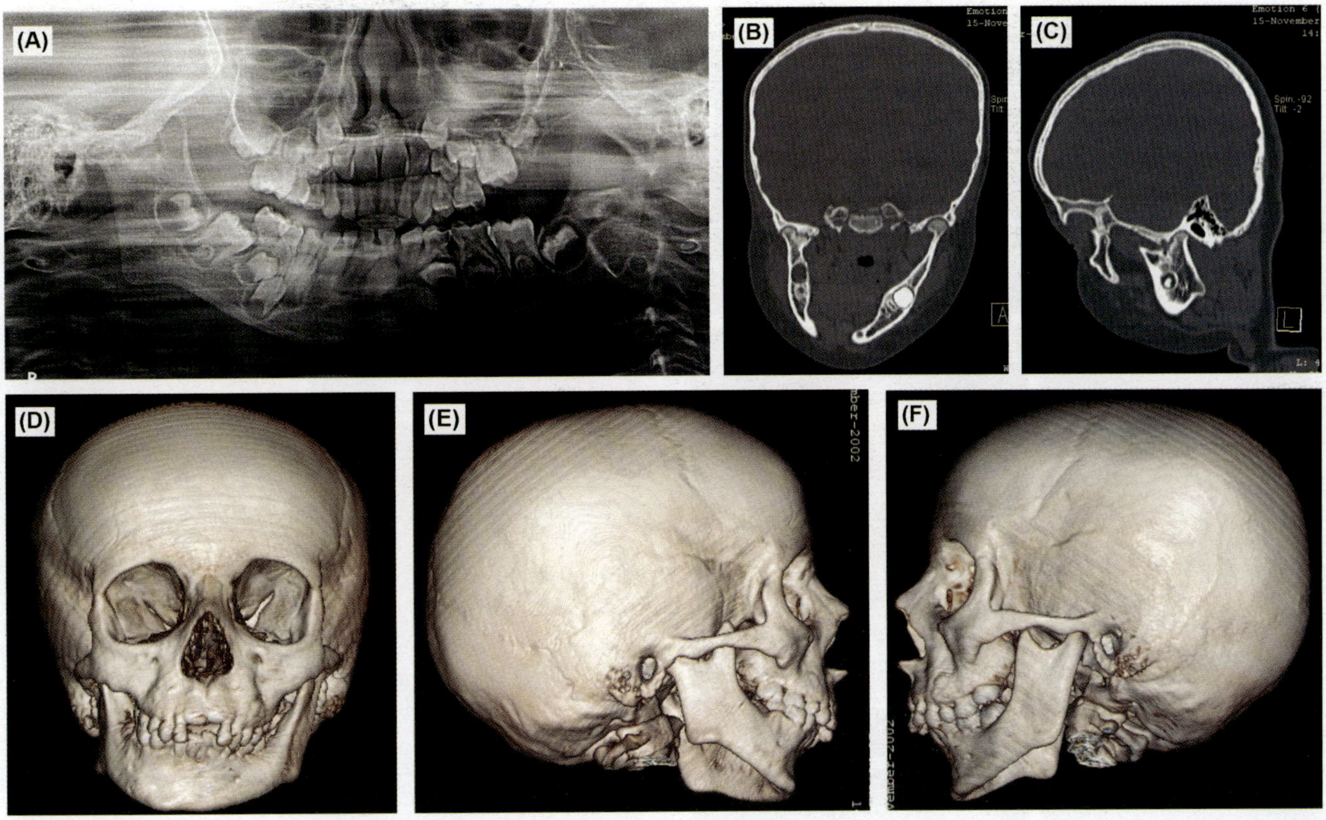

Figure 38.5 Unilateral ankylosis. (**A**) OPG showing right side ankylosis. (**B** and **C**) Coronal and sagittal section showing right ankylosis with elongation and shift of left mandible. (**D–F**) 3D CT frontal, right and left side.

mouth opening. In the past, *blind nasal intubation, retrograde intubation and tracheostomy* were performed, but with significant morbidity. Nowadays, fibreoptic-assisted nasotracheal intubation has become the gold standard and most acceptable method to administer anaesthesia for TMJ ankylosis patients for ankylotic surgery. Emergency tracheostomy may be required if obstructive sleep apnoea is severe and in bilateral ankylotic release without ramus height reconstruction.

SURGICAL ANATOMY

The *facial nerve* exists from the skull at the stylomastoid foramen, and divides into temporofacial and cervicofacial branches. The temporal branch emerges from the parotid gland and crosses the zygoma to the forehead. Damage to the temporal nerve during surgery results in inability to raise the eyebrow and ptosis of the brow. Damage to the zygomatic branch manifests as paralysis of the orbicularis oculi muscle.

Distance between the external auditory meatus to the bifurcation of the facial nerve = 1.5 to 2.8 cm

Distance between the postglenoid tubercle to the bifurcation = 2.4 to 3.5 cm

The point at which the upper trunk crosses the zygomatic arch = 8 to 35 mm anterior to the bony external auditory canal (EAC) (refer Chapter 35, Fig. 35.8).

The *auriculotemporal nerve* courses along the medial side of the neck of the condyle and turns superiorly, running over the zygomatic root of the temporal bone. Care must be taken to avoid injury to this nerve during preauricular exposure to TMJ.

ECA branches into the superficial temporal artery and the internal maxillary artery. The *internal maxillary artery* runs medial to the sigmoid notch. The most commonly injured artery during surgery is the middle meningeal branch of internal maxillary artery.

SURGICAL APPROACHES TO TEMPOROMANDIBULAR JOINT

Ideally, an approach should accomplish the following:

- Maximise the area of exposure for the specific procedure
- Prevent injury to the branches of the facial nerve
- Avoid damage to the major blood vessels
- Avoid damage to the parotid gland
- Cosmetic wound closure by utilising the natural skin creases.

The classic ***surgical approaches*** to the TMJ are as follows:

a. Preauricular approach:
   i. Dingman's preauricular approach
   ii. Blair inverted hockey stick
   iii. Thoma
   iv. Al-Kayat and Bramley
   v. Popwich's modification
   vi. Coronal extension of preauricular
b. Endaural approach (Lemport's)

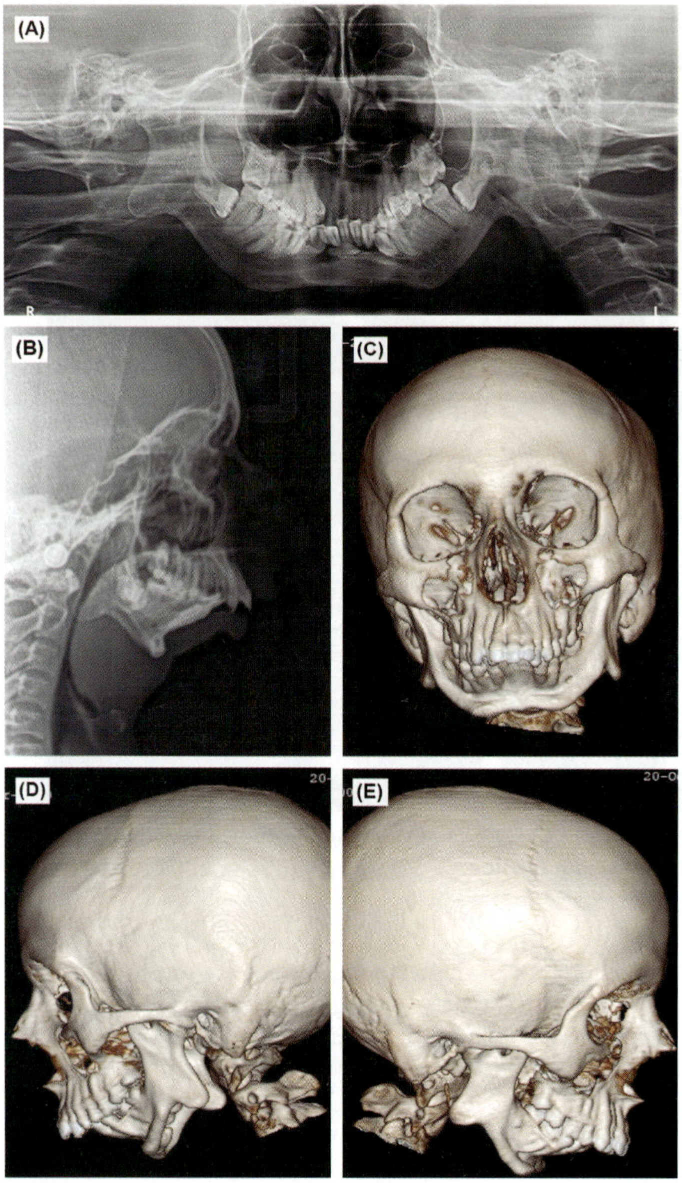

Figure 38.6 Bilateral ankylosis. (**A** and **B**) OPG and lateral cephalogram showing bilateral ankylosis. (**C–E**) 3D CT images with ankylosis on both right and left side and convex profile.

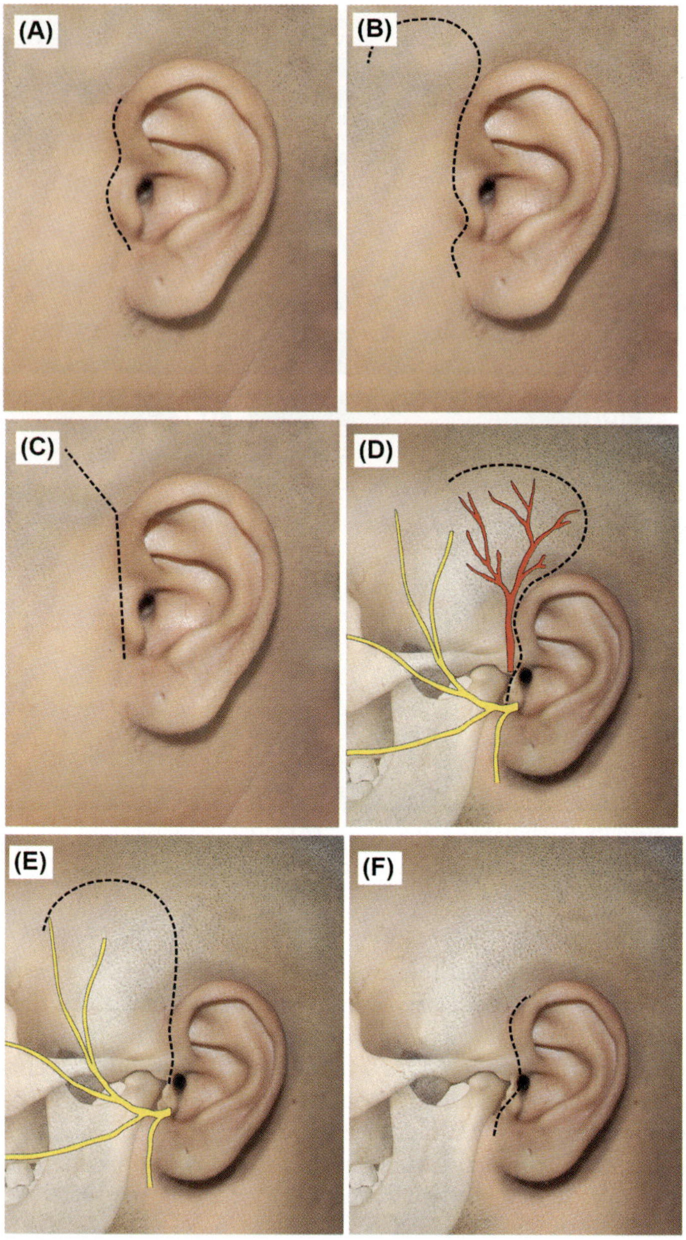

Figure 38.7 Preauricular approaches. (**A**) Dingman. (**B**) Blair's inverted hockey stick. (**C**) Thoma. (**D**) Al-Kayat and Bramley. (**E**) Popwich's modification. (**F**) Endaural.

c. Postauricular approach
d. Rhytidectomy
e. Retromandibular/postramal approach (Hind's)
f. Submandibular approach (Risdon's)
g. Coronal/bifrontal approach
h. Capsular incisions
i. Intraoral.

a. Preauricular approaches

i. Dingman's preauricular approach

It is a gold standard approach for TMJ and often used by oral and maxillofacial surgeons with many variations.

Layers of dissection

An incision of approximately 3–4 cm in length is made along the course of the helix, in front of the tragus, till the ear lobule (Fig. 38.7A). An incision is made through the skin and subcutaneous tissue to the superficial temporal fascia. The superficial temporal artery and vein run above the fascial layer and branches of the facial nerve run deep to it. An oblique incision is made through the superficial temporal fascia for about 2 cm above the zygomatic arch, and blunt dissection is done to reach the zygomatic arch. The periosteum of the zygomatic arch is incised, and blunt dissection is done above and below the zygomatic arch along the external auditory meatus to reach the articular capsule. The flap should be reflected anteroinferiorly. An incision through the joint capsule opens into the upper joint space, and an additional incision of the lateral collateral ligament of the TMJ disc enters the inferior joint space. Once the TMJ has been repaired, a layer wise closure is needed.

ii. Blair

It is similar to the Dingman's incision in preauricular fold, but in the region of the zygomatic arch it bends like a hockey stick (Fig. 38.7B). The disadvantages include the possibility of scar formation and damage to the frontal branch of facial nerve.

iii. Thoma

The incision in the preauricular fold is vertical limb but angulated at 45 degrees near the bifurcation of the superficial temporal vessels in the hairline (Fig. 38.7C).

iv. Al-Kayat and Bramley

The incision resembles a reverse question mark, starting superiorly from the scalp in the temporal region, curves backwards and downwards and extends inferiorly to the tragus (Fig. 38.7D). The superficial layer of the temporalis fascia is identified and incised at 45 degrees anterosuperiorly, at the root of the arch to avoid injury to the facial nerve branches. Advantage of this incision is the excellent access to the TMJ without any damage to important anatomical structures and also cosmetically acceptable.

v. Popowich's modification

This approach also gives excellent visibility of the joint with safety. It is longer and wider than the conventional preauricular incision. Superiorly, it begins about a pinna's length away from the ear within the hairline, curves backward and downward well posterior to the main branches of the temporal vessels, till it meets the upper attachment of the ear (Fig. 38.7E).

vi. Coronal extension

The preauricular incision is extended anterosuperiorly over the scalp when a large area of exposure (the anterior cranial vault, forehead, and upper and middle regions of the fascial skeleton) is required. It avoids visible fascial scars. Hemicoronal or bicoronal approaches are used in very complicated cases and extensive surgeries in the upper and midface regions.

b. Endaural approach

It is a cosmetic modification of the preauricular approach. Here skin incision is incorporated behind the prominence of the tragus. Care must becv taken not to damage the tragal cartilage as it may result in poor wound healing. Once the skin flap with tragus is reflected, the dissection is same as preauricular incision (Fig. 38.7F).

Disadvantage: Potential for perichondritis and cartilage damage.

c. Postauricular approach

In the postauricular approach, the incision is made posterior to the ear and involves sectioning of the external auditory meatus (EAM). The incision is made 3–4 mm posterior to the auricle and extends towards the mastoid process (Fig. 38.8A). The superior portion may be extended into the hairline for additional exposure.

Advantage: Low risk of facial nerve injury and cosmetic superiority

Disadvantage: Auricular stenosis.

d. Rhytidectomy approach/facelift approach

It is a combination of preauricular, retromandibular and postauricular incision. It is indicated when an extensive exposure of the joint is required. Incision begins from the front of the ear extending into the hairline above and curves around the bottom of the ear below and then behind it, usually ending near the hairline on the back of the neck (Fig. 38.8B and C).

Advantage: Minimally visible facial scar and good access to the entire posterior border of the mandible

Disadvantage: The possibility of damage to the facial nerve.

e. Retromandibular (Hind's) approach

Indicated for surgeries involving the condylar neck or ramus of mandible. The incision is placed vertically behind the posterior

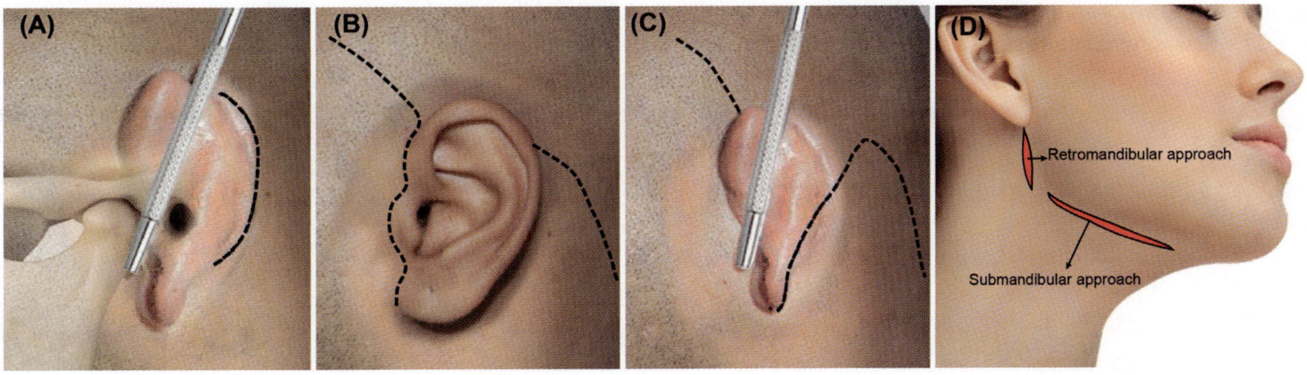

Figure 38.8 (**A**) Postauricular. (**B** and **C**) Rhytidectomy (**D**) Retromandibular and submandibular approaches.

border of ramus. The incision is a curvilinear line of approximately 5 cm long and 2 cm distal to the inferior point of mandibular angle (Fig. 38.8D).

Layers of dissection are through the skin, subcutaneous tissue, platysma, and superficial musculoaponeurotic system (SMAS) layer. A vertical incision is made through the SMAS layer into the parotid gland. Blunt dissection is continued through the parotid gland parallel to the direction of the facial nerve branches towards the posterior border of mandible.

Advantage: Good accessibility to the condylar neck and subcondyle area

Disadvantage: Limited access to the TMJ space and anteromedial side of TMJ.

f. Submandibular (Risdon's) approach

Indicated for approaching the mandibular angle, body and low subcondyle region. Incision must be placed within the skin tension line 1.5–2 cm below the mandibular inferior border (Fig. 38.8D).

Layers of dissection:

- Skin
- Subcutaneous tissue
- Sharp division of platysma muscle exposing the superficial layer of deep cervical fascia, which forms the capsule around the submandibular gland
- The most important step is dissection through the superficial layer of deep cervical fascia, as the facial artery and vein and the marginal mandibular nerve traverse this layer
- Facial artery and vein need to be ligated if the area of interest is anterior to the masseteric notch
- Division of the pterygomasseteric sling
- Submasseteric dissection till the inferior border of mandible is exposed
- Repair followed by a layer wise closure

Advantage: Ability to retract the mandibular angle, during reduction of condyle fracture

Disadvantage: Limited access to the high condyle region and joint spaces.

g. Coronal/Bifrontal approach

This approach provides excellent access to the NOE complex, lateral orbital rim, zygoma, and its arch with almost no complications. The scar is invisible as it is hidden within the hairline.

Technique: A strip of hair is removed across the superior aspect of the head, in the area of the incision. The incision is placed from the preauricular area on one side, extending transversely over the skull vault, crossing the midline, to the opposite side, behind the hairline. Inferiorly, it can be extended to the anterior border of the helix to provide improved access to the TMJ area and zygomatic arch.

The incision is made using a blade through the skin, subcutaneous tissue, and the galea. The flap is elevated in a subgaleal plane, just beneath the pericranium. In the anterior region, superior to the supraorbital ridges, the dissection is carried out sub-periosteally, using a blunt periosteal elevator or finger dissection. On the lateral aspect of the skull, the pericranium inserts into the temporal fascia. The superficial layer of temporal fascia is now incised for about 2 cm, where it encounters an area of fat and areolar tissue. Further dissection inferiorly provides access to the zygomatic arch. A periosteal incision is then made along the superior aspect of the arch to expose the TMJ region. The superficial flap is reflected with the temporal branch of the facial nerve using this technique.

After TMJ surgery, the flap is replaced, and the wound is closed in layers: the temporal fascia, galea, and skin. The skin sutures or staples are removed in 7 to 10 days.

h. Capsular incisions

The articular surfaces (superior and inferior joint spaces) are approached through an incision on the capsular ligament. Horizontal incisions on the capsule can be made at different locations; above and below the disc, or over and below the lateral rim of the glenoid fossa. A T-shaped incision can also be made on the capsule over the insertion of lateral condyle (Fig. 38.9).

Disadvantage: Closure of the capsule is often difficult.

i. Intraoral incision

An intraoral approach is achieved by making an incision along the external oblique ridge. A subperiosteal dissection is done medially and laterally along the mandibular ramus to reach the coronoid process and condylar neck.

Advantages: Decreased facial and auriculotemporal nerve injury and avoids scar formation

Limitations: Limited access to the structures superior to the condylar neck.

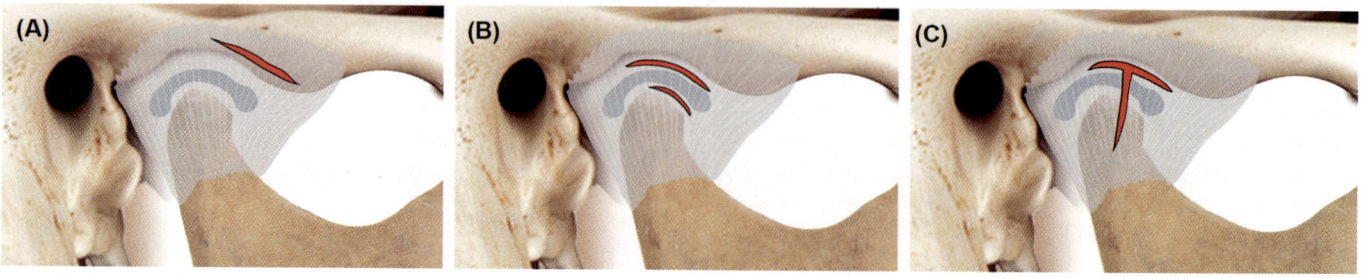

Figure 38.9 Capsular incisions at various locations. **(A)** Horizontal incision over the lateral rim of the glenoid fossa. **(B)** Horizontal incisions above and below the disc. **(C)** T-shaped incision.

BOX 38.1 Aims and Objectives of Surgery

1. Release of ankylosed mass and creation of a gap to mobilise the joint.
2. Creation of a functional joint.
3. To reconstruct the joint and restore the vertical height of the ramus.
4. To prevent recurrence.
5. To restore normal facial growth pattern.
6. To improve aesthetics and rehabilitate the patient.

TREATMENT PROTOCOL

The management strategy for TMJ ankylosis is dependent on the stage of ankylosis, the associated deformity, and the age of presentation. Definitive management of TMJ ankylosis is total removal of the ankylotic mass, minimise the incidence of re-ankylosis and produce satisfactory movement of the joint. The concept is to create a nonunion between the osteotomised bone ends (Box 38.1).

The well-known and widely followed protocol for managing TMJ ankylosis is the one proposed by Kaban and his colleagues in 1990. Their strategy reduces the risk of re-ankylosis and provides satisfactory movement in the TMJ.

KABAN'S PROTOCOL FOR THE MANAGEMENT OF TEMPOROMANDIBULAR JOINT ANKYLOSIS

The well-known and widely followed protocol for managing TMJ ankylosis is the one proposed by Kaban (Box 38.2).

Gap arthroplasty or aggressive resection of the ankylotic mass

A gap of at least 1–1.5 cm should be produced between the cut bone ends (temporal and mandibular bone). This procedure is known as aggressive excision of the ankylotic mass or gap arthroplasty. The medial side of the ankylosed bone mass or ramus requires special attention as an old malunited fragment can be seen attached to the medial side.

Ipsilateral coronoidectomy

In many cases, the ankylosis may involve the coronoid process also. After gap arthroplasty, coronoidectomy on the same side of ankylosis can be implemented either through the same incision or separately from an intraoral incision. It can be accomplished by cutting the coronoid process at the level of sigmoid notch till the anterior border of ramus. It is followed by dissection and stripping of the temporalis muscle attachment (temporalis myotomy). If necessary, the fibres of masseter and medial pterygoid can also be stripped off. After ipsilateral coronoidectomy, the mouth opening should be assessed. If the maximum mouth opening is larger than 35 mm, then there is no requirement for contralateral coronoidectomy to be performed.

BOX 38.2 Protocol for Management of TMJ Ankylosis

Kaban, Perrot, and Fisher Protocol for Management of TMJ Ankylosis (1990)

a. Aggressive resection of the ankylotic segment.
b. Ipsilateral coronoidectomy.
c. Contralateral coronoidectomy, if necessary.
d. Lining of the joint with temporalis fascia or cartilage.
e. Reconstruction of the ramus with a costochondral graft.
f. Rigid fixation of the graft.
g. Early mobilisation and aggressive physiotherapy.

Kaban's Modified Protocol for the Management of TMJ Ankylosis in Children (2009)

a. Aggressive excision of fibrous and/or bony mass.
b. Coronoidectomy on affected side.
c. Coronoidectomy on opposite side if steps 1 and 2 do not result in maximal interincisal opening (MIO) of 35 mm or to point of dislocation of opposite side.
d. Lining of joint with temporalis fascia or the native disc, if it can be salvaged.
e. Reconstruction of ramus condyle unit (RCU) with either distraction osteogenesis (DO) or costochondral graft (CCG) and rigid fixation.
f. Early mobilisation of jaw. If DO used to reconstruct RCU mobilise day of surgery; if CCG used, early mobilisation with minimal intermaxillary fixation (not >10 days).
g. Aggressive physiotherapy.

Contralateral coronoidectomy

If the maximal interincisal opening measured is less than 35 mm after an ipsilateral coronoidectomy, a contralateral coronoidectomy is performed using an intraoral approach.

Lining of temporomandibular joint

At the site of the gap arthroplasty, the temporalis fascia is placed in an intermediate position between the cut ends of the bone. Alternately, various authors have suggested the utilisation of an undamaged disc, if identified during the process of resection of ankylosed mass or cartilage from a number of different sources (e.g. auricular). Intermaxillary fixation (IMF) is performed in order to establish occlusion after the removal of the ankylotic mass, coronoidectomy and lining of the joint.

Reconstruction

The ramus is reconstructed using a costochondral graft (CCG).

Rigid fixation

The reconstructed graft is rigidly fixed using plates and screws.

Early mobilisation

Early mobilisation and vigorous physiotherapy for a period of at least 6 months after surgery are highly recommended to prevent re-ankylosis.

SURGICAL TECHNIQUES FOR TEMPOROMANDIBULAR JOINT ANKYLOSIS

Though a variety of techniques have been advocated, the basic methods for ankylosis release includes:

- Condylectomy
- Gap arthroplasty
- Interposition arthroplasty.

Condylectomy

In 1854, *Humphrey* was the 1st person to advocate the procedure known as condylectomy. It is indicated in cases with *fibrous ankylosis*, where the articular space has not been completely eliminated. The condyle is exposed by preauricular incision and the condylar head is located and identified. It is important to maintain the integrity of the vital structures that are located on the medial aspect of the joint. These structures include the internal maxillary artery and the auriculotemporal nerve. The condylar head is resected by making horizontal cuts and the fibrous adhesions are then contravened to complete the procedure. The remaining stump of the condyle is smoothened and the wound is closed in layers. Unilateral condylectomy can often cause the mandible to shift towards the operated side on opening the mouth. In bilateral condylectomy, patients will have an anterior open bite.

Indications:

- Severe arthrosis
- Various types of arthritis
- Malunited condylar fractures with limitation of motion and pain during mastication
- Fibrous ankylosis where the articular space has not been completely eliminated

Disadvantages:

- Loss of vertical height of the ramus
- In case of bilateral condylectomy, it may create an anterior open bite
- In unilateral cases, there may be deviation of the jaw on mouth opening.

Gap arthroplasty (Figs. 38.10–38.12)

In severe *bony ankylosis*, a large thick area of bone deposition completely obliterates the whole joint, including the sigmoid notch and the coronoid process. Gap arthroplasty is complete removal of a segment of bone to remove the ankylotic mass, and creating a gap between the temporal and mandibular ends of bone. It is a simple bone division to separate the ramus from the cranial base, which will result in the formation of pseudoarthrosis.

- Patients are operated under GA and the ankylotic mass is exposed using a preauricular approach
- The width of bone removal is crucial and there are different opinions regarding the amount of bone to be removed. Several authors recommend a *minimum gap of 1 cm*, to prevent re-ankylosis
- The upper and lower osteotomy cuts are marked on the bone planned for removal. If the joint normal architecture is maintained, the lower osteotomy cut is placed just below the sigmoid notch. In cases where the normal architecture is not clear, the cut is placed 1.5 cm below the lower border of zygomatic arch. The osteotomy cuts are completed using a bur, saw, piezoelectric unit or osteotome, and the ankylotic mass is removed
- Care is taken to prevent injury to the internal maxillary artery and venous plexus. The ipsilateral coronoid process is also removed
- After complete resection, the jaw is mobilised and the maximum interincisal opening (MIO) achieved is measured, which should be greater than 35 mm

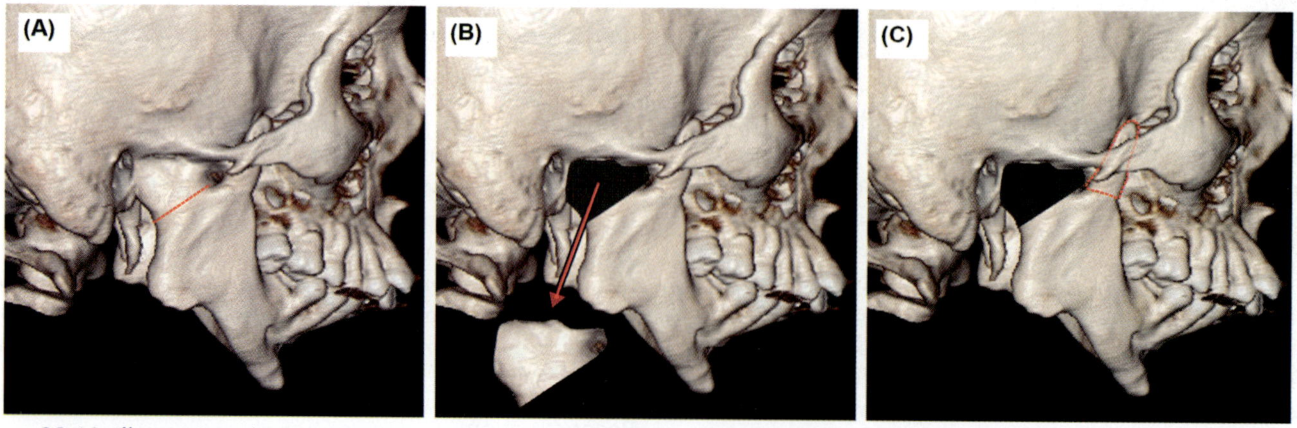

Figure 38.10 Illustration showing gap arthroplasty. (**A**) CT scan showing ankylosis on the right side. A marking is made on the amount of bone to be removed. (**B**) An osteotomy cut is made on the bone and the ankylotic mass is removed. The remaining condylar stump is reshaped to achieve a rounded contour. (**C**) Markings for ipsilateral coronoidectomy.

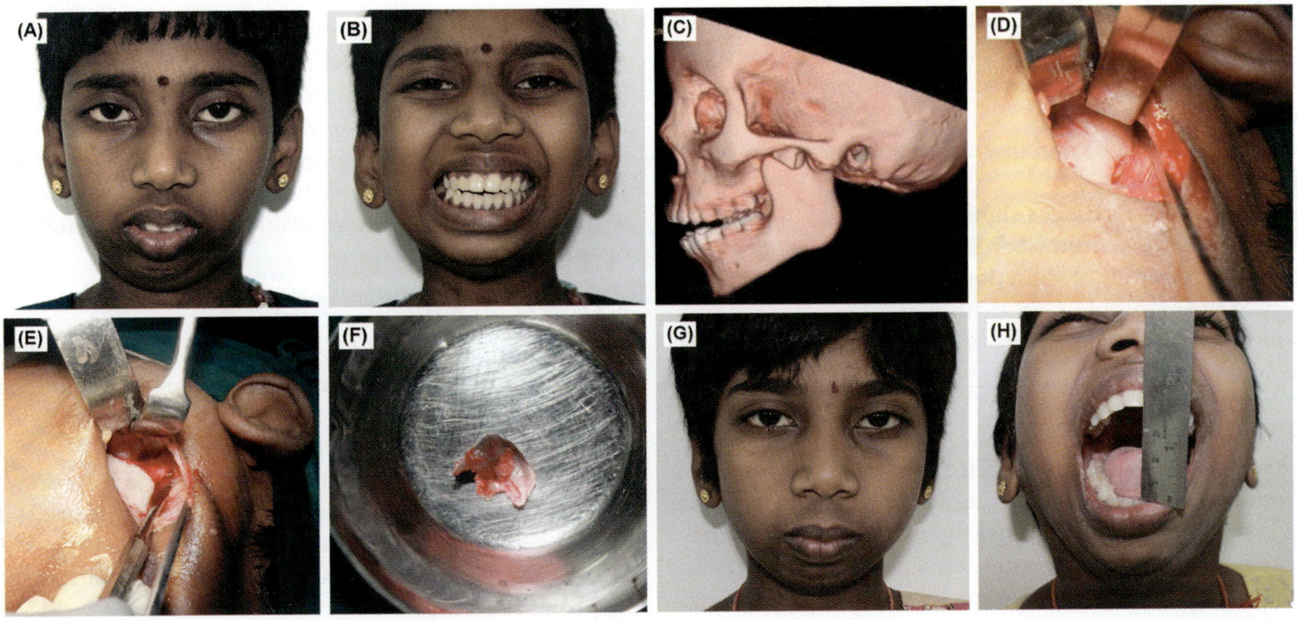

Figure 38.11 Unilateral gap arthroplasty. (**A–C**) Preoperative view showing left TMJ ankylosis with 2–3 mm of mouth opening. (**D–F**) Intraoperative view showing gap arthroplasty with excised specimen. (**G** and **H**) Postoperative view with almost 40 mm of mouth opening.

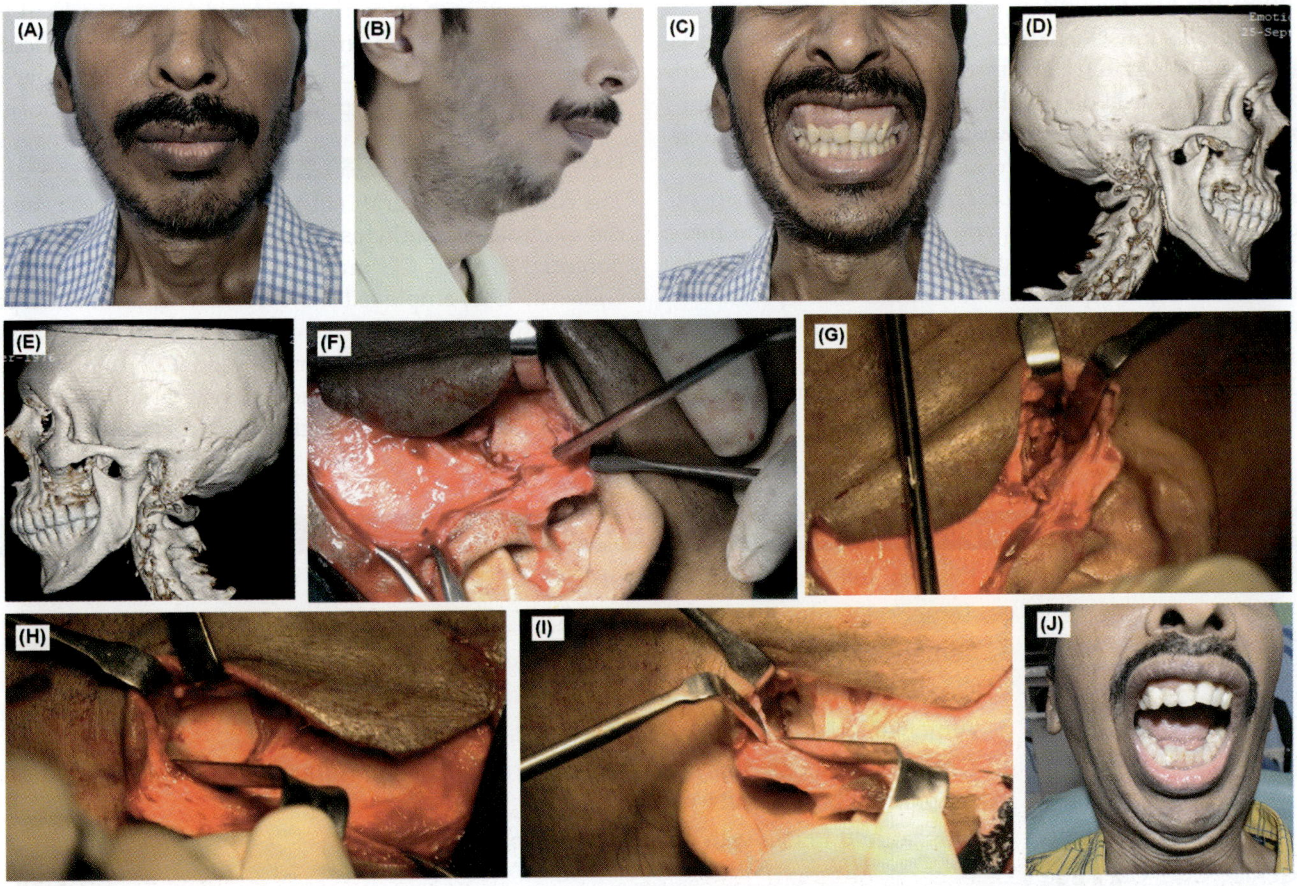

Figure 38.12 Bilateral gap arthroplasty. (**A–C**) Preoperative view of a patient with bilateral TMJ ankylosis and nil mouth opening. (**D** and **E**) CT scan showing TMJ ankylosis on the right and left side. (**F**) Right side ankylosis was exposed using preauricular incision. (**G**) The ankylotic mass was excised using bur and a gap is created between the ramus and cranium. (**H** and **I**) The same procedure is repeated on the left side ankylosis. (**J**) Postoperative with adequate mouth opening.

- In cases with long standing ankylosis and MIO <35 mm, complete dissection of the masseter attachment from the zygomatic arch and an opposite side coronoidectomy may be required
- An intact disc can be mobilised and repositioned into the new glenoid fossa.

Judicial amount of tissues should be removed, to prevent reunion of the osteotomised segments or re-ankylosis. Unnecessary removal of functional muscles restricts the mobility of the mandible. Gap arthroplasty may cause ramus shortening, malocclusion, open bite, obstructive sleep apnoea and re-ankylosis.

Interposition arthroplasty

Gap arthroplasty with a soft tissue placed between the cut ends are known as interpositional arthroplasty. The bony margins of gap arthroplasty have high osteogenic potential and may promote reunion of the osteotomised segments or re-ankylosis. Hence it is necessary to introduce an interpositional material between the two bone margins and create pseudoarthrosis (Table 38.5).

Autogenous interpositioning materials are the most commonly used materials.

a. Temporalis muscle flap

The temporalis muscle flap is the commonest interpositional material used in the treatment of ankylosis. A pedicled temporalis myofascial flap of about 5 × 2 cm is raised supraperiosteally and taken either over/under the zygomatic arch and sutured medially and posteriorly.

Advantages: Its ease of elevation, proximity to the site of surgery, reliable blood supply, and camouflage of the incision within the hairline. In addition, the fan-shaped muscle itself and the deep temporal fascia over it forms a protective covering.

Disadvantages: Extended incision, increased chances of facial nerve injury, temporal hollowing and myofascial pain (Fig. 38.13).

b. Autogenous fat

In 1914, Murphy reported the usage of autogenous fat for interpositioning and Rattan V (2006) has published reports favouring the use of fat grafts in the TM joint after release of ankylosis. Dimitroulis postulated that the fat grafts are fragile when used alone, whereas, when it is placed along with the dermis, it is more stable and easy to handle in the operative site.

c. Dermal fat graft

The abdominal dermal fat graft of around 7 × 3 cm is harvested from the suprapubic area using an elliptical incision. The graft is then folded onto itself with the dermis surfaces apposed and secured into the gap (Fig. 38.14).

Advantage: Reduced rate of re-ankylosis and infection, minimal donor site morbidity, easy sculpting of graft, minimal heterotopic calcification and the hidden scar

Disadvantage: Since it is a nonvascularised graft, it may be prone to resorption.

d. Buccal fat pad graft

Incision through the anterior most part of the coronoid stump or along the anterior border of ramus exposes the yellowish buccal pad of fat. Since the buccal fat pad (BFP) is in close approximation to the coronoid process and tendon of the temporalis. The main advantage of BFP is its vascularity, which would maintain the volume of fat for a longer duration with minimal resorption.

e. Costochondral grafts

The costochondral graft (rib) has been found to be the material of choice for ankylosis in growing children. The growth potential of the CCG makes it an ideal choice for children. Gillies in 1920 employed the CCG in TMJ reconstruction.

This rib cartilage has structural and physical properties similar to that of the condylar cartilage. When a replaced CCG is subjected to functional movements, it can function both histologically and physiologically as a normal mandibular

TABLE 38.5 Common Interpositional Grafts used in TMJ Ankylosis

Autogenous	Skin	Dermis, full thickness skin graft
	Muscle	Temporalis, pterygomasseteric sling
	Fascia	Temporalis, fascia lata, dura
	Fat	Groin, buccal, dermal
	Cartilage	Auricular, costochondral graft, iliac crest cartilage
	Bone	Coronoid process, ankylotic mass, sternoclavicular, ramus osteotomy pedicled graft, metatarsal bone grafts
	Combined	Muscle and fascia with or without periosteum
Allogenic	Cartilage (costal cartilage), dura	
Alloplastic	Metallic (titanium, gold and tantalum), silastic, acrylic	
Xenograft	Collagen, cartilage	

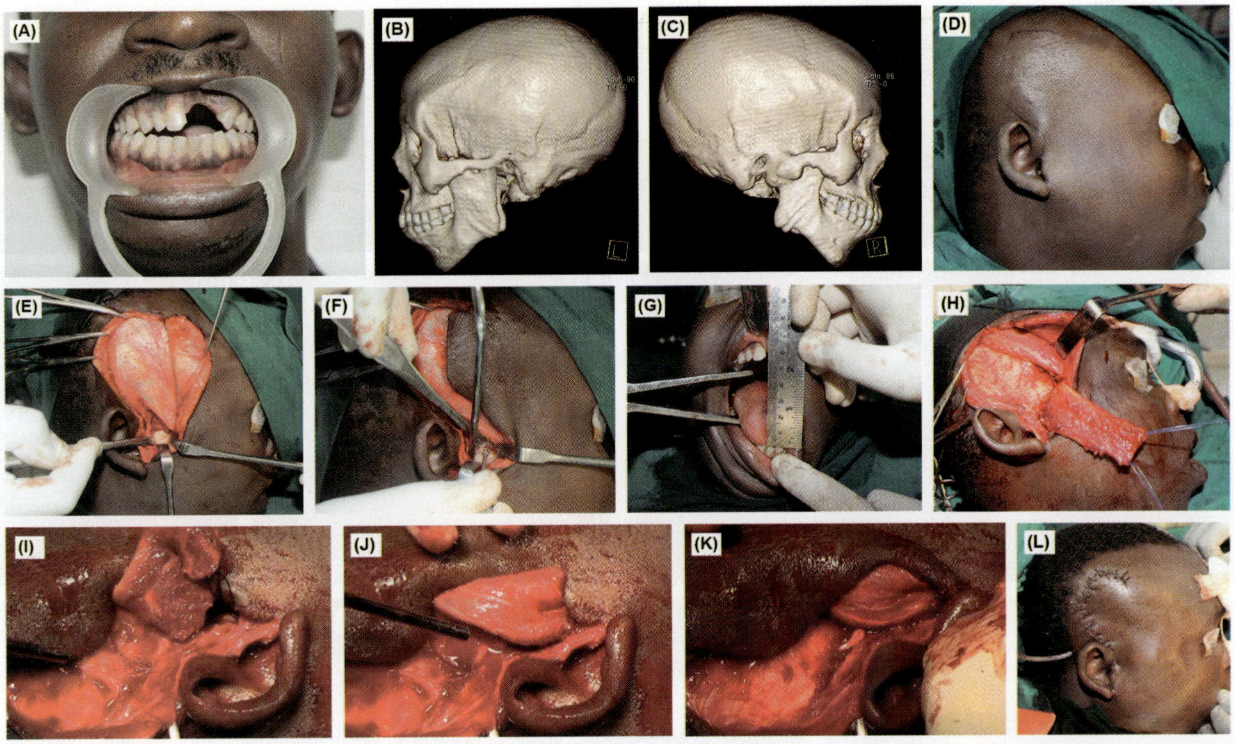

Figure 38.13 Temporalis muscle flap as interpositional material. (**A**) Preoperative view of patient with right TMJ ankylosis. (**B and C**) CT scan showing left & right TMJ ankylosis. (**D**) Intraoperative view with marking of preauricular incision. (**E**) Flap is raised and the ankylotic mass is exposed. (**F**) Removal of ankylotic mass using bur. (**G**) Intraoperative mouth opening is checked and is about 55 mm. (**H**) Raising of temporalis muscle flap for using it as interpositional graft. (**I–K**) The flap is help by a suture and rotated under the zygomatic arch. It is then secured in the gap created on removal of the ankylotic mass. (**L**) Closure of the surgical wound.

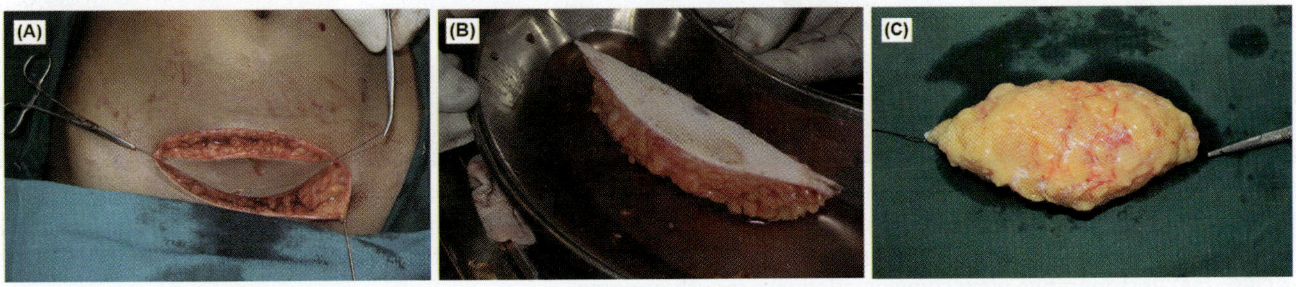

Figure 38.14 Dermal fat graft. (**A**) Harvesting of abdominal dermal fat graft using an elliptical incision. (**B and C**) The obtained graft with the skin and fat surfaces.

condyle. The cartilaginous portions of the CCG adapt well to function by reproducing the condylar morphology. Thus, with the growth of the CCG, good functional and aesthetics can be achieved.

Advantages: Biological compatibility, simple work technique, accessibility, functional adaptability, cartilaginous articulating surface, biologic remodelling and minimum donor site morbidity for the patient.

Complications: Donor site morbidity such as pneumothorax, pleuritic pain and the unpredictability of fate of the graft. Other potential problems of this graft include fracture, further ankylosis, and the variable growth behaviour of the graft. The rate of re-ankylosis is higher in adult patients, especially in individuals with multiple previous operations.

The costochondral junction, also known as the rib growth-steering centre, is expected to develop in length that is equivalent to the normal side of the mandible. However, the graft has a propensity to grow in an unpredictable manner, which can subsequently lead to a deviation of the chin as well as mandibular prognathism (Fig. 38.15).

f. Auricular cartilage

The auricular cartilage is harvested through a 3–4 cm incision on the posterior auricle. The graft is convex and can fit the anatomy

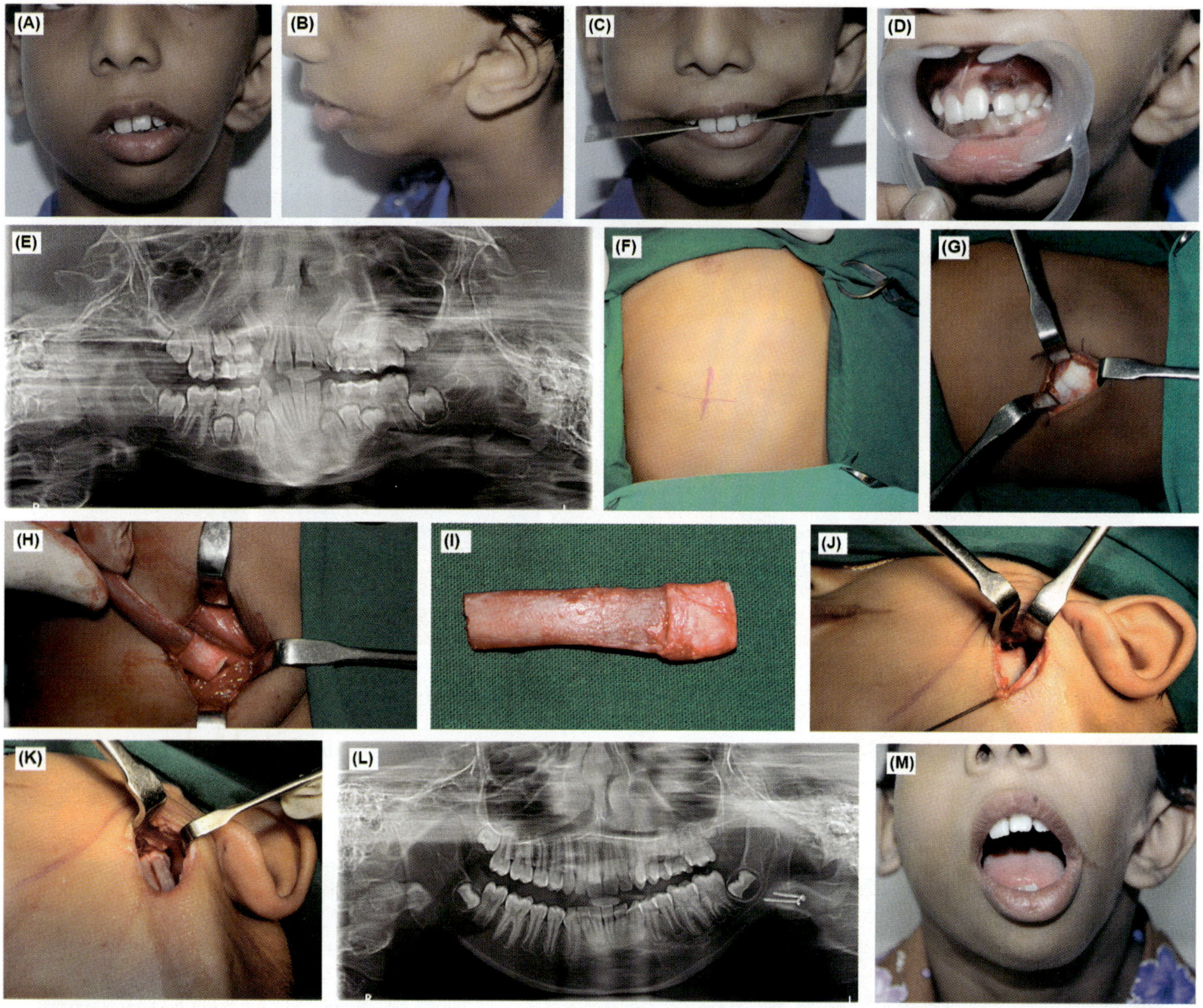

Figure 38.15 Costochondral graft as interpositional material. **(A–D)** Preoperative view of a patient with left TMJ ankylosis. **(E)** OPG showing left ankylosis. **(F–I)** Obtainment of the costochondral graft from the rib. **(J)** Through submandibular incision, the ankylosis is released using bur. **(K)** The costochondral graft is placed and secured into the left side ramus and condyle region. **(L)** Postoperative OPG. **(M)** Postoperative view showing adequate mouth opening.

of the fossa well. The graft is inserted into the appropriate position between the condyle and fossa and sutured firmly to the surrounding soft tissues. The graft appeared to be resistant to pressure and its smooth surface allowed sliding motion.

Advantages: Harvesting of the graft in the same surgical field, viable and its adaptability to the articular fossa

Disadvantages: Difficulty in stabilisation of graft, excessive elasticity and thinness, with susceptibility to perforation or fracture of the graft. Moreover, the ear cannot yield enough cartilage to cover large ankylosis defects without losing its dimensional stability.

POSTOPERATIVE PHYSIOTHERAPY

Early aggressive physiotherapy is often required to maintain a functional MIO postoperatively. It is also important to disrupt adhesions and soft tissue contractions that may occur postoperatively.

The use of mechanically assisted mandibular motion devices as well as manual exercisers, tongue blades, and finger-stretch exercises have all been reported as various rehabilitation therapies. It is also essential to continue physical therapy even after achieving adequate mouth opening to prevent subsequent relapse (Fig. 38.16).

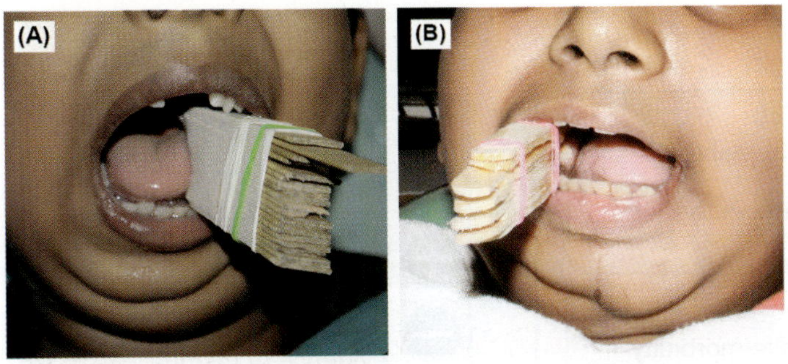

Figure 38.16 Rehabilitation exercises using sticks.

RAMUS CONDYLE UNIT RECONSTRUCTION (Fig. 38.17)

TRANSPORT DISTRACTION OSTEOGENESIS

A small percentage of autogenous grafts may fail or cause re-ankylosis. As a result, transport distraction osteogenesis can be used to reconstruct the ramus condyle unit, particularly in children with re-ankylosis. By compressing the connective tissue between the transport segment and the glenoid fossa, it forms a fibrous/pseudo-disc. The distractor can be fixed with an L-shaped ramus osteotomy.

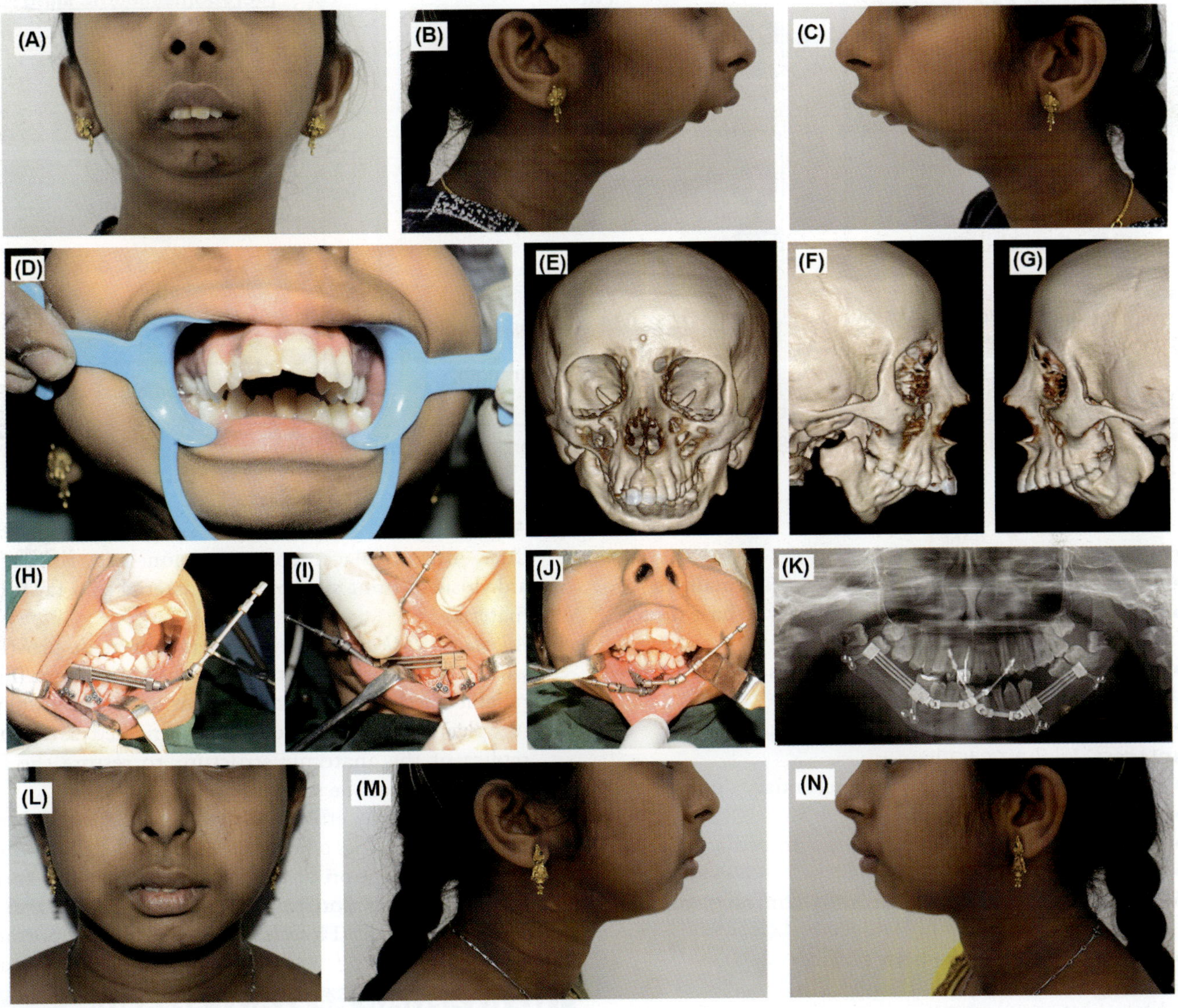

Figure 38.17 Distraction osteogenesis in the reconstruction of mandible after ankylotic release. **(A–D)** Preoperative view showing bilateral ankylosis with bird facies and severe Class II malocclusion. **(E–G)** CT scan showing decreased mandibular length and height after ankylotic release. **(H–J)** The osteotomy cuts are made and intraoral distraction device is fixed bilaterally. **(K)** OPG taken post distraction showing the intact distraction device and the newly formed bone. **(L–N)** Postoperative picture after removal of the distraction device.

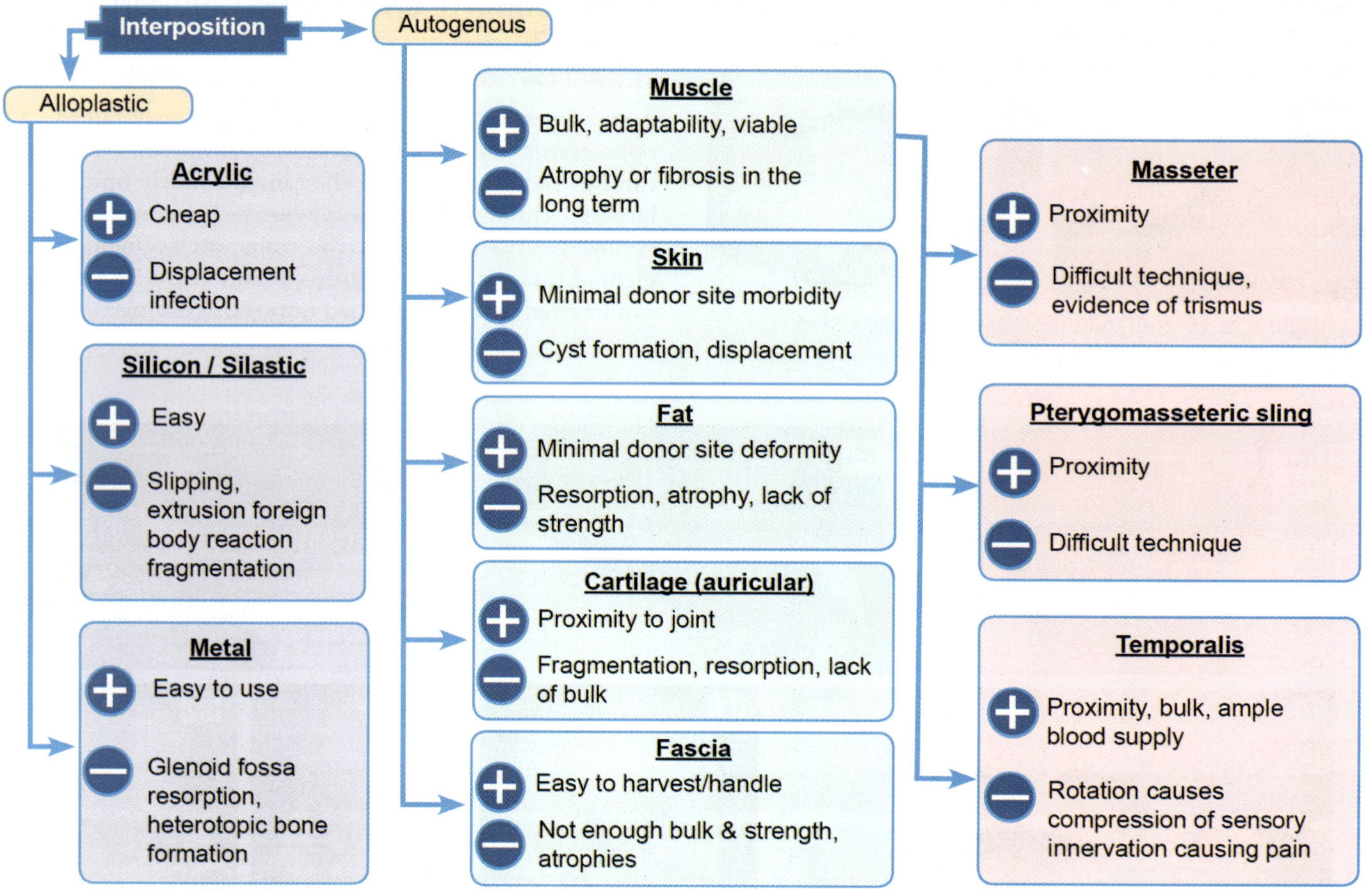

Flowchart 38.2 Materials used for interpositional arthroplasty.

ALLOPLASTIC MATERIALS

Indications:

- Re-ankylosis with severe anatomic abnormalities
- Autogenous graft failure in patients who have undergone multiple operations
- Destruction of autogenous graft tissue by underlying pathology
- Severe inflammatory joint disease

Advantages:

- There is no requirement for a secondary donor site
- Surgery time is reduced
- Physical rehabilitation may begin immediately
- Immediate jaw function
- Mimics the typical anatomic contours of the structures
- Better adapted to the bony surfaces

Disadvantages:

- Material wear and failure
- Long-term stability
- Inability to follow the patient's growth.

Materials used:

Silastic: It is no longer recommended as an interpositional material due to its tendency to slip from the impacted site, fragmentation and re-ankylosis of joint

Acrylic: The usage of acrylic is simple and safe procedure. But displacement, extrusion and risk of re-ankylosis did not support this material as a favourable material

Alloplastic TMJ prosthesis: It is a custom-made prosthesis with a fossa component and ramus component. It is a reliable method to treat recurrent ankylosis in adults. Alloplastic TMJ prosthesis are fabricated as an exact replica of the anatomic structure, to restore the form and function of the structure.

The potential side effects of the alloplasts are infection, postoperative pain, loss of joint mobility due to development of adhesions, resorption or erosion of glenoid fossa, foreign body or allergic reaction to implant components and displacement of implant (Flowchart 38.2).

MANAGEMENT OF FACIAL DEFORMITY SECONDARY TO TEMPOROMANDIBULAR JOINT ANKYLOSIS

Reduced ramus length, chin deviation, bird face deformity, retrognathic mandible and occlusal cant are all common secondary deformities associated with TMJ ankylosis. Surgical correction of postankylotic secondary deformities has always been a challenge for surgeons. Orthognathic surgery (a variety of osteotomies) can help with postoperative asymmetry and achieving a more stable occlusion. Distraction osteogenesis has recently been shown to be an effective method of correcting secondary deformities in the face. TMJ ankylosis is sometimes linked to obstructive sleep apnoea, necessitating treatment for both conditions.

COMPLICATIONS OF TMJ ANKYLOSIS SURGERY

- Haemorrhage (damage of any superficial temporal vessels, transverse facial artery, inferior alveolar vessels and internal maxillary artery, pterygoid plexus of veins, etc.)
- Damage to the external acoustic meatus, the parotid gland (salivary gland fistula), the auriculotemporal nerve (Frey's syndrome), the zygomatic and temporal branch of facial nerve, the teeth
- Infection
- Open bite
- Re-ankylosis (recurrence).

FALSE ANKYLOSIS

False ankylosis is restriction of mandibular movement due to extraarticular joint abnormalities. This type of ankylosis can also be considered as trismus. False ankylosis can result from one of the following reasons:

- **Muscular trismus**—pericoronitis, infection involving the masticatory spaces
- **Muscular fibrosis**—long standing dysfunction like arthritis and myositis
- **Myositis ossificans**—progressive ossification of muscles after injury or haematoma formation
- **Tetany**—hypocalcaemia causes the spasms of muscles
- **Tetanus**—acute infectious disease presenting with lockjaw due to persistent muscle spasm
- **Neurogenic causes**—epilepsy, brain tumour and haemorrhage in medulla oblongata
- **Trismus hystericus**—disease of psychogenic origin
- **Drug-induced spasms**—like strychnine poisoning.

TRISMUS

***Trismus** is defined as a prolonged, spasm of the jaw muscles by which normal opening of the mouth is restricted.* Trismus is also commonly referred to as 'lockjaw' and is usually due to sustained tetanic spasm of the muscles of mastication. It is restriction in the range of motion of the jaws.

Trismus is a bilateral condition due to elevated tone mediated by the efferent section of the trigeminal nerve's reflex arch. It is usually transitory and disappears in less than 2 weeks, but persistent trismus can arise and interfere with daily tasks such as eating and speaking.

The normal range of mouth opening is 40–60 mm. Trismus is characterised as a mouth opening of less than 40 mm. Trismus has been assessed by other authors based on the visual evaluation of mouth opening (Box 38.3).

BOX 38.3 Grading of Trismus

Group	Mouth Opening
I	>35 mm
II	25–35 mm
III	15–25 mm
IV	2–15 mm

AETIOLOGY

Trismus can be caused or predisposed to by a number of factors. Few studies categorised TMJ aetiology into intraarticular and extraarticular aetiologies based on TMJ involvement.

The various causes of trismus are depicted in Table 38.6.

CLINICAL PRESENTATION

Patients present with a restricted mouth opening and sometimes associated with pain while opening the mouth. Patient complaints are related to the cause of trismus. A complete clinical examination is necessary to identify the cause. Trismus is frequently diagnosed clinically. CT scans and other imaging act as adjuvants in identifying the aetiology (trauma, fractures, haematomas, etc.).

MANAGEMENT OF TRISMUS

Management of trismus is directed towards treating the aetiology and mostly involves symptomatic treatment, which is followed by physiotherapy. Long-term trismus may necessitate surgical procedures to achieve adequate mouth opening (Table 38.7).

Applying moist towels to the affected area for 15–20 min/h is heat therapy. Analgesics such as aspirin are usually sufficient for pain management. A narcotic analgesic may be required if the pain is severe. A muscle relaxant, such as diazepam, in doses ranging from 2.5 to 5 mg three times per day, may also be prescribed. After the acute phase has passed, the patient should perform mouth opening exercises for 5 min every 3–4 h. If the trismus is caused by an infection, antibiotics can be prescribed for 5–7 days. If the trismus does not resolve within 2–3 days, the patient may need surgical intervention.

TABLE 38.6 Aetiology and Differential Diagnosis of Trismus

A. **Intraarticular** 1. Ankylosis 2. Arthritis synovitis 3. Meniscus pathology	4. **Dental treatment related** • Local anaesthetic injection injury • Post extraction (e.g. 3rd molar removal, TMJ surgery)
B. **Extraarticular** 1. **Congenital** • Trismus pseudocamptodactyly syndrome • Hypertrophy of coronoid • Haemifacial microsomia • Birth injury	5. **TMD** • Trauma to TMJ on wide or prolonged opening of mouth • Myofascial muscle spasm (MPDS) • Internal derangement • TMJ ankylosis (fibrous and bony)
2. **Infection** **Odontogenic** • Pulpal • Periodontal • Pericoronal **Nonodontogenic** • Tetanus • Tonsillitis and peritonsillar abscess • Parotid abscess • Brain abscess • Mumps • Septic arthritis • Cancrum oris • Osteomyelitis of the mandible and temporal bone • Abscesses of the submasseteric, lateral pharyngeal, pterygomandibular, submandibular and temporal spaces	6. **Neoplastic/tumours** • Tumours of the TMJ and surrounding structures (e.g. osteochondroma) • Tumours of the oropharynx (Trotter's syndrome) • Metastatic disease of the mandible and infratemporal fossa 7. **Radiation and chemotherapy** • Osteoradionecrosis • Post radiation fibrosis 8. **Inflammatory/chronic reactive** • Degenerative joint disease • Rheumatoid arthritis • Systemic sclerosis • Submucous fibrosis • Myositis ossificans 9. **Neurogenic** • Tetanus • Parkinsonism • Status epilepticus • Hypocalcaemia, hypomagnesaemia, respiratory alkalosis
3. **Trauma (acute)** • Fractures of mandible, zygomatic or temporal bones • Haematomas in the joint or muscle of mastication • Paradoxical muscle spasm following head injury • Anterior dislocated meniscus	10. **Drug induced** • Extrapyramidal reaction (facial dyskinesia) • Strychnine poisoning • Adverse effects of medications (phenothiazine, succinylcholine, Tricyclic antidepressants (TCA), halothane)

TABLE 38.7 Management of Trismus

Acute Phase	After Acute Phase	Long-Term Trismus (Surgery)
• Heat therapy • Analgesics—NSAIDs • Muscle relaxants—diazepam • Soft diet	• Stretching exercises (mouth opening and lateral movements, chewing gums) • Intensive physiotherapy (using commercially available devices)	• Coronoidectomy • Tissue release • Free flap reconstruction

Chapter 39

Growth Disorders of Temporomandibular Joint

OUTLINE

INTRODUCTION AND DEVELOPMENT OF TEMPOROMANDIBULAR JOINT

Temporomandibular joint (TMJ) morphology is typically underdeveloped at birth. TMJ develops at 7 weeks intrauterine. At about 10 weeks, the mandibular condyle area forms bone and cartilage, concluding disc morphogenesis. At the time of birth, fibrous connective tissue covers the condyle and temporal bone articular surfaces. Under functional forces, this tissue becomes fibrocartilage. Remodelling of the bones occurs when the condyle and temporal fossa develop. Condyle growth disorders may arise prenatally or postnatally. Congenital or acquired condyle defects may occur. Congenital defects might result from systemic conditions in the 10th week, and trauma, infection, or rheumatoid arthritis might cause them by the 14th week. Depending on the tissues involved, masticatory system disorders are classified as bone or muscle disorders (Box 39.1). The different stages of incomplete development are called agenesis, aplasia, and hypoplasia. Agenesis and aplasia are seldom used interchangeably to denote organ absence or failure to develop. Hypoplasia is organ underdevelopment.

BOX 39.1 Classification of Growth Disorders of bone and muscle

I. Congenital and developmental bone disorders:
- **A.** Agenesis (no growth)
- **B.** Hypoplasia (insufficient growth):
  - **1.** Unilateral condylar hypoplasia
  - **2.** Bilateral condylar hypoplasia
- **C.** Hyperplasia (excessive growth)
- **D.** Neoplasia (uncontrolled destructive growth)

II. Congenital and developmental muscle disorders:
- **A.** Hypotrophy (weakened muscle)
- **B.** Hypertrophy (increased size and strength of the muscle)
- **C.** Neoplasia (uncontrolled, destructive growth)

GROWTH DISORDERS OF BONE

Aetiology

Bone growth disorders have unknown causes. Though trauma is a leading cause, juvenile arthritis, hormonal imbalance (parathyroid hormone), and radiation may also cause it. Trauma may produce condyle hypoplasia or hyperplasia, causing uneven mandibular growth and corresponding malocclusion.

Clinical presentation

- Clinical asymmetry from growth disruption
- Structural changes
- Alteration of function
- Pain is usually not present but can be secondary to structural changes
- CT scans show bony changes in the TMJ region.

Treatment

Generally, the treatment of bone growth disorders is specific to each patient's structural changes and should be aimed at restoring function without traumatising the associated structures.

AGENESIS OR APLASIA (CONDYLE)

It is defined as lack or defective growth in the skull or mandibular bones. Condylar agenesis is congenital nonformation of condyle. These defects have no condyle, no articular disc or eminence since birth. It can be caused by mechanical trauma during active growth, infection or inflammatory process at the TMJ area or as manifestation of syndromes. For example, mandibular anomalies such as hemifacial microsomia.

Clinical presentation of condylar aplasia

- Congenital
- Usually unilateral
- Deviation of mandible towards the affected side
- Unaffected side is flat and long
- Severe malocclusion
- Often with ear abnormalities
- Bilateral aplasia presents with lack of facial asymmetry, micrognathia and short mandible
- Isolated condylar aplasia is very rare and is often associated with other soft tissue or skeletal malformations (ear, temporal bone, angle of mouth, zygoma).

Radiographs show ill-defined or rudimentary glenoid fossa, no condyle or no articular disc.

Treatment

It requires a multidisciplinary approach involving oral surgeon, plastic surgeon, and orthodontist. Surgical reconstruction with costochondral graft can be done to establish an active growth centre, preferably before the growth spurt and orthognathic surgery at the end of the growth period. Krogstad suggested the use of an orthodontic activator which promotes the formation of mandibular condyle.

HYPOPLASIA

It is low or incomplete growth of bones which is milder than aplasia. For example, craniofacial anomalies such as Treacher Collins' syndrome, Morquio's syndrome and Proteus' syndrome.

CONDYLAR HYPOPLASIA

Condylar hypoplasia is the underdeveloped or defective formation of the condyle, resulting from congenital, developmental or acquired diseases affecting the growth of the condyle. It may occur at birth (congenital) due to pharyngeal 1st and 2nd arch malformation, or it may result from trauma, infection or irradiation during the growth period (acquired). Condylar hypoplasia can occur unilaterally or bilaterally.

Unilateral condylar hypoplasia

Clinical presentation (Figs. 39.1)

- Facial asymmetry
- Shortened mandibular vertical height on the affected side
- Deviation of the chin towards the affected side
- Deviation of the mandible on mouth opening towards the affected side
- Elongated body of mandible and flat face on the unaffected side
- Malocclusion
- Antegonial notching

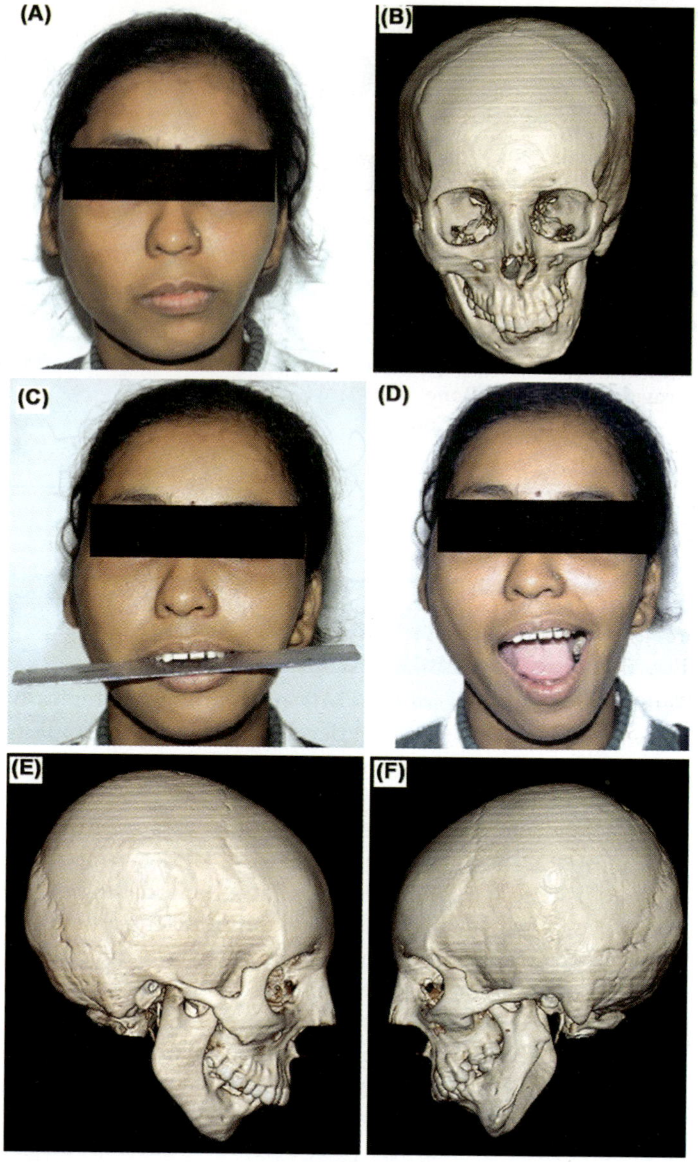

Figure 39.1 Unilateral condylar hypoplasia (craniofacial microsomia syndrome). **(A)** Condylar hypoplasia on the left side. **(B)** Left condylar hypoplasia, deviation of chin and occlusal canting seen. **(C)** Occlusal cant. **(D)** Deviation of mouth towards the affected side. **(E)** Normal right side of the mandible. **(F)** Hypoplastic condyle with reduced mandibular vertical height on the left side.

- Occlusal cant
- TMJ dysfunction.

Isolated condylar hypoplasia is extremely unusual, and generally occurs in association with other facial abnormalities (eye, ear, etc.) or as a feature of a syndrome. Some of the common syndromes associated with hemimandibular hypoplasia are: Goldenhar–Gorlin syndrome, 1st and 2nd brachial arch syndromes, craniofacial microsomia (Fig. 39.1), Dyke–Davidoff–Masson syndrome and femoral-facial syndrome.

Bilateral condylar hypoplasia

Clinical features

- Micrognathia or small mandible
- Bird-like face
- Retruded chin with a small mandibular arch
- Respiratory distress due to obstruction of the pharyngeal airway by falling back of the tongue
- Class II malocclusion
- Deepened antegonial notch
- TMJ dysfunction.

Radiographic appearance

- The structure and shape of condyle may be normal but diminished in size
- Proportionally small mandibular fossa
- Condylar neck may be short, thin or elongated
- Decreased vertical height of the mandibular body
- Degenerative changes in the affected joint.

Syndromes associated with bilateral condylar hypoplasia are Pierre Robin's syndrome, Treacher Collins' syndrome (Fig. 39.2), Nager's syndrome, Townes–Brocks syndrome, branchiootorenal syndrome, branchiooculofacial syndromes, and Stickler's syndrome. Deficiencies in the condyle can range from hypoplasia to aplasia in conditions such as craniofacial microsomia, thalidomide embryopathy, and Treacher Collins' syndrome. In Nager–de Reynier syndrome, the condyle may be aplastic or dysplastic (Table 39.1).

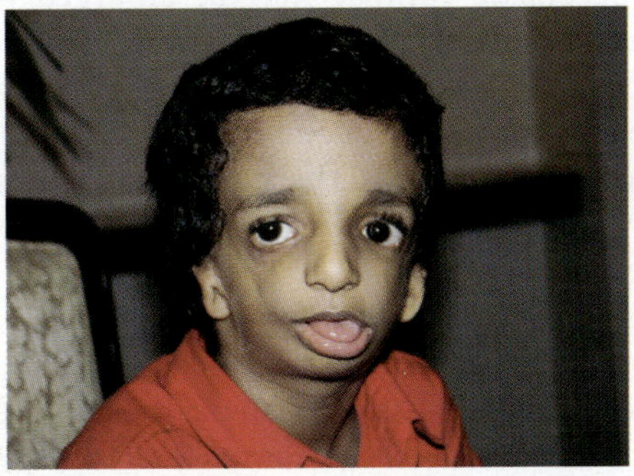

Figure 39.2 Bilateral condylar hypoplasia (Treacher Collins' syndrome).

TREATMENT OF CONDYLAR HYPOPLASIA

The treatment of condylar hypoplasia varies depending on the age of the patient, type and severity of the facial abnormalities. Various treatment modalities have been proposed for treating condylar hypoplasia, which include the following:

- In the growing phase, *functional appliances* are helpful in correcting or reducing the deformities
- In young growing children, *growth centre transplantation* (reconstruction of TMJ with costochondral graft) or *mandibular distraction osteogenesis* may be required to correct the facial asymmetry (Fig. 39.3)
- After the growth phase, skeletal deformities can be corrected by *orthognathic surgery*
- *Orthodontic treatment* for dental corrections.

GROWTH CENTRE TRANSPLANTATION

Ideally, successful rehabilitation of individuals with condylar abnormalities should have a TMJ that is structurally and functionally adequate. In addition, when dealing with severe condylar dysplasia in young growing individuals, treatment objectives should be directed at establishing a region where adaptive growth can occur. The most common method for achieving the desired result is the insertion of a cartilaginous graft into the osteotomy site. Costochondral rib grafts (costochondral junction of the 5th, 6th or 7th rib) are most suitable for this purpose as they can be transplanted as growth centre replacements to achieve mandibular growth.

DISTRACTION OSTEOGENESIS

Distraction osteogenesis may extend the jaw and create new bone without bone grafting or donor site morbidity. They

TABLE 39.1 Various Syndromes Associated with Hypoplasia and Their Traits

Syndromes	Skeletal Traits	Other Traits
Hemifacial microsomia (1st and 2nd branchial arch syndrome)	Underdevelopment of TMJ and ramus	Underdevelopment of ear, muscles and cardiac anomalies
Goldenhar's syndrome (Oculoauriculovertebral syndrome)	Severe form of microfacial microsomia	Fused spine and eye tumours
Treacher Collins' syndrome (Mandibulofacial dysostosis)	Hypoplasia of mandible, zygomatic arch, condyle and coronoid process	Underdevelopment of ear, eyes and hearing loss
Hallermann–Streiff syndrome (HSS) (Oculomandibulodyscephaly)	Hypoplasia of mandible, ramus, missing condyle, bird face, dyscephalia	Skin atrophy, dental anomalies, cataract, microphthalmia
Morquio syndrome	Abnormal development of bones, prominent lower face	Cardiac, ocular, respiratory, hepatic abnormalities and enamel hypoplasia
Proteus syndrome	Atypical growth of bones, cranial hyperostosis	Skin thickening, vascular anomalies, verrucous epidermal naevus

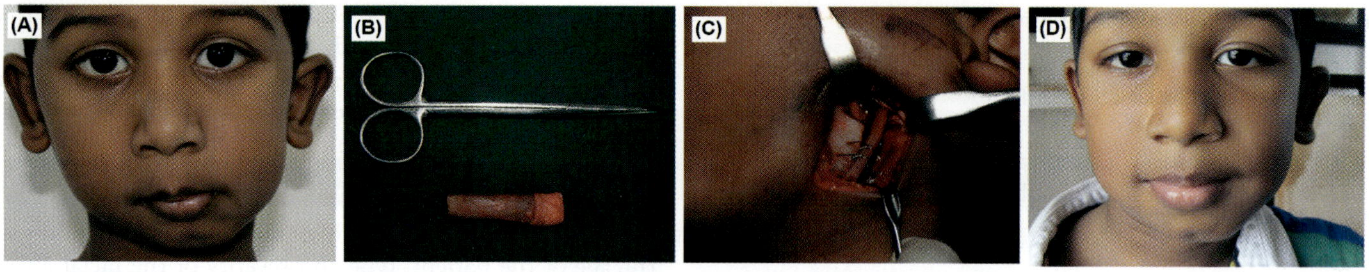

Figure 39.3 Treatment of condylar hypoplasia. (**A**) Unilateral condylar hypoplasia—preop. (**B**) Costochondral graft. (**C**) Placement of costochondral graft in the ostectomy site. (**D**) Two years after costochondral growth centre transplantation.

help mandibular lengthening devoid of relapse. New multi-directional buried intraoral distraction devices have solved several hurdles with improved vector control, occlusion, and aesthetics.

ORTHOGNATHIC SURGERY AND ORTHODONTICS

A combination of maxillary and mandibular osteotomies can be performed to correct the skeletal deformity (facial asymmetry) caused by the condylar hypoplasia after cessation of growth. Bilateral sagittal split osteotomy (BSSO) is the workhorse osteotomy of traditional mandibular advancement surgery for correction of micrognathia. Le Fort I osteotomy with derotation to correct the occlusal cant, followed by vertical ramus osteotomy and genioplastic procedures, which yields good symmetry and aesthetic results.

HYPERPLASIA

It is extensive growth of bones in congenital or acquired form, for example, condylar hyperplasia.

CONDYLAR HYPERPLASIA

Condylar hyperplasia (CH) is bone disorder characterised by increased growth of the condyle, which was 1st described by *Robert Adams.*

Aetiologic factors

It can be caused by trauma, infection, hormonal influence, intrauterine factors, heredity, and hyper vascularity. It can be due to overactive cartilage, resulting in increased thickness of the cartilaginous and precartilaginous layers. It is usually unilateral.

Clinical features

CH is more common in females and is frequently detected before the age of 20 years. It may progress slowly or rapidly and tends to be arrested with termination of skeletal growth.

- Increase in facial height on the affected side
- Mandibular asymmetry depending on the degree of condylar enlargement
- Deviation of the chin to the unaffected side
- Increase in the vertical dimension of the ramus, body or alveolar process on the affected side
- Malocclusion
- Posterior open bite on the affected side
- Cross bite on the contralateral side
- On the affected side, the lower border of the mandible is convex
- Problems with mastication or speech
- TMJ dysfunction (deviated mandibular opening)
- Bilateral condylar hyperplasia can cause prognathism
- Unilateral condylar hyperplasia causes facial asymmetry.

Radiographic features

- The hyperplastic condyle may be enlarged with a relatively normal shape or with an altered shape (e.g. elongated, conical, spherical, lobulated) or irregular shape
- It appears more radiopaque because of the additional bone volume. However, the cortical thickness and trabecular pattern of the enlarged condyle are normal
- Enlarged glenoid fossa
- Secondary degenerative changes
- Longer and thickened condylar neck
- Forward bending of the elongated condylar head and neck
- No increase in height of ramus or length of body of mandible.

Diagnostic methods for condylar hyperplasia

The goal of the diagnosis of condylar hyperplasia is to determine the activity and morphology of the condyle affected. CT scans help to recognise the pathology and condylar morphology. The bone metabolism or the presence of condylar hyperactivity can be provided by nuclear imaging. The different types of nuclear imaging includes *planar scintigraphy, single-photon emission computed tomography (SPECT) and positron emission tomography (PET).* Bone scintigraphy can identify a change in bone metabolism but is limited in differentiating various conditions.

Treatment

Treatment before completion of condylar growth limits the severity of mandibular deformation. Treatment after completion of growth helps to avoid relapse and additional interventions. A technetium bone scan helps in determining the active growth of the condyle. Treatment is a combination of *condylectomy, orthognathic surgery and orthodontics.* Condylectomy removes the source of abnormal growth, whereas orthognathic surgery and orthodontics are done to correct the functional and aesthetic defects.

Obwegeser and Makek (1986) differentiated hyperplasia into three categories based on the asymmetry and predominant growth vector:

(i) Type I—Hemimandibular elongation (HME)
(ii) Type II—Hemimandibular hyperplasia (HMH)
(iii) Type III—Combination of types I and II.

HEMIMANDIBULAR ELONGATION (TYPE I)

It is characterised by excessive growth of the mandible in a horizontal vector/horizontal displacement of the mandible. The condyle is usually unaffected, but the neck appears malformed and slender, and the ramus is elongated, which is the basis for referring as hemimandibular elongation.

Clinical findings (Fig. 39.4A–C)

- Midline shift to the contralateral side
- Chin deviation towards the unaffected side
- Mild mandibular protrusion
- Posterior cross bite
- Lip line slopes down towards the affected side
- The occlusal plane sometimes slopes upwards to affected side.

Radiographic features (Fig. 39.4D)

The unilateral HME can be noticed using orthopantomogram (OPG), 3DCT of skull and posteroanterior (PA) cephalogram in an opened mouth position.

Treatment

- High condylectomy and orthognathic surgery:
  If the asymmetry is minor, no high condylectomy is required, and simply orthognathic surgery is used to address the asymmetry. High condylectomy is a procedure in which the condylar head is shaved for roughly 2–3 mm, removing overly developing condylar cartilage. Remodelling of the excised condylar head and formation of new articulating cartilage are said to be seen following high condylectomy. As a result, orthognathic surgery should not be done concurrently with, or even soon after, condylectomy. It is advisable to postpone orthognathic surgery until mandibular development has stopped
  In the fully developed condition following any presurgical orthodontics, spatial correction is required
- In the simpler cases where there is no cant of the occlusal plane, a bilateral mandibular ramus osteotomy is usually sufficient to achieve a reasonable result. In addition, a genioplasty is sometimes necessary to achieve symmetry of the chin
- In patients with occlusal cant, the maxillary occlusion plane can be corrected using a Le Fort I osteotomy in addition to the mandibular surgery.

HEMIMANDIBULAR HYPERPLASIA (TYPE II)

It is characterised as excessive growth of the mandible in a vertical vector. It is associated with three-dimensional enlargement of one side of the condyle, condylar neck, the ramus and body of the mandible. The growth terminates exactly at the symphysis region. Hyperplasia usually commences before puberty. The condyle often appears enlarged, with a deformed head and a thickened or elongated neck of the condyle. HMH is a more aggressive condition than HME, progressing more rapidly and resulting in considerably more anatomical distortion.

Clinical findings (Fig. 39.5)

- Increased height of the mandible on the affected side
- Rotated face appearance with sloping rima orbis
- Unilateral downward projection of the ramus and angle of the mandible on the affected side
- Enlargement of the condyle, condylar neck, ascending ramus and the body
- The abnormal growth terminates precisely at the symphysis, giving rise to a sharp demarcation at that site
- No chin deviation
- No midline shift
- Open bite on the affected side
- Downward cant due to supra eruption of maxillary teeth on the affected side for compensation
- Downward growth of the mandible
- On the ipsilateral side, the maxillary alveolar bone also grows excessively to maintain occlusion
- Pain in the affected TMJ region is common.

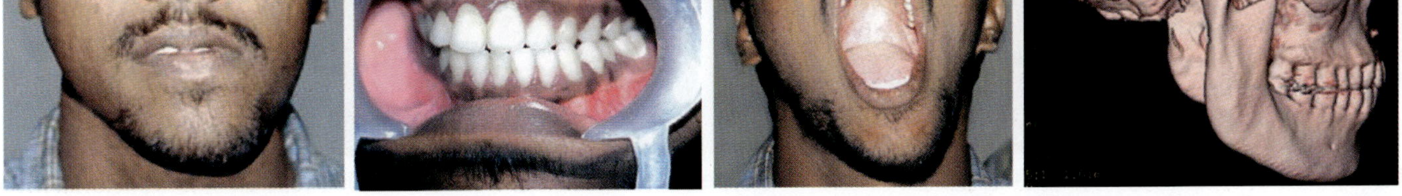

Figure 39.4 Hemimandibular elongation. **(A)** Increased vertical growth on the right side. **(B)** Contralateral cross bite. **(C)** Deviation of the mouth on opening towards the normal side. **(D)** CT image showing condylar hyperplasia.

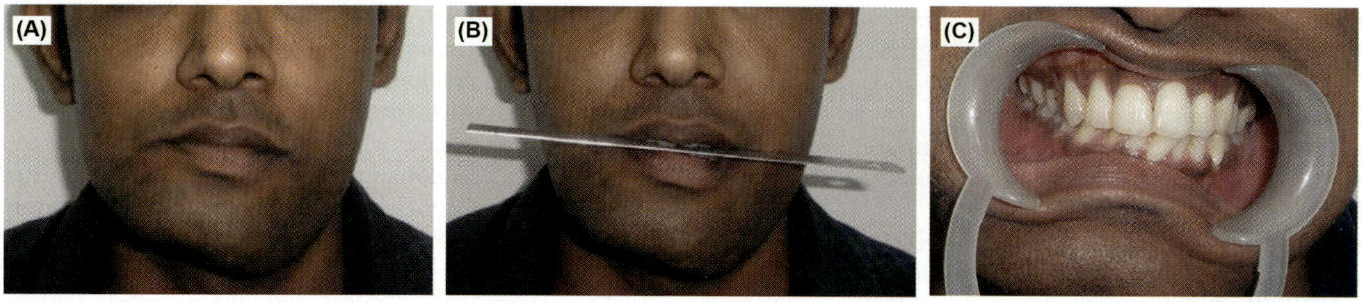

Figure 39.5 Hemimandibular hyperplasia. (**A**) Hemimandibular hyperplasia on the left side—note the bowing of the inferior border of the mandible on the left side. (**B**) Occlusal cant on the left side. (**C**) Downward growth of the maxillary and mandibular teeth on the left side.

Radiographic features

Asymmetry and bone density can be measured using CT and MRI scans, which are recommended to assess the occurrence of active growth.

- Increase in length of the ramus and increased height of the body of the mandible (distance between the tooth roots and inferior alveolar nerve canal)
- Enlarged condylar head with elongated and thick condylar neck
- Vertical downward displacement of the lower border of the mandible
- Rounded angle of mandible
- Inferior alveolar canal is displaced towards the lower border of the mandible
- Clear demarcation of the anomaly at the symphysis region.

Management

Treatment should be based on the degree of asymmetry, malocclusion, growth activity of the condyle and the patient's age. Treatment is primarily surgical and followed by orthodontics to correct occlusion. Condylar surgery (condylotomy, condyloplasty) during the growth period will arrest or retard the growth, thus limiting the amount of secondary anatomical distortion.

The treatment protocols are as follows:

1. High condylectomy to arrest the condylar growth
2. Articular disc repositioning
3. Concomitant orthognathic surgery:
   - Intraoral vertical ramus osteotomy
   - Maxillary Le Fort I osteotomy
   - Mandibular contouring.

If at the time of diagnosis, the maxilla is also affected, then two jaw surgeries may be necessary. The *orthodontic treatment should precede* and follow the surgical treatment for the end-stage corrections. The secondary canting of the maxillary plane can be corrected by means of a Le Fort I osteotomy. The bowing of the lower border of the mandible is resected intraorally. Care must be taken to determine the exact position of the mandibular canal prior to operation; it can be accurately marked out and the neurovascular bundle dissected prior to the completion of the horizontal osteotomy. A compensatory sliding genioplasty will sometimes be necessary in addition to other mandibular surgical procedures.

COMBINATION OF TYPES I AND II (HEMIMANDIBULAR ELONGATION AND HYPERPLASIA)

It is possible to have a combination of HMH on one side and HME on the other side (Fig. 39.6).

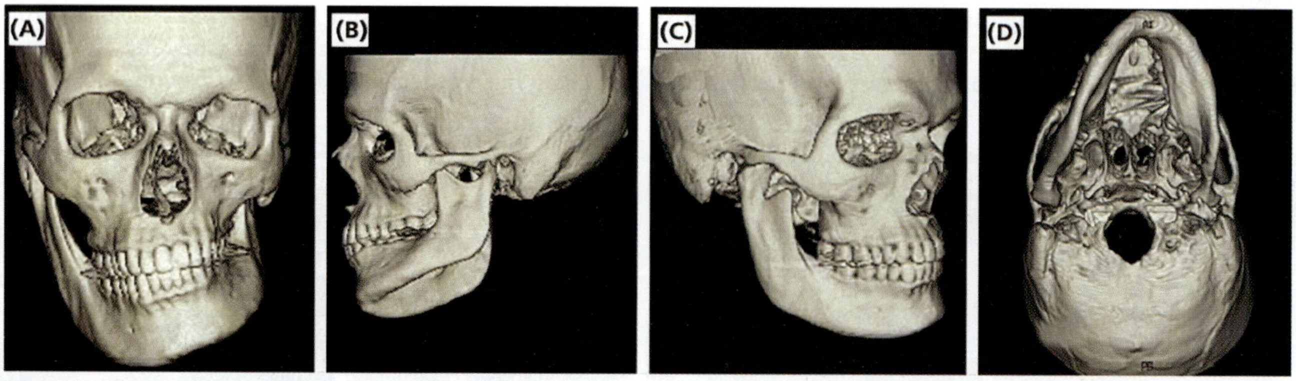

Figure 39.6 3D CT showing combinations of hemimandibular hyperplasia and elongation. (**A**) Hemimandibular hyperplasia and elongation on the right side. (**B**) Left side normal. (**C**) Right side hyperplasia and elongation of the mandible. (**D**) Base of the skull—notice the hyperplasia and elongation of the mandible on the right side.

BOX 39.2 TMJ Benign Tumours Arising from Bone

- Osteochondroma
- Chondroma
- Chondroblastoma
- Synovial chondromatosis
- Osteoma
- Osteoid osteoma
- Osteoblastoma
- Giant cell tumour
- Haemangioma
- Lipoma
- Ossifying fibroma

The clinical features are as follows:

- Chin deviation towards contralateral side with a sloping rima oris
- Midline shift
- Possible open bite and/or cross bite
- Excessive growth in vertical and horizontal vectors
- Enlarged condylar head, neck and ramus
- Irregularly shaped condylar head, neck and/or ramus.

NEOPLASIA

Neoplasia is abnormal and excessive tissue proliferation. Neoplasms that arise from the TMJ are extremely rare and may be benign or malignant (Box 39.2). TMJ tumours may arise from three potential sites:

1. Intrinsic tissue of TMJ
2. Extension of tumours from adjacent tissues such as parotid gland
3. Distant metastatic spread to the joint.

Clinical features

The majority of tumours manifest unilaterally with preauricular oedema and TMJ dysfunction including discomfort, trismus, malocclusion and mandibular deviation to the afflicted side.

Depending on the kind of tumour, radiographs may reveal a normal-sized condyle, an enlarged condyle, or bone disintegration.

Treatment

Alternative treatments for benign TMJ tumours include curettage, resection or excision, and cryotherapy. Resection may be followed with TMJ reconstruction, which has a significant impact on facial symmetry, TMJ function, and the patient's postoperative quality of life. Surgery remains the most important therapeutic option for malignant tumours. Surgery with chemotherapy used as adjuvant therapy for advanced-stage tumours and metastatic disease.

GROWTH DISORDERS OF MUSCLE (CONGENITAL AND DEVELOPMENTAL)

Muscle disorders can be broadly divided into three categories:

- Hypotrophy (muscle weakening), for example, muscular dystrophy, myasthenia gravis and multiple sclerosis
- Hypertrophy (over development), for example, prolonged bruxism
- Neoplasms (uncontrolled, destructive growth), for example, rhabdomyoma.

Aetiology

Muscle disorders are associated with several causes. Muscular dystrophy is often a set of genetic disorders, while hypertrophy is frequently caused by overuse. The pathogenesis of neoplastic muscular diseases is unknown and additional research is required. Neoplasms of the masticatory muscle are relatively rare and may be benign or malignant.

Clinical characteristics

Muscular hypotrophy is often difficult to diagnose and commonly presents with a feeling of muscle weakness. Hypertrophic muscles rarely produce any symptom but can be observed as large muscle (masseter) or concerned with aesthetics. Patients are generally unaware of the disorder as they produce slow changes. The mandibular movement is likely to be present within the normal range.

Neoplasms of the jaw muscles are apparent as a hard, well-circumscribed, slow-growing, painless, palpable mass in one of the muscles. They typically appear in the palate, tongue, floor of the mouth, larynx, throat or uvula. The malignant tumours metastasise rapidly and usually interfere with jaw function.

Treatment

Muscle disorders should be treated according to the severity of the condition. The goal of therapy is to restore function and appearance while minimising trauma to the surrounding tissues. A stabilisation appliance is the best way to address hypertrophy caused by bruxism. Botulinum toxin-A injections diminish the size of the masseter and temporalis muscles. The presence of neoplastic activity is aggressively addressed.

Section XI

Neurological Disorders of Maxillofacial Region

Chapter

40

Sensory and Motor Disturbances of the Orofacial Region

OUTLINE

Allodynia: Pain caused to a stimuli, which usually does not provoke pain.

Analgesia: Absence of pain to stimuli, which normally causes pain.

Causalgia: Chronic progressive disease causing persistent burning pain. Following nerve injury, allodynia and hyperpathia may occur; initially, there is vasomotor and pseudomotor dysfunction, which later progresses to atrophic changes.

Dysaesthesia: An obnoxious, abnormal sensation, may be spontaneous or evoked.

Hyperaesthesia: Elevated response to stimuli, this excludes response of special senses.

Hyperalgesia: An exaggerated response to normally painful stimuli.

Hyperpathia: A symptom associated with some neurological disorder characterised by elevated response to stimuli mainly when the stimuli is of high threshold and repetitive in nature.

Neuralgia: Pain in the areas specific to the nerve supply.

Neuritis: Inflammation of the nerve or nerves.

Neuropathy: Any changes in a nerve that creates a pathologic or functional dysfunction.

Nociception: Pain perception resulting from stimulation of nociceptors.

Nociceptor: A sensory receptor that responds to any damaging stimuli or normal stimuli, which may become damaging if it is prolonged.

Paraesthesia: Tingling or pins and needle sensation caused usually due to incomplete reinnervation.

Pain threshold: The lowest stimuli potential at which the pain is perceived by the individual.

Pain tolerance level: The highest stimuli potential that the subject can tolerate.

SENSORY DISTURBANCES OF THE FACE

Sensory disturbances of the face and jaws are altered or impaired sensations like paraesthesia or dysaesthesia caused due to injury to the trigeminal nerve, which transmits the sensations of the face (Refer Chapter 42, Fig. 42.2). **Classification of disorders of the nerve** are depicted in Box 40.1.

ANATOMY OF THE PERIPHERAL NERVE

Neuron is an excitable cell, which consists of nerve cell body and all its processes that is specialised for reception of stimuli and conduction of the nerve impulses. They vary in size and shape, but each possesses a cell body from whose surface projects one or more processes called neurites. The neurites are further classified into axons and dendrites.

PARTS OF THE NEURON (Figs. 40.1 and 40.2)

1. **Nerve cell body:** It is a mass of cytoplasm in which the nucleus is embedded. It is bounded externally by a plasma membrane
2. **Dendrites**: The nerve cell has five to seven processes called dendrites that extend outward from the cell body and arborise extensively
3. **Axon**: A neuron has a long fibrous axon that originates from the axon hillock of the cell body

BOX 40.1 Classification of Disorders of the Nerve

1. **Traumatic injuries**
   a. Neurapraxia
   b. Axonotmesis
   c. Neurotmesis
   d. Traumatic neuroma
2. **Inflammation**
   a. Neuritis
3. **Neuralgias**
   a. Trigeminal nerve neuralgia
   b. Bell's palsy
   c. Glossopharyngeal neuralgia
   d. Sphenopalatine neuralgia
4. **Specific types of injuries**
   a. Injection injuries
   b. Irradiation
   c. Compression neuropathies
5. **Tumours**
   a. Benign and malignant

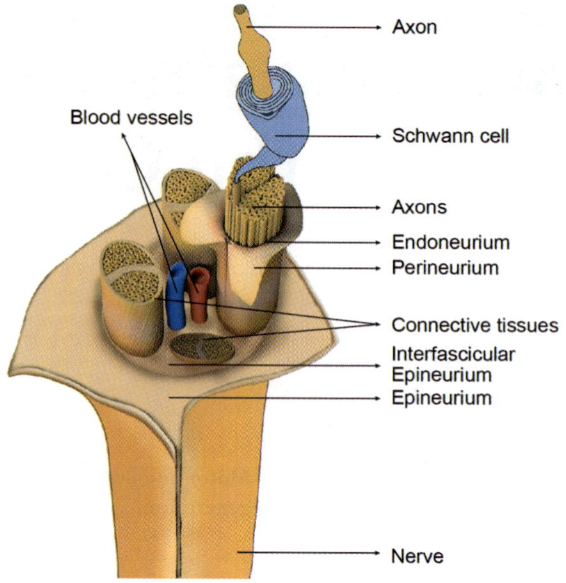

Figure 40.1 Nerve anatomy.

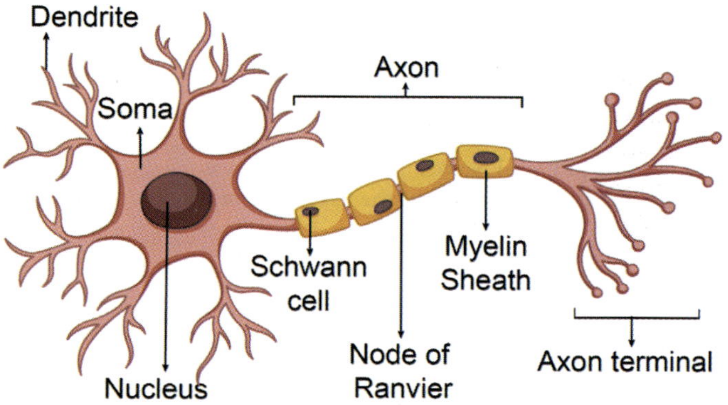

Figure 40.2 Multipolar neuron.

4. **Axon hillock:** Thickened area of the cell body
5. **Initial segment:** The 1st portion of the axon
6. **Synaptic knobs:** The axon is divided into terminal branches, each ending in a number of synaptic knobs. They contain synaptic vesicles or granules, which contain synaptic transmitters, which are secreted by the nerves and stored
7. **Myelinated neurons:** Outside the CNS, the axon is myelinated, that is the axon acquires a sheath of myelin, a protein-lipid complex made up of many layers of the cell membrane of Schwann's cells
8. **Nodes of Ranvier:** The myelin sheath envelops the axon except at the endings and nodes of Ranvier. They are periodic 1 mm constrictions that are about 1 mm apart
9. **Epineurium:** The epineurium is the outermost covering of a peripheral nerve. The epineurium is made of areolar connective tissue and has numerous blood vessels, which supply the peripheral nerve. Though highly dense collateral supply is provided to the nerve, disruption in blood supply may occur causing many kinds of nerve injuries

TABLE 40.1 Types of Nerve Fibres

Fibre Types		Diameter (mu)	CV (m/s)	Functions
A	α	12–20	100	Proprioception, somatomotor
	β	5–12	30–70	Touch, pressure
	γ	3–6	15–30	Motor to muscle spindle
	δ	2–5	12–30	Pain especially cold, touch
B		<3	3–15	Preganglionic autonomic
C		0.4–1.2	0.5–2	Thermal pain, mechanoreceptor
		0.3–1.3	0.7–2.3	Postganglionic autonomic

10. **Nerve fibres:** Nerve fibres occupy 25%–75% of the cross-section of a nerve. The composition of nerve fibre in a nerve varies depending on the type and location. They may be myelinated or unmyelinated. The myelinated nerve fibres are thicker (2–25 mm) than the unmyelinated fibres (0.2–3 mm). The types of nerve fibres are presented in Table 40.1
11. **Fascicles:** Clusters of nerve fibres, which form bundles are called fascicles. The fascicle is covered by perineurium. From the surgical aspect, the perineurium is the smallest structure in peripheral nerve where the sutures are placed. Fascicular diameter ranges from 0.04 to 3 mm. Fascicles are organised as a single fascicle or in bands as they course along the nerve. The fascicles are embedded in epineural connective tissue and epifascicular interfascicular epineurium. Peripheral nerves are classified as monofascicular, oligofascicular and polyfascicular. Monofascicular nerves such as the terminal branches of digital nerves have one main fascicle with many small nerve fibres. They are generally either pure sensory or pure motor in function. Oligofascicular nerves have less number of fascicles and may be pure or mixed with both sensory and motor functions. Example: Ulnar nerve at the elbow. Polyfascicular nerves consist of a number of minute fascicles. Example: Radial nerve in the upper arm.

TRAUMATIC NERVE INJURIES

Nerve injury can be caused due to direct or indirect trauma like in fracture and iatrogenic causes like compression or stretching of the nerve during extraction, implant placement, bone grafting, orthognathic surgery, laceration or chemical injuries caused during procedures like chemical irrigation in infected lesions or local infiltration of anaesthetics. It can be as mild as just inflammation of the nerve–neuritis or more severe nerve injury.

NEURITIS—INFLAMMATION

'Neuritis' is the term applied to describe inflammation of a peripheral nerve, mostly associated with degenerative changes in nervous tissue. Multiple neuritis or polyneuritis is a disease, which symmetrically affects most of the peripheral nerves simultaneously.

Types: (1) Localised and (2) multiple/polyneuritis

Aetiology:

1. Localised:
    a. Exposure to cold
    b. Following trauma to a nerve
    c. Stretching of a nerve
    d. Nerve may share extension of neighbouring inflammation
    e. Vascular lesions, for example, occlusion of a blood vessel or haemorrhage into the nervous tissue
2. Generalised:
    a. Infection–due to invasion of microorganisms
    b. Toxic–metallic or chemical poisoning, alcoholic
    c. Metabolic–vitamin deficiencies, pernicious anaemia
    d. General disorders–gout, rheumatism, tubercle, carcinoma
    e. Autoimmune diseases in which the body's natural defences attack the peripheral nerves, for example, systemic lupus erythematosus (SLE), idiopathic peripheral neuropathy (in case of autoimmune diseases, the peripheral nerves are damaged by the auto antibodies)
    f. Diabetes mellitus
    g. Toxaemia of pregnancy.

Signs and symptoms of neuritis

- In localised neuritis, the patient complains of pain of boring character along the course and distribution of the nerve
- On examination, the involved region is slightly erythematous and sensitive to pressure; oedema and painful muscular movement along the affected nerve
- Numbness, loss of tactile function is noted as the disease progresses, finally resulting in muscular atrophy
- Degeneration occurs in the nerve or nerve sheath
- Mild cases such as exposure to cold or injury may recover in a few days
- Severe cases such as those damaged by the pressure of an unreduced fracture may last for months.

CLASSIFICATION OF NERVE INJURIES—MOTOR AND SENSORY

SEDDON'S CLASSIFICATION (1943)

H. J. Seddon propounded that the clinical symptoms caused depend on the extent of nerve damage. He coined the terms neuropraxia, axonotmesis and neurotmesis in 1942 with Prof. Henry Cohen and gave a complete description of the classification in 1943. A summary of the classification compared with the Sunderland's classification is described in Table 40.2.

TABLE 40.2 A Summary of the Classifications of Nerve Injuries, their Pathology and Prognosis has been Described

Seddon's Classification	Neuropraxia	Axonotmesis	Neurotmesis		
Illustration depicting Seddon's classification	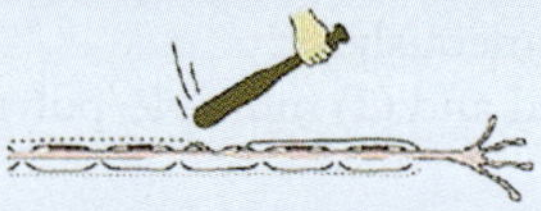	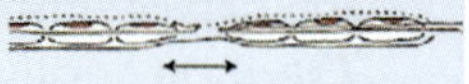	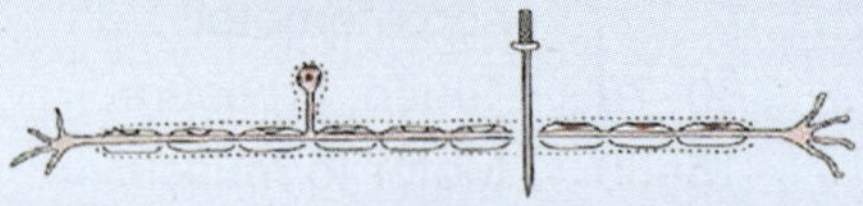		
Sunderland's classification	**1st degree—myelin**	**2nd degree—axon**	**3rd degree—endoneurium**	**4th degree—perineurium**	**5th degree—epineurium**
Illustration depicting Sunderland's classification	1st degree 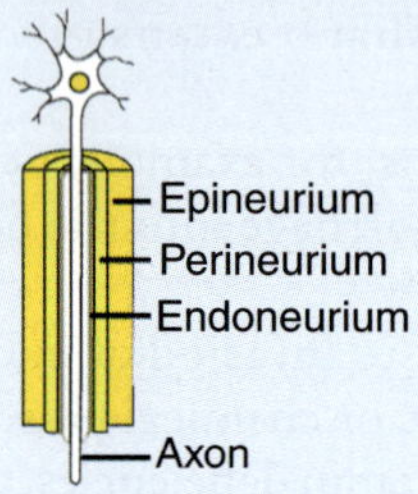	2nd degree 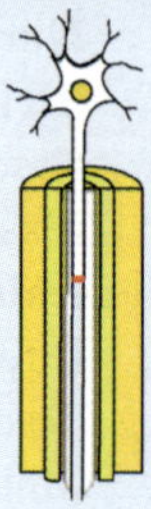	3rd degree 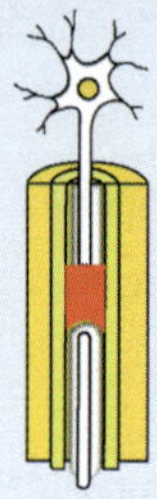	4th degree 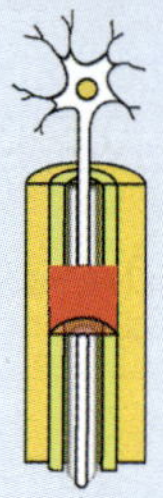	5th degree 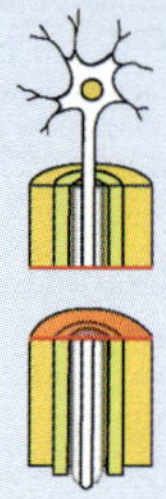
Pathology of nerve sheath	Myelin injury	Endoneurium tube is still intact Intact epineurium and perineurium	Neural tube is disrupted. Loss in continuity of the endoneurium	Epineurium remains intact Perineurium, endoneurium	Interrupted endoneurium, perineurium and epineurium
Axon	Intact but disruption of axons	Disrupted	Axonal destruction	Axon disrupted	Disruption of axons
Wallerian degeneration	No Wallerian degeneration occurs	Partial Wallerian degeneration occurs on distal axon from the site of injury	Partial Wallerian degeneration occurs	Partial Wallerian degeneration occurs	Complete Wallerian degeneration occurs
Conduction block	Transitory conduction block caused by cessation of axoplasmic flow	Prolonged conduction block	Prolonged conduction block	Prolonged conduction block	Permanent conduction block
Prognosis	Good prognosis Excellent recovery	Full recovery Expected	Poor prognosis Surgery may be required. If regeneration occurs, there will be high incidence of synkinesis (abnormal mass movement of muscles which do not normally contract together)	Poor functional outcome with higher risk for synkinesis Surgery usually required	Surgery required Little chance of regeneration Risk of neuroma formation
Recovery type and time	Complete recovery Within 24 h to 8 weeks Type I 1st degree—24 h Type II 1st degree—1 to 2 days Type III 1st degree—1 to 2 months	Partial recovery can take 2–4 months improves over 8–10 months and complete recovery 12 months	Partial recovery can take months	Partial recovery can take months	Poor recovery—if recovery can happen begins at 3 months

Neuropraxia

In neuropraxia, there is a break in impulse transmission down the nerve fibre and recovery takes place without Wallerian degeneration. It is described as a mild, temporary injury of the nerve. There is no axonal degeneration or demyelination distal to the site of injury. The aetiologic injury for neuropraxia are tractional forces to the nerve like retraction, compression, direct blunt injuries, intermittent or sudden compression, intermittent exposure to freezing temperatures or interfascicular oedema. Anoxia due to intermittent blood supply of epineurial or endoneurial blood vessels can cause a temporary conduction block, that is loss of sensation and motor function. Spontaneous complete recovery of the sensations occurs within 24 h or up to 4 weeks. Surgical intervention is not required for neuropraxia.

Axonotmesis

This is a more significant injury as there is a disruption in the continuity of some of the axons. The injured axons undergo Wallerian degeneration. Usually, there are no other disruptions, the epineurium, perineurium and endoneurium are not injured in axonotmesis. Conduction block prolongs until regeneration of the affected axons. The aetiologic injuries include direct blunt injury, combined traction and compressive forces causing friction, exposure to freezing temperatures. Local chemical poisoning (injection of certain drugs) and crush injuries. Proximal lesion may grow distally as fast as 2 to 3 mm/day and distal lesion as slowly as 1.5 mm/day.

Anterograde (Wallerian) ascending degeneration of axons—when an axon of the central nervous system is severed—**axotomy**, its distal (ascending) segment, being separated from its cell body, quickly degenerates and disappears and its investing myelin sheath undergoes a slower breakdown into simpler lipids that are eventually catabolised. This process is called anterograde or **Wallerian degeneration** (Fig. 40.3). It occurs on the axon distal to the site of damage (farther from the cell body). *Stage 1 Axonal degeneration:* The axon swells up, becomes irregular and breaks down into fragments. *Stage 2 Myelin clearance:* These fragments—debris are digested by the surrounding Schwann's cells and macrophages. This process takes up to 1 week for complete destruction of the affected part of the axon.

Neurotmesis

Aetiologic injury is cut wounds, bullet wounds, iatrogenic injury with bone drills or saw, retraction and tractional forces to the nerve, direct blunt injury, crush injury and local chemical poisoning. The epineurium, perineurium and endoneurium are injured in neurotmesis at varying degrees depending on the injury. Complete Wallerian degeneration occurs distal to the injury. Permanent conduction block occurs (loss of sensation and motor function). The proximal part of the nerve becomes a scar—a nerve stump. Without surgical intervention, rejoining of the proximal segment with the distal segment and recovery is not possible.

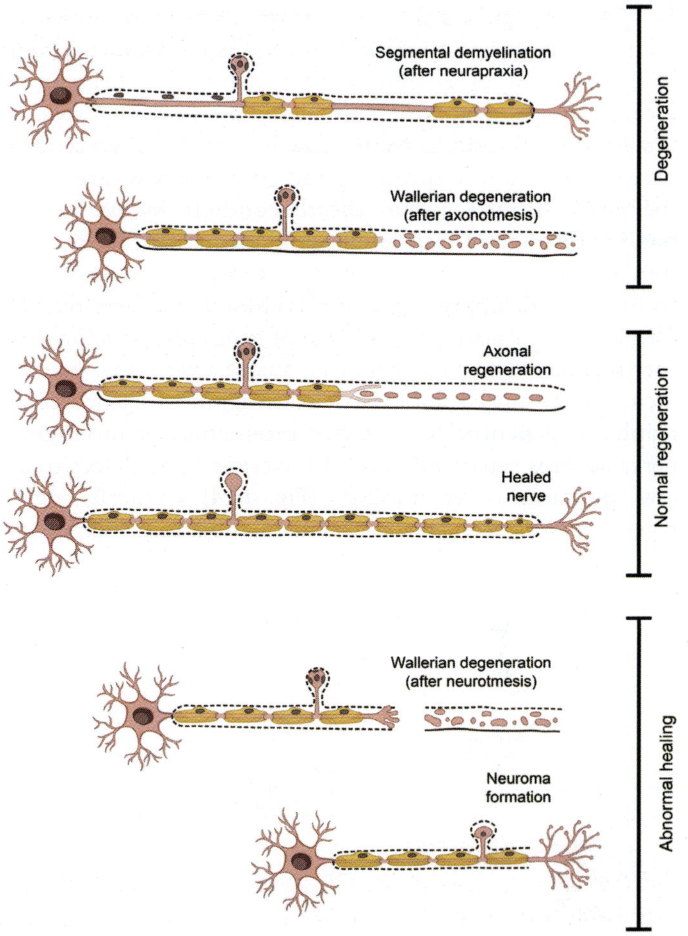

Figure 40.3 Response of the nerve fibre to different types of injuries.

PHYSIOLOGY OF NERVE HEALING—REGENERATION

The Schwann's cells surround both myelinated (one Schwann's cell per nerve fibre) and unmyelinated (one Schwann's cell per several nerve fibres) nerves, and they play a major role in nerve survival and regeneration following injury. The myelin sheath does not survive a nerve injury, but the Schwann's cells do and they provide a supportive role in the production of neurotropic factors (such as nerve growth factor) that enhance neural recovery. Nerve healing involves both degeneration and regeneration. The nerve cell body responds with an increased metabolic phase with a heightened production of RNA (protein synthesis) and breakdown of **Nissl's substance** for export from the cell body with the accumulation of particulate cellular debris. Within days, axonal sprouts begin to bud and extend from the proximal nerve stump in the area of injury. Each axon may have as many as

50 collateral sprouts from the proximal nerve stump with random orientation towards the distal nerve stump. A high level of activity of Schwann's cells occurs, which begin to form new myelin 'conduits' in anticipation of the arrival of the new axonal sprouts. Nerve growth factors produced influence the direction of sprouting and guide the new axons into the newly formed myelin sheath conduits known as the **bands of Büngner** in the event spontaneous neural regeneration will occur. If one or more of the reparative processes fail to occur at the appropriate time and location, there may be formation of a neuroma and lack of spontaneous neurosensory recovery. This failure may be due to a variety of reasons including advanced local tissue scarring, insufficient neurotrophic and neurotrophic factor production or misaligned nerve stumps separated beyond the critical size defect to allow spontaneous reconnection (Fig. 40.4). Clinically, nerve regeneration is monitored by electroneurographic diagnostic studies or electroneurography (ENoG), which is a neurological noninvasive test. The patient also presents with a tingling sensation on percussion over the divided nerve in the area supplied by the injured peripheral nerve called **Tinel's sign**.

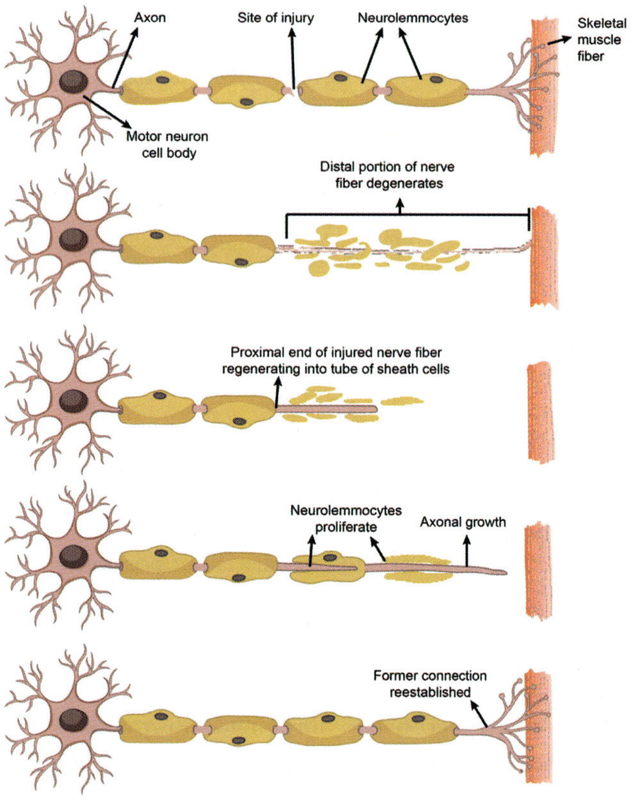

Figure 40.4 Neural wound healing mechanisms.

NEUROPATHIC EVENTS AFTER NERVE INJURY

Neuropathic events after nerve injury manifest clinically as anaesthesia dolorosa, causalgia, allodynia and hyperpathia. Pathological events that follow nerve injury are as follows:

1. Collateral macro-sprouting
2. Peripheral neuroma
3. Cervical sympathetic pathosis
4. Central pathosis.

Neuromas

A neuroma is caused due to local injury to peripheral nerves, which presents as a painful, submucosal bump. Most neuromas are surgically excised. Neuroma is not classified as a tumour; it is only a series of changes taking place after a local injury to the peripheral nerve. They are the consequences of disrupting a peripheral nerve during surgery or trauma. After recovery, the regenerated nerve fibres arrange themselves in a disorganised manner as they are unable to penetrate into the severed nerve sheath. This results in the formation of a painful disorganised mass in the area of injury. Nerve regeneration is stimulated by Schwann's cells and trophic factors as nerve growth factors. There is exaggerated expression of these trophic factors in neuroma formation. The result is stump neuroma or amputation neuroma.

Histological features of traumatic neuromas include presence of clusters of small peripheral nerve fibres, a feature which differentiates it from neurilemmoma and neurofibroma. Traumatic neuroma is surgically excised. Recurrence is rare and there is no risk of malignant transformation.

Types of neuromas

Neuromas are classified by gross morphology into the following types:

- Amputation (stump) neuroma—seen in 5 degrees Sunderland's nerve injury
- Neuroma-in-continuity (central or fusiform neuroma)—seen in 4 degrees nerve injury
- Eccentric neuromas are of three types on the inferior alveolar nerve—lateral exophytic neuroma, lateral adhesive neuromas and stellate neuroma (Fig. 40.5).

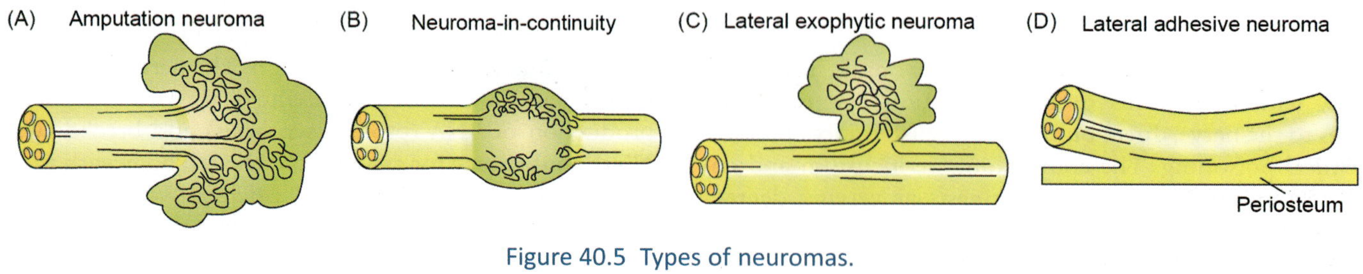

Figure 40.5 Types of neuromas.

PATIENT EVALUATION

HISTORY TAKING

Proper history plays an important role in diagnosis. The patient with nerve injury presents with chief complaints such as difficulty in mastication, speech and maintaining oral hygiene. They may present with decreased taste sensation, drooling, lip, cheek, tongue biting, altered sensation and numbness, all these leading to decreased sensation of self-confidence. The patient presents with a history of trauma or a surgical procedure at or near the site of nerve injury. The symptoms are progressive in nature and the process of recovery may have started, indicated with Tinel's sign.

ASSESSMENTS USED IN NERVE INJURY

1. Questionnaire for quantitative assessment of posttraumatic trigeminal neuropathy: It has a scoring chart, which can be used to compare the recovery at every patient review
2. Questionnaire for assessment of functional impairment: Difficulty in functions like smiling, swallowing and talking are listed out and scores are given to rate the functional impairment as 0%—none, 25%—mild, 50%—moderate, 75%—severe, 100%—total functional impairment
3. Questionnaire for assessment of pain and discomfort: Various questions related to pain are asked and scoring of which as 0%—no discomfort, 25%—mild pain, 50%—moderate pain, 75%—severe pain and 100%—intolerable pain.

These assessments and history taking provides with two categories of patients that helps in treatment plan (Flowchart 40.1).

CLINICAL EXAMINATION

Patients presenting with paraesthesia undergo clinical neurosensory testing (NST), which helps in the treatment planning. It should be performed within 2 weeks from nerve injury, and with the baseline finding, a follow-up can be performed. The disadvantage of NST is the tests being subjective, results can differ with every individual.

CLINICAL NEUROSENSORY TESTING FOR PERIPHERAL NERVE INJURIES

These tests are performed on the patient in a calm room without any photogenic or sound stimulation. The pain-free normal side is used as control for the tests. NST for paraesthesia is divided into three levels as explained in the illustration (Fig. 40.6).

MANAGEMENT

Early treatment in acute nerve injury prevents chronic refractory neuropathies. Dysfunctional sensory defects should be treated within 90 days. Early nerve injury is treated by removing the aetiologic factor causing secondary nerve injury and

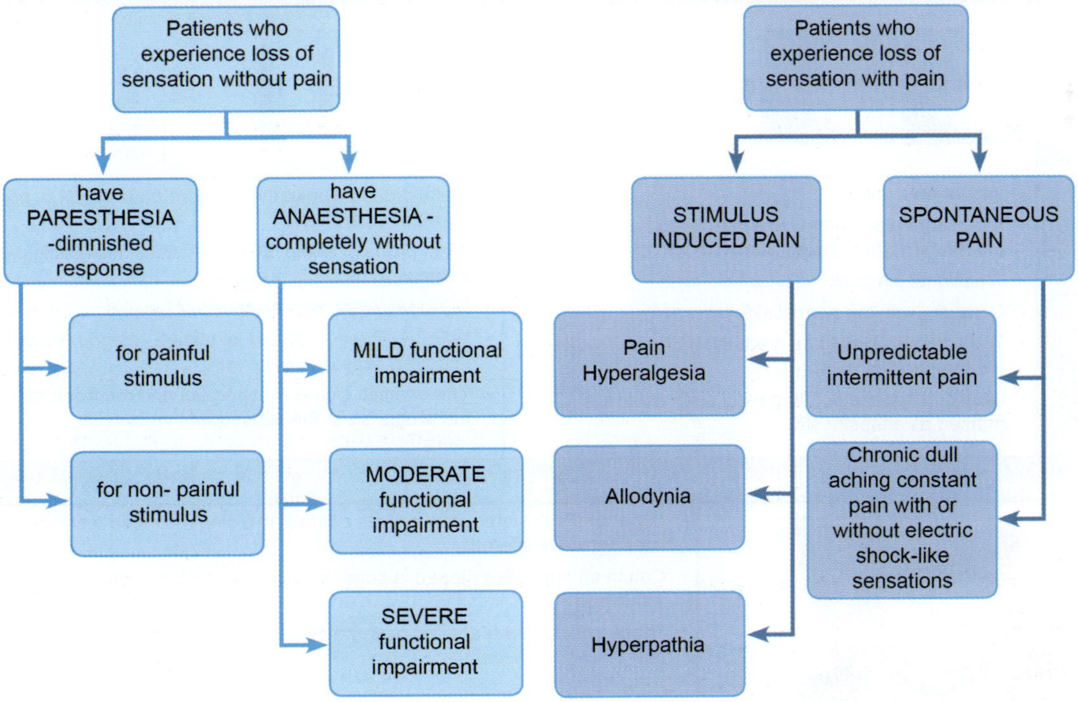

Flowchart 40.1 Two types of patients derived from history taking and questionnaires. Patients without pain can present with paraesthesia and anaesthesia and those with pain presenting with pain hyperalgesia—an exaggerated sharp pain response, allodynia—pain caused to stimulus, which usually does not provoke pain and hyperpathia—a symptom associated with some neurological disorder characterised by elevated response to stimuli, mainly when the stimuli is of high threshold and repetitive in nature.

	TACTILE BRUSH STROKE DETECTION		**TWO - POINT DISCRIMINATION**
	Step 1	**Step 2**	**Step 3**
Level A Evaluation by Tactile Brush stroke and two-point discrimination	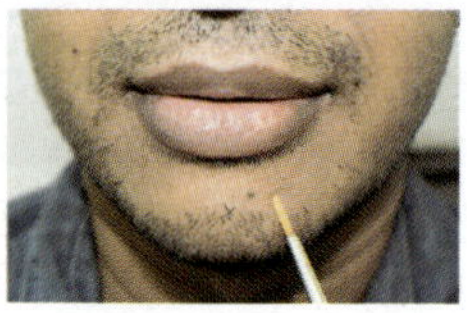	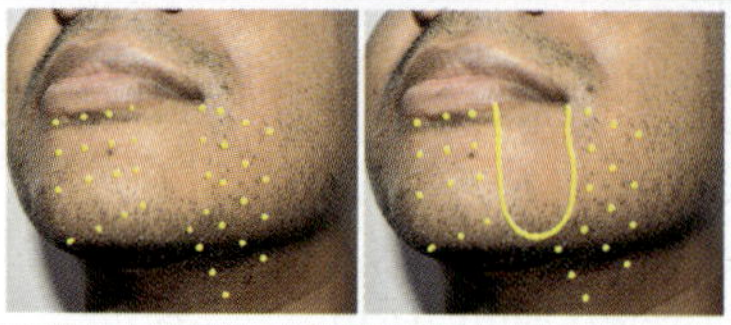	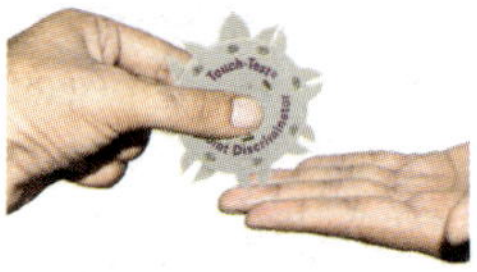
	• Soft camel brush (0.75 x 0.5 cm) is stroked in all four directions • Brush is moved from unaffected area to affected area • Patient indicates when the brush can no longer be felt • Topographic recording is marked with skin pencil as grids	**ABNORMAL SENSATIONS** • A dot is marked in the centre of each grid • The patient has to identify the direction of the brush atleast 12 out of 15 times • If not, it is marked as decreased sensation	• A two- point anesthesiometer or Boley gauge - caliper is used to determine the degree of tactile sensitivity. • The distance between the points are increased in an increament of 2 mm untill the patient can differentiate the two points
Level B Evaluation by contact detection using a Semmes-Wienstein filament also called Von Frey's hair fibres	**Static light touch detection**	**Touch detection**	**Brush direction discrimination**
	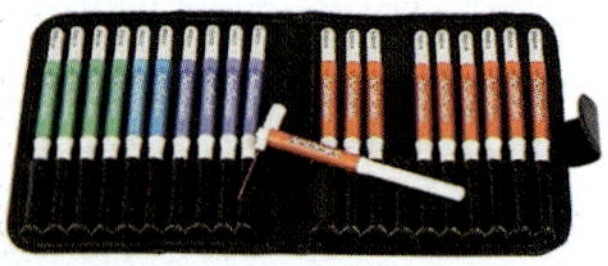	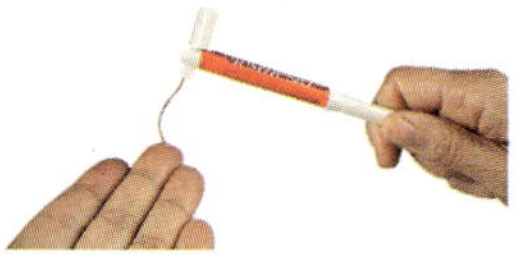	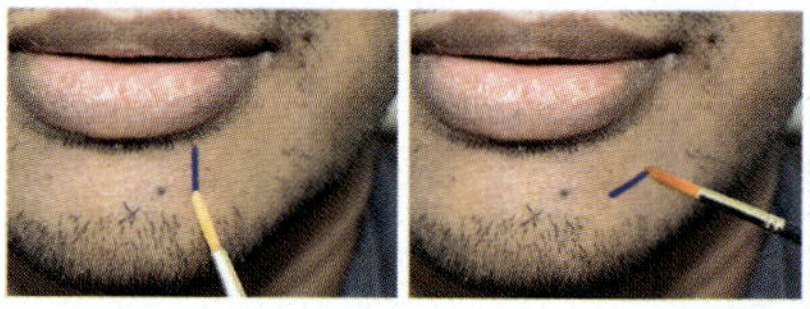
	• Level of contact is determined by Semmes- Wienstein filaments or Von Frey's hair filaments	• The patient is blindfolded and notifies when touch sensation is felt • The filament is placed perpendicular to the skin tested and pressed until the filament bends for 1 - 1.5 seconds	• A small soft brush is used to stroke the skin tested over 1 cm area • The patient has to discriminate the area and direction of sensation
Level C Evaluation by response to mecahnical noxious stimuli and thermal noxious stimuli	**Response to mechanical noxious stimuli**	**Response to thermal noxious stimuli**	
	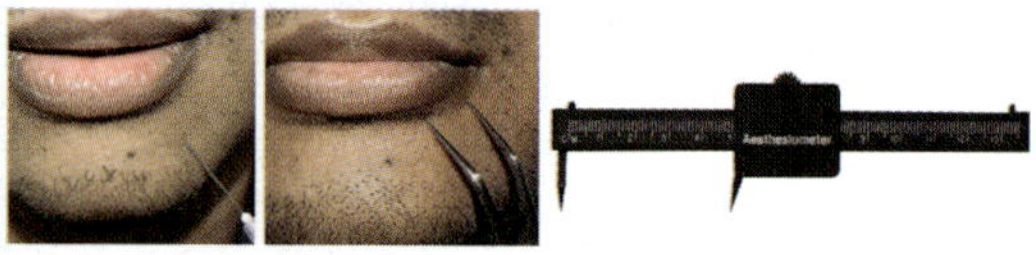	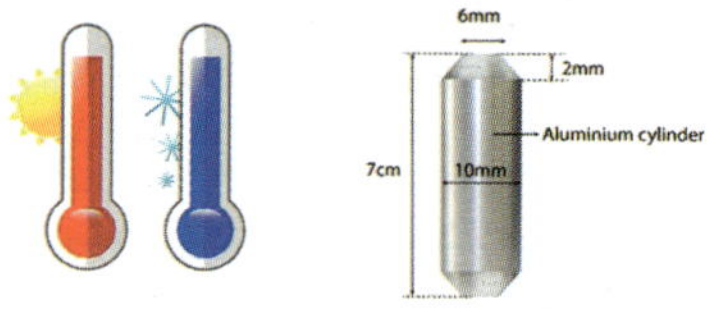	
	• Instruments used • A pressure algometer with a needle and an orthodontic strain gauge with 15 to 150 gms of force • Traditional pin prick • Compare with the normal side • The pressure should be gradually increased to note the threshold of pain • Lack of response at 100 gms of pin pressure is marked as anaesthesia	• Metal probes dipped in hot (more than 40° C) or cold (less than 20° C) are used • A hot probe of about 50° C will cause intolerable pain but no damage to tissue is present • NORMAL response - diagnosis of Level B • IMPAIRED response to Hot stimuli - diagnosed as severely impaired sensation at Level C • The affected skin is mapped out and recorded for analysing the prognosis in the subsequent visits	
Final clinical neurosensory test for lingual nerve damage			
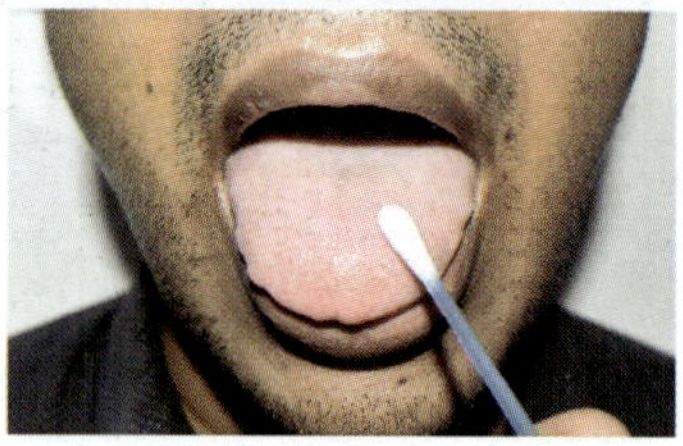	• Sugar and salt water breakers are offered as a single-blinded test (Patient does not know which is offered) • Cotton tip applicator dipped in sugar solution first and then salt solution after rinsing with water • These solutions are applied over the affected area and affected area are mapped out		

Figure 40.6 The neurosensory tests for paraesthesia may be broken down into three different levels based on the severity; levels A–C. Lingual nerve neurosensory test has also been illustrated.

by creating an optimal environment for nerve regeneration. The surgical re-suturing of a divided nerve is called neurorrhaphy. It should not be performed when an active infection is present. Any offending agent like implant, foreign body or bony fragments should be removed from impinging the nerve to allow recovery.

MEDICAL MANAGEMENT (TABLE 40.3)

SURGICAL MANAGEMENT

The repair requires magnification of the surgical site with 3× or 6× surgical loupes or with an operating microscope for the proper alignment and anastomosis of nerve segments. The timing of repair plays a vital role and the techniques for microsurgical repair are discussed subsequently (Box 40.2).

TIMING OF NERVE REPAIR

Primary or immediate repair:

- The repair is done immediately after injury usually an iatrogenic injury, which is during surgical procedures like orthognathic, implant, reconstruction, impaction surgeries and trauma

TABLE 40.3 Medical Management

Type of Medication	Mechanism of Action	Systemic Medication for Acute Nerve Injury and Neuropathic Pain	Topical Medication for Neuropathic Pain
Anaesthetic	To minimise pain	Local anaesthesia—nerve blocks—2% lidocaine	5% Lidocaine gel or transcutaneous patch, 20% Benzocaine gel, 2.5% Prilocaine
Corticosteroids	Nerve injury causes perineural inflammation during the 1st week It is decreased by corticosteroids	Dexamethasone 8–12 mg/day	-
Rapid acting anticonvulsants	To protect the CNS	Clonazepam 2–10 mg/day	-
Neuropeptides	Decreases reaccumulation of substance P, thus hinders transmission of pain impulses to the brain	-	0.025% Capsaicin cream
NSAIDs—nonsteroidal antiinflammatory drugs	Inhibition of the enzyme COX—cyclooxygenase	Diclofenac 150 mg/day Ketorolac 60 mg/day	Ketoprofen or Diclofenac 10%–20% PLO base
Sympathomimetics	-	-	Clonidine 0.01% PLO base or patch
N-methyl-D-aspartate receptor antagonist	Inhibits dopamine and serotonin reuptake	Ketamine 10–25 mg TDS	Ketamine 0.5% PLO base
Anticonvulsants	-	Carbamazepine - initial dosage 200 mg, then maintain at 600mg. Maximum dosage 1200mg/day	Carbamazepine 2% PLO base
Tricyclic antidepressants	Blocks serotonin and norepinephrine reuptake	Amitriptyline initial dose 10 mg gradual increase to maximum dose of 150 mg	Amitriptyline 2% PLO base
Muscle relaxants—antispasmodics	A synthetic derivative of GABA inhibitory neurotransmitter	Baclofen initial dose 5 mg BD or TDS	Baclofen 2% PLO base
Opioids	Selective action on opioid receptor and inhibition of norepinephrine and serotonin reuptake	Tramadol 50–100 mg (initial dose) up to 400 mg/day	-

PLO base—pluronic lecithin organogel base is a cream with smooth consistency and stability at room temperature and cooler temperatures. PLO base creams delivers the drugs transdermally better than PLO gel.

BOX 40.2 Microsurgical Techniques for Nerve Repair

Decompression.

Excision of traumatic neuroma.

Internal neurolysis or nerve combing.

Direct re-anastomosis—microsuture repair with neurorrhaphy.

Interpositional graft repair for nerve tissue loss.

- Axonal regeneration is better and may be complete by the 3rd week
- No formation of neuroma or scar can occur when performed correctly
- Surgical loupes are used for this procedure for epineural suturing and alloplastic tubes can help as a guide for nerve regeneration

Delayed primary repair:

- Performed a few weeks after injury after the surgical site has recovered. The procedure is planned for proper nerve exposure and microsurgical repair

Secondary nerve repair:

- Prognosis is much lesser
- Schwann's cell scarring and intraneural and extraneural collagen deposition is increased
- The repair becomes more difficult.

INDICATIONS

- For more than 2 to 3 months after injury
- Neuropathic pain that cannot be treated by medical therapy
- When nerve severance occurs and immediate repair is possible
- For removal of foreign bodies impinging on it or around it
- Nonresponsive anaesthesia or hypoaesthesia
- Presence of neuroma.

CONTRAINDICATIONS

- Signs of improvement by clinical NST
- Spreading regional dysaesthesia
- Secondary hyperalgesia
- Intensifying deafferentation pain
- Presence of infection and/or inflammation
- Medically compromised patients with severe complications for GA
- Delayed nerve repair.

SURGICAL EXPOSURE

Surgical approach to most nerve injuries in the faciomaxillary region are repaired by intraoral approach.

- The **infraorbital nerve**—intraoral maxillary vestibular approach
- **Lingual nerve**—incision on the lingual aspect of the premolars and molars extending superiorly along the internal oblique ridge of the mandibular ramus
- **Mental nerve**—transoral approach—sulcular incision
- **Inferior alveolar nerve**—transoral approach, submandibular approach.

MICROSURGICAL TECHNIQUES FOR NERVE REPAIR

DECOMPRESSION

Decompression is performed when the injured nerve needs to be released from the offending agent like foreign bodies—implant, tooth, bone fragments. Types 1 and 2 Sunderland's injuries are best indicated for decompression. A protective barrier like polyglycolic acid (PGA), collagenous neurocuffs and other alloplastic material can be placed over the injured area of the nerve. After decompression, the injured nerve is inspected for discontinuity, neuromas, loss of vascularisation and for intraneural scarification. This is performed after stabilising the proximal and distal ends with umbilical tapes.

EXCISION OF TRAUMATIC NEUROMA

Traumatic neuroma is excised from the nerve with a Beaver blade 3 mm proximal and distal to the neuroma. Confirmed diagnosis of neuroma is obtained by histopathological examination, which also shows the excision ends with normal herniation of intact fascicles from the epineural nerve endings. The proximal and distal ends are excised at 1 mm thickness till normal fascicles are visualised under frozen sections. The discontinuity defect caused by the excision of the neuroma can be corrected with nerve grafts.

INTERNAL NEUROLYSIS OR NERVE COMBING

For Sunderland types 2 and 3 injuries with mild internal fibrosis, internal neurolysis (nerve combing/neurocombing) has a good prognosis, where the epineurium is incised open and the trigeminal nerve fibres are surgically separated into those from the pons and fibres from the porus trigeminus to remove the scar tissue or the fibrosis around or between the fascicles.

DIRECT RE-ANASTOMOSIS—MICROSUTURE REPAIR WITH NEURORRHAPHY

Short span nerve gap (10–15 mm): Direct re-anastomosis is possible in lingual nerve without autogenous nerve grafting or 'guided nerve regeneration' (GNR). GNR is performed with an alloplastic tube (polytetrafluoroethylene, PGA, silicone, laminin gel collagen) or autogenous tissue like fascia or vein grafts. However, 10–15 mm nerve gap cannot be re-anastomosed in infraorbital, mental and inferior alveolar nerve injury.

INTERPOSITIONAL GRAFT REPAIR FOR NERVE TISSUE LOSS

For greater than 15–20 mm gaps, direct neurorrhaphy is not possible and so autogenous nerve graft from the greater auricular nerve, medial antebrachial cutaneous nerve of the

BOX 40.3 Materials for Entubulation (Conduit) Repair

Autogenous materials:

a. Collagen

b. Muscle

c. Fascia

d. Vein

Alloplastic materials:

a. Polyglycolic acid

b. Polyester

c. PTFE—polytetrafluoroethylene

d. ePTFE—expanded polytetrafluoroethylene

e. Silicone, polymeric silicone

Allogeneic materials:

a. Cadaveric nerve allograft

forearm or the sural nerve of the lower limb can be used as donor graft sites.

POSTOPERATIVE MANAGEMENT AND PROGNOSIS

1. A course of antibiotics is given through the i.v. route
2. Analgesics and fluids are monitored and given appropriately
3. Suture removal over skin is removed after 7 days.

RECENT ADVANCES—NERVE REGENERATION

When nerve injury causes a loss of nerve tissue or when the severed ends cannot reach to be re-anastomosed, a nerve graft is used to replace the nerve deficit. This leaves the donor nerve as a defect. To overcome this, tissue engineering with bioresorbable nerve regeneration guidance conduits are utilised. These are placed around the proximal and distal severed ends by suturing as shown in the figure. These conduits form a path for the nerve to regenerate. The modifications of these conduits are biodegradable polymers, micropatterning polymer surfaces with peptides for controlled release of drugs (Box 40.3). This encourages cell adhesion and axonal outgrowth (Fig. 40.7).

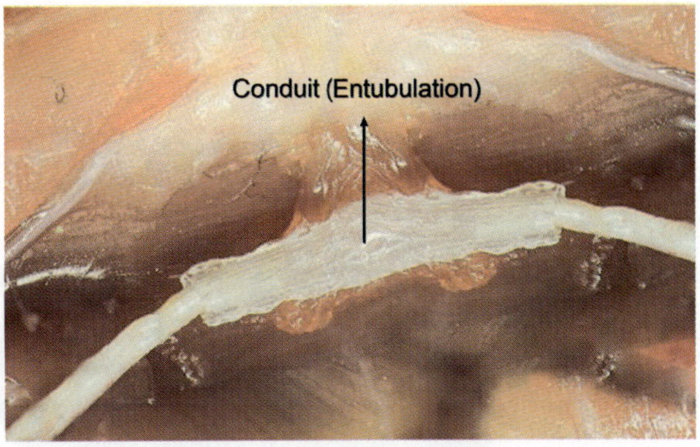

Figure 40.7 Nerve guidance conduits allows regeneration of nerve.

MOTOR DISTURBANCES OF THE FACE

ANATOMY OF FACIAL NERVE

The facial nerve consists of a motor and a sensory part, the latter being frequently described under the name of the nervus intermedius (pars intermedii of Wrisberg).

Branches of facial nerve transmit a combination of sensory, motor and parasympathetic fibres (Fig. 40.8).

COURSES

- Intracranial course
- Extracranial course.

Intracranial course of facial nerve

The nerve arises from the lateral part of the lower border of the pons and begins as two roots: a large motor root and a small sensory root (the part of the facial nerve that arises from the sensory root is sometimes known as the intermediate nerve). Along with the eight cranial nerve, the two roots enter the internal acoustic meatus.

In the meatus, the motor root lies over a groove in the 8th nerve and the sensory branches passes between them. The roots leave the internal acoustic meatus, and enter into the facial canal, which is a 'Z' shaped structure. Within the facial canal, the two roots fuse to form the facial nerve and then the nerve forms the geniculate ganglion (a ganglion is a collection of nerve cell bodies) at the anteroposterior part of promontory.

Later, they give rise to the greater petrosal nerve (parasympathetic fibres to glands), the nerve to stapedius (motor fibres to stapedius muscle) and the chorda tympani (special sensory fibres to the anterior two-thirds tongue).

Extracranial course

The facial nerve exits the skull through the stylomastoid foramen and passes near the lateral border of the styloid process.

The 1st extracranial branch to arise is the posterior auricular nerve. It provides motor innervation to some of the muscles around the ear. Immediately distal to this, motor nerve branches arise to innervate the posterior belly of the digastric muscle and the stylohyoid muscle.

The main trunk of the nerve, now termed the motor root of the facial nerve, continues anteriorly and inferiorly into the parotid gland within the parotid gland. The nerve terminates by dividing into five branches: temporal branch, zygomatic branch, buccal branch, marginal mandibular branch, cervical branch (Table 40.4).

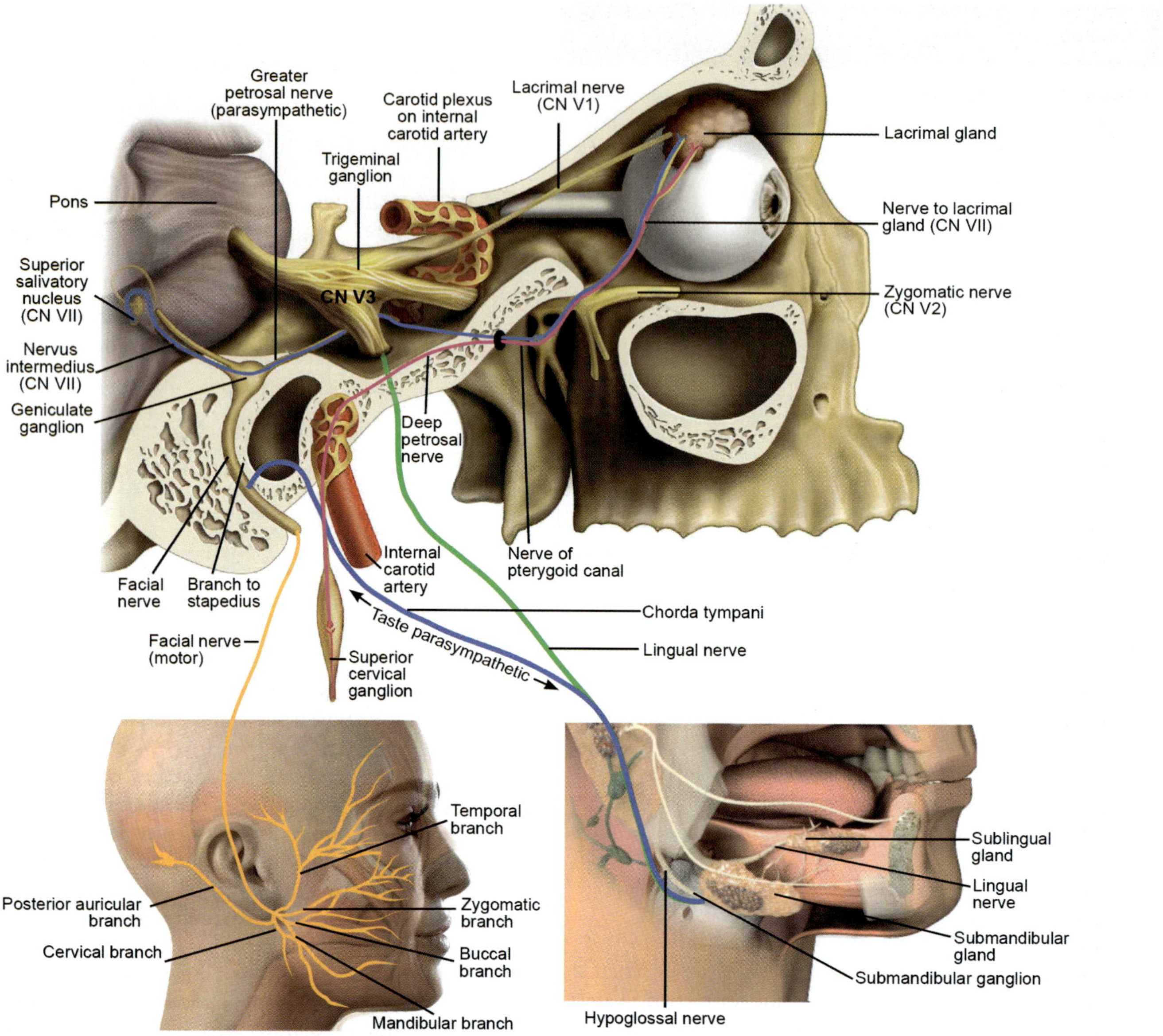

Figure 40.8 Facial nerve anatomy.

FUNCTIONAL COMPONENTS OF THE FACIAL NERVE

The facial nerve has three functions: (i) maintaining the muscle tone without which the facial tissues will droop; (ii) facial muscular activity such as closing the eyes or labial movement; and (iii) emotional expression. The functional components of the nerve are illustrated in Fig. 40.9. To provide a correct diagnosis and management of patients with acute facial nerve paralysis, a vivid understanding of the anatomy and function of the facial nerve is essential.

MOTOR FUNCTIONS

- Nerve to stapedius—supply the stapedius muscle in the middle ear
- Posterior auricular nerve—intrinsic and extrinsic muscles of the outer ear. It also supplies the occipital part of the occipitofrontalis muscle
- Nerve to the posterior belly of the digastric muscle—innervates the posterior belly of the digastric muscle
- Nerve to the stylohyoid muscle—innervates the stylohyoid muscle
- Temporal branches—it passes over the zygomatic arch to the temporal region and supplies the auricularis anterior and superior, the frontalis, the orbicularis oculi and the corrugator supercilii
- Zygomatic branches—course over the zygomatic, supplies the orbicularis oculi
- Buccal branches—they are larger than other branches; it divides mainly into deep and superficial branches. Superficial branches run over the muscles of the face and supply them. The deep branches run beneath the zygomaticus. It supplies the zygomaticus, the quadratus labii superioris, the buccinator and the orbicularis oris

TABLE 40.4 Facial Nerve Branches and Ganglia Associated with it

Facial Nerve Branches:

1. Branches within the facial canal
   a. Nerve to stapedius
   b. Chorda tympani
   c. Greater petrosal nerve
2. At the stylomastoid foramen
   a. Posterior auricular
   b. Posterior belly of digastric
   c. Stylohyoid
3. On the face-terminal branches within the parotid gland
   a. Temporal
   b. Zygomatic
   c. Buccal
   d. Marginal mandibular
   e. Cervical
4. Communicating branches—communicate with the sensory nerve distributed in its origin

Ganglia Associated with the Facial Nerve:

1. Geniculate ganglion
2. Pterygopalatine ganglion or sphenopalatine ganglion
   Branches that arise from this flat ganglion are:
   a. Orbital branches
   b. Palatine branches
   c. Nasal branches
   d. Pharyngeal branches
3. Submandibular ganglion

- Mandibular branch—it runs down the platysma and supplies the platysma and the muscles of the lower lip and chin
- Cervical branch—it pierces from the apex of the parotid, courses downward in the neck and supplies the platysma.

SPECIAL SENSORY FUNCTIONS

The chorda tympani branch of the facial nerve is responsible for innervating the anterior two-thirds of the tongue with the special sense of taste.

Parasympathetic functions

Greater petrosal nerve combines with deep petrosal nerve to form the nerve of the pterygoid canal, which then passes through the pterygoid canal to enter the pterygopalatine fossa, and synapses with the pterygopalatine ganglion. Branches from this ganglion then go on to provide parasympathetic innervation to the mucous glands of the oral cavity, nose and pharynx, and the lacrimal gland.

Chorda tympani combines with the lingual nerve (a branch of the trigeminal nerve) in the infratemporal fossa and forms the submandibular ganglion. Branches from this ganglion travel to the submandibular and sublingual salivary glands.

FACIAL PALSY

FACIAL NERVE PATHOLOGY

Facial nerve injury leads to facial palsy or Bell's palsy. **Facial palsy or facial paralysis** is weakness or total flaccidity of the muscles on the face causing functional and aesthetic defects. **Bell's palsy** is an idiopathic paralysis of the facial nerve of sudden onset. The name was coined after Sir Charles Bell who demonstrated the separation of the sensory and motor innervations of the face. **Facial paresis** is weakness of the muscles of the face causing partial dysfunction.

CLASSIFICATION OF FACIAL PALSY (Table 40.5)

I. Based on the anatomical level of destruction or lesion, facial palsy can be classified as:
   1. Central or cerebral facial palsy:
      - It is caused by a supranuclear lesion that occurs in fibres passing from the cortex through the

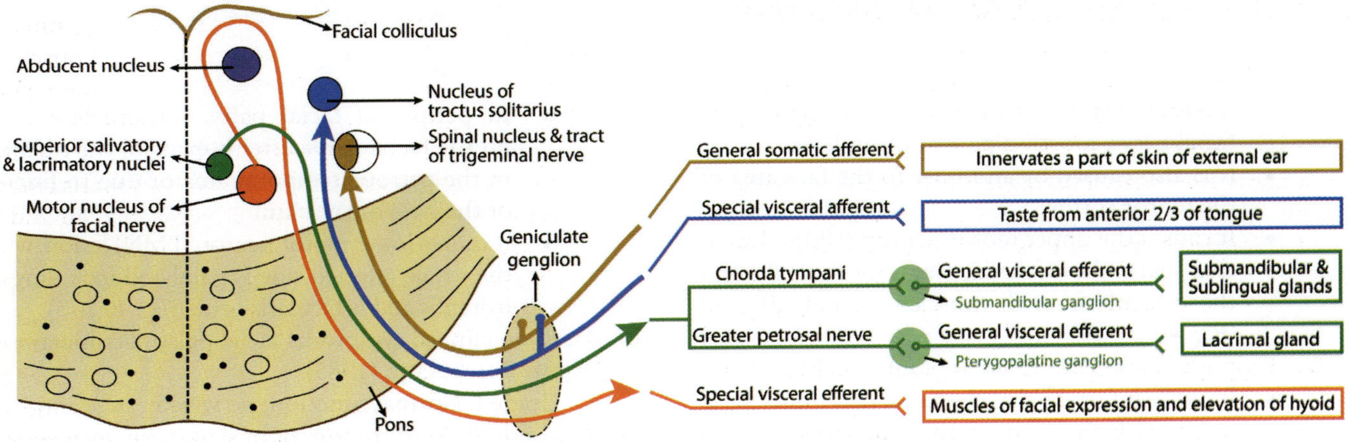

Figure 40.9 Functional components of the facial nerve. General somatic afferent (GSA), special visceral afferent (SVA) and special visceral efferent (SVE) from the nuclei to the organ of innervation are illustrated.

TABLE 40.5 Classification of Facial Palsy Based on Aetiology

Congenital facial paralysis	• **Newborn facial paralysis** is a rare disorder (0.23% of live births). • **Moebius' syndrome** is a rare neurological disorder characterised by absence of facial expression, lack of lateral movement of the eyes and may have limb abnormalities, the facial symptoms are mainly due to underdeveloped abducent and facial nerve. • **Dysgenesis of the intratemporal facial nerve**—a rare cause of isolated newborn facial paralysis
Intracranial causes	• Stroke and vascular abnormalities • CNS degenerative disease • Tumours of the intracranial cavity • Trauma • Congenital defects or agenesis
Intratemporal causes	• Infection (bacterial/viral/fungal) • Cholesteatoma • Trauma—blunt temporal bone fracture, fracture of the temporal bone, gunshot wounds • Tumour of the middle ear invading the facial nerve canal
Extracranial	• Bell's palsy • Ballistic injuries or laceration on the face involving the facial nerve • Otitis media • Ramsay Hunt's syndrome • Sarcoidosis • Lyme disease • Marcus Gunn's or jaw-winking syndrome • Crocodile tear syndrome • Primary tumour of the facial nerve or salivary gland tumour invading the facial nerve • Melkersson–Rosenthal syndrome
Iatrogenic	• **Birth trauma**—difficult delivery leading to facial oedema, injury along the extracranial course of the nerve and haemotympanum are elicited • Orthognathic surgery • TMJ surgeries—preauricular approach, TMJ arthrotomy/arthroscopy • Parotid gland surgeries • Other minor surgical procedures in the area of facial nerve
Transient facial palsy due to pterygomandibular nerve block	Occurs when the needle is penetrated too far behind during a pterygomandibular nerve block • **Acute transient facial palsy:** The LA solution deposited can be near the parotid gland, thus anaesthetising the facial nerve until the anaesthetic duration • **Delayed transient facial palsy:** The vasoconstrictor in the LA solution can cause ischaemic paralysis of the nerve exiting the stylomastoid foramen leading to neuropraxia or injury of a greater degree

internal capsule and to the motor nucleus of the facial nerve, mostly a part of hemiplegia
- It is also caused by an injury to the face area of the motor cortex
- It causes the upper motor neuron (UMN) lesion that spares the forehead, that is the frontalis and the orbicularis oculi muscles are not affected (Fig. 40.10A)

2. Peripheral facial palsy (nuclear or infranuclear lesion):
   - In nuclear facial palsy, the facial nerve nucleus is damaged by a lesion in the pons affecting the motor nucleus
   - In peripheral facial palsy, infranuclear lesion on the facial nerve after it exits all the nuclei or in the petrous temporal area or due to fracture of the base of the skull
   - It causes lower motor neuron (LMN) lesion, where the whole affected side is paralysed including the frontalis and orbicularis oculi (Fig. 40.10B)

II. Based on clinical symptoms facial palsy classification by House–Brackmann (1985):
- Grade I: Normal function; no weakness
- Grade II: Mild dysfunction; synkinesis may be present; mild asymmetry

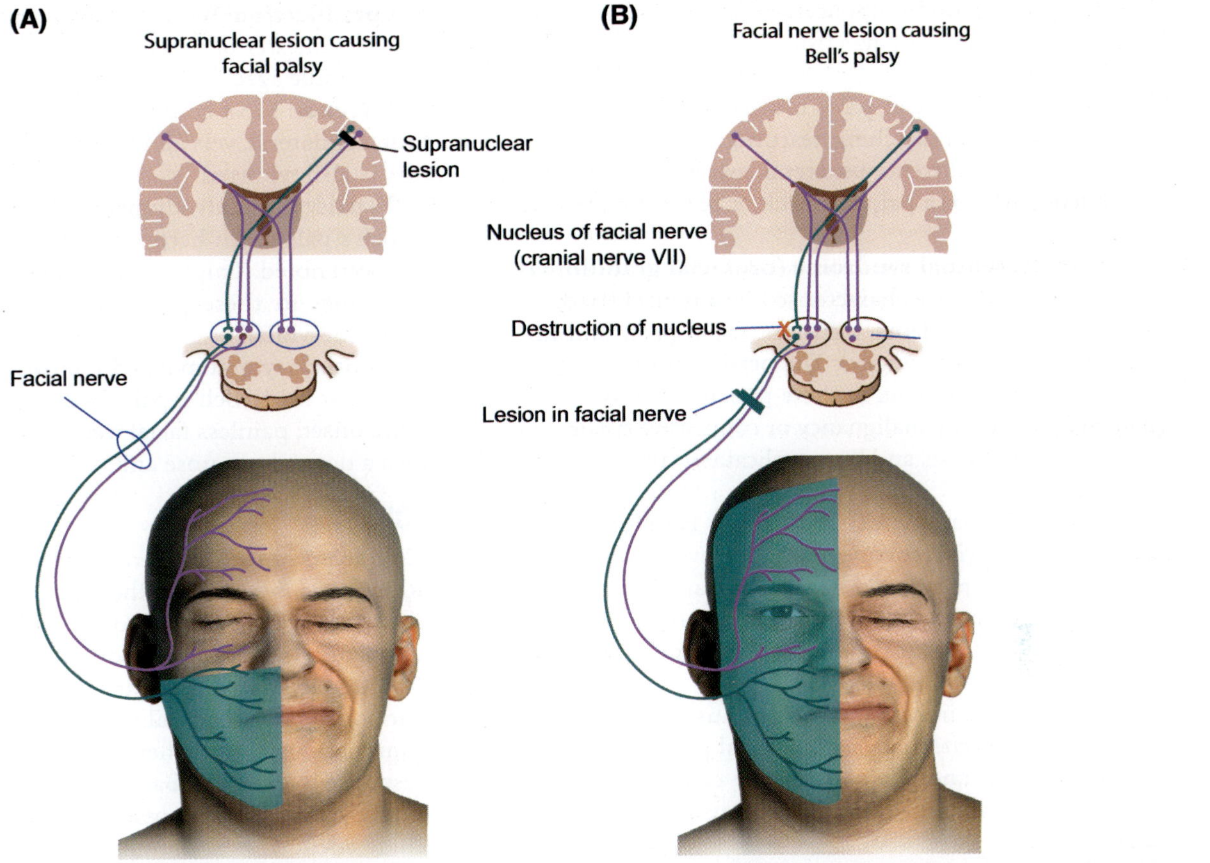

Figure 40.10 Aetiology of facial palsy. (**A**) Supranuclear lesion causing UMN palsy. (**B**) Facial nerve lesion causing LMN palsy.

- Grade III: Moderate dysfunction; weakness is present; asymmetry with contracture; hemifacial spasm may or may not be present
- Grade IV: Moderately severe dysfunction; disfiguring weakness; obvious asymmetry; severe synkinesis; lack of forehead muscle movement and incomplete eye closure
- Grade V: Severe dysfunction; asymmetry at rest; slight facial movement
- Grade VI: Total paralysis; complete absence of muscle tone

CAUSES OF FACIAL PALSY

Trauma is a common cause of facial nerve paralysis. Immediate assessment of soft tissue trauma provides the clinician with the appropriate surgical intervention. Eighty per cent of the temporal bone fractures are longitudinal fractures, that is along the longitudinal axis of the temporal bone causing an external auditory canal disruption, temporomandibular (TM) rupture and ossicular damage or haemotympanum. Facial nerve injury at the peri-geniculate region occurs in ~20% of these fractures. Ballistic temporal bone injury causes facial paralysis in 50% of cases due to the force of the bullet or the fragmented bones

Herpes zoster oticus (Ramsay Hunt's syndrome) is a disease of the facial nerve, caused by reactivation of the inert varicella zoster virus in the geniculate ganglia, occurs when cell-mediated immunity is depressed. Patient usually presents with pain in the ear, followed by LMN paralysis. Vesiculation in the external ear, loss of tears due to involvement of the greater superficial petrosal nerve and loss of ipsilateral taste are characteristic features. There may also be unilateral perceptive deafness, tinnitus and vertigo due to involvement of the 8th nerve. Initial symptoms are similar to Bell's palsy, but pain is more severe. Characteristic herpetic eruptions occur over the palate, concha and external auditory canal. Other features include severe otalgia, facial paralysis and facial numbness. Patient may have sensorineural hearing loss (SNHL). When the vestibulocochlear nerve is involved, patient complains of vertigo, tinnitus and vomiting. Treatment includes steroids, valacyclovir 1 g per oral t.i.d. and proper eye care

Otitis media is the most common feature preceding facial nerve palsy. Chronic otitis media may cause facial palsy; this may be due to prolonged inflammation, osteitis compressing the facial nerve or secondary to cholesteatoma. Good eye care, irrespective of the line of management is essential with periodic application of natural tear eye drops and protection of eyes from dust by wearing safety goggles

Tumours—when the facial palsy evolves slowly over more than 3 weeks, facial twitching, features of adjacent cranial nerve deficits, recurrent ipsilateral involvement, associated adenopathy or a palpable neck or parotid mass may occur

Melkersson–Rosenthal syndrome (orofacial granulomatosis) is a rare disease characterised by a typical triad; recurrent orofacial oedema, recurrent facial palsy and lingua plicata (fissured tongue). The persistent or recurrent nonpitting facial oedema in these patients cannot be explained by infection, malignancy or connective tissue disorder. Facial paralysis and lingua plicata occurs in half of the patients

Sarcoidosis—one variant of sarcoidosis, Heerford's disease, is characterised by uveitis, mild fever, nonsuppurative parotitis and cranial nerve paralysis. Facial nerve is the most commonly involved cranial nerve and paralysis usually starts abruptly days to months after the parotitis

Lyme disease is an infectious disease caused by the tick-borne bacteria *Borrelia burgdorferi*. Facial paralysis (unilateral or bilateral) and deafness are the characteristic features of the disease. The facial paralysis usually recovers as normal

Marcus Gunn's or jaw-winking syndrome—this rare condition may be congenital or posttraumatic. This is characterised by ptosis or palpebral movement (winking) stimulated by mandible movement as chewing

Crocodile tear syndrome—misdirection of nerve fibres post injury to the proximal part of the facial nerve. These fibres attach from the geniculate ganglion to the lacrimal gland instead of the submandibular gland. The patient tears up instead of salivating while eating.

BELL'S PALSY

- It is defined as the idiopathic paresis or paralysis of the facial nerve of sudden onset (unilateral lower motor neuron paralysis of sudden onset, not related to any other disease elsewhere in the body) (Box 40.4)

BOX 40.4 Bell's Palsy Pneumonic

- Blink relfex abnormal
- Earache
- Lacrimation
- Loss of taste
- Sudden onset
- Painless
- Acute
- Lower motor neurone (distribution of facial weakness)
- Systemically well
- Your examination is otherwise normal

- **Sex predilection:** Women (mostly in pregnant women in the 3rd trimester of pregnancy)
- **Age**: Middle aged
- **Recurrence**: Most commonly in diabetics
- **Side**: Unilateral, very rarely bilateral. Positive family history is also reported
- Bell's palsy is mainly idiopathic. However, an association of Bell's palsy with herpes simplex virus (HSV) infection has been noted. This is suggested by the presence of HSV antibodies in these patients when compared to unaffected individuals
- **Diagnosis**: A symptom-based approach in internal medicine
- A patient with Bell's palsy will typically present with acute onset, painless facial weakness (LMN distribution) with a normal ear, nose and throat (ENT) examination.

AETIOLOGY

1. Cold hypothesis: Exposure to extreme cold
2. Rheumatic hypothesis: Rheumatic swelling might press the nerve against the wall of the fallopian canal
3. Ischaemic hypothesis: Vasospasm due to cold, anoxia, CO_2 excess, injury, toxic drugs, allergy, hormonal influence, vasomotor instability
4. Immunological hypothesis: Cell mediated autoimmune response to Guillain–Barre syndrome causes Bell's palsy
5. Viral hypothesis: The possible viral aetiological agents include adenoviruses, mumps and the herpes virus family (herpes simplex virus 1, herpes simplex virus 2 and Varicella-zoster virus).

CLINICAL FEATURES OF BELL'S PALSY

Before testing the function of the nerve, one should compare the facial expression and movement between the two sides of the face (Fig. 40.11).

1. Sudden onset:
   a. Acute onset causing abrupt loss of muscle control

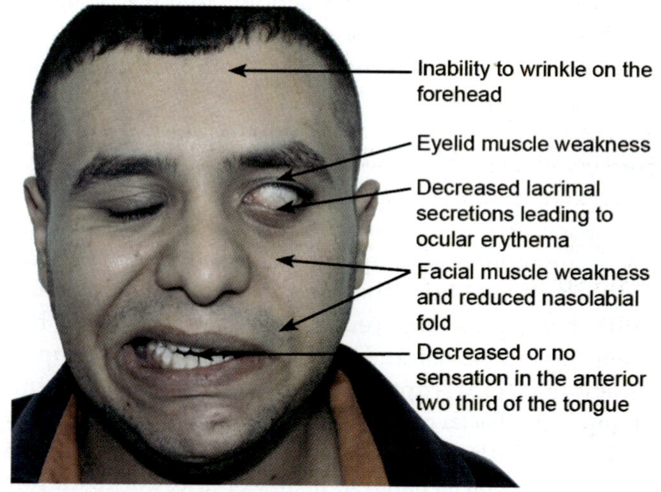

Figure 40.11 Clinical signs and symptoms of facial palsy illustrated.

   b. Bell's palsy develops over hours to days. The peak involvement usually happens within several days, thus caused as an acute but slow onset
   c. Mild pain behind the ear is common at onset as is a subjective sensation of 'numbness' on the affected side (due to altered sensation)
2. **Unilateral involvement—LMN type seen in Bell's palsy,** as opposed to UMN type seen in supranuclear (central) lesions (Table 40.6)
3. Eyes:
   a. Impaired blinking—inability to blink or close the eyes, tearing and dry eyes
   b. **Bell's sign:** Eyeball rolls up as patient attempts to close eyes. Thus, the pupil rolls up and only the white sclera of the eye is visible. Bell's sign or phenomenon occurs in peripheral lesion
   c. Increased lacrimal secretions as the eye is partially opened
   d. Epiphora—watering of eye (loss of closure of eyelid)
   e. Inability to raise eyebrows
   f. Widening of the palpebral fissure
4. Sagging cheek—facial droop and difficulty in making facial expressions, like smiling
5. Flattening of the nasolabial crease (characteristic features of facial palsy)
6. Forehead remains mask-like; all creases are smoothened out
7. Inability to wrinkle forehead on the affected side
8. Intraoral:
   a. Papillitis of the fungiform papillae of the affected side, speech may be slurred
   b. Diminished taste sensation in anterior two-thirds of the tongue
   c. When tongue is protruded, it deviates towards the unaffected side
   d. Drooling of saliva as the corner of the mouth droops
   e. Lips cannot be pursed, thus patient cannot whistle
   f. Inability to puff cheek and hold air or water
   g. Weakness around mouth impairs speaking (slurred), eating (food collects down between gum and cheek; then it gets pushed out through the paralysed side of the lips
9. Hyperacusis—exaggerated sound in the affected side (hyperacusis) due to the paralysis of stapedius muscle, but also occurs independently
10. The ala nasi does not move during respiration
11. Tip of the nose is deviated to the unaffected side
12. **Histrionic spasms may occur**—they are uncontrollable sudden twitching of the face caused by the muscles
13. **Degree of Bell's palsy**—the grade is determined as per *House classification system*, depending on the extent of voluntary movement (Table 40.7).

CLINICAL EXAMINATION AND DIAGNOSTIC TESTS

Following basic functions are examined in the clinical examination:

1. Raising the eyebrows to test frontalis corrugator activity
2. Tightly closing the eyes for orbicularis oculi sphincter function (Fig. 40.12)
3. Asking the patient to grin or smile, to examine the retractor muscles acting on the angles of the mouth

TABLE 40.6 Differences between Upper Motor Neuron (UMN) and Lower Motor Neuron (LMN) Type of Facial Palsy

UMN Type	LMN Type
Upper face is unaffected, only lower half of the face is affected, that is eyes can be closed, forehead can be wrinkled but patient presents with inability to smile due to weakness of lip and buccinator.	Both upper and lower half of the face is affected.
Emotional movements not affected in unilateral cases In bilateral lesions, the whole lower half of the face is paralysed; hence, affecting emotional movements.	Emotional movements are lost.
Bell's phenomenon is absent.	Bell's phenomenon is present.
No atrophy of facial musculature.	Fasciculation/atrophy on the affected side.
Taste sensation retained.	Taste sensation may be lost.
Corneal reflex not affected.	Corneal reflex absent.
Hemiplegia associated with ipsilateral hemiplegia or hemiparesis or monoplegia.	Hemiplegia may be an isolated phenomenon, in case associated with hemiplegia, it is always crossed.
Plantar response-extensor on the paralysed side of the face.	Plantar response-flexor on the paralysed side of the face, may be extensor on the opposite side.
Examples: cardiovascular accident, CNS neoplasm, multiple sclerosis.	Examples: Bell's palsy, Lyme disease.

TABLE 40.7 Degree of Voluntary Movement in Facial Paralysis

Grade	Description
I	Normal facial movements; no synkinesis
II	Mild deformity, mild synkinesis, good forehead function, slight asymmetry
III	Obvious facial weakness, frontalis activity present, good eye closure, asymmetry, Bell's phenomenon present
IV	Obvious weakness, increasing synkinesis, no forehead motion
V	Very obvious facial paralysis, cannot close eye
VI	Complete facial paralysis

4. Taste may also be tested
5. Patient is asked to blow out air, hold air in mouth and whistle.

Any patient presenting with facial paralysis should undergo formal audiological testing, including pure tone, air and bone conduction, speech discrimination, reflexes and tympanometry. If asymmetry is found on the audiogram, an auditory brainstem response (ABR) and/or MRI should be obtained (Table 40.8).

PROGNOSIS

Prognosis for Bell's palsy is generally good; with 85%–90% of the patients fully recovering within 1 month. Other 15% show no signs of recovery for 3–6 months due to complete degeneration. Complications are higher in those where the recovery is slow. The degree of paralysis determines the prognosis for the patient. Incomplete paralysis has good prognosis than the complete paralysis.

MANAGEMENT OF BELL'S PALSY

Treatment of Bell's palsy is variable, ranging from observation to surgical decompression. Physiotherapy is started immediately with 10–20 repetitions per day to prevent muscle atrophy and maintain muscle tone. It also consists of facial massages, heat therapy and electric stimuli with galvanism. To prevent corneal ulceration, topical ointment, methyl cellulose lubrication during daytime, lacrilube ointment before sleeping and eye patch or cotton pad are used. Oral ulcers, abrasions while mastication and inability to drink are prevented by using straw and soft diet. Patient is advised to cover the eyes with protective goggles when going outside. Oral prednisone in a divided dosage of 1 mg/kg/day may be prescribed to minimise degeneration, to relieve pain and help in early recovery (Table 40.9).

SURGICAL MANAGEMENT OF NERVE INJURIES

Surgical management is divided into two major sections:

A. Primary management describes immediate clinical practice with respect to acute extracranial facial nerve injuries
   1. Surgical decompression:
      a. Internal decompression
      b. External decompression

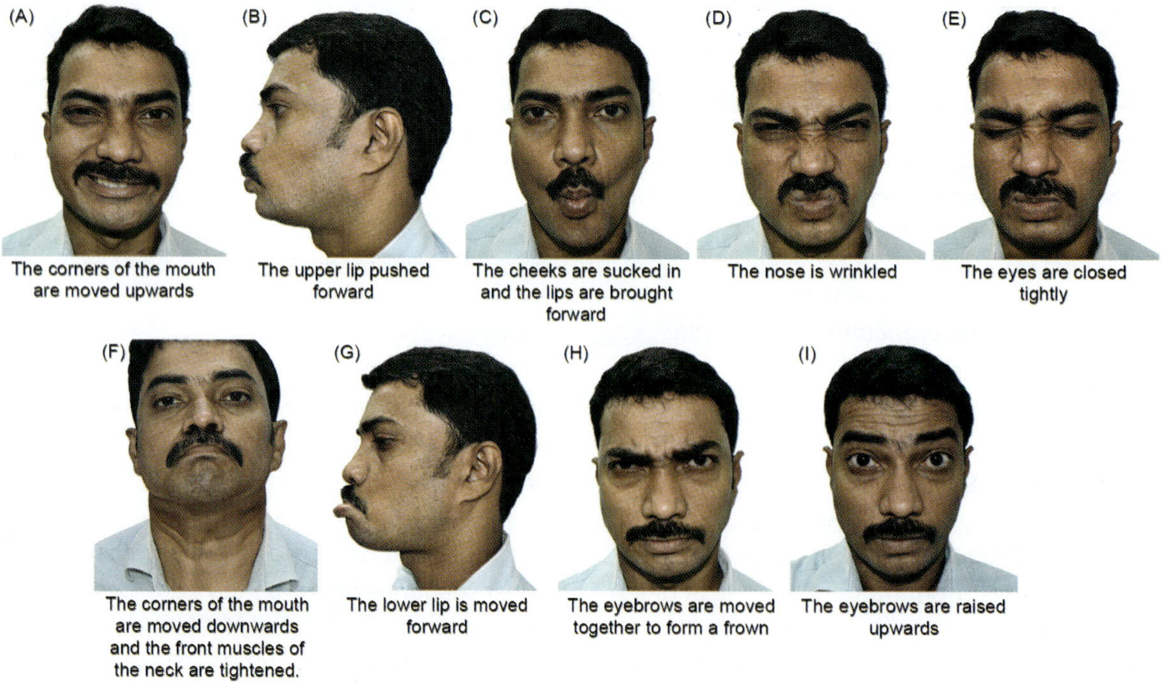

Figure 40.12 Clinical examination of facial palsy.

TABLE 40.8 Diagnostic Tests for Bell's Palsy

Topognostic testing	This includes tests to determine the level of lesion indicated by loss of function in branches distal to injury.		
	Test	**Nerve Tested**	**Function Assessed**
	Schirmer's test for lacrimation (Greater superficial petrosal nerve)	Greater superficial petrosal nerve	Rate of lacrimation
	Stapedial reflex test	Stapedial branch	Hyperacusis
	Taste testing	Chorda tympani nerve	Loss of taste
	Salivary flow rates and pH	Chorda tympani nerve	Salivary flow rate
Electrophysiologic tests	These tests are of significance in patients with complete paralysis for determining prognosis for return of facial function and when decompression surgery is considered		
Imaging studies	• Facial bone CT scan or plain radiographs: Potential causes like petrous bone fractures or bony metastasis can be detected. • CT brain: In stroke, multiple sclerosis or acquired immunodeficiency syndrome (AIDS); CNS involvement is considered. • MRI: Neoplasm of the temporal bone, brain, parotid gland or other structure. MRI images the course of the facial nerve through the temporal bone as well as extracranial course in face and glands.		

TABLE 40.9 Medical Management of Bell's Palsy

Patient seen within 2 to 3 weeks of onset of palsy (not of use after 3 to 4 weeks)	Oral steroids within 72 h of onset—prednisolone 1 mg/kg/day for 10–14 days and then gradually tapered
Nerve regeneration	Vitamin B complex (B1—antioxidant, B6—balances nerve metabolism, B12—maintains myelin sheaths)
Viral infection	Acyclovir 200–400 g five times a day Valacyclovir 1000 mg three times a day

2. Direct facial nerve repair—neurorrhaphy
3. Nerve grafts—graft neurorrhaphy:
   a. Great auricular nerve
   b. Sural nerve
   c. Medial antebrachial nerve
   d. Cross-facial nerve grafting
4. Nerve transposition:
   a. Branch of facial nerve
   b. Hypoglossal nerve

B. Delayed or secondary interventions aimed at facial reanimation or aesthetic improvements
   1. Static suspension procedures
   2. Dynamic neuromuscular transfers
   3. Lateral tarsorrhaphy.

PRIMARY MANAGEMENT

SURGICAL DECOMPRESSION

INTERNAL DECOMPRESSION

It is hypothesised that the facial nerve may undergo pathological compression injury due to oedema at the facial canal (fallopian canal). Surgical decompression may decrease oedema and allow axoplasmic flow. This procedure is usually carried out through the middle fossa approach. It is preferred within 2 weeks, that is before irreversible damage occurs to nerve fibres. It is not performed in the single hearing ear.

EXTERNAL DECOMPRESSION

The epineural sheath is released from the surrounding scar tissues.

NEURORRHAPHY

Indications: Direct neurorrhaphy is especially indicated when sharp precise lacerations of the facial nerve have occurred. Example: razor blade, knife or glass injury.

Technique:

- Direct repair of the facial nerve should be accomplished by a skilled microsurgeon under optimal conditions. Partial parotidectomy is often required to gain adequate exposure for nerve anastomosis. Bipolar cautery is used where necessary within close proximity to the nerve. A bloodless field is required to achieve appropriate visualisation of the nerve ends.

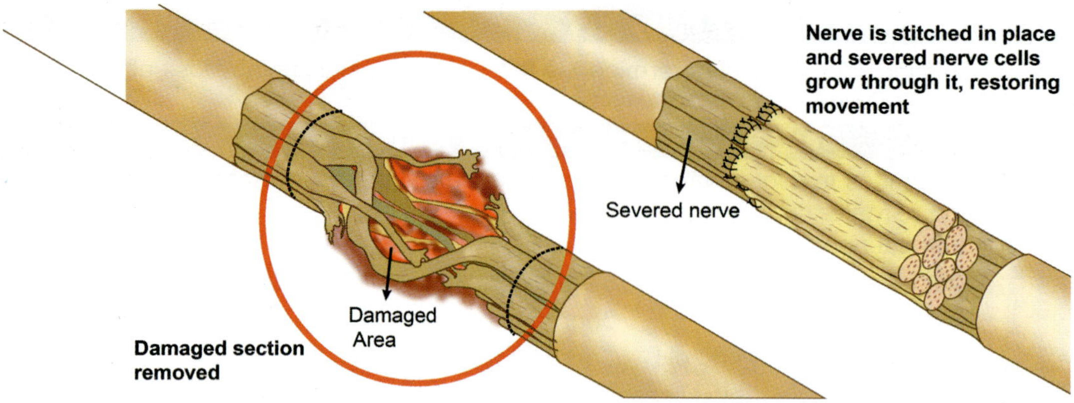

Figure 40.13 Neurorrhaphy; the cut ends of the damaged nerve is sutured together.

The proximal nerve must be identified by visual inspection. Orientation and depth are key features used to identify the nerve (Fig. 40.13)

- Identification of the nerve: High levels of magnification and trimming of the nerve allow characterisation of the structure at the proximal end. These procedures and electrical stimulation can be used within 3 days of transection for confirmation of the nature of the distal segment
- Suturing of the nerve: The identified segments must be minimally dissected to preserve blood supply to the remaining nerve segments. The nerve ends are carefully and completely trimmed. Direct simple perineural sutures are used to achieve approximation. Careful coaptation is necessary to prevent scar tissue ingrowth during the time of axonal regeneration. Nylon or prolene sutures (10-0) are typically used. A surgeon's knot and two additional square throws are adequate. The ideal anastomosis uses a minimal number and volume of suture to limit the inflammatory response to these materials. A taper-cut needle has the advantage of being easy to pass while causing minimal trauma to the nerve. Generally, needles in the range of 50–75 μm are most applicable.

GUIDED NERVE REGENERATION

Placement of a conduit is utilised to guide axonal sprouting and regeneration across a nerve gap from proximal to distal portions of a nerve. This technique is successful only in short nerve gaps (<3 cm) when used in peripheral trigeminal nerve repairs. An alloplastic nerve conduit (polyglycolic acid or polytetrafluoroethylene) has been used with limited success in facial nerve injuries, but only in minimal nerve gaps.

GRAFT NEURORRHAPHY

Indications: The procedure of nerve grafting is identical to that of direct nerve repair with the exception of requiring an additional anastomosis for each nerve branch treated. Autogenous nerve grafts remain the standard when all other treatments are compared. Generally, nerve grafting is required following avulsive type injuries.

Common donor sites:

1. Greater auricular nerve—used when total length of nerve graft required is small
2. Sural nerve—used following extensive injuries or resections of multiple facial nerve branches
3. Antebrachial cutaneous nerve (recently)—structure in the proximal forearm involves many branches that are often suitable to the replacement of multiple branches of the facial nerve.

Reproducible result of nerve graft reconstruction of facial nerve defects can be best appreciated by comparing the procedure to immediate grafting of the facial nerve in radical parotidectomy.

GREAT AURICULAR NERVE

- Great auricular nerve is easily identified in relation to the external jugular vein (posterior and parallel)
- **Surface marking:** A useful additional external reference is produced by dropping a perpendicular line at the midpoint of a line drawn from the mastoid to the angle of the mandible. A cervical skin crease is used to camouflage the donor site incision
- **Technique**: The degree of elevation of skin platysma flaps along the superficial plane of the superficial layer of the deep cervical fascia depends on the length of nerve required. In general, a maximum useful nerve length is 6–8 cm. The nerve is isolated posterior to the jugular vein and dissected to its entrance into the parotid. Branching of the nerve can prove useful in the nerve defect site and this should be used to its full advantage. Proximal dissection of the nerve is typically limited by the passage of the nerve deep to the posterior border of the sternocleidomastoid muscle (Fig. 40.14A).

SURAL NERVE

- Sural nerve is the branch of tibial nerve arising in the middle of the popliteal fossa. It supplies the skin of the lower half of the back of the leg and the entire lateral border of the foot up to the tip of the little toe. The greatest advantage of using sural nerve in facial nerve grafting is its abundant length. As

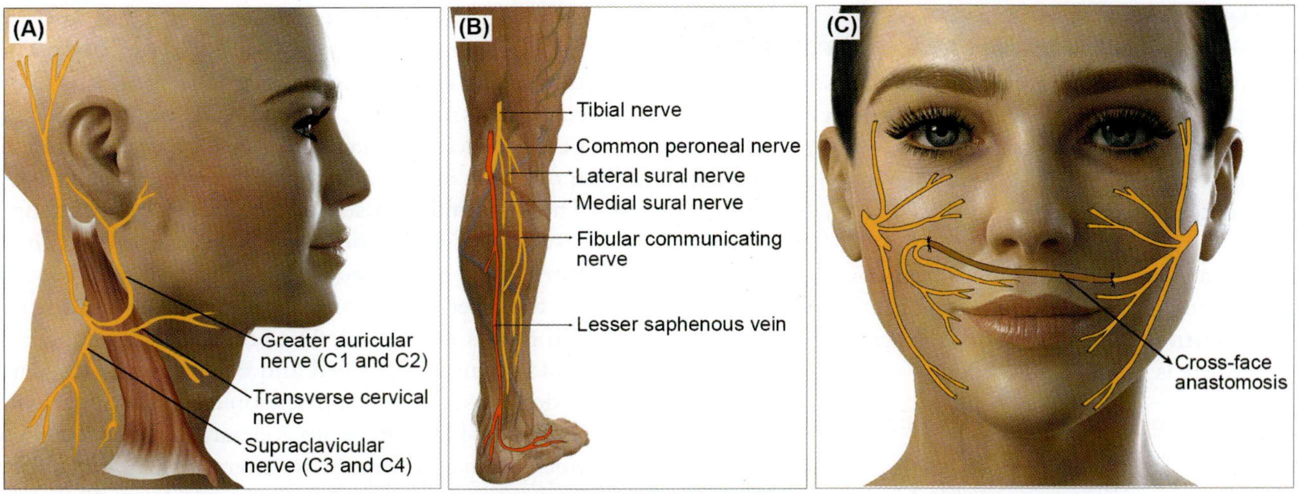

Figure 40.14 (**A**) Greater auricular nerve. (**B**) Sural nerve. (**C**) Cross-facial anastomosis.

much as 40 cm of nerve is available for harvest, the diameter of the nerve is comparable to that of most cranial nerves. Ideal use is in the case of multiple facial nerve defects in separate branches of the facial nerve or in extracranial defects involving the facial nerve trunk only (Fig. 40.14B)

- **Indication**: Cases in which the defect originates at the trunk and extends to multiple branches are most well suited to reconstruction with either the greater auricular nerve or antebrachial cutaneous nerve. A branching pattern of the sural nerve can be harvested from its extreme distal course, but this requires incision and dissection across the ankle joint
- **Technique**: The sural nerve segment that is typically harvested is the distal portion of the lower leg after the point at which it becomes superficial to the muscular fascia overlying the gastrocnemius. In this position, it is easily identified adjacent (medial) to the lesser saphenous vein posterior to the lateral malleolus. Serial small horizontal incisions or a single longitudinal incision is used. Particular attention should be given to management of the proximal nerve stump. This should be placed into a pocket within the adjacent muscle and secured by suture
- **Complication**: Neuroma formation on a superficially located nerve stump can be a source of considerable patient discomfort.

MEDIAL ANTEBRACHIAL CUTANEOUS NERVE

The medial antebrachial cutaneous nerve can be harvested from the upper extremity with minimal morbidity. It originates from the medial cord of the brachial plexus in a majority of cases (78%). Due to its proximity to the basilic vein, the nerve is relatively easy to identify. Near the antecubital fossa, the nerve typically divides into the anterior and posterior branches.

Indications: The anterior branch is most useful for facial nerve reconstruction because it has multiple branches suitable for the replacement of the facial nerve.

Technique: Harvest of the medial antebrachial cutaneous nerve is accomplished by making a cutaneous incision parallel to the plane formed by the fascial plane separating the biceps and triceps muscles. The depths of incision and dissection must remain within the subcutaneous plane. The nerve is easily found along the course of the basilic vein. It is appropriate to dissect the nerve distally to the point of numerous branches to identify a pattern and size most consistent with the demands of the facial nerve defect.

CROSS-FACIAL NERVE GRAFTING

The use of the normal facial nerve on the uninjured side has obvious useful clinical indications. In such cases, patient re-education to achieve nerve stimulation is not required. The principle is really quite simple. A branch of the normal facial nerve is sacrificed (a buccal branch being the most appropriate) and a sural nerve graft is passed through a subcutaneous tunnel to allow either neurorrhaphy or to serve as a nerve conduit to use in conjunction with or without a microvascular neuromuscular transfer at the opposite side (Fig. 40.14C).

NERVE TRANSPOSITION

Two situations exist wherein nerve transposition can prove exceptionally useful:

- The 1st such condition is when there has been isolated segmental injury to a crucial (mandibular or zygomatic) branch of the facial nerve. In such cases, transposition of a less critical ***segment of the facial nerve*** (frontal, cervical) can be accomplished and direct anastomosis can be completed to the distal portion of the injured nerve
- The 2nd of these conditions is that in which extreme proximal facial nerve is injured. ***The hypoglossal nerve*** can be transposed and sutured to the trunk of the distal facial nerve. In these cases, the major drawback is mass movement of the face, but the outcome compares favourably with that of microvascular neuromuscular transfer and cross-facial nerve grafting. Facial movements can be assessed through tongue movements.

SECONDARY MANAGEMENT

Late reconstruction of facial nerve injuries is sometimes required. In such cases, the surgeon must weigh carefully the benefit of each modality of treatment in order to select the most appropriate reconstruction for each individual patient. Static procedures are advantageous due to their simplicity and single surgical intervention. Complex neuromuscular reconstructions require multiple procedures and a long interval of healing prior to extensive re-education and rehabilitation. It is critical to ensure that the anticipated outcome of each procedure is clearly understood.

TEMPORALIS LENGTHENING WITH FASCIA LATA (Figs. 40.15 and 40.16)

- A 2 cm wide strip is prepared behind the level of the helix insertion on the paralysed side. The incision lines are made in the temporal region and brought backwards, forwards and downwards in the preauricular region, extending inferiorly as far as the level of the tragus

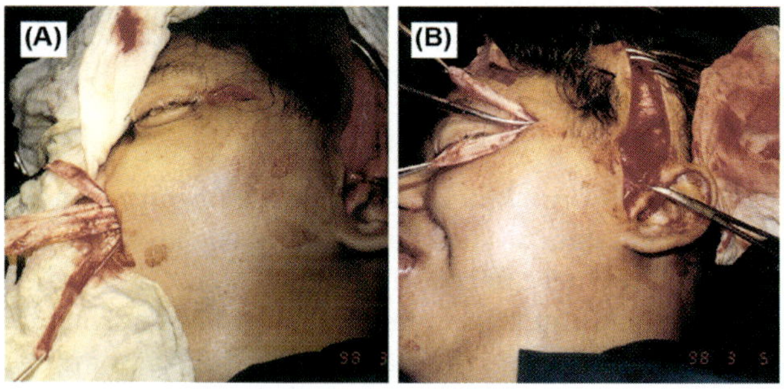

Figure 40.15 (**A** and **B**) Temporalis lengthening using fascia lata for facial palsy.

- Skin and subcutaneous tissue are elevated to reveal the temporoparietal fascia and the zygomatic arch. The portion of the arch measuring about 18 mm lying above the temporalis muscle is excised with bone drills and left pedicled to the masseter. This procedure allows free movement of the muscle during excursions
- The temporalis muscle is then traced inferiorly up to its attachment in the coronoid. To release its attachment, an intraoral coronoidotomy is planned. An incision is made on the external oblique ridge intraorally and the ascending ramus is exposed. The coronoid with its tendinous attachment is identified and osteotomy of the coronoid is done just below the insertion of the temporalis
- The bulk of the temporalis is elevated extraorally taking care not to damage the maxillary artery or mandibular nerve
- To harvest the required fascia lata graft, an 'S'-shaped incision is made over the lateral aspect of the thigh. This curved incision prevents undue scar contraction and muscle herniation. The broad sheet of the fascia lata over the costus lateralis muscle measuring about 6 × 12 cm is stripped away
- Advantage of using fascia lata is primarily based on the fact that it does not require a lot of blood supply for its survival. The fascia is then carefully stitched to the ends of the temporalis in an overlay fashion with 2-0 ethilon and secured tightly
- A vertical incision is made at the site of the new nasolabial groove, more medial than the original, keeping in mind the lateral drift, which proceeds due to loss of muscle tone. A tunnel is created subdermally between the nasolabial and preauricular incisions. The ends of the fascia with the attached muscle are passed through the tunnel and brought out at the nasolabial incision. At this juncture, the broad sheet is divided into a narrow upper and a lower strip leaving the middle strip broader

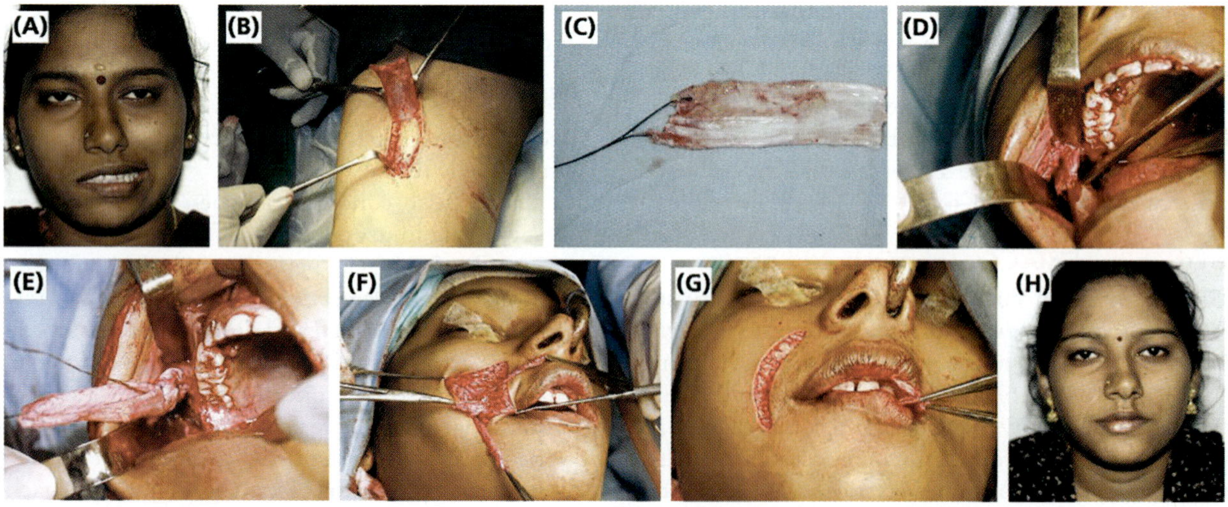

Figure 40.16 Facial reanimation with temporalis lengthened with fascia lata. (**A**) Preoperative photograph. (**B**) Harvesting fascia lata from the lateral aspect of the thigh. (**C**) Harvested fascia lata. (**D**) Intraoral coronoidectomy to release temporalis from its insertion. (**E**) Fascia lata sutured to the temporalis. (**F**) Fascia lata divided into three strips; central strip wound around the modiolus. (**G**) Upper and lower strips of the fascia lata tunnelled to the upper and lower lip. (**H**) Postoperative photograph.

- The upper strip is then again tunnelled subdermally to a smaller vertical incision, lateral to the contralateral philtral column of the upper lip. Similarly, the lower narrow strip is tunnelled into the lower lip and affixed to the dermis at the point lateral to the midline of the unaffected side, the broad middle sheet is then passed around the partially atrophied orbicularis oris muscle, which thereby acts as a sling at the angle of the mouth. All these transfers are made as tight as possible
- **Blair's procedure—with four strips of fascia lata:** One strip at the angle of the mouth; another attached to the tissue at the nasolabial fold; the other two attached to the upper lip and the lower lip.

REGIONAL MUSCLE TRANSPOSITION

In patients with facial drooping, regional muscle transfer can be done with the temporalis, masseter or the platysma muscles. The surgical technique is similar to the fascia lata procedure, but performed only with muscle.

LABBE'S TECHNIQUE—TEMPORALIS LENGTHENING WITHOUT FASCIA LATA

- The incision is made at the temporal region, just within the hairline about a pinna's length above the ear. It is then taken in a curve backwards and downwards well behind the main branches of the temporal vessels to the upper most skin attachment of the pinna. The incision is then made anterior to the tragus and then moved endaurally. At this point, the incision is made across the notch between the helix and the tragus and passed posterolateral to the tragus, in the anterior wall of the external auditory meatus where it can be cosmetically concealed. The incision line is then traversed inferiorly within the external auditory meatus, adjacent and parallel to the tragus till its inferior border and finally out again to the skin crease in front of the lobe of the ear
- Using blunt and sharp dissection, superficial fascia and preauricular fascia are lifted as parts of the skin flap. At the level of the tragus, the skin is dissected off the cartilage of the tragus and its continuation of the cartilage of the external auditory canal
- An incision is made on the superficial temporal fascia parallel to the zygomatic arch continuing inferiorly between the two layers of the temporalis fascia
- Subperiosteal dissection on the zygomatic arch is done by sweeping movements of the elevator connecting both zygomatic and external orbital rim dissections
- The exposed zygomatic arch is sectioned and shifted inferiorly, attached to the masseter muscle
- Intraoral coronoidotomy is done
- Temporalis aponeurosis is incised 1 cm below the temporal crest to leave a strip of tissue for the final suturing of the muscle
- The entire muscle is dissected off the squamous temporal bone by an elevator
- A 4 cm incision is made in the nasolabial crease excising skin in elderly. A subcutaneous tunnel is made in the fat plane connecting the nasolabial crease to the temporal region
- The coronoid process with the temporalis tendon is guided into the tunnel
- The coronoid process is dissected off the muscle and removed
- The temporalis tendon, spread 3 to 4 cm wide, sutured to the perioral muscles
- The temporalis muscle body is then stretched and sutured to the aponeurotic strip on the anterior portion of the crest. The traction of the muscle before its fixation, creates an overcorrection of the paralysed side. The zygomatic arch is refixed
- Contralateral myectomies are almost always necessary for better symmetry, done by intraoral approach (Fig. 40.17).

STATIC SUSPENSION

- The utilisation of static procedures following facial nerve injury is the oldest of the accepted methods of secondary management of facial nerve injuries. Static suspension of the face can achieve acceptable reconstruction of the nasolabial fold and labial commissure that hide the deformity, except during facial animation
- Autogenous tissue is preferred for facial suspension. Most commonly, the **fascia lata** is used. The fascia is harvested as a wide strip that can then be adapted to provide a number of sites of inset for the suspension. The flaccid **facial musculature** can also be suspended to the zygoma using sutures
- The superior portion of a face-lift incision is used with subcutaneous dissection accomplished to the sites of planned inset. Separate incisions at the insertion sites are required to secure the fascia to the dermis. Permanent sutures are used to secure the fascia at these distal sites 1st. Appropriate tension is then placed on the graft and it is sutured to the superficial musculoaponeurotic system (SMAS) or temporal fascia. It is generally preferable to apply tension in such a manner so as to place the nasolabial fold, oral commissure and lips in a position approximating the midpoint of a smile. Allowances must be made for the relaxation that occurs as a result of gravitational effects and skin creep. Patients must be aware of this prior to surgery because the immediate postoperative appearance can resemble that of a snarl
- Previous methods that attempted to use temporalis muscle and fascia were reported to result in animation of the face. The true outcome of such cases was generally equal to that of static suspension because preservation of the neurovascular supply to the muscle and achieving appropriate relaxed tension were extremely difficult (Fig. 40.18).

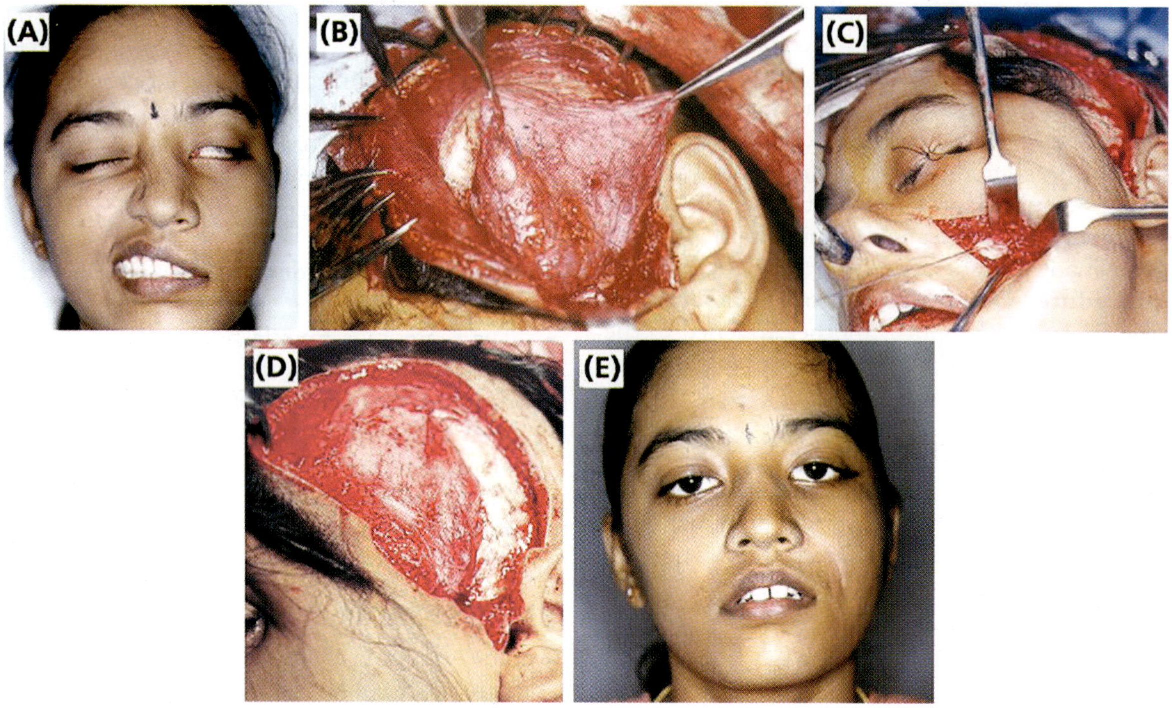

Figure 40.17 Facial reanimation with temporalis lengthened without fascia lata (Labbe's technique): (**A**) Preoperative photograph. (**B**) Temporalis muscle harvested from the temporal fossa. (**C**) Once coronoidectomy is done, the temporalis is tunnelled to the extraoral incision at the nasolabial crease and sutured to the paralysed zygomatic major muscle. (**D**) Temporalis repositioned and is sutured back to the temporal fascia in the temporal fossa. (**E**) Postoperative photograph.

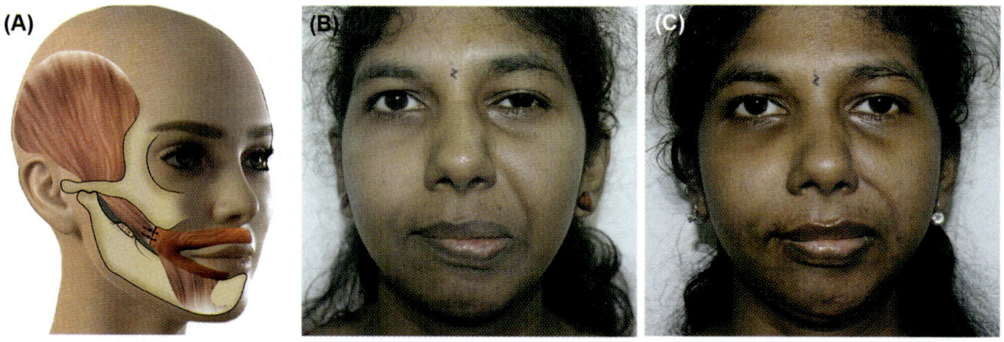

Figure 40.18 (**A**) Static suspension. (**B**) Preoperative photograph. (**C**) Postoperative photograph.

NEUROMUSCULAR TRANSFER

- The gracilis muscle has been popularised for dynamic facial reanimation. Other muscles used for this purpose include serratus anterior and pectoralis minor. A significant decrease in the muscle bulk can be achieved by selectively harvesting of that portion of the muscle innervated by the anterior branch of the obturator nerve. Intraoperative identification of this portion of the muscle is easily accomplished by selective use of a nerve stimulator. This procedure often follows an initial cross-face facial nerve graft procedure. The muscle is inset in a manner much the same as that of static suspension
- Correction must be made for the contraction of the muscle following transection in the process of the transfer. This is commonly accomplished by marking the muscle with vascular staples at predetermined lengths prior to transection. The muscle is then stretched to its original dimension at the time of inset. Microvascular anastomosis is accomplished using the facial artery and vein as recipient vessels
- In most cases, neural anastomosis is accomplished to a cross-face facial nerve graft. Experience with this procedure is necessary to achieve an acceptable result. Indications for this procedure are rare (Fig. 40.19A and B).

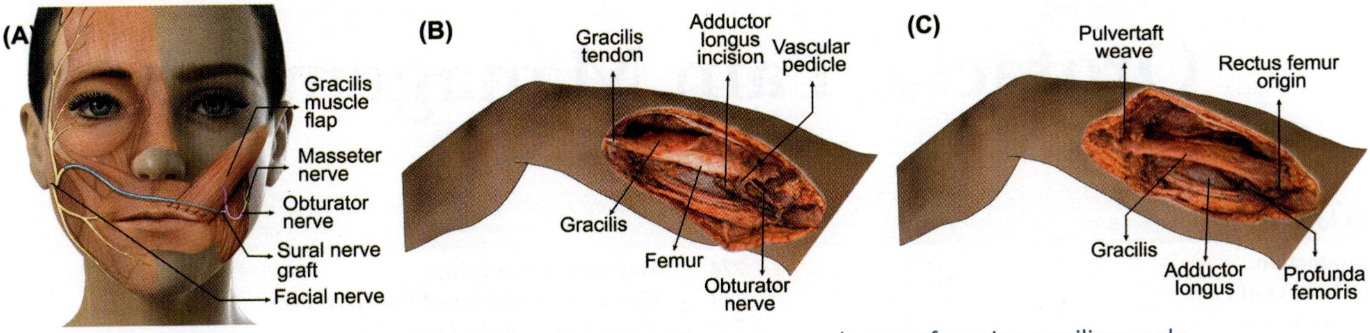

Figure 40.19 (**A** and **B**) Facial reanimation with neuromuscular transfer using gracilis muscle.

MCLAUGHLIN'S TARSORRHAPHY

In long-term facial palsy patients, the eyelid remains open and may droop subsequently. To protect the cornea, lateral tarsorrhaphy can be performed. The lateral 3rd of the upper eyelid and lower eyelid at the grey line are split and the posterior lamellae are sutured with interrupted 5-0 vicryl suture and the overlying skin with interrupted 6-0 vicryl or gut sutures in a layered fashion (Fig. 40.20).

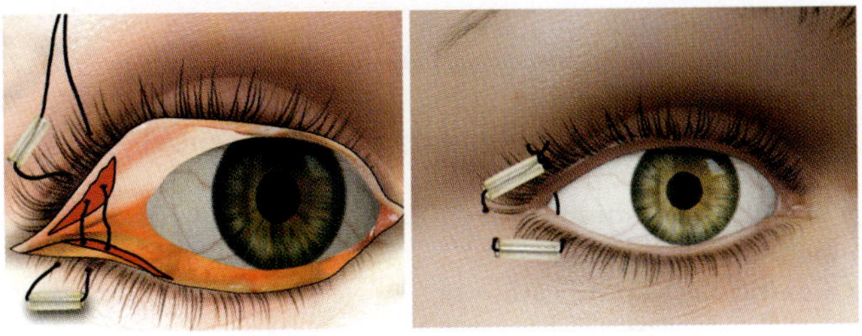

Figure 40.20 McLaughlin's tarsorrhaphy.

Chapter 41

Orofacial Pain Management

OUTLINE

INTRODUCTION

Pain is defined as an unpleasant sensory, emotional and motivational experience associated with potential or actual tissue damage, which requires consciousness. Pain is a localised sensation that occurs as a result of noxious stimulation, mediated by specialised neural structures made for that purpose. Pain functions as a defence mechanism against injury.

Orofacial pain (OFP) refers to pain that is associated with the soft and hard tissues of the face, head and neck. OFP can impair the quality of an individual's life. Chronic pain in the orofacial structures limits the ability to chew, compromises the speech and eventually affects the emotional component of the individual.

THEORIES OF PAIN

SPECIFICITY THEORY

A noxious stimulus evokes pain from specific 'pain receptors' to regions in the central nervous system (CNS) that process only pain-related signals.

INTENSIVE OR SUMMATION THEORY

It proposes that noxious stimulation activates several different types of receptors, and the summation of these signals in the central nervous system leads to pain.

PATTERN THEORY

It proposes that the noxious stimulus produces a pattern of signals that is important for the recognition of pain and its distinction from other sensations.

GATE CONTROL THEORY

A large amount of interactions exist between nociceptive and non-nociceptive inputs to the CNS. According to gate control theory, there is a potential for inhibition of nociceptive transmission in the CNS by the low-threshold mechanosensitive afferent inputs. This 'gating' of nociceptive transmission in the spinal cord and brainstem could be provoked by controls descending from brain centres.

The recent advances in anatomic, physiologic, neurochemical, molecular, pharmacologic, and behavioural research have pointed pain as a high level of neural integration and involvement of multiple factors.

PAIN TERMS

Acute pain—the pain is sharp but subsides soon. It is protective and it warns us from the upcoming tissue damage.

Persistent pain—pain that lasts for a few days or a few weeks. It can also be protective as it enforces us to give rest to the injured part and avoid further damage.

Chronic pain—pain that lasts for at least 3–6 months after an injury and has apparently healed. It is considered as a nonprotective pain (Flowchart 41.1).

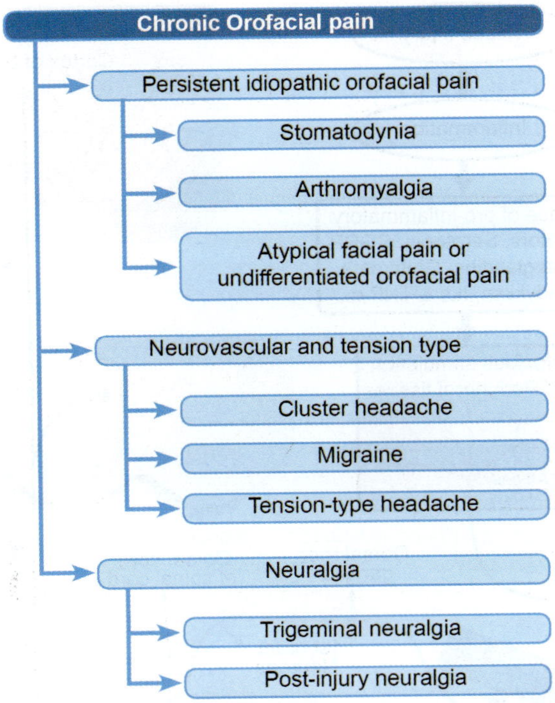

Flowchart 41.1 Classification of chronic orofacial pain.

CLASSIFICATION OF OROFACIAL PAIN

CLASSIFICATION OF OROFACIAL PAIN CONDITIONS BY AMERICAN ACADEMY OF OROFACIAL PAIN GUIDELINES (DE LEEUW AND KLASSER 2013) (Flowchart 41.2)

1. Vascular and nonvascular intracranial causes of orofacial pain:
   - Headache associated with vascular/nonvascular intracranial disorders
2. Primary headache disorders:
   - Migraine
   - Tension-type headache
   - Cluster headache and other trigeminal autonomic cephalgias
3. Neuropathic pain:
   - Episodic neuropathic pain
   - Continuous neuropathic pain
   - Dysaesthesia
4. Intraoral pain disorders:
   - Odontogenic pain
   - Nonodontogenic pain
   - Oral mucosal pain
5. Temporomandibular disorders:
   - Temporomandibular joint (TMJ) disorders
   - Masticatory muscle disorders
6. Extracranial causes of OFP and headaches:
   - Pain stemming from tissues or organs in the head and neck
   - Pain stemming from systemic disease

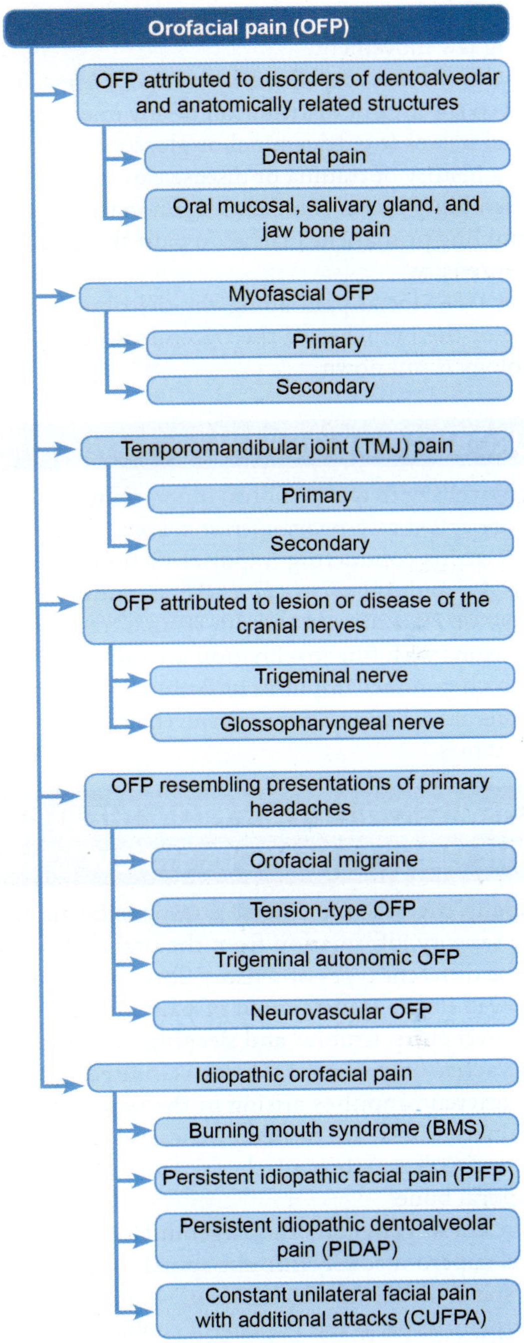

Flowchart 41.2 International classification of orofacial pain (ICOP).

7. Cervicogenic mechanisms of OFP and headaches:
   - Common cervical spine disorders.

INTERNATIONAL CLASSIFICATION OF OROFACIAL PAIN

OFP attributed to disorders of *dentoalveolar structures*—pain is caused by injury to the tooth pulp, periodontium, gingiva, oral mucosa, salivary glands, or jawbone tissue.

Myofascial OFP—pain associated with masticatory muscles with or without functional impairment.

TMJ pain—pain around the TMJ region that occurs at rest or during jaw movement.

OFP due to the *disease of cranial nerves or any lesion*—pain confined to the area of distribution of any one of the sensory cranial nerves (e.g. trigeminal or glossopharyngeal nerve) with a history of trauma or disease causing nerve injury.

OFP resembling *primary headaches*—pain in the orofacial area, resembling primary headaches in pain character, duration and intensity.

Idiopathic OFP—facial pain along the distribution of one or more of the branches of the trigeminal nerve, where the aetiology is unknown.

NEUROBIOLOGY OF PAIN

The nerve cells with axons (fibres) innervating the peripheral tissues are called as *primary afferent neurons* (sensory). Large-diameter axons conducting impulses (action potentials) are called as *A-α* and *A-β afferent fibres.* They conduct impulses in the range of 70–120 m/s and 30–70 m/s, respectively. The smaller axons with fine myelination are called as A-δ *afferent fibres,* which conduct impulses at 3–30 m/s. The unmyelinated axons are called as *C-fibre afferents* that conduct impulses at 0.5–3.0 m/s.

TRANSMISSION OF PAIN FROM THE PERIPHERY TO THE CENTRAL NERVOUS SYSTEM

Peripherally, the trigeminal nerve is responsible for transmitting the sensory information from the oral and facial structures. The different types of sensory fibres (nociceptors) that are involved in the transmission of pain are: A-δ fibres, A-β mechanoreceptors, C-fibres and sleeping nociceptors, which becomes active only when the tissue is injured.

- The afferent impulses arising in the periphery (oral and facial structures) are carried by these sensory fibres (A-δ, A-β and C-fibres) through the trigeminal ganglion in the temporal bone
- From these ganglion, the trigeminal nerve arises and travel supero-medially into the spinal cord
- The spinal cord (trigeminal nucleus), which is located in the brainstem, serves as the 1st point of contact between the peripheral nociceptors and the central nervous system (CNS)
- Through the spinothalamic tract and many other ascending pathways, nociceptive information (sensory information) is transferred from the spinal cord, through the pons and thalamus into the somatosensory cortex of the brain.

PERIPHERAL SENSITISATION OF OROFACIAL PAIN

Pain arising from peripheral sources are mediated by the sensory receptors and ***primary sensory neurons***/primary afferent neurons, constituting the peripheral pain pathway. A-δ and *C-fibre* afferents terminate in the peripheral tissues as free nerve endings, thus forming the peripheral basis for pain. A-δ and *C-fibre* act as nociceptor/sense organ, which are activated by ***noxious stimulation of peripheral tissues*** and produce action potentials that are conducted along the fibres to the CNS.

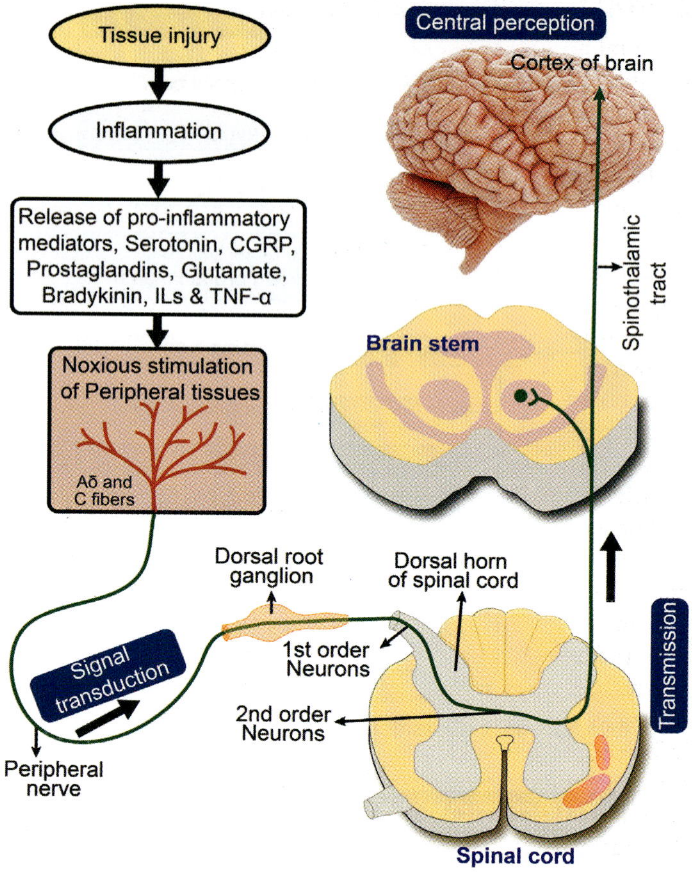

Figure 41.1 Peripheral sensitisation of orofacial pain.

In addition to noxious stimulation, the tissue injury activates the primary afferent neurons and nonneuronal cells to ***release pro-inflammatory mediators*** such as serotonin, glutamate, calcitonin gene-related peptide (CGRP), bradykinins, prostaglandins, interleukins and TNF-α. They increase the responsiveness to subsequent stimulation by acting on the peripheral terminal of nociceptor (Fig. 41.1).

CENTRAL SENSITISATION

Because of the increased peripheral activation that occurs when a tissue or nerve is damaged, *neurons in the spinal cord and brain go through long-term alterations.* This process is known as central sensitisation. These alterations produce significant changes in the neurons, which includes: lowering of activation thresholds, expansion of receptive field size, and an increase in spontaneous activity.

The ***mechanisms*** involved in the development of central sensitisation are: (1) stimulation of N-methyl-D-aspartic acid (NMDA), a glutamate receptor; (2) loss of inhibitory control and interactions among microglia, astrocytes and spinal cord neurons. The central sensitisation of pain pathway may also result from alterations in the brainstem. Thus, *central sensitisation contributes to the development of persistent or chronic pain.*

CENTRAL NOCICEPTIVE PATHWAYS

The oral and masticatory areas are innervated by the 5th (trigeminal), 7th, 9th and 10th cranial nerves, as well as the 1st, 2nd and 3rd cervical spinal nerves. Additionally, the visceral nerves actively contribute to the mediation of painful sensations (Fig. 41.2).

The *trigeminal nerve* innervates the majority of facial structures including skin, intraoral mucosa, teeth, cranial vessels, muscles, deep tissues and TMJ. Primary afferent neurons enter the dorsal horn of the spinal cord, where they transmit impulses to 2nd order neurons. This process of action potential transfer from a 1st order neuron to a 2nd order neuron is known as *transmission*. These 2nd order neurons traverse the spinal cord to reach either the neospinothalamic tract (NST) or the paleospinothalamic tract (PST). The NST carries Aδ inputs (fast pain) straight to higher centres, while the PST mostly carries delayed C-fibre nociception and goes via several other centres before reaching the brain.

The dorsal horn of the spinal cord receives descending neural pathways from the higher centres. These neurons are important in the transmission of nociception, or pain because they have the ability to suppress ascending neural input to higher centres. Central sensitisation refers to the overall effect of these inputs as well as the local response of interneurons. Thus, the information carried by the 2nd order neuron to the higher centres is a cumulative result of interactions between the primary afferent neuron, interneurons and descending neurons, rather than just that of the primary afferent neuron.

In the higher centres, nociceptive impulses are processed. Supraspinal structures make up the higher centres (thalamus, cortex and limbic structures). The beginning of a person's suffering and pain-behaviour is only at this level (Fig. 41.3).

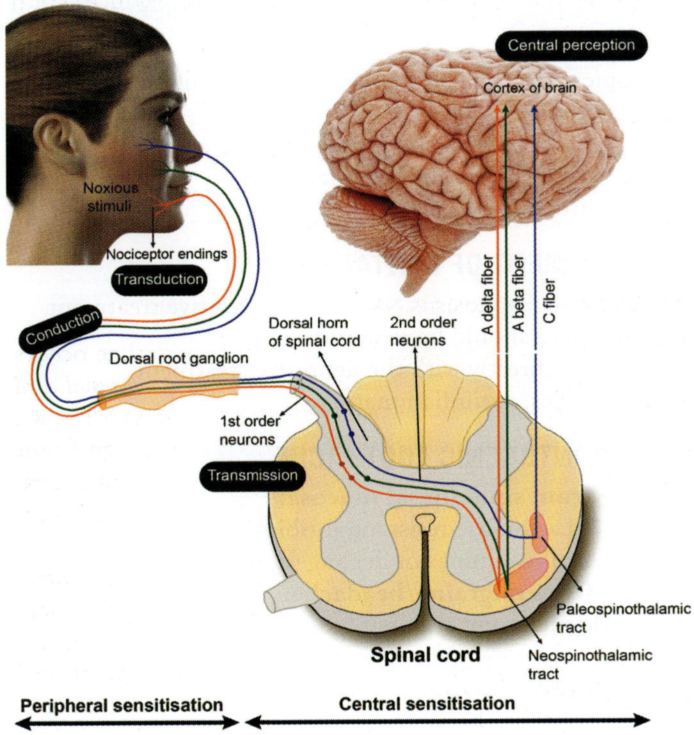

Figure 41.2 Central nociceptive pathway.

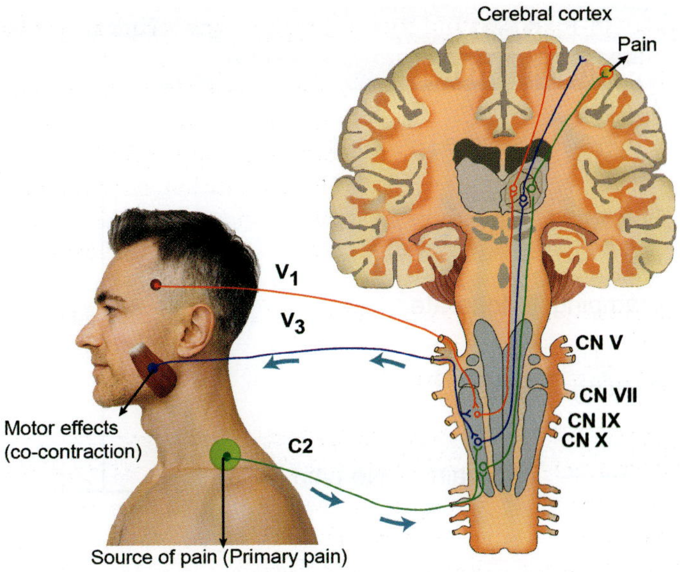

Figure 41.3 The efferent neurons affecting the muscle.

Constant afferent nociceptive input can excite the central efferent neurons (motor). The efferent neuron affects the muscle innervated by resulting in co-contraction of the muscle or the development of myofascial trigger points.

MEASUREMENT OF PAIN

Pain measures should be extremely valid, reliable and allow for comparison across treatments.

- *Pain threshold:* It is defined as the average point at which the patient starts to feel the pain
- *Pain tolerance:* The greatest level of pain that a patient can tolerate
- *Pain scales:*
  - **Nominal scale:** Describes the quality of pain
  - **Ordinal scales:** Describes the level of pain based on a given dimension (numbers, images, verbal labels). Pain experience according to discrete categories
  - **Magnitude estimation scales:** Level of pain experienced is represented on a continuum (VAG—visual analogue scale or numeric scale) (Table 41.1).

CLINICAL PRESENTATION OF OROFACIAL PAIN

There are four categories of pain:

1. Nociceptive pain

The pain is associated with tissue injury, pressure, heat or chemical stimulation. It can be easily identified and explained.

2. Inflammatory pain

Tissue injury triggers a painful inflammatory response. Prostaglandins, bradykinins and other chemicals generated by

TABLE 41.1 Types of Pain Scales

Nominal	Ordinal	Magnitude Estimation	
Burning	Very severe	The most pain imaginable	100
Dull	Severe		
Cramping	Moderate		50
Pricking	Mild		
———	No pain	No pain	0

the inflammatory process are mostly responsible for the pain. This function is considered protective.

3. Neuropathic pain

The pain arises from abnormalities in the neural structures and not from the peripheral or deep structures. Neuropathic pains are often difficult to diagnose and may mislead the treatment.

4. Dysfunctional pain

The aetiology of the pain is within the CNS, centrally mediated pain. The pain may have spontaneously begun with no apparent initiating event (e.g. fibromyalgia).

The information about the pain is gathered by the detailed history and clinical examination that helps us in locating the source of pain and determine proper diagnosis of pain. The history of a patient with pain should include location, onset, quality, behaviour of pain, intensity, frequency, aggravating factors, improving factors, stress, medications and previous treatments. Proper clinical examination is recommended to identify the source of pain. If the information gained through clinical examination is not enough to identify the pain, then local anaesthetic blocks, imaging and laboratory tests may be needed (Table 41.2).

MANAGEMENT OF OROFACIAL PAIN

Orofacial pain management is described in Table 41.3.

MANAGEMENT OF MUCOSAL PAIN (SUPERFICIAL SOMATIC PAIN)

The following are the therapeutic options for pain arising from the mucosal or cutaneous areas:

- Analgesics, antiinflammatory, antibiotics and antimicrobials
- Identification and treatment of aetiology
- Elimination of all oral irritants and good oral hygiene
- Astringent mouth rinses

TABLE 41.2 Quality of Pain and the Secondary Symptoms Associated

Category of Pain	Quality of Pain	Secondary Symptoms
Musculoskeletal	• Dull aching • Pressure • Tight or stiff • Occasionally sharp • Depressing	• Hyperalgesia • Allodynia • Referred from distant sites • Worsens with function
Neurovascular pain	• Throbbing • Pounding • Stabbing • Rhythmic	• Worsens by physical activity or with increasing intracranial pressure • Sensitivity to light or sound • Nausea or vomiting
Neuropathic pain	• Shooting • Burning or itchy • Cutting • Like electric shock	• Numbness • Hyperalgesia • Paraesthesia • Dysaesthesia
Psychogenic pain	• Descriptive	• Complaint patterns does not match any of the sensory supply

- Topical therapy—lidocaine cream, dexamethasone, antihistamines
- Elimination of saliva—depressing drugs
- Chewing of gum to stimulate salivary flow or salivary substitutes.

MANAGEMENT OF DENTAL PAIN

- Accurate diagnosis is essential for effective treatment
- The cause should be removed
- Proceed directly with the definitive treatment
- Analgesics, antiinflammatory.

NONODONTOGENIC TOOTHACHE

Arising from sinus/nasal mucosa:

- β-Lactamase-resistant antibiotics
- Antihistamines or decongestants

Arising from migraine/headache:

- Identify and eliminate the triggering factors
- Environmental triggering factors should be avoided
- Stress relaxation
- Triptans, beta-blockers, calcium channel blockers, Tricyclic antidepressants (TCA).

TABLE 41.3 Therapeutic Modalities Available for the Management of Orofacial Pain

1. **Pharmacotherapy**
   - Analgesics
   - Antiinflammatory
   - Muscle relaxants
   - Anaesthetic medications
   - Anxiolytics
   - Antidepressants
   - Anticonvulsants
   - Vasoactive medications
   - Norepinephrine blockers
   - Antihistamines
2. **Physical treatment modalities**
   - Massage
   - Spray and stretch techniques
   - Joint mobilisation
   - Counter stimulation
   - Thermal therapy
   - Coolant therapy
   - Ultrasound
   - Phonophoresis
   - Iontophoresis
   - Electrogalvanic stimulation
   - TENS—transcutaneous electrical nerve stimulation
   - Laser
3. **Occlusal therapies**
   - Interocclusal appliance
   - Occlusal corrections
4. **Psychological therapy**
   - Counselling
   - Stress reduction training
   - Physical self-regulation

MANAGEMENT OF INFLAMMATORY PAIN

- Nonopioid analgesics
- COX-2 inhibitors
- Combination analgesics.

MANAGEMENT OF MUSCLE PAIN DISORDERS (MYOSPASM, MYOFASCIAL PAIN, FIBROMYALGIA)

- Patient education and self-care:
  a. Restrict mandible use within painless limits
  b. Application of moist heat or cold over the sore joint or muscles
  c. Food should be chewed on both sides of the back teeth
  d. Keep the tongue up, teeth apart and jaw muscles relaxed
  e. Avoid oral habits that put strain on the jaw and neck (clenching, biting lips)
  f. Balance and relaxed position of the head, neck and shoulders by keeping the head up, chin in, and shoulders down and back
  g. Stress relaxation and breathing exercises
  h. The events that trigger the pain should be identified and avoided
  i. Adequate night sleep
- Analgesics, antiinflammatory, muscle relaxants, tricyclic antidepressants, corticosteroids
- Therapeutic exercises and other modalities include ultrasound, phonophoresis, iontophoresis, diathermy, electric stimulation and laser therapy
- Intraoral splints and dental treatment
- TMJ surgery.

MANAGEMENT OF NEUROPATHIC PAIN

- Opioids: Morphine, fentanyl, tramadol, etc
- Amitriptyline, imipramine
- Nontricyclic antidepressants: Duloxetine
- Anticonvulsants: gabapentin, pregabalin
- Topicals: lidocaine
- NSAIDs: ibuprofen, naproxen.

Drugs for trigeminal neuralgia: carbamazepine, oxcarbazepine, phenytoin, baclofen, clonazepam, gabapentin and valproic acid.

TEMPOROMANDIBULAR JOINT PAIN (INTERNAL DERANGEMENT DISORDERS) (REFER TO CHAPTER 37)

- Decrease load on the TMJ
- Softer foods, slow chewing with small bites
- Moist heat or ice applied over the joint
- Physical exercises
- Analgesics and antiinflammatory
- Occlusal appliance.

CONCLUSION

OFP treatment remains problematic for many. OFP has biological, psychological and social effects; as a result, it should always be carefully evaluated to determine the correct diagnosis and therapy.

Chapter 42

Trigeminal Neuralgia and Other Orofacial Neuralgias

OUTLINE

NEURALGIA

A simple definition of neuralgia can be 'pain which follows the paths of specific nerves'.

TRIGEMINAL NEURALGIA

Trigeminal neuralgia (TN), also called *tic douloureux*, is the most common of the cranial neuralgias and chiefly affects individuals older than 50 years of age. Other names: trifacial neuralgia, Fothergill's disease, Tic douloureux–*Tic*–a sudden, spasmodic, painless, involuntary muscular contraction, especially involving the facial muscles. *Douloureux–painful.* **International Association for the Study of Pain (IASP)** defined TN as '*sudden usually unilateral severe brief stabbing recurrent pain in the distribution of one or more branches of the Vth cranial nerve*'. According to **International Headache Society (IHS)**, TN may be defined as '*painful unilateral affliction of the face characterized by brief electric shock like pain limited to the distribution of one or more divisions of trigeminal nerve*'.

ANATOMY

It is the largest cranial nerve. Its sensory part supplies to the face, greater part of scalp, teeth, oral and nasal cavities (Fig. 42.1). Its motor part supplies the muscles of mastication.

It divides into three branches: ophthalmic, maxillary and mandibular (Flowchart 42.1, Fig. 42.2).

COURSE

The trigeminal nerve is continuous with the ventral surface of the pons, by a small motor root and a large sensory root. The fibres of the sensory root arise from the cells of the trigeminal (semilunar or gasserian) ganglion. This ganglion occupies a recess (Meckel's cave) in the dura mater. The ganglion is crescent shaped. The other nuclei are the sensory nucleus, motor nucleus and spinal nucleus. The branches of the unipolar cells of the ganglion are divided into peripheral and central branches. The peripheral branches are grouped to form the ophthalmic and maxillary nerves and the sensory part of the mandibular nerve. The central branches constitute the sensory root, which leaves the ganglion backwards and medially to enter the pons.

Ophthalmic nerve

It is the superior and smallest division of trigeminal nerve, wholly sensory, gives branches to the eyeball, lacrimal gland, conjunctiva and part of the mucous membrane of nasal cavity, skin of the nose, eyelids, forehead and scalp. It arises from the anteromedial part of the trigeminal ganglion and passes forwards in the cavernous sinus close to its lateral wall and below the oculomotor and trochlear nerves. Just before entering the superior orbital fissure, it divides into three branches, that is lacrimal, frontal and nasociliary.

Maxillary nerve

The maxillary nerve is a true sensory nerve. It originates in the middle of the trigeminal ganglion and passes horizontally forward along the lateral wall of the cavernous sinus. It exits the skull through the foramen rotundum into the pterygopalatine fossa. It exits the pterygopalatine fossa to enter the orbit through the inferior orbital fissure. Within the orbit, it continues as infraorbital nerve, occupying the infraorbital groove and canal. It exits the orbit through the infraorbital foramen as labial, palpebral and nasal branches.

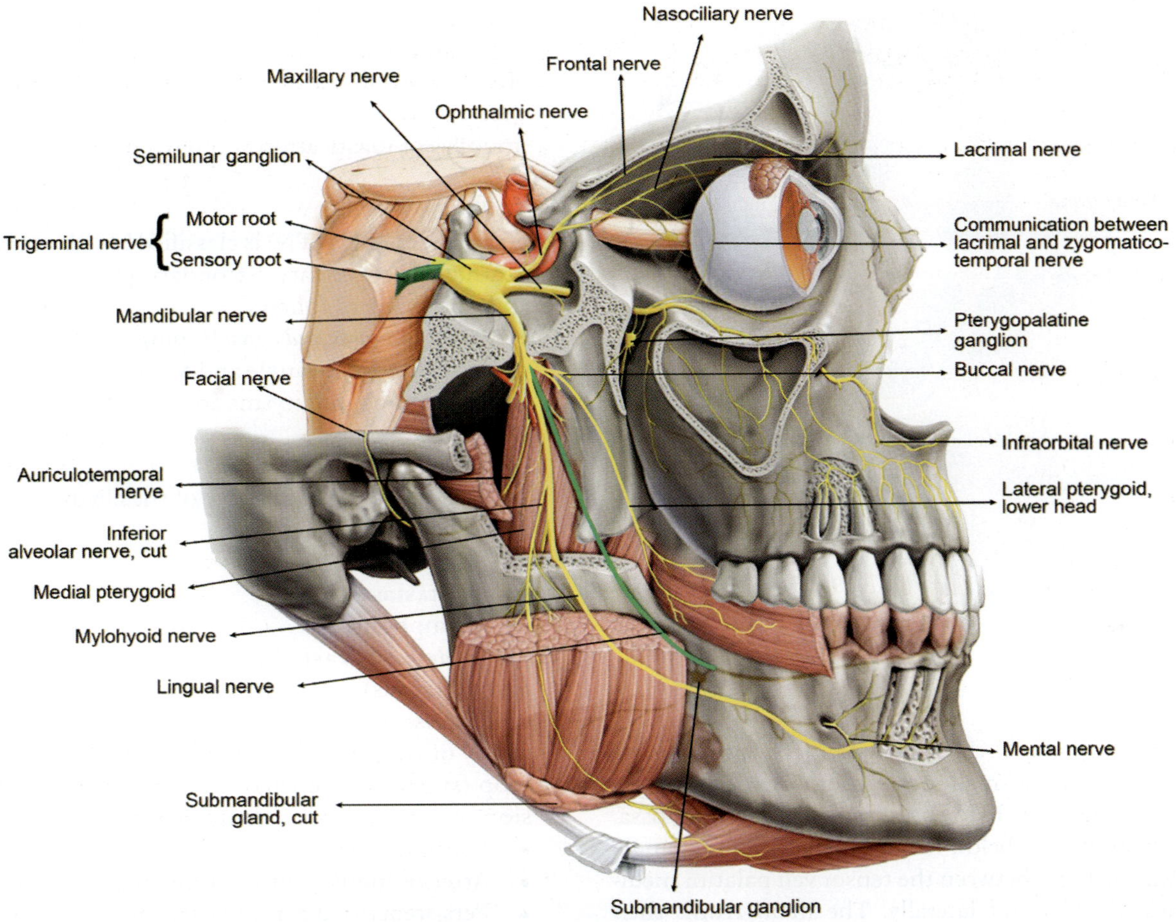

Figure 42.1 Distribution of sensory fibres to each division.

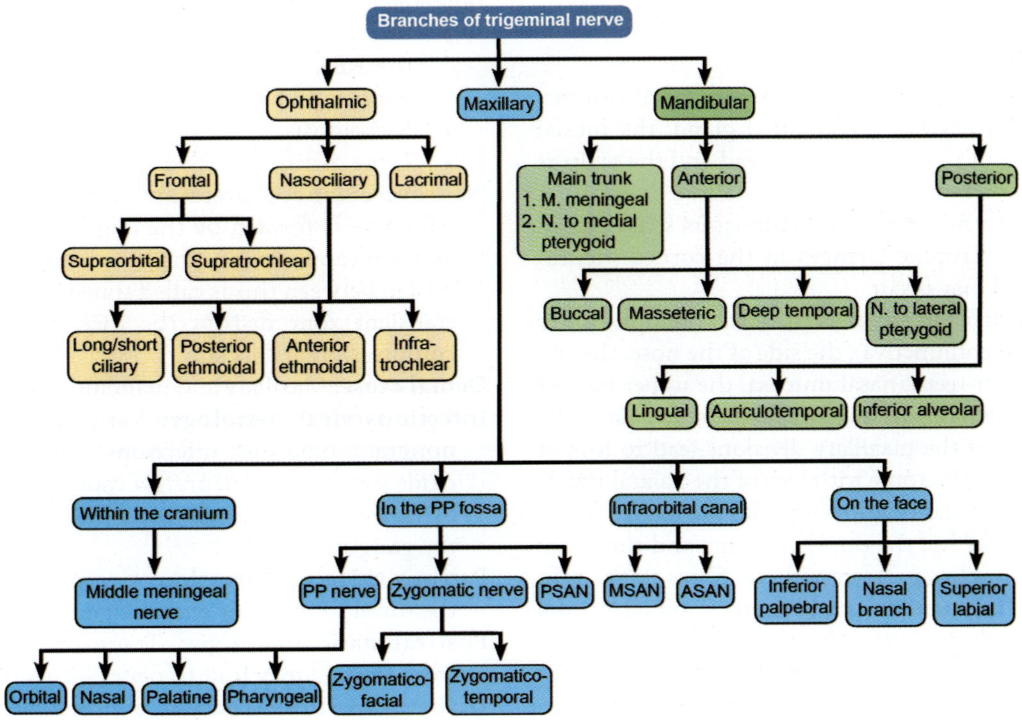

Flowchart 42.1 Branches of trigeminal nerve. ASAN, anterior superior alveolar nerve; MSAN, middle superior alveolar nerve; PP, pterygopalatine; PSAN, posterior superior alveolar nerve.

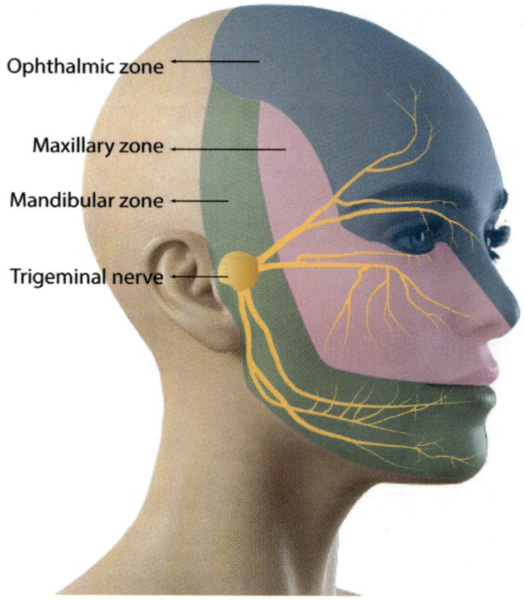

Figure 42.2 Branches of trigeminal nerve.

Mandibular nerve

It is the largest division of the trigeminal nerve and consists of a large sensory and a small motor root. The nerve passes through the foramen ovale to enter the infratemporal fossa. The two roots unite just below the foramen, forming a single main trunk, which lies between the tensor veli palatini medially and lateral pterygoid laterally. The main trunk then divides into a small anterior and a large posterior trunk providing branches to the tongue, mandible, all muscles of mastication, etc.

Applied anatomy

- The ophthalmic division supplies the skin and conjunctiva of the upper eyelid, the lacrimal gland, the mesial part of the skin of the nose, the forehead and the scalp as far as the vertex. Lesions of the ophthalmic division result in loss of corneal reflex and cutaneous sensation in its dermatome. Trophic changes in the cornea (neuropathic keratitis) may occur
- The maxillary division supplies the cheek, temple, lower eyelid (skin and conjunctiva), the side of the nose, the upper lip, the upper teeth, nasal mucosa, the upper part of the pharynx, the hard palate, part of the soft palate, the tonsils. Lesions of the maxillary divisions lead to loss of sensation in its dermatome with loss of the palatal reflex
- The 3rd or mandibular division supplies the lower part of the face, the lower lip, the ear, the tongue and the lower teeth. It also supplies parasympathetic fibres to the salivary glands. The mandibular division is joined by the motor root which innervates the muscles of mastication. The motor root originates from a small nucleus, medial to the main sensory nucleus and partly from nerve cells scattered around the cerebral aqueduct. Lesions of this division lead to diminished salivary and lacrimal secretions and trophic ulcers of the mouth, nose and cornea. Taste is spared though loss of general sensation in anterior two-thirds of the tongue occurs. Weakness of the muscles of mastication is often a prominent feature.

AETIOLOGY

Trigeminal neuralgia (TN) is classified based on the aetiology: idiopathic and secondary. Secondary TN is due to secondary lesions, which are as follows:

Intracranial tumours and cysts: Impingement of meningiomas of cerebellopontine angle and Meckel's cave, arteriovenous malformations, aneurysms and vascular compressions can cause TN

- Acoustic neurinoma
- Chondroma at the level of the clivus
- Pontine glioma
- Epidermoid cyst
- Metastases
- Lymphoma

Vascular defects: **Vascular causes** (intracranial vascular compressions)–vascular compression is the most common cause of TN. Distortion of the root entry zone (REZ) of the trigeminal nerve at the pons by an arterial loop (superior cerebellar artery) or by venous compression by arteriovenous malformation

- Pontine infarct
- Arteriovenous malformation in the vicinity
- Persistence of a primitive trigeminal artery
- Pulsatile compression by the adjacent superior cerebellar artery (more rarely, anteroinferior artery)

Inflammatory causes:

- Multiple sclerosis (MS): Presence of sclerotic plaque at the REZ of the trigeminal nerve (mostly young patients with bilateral involvement)
- Sarcoidosis
- Lyme disease neuropathy

Neurovascular compression: Myelin sheath of the trigeminal nerve is formed by the oligodendrocytes in the CNS and Schwann's cells in the peripheral nervous system. The area in between this is called transient zone. Defects in the transient zone disrupt the REZ causing neurovascular compression at this site

Dental cause: Maxillary and mandibular divisions are affected

Infections/viral aetiology: Various granulomatous and nongranulomatous infections. Aetiological factors include postherpetic neuralgia caused by a previous history of varicella infection and the presence of viral lesions in the ganglion

Petrous ridge compression: Compression of the nerve at the dural foramen or over the petrous tip can cause TN

Posttraumatic neuralgia: Traumatic neuroma resulting from trauma may lead to neuralgic pain

Diabetes mellitus: Diabetic neuropathy manifests with a neuropathic pain that feels as a bilateral hot, burning, electric and pins and needles sensation. Hyperglycaemia can aggravate nerve damage.

AETIOLOGICAL THEORIES

1. **Diseases-related theory:** Vascular diseases, rheumatism, MS, diabetes mellitus and others
2. **Direct trauma to the nerve:**
   a. *Allergy* due to odontogenic inflammation and otolaryngological pathology may impact the TN's periphery
   b. *Compression syndrome hypothesis*—narrowing of the nerve osseous canals due to trauma. In this the central part of TN can get affected due to *compression hypothesis* at the REZ. Causes for this compressions maybe:
      i. Arteriovenous malformation
      ii. Vestibular schwannoma
      iii. Meningiomas
      iv. Epidermoid cysts
      v. Tuberculomas
      vi. Other cysts and tumours.

PATHOPHYSIOLOGY

The mechanism of pain production remains controversial. TN is typical of neuropathic pain where the mechanism of pain is altered. The small and large nerve fibres are altered such that they can be easily triggered by minimal stimuli such as vibration. Demyelination of the REZ of the nerve fibres, where the peripheral and central nerve myelin sheath meet, causes uncontrolled firing of small unmyelinated trigeminal nerve fibres. Lack of inhibitory inputs from large myelinated nerve fibres cause prolonged excitation of the smaller trigeminal fibres to the stimuli. Involvement of the central nervous system is also suggested due to the delay between stimulations. Pathogenesis of idiopathic TN is unclear. Studies have suggested that the compression of the artery or vein over the ganglia or nerve causes ectopic impulses, resulting in pain. Most commonly, the superior cerebellar artery is the compressing artery. Compression causes demyelination of the trigeminal roots at these sites. Reactivation of the herpes simplex virus (HSV) has also been suggested, but may not be the sole causative factor.

CLASSIFICATION

1. By IASP (Table 42.1)
2. By IHS (Table 42.2)
3. Burchiel's classification (Box 42.1).

CLINICAL FEATURES

1. TN is a chronic condition, though symptoms may not be present for a few months
2. It typically manifests as a sudden unilateral, intermittent, paroxysmal, sharp, shooting, lancinating, 'electric shock' like pain
3. The pain is lightning like, sudden in onset, lasts a few seconds and there are numerous episodes of this typical pain; the patient may describe it as a continuous pain

TABLE 42.1 Classification Proposed by International Association for the Study of Pain (IASP)

Classical **TN**	Caused by vascular compression of the trigeminal nerve root, resulting in morphological changes of the root
Secondary **TN**	Caused by major neurological disease, for example, a tumour of the cerebellopontine angle (TN attributed to space-occupying lesions) or **MS**
Idiopathic **TN**	No apparent cause

TABLE 42.2 Diagnostic Criteria Proposed by IHS (International Headache Society)

Criteria	Classic	Symptomatic
Criteria A	Paroxysmal attacks of pain lasting from a fraction of a second to 2 min, affecting one or more divisions of the trigeminal nerve, and fulfilling criteria B and C.	Paroxysmal attacks of pain lasting from a fraction of a second to 2 min, with or without persistence of aching between paroxysms.
Criteria B	Pain has at least one of the following characteristics: • Intense, sharp, superficial or stabbing • Precipitated from trigger zones or by trigger factors	Pain has at least one of the following characteristics: • Intense, sharp, superficial or stabbing • Precipitated from trigger zones or by trigger factors
Criteria C	Attacks are stereotyped in the individual patient.	Attacks are stereotyped in the individual patient.
Criteria D	There is no clinically evident neurologic deficit.	A causative lesion, other than vascular compression has been demonstrated by special investigations and/or posterior fossa exploration.
Criteria E	Not attributed to another disorder.	

BOX 42.1 Burchiel's Classification of Facial Pain

Spontaneous Onset

- TN Type 1 (classic TN)

  >50% episodic pain
- TN Type 2 (atypical TN)

  >50% constant pain

Trigeminal Injury

- Symptomatic TN (multiple sclerosis)
- Trigeminal neuropathic pain (posttraumatic)
- Trigeminal deafferentation pain (Radiofrequency (RF) lesion, Gamma knife radiosurgery (GKR), etc.)
- Postherpetic facial pain
- Secondary TN
  - Tumours, aneurysm, arteriovenous malformation (AVM), etc.
- Atypical facial pain (somatiform pain disorder)

4. The pain can occur hundreds of times in a day or over weeks or months. It can also stop sometimes with pain-free intervals for years. It can undergo remission sometimes too
5. The pain is so severe that it prevents eating or drinking. The nerves affected are usually stereotyped for a particular patient and lie within the sensory distribution of the trigeminal nerve
6. The attack is precipitated by touching the superficial trigger points
7. Refractory period between each episode is very short, may be 1 or 2 min
8. After the episode, a bothersome sensation is present over the region
9. Mandibular or maxillary divisions are commonly involved, while the ophthalmic division is the least affected
10. Although bilateral cases have been reported, pain is invariably unilateral and does not shift sides. **Trigger points:**
    a. V1—supraorbital ridge of the affected side
    b. V2—skin of the upper lip, ala nasi or cheek or on the upper gums
    c. V3—lower lip, teeth or gums of the lower jaw, rarely the tongue
11. The various stimuli precipitating the episode:
    a. Touching, shaving, applying makeup
    b. Applying heat or cold to the cheek
    c. Exposure to cold wind/breeze on the face
    d. Gum chewing
    e. Eating, chewing or biting into food
    f. Yawning
    g. Speaking, smiling, swallowing
    h. Wind blowing on the face
    i. Gustatory stimuli and vibration
12. Stimuli vary with patients and are consistent for each patient
13. Pain is easily described using the 'SOCRATES' assessment tool (Table 42.3)
14. Attack do not occur during sleep is one of the characteristic of the disorder (Flowchart 42.2).

DIAGNOSIS

The diagnosis of TN is purely clinical. Haematological investigations at regular intervals are important in patients on drug therapy. Radiologic investigations are important. Secondary TN (e.g. MS, cysts and vascular pathologies) can be ruled out with the help of MRI. Sensory testing is not done routinely, but quantitative sensory testing (QST) and evoked potentials may play an important role in differentiating between symptomatic and idiopathic TN. Sweet's diagnostic criteria:

1. It is paroxysmal
2. It may be provoked by a light touch to the face
3. It is confined to trigeminal distribution
4. It is unilateral
5. The clinical sensory examination is normal.

TABLE 42.3 SOCRATES Assessment Tool

Site/localisation	Can the pain be localised to a specific area?
Onset	Sudden or gradual? When—day/night/spontaneous?
Characteristic of pain	Sharp, stabbing and dull ache
Radiation	Does the pain radiate elsewhere?
Associated signs and symptoms	Any associated signs or symptoms?
Timing/duration	Seconds/minutes/hours? (Constant, paroxysmal-recurrent and slowly/rapidly progressive)
Exacerbating or relieving factors	Does anything make it better/worse?
Severity	How intense is the pain? Scale 1–10

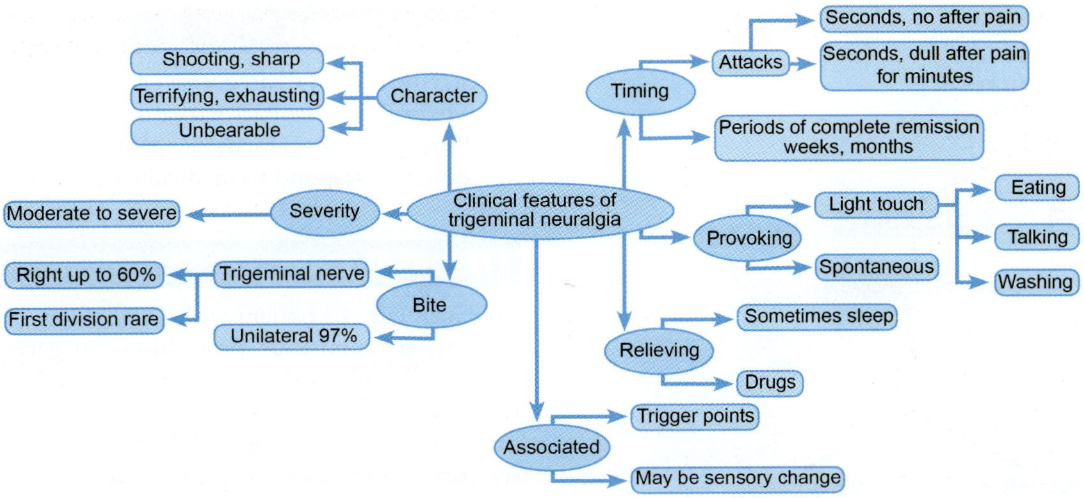

Flowchart 42.2 Important clinical features of trigeminal neuralgia.

DIFFERENTIAL DIAGNOSIS

Differential diagnosis for TN is important as failure of right diagnosis can lead to wrongful treatment (Table 42.4).

INVESTIGATIONS AND DIAGNOSTIC TESTS

IMAGING

- Intraoral periapical (IOPA) radiograph and orthopantomogram (OPG) for differential diagnosis
- Cranial CT to rule out maxillary sinus pathologies
- Imaging studies are indicated to differentiate idiopathic TN from secondary TN
- Magnetic resonance imaging (MRI) is preferable over CT due to its better resolution of the posterior fossa
- MRI can identify MS plaques and tumours like pontine gliomas
- Magnetic resonance tomographic angiography (MRTA) can locate a vascular compression
- Advanced techniques enable to view enlarged sections of the pontine area that can manifest a neurovascular conflict (e.g. the posteroinferior cerebellar artery compresses the trigeminal root). Though the vascular abnormalities are noted by conventional angiogram, its relation with the underlying trigeminal nerve cannot be appreciated.

OTHER TESTS

- Clinical neurological testing with a blink reflex study. Bilateral delay in response to the stimulation on the affected side reveal a lesion in the trigeminal nerve, whereas a normal blink reflex is seen in idiopathic TN
- A diagnostic injection of local anaesthetic agent into the patient's trigger zone should temporarily eliminate all pain.

Positive: Sensitive trigger zones in the peripheral areas are blocked and the patient will be completely relieved of pain, even for a prolonged duration. Selectively blocking the nerve ending with local anaesthetic infiltration (2% xylocaine; 1:80,000 concentration) is valuable in the determination of the affected periphery (Flowchart 42.3).

TABLE 42.4 Differential Diagnosis of Trigeminal Neuralgia

Diagnosis	Important Features
Dental infection or cracked tooth	Well localised to tooth; local swelling and erythema; appropriate findings on dental examination.
Temporomandibular joint pain	Often bilateral and may radiate around ear and to neck and temples; jaw opening may be limited and can produce an audible click.
Persistent idiopathic facial pain (previously 'atypical facial pain')	Often bilateral and may extend out of trigeminal territory; pain often continuous, mild to moderate in severity and aching or throbbing in character.
Migraine	Often preceded by aura; severe unilateral headache often associated with nausea, photophobia, phonophobia and neck stiffness.
Temporal arteritis	Common in elderly people; temporal pain should be constant and often associated with jaw claudication, fever and weight loss; temporal arteries may be firm, tender and nonpulsatile on examination.

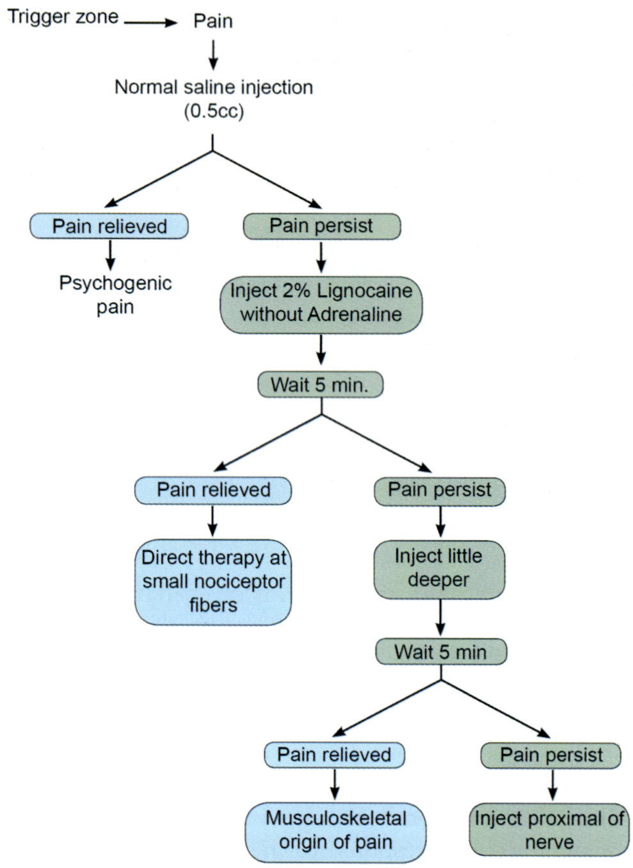

Flowchart 42.3 Local anaesthetic diagnostic test.

MANAGEMENT

Management can be categorised as:

1. Medical care: Palliative treatment and drugs
2. Surgical management is recommended if the patient does not respond to medical treatment.

MEDICAL CARE

Management of a patient with TN includes pharmacological therapy, percutaneous procedures, surgery and radiation therapy. Usually, the 1st line of treatment is pharmacological therapy. Initially, the patient responds well, but prolonged drug therapy may become ineffective. Some patients are refractory to any type of treatment. Treatment is custom-made for each patient depending on the patient's age, general condition. Removal of the primary cause is necessary in case of secondary TN.

Carbamazepine (tegretol, carbatrol) remains the standard drug of choice for TN. Phenytoin (dilantin) is not as effective as carbamazepine, but sometimes a patient may respond to it and not to carbamazepine. The dose varies with patients. Baclofen has been used successfully in the literature. Clonazepam (klonopin) is moderately effective but is not used due to its adverse effects (e.g. sedation) and dependence. Amitriptyline (elavil), gabapentin (neurontin), lamotrigine (lamictal) are other drugs which are useful in the treatment of TN (Table 42.5).

TABLE 42.5 Medical Management of Trigeminal Neuralgia

Drugs	Initial Doses	Maintenance Doses	Adverse Effects
Carbamazepine (CBZ)—Tegretol ***Drug of choice***	200 mg/day	400–1200 mg/day	Sedation, dizziness, cognitive impairment, headache, GI symptoms, allergic rash, leukopaenia, folate deficiency, hyponatraemia (20% of patients), several drug interactions, warfarin
<u>National Institute for health and Care Excellence (NICE) Guidelines for the use of carbamazepine</u> A total of 100 mg up to twice per day, increasing 100–200 mg every 2 weeks until pain has been relieved. A total of 200 mg three of four times per day (600–800 mg daily) for persistent pain. A total of 1600 mg maximum dose per day. When the neuralgic pain is in remission, the dosage is gradually reduced. A low dose for maintenance can be given. In most cases, CBZ can be discontinued until a further episode occurs.			
Oxcarbazepine (OXC)	300 mg/day	600–1200 mg/day	Better tolerated than CBZ, sedation, dizziness, cognitive impairment, hyponatraemia, rash
Phenytoin (PHT)	300 mg/day	200–400 mg/day	Sedation, ataxia, behavioural change, cognitive impairment, lymphadenopathy, osteopaenia, acne, gingival hypertrophy, rash, folate deficiency, liver failure, several drug interactions
Lamotrigine (LTG)	25–50 mg/day	200–400 mg/day	Allergic rash (necessitates immediate discontinuation), sedation, dizziness, headache, ataxia, significant interact with other anticonvulsants

Table 42.5 Medical Management of Trigeminal Neuralgia—cont'd

Drugs	Initial Doses	Maintenance Doses	Adverse Effects
Baclofen (BAG)	10 mg/day	30–80 mg/day	Sedation, ataxia, fatigue, GI symptoms, muscle weakness
Gabapentin	300 mg TID	1800 mg	Sleepiness, dizziness, fatigue, tremor, nervousness muscle ache, dry mouth or sore throat, swelling of hands or feet
Clonazepam	0.5 mg TID	4–20 mg	Drowsiness, dizziness, weakness, unsteadiness, depression, loss of orientation, headache, sleep disturbances, diarrhoea, constipation and blurred vision
Topiramide	50 mg QD	200 mg BID	Anxiety, ataxia, confusion, diarrhoea, diplopia, dizziness, drowsiness, dysphasia, fatigue, lack of concentration, memory impairment, nausea, nervousness, paraesthesia, psychomotor disturbance, speech disturbance, depression, visual disturbance, weight loss

SURGICAL MANAGEMENT

OPEN OPERATIONS

MICROVASCULAR DECOMPRESSION (MVD)

This therapy has virtually supplanted all other open procedures, and it is the 1st line treatment in many centres for patients with refractory pain and who can endure surgery.

The patient is placed in the lateral position and the trigeminal nerve-pons junction is approached through a 5 to 6 cm retromastoid incision on the affected side. A small craniotomy or craniectomy is made up to the confluence of the transverse and sigmoid venous sinuses to reach the posterior cranial fossa. This represents the junction of the tentorium and the petrous temporal bone. An opening is made in the dura up to this junction and the cerebellum is retracted gently while cerebrospinal fluid (CSF) is aspirated. Under the microscope, the right-angled corner between tentorium and petrous is identified and followed medially. The petrosal vein is encountered next and may be safely divided. Just medial to this, the trigeminal nerve root will come into view. The root is examined closely and arachnoid adhesions are divided. In most cases, a compressing vessel will be seen medial to the nerve at the root entry zone—the area where its rootlets enter the pons. This is usually a branch of the ***superior cerebellar artery***. It may also be ***anterior inferior cerebellar artery, posterior inferior cerebellar artery, vertebrobasilar artery*** or ***venous compressions*** which are more common with atypical TN or it may be ***combined arterial and venous compressions***. Any artery encountered in this region must be treated with the utmost care as most are end vessels and obstruction or division results in a stroke. The offending vessel is carefully dissected away from the nerve, upon which a groove is often seen where it has been compressed. A piece of Teflon may be placed to keep the nerve and the offending artery apart (Fig. 42.3).

If it is possible to displace the vessel permanently—if for instance, it is a loop and may be displaced lateral to the nerve—this is done, but more commonly the vessel is merely dissected off the nerve and then separated permanently from it by the interposition of an inert material such as Teflon wool. It is important to avoid kinking the artery as this may obstruct or compromise blood flow. Before this is done, a thorough search of the length of the nerve must be carried out to ensure that there are no other compressive vessels. If no artery is found but a vein is compressing the nerve, this should be treated similarly, although the chances of complete cure of symptoms are less good. After meticulous haemostasis, retraction is withdrawn and the craniotomy is closed. The patient is closely observed overnight and may usually be discharged within 3–5 days.

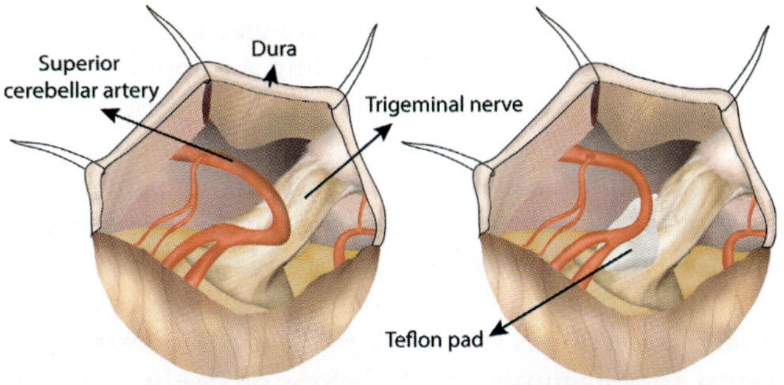

Figure 42.3 Microvascular decompression through a keyhole retromastoid by an endoscope or microscope. Teflon pad placed between the nerve and artery to decompress the nerve for normal function.

Advantages

It is the best nondestructive procedure for the treatment of TN. Risk of facial sensory loss or postoperative dysaesthesias or anaesthesia dolorosa is low. It treats the primary underlying pathology, the vascular compression most commonly on the superior cerebellar artery. MVD has the best long-term results.

Disadvantages

It is a major surgery. It cannot be performed on patients with medical comorbidities. The procedure can cause other complications like bacterial meningitis, aseptic meningitis, CSF leak, cranial nerve deficits, diplopia, sensory loss or dysaesthesias, facial weakness, hearing loss and stroke.

Trigeminal root section

This is rarely used nowadays, although it enjoyed popularity as the standard operation for TN from its introduction in the early 1900s by Frazier until the 1950s. This operation was originally performed via a subtemporal, extradural route, exposing the ganglion and dividing the sensory root—sparing the motor root—as close to the brainstem as possible. Although this inevitably caused facial numbness, often involving the ophthalmic division of the nerve and rendering the patient liable to keratitis, particularly when the greater superficial petrosal nerve was damaged, it was nevertheless extremely successful at relieving neuralgia. In 1932, Walter Dandy published data recommending an approach to the root in the posterior fossa, dividing it only partially and affording pain relief with considerable preservation of sensation. More importantly, he later suggested that pain might be caused by an aberrant artery compressing the root at its entry zone—the basis of TN as it is understood today.

In cases refractory to percutaneous techniques or MVD, partial root section is still occasionally used. It is essential to confirm the diagnosis of TN before proceeding, as other types of facial pain may be exacerbated or, at best, not react. It is most frequently performed when a re-exploration for recurrent neuralgia reveals no vascular compression.

Potential hazards of posterior fossa surgery include cranial nerve damage (5th, 7th or 8th) from excessive retraction or manipulation; vascular damage, particularly to perforating vessels; and postoperative haemorrhage causing cerebellar or brainstem compression. These are extremely rare in experienced hands.

CENTRAL PROCEDURES

Surgical lesions of the brainstem or sensory tracts have an uncertain place at present in the treatment of facial pain and probably no place in trigeminal neuralgia. Tractotomy and dorsal root entry zone (DREZ) lesions have been performed for desperate patients with good results when conducted with care, although potential complications are many and pain relief is unpredictable. Electrical stimulation of central target areas rather than destruction is currently being evaluated, and has had some success in otherwise intractable facial pain.

PERCUTANEOUS GANGLION PROCEDURES

These procedures advocate percutaneous approaches to the trigeminal ganglion via the foramen ovale. Alcohol was the most commonly used neurolytic agent. But nowadays, three main techniques remain in common use: (i) thermocoagulation, (ii) glycerol injection and (iii) balloon compression.

PERCUTANEOUS RADIOFREQUENCY THERMOCOAGULATION RHIZOTOMY

The needle used here has an insulated shaft and a bore sufficient for the passage of a radiofrequency electrode. It is reusable and therefore must be kept well sharpened. An indifferent electrode is usually a simple hypodermic needle inserted obliquely into the skin of the forehead. Once the radiofrequency needle is in the foramen ovale, it is advanced into the trigeminal ganglion. When it is correctly placed, CSF should emerge on removal of the stylet as the ganglion contains CSF. The electrode is inserted just beyond the tip of the needle and low amplitude current is applied using a lesion generator. The patient, who must be awake and cooperative at this point, is asked to specify where the stimulation is felt on the face. A photograph of a face held in front of the patient helps in this mapping. The position of the electrode is adjusted sequentially until stimulation is felt in the normal distribution of the patient's TN. The patient is anaesthetised and thermocoagulated with 0.2–1 V. This is repeated for 45–90 s cycles at 60°C–90°C until the sensory mapping presents without pain.

PERCUTANEOUS GLYCEROL INJECTION RHIZOTOMY

This procedure can be performed under local anaesthesia, but it is difficult as the patient head position on the operating table has to be kept still and flexed for some time afterwards. A 16 G spinal needle is used and is inserted through the foramen ovale into the ganglion until CSF is obtained on withdrawal of the stylet. The patient is made to sit up, supported with the head fixed. A modified dental chair is useful. In this position, an injected fluid with a higher specific gravity than CSF will lie within the ganglion or in Meckel's cave or preferably outline the inside of the ganglion.

Adjustment of the needle will be required if the contrast is extradural or if it diffuses rapidly away from the cave. The contrast is evacuated and replaced with 0.1–0.4 mL of pure glycerol. The patient is transferred back to the ward with the head to be maintained in the same position for at least 2 h. This method is well tolerated with complications such as meningitis, Cranial nerve (CN) palsies, local haematomas and permanent masseter weakness.

PERCUTANEOUS BALLOON COMPRESSION OF TRIGEMINAL NERVE

Although this is the easiest of the three procedures, it still necessitates general anaesthesia. A 4 FG Fogarty's catheter is used, the balloon being primed with X-ray contrast medium from a 1 mL syringe. A 12-gauge spinal needle is required. In this case, it is advanced only just into the foramen ovale and the balloon catheter passed through it. This should be discernible on image intensification. If the needle is passed too far, the balloon will pass intracranially rather than into the ganglion and if not far enough, it will be extradural or will not pass. When inflated, the balloon should take on the shape of Meckel's cave and should appear pear shaped. No more than 0.75 mL of contrast should be injected and prior to full inflation, the needle should be withdrawn slightly to prevent the balloon bursting on it. If the balloon takes on a regular oval shape, it means it is not within the cave and should be repositioned. The balloon should remain inflated for 1–6 min.

Complications

Hazards common to all percutaneous procedures relate to haemorrhage caused by inappropriate placement of the needle, usually in the foramen lacerum and thus the basal carotid artery or by the needle transgressing a vessel in its appropriate trajectory. Extracranial haemorrhage can result in facial swelling or bruising, but it is rarely a serious condition. Intracranial bleeding is rare but may cause all the symptoms and complications of subarachnoid haemorrhage. Progressive and gentle manipulation of the needle, particularly once the foramen ovale is entered, with frequent radiologic checks, helps to reduce the incidence of untoward events. Infective complications are so rare that few surgeons use antibiotic prophylaxis.

PERCUTANEOUS (GAMMA KNIFE) STEREOTACTIC RADIOSURGERY

Stereotactically focused radiotherapy—provided either by an adapted linear accelerator or by the so-called '*Gamma Knife*' has increasingly found a place in the treatment of vascular lesions and tumours. The mechanism of action here is clear. However, when aimed at the trigeminal nerve's REZ, radiosurgery has been shown to be effective in lowering or eliminating the symptoms of TN. It is unclear how long this effect will continue or why it exists, but it is likely that, like many of the treatments mentioned above, it produces focal damage to the root and disrupts the 'short circuits' that induce neuralgia.

NEEDLE PLACEMENT RHIZOTOMY

The technique of needle placement is common to all of these. Although the pioneering operations were performed free hand, image intensification or hardcopy radiographs are almost universally employed now for visualisation of the position of the foramen and later for confirmation of the depth of penetration and the position of any contrast medium used.

Approaches

Anterior approach is more commonly used. The patient lies on a radiolucent table with the neck well extended. The foramen ovale is best visualised with the X-ray tube placed in a submentovertex projection.

The entry point for the needle is about 15 mm lateral to the angle of the mouth. It is best to infiltrate the skin and cheek with local anaesthetic even if the procedure is done under general anaesthesia, as the needle is less likely to penetrate the buccal mucosa if the cheek is swollen. The needle is initially directed slightly laterally for the same reason and then towards the foramen. *The position of this is determined from surface markings*: it lies in the base of the skull at the intersection of a sagittal plane through the inner canthus of the ipsilateral eye and a coronal plane through the zygoma 2.5 cm anterior to the tragus. The lateral pterygoid is usually just medial to the line.

Engagement of the needle in the foramen is best confirmed by biplanar radiology, but some clinical signs may be apparent. If insufficient local anaesthetic is used in local anaesthesia cases, penetration of the mandibular nerve will be extremely painful. Even careful local anaesthetic administration at this point does not usually make the remainder of the procedure painless. In general anaesthesia cases, fibrillation of the ipsilateral masseter may be apparent as the nerve is entered.

PERIPHERAL NERVE SURGERY

This surgery is done very close to the area where the trigger area is located: cryotherapy, alcohol block, laser and neurectomy. These give short-term pain relief and cause few complications. Many patients, however, need to continue the medication. They are now rarely used and are only suitable when other procedures are not possible.

NEURECTOMY

Infraorbital neurectomy is a simple procedure performed for temporary pain relief as the pain free period lasts only up to 24 months; after which recurrence occurs. The infraorbital nerve is approached through the maxillary vestibular incision. The nerve is sectioned off with diathermy to prevent further touch sensations. The use of bone wax to seal the infraorbital nerve canal has shown a longer duration of pain free period up to 5 years (Fig. 42.4).

Ginwalla's approach for inferior alveolar nerve neurectomy has also been performed without lasting results. This procedure can be performed under local anaesthesia, an inverted 'Y' incision is made on the anterior and medial aspect of the ramus (Fig. 42.5A). The mucoperiosteal flap is

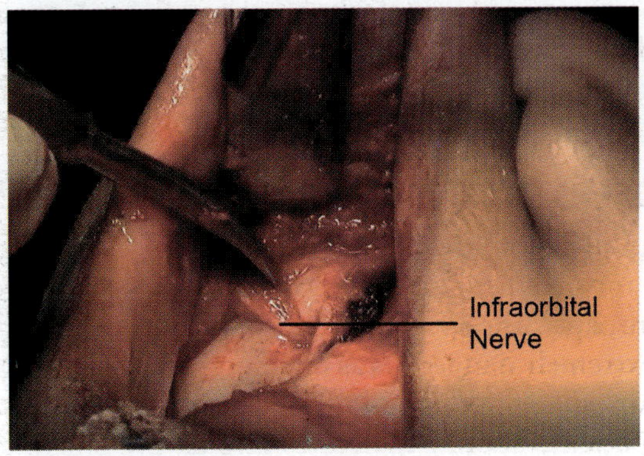

Figure 42.4 The maxillary vestibular incision is used to access the infraorbital nerve.

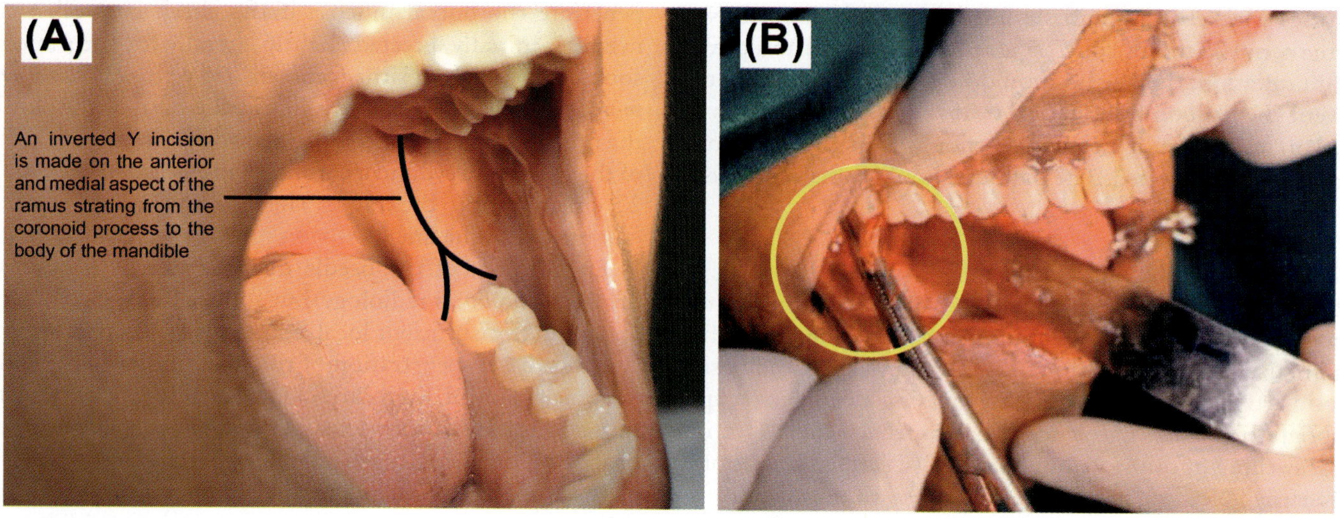

Figure 42.5 (**A**) An inverted 'Y' incision is made on the anterior and medial aspect of the ramus. (**B**) Ginwalla's technique of peripheral neurectomy.

raised by dissecting the temporalis superiorly, medial pterygoid and buccinator laterally. The periosteum is raised to access the lingula in the pterygoid space. Once the inferior alveolar nerve is identified, it is clamped and knotted on either side with heavy black linen thread like 2-0 silk. The distal end is held with the haemostat and the proximal end retracts upward after it is sectioned off with diathermy. Another incision is placed on the buccal sulcus and the mental foramen is exposed. The distal end is wound around and avulsed from the mandibular nerve canal. The haemostat is removed and the entire nerve length end is avulsed out through the mental foramen. The mental foramen is sealed with bone wax or titanium screws. While the advantages are that this procedure can be performed in older patients and patients with comorbidities and patients who do not want to undergo a major surgery without risk of complications, the major disadvantage of this procedure seen in literature is the reversal of the neurectomy as quickly as 30 days (Fig. 42.5B).

OTHER PERIPHERAL SURGERIES

Cryotherapy, peripheral alcohol block (0.5–1 mL of absolute alcohol), radiofrequency coagulation, chemical neurolysis with lignocaine mixed with streptomycin and tetracaine can be used for peripheral neurolysis.

POSTOPERATIVE CARE

All surgical procedures carry a risk of sensory loss. While this may be inconvenient when affecting the 2nd or 3rd trigeminal divisions, anaesthesia of the 1st division and thus of the cornea is extremely dangerous as unrecognised scarring can lead to blindness.

All patients should therefore have an eye shield applied until they are cooperative enough for corneal sensation to be tested. If sensation is absent and fails to return, special glasses with side panels should be worn and the patient instructed about appropriate eye care.

Routine clinical observations are sufficient for patients following percutaneous procedures and they can usually be allowed to return home the same or the following day. Open procedures carry more serious risks. Observation in an intensive care or high dependency unit is recommended as the development of a posterior fossa haematoma, while exceedingly rare, is a life-threatening emergency. The patient will often have headache or will be dizzy or nauseated for a day or two, and will not usually be discharged until the 3rd or 4th postoperative day.

If the procedure eliminates pain, medication may be withdrawn immediately although some patients prefer a gradual withdrawal.

ANAESTHESIA DOLOROSA

This is a condition in which a localised area, usually in the face has severe pain and numbness. It occurs mainly after an injury to the trigeminal nerve. The pain is continuous, burning, gnawing or pricking type. The commonest cause is traumatic injury to the trigeminal nerve during surgery. The pain is usually refractory to medications. Surgical interventions including focused injury to the brainstem (tractotomy of the nucleus caudalis), deep brain stimulation and premotor cortex stimulation have shown poor prognosis.

GENICULATE NEURALGIA

This rare condition is characterised by severe pain in and around the ears. The pain is pricky, flickering or shooting type. Sometimes, it may be associated with trigeminal or glossopharyngeal neuralgia. Women are more affected than men, usually in their 2nd or 3rd decades. Cold, noise, swallowing or touch may trigger an episode. Other related symptoms include increased salivation, bitter taste, tinnitus and vertigo.

Aetiology

Geniculate neuralgia (GN) is mainly caused by the compression of the somatic sensory branch of the facial nerve and sometimes V, VIII, X nerves. The signals sent along the nerve are altered and interpreted by the geniculate ganglion. Occasionally, GN may be followed by herpes zoster oticus (Ramsay Hunt syndrome), where cold sores occur on the ear drum or ear. Facial paresis (weakness), tinnitus, vertigo and deafness may be present.

Treatment

Medical therapy is seen to be less effective in patients with GN than in TN. Microvascular decompression of the glossopharyngeal and vagus (9th and 10th) cranial nerves is indicated when all therapy fails. Intracranial rhizotomy of the 9th nerve and upper $1/3^{rd}$ of the vagus has shown 85% success rate in the literature. But it poses a 20% risk of swallowing dysfunction. Percutaneous glossopharyngeal rhizotomy is used rarely.

SPHENOPALATINE NEURALGIA (SLUDER'S NEURALGIA)

- A neuropathic disorder consisting of neuralgic, motor, sensory and gustatory involvement of the sphenopalatine ganglion is more common in women (2:1) than men
- The features are unilateral headache behind the eyes with pain in the upper jaw or soft palate, with occasional aching in the back of the nose, the teeth, the temple, the occiput or the neck
- The pain is associated with nasal and/or sinus congestion, swelling or redness of nasal mucous membranes, tearing and redness of the face
- Sphenopalatine neuralgia has similar features of cluster headache. In case of Sluder's neuralgia, the duration of pain is longer and is associated with inflammation of the mucosa
- Ganglion blocks provide intermediate pain relief, either by intranasal or direct technique. Removal of the primary cause of Sluder's neuralgia, if evident, is required.

PARATRIGEMINAL NEURALGIA OF RAEDER

- Paratrigeminal neuralgia of Raeder is a syndrome characterised by unilateral, intense throbbing pain in the face along the region of the ophthalmic division of the trigeminal nerve, associated with eye and skin changes (oculosympathetic palsy). Other findings include drooping of the eyelid and contraction of the pupil (miosis). The symptoms are more pronounced in the morning. In the case of chorda tympani (branch of VII cranial nerve) involvement, the patient complains of altered taste sensation (dysgeusia)
- Group I: Patients with symptomatic paratrigeminal neuralgia usually have multiple parasellar cranial nerve defects, including tumours and lesions. A neuropathic quality of pain is present
- Group II: The migrainous form with oculosympathetic palsy is of unknown cause, but may be associated with upper respiratory infection, pneumonia, otitis media, chronic sinusitis and dental abscess.

Section XII

Dentofacial Deformities

Chapter
43

Orthognathic Surgery

OUTLINE

INTRODUCTION

The word 'orthognathic' comes from the Greek word 'ortho' meaning to straighten and 'gnathia' meaning jaw. Orthognathic surgery thus means to straighten a jaw. Orthognathic surgery is defined as 'the art and science of diagnosis, treatment planning and execution of treatment to correct musculoskeletal, dento-osseous and soft tissue deformities of the jaws and associated structures'.

Various features of a human face put together in different proportions give a diverse variety. Dentofacial deformity refers to any deviation from the normal and accepted facial proportions and dental relationships bring about unpleasant facial appearance, mental depression and decreased level of confidence for the patient. Dentofacial deformities affect approximately 20% of the population.

Patients with dentofacial deformities may demonstrate varying degrees of functional and aesthetic compromise.

Such malformations may be isolated to one jaw or may involve multiple craniofacial structures. They may be expressed to varying degrees in the horizontal, vertical and transverse facial planes. Dentoalveolar abnormalities may deceive the observer as a skeletal abnormality. Thus differentiating dentoalveolar deformity from skeletal abnormality becomes a diagnostic challenge, before planning an orthognathic surgery.

Envelope of discrepancy (profit)

It shows how much of change can be produced by various treat ment modalities in three planes of space (i.e. anteroposterior, vertical and transverse planes).

Many patients with severe dentofacial deformities (Table 43.1) can benefit from corrective orthognathic treatment. With the advent of distraction osteogenesis, orthognathic surgery has become a secondary option for hypoplasia/deficiency. But orthognathic surgery remains the prime surgical treatment in managing skeletal excess efficiently. Osteotomy refers to simple bone cut whereas osteotomy means the removal of a portion of the bone. The fundamental biology behind orthognathic surgery is that the maxillary and mandibular bones are intentionally sectioned and repositioned at the desired sites to correct the dentofacial deformities (Fig. 43.1).

Indications for orthognathic surgery:

- Very severe dentoalveolar problems that cannot be corrected by orthodontics alone
- Severe class II, class III and transverse skeletal discrepancies
- Vertical discrepancies: Long face and short face
- Congenital craniofacial syndromes
- Facial asymmetry.

Timing of surgery

As a general rule, early jaw surgery has an inhibitory effect on further growth, hence surgery should be delayed in patients who have excessive growth problems and can be considered earlier for patients with growth deficiencies but not before adolescent growth spurts (Table 43.2).

CLASSIFICATION

MAXILLARY DEFORMITIES (Figs. 43.2–43.4)

I. Maxillary prognathism

- Short hypotonic lip with poor lip seal
- Increased lower facial height
- Patient has a convex profile
- Most of the patients have abnormal muscle activity, for example, abnormal buccinators activity results in a constricted, narrow upper arch leading to posterior crossbite
- The mentalis muscle may be hyperactive giving a prominent chin button
- Increased overjet, overbite and curve of Spee
- The molar relation may be Angle's class II malocclusion.

TABLE 43.1 Classification of Dentofacial Deformities

Skeletal Deformity	Description	Underlying Skeletal Problem
Angle's class II	Short mandible in anterior–posterior plane	1. Maxillary hyperplasia in anterior–posterior plane
Angle's class III	Long mandible in anterior–posterior plane/short maxilla in anterior–posterior plane	1. Maxillary hypoplasia in anterior–posterior plane or 2. Mandibular hyperplasia in anterior–posterior plane or 3. Combination
Vertical maxillary excess (VME)	Long maxilla in vertical plane	1. Vertical maxillary hyperplasia
Bimaxillary protrusion	Proclined anterior bimaxillary alveolus	1. Bimaxillary dentoalveolar hyperplasia in anterior–posterior plane
Open bite	Nonoccluding anterior teeth	1. Reverse curve of Spee or 2. Posterior vertical maxillary excess 3. Short mandibular ramus or 4. Combination
Facial asymmetry	Deviated jaw/chin	1. Unilateral condylar hyperplasia or 2. Unilateral mandibular hyperplasia or 3. Chin deviation

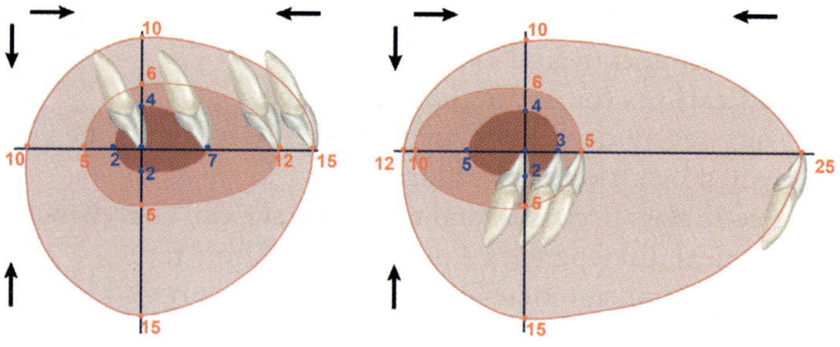

Figure 43.1 Envelope of discrepancy.

II. Maxillary retrognathism or hypoplasia

- Sagging upper lip giving an old look
- Deficient paranasal prominence
- Concave facial profile
- Angle's class I or class III malocclusion
- Incisors in edge to edge or with reverse overjet
- If associated with zygoma hypoplasia, zygoma prominence will be diminished with scleral show.

III. Transverse maxillary deficiency

- Most common skeletal deformity associated with maxillary vertical and anteroposterior hypoplasia
- Unilateral or bilateral posterior crossbite
- Crowded, rotated and palatally or buccally displaced teeth
- Narrow and tapering maxillary arch form—hourglass-shaped high, narrow palatal arch.

TABLE 43.2 Timing of Surgery

Nature of Problem	Recommended Time of Orthognathic Treatment
• Maxillary excess	After growth completion
• Maxillary deficiency	Maxillary advancement may be delayed till adolescent growth spurt
• Mandibular excess	Treated best when growth is completed, assessed by hand-wrist radiograph or serial cephalometric tracing
• Mandibular deficiency	Girls: 14–16 years Boys: approx. 18 years
• Asymmetry	Early surgical intervention recommended only when abnormal growth worsens the existing situation
• Long face	Early surgery not recommended
• Short face	Similar to mandibular deficiency problem

MANDIBULAR DEFORMITIES (Figs. 43.5–43.7)

I. Mandibular prognathism

- Increased lower facial height with prominent chin
- Oblique mandibular plane
- The patient usually has a concave profile
- Angle's class III malocclusion
- Posterior crossbites are common due to narrow and short upper arch but broad lower arch.

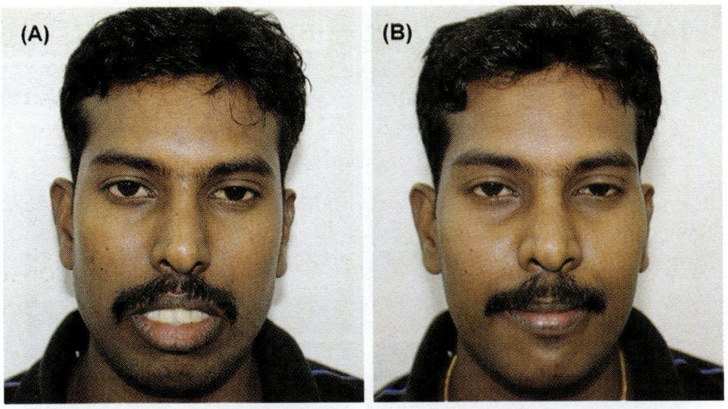

Figure 43.2 (**A**) Preoperative view showing short upper lip and maxillary excess. (**B**) Postoperative view.

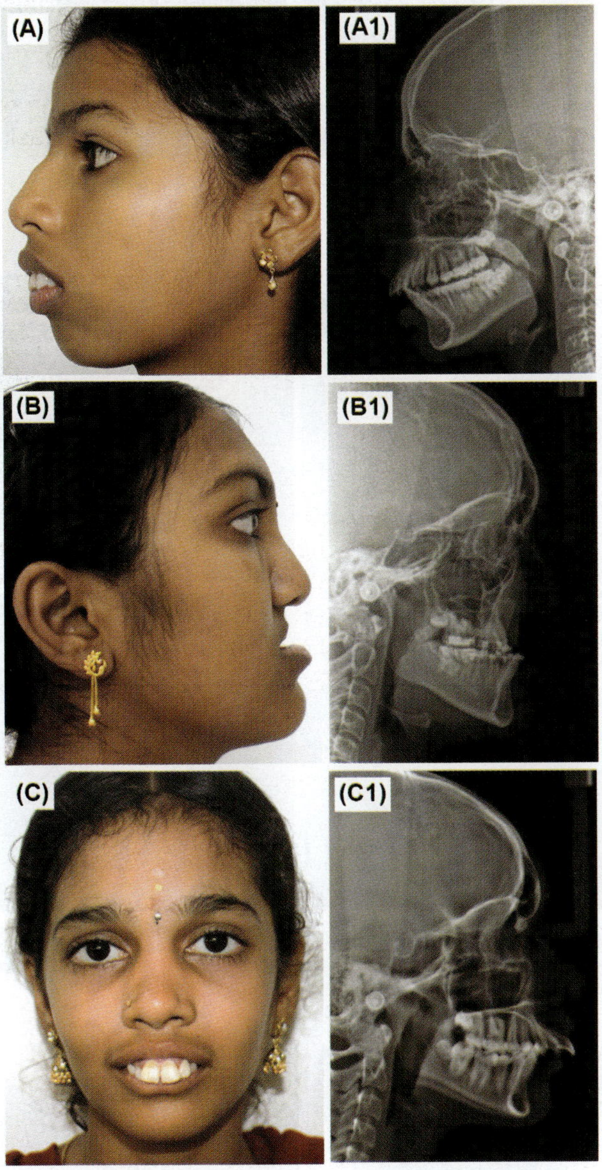

Figure 43.3 (**A**, **A1**) Maxillary anteroposterior excess. (**B**, **B1**) Maxillary anteroposterior deficiency (cleft). (**C**, **C1**) Vertical maxillary excess.

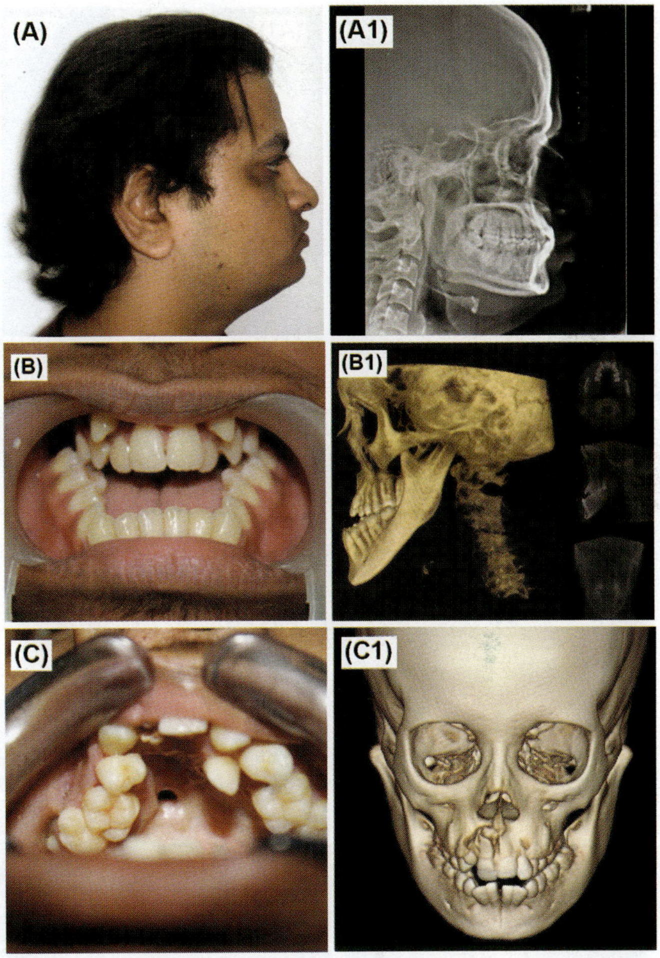

Figure 43.4 (**A**, **A1**) Vertical maxillary deficiency. (**B**, **B1**) Combination of anterior–posterior and transverse maxillary deficiency. (**C**, **C1**) Transverse maxillary deficiency.

II. Mandibular retrognathism

- Reduced lower facial height
- Posteriorly positioned chin
- Convex profile
- May be associated with obstructive sleep apnoea
- Angle's class II malocclusion.

COMBINED DEFORMITIES

I. Skeletal anterior open bite

- The patient often has a long and narrow face
- Lower facial height is increased
- Short upper lip with excessive show of maxillary incisors
- A steep mandibular plane angle
- Cephalometric examination shows:
  - i) A downward and forward rotation of the mandible
  - ii) In some patients, an upward tipping of the maxillary skeletal base can be observed
  - iii) Another common feature is a posterior vertical maxillary increase.

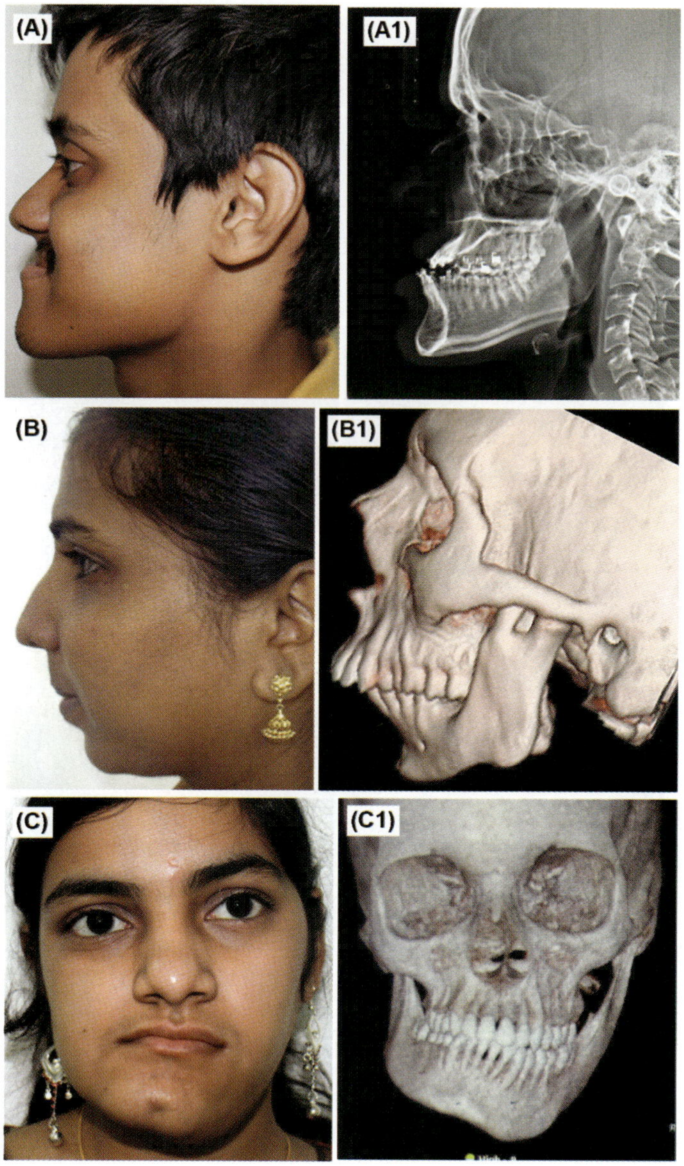

Figure 43.5 (**A, A1**) Mandibular anteroposterior excess. (**B, B1**) Mandibular anteroposterior deficiency. (**C, C1**) Hemimandibular elongation.

II. Skeletal deep bite

Skeletal deep bites are usually of genetic origin. Forward and upward rotation of the mandible with or without downward and forward inclination of the maxilla results in this skeletal deep bite.

- Reduced anterior facial height
- Horizontal growth pattern of the face
- A reduced interocclusal clearance (freeway space)
- A cephalometric examination reveals that most of the horizontal cephalometric planes such as mandibular plane, Frankfort horizontal (FH) plane and sella-nasion (S-N) plane are parallel to each other.

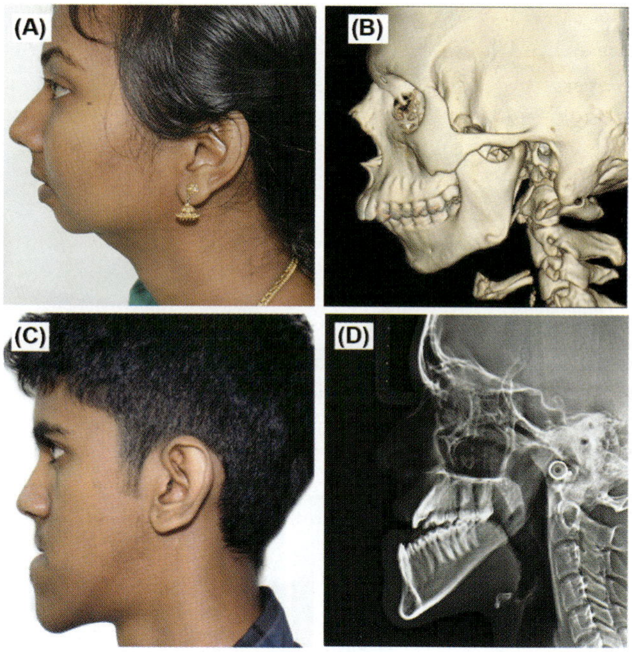

Figure 43.6 (**A** and **B**) Genial deficiency—microgenia. (**C** and **D**) Genial excess.

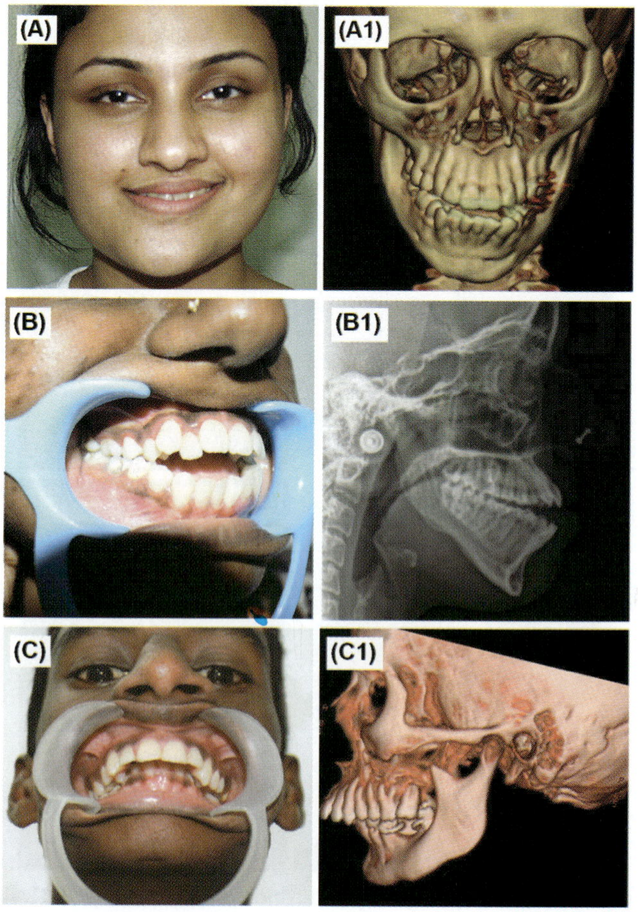

Figure 43.7 (**A, A1**) Genial asymmetry. (**B, B1**) Open bite. (**C, C1**) Deep bite.

DIAGNOSIS AND TREATMENT PLANNING

The overall patient management entirely depends upon the thorough evaluation and diagnosis of the deformity. Any failure on the side of the clinician to recognise the major functional and aesthetic problems might have undesirable and complicated outcomes.

Diagnosis and treatment planning for any orthognathic case is established through proper interaction and communication of both orthodontist and maxillofacial surgeon (Table 43.3 and Flowchart 43.1).

PATIENT EVALUATION

It includes thorough evaluation and diagnosis for overall patient management. The sequence in evaluating a patient for orthognathic surgery should follow the below four main areas:

I. Patient concerns or chief complaints
II. Clinical evaluation

TABLE 43.3 Typical Presentation of Maxillofacial Deformities

		Clinical Features	Skeletal Assessment	Dental Assessment
Maxilla	Sagittal deficiency (anterior–posterior plane)	• Concave facial profile • Retrusive upper lip • Acute nasolabial angle • Alar base narrow • Lack of dental display	• SNA decreased • SNB normal • ANB decreased	• SNA decreased • SNB normal • ANB decreased
	Sagittal excess (anterior–posterior plane)	• Convex facial profile • Obtuse nasolabial angle	• SNA increased • SNB normal • ANB increased	
	Vertical excess (long face syndrome)	• Convex profile • Lower facial height increased • Alar base constricted • Nasolabial angle obtuse • Excessive gingival show • Excessive incisor show • Lip incompetence • Mentalis strain with lip closure • Chin vertically long, retruded	• Lower facial height increased • SNA decreased • SNB decreased • ANB increased • Mandibular plane angle steep • Palatal occlusal plane increased	• Class II, class I • Anterior open bite • Maxillary arch constricted • Curve of Spee, flat-accentuated • Dental crowding
	Vertical deficiency (short face syndrome)	• Concave facial profile • Lower facial height decreased • Nasolabial angle acute • Alar base widened • Lack of incisor show • Chin protruded	• Lower facial height decreased • SNB increased • ANB negative • Palatal occlusal plane decreased • Edentulous appearance	• Class II, class I • Deep bite • Crowding • Curve of Spee is reverse • Mandibular plane angle-acute
Mandible	Deficiency	• Convex profile • Retruded chin • Deep labiomental crease • Lower lip everted • Mentalis strain with lip closure	• SNA normal • SNB decreased • ANB increased • Ar-Gn decreased	• Class II • Mandibular incisors proclined • Maxillary incisors retroclined • Curve of Spee accentuated
	Excess	• Concave profile • Midface appears deficient • Lower 3rd broad • Lower lip thin	• SNA normal • SNB decreased • ANB decreased	• Class II • Maxillary incisors proclined • Mandibular incisors retroclined

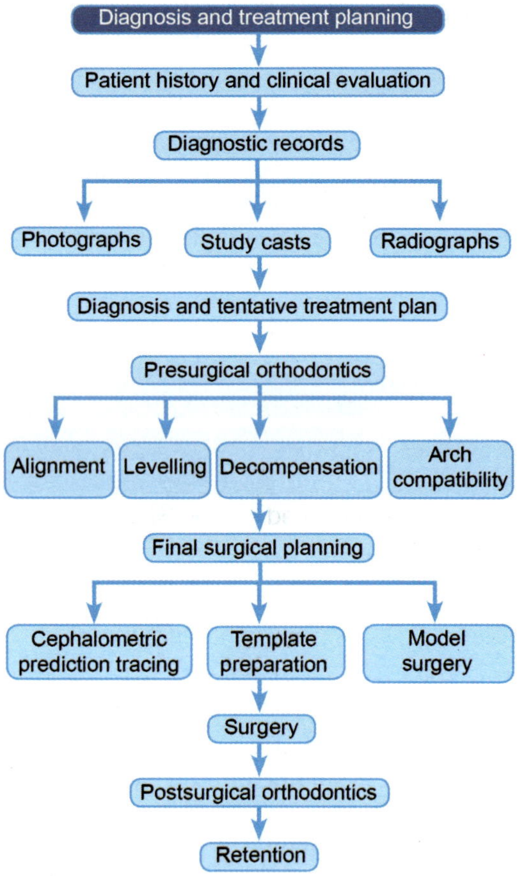

Flowchart 43.1 Diagnosis and treatment planning.

III. Radiographic and imaging analysis
IV. Dental model analysis.

I. Patient concerns

Most of the patients get satisfied with the treatment outcome based on their initial perceptions and their concerns prior to surgery failing, which will affect the psychological health of the patient. Every patient's chief concerns should include the following questionnaire which helps in developing a preliminary problem list, and helps identify patients with unrealistic expectations:

- What are your concerns or problems?
- Have you had previous treatment and what was the outcome?
- Why do you want the treatment?
- What are your expectations from the treatment?

II. Clinical evaluation

Clinical evaluation for orthognathic surgery includes:

- Patient history
- Clinical photographs
- Patient preparation for dentofacial examination
- Dentofacial evaluation.

PATIENT HISTORY

A thorough medical and dental history, physical examination and laboratory investigation should be done to rule out or identify patients with airway problems, connective tissue or autoimmune diseases, bleeding disorders or other pathologic conditions that may preclude or modify surgery.

CLINICAL PHOTOGRAPHS

- Essential for documentation and can be used for photometric analysis
- Also to obtain soft tissue landmarks for angular and linear measurements.

PATIENT PREPARATION FOR DENTOFACIAL EXAMINATION

Before proceeding with the patient's facial evaluation, it is important to seat the patient in the following position:

- **Sitting upright in** a straight-backed chair
- **The pupillary plane** should be parallel to the floor
- **Natural head position**: It is the most important factor in which the patient's head is positioned in a way that the clinical FH plane (defined as the line from the tragus of the ear to the bony infraorbital rim) is parallel to the floor. Most standardised measurements throughout the treatment are obtained in this position only
- Centric relation—usually the patient is asked to position the tongue at the most posterior aspect of the palate while gently closing the teeth together
- Lips should be relaxed as it allows in evaluating the vertical facial height, tooth to lip measurements, lip incompetences and coincidences of the dental midlines.

DENTOFACIAL EVALUATION (Table 43.4)

The goals of dentofacial examination are to evaluate and document the following problems:

- Extraoral examination (macro and miniaesthetics)
- Intraoal examination (microaesthetics)
- Functional examination.

Extraoral examination

General

Any temporomandibular joint (TMJ) dysfunction or pathosis should be detected prior to surgery. Any nasal trauma, nasal airway obstruction, allergies, sinus problems, predominant mouth breathing, etc. are evaluated.

Macroaesthetics

The facial features for macroaesthetic examination are evaluated from the frontal and lateral profile views as listed in Flowchart 43.2.

Miniaesthetics (*Fig. 43.14*)

The miniaesthetic examination includes the following features:

1. Vertical characteristics of the smile:
    - Lip-tooth-gingival relationships

TABLE 43.4 Facial Aesthetics

Macroaesthetics 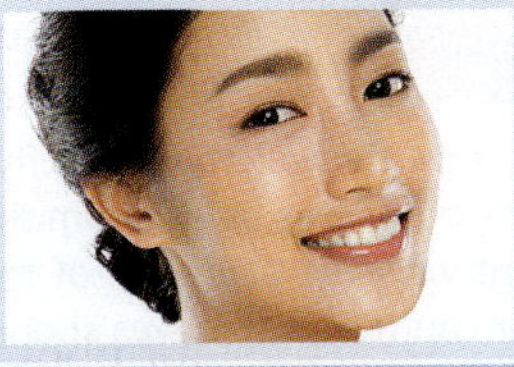	• Profile • Vertical Proportions • Lip fullness • Chin projection • Nasal projection • Ear size
Miniaesthetics 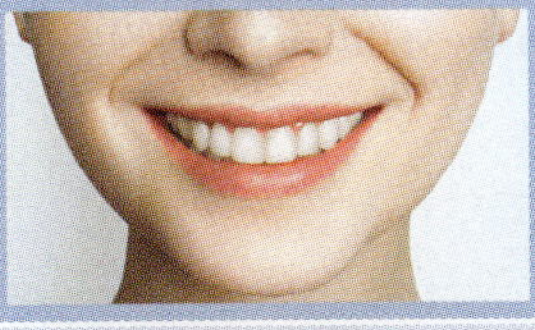	• Incisor display • Transverse smile • Smile symmetry • Crowding • Smile arc
Microaesthetics 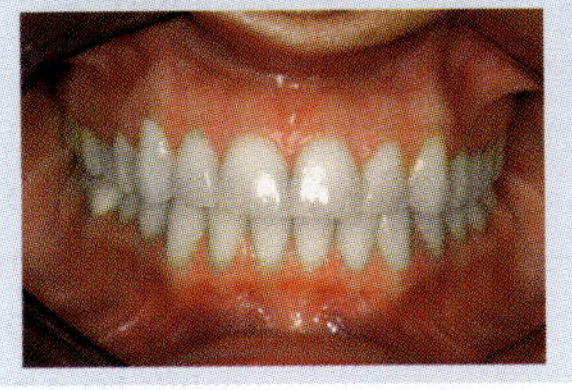	• Gingival heights • Triangular holes • Emergence profiles • Spacing • Tooth shade • Tooth shape • Incisor angulations

- Gingival display on smile
- Philtrum height
- Clinical crown height
- Maxillary incisors inclination

2. Transverse characteristics of the smile (Fig. 43.17):
    - Arch form
    - Buccal corridor
    - Cant of the transverse occlusal plane
    - *Lower lip, chin, throat angle:* It is the angle between a line drawn from the lower lip to the soft tissue pogonion and a line drawn tangentially to the soft tissue contour below the body of the mandible. The normal angulation is 110 degrees ± 8 degrees. A large angle indicates recessive chin while low angulation suggests an excessive chin.

Intraoral examination

Microaesthetics

- Occlusal relationship
- Anterior deep bite or open bite
- Anterior overjet and any crossbite
- Health of the dentition
- Tooth size discrepancies
- Curve of Wilson & Curve of Spee
- Dental crowding or spacing
- Missing and carious teeth
- Periodontal evaluation
- Transverse, vertical and anteroposterior discrepancies
- Anatomical, functional tongue abnormalities
- Attrition.

Macroaesthetics

- **Frontal view**
    - **1. Vertical proportions** (Fig. 43.8)
    - **2. Transverse proportions** (Fig. 43.9)
        - a. Rule of fifths
        - b. Nasal Anatomy
            - Dorsum
            - Nasal tip
            - Columella
            - Alar base
        - c. Eyes intercanthal distance (Fig. 43.10)
    - **3. Transverse symmetry** (Fig. 43.11)
        - a. Nasal tip to mid-sagittal plane (MSP)
        - b. Maxillary dental midline to MSP
        - c. Mandibular dental midline to symphysis
        - d. Maxillomandibular asymmetry
        - e. Chin asymmetry
    - **4. Lips** (Fig. 43.12)
        - Upper lip length
        - Lower lip length
        - Competency
- **Profile view**
    - **1. Facial profile** (Fig. 43.13)
        - a. Convex
        - b. Concave
        - c. Straight
    - **2. Facial divergence**
        - a. Anterior
        - b. Posterior
    - **3. Lip form**
        - a. Size
        - b. Projection
        - c. Mentolabial sulcus
    - **4. Nasolabial angle** (Fig. 43.15)
    - **5. Chin projection** (Fig. 43.16)
    - **6. Chin to throat angle**

Flowchart 43.2 Macroaesthetics examination.

Oral examination helps to find out functional and aesthetic deformities of the dentofacial structures.

Extraoral examination

Any TMJ dysfunction or pathosis should be detected prior to surgery. Any nasal trauma, nasal airway obstruction, allergies, sinus problems, predominant mouth breathing, etc. are evaluated.

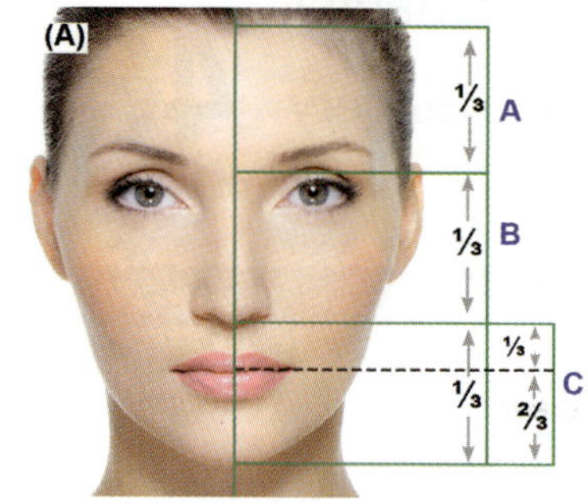

Figure 43.8 (**A**) Vertical proportions of frontal view. (**B**) Vertical proportions of profile view. A, Upper facial 3rd—from the hairline to the glabella. B, Middle facial 3rd—glabella to subnasale. C, Lower facial 3rd—subnasale to soft tissue menton. All the facial 3rd proportions should be in 1:1:1 ratio.

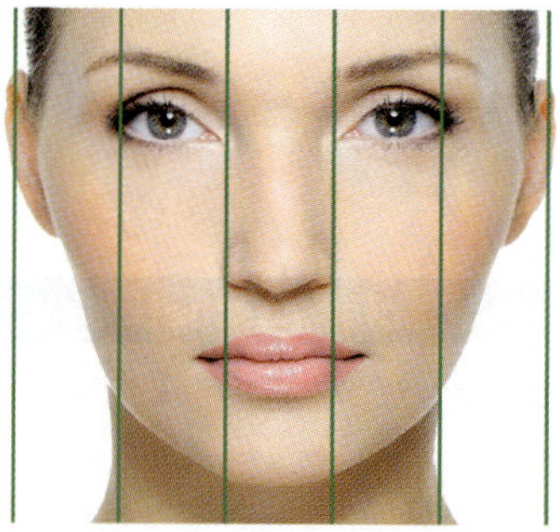

Figure 43.9 Rule of five. The face is divided sagittally into five equal parts from helix to helix of the outer ears. A line from the inner canthus should be coincident with the alar base of the nose. A vertical line from the outer canthus of the eyes should be coincident with the gonial angles of the mandible. The outer two-fifths of the face is measured from the lateral canthus to the lateral helix, which represents the width of the ears.

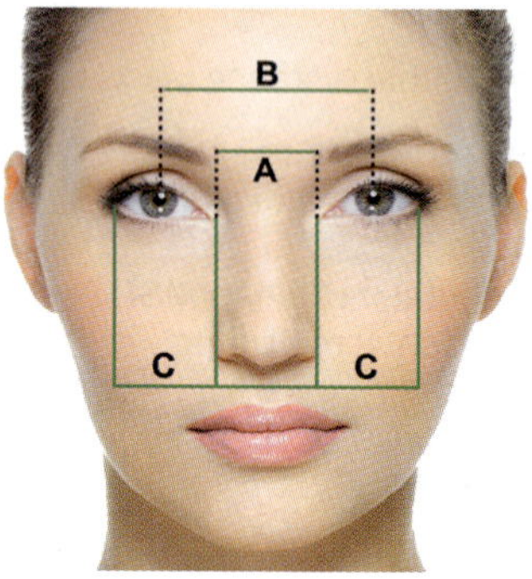

Figure 43.10 Transverse proportions. (**A**) Intercanthal distance—35 ± 3 mm. (**B**) Interpupillary distance—65 ± 3 mm. (**C**) The palpebral fissure width should be equal to the intercanthal distance.

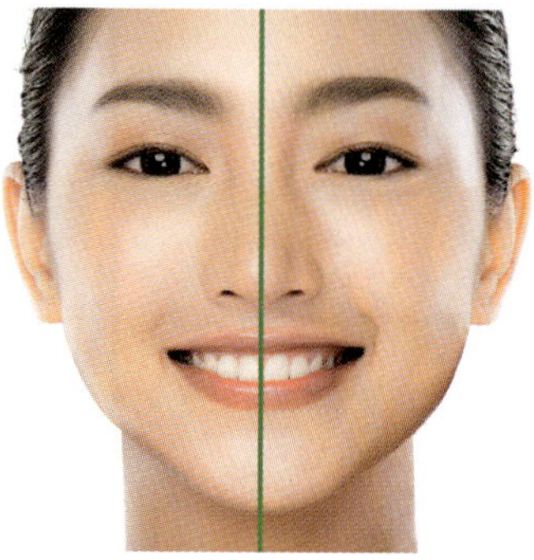

Figure 43.11 Transverse symmetry. The nasal, maxillary, mandibular and chin midlines are assessed in relation to the midsagittal plane (MSP). Left to right facial symmetry is assessed.

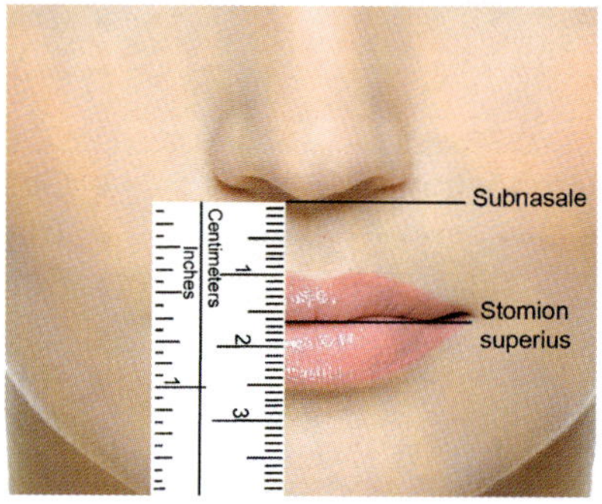

Figure 43.12 Upper lip length. Measured from the subnasale to stomion superius. Normal value for males 22 ± 2 mm and for females 20 ± 2 mm, and upper lip should be one-3rd the length of the lower facial 3rd.

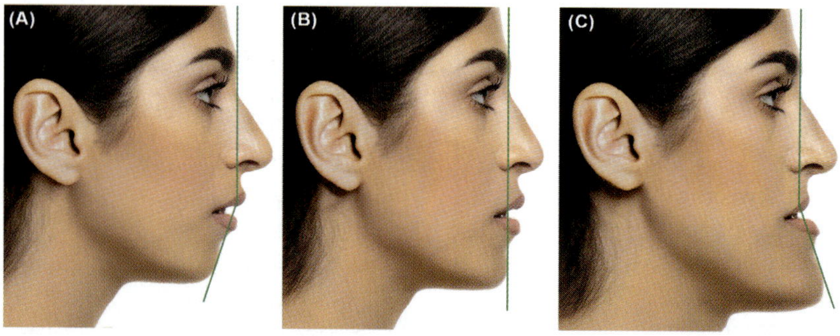

Figure 43.13 Facial profile analysis. (**A**) Convex profile. (**B**) Straight profile. (**C**) Concave profile.

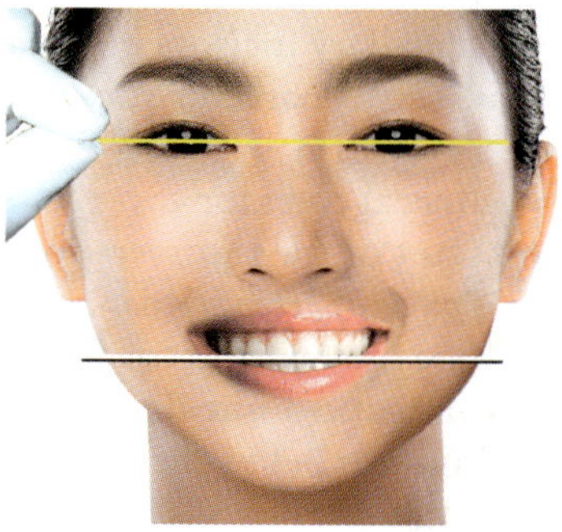

Figure 43.14 Transvere occlusal plane. It should be parallel to the interpupillary plane and any changes usually indicate infraorbital hypoplasia, orbital dystopia or exophthalmos.

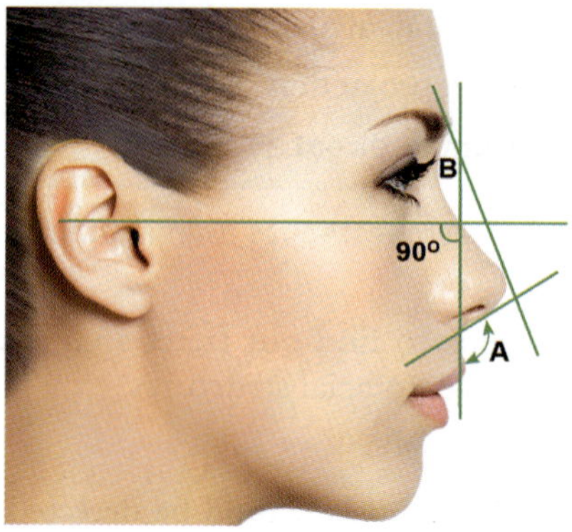

Figure 43.15 (**A**) The normal nasolabial angle is 90–105 degrees. (**B**) The normal nasal projection angle with a line tangent to the dorsum of the nose and the angle created by the line perpendicular to Frankfort horizontal should be 36 degrees for males and 34 degrees for females.

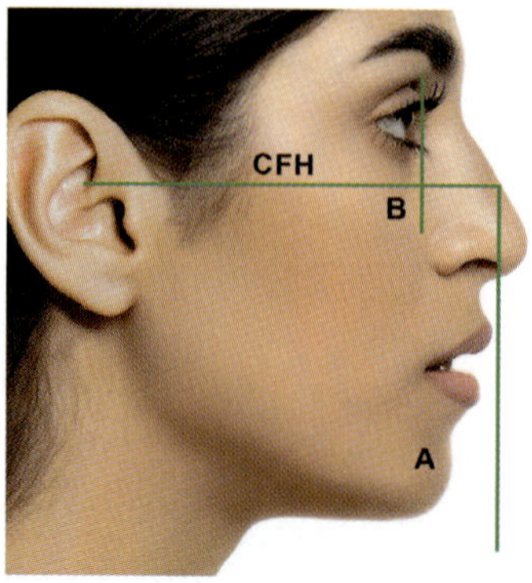

Figure 43.16 Chin projection. (**A**) A line perpendicular to the clinical Frankfort horizontal (CFH) plane through subnasale should be 3 ± 3 mm anterior to the chin. (**B**) A line tangent to the globe should fall on the infraorbital soft tissues ±2 mm.

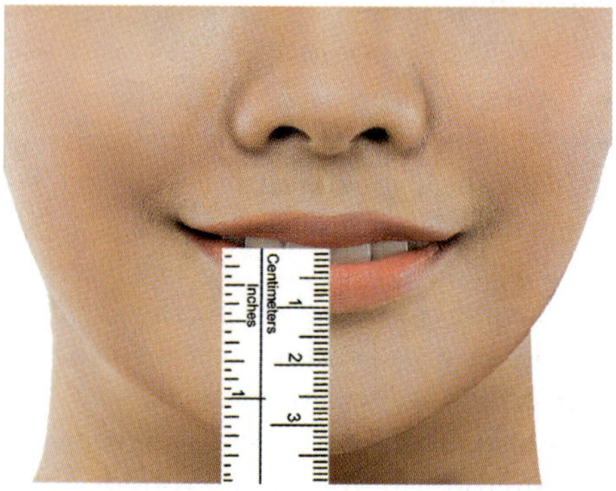

Figure 43.17 Incisor display. Normal upper tooth to lip relationship should expose 2.5 ± 1.5 mm of incisal edge with the lips in repose.

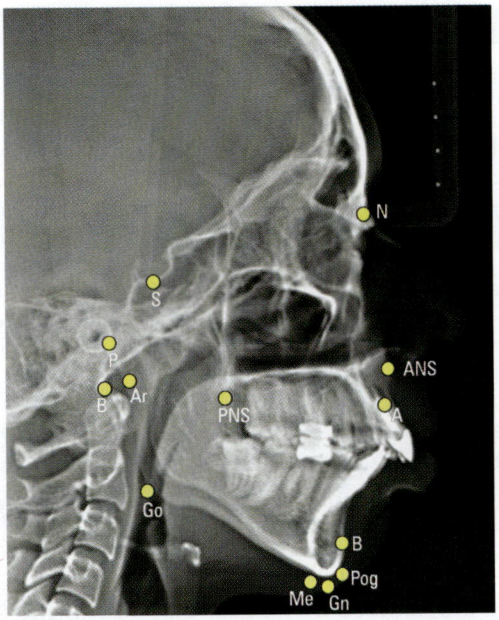

Figure 43.18 Important landmarks on a lateral skull radiograph for cephalometric analysis.

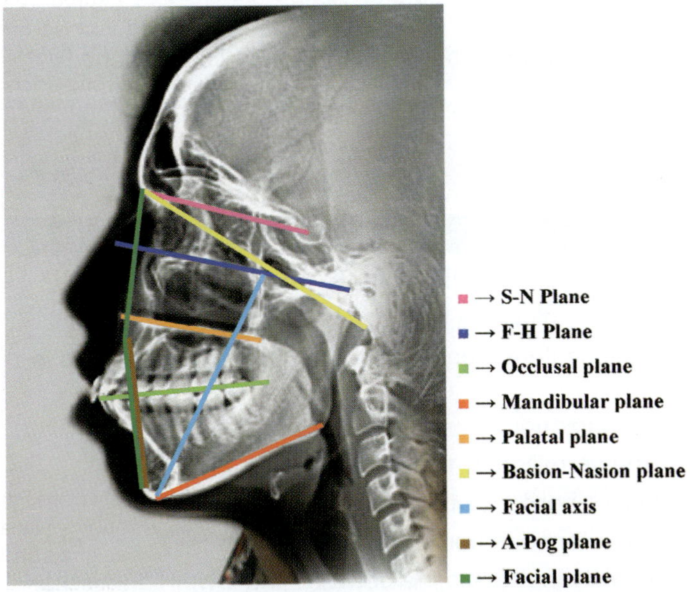

Figure 43.19 Important planes on a lateral skull radiograph for cephalometric analysis.

III. Radiographic and imaging analysis

Cephalometric analysis can be an aid in the diagnosis of skeletal and dental problems and as a tool for simulating surgery and orthodontics. A number of cephalometric analyses are commonly used for orthodontic case analysis. These analyses are primarily intended to reposition the misaligned teeth with the existing skeletal pattern.

For the purpose of cephalometric analysis, following landmarks of planes on the lateral skull radiograph are essential (Figs. 43.18 and 43.19).

Cephalometric hard and soft tissue landmarks (Tables 43.5 and 43.6)

Cranial base

The base line for comparison of most of the data in this cephalometric analysis is a constructed plane called horizontal plane (HP). It is constructed by drawing a line 7 degrees from the line SN. It is a substitute to Frankfort plane. Most of the measurements are made from projections either parallel or perpendicular to horizontal plane. The length of the cranial base is measured from Ar to N and parallel to HP.

Horizontal skeletal profile analysis (Fig. 43.20A and B)

Horizontal skeletal profile analyses are made parallel to HP. These are very important because most surgical corrections are primarily made in the anteroposterior direction.

Degree of skeletal convexity

The angle of facial convexity is measured by the angle formed by the line NA and the line from A to Pog. The N-A-Pog angle gives an indication of the overall facial convexity, but does not specify the diagnosis that whether the maxilla or the mandible is at fault.

A positive angle of convexity denotes convex face and a negative angle denotes concave face. A clockwise angle is positive (+), a counter clockwise angle is negative (-).

A line perpendicular from HP is dropped through N. Horizontal position of A is measured from this perpendicular line. This measurement describes the apical base of the maxilla in relation to N and enables to determine if the anterior part of the maxilla is protrusive or retrusive. Similarly, position of point B from this perpendicular line describes the horizontal position of the apical base of the mandible in relation to N. When inferior anatomical landmark is measured in relation to the superior structure, the positive sign (+) denotes anterior and the negative sign (-) denotes posterior.

Thus, these measurements are useful in the planning of treatment of maxillary or mandibular advancement or reduction.

N-Pog is measured in the same manner as NA and NB and indicates the prominence of the chin. These measurements determine if there is horizontal genial hyperplasia or hypoplasia and useful in the planning of treatment as augmentation and reduction genioplasty, anterior mandibular horizontal advancement or reduction and total mandibular horizontal advancement or reduction.

Vertical skeletal profile analysis (Fig. 43.21)

Vertical skeletal discrepancy may reflect anterior, posterior or complex dysplasia of the face. Therefore, vertical skeletal cephalometric measurements are divided into anterior and posterior components.

- *Anterior component:* The anterior component is subdivided into measurements of: (1) the middle 3rd facial height [distance from N to anterior nasal spine (ANS)]

TABLE 43.5 Landmarks of Hard Tissue on Cephalograph

SELLA (S)	The centre of the pituitary fossa
NASION (N)	The most anterior point of the nasofrontal suture in the midsagittal plane
ARTICULARE (Ar)	The intersection of the basisphenoid and the posterior border of the condyle mandibularis
PTERYGOMAXILLARY FISSURE (PTM)	The most posterior point on the anterior contour of the maxillary tuberosity
SUBSPINALE (A)	The deepest point in the midsagittal plane between the anterior nasal spine and prosthion, usually around the level of and anterior to the apex of the maxillary central incisors
POGONION (Pog)	The most anterior point in the midsaggital plane of the contour of the chin
SUPRAMENTALE (B)	The deepest point in the midsagittal plane between infradentale and Pog. Usually anterior to and slightly below the apices of the mandibular incisors
ANTERIOR NASAL SPINE (ANS)	The most anterior point of the nasal floor; the tip of the premaxilla in the midsagittal plane
MENTON (Me)	The lowest point on the contour of the mandibular symphysis
GNATHION (Gn)	The midpoint between Pog and Me, located by bisecting the facial line N-Pog and the mandibular plane (lower border)
POSTERIOR NASAL SPINE (PNS)	The most posterior point on the contour of the palate
MANDIBULAR PLANE (MP)	A plane constructed from Me to the angle of the mandible (Go)
NASAL FLOOR (NF)	A plane constructed from PNS to ANS
GONION (Go)	Located by bisecting the posterior ramal plane and the mandibular plane angle

TABLE 43.6 Landmarks of Soft Tissue on Cephalograph

GLABELLA (G)	The most prominent point in the midsagittal plane of the forehead
COLUMELLA POINT (Cm)	The most anterior point on the columella of the nose
SUBNASALE (Sn)	The point at which the nasal septum merges with the upper cutaneous lip in the midsagittal plane
LABRALE SUPERIUS (Ls)	A point indicating the mucocutaneous border of the upper lip
STOMION SUPERIUS (Stms)	The lower most point of the vermilion of the upper lip
STOMION INFERIUS (Stmi)	A point indicating the superior border of the lower lip
LABRALE INFERIUS (Li)	A point indicating the mucocutaneous border of the lower lip
MENTOLABIAL SULCUS (Si)	The point of greatest concavity in the midline between the lower lip and the chin (Pog′)
SOFT TISSUE POGONION (Pog′)	The most anterior point of soft tissue chin
SOFT TISSUE GNATHION (Gn′)	The constructed point between soft tissue pogonion and the soft tissue menton; can be located at the intersection of the subnasale to soft tissue pogonion line and the line from C to Me′
SOFT TISSUE MENTON (Me′)	The lowest point on the contour of the soft tissue chin; found by dropping a perpendicular from horizontal plane through menton
CERVICAL POINT (C)	The inner most point between the submental area and the neck located at the intersection of lines drawn tangent to the neck and submental areas

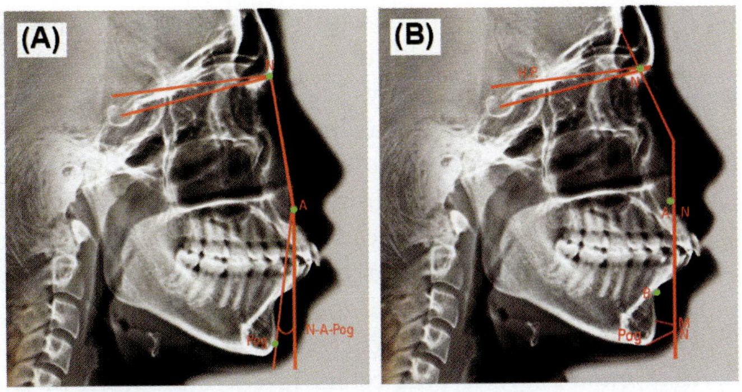

Figure 43.20 (**A**) Horizontal skeletal angle of convexity. (**B**) Horizontal skeletal profile.

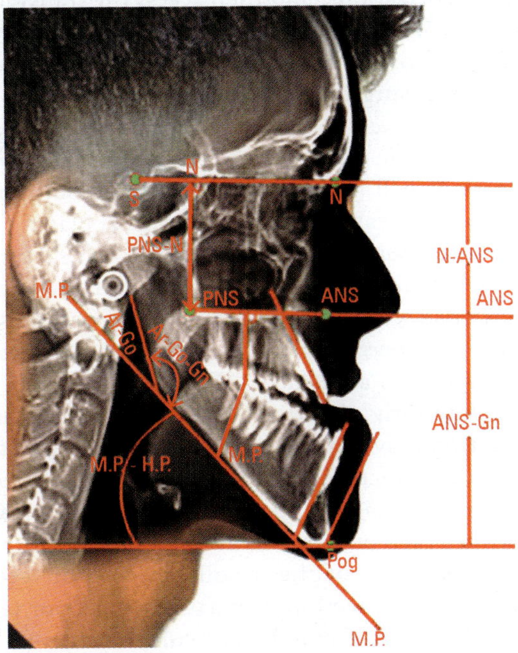

Figure 43.21 Vertical skeletal and dental measurements.

that is measured perpendicular to HP and (2) the lower 3rd facial height which is a measurement from ANS to Gn and is measured perpendicular to HP

- *Posterior component:* Posterior maxillary height is the length of a perpendicular line dropped from HP intersecting the posterior nasal spine (PNS). The divergence of the mandible posteriorly is shown by the mandibular plane angle (MP-HP), which is the angle formed between Go, Gn and HP. This angle helps in relating the posterior facial divergence with respect to the anterior facial height.

Vertical skeletal measurements help in the diagnosis of anterior, posterior and total maxillary hyperplasia or hypoplasia and also clockwise or counter clockwise rotation of the maxilla and mandible.

Surgical correction of these problems includes total maxillary vertical advancement or reduction, anterior maxillary vertical augmentation or reduction, posterior maxillary vertical augmentation or reduction, combination of anterior and posterior maxillary vertical augmentation or reduction and mandibular ramus rotation and ramus height reduction.

NORMAL CEPHALOMETRIC VALUES (Table 43.7)

Tracing for cephalometric studies (Fig. 43.22): The tracing should be made under suitable conditions—a darkened room, a well-illuminated viewing screen blanked off with a card to leave a window just large enough for the radiograph, a good quality tracing sheet fixed to the radiograph with clear adhesive tape and a hard pencil are required. Radiograph should be oriented with the Frankfort plane (or HP plane) parallel to the bottom edge of the screen, because a number of landmark definitions depend on head orientation

Interpretation of tracing: By comparison of angular measurement with normal values, one can interpret the results of analysis to give a diagnosis of the patient's presenting skeletal pattern. Comparison of the findings from

TABLE 43.7 Normal Cephalometric Values

	Variable	Normal	Increased	Decreased
1.	SNA	82 degrees	Prognathic maxilla	Retrognathic maxilla
2.	SNB	80 degrees	Prognathic mandible	Retrognathic mandible
3.	ANB	2 degrees	Class II skeletal pattern	Class III skeletal pattern
4.	Occlusal plane	14 degrees	Clockwise rotation of occlusal plane	Counterclockwise rotation of occlusal plane
5.	Mandibular plane	32 degrees	Vertical growth pattern	Horizontal growth pattern
6.	U incisor to NA (angular)	22 degrees	Upper incisor proclination	Upper incisor retroclination
7.	U incisor to NA (linear)	4 mm	Upper incisor proclination	Upper incisor retroclination
8.	L incisor to NB (angular)	25 degrees	Lower incisor proclination	Lower incisor retroclination
9.	L incisor to NB (linear)	4 mm	Lower incisor proclination	Lower incisor retroclination
10.	Interincisal angle	132 degrees	Retroclined incisors	Proclined incisors
11.	'S' line	0 mm	Protrusive lips	Retrusive lips

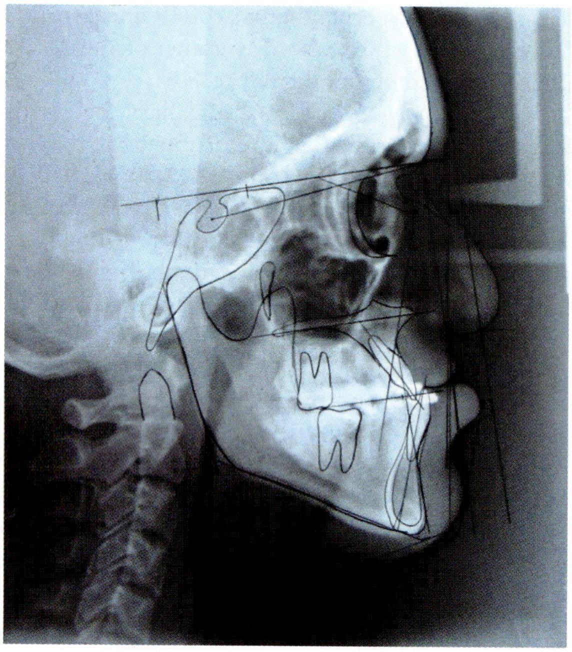

Figure 43.22 Lateral cephalogram showing cephalometric tracing done for Burstone's analysis.

the original and the final cephalometric radiographs will allow us to assess the outcome of treatment.

Apart from cephalometric studies, CT scanning and MRI are also used extensively.

IV. Dental model analysis (Fig. 43.23)

Proper model analysis improves understanding and development of the presurgical orthodontic goal. There are 10 basic dental model evaluations that should be made:

1. *Arch length:* The arch length measurement should correlate with the width of the teeth and availability of alveolar bone. These measurements give an idea whether the tooth needs to be extracted or not
2. *Tooth size analysis:* It refers to the correlation of the mesiodistal width of the upper teeth to that of the lower teeth. This is primarily seen in the anterior six maxillary and mandibular teeth

   Bolton's analysis: Total width of six upper anterior teeth = 1.3 × total width of lower six anterior teeth. Average is 77.5 ± 3.5. This analysis helps in determining disproportion in size between maxillary and mandibular teeth
3. *Tooth position in context of orthognathic analysis:* This refers primarily to the angulation of the maxillary and mandibular incisors relative to the basal bone. This analysis determines whether extractions are necessary, whether spaces need to be created and what kind of mechanics should be used for teeth correction
4. *Arch width analysis:* This refers to the evaluation of the intraarch width between the maxilla and mandible. This is best analysed by holding the models in the occlusal position that is to be achieved with the orthodontic and surgical corrections, and then access the transverse relationship. Arch width analysis is helpful in determining presurgical orthodontic mechanics as well as selecting appropriate surgical procedures
5. *Curve of occlusion:* This has a significant influence on whether it can be corrected orthodontically whether extractions will be necessary or whether surgical intervention is indicated to level the occlusal plane
6. *Cuspid-molar position:* This dictates the occlusal functions. It is preferable to have class I cuspid-molar relation
7. *Overbite and overjet relationship*
8. *Tooth arch symmetry:* There might be significant asymmetry within each arch such as cuspid on one side may be more anteriorly placed than the cuspid on other side. Correction may require special orthodontic mechanics, unilateral extraction or additional surgical procedures
9. *Buccal tooth tipping* (comparison of right and left symmetry within each other): This evaluates the position of the occlusal surfaces of the maxillary posterior teeth, in a medial-lateral direction. If maxillary posterior teeth are tipped buccally, it may be difficult to achieve a proper occlusal relationship
10. *Missing, broken down or crowned teeth:* This may influence treatment designs. If a tooth is nonrestorable and requires extraction in a potential osteotomy location, the extraction space may need to be closed orthodontically or the space maintained.

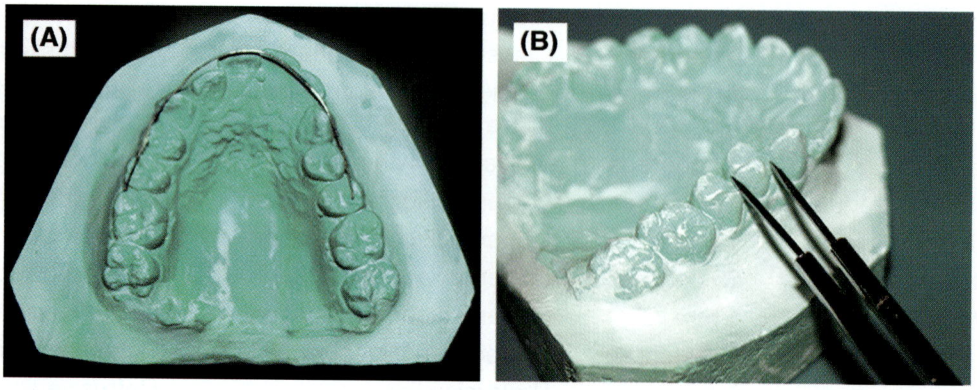

Figure 43.23 (**A** and **B**) Dental model analysis.

PRESURGICAL ORTHODONTICS

The orthodontist is responsible for moving the teeth to a more desirable position over the basal bone in preparation for surgical repositioning in all the three planes—anteroposterior, vertical and transverse. It facilitates the planned skeletal and facial correction.

The basic presurgical orthodontic goals are as follows:

- Position the long axis of the maxillary central incisors so that the final position would be approximately 22 degrees to the NA line, with the labial face of the incisors 4 mm anterior to that line
- Position the mandibular central incisors so that final position will be approximately 20 degrees to the NB line, with the labial face of the incisors 4 mm anterior to that line
- *Aligning*: Align and position the teeth over the basal bone
- *Levelling*: Avoid excessive intrusion or extrusion of the teeth
- *Decompensate teeth*: Also called as *'reverse orthodontics'* and it is one of the major goals in presurgical orthodontics. Establish the anteroposterior position of incisors and usually worsens the malocclusion to fully reveals the skeletal discrepancies
- *Adjust the tooth size discrepancies:* Done by recontouring the interproximal contact areas or by closing or opening the spaces between the maxillary or mandibular anterior teeth
- *Correct the rotated teeth*
- Avoid class II and class III mechanics (unless required for dental decompensation)
- Avoid orthodontic movements that can be performed more predictably with surgery
- *Arch compatibility*: It is the last step done in which the transverse arch width discrepancies are corrected with stable and predictable orthodontic movements through orthodontic camouflage or surgery.

Advantages

- Relapse tendencies are controlled
- Total treatment time is reduced
- Results in proper intraoperative interdigitation
- Allows quick and easy postsurgical orthodontic correction
- Allows effective surgical correction
- Improves results in terms of stability and occlusion.

Presurgical aids in orthodontics

While performing orthognathic surgery, if any surgical procedure is considered to help the treatment, it is known as surgical aid to orthodontics. Following are some of the common surgical aids to orthodontic treatment:

1. Serial extraction
2. Therapeutic extraction
3. Removal or surgical exposure of unerupted teeth
4. Extraction of submerged deciduous molars, removal of odontomes
5. Correction of diastema
6. Corticotomy.

POSTSURGICAL ORTHODONTICS

Four to six weeks after the surgery, when the surgeon confirms the satisfactory healing, the stabilising arch wires are replaced by light arch wires and occlusion is allowed to settle.

Goals

- Closure of residual spaces
- Root parallelling at the extraction sites
- Maximum interdigitation
- Finer tooth alignment
- Retention of the reoriented oral musculature to prevent relapse
- Aggressive postsurgical orthodontics if the occlusion is not perfect initially postsurgery, the surgeon and/or orthodontist must aggressively apply the appropriate elastic mechanics
- Ideal overbite and overjet
- To stabilise the results obtained through the surgery
- Changing arch wires
- Final positioning of the teeth usually takes 3–12 months or sometimes longer depending on the orthodontic requirements
- Orthodontic retainers to provide transverse support to the width of the maxillary and mandibular dental arches and maintain the dental alignment.

MODEL SURGERY

Model surgery is the dental cast version of cephalometric prediction of surgical results. When the teeth are highly irregular or when the maxillary and mandibular arch forms are incompatible, model surgery is impossible without simulating the presurgical orthodontic treatment. In this case, a diagnostic setup is done 1st and then the setup models are moved as they might be at surgery.

In its simplest form, model surgery requires nothing more than articulating the pretreatment casts by hand in a possible postsurgical position. Mandibular advancement can be simulated, for instance, by sliding the lower cast forward relative to the upper cast. It is easier to study the possible tooth relationship if the casts are mounted temporarily on arbitrary articulators so that they are held in the desired position. The better the occlusion without any tooth movement, it is easier to articulate the casts by hand and vice versa.

Purpose

- To determine the magnitude and direction of skeletal movements
- To determine the size and shape of the osteotomies especially interdentally
- To provide a splint for surgical correction
- To provide a comparative reference to the occlusal result actually achieved as noted on release of intermaxillary fixation.

Indications

Model surgery is used in double jaw surgery, as well as single jaw surgery where unoperated jaw will act as a template.

Advantages

- The simulation of the patient's facial structure functionally and spatially in three dimensions
- The surgeon can correlate the relevant information and arrive at the surgical prediction in three dimensions
- Model surgery gives an accurate 1:1 replica of the patient's dentition allowing an increased accuracy in prediction, when compared to the 10% discrepancy seen in cephalometric distortion
- Model platform and block is capable of accurately measuring articulator mounted models in three planes of space, which allows the surgeon to carry out accurate model surgery movements on a full-sized anatomic articulator.

Disadvantages

- Condyles are never perfectly symmetrical; therefore, the model surgery performed on the mounted casts give slightly inaccurate readings
- There can be errors related to the actual model orientation itself
- There can be measurement errors related to instruments and perspective.

SURGICAL SPLINTS

Surgical splints are also known as occlusal wafer splints. They are utilised in the operating room to position the teeth and add to stabilisation. They are used during the surgery as well as postsurgically.

Advantages

1. Provide a clearly visualised goal for the surgeon at the operating table
2. Aids in positioning bone fragments correctly to aid healing
3. Possible to put teeth in a planned position at surgery, even if they do not interdigitate perfectly without a splint
4. Surgical splints are utilised in the following procedures
   - Maxillary surgery
   - Mandibular ramus surgery
   - Segmental jaw surgery
   - Dual jaw surgery.

Construction of splints

The splint is made on the casts as they have been related by model surgery. After they have been checked by the surgeon and orthodontist, the following steps are undertaken:

1. Stabilise cast with plaster or stone, so that no shift occurs as splint is fabricated
2. Articulator is opened to allow for enough thickness of splint material
3. Self-curing acrylic is formed into the desired U-shaped configuration. Care is taken to avoid rolling the acrylic excessively, as this causes cracks and bubbles
4. Lay the U-shaped roll of uncured acrylic on the lower occlusal surface. The casts are then closed onto it. At this point, the casts must be firmly secured to the articulator. If the casts shift, splint dictates wrong position at surgery
5. While the acrylic is still soft, scissors/scalpel is used to trim the excess on the labial aspect. Ensure that it does not tear away while carrying out this procedure
6. After the acrylic has cured, a semitrimmed splint with occlusal indentations is obtained
7. Trim away excessive bulk labially and lingually with burs. Buccal aspect of splint must be contoured to avoid interference with orthodontic appliances and to allow visual determination of proper seating during surgery. The acrylic should be relieved on lingual aspect of anterior teeth and distal aspect of buccal segment cusp tip to allow a smooth arc of closure
8. Trim occlusal surfaces so that only shallow occlusal indentations remain
9. Finally, place bur holes along labial and buccal surface for attaching splint to the arch wires
10. Routine finishing and polishing must be carried out for patient's comfort and maintenance of oral hygiene.

TREATMENT OF DENTOFACIAL DEFORMITIES

- To reposition bone and dentoalveolar segments into normal relationship
- To provide best functional aesthetic results along with stability.

Mild deformities can be corrected using orthodontic tooth movement. For severe skeletal deformities, there are three options: (1) growth modification, (2) orthodontic camouflage and (3) orthognathic surgery.

Growth modification

Growth modification can be achieved in children, in whom the growth potential is still present, through: (1) orthopaedic appliances like head gear, chin cup and (2) myofunctional appliances.

Orthodontic camouflage

When the skeletal deformity is very mild and any further change is not expected, orthodontic camouflage should be considered. Establishing normal overjet and overbite can compensate a few discrepancies, for example, in case of mild skeletal class II malocclusion, the maxillary teeth can be retracted and the mandibular teeth slightly proclined to camouflage the skeletal deformity. Camouflage should not be done at the expense of undesirable facial aesthetics though there might be some compensation of the same. The utmost significance in orthodontic camouflage is given to the ultimate facial aesthetics and occlusional stability.

ORTHOGNATHIC SURGERY

The fundamental goal of orthognathic surgery is to reposition basal bone and the dentoalveolar segments into normal relationship and to provide best functional aesthetic results along with stability (Box 43.1).

Guidelines for performing osteotomy

- Bell in 1975 proved that the blood supply to the osteotomised segment will be maintained adequately, if at least one soft tissue pedicle is preserved intact. Therefore, the design of the soft tissue incision should be such that it follows Bell's principle
- The neurovascular bundle should be preserved during the osteotomy cut
- The cut should be done under constant irrigation in order to avoid necrosis of the tissues due to excessive heat produced by the micromotor
- The cut for subapical surgery should be a minimum of 4–5 mm away from the root apex, and for that matter any osteotomy cut should not jeopardise the integrity of the periodontal ligament of any tooth
- The osteotomised portions should be well approximated without any bony or soft tissue interference.

BOX 43.1 Maxillary Surgeries

1. **Segmental Osteotomy of the Maxilla**
   a. Single tooth osteotomy
   b. Corticotomy
   c. Surgically assisted rapid maxillary expansion (SARME)
   d. Anterior segmental maxillary osteotomy
      - Wassmund's technique
      - Wunderer's technique
      - Epker's anterior maxillary osteotomy
      - Cupar's technique
   e. Posterior subapical osteotomy of maxilla
      - Kufner
      - Schuchardt
      - Perko and Bell
2. **Total Maxillary Osteotomy**
   a. Le Fort I
   b. Le Fort II
   c. Le Fort III

MAXILLARY OSTEOTOMY PROCEDURES

From 1969 to 1975, Bell carried out extensive research studies on rhesus monkeys and performed many maxillary osteotomies which led to its popularity. He experimented and studied revascularisation and bone healing of the various osteotomy procedures. He proved that if at least one soft tissue pedicle is preserved intact, blood supply to the osteotomised segments can be maintained. This was the biological basis for many maxillary osteotomies.

SINGLE TOOTH OSTEOTOMY (Fig. 43.24A–C)

Single tooth osteotomy is used for correction of tooth malposition, dental ankylosis, or closure of a diastema. Because soft tissue pedicle to the dentoalveolar segment is relatively small, some surgeons have been reluctant to use this technique for fear of compromising vascular supply and causing ischaemic necrosis of the involved segment. Benefits of this surgical technique are a reduction in treatment time and a lower incidence of dental relapse when compared with conventional orthodontic therapy. Drawbacks of the procedure include injury to the adjacent teeth, periodontal compromise of the treated tooth or adjacent tooth and devitalisation of teeth. These factors lead to pulpal necrosis, colour change, root resorption and possibly the need for endodontic therapy.

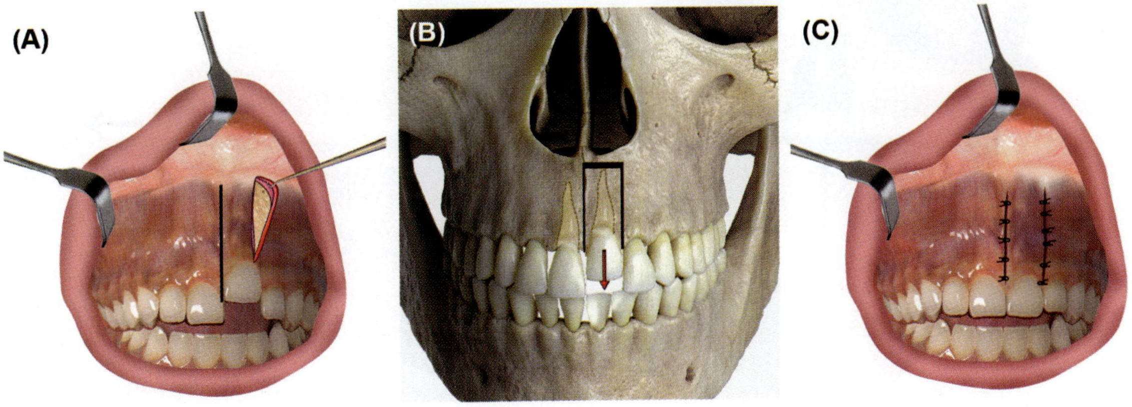

Figure 43.24 Single tooth osteotomy for repositioning superiorly positioned central incisor. (**A**) Incision. (**B**) Osteotomy cut. (**C**) Repositioning.

SURGICALLY ASSISTED RAPID MAXILLARY EXPANSION (Fig. 43.25)

Rapid maxillary expansion is a technique used in treating transverse maxillomandibular discrepancy. It was 1st described in 1860 by Angell and later reintroduced by Haas in 1961. The surgically assisted rapid maxillary expansion (SARME) procedure is a combination of distraction osteogenesis and controlled soft tissue expansion. SARME is successful in children prior to suture closure. It is best performed before the transverse maxillary growth ceases and the maxillofacial suture closure which is at skeletal age 14–15 years in females and 15–16 years in males. The expansion is achieved usually by using jackscrew appliances, mostly the Hass and Hyrax appliances.

Indications

- Transverse maxillary deficiency >5 mm discrepancy and with unilateral or bilateral posterior skeletal crossbite that may result from one of the following maxillomandibular combinations
    i. Narrow maxilla and normal mandible
    ii. Normal maxilla and wide mandible
    iii. Narrow maxilla and wide mandible
- Failed orthodontic expansion
- Large amount of expansion or preference to avoid potential increased risk of segmental osteotomies
- Presence of significant buccal gingival recession in the canine bicuspid region of the maxilla or very thin and delicate gingival tissues
- Nasal stenosis.

Technique

- It is also called a subtotal Le Fort I maxillary osteotomy
- The mandibular dentition should be decompensated before surgery to allow assessment of the amount of transverse expansion necessary and to prevent postexpansion relapse
- The appliance must be placed preoperatively and the appliance key must be present in the operating site to allow intraoperative activation
- A horizontal incision is made in the maxillary vestibule from the 2nd molar region of one side to the same area on the opposite side
- Bilateral maxillary osteotomy from the pyriform rim to the pterygomaxillary fissure
- Release of the nasal septum to prevent septal deviation during expansion
- Midline palatal osteotomy extending interdentally between the maxillary incisors and from the ANS to the PNS
- Osteotomy of the lateral nasal wall anteriorly of about 1.5 mm
- Bilateral release of the pterygoid plates
- Activation of the appliance with a total widening of 1–1.5 mm with evaluation for symmetric expansion, and the surgeon should check that the both maxillae are adequately mobile
- Soft tissue closure including alar base cinch and V–Y closure to control the soft tissues of the nasal base and upper lip.

Following the surgery, the maxilla should remain stationary for at least 5 days before initiating the expansion at a rate of 0.5 mm/day. Expansion greater than this may cause gingival recession on the mesial side of the central incisors.

Complications

Intraoperative complications are similar to those that occur in Le Fort I osteotomy like:

- Intraoperative haemorrhage
- Pain and discomfort due to tightness at the nasal root—glabellar area and posterior orbit
- Devitalisation of the teeth
- Gingival recession on the mesial side of the central incisors.

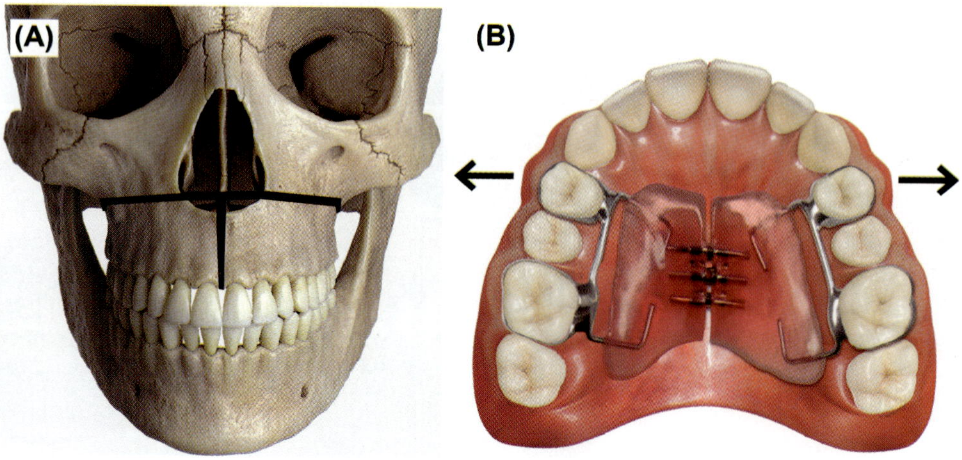

Figure 43.25 Surgically assisted rapid maxillary expansion (SARME). **(A)** Frontal view of the completed SARME. **(B)** Palatal view of the Hass expansion device in place with the vectors of expansion demonstrated.

ANTERIOR SEGMENTAL MAXILLARY OSTEOTOMY (FIG. 43.26)

Segmental maxillary surgery was performed for many years before total maxillary osteotomy became popular. In 1921, Cohn Stock performed the 1st maxillary segmental osteotomy. He performed a wedge-shaped osteotomy through transverse palatal incisions; followed by a greenstick fracture of the anterior maxillary segment that was retracted, but the segment relapsed in 4 weeks duration. Later, this procedure was modified with variations in incision designs depending on the desired osseous movements.

Indications

- To correct the protrusion of the maxillary teeth with normal incisor axial inclination to the alveolar bone

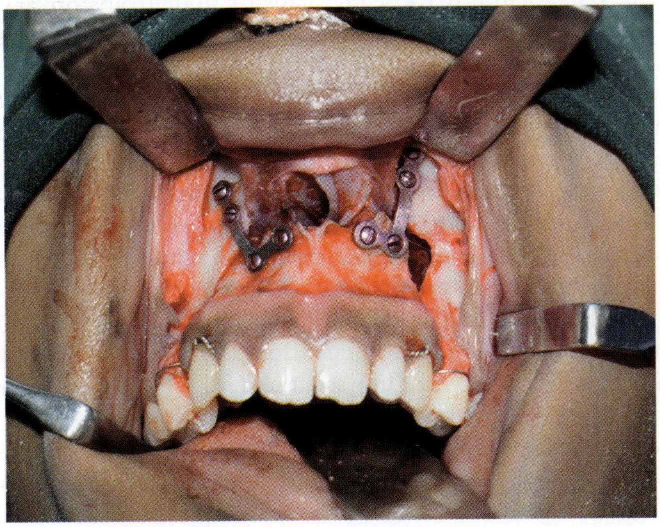

Figure 43.26 Anterior maxillary osteotomy.

- To correct the anterior open bite provided vertical maxillary excess is not present
- Correction of premaxilla in a vertical plane as required in anterior deep bite or open bite
- When orthodontic therapy cannot be accomplished for the retraction of the maxillary teeth as in pathological resorption or dental ankylosis
- To improve facial appearance in prognathic maxilla with competent lips and adequate lip length.

Technique

Wassmund's technique (Fig. 43.27)

- In 1935, Wassmund described a technique for maxillary osteotomy which was used widely and is used to this day with slight modification
- A vertical incision is made between the canine and premolar extending to the nasal floor and mucoperiosteum is reflected posteriorly and superiorly. While reaching the apical region of the canine, reflection is carried out to the inferolateral border of the nasal pyriform aperture. The mucoperiosteum of the pyriform aperture is reflected using a free elevator
- If planned, 1st premolar is extracted at this stage. A midline sagittal incision on the palate gives better visibility and access to the palatal midline for performing the palatal osteotomy. The palatal mucosa is reflected by tunnelling past midline and care is taken not to injure the anterior palatine vessels
- The bony cut is made on the buccal aspect of the alveolus using bur or reciprocating saw. The cut is taken vertically upwards and turned medially to the pyriform aperture so that 3–5 mm of intact bone remains above the apex of the canine tooth
- Next step is transpalatal osteotomy of the palatal bone from the alveolus of one side to that of the other side.

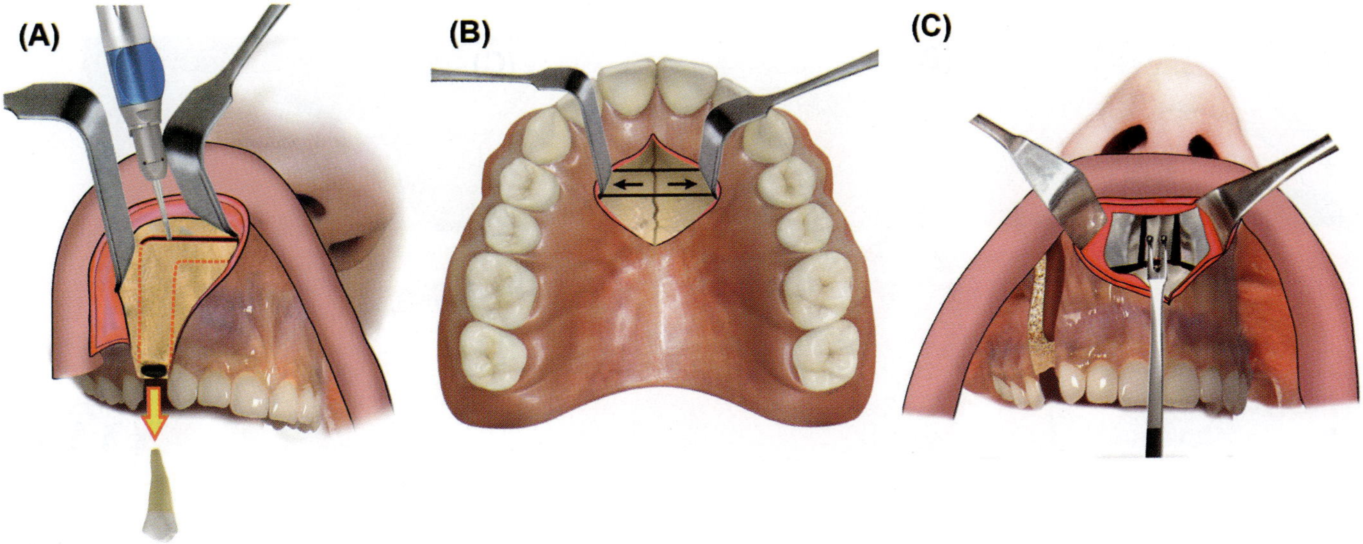

Figure 43.27 Wassmund's technique. (**A**) Buccal bone cut. (**B**) Exposure of the palate. (**C**) Separation of the nasal septum.

Care should be taken not to injure the palatal soft tissues. Towards the midline, palatal bone is hard to cut due to difficult access and increased thickness of the bone. This region can be cut through a midpalatine incision in the anteroposterior direction

- Now, the maxillary segment has to be separated from the nasal septum. Sometimes this can be done through finger pressure. Usually a vertical incision is placed over the ANS. Reflection of mucoperiosteum is done from the nasal spine and cartilaginous nasal septum. The septum is separated from the anterior maxillary segment using a nasal osteotome
- At this stage, dentoalveolar segment can be split in the midline, if required. This is done by tunnelling and using a straight fissure bur and an osteotome. This is useful in cases of closure of diastema and minor adjustments in apposition of the canine
- The folds on the soft tissue are checked to ascertain that there is no hindrance to proper blood flow. Soft tissue is closed using 3-0 catgut.

Wunderer's technique (Fig. 43.28)

This technique (1963) is suitable especially when 2nd premolar is to be extracted. The labial approach is same as that of the Wassmund's procedure. The palatal surgery is started once the buccal part of the surgery is completed.

In Wunderer's technique, a transverse palatal cut anterior to the planned osteotomy site is made. Then the soft tissue is raised posteriorly a little behind the planned osteotomy site. The osteotomy is now performed. In the midline, bone is little harder but access to the palate is very good and the cut can be done as far posteriorly as the 2nd molar. Anterior segment can be mobilised and separated from the nasal septum, once the bony cuts are completed. It is then positioned and fixed using prefabricated occlusal splint and soft tissue closure is done.

It is similar to Wassmund's technique except for palatal exposure by transverse palatal incision with margins away from osteotomy site.

Epker's anterior maxillary osteotomy

In this technique, either the 1st or the 2nd premolars are to be extracted. A transverse incision is made in depth of the sulcus from behind the planned osteotomy site to the opposite side. Subperiosteal dissection is done only superiorly. The pyriform aperture is exposed and nasal mucoperiosteum is dissected on the lateral wall and floor. The cartilaginous nasal septum is elevated from the vomerian groove in the anterior nasal crest of the maxilla.

The dissection is carried out for about 15 mm posteriorly. Subapical osteotomy is done leaving 3–5 mm of healthy bone above the teeth apices. The vertical osteotomy is done after tunnelling the mucoperiosteum at the interdental region; all bone cuts including those of palate are done from labiobuccal side. When this alveolar osteotomy is done, care should be taken not to injure the palatal tissues. For this, a finger should be kept in the palatal area, which helps to feel the bur perforating the bone. After completion of the subapical and alveolar osteotomy, a midline osteotomy is done if necessary, like in cases of midline diastema and in cases where the intercuspid distance has to be increased. About 15 mm of anterior portion of nasal crest of the maxilla is removed for better visualisation in the transpalatal osteotomy.

With a straight osteotometranspalatal osteotomy is completed and the anterior maxilla is down fractured. The palatal mucoperiosteum is carefully separated from the palate posterior to the osteotomy site. With a large round bur the required ostectomy is done. The osteotomy sites are inspected for any bony protuberances and intermaxillary fixation is done using arch wire on previously applied orthodontic gadgets. Intermaxillary fixation is required for a period of 1–2 weeks only.

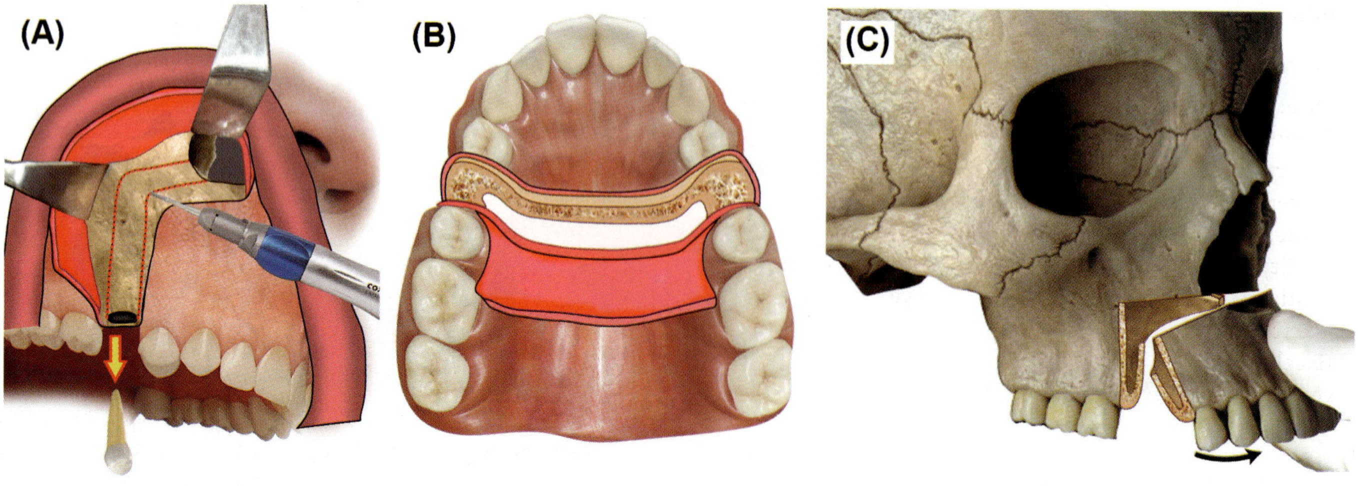

Figure 43.28 Wunderer's technique for repositioning anterior segment. (**A**) Buccal bone cut. (**B**) Transpalatal incision made; flap elevated and palatal cut made. (**C**) Maxillary segment separated.

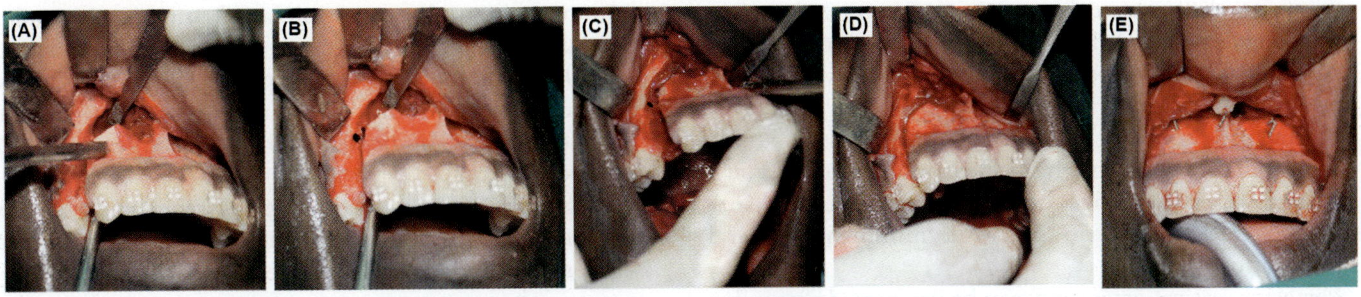

Figure 43.29 **(A–E)** Cupar's anterior maxillary osteotomy.

Cupar's anterior maxillary osteotomy (*Fig. 43.29*)

It is a minor version of total maxillary osteotomy down fracture technique. A buccal vestibular incision is created, allowing direct access to the anterior lateral maxillary walls, pyriform aperture, nasal floor and septum. Sequence of osteotomies is operator dependent, but general procedure involves completion of the vertical buccal and horizontal osteotomies.

The nasal mucosa is elevated from the superior surface of the maxilla. Nasal septum is 1st released from the maxillary crest. Horizontal osteotomy is performed followed by vertical osteotomy, which is performed bilaterally between the teeth. Through this vertical cut, transpalatal osteotomy is completed with either a reciprocating saw or an osteotome. A finger is placed on the palatal mucosa to palpate the osteotome in an attempt to protect the palatal tissue from injury by the osteotome.

The transpalatal osteotomy is now completed under direct visualisation from above, allowing excellent access to the nasal crest of the maxilla and midpalatal bone for osseous recontouring.

Occlusal stent stabilisation, osseous wiring, skeletal fixation, rigid internal fixation or a combination of these methods completes fixation of the anterior maxillary osteotomy (AMO).

Advantages

- Direct access to the nasal structures to allow for manipulation of the cartilaginous septum, thus preventing any deformities due to buckling
- Preservation of blood supply through an excellent palatal pedicle
- Ability to remove bone from the palate under direct visualisation after the anterior maxilla has been down fractured
- Excellent access to the superior maxilla for reduction of vertical maxillary excess or bone grafting
- Easy placement of rigid internal fixation.

POSTERIOR SEGMENTAL MAXILLARY OSTEOTOMY

Posterior maxillary osteotomy (PMO) was originally described in 1959 by Schuchardt as a two-stage procedure for the correction of open bite deformities. Indications cited for PMO today are more extensive.

Indications

- Posterior maxillary alveolar hyperplasia
- Total maxillary hyperplasia (when combined with AMO)
- Spacing in the dentition that can be closed by anterior repositioning of the posterior segment
- Transverse excess or deficiency
- Posterior open bite
- Correction of posterior crossbite.

Surgical technique

- PMO is most commonly performed as a single-stage procedure through a buccal vestibular incision extending from the canine region to that of the 2nd molar below the zygomatic buttress
- Alternatively, vertical incisions in the region of the anterior and posterior osteotomies can be created and combined with a parasagittal palatal incision
- If indicated, dental extraction is carefully performed to preserve alveolar bone
- The palatal osteotomy is generally performed transantrally through the buccal horizontal osteotomy
- A palatal incision is generally not required unless medial movement of the maxillary segment greater than a few millimetres is planned, or the mobilised segment will not be able to be positioned appropriately. In this case, a parasagittal incision can be created away from the area of the planned osteotomy. Reflection of the palatal flap to remove bone under direct visualisation must be done with caution in order to preserve the palatal vasculature
- Horizontal buccal osteotomy is completed at least 5 mm above the apices of the teeth using either rotary instrumentation or a reciprocating saw from the location of the anterior vertical osteotomy to the maxillary tuberosity. An appropriate amount of bone is removed when performing the osteotomy to allow for superior repositioning of the posterior maxillary segment
- Vertical osteotomy can then be performed through an extraction site or space created orthodontically using a

fine fissure bur or spatula osteotome. Care must be taken to preserve at least 1 mm of bone support along the root surfaces of the adjacent teeth in order to prevent a periodontal defect

- Palatal osteotomy is usually performed with a curved osteotome placed through the horizontal osteotomy site, with the operator's finger on the palatal tissues to ensure complete osseous sectioning while minimising palatal perforation
- Posterior vertical osteotomy can be performed through a 3rd molar extraction site or by pterygomaxillary separation. With the latter technique, a subperiosteal tunnel is created posteriorly to localise the pterygomaxillary junction in a manner similar to that used during the total maxillary osteotomy
- The disjunction is then completed using a curved osteotome oriented in an anterior, inferior and medial direction. Posterior dentoalveolar segment is down fractured with finger pressure and previously inaccessible regions, such as the medial and posterior extents of the osseous segment, are recontoured if indicated
- Posterior segment is positioned into the acrylic splint derived from model surgery and the mandible is rotated into position to ensure that there are no occlusal interferences
- In most circumstances, miniplate fixation is adequate, although skeletal fixation, direct osseous wiring or the surgical stent alone can be used, provided there is adequate bone contact and sufficient number of teeth for stability
- Bone grafts are indicated if there are large gaps at the osteotomy site
- If rigid fixation is not used, surgical stent should be maintained for 3–6 months or replaced by a retentive orthodontic appliance to prevent relapse of the segments.

Variations of posterior segmental maxillary osteotomy

1. In 1970, Kufner made only a horizontal incision above the apices of the involved teeth, gaining access to the palatal aspect
2. Perko in 1972 and later Bell in 1975 made a hockey stick incision along the midline of the palate as far forwards as the incisive papilla, and then carried it out laterally anterior to the proposed osteotomy site.

LE FORT I OSTEOTOMY (Figs. 43.30 and 43.31)

In 1972, Martin Wassmund introduced a surgical procedure for moving the entire maxilla. This operation, which has been since called Le Fort I osteotomy or total maxillary osteotomy, was 1st used to correct open bite. The maxilla was not

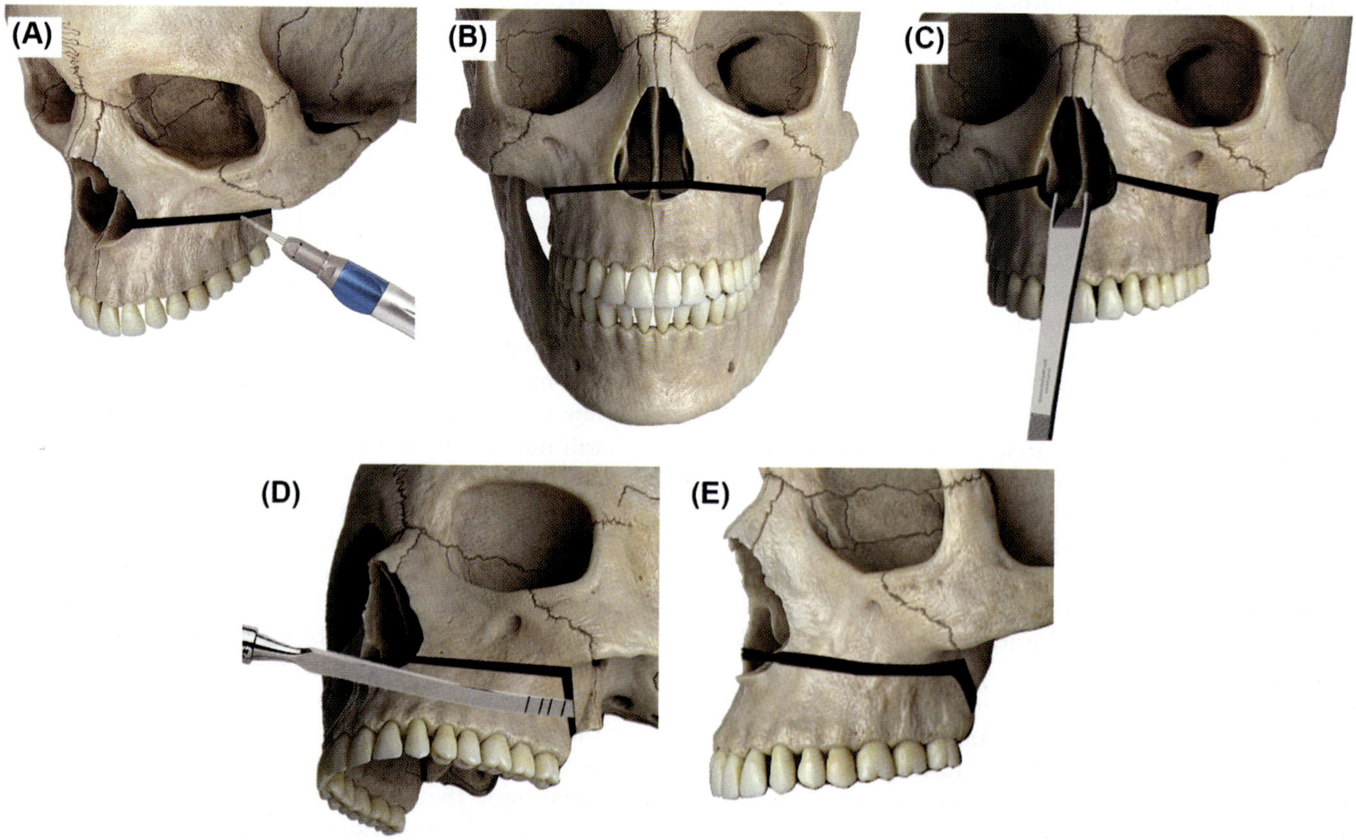

Figure 43.30 Le Fort I osteotomy. (**A**) Osteotomy cut. (**B**) Osteotomy cut completed on both sides. (**C**) Nasoseptal osteotome used to separate the nasal septum from maxilla. (**D**) Separation of maxilla from pterygoid plate. (**E**) Completely separated maxilla.

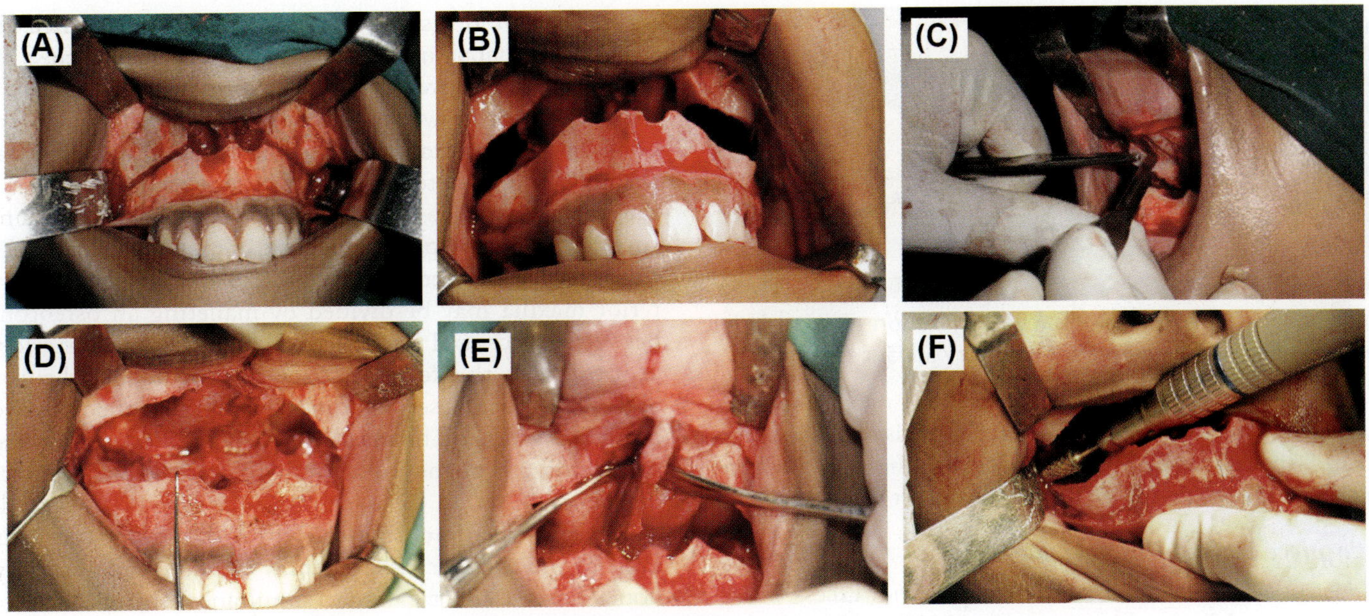

Figure 43.31 **(A–F)** Intraoperative pictures showing Le Fort I osteotomy.

completely sectioned from its bony attachments initially but as time elapsed and with increase in clinical experience, evolution of sound surgical and biological principles, surgeons became more aggressive and complete mobilisation of the maxilla and adequate fixation was accomplished.

Le Fort I osteotomy has become the workhorse of orthognathic surgical procedures. It can be used to correct a variety of maxillofacial problems.

Indications

- Vertical maxillary excess
- Vertical maxillary deficiency
- Anterior–posterior maxillary deficiency (maxillary hypoplasia)
- Facial asymmetry.

Surgical technique

The procedure is performed under general anaesthesia, preferably hypotensive anaesthesia. Lidocaine 2% with 1:100,000 epinephrine is infiltrated into the mucosal tissues of the upper lip. A horizontal incision is made in the maxillary vestibule from the 2nd molar region of one side to the same area on the opposite side. A mucoperiosteal flap is raised to expose the anterior nasal floor, pyriform aperture, lateral walls of the maxilla, zygomatic crests and pterygomaxillary junction. A nasoseptal osteotome is used to separate the nasal septum from the maxilla. The bone is sectioned 4–5 mm above the apices of teeth extending from the lateral part of the pyriform rim posteriorly across the canine fossa and through the zygomatic maxillary crest. The anterior, posterior and inferior parts of the lateral nasal wall can be sectioned transantrally under direct vision. Posterior aspect of the lateral maxilla and the posterolateral antral wall is cut by malleting a spatula osteotome posteriorly until contact is made with the dense perpendicular plate of the palatine bone. Final step then involves pterygomaxillary disjunction by using a (obwegeser-pterygoid-osteotome) medially and anteriorly into the pterygomaxillary suture to separate the maxillary tuberosity from the pterygoid plates. The maxilla is down fractured by inferior pressure against the anterior portion of maxilla and forward pressure against the tuberosity. This can be facilitated by use of Tessier's mobilisers or Rowe maxillary disimpaction forceps. The maxilla is then wired into occlusion by using a splint with intermaxillary fixation. Stabilisation of the maxilla is then achieved by interosseous wires or miniplate fixation done at the nasal and zygomaticomaxillary buttresses of the proximal and distal segments. These two sites have buttress bone to symphysis fixation.

When large osseous gaps are created at the ostectomy sites, bone grafts are laid across them for added stability and rapid union. Lateral walls of the maxilla and the zygomatic buttress are two critical areas. Autogenous corticocancellous bone harvested from the iliac is most commonly used.

Modifications of the Le Fort I osteotomy

Many technical modifications of the Le Fort I osteotomy are feasible to facilitate anteroposterior, vertical, or horizontal movements of the anterior and posterior portions of the maxilla. The level of the osteotomy cut can also be varied according to individual patient needs (Figs. 43.32–43.34).

Segmenting the maxilla

Transverse discrepancies between the dental arches, vertical steps in the maxillary occlusal plane and space remaining in the maxillary arch are indications to segment the maxilla. When segmenting the maxilla, two paramedian osteotomies and one

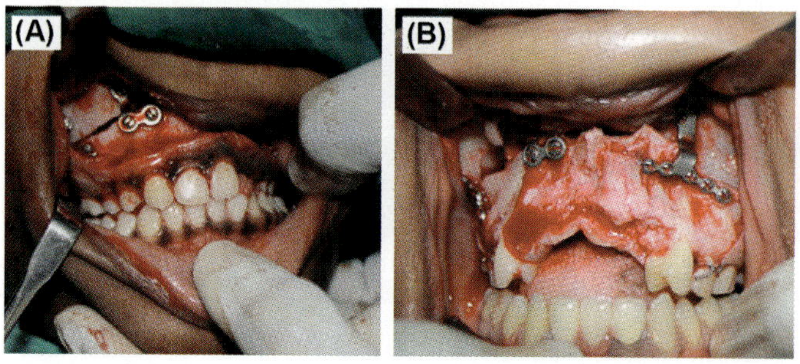

Figure 43.32 Le Fort I osteotomy. (**A**) Fixation after superior repositioning. (**B**) Fixation after maxillary advancement.

transverse osteotomy are used. Once mobilisation is accomplished, the palatal soft tissues pedicled to the island of bone may be relaxed to permit expansion and/other manoeuvres.

Two-piece Le Fort I osteotomy

In case of extreme vertical and anteroposterior excess, a classical Le Fort I in combination with AMO may be required (Fig. 43.35A–D).

In cases of transverse horizontal maxillary deficiency, maxillary expansion can be achieved by segmenting the maxilla after a conventional Le Fort I osteotomy. With the maxilla in the down fractured position, the midpalatal bone or parasagittal palatal bone can be osteotomised through appropriate interdental space transpalatally. 1st, the thick part of the anterior maxilla is sectioned with a fissure bur, then the palatal cuts are completed. The bone is then completely sectioned by the use of an osteotome. Anterior maxilla may be divided by malleting an osteotome between the central incisors and then directed posteriorly as it transects the deeper portion of the midpalatal suture and splits the interseptal bone. This step is done in case of midline diastema. The maxilla is then divided into two segments and can be moved laterally to correct the horizontal deficiency.

The most common indication for this technique is the need to move the maxilla laterally by more than 8 mm in noncleft cases, and the need to simultaneously repair an oronasal fistula, graft alveolar clefts and expand the palate in cleft palate patients.

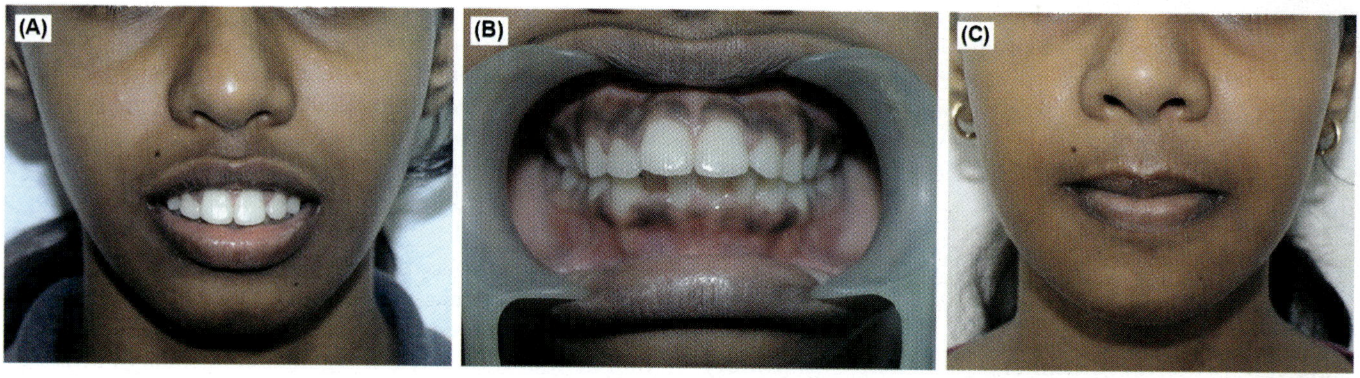

Figure 43.33 Le Fort I osteotomy. (**A–C**) Preoperative and postoperative views.

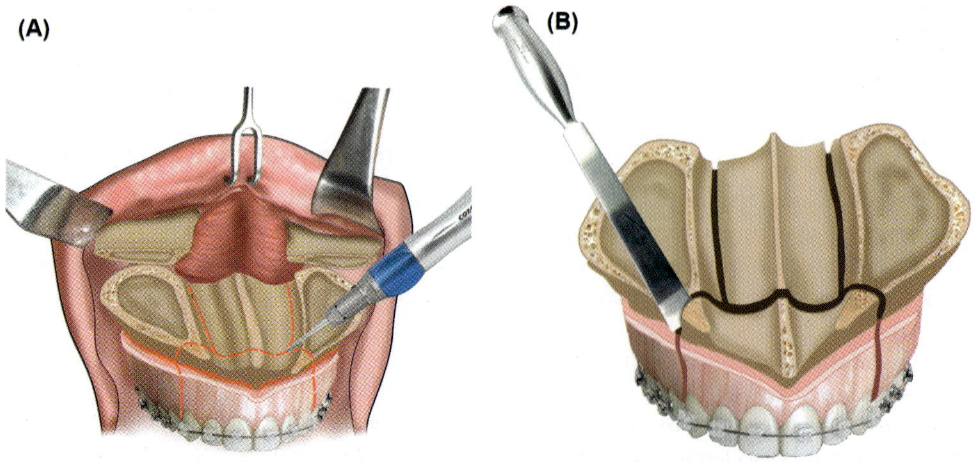

Figure 43.34 Segmenting of the maxilla. (**A**) Two paramedian osteotomies and one transverse osteotomy lines. (**B**) Maxilla segmented into four pieces.

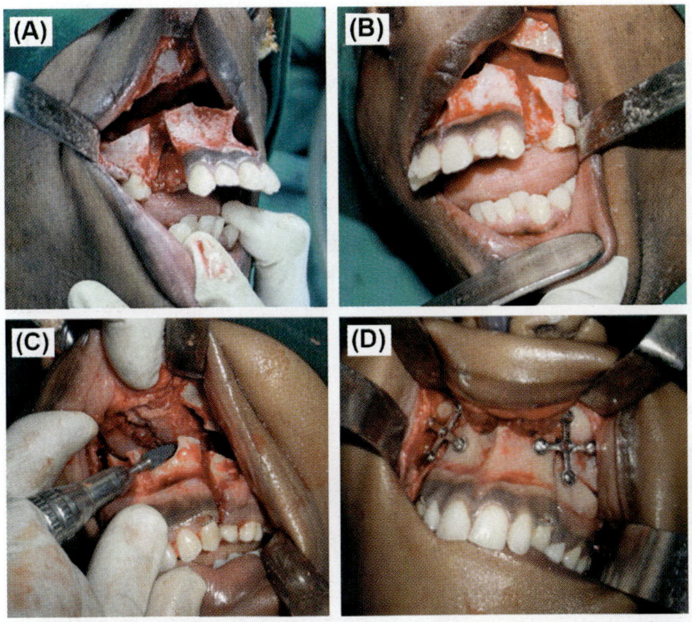

Figure 43.35 **(A–D)** Le Fort I with anterior maxillary osteotomy.

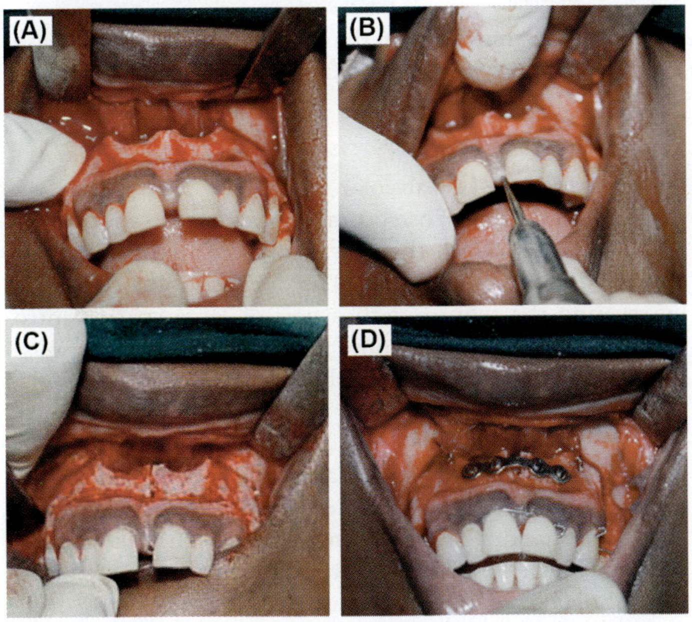

Figure 43.36 **(A–D)** Le Fort I with midline osteotomy.

Quadrangular Le Fort I osteotomy (Fig. 43.36)

1st described by Obwegeser as a Le Fort I osteotomy in which the osteotomy was placed as high as possible, from the tuberosity area around the whole maxilla, staying just beneath the infraorbital foramen.

This modification of Le Fort I osteotomy is indicated in patients with maxillary zygomatic horizontal deficiency, class III skeletal malocclusion and normal nasal projection. Coexisting vertical maxillary excess or deficiency or maxillary transverse deficiency can be treated with quadrangular Le Fort I osteotomy.

Surgical procedure: The incision is same as that for a conventional Le Fort I osteotomy. The maxillary exposure is done superiorly to visualise the infraorbital nerve and infraorbital rim, the lacrimal fossa medially and lateral orbital rim laterally. Anterior body of the zygoma is also exposed to varying degrees, depending on the necessity. Septal cartilage is detached from the maxillary crest anteriorly and the vomer is detached from the palatal midline posteriorly with a fine chisel. The bone cuts are then made starting from the pyriform rim at the level of the infraorbital nerve and extending laterally just inferior to the infraorbital foramen to the zygoma body. At this point, the cut makes a right angle and proceeds inferiorly through the buttress and lateral antral wall to the pterygopalatine fissure. Posterior osteotomy cut is completed just anterior to the pterygoid plate with a fine chisel. The same line of osteotomy cut is performed on the other side and all bone cuts are checked for completeness. The maxilla is then down fractured with finger pressure on the anterior maxilla and forward pressure on the tuberosity region. The mobilised maxilla is then secured to the mandible with a prefabricated splint and intermaxillary wires.

LE FORT II OSTEOTOMY (Fig. 43.37)

Severe paranasal hypoplasia extending to the infraorbital rims necessitates a Le Fort II osteotomy as described by Henderson and Jackson (1973), but it should be understood that this is not a common occurrence.

Exposure is gained through a bicoronal incision or bilateral paranasal incisions. The former is a more extensive procedure, possibly entailing medial canthal disruption; the latter results in potentially visible external scar. Intraoral access was also described for Le Fort II osteotomy.

The medial orbital floor, infraorbital rim, medial orbital wall and lacrimal sac are exposed in a subperiosteal plane. Medial canthal tendons are left undisturbed. An osteotomy is made with a side-cutting bur, down the medial orbital wall behind the lacrimal groove. It is extended medially to the infraorbital nerve area through the orbital floor, over the anterior maxilla and caudally as far as possible. Aufricht retractor is inserted from one paranasal incision to the other to retract the dorsal nasal skin and the osteotomies are connected at the nasal dorsum using a reciprocating saw. Any unconnected areas are cut with a fine osteotome; exposure for the osteotomies is improved with the bicoronal approach. Through a posterior buccal sulcus incision, osteotomy cuts are located and are extended across the maxillary tuberosities to the pterygomaxillary fissures. Maxillary tuberosities are separated from the pterygoid plates with a curved osteotome. To complete the osteotomy, a curved osteotome is placed in the transverse cut across the nasofrontal junction and is driven posteriorly and inferiorly to separate the vomer from the anterior skull base. Mobilisation of the maxilla is achieved as in the Le Fort I procedure.

Management of the fistula, bone grafting of the cleft, fixation and postoperative management differs little from

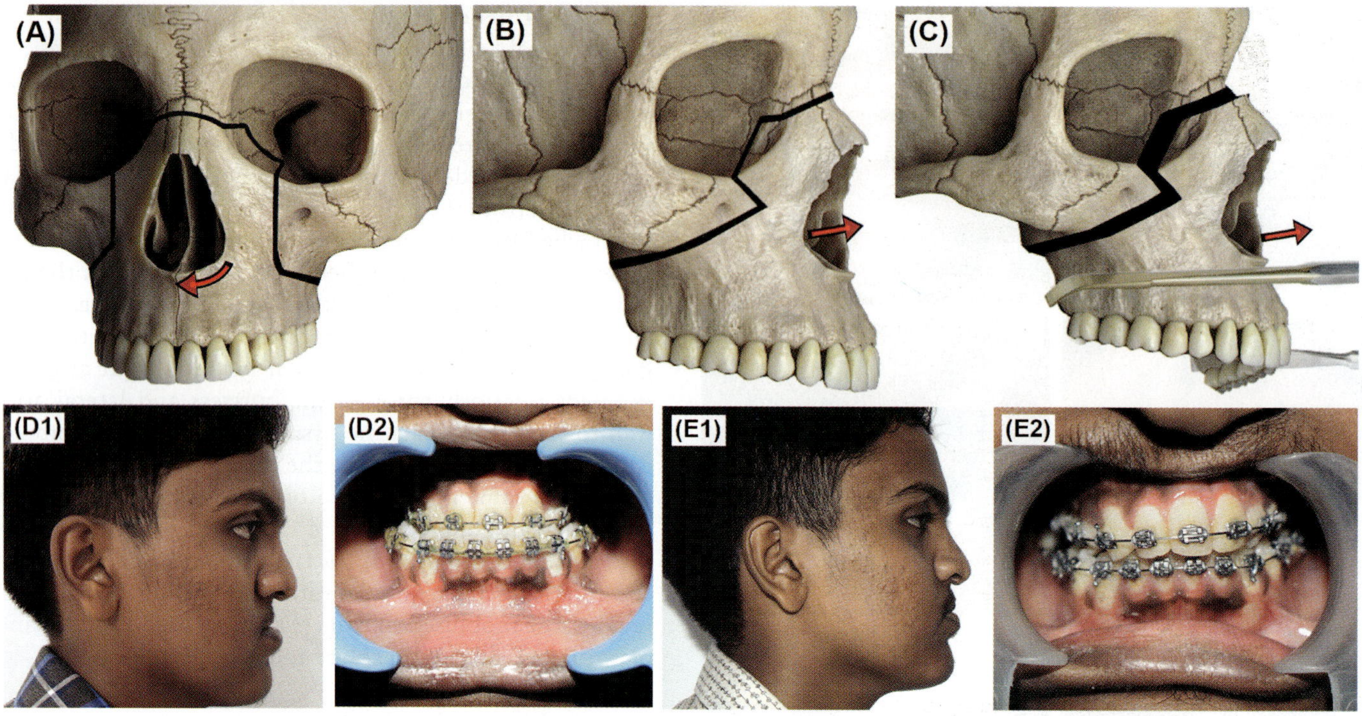

Figure 43.37 Le Fort II osteotomy. (**A** and **B**) Osteotomy cut. (**C**) Separation of the maxilla from the pterygoid plate and mobilisation. (**D1** & **D2**) Preoperative profile view and Occlusion. (**E1** & **E2**) Postoperative profile view and Occlusion.

the Le Fort I osteotomy. The infraorbital rim defects are accurately bone grafted through the paranasal incisions. Anterior osteotomy sites are filled with inlay and onlay bone grafts using the buccal sulcus approach. Split cranial bone grafts are readily available when a coronal approach is used (Jackson, Pellett and Smith, 1983). Wire or multiple screws and miniplates placed from the frontal bone to the nasal skeleton provide secure fixation of the central maxilla to the skull. If nasal height is lacking, a split cranial bone graft can be placed beneath the dorsal nasal skin and secured with two screws or wire to provide a cantilever type of dorsal graft.

LE FORT III OSTEOTOMY (Fig. 43.38)

Gillies and Harrison (1950–1951) reported the 1st high maxillary (a modified Le Fort III) osteotomy in a patient with craniofacial dysostosis. Through external incisions they performed transverse osteotomies that separated the nasal bones from the frontal bones. Osteotomy of the orbital floor was placed immediately within the infraorbital margin and extended across the floor of the orbit to the medial orbital wall anterior to the lacrimal groove. Osteotomies were also performed through frontal processes of the maxilla to diminish the width of the nose. Temporal process of the zygoma was divided on each side. An osteotome was then introduced into the pterygomaxillary junction. Anterior to the greater palatine foramen, an incision was made transversely across the mucoperiosteum of the hard palate, extending laterally and posterior to the alveolar ridge. The hard palate was divided and the line of osteotomy was rejoined at the pterygomaxillary junction. In this way, spatial relationships of the soft palate were undisturbed. The operation was completed by severing the septum with a pair of large scissors introduced through the osteotomy line at the root of the nose. Intermaxillary fixation was established.

MANDIBULAR OSTEOTOMY PROCEDURES

An abnormal occlusion with class III molar relation with reverse incisal overjet is most commonly due to excessive growth of mandible. In these cases, mostly an obvious facial deformity will be evident. Facial features associated with mandibular excess include prominence of the lower 3rd of the face, particularly in the area of the lower lip and chin in anteroposterior and vertical dimension.

Mandibular excess was one of the 1st dentofacial deformities recognised as being best treated by a combination of orthodontics and surgery. Although, surgical techniques for the correction of mandibular excess were reported as early as the late 1800s, widespread use of currently accepted technique began in the middle of this century.

Initially techniques for the treatment of mandibular prognathism dealt with the deformity by removing sections of bone in the body of the mandible, which allowed the anterior segment to be moved posteriorly. Subsequently, osteotomy techniques performed in ramus of the mandible were popularised by Caldwell and Letterman. In this technique, lateral

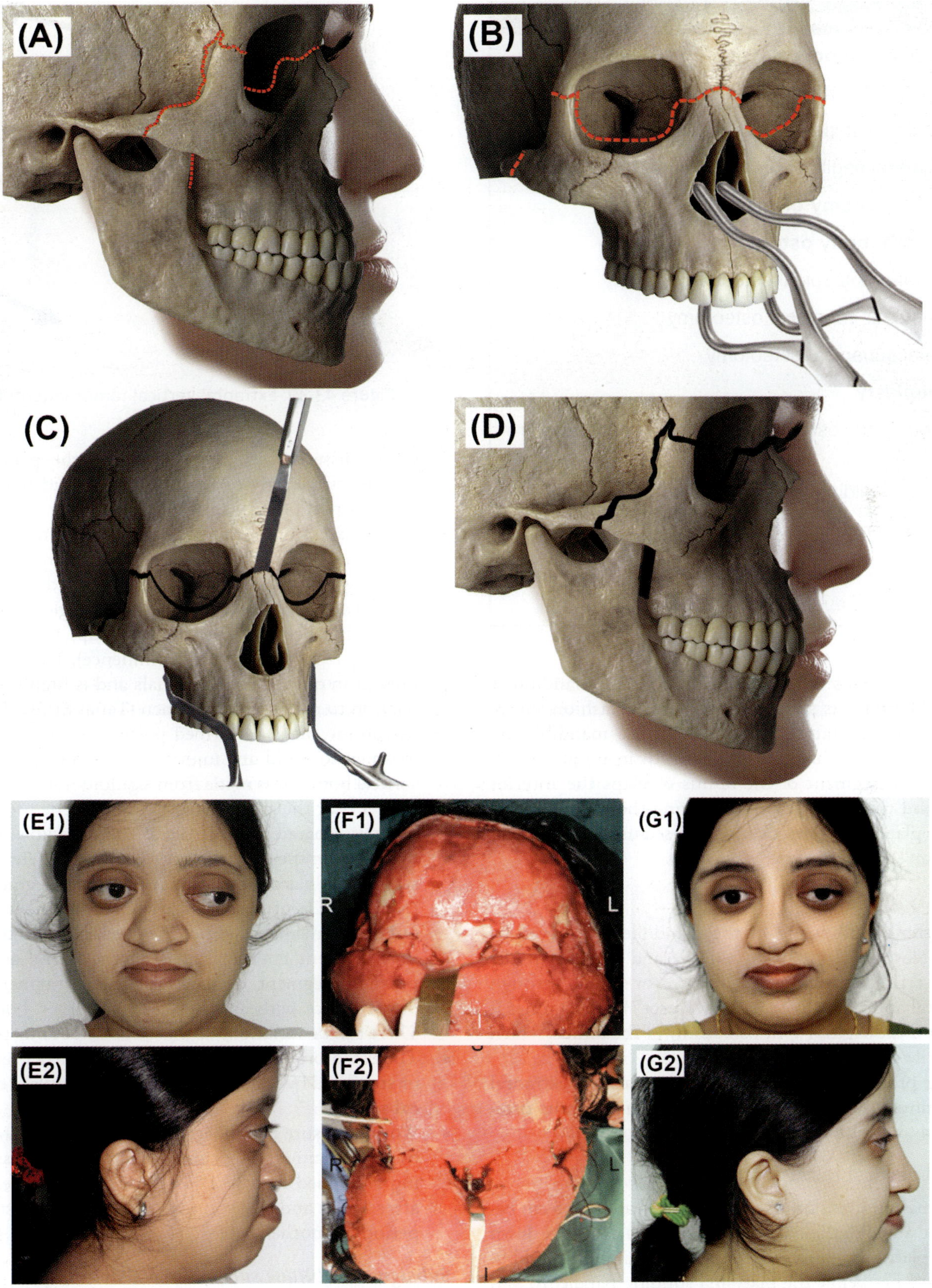

Figure 43.38 Le Fort III osteotomy. (**A–D**) Mobilisation and bone graft. Scan to play Crouzon's syndrome correction with Le Fort III midfacial advancement. (**E1** & **E2**) Preoperative views. (**F1** & **F2**) Le Fort III osteotomy intraoperative view. (**G1** & **G2**) Postoperative views.

BOX 43.2 Mandibular Surgeries

1. **Ramus osteotomy**
   a. Extraoral vertical ramus osteotomy (EVRO)
   b. Intraoral vertical ramus osteotomy (IVRO)
   c. Bilateral sagittal split osteotomy (BSSO)
2. **Body osteotomy of mandible**
3. **Subapical body osteotomy**
   a. Anterior subapical osteotomy
   b. Posterior subapical osteotomy
   c. Total subapical osteotomy
4. **Genioplasty**
   a. Horizontal osteotomy with anteroposterior reduction
   b. Double sliding horizontal osteotomy
   c. Vertical reduction genioplasty
   d. Tenon technique
   e. Alloplastic augmentation

aspect of the ramus is exposed through a submandibular incision, the ramus is sectioned in a vertical fashion, entire body and anterior ramus of section of the mandible are moved posteriorly, which places the teeth in proper occlusion. Proximal segment of the ramus overlaps the anterior segment and the jaw is stabilised during the healing phase with bone plates or screws, or immobilised using intermaxillary fixation (Box 43.2).

RAMUS OSTEOTOMY

Anteroposterior movement of the mandible is achieved by ramus osteotomy. In 1954, Caldwell and Letterman described a vertical subsigmoid osteotomy (or ramus) through an extraoral approach. In 1957, Obwegeser H and Trauner R put forward the sagittal split osteotomy of the ramus, which was versatile in technique.

Various procedures of ramus osteotomy are: (1) extraoral vertical ramus osteotomy, (2) intraoral vertical ramus osteotomy and (3) sagittal split osteotomy.

Extraoral vertical ramus osteotomy (Fig. 43.39)

- A submandibular skin incision is placed about 1.5 cm below the angle of the mandible. Incision is extended down to the platysma which is then divided. Marginal mandibular nerve lies below the platysma running parallel to and often below the lower border of the mandible crossing the facial vessels superficially as it passes upwards. After identification and protection of marginal mandibular nerve, dissection is carried out and the periosteum is reflected superiorly to the level of sigmoid notch on the lateral aspect of the ramus

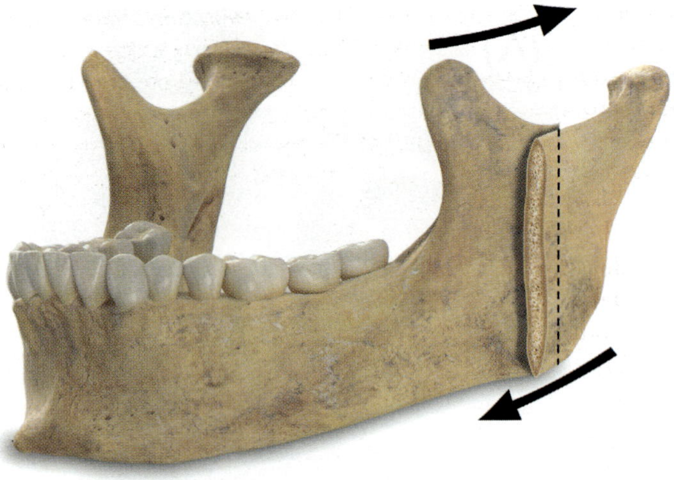

Figure 43.39 Extraoral vertical ramus osteotomy.

- Lateral aspect of the ramus is inspected for the small bulge to identify the position of mandibular foramen. This small bulge was 1st described by Caldwell and Letterman in 1984. Later, this landmark gained surgical significance with Alling, Behrman (Behrman's bump), Hall et al., Levine and Topazian (antilingual prominence). This landmark is present in only some individuals and is highly variable in relation to mandibular foramen (Tanas Study, 1979). The osteotomy cut is performed posterior to the mandibular foramen to avoid any injury to the mandibular nerve. A vertical bony cut is made from sigmoid notch to the lower border near the angle of the mandible. The proximal segment is separated from rest of the mandible and is detached from the medial pterygoid muscles. This proximal segment is placed laterally on the distal segment of the mandible. Decortication of the distal segment is carried out on the medial aspect of the overlap area and the proximal segment is decorticated on the lateral aspect. The proximal segment overlaps the distal fragment on the outer aspect with intraosseous wiring or bone plates. There can be variations of this basic osteotomy procedure.
- The osteotomy site may be left to become a pseudo-joint or stabilised by transosseous wire or miniplate or bicortical screws
- Wound closure is done in layers. The skin may be closed by monofilament 6-0 or smaller sutures. A pressure dressing is applied for the 1st 24–48 h. Sutures are removed after 5 days and the wound supported by steristrips for a period of another 1 week.

Subsigmoid oblique subcondylar osteotomy

This was 1st advocated by Robinson and Hinds in 1955. The cut is extended from the sigmoid notch to the posterior border. After subsigmoid vertical cut, the condylar segment is overlapped on the ramus of the distal (tooth bearing) segment. It is stabilised by transosseous wiring. Depending on the amount of posterior replacement, sectioning of the coronoid process is determined. These procedures can also be used for advancement of mandible along with the use of bone grafts fitted between the distal and proximal segments.

Advantages

- Adequate access
- Adequate control of bony fragments
- Good surface contact between the bony fragments
- Minimal relapse tendency
- Gonial angle contour can be changed
- No loss of teeth or arch size.

Disadvantages

- Scar formation due to extraoral incision. If the patient has keloid tendency, then this approach is contraindicated
- Potential damage to the mandibular branch of facial nerve
- Bleeding may occur due to injury to the retromandibular vein or masseteric artery where it crosses laterally through the sigmoid notch
- Applicable only for mandibular setback and not advancement.

Intraoral vertical ramus osteotomy (Fig. 43.40)

- Introduced by Caldwell and Letterman in 1954
- The incision is similar to that of sagittal split osteotomy where anterior border of the ramus is exposed. Lateral border is exposed by subperiosteal dissection. The pterygomassetric sling at the inferior and posterior border is stripped
- If fixation is planned, medial aspect of the ramus above the lingula is dissected subperiosteally to the posterior border. The width need only be enough to pass the wires
- Osteotomy in this case extends from the sigmoid notch to the inferior border, behind the entry of the mandibular nerve into the mandible. An appropriate mandibular posterior border retractor as Bauer or channel retractor is used to engage posterior border and retract soft tissue laterally
- An oscillating saw at 30 degrees angulation is used to do the vertical cut and care should be taken to orient the cut such as to prevent injury to the soft tissues. After osteotomy is completed, condylar segment is overlapped laterally over the mandible. To facilitate tension-free placement of the condylar segment, the medial pterygoid attached to the medial aspect may be stripped in anterior region of the segment
- The proximal segment must always overlap the distal laterally. In cases of medial overlap, the pharyngeal air space may be narrowed postoperatively. If this occurs, immediately reshift the patient to the operating table for correcting the position of proximal segment.

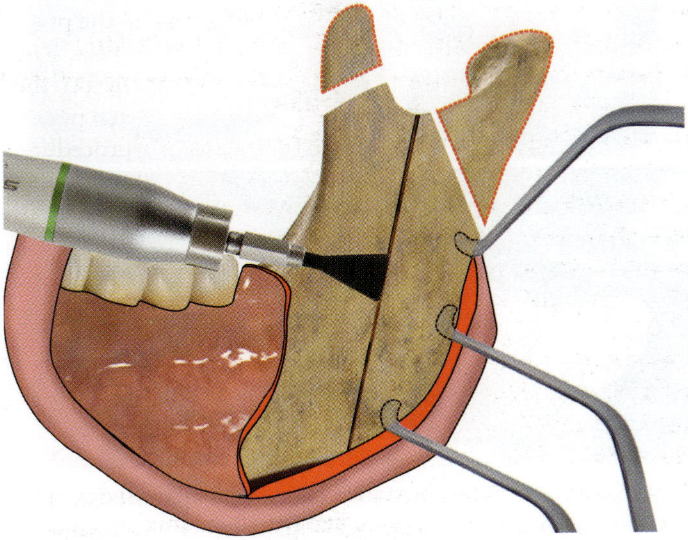

Figure 43.40 Intraoral vertical ramus osteotomy.

Advantages

- No external scar
- No risk of injury to the marginal mandibular nerve.

Disadvantages

- Difficulty in visualisation of and access to the area
- Applicable only for mandibular setback.

Bilateral sagittal split osteotomy (Figs. 43.41 and 43.42)

Bilateral sagittal split osteotomy (BSSO) can be used to correct both mandibular prognathism as well as retrognathism. It is the most versatile mandibular osteotomy.

The BSSO as introduced by Obwegeser and Trauner in 1957 has undergone many modifications over the years.

Technique

- An incision is placed over the anterior aspect of the ramus, running down the midramus over the external oblique ridge till the 1st molar tooth region. The incision then curves down to the buccal vestibule
- Retracting the tissues buccally, before the placement of incision, prevents exposure of the buccal pad of fat which is an unwanted interference during surgery
- Mucoperiosteal flap elevation is done above the lateral aspect of the mandible at the molar region until the inferior border
- Medial periosteal elevation is done very carefully. Level of lingula and mandibular foramen is ascertained as it is usually in the deepest concavity of the anterior border of the ramus. The dissection should be above the mandibular foramen and, using an elevator, lingula is exposed subperiosteally
- Osteotomy is done by cutting the cortical bone above the lingula. The cut extends just posterior the mandibular foramen. Cut is taken anteriorly to anterior border of the

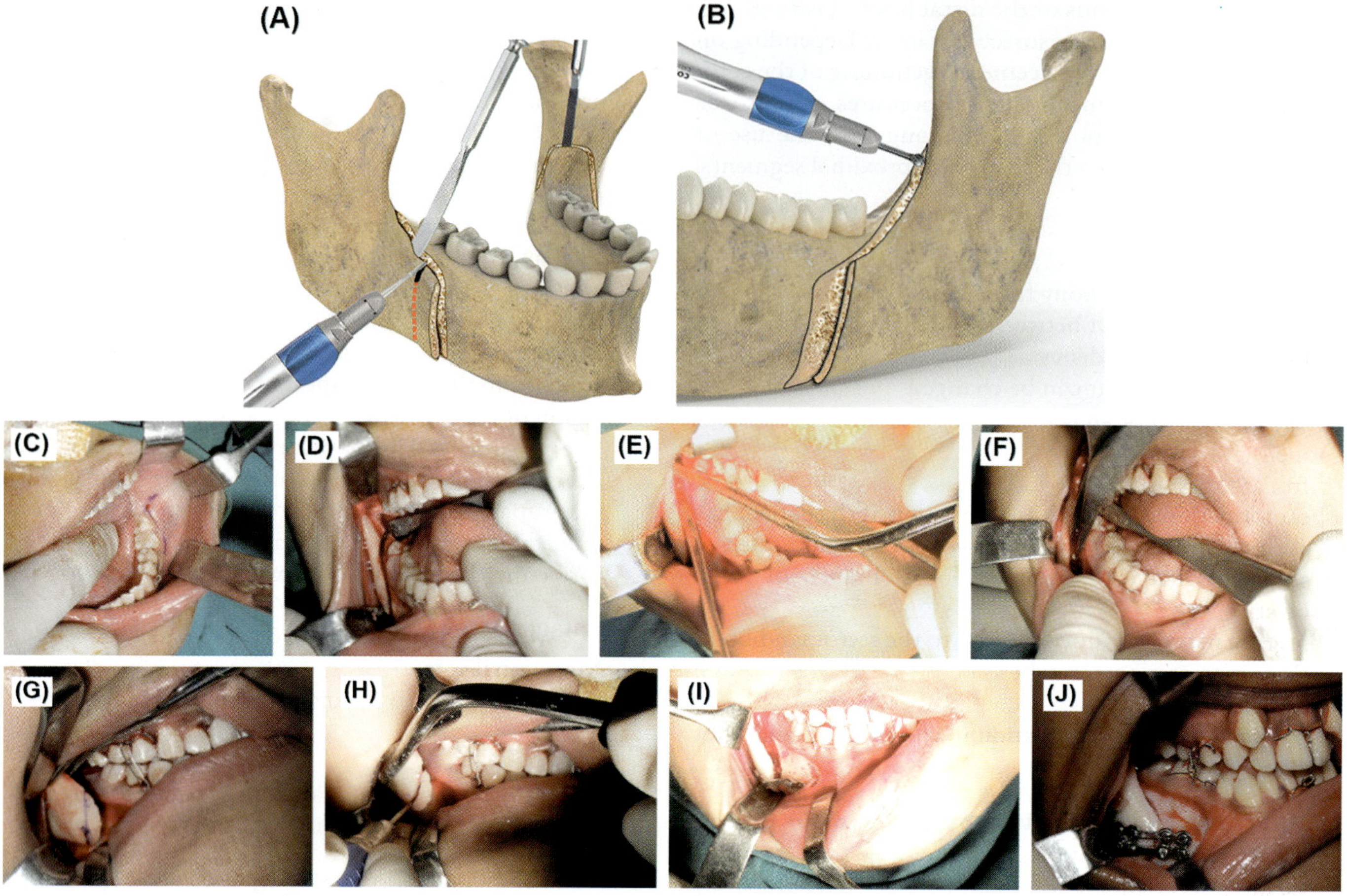

Figure 43.41 (**A–J**) Bilateral sagittal split osteotomy (BSSO).

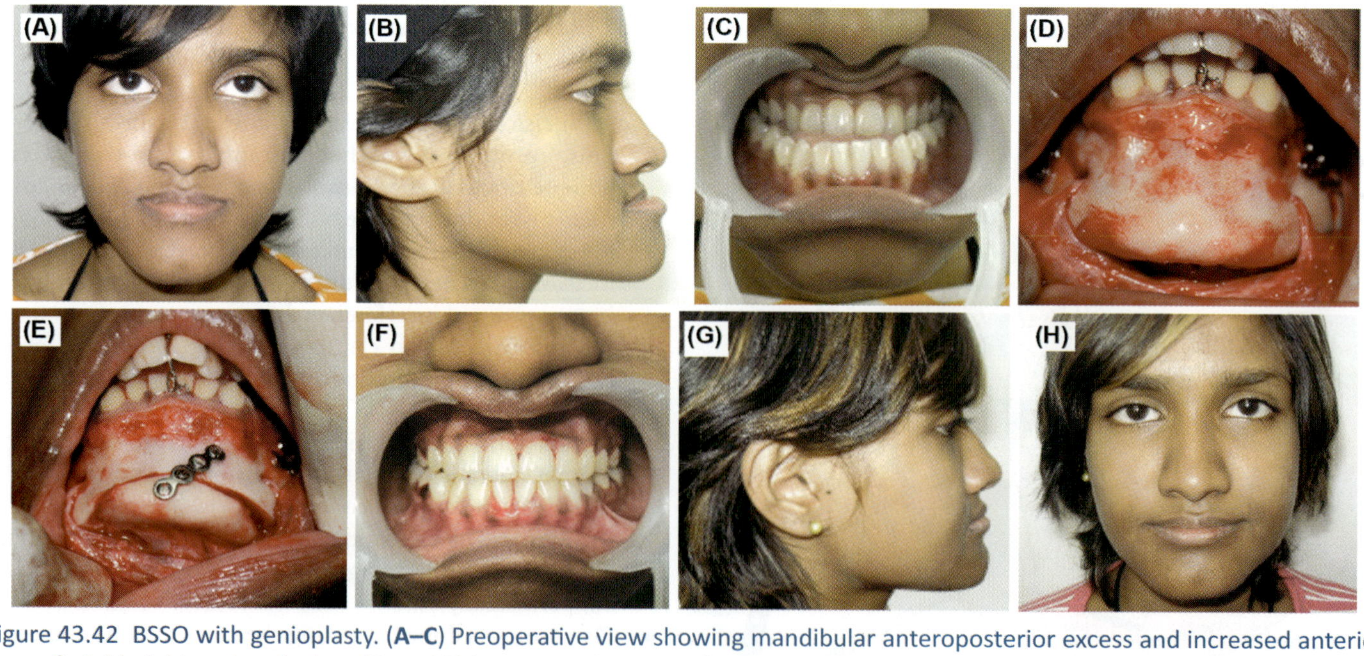

Figure 43.42 BSSO with genioplasty. (**A–C**) Preoperative view showing mandibular anteroposterior excess and increased anterior lower facial height and occlusion. (**D** and **E**) Intraoperative view showing BSSO with reduction genioplasty. (**F–H**) Postoperative view and occlusion.

ramus of the mandible and is then continued along external oblique ridge to the 2nd molar region over the lateral cortical plate. A vertical cut is made in this region; the depth of the cut should be kept minimal here; just enough to reach the cancellous bone. This cut should include the inferior border to control the splitting. After cortical cut is completed, a small spatula osteotome is malleted to the site from the medial cut to vertical cut. Osteotome should be directed laterally to prevent injury to the neurovascular bundle. During the process of splitting, neurovascular bundle is visualised and care should be taken to maintain it to the distal fragment

- This procedure is repeated on the opposite side
- Sagittal split osteotomy can be used for both advancement and backward positioning of the mandible
- In cases of mandibular advancement, medial pterygoid muscle is separated from the inferior border of the distal segment with periosteal elevator. When the mandible is set back the medial pterygoid and masseter may have to be stripped to prevent the displacement of the condylar segment posteriorly. When condylar segment overlaps the medial tooth bearing segment, overlapping part is excised and condylar segment is allowed to be on the cancellous part without any tension, taking care that the proximal segment with condyle is in its anatomic position in the glenoid fossa. This is the most important step during fixation to prevent condylar sag
- Rigid internal fixation using plates and screws or lag screws is the best way of fixation
- Other methods are lower border wiring, upper border wiring and circum-ramus body wiring.

Wound closure

Wounds are well irrigated with saline and haemostasis achieved followed by 3-0 chromic catgut or vicryl.

Postoperative sequelae

- Oedema may be expected, which resolves in 2 weeks
- Diminished sensation of lips may be experienced by some patients, mainly due to injury to the inferior alveolar nerve. More than two-thirds of the patients experience some sensory deficit even after 1 year. But most of the patients are satisfied with the overall result and adjust to the sensory deficit.

Complications

- Injury to the neurovascular bundle
- Malpositioning of the condylar segment (proximal)
- Bad split, multiple undesirable splits
- Excessive bleeding.

Injury to inferior alveolar neurovascular bundle

Continuity of neurovascular bundle should be maintained throughout the process. If mistakenly the nerve is transected, the cut ends should be microanastomosed.

Malpositioning of condylar segment

Care should be taken while wiring the segment. Improper transosseous wiring can pull or push the condylar segment to an untoward position. When the maxillomandibular fixation (MMF) is released, an open bite is the most common presentation requiring surgical recorrection.

Bad splits

Wrong splits may occur at the lingual cortical plate. Poor split may occur at the condylar segment. This poor split is usually due to the removal of the last molar at the time of surgery. Therefore, it is advisable to remove the 3rd molar 6 months before the surgery. The main reason for poor split is the use of wrong fulcrum on the lateral segment.

Excessive bleeding

Bleeding can occur from the inferior neurovascular bundle, facial vessels, medullary bed and rarely from retromandibular vein. Except for the facial vessels, bleeding can be controlled by local measures. But in case of facial vessels, they have to be identified and ligated. Using channelled retractor with the cup to hold the inferior border prevents injury to the facial vessels to a great extent.

Advantages

- Greater flexibility in repositioning the distal tooth bearing segment
- Better cancellous bone contact which enhances healing
- No external scar and injury to the marginal mandibular nerve
- Minimum alteration in the position of condyles and the muscles of mastication.

Disadvantage

Chances of injury to the inferior alveolar nerve are greater.

Modifications

- *Trauner and Obwegeser (1957)* made a horizontal cut just above the mandibular foramen on the mesial side of ramus. The vertical cut was taken down the anterior border of ramus of the mandible. An oblique cut was made through the lateral cortex towards angle of the jaw. It is a good technique for mandibular setback but had poor bone contact with mandibular advancement. Aseptic necrosis of angle due to extensive stripping of the pterygomasseteric sling may occur
- *Dalpont (1961)* modified the sagittal split by advancing the oblique cut towards the molar region and making the vertical cut through the lateral cortex. The main problem with setbacks was interference between the retropositioned distal fragment and the mastoid process where occasional pressure on the facial nerve may occur as well
- *Hunsuck (1968)* shortened the cut through the medial cortex of the ramus by taking it only as far as the mandibular foramen, which prevented occasional shattering of the ramus in mandibular setbacks

- *Bell and Schendel (1977) and Epker (1978)* made an anterior vertical cut, through which whole of the lower border was sectioned through and through using a bur. The split is kept more laterally by directing fine osteotomes down the inner surface of the lateral cortex to produce easier splitting and greater protection for the inferior dental nerve. Blood supply to the ramus is preserved as the need to strip the pterygomasseteric sling is eliminated.

MANDIBULAR BODY OSTEOTOMY

Blair (1907) was the 1st person to describe body osteotomy of the mandible. It can be performed between adjacent teeth, through preexisting edentulous space or through the extraction sites.

There are three types of body osteotomies. They are: (1) anterior body osteotomy, (2) posterior body osteotomy and (3) midsymphysis osteotomy.

Anterior body osteotomy (Fig. 43.43)

Anterior body osteotomy is a common term used for the osteotomies performed anterior to the mental foramen.

Procedure

Small vestibular incisions are made bilaterally leaving attached gingiva intact in the 1st or 2nd premolar regions. Superiorly, mucoperiosteal tunnelling is carried out till the alveolar crest and inferiorly till the inferior border of the tooth to be extracted. Mental nerve and its branches should be taken care of to avoid injury. Lingually, a periosteal elevator is inserted through the extraction site subperiosteally to protect the lingual soft tissue during osteotomy cuts. Vertical osteotomy cut is started in the socket at the alveolar margin, involving both buccal and lingual cortices, going towards the inferior border. Entire extraction socket should be utilised and cuts are made parallel to each other or slightly convergent from buccal to lingual for better approximation.

To prevent periodontal defects, care should be taken not to remove excessive crestal bone. Same procedure is repeated on the opposite side. If some bony interference is present, immediately occlusal splint is tried and osteotomy cuts are modified. Once accurate fit of the occlusal splint is achieved, fragments are stabilised at the superior margin by passing figure-of-eight wires around the necks of the canine and premolar and inferiorly by using miniplate fixation or intraosseous wiring. Wound is closed in a single layer. Modified step osteotomy is preferred over straight vertical osteotomy, to avoid damage to the mental nerve and to have better bony contact.

Posterior body osteotomy (Fig. 43.44)

Thoma (1943) described the Y-shaped and trapezoid ostectomy of the posterior body of the mandible to correct open

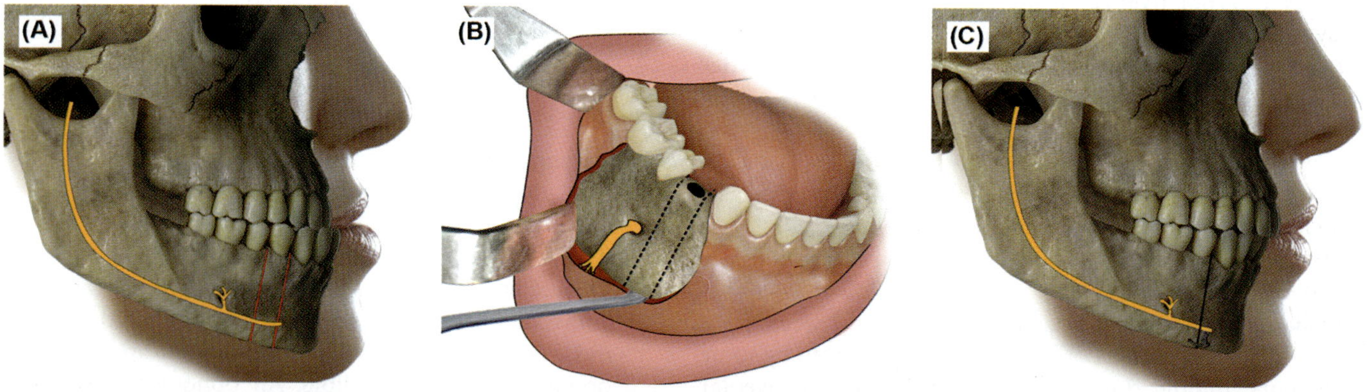

Figure 43.43 (A–C) Anterior body osteotomy.

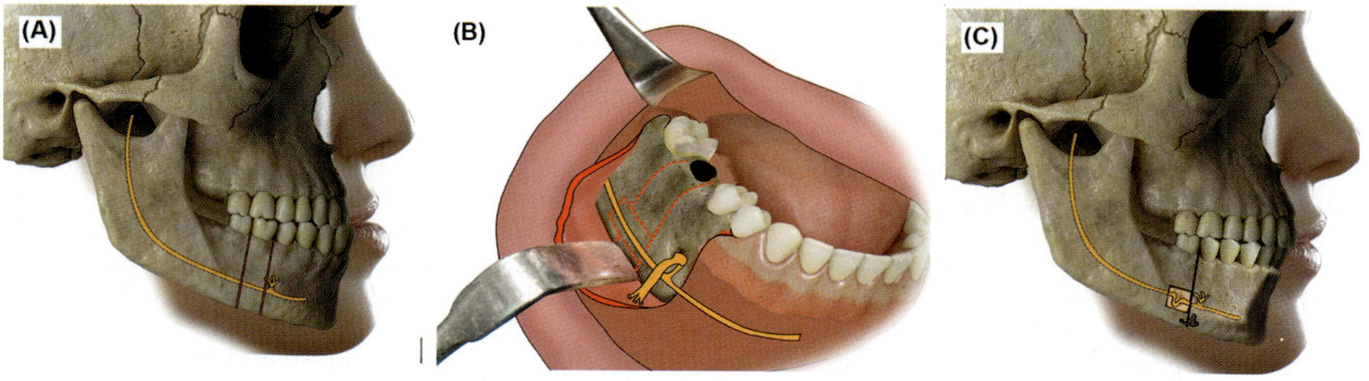

Figure 43.44 (A–C) Posterior body osteotomy.

bites. Posterior body osteotomy is a term used for the osteotomies performed posterior to the mental foramen. Here the preservation of neurovascular bundle is of utmost importance. It is not commonly used nowadays.

Procedure

- Make two vestibular incisions, one tooth anterior and one tooth distal to the osteotomy site. The distal incision can be extended posteriorly up to the external oblique ridge for more relaxation
- The cut is started superior to the neurovascular bundle and finished through both the cortices
- At the level of the neurovascular bundle, small window is made by removal of only external cortex and thus exposing the neurovascular bundle
- The nerve hook is inserted to pull the bundle towards buccal side and lingual osteotomy cut is completed
- Then neurovascular bundle is retracted gently upward, so that the inferior border cut can be completed through and through
- Same procedure is repeated on the other side and the fragments approximated in such a way that the neurovascular bundle is not damaged
- The occlusal splint is fitted properly and the osteotomised segments fixed with either intraosseous wiring or bone plating at the inferior border.

Midsymphysis osteotomy

Midsymphysis osteotomy can be used to widen or narrow the anterior arch width. If it is combined with posterior or anterior body osteotomy, then complete vestibular incision can be planned.

Procedure

An incision is placed posterior to the mental foramen. A mucoperiosteal flap is elevated from the cervical region of the anterior teeth. The mucoperiosteum on the lingual side is tunnelled with the periosteal elevator. Osteotomy is done using a reciprocating saw or a fissure bur. In case of narrowing of the mandible, a space must be created in the midline by orthodontic means or extraction of a tooth. Two vertical osteotomy cuts are given. In case of expansion, bone grafting is advised to fill the gap. Care is taken to place the osteotomy cuts without damaging the roots of the teeth.

SEGMENTAL SUBAPICAL MANDIBULAR SURGERIES

Segmental subapical mandibular surgeries can be used to reposition the anterior, posterior or entire mandibular dentoalveolar segment.

Anterior subapical mandibular osteotomy

Hullihen (1949) was the 1st person to perform an anterior subapical osteotomy to correct an anterior open bite. Hofer (1942) and Kole (1959) popularised the subapical technique for mandibular horizontal deficiency and excess.

Indications

- To advance or retrude the lower anterior segment
- To close anterior open bite.

Procedure

- An incision in the lower lip approximately 15 mm from the vestibule. Incision extends from 1st bicuspid of one side to 1st biscuspid of the opposite side. Anterior mandible is degloved to the inferior border
- Dissection proceeds posteriorly along the inferior border until the mental neuromuscular bundle is visualised
- Osteotomy can be accomplished with rotatory instruments or with appropriate microsaws. After the vertical cut is completed, a horizontal cut is made connecting the vertical cuts 5 mm below the apices of the anterior mandibular teeth. Remainder of the osteotomy is completed using a thin osteotome or a spatula chisel
- *Modified osteotomy*—a midline osteotomy may be incorporated in case of midline diastema (Fig. 43.45)
- *Extended osteotomy*—sometimes the osteotomy may be extended into existing edentulous spaces if feasible (Fig. 43.46)
- Cut segment can now be mobilised with gentle pressure at the osteotomy site to the desired position
- Closure is done in a layered fashion submucosally using resorbable 4-0 chromic sutures followed by vertical

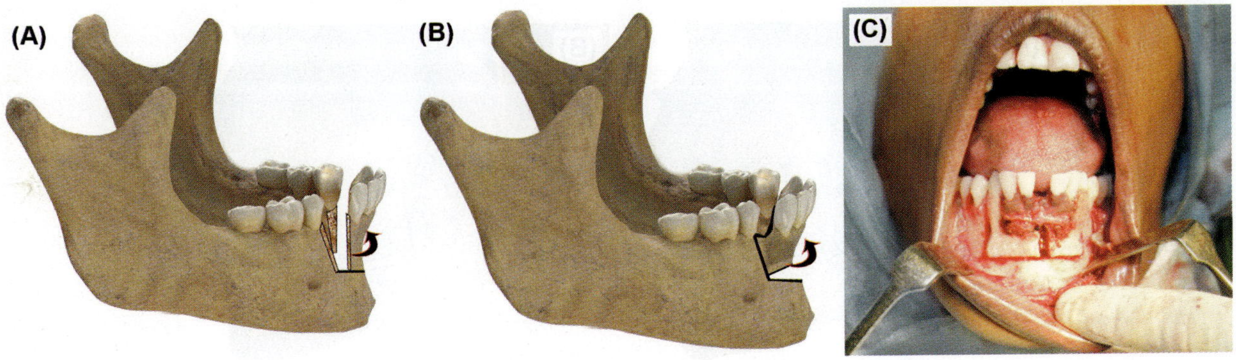

Figure 43.45 Anterior subapical with midline osteotomy. (**A–C**) Anterior with midline split, mandibular subapical osteotomy.

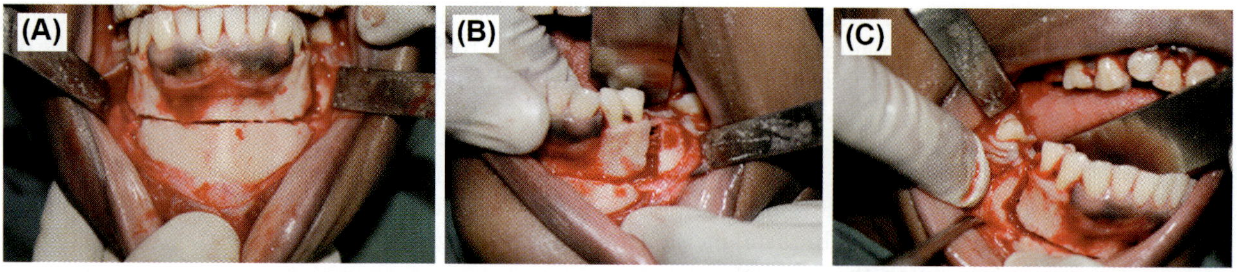

Figure 43.46 Extended anterior subapical osteotomy. (**A–C**) Anterior mandibular extended subapical osteotomy utilising the edentulous space.

mattress sutures to close the mucosal layer. Then external pressure is applied for 5–7 days to prevent oedema and haematoma formation.

Kole's modification: Kole modified by excising a horizontal wedge of bone from symphysis and inferior border of mandible to shorten facial height.

Posterior subapical mandibular osteotomy (Fig. 43.47)

This technique is used rarely, as it is technically difficult and there is a high risk of injury to the inferior alveolar neurovascular bundle. But with the proper acquired skill, it can be used successfully.

Procedure

- A horizontal vestibular incision is made and mucoperiosteal flap reflected slightly upward and downward till the inferior border of the mandible
- Here the anterior vertical cut is taken in the area of extracted or missing 1st premolar or 1st molar, and 2nd vertical cut is placed behind the last existing molar. The horizontal cut is taken below the apices of the teeth, protecting the neurovascular bundle
- Both the vertical cuts are carried out from the alveolar crest till above the level of neurovascular bundle
- The portion of the buccal cortex that overlies the nerve bundle is removed. This window should extend several millimetres posterior to the distal vertical cut. The window is made in such a way that the cut extends only in the buccal cortex and the bone is removed with osteotome and saved
- After identification and protection of the nerve bundle, lingual cortex is osteotomised
- Both vertical cuts are also completed till the horizontal cut level and entire segment is mobilised with the osteotome in the desired position
- The segment can be stabilised by fixing the occlusal splint and by placing a circum mandibular wire over the splint. The outer cortical bony plate, which was saved, should be fitted prior to suturing.

Total subapical mandibular osteotomy (Fig. 43.48)

This technique is again not performed routinely, as it is technically difficult and there is a high risk of damage to the neurovascular bundle.

Indications

- To reposition the entire mandibular dentoalveolar segment either anteriorly, posteriorly or superiorly
- For lengthening of lower 3rd of the face.

Procedure

- Circumvestibular incision is made from the retromolar area of one side of the mandible to the opposite side; care should be taken to identify the mental neurovascular bundle which is skeletonised with blunt dissection to avoid damage
- The buccal cortical bone above and below the neurovascular canal is cut with a fissure bur, and then removed with an osteotome. Vertical reference marks are made anteriorly and posteriorly on the buccal cortical bone

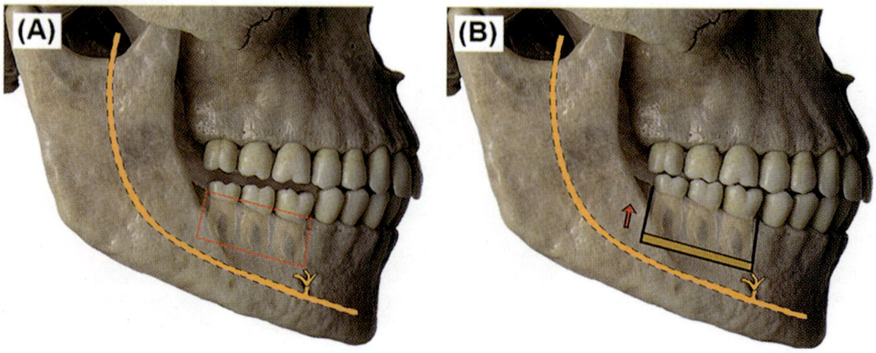

Figure 43.47 (**A** and **B**) Posterior subapical mandibular osteotomy for superior repositioning.

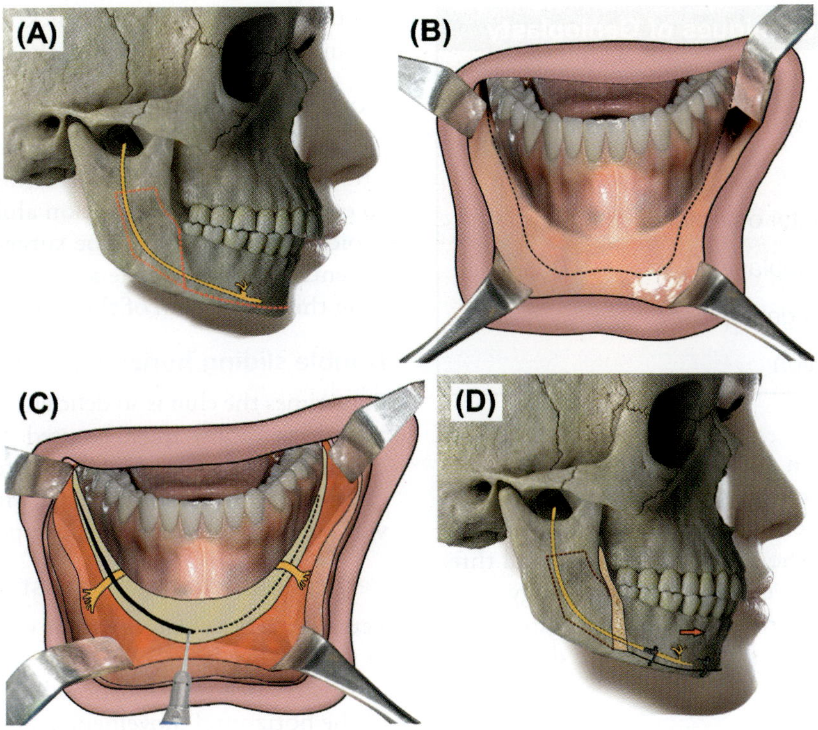

Figure 43.48 (**A–D**) Subtotal mandibular osteotomy.

before making the horizontal cut. Reciprocating and oscillating saws are most commonly used

- After exposing the neurovascular bundle through lateral cortical osteotomy, horizontal osteotomy can be completed safely by positioning it between the apices of the teeth and inferior alveolar neurovascular bundle
- Design of the osteotomy varies depending on the desired movement of the dentoalveolar segment
- When advancement is required oblique osteotomy is performed in the retromolar region in order to increase contact surface area between the osteotomised bone segments. In advancement cases, care should be taken not to overstretch the nerve. It can tolerate 3–6 mm of stretching. When dentoalveolar component is to be posteriorly repositioned, bone is removed via a vertical osteotomy in the 3rd molar region
- Segmentalisation of the alveolus is completed by performing the vertical osteotomy through an extraction site or between adjacent teeth using a sagittal saw or fine osteotome.

GENIOPLASTY (Fig. 43.49)

Genioplasty is the surgical technique used to alter the size, morphology, position and projection of the bony chin with concomitant changes in the surrounding soft tissues. Otherwise known as mentoplasty, chin surgery is commonly combined with other orthognathic procedures. About 15% of all dentofacial deformities primarily involve the chin. Genioplasty can be used as a single procedure or it can be used as an adjunctive procedure along with other major osteotomies of the jaw bone.

In 1942, Hofer was the 1st to describe osteotomy of the anterior lower border of the mandible via an extraoral

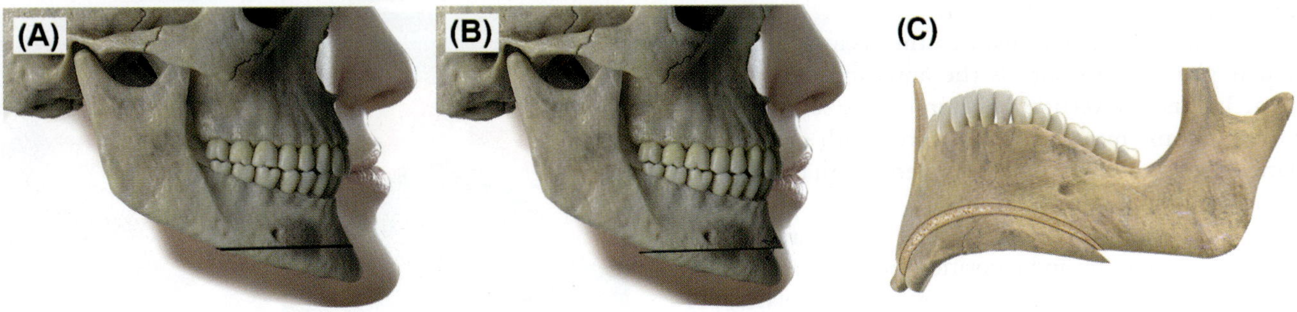

Figure 43.49 (**A–C**) Genioplasty.

BOX 43.3 Different Techniques of Genioplasty

- Horizontal osteotomy with advancement
- Horizontal osteotomy with anteroposterior reduction
- Tenon technique
- Double sliding horizontal osteotomy
- Vertical reduction genioplasty
- Vertical augmentation genioplasty
- Alloplastic augmentation

submental incision. Later, in 1957, Trauner and Obwegeser described intraoral approach or labial sulcular incision, to the osteotomy of the anterior mandibular lower border.

Deformities of the chin should be considered in all three planes—AP, vertical and transverse, as the morphology of the symphysis region is highly variable in different individuals, even with the same basic types of dentofacial deformities (Box 43.3).

Horizontal osteotomy with advancement

- A bidirectional incision is placed just above the depth of the vestibule and extended bilaterally till the canine region approximately. Once mucosa has been incised, it is undermined, where upon the mentalis muscle is divided on a bevel inferiorly towards the bone. Reflection of the periosteum from the anterior mandible can be accomplished
- Periosteum should be left intact on the inferior border and a minimum of 5–10 mm of periosteum should be maintained in the midpoint of the anterior mandible so that soft tissue support and blood supply are maintained
- To facilitate repositioning following any asymmetric or symmetric movements with anterior, posterior or vertical changes, midline and paramidline orientation lines should be inscribed in the bone with a small bur
- It is important to inscribe the proposed line of osteotomy at a level approximately 5 mm below the canine root as well as 10–15 mm above the inferior border. The orientation of the osteotomy should extend proximally 4–5 mm below the lowest mental foramen
- More parallel the osteotomy with the occlusal and mandibular plane, more pure is the anteroposterior movement. In case of vertical shortening, osteotomy angle should become more acute compared with mandibular plane. The osteotomy can be completed with the reciprocating oscillating saw
- Upon completion of osteotomy, different techniques can be utilised to stabilise and reposition the inferior fragment including unicortical or bicortical wires, bone plates, prebent chin plates or lag screws. While using transosseous wiring, degree of advancement available can be limited to the overall symphyseal thickness and this must be determined before deciding on the method of stabilisation.

Horizontal osteotomy with anteroposterior reduction

The surgical procedure is same as that for advancement, but proximal tips of the mobilised fragments should be reduced to ensure a smooth transition along the inferior border and avoid palpable 'wings'. The surgeon must also consider the potential changes in the anterior vertical height when planning the orientation of the osteotomy.

Double sliding horizontal osteotomy

Sometimes the chin is so deficient that the double sliding horizontal osteotomy must be used. Surgical technique involves creation of the stepped intermediate wafer of bone between the inferior fragment and mandible, which is also advanced to provide bony contact between the upper and lower fragments.

Vertical reduction genioplasty (Figs. 43.50 and 43.51)

Vertical height changes can be effected during advancement or setback by altering the angle of the osteotomy. Magnitude of this change is proportional to the amount and direction of the horizontal movement. Approximately, 3–5 mm of vertical change can be obtained. If in case a greater shortening of the chin is required, with or without anteroposterior movement, a wedge reduction is indicated and this can be accomplished using the tenon technique. It is often easier to remove the wedge from the superior tables fragment but intraoperative care is important to avoid sectioning tooth roots and still leaving an adequate inferior fragment.

Tenon technique

In 1974, Michelet and associates described this technique. Here, symmetry is ensured by the tenon and the visual

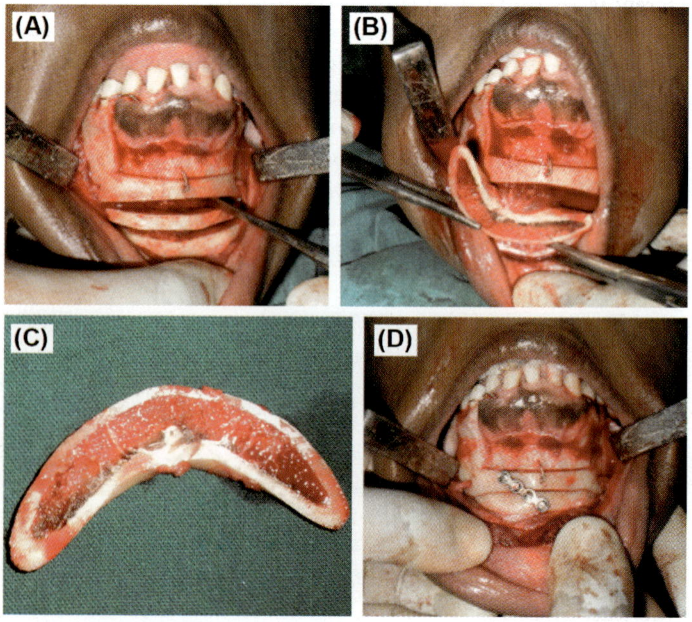

Figure 43.50 Vertical reduction genioplasty. **(A–D)** Anterior mandibular subapical osteotomy with reduction genioplasty.

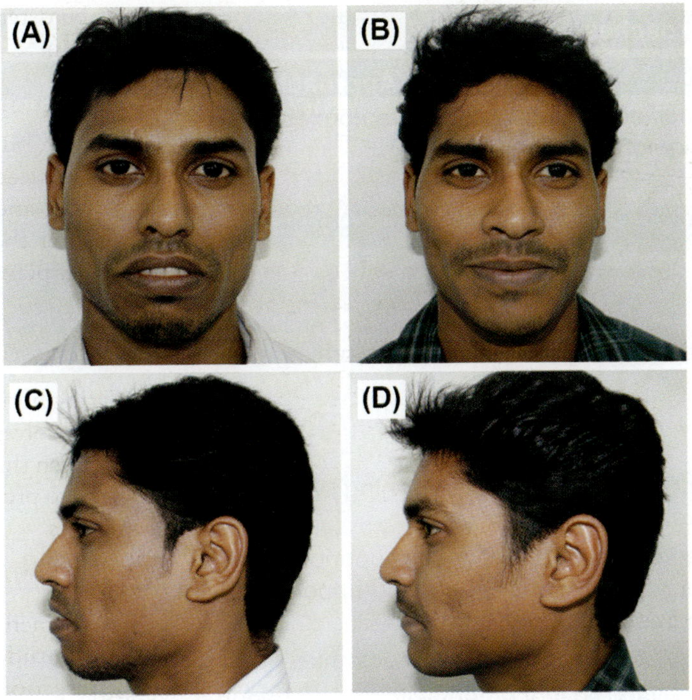

Figure 43.51 (**A**) Preoperative frontal view showing incisal exposure at rest, short upper lip, hyperactive mentalis muscle and increased lower facial height. (**B**) Postoperative view showing improved facial appearance. (**C**) Preoperative profile view showing increased lower facial height, everted lower lip from hyperactive mentalis muscle. (**D**) Postoperative view showing altered facial proportion, aesthetic nasolabial angle and mentolabial sulcus. Note the improved chin prominence from autorotation of mandible.

inspections of the proximal extensions. Only a single lag screw is required for stabilisation. But amount of advancement is limited by the overall thickness of the anterior mandible. Surgical procedure is almost the same as that described previously. A U-shaped monocortical osteotomy is created centrally on the symphysis. Lateral extension should be below the mental nerves, which connect to the superior aspects of the tenon corticotomy. Full thickness osteotomies are completed on the lateral extensions and only through the lingual cortex on the superior of the tenon. Resulting full thickness bone behind the tenon facilitates the mortising of the tenon and lag screw fixation. When posterior movement is desired, the 'U' is inverted and osteotomy is completed with mortising of the tenon, which is now on the inferior fragment, into the mandible.

Vertical augmentation

Vertical augmentation is indicated when lower facial height is to be increased. In such cases, the deficit is especially in the mandibular alveolus or in the symphysis. Vertical augmentation is accomplished by interpositional grafting or alloplastic implant placement between the osteotomised segments following osteotomy of the mandible. Autogenous bone and hydroxyapatite are the most commonly used materials.

Alloplastic augmentation

Alloplasts are used for anteroposterior, vertical or more importantly lateral augmentation. The products of osseous genioplasty include possibility of asymmetric advancement and inadvertent narrowing of the anterior mandible with large advancements. Use of alloplast with lateral extensions can eliminate this problem. There are various techniques used for insertion of an alloplast. Placement through the submental floor can be combined with open lipectomy or liposuction. Intraoral surgical approaches include a vestibular incision or a midline vertical incision with a tunnelling technique. Implants can be used to lengthen the anterior mandibular dimension by extending below the anterior mandibular border as well as to augment the parasymphyseal region to a greater extent than the single piece osseous genioplasty. Implants should be stabilised with transosseous wires or position screws to ensure immobility.

Chin implants are usually placed in a subperiosteal pocket that requires no fixation except for the surrounding soft tissue pressure which holds them in place.

Soft tissue closure

It is essential that the mentalis muscle is approximated accurately. Incision should be closed in two to three layers and a pressure dressing is applied to minimise haematoma formation.

Complications

- Prolonged neurosensory changes attributable to direct nerve injury or traction neurapraxia
- Excessive resorption of bone or avascular necrosis of the mobilised segment can occur. This can be avoided by maintaining a broad vascularised soft tissue pedicle
- Haemorrhage and airway compromise are rare complications
- Chin ptosis results from inferior redraping of soft tissues of the chin. Signs include flattening of labiomental fold, excessive lower tooth display and lip incompetence. Usual cause is total stripping of mentalis muscle and improper reattachment
- Bone resorption under alloplasts can take place
- Devitalisation of teeth may result from compromise of pulpal blood flow. Therefore, it is recommended that osteotomies be carried out 5 mm below the longest tooth root.

DENTOFACIAL DEFORMITIES AND COMMON SURGICAL APPROACHES

Dentofacial deformities and common surgical approaches are depicted in Tables 43.8 and 43.9.

COMPLICATIONS IN ORTHOGNATHIC SURGERY

- Complications due to osteotomy procedure (Table 43.9)
- Complications based on time frames.

TABLE 43.8 Dentofacial Deformities and Surgical Approaches

Dentofacial Deformities	Surgical Approaches
Class II division 1 malocclusion with normal overbite—characterised by maxillary excess and mandibular deficiency	• Modified sagittal ramus osteotomies • Augmentation genioplasty
Class I division 1 deformity with deep bite—characterised by maxillary excess and mandibular deficiency with excessive overlapping of the maxillary teeth over the mandibular teeth	• Modified sagittal ramus osteotomies
Class II division 2 deformity—maxillary excess with mandibular deficiency with the presence of lingually inclined upper central incisors and labially tipped upper lateral incisors overlapping the central incisors	• Modified sagittal ramus osteotomies
Vertical maxillary excess without open bite	• Le Fort—superior repositioning of the maxilla • Augmentation genioplasty
Class II deformity with open bite	• Segmental total subapical superior maxillary repositioning • Surgical control of nasal and upper lip aesthetics • Augmentation genioplasty
Mandibular prognathism	• Class III sagittal ramus osteotomies
Maxillary deficiency	• Maxillary advancement with simultaneous maxillary expansion and autogenous bone grafting
Class III deformity with open bite	• Superior repositioning of the maxilla with mandibular setback and possible genioplasty
Midface dentofacial deformity	• Modified Le Fort III osteotomy
Bimaxillary protrusion with or without open bite	• Posterosuperior maxillary repositioning with mandibular setback and bony augmentation genioplasty
Class I vertical maxillary excess with or without open bite	• Superior repositioning of maxilla with possible genioplasty
Transverse maxillary deficiency	• Bilateral combined orthodontic surgical expansion of total maxilla
Asymmetric class II dentofacial deformity	• Modified or reverse sagittal ramus osteotomies with optional genioplasty
Asymmetric class III dentofacial deformity	• Asymmetric mandibular setback with optional genioplasty

TABLE 43.9 Complications Due to Osteotomy Procedure

Maxillary Osteotomies	Mandibular Osteotomies	Genioplasty
• Haemorrhage • Dental trauma • Poor down fracture • Mobilisation • Soft tissue injury • Positioning problems • Stabilisation • Unaesthetic soft tissue changes • Nerve injury • Airway compromises	• Nerve injury • Poor osteotomy splitting • Poor segment alignment • Bleeding • Impacted wisdom teeth • Condylar positioning • Dental trauma • Stabilisation • Mobilisation	• Nerve injury • Dental trauma • Mobilisation • Stabilisation • Mandible fracture • Unaesthetic soft tissue changes • Bleeding

Chapter 44

Distraction Osteogenesis

OUTLINE

INTRODUCTION

Distraction osteogenesis (DO) is a biological process in which the osteotomised bone segments are gradually separated by incremental traction, resulting in the spontaneous formation of new bone. Callus tissue that forms in the gap between the osteotomy borders eventually mineralises, creating a new bony bridge.

The principle of DO is based on 'tension-stress', which states that the bone traction (tension) generates stress and results in the stimulation of new bone, in a direction parallel to the vector of distraction.

Most commonly, the bone is fractured by a corticotomy and then the fractured fragments are separated from each other using a special device (distractor) at a rate of 1 mm/day, following 5–7 days of latency period.

Corticotomy is an osteotomy of the bone cortex, preserving the local vascularity of both periosteum and medullary canal.

Latency period is the immobilisation period, after a corticotomy, during which the initial fracture healing repair bridges the fragmented bone surfaces.

Rate of distraction is the number of millimetres per day at which the bone surfaces are distracted apart (The usual rate is 1 mm/day.)

Rhythm of distraction is the number and amount of increments in which the 'rate of distraction' is achieved. (The bone can be distracted at a rhythm of 0.25 mm four times a day to achieve the rate of 1 mm/day, that is 4 × 0.25 mm = 1 mm).

Transformation osteogenesis is the change of nonosseous interpositions (e.g. fibrocartilage in nonunions, synovial cavities in pseudoarthrosis or muscle/fat in delayed unions) into normal bone by combined compression and distraction forces, sometimes supplemented by a corticotomy.

Bone transportation is the regeneration of segmental bone defects by combined distraction and transformation osteogenesis.

Healing index is the number of months taken for the treatment (from operation to complete consolidation) for each centimetre of new bone length.

Oral surgeons encounter clinical situations where bone growth or augmentation is necessary as part of the treatment., For example, loss of bone tissue due to tumour resection or avulsive trauma, resorption of the edentulous alveolar arches beyond capacity for prosthetic rehabilitation, hypoplasia of the maxilla or mandible hampering occlusion and appearance. The simplest solution in such circumstances, where bone augmentation or development is required, is to employ a bone graft.

According to the (donor) site of origin, a graft can be autogenous (harvested from one's own body), allogenous (harvested from the same species), alloplastic (synthesised), etc. The autogenous grafts produce the best results with the lowest rates of rejection when compared to all other types of grafts. However, harvesting autogenous bone graft from the patient's body requires a 2nd site of surgery and is constantly associated with some morbidity at the donor site. Added to the morbidity of harvesting a large graft and its questionable survival, soft tissue tension due to acute stretching over the augmented bone has also posed problems during graft procedures, limiting their applications. A technique which can avoid these problems but provide native bone augmentation was developed by orthopaedic surgeons for long bones which was later adapted for use in the maxillofacial skeletal defects. This technique was termed '*distraction osteogenesis*'.

HISTORY OF DISTRACTION OSTEOGENESIS

The discovery of distraction osteogenesis technique was 1st attributed to Codivilla in 1905, who described a femur osteotomy and intense pull to elongate the bone (Table 44.1).

However, ***Ilizarov*** is named as the ***'father of distraction'*** since he laid down the biologic principle for regenerating hard and soft tissues, which was further developed as '*a law of tension stress effect*'. He popularised the technique in orthopaedic surgery in the 1970s.

Codivilla in 1905 introduced bone lengthening by ***osteotomy of the femur*** and proposed that bone and its surrounding soft tissues could be lengthened by gradual distraction of the osteotomised fragments. He applied intermittent pulls to the osteotomised femur while the limb was in a plaster cast.

In the 1950s, Ilizarov designed a ***circular external fixation device***, which is still used. This circular fixation device can immobilise and apply traction on the bone segments to which it is attached. He proved that on applying gradual tensile forces to fractured bone fragments, new bone can be regenerated and length of the bone can also be increased.

He developed a theory named '*The Laws of Tension Stress*'. He stipulated the biological principles of distraction—namely '*The Ilizarov Effects*', which describes the effect of tension stress on the regeneration of tissues. Usage of distraction on long bones was thus initiated and developed successfully by Ilizarov and the concept soon became popular and published.

BIOLOGICAL ASPECTS IN DISTRACTION OSTEOGENESIS

The 1st description of the biological basis of the distraction gap healing was published by *Ilizarov*. After an osteotomy, the distractor device is activated, which results in the creation of a gap and 'regenerate' between the bone segments. *Histologic analysis* of the 'regenerated bone' revealed the presence of four different zones (Fig. 44.1):

1. ***Stage of fibrous tissue (central area):*** It consists of highly organised, longitudinally aligned collagen strands with spindle-shaped fibroblasts and undifferentiated mesenchymal cells all over the matrix.

TABLE 44.1 History at a Glance

14th century	Guy de Chauliac applied continuous traction for fracture reduction
1847	Malgaigne described the concept of external fixation
1905	Codivilla proposed that bone and its surrounding soft tissue could be lengthened by gradual distraction
1921	Putti designed unilateral device for femoral lengthening
1927	Abbot replaced the multiple cast with pins inserted on the femur and used springs to aid in distraction
1927	Rosenthal (coined the term distraction osteogenesis) tried distraction osteogenesis in the craniofacial skeletal level
1939–45 (World War II)	Treatment of congenital anomalies using distraction osteogenesis
1948	Allan incorporated a screw device that more accurately controlled the rate of distraction
1954	Ilizarov established principles to maximise the osteogenic outcome and produce ideal soft tissue response
1973	Snyder et al.,—mandibular lengthening in canine animal model. Karp et al., McCarthy et al.,—clinical investigations—proved normal osseous formation in the elongated area
1984	Kutsevliak and Sukachev experimental 1.2 cm lengthening of a normal canine mandible using the Ilizarov's principles
1989	McCarthy et al.—1st successful extraoral distraction in human mandible
1995	Polley and Figuera—rigid external distractor for midface
1996	Chin and Toth—1st alveolar distraction
1999	Molina and Ortiz-Monasterio—1st simultaneous distraction

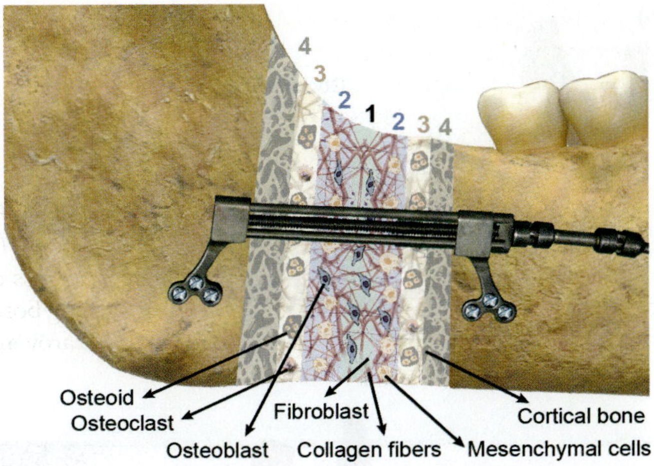

Figure 44.1 Histological zones of regeneration (Stages 1- 4).

2. ***Stage of extending bone formation:*** Fibroblast and undifferentiated mesenchymal cells are in continuity with the *osteoblasts*. These osteoblasts are derived from the fibroblastic cells that have undergone a transformation and are longitudinally oriented between the collagen bundles.
3. ***Stage of bone remodelling:*** It consists of fields of bone resorption and apposition with increased number of *osteoclasts*.
4. ***Stage of mature bone:*** It shows compact cortical bone close to the nondistracted areas with thicker bony spicules.

The initial process of healing in DO is similar to fracture healing. The sequence of healing in DO involves inflammation, formation of soft callus, gradual traction of the soft callus, formation of hard callus and remodelling.

The healing process in DO differs from that of a fracture repair in two key ways: (1) it has the benefit of controlled microtrauma and (2) the *ossification mechanism is membranous* rather than endochondral.

According to Bouletreau et al., a variety of growth factors such as cytokines, extracellular matrix (ECM) proteins are involved in the production, mineralisation and maturation of bone tissue at the distraction gap. TGF morphogens, angiogenic factors and inflammatory mediators are the prime mediators to induce healing in DO.

CLASSIFICATION OF DISTRACTION OSTEOGENESIS TECHNIQUES (Flowchart 44.1)

A. Depending on the location at which tensional stress is created, distraction can be categorised as:

Callotasis refers to gradual elongation of the reparative callus that is formed around the bone segments disrupted by osteotomy. It comprises five sequential phases: osteotomy, latency, distraction, consolidation and remodelling.

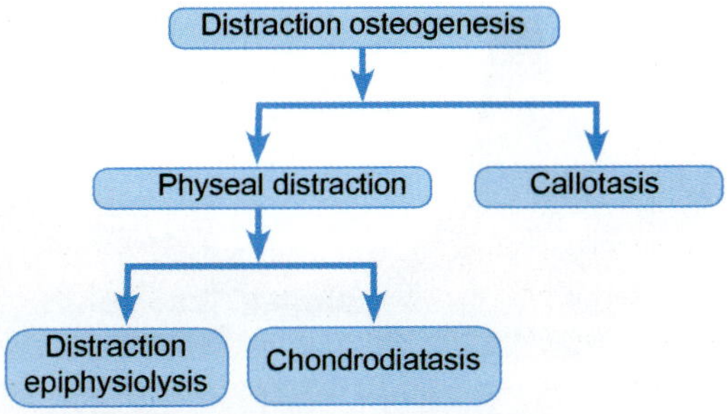

Flowchart 44.1 Classification of distraction osteogenesis.

Physeal distraction refers to the process of distracting the *bone growth plate*. This process can be achieved by:

- *Distraction epiphysiolysis,* where the separation occurs at a rate of 1–1.5 millimetres per day and ultimately leads to bone formation. This increased tension between the growth plates ultimately results in fracture of the physis.
- *Chondrodiatasis,* in which the separation occurs at a rate of less than 0.5 millimetres per day. The stretching of the growth plate occurs without any fracture.

B. According to the number of sites of neo-osteogenesis and bone fragments involved,

Monofocal: The surgical fracture creates a 'distraction gap' for unilateral traction of the separated bone segments. In this, one fragment is considered fixed and the other mobile. It involves separation of two bony segments across a single osteotomy and is commonly used to lengthen abnormally shortened bones.

Bifocal: Reconstruction of a segmental defect by sectioning a bone segment along the proximal end of the defect and then transporting it across the defect to the distal end of the defect. The segment of bone that is moved across the defect is called the 'transport disc'. Reconstruction by bifocal transport distraction is frequently used in segmental mandibular resections.

Trifocal: In cases where larger segment needs to be reconstructed, especially one that crosses the midline, two segments of bone (transport discs) are sectioned from both ends of the continuity defect and moved towards each other until they meet in the middle. This expedites reconstruction of large bone defects using transport distraction since the time taken for a single disc to travel the entire distance is halved. This also overcomes the problem of premature consolidation in long distractions.

In a similar way, multiple transport discs can be used for creating the mandibular arch form. Since distraction can create only linear bone, in order to create a curved mandibular bone, multiple transport discs can be created, each angulated from each other at a small degree, to produce multiple straight lines that can on the whole, resemble an arch (Fig. 44.2).

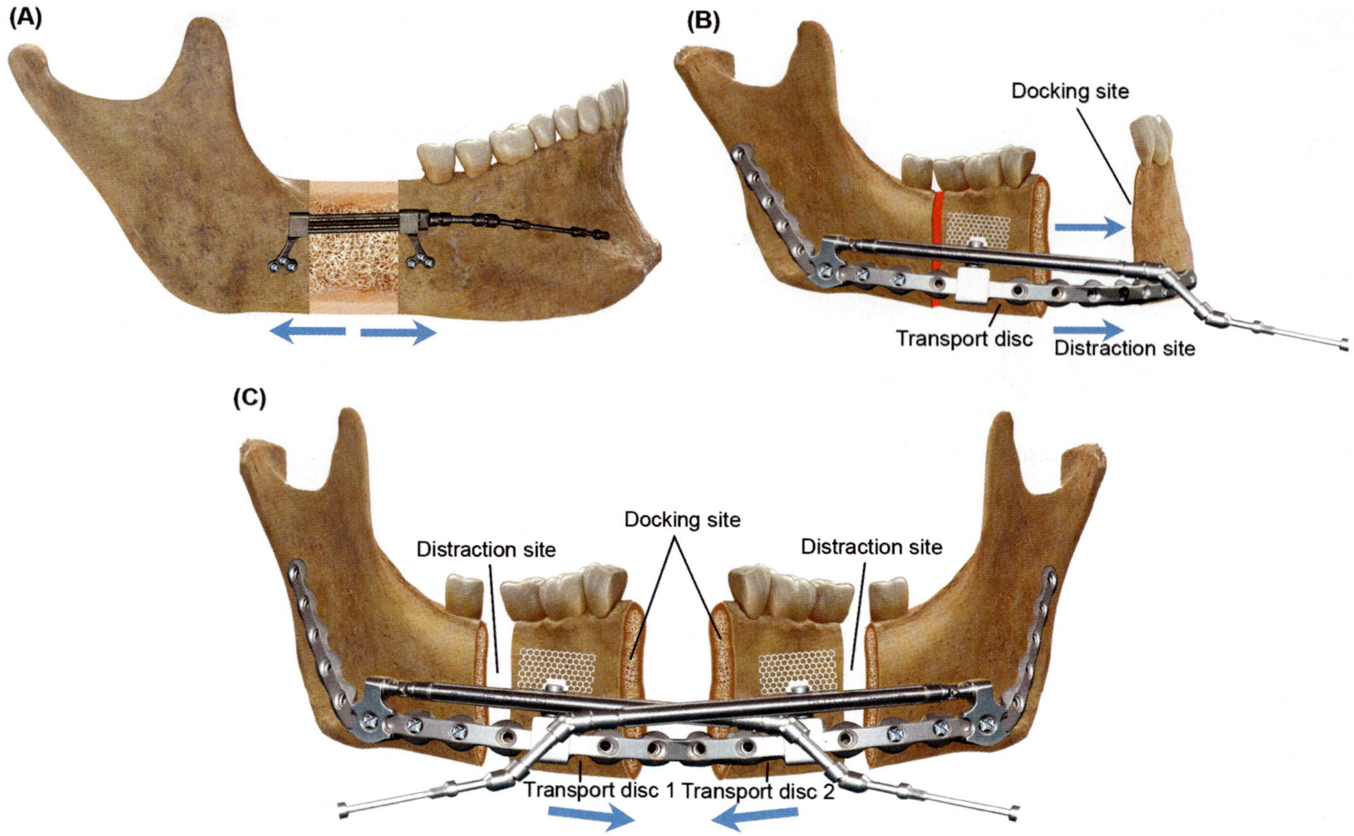

Figure 44.2 Modalities of distraction osteogenesis. (**A**) Unifocal distraction (unilateral lengthening). (**B**) Bifocal distraction (unilateral transport of one bone segment to fill a defect). (**C**) Trifocal distraction (transport of two bone segments bilaterally to reconstruct the defect).

PRINCIPLES OF DISTRACTION OSTEOGENESIS

Osteogenesis is a biological process that refers to the development of bone between the surfaces of bone segments that are gradually separated by incremental traction. The process of distraction is based on the principle of *'tension stress'*, which states that the gradual application of tensile forces should stimulate histogenesis. Bone traction produces tension and induces the formation of new bone in a direction that is parallel to the vector of distraction. Clinically, DO involves four phases after surgical osteotomy (Tables 44.2 and 44.3, Fig. 44.3, Flowchart 44.2).

PHASES OF DISTRACTION

OSTEOTOMY OR CORTICOTOMY AND PLACEMENT OF A DISTRACTION DEVICE

It is a process of creating an *osteotomy in the cortical layer of bone* to separate the segments while keeping the medulla and periosteum's blood supply intact. It can be done using burs with constant irrigation and minimal thermal injury to the bone. The osteotomy produces an initial defect of about 1 mm. The *distraction device is fixed to the bony segment* using pins or screws.

LATENCY PHASE

It is the period from the bone division (corticotomy) to the beginning of device activation. This allows for primary healing and formation of fibrous tissue (*primary bone callus*) between the osteotomy surfaces. According to Ilizarov's distraction protocol, the *latency period is about 5–7 days*. There is a wide range of latency period reported in the literature, from 0 to 14 days. In young patients, a minimum latency period of 2–5 days is recommended.

If the latency period is too short, the regenerate was found to have increased fibrous tissue and less bone density, resulting in poor osteogenic response and decreased vascularity. If the latency period is too long, the callus will calcify and result in failure of distraction.

DISTRACTION/ACTIVATION PHASE

During this period, the two osteotomised segments are moved apart, usually at the *rate of 1 mm/day* till the desired length is achieved. The traction force delivered by the distractor induces new cell formation at the distraction gap, in a direction parallel to the vector. Chin and Toth employed a distraction rate of up to 3 mm/day, while Ramchiel et al. used a rate of 2 mm/day. The most widely recommended

TABLE 44.2 Phases of Distraction Osteogenesis and their Biological Processes

Osteotomy	• Mechanical dividing of the bone (osteotomy) as atraumatically as possible • Recruitment of osteoprogenitor cells, followed by osteoinduction
Latency phase (1–7 days)	• Process of normal bone healing occurs • It is the period from bone division to commencement of traction • Haematoma formation is followed by bone end necrosis, angioinvasion and a cellular inflammatory phase that lasts 1–3 days before soft callus formation
Distraction phase	• Traction forces are applied to the osteotomised bone segments, gradually but steadily increasing the intersegment gap • The soft callus is stretched. Stimulation of cellular alterations, angiogenesis and fibroblast proliferation at the 2nd week of distraction. Recruitment of osteoblasts followed by intramembranous ossification.
Consolidation phase	• Period between the end of the distraction and the removal of the device • The distraction regenerate undergoes *complete mineralisation,* which ranges from 8–12 weeks
Remodelling phase	• Six weeks after consolidation complete remodelling takes place • Enlargement of the Haversian system and osteoclastic resorption

TABLE 44.3 Factors that Affect Bone Healing Process during DO

Local Factors	Systemic Factors	Distraction Factors
• Osteoprogenitor supply • Blood supply • Infection • Soft tissue scarring • Bone stock • Prior radiation therapy	• Age • Metabolic disorders • Vitamin D deficiency • Connective tissue disease • Steroid therapy • Calcium deficiency	• Rate of distraction • Frequency of distraction • Latency period • Rigidity of fixation • Adequate consolidation period • Length of regenerate

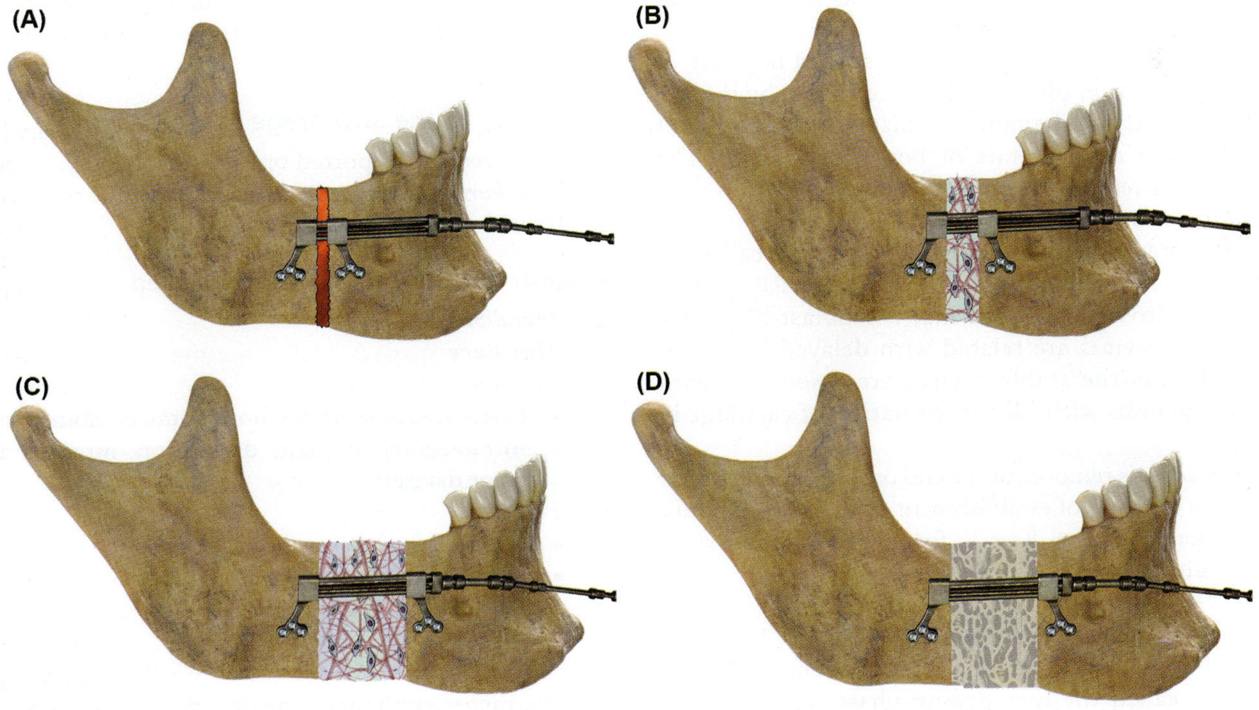

Figure 44.3 Phases of distraction osteogenesis. (**A**) Osteotomy and latency period. (**B**) Distraction period with increase in the gap, (**C**) Consolidation period. (**D**) Remodelling phase.

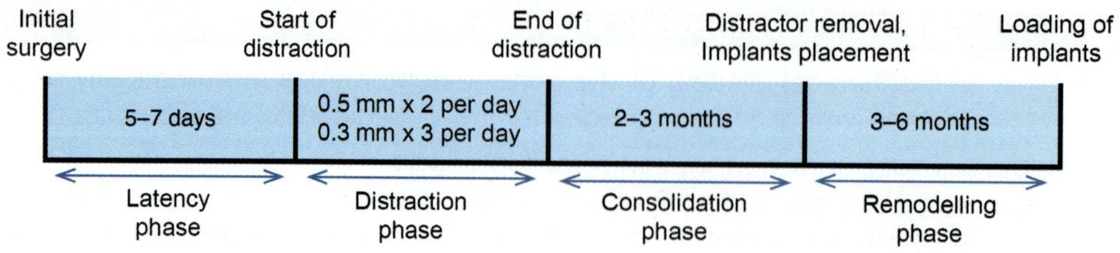

Flowchart 44.2 Distraction protocol.

frequency of activation is 2–4 times per day with a target of 1–1.5 mm distraction per day.

The two important variables in distraction phase are as follows:

Rate: Amount of distraction per day or the length of bone distracted per day—1 to 2 mm/day.

Rhythm: Frequency of activation of the distraction device or the number of distractions per day—2 to 4 times a day.

It is considered clinically appropriate to have a rate and rhythm of 0.25 mm four times a day or 0.5 mm twice a day. Increasing the number of rhythm to many cycles per day reduces the amount of damage on the bone and soft tissue and also raises the patient's level of comfort.

CONSOLIDATION OR STABILISATION PERIOD

It is a period of immobilisation during which the fragments are stabilised in their ideal position, and the stretched *callus or newly formed bone within the distraction gap is allowed to mature and mineralise.* The distractor device is inactivated with acrylic resin and is used as a rigid fixation device. The consolidation period ranges from 4 to 12 weeks with a mean of about 8 weeks.

Clinically, the consolidation period should be twice as long as the activation phase, and is determined by the age of patient, location and amount of distraction, volume of callus generated and the rate of bone metabolism. The maxillary bones require longer time for consolidation than the mandible.

Several 'osteoinductors' have found in the callus to accelerate the consolidation such as BMP-2, PRP, growth hormones, chitosan, mesenchymal osteoblast-like cells, etc. Unstable devices are related with delayed bone formation, whereas the stable devices are associated with direct osteogenesis without the formation of cartilage in between.

The distractor is removed at the end of this stage and after radiographic evidence of establishment of the osseous continuity. It generally takes 6–8 weeks for the radiographic signs of bone healing to be seen.

REMODELLING PHASE

The period of bone remodelling after the removal of the distractor is called the remodelling phase. It starts with full functional muscle load followed by continuous shrinkage and remodelling. In most cases, functional therapy and/or orthodontic treatment are required to correct an open bite, establish a functional occlusion, and maintain the results obtained.

DISTRACTOR DEVICE

Distractor is the device that pushes the two osteotomised bone segments apart from each other to stimulate bone formation by stretching the fibrous connective tissue, which is formed after 5 days of latency. The distractor must also hold the segments rigidly until the bone consolidation is complete.

CLASSIFICATION OF DISTRACTION DEVICE/ DISTRACTORS

According to the relation with the skin surface

External: The distraction devices are extraoral. Percutaneous pins connected to fixation clamps externally secure the external devices to the bone. When activated, a distraction rod pushes the fixation clamps and the associated bone segments apart, producing new bone (Fig. 44.4A and B).

Internal: The distraction devices are placed subcutaneously or intraorally (within the oral cavity). Distraction appliances can be bone-borne, tooth-borne or hybrid depending on its attachment to the bone, tooth or both teeth and bones (Fig. 44.4C and D).

According to the anchorage tissue

- ***Tooth-borne***—supported only by teeth
- ***Bone-borne***—anchored exclusively on bone tissue
- ***Hybrid***—fixed to both bone and teeth

According to the site where it is used

a. ***Mandibular***
b. ***Maxillary***
c. ***Alveolar***
    - Extraosseous (vertical, horizontal, combined)
    - Intraosseous (implant distraction, internal replacement device)
d. ***Palatal***
    - Transverse
    - Posterior
e. ***Craniofacial***

According to the vectors of movement

The distractor appliance is designed to move the bone segments away from each other. Unlike long bones, the facial bones are curved, and therefore it is not always enough to

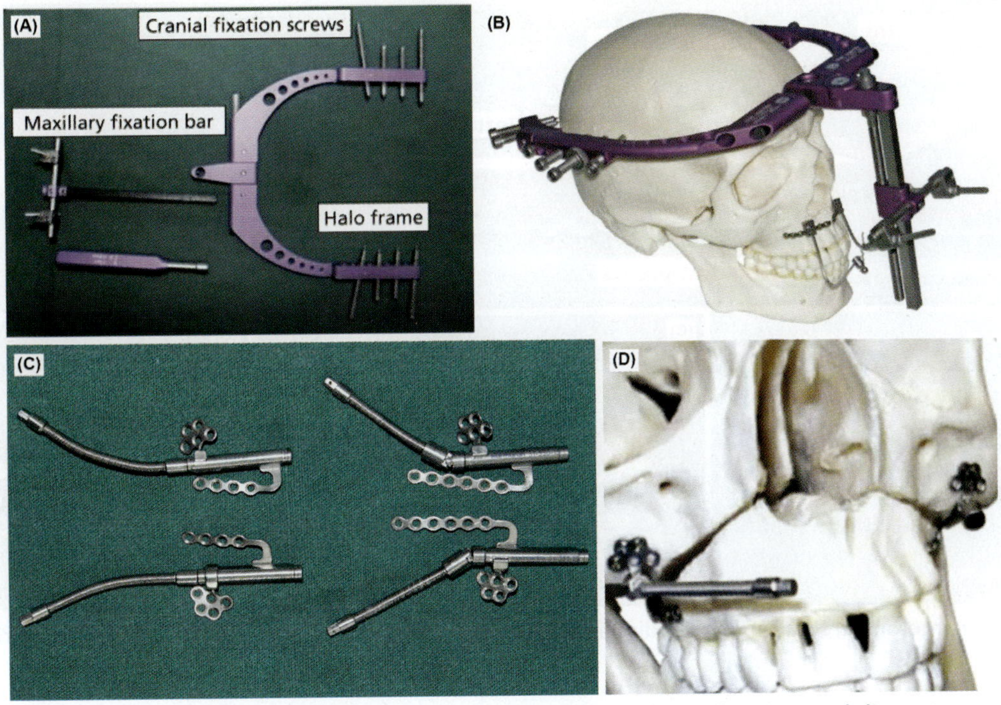

Figure 44.4 (**A** and **B**) Rigid external distractor. (**C** and **D**) Maxillary internal distractors.

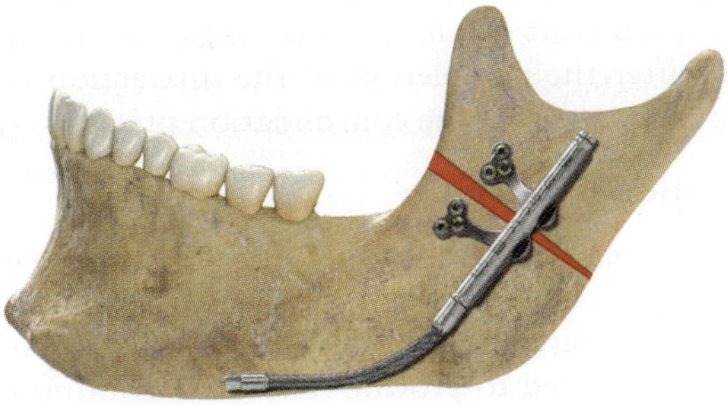

Figure 44.5 Univector distractor.

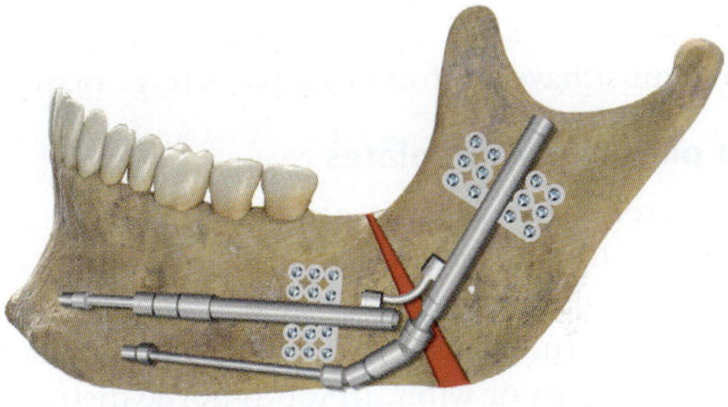

Figure 44.6 Bivector distractor.

just move the bone segments apart from each other in a straight line, to achieve the desired reconstruction. Therefore, the distractors of the maxillofacial region are designed, not just to move the host bone fragments apart but also to change the direction of the movement in order to achieve a curvilinear path. The capacity of the distractor to change direction is named as the 'vector' of the distractor.

a. ***Univector or unidirectional:*** The distractor has the capacity to move the host bone segments in just one direction (Fig. 44.5).
b. ***Bivector or bidirectional:*** The distractor has the capacity to move the host bone segments in two directions (Fig. 44.6).
c. ***Multivector or multidirectional:*** The distractor has the capacity to move the host bone segments in multiple directions (Fig. 44.7).

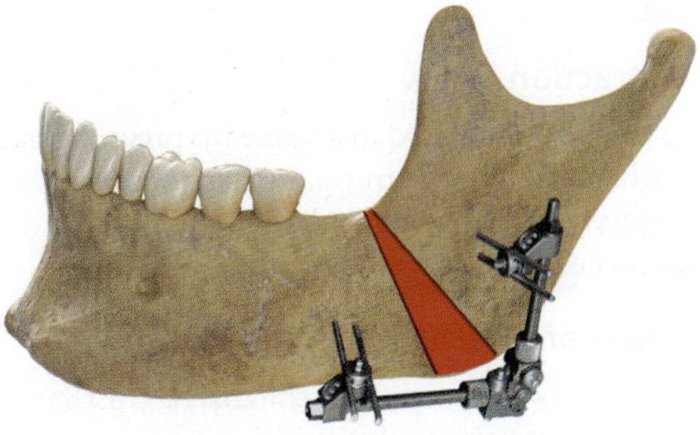

Figure 44.7 Multivector distractor.

Depending on the type of distractor material

- Bioresorbable device: It is commonly used in infants with congenital disorders.
- Nonresorbable metallic devices (titanium, stainless steel).

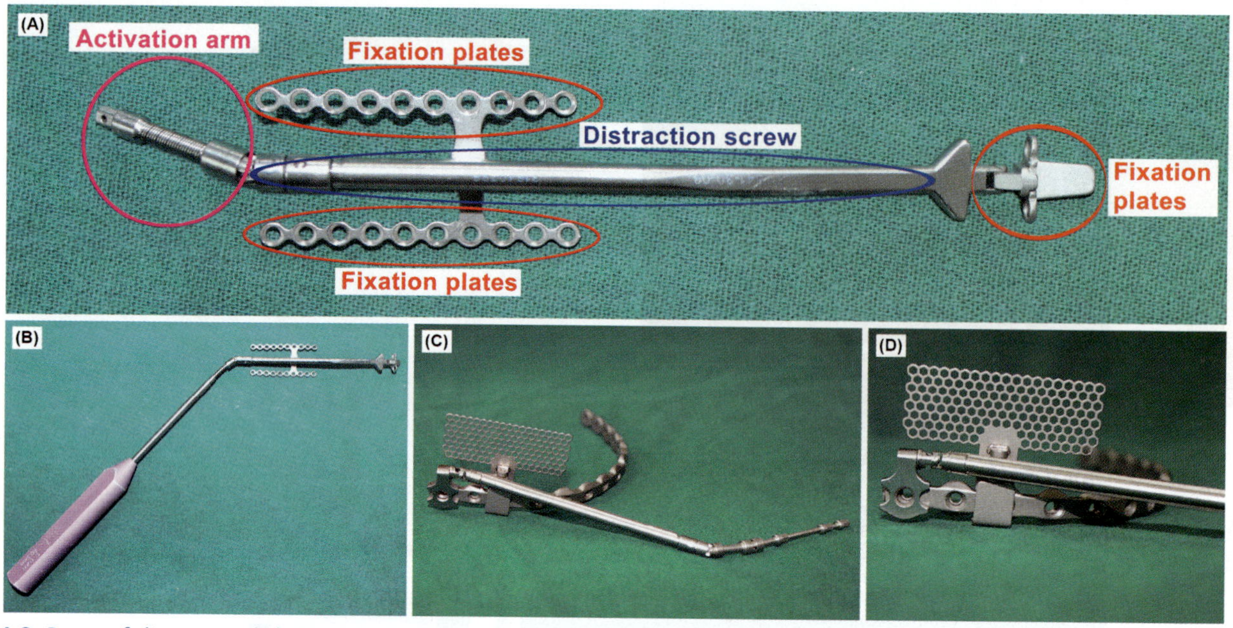

Figure 44.8 Parts of distractor. (**A**) Fixation plates, distraction screw and activation arm. (**B**) Activation screwdriver. (**C** and **D**) Stabilisation arm.

PARTS OF DISTRACTOR

Although distractors are designed as per requirement, every distractor must have the following parts (Fig. 44.8):

1. Foot plates/fixation plates

The distractor is fixed to the osteotomised bone segments using these plates and screws. In some cases, wires may also be used. The fixation plates vary depending on the type of distractor used. In external distractors, the fixation can be achieved using pins or wires. In tooth-borne distractors, the distractor can be fixed using bands to the teeth. The anchorage in transpalatal distractors is via jagged surfaces rather than screws.

2. The distraction screw

It consists of a screw, encased in a sleeve (to prevent tissue catching) that, when rotated, can move the two foot plates apart.
Clockwise movement: Moves the plates apart.
Anticlockwise movement: Moves the plates together.

3. Activation arm

The activation arm is the part of the distractor that is placed externally for activation. Intraoral placement requires a piercing of the mucosa inside the mouth, while extraoral placement requires a piercing of the skin. This activation arm when rotated will rotate the distraction screw in a calibrated manner to move the osteotomised segments apart. Usually one full turn is calibrated to bring about a movement (distraction) of 0.5 mm. This may vary according to the distractors. The activation arm could be flexible or rigid depending upon the ease of the surgeon. The activation arm in some distractors are made detachable so that it can be removed after the completion of the distraction phase, at the commencement of the consolidation phase.

4. Activation screwdriver

The activation screwdriver should fit the activation arm precisely. The device when turned will rotate the activation arm to deliver the desired distraction. Motorised distractors have also been developed to provide calibrated, continuous, uniform microtraction, eliminating the need for daily incremental rotation using screwdrivers.

5. Stabilisation arm

In a few situations, especially in long distractions, additional component may be required to stabilise and guide the distractor in its vector. For example, in transport distractors using plate as guide, an extra arm is used to guide the distraction fragment all the way around the reconstruction plate.

6. Vector manipulating knobs (Fig. 44.9)

One of the main complications in the application of DO technique to the facial skeleton is the complex shape of the bones involved. Therefore, the vector must be predetermined. In some cases, it may not be practically feasible to place the distractor at a desired angulation to the osteotomy. There may also be a need to manipulate the callus to obtain the desired shape. In such cases, an additional component that can change the orientation of the distraction vector is required. Advanced distractors may have this incorporated in the design.

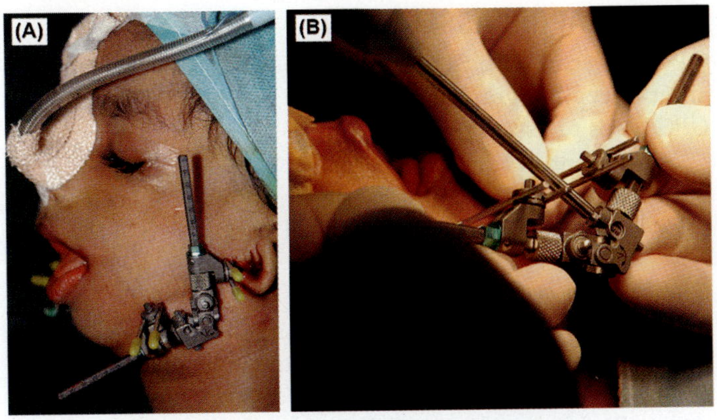

Figure 44.9 Vector manipulating knobs.

DISTRACTION PROTOCOL (RATE AND RHYTHM OF DISTRACTION)

Determination of ideal rate of distraction depends on many factors.

- The maximum rate at which bone growth can be induced without fracturing the callus as well as regeneration of nerve and soft tissue.
- Ilizarov suggests that a *distraction rate of 1 mm a day in four increments of 0.25 mm* each offers better results.
- Although the majority of the authors agree with the distraction rate of 1 mm/day, Chin and Toth used a distraction rate of up to 3 mm/day and Ramchiel et al. established a rate of 2 mm/day. Regarding the frequency of activation, twice daily of 0.5 mm increments appear to be the most accepted method.
- Excellent bone regeneration and a favourable soft tissue response have been reported with a rate of distraction of 1 mm/day performed at a highly fractionated, continuous rhythm.
- Bone tissue can effectively withstand both tensile and compressive loads, with a tensile strength of 12,000 psi and a compressive strength of 15,000 psi. However, muscles and nerves cannot take that amount of tensile pressure.
- *A slower rate of distraction provides better muscle adaptation* to bone lengthening.
- Abnormalities have been detected in muscles lengthened at a rate higher than 0.7 mm/day. Rapid rates of distraction were associated with gross changes including disorganisation of muscle structure, necrosis and significant accumulation of connective tissue in the interstitium.
- *Normal muscle regeneration was evident only with a rate of 0.4 mm/day*. Although muscle adaptation requires a slower rate of distraction than the bone, premature consolidation of the bone regeneration may occur at a rate below 0.5 mm.
- To balance bone and soft tissue regeneration, an empirical optimal distraction rate of 0.75–1 mm/day is currently practiced worldwide.

INDICATIONS FOR DISTRACTION OSTEOGENESIS

- Reconstruction of posttraumatic deformities
- Reconstruction of resorbed alveolar bone (alveolar height and width)
- Reconstruction of postresection segmental defects (oncologic or aggressive cyst)
- Mandible for:
  - Unilateral distraction of ramus, angle and body, for example hemifacial microsomia
  - Bilateral advancement of the body of mandible, for example severe mandibular hypoplasia as in Pierre Robin syndrome, Treacher Collins syndrome, etc.
  - Vertical distraction of the alveolar segments
  - Horizontal distraction across the midline
  - Widening of the narrow mandibular arch
  - Transport DO—for reconstruction of neocondyle and temporomandibular joint (TMJ)
- Maxilla for:
  - Complete midface advancement, for example Crouzon syndrome, Pfeiffer syndrome
  - Advancement of maxilla at Le Fort I level
  - Closure of alveolar cleft associated deformities in lip and palate
  - Expansion of constricted palate
  - Rapid canine retraction
  - Correction of velopharyngeal insufficiency (VPI) by palatal distraction
  - Zygomatic distraction
- Craniofacial DO
  - Sutural expansion in craniosynostosis
  - Facial asymmetry
  - Patients with severe obstructive sleep apnoea (OSA)
- Sites of previous bone graft failure
- Insufficient soft tissue coverage
- The patient is not indicated for bone graft

CONTRAINDICATIONS

- Generalised bone disorders such as osteoporosis, osteogenesis imperfecta, osteopetrosis, etc.
- Poor patient compliance
- History of poor fracture healing (fibrous dysplasia, hyperparathyroidism)
- Aggressive jaw tumour: Primary resection should be followed by 1 year disease-free interval
- Preexisting TMJ disorders: Chances of worsening of the problem
- Patient reluctant for multiple surgeries and long duration treatment strategy of DO

ADVANTAGES

- It avoids 2nd site of surgery for bone harvest
- It avoids graft rejection, incompatibility, foreign body reaction, etc.
- It augments native bone
- Soft tissue around the bone is also regenerated

- There has been evidence of nerve growth at the distracted site
- It can be used to increase the length as well as the breadth
- Even grafted bone can be distracted
- It does not hamper bone growth when performed in growing children
- Relapse rate is much less compared to conventional bone graft and orthognathic surgery due to simultaneous soft tissue histogenesis

DISADVANTAGES

- Patient compliance is necessary for the device as well as the longer duration of treatment (consolidation period)
- May require at least two surgeries; however, biodegradable ones are being developed to eliminate the need for the removal of the distractor
- Device failures are common
- Technique sensitive
- Requires meticulous treatment planning
- External devices can cause scarring
- Infection
- Improper consolidation or failure to consolidate may worsen the condition

TREATMENT PLANNING

The goals of treatment planning include:

- To increase the vertical dimension in hypoplastic ramus of mandible
- Re-establishing the bigonial width (transverse position) of the ramus
- To increase the anteroposterior projection of the mandibular body and symphysis
- To restore the dentoalveolar relations
- Levelling of the occlusal plane
- Correction of any asymmetry
- To increase the chin projection

PREOPERATIVE ASSESSMENT

CLINICAL EXAMINATION (Fig. 44.10)

The patient is examined similar to that of orthognathic or craniofacial surgery and the following details are recorded:

- Identify the deficiency (skeletal or soft tissue)
- Location and extent of the defect/lesion
- Any soft tissues abnormalities
- Availability of healthy bone for distraction
- The position of the chin, inferior border and angle of mandible
- Mandibular functions such as excursions, interincisal mouth opening
- TMJ function
- Occlusion
- Occlusal plane or cant
- Nerve functions (motor and sensory)

RADIOGRAPHIC ASSESSMENT

OPG, CT scan with 3D reconstruction, lateral and postero-anterior cephalogram are used in the planning of distraction.

OPG helps to assess the:

- Extent of the lesion or defect
- Shape and size of condyle
- Position of partially erupted teeth, roots and tooth follicles

Cephalogram

- Important landmarks such as orbital rims, pyriform aperture, maxilla, mandible and occlusal plane
- Degree of skeletal deformity/asymmetry
- Position and type of distractor

CT scan

- A detailed description of the defect/lesion
- Outcome of distraction

MODEL ANALYSIS

Stereolithographic model:

- Presurgical planning, which includes the extent/margins of the defect
- Designing (location and length) of the distraction segment
- Customisation of the distraction device
- Amount of distraction needed
- Outcome of distraction can be predicted
- Mock surgery

  In recent years, the development of software and stereolithographic models have made it easier to customise the distraction device.

  This software also permits the preparation of surgical templates that aid in surgical planning, localisation of the device and controlling the 3D movement.

Dental casts:

- Assessment of occlusion
- Construction and adaptation of the distraction device

SELECTION OF DISTRACTION DEVICE

Unidirectional devices can correct discrepancies in linear direction only, whereas the *multidirectional distraction* devices allow manipulation of bone segments in multiple planes of space (Table 44.4).

EXTERNAL DISTRACTOR DEVICES

Advantages:

- It permits bone distraction in three dimensions
- During distraction process, the direction or vector of distraction can be easily adjusted
- It allows for larger distraction length (40 mm or greater)

Disadvantages:

- Possibility of facial scar
- The increased distance between the distractor and the bone leads to greater risk for pin loosening/displacement at the pin-bone interface
- The sites of percutaneous pin require patient care

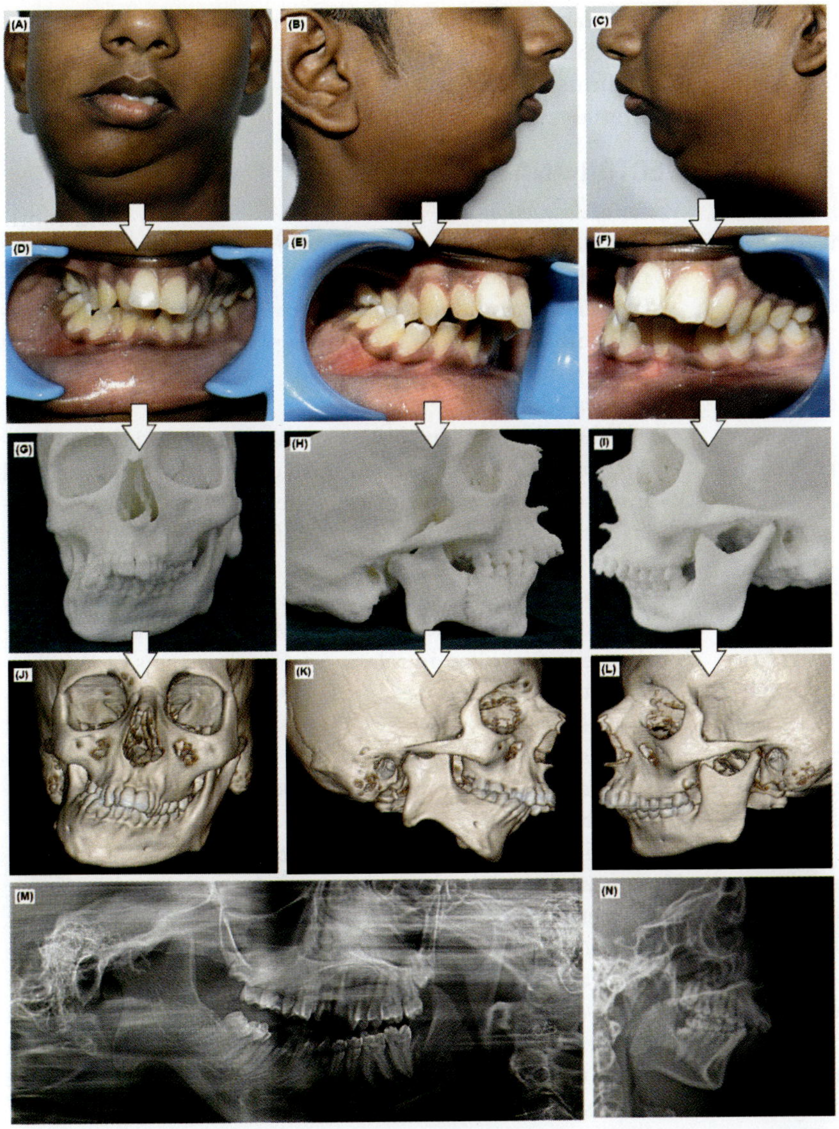

Figure 44.10 Clinical examination. (**A–C**) Preoperative extraoral assessment of a patient exhibits skeletal and soft tissue deformity in the right lower jaw, with deviation of jaw towards the right side, facial asymmetry, retruded chin and convex profile. (**D–F**) Intraoral assessment showing occlusal cant, cross bite on the right side, midline shift, crowing on anterior teeth and increased overjet.

(**G–I**) Stereolithographic model of the same patient displaying defect on the right side of mandible.

Radiographic assessment. (**J–L**) CT scan reveals deviation of lower jaw towards the right side. decreased ramus height and body length with deformed condyle on the right side. (**M**) OPG presents with deformed condyle, prominent antegonial notch, and decreased ramus height on the right side of mandible. (**N**) Lateral cephalogram reveals convex profile with retruded mandible and proclined upper anteriors.

TABLE 44.4 Comparison between External and Internal Devices

	External	Internal
Osteotomy	Osteotomies are easier to perform and pins can be placed in a wider range of anatomical structures	Depends on the local anatomy and dimension of the device
Placement	Easy to place	Placement of the device is restricted due to the lack of subperiosteal space
Distraction length	Longer distance of distraction	Limited distance
Patient compliance	Uncomfortable	More comfortable and safer
Distraction vector	Unpredictable	More predictable
Distractor stability	Possibility of pin loosening	More stable
Facial nerve damage	Less risk	Greater risk
Infection	More chance of infection	Less chance of infection
Device removal	Easy removal by unscrewing the pins	Requires 2nd surgery to remove the distractor
Facial scars	Visible	Less visible

- Increased risk for nerve damage
- Higher chance of infection
- Chances for negative psychosocial effects
- Need for special care, especially children

INTERNAL DISTRACTOR DEVICES

Advantages:

- As the distractor is in close proximity to bone, higher quality of distraction can be obtained
- Absence of facial scars
- Patient's social life remains unchanged

Disadvantages:

- Maximum length of distraction is limited to 25 mm or less.
- The direction of the distractor cannot be altered during distraction
- Device removal necessitates 2nd surgery

Douglas et al., advocated bone-anchoring devices rather than the tooth-borne devices, as the tooth-borne devices can cause undesirable dental movements.

The *selection of distractor* depends on the following factors: site of distractor fixation, vector of distraction, magnitude of movement, patient's age, comorbidities and surgeon's preference. In terms of distractors, there is a *strong preference for internal devices* (Fig. 44.11), except in cases where this is impracticable due to anatomical constraints or case characteristics.

The length of distraction device should be at least two times longer than the length of distraction required.

AMOUNT OF DISTRACTION

The amount of distraction needed can also be calculated by using a formula. It is done by drawing a triangle, the two sides of which represents the length of mandibular body and ramus present. The angle formed between these two sides is the gonial angle and the 3rd side indicates the amount of distraction.

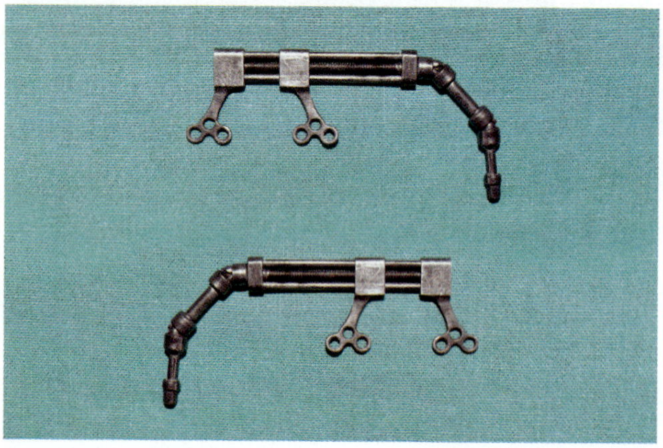

Figure 44.11 Intraoral distraction device. The patient has been planned for unidirectional distraction of the body of mandible using an intraoral distractor. It is planned to use a distractor with a vertical vector and a fixation point on the body of mandible around the 2nd molar region.

$$\textbf{Distraction amount} = \textbf{Dc} + \textbf{Dr} - \textbf{2(Dc} \times \textbf{Dr) cos A}$$

Dc: Corpus or body deficiency
Dr: Ramus deficiency
A: Gonial angle

VECTOR ANALYSIS

Vector of distraction

It is defined as the *positioning of the distraction device* on the maxilla or mandible at the time of surgery or movement in a distraction device. The vector of distraction has a direct influence on the morphology and orientation of the *newly formed bone* by distraction.

Assessment of vector

The key elements in *positioning* the distraction device (vector) are the neuromuscular envelop, skeletal anatomy and intercuspation of dentition. These factors directly influence the bone regenerate (newly formed bone).

Types of vector

The placement of the device can be described as vertical, horizontal and oblique. The orientation or position of the device is described in relation to the long axis of the skeletal component, for example posterior border of the ramus, inferior border of the body of mandible or occlusal planes (Fig. 44.12).

Vertical vector: The device is placed perpendicular to the body of the mandible. It results in increase in the vertical dimension of the mandibular ramus.

Horizontal vector: The device is oriented parallel to the inferior border of the body of mandible or the occlusal plane. It produces sagittal or anteroposterior projection of the body and symphysis of mandible.

Oblique vector: The device is oriented at the bisector between the horizontal and vertical vectors. It results in increase in both the vertical and anteroposterior projection of the ramus and body of mandible.

For cases requiring simultaneous lengthening of mandibular ramus and body, the direction of distraction can be calculated by using the formula.

$$\text{Pin placement angle} = 180 - \text{Gonial angle} \times \frac{\text{Ramus deficiency}}{\text{Total deficiency}}$$

It is the angle formed between the distraction vector and the mandibular plane.

The following variables appear to influence the clinical outcome of DO:

- Type of distraction device and its vector of distraction
- Planning of osteotomy area
- Surgical technique and device placement
- The bone regenerate formed during and after distraction

SURGICAL PROCEDURE (Figs. 44.13–44.16)

a. Operative/surgical phase
   i. Surgical approach
   ii. Osteotomies and device fixation
   iii. Primary closure

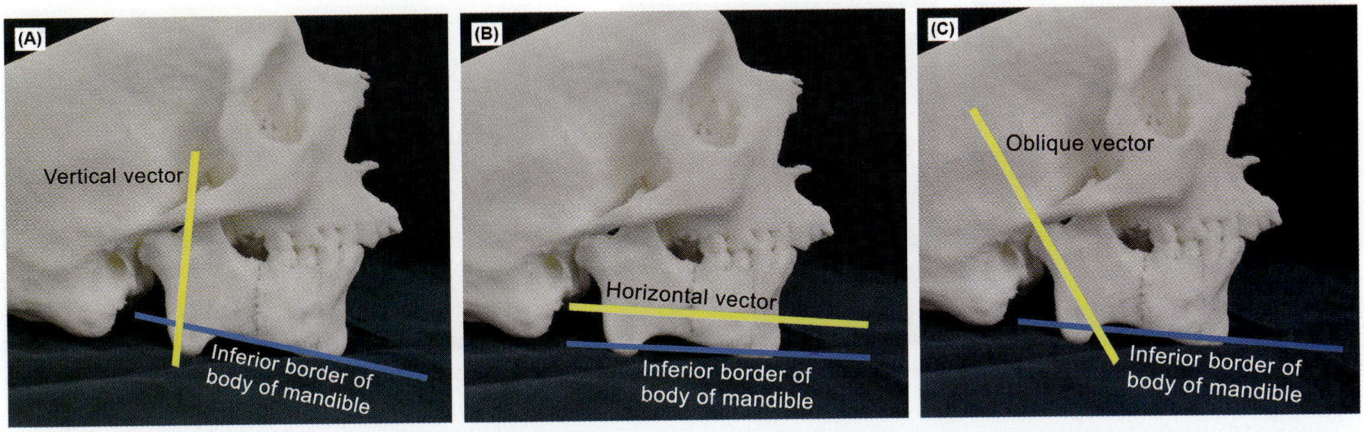

Figure 44.12 Vector of distraction. (**A**) Vertical vector. (**B**) Horizontal vector, (**C**) Oblique vector.

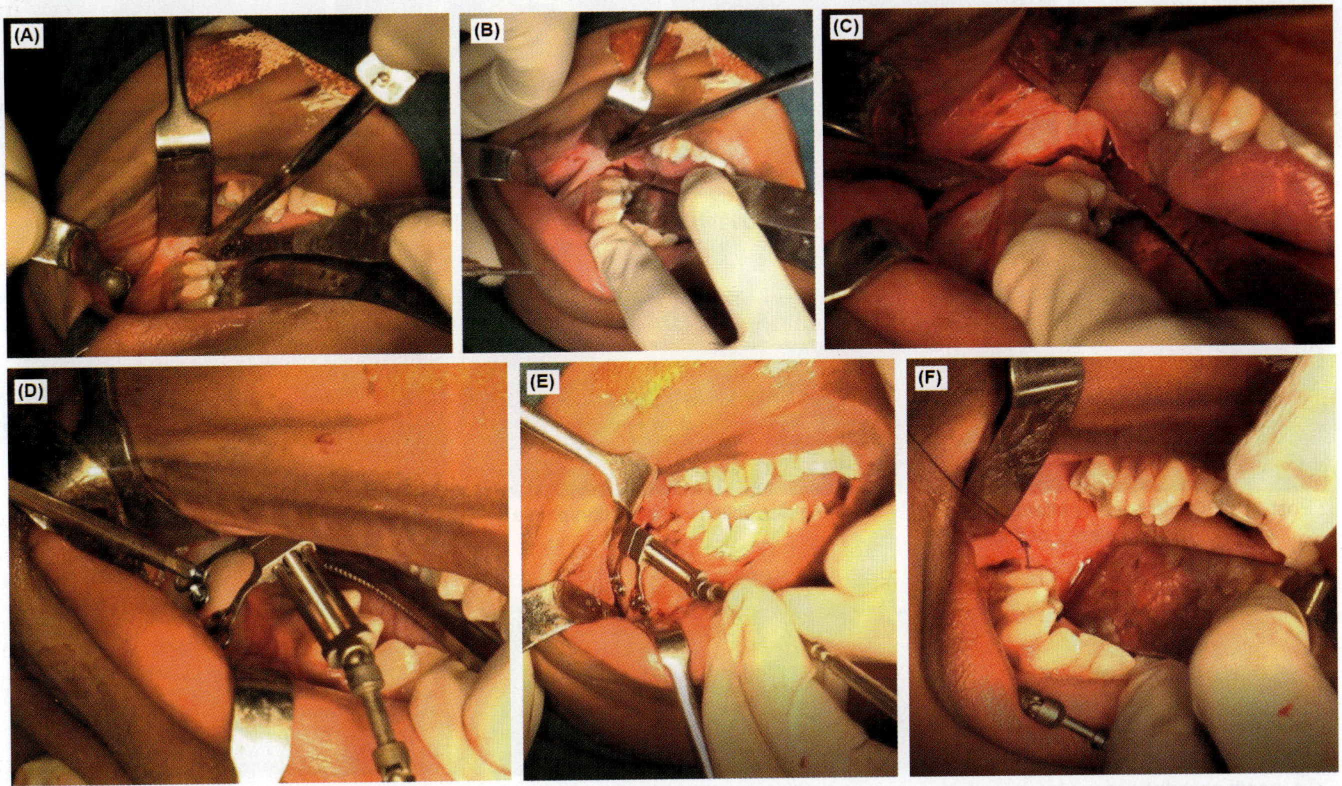

Figure 44.13 Surgical procedure of fixation of the intraoral distractor. (**A**) The bone site is exposed by vestibular incision and subperiosteal dissection. (**B**) A vertical osteotomy is placed on the site planned for positioning of the device using bur and saline. (**C**) The osteotomy is completed and the bony segments are separated using an osteotome. (**D**) The intraoral distraction device is fixed to bone using screws. (**E**) Activation of the distractor is done to check the free movements of the bony segments. (**F**) Primary closure of the mucosa using vicryl.

b. Lag or latency phase
c. Distraction phase
d. Consolidation phase
e. Distractor removal

Depending on the size of the defect and the type of distractor planned for fixation, the bone site can be approached through an *extraoral or intraoral incision*. The dissection can be performed in a *subperiosteal plane* while nerves are preserved. The surgical procedure should be nontraumatic and should preserve both the soft tissues and the periosteum's blood supply.

The bone is *osteotomised* at the site planned for positioning the device, using low-energy osteotomy, or by surgical burs and chisels. Osteotomies can be performed in a variety of orientations, including angulated, reverse L-shaped or vertical. Care is taken to avoid drilling at the unerupted tooth follicles.

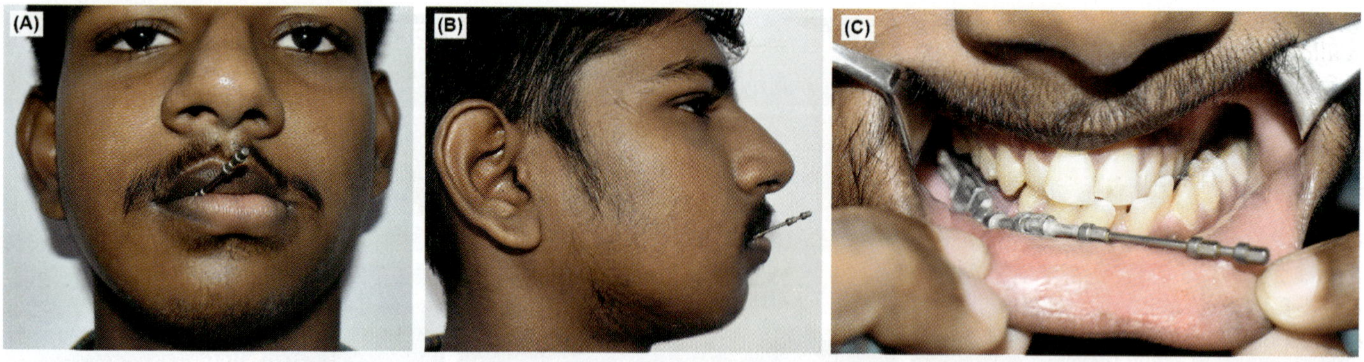

Figure 44.14 (**A–C**) Postoperative pictures after completion of distraction.

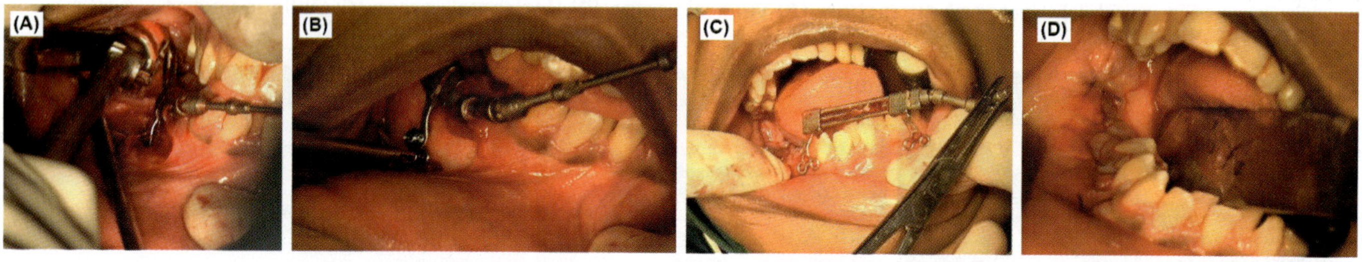

Figure 44.15 (**A–D**) Surgical removal of the distractor and closure of the wound.

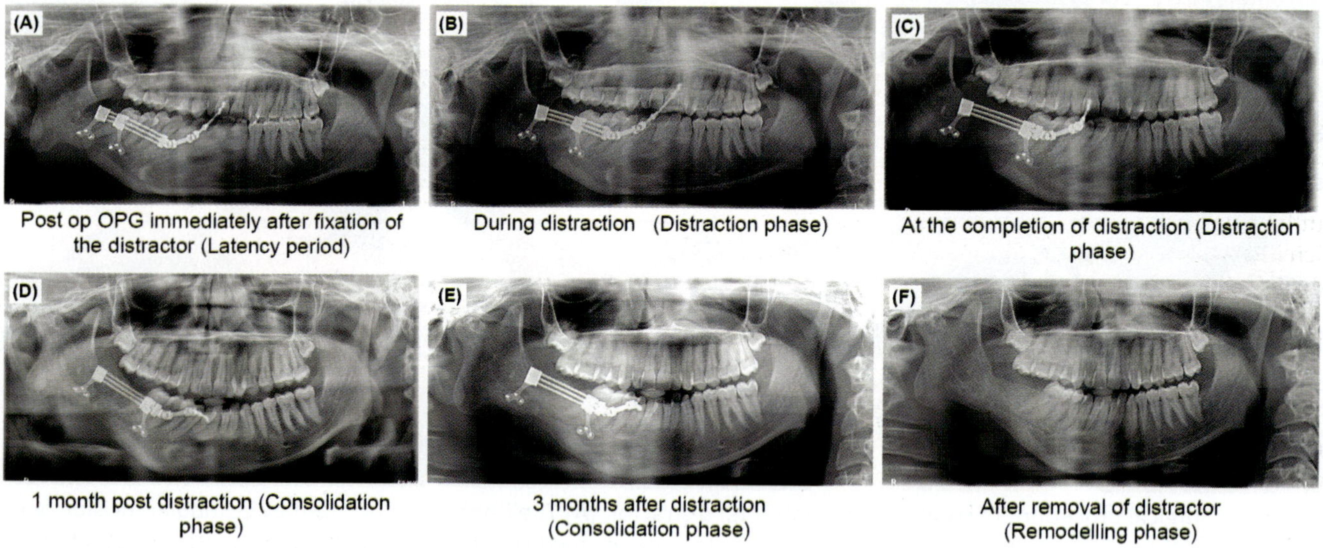

Figure 44.16 Radiographic assessment of the distraction process using an Orthopantomogram (OPG).

It is recommended to *position the distractors* before completing osteotomy in order to have a control over the orientation of the distractor. On the bone, drill holes are produced for fixing the device; the location of these holes relies on the orientation of the device or the vector of distraction. These drill holes are irrigated with saline and the distraction device is fixed on either side of the bone cut using screws or pins.

The *osteotomy is completed* using an osteotome and by separating the bony segments. A complete osteotomy should allow the mandible to move freely. It is essential to confirm that the osteotomy is complete because a greenstick fracture will not cause distraction.

The flaps are replaced and *primary closure* is achieved using nylon or vicryl, with the distractor arm protruding in the vestibule.

It is followed by the 2nd latency phase, which is generally around 7 days after fixation of the device. In this period, the distractor is not activated and the bone is allowed for initial healing.

In the 3rd distraction phase, the device is activated at a rate of 1 mm/day (0.5 mm twice a day) till the desired length is achieved. The fixation of the device on either side of the bone cut allows for gradual separation of the two segments allowing the formation of new bone in the gap. The distraction progress is monitored by the change in relationship of occlusion, level of occlusal plane and chin point. Generally, it is advisable to over-correct the deformity especially in growing children.

In the consolidation phase, the device is kept inactive and the bone is allowed to heal, which is approximately 8 weeks.

In a 2nd surgical procedure, the distraction device is removed following the consolidation period. The removal of device is recommended only after a radiographic evidence of a cortical outline or mineralisation of the new bone is seen. After the device is removed, orthodontic correction of teeth can be performed to correct the occlusion. If necessary, splints can be utilised to retain the position of newly formed bone.

After consolidation, the newly formed bone can be manipulated by using any of these methods; elastic traction, maxillary expansion, bite blocks, stabilisation appliances or orthodontic treatment.

THE FACTORS THAT INFLUENCE THE SUCCESS OF DISTRACTION OSTEOGENESIS INCLUDE

Device-related factors

It affects the characteristics of distractor and the stability of fixation. These factors include distractor design, vector and orientation of the device, rigidity of fixation and the number, length, and diameter of fixation pins.

Tissue-related parameters

It influences the quality of generated distraction tissue, which includes the structure, density and regenerative ability of the bone.

Dental aspects

It involves orthodontic treatment performed before and after the distraction, as well as the positioning and orientation of the distractor, distraction splints and functional loading of the newly created bone.

Biological parameters

- Lower power osteotomy with maximum preservation of tissues and blood supply
- Adequate latency period
- Optimal rate and rhythm of distraction
- Sufficient consolidation time

APPLICATIONS OF DISTRACTION OSTEOGENESIS IN MAXILLOFACIAL SURGERY

MIDFACE AND MAXILLARY DISTRACTION

The DO is used in maxilla and midface mainly for the correction of *maxillary hypoplasia due to cleft maxilla or craniofacial syndromes* such as Crouzon and Apert. In cleft patients, correction of hypoplastic maxilla is difficult due to the presence of scarring from previous surgeries in the lip, hard and soft palate. In addition, the conventional Le Fort I orthognathic surgery in cleft patients have a high tendency to relapse, if the movement is over 10 mm. But DO enables controlled soft tissue expansion, which ultimately helps to reduce this problem.

Maxillary or midface distraction can be performed with an *external or internal device*. Rigid external distractor (RED) is effective for craniofacial or midface distractions. RED allowed for full correction of midface deficiency, which includes both skeletal and soft tissue deficiencies. For intraoral devices, two distractors are fixed on each side with the zygomatic buttress as anchorage.

Maxillary *skeletal transverse defects* are best corrected using the *Miniscrew-assisted rapid palatal expansion (MARPE)* operation, which uses a miniscrew implant assisted rapid palatal expansion. Adults with a severely narrowed and crowded maxillary arch may also benefit from the MARPE.

The surgical procedure includes osteotomies at different levels depending on the deficiency. For forward distraction or lengthening of the maxilla, the osteotomy is horizontal, whereas for forward and downward displacement of the maxilla, the osteotomy is oblique or step osteotomy can be performed.

DISTRACTION FOR MANDIBULAR DEFICIENCY

DO can be used in mandible for the treatment of hypoplastic mandible, maxillofacial asymmetry or widening of mandible. Unilateral or bilateral deficiencies in mandible can also be treated with mandibular distraction.

Initially, *external distraction devices* were used in the distraction of mandible. Though they offer greater distraction length, they are less comfortable to the patients and cause facial scarring. In later years, *internal devices* that are smaller and applied directly to the bone were developed. The primary benefits of internal devices were a predictable lengthening and invisibility to the patients.

The distraction devices used for mandible deficiencies can be classified as (1) unidirectional, (2) bidirectional and (3) multidirectional. Unidirectional devices extend the mandible in a single direction. Bidirectional devices lengthen the ascending ramus and the body of mandible simultaneously by creating two distraction sites. Multidirectional devices may enable an additional transverse horizontal correction, especially at the gonial angle. They also repair the deformities in the ramus, body and angle of the mandible.

Distraction devices with curvilinear, motorised and hydraulic devices have also been developed recently. They allow for better control of vector.

In patients with transverse deficits, Guerrero used an intraoral tooth-borne hyrax-type device for midsymphyseal mandibular widening.

The surgical procedure includes mandibular osteotomies at the following sites:

- Ramus osteotomy
- Oblique osteotomy at the angle of mandible
- Mandibular body osteotomy

DISTRACTION OSTEOGENESIS IN OBSTRUCTIVE SLEEP APNOEA (OSA) SYNDROME

In OSA, patients present with severely hypoplastic and retruded mandible which causes posterior collapse of the tongue and lead to airway obstruction. These patients often require a permanent tracheostomy to prevent airway obstruction. In such cases, mandibular DO offers a promising technique by increasing the distraction length of up to 25 mm and eliminating the need for a tracheostomy.

RECONSTRUCTION OF JAWS (TRANSPORT DISTRACTION OSTEOGENESIS)

Transport distraction osteogenesis (TDO) is a technique used for correcting long bone defects resulting from trauma, oncologic resection or congenital anomalies. A distraction device is used to gradually move an osteotomised bone segment (the transport disc) across the defect in the bone. New bone tissue is created across the defect, as the transport bone segment advances. On reaching the opposite side host bone segment, the intervening fibrous tissue between the transport and the host bone segments is removed surgically and the docking site is compressed.

The transport distraction can also be used to establish a neocondyle and TMJ in patients with severe joint ankylosis.

ALVEOLAR RECONSTRUCTION

Alveolar distraction osteogenesis (ADO) is a procedure in which a transport segment is used to increase the alveolar crest for placement of implants, cosmetic or functional reasons.

ADO can be used for minor alveolar deficiencies such as alveolar cleft to severe bone deficiency resulting from trauma, periodontal disease or resection of tumours. Elongation of the deficient alveolus in both the horizontal and vertical planes can be achieved by ADO. It is crucial to ensure that the transport segment's lingual or palatal mucosa remains intact during distraction. It is possible to increase the alveolar bone height of up to 16 mm with ADO.

The advantage of ADO includes the simultaneous expansion of both bone and soft tissue without any donor site morbidity. The alveolar crestal bone remains cortical and mature.

The alveolar distraction device can be unidirectional, bidirectional or horizontal. It can also be divided into extraosseous, intraosseous devices or distraction by implants.

The surgical procedure includes two vertical and one horizontal osteotomies to create a transport segment with the mucosa intact.

CRANIOFACIAL DISTRACTION

DO has been successfully applied for the treatment of patients with craniofacial deformities such as Crouzon syndrome, Apert syndrome, Pfeiffer syndrome as well as midface abnormalities secondary to craniofacial anomalies. These patients may suffer from functional problems associated to increased intracranial pressure (ICP), severe exorbitism and OSA secondary to the early fusion of cranial sutures.

Distraction of the cranium and midface can be accomplished with a variety of external and internal devices. In severe cases, it may be necessary to begin the treatment as early as 1 year.

The surgical procedure involves Le Fort III or Le Fort IV osteotomy with internal or external distractor producing simultaneous midface and forehead distraction.

COMPLICATIONS OF DISTRACTION OSTEOGENESIS

PK's classification of complications of maxillofacial distraction osteogenesis (Table 44.5).

Patient counselling: It is necessary to counsel and encourage the patient and family about the length of treatment, device activation, oral cleanliness and a balanced diet.

Improper vector: Improper vector may result in anterior open bite, condyle resorption and TMJ disorders ultimately leading to failure of the surgery. It can be managed by proper surgical planning and proper positioning and orientation of the distraction device.

TABLE 44.5 PK's Classification

Planning Phase	Intraoperative/Surgery Phase	Distraction Phase	Postdistraction/ Consolidation Phase
• Improper patient selection and counselling • Improper vector planning • Errors in device selection	• Tooth injury • Neurosensory dysfunction • Incomplete osteotomy • Fracture of bone • Excessive bleeding • Device-related problems (e.g. fracture and unstable placement)	• Device failure • Pain • Premature consolidation • Interference due to device • Infection • Malnutrition	• Infection • Hypertrophic scar • Incomplete ossification • Fracture of regenerate • Relapse • TMJ disorders • Malunion • Persistent nerve damage

Tooth injury: The presence of impacted tooth buds in the line of osteotomy is at the risk of injury. Preoperative osteotomy site planning using virtual models or oblique osteotomy design can be done to avoid tooth injury.

Incomplete osteotomy: It may lead to failure in obtaining the amount of distraction. Incomplete osteotomy manifests as pain in the osteotomy site, failure in activation of device or loosening of the fixation screws. To avoid this, the distractor should be activated intraoperatively to ensure the osteotomy is finished. Few cases may require re-surgery to complete the osteotomy.

Fracture of bone: Unfavourable fractures of the bone can result from incomplete osteotomy or excessive force delivered during completion of osteotomy. It can be prevented by appropriate use of osteotome, controlled force and complete osteotomy.

Device failure: It includes device breakage and loosening of the screws or pins. It often requires 2nd surgery to replace the failed device.

Premature consolidation: Generally, mineralisation of the newly formed bone begins from the outer margin towards the centre. Premature consolidation can arise from inadequate rate of distraction and excessive compressive forces on one side leading to early contact between the segments. The daily rate and rhythm of distraction should be increased or re-surgery should be performed in case of incomplete distraction of jaws.

Overstretching of the soft tissues: It can be due to inappropriate distraction forces and compression by the device. The degree of damage to the soft tissues such as blood vessels, peripheral nerves and skeletal muscles can vary. Muscle overstretching can limit the amount of distraction. It may require 2nd surgery and active joint motion therapies.

Infection: It is the most common complication that can occur at any phase of distraction. It can arise due to inadequate fixation of device, poor oral hygiene maintenance and prolonged retention of the activation port. Proper oral hygiene maintenance, appropriate antibiotics, stable fixation and adequate care of the device are the measures that can be taken to avoid infection.

Hypertrophic scar: These are developed in extraoral devices. It can be minimised by using transcutaneous pins in an area where the scar is less visible.

Relapse: It is common and can result from increased rate of distraction, osteotomy cuts placed near the muscle attachment or from increased reflection of the periosteum. It can be avoided by following appropriate rate and rhythm of distraction.

TMJ disorders: It is noticed in patients undergoing mandibular distraction having preexisting condylar pathologies. It is managed by ensuring occlusal harmony from the beginning of planning phase.

CONCLUSION

In cases of moderate to severe bone deficiencies in the mandible, maxilla and midface, DO is proved to be an effective and well-established technique in the regeneration of bone and soft tissues. DO also contributes to the long-term stability to the newly formed bone. The DO of the craniofacial skeleton has replaced many of the conventional orthognathic procedures. Hence, DO can be considered as a gold standard treatment with a wide range of applications in maxillofacial skeleton.

The following are cases treated by DO (Cases 44.1–44.3). Each case and the distractor used are unique.

CASE 44.1 Tooth-Borne Palatal Distraction

Indication: Constricted maxilla

Vector: Univector

Device: Transpalatal tooth-borne custom made distractor

Osteotomy site: Midpalatal

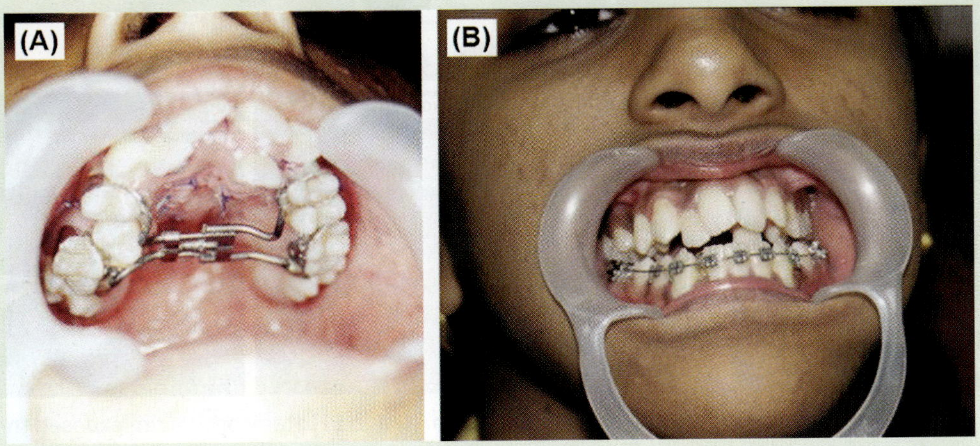

(**A**) Constricted maxillary arch. Expansion device placed after midpalatal osteotomy. (**B**) Expanded arch showing correction of crossbite.

CASE 44.2 Correction of Mandibular Micrognathia Using Intraoral Mandibular Distractor Bilaterally

Indication: Micrognathia

Device: Intraoral horizontal ramus distractor

Vector: Univector

Osteotomy site: Mandibular body

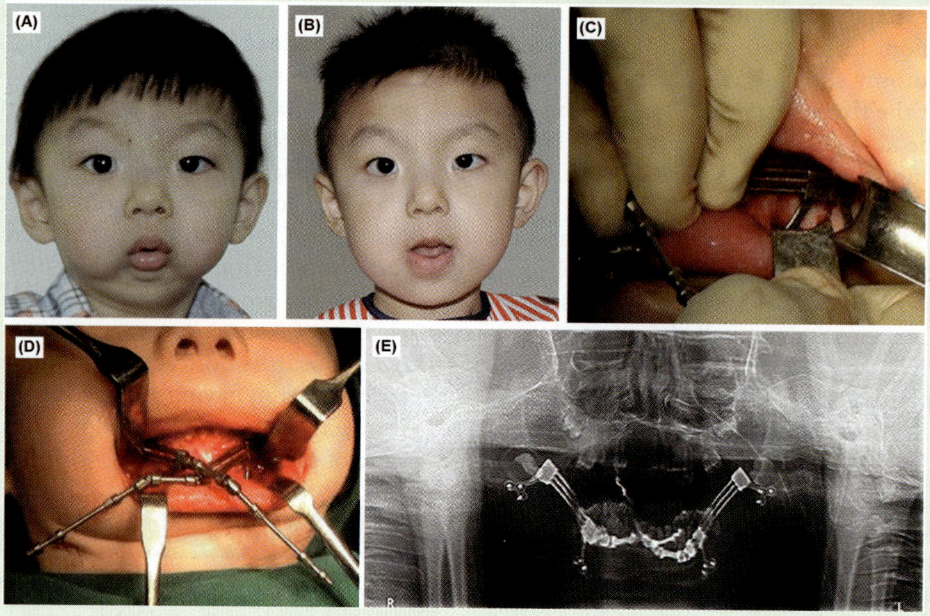

(**A**) Preoperative profile: A boy with Pierre Robin syndrome with micrognathia causing severe respiratory problems and sleep apnoea. Preoperative facial appearance lip incompetence with inability to place tongue within the mouth. (**B**) Postoperative view showing mandibular lengthening. (**C** and **D**) Fixation of intraoral mandibular distractor at the body of mandible. (**E**) Postoperative OPG.

CASE 44.3 Craniofacial Distraction

Indication: Midfacial hypoplasia due to Crouzon syndrome

Device: Kawamoto craniofacial internal distractor

Vector: Univector

Osteotomy: Le Fort III

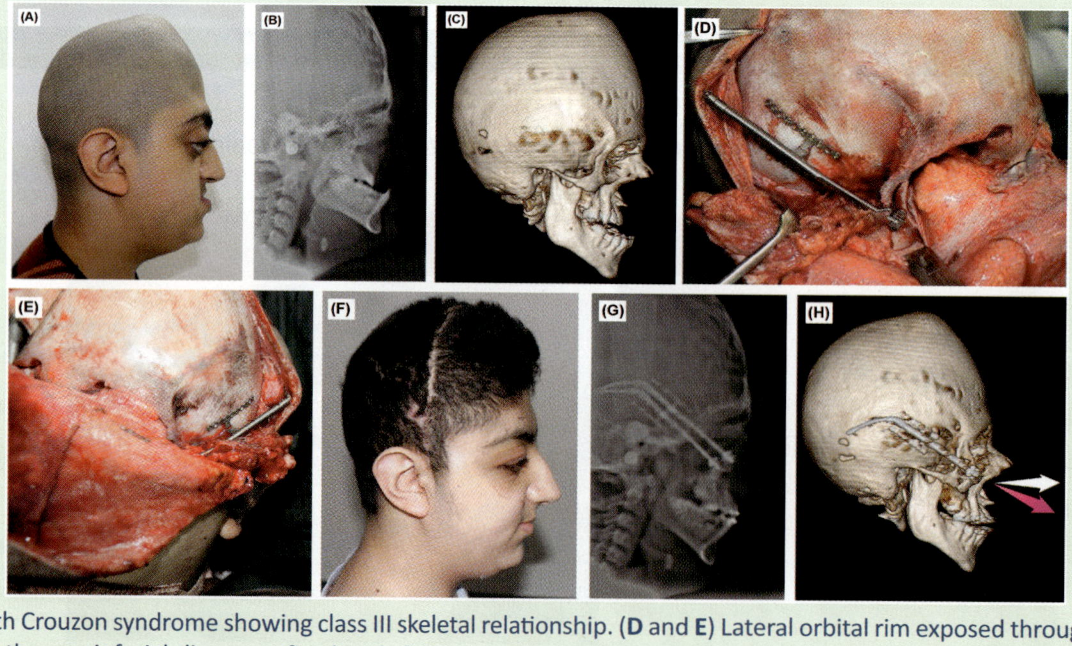

(**A–C**) Teen with Crouzon syndrome showing class III skeletal relationship. (**D** and **E**) Lateral orbital rim exposed through a bicoronal approach and the craniofacial distractor fixed with fixed plate on the cranium and the movable plate on the lateral orbital rim after Le Fort III osteotomy. The activator placed transcutaneously on the cranium. (**F–H**) Facial profile and skeletal relationship after completion of distraction. (Scan to play Le Fort III advancement with internal distractors for Crouzon syndrome.)

Chapter 45

Orofacial Cleft

OUTLINE

INTRODUCTION

Congenital deformities

The abnormalities in the appearance or function that occur due to unusual occurrence(s) in the embryological developmental sequence during the prenatal period.

Cleft lip

A congenital deformity that presents as an abnormal lack of continuity of the lip musculature, lip skin and the mucous membrane. The unusual breach can extend from the base of the nose to the free margin of the lip. The deformity may range from a simple notch at the free margin to a complete disjointed lip that also results in a nasal deformity. This most commonly occurs in the upper lip (Fig. 45.1A and B).

Simonart's band

In some complete clefts, the nasal floor on the cleft side is sometimes bridged by skin giving an appearance of an intact nasal sill. This band of skin is termed Simonart's band (Fig. 45.1 C).

Microform cleft

A mild abnormality of the (upper) lip that may or may not be due to an aberrance or discontinuity in the lip musculature. It may manifest as a ridge-shaped philtral column (Fig. 45.1 D).

Cleft palate

An abnormal discontinuity in the palatal musculature, mucous membrane with or without involvement of the hard palate that may extend from the uvula to the alveolus (Fig. 45.1 E).

Isolated cleft palate

Isolated cleft palate is an isolated finding which is both genetically and embryologically distinct from cleft lip with or without cleft palate. Isolated cleft palate rarely occurs in members of the same family. This suggests that the major causative genes for nonsyndromic cleft lip differ from those resulting in isolated cleft palate, although these defects may share one or two susceptibility genes of smaller effect. Both types of clefts are formed due to genetic aberrations and are inheritable (Fig. 45.1F).

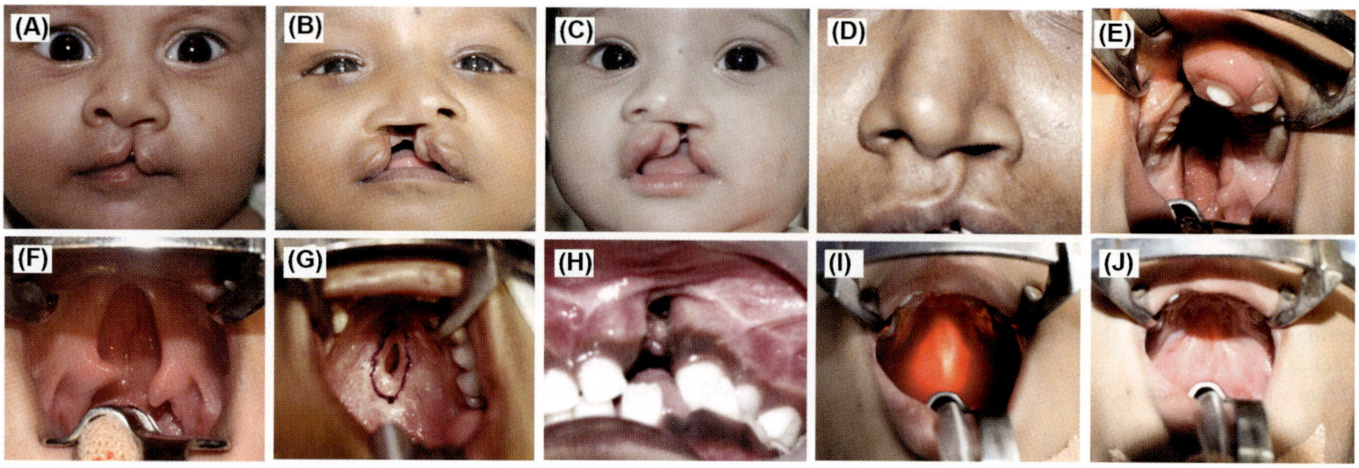

Figure 45.1 **(A)** Incomplete cleft lip. **(B)** Complete cleft lip. **(C)** Simonart's band. **(D)** Microform cleft lip. **(E)** Complete cleft palate. **(F)** Isolated cleft palate. **(G)** Palatal fistula. **(H)** Alveolar cleft (yellow arrow) with oronasal fistula (white arrow). **(I** and **J)** Submucous cleft.

Palatal fistula

A breach in continuity of the palate that results in an abnormal communication between the nasal cavity and the oral cavity. It can also be of traumatic or oncogenic origin (Fig. 45.1G).

Oronasal fistula

An abnormal breach in continuity on the floor of the nose that forms a communication between the anterior nasal airway and the buccal sulcus (Fig. 45.1H).

Alveolar cleft

An abnormal breach in the continuity of the alveolar bone of the maxilla occurring most commonly in the region between the lateral incisor and canine that may manifest as a simple notching of the alveolus to a complete discontinuity resulting in a fistulous tract between the nasal floor and the mouth (Fig. 45.1H).

Submucous cleft

A cleft or discontinuity that is present only in the palatal musculature without any breach of mucous membrane (Fig. 45.1I and J).

Velopharyngeal incompetence (VPI)

In velopharyngeal insufficiency, the velopharyngeal closure is compromised, which is essential for clear speaking. The contraction of the levator veli superioris muscle causes a posterior and superior displacement of the soft palate, which results in the production of audible sound. The pharyngeal walls must also move inward and forward for the velopharynx to close. This happens when the superior pharyngeal constrictor contracts. All these muscle functions are compromised in patients with cleft palate and VPI, thus causing a nasal twang in their speech. This condition is often found in patients with cleft palate.

Nonsyndromic cleft lip and palate

A 'non-syndromic' cleft is so termed when the affected individual has no other systemic or physical problems or any evidence of delay in motor or cognitive development. Nonsyndromic cleft is thought to be a complex or multifactorial trait and is not attributable to any single gene. It is an effect of both environmental and genetic factors (Fig. 45.2A and B).

Syndromic cleft lip and palate (CLP)

- CLP is most frequently an isolated anomaly
- May be associated with other congenital defects
- 24% of cases are associated with cardiovascular disorders
- 33% of cases are associated with malformations of the upper or lower limbs or the vertebral column
- Cases with associated malformations are more likely to have combined cleft lip and palate or an isolated cleft palate than a cleft lip alone
- 15% of all associated malformations are multiple and syndromic including those due to teratogens
- In association with other congenital anomalies like
- Cardiac anomalies,
  a. Clubbing
  b. Spina bifida
  c. Mental retardation
  d. Meningocoele
  e. May occur as part of a syndrome, only 3% of the cleft population
  f. In most cases, CLP occurs as a singular deformity without any associated anomalies.
- Approximately, 3% of all clinical cleft population are affected by syndromic clefts. ***Syndromic cleft*** is when the child presents with an orofacial cleft as a part of a syndrome. Most of these group of patients have identifiable syndromes. There are over 400 syndromes associated with cleft lip or palate, which may be due to single gene disorder and therefore follow a Mendelian inheritance.

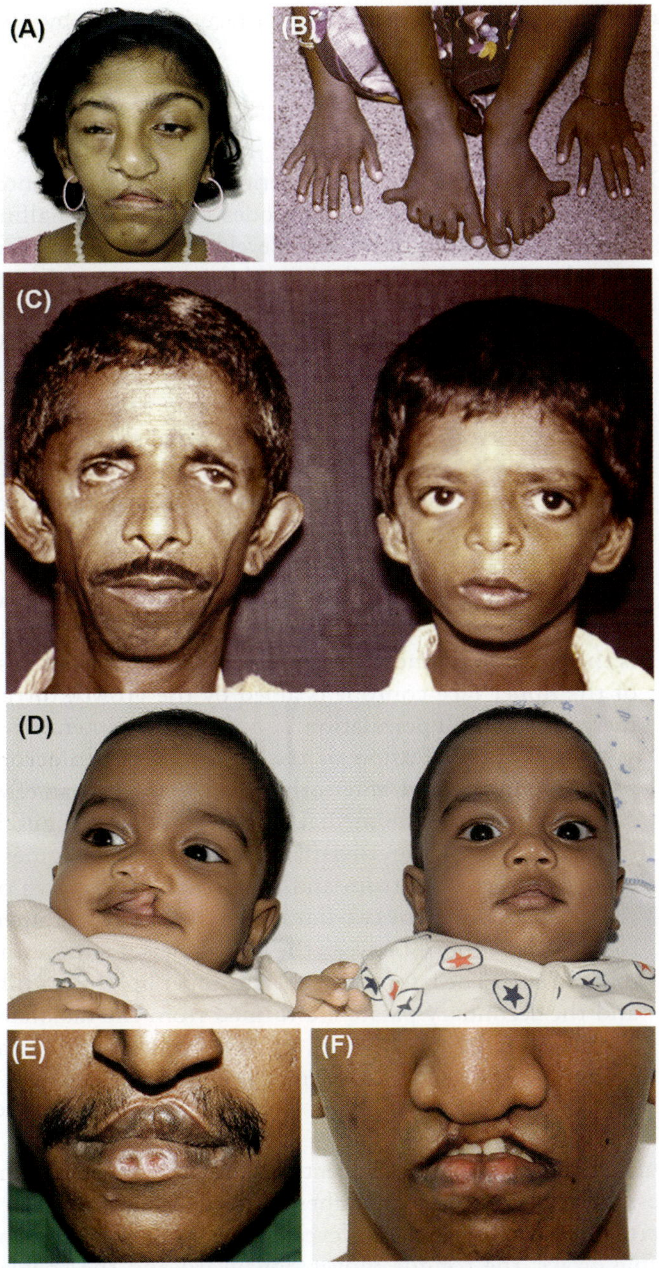

Figure 45.2 (**A**) Goldenhar syndrome: with bilateral cleft lip, macrostomia, strabismus, coloboma and ear deformity. (**B**) Polydactyly occurring with cleft. (**C**) Treacher Collins syndrome: inheritable condition with absence of zygomatic arch, micrognathism, cleft palate, low set ears. (**D**) Twins are more likely to be concordant for Cleft Lip/Palate, here one twin is affected. (**E** and **F**) Van der Woude syndrome: congenital lip pits.

Some of the common syndromes associated with Cleft Lip/Palate are depicted below.

- **Syndromes associated with cleft lip and palate:**
  1. *Chromosomal syndromes*
     a. Trisomy 13
     b. Trisomy 18
     c. Velocardiofacial syndrome (22q11.2 deletion)
  2. *Non-Mendelian syndromes*
     a. Pierre Robin sequence
     b. Goldenhar syndrome (Fig. 45.2A)
  3. *Mendelian syndromes*
     a. Ectrodactyly-ectoderm
     b. Dysplasia-clefting syndrome (AD)
     c. Gorlin syndrome (AD)
     d. Oto-palato-digital syndrome (XL)
     e. Oral-facial-digital syndrome (XL) (Fig. 45.2B)
     f. Smith-Lemli-Opitz syndrome (AR)
     g. Stickler syndrome (AD)
     h. Treacher Collins syndrome (AD) (Fig. 45.2C)
     i. Van der Woude syndrome (AD) (Fig. 45.2E and F)
  4. *Teratogenic syndromes*
     a. Foetal alcohol syndrome
     b. Foetal phenytoin syndrome
     c. Foetal valproate syndrome.

AD, Autosomal dominant; *AR*, autosomal recessive; *XL*, X-linked inheritance.

PREVALENCE

- Cleft lip is the most common congenital deformity of the face
- WHO reports a child with cleft is born every 2½ min
- In 2012, prevalence of 1 in 700 live births
- In India, a study in 2001 at Andhra Pradesh shows an incidence of 1.09 in 1000 live births
- This is significantly less than the Caucasian and Filipino population
- But significantly higher than in African population.

AETIOLOGY OF ORAL CLEFT

- **Multifactorial aetiology**
- Genetic factors
- Environmental factors
- Inheritability
- Syndromic aetiology.

GENES

Four categories of genes for which there are results suggestive of a genetic susceptibility to orofacial cleft formation are as follows:

1. Genes expressed in a **particular area** or period of the palatine arch development, such as the
   a. Transforming growth factors alpha and beta (TGF alpha, TGF beta 2, TGF beta 3)
2. Genes linked to the pathogenesis without direct involvement
   a. Retinoic acid receptor (RAR)
   b. Methylene tetrahydrofolate reductase (MTHFR) receptor
   c. Folate receptor 1 (FOLR1)

3. Genes or locus identified in experimental animals—Homeobox gene (HOX7)
   a. Homeotic genes MSX-1 and MSX-2
4. Genes involved in the interaction with xenobiotics metabolism
   a. Cytochrome P-450.

ENVIRONMENTAL FACTORS

- Folic acid deficiency—depending on the maternal or embryo genotype
- Folic acid supplementation before and during conception has become mandatory to prevent neural tube defects
- Advanced maternal age
- Excess retinoic acid
- Consanguinity of marriage—phenotypic expression of the genotype
- Teratogenic agents
  a. Smoking
  b. Alcohol intake (ethyl alcohol)
  c. Drugs: Phenytoin, diphenyl hydantoin, methotrexate, aminopterin, retinoids and sodium valproate
  d. Pesticides such as dioxin
  e. Hyperthermia during pregnancy.

INHERITABILITY

- If the 1st child has a cleft, the chance of the 2nd child also being affected with cleft lip or palate is around 30–40 times the risk.
- Monozygotic twins (identical and therefore sharing the same genes) are far more likely to be concordant for Cleft Lip/Palate (where either both are affected or both unaffected).
- For monozygotic twins, the concordance rate is 25%–40%.
- For dizygotic twins (only half of their genes in common), the concordance rate is 3%–6%.

EMBRYOLOGY

DEVELOPMENT OF THE FACE (4TH TO 8TH WEEK IUL)

The developmental inception of the human head is from the branchial arch system, which begins at the ***4th week*** intrauterine life (IUL). The ectodermal layer formed ***at 3rd week*** will now differentiate to surface ectoderm and neural ectoderm and the most important interface of both the neural crest cells (NCC). By the end of the ***4th week of IUL***, the facial structures start developing by five facial prominences around the stomodeum. The stomodeum is the future oral cavity. The five processes are the single unpaired frontonasal process, the paired maxillary process and the paired mandibular process. By the ***6th week***, the medial nasal processes from the frontonasal process fuse to form the upper lip and the mandibular processes fuse to form the lower lip. Mesenchymal migration and fusion of the facial prominences occurs within ***4 to 8 weeks IUL***, and a distinctly human face is formed by ***10th week IUL***.

MORPHOGENESIS OF THE LIP AND PRIMARY PALATE (4TH WEEK TO 8TH WEEK IUL)

Day 24 to day 33—The lateral inferior aspect of the frontonasal process is where nasal placodes 1st appear, signalling the beginning of central face development. At the placodes border, mesenchyme derived from the neural crest rapidly accumulates and multiplies. The lateral and medial rims expand outwards to form a pit or a groove. As the lateral and medial processes develop, the nasal pit deepens. The maxillary process of the 1st branchial arch forms its bottom border. When the medial surface of the lateral processes meets the lateral surface of the medial processes, the definitive formation of the primary palate begins. The apposed epithelia form an epithelial seam that is almost immediately obliterated by autolysis and replaced by mesenchyme. An epithelial seam is formed as the medial processes come together, and this mesenchyme is then autolysed and replaced. The eventual smoothness of the upper face contour is aided by the growth of the mesenchymal cell population.

Day 40 to day 48—Fusion of the lateral processes occurs more superiorly and anteriorly with the medial process. At the same time, the medial processes merge with each other to form the intermaxillary segment. This segment gives rise to the philtrum and the premaxilla, an area of the palate bounded by two lines from the incisive foramen to the alveolar bone between the lateral incisor and canine on each side. The lateral parts of the upper lip, the maxilla and the secondary palate are formed from the maxillary processes. By the 14th week of development, the facial contour of the new-born is virtually complete (Figs. 45.3).

MORPHOGENESIS OF THE SECONDARY PALATE

Palatal shelves are two projections of the maxillary processes of the 1st branchial arches. Initially, these shelves are vertical on each side of the developing tongue. As the mandible grows, the tongue moves downward and the shelves become horizontal and grow towards each other. Cleft palate, which is often associated with cleft lip, is thought to be a secondary malformation caused by the tongue. In the ***8th week*** of development, the shelves have grown large enough to approximate each other and fuse anteriorly. Fusion is complete by the ***17th week*** of embryonic life. These shelves fuse with the primary palate and nasal septum, a downgrowth of the merged medial processes. During fusion, the epithelia form an epithelial seam that breaks down and allows mesenchymal continuity. Potential possibilities for developmental failure:

1. A structural abnormality within the shelves can prevent their movement to the final horizontal position
2. Narrow palatal shelves and thus unable to meet each other in the midline

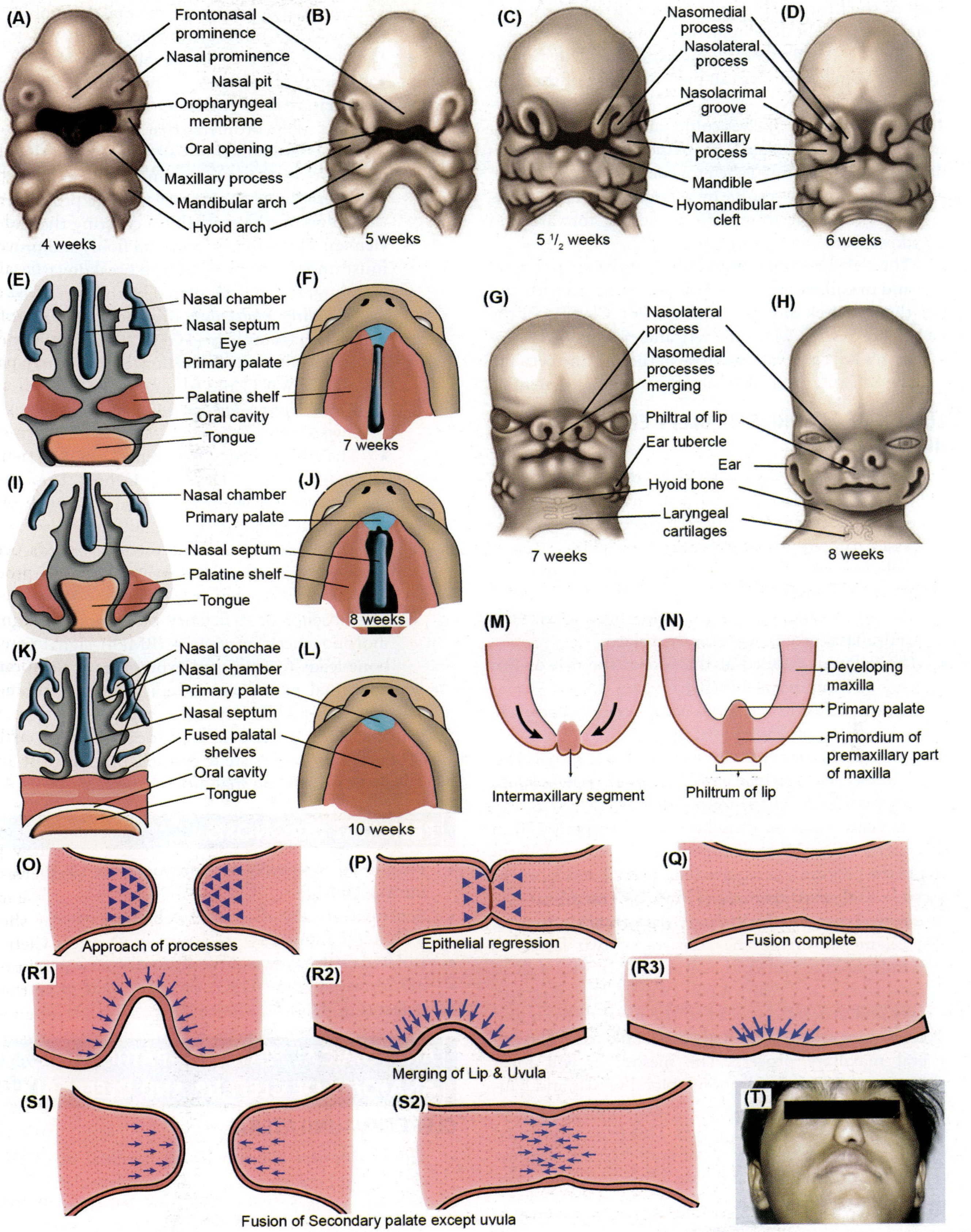

Figure 45.3 (**A-L**) Development of face and palate at every week (**M-N**) Development of the lip (**O-S2**) Evolution of theories of cleft embryo pathogenesis (**O-Q**) His's theory (**R1-S2**) Stark's theory (**T**) Hemiarhinia with cleft palate.

3. Lack of shelf force can delay horizontalisation, missing fusion at the right developmental time
4. Interference for downward movement of the tongue from between the shelves can prevent fusion of the palatal shelves
5. The epithelia of the shelves could fail to fuse for cellular and molecular reasons. The pathogenesis of human palatal and lip clefting is heterogeneous
   a. The lip defect results in a large premaxilla, thus preventing the tongue from moving forward and downward
   b. The cleft lip results from failure of the medial nasal and maxillary processes to fuse between the 4th and the 6th week of foetal development. Clefting of the palate results when the left and right palatal processes fail to elevate and fuse in the midline between the 8th and the 12th week of foetal development.

EVOLUTION OF THEORIES OF CLEFT EMBRYO PATHOGENESIS

1. **Fusion of process—Classical theory of Dursy and His:**
   - Wilhelm His (1874) stated that the mid-portion occupied by the oral cavity is formed from five processes: the frontonasal process, the paired palatal shelves from the two maxillary processes and two mandibular processes
   - The palatal shelves fuse with each other and with the frontonasal process to form the palate
   - The palate is formed at the end of the 6th or 7th week of Intrauterine life (IUL)
   - Failure of fusion results in complete or incomplete cleft of lip, alveolus and palate
2. **Fleischmann's theory** is that '*cleft palate is the arrest of the disappearance of the epithelial membrane, which remains intact, not penetrated by the adjacent mesoderm*'
3. **Victor Veau** based on Fleischmann's theory noticed in specimens of embryo that penetration of mesoderm across the process was required for normal development
4. **Mesodermal reinforcement of branchial membranes—conceptual sequence by Richard Stark (Stark's theory):** The bilamellar membrane consists of two layers of ectoderm called an epithelial wall (epithelial wall of Hochstetter and Veau). A part of mesoderm migrates over and around the head to the nasal dorsum and central lip and another part bilaterally from the lateral maxillary process. The mesoderm will form bone, cartilage, muscle, nerve, blood vessels and lymphatics. If the mesoderm layers fail to bolster early or rapidly, cleft formation occurs. This process is called mesodermal reinforcement of branchial membranes
   - Failure of mesodermal delivery from the migratory route over the head results in:
     - Forebrain maldevelopment or arhinencephaly, in which at least the olfactory lobes are deficient and there will be associated medial cleft of the lip
   - Mesodermal deficiency of the malar region
     - Treacher Collins syndrome
   - Deficiency in the 1st branchial arch
     - Macrostomia, hemignathia, preauricular tags, etc
5. **Neuromeric theory (Michael Carstens):** The human embryo has the neuromeres that consists of NCC; these cells prompt development of all structures of the embryo
   - The lip closure requires a mesenchymal 'flow' from the lateral lip elements towards the prolabium. For this to occur, the epithelium covering the lateral lip element, the skin bridge (nasal floor) and prolabium must undergo a gene-induced breakdown
   - This interaction is regulated by the expression of:
     - ***Signaling molecules:*** Members of transforming growth factor beta (TGFβ), fibroblast growth factor (FGF), sonic hedgehog (SHH), Wingless/Integrated (WNT) and tumour necrosis factor (TNF)
     - ***Transcription factors:*** Msx1, Pax9, Osr2, Runx2, Twist-1, etc
     - The three hedgehog genes are SHH, Indian hedgehog and Desert hedgehog. They play an important role in craniofacial development by maintaining epithelial stability
   - For the mesodermal facial processes to fuse as they come into proximity to each other, there must be epithelial breakdown at their leading edges
   - The absence or deficiency of an appropriate Bone morphogenetic protein 4 (BMP4) signal from the bone leads to restricted expression of SHH causing abnormal persistence of epithelium and failure of mesenchymal fusion
   - If a bony cleft is present, a local reduction in BMP4 will lead to persistent epithelialisation of the facial processes and an inability to fuse.

PRENATAL DIAGNOSIS

- Diagnosed prenatally by ultrasound at 13–16 weeks of intrauterine life
- Sensitivity to the diagnosis is highest when associated with other anomalies
- Isolated cleft palate is difficult to diagnose prenatally
- 3D ultrasonogram (USG) provides clear picture of the defect (Fig. 45.4).

ANATOMICAL FEATURES—PATHOLOGICAL ANATOMY OF CLEFT LIP AND CLEFT PALATE

CLEFT LIP—UNILATERAL

- The anatomical abnormality is minimal in incomplete cleft lip and maximum in wide complete cleft lip
- There is a characteristic skeleton deformity due to the abnormal growth of the skeleton in pre- and postnatal period, which accentuates the original deformity due to embryological failure (Fig. 45.5)

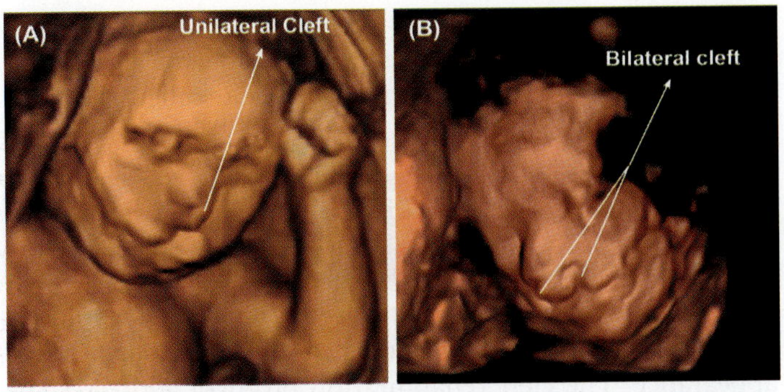

Figure 45.4 3D USG of unilateral and bilateral cleft lip.

- **Nose**
  a. The premaxilla is externally rotated
  b. The lateral segment is retroposed
  c. Nose is rotated towards the normal side
  d. The columella is deviated as it is shorter on the affected side
  e. The nasal floor is completely cleft and the nostril is transversely placed on the cleft side
  f. The septum is deflected
  g. The caudal end of the septum is detached from the vomerine groove
- **Lip**
  a. Orbicularis oris of the lips are unable to balance each side
  b. The orbicularis oris during development fail to meet the muscle fibres from the opposite side
  c. It turns upwards instead due to the cleft, it inserts partially into the lip margin with some fibres extending up towards the anterior nasal spine and base of columella medially and the alar base laterally. The labial vessels also pass upwards in the margins of the cleft.

CLEFT LIP—BILATERAL

In bilateral cleft lip cases, central frontonasal segment is not attached to the maxilla and so there is marked forward projection of the premaxilla (Fig. 45.6).

The abnormal forward projection of the premaxilla is due to a marked forward position of the alveolar bone and the hypoplastic maxilla on both sides.

Nose:

- The nasal deformity is symmetrical when the cleft is symmetrical on both sides
- The septum is straight
- The columella is absent
- Thus, there is no columella-labial angle
- The base of the ala is flared
- Nostril floor is absent
- Bilaterally longer lateral crura and short splayed medial crura
- The nasal tip is flat with wide separation of the medial crura

Lip

- Embryonically, mesenchyme does not penetrate the processes from either side
- As no muscle develops from the medial nasal process
- Muscle is absent behind the prolabium skin

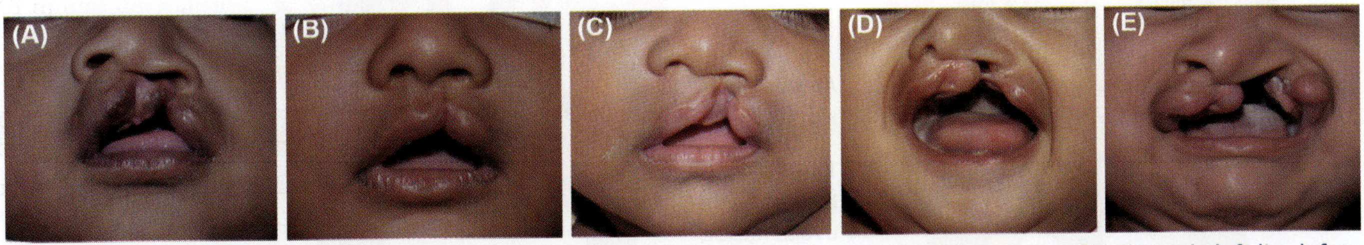

Figure 45.5 (**A**) Unilateral cleft lip and palate—showing all characteristic features. (**B–E**) Spectrum of unilateral cleft lip deformities. (**B**) Microform unilateral cleft lip. (**C**) Incomplete unilateral cleft lip. (**D**) Complete unilateral cleft lip and alveolus. (**E**) Complete unilateral cleft lip and palate.

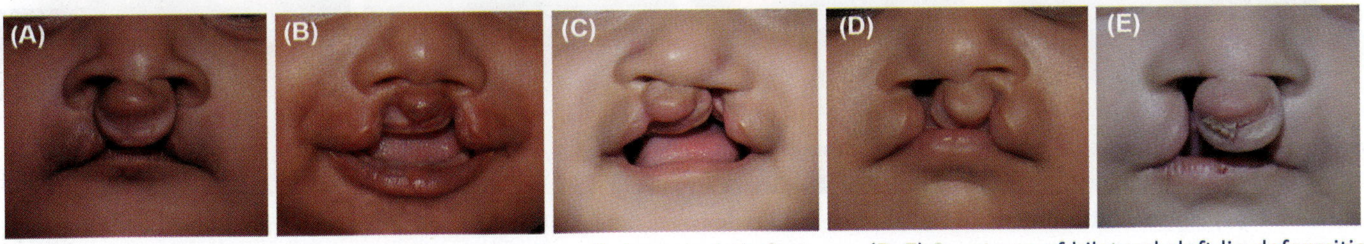

Figure 45.6 (**A**) Bilateral cleft lip and palate—showing all characteristic features. (**B–E**) Spectrum of bilateral cleft lip deformities. (**B**) Bilateral incomplete cleft lip. (**C**) Microform right and complete left bilateral cleft lip. (**D**) Complete left and incomplete right bilateral cleft lip and alveolus. (**E**) Complete bilateral cleft lip and palate.

- Hair follicles are also absent
- The abnormal insertion of the orbicularis oris pulls the medial and lateral crura of the alar cartilage outwards.

CLEFT PALATE—HARD PALATE

The vomer bone is the perpendicular bone in the nasal cavity that attaches to the superior surface of the hard palate (palatal shelf) in a normal individual. In unilateral cleft, the vomer is joined to the palatal shelf on the noncleft side, along its medial edge. The palatal shelf on the cleft side is smaller in width and the vomer does not join with it, forming the cleft.

CLEFT PALATE—SOFT PALATE

The abnormal velar musculature in cleft was 1st described by Veau (1931). The tensor muscle after passing around the hook of hamulus forms a thick fibrous triangular insertion into the lateral and posterior edge of the hard palate and palatal aponeurosis. The levator, palatopharyngeus and palatoglossus, unable to meet in the midline, pass more anteriorly to be inserted into the margins of the cleft, the oral and nasal mucosa, the abnormal palatal aponeurosis and into the back of the hard palate. Near the midline, the levator and palatopharyngeus fuse to form what Veau called the 'cleft muscle' (Fig. 45.7).

CLINICAL FEATURES—PROBLEMS FACED BY CLEFT CHILDREN

A child born with cleft lip with or without palate would experience the following problems in addition to abnormal appearance. The cleft rehabilitation protocol addresses the same without causing any damage to their potential to grow normally. The protocol aims to provide these children a normal quality of life as possible.

1. Feeding problems
2. Associated systemic anomalies
3. Speech
4. Ear infections
5. Malocclusion and maxillary growth retardation
6. Scarring
7. Cosmetic defect–abnormal appearance.

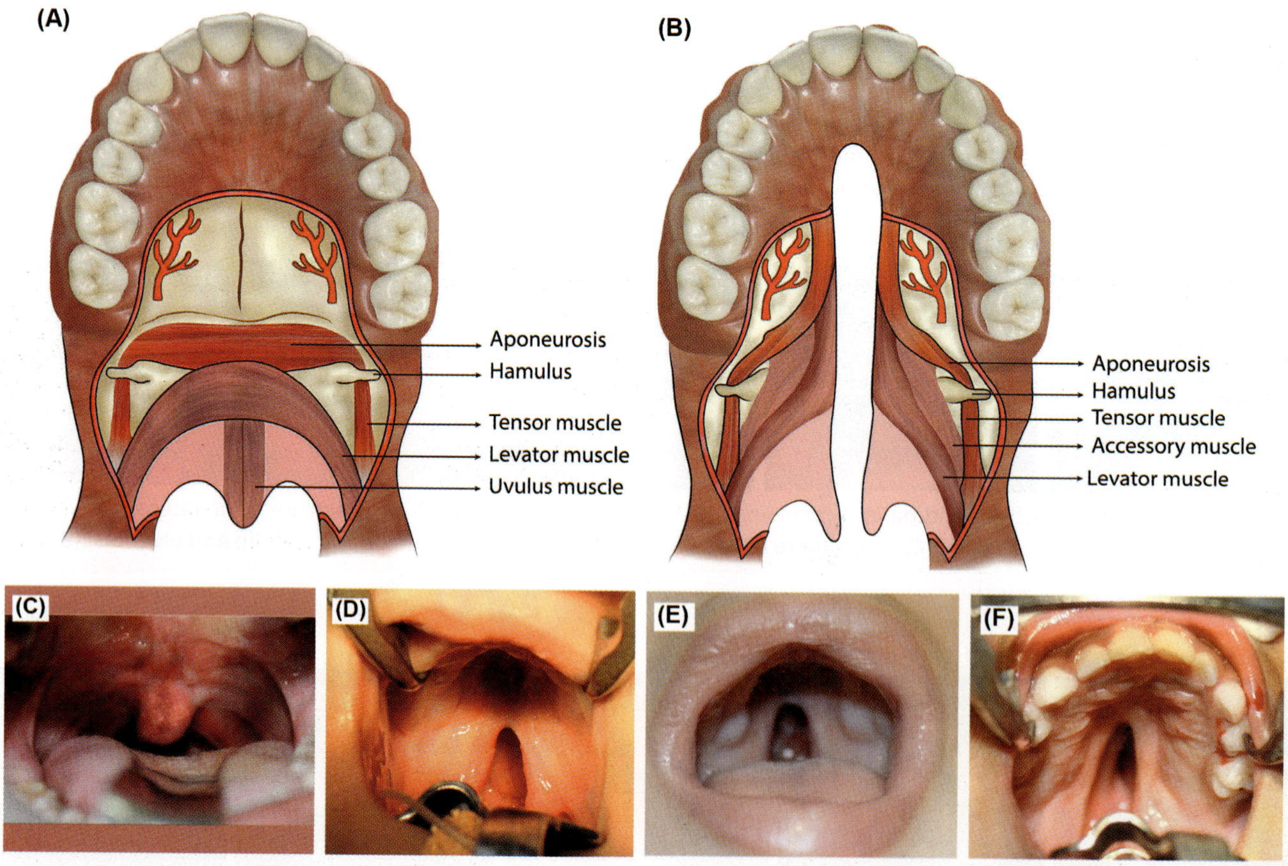

Figure 45.7 (**A**) Normal attachments of the important muscles of the soft palate, the tensor veli palatini, levator veli palatini and uvulus muscles. The palatal aponeurosis is also seen. (**B**) Abnormal attachments of the same muscles in cleft palate. The variation in attachments can be noted. (**C–F**) Spectrum of cleft palate. (**C**) Bifid uvula. (**D**) Cleft of the soft palate. (**E** and **F**) Cleft of the hard and soft palate.

Feeding problems and regurgitation

- In order to suckle milk, the baby needs to create an air-tight seal around the mother's nipple with the lips and exert negative pressure to express the milk. An associated cleft palate can cause regurgitation of fluids causing respiratory problems
- The other difficulties and the cycle of events due to these difficulties have been briefed in Flowchart 45.1. Despite these problems, many children with cleft learn to suckle but are unable to exert adequate pressure due to:
  a. the loss of muscle continuity in the lip and
  b. the communication between mouth and nose in a cleft in the palate
- **Temporary management:**
  a. These children need to be burped more often
  b. The feeding posture should be more upright to prevent regurgitation (Fig. 45.8)
  c. Feeding plate or palatal obturators are of use if delivered a few days after birth
  d. A feeding consultant can train the parents to tape the cleft lip together in order to provide lip seal and thereby provide more suction pressure
  e. If all fails, the children have to be trained on the bottle
  f. The nipple hole of feeding bottle can be enlarged to enable the child to extract more milk with less pressure
  g. Special feeding bottles have been designed for cleft children to provide nutrition till the baby's weight is adequate for performing the cleft lip repair surgery
  h. Few children may need a feeding tube if aspiration is not preventable and proves to be life threatening
- **Permanent management:**
  a. The suckling problem will be solved once the surgical lip correction has been completed at 3 months of age. Regurgitation will minimise after primary palatal repair at 9 months of age. The children can be weaned normally.

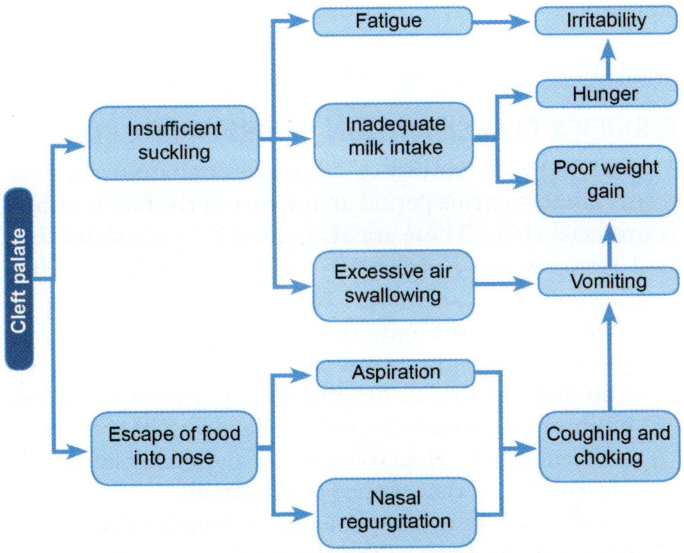

Flowchart 45.1 Feeding difficulties and the cycle of events leading to poor weight gain.

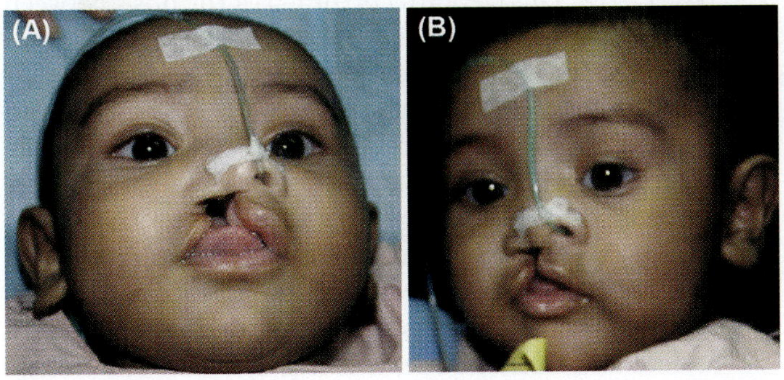

Figure 45.8 Feeding tube to prevent regurgitation and subsequent lung infection.

Associated deformities

Children with associated deformities of the CVS in velo-cardio-facial syndrome will require cardiac intervention. In Pierre Robin's syndrome, airway problems like obstructive sleep apnoea due to severe micrognathia require mandibular expansion or tracheostomy prior to the primary lip/palate surgery.

Speech

Even after palatal repair, speech may be affected. This may be attributed to several factors:

- Velopharyngeal incompetence (VPI) causing hypernasality
- Oronasal fistula (ONF) causing a nasal twang

VPI and ONF can be corrected surgically. Physical obstructions can be cleared surgically or orthodontically. Cleft children should be under the care of a speech therapist till the improper speech patterns are rectified.

- Malocclusion
- Lip incompetence causing problems in pronunciation
- Hearing disability causing impaired speech learning
- Learning disability, etc.

Ear infection

Cleft children are susceptible to ear infection, otitis media. The malposition of the Eustachian tube results in more frequent middle ear infection. Some children may require myringotomy to prevent hearing loss.

Malocclusion

It may occur due to missing lateral incisor, impacted canine and failure of maxilla to grow or due to maxillary arch collapse. A combination of orthodontics, orthognathic surgery and distraction are warranted to correct the maxillary hypoplasia that develops after palatal repair. Missing teeth can be replaced using implant supported prosthesis.

Maxillary growth retardation

Decreased maxillary growth in cleft children is the most common problem encountered which accentuates as the child grows. Both anteroposterior and transverse growth of the maxilla is restricted in children with cleft palate necessitating procedures to bring the dental arch into Class I alignment.

They often present with:

1. Severe Class III skeletal malocclusion
2. With or without collapse and posterior crossbite

This maxillary growth discrepancy is attributed to the following reasons:

1. Early surgical manipulation of the periosteum of the hard palate or the vomer
2. Intrinsic deficiency of growth of the cleft maxilla
3. The inter-arch discrepancy that exists at birth
4. Discontinuity between the maxillary growth center and the cleft maxillary segment

Management of maxillary hypoplasia:

1. Early presurgical orthopaedic alveolar moulding to bring the alveolar arches to a favourable position before primary repair
2. Early premaxillary set back to correct extremely prognathic premaxilla
3. Pre- and postsurgical orthodontics to bring the teeth in favourable alignments
4. Palatal expansion
5. Orthognathic surgery
6. Distraction osteogenesis.

Cosmetic defects

Lip defect, nasal deformity (deviated nose in case of unilateral complete cleft lip and palate (UCLP); flat and broad nose in case of bilateral cleft lip and palate (BCLP)), maxillary hypoplasia and collapse, missing lateral incisor/canine. The lip is primarily repaired in early childhood. If the scar is not aesthetic, it can be revised again after puberty. The nasal defect is repaired primarily during the primary lip surgery and the secondary finite revision surgery is performed after the skeletal hypoplasia is corrected.

CLASSIFICATIONS OF ORAL AND FACIAL CLEFTS

KERNAHAN'S MODIFICATION (1971)

The striped Y classification: The involved area is filled in by pen and provides graphic demonstration of the site and extent of cleft involvement. The arms of the Y represent the primary palate (the lip, alveolar process to the incisive foramen) and the stem of the Y represents the secondary palate, posterior to the incisive foramen. Stippling the appropriate segments is employed to show the extent of gross clefts; and the horizontal lines, possible submucous Simonart's bands. Areas 1 and 4 represent the right and left sides of the lip, areas 2 and 5 represent the right and left alveolus, areas 3 and 6

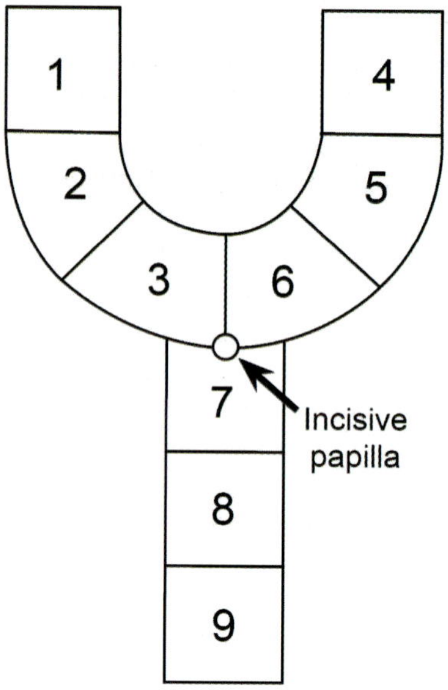

Figure 45.9 Kernahan's classification.

represent the right and left sides of the primary palate. Areas 7 and 8 represent the hard palate and area 9 represent the soft palate. The circle represents the incisive papilla (Fig. 45.9).

TESSIER'S CLASSIFICATION OF OROFACIAL CLEFTS

A breach in the continuity of soft tissues or hard tissues that occurs at intrauterine period at any part of the face is termed as orofacial clefts. These are also called Tessier's clefts since Paul Tessier was one of the 1st to classify them (Fig. 45.10).

1. *Tessier 0–14*: This midline cleft involves the median encephalocoele, the ethmoid (duplication of the crista galli), the nose (duplication/pneumatisation of the septum and columella), maxilla and lip. Absence of prolabium of lip, premaxilla, columella giving impression of arhinencephaly. Hypertelorism or hypotelorism may be present due to the absence of premaxilla
2. *Tessier 1–13:* It is a paramedian craniofacial cleft that separates the dome of the alar cartilage and the lip as in cleft lip. It affects the frontal bone causing hypertelorism, the olfactory groove of the cribriform plate, the nasal bones and the alveolar bones
3. *Tessier 2–12:* This cleft affects the ala of the nose, between the summit and the base of the ala of the nose, the alar cartilage on the lip. On the skeleton, it traverses the lateral mass of the ethmoid. The glabella is flattened and the frontal sinus is enlarged. Nasal hemiatrophy, the supernumerary nostrils and the proboscis lateralis are probably of different degrees and forms the same paracentral defect. *Tessier 12* is located medial to the medial canthus. The frontal process of the maxilla is flat (telecanthus). The cleft crosses the lateral mass of the ethmoidal and frontal bone, which is also flat. The frontal sinus is enlarged. On the soft tissue, there is a coloboma of the root of the eyebrow)

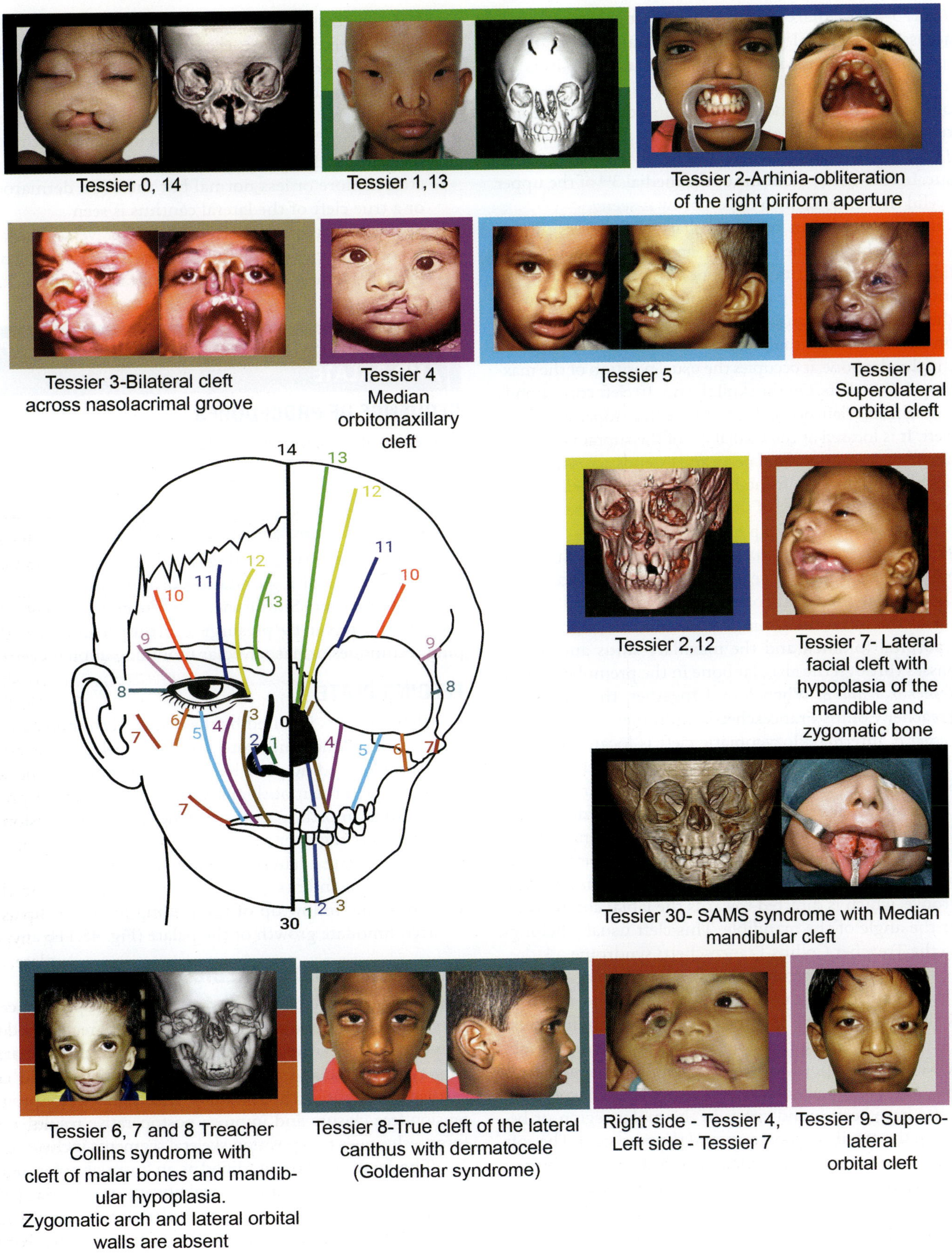

Figure 45.10 Tessier's classification of orofacial clefts.

4. *Tessier 3–11:* Medial orbitomaxillary cleft passes obliquely across the lacrimal groove. The frontal process of the maxilla and the medial wall of the maxillary sinus are affected. The cleft traverses across the lacrimal segment of the lower eyelid and passes around the alar base and traverses the lip and alveolar ridge like a cleft lip. *Tessier 11 is a* superomedial orbital cleft involving only soft tissue. In this cleft, coloboma of the medial 3rd of the upper eyelid that extends into the eyebrow is seen
5. *Tessier 4–10:* Median orbitomaxillary cleft passes almost vertically through the lacrimal segment of the inferior eyelid, the infraorbital rim and floor of the orbit (medial to the infraorbital nerve); it passes through the maxillary sinus in the cheek (causing an extrophy of the sinus) and continues on the lip between the philtral crest and commissure. On the alveolar bone, it occupies the usual position of the maxillopalatine clefts. On the skull the no. 10 cleft corresponds to the facial cleft no. 4. *Tessier 10.* Central superior orbital cleft. It is located at the medial 3rd of the supraorbital rim, lateral to the supraorbital nerve and extends across the roof of the orbit and the frontal bone (encephalocoele). Coloboma of the medial 3rd of the upper eyelid is present and it continues to join the scalp hairline
6. *Tessier 5:* Lateral orbitomaxillary cleft traverses the lower eyelid and cheek; it appears as a groove and extends to the lip near the labial commissure. On the skull, it traverses the infraorbital rim, the maxilla lateral to the infraorbital foramen and the maxillary sinus and finally passes through the alveolar bone in the premolar region.
7. *Tessier 6, 7 and 8:* When found together, they form the Treacher Collins-Franceschetti syndrome
8. *Tessier 6:* Intermaxillozygomatic cleft is located between the maxilla and malar bone and opens into the inferior orbital fissure; it does not involve the alveolar bone but the posterior portion of the maxilla is underdeveloped. The palate is high-vaulted with a relative choanal atresia. The coloboma of the lower eyelid is located between the medial and lateral thirds. On the cheek, there is a vertical groove, which is directed towards the labial commissure or the angle of the mandible. This cleft usually belongs to the Treacher Collins-Franceschetti syndrome
9. *Tessier 7:* Temporozygomatic cleft. The zygomatic arch is absent or atrophic, the ascending ramus of the mandible is short, the condyle and the coronoid are often absent. The absence of the coronoid is associated with the absence of the temporal muscle. The height of the maxilla is reduced and the alveolar wall is hypoplastic. Incomplete clefts have been found either in the molar region or between the maxillary tuberosity and the pterygoid. The soft tissue anomalies include microtia and atrophy or absence of the temporal muscle. This cleft corresponds to Treacher Collins-Franceschetti syndrome and also to hemifacial microsomia (Otomandibular syndrome).
10. *Tessier 8:* Frontozygomatic cleft. It is common in Treacher Collins-Franceschetti and Goldenhar syndromes. The bony defects predominate in the Treacher Collins-Franceschetti, whereas the soft tissue malformations are more marked in the Goldenhar syndrome. In Treacher Collins-Franceschetti, there is the absence of the malar bone, lateral border of the orbit, which is formed by the greater wing of the sphenoid and it extends both anteriorly and medially. In the Goldenhar syndrome, the skeleton is more or less normal but there is a dermatocoele or a true cleft of the lateral canthus is seen
11. *Tessier 9:* Superolateral orbital cleft. It traverses the lateral 3rd of the upper eyelid and the superolateral angle of the orbit. It is the cranial equivalent of facial cleft no. 5.

MANAGEMENT OF PATIENTS WITH CLEFT LIP AND PALATE

SEQUENCE OF PROCEDURES

Sequence of procedures for cleft lip and palate patients is described in Table 45.1.

PRIMARY MANAGEMENT

The child's difficulty in feeding is managed by a feeding plate that prevents nasal regurgitation of milk and allows easier intake of nutrition. Simultaneously, the child is prepared for the cleft lip repair by presurgical orthopaedics with strapping techniques or nasoalveolar moulding appliances.

FEEDING PLATE

- Cleft palate is repaired by the 9th or 10th month, regurgitation of the fluids into the nose while feeding is very common, feeding plate helps to create and hold negative pressure in the mouth and serves as an obturator
- It also is an orthopaedic appliance to mould the alveolar fragments together
- Usually, plates delivered before 48 h from birth are best accepted by infants
- A monthly follow up of the feeding plate is essential to accommodate growth of the palate (Fig. 45.11E and F).

PRESURGICAL ORTHOPAEDICS

Primary lip and palatal surgery depends on preoperative deformity. Wider the cleft, more displaced the nose, greater the deformity and postoperative outcome. Between birth and primary lip surgery, the alveolar fragments supporting the lip and nasal cartilages can be orthopaedically manipulated to promote tension-free closure and improve postoperative results. Active force techniques to reposition skeletal segments include:

1. **The feeding plate** modified as an 'intra-alveolar moulding plate': The feeding palatal obturator with additional thickness of acrylic anterior to the alveolar ridge that is protruding and space posterior to the arch to allow the pressure while suckling to mould the arches into a more normal position

TABLE 45.1 Sequence of Procedures

Age	Treatment	Rationale
At birth	Feeding plate	Sucking milk
2–3 months	Lip repair	Feeding and appearance
9–11 months	Palate repair	Sealing the communication gap between the mouth and nose to enhance feeding and speech
3 years	Premaxillary setback (in case of bilateral cleft)	Creation of labial vestibule (space between lips and upper front teeth), speech and aesthetics
3+ years	Pharyngoplasty (if needed) Speech therapy	Correction of nasal sounding speech (by preventing escape of air through the nose) Improving pronunciation
4–5 years	Cleft alveolar bone closure using BMP	Closing alveolar cleft and enabling normal teeth eruption
or		
7–9 years	Cleft alveolar bone closure with bone grafting	Closing alveolar cleft and enabling normal teeth eruption
13 years	Cleft orthodontics (correction of malaligned teeth)	Normal positioning of teeth
14–16 years	Rhinoplasty (nose correction)	Aesthetics
Depending upon the severity of the cleft, these procedures may be performed	Distraction osteogenesis	Upper jaw advancement
	Orthognathic surgery (jaw correction surgery)	Aesthetics
	Secondary corrections	Aesthetics

2. **Strapping** of the lips or the premaxilla using rubber bands: Pressure across the lips may contribute to some moulding (Fig. 45.11G and H)
3. **Head gear** like appliances
4. **Nasoalveolar moulding appliances**
5. **Lip adhesion.**

NASOALVEOLAR MOULDING

Nasoalveolar moulding (NAM) is based on the physiological levels of hyaluronic acid, which was found to be high in infants' blood. This may contribute to the elasticity of the nasal cartilages in the neonatal period. Presurgical nasoalveolar moulding is the technique by which the alveolus and the nasal cartilages are moulded into a more favourable position.

Nasoalveolar moulding—unilateral cleft lip

The nose is asymmetric at the alar base with a tilted columella and a flattened, concave and depressed lateral crus. The aim of presurgical NAM is to align and bring the alveolar cleft segments as close together as possible for achieving good surgical correction of the nasal cartilage and soft tissue deformity. This is accomplished by adding a nasal stent to the labial vestibular flange of a conventional intraoral moulding plate. The nasal stent and alveolar moulding plate are adjusted over a period of 3 months to achieve nasal and alveolar symmetry. The nasoalveolar orthopaedic appliance is retained in position with surgical tapes and elastics applied to the cheeks and cleft lip segments (Fig. 45.11A&B).

Nasoalveolar moulding—bilateral cleft lip

The bilateral cleft lip nasal deformity presents with a short or absent columella and an excessively wide prolabium. In the method of NAM and columella elongation, the posterior lateral alveolar ridges are moulded to an appropriate width to accept the premaxilla between them. The premaxilla is then retracted by using the moulding plate in conjunction with external tape and elastics. Bilateral nasal stents are extended into the nostril aperture from the vestibular flange of the intraoral moulding plate. A band of soft acrylic presses against the nasolabial fold. The combined effect of pushing the nasal tip forward and pressing back on the nasolabial fold results in gradual tissue expansion and lengthening of the columella (Fig. 45.11C&D).

LIP ADHESION

- Partial suturing of the cleft lip segments in order to manipulate the fragments nearer to each other is called lip adhesion
- This invasive surgical procedure is performed at 2 weeks of age
- Primary complication is dehiscence of the wound

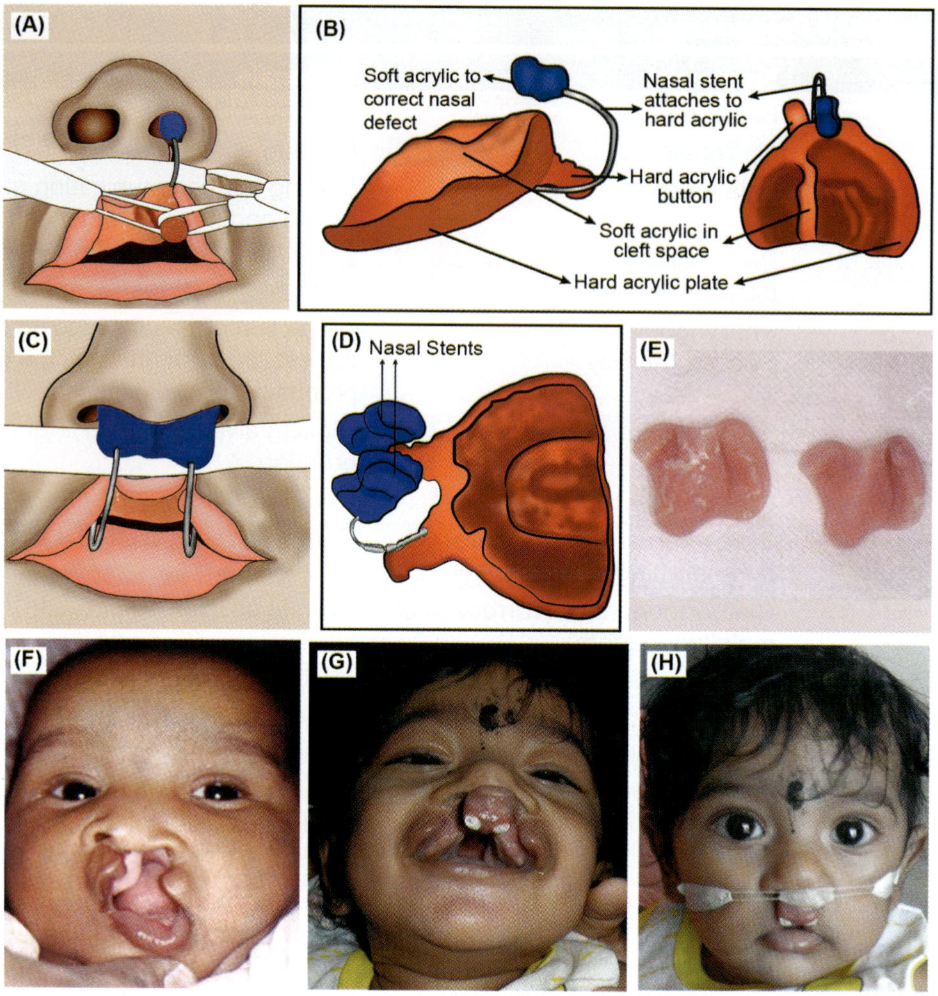

Figure 45.11 Presurgical nasoalveolar moulding (NAM) techniques by which the alveolus and the nasal cartilages are moulded to a more favourable position. (**A**) Unilateral nasoalveolar moulding appliance and strapping in situ. (**B**) Parts of a unilateral NAM appliance marked. (**C**) Bilateral nasoalveolar moulding appliance and strapping in situ. (**D**) Bilateral NAM appliance (**E**). Feeding plate or Hotz plate assists in feeding the child without nasal regurgitation and can be used as an orthopaedic appliance for moulding the cleft segments to a more favourable symmetric position before performing lip repair. (**F**) Feeding plate in a case of UCLP. (**G** and **H**) Strapping of bilateral cleft lip using rubber bands to orthopaedically manipulate the prognathic premaxilla to a more favourable position before lip surger y. It also assists in decreasing the width of the cleft and in bringing the lip segments closer to each other.

- Leads to scarring, which can affect the cosmetic result of the primary lip repair.

LIP REPAIR

Surgical approximation of the cleft lip segments has been tried for many centuries. The early techniques used were only a straight-line closure, resulting in scarring which made the repaired lip look shorter. The muscle position was ignored. Rose (1833) used curved incisions with concavities apposed and Thompson (1912) used straight incisions running obliquely across the lip to gain length. Tennison's triangular flap used two z-plastys to achieve equal flaps to achieve the philtral length. The aims of cleft closure now are to obtain good muscle alignment, an acceptable scar and an evenly balanced lip.

The 'rule of 10s' to determines the timing of cleft lip surgical repair states that the child should weigh at least 10 pounds, haemoglobin of 10% and an age of at least 10 weeks. Most of the surgeons prefer to undertake the surgery only when the child is older, usually between 3 and 6 months (Box 45.1).

UNILATERAL CLEFT LIP REPAIR

The most popular technique based on which the rest of the modifications are based on is the Millard's rotation advancement repair. The cleft lip presents with a defect involving the nasal sill, the alar base, the philtral columns, the philtral dimple, the Cupid's bow, the white roll and the vermillion. These parts can be noted on the surface anatomy illustration in Fig. 45.12A.

BOX 45.1 Rule of 10's for Timing of Cleft Lip Surgery

Rule of 10's for Cleft Lip

- 10 pounds of weight
- 10 g of Hb
- 10 weeks of age
- 10,000 TLC

MILLARD'S ROTATION ADVANCEMENT REPAIR

Advantages

- It is a technique that allows variation as the surgeon progresses with the operation
- The resultant scar follows natural lines in the lower half of the lip and provides a scar that is simple to revise
- Preserves the Cupid's bow and philtral dimple
- Preserves pleasing outward pointing of the lower portion of the lip
- Method is a highly flexible one, which permits constant modification
- The lip is tightest in its upper part, where it should be and has more fullness in its lower portions, where these features are desirable.

Disadvantages

- Difficult to get adequate rotation and optimal lateral flap in wide cleft lip
- In order to obtain a suitable flap, it may be necessary to take off too much of lateral vermilion, thereby causing noticeable asymmetry of Cupid's bow.

Long-term follow-up of the techniques have proven that geometric alignment of the lip segments alone is not sufficient. In order to achieve functional repair, muscle alignment repair is very important to achieve an aesthetic as well as a functional lip. The results of a repaired cleft lip, which may look excellent is not constant, until the muscles within it are properly aligned. Therefore, it is important to get good muscle union. If this is achieved, the alignment of the lip will be satisfactory both aesthetically and functionally and the skin scar will not be unsightly.

PROCEDURE

Under General anesthesia (GA) with a noncuffed oral Ring-Adair-Elwyn (RAE) tracheal tube positioned midline and fixed to the lower lip. Prior to local anaesthesia (LA) infiltration, the anatomic landmarks are marked with methylene blue dye. The measurements are measured and marked onto the affected side to guide the surgeon in creating a symmetric lip.

Markings for unilateral cleft lip repair (Fig. 45.12B):

1. Point 1 is the centre point of the Cupid's bow (lowest point)
2. Point 2 is the normal peak of the Cupid's bow (highest point) on the normal side
3. Point 3 is the medial peak of the affected Cupid's bow. It is the mirror image of Point 2 on the affected Cupid's bow
4. Point 4 is the midpoint of the alar base on the normal side
5. Point 5 is the midpoint of the columella
6. Point 6 is the oral commissural point of the normal side (corner of the mouth)
7. Point 7 is the oral commissural point of the normal side (corner of the mouth)
8. Point 8 is the lateral peak of the affected Cupid's bow. This point is marked at the widest part of the vermillion on the cleft affected side. The peak of the Cupid's bow is divided into the medial and lateral peak by the cleft deformity
9. Point 9 is the medial tip of the advancement flap from the cleft side
10. Point 10 is the midpoint of the alar base on the cleft side
11. Point 11 is the lateral point of the alar base on the cleft side
12. Point 12 is the extent of the alotomy incision on the cleft side
13. Point 'X' is the extent of the back cut incision for the 'C' flap
14. Millard also stated a few points that has to be included in the marking for determining Point 8 and for geometric symmetry of the cosmetic outcome
    a. Point 1 to 2 = point 1 to 3 = 2 - 4 mm
    b. Point 2 to 6 = point 8 to 7 = approximately 20 mm
        i. This rule of distance is unreliable and therefore not followed in the modification techniques as there is unequal tension of the underlying orbicularis muscle
        ii. The peak on the cleft side, point 8, is placed in level with Point 2, where the dry vermilion is widest and the white roll above is well developed. The white roll and dry vermilion taper off medial to this point
        iii. Point 8 is determined by the surgeon based on modifications and techniques followed
    c. Point 2 to 4 = Point 8 to 10 = 9–11 mm
        i. This rule of distance is also unreliable according to literature
    d. Point 3 to 5 + X (curved distance) = Point 8 to 9
        i. This marking is the line that determines the border between the R and C flaps, this determines the philtral length—the new philtral column on the cleft side
15. Two key elements are involved in the markings:
    a. The placement of the ***final position of the new Cupid's bow peak (point 8)***
    b. The ***vertical length of the philtral column (length of the points 3-5-X)*** to be created on the cleft side.

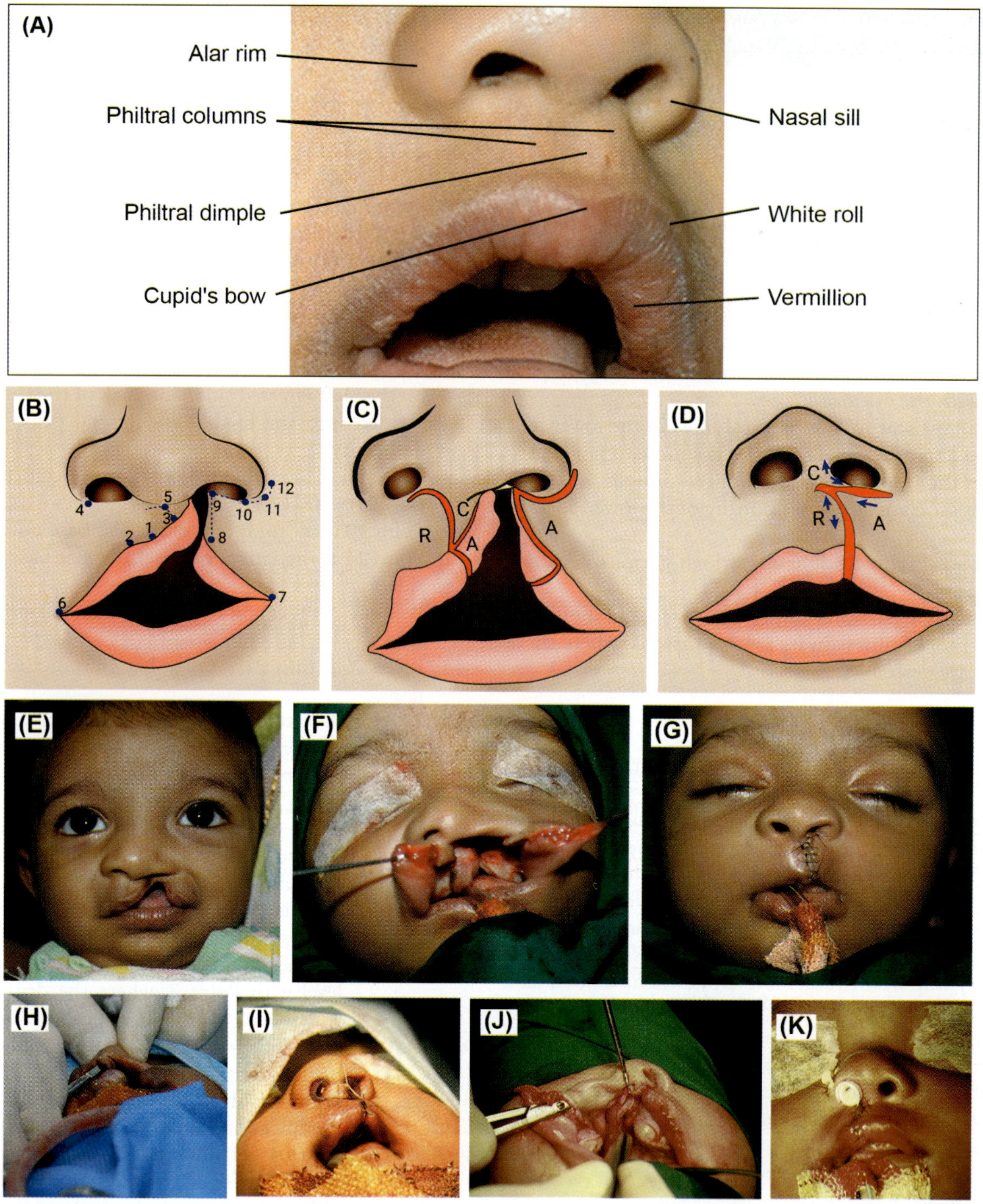

Figure 45.12 (**A**) Surface anatomy of the lip and nose. (**B–D**) Millard's classical technique. (**B**) Illustrates markings of the anatomic landmarks used in Millard's cleft lip repair. (**C**) The five major flaps of the Classical Millard's Technique. (**D**) Final positions of the flaps created. (**E–G**) Millard's rotation advancement repair (Scan to play unilateral cleft lip correction surgery). (**H**) Delaire's technique—separating the superficial nasolabial musculature including lip levators from the deeper orbicularis muscle and their concomitant anatomical repositioning. (**I**) Primary closure. (**J**) Primary rhinoplasty—dissection of the malpositioned alar cartilage with anatomical repositioning of the nasal septum (**K**) Primary closure.

Drawing the flap based on the markings (Fig. 45.12C):

Incision lines that produce the flaps involved in the lip reconstruction are:

1. ***Inferior rotation flap (R) from the normal lip***
2. ***The medial advancement flap (A) from the cleft lip***
3. ***The columellar base flap (C)***
4. ***Pared medial mucosal flaps (m)***
5. ***Pared lateral mucosal flap (l) lip elements***
6. Flaps that refine the surgical correction
   a. ***A white roll flap***
   b. ***A vermilion triangular flap*** to allow for a smoother transition at the vermilion cutaneous junction and at the vermilion contour.

CONCEPT OF MILLARD'S TECHNIQUE (Fig. 45.12B–G)

Correcting the tilted Cupid's bow—use of 'R' flap and 'C' flap

In a unilateral cleft lip, the Cupid's bow is tilted. The tilted Cupid's bow is rotated downward to attain normal tilt by following a curved incision extending under the columella (Point 3-5-X). This allows rotation of the misplaced Cupid's bow and philtral dimple into a normal position. This curved incision also allows the philtral length to be elongated to match the length between point 8 and 9.

Inferior rotation of the R flap

Incision for the R and C flap should be deep enough to involve the layers of the skin, subcutaneous tissue, muscle, fibrous attachments to the anterior nasal spine and the labial mucosa. An additional back cut of about 1 to 2 mm is required for the C flap to allow inferior rotation of the R flap.

C flap

The C flap created above the R flap is attached to the alar base of the cleft side thus forming the nasal sill.

The m and l flaps

The skin or mucosa is dissected from the muscle at the margins of the cleft. This procedure of splitting the skin from the muscle is called paring. These pared flaps are named the m and l flaps. The l flap is inserted as the nasal vestibule lining and the m flap as a part of the oral vestibule lining.

The A flap

The A flap from the affected side is advanced into the gap between the R and C flaps. The incision along the length of points 10, 11 and 12 at the alar base is called the alotomy incision. Alotomy incision extent (Point 12) on the skin is kept minimal and the subcutaneous release at the alar base to the piriform margin of the maxilla is made to mobilise the ala at the subperiosteal level and allow it to be repositioned, creating a large gap to be filled by the A flap.

Suturing

The 1st layer to be sutured is the oral labial layer of the mucosa, so the m and l flaps are sutured. This is followed by suturing of the orbicularis oris muscle and then the skin. The white roll is 1st sutured followed by the skin and then the vermillion. Common sutures to approximate the skin edges are:

- Nylon sutures–Ethilon 6-0 or 5-0 size can be used. Removed after 7 days
- Cyanoacrylate-type adhesive can be used over these dermal sutures
- The cleft alar cartilage can be transfixed with sutures and a nostril stent.

DELAIRE'S TECHNIQUE OF MUSCULAR RECONSTRUCTION (FUNCTIONAL REPAIR)

Millard's technique often resulted in smaller nostrils due to lack of muscular approximation. Delaire proposed an enhancement to this technique. He stated a wide dissection of the lateral lip and the nasal elements, muscular approximation of the lip and the nose is also performed presenting with a symmetric nose and highly functional upper lip.

Advantages: Unlike Millard's classical technique, this technique avoids incisions that cross sensitive areas like the columellar base and alar rims (flap C and alotomy incision). Delaire's technique also restores the nasal and labio-maxillary muscle function (Fig. 45.12H and I).

NOORDHOFF'S TECHNIQUE

The Noordhoff's modification of Millard's rotation advancement cheiloplasty technique of lip repair is focused on simultaneous primary nasal repair along with lip repair.

PRIMARY UNILATERAL CLEFT NOSE REPAIR

There are two schools of thoughts for nose correction in unilateral cleft lip. The nose correction surgery is performed after adolescence to prevent any growth disturbance due to stripping of the perichondrium. However, a few surgeons have advocated concurrent, early nose repair. This was criticised for the development of secondary scar contracture and stenosis. However, less invasive and more effective techniques are now employed for primary nose repair along with the lip.

1. **McComb**'s technique had no incisions in the nasal lining to avoid nasal stenosis (Fig. 45.12J and K)
2. **Thompson's technique** with the addition of a primary nasal correction through intranasal incisions and dissection between the upper lateral cartilages and lower lateral cartilage
3. **Bardach**'s technique corrected the nasal floor, important for nostril symmetry and alar base elevation
4. **Salyer** (1986) used bolster sutures and stents to assist in the correction
5. **Turdek et al.** (1997) advocated primary septal cartilage repositioning to decrease nostril asymmetry.

BILATERAL CLEFT LIP REPAIR

The forward projection of the prolabium and premaxilla on the vomer at the nose's tip is difficult to treat. When the premaxilla is normal or moderately protruding, the lip can be repaired easily. Due to tension, excessive protrusion can cause wound dehiscence or scar spread. Before primary lip repair, early orthopaedics and elastic pressure should be considered. In cases of late lip repair where the premaxilla has grown to disproportionate levels and cannot be managed orthopaedically, the premaxilla is surgically sectioned posterior to the premaxillary–vomerine line to minimise maxillary growth retardation.

TECHNIQUES

A bilateral cleft lip repair must restore the orbicularis muscle circumorally for the upper lip to function properly. A deep upper buccal sulcus should be created, which separates the lip from adhesion to the premaxilla. This allows normal function, growth and development of the muscles. A few techniques of bilateral lip repair are as follows:

1. Straight-line closure (Veau III operation)
2. Adaptation of Tennison's unilateral cleft lip repair
3. Millard's repair of complete and incomplete bilateral clefts
4. Skoog's techniques
5. Manchester's method
6. Barsky (Veau II)
7. Paul Black's technique (Fig. 45.13A–F).

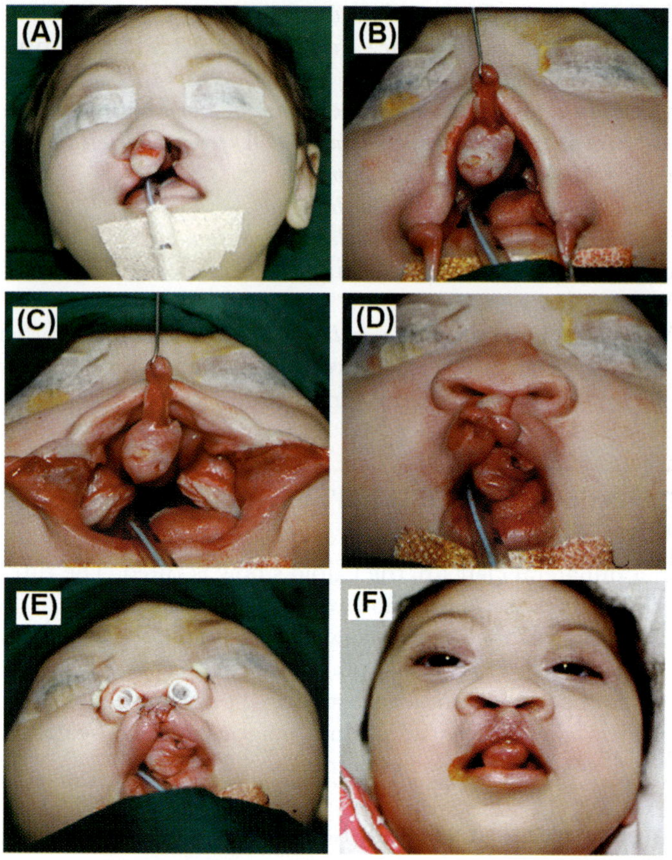

Figure 45.13 (**A–F**) Paul Black's technique of bilateral lip repair.

PRIMARY BILATERAL CLEFT NOSE REPAIR

1. **Delayed 'columellar lengthening':** By transferring tissue from the broad prolabium or the nasal floor (Cronin and Upton, 1978)
2. **Broadbent and Woolf (1984):** Medial advancement of the alars combined with excision of skin from the broad tip
3. **McComb's V–Y primary nasal repair**: A cutaneous incision to approximate the splayed alar cartilages and narrowing the nasal tip by cutaneous V–Y plasty
4. **Mulliken's technique** for repositioning the alar domes and reorganising the nasal soft tissues. The nostril flare when cleft children smile can be prevented by securing the alar bases to the underlying orbicularis muscle to mimic the action of depressor labii inferioris alaeque nasi muscle
5. Dissecting the anterior surface of the middle crura and correcting the displaced alar cartilages through open rhinoplasty improved the nasal tip by lifting the prolabium and columella.

Primary nasal surgery is therefore done based on the necessity of the situation, viewing the existing structural deformity, the growth potential and the muscular action.

PALATE REPAIR

The hard palate is supported by bony shelves with mucosal coverings, while the soft palate consists of muscle with mucosal covering. Early repair of the cleft of the hard and soft palate is undertaken with two main objectives: to make the process of eating and drinking easier by preventing the regurgitation of food through the nose and to correct and improve speech by the time the child starts to speak. The most significant goal in surgical reconstruction of the palate is providing a normal anatomical environment for the development of normal speech.

TIMING OF REPAIR

- As an early closure of the clefted palate improves the development of speech and hearing due to an improved ventilation of the Eustachian tubes, the time of surgery has been brought forward continuously
- **The favoured patient age for palatal closure is between 9 and 12 months of age.**

PROCEDURES

Anatomic basis for cleft palate repair is that in the cleft condition, muscles of the palate are hypoplastic and have abnormal insertions on the posterior edge of hard palate and along the margins of hard palate cleft. This abnormal insertion contributes to the overall shortness of the palate, and due to the fact that the levator sling cannot be created, may result in inability of the palate to reach the posterior pharyngeal wall and achieve velopharyngeal competence. Thus, unless these muscles are carefully detached from their abnormal insertions, rotated medially and realigned in the midline to recreate the levator sling, correct muscle function is impossible. The different techniques followed are as follows:

I. Von Langenbeck operation
II. V–Y pushback palatoplasty (Kilner–Wardill)
III. Furlow double opposing Z-plasty
IV. Anterior vomer flap (Veau)
V. Intravelar veloplasty.

VON LANGENBECK OPERATION

It is an established procedure that includes the elevation of large mucoperiosteal flaps from the hard palate. It is a side-to-side approximation of the cleft margins of both the hard and soft palate with detachment of the levator muscles from their bony insertions and use of long, relaxing incisions laterally to close the hard palate without tension. It does not include a lengthening manoeuvre.

WARDILL–KILNER–VEAU OPERATION

To increase the anteroposterior length of the palate at the time of primary palatoplasty, various mucoperiosteal flap manoeuvres in the hard palate have been recommended. A V–Y lengthening operation is done in the tissues of the mucoperiosteum of the hard palate. The rigid mucoperiosteum probably maintains the length that is achieved, although a similar amount of lengthening must be obtained in the nasal mucosa of the soft palate. This V–Y pushback palatoplasty includes lateral relaxing incision and bilateral island flaps based on the posterior palatine arteries (Fig. 45.14A–H).

SECONDARY CORRECTIONS

Secondary surgery is mandatory in some cases because certain cosmetic and functional defects cannot be assessed fully or managed before the cessation of growth. Also, secondary surgery can overcome the shortcomings of the primary surgery. For example, adult nose shape develops in the teens. For instance, the contour of an adult nose develops during the teen years. The nose shape that was inherited is overlaid on an unknown degree of underdevelopment of the underlying maxillary bone, which is caused by both the cleft and the corrective surgery, an unknown amount of nasal deformity can result. It is clear that the final correction cannot take place before these factors have reached a stable state. It must also await corrective movements on the underlying bone and teeth, which may be undertaken by the orthodontist in the early teens and major surgery on the maxilla, which may be undertaken in the late teens. It has been considered that operation on certain tissue earlier may impair its growth potential by damaging its blood supply or restricting its growth by scar tissue.

CLOSURE OF PALATAL FISTULAE

The fistula may be present in front of, through or behind the alveolus or in the main hard palate.

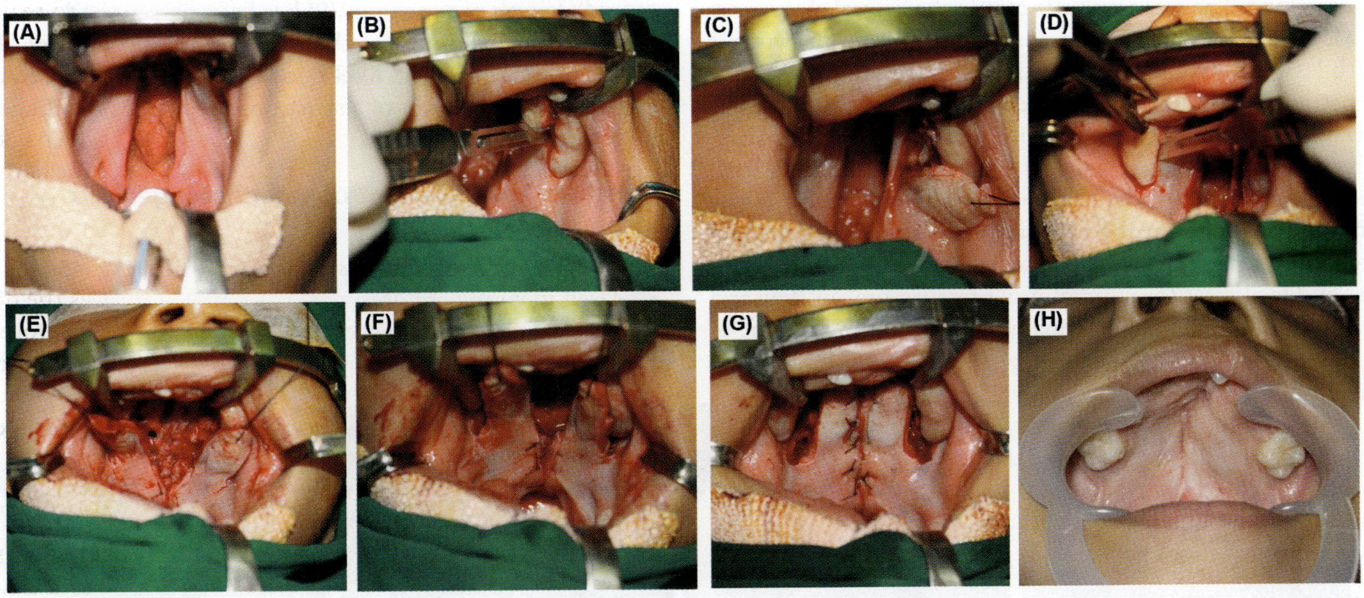

Figure 45.14 The Wardill–Kilner's technique of primary cleft palate repair. **(A)** Intraoperative view of the defective cleft palate. **(B–D)** A V–Y lengthening results in a lengthened palate with an exposed area of bone at the sides that gradually granulates and epithelises. The levator muscles are detached, reoriented and sutured either end-to-end or in an overlapped position. **(C and D)** Incision and raising of the palatal flaps on both sides. **(E)** Closure of nasal layer and muscle approximation. **(F)** Oral layer closed (double layered closure), raw areas packed with tincture benzoin. **(H)** Postoperative view after 10 years of follow-up (scan to play palatoplasty—Cleft palate surgery).

SYMPTOMS

- Increased nasalance in speech with articulatory difficulty
- Regurgitation of fluids into the nose
- Halitosis
- Increased incidence of ear and paranasal sinus infections.

TIMING OF CLOSURE

When it comes to the timing of the procedure, closure of a fistula may be done at any age and probably the sooner the better, provided that it is causing symptoms and suitable tissues are available.

PROCEDURE

The simplest method of closure is with the palate tissue adjacent to the fistula. This can be made to provide a lining for the nose from one side of the fistula, the tissue 'flap' being hinged on the scar at the cleft margin. The oral layer is made by sliding a flap of mucosa sideways across the hole (Fig. 45.15A–D). In cases of large, persistent palatal fistula, a tongue flap or a temporalis flap is used. Palatal obturators have also been used in cases where the blood supply of the palate is compromised beyond capacity for repair.

VELOPHARYNGEAL INCOMPETENCE

VPI is the term used when the patient is diagnosed as being unable to raise the velum to meet the posterior pharyngeal wall to seal the nasal airway during speech.

NORMAL VELOPHARYNGEAL FUNCTION

Velopharyngeal closure is a sphincteric valving operation essential for normal speech, whistling, blowing, swallowing and sucking. The main muscles of velopharyngeal closure are the levator veli palatini, uvulus muscle and palatopharyngeus with lesser contribution from superior fibres of the superior constrictor. Velopharyngeal mechanism for speech requires the upward and backward movement of the soft palate, which is called valving. Valving occurs simultaneously with medial movement of the lateral and posterior aspects of the pharyngeal walls causing a sphincteric action. This activity creates a seal that effectively separates the nasal and oral cavities and facilitates the supraglottal pressure, oral air flow and resonance necessary for adequate speech. This movement of the soft palate and posterior wall of the pharynx can be assessed using lateral cephalogram.

THE VELOPHARYNGEAL DEFECT

In velopharyngeal dysfunction, air resonates in the nose and nasopharynx. This is called hypernasal resonance. Frequently, air can be heard hissing, bubbling or snorting from the nose.

Patients may grimace by using their nasal or facial musculature in an attempt to prevent air escaping down the nose.

To achieve good speech, it is significant to surgically create the palate to be long enough to close off the velopharyngeal port instead of merely closing the palatal defect. The most common causes of VPI are as follows:

- Cleft of the secondary palate
- Scarred palate preventing muscular action of the palatal elevators
- Short palate
- Presence of a palatal fistula or fistulae
- Submucous cleft palate
- Neuromuscular abnormalities (congenital or acquired)
- Adenoidectomy
- Congenital VPI of unknown aetiology.

TREATMENT

Following primary cleft palate surgery, secondary techniques for the correction of VPI include palatal lengthening procedures, pharyngeal flaps, augmentation of posterior pharyngeal wall with soft tissues or implants, sphincteric reconstruction and prosthetic obturators.

The age of the patient, aetiology of VPI (congenital vs acquired), length of time that VPI has been present and general intellectual capabilities of the patient can all influence the choice of treatment and likelihood of success. Surgical treatment should form part of a strict protocol and the following options are recommended.

Prosthetic management of velopharyngeal incompetence

The palatal lift procedure using **speech bulb** (Fig. 45.16):

- Used in young children
- To aid in developing speech

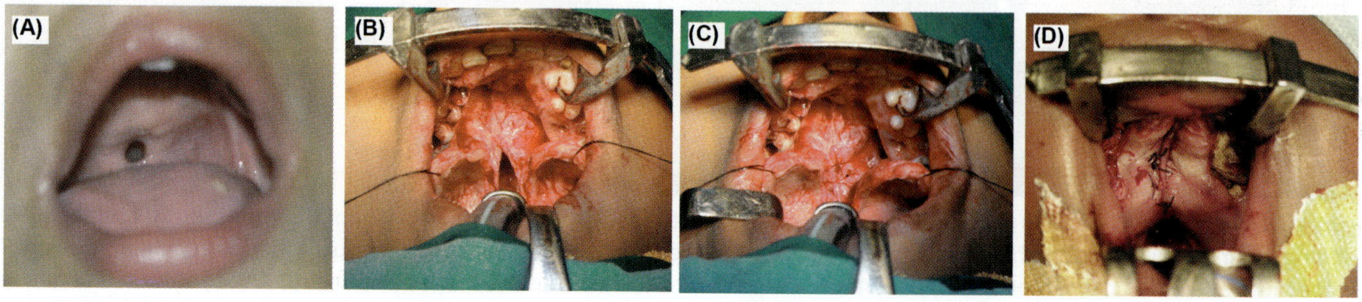

Figure 45.15 **(A)** Palatal fistula. **(B)** Raising a mucoperiosteal flap from the hard palate. **(C)** Closure of oral layer in V–Y fashion. **(D)** Packing the exposed palatal bone area with gauze soaked with a haemostat.

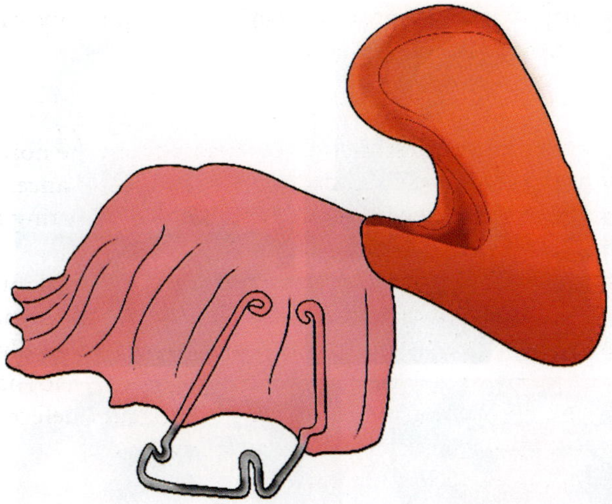

Figure 45.16 Speech bulb used in velopharyngeal incompetence.

- In adults to compensate soft tissue
- It elevates the soft palate
- It is a temporary treatment of VPI
- Only above age of 4–5 years
- With active speech therapy is started at this age.

Speech bulb is advisable before any surgical intervention for VPI. It aids in proper articulation of the speech and reduces hypernasality. If this fails, surgery should be considered.

Surgical management of velopharyngeal incompetence (pharyngoplasty)

VPI is usually corrected surgically. The aim of the operation is to close the velopharyngeal aperture but leaving a sufficient resting gap to permit nasal resonance to occur normally on the sounds 'm', 'n' and 'ng', to allow comfortable nasal breathing while eating and sleeping and normal drainage of the nasal cavity. Surgical correction of VPI is not a new concept. In the 16th century, Pierre France (1561) indicated an awareness of connection between cleft palate and poor speech. During the 19th century, surgical procedures were developed that are still being used in modified forms (Fig. 45.17A–D).

Closure of palatal fistula

Fistulae that are symptomatic or potentially symptomatic should be closed. Unfortunately, palate re-repair is inappropriate for some patients, particularly those whose VPI is not due to a cleft and those with severe tissue deficiency. For those patients whose palatal function cannot be adequately improved, a number of operations have been devised, which alter the shape of the nasopharynx to reduce its size and make the closure easier. These operations are collectively called pharyngoplasties.

Revision of palatoplasty and velar lengthening

Inadequate movement of the entire soft palate, but normal movement of the pharyngeal musculature implies an incomplete, limited or complete absence of restoration of muscle continuity at the time of primary surgery. Revision of palatoplasty must be the procedure of choice. This approach has the additional benefit of lengthening the palatal soft tissues.

Pharyngeal surgery

Despite the evidence that revision palatoplasty might be more appropriate in the 1st instance, pharyngeal surgery with or without palatal lengthening remains a popular 1st-line method of managing VPI. Two surgical techniques are followed depending on the abnormality found: posterior or lateral pharyngeal wall surgery.

Posterior (flap) pharyngoplasty

Posterior pharyngeal flap surgery is well established, with a long history dating back into the 19th century. These procedures may be superiorly or inferiorly based. The superiorly based flap is more popular, with its base at the level of the tubercle of the atlas and its insertion into the soft palate at predetermined points.

Lateral (sphincter) pharyngoplasty

The concept of surgical creation of a dynamic sphincter pharyngoplasty to provide velopharyngeal closure rather than a pharyngeal flap to control the size of pharyngeal orifice was 1st introduced by Hynes in 1950 (Fig. 45.17E–J). The sphincter is formed from the posterior tonsillar pillars, which are raised, including the palatopharyngeus, rotated and sutured end to end. This procedure is designed to reduce the size of the lateral ports and tighten the central area.

SPEECH THERAPY

If the cleft palate repair had not significantly contributed to the improvement of speech, then a secondary surgery in the form of pharyngoplasty would be required, which could improve articulation of speech; however, it is also speech therapy, which can directly improve articulation and communication skills.

If significant velopharyngeal insufficiency persists following primary repair of the palate, there may be nothing a speech therapist could do to improve the articulation to any significant extent. If on the other hand, there is velopharyngeal sufficiency for speech, no gross collapse of the alveolar arch and disturbance to maxillofacial growth is minimised, it is much easier for the speech therapist to effect speech changes.

CLOSURE OF ALVEOLAR CLEFT

1. Gingivoperiosteoplasty
2. Primary bone grafting
3. Secondary alveolar bone grafting
4. Alveolar distraction.

GINGIVOPERIOSTEOPLASTY

Stripping of periosteum from the bone is avoided till bone growth is complete for fear of losing growing potential. However, a few surgeons practice a form of early alveolar cleft

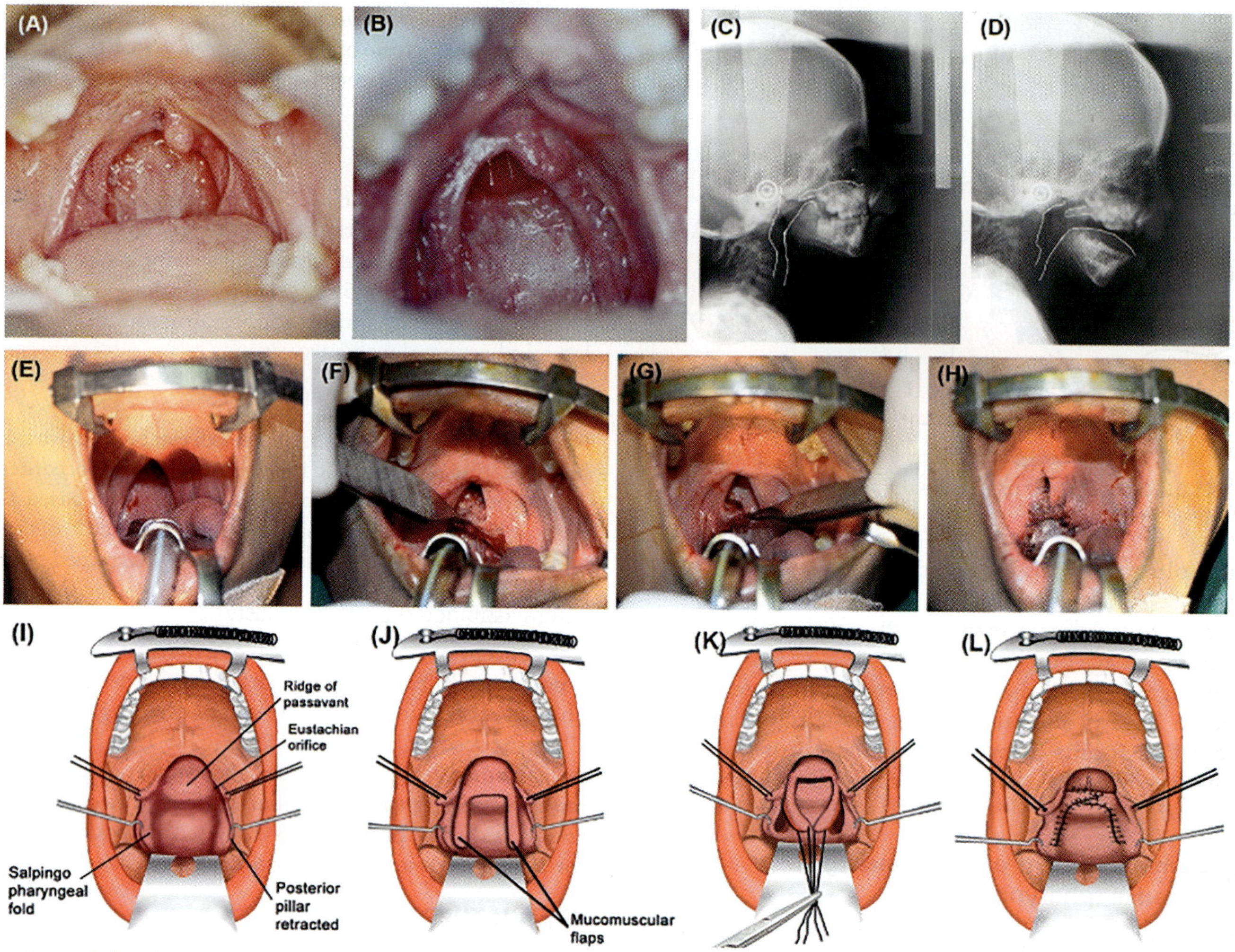

Figure 45.17 (**A**) Velopharyngeal incompetence. Movement and elevation of palate limited by scarring. (B) Elevation of the posterior wall of the pharynx, the Passavant's ridge while the patient attempts to speak. The soft palate being short is unable to close the velopharyngeal port resulting in VPI. (**C** and **D**) Lateral cephalometric X-ray of a bilateral cleft child at rest and during phonation. Note the inability of the velum to raise to close the velopharyngeal port resulting in VPI. (**E–H**) Hynes pharyngoplasty—clinical pictures. (**I–L**) Illustration of Hynes pharyngoplasty.

repair by suturing the periosteum of the cleft alveolar ridges together.

PRIMARY BONE GRAFTING

The maxilla with cleft has a bony deficiency at the canine-lateral incisor region. This may be accompanied by a hypoplastic or absent lateral incisor. Lack of bone at the anterior maxilla results in:

1. Lack of bone for permanent canine eruption or orthodontic treatment
2. Oronasal fistulae
3. Unequal distribution of the growth, which leads to:
    a. Premaxillary protuberance in bilateral cleft
    b. Lateral segments collapse in bilateral cleft
    c. Collapse of the maxillary alveolus on the cleft side
    d. Unequal anteroposterior position of maxillary alveolus of cleft side and noncleft side in unilateral cleft
    e. Midfacial growth retrusion
    f. Hypoplastic piriform aperture
    g. Poor arch forms
    h. Inadequate alveolar bone.

Bone or bone substitutes can be used to prevent these sequelae by alveolar bone grafting. This eliminates oronasal fistula, creates bone support for tooth eruption and restructures the hypoplastic piriform aperture. Depending on when the surgery is performed, alveolar bone grafting can be primary, early secondary or secondary. Children under 2 years undergo primary bone grafting. Between 2 and 5 years old, early secondary bone grafting is performed. Secondary bone grafting is performed after age 5. Early stripping of the maxillary periosteum, especially the premaxillary-vomerine suture, can slow growth. Few surgeons recommend primary bone grafting. Primary bone grafting stabilises the maxillary arch and obliterates alveolar oronasal fistula (nasal fluid escape and improved oral hygiene). Since the iliac crest in children under 5 years is cartilaginous, the rib is used. With rhBMP-2, graft harvesting can avoid a 2nd (donor) site morbidity. Premaxillary setbacks are performed in bilateral clefts with protrusion.

Secondary alveolar bone grafting in the mixed dentition, before the eruption of permanent canine, is the treatment for residual alveolar defect in cleft lip and palate patients, generally between the age of 7 and 11 years.

GOALS OF SECONDARY ALVEOLAR BONE GRAFTING

1. Stabilisation of maxillary arch
2. Closure of vestibular and palatal oronasal fistulae
3. Provision of bone to allow eruption of the permanent lateral incisor and canine teeth, but also maintenance of adequate bone about the root of the permanent central incisor adjacent to the cleft
4. Provision of support for the soft tissue nasal base and reconstruction of the hypoplastic piriform aperture
5. Provision of suitable bony architecture of the premaxilla and anterior face of the maxilla on the cleft side to support accurate nasolabial muscle reconstruction
6. Provision of adequate bone stock for ultimate placement of osseointegrated implant
7. To provide better periodontal support for teeth bordering the cleft.

BONE GRAFTING

Autogenous cancellous bone graft can repair osseous defects quickly as it is an osteogenic material. In cancellous bone grafts, viable cells are transplanted and early revascularisation occurs within 1 week and full revascularisation within 3 weeks. A watertight repair of the palatal cleft, nasal lining and anterior alveolus soft tissue is important. Maintaining cell viability before transplantation requires an atraumatic surgical method, avoiding heat generation during graft harvesting and storing bone particles in a saline-soaked sponge to prevent desiccation. Recently, rhBMP-2 soaked in absorbable collagen sponge has replaced bone. Using tension and stress, distraction osteogenesis of the alveolar bone creates new intramembranous bone and soft tissue. Distraction osteogenesis creates bone and soft tissue similar to the adjacent. This procedure corrects hard and soft tissue abnormalities, generating enough bone for implants.

Surgical Procedure

In older patients, iliac bone has been most frequently used since it is a rich source of purely cancellous bone. In children under the age of 9–10 years, one cannot expect to find large amounts of cancellous iliac bone, since apophysis of the iliac crest is still largely cartilaginous. The cancellous bone is harvested through a short incision over the iliac crest. A trapdoor of cortical bone is raised, hinged on the inner edge of the crest. By means of a small gouge and sharp spoon, thin slivers of cancellous bone are removed, leaving the inner and outer cortical plates intact. The cortical lid is replaced and held in position by absorbable sutures.

The cleft area is widely exposed through incisions along the edges of the cleft, midway between the palate and the nasal floor. Superiorly based flaps are developed for nasal lining and inferiorly based flaps are reflected caudally for closure of the palate. All soft tissues within the cleft are completely removed. The nasal layer suturing is completed and then the palatal mucoperiosteal flaps are brought together with everting mattress sutures.

This leaves a well-defined pear-shaped cavity. The cancellous bone is now packed into the alveolar defect, with a layer of bone chips also placed subperiosteally on the front of the hypoplastic maxilla and under the alar base and nostril sill. The bone grafts are then covered by suturing together the lateral and medial flaps and across the ridge of bone grafts to the palatal mucoperiosteum (Fig. 45.18).

ORTHODONTIC TREATMENT

1. The aim of orthodontic treatment is to provide a dentition that is in proper alignment and function properly. The anterior maxillary dentition should be symmetrical at the facial midline. This arrangement facilitates and improves the quality of the orthognathic surgery
2. Orthodontic treatment takes place at three different stages depending upon the severity of the cleft. The stages are:
   i. Functional orthognathic treatment in infants—nasoalveolar moulding
   ii. Anterior crossbite correction in mixed dentition
   iii. Orthodontic treatment of the permanent teeth during adolescence before treatment of the orthognathic deformity by surgery
3. Early orthodontic treatment involves orthopaedic movement of the alveolar or dentoalveolar arches before the primary surgeries. The purpose of this treatment is to align the lateral dentoalveolar arches and to reposition the premaxilla in case of bilateral cleft lip. Palatal plate and headgears are used for this purpose
4. Orthodontic treatment during mixed dentition period is most often neglected. Minor crossbites occur quite often and deciduous lateral incisor may be absent or hypoplastic. This tooth should be maintained as an extraction may widen the existing cleft, thus make the treatment procedure difficult.
5. A removable appliance with Adams clasp for retention and Z-spring or anterior expansion screw to move the incisors may be used. Functional appliances such as bite plane or Frankel's appliance may also be chosen.
6. Expansion of the arches is better performed before bone grafting since expansion of the palatal arches can open up palatal fistulae.
7. Secondary alveolar bone grafting facilitates canine eruption and it should be performed before final orthodontic alignment (Fig. 45.19A and B). Minor orthodontic tooth movement such as crossbite may be required before the surgery.

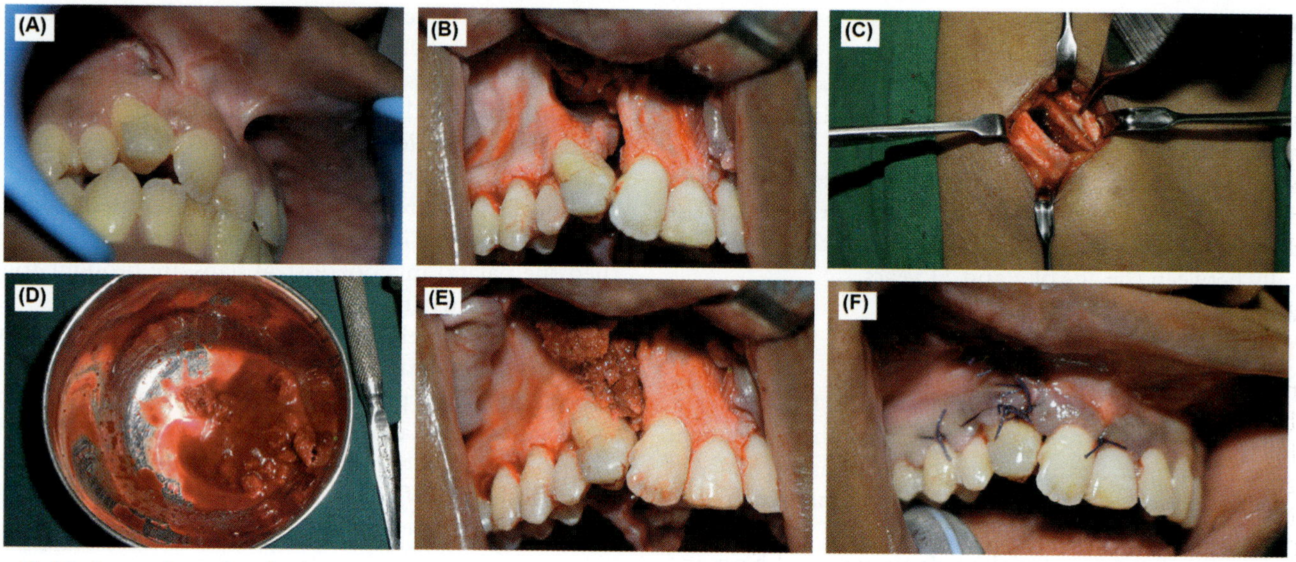

Figure 45.18 Secondary alveolar bone grafting for alveolar cleft repair using cancellous iliac bone graft. (**A**) Oronasal fistula distal to the central incisor and medial to canine. (**B**) Mucoperiosteal flap raised to expose the alveolar cleft. (**C** and **D**) Harvesting the iliac cancellous bone graft. Skin incision placed 1 cm posterior to the anterior superior iliac spine along the iliac tubercle. Layer wise dissection done followed by the periosteal incision. Anterior posterior and medial osteotomy done raising a laterally based osteoplastic flap exposing the cancellous marrow. Cancellous bone marrow harvested using a bone scoop. (**E**) After dissection and closure of the nasal and palatial lining, the bone graft is augmented into the defect. (**F**) Postoperative view.

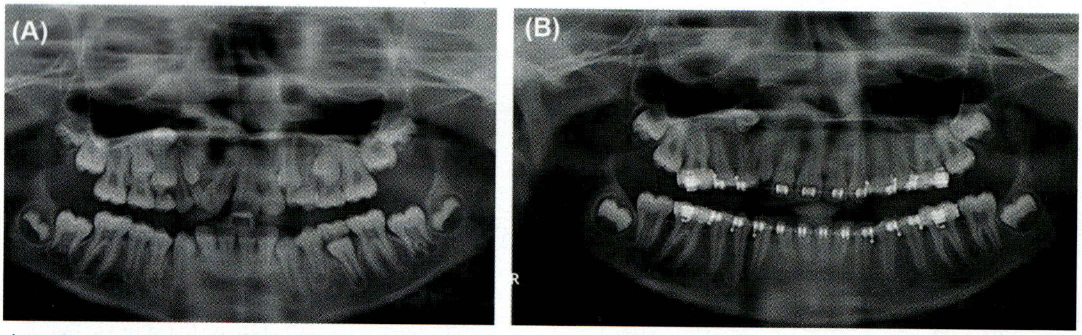

Figure 45.19 (**A**) Orthopantomogram (OPG) of a unilateral cleft child showing right alveolar cleft, retained deciduous right maxillary lateral incisor with impacted right maxillary permanent canine and microform right maxillary lateral incisor. (**B**) After grafting the alveolar cleft with rhBMP-2, orthodontic treatment done. Note the eruption of the lateral incisor through the graft and achievement of arch form (all permanent teeth except the impacted maxillary canine).

ORTHOGNATHIC SURGERY

Many children who have undergone the repair of a cleft lip and palate develop an increasing deformity of the facial structures as they grow, particularly as they pass through adolescence. This is particularly due to underdevelopment of the maxilla and relatively greater growth of the mandible, which leads to a concave facial profile and disproportion between the height of the middle and lower thirds of the face. These deformities can be corrected through orthognathic surgery. Usually this involves a maxillary osteotomy at Le Fort I level. Less often, osteotomy at a higher level may be needed, combined with mandibular or genial osteotomies.

Maxillary hypoplasia can give rise to increasing psychosocial problems, difficulties in mastication, pain and speech abnormalities, all of which would make early surgical correction desirable. Unfortunately, extensive surgery to the maxilla at an early age may cause damage to unerupted teeth, contribute to retardation of future maxillary growth or create an ideal occlusion, which is later disrupted by disproportionate maxillary and mandibular growth. For these reasons, orthognathic surgery is usually delayed until facial growth is complete.

DISTRACTION OSTEOGENESIS IN CLEFT MAXILLARY HYPOPLASIA

Patients affected with cleft present with maxillary hypoplasia, thus presenting with a concave facial profile. The profile is corrected to a straight profile with midface advancement techniques like distraction osteogenesis. Refer to Chapter 44 on Distraction Osteogenesis. It is ideal due to three-dimensional hard and soft tissue reconstruction, with excellent outcome, without the need of bone and soft tissue grafting. It is a well-accepted modality for a predictable correction of osseous deficiencies with vascular bone in patients with cleft deformity and provides a safe and effective method of bone lengthening (Fig. 45.20).

RHINOPLASTY

NOSE REVISION

The nasal deformity is enormously important. It almost invariably becomes worse with age. This deformity is very complex in its three-dimensional components and is widely considered to be difficult or impossible to correct perfectly. If a deficiency of bone, cartilage, skin or mucosal lining is present. Grafts are harvested as:

- Rib graft
- Iliac graft
- Nasal septum
- From the concha of the ear
- Skin can be taken from the back of the ear
- Mucosa from the nasal septum
- Mucosa from the buccal mucosa.

NOSE TIP

Secondary corrections of the nose include balancing operations of the nasal tip. On the cleft side, the nasal tip will not project forward and the nostril-rim will hang down. When viewed from below, the nostril apex and the alar base will be pushed inward.

NASAL SEPTUM

- The septal cartilage is convex in unilateral cleft patients towards the normal side
- Various techniques to straighten the septum are used
- The nasal correction is done after orthodontic and orthognathic correction of the maxilla and mandible (Fig. 45.21).

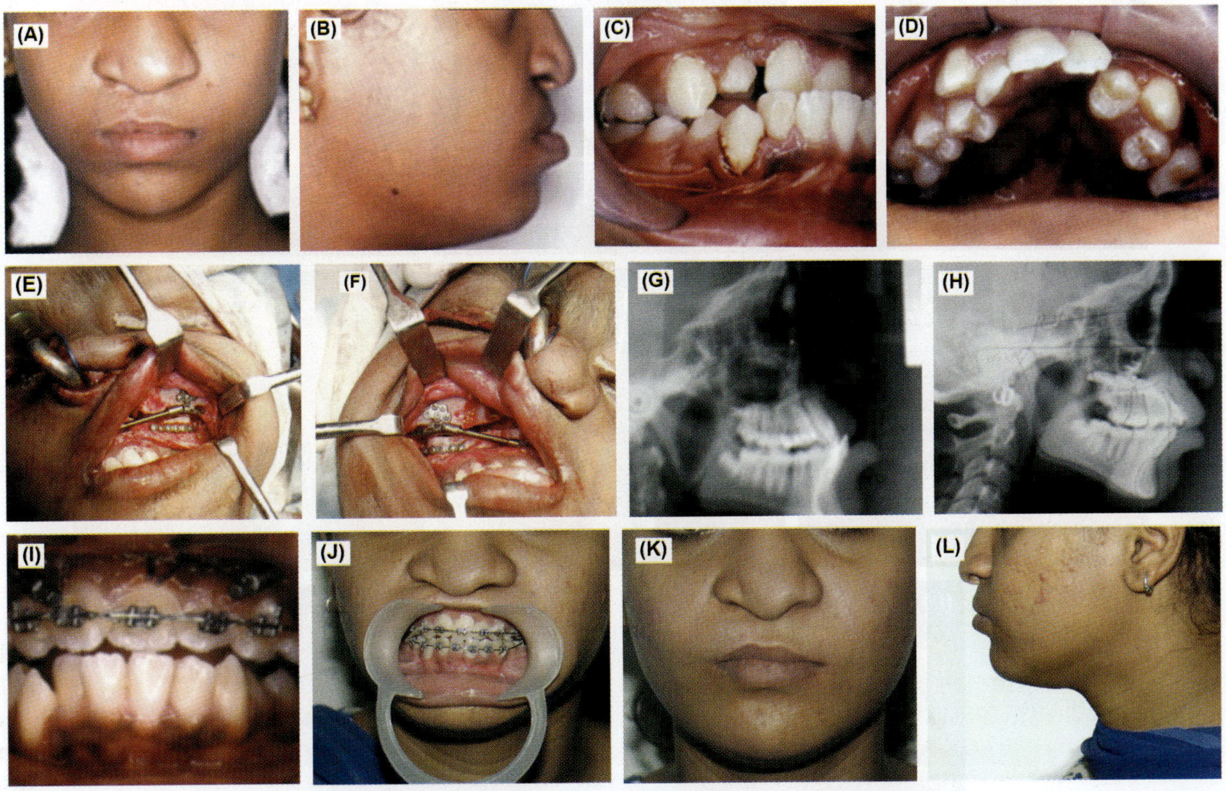

Figure 45.20 Internal maxillary distraction. (**A–D**) Unilateral cleft lip and palate facies: maxillary hypoplasia, concave facial profile, skeletal class III malocclusion, collapsed maxillary arch. Postalveolar bone grafting, planned for presurgical orthodontics and internal maxillary distraction. Presurgical orthodontics initiated before distraction. (**E**) Exposure of the maxilla through a vestibular approach. Le Fort I osteotomy performed and the internal maxillary distraction device fixed to the anterior surface of the zygoma. The internal distractor fixed to the osteotomised maxilla (left). (**F**) The internal distractor fixed to the osteotomised maxilla (right). The activating arm exposed intraorally in the buccal sulcus. Removal of distractor device after complete consolidation was performed. (**G and H**) Comparison of lateral cephalogram showing change in skeletal relation from class III to class I. (**I**) Postdistraction occlusion showing achievement of class I incisor relationship. (**J**) Postdistraction orthodontics continued for dental arch alignment. (**K**) Postdistraction facial appearance. (**L**) Postdistraction facial profile.

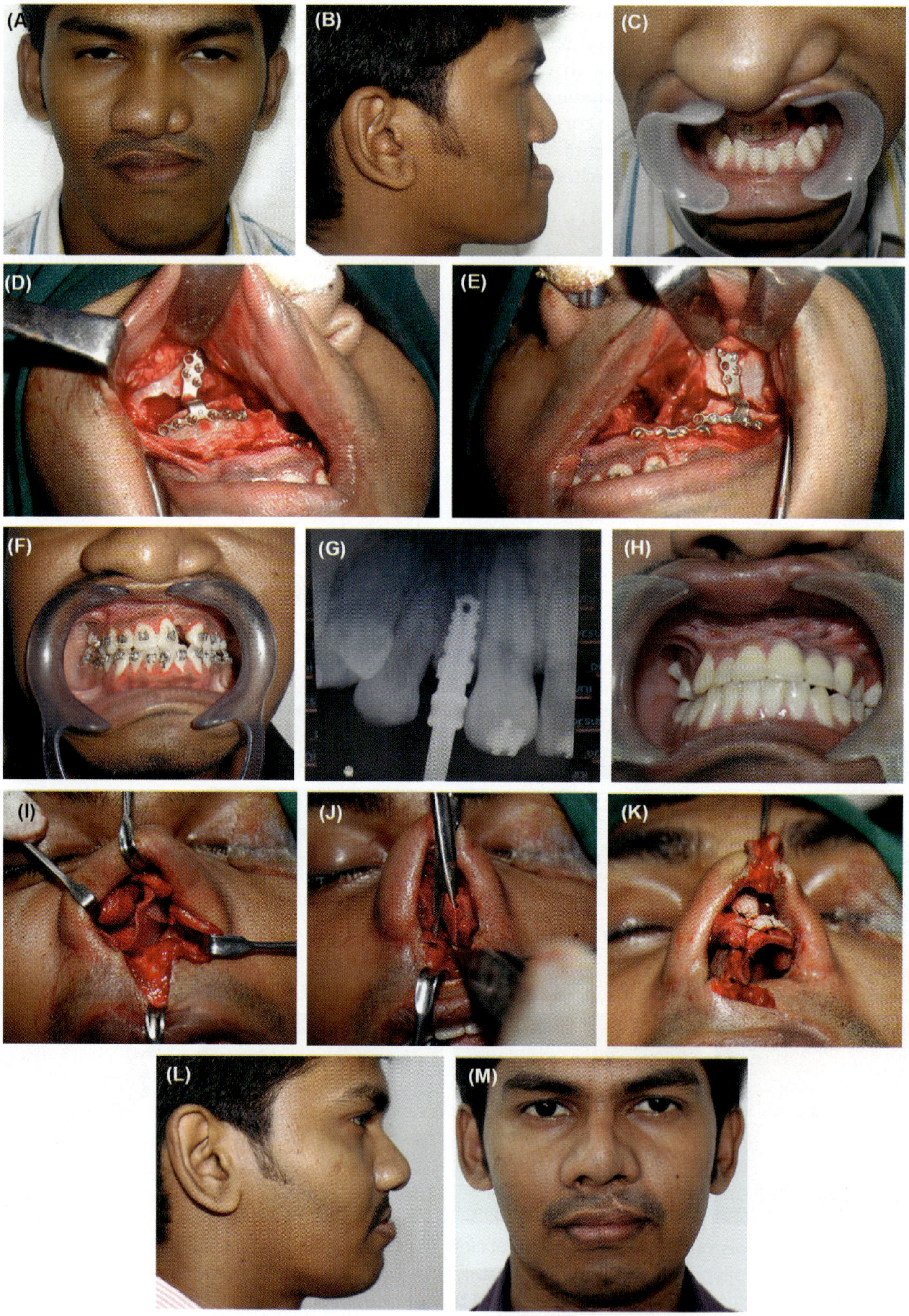

Figure 45.21 (**A–C**) Preoperative view showing hypoplastic maxilla in skeletal class III with depressed cleft left ala and concave profile. Note the reverse overjet and class III incisor relation. (**D** and **E**) Le Fort I osteotomy and maxillary advancement fixed using titanium miniplate. (**F**) Occlusion at the end of surgery and postsurgical orthodontics showing class I incisor relation and missing 22. (**G** and **H**) Missing 22 replaced with implant supported prosthesis. (**I**) Open rhinoplasty via transcolumellar incision and infracartilaginous incisions exposing the deviated nasal septum. (**J** and **K**) Caudal septal resection, dorsal and alar augmentation with costal cartilage grafts. (**L** and **M**) Postoperative appearance showing change in facial and nasal profile to straight profile and aesthetic nasal projection.

LIP SCAR REVISION

Abnormalities after cleft lip repair can be corrected by various techniques. The most common being asymmetry of the Cupid's bow. Short philtral length correction by Millard (Fig. 45.22).

- Residual lip length discrepancy can be corrected with an inferior Z-plasty or a triangular flap
- Many techniques are followed for the correction of these deformities like:
  a. V–Y advancement flap
  b. Kapetansky's pendulum flaps
  c. Abbe flap, etc.

ABBE FLAP FOR SHORT COLUMELLA

Deformity:

- Lack of tissue and short appearance of the upper lip
- Normal lower lip may look protuberant
- In the cleft patients, maxillary hypoplasia is a common finding. The upper lip usually lies on the bony maxilla, which lacks the proper amount of forward projection
- Lack of normal Cupid's bow after lip repair

Procedure: A wedge of the full thickness flap from the lower lip to the upper lip is transferred.

- This flap is sutured to the upper lip and forms a bridge of tissue that carries the vascular pedicle for the full thickness flap

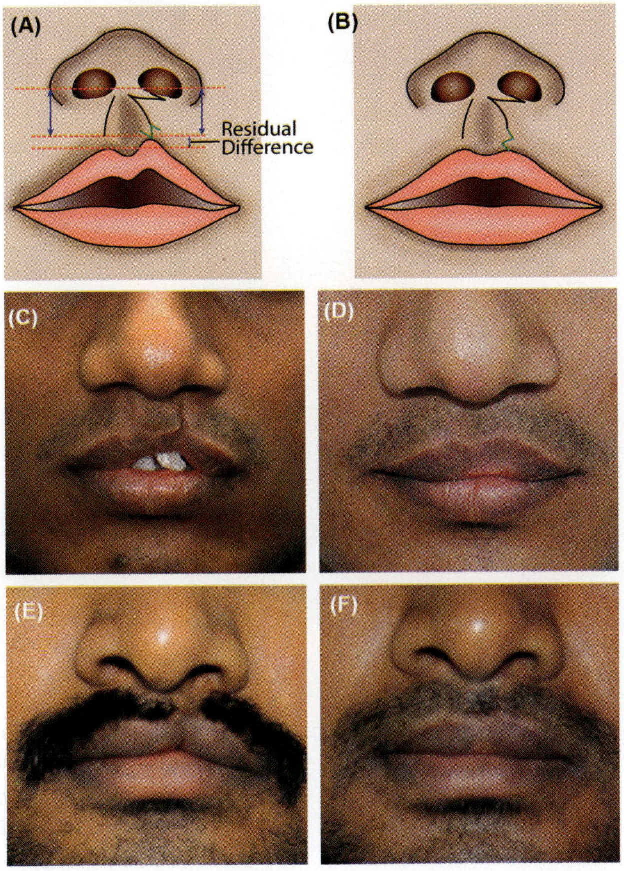

Figure 45.22 Millard's rotation advancement repair.

- This remains in place for 10–14 days while the tissue picks up new blood supply, after which the bridge is divided and both top and bottom lip scars completed.

PROSTHESIS FOR CLEFT PATIENTS

The usual prosthetic treatment is replacement of a tooth or teeth in the line of the cleft. If the anterior segment of a complete bilateral cleft has not been surgically stabilised, fixed prosthetics should be considered. Unrepaired clefts are usually restored using a combination of fixed and removable appliance.

Infant feeding prosthesis (palatal plate): The purpose of this prosthesis is to provide a normal contour to the defective alveolar process and palate. Thus, tongue can flatten and press the nipple into the palate during normal suckling movements, for example, palatal plate (Fig. 45.11).

HEAD GEARS

They are used during the growth period to intercept or correct the malocclusion as well as to distalise the maxillary dentition or maxilla itself. They derive anchorage from the cervical or cranial regions.

PHARYNGEAL OBTURATORS

This is a device that prevents air from escaping into the nasal cavity by sealing off the posterior pharyngeal wall during speech, for example, speech bulb. It is composed of three components: (i) maxillary appliance (ii) a palatal extension and (iii) a nasopharyngeal section.

The maxillary appliance acts as a source of retention and resists the dislodging forces of the nasopharyngeal section. The palatal extension is the connection between the maxillary appliance and the nasopharyngeal section. It is usually constructed as a loop so that the nasopharyngeal section will not rotate on it. The nasopharyngeal section of the obturator acts to separate the oral and nasal cavity (Fig. 45.10).

FIXED AND REMOVABLE PARTIAL DENTURES

The fixed partial denture is used to replace and restore the missing teeth by using the support of adjacent teeth. Removable prosthesis is usually a modified partial denture, which restores the teeth and associated alveolar and supporting structures to achieve an aesthetic and functional result.

DENTAL IMPLANTS

For cleft palate patients, restoration of the single missing tooth to provide an abutment for small bridges appears to be the primary indication for implants (Fig. 45.21F–H). Considering the increasing number of dental implants used in the general population, this treatment modality will undoubtedly play a role in prosthodontic consideration of the treatment of the cleft patients.

Section XIII

Maxillofacial Trauma

Chapter 46

Emergency Management of Trauma Patients and Soft Tissue Injuries

OUTLINE

INTRODUCTION

Maxillofacial injuries are relatively a common form of trauma in everyday life, so it is essential for us to know the primary care and definitive management of these injuries. Maxillofacial injuries can be simple or complex with missing tissues. Early treatment and rehabilitation of these injuries help us to restore form and function.

Road traffic accidents (RTA) are considered to be the primary cause of maxillofacial trauma. The other causes are assaults, falls, sport injuries, gun shots, war injuries, work-related injuries, burns and animal bites.

Trauma to the midface and mandible can cause airway obstruction. Severe trauma can lead to death. Death from trauma has a trimodal distribution and follows the following patterns:

i. The 1st peak of injury is within seconds or minutes of the incident happening due to the injuries to the brain, brain stem, high spinal cord, heart and great vessels. The survival possibility is very remote
ii. The 2nd peak occurs few minutes to hours after the incident. The 1st 60 minutes following trauma is the most critical period that determines the patient outcomes and is called as the "golden hour". Because these patients can be saved if rapid assessment and management of their injuries are done. For example, extradural haematomas or haemopneumothorax. After this period, there will be a significant increase in the mortality and morbidity of the patient
iii. The 3rd peak occurs days or weeks after the injury and occurs due to pulmonary embolism, multiple organ failure or sepsis.

The initial evaluation of the injuries and the stability of the patient's vital signs are assessed, and treatment priorities are established. In critical injuries, a sequential treatment priorities must be established on the basis of overall patient assessment. Generally, injuries can be divided into three categories:

- *Severe injuries* are life-threatening injuries, which involve the vital physiologic functions and are associated with traumatic deaths
- *Urgent injuries* offer no immediate threat to life. The vital signs of these patients are stable and may require surgical intervention or repair
- *Nonurgent injuries* are not immediately life-threatening. The exact nature of the injury may not become apparent initially and may require significant evaluation.

In a trauma patient, emergency care aims to identify life-threatening injuries, resuscitate vital functions and offer lifesaving measures until definitive care can be provided.

ASSESSMENT OF SEVERITY OF INJURY

Sorting patients based on the severity of their injuries, the need for treatment, and the available resources is known as triage. The primary goal of triage is to promptly and accurately identify patients with life-threatening injuries and manage them with the available resources. Many *scales and scoring systems* help us in predicting outcomes based on

TABLE 46.1 Adults Glasgow Coma Scale

Eye Opening (E)	Verbal Response (V)	Motor Response (M)
Spontaneous = 4	Oriented = 5	Obeys = 6
To speech = 3	Confused conversation = 4	Localises = 5
To pain = 2	Inappropriate words= 3	Withdraws = 4
Nil = 1	No words only sounds = 2	Abnormal flexion = 3
	Nil = 1	Extensor response = 2
		Nil = 1
Total Score = E + M + V Minimum = 3, Maximum = 15		

TABLE 46.2 Paediatric Glasgow Coma Scale

Eye Opening (E)	Verbal Response (V)	Motor Response (M)
Spontaneously = 4	Age appropriate verbalisation = 5	Obeys commands = 6
To voice = 3	Cries but consolable, irritable, uncooperative, inappropriate interaction = 4	Localising pain = 5
To pain = 2	Moaning, inconsistently consolable = 3	Withdrawal from pain = 4
None = 1	Inconsolable, agitated, unaware of the environment = 2	Flexion to pain = 3
	None = 1	Extension to pain = 2
		None = 1

several criteria. This sorting can be performed either by the paramedic team at the accident site or at the hospital.

GLASGOW COMA SCALE (GCS)

GCS was 1st described by *Teasdale and Jennett* in 1974 to quantify the severity of head injury. The patient is assessed by using three variables: best motor response, best verbal response and eye opening. The eye opening indicates the function of brainstem activity. Motor response reflects the level of central nervous system (CNS) function and verbal response shows the ability of CNS to integrate information.

The disadvantage of GCS is that it does not take into account diffuse metabolic processes or intoxication (Tables 46.1 and 46.2).

Inference for Glasgow Coma Scale score

GCS total score = 3 to 15

GCS score of 8 or less—Patient is in coma.

GCS score of 3-8—Severe head injury and requires urgent management.

They have higher mortality rates.

Higher scores represent increased degree of consciousness.

Letter T designates—patient was intubated at the time of the examination.

A head injury patient with GCS score of 13–15 is considered as mild, with GCS score of 9–12 as moderate, GCS score of <8 as severe.

TRIAGE COLOUR CODING

Maxillofacial injuries can be broadly placed into groups depending on the urgency of the treatment required (Table 46.3).

TABLE 46.3 Triage Colour Coding

Group	Colour Coding	Description
Group 1	Red	Requires intervention within few minutes. Needs immediate lifesaving management.
Group 2	Yellow	Requires intervention within few hours. Patient is stable but needs urgent management.
Group 3	Green	Requires intervention within few days. Patient is stable and the treatment can be done in a day or two.
Group 4	Black	Requires intervention within few weeks. Treatment can be delayed for many days.

REVISED TRAUMA SCORE

In 1989, Champion developed the revised trauma score to assess the extent of injury to vital systems, the severity of injury and the treatment required for the patient. It quantifies the physiological status of the patient's neurological, cardiovascular and respiratory system. Lower score represents increased severity of injury (Table 46.4).

ASSESSMENT PRINCIPLES - ATLS

Once the patient with major trauma reaches the hospital, initial assessment should follow the Advanced Trauma Life

TABLE 46.4 Revised Trauma Score

Glasgow Coma Scale	Systolic Blood Pressure (mm Hg)	Respiratory Rate	Coded Value
13–15	>89	10–29	4
9–12	76–89	>29	3
6–8	50–75	6–9	2
4 or 5	1–49	1–5	1
3	0	0	0

Support (ATLS) protocols. It is important to record every detail of the patient, as it means the difference between life and death.

PRIMARY SURVEY AND RESUSCITATION

During the primary survey, life-threatening conditions are identified and treated without delay. The vital signs are stabilised. The sequence of this primary survey constitutes the ABCDEs of trauma (Flowchart 46.1).

A—Airway maintenance with cervical spine control
B—Breathing and ventilation
C—Circulation with haemorrhage control
D—Disability and neurological status
E—Exposure and environmental control

Simultaneously, patient should be monitored for pulse oximetry, electrocardiogram (ECG), blood pressure (BP), blood investigations, chest and pelvic radiographs.

A—AIRWAY MAINTENANCE WITH CERVICAL SPINE CONTROL

The highest and foremost priority in a maxillofacial trauma patient is the establishment and maintenance of a patent airway. *The obstruction of upper airway can be due to:*

- Bleeding from the oral structures
- Aspiration of foreign bodies

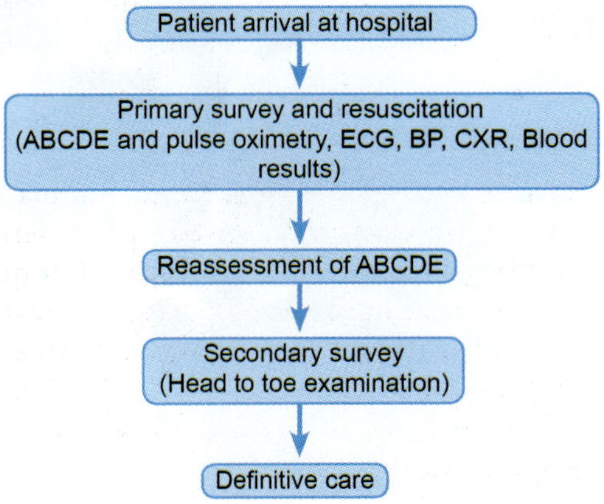

Flowchart 46.1 Management of a trauma patient (ATLS protocol).

- Tongue fall back
- Fractures of maxilla, mandible, trachea or larynx
- Soft tissue oedema of the face
- Regurgitation of stomach contents
- Cervical spine injury.

Maxillofacial injuries that cause airway obstruction are:

- Bilateral fracture of anterior mandible producing tongue fall back
- Midface fracture causing downward and backward displacement of maxilla into the nasopharynx
- Haemorrhage from open wounds or severe nasal bleeding
- Soft tissue swelling and oedema
- Aspiration of fractured teeth, bone fragments, blood, vomitus, foreign bodies or dentures.

SIGNS OF AIRWAY OBSTRUCTION

The early signs of airway compromise are tachypnoea (>25 per min) or inability to enunciate words or sentences. An inappropriate response or failure to respond suggests an altered level of consciousness, airway compromise or both. Patients with altered level of consciousness are at potential risk of airway compromise and aspiration.

Pulse oximetry can be used to detect inadequate oxygenation. An abnormal, noisy breathing (snoring, gurgling and stridor) indicates partial obstruction of the pharynx or larynx. Voice hoarseness suggests laryngeal obstruction.

AIRWAY MANAGEMENT

The primary aim of airway management is to achieve airway patency and adequate ventilation (oxygenation) quickly. This can be accomplished by *airway maintenance techniques, definitive airway or surgical airway.* In addition, the cervical spine should be protected in all trauma patients.

Airway management can be summarised as:

- Recognise the airway obstruction
- Place the patient in a semiprone position with the head slightly lowered (Trendelenburg's position)
- Head tilt and chin-lift, oropharyngeal airway or jaw-thrust procedure can be performed to re-position the tongue and open the airway (refer to Chapter 8, page number 99)
- Suctioning is done to clear the pharynx and oral cavity
- Nasopharyngeal/oropharyngeal tube can be used to maintain the airway patency
- The cervical spine (C-spine) needs to be protected and stabilised. Cervical collar can be placed until the C-spine injury is ruled out. The C-spine can be maintained in a neutral position using a backboard, bindings and head immobilisers
- Definitive airway management by oral or nasal intubation is necessary if the patient is unconscious or with altered consciousness. It allows for adequate ventilation and higher concentrations of oxygen (refer to Chapter 12)
- If intubation is not possible, airway patency is accomplished surgically by cricothyrotomy/tracheostomy
- Oxygen administration/artificial ventilation.

CERVICAL SPINE INJURY

It is very important to recognise the cervical spine injury and prevent any movement of the C-spine while attempting to achieve a patent airway. Therefore, the patient's head and neck should **not be hyperextended or hyperflexed** to establish or maintain an airway. *It is better to assume a cervical spine injury in any patient especially with a blunt injury above the clavicle unless proven otherwise.* Cervical injury can be excluded by appropriate radiographs. Until then, a hard cervical collar should be worn and supported by a sandbag and a tape (Fig. 46.1).

If airway obstruction is due to a displaced or impacted fractured maxilla, restoration of its normal position can be carried out by digital disimpaction of the maxilla. This is done by placing the index and middle fingers in the posterior choanae and drawing the maxilla upward and forward, while maintaining countertraction on the forehead.

B—BREATHING AND VENTILATION

After establishment of an adequate airway, *breathing (pulmonary status)* of the patient should be evaluated.

Evaluation of patient's breathing involves:

i. Inspection of the chest wall movements during breathing
ii. Auscultation for breath sounds and air movements
iii. Palpation and percussion to detect chest injuries, diaphragmatic excursions and any signs of air or blood in the pleural space
iv. Plain chest X-ray, pulse oximetry and arterial blood gas help us in assessing the breathing.

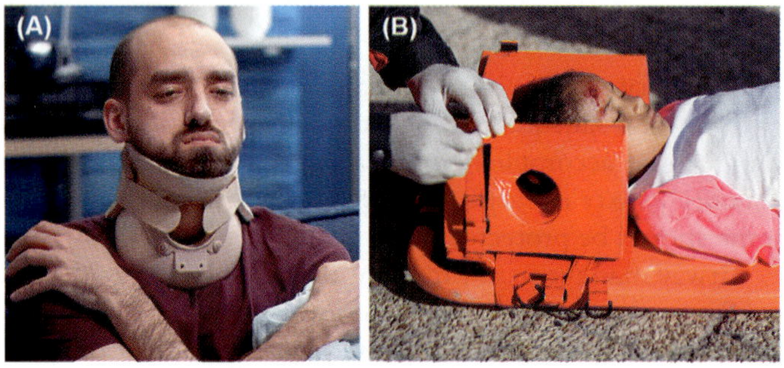

Figure 46.1 (**A**) Hard collars (**B**) block and straps.

Ventilation is the exchange of air between the lungs and the atmosphere that allows oxygen to be exchanged for carbon dioxide in the lungs. In trauma patients, establishing an adequate airway alone does not guarantee sufficient ventilation. The chest wall, lungs, and diaphragm should all function adequately to ensure proper ventilation. Any injuries to the lungs or chest wall, such as pneumothorax, flail chest or haemothorax can lead to impaired ventilation. Shallow breaths, tachypnoea, anxiety, hypoxaemia, hypercarbia, cyanosis, bradycardia, tachycardia, hypertension and/or hypotension are all signs of inadequate ventilation.

Inadequate ventilation can be managed by a secure airway and artificial ventilation.

- As a general rule, it is recommended to administer *high-flow oxygen by mask* to all patients in order to avoid the development of hypoxaemia
- Artificial ventilation can be provided by an *Ambu bag*, bag-valve mask or *mechanical ventilators* till the chest status is evaluated (Fig. 46.2)
- The causes of inadequate ventilation should be identified quickly and treated
- *Open pneumothorax* is defined as a defect in the chest wall allowing air to move in and out of the pleural cavity with each respiration. Initially, it is managed by covering the defect with a *sterile occlusive dressing* (petrolatum gauze), followed by closure of the wound in the operating room. A chest tube can be placed at a distant site on the affected chest wall
- *Closed pneumothorax* or pneumothoraces can be treated with a regular chest tube (*tube thoracostomy*) or needle insertion. The chest tube is usually placed at the 5th intercostal space

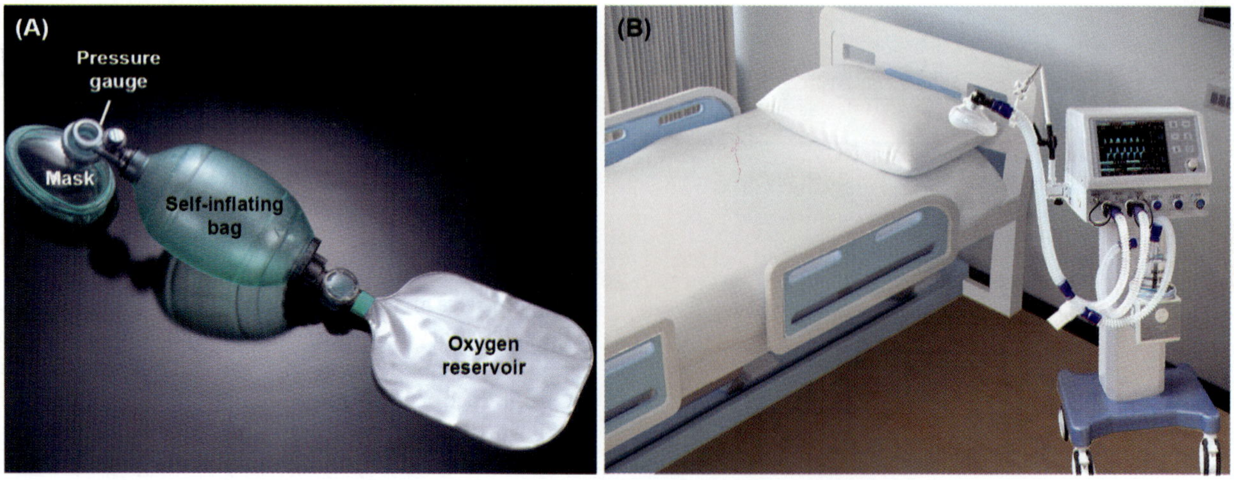

Figure 46.2 (**A**) Ambu bag (**B**) mechanical ventilator.

- *Tension pneumothorax* is defined as a progressive increase of intrapleural pressure. It develops when the air that enters the pleural cavity on inspiration cannot escape on expiration. If a tension pneumothorax is suspected, the positive intrapleural pressure should be released as quickly as possible. The pressure can be released by inserting a *large-bore needle* (14–16 gauge) through the 2nd or 3rd intercostal space into the affected hemithorax. This quickly converts the tension pneumothorax to a pneumothorax, which can be treated with the placement of a chest tube (Fig. 46.3)
- *Haemothorax* is the collection of blood in the pleural cavity. Treatment of a haemothorax consists of the restoration of circulating blood volume with transfusion of fluids or blood products, control of the airway, ventilation, and drainage of the accumulated blood from the pleural cavity. A *large chest tube* should be inserted in the 5th or 6th intercostal space in the mid-axillary line. The chest tube should be connected to an underwater seal and suction. Thoracotomy for intrathoracic bleeding is indicated
- *Flail chest* occurs when there are multiple rib fractures. Recommended management of flail chest involves pain management, supplemental oxygen and ventilation
- *Oxygenation:* After the establishment of a patent airway and sustained breathing, the patient should be given supplemental oxygen through a facemask or endotracheal tube.

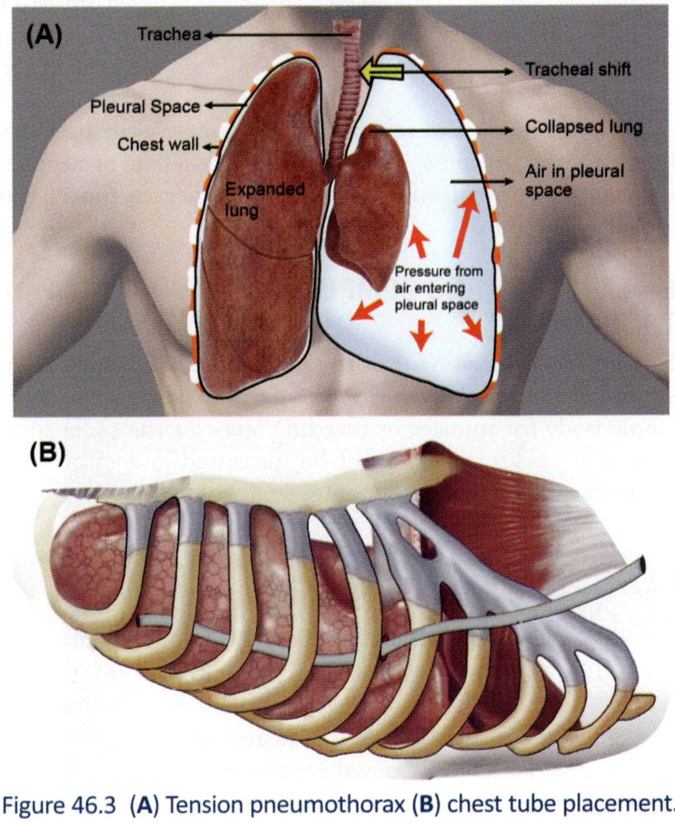

Figure 46.3 **(A)** Tension pneumothorax **(B)** chest tube placement.

In *maxillofacial injuries*, patients might develop breathing problems, following aspiration of teeth, dentures, vomit and other foreign materials. To exclude the presence of teeth and dentures in pharynx or lower airway, chest X-ray and soft tissue views of the neck should be taken. Unfortunately, acrylic is not obvious on a radiograph, and an endoscope can help to identify and remove denture fragments or foreign bodies. Occasionally CT scanning or fibreoptic endoscopy may be necessary.

C—CIRCULATION WITH HAEMORRHAGE CONTROL

After establishment of an adequate airway and breathing, the cardiovascular system of the patient must be assessed and a baseline circulation should be quickly restored. In a trauma patient, loss of blood can lead to hypovolaemia and decreased tissue perfusion.

The haemodynamic status (*blood volume and cardiac output*) can be assessed by:

- **Pulse:** Should be checked in central arteries such as the femoral and carotid arteries. The pulse rate is a more sensitive measure of hypovolaemia and cardiac rate. *Rapid and irregular pulse* indicates hypovolaemia and cardiac hypoxia
- **Respiratory rate:** *Tachypnoea* occurs as a physiologic response to the tissue's requirement for extra oxygen
- **Blood pressure:** When there is significant blood loss (>30% of blood volume), the *blood pressure will drop* below the baseline level
- **Skin colour:** It is the more reliable indicator of poor tissue perfusion. A *grey, pale ash tone of skin* indicates hypovolaemia
- **Urinary output:** Decrease in intravascular volume is immediately reflected as decreased urinary output. The normal urine output for adults is 0.5 mL/kg/h and 1 mL/kg/h for children. A decrease of urinary output to *less than 30 mL/h* indicates hypovolaemia
- **Acid-base balance:** In early haemorrhagic shock, there is an initial respiratory alkalosis, followed by metabolic acidosis
- Hypovolaemia due to blood loss can cause flat neck veins.

Management

The initial step in managing haemorrhage is to minimise the blood loss by identifying the source of bleeding and to stop them. Bleeding can be external or internal.

- *External bleeding* can be controlled by direct manual pressure on the wound and bandages. Scalp and skin wounds are best managed by immediate closure with sutures
- *Internal bleeding* can occur in areas such as chest, abdomen, retroperitoneum, pelvis and long bones. They can be identified by chest X-ray, pelvic X-ray, ultrasound or CT scans
- Only external haemorrhage is controlled in the primary survey. The internal haemorrhage is addressed only when the haemorrhage has damaging effects on the

cardiovascular or pulmonary system. Slow internal haemorrhage can be controlled by splinting, casting, and fixation of fractures, natural mechanism of clot formation or by open exploratory surgery

- When the bleeding has stopped, the fluid that was lost must be replenished. Initial intravenous resuscitation fluid used commonly is *1–2 L of Ringer's lactate (RL) solution or normal saline*. The patient's response is assessed by the urine output, mental status and vital signs
- If the systolic BP does not raise, the patient requires additional fluid or blood. Ideally, the patient should be given *whole blood* that has been properly typed and cross-matched. The transfusion of blood restores the intravascular oxygen-carrying capacity. *Fresh frozen plasma* is frequently used as a volume expander. If the patient does not respond to initial fluid resuscitation and blood transfusions, surgical intervention is required to control haemorrhage. Adequate resuscitation is achieved only when adequate oxygenation, circulation and urine output are restored.

Maxillofacial area

The majority of the fractures of the facial skeleton are *closed injuries* and severe haemorrhage is unusual. When there are extensive soft tissue lacerations (missile injuries or assaults), they require urgent attention, as local blood loss can be considerable.

Epistaxis (*nasal bleeding*) of some degree is an inevitable consequence of injury to the central middle 3rd of the face. It usually stops spontaneously or is easily controlled by *packing* the nose through anterior nares using the *ribbon gauze soaked in saline or adrenaline 1:1000 strength*. Profuse haemorrhage into the nasopharynx from terminal branches of maxillary artery can occur in Le Fort I, II or III fractures. This is potentially life-threatening, both in terms of blood loss and breathing obstruction. A postnasal pack is needed in such extreme situation.

D—DISABILITY DETERMINED BY A BRIEF NEUROLOGICAL EXAMINATION

After the establishment of the airway and stabilisation of the cardiovascular system, a neurological examination is done to evaluate the level of consciousness and pupillary size and reaction. A rapid neurological assessment is necessary to quickly identify any CNS problems that require immediate intervention or additional investigations. To assess the patient's level of consciousness, the AVPU mnemonic can be used:

A: Alert
V: Responds to **vocal** stimuli
P: Responds only to **painful** stimuli
U: Unresponsive

In the unconscious patient, differential diagnosis has to be established regarding the cause of unconsciousness. A baseline of the neurological status is established in the primary survey, whereas a more detailed quantitative neurologic examination is done in the secondary survey.

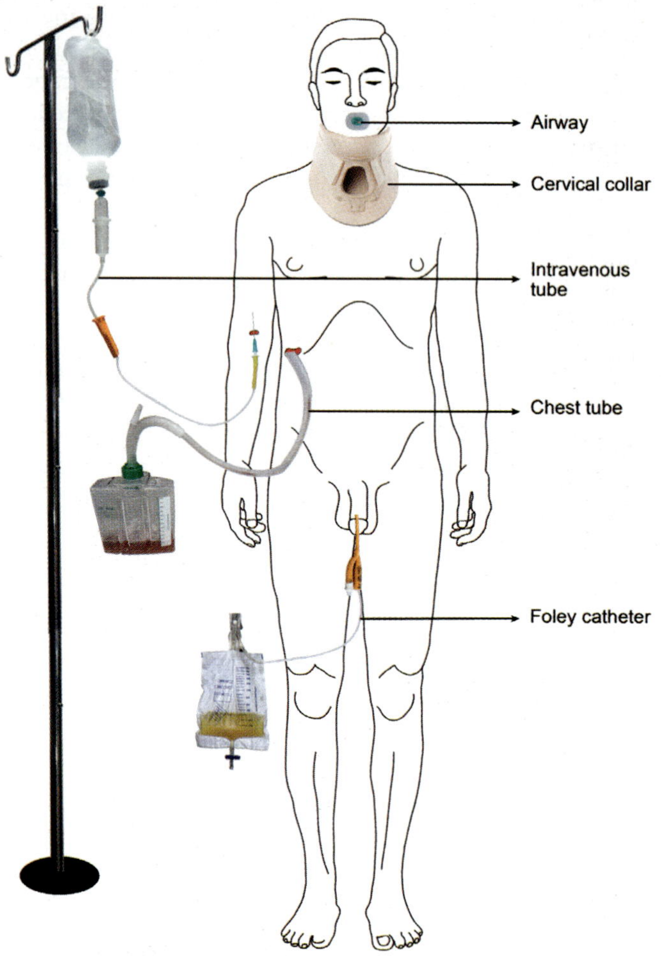

Figure 46.4 Primary survey of a patient.

GCS is a quick and reliable way to quantify the patient's level of consciousness. The neurologic assessment also includes the examination of pupils, cranial nerves, motor and sensory function.

E—EXPOSURE AND COMPLETE EXAMINATION OF THE PATIENT

It is the final component of the primary survey. The patient should be completely exposed to facilitate examination of whole body for injuries or bleeding sites. At the same time, patient's temperature should be measured and efforts are taken to avoid hypothermia (Fig. 46.4).

SECONDARY SURVEY (COMPLETE EXAMINATION OF THE PATIENT)

Secondary survey is a complete examination of the trauma patient from head to toe, which includes a thorough history and physical examination. A brief history should be obtained from the patient, family members or other victims at the site of injury.

In secondary survey, the patient's vital signs should be continuously monitored and any other life-threatening problems which were not evident in the primary survey should also be assessed.

HISTORY TAKING

The clinician should know the cause of the trauma, which will alert him/her regarding the type of injury. For example, trauma caused due to sharp objects may result in penetrating injuries, and blunt trauma is most likely to result in a fracture of the facial skeleton.

A mnemonic that is helpful in the immediate assessment of the patient is AMPLE:

A: Allergies
M: Medications
P: Past illness
L: Last meal
E: Events leading to the injury

It is also necessary to enquire about the patient's last meal for two reasons:

1. Alcoholic drink—causes altered sensorium, thus GCS is not applicable
2. Decreases the gut mobility and tendency to vomit from trauma contraindicates general anaesthesia.

Therefore, nasogastric suction and techniques to prevent vomiting or aspiration must be employed during intubation and/or anaesthesia. Extreme caution must be exerted during the insertion of nasogastric tube in patients with Le Fort II and III injuries as the tube may penetrate the anterior cranial fossa if it is passed injudiciously.

REVIEW OF SYSTEMS

All segments of the body from head to toe (head and skull, maxillofacial area, neck, chest, spinal cord, abdomen, extremities, musculoskeletal and neurological system) should be inspected, palpated, percussed or auscultated to provide the patient's current situation.

HEAD AND SKULL

Primary examination involves lacerations, abrasions, contusions and fractures of cranium. Intracranial lesions such as cerebral contusions and intracranial bleeding (epidural, subdural and intracerebral haematomas) should also be evaluated. Other than these injuries, hypoxia or ischaemia to brain, visual acuity, pupillary size and ocular entrapment should also be examined.

CT scans provide a rapid and accurate assessment of intracranial injury. It helps us in identifying the intracranial haemorrhage, skull fractures, contusion, brain shift, hydrocephalus and foreign bodies. The GCS scoring can be used to grade the consciousness and functional capacity of the cerebral cortex.

CHEST

The primarily assessed problems such as pneumothorax, haemothorax, flail chest and cardiac tamponade should be treated accordingly. The secondary assessment involves an upright chest X-ray to find the presence of air, fluid, midline shift or thoracic injuries. If a chest injury is suspected in an X-ray, then a CT scan should be obtained.

MAXILLOFACIAL AREA

Maxillofacial injuries can cause airway obstruction by the blood and secretions, arising from soft tissue injuries, midface and/or mandibular fracture. The maxillofacial examination can be proceeded in the following order: Soft tissues, Nerves and Skeleton.

Soft tissue examination

A careful examination of any lacerations, contusions, swelling, abrasions and penetrating injuries should be done. The clinician should also rule out that the penetration injuries have not affected any vital structures. Soft tissue injuries in maxillofacial region can reflect other associated or underlying injuries such as:

- Penetrating wounds of soft palate may extend into the middle cranial fossa
- Orbital injuries manifest as subconjunctival haemorrhage
- Temporomandibular joint (TMJ) or middle cranial fossa injuries manifest as bleeding from external auditory canal
- Basilar skull fractures may result in cerebrospinal fluid (CSF) otorrhoea
- The presence of septal haematoma indicates nasal septal fracture
- CSF rhinorrhoea indicates skull base fractures
- Ecchymosis behind the ear also known as Battle's sign indicates middle cranial fossa fracture
- Bilateral periorbital ecchymosis (raccoon eyes) is commonly seen in anterior cranial fossa fracture
- Subcutaneous emphysema indicates injuries at the upper airway such as maxillary sinus, frontal sinus, orbital roof and medial wall
- Stensen's and Wharton's ducts must be evaluated for patency and salivary flow
- Sublingual haematoma is the most common sign of mandibular fracture
- A laceration of the hard palate is usually associated with paramedian fractures of the palate.

Skeletal examination

Inspectory findings such as facial asymmetry, swelling and discolouration may indicate a bony or soft tissue injury. The palpation of the bony landmarks should begin from supraorbital, lateral and infraorbital rims, malar eminences, zygomatic buttress and arch, nasal bone, maxilla and mandible. Any step deformity or irregularities along the bony margin and mobility of the fragments are suggestive of a fracture. Numbness over the area of distribution can also occur in relation to the fracture area.

- Limited mouth opening or deviation of more than 6 mm indicates trismus secondary to mandible or condyle fracture, or a preexisting TMJ disorder

- Limited mouth opening or an anterior open bite with preauricular pain is suggestive of bilateral subcondylar fracture
- Deranged occlusion and mobility of the fragments are pathognomonic of mandibular fracture
- Occlusal derangement with class III open bite indicates maxillary fracture. Movement of the maxilla as a whole within the soft tissue is suggestive of maxillary fracture. Lack of mobility of the maxilla does not rule out a maxillary fracture, as the maxilla could be impacted into the cranial base
- Displacement at the lateral wall of orbit, diplopia and step deformity at the zygomatic buttress may disclose a zygomaticomaxillary complex (ZMC) fracture
- Combination of nasal deviation, obtuse medial canthal angle, increased intercanthal distance (beyond 32 mm) and flattened nasal bridge is indicative of naso-orbito-ethmoid (NOE) complex fracture
- Nasal bleeding, CSF rhinorrhoea and septal haematoma are associated with nasal fracture
- The teeth should be evaluated for mobility, fractures, displacement and missing.

Neurological examination

The nerves commonly injured in maxillofacial trauma are:

- *Inferior alveolar nerve:* It is frequently injured in mandibular fractures and may result in lip paraesthesia on the affected side, which may be permanent
- *Lingual nerve:* This nerve is less commonly injured. Injury to lingual nerve results in paraesthesia of the anterior two-thirds of the tongue
- *Infraorbital nerve:* It is commonly associated with fractures of ZMC, Le Fort II and orbital floor as the fracture line involve the inferior orbital fissure
- *Optic nerve:* Injury to this nerve results from fractures surrounding the optic foramen. Early identification of the injury and decompression of the optic nerve may salvage the patient's vision
- *Oculomotor nerve:* Presence of dilated pupil indicates oculomotor nerve damage, which usually results from increased intracranial pressure due to intracranial nerve compression
- *Abducent nerve:* Injury to the abducent nerve results in lateral rectus muscle dysfunction on lateral gaze
- *Olfactory nerve:* Injury to this nerve results from midface fracture involving the cribriform plate of ethmoid. Anosmia resulting from damage to the olfactory nerve is usually permanent
- *Facial nerve:* Damage to this nerve is common in parotid injuries and condyle fractures.

NECK

The neck should be examined for the presence of air in the soft tissue that may be a result of tracheal damage or pneumothorax. An expanding oedema or haematoma in the neck should be closely observed as it may cause airway compromise. The sensory and motor functions of cranial nerves, cervical and the brachial plexus should also be evaluated. Tracheal, laryngeal or oesophageal injury requires immediate surgical intervention.

ABDOMEN

Penetrating wounds in the abdomen must be identified and managed safely by laparotomy or surgery. If required, a nasogastric tube can be passed into the stomach to remove the gastric contents. Plain films are of limited use in abdominal trauma. Ultrasonography or focused assessment with sonography has become an integral diagnostic measure for abdominal trauma.

GENITOURINARY TRACT

The patient should be examined for contusions, lacerations, haematomas and urethral bleeding. In patients with perineal haematoma, Foley's catheter should be avoided. Pelvic fractures can be identified by the presence of ecchymosis over iliac, pubis or scrotum. Control of haemorrhage and fluid resuscitation is the primary management of pelvic fracture.

EXTREMITIES

Fractures of pelvic bone, femur and multiple fractures of long bone are important as they are extremely difficult in identifying the primary site of bleeding. These fractures may lead to life-threatening blood loss and are the major cause of hypovolaemic shock. Blood loss in a closed fracture for pelvis is 1–5 L, femur 1–4 L and for arm fracture 0.5–1 L. Direct pressure and splints should be used as quickly as possible to control haemorrhage. Fractures of long bones are usually associated with fat embolism and Acute respiratory distress syndrome (ARDS).

With an early aggressive management of haemorrhagic shock, fluid and electrolyte therapy and prompt surgical treatment, severely injured patients can be stabilised.

IMAGING OF MAXILLOFACIAL INJURIES

Plain radiographs are 'gold standard' in maxillofacial trauma. Management of maxillofacial injury is rarely an emergency, and definitive management can be deferred until radiographs of diagnostic quality can be obtained and a treatment plan can be formulated.

Radiographs which are ideal in mandibular fracture are:

- Panoramic radiograph (Orthopantomograph [OPG])
- Posteroanterior view of mandible (PA mandible)
- Townes view of mandibular condyle
- Lateral view of skull.

For evaluation of maxillary fractures:

- Waters sinus view (paranasal sinus [PNS] view)
- PNS view for maxillary, zygomatic, nasal and periorbital regions.

CT scans (computed tomography) in the coronal, sagittal and axial planes provide the extent of maxillofacial injuries.

3D reconstruction of CT scans can also be of assistance, particularly in fractures involving severe frontal bone and NOE injuries. However, magnetic resonance imaging is of little benefit in the assessment of traumatised patients. Arteriography is indicated in patients with severe bleeding that is difficult to control and in patients with penetrating injuries that involve major vessels.

SOFT TISSUE INJURIES

INTRODUCTION

'Soft tissue' refers to all the nonbony structures such as fat, muscles, nerves and blood vessels. Soft tissue injuries are commonly encountered in the emergency department. Facial soft tissue injuries may be isolated or associated with additional injuries. The wounds can be limited to superficial tissues or can involve deeper structures such as facial bones, nerves, glands and dentoalveolar structures. The most common causes of soft tissue trauma are motor vehicle accidents, falls, sports, industrial accidents and bites.

The management of soft tissue injuries often poses a challenge to the surgeon because of the specialised nature of facial tissues and their aesthetic importance. Understanding the mechanism of injury and the anatomy of the region is essential for satisfactory management.

CLASSIFICATION OF SOFT TISSUE INJURIES

CDC CLASSIFICATION OF SURGICAL WOUNDS

Centers for Disease Control and Prevention (CDC) 1999

- Clean wound—75% of surgical wound
- Clean contaminated wound
- Contaminated wound
- Dirty or infected wound.

Clean wound shows no signs of infection. Clean-contamination wounds show no signs of infections but are at increased risk of becoming infected. Contaminated wound is where an outside object has come into contact with the skin and has a high risk of infection, for example, gunshot wound. Dirty wounds have already been exposed to faecal material and have a high bacterial load.

BASED ON THE MECHANISM OF INJURY

1. Mechanical or physical injuries:
   (a) When injury is caused by a blunt force:
      - Abrasions
      - Contusions
      - Lacerations
   (b) When injury is caused due to sharp force:
      - Incised wounds
      - Chop wounds
      - Stab/punctured wounds
2. Thermal injuries:
   - Due to excessive cold: for example, frostbite
   - Due to moist heat: for example, burns and scald wounds
3. Chemical injuries:
   - Corrosive acids
   - Corrosive alkalis
4. Miscellaneous:
   - Electrical injuries
   - Lightening injuries
   - X-radiation injuries
   - Radioactive injuries
5. Explosions and blast injuries.

BASED ON THE COMMUNICATION OF INJURY WITH THE EXTERNAL ENVIRONMENT

In general, soft tissue injuries can be classified as *open or closed wounds.* A closed wound is where the damage occurs to the underlying tissue and/or structures without breaking the skin. Open wounds occur through a break in the skin, exposing the underlying structures to the external environment.

BASED ON THE FACIAL SUBUNITS INVOLVED/ LOCATION OF WOUND

Major facial subunits are: scalp, forehead, periorbital region, nose, cheek, perioral region, auricle, lip, tongue, parotid duct and neck.

BASED ON ADDITIONAL INJURIES

- *Injury to the nerve:* Nerve injuries are more common in open wounds. The most commonly injured nerves in the facial region are the facial nerve and the trigeminal nerve
- *Injury to arteries and veins:* The face is a highly vascular region, hence even a small injury leads to significant bleeding
- *Injuries to parotid duct:* The parotid duct injury can be cumbersome and leads to parotid fistula.

RANK AND WAKEFIELD CLASSIFICATION

Tidy wounds—These wounds are due to sharp instruments and contain no devitalised tissue. They can be closed primarily, for example, surgical incisions and knife wounds.

Untidy wounds—They are from tearing, crushing or vascular injury and contain devitalised tissue. The untidy wounds are best treated by wound excision.

LEGAL CLASSIFICATION

- Simple injuries
- Grievous injuries
- Dangerous injuries.

COMMON SOFT TISSUE INJURIES/BASED ON THE TYPE OF INJURY

- Abrasions
- Contusions
- Incised wounds
- Laceration

- Stab or puncture wounds
- Crush injury
- Avulsion injuries
- Burn injury
- Bites.

Common soft tissue injuries and its management

Abrasion (Gravel rash)

It is characterised by superficial injuries that denude the surface epithelium and occasionally involve the deeper layers. It is caused by friction between a hard, irregular surface and soft tissue. Abrasions are painful, as they remove the epithelial layer and papillary layer of the dermis, leaving the reticular layer exposed to nerve endings. Bleeding from the superficial capillaries is usually mild and can be controlled with gentle pressure (Fig. 46.5).

Management

- The abraded areas should be thoroughly *cleansed* using mild soap and copious saline irrigation
- All foreign materials must be removed. If these particles remain within the tissue, it results in growth of new epithelium over the contamination known as *'traumatic tattooing'*. This foreign material gives a bluish discolouration to the skin that remains as a permanent discolouration
- After the wound is cleaned, a thin layer of topical antibiotic ointment (bacitracin) or sterile gauze dressing or antibiotic-coated cellulose acetate gauze can be applied. Superficial injuries generally heal with local wound care measures
- In case of deep abrasion, loose bandages can be applied. Few deep abrasions of the skin surface might require skin grafting
- Abrasions of the oral mucosa regenerates rapidly and no treatment is required.

Contusion/Bruise

It indicates tissue disruption and rupture of small blood vessels without destruction of the superficial layer of skin. It results in submucosal haemorrhage and presents as areas of ecchymosis (purplish discolouration). Contusions are frequently caused by blunt trauma without breech of the overlying skin. When a contusion is evident in a facial fracture, one should always look for an associated osseous fracture (Fig. 46.6).

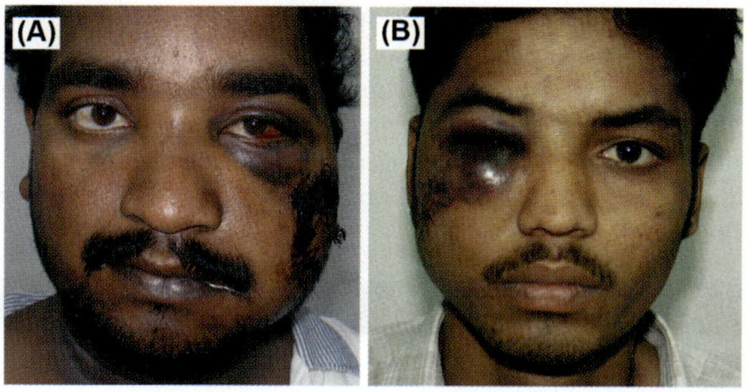

Figure 46.6 **(A & B)** Contusions injuries.

Management

- If the contusion is small and seen early, application of ice or pressure dressing may constrict the blood vessels and thereby decrease the amount of haematoma that forms
- Small haematomas usually resorbs without treatment and necessitate no surgical treatment
- If the haematomas are expanding, an artery might be involved within the wound and might require surgical exploration and ligation of the vessel
- Large haematomas should be drained immediately to avoid the development of permanent pigmentary changes and atrophy of the subcutaneous tissues
- Needle aspiration can be done in cases of liquefaction of the clot, which typically occurs around 10 days of postinjury
- Haematomas of the tongue, floor of mouth or neck may be a potential for airway compromise.

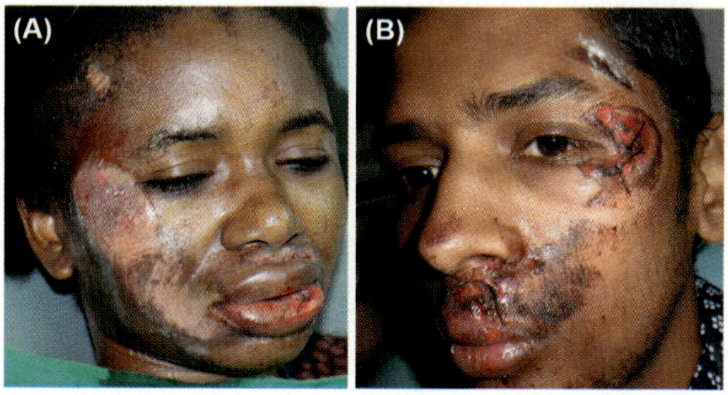

Figure 46.5 **(A & B)** Abrasive injuries on the face.

Lacerations

Laceration can be explained as a tear in the epithelial and subepithelial tissues. The most frequent type of soft tissue injury, usually caused by sharp objects like knives, glass, etc. Sharp objects usually create clean wounds with clean, straight edges that are easy to repair and produce a fine scar. Few lacerations may extend deep into the tissues and disrupt nerves, vessels, muscles and other vital structures (Fig. 46.7).

Management

The treatment of any laceration is similar to that of a surgical incision: re-approximation of deep tissue, dermis with a tension-free closure, precise apposition of epidermal edges, and an everted skin closure. After adequate anaesthesia, surgical management of lacerations involves four major steps: *Cleansing of the wound, debridement—removal of devitalised tissue, haemostasis and closure*.

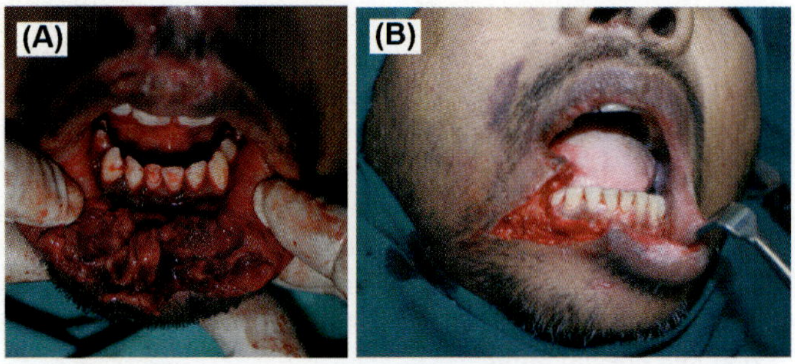

Figure 46.7 (**A** and **B**) Lacerations in lip.

Small lacerations do not need sutures for their closure, as these wounds can heal well by secondary intention. Deep lacerations are closed by sutures in layers. Laceration of gingiva, alveolar mucosa or floor of mouth is closed in one layer. Laceration of the tongue or lips is closed in different layers using resorbable sutures.

Avulsion injuries

These are characterised by significant tissue loss. It can also mean complete loss of some body parts such as eyelids, parts of ear, etc. Avulsion injuries in face are relatively uncommon and occurs exclusively in gunshot or sharp-edged large weapons (Fig. 46.8).

Management

The management of these wounds depends on the location and extent of the missing tissue. Treatment ranges from direct closure, local flaps to microsurgical free tissue transfer, depending on the size and location of the defect. Early treatment avoids contracture of the wound and decreases the risk of infection.

- For small defects, undermining of the surrounding tissues provides primary closure without tension on the wound margins
- If a significant amount of soft tissue is missing and primary closure is not possible, other options such as skin grafts, local flaps or free tissue transfer should be considered
- In few circumstances, the defect can be initially covered with a split-thickness skin graft, followed by facial reconstruction at a later stage (e.g. tissue expansion).

Animal and human bites

Dog bites are more common among human beings. Bites are potentially serious injuries, as they are prone to infections when not properly treated.

Infections from dog bites are polymicrobial, containing aerobic and anaerobic organisms, which includes *Pasteurella multocida, Staphylococcus aureus, Streptococcus viridans, Capnocytophaga canimorsus* and oral anaerobes. Human bites are often complicated by *Eikenella corrodens.* In cat bites, the most frequent pathogen being *P. multocida* and *Pasteurella septica. The infections caused by a cat bite is two times more dangerous than the infection caused by a dog bite.* The effect of dog bites can vary from a simple puncture wound, irregular tears to missing some part of tissues.

Management

Management of bite injuries involves copious irrigation and debridement to reduce infection and primary closure. The patient should be followed up for 24–48 h after the initiation of therapy to monitor the wound for any signs of infection.

Antibiotic prophylaxis for animal bites: Amoxicillin clavulanate is the current drug of choice for infections presenting within 24 h of injury. For wounds that are present after 24 h of injury, dicloxacillin or cephalexin is suggested.

The wounds are sutured primarily to reduce the risk of infection. But in extensive crushing of the tissue or extensive oedema, delayed closure is preferred. Rabies prophylaxis should be given for bite wounds that occur in an unprovoked domestic dog or cat that exhibits bizarre behaviour or an attack by a wild animal such as a raccoon, bat or fox.

Crush injuries

Prolonged or excessive force on any region can lead to crush injury. When head, face and neck are involved, the consequences can be disastrous. Crush injuries are frequently associated with devitalised tissue, leading to tissue necrosis and poor wound healing.

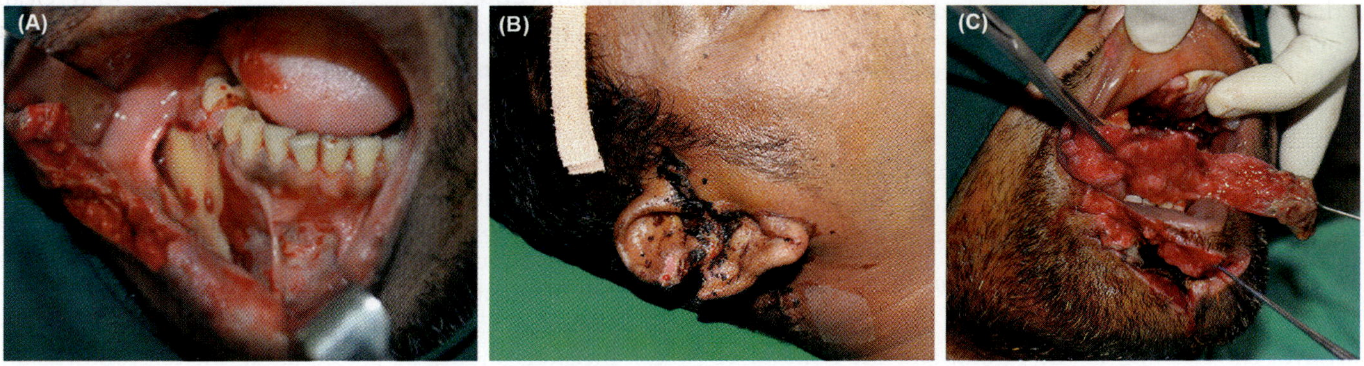

Figure 46.8 (**A–C**) Laceration with soft tissue loss.

Burn injuries

These are injuries to the tissues caused by friction, heat, electricity, radiation or chemicals. Skin cells die as a result of severe damage from burns. They are highly painful and require specific treatment.

GENERAL MANAGEMENT OF SOFT TISSUE INJURIES

1. Generally, many patients with soft tissue trauma present with multiple injuries, hence their initial management should be focused on establishing the airway, controlling haemorrhage and *stabilisation of the patient* (ATLS protocol) before evaluation of the facial soft tissue wounds
2. If there is significant oedema or oral bleeding, soft tissue trauma can contribute to airway compromise or circulatory compromise. *Haemorrhages* that are associated with facial injuries are usually controlled with local measures such as pressure, clamping, ligation or electrocautery of the bleeding vessels
3. Once the patient is stabilised, the patient's history regarding the *time and mechanism of injury* is obtained. This helps in assessing the risk of contamination and the possibility of associated injuries
4. Patient's status regarding their *tetanus immunisation* is an essential part of the medical history. Whether the patient has had an initial tetanus immunisation, and the last date of the tetanus toxoid booster should be recorded. Although the wounds might appear clean, the patient can still be at risk and may require tetanus prophylaxis
5. Preinjury photographs, if available, are a useful tool in identifying preexisting facial morphology and/or deformities
6. After obtaining the patient's information, an *initial examination* of the soft tissue injury is performed to assess the *quality of the wound* and nerve function. All wounds should be evaluated for the size, depth and status of the wound base
7. The *wounds should be kept moist* during the assessment period or until the final management. Bone and neurovascular structures are dressed with nonadherent dressings such as *xeroform gauze with or without bacitracin* ointment. Abrasions or burns are dressed with Adaptic gauze and Bacitracin or silver sulfadiazine. Deeper wounds that cannot be closed can be packed with gauze soaked in normal saline or iodoform
8. Antibiotics should be administered within 3 h of injury, as it is considered to be the 'golden period' for effective antibiotic use.

Antibiotics are indicated in circumstances such as grossly contaminated wounds, lacerations, bite wounds, and patients with systemic disease that compromises healing.

Wound debridement/wound excision or toileting of the wound

It involves the cleaning of the wound and the removal of foreign bodies. Debridement is the removal of devitalised tissue, tissue stained with dirt, necrotic tissue, or other particles. *Initial cleaning* of the wound should be done with a gentle soap (e.g., ivory soap) or a *diluted betadine*. These agents reduce bacterial counts.

- Materials such as *alcohol, hydrogen peroxide, benzalkonium chloride and hexachlorophene* should not be used directly over the open wound, as these materials are toxic to the cells. They can be used to clean around the wound along with a balanced salt solution such as *lactated Ringer's solution and normal saline*
- Hydrogen peroxide should not be used routinely to clean wounds, as it would impede wound healing. Three per cent hydrogen peroxide diluted 1:1 does not harm the wounds, but its bactericidal effectiveness is compromised. Antiseptics containing *iodophor or chlorhexidine* are active against a broad spectrum of organisms and can be used over the skin
- *Hair* is usually not removed since its presence serves as a guide to good anatomical reconstruction. For lacerations involving the scalp, mustache or beard, the area should be shaved for adequate debridement and repair. Wounds involving the eyebrows or hairline should not be shaved but cropped closely with scissors to provide a landmark for accurate repositioning of the soft tissues during closure
- *Abrasive wounds* containing materials such as dirt, glass or other debris can be cleaned by using a surgical scrub or detergent soap to remove the foreign material. The residual grease that cannot be removed with routine scrubbing can be removed using *polymyxin B sulfate ointment* and copious irrigation with a balanced salt solution. The wound should be completely cleaned from all the materials, as any contaminant can act as a source of infection
- *Excision of the wound edges* is not advised unless the tissues are obviously crushed and nonviable.

Wound closure

Wound closure is indicated for meticulous alignment of the tissues. In facial wounds, the layer wise closure is done to provide anatomic alignment, prevent dead space and excessive scarring of the wounds. Ideally, the facial soft tissue injuries should be closed as early as possible.

Timing of repair

Uncomplicated clean wounds are repaired by *primary closure* within 24 h of injury. *Delayed primary closure* is done in dirty, infected wounds or unrepaired wounds (Table 46.5).

A primary wound closure should not be attempted when there is any evidence of wound infection such as swelling, erythema, warmth or pus drainage.

Basic principles/guidelines for closure of facial wounds:

a. Gentle handling of the injured tissues, with minimal debridement and clean wound
b. Complete haemostasis
c. Incisions should be placed along the tension lines and natural folds of the skin

TABLE 46.5 Timing of Wound Closure is Directly Correlated with the Risk of Infection

Wounds	Timing of Closure
Wounds with a high risk of infection	6–8 h
Low risk of infection (head and neck area)	18–24 h
After 24 h	Packing of the wounds and secondary repair 4–8 days

d. The skin margins must be relaxed without tension
e. Fine sutures should be used and removed as early as possible
f. The wound edges should be everted
g. Dead space must be obliterated
h. The tissues should be closed in layers
i. The scar tissue must be allowed to mature before revision procedures (Figs. 46.9 and 46.10)
   - Clean wounds should be closed *within 12 h of injury* with accurate repositioning of the tissues. If the wound edges are ragged, judicious trimming of the edges helps in accomplishing a neat edge for accurate closure of the wound
   - Common methods for closing wounds include ***suturing, adhesives and staples***. It is always preferable to suture all complex facial lacerations. All deep lacerations should be re-approximated by layered closure to eliminate the dead space
   - *Tissue adhesives* with octylcyanoacrylate can be used to treat noncrushed lacerations within 6 h after injury. Tissue adhesives can be applied quickly and are useful, especially in children. But accurate alignment of the skin edges is difficult and its use is avoided in complex lacerations of the face
   - *Staples* have been primarily used for closing surgically created incisions, but they can be used for traumatic lacerations also. Staple closure is ideal for linear, sharp lacerations of the extremities, trunk and scalp. It can also be used for temporary closure of superficial lacerations or for rapid haemostasis during life-threatening conditions. The advantages of stable include: rapidity, good cosmesis, resistance to infection and less wound inflammatory response. The disadvantage is that it requires a special removal device and is uncomfortable for the patient during removal
   - Ideally, the facial fractures should be reduced and stabilised before final closure of the soft tissues, as the wounds provide access to the fracture site and the closure might get damaged during fracture reduction
   - If the bony repair is to be delayed, it is optimal to close the lacerations initially. The wounds can be re-entered and revised when the fracture site is to be accessed.

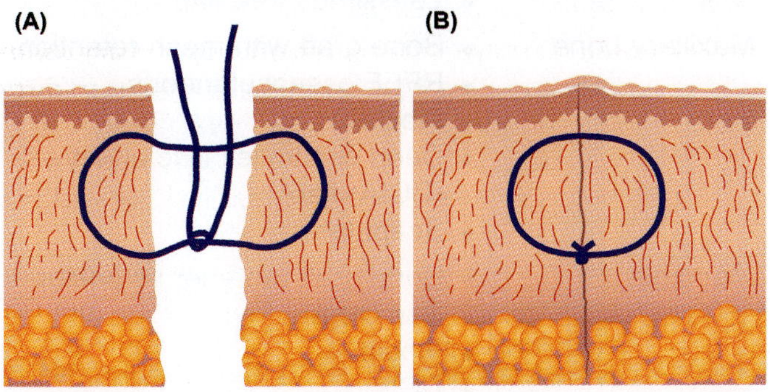

Figure 46.9 (**A**) The use of deep sutures to re-approximate the wound edges (**B**) Allows for an even and everted skin edges.

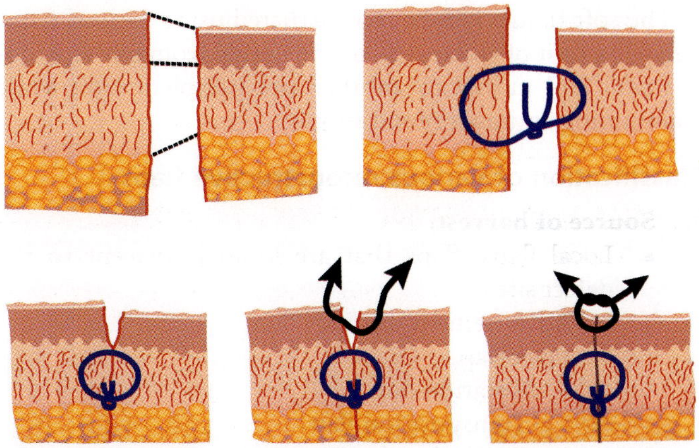

Figure 46.10 (**A**) The management of the wounds in an uneven thickness of the dermal edges. (**B**) Layer-wise closure 1st involves the placement of deep sutures to realign the deep tissues. (**C**) After closure of the deep tissues, the uneven dermal tissues should be corrected. (**D**) It is done by placing the dermal suture more deeply through the thinner edge and more superficially at the thicker dermal edge. (**E**) It helps to bring the epidermal edges together in an even manner.

Reconstruction/Management of tissue loss

Reconstruction is done in extensive degloving injuries. Tissue loss is relatively uncommon and mostly the tissues are displaced rather than loss. The options for primary management of tissue loss involve:

- Immediate replacement of the avulsed tissue as a free graft
- Dressing of the wound and allowing it to heal by secondary intention
- Direct closure with an acceptable tension
- Partial or full thickness skin graft
- Reconstruction with a free composite graft
- Local or regional flap
- Avulsion of ear, nose or scalp: replantation of the parts using microsurgical techniques.

The soft tissues can be reconstructed using various flaps. A flap is a unit of tissue that is transferred from one site (donor site) and moved to another site (recipient site) while maintaining an intact blood supply.

Classification of various reconstructive flaps

i. **Source of harvest:**
- Local flaps—flaps that are located adjacent to the defect site
  - Advancement or hinge flap
  - Pivot flap
    - Rotation flap
    - Transposition flap
    - Interpolated
    - Island flap
- Regional flaps—located at the same region
  - Axial pattern flap
  - Random pattern flap
    - Rhombic
    - Bilobed
    - V–Y
    - Z-plasties
    - W-plasties
- Distant flaps—region away from the wound
- Free flaps—flaps have their own blood supply and connected to the defect using microvascular technique. It requires detachment of the feeding vessels and transfer of the flap to the recipient site

ii. **Based on the composition of flap/types of tissues present:**
- Dermal/cutaneous flaps
- Fascia flaps
- Muscle flaps
- Tendon flaps
- Bone flaps
- Various combinations

iii. **Based on the blood supply:**
- Axial flaps
- Random flaps
- Pedicled flaps

iv. **Based on the mode of transfer of flap:**
- Rotational—A flap pivoting onto the defect
- Transpositional—A flap that moves laterally around the defect
- Advancement—A flap moved forward into the wound defect
- Interpolational—A flap undermined to reach the area

v. **Based on the thickness of the flap:**
- Full thickness flap
- Partial thickness flap.

Local or regional flaps provide a one-stage repair of the avulsive defects. The basic flaps used for facial reconstruction are advancement, rotational, transpositional and microvascular anastomotic flaps (Table 46.6).

TABLE 46.6 Reconstructive Flap Options for Site-Specific Defects

Lip	• Abbe flap (cross lip) • Facial artery musculomucosal (FAMM) flap • Radial forearm free flap (RFFF) • Anterolateral thigh (ALT)
Nasal tip	• Nasal flap • Paramedian forehead • Bilobed
Total nasal defects	• Paramedian forehead • Prefabricated flap
Eyebrow	• Subcutaneous island pedicle flap • Free scalp graft • Pedicle superficial temporal artery scalp flap
Ear	• Re-anastomosis of avulsed ear if adequate vessels remain • Temporoparietal fascia flap coverage of rib
Cheek (through and through)	• Double island pectoralis major myocutaneous flap • RFFF • ALT • Combination of free tissue and local flap • One flap with a skin graft for the exposed surface
Cheek	• Cervicofacial • Submental island flap • RFFF • ALT • Rectus abdominis
Scalp	• Rotation flaps • Ortichochea (banana peel) flap • ALT • RFFF • Latissimus free flap
Maxillary bone	• Bone graft with mesh retention • RFFF osseocutaneous • Fibula • Deep circumflex iliac artery (DCIA) flap • Scapula
Mandible	• Bone graft (anterior vs posterior iliac crest) • Fibula • DCIA • RFFF (osteocutaneous)

Graft failure

The most common reasons for graft failure are the formation of haematoma and failure of immobilisation. Improper orientation of the grafted tissue, such as securing a graft upside down or wrong side down, may also lead to graft failure.

Wound dressing

Wound dressings are sterile pad over the wounds. The dressings should be clean and provide a warm and moist environment for successful wound healing. The wounds must be applied with antibacterial ointments to keep it free from bacteria and adequate lubrication. The dressings are also needed to be changed frequently to keep the wound free from bacteria.

Uses of dressing:

- Prevention of bacterial contamination
- Protection of wound from outside environment
- Absorption of exudate
- Facilitates haemostasis
- Relieves pain in few cases.

The various types of dressing that are available are listed in Table 46.7.

TABLE 46.7 Types of Wound Dressing Materials	
Materials	**Indications**
Gauze	Dry dressing—It can be used as secondary dressing over another material
Tegaderm	For surgical incisions
Hydrogels/polymeric films	Wounds with mild exudates
Hydrocolloids	Wounds with light to heavy exudates
Antimicrobial dressing	Skin graft donor sites, superficial burns and abrasions
Collagen dressing	Chronic nonhealing wounds/ burn wounds

TYPES OF WOUND HEALING

a. **Primary closure and healing by primary intention:** Primary closure refers to direct apposition of the wound edges and healing of the wound is by primary intention. It favours in early return to function, with minimal scarring and loss of skin. Clean wounds treated within 24 h heal primarily. Ideally, the wounds should be closed without tension. Deep lacerations are closed in layers, eliminating 'dead space'

b. **Secondary closure**—It is indicated in wounds where the edges cannot be approximated and the healing is by secondary intention. The healing occurs from the bottom of the wounds to upwards and the defect is filled with granulation tissue, creating more scar tissue. The wound is left open, treating it with frequent dressings and allowing it to heal by secondary intention and wound contracture

c. **Delayed primary closure**—It is also known as tertiary intention. It is usually a combination of primary and secondary intention. It is indicated in patients with extensive soft tissue oedema, subcutaneous haematoma, crushing injuries, devitalised wound edges, dog bites or lacerations with foreign bodies. The wound is 1st cleaned and observed for a few days (usually 3–5 days) to ensure that no infection is apparent and then closed surgically. Primary closure is delayed to allow our immune response to control infection.

COMPLICATIONS

Complications in wound healing can be due to various factors such as foreign bodies, haematoma, radiation, smoking, diabetes, malnutrition and steroids. The common complications are:

- Delayed healing
- Infection
- Chronic inflammation
- Over repair
- Scar formation.

Delayed healing

Soft tissue wounds normally heal in three phases, which include the inflammatory phase, proliferative phase and maturation phase. Delayed healing may be due to prolongation or failure of any of these phases.

Infection

Wound healing and host resistance are hampered when bacteria are present. Bacterial growth is aided by the presence of foreign objects, sutures, haematomas and necrotic tissue. Antibiotics along with operative management help to reduce the bacteria and promote wound healing.

Chronic inflammation

Wounds with long-standing bacteria fail to progress through the phases of wound healing. Generally, for chronic wounds, systemic antibiotics are not indicated. Enzymatic debridement and silver releasing hydroalginate dressings favour chronic wound healing.

Scar formation

One of the most common complications is 'abnormal wound healing', which presents as keloid and hypertrophic scars. These are proliferative scars with excessive collagen deposition. The most common treatment for keloids is intralesional injection of steroids. Electron beam radiation after surgical excision of keloids has been used to prevent recurrence. Various other modalities used to decrease the recurrence of keloid include cryotherapy, 5-fluorouracil, laser therapy and intralesional bleomycin.

Chapter 47

Basic Principles in the Management of Maxillofacial Trauma

OUTLINE

INTRODUCTION

Maxillofacial injuries are complex and require multidisciplinary care for its successful management. In brief, the treatment involves primary survey, resuscitation of vital functions, stabilisation of the patient followed by 2nd survey and definitive care. The important role of a maxillofacial surgeon in facial injuries is to restore the maxillofacial skeleton and soft tissues to their pretraumatic positions, both functionally and aesthetically. Restoration of form and function remains the ultimate goal of facial fracture repair. Although the principles of basic treatment remain unchanged, there have been significant advances in the methods of fixation. This chapter describes the various techniques that have evolved and are used for treating facial bone fractures.

BIOLOGY OF BONE AND FRACTURE HEALING

ANATOMY OF BONE

Bone is the main constituent of the human skeletal system and serves multiple purposes. It is metabolically highly active in regulating the serum electrolytes—calcium and phosphate. The human skeleton has 80% cortical bone and 20% trabecular bone. The cortical bone is dense and solid, surrounding the marrow space, whereas the trabecular bone is composed of trabecular plates and rods interspersed in the bone marrow. The cortical bone contains a basic construction unit called as osteon or Haversian system, whereas the trabecular bones have no osteons (Fig. 47.1 and Box 47.1).

FRACTURE/WOUND HEALING

A fracture is defined as a breach in the structural continuity of the bone cortex, along with injury to the surrounding soft tissues.

Any fracture develops a tissue response to remove tissue debris, to reestablish the vascular supply and to produce a new skeletal matrix. The bone regenerative process aims in restoring the structural and mechanical integrity of the fracture to the preinjury levels, similar to the surrounding bone. *Bone healing can be broadly classified as primary or secondary healing.*

PRIMARY HEALING/DIRECT FRACTURE HEALING

The reestablishment of the cortex or healing without callus formation is called as primary bone healing. Primary bone healing requires excellent anatomic reduction, minimal gap between the fragments, rigid fixation, minimal or no mobility of the fracture segments and good vascular supply at the fracture site. *It allows for direct reestablishment of the cortical bone.*

The primary/direct healing of the fracture occurs by direct remodelling of the lamellar bone, Haversian canals and blood vessels. Osteoclasts migrate to the fracture site and widen the Haversian systems, allowing osteoblasts to produce bone matrix—osteoid, which is eventually calcified into an organised *mature lamellar bone*. This cortical bridging takes 8 weeks and is completed in 16 weeks.

The formation of new bone (lamellar bone) along the fractured site in a cortical bone fracture occurs in two ways:

i. Gap healing.
ii. Contact healing.

GAP HEALING

Gaps are primarily filled with woven bone, which is then subsequently remodelled into lamellar bone—gap healing.

Even with rigid fixation, a perfect anatomic reduction rarely exists and small gaps do occur due to the deforming forces of the muscles. When the gaps are less than 800 μm to 1 mm, the fracture site is primarily filled by osteoblasts and then *by lamellar bone oriented perpendicular to the long axis*. This initial process of formation of lamellar bone takes over a period of 8 weeks, but the perpendicularly oriented lamellar

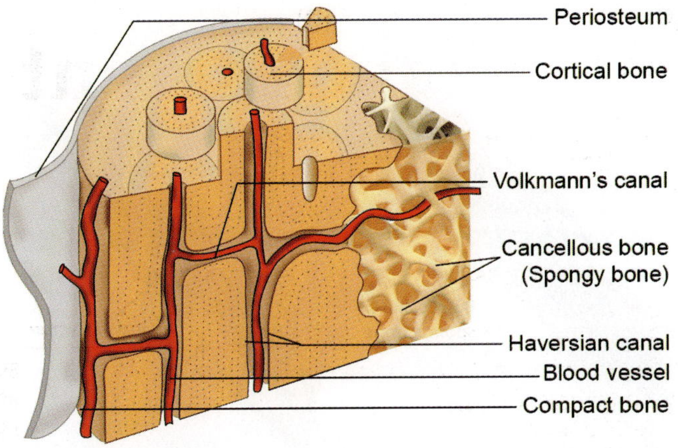

Figure 47.1 Anatomy of bone.

BOX 47.1 Bone Composition

1. Cells—osteocytes, osteoblasts, osteoclasts
2. Extracellular matrix
   a. Organic (35%)—collagen (type I), osteocalcin, osteonectin, proteoglycans, glycosaminoglycans
   b. Inorganic (65%)—primarily hydroxyapatite

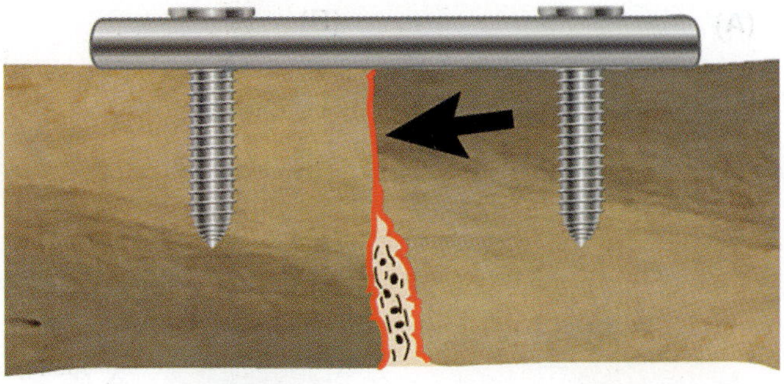

Figure 47.2 Contact and gap healing.

bone is weak and requires *secondary osteonal reconstruction* to reorient the lamellar bone longitudinally. Thus, in gap healing, gaps are filled by appositional bone formation followed by remodelling.

CONTACT HEALING

Healing of the fracture ends with lamellar bone immediately is known as contact healing.

When the gap between the bone ends is less than 0.01 mm and the interfragmentary strain is less than 2%, the fracture unites by contact healing. In these conditions, *cutting cones* consisting of osteoclasts are formed across the fracture site. These cutting cones generate longitudinal cavities at a rate of 50–100 mm/day. Osteoblasts fill these cavities with *Haversian system*, resulting in formation of *longitudinally oriented lamellar bone* and bony union. Remodelling of the lamellar bone results in healing without callus formation. Thus in contact healing, consolidation is achieved through Haversian remodelling alone.

Both gap and contact healing attempts to reestablish the anatomically correct position of the bone by the formation of competent lamellar bone (Fig. 47.2).

SECONDARY HEALING/INDIRECT FRACTURE HEALING

Secondary bone healing occurs through a process of *remodelling and intermediary callus formation* (Flowchart 47.1). It consists of a combination of intramembranous and endochondral ossification, but the end product is the same mature bone (lamellar) that is formed by primary healing.

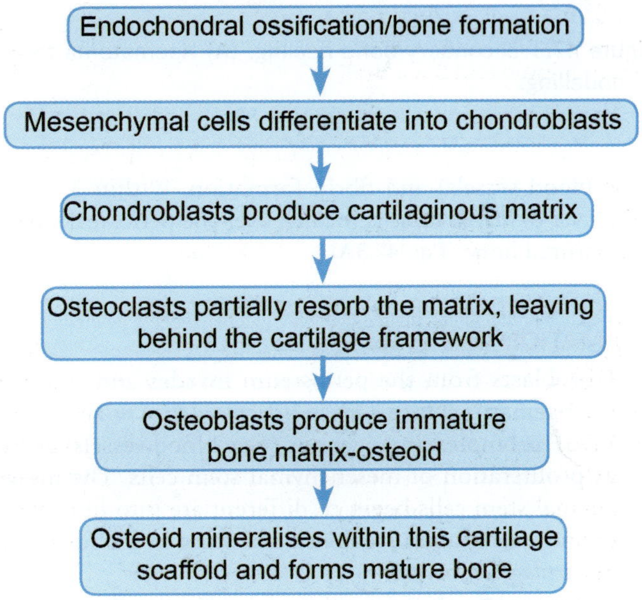

Flowchart 47.1 Secondary bone healing.

Secondary bone healing is the most common form of fracture healing and does not require anatomical reduction or rigid fixation. It takes an average of 4–6 weeks for initial healing and involves the following four phases: *(i) initial stage, (ii) cartilaginous callus, (iii) bony callus and (iv) remodelling.*

INITIAL STAGE/INFLAMMATION (1–5 DAYS)

This stage begins immediately following the fracture. The periosteum and the blood vessels supplying the bone are ruptured and a *haematoma* is formed throughout the fracture. This vascular compromise causes necrosis of bone at the fracture edges initially. It is followed by an inflammatory process by the macrophages, monocytes, neutrophils, platelets and inflammatory cytokines (TNF-α, BMP_s, IL). They act together and remove the damaged and necrotic tissue from the fractured site. Cytokines like vascular endothelial growth factor (VEGF) stimulate healing by enhancing angiogenesis

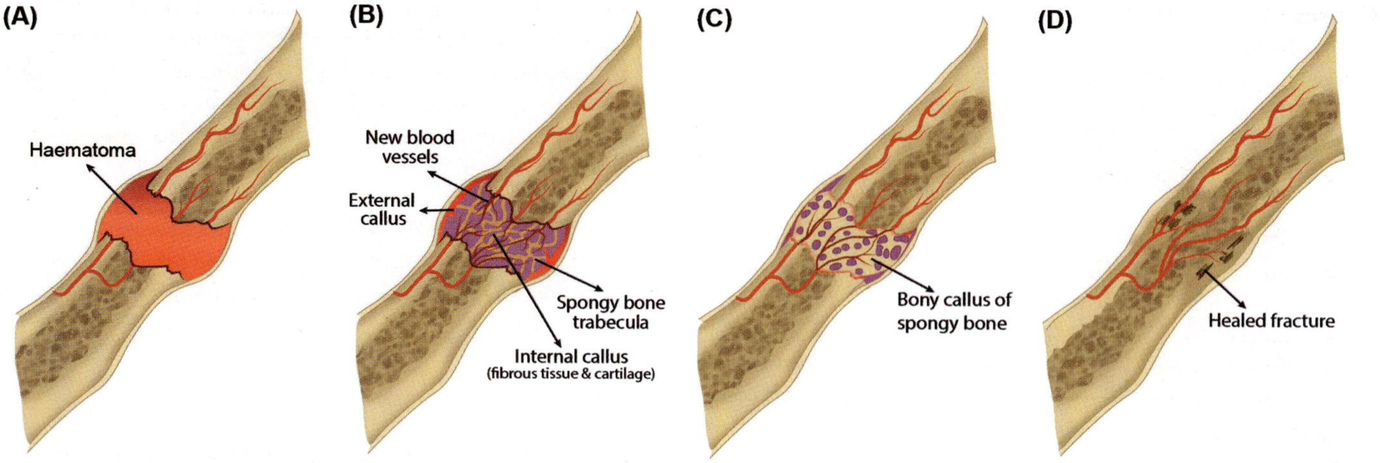

Figure 47.3 Secondary bone healing. **(A)** Haematoma formation. **(B)** Soft callus formation. **(C)** Hard callus formation. **(D)** Bone remodelling.

(new blood vessels) and fibrin formation. Within 3 days, a thin layer of *fibrous tissue* is formed over the periosteal surface of fractured bone (Fig. 47.3A).

FIBROCARTILAGINOUS CALLUS (SOFT CALLUS) FORMATION (2–3 WEEKS)

- Fibroblasts from the periosteum invades and colonises the haematoma into a *fibrin-rich granulation tissue*
- VEGF promotes angiogenesis (new blood vessels) as well as proliferation of mesenchymal stem cells. The mesenchymal stem cells begin to differentiate into fibroblasts, chondrocytes and osteoblasts resulting in the formation of *cartilaginous matrix*
- Subsequently, the haematoma is replaced with soft callus (*cartilaginous tissue*). This soft callus makes the *fracture site more stable* by increasing the strength and stiffness of bones and by eliminating the mobility across the fracture (Fig. 47.3B).

HARD CALLUS (BONY CALLUS) FORMATION (11–28 DAYS)

This stage involves the conversion of soft callus (cartilaginous tissue) into *bony callus/woven bone* through endochondral ossification. It starts from the periphery moving towards the centre and typically takes 3–4 weeks following injury. At the end of this phase, the soft callus is replaced with a *hard, calcified callus of immature bone (endochondral bone)* (Fig. 47.3C).

REMODELLING (MONTHS TO YEARS)

It is a stage of return of the osseous tissue to its preinjury state. The hard callus (woven bone) is remodelled into a *mature lamellar bone* (normal bone). The remodelling process is a balance of hard callus resorption by osteoclasts and lamellar bone deposition by osteoblasts. Though this process is initiated as early as 3–4 weeks, it may take years to be completed and to achieve a fully regenerated bone.

Bone healing occurs according to Wolff's law. He proposed that remodelling of a bone occurs in response to physical stresses from the soft tissue envelope and the muscles. Bone deposition occurs at the sites subjected to stress and bone resorption takes places at sites with little stress. It requires 4–6 months of remodelling of the mandible for the bone to reach its full load-bearing state (Fig. 47.3D).

Factors influencing fracture healing

Multiple factors affect the fracture healing, which can be broadly categorised into local and systemic (Table 47.1).

COMPLICATIONS IN BONE HEALING

1. Nonunion
2. Delayed union
3. Malunion
4. Osteomyelitis.

NONUNION

Nonunion is defined as a fracture in which the healing is delayed for more than 8 weeks. Clinically, the fracture lacks healing and the fragment is mobile.

TABLE 47.1 Factors that Affect Fracture Healing

Local Factors	Systemic Factors

• Blood supply
• Infection
• Fracture characteristics such as:
  • Excessive movement
  • Malalignment
  • Extent of damage
  • Soft tissue conditions
	• Age
	• Anaemia
	• Endocrine disorders—diabetes, parathyroid, etc.
	• Steroid
	• Malnutrition
	• Smoking

Causes of nonunion:

- Infection
- Improper reduction
- Inadequate immobilisation
- Interposition of soft tissue
- Delayed treatment
- Comminuted fractures
- Severe atrophic fractures
- Immunosuppression
- Inadequate blood supply
- Loss of bone or soft tissue
- Smoking and alcohol abuse
- Poor patient compliance.

Diagnostic considerations:

Clinically:

- Deformity at the fracture site
- Mobility of the fragment
- Persistent pain at the fracture site.

Radiographic findings

A persistent radiolucent line at the fracture or irregular radiolucency with mottled fracture ends. In later stages, the bone ends show rounding off and sclerosis of the ends, a condition referred as eburnation.

Types of nonunion

- Hypertrophic nonunion
- Atrophic nonunion
- Oligotrophic nonunion.

Management

The management of nonunion needs to be individualised and varies depending upon the factors that contributed to nonunion.

- Any infection present at the site needs to be controlled
- Debridement—of fibrous tissue, necrotic bone or failed hardware from the fracture site
- Immobilisation—the fracture is then stabilised with any form of rigid fixation (external or internal)
- Bone grafting—few cases may require bone grafting to fill the continuity defects.

In simple cases, healing becomes evident within 3 months.

DELAYED UNION

Delayed union occurs when a bone fails to unite within an anticipated time. Healing is considered delayed when the union takes longer than normally expected. Some authors have used the term *inadequate union* or *fibrous union* for delayed union. Though the healing process is still continuing, the outcome is uncertain.

Management

No active intervention is necessary in the short term. A fracture in which fibrous union has occurred will frequently progress to slow bony consolidation during the ensuring 12 months after injury. Fibrous union may be an acceptable result in an elderly edentulous patient. However, in a younger dentate, individual prosthetic replacement of missing teeth is impractical if any mobility at a fracture site remains and at some point nonunion has to be accepted and treated.

MALUNION/MALOCCLUSION

It is defined as healing of the bone in an abnormal position. It happens when the bone fragments are placed in an unsatisfactory position.

Causes:

- Mostly due to insufficient reduction
- Improper stabilisation—movement of the bone before complete healing has taken place
- Noncompliance of the patient.

Types:

- Simple—skeletal malalignment
- Complex—skeletal malalignment with soft tissue abnormality.

Clinically:

- Functional limitation
- Pain
- Deformity—bone being shorter than normal, twisted or bent.

Management:

- Osteotomy at the site of original fracture site and realignment of the fracture to its anatomically correct position. It is done to correct the malalignment
- Followed by stable fixation.

Malunion in mandibular fracture

Malunion in mandible is often due to inadequate anatomic reduction, poor adaptation of fixation plate and inadequately established occlusion.

Clinically, it is often diagnosed with malocclusion. Dental models can be used to study and plan the occlusion.

Management (Table 47.2)

- Resurgery to correct the malalignment
- Minor occlusal corrections are treated with orthodontic appliance.

BASIC PRINCIPLES IN THE TREATMENT OF A FRACTURE

The basic principles to ensure adequate treatment of fractures are as follows:

1. Anatomic reduction
2. Stable fixation
3. Immobilisation of fragment
4. Establish and preserve the occlusion
5. Early return of function
6. Avoidance of complications.

TABLE 47.2 Management of Early and Late Malunion

Early Malunions	Late Malunions
• Surgical approach is similar to the primary treatment • Removal of old hardware ↓ Occlusion is achieved ↓ MMF ↓ Fracture reduction and new fixation	• Surgical approach is based on type of osteotomy • Mock surgery can be done using study models • Osteotomy and refracture of the mandible ↓ Occlusion is achieved using surgical splints ↓ MMF ↓ New rigid fixation (bone grafts, if necessary)

TABLE 47.3 Indications and Contraindications of Closed Reduction

Indications	Contraindications
• Favourable, closed fractures with full dentition. • Grossly comminuted fractures. • Minimally displaced fractures. • Fractures exposed due to significant loss of overlying soft tissue. • Edentulous mandibular fractures. • Mandibular fractures in children with developing dentition. • Infected fractures.	• Severe asthma, respiratory disorders. • Chronic obstructive lung disease. • Gastrointestinal disorders. • Psychiatric or neurological problems. • Mentally retarded patients. • Seizures.

COMMONLY USED TERMS

OPEN REDUCTION

The exposure, reduction and fixation of the fracture under direct visualisation is known as open reduction. It involves exposure of the fracture through a surgical incision or the laceration and directly exploring the fracture site.

CLOSED REDUCTION

It refers to no direct visualisation of the fracture site. In closed reduction, the reduction and fixation are blind, which is achieved indirectly. In maxillofacial surgery, the most common and reliable method of closed treatment is Intermaxillary fixation(IMF)/Maxillomandibular fixation (MMF) IMF relies on the correct/preinjury positioning of the teeth.

CONSERVATIVE MANAGEMENT

It means no treatment of any kind, no surgical treatment. It can be considered as *wait and watch*, *nonsurgical* or *closed* treatment.

REDUCTION

CLOSED REDUCTION

It is an indirect or blind reduction of the fracture. The fracture fragments are aligned without surgery. In this method, reduction is done using the teeth position, palpation of the fragment, and postoperative radiographs as guides to check the accuracy of reduction. Closed reduction of mandible relies on teeth (occlusion), whereas the upper facial fractures (isolated zygoma, orbital or nasal fractures) relies on palpation of the fragment. Indications and contraindications of closed reductions are (Table 47.3) as follows:

Advantages:

- Simple to treat
- Less traumatic procedure
- Preserves the vascularity of the trauma site
- Less expensive
- Less operator sensitive
- Reduced risk of nerve injury and occlusal dysfunction.

Disadvantages:

- It requires a significant period of immobilisation as well as closure of the oral cavity
- Requires intact dentition
- Noncompliance of patient
- Reduced mouth opening
- Malocclusion
- Deviation on opening
- Temporomandibular joint (TMJ) pain and clicking.

Techniques of closed reduction:

Reduction by manipulation

The fracture fragments can be reduced by closed manipulation using instruments. The segments are reduced into occlusion.

Rowe's disimpaction forceps can be used to disimpact the fractured maxilla and bring it to occlusion. Maxilla with midpalatal split can be reduced by *Hayton William's forceps*. *Walsham's forceps* can be used to manipulate certain nasal fractures. *Asch's forceps* is used for septal fracture reduction (refer Chapter 52) (Figs. 47.4 and 47.5). Bristow's elevator, Rowe's elevator, Stacey bone hook and Carroll Girard device are the most commonly used instruments for indirect reduction of zygoma without exposure of the fracture site (Table 47.4).

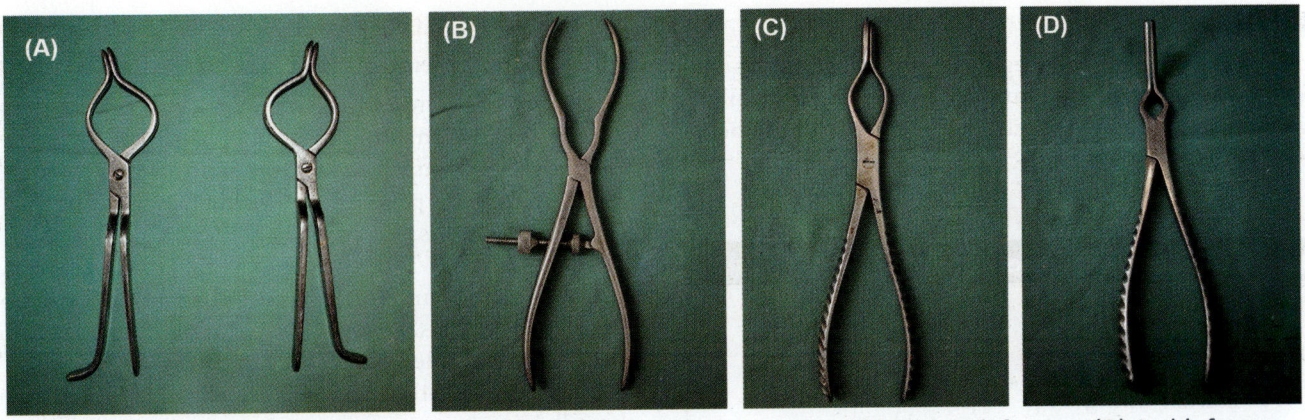

Figure 47.4 (**A**) Rowe's disimpaction forceps. (**B**) Hayton William's forceps. (**C**) Walsham's forceps. (**D**) Asch's forceps.

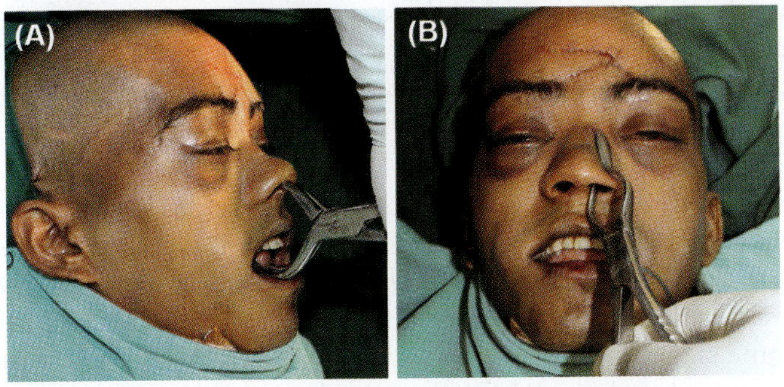

Figure 47.5 (**A**) Closed reduction of maxilla using Rowe's disimpaction forceps. (**B**) Nasal reduction using Walsham's forceps.

TABLE 47.4 Closed Reduction Devices

Maxilla	• Rowe's disimpaction forceps • Hayton-Williams' forceps • Walsham's forceps • Asch's forceps
Mandible	Intermaxillary fixation (IMF)
Zygomaticomaxillary complex (ZMC)	• Bristow's elevator • Rowe's elevator • Stacey bone hook • Carroll Girard device

Reduction by traction

Intraoral traction

It involves fixation of prefabricated arch bars to the maxillary and mandibular arches and traction of the segments to normal occlusion using elastics.

Extraoral traction

It involves anchorage from the intact skull for traction. The process of traction is extremely slow and the patient is encouraged to open and close the mouth to facilitate the elastic traction. After achieving satisfactory occlusion, elastics are removed and IMF is done with wires.

OPEN REDUCTION

Open reduction refers to exposure of the fracture through a surgical incision and reduction of the fracture under direct vision. Open reduction can produce excellent outcomes with low morbidity. For exposure of the fracture, an appropriate approach is selected by the surgeon based on the severity and location of the fracture. After adequate exposure of the fracture, the segments are reduced by various methods, including bone reduction forceps, manual anatomic reduction and a combination of these. The reduced segments are stabilised by internal fixation using wires, plates or screws. The open reduction and internal fixation (ORIF) has become the gold standard in maxillofacial injuries.

Indications:

- Displaced and unfavourable fractures
- Severely displaced edentulous fracture
- Unstable fractures or those with rotation or angulation
- Multiple fractures of the facial bones
- Midface fractures with displaced bilateral condylar fractures
- Edentulous maxilla opposing a mandibular fracture
- The presence of concomitant head trauma
- Delayed treatment of displaced fractures
- Malunited fractures
- Systemic conditions contraindicating IMF
- Cases with failed closed reduction.

Advantages:

- Allows for direct visualisation and reduction of fractured bone segments
- Restoration of the patient's preinjury occlusion
- Superior stabilisation of the fracture line
- Bony healing in a shorter period of time
- Early return to normal jaw function.

Disadvantages:

- Infections are more likely
- Few may be associated with increased morbidity due to changes in the vascularity at the time of surgery
- Risk of neurovascular damage.

FIXATION

In this, the reduced fracture segments are fixed to their anatomical position. Adequate fixation allows for early mobilisation and return to normal function. The fractured fragments can be fixed by direct or indirect methods (Box. 47.2).

BOX 47.2 Fixation Methods

Indirect/closed fixation

- **a)** IMF/MMF
  - Dental wiring
  - Arch bars
  - Intermaxillary fixation (IMF) screws
  - Splints
  - Bonded orthodontic brackets
- **b)** Suspension wires
  - Frontal—central or lateral
  - Circumzygomatic
  - Zygomatic buttress
  - Infraorbital
  - Pyriform aperture
- **c)** External fixation
  - Craniomandibular
    - **a.** Box frame
    - **b.** Halo frame
    - **c.** Plaster of Paris head cap
  - Craniomaxillary
    - **a.** Supraorbital pins
    - **b.** Zygomatic pins
    - **c.** Halo frame

Direct/internal fixation

- **a)** Nonrigid fixation
  - Transosseous wiring
- **b)** Semi-rigid fixation
  - Miniplates
- **c)** Rigid fixation
  - Compression osteosynthesis (DCP, EDC and lag screw)
  - Noncompression osteosynthesis (locking plate, reconstruction plate and THORP)

INDIRECT/CLOSED FIXATION

Intermaxillary fixation (IMF/MMF)

It refers to reduction of the maxilla and mandible into occlusion (maximum intercuspation) with the aid of wires. The dentition is used as a stable point. MMF is the basic and fundamental principle in the management of the maxillofacial fractures. It serves as a cornerstone, providing a stable base from which the facial form and function can be restored. It helps in reestablishing the patient's premorbid occlusion and also assists in reduction and fixation of simple and complex facial fractures.

A variety of MMF techniques are available, which includes the following:

1) Dental wiring
2) Arch bars
3) IMF screws
4) Splints
5) Bonded orthodontic brackets.

Dental wiring (1918–1968)

It is used when the patient has a complete or almost complete set of suitable teeth. The most commonly used wire is soft *stainless-steel wire of gauge 24 G (0.45 mm). The wire should be stretched to about 10% before use.* If not done, the wires will become slack (loose) in a few days. Overstretching of the wire makes it brittle and difficult to work.

Various techniques of wiring have been followed:

- Direct interdental wiring (Gilmer's wiring)
- Interdental eyelet wiring (Ivy's loop method)
- Continuous or multiple loop wiring
- Risdon's wiring
- Bridle wire.

Direct interdental wiring (Gilmer's wiring)

Dr. Thomas Gilmer of Chicago (1881) was the 1st person to advocate IMF for complex maxillomandibular fractures through dental bands or wires fastened directly to the necks of teeth. It provides a simple and rapid method of immobilisation of the jaws.

Technique

A prestretched wire of 15 cm in length is taken and the middle portion of the wire is twisted around a tooth. The free ends of the wire are twisted together to form a 3 cm plaited tail. Similarly, other teeth in the upper and lower jaw are also twisted with wires. The fracture is reduced and the plaited ends of the wire in the upper and lower jaws are twisted together.

The disadvantage of this technique is that the IMF wires are connected to the teeth itself. Hence, it is difficult to release the IMF connection without stripping off all the fixation (Fig. 47.6A).

Interdental eyelet wiring (Ivy's loop method)

Robert Ivy (1918) used eyelets between two teeth in the upper and lower jaw. Around five eyelets in each jaw, and a 3rd tie

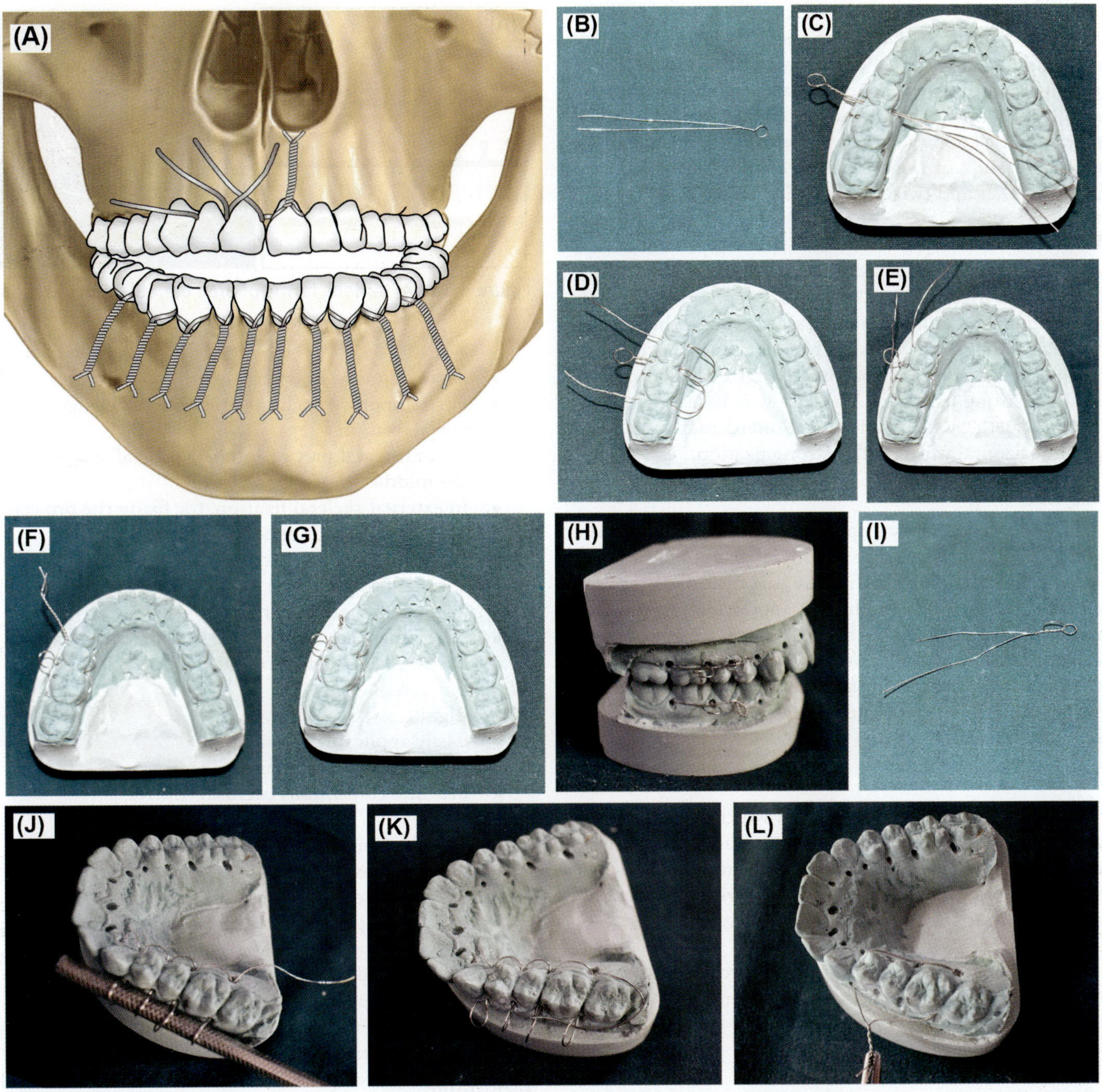

Figure 47.6 (**A**) Gilmer's wiring. (**B–H**) Interdental eyelet wiring (Ivy's method). (**I**) Williams' modification of Ivy's loop. (**J** and **K**) Multiple loop wiring. (**L**) Bridle wire.

wire was passed through the eyelets of the upper and lower jaw and twisted tightly for complete immobilisation.

Eyelets are formed by making a *loop (3 mm diameter)* at the centre of each wire, *with three or four twists*. The edges of the wire are trimmed off to uniform lengths with sharp points, so that it can be passed through the interproximal area smoothly. Tie wires are generally tightened in the molar area, 1st on one side and then on the other side, and then in the incisor area. It offers excellent reduction and immobilisation, and IMF can be released by removing the tie wires alone (Fig. 47.6B–H).

Continuous or multiple loop wiring

Colonel Roy A. Stout described this technique of wiring in which blocks of teeth (posterior part) in either jaw is wired and elastic traction is used to reduce the fracture. A piece of wire is adapted to the buccal surface of the teeth, and the other end is brought distally to the 2nd molar and taken around the teeth on the lingual side. It is then passed through the interdental space and around the buccal wire of the remaining teeth in a sequential manner enclosing a quadrant. The loops formed are twisted to form eyelets. Finally, the ends of the wire lying on the buccal side are pulled together and twisted (Fig. 47.6J and K).

Risdon's wiring

Risdon of Toronto proposed a heavier form of continuous wiring. In this method, the 2nd molars are chosen for anchorage on either side. A long wire is passed around the neck of 2nd molar and both the ends are brought to the buccal side. The ends are twisted for the entire length till the midline forming a strong base wire. The base wire is secured to the individual teeth by using additional interdental wires. This type of horizontal wiring offers strong fixation.

Bridle wire

It was first advocated by Hippocrates for reduction of the mandibular fractures. A single wire is placed around the necks of the teeth adjacent to the fracture, the fracture is reduced manually and the wire is tightened approximating the fracture. In case the adjacent teeth are loose, decayed or avulsed, the nearest stable teeth is chosen. This helps in temporary stabilisation of the fragment and prevents further soft tissue damage, mobility of the fragments, and protects the airway (Fig. 47.6L).

Arch bar

Arch bars are flat stainless-steel bars, which are secured to teeth to encourage jaw healing in correct alignment. These arch bars are available in suitable lengths and have hooks or notches to assist in maintenance of IMF wires. There are different types of arch bars (Table 47.5 and Fig. 47.7).

Uses:

- Dentoalveolar fractures requiring arch stabilisation
- At the alveolar level it acts as 'tension band'
- For MMF
- In undisplaced fractures
- Closed reduction of fractures

TABLE 47.5 Types of Arch Bar

Prefabricated	Custom made (prepared individually for a specific patient)
• Jelenko • German silver bar • Erich	• Acrylic • Cast silver • Schuchardt's acrylic arch bar • Stanhope's modification of Schuchardt • Directly bonded arch bar

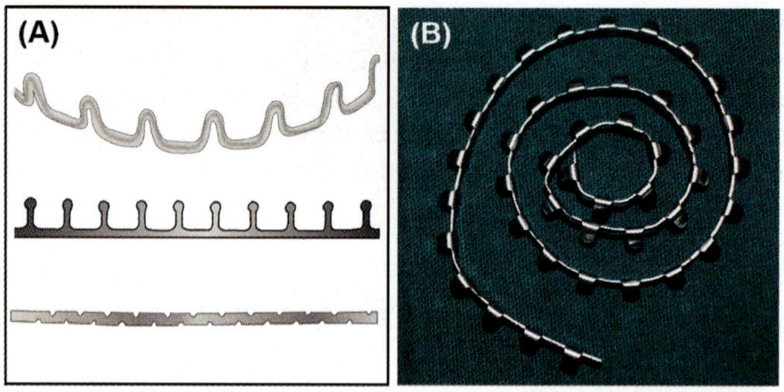

Figure 47.7 (**A**) Various forms of arch bar. (**B**) Erich's arch bar.

- As an adjuvant in open reduction of fractures
- For temporary occlusal orientation during rigid internal fixation
- As an integral part of internal skeletal suspension in the middle 3rd of the fractures
- In external skeletal fixation, for fixing the projection bar, custom-made arch bars are needed
- For using elastics to correct minor occlusal discrepancy and to guide the mandibular motion, especially in subcondylar fractures
- When there are insufficient teeth for eyelet wiring
- Discontinuity defects requiring occlusal control.

Advantages:

- Rigid
- Easily applicable and adaptable
- Prefabricated or custom-made
- Provides continuous occlusal control.

Disadvantages:

- Difficulty in oral hygiene maintenance
- Lip or gingival injury
- Risk of penetrating injury to the surgeon
- Improper application can result in fracture displacement or tooth movement
- Not applicable for edentulous arch spans
- Prolonged operating time
- Interference with computed tomography (CT) imaging/ Magnetic resonance imaging (MRI).

Technique

Arch bar adaptation

Arch bars are cut to the required length, bent and adapted to the dental arch. Stainless steel ligature wires of 0.45 mm or 0.35 mm of 6 inch (15 cm) can be used to adapt the arch bar. The fracture fragment is reduced and arch bar is adapted.

Securing arch bar

The arch bar should be oriented with the open hooks facing the gums. Using individual wires, the arch bar is tied to each tooth, from midline to successive teeth on each side moving backwards to the 3rd molar. This way helps in preventing minor discrepancies in wiring and produces close adaptation of the bar to the dental arch. *Each wire is passed over the arch bar mesially, around the tooth and under the bar distally (over/under technique)*. The two ends are apically pulled and twisted together. The twisted wire is then cut and tucked into position towards the bar without irritating the tissues.

Maxillomandibular fixation

IMF is achieved using wires or orthodontic elastic bands between the fleets of the upper and lower arch bar. Before tightening the wires, the occlusion should be checked and any tongue impingement relieved. The wires are then pulled, tightened and cut in such a way, that the sharp ends of the wire are twisted and angled into the interdental area to avoid any soft tissue injury.

Intermaxillary fixation screws (MMF/IMF screws)

The use of *cortical bone screw fixation* for treating mandibular fractures was 1st introduced by Karlis and Glickman. The self-tapping intermaxillary screws were 1st introduced by Arthur and Berardo in 1989 and later modified by *Carl Jones*.

Uses:

- MMF screws act as bone anchors during the establishment of occlusion
- It shortens the way to achieve IMF.

Screw design:

IMF screws are made of stainless steel/titanium. The screw head is elongated with two holes where the wire can be passed for IMF and a pointed tip. They are *self-drilling and self-tapping screws*. Self-tapping screws require pilot holes or predrilling during placement, whereas self-drilling screws does not need pilot holes (Table 47.6 and Fig. 47.8).

Screw site selection:

The anatomical site for the placement of MMF screws is chosen with respect to the fracture location, dentition and the availability of bone around the fracture line. The *anterior vestibular regions as well as the canine and premolar regions* of both jaws are considered as ideal, because these areas are conveniently accessible and supply an appropriate bone stock away from the tooth root (Table 47.7). OPG (Orthopantomogram) and CT scans act as a guideline in bypassing the tooth roots, maxillary antrum, mandibular canal or mental foramen with preciseness.

IMF screws can provide *'4-point' fixation* in these regions.

Areas to be avoided:

- Alveolar process close to the tooth roots
- Densely approximated dental roots (molars and lower anteriors)
- Interradicular spaces of the mandibular or maxillary molars
- Soft tissue coverage:
  - The lower vestibular sulcus height is decreased due to the muscle attachment, which may bury the screw head into the mucosa. To avoid this, the screw is pierced angulating downward onto the mental protuberance
  - The soft tissues in the mandibular premolar region surround the mental foramen, hence must be avoided.

Technique:

- Screw placement can be done under local or general anaesthesia
- MMF screws are inserted in two ways: Either through a perforation of the *closed mucosa (transmucosal)* or an *open approach exposing the bone* surface. The puncture can be placed with an electrocautery needle, a No. 11-blade or a 1-mm punch
- Holes are drilled with a slow-speed handpiece under copious irrigation directly through the thin mucoperiosteal layer for self-tapping screws. Self-drilling screws are driven into the bone by hand without any preparation
- The MMF screws are inserted till the screw tips penetrate the inner cortical layer. The screw heads should not be submerged into the mucosa and the stability of each individual screw is checked. A minimum of four screws are required for IMF
- After achieving the required occlusion, the ends of the tie wire are passed through the holes in the screw heads of the upper and lower jaw and twisted tightly

TABLE 47.6 IMF Screw

Material	Size (Head Diameter)	Thread Diameter	Length
Stainless steel/titanium	4–5 mm	2 mm	6–12 mm

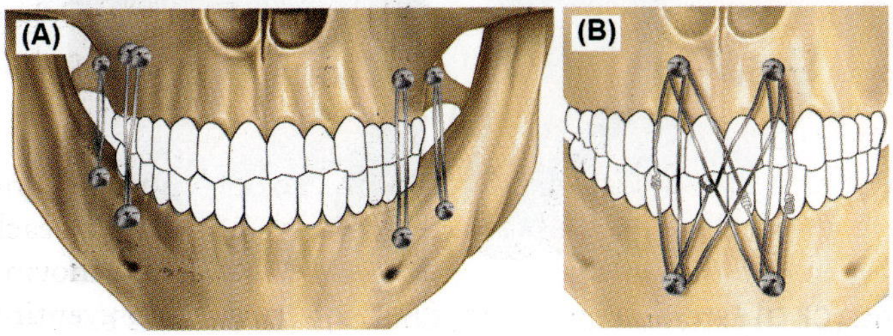

Figure 47.8 (**A** and **B**) Maxillomandibular fixation using IMF screws.

TABLE 47.7 Safe Areas for IMF Placement

Anterior maxilla	Pyriform rim below the nasal spine and above the dental apices
Anterior mandible	Symphysis and parasymphysis area underneath the incisor and canine root apex
Posterior maxilla	Zygomatico maxillary crest
Posterior mandible	Solid buttress bone on the mandibular outer cortex

- Removal of MMF screws after completion of therapy can be done with a screwdriver.

Indications:

- Emergency cases
- In contagious patients, as an alternative to arch bars
- Simple fractures of fully dentate mandible/maxilla
- For orthognathic or reconstructive surgery
- Alveolar process fractures
- In palatal fractures, to prevent the arches from tilting, collapsing or widening
- In complete edentulism, IMF screws can be placed through the existing dentures.

Contraindications:

- Severely comminuted and displaced fractures
- Unstable segmented fractures
- Children with tooth buds
- Patients with multiple mobile teeth
- Severe atrophied bone and highly pneumatised maxillae
- Pathologically affected bone
- Congenital or acquired bleeding disorders
- In patients where MMF is generally contraindicated such as epilepsy, chronic alcoholism, obstructive airway disease, psychiatric disorders, gastric reflux and anorexia.

Advantages:

- The simplicity of the procedure
- Shorter operating time, cost-effective
- Minimal amount of hardware in the oral cavity
- Improved comfort and oral hygiene
- Suitable for application in patients with extensive prosthodontic restorations
- Compatible with open reduction
- Painless and fast removal.

Disadvantages:

- Technique sensitive
- Risk of injuring tooth roots
- Soft tissue burying of screw heads
- Loosening of screw
- Interference with the upper incisor edges
- Lack of tension band effect
- Interference with internal fixation plates

Splints (1866–1918)

Splints are used to stabilise the upper and lower jaws in normal occlusion. Till the beginning of the 20th century, dental splints were the mainstay in closed treatment of fractures. In 1868, *Gunning* introduced dental splints made of *vulcanite* for treating fractures of the jaw. However, these were contraindicated in fractures posterior to the teeth as they often resulted in open bite. *G.V. Black combined vulcanite splint with circumferential wiring* of the bone to immobilise an edentulous mandibular fracture. In late 19th century, *Simon P. Hullihen* described a *continuous dental splint* made of metal, vulcanite, celluloid or hard rubber, which was moulded over a plaster or metal reproduction of the dentures.

The development of dental casts enabled the use of metal splints such as silver or aluminium in treating maxillofacial injuries. The making of splints, however, generally took several days and often resulted in unfavourable outcomes for patients, such as nonunion or malunion. Polymer (methyl methacrylate) was 1st used in 1940 for oral splints in the treatment of jaw fractures.

Types of splints

Extraoral splints

These splints surround externally and support the broken bone (head bandaging, halo appliance and chin cap). The head/chin strap is one of the oldest types and are used only for temporary immobilisation in exceptional situations. They are insufficiently stable and can obstruct breathing if it slips (Fig. 47.9C&D).

Intraoral splints

These splints are attached to the teeth (cap splints) or are placed on the edentulous jaw in a similar fashion to a prosthesis (denture splinting).

Cap splints

Cap splints are made of acrylic and cover the teeth completely.

Indications

- Extensive and advanced periodontal disease
- Fractures with substantial soft-tissue loss, splints helps in retaining the remaining tooth-bearing segments and soft tissue healing

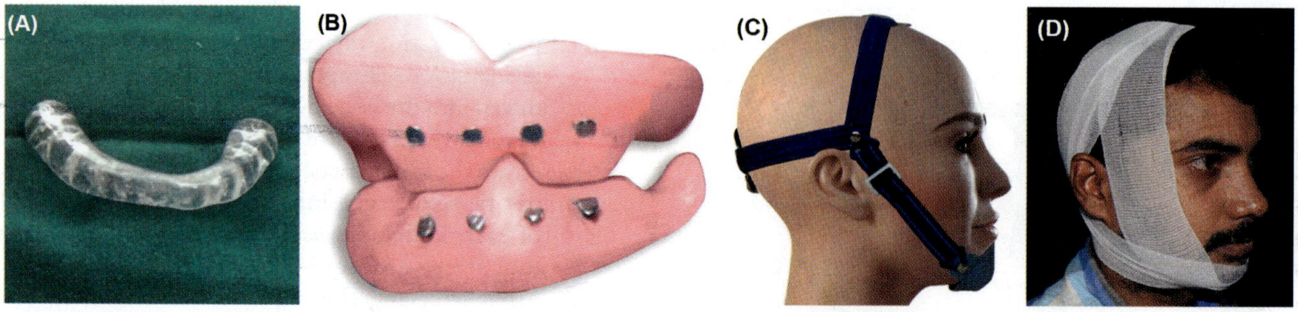

Figure 47.9 **(A&B)** Intraoral splints - **(A)** Cap splint; **(B)** Gunning's splint. **(C&D)** Extraoral splints - **(C)** Chin cap; **(D)** Barton's bandage

- Splinting of luxated teeth
- Extraoral fixation of complicated fractures.

The cap splints can be fabricated either by taking impression of the jaw or with the help of an articulator. These splints can be secured to the teeth either by cement, circumferential wiring or with osteosynthetic screws (Fig. 47.9A).

Denture splints

In edentulous patients, *Gunning splints* and *denture splints* are routinely used for reduction and stabilisation of the fractured segments (refer Chapter 49). In denture splints, the patient's denture can be used for immobilisation. These dentures are securely fixed using circumferential wiring of the mandible or by suspension wiring firmly fixed to the maxilla and then connected to each other with wire ligatures (Fig. 47.9B).

Combined extraoral and intraoral splints

Extraoral splinting is combined with intraoral splinting.

Bonded modified orthodontic brackets

Fractures with minimal displacement can be immobilised using orthodontic brackets on the teeth and intermaxillary elastic bands. Small hooks are welded to the orthodontic brackets and bonded to the selected teeth in each jaw with composite resin. IMF is then achieved by elastic bands applied to the hooks.

Skeletal wiring/suspension wires

In 1980s, suspension wires with MMF were commonly used for immobilisation of midface fractures. Wires were dropped down from the orbit, zygoma or stable bone structures adjacent to or above the fractured site, to suspend the occluded tooth-bearing segment.

Indications

- Closed reduction of edentulous or partially dentate patients
- Children with primary or early mixed dentition
- Panfacial trauma or complex wounds
- Gunshot injuries.

Disadvantages:

- Three-dimensional stability not obtained. Suspensory wires create only a vertical vector, which precludes control of sagittal direction—a major limitation
- Tightening of the suspension wire forces the midface towards the cranial base, which results in vertical shortening and retruded midface
- Incomplete fixation of fracture fragments
- Insufficient visualisation of fracture
- Patient discomfort.

Skeletal suspension wiring techniques:

- Circumzygomatic
- Zygomatic buttress
- Frontal—central
- Frontal—lateral
- Infraorbital
- Pyriform aperture suspension.

Central (frontal suspension)

This technique was introduced by *Kufner* and is of minimal significance (Fig. 47.10A).

Lateral (Adam)

The zygomatic process of the frontal bone is exposed through an incision made in the lateral 3rd of the eyebrow just above the frontozygomatic suture. *A hole is drilled 5 mm above the frontozygomatic suture in the posterior direction towards the infratemporal region*. Stainless steel wire of 0.5 mm diameter is passed through this hole. Using an *awl*, the wire is passed beneath the zygomatic arch to enter into the *buccal sulcus* intraorally where it is secured to the arch bar (Fig. 47.10B).

Circumzygomatic suspension

The zygomatic arch is used as the stable bone for suspension. The wire is passed as a sling around the arch using a bone awl. The free ends are exited through buccal vestibule opposing the 1st molar and fastened to maxillary and/or mandibular arch bars.

An awl is introduced extraorally at the junction of zygomatic and temporal bone medial to the zygomatic arch in a downward and forward direction into the buccal sulcus intraorally. A 0.5 mm diameter stainless steel wire is attached to the tip of the awl and the instrument is withdrawn to lie just above the zygomatic arch without emerging out from the skin. Now the instrument is passed on the lateral aspect of the zygomatic arch in the same direction as previously mentioned. The free ends of the wire are secured to the arch bar (Fig. 47.10C).

Zygomatic buttress suspension

A 3 cm incision is made in the region of premolar and molar in the depth of the vestibular sulcus. Blunt dissection is done to expose the inferior border of the zygomatic buttress. Using a bur, a hole is drilled on the *zygomatic buttress and a 0.5 mm diameter stainless steel wire* is passed through it. The two ends of the wire are then attached to suitable loops of the arch bar.

Infraorbital

A 3 cm vestibular incision is made in the region of the canine and dissected subperiosteally to expose the inferior orbital margin lateral to the infraorbital foramen. Using a bur, a hole is drilled in an *upward and posterior direction*; and the wire is passed through the hole, withdrawn into the mouth and attached to the arch bar (Fig. 47.10D).

Pyriform aperture

A 2 cm transverse incision is made in the upper labial sulcus above the lateral incisor tooth and the *pyriform aperture* of the

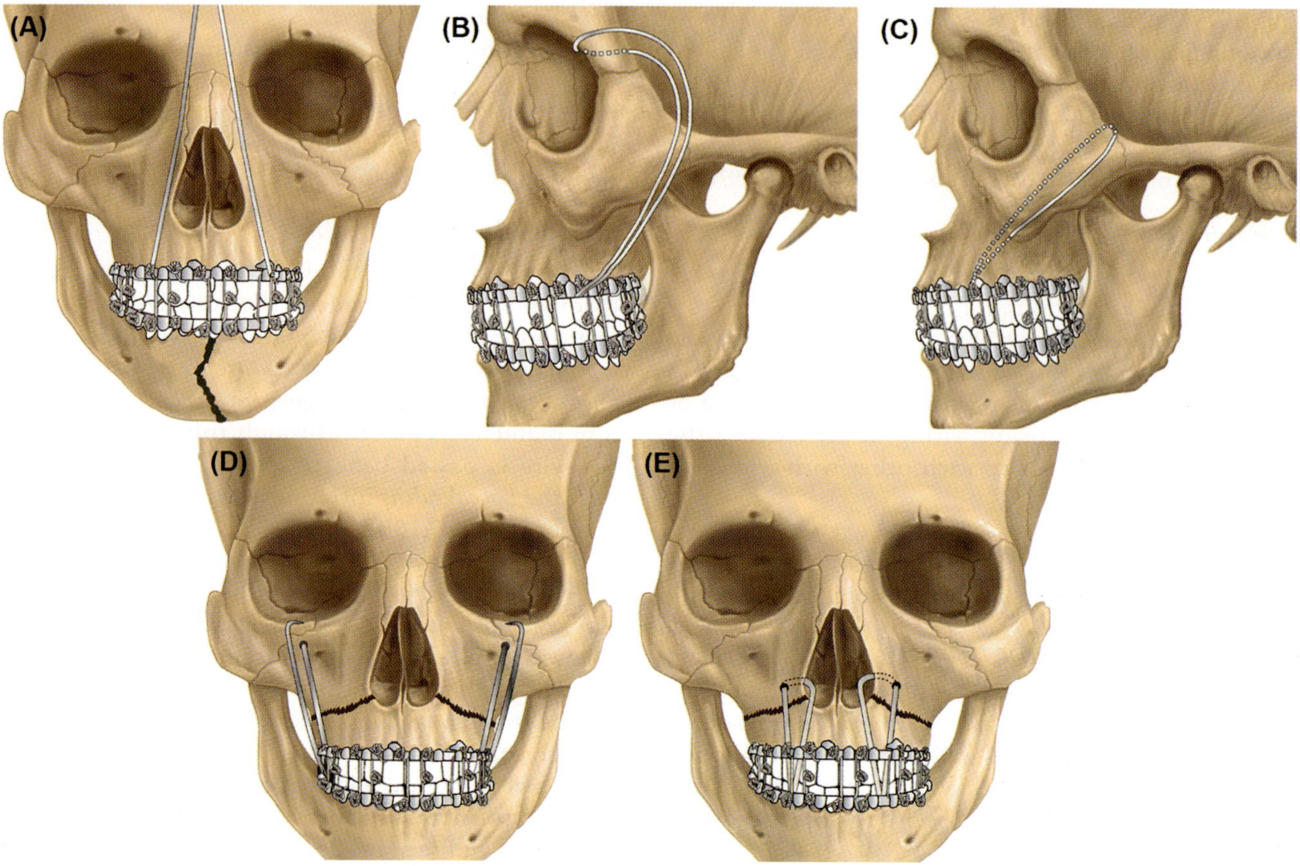

Figure 47.10 (**A**) Frontal suspension. (**B**) Adam's suspension. (**C**) Circumzygomatic suspension. (**D**) Infraorbital suspension. (**E**) Pyriform aperture.

nose is exposed by elevating the periosteum. The nasal mucosa is elevated and protected using a periosteal elevator. A hole is drilled 1 cm away from the free margin of the pyriform aperture from the medial to lateral side. A wire is passed through this hole and the ends are tied to the arch bar (Fig. 47.10E).

Per alveolar suspension

A Gunning's type of splint is used and the position of holes on the palatal aspect of the splint is marked on the underlying palatal mucosa. *Per alveolar awl* is passed through the alveolus in the buccal sulcus, piercing the palate at the marked position. Using an awl, the wire is passed through this hole on the palatal surface and withdrawn through the buccal sulcus. The two ends of the wire are twisted over the Gunning's type splint and turned over.

External fixation

External fixation is a method by which the bone segments are held in place by percutaneous wires attached to an external frame (e.g. box frame, halo frame and plaster of paris head cap) (Box 47.3 and Fig. 47.11).

Craniomaxillary fixation—fixation of upper jaw to the cranial vault using rods and universal joints.

BOX 47.3 External Fixation Methods

Craniomaxillary fixation

- **a.** Supraorbital pins
- **b.** Zygomatic pins
- **c.** Halo frame

Craniomandibular fixation

- **a.** Box frame
- **b.** Halo frame
- **c.** Plaster of Paris head cap

Craniomandibular fixation—fixation of mandible to the cranial vault with the middle third sandwiched between them.

Indications:

- Extensively comminuted fractures
- Infected fracture line
- Severely atrophic mandibles
- Edentulous mandibular fractures
- Severe soft tissue injury

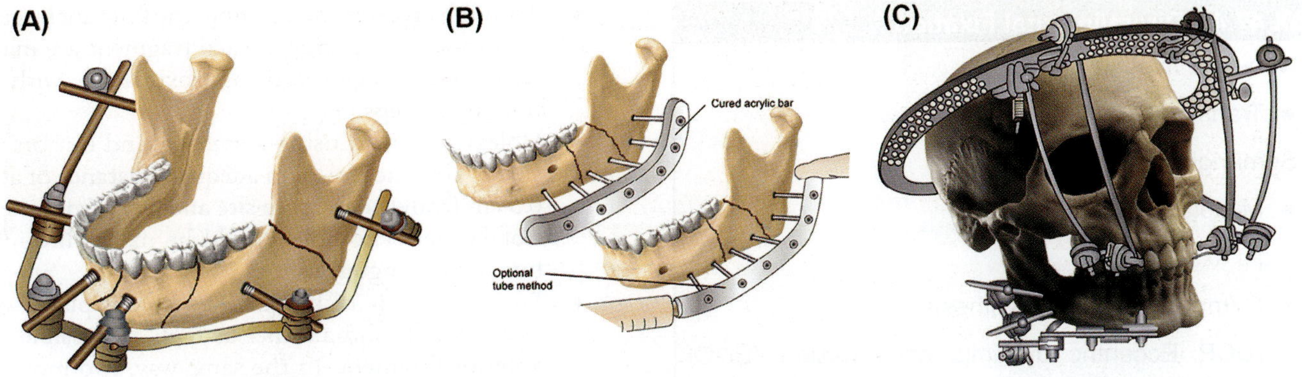

Figure 47.11 (**A**) External pin fixation. (**B**) Joe Hall Morris' appliance. (**C**) Halo frame.

- Complex Le Fort fractures
- Medically unstable patients for major surgeries.

External pin fixation consists of stainless steel or titanium pins screwed into the prepared holes of bones. After reduction, these pins are linked by a connecting rod to the universal joints. These rods are also attached to the lower cap splints. This type of fixation is not rigid and often supplemented with IMF.

Bone clamps

The fracture segments are secured by clamps attached to the lower border of the mandible and from these clamps the pins project, which are connected by external rods as in the case of external pin fixation. This system, best known as *Brenthurst splint*, was used in the past and is rarely used now.

Kirschner's wires

After reduction, the wire is passed from the fracture side cortex and passed through the medullary cavity of the undamaged bone on the other side of the fracture.

Halo frames

It is mainly indicated for supraorbital fractures requiring a higher point of fixation in the cranium. It consists of a circular frame, which encircles the head and is attached to the skull by means of four pins. The screw pins engage only the outer table of the skull. The halo is linked to the anterior projection bar of cap splint by stainless steel rods and universal joints (Fig. 47.11C).

Disadvantage—it projects backwards from the head and prevents the patient from lying down comfortably on the back of the head.

Box frame

The box frame is a rigid form of craniomandibular fixation. Two pins are inserted into the supraorbital and mandible regions, respectively. These four pins are connected by rods and universal joints. It does not require an anterior connecting bar.

Plaster of Paris head cap

Use of plaster of Paris as a head cap is being replaced by the recent techniques. This is useful in cases where there is extensive fracture of the cranial vault that cannot be managed by halo frames or pins. The construction of the head cap should be accurately fitting and comfortable since an ill-fitting or uncomfortable head cap may not serve the purpose. To construct a head cap, plaster of Paris bandage is immersed in water. The 1st bandage is surrounded tightly around the head. The 2nd bandage is applied higher up in the forehead surrounding the occiput. Now, a retention framework is attached to it by means of a 3rd bandage.

This method is used for patients with fractures involving the middle 3rd along with cranial vault where the halo frame cannot be applied. It can also be used for patients who are contraindicated for general anaesthesia because of trauma to the chest or other reasons. Alternately, plaster of Paris head-chin cap can also be applied wherein the fractured maxilla is suspended in between the skull and the mandible.

DIRECT/INTERNAL FIXATION (ORIF)

Internal or direct fixation refers to placement of stainless steel wires, rods, plate, screws or other hardware directly onto the bones for stabilisation of the fracture. Internal fixation can be rigid or nonrigid depending on the nature of the fracture and the type and strength of hardware placed (Box 47.4).

Nonrigid fixation

It is the fixation that allows movement between the bone fragments along the fracture line (interfragmentary motion). Nonrigid fixation serves only in approximating/realigning the fracture fragments and prevents their displacement by the muscles. It usually requires a short duration of supportive MMF for adequate stabilisation of the fractures. The healing of the fracture occurs by secondary intention.

Transosseous wiring

In 1847, Fauchard and Buck commenced the use of transosseous wiring with silver wires. Transosseous wiring refers to direct wiring across the fracture line, which can be done through

BOX 47.4 Direct/Internal Fixation
1. Non-rigid fixation
• Transosseous wiring
2. Semi-rigid fixation
• Miniplates
3. Rigid fixation
• Compression osteosynthesis
(DCP, Eccentric dynamic compression (EDC) and lag screw)
• Noncompression osteosynthesis
(locking plate, reconstruction plate and THORP)

an intraoral or extraoral approach. It is affordable, easy to use and biologically well tolerated by the patients. Most of the time, it is associated with IMF. It is an effective method of fixation for angle of mandible fracture. In the midface, it can be done at the frontonasal suture, orbital rim, zygomatico-maxillary sutures, zygomatic bone and alveolus (Fig. 47.12).

Indications:

- Closed reduction is impossible
- Unfavourable edentulous fractures
- Inadequate teeth for MMF
- Complex fractures.

Advantages:

- Economical
- Patient compliance
- Minimal equipment.

Disadvantages:

- It does not provide three-dimensional stability
- Micro movement at the fracture site
- It may result in nonunion, malunion or delayed union
- It may take longer period to regain the preinjury mouth opening.

Technique:

- Transosseous wiring is commonly done at the angle of mandible and symphysis region
- Through an extraoral incision, the fracture fragments are exposed. The ends of each fragment are manipulated and brought into approximation with bone holding forceps
- Holes are drilled using a small round bur on either side of the fracture at an adequate distance of at least 0.5 cm from the fracture site and away from the inferior border. The hole should be made through the buccal and lingual cortex
- For a four-hole technique, one hole is placed at the lower border and another as high as possible in the anterior fragment. In the same way, two more holes are made in the posterior fragment
- One wire is passed into the No. 1 hole of the anterior fragment from the buccal to lingual cortex and from the lingual to buccal cortex at the posterior fragment (No. 4 hole). Then another wire is passed through the No. 2 hole and brought out from the No. 3 hole. Both these wires are twisted individually in a crisscross manner after approximating the fragments
- Usually a single lower border wire is not sufficient to stabilise the fractured segments, especially when the fracture line is oblique. These segments tend to override. In such cases, a figure-of-eight wiring along with the conventional wiring is done
- Wound closure is done in layers. IMF is done postoperatively for additional stability.

Transosseous wires can be applied on the upper border or the lower border of the mandible depending upon the type of fracture.

Upper border (alveolus)—mandibular angle or edentulous body fracture.

Inferior border—grossly displaced angle fracture, edentulous fracture and malunited fractures. With the methods and materials available today, *nonrigid fixation is no longer in use.*

Semi-rigid fixation

Semi-rigid fixation refers to the fixation of fracture fragments with noncompression miniplates that provide some degrees of rigidity, though not sufficient enough for the jawbones to withstand masticatory forces. It usually requires a short duration of supportive MMF for immobilisation.

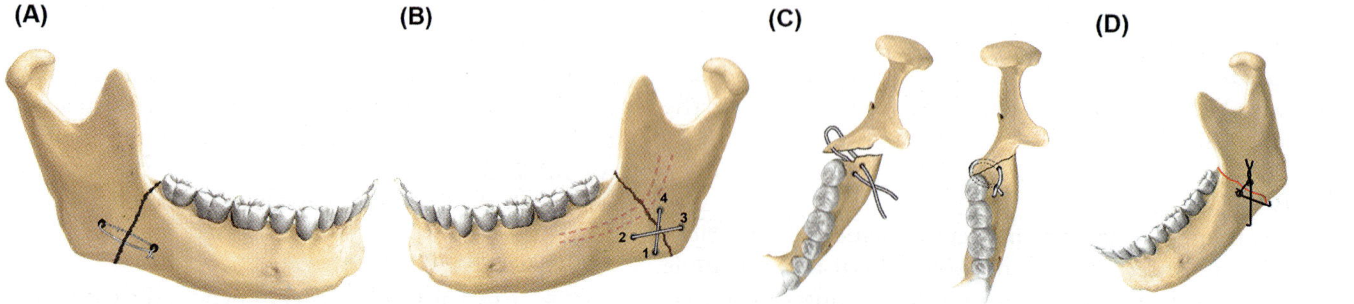

Figure 47.12 Various types of transosseous wiring. (A) Simple transosseous wiring. (B) Figure-of-eight wiring. (C) Transosseous wiring of the upper border of the mandible. (D) Lower border wiring: Hayton-Williams' modification.

Champy's line of osteosynthesis

In the early 1970s, Michelet et al., first applied Vitallium miniplates for mandibular fractures and reported favourable clinical outcomes. Champy et al., modified Michelet's technique and provided a biomechanical basis for the treatment. He advocated 'semi-rigid fixation' with miniplates based upon the ideal lines of osteosynthesis. *The ideal lines of osteosynthesis are the lines of maximum tensile stress*, extending from the oblique ridge along the base of the alveolus to the mental foramen. Champy hypothesised that a single miniplate, placed at the ideal line of osteosynthesis, is sufficient enough to cope with the tensile stresses and also provide adequate stabilisation of the mandibular fractures and achieve predictable union (Fig. 47.13).

Under function, the mandible exhibits tensile forces at the superior border and compression at the inferior border of mandible. *The displacement of the fragments is caused by the tensional forces along the upper border. Hence, Champy's method of monocortical miniplate fixation at the superior border provides enough stability* to withstand the tensile forces and also favour osteosynthesis.

The *monocortical, noncompression, miniplates* can be inserted intraorally and are fixed with monocortical mini screws. When placed along the Champy's line of osteosynthesis, they achieve maximum stability and osteosynthesis. This osteosynthesis is achieved by neutralising undesirable tensile forces, while retaining favourable compression forces during function. He believed that compression plates are unnecessary because the masticatory forces produce a natural strain of compression along the inferior border of the mandible. This stability is achieved by *load-sharing fixation* and these plates are commonly used in simple fracture patterns having an acceptable amount of bone stock.

Areas of plate application

Champy calculated the forces applied to these plates under physiological strain and produced the most desirable shape of minimum thickness and reasonable malleability to neutralise the harmful tension forces that cause displacement of the fracture segments.

- For fractures anterior to the mental foramen or 1st premolar, two plates separated by 4–5 mm are required to prevent the torsional movements at the symphysis region. The inferior plate is adapted 1st, followed by the sub-apical one
- For fractures posterior to the mental foramen (1st premolar), a single plate placed below the dental roots and above the inferior alveolar nerve is sufficient
- For fractures of the angle region, a single miniplate can be applied on the superior border along the external oblique ridge and ascending ramus with at least two screw holes on each side.

Noncompression miniplates

Original Champy's miniplates were made with stainless steel, but currently titanium plates are also available. Miniplates are available in various sizes and shapes with self-tapping monocortical screws. The plates usually used are of 2–2.5 mm thickness and the screws available are in various lengths of 4, 6, 8 and 10 mm. Miniplates and screws provide three-dimensional stability of the fragment and also resist the rotary and anteroposterior movement of the fractured segment (Fig. 47.14).

Principles in application of miniplates for fixation of mandibular fractures

- Plates are slightly overbent to adapt closely on the lingual aspect of fracture
- Recontouring of the bony irregularities may facilitate better plate adaptation

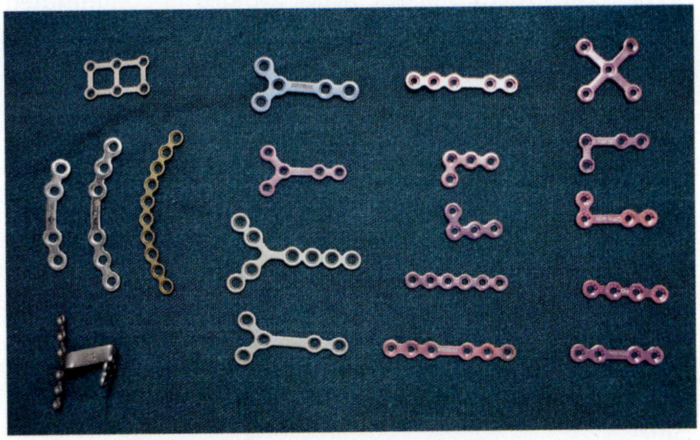

Figure 47.14 Miniplates.

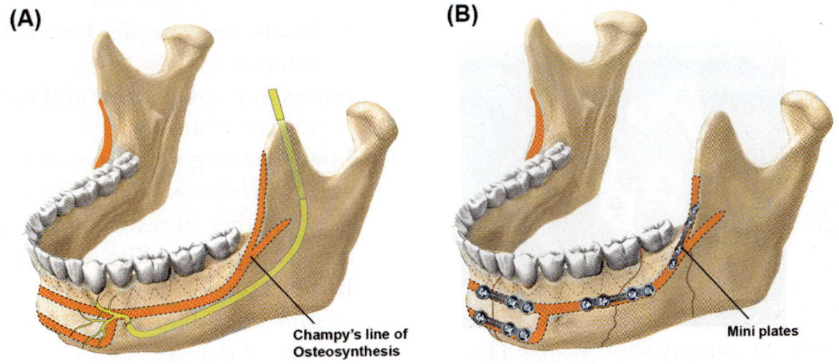

Figure 47.13 (**A**) Champy's line of osteosynthesis. (**B**) Miniplates along the Champy's line.

- Poor plate adaptation can cause fracture displacement during tightening of the screws
- Proper plate positioning minimises the chance of piercing the mandibular canal with a drill or screw
- Screw holes are prepared under irrigation using a drill guide to facilitate proper preparation of the bone
- Loose screws must be replaced with an emergency screw; if the emergency screw also slips, it must be removed and the plate hole must be left empty, or a longer plate can be used.

Advantages

- Monocortical application
- Can be applied by intraoral approach
- Functionally stable
- Biomechanically favourable
- Decreased operating time
- Easily adaptable and easy placement
- Postoperative dental correction is reduced
- Intermaxillary fixation is not necessary
- The side effects are greatly reduced
- Early mobilisation, less discomfort and not palpable by the patient.

Complications

- They are not as rigid as dynamic compression plate (DCP) or reconstruction plates, hence avoided in comminuted or infected plates
- Exposure of miniplates
- Sensory abnormalities
- Delayed or deformed union
- Widening of intergonial space at the angle region
- Infection
- Loose screws
- Granulation tissue formation
- Difficulty in removal of screws.

3D miniplates

The 3D miniplate is a misnomer as the plates are not three dimensional, but hold the fracture fragments rigidly by resisting the forces in three dimensions, namely shearing, bending and torsional forces (Fig. 47.15A).

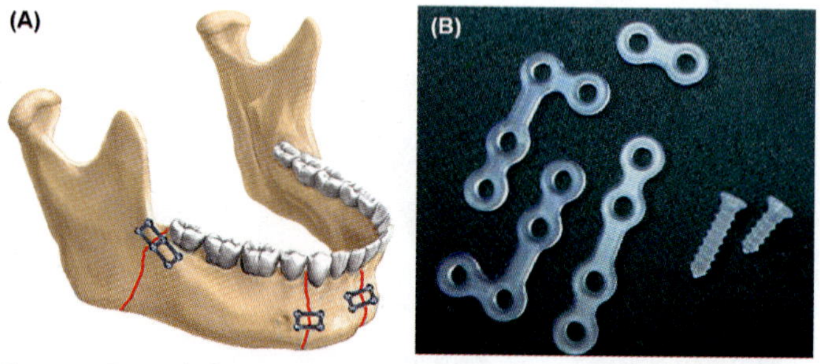

Figure 47.15 **(A)** 3D miniplates at various sites in mandible. **(B)** Resorbable miniplates.

The basic concept is that the geometrically closed quadrangular plate secured with bone screws creates stability in three dimensions. This stability is attained by its configuration and not by its thickness or length.

Resorbable miniplates

Materials used for bioabsorbable miniplates are as follows:

- Polydioxanone
- Polyglycolic acid
- Polylactic acid.

These resorbable plates does not have to be removed as they usually get resorbed over a period of 2–4 years (Fig. 47.15B).

Advantages

- Provides strength when necessary and then degrades over time without harming the structures
- No need for an additional removal surgery
- Blending pliers are not necessary.

Disadvantage

The strength is inadequate to provide clinically acceptable rigid fixation.

Concept of functional stability

Functional stability occurs where the interfragmentary movement between the fracture segments is balanced by the external forces and also allows healing of the fracture.

An example, of functional stability is Champy's technique of single miniplate adapted to the superior border of angle fracture. This technique is functionally stable as it allows healing of the mandible even in the presence of interfragmentary motion and the pull of the pterygomasseteric sling and suprahyoid muscles.

Functional stability is provided by the internal fixation systems in two ways:

1) **Load-sharing stability**—it is any form of internal fixation that is *insufficiently* stable to bear all the functional loads applied across the fracture. The fixation system requires additional stabilising forces to achieve functional stability, that is the functional *load is shared between the hardware and the apposed (bone) cortices* along the fracture site (Fig. 47.16A).

   Indications—simple linear fractures and mandible fracture.

   For example, lag screw and miniplate fixation (stainless steel or titanium).

2) **Load-bearing stability**—the functional stability is provided *solely by the fixation system*. The hardware is of sufficient rigidity to resist all functional forces until osseous union is achieved (Fig. 47.16B).

   Indications—comminuted mandibular fractures, atrophic mandibular fractures and fractures with segmental defects.

   For example, reconstruction plate.

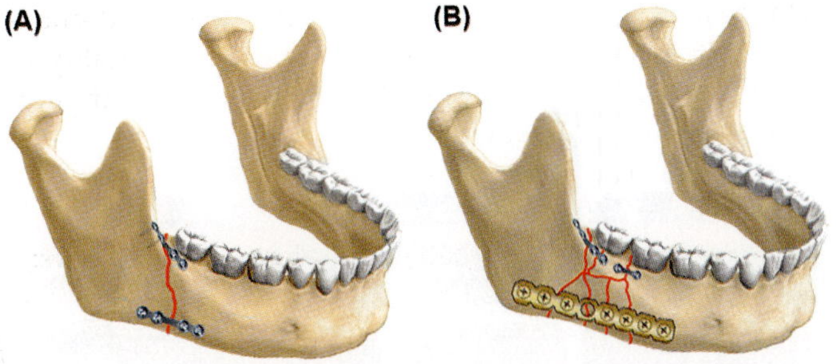

Figure 47.16 Functional stability. (**A**) Load-sharing fixation. Fixation is applied both at the inferior and superior border. (**B**) Load-bearing fixation—functional stability is provided by reconstruction plate at the lower border and secondary fixation at superior border.

Rigid internal fixation

Any kind of internal fixation that is strong and limits interfragmentary motion across the fracture while engaging the skeletal structure to movement is considered to be rigid internal fixation (RIF). RIF is defined as 'any form of internal fixation that is rigid'. It refers to the direct method of fixation where the hardware used for implant provides sufficient rigidity for the jaw bone to withstand masticatory stress. The bone heals by *primary or direct bone union* without callus formation.

Principles of rigid internal fixation (RIF)

In 1950s, (Arbeitsgemeinschaft für Osteosynthesefragen/ Association for the study of internal fixation) proposed these biomechanical principles in achieving RIF, which included the following:

1. Accurate anatomical reduction
2. Functionally stable fixation of the fragments
3. Atraumatic operative techniques in preserving the vitality of bone and soft tissues
4. Early and active functional mobility.

Accurate anatomical reduction of bone fragments

The term complete anatomic approximation refers to reduction of both occlusal and basal regions. In closed reduction, only occlusal reduction is achieved and not the basal reduction.

Functionally stable fixation of the fragments

Absolute stability refers to absence of relative motion between the plates and the bone, and also between the bone ends. The relative motion can be prevented by anchoring the free end plate with a single screw that is inserted under tension. Other screws should be placed under minimal tension, which finally results in direct bony union of the fracture.

Preserving the blood supply (vascularity)

An atraumatic surgical technique is an essential preventive measure to avoid poor healing and infection.

Early, active and pain-free mobilisation

Immediate, pain-free, oral opening is so critically important, which makes open reduction superior to conventional IMF. Advantages are prevention of tracheostomy, normal food intake and the patient's ability to speak and interact socially. *Rigid fixation techniques* depends on *two-point fixation:*

- A *stabilising unit* (plating at the inferior border)
- *A tension band* (like a miniplate or arch bar superior to the stabilising unit, except a load-bearing reconstruction plate).

Examples of RIF are as follows:

- Compression plate and arch bar
- Reconstruction plate
- Two bone plates
- Two lag screws.

Types of rigid internal fixation (RIF)

1. Compression osteosynthesis:
   a. DCP
   b. EDC
   c. Lag screw.
2. Noncompression/fixation osteosynthesis:
   a. Locking plate
   b. Reconstruction plate
   c. Titanium-coated hollow screw and reconstruction plate (THORP).

Compression osteosynthesis

The goal of *compression osteosynthesis* is to establish absolute stability across a fracture. It is defined as 'complete *elimination of movement between the fractured segments of bone and zero mobility of hardware against the bone*'.

Compression of the fracture segments generates friction across the segments and minimises the gap between them. Linear compression between the segments counteracts the torsional forces produced by the masticatory apparatus and prevents interfragmentary motion. Traction forces perpendicular to the fracture are maintained by the plate by sharing the load.

Mechanics of compression osteosynthesis (Flowchart 47.2):

Compression of fractured bony segments enhances successful primary healing in two ways:

1. *Generation of preload*
2. *Friction.*

Generation of the *preload is the force generated across the fracture by the fixation system.* Preload provides absolute stability of the loaded mandible.

Friction is produced by compression of the fractured bone segments. This friction reduces the fracture mobility, thereby increasing the fracture stability.

Fixation methods for compression osteogenesis

Several methods of fixation have been developed to provide compression osteogenesis, they are as follows:

i. DCP
ii. Eccentric dynamic compression plates (EDCP)
iii. Lag screw osteosynthesis.

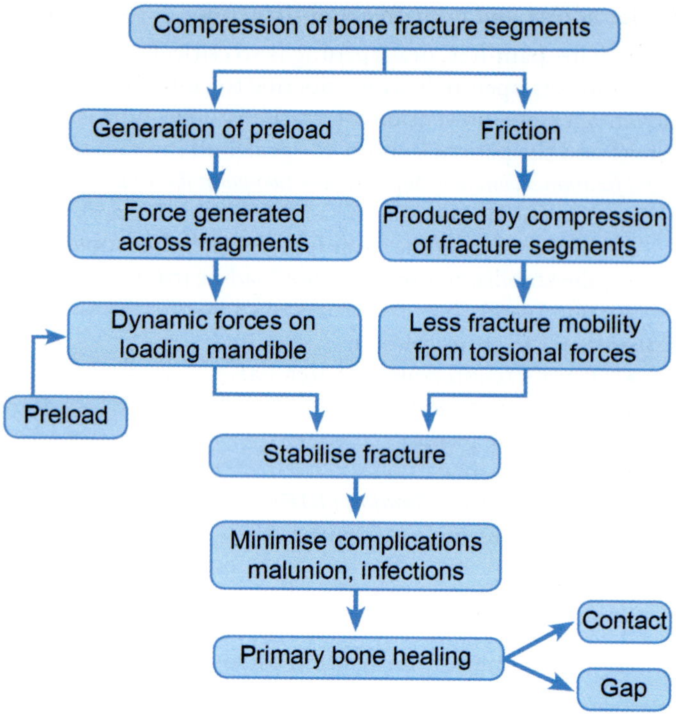

Flowchart 47.2 Mechanics of compression osteosynthesis.

Compression plates are designed such that the proper placement of the screws will result in a *relative motion between the plate and screws that will force the bony fragments together*, compressing them across the fracture line (Fig. 47.17). To accomplish this, the plate is designed with elliptical or oblong holes and screws with a large head to overlap the metal of the plate. When the screw is placed into the bone, it forms a 'screw-bone unit'. Thus, any relative motion between the plate and the screw will bring the bone along with screw. When the screw is tightened, it moves relative to the plate until the screw is seated completely in the plate hole. The bones will be compressed even further against one another if the screw in the opposite fragment is tightened. To increase the stability of the fixation, additional screws can be placed neutrally. Thus, compression plates provide compression osteosynthesis by *bringing the fractured margins closer together and compressing them* and also impart additional stability by increasing the frictional interlocking between them.

Indications

- In fractures with minimal obliquity and sound bony buttresses
- All mandible fractures except in fractures with bone loss
- Absolute rigidity across the fracture is desired
- Noncompliant patient who is likely to chew on the fracture side
- Patients where IMF is not recommended
- Presence of local soft tissue infection and no bone infection.

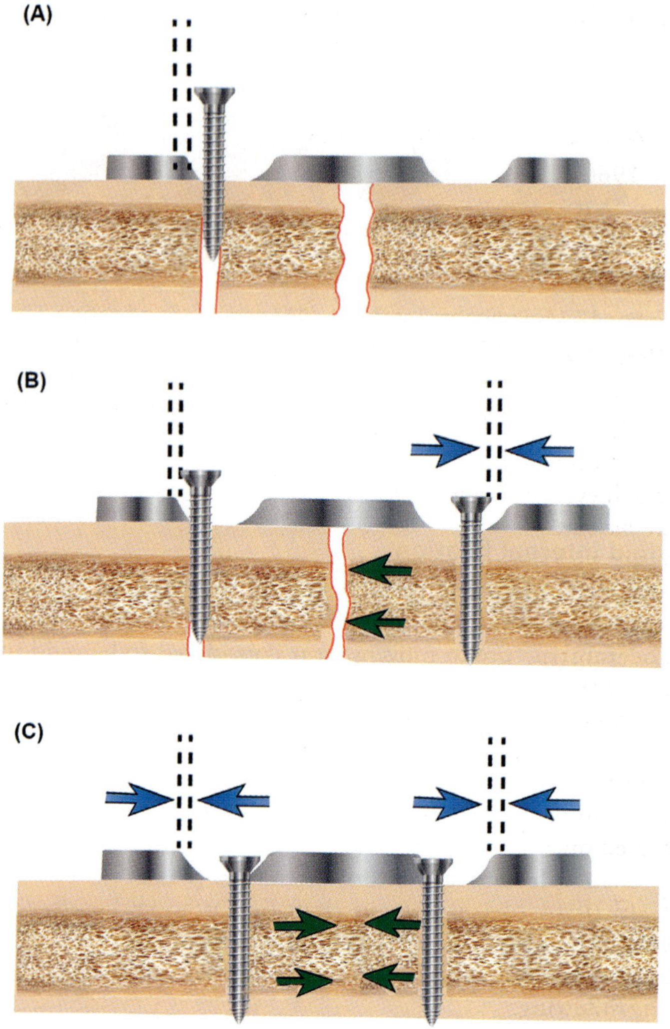

Figure 47.17 Compression plates. (**A**) Placement of screw at the distal end of the hole. (**B**) On tightening of the screw, the fragments move closer to each other. (**C**) Screw tightening is completed and the two bone fragments are compressed together.

Contraindications

- Inadequate bony buttressing at the fracture site (atrophic edentulous mandible fracture, comminuted and complex fractures)
- Simple fractures with an extreme oblique pattern
- Bone loss
- Presence of bone infection (osteomyelitis).

Advantages

- Low incidence of malunion
- Stable internal fixation
- No need for external immobilisation/IMF
- Early functional mobility.

Disadvantages

- Fractures heal by primary healing, which is a long and slow process
- Sometimes, microscopic fracture lines act as stress raisers and can initiate fatigue crack

- Rarely, loss of bone mass occurs at the subcortical bone, leading to osteoporosis and secondary bone fracture.

i. Dynamic compression plate

In 1960s, Luhr introduced Vitallium compression plating. During the early 1970s, Schmoker and Spiessel developed dynamic compression plate for the mandible, which used *eccentrically placed screws to generate compression* (Fig. 47.18).

Plate design

Principle of dynamic compression plate—spherical gliding principle.

The DCP is a narrow or broad *straight plate with ramped holes* facing outward. The screw holes and the screws are designed to achieve a congruent fit. The *screw holes* of DCP shapes like an *inclined transverse cylinder*. The *screws* used are *bicortical screws* with 'ball-headed' and spherical shoulder to fit in all positions. Minimum of two screws on each side of the fracture is required, with the outer holes acting as passive screw. The number of holes vary with the type of fracture. The use of more screws increases the stability of the plate and decreases the risk of screw loosening.

Eccentric drilling for compression

The compression plate is adapted and eccentric holes are drilled on either side of the fracture using drill guides.

Technique of compression plating

DCP is designed such that the compression can be achieved by appropriate positioning of the screw relative to the plate (Fig. 47.19).

- If the screw placed at the *height of an inclined plane* moves as it is tightened, it is called a *compression screw*. If the screw is placed at the *lowest point in the hole* so that it does not create compression when it is tightened, it is termed a *static or passive screw*. A DCP should have at least one compression hole in each fragment of the fracture; usually placed proximal to the fracture line.

Additional tension band

For mandible, the tension is on the alveolar (upper) side and compression is on the inferior border. Therefore, to achieve stability a compression plate should be placed in the alveolar region. Owing to the anatomical constraints and location of inferior alveolar nerve, the DCP should always be placed at the inferior border of the mandible (Fig. 47.20). However, DCP alone at the base of the mandible is insufficient to stabilise and can cause distraction at the alveolar side leading to infection, pseudo arthrosis and malocclusion. To overcome these problems, an IMF or arch bar or miniplates are applied on the alveolar border and DCP at the inferior border (tension band principle).

ii. Eccentric dynamic compression plate

DCP provides fixation at the inferior border of the mandible, but requires an additional tension band at the upper border to prevent splaying. In order to avoid the tension band or when a tension band cannot be applied, the EDCP is recommended. The EDCP works on the principle of *activation of compression holes in two different planes.*

Indications:

- Edentulous patient
- Fractures with the presence of an impacted 3rd molar
- Presence of avulsed bone near the alveolar site
- Teeth that are inadequate for IMF
- Patients with multiple fixed bridges
- Patients who cannot tolerate IMF.

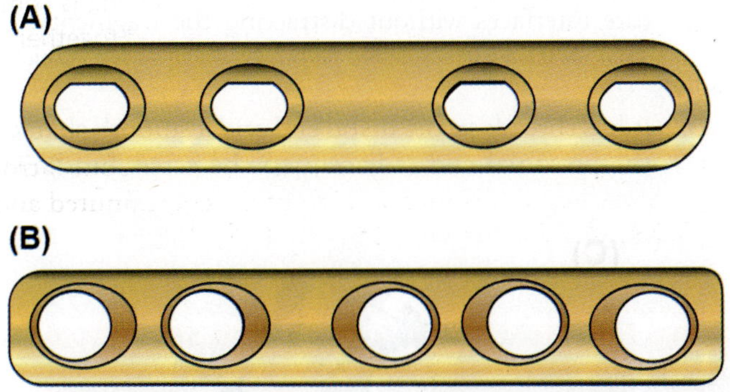

Figure 47.18 (**A & B**) Dynamic compression plate.

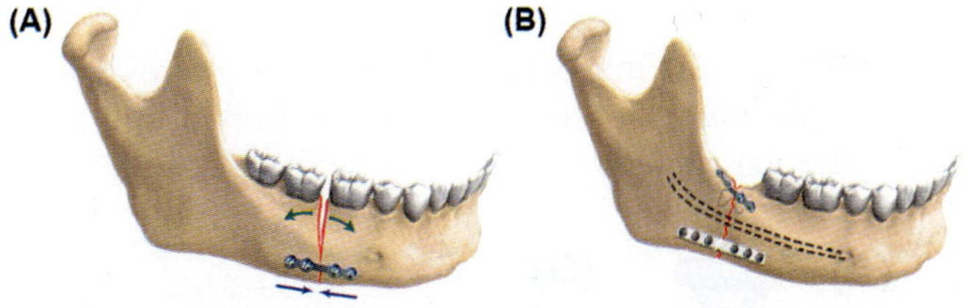

Figure 47.20 (**A**) DCP at the inferior border causing a gap at the superior border. (**B**) DCP at the lower border and miniplate at the superior border acting as tension band.

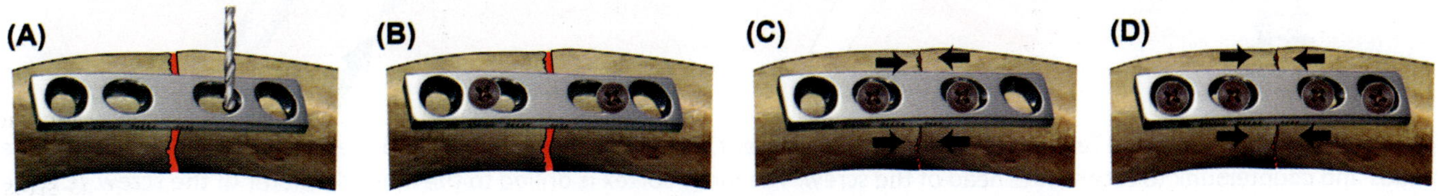

Figure 47.19 (**A-D**) Technique of compression plating. DCP showing the eccentrically placed screws and static screws in position.

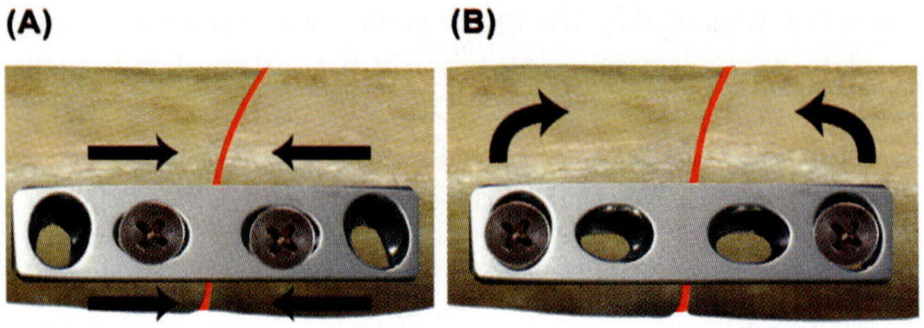

Figure 47.21 (**A**) Inner hole positioned horizontally, compresses the lower border. (**B**) Outer hole superiorly placed (eccentrically placed holes) compresses the alveolar border.

Design:

In 1973, Schmoker, Niederdellmann and Schilli simultaneously developed a plate incorporating the principle of eccentric dynamic compression. The design of this plate represents a *method of producing compression at the superior border of the fractured mandible.*

It consists of an *inner hole similar to the DCP and two outer eccentric compression holes* that are aligned at an angle oblique to the long axis of the plate. The design of inner holes are such that it produces compression across the fracture site whereas activation of the outer holes produces a rotational movement of the fracture segments and establishes compression at the superior border of the mandible (Fig. 47.21).

The EDCP is applied using the same screws, drills and taps as those used with the DCP. The screws are placed in the inner holes 1st followed by the outer eccentric holes to achieve compression at the superior border.

The goal of the EDCP is to1st establish longitudinal compression across the fracture at the inferior border and then to rotate the fragments around the screws to achieve additional compression at the level of the alveolus.

Advantages:

- Even distribution of forces along the length of fracture
- The fracture line is brought completely into dynamic compression, both at the inferior border and at the alveolar ridge
- Early return to function
- IMF and its associated difficulties are avoided.

Disadvantages:

- Technique sensitive
- It cannot be used to treat severely comminuted fractures
- Not recommended for condylar fractures
- Compound fractures are a relative contraindication due to infection.

iii. Lag screws

Lag screw osteosynthesis is a compression technique that can be carried out by using either *true lag screws or a lag technique with long bone screws.*

Lag screw was 1st introduced by Brons and Boering in 1970, who cautioned that at least two screws are necessary to prevent rotational movement of the fragments in oblique fractures of the mandible (Figs. 47.22 and 47.23).

Indication:

- Oblique mandibular fractures except the condyle
- Overlapping of the bone fragments
- Extra stabilisation is required
- Refixation of temporary mandibular osteotomy.

Principle:

- The premise of this technique is its *ability to engage and pull or lag the distal cortex towards the proximal cortex across a fracture.* This method provides a high degree of compression resulting in very stable fixation
- A screw that glides through the cortex of one fragment and engages the *cortex* of the opposite fragment with its threads, draws the fragments together and compresses them when tightened. Gliding holes and thread hole must be coaxial
- It necessitates careful orientation of the screws to the fracture line. The correct placement of the screws helps distribute the compressive forces evenly across the fracture interfaces without distracting the fragments. *The screw should always be drilled perpendicular to the line of fracture*

Design:

- It has threads in the distal end and a smooth shank at the proximal end (adjacent to the screw head). The

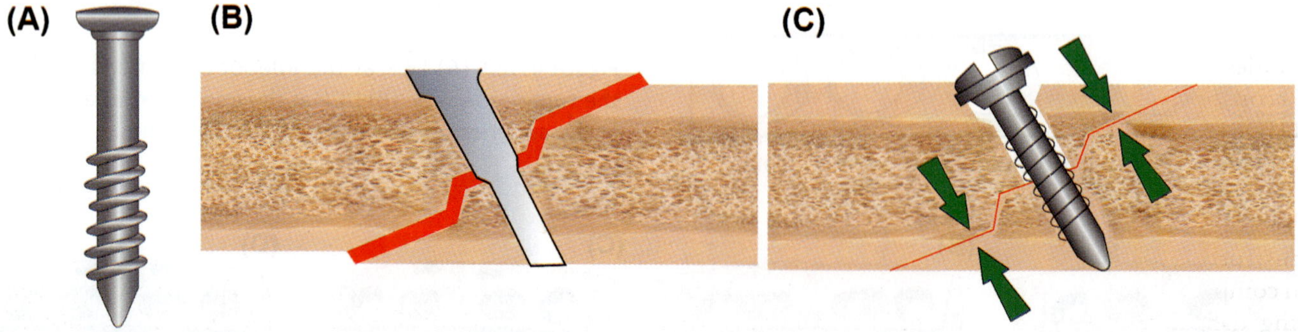

Figure 47.22 (**A**) Lag screw. (**B**) Technique of lag screw placement. The outer cortex is drilled to the external diameter of the screw threads and countersunk to receive the head of the screw. The inner cortex is drilled to the inner diameter of the screw. (**C**) Screw tightening creates compression of the bony interfaces.

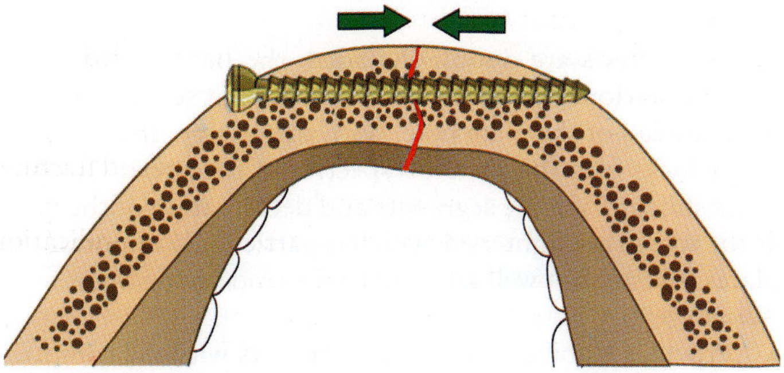

Figure 47.23 Lag screw fixation of mandibular symphysis fracture.

distal end gains purchase of the most distant osseous fragment while the proximal fragment fits passively. *The principle of lag screw fixation is that the threaded part of the screw glides through the 1st fragment and catches in the 2nd bone fragment.*

Advantages:

- It can be applied more rapidly
- It obviates the need for a bone plate adaptation
- Minimal displacement of bone segments
- It directly traverses the fracture line, and when properly used, lag screw fixation offers the *most rigidity of all rigid fixation techniques*. It is possible to achieve between 2000 and 4000 N of compressive force when using lag screw, compared with the 600 N achieved with prebent compression plates
- Lag screw can also be used to stabilise bone grafts
- It can be used in conjunction with a noncompression plate or compression plate
- Less hardware.

Disadvantage: Technique sensitive—screw must be placed perpendicular to fracture.

Complications of compression plating:

- Infection
- Malocclusion
- Nerve injury
- Tooth root injury
- Pain, palpability and cold intolerance in a few cases.

Noncompression osteosynthesis/fixation osteosynthesis

It includes the following:

- Reconstruction plates
- THORP
- Locking plates.

Mandibular reconstruction plate

Reconstruction plates are thicker and have a longer span when compared to other plates. Hence, they are used in load-bearing defects and reconstruction of the mandible. This larger dimension of the reconstruction plate provides increased strength and stabilises the fragments against functional displacement.

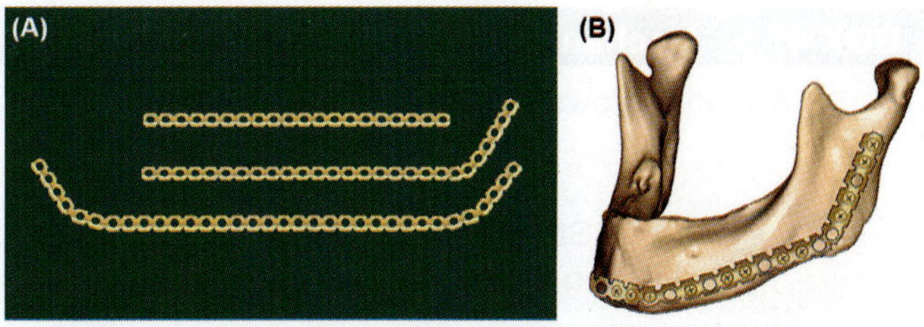

Figure 47.24 Various types of reconstruction plate.

The reconstruction plate is bendable, contains many holes for fixation points and is strong enough to stabilise a defective area in the mandible (Fig. 47.24).

Indications:

- Oblique fracture
- Comminuted fractures
- Loss of bone fragments in fracture
- Atrophic edentulous mandible fracture
- Severely displaced angle fracture
- Questionable postoperative compliance
- Patient where MMF is undesirable.

Advantages:

- Rigid fixation with load-bearing properties
- Lower incidence of infection
- Increased stability
- Temporary stabilisation of fragments
- Edentulous and comminuted fractures.

Technique:

- The reconstruction plate is adapted to the bone and pilot holes are drilled in the sound bone. Then the holes are tapped with the appropriately sized tap and screws are inserted. All screws are positioned neutrally
- It is suggested to place *at least three screws* in each of the fractured segments, and if an osseous gap is being bridged, it is suggested that at least four screws be placed in each segment.

Disadvantage:

- Distraction of the bone segments, resulting in malocclusion or segmental splay
- Loosening of the screws or fracture of the plate
- Difficulty in adaptation to the contours of the mandible.

Titanium-coated hollow screw and reconstruction plate

The standard reconstruction plate has been observed with problems such as screw loosening, plate mobility and instability of the bone segments.

In order to improve and prevent these complications, a modification was developed by Raveh (1981) called THORP. It combines the properties of *an external fixation system and an internal osteosynthesis*, converting the system into an internal fixation device. The modifications over the standard plates were as follows:

- Screws and plates were made with titanium for superior biocompatibility and osseointegration

BOX 47.5 Mechanism—THORP

Anchor screws osseointegrate with bone

↓

↑Stability over time
↓Friction with the hole in plate

↓

↑Stability to plate and fracture segments
↓Bone resorption

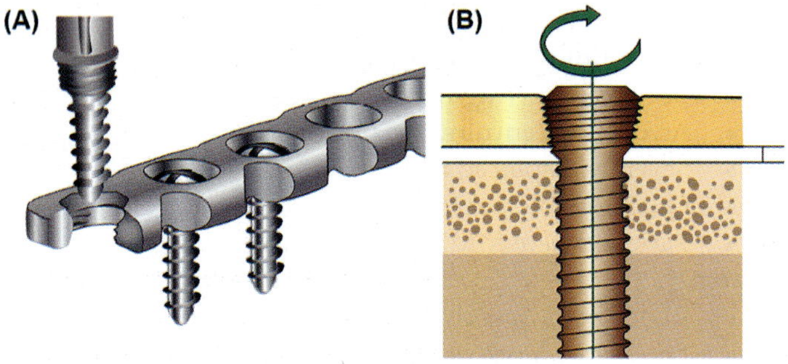

Figure 47.25 Locking plate-screw system.

- The cylindrical screw head and the head-expanding bolt were designed to fit snugly into the plate holes to ensure rigid fixation between screw and the plate.

Unlike standard reconstruction plate, *THORP stability is based on the osseointegration of titanium screws and the rigid fixation of the head and screws to the plate.*

The THORP system has a plate thickness of *3.0 mm, and a 4.0 mm screw diameter* with special locking screws. Although the procedures for placing the plate are indistinguishable to those used for conventional reconstruction plates, the holes drilled and screws utilised are wider (Box 47.5).

Disadvantage: The screws and plate osseointegrate with bone, making its removal difficult.

Locking plates

These plates achieve stability by *locking the screw to the plate*. They are useful in securing plates that cannot be perfectly adapted to fractures or if bone quality is poor (Fig. 47.25).

Design

Locking screws are double-threaded; the head of the screw has an additional larger diameter thread that secures into the inner thread of the plate hole. With this design, the screw actually locks into the plate irrespective of the bone. This prevents shifting of bone segments and deformation of the plate as the screws are tightened, which is particularly important in plates that are not well adapted to the underlying bone.

Advantage:

- Provides stabilisation of the segments without compression of the bone
- Loosening and extrusion of the screw from the plate is prevented
- Reduced chance of infection and nonunion
- Greater amount of stability than the standard nonlocking screws
- It resists mechanical yielding.

Locking plate-screw systems are considered whenever noncompression plates are used for a fracture. Modern plating systems are designed with fracture plates that accept standard bone and locking screws.

CONCLUSION

Many fixation methods have been used in the treatment of maxillofacial fractures with great success. The main objectives of the fixation is to reestablish preinjury aesthetics, normal masticatory function and proper occlusion. For conservative management of fractures, MMF can be done with the help of arch bars, wiring and cap splints, and in edentulous patients by Gunning's splints. ORIF can be carried out with the help of miniplates, 3D plates, compression plates, locking plates and reconstruction plates. Different plating systems and wiring techniques make the management of the maxillofacial fractures with high success rate.

IMMOBILISATION

It is prevention of any movement of the bone after realignment or stabilisation of the reduced fragment until the bony union takes place. It can be achieved by fixation devices, wires, arch bars and IMF. Immobilisation period varies depending on the type of fracture, fracture location, severity of fracture, presence of infection, method of fixation used, age and general health of the patient. Immobilisation period ranges from 3 to 4 weeks for maxillary fractures and 3 to 6 weeks for mandibular fracture.

Chapter 48

Dentoalveolar Fracture

OUTLINE

INTRODUCTION

The term 'dentoalveolar injury' describes fractures involving the teeth and surrounding bone without extension to the basal bones of maxilla or mandible. It can occur either as an isolated clinical entity or in conjunction with other injuries. They involve the soft tissues, teeth and associated bone and commonly occur in the age group of 8–12 years.

AETIOLOGY AND RISK FACTORS

Dentoalveolar injury caused by trauma is the foremost aetiological factor that leads to significant loss of teeth. These injuries are most commonly due to motor vehicle accidents, sports injuries, assaults, falls and industrial accidents in adults while self-fall and assaults are the most common cause in young children.

Dentoalveolar injuries can result from either a direct trauma to the teeth or an indirect trauma causing the mandible to forcibly close against the maxillary dentition. Direct trauma is inferential with injury to the maxillary incisor teeth, whereas indirect trauma often results in crown fracture and crown-root fracture with or without soft tissue injury.

The other factors that increase the risk of dentoalveolar injuries are as follows:

- Uncoordinated movements or sports activities in children
- Amount, direction and the location of force:
  a. *Low velocity impact:* Dentoalveolar fracture
  b. *High velocity impact:* Dental fracture
  c. *Indirect injury:* Blow to chin
- Prognathic maxilla and mandible
- Proclined incisors
- Teeth at the risk of avulsion due to poor periodontal health
- Extreme biting force during a seizure or drug abuse
- Jaw position during trauma (occluded or open mouth)
- Malocclusion
- Type of object:
  a. Sharp: Clean crown fracture
  b. Blunt: Root fracture, luxation.

CLINICAL FINDINGS

HISTORY

A complete history of the place, mechanism and time of injury should be obtained for accurate diagnosis and appropriate treatment. The patient's general health, any systemic diseases as well as the medications taken by the patient should also be recorded.

CLINICAL EXAMINATION

Examination of the face should be done in a systematic sequence (outside - inside) to achieve the desired management protocol.

Soft tissue examination

The soft tissues should be inspected for:

- Facial asymmetry
- Haematoma or ecchymosis
- Contusion, abrasion or laceration
- Any embedded foreign bodies or tooth fragments
- Damage to the vital structures such as submandibular duct, blood vessels and nerves
- Associated dentoalveolar injuries or fractures.

'Degloving injury' and tears are more common in the mandibular anterior region.

Damage to teeth

A detailed examination of the teeth should be performed after cleaning up any foreign bodies, blood and debris. The teeth should be examined for:

- Missing tooth or tooth fragments
- Abnormal mobility of the teeth
- Tooth displacement/dislocation
- Crown or crown-root fracture
- Exposure of the pulp chamber
- Root fractures
- Occlusal derangement
- Vertical split or a horizontal fracture of the tooth structure.

Mobility of a tooth should be tested in both the horizontal and axial directions. Movement of adjacent teeth is a typical sign of alveolar fracture when the mobility of a single tooth is tested. Derangement of occlusion is indicative of the fracture involving the dentoalveolar structures, jaws or displaced teeth.

Alveolar fractures

- Bimanual palpation of the maxillary and mandibular dentition should be done to assess for mobility or detect any discrepancy in the alveolar bone
- Fractures of the alveolus may or may not be associated with injury to the teeth and jaw
- Alveolar fractures are more commonly associated with mandibular fractures
- *Crepitations, step deformity and malocclusion* are the common findings of fractures involving the bone
- Blood-tinged saliva is a common finding of alveolar fracture with associated gingival tear
- Posterior open bite may occur with fractures of the anterior alveolar process.

Pulp testing and percussion test

Percussion test

It is performed by gently tapping the tooth with the blunt end of an instrument. A positive response (pain on percussion) is indicative of damage to the periodontal ligament. Dullness on percussion can be indicative of a luxated tooth, fractured tooth or alveolar bone fracture. An uninjured tooth will have a solid, metallic sound, whereas a luxated tooth produces a dull sound.

Pulp testing—vitality test

The degree of tooth injury can be evaluated through the pulp vitality test. The vitality test registers the conduction of stimuli to the sensory receptors of the dental pulp. A positive response indicates that the pulp is alive, whereas a negative response indicates dead pulp. Following injury, the tooth may be in a state of shock and may give a false response. Pulp testing should therefore be performed only during the subsequent visits.

Some of the methods of pulp testing are as follows:

i. *Thermal test* using gutta-percha, ice, ethyl chloride and carbon dioxide
ii. *Electric vitality testing:*
   The tooth is subjected to an increasing intensity of electric current to stimulate a pulpal response. It is influenced by a number of factors including the stage of eruption of the tooth, the presence of a restoration and the ability to isolate the tooth from saliva
iii. *Laser Doppler flowmetry (LDF):*
   It is a new pulp testing apparatus. It employs a laser beam directed at the pulp, which in turn produces a shift in the Doppler's frequency. It is a more reliable method of assessing pulp vitality.

RADIOGRAPHIC FINDINGS

The radiographs should provide information regarding injuries of the crown, root, periodontal ligament and bone. Radiographs for dentoalveolar fracture include the following:

- Intraoral periapical (IOPA) radiograph
- Orthopantomogram (OPG)
- Occlusal radiographs
- Cone beam computed tomography (CBCT)
- Conventional computerised tomography (CT) scan.

IOPA—it provides vital information about root fractures and dislocation of teeth. The relative position of an avulsed tooth within the alveolar bone can also be assessed. Occlusal radiographs help in the diagnosis of root fractures and displaced teeth. **OPG** illustrates fractures of the maxilla and mandible as well as fractures of the alveolar ridge and teeth. **CBCT** is useful for diagnosis of fractures of the alveolar bone, teeth and jaw with high resolution. **CT** scans have limited use for dentoalveolar fractures, but remain the gold standard for facial bone fractures.

Any missing teeth at the time of injury can be aspirated, swallowed or displaced into tissues. Hence, radiographic examination of the head, neck, chest and abdomen is necessary to rule out the presence of any teeth or fragments in these tissues.

CLASSIFICATION

Many classification systems have been developed for the traumatic injuries of the teeth and its supporting structures. The most common systems used for dentoalveolar injuries are by Ellis, Sanders and Andreasen (Table 48.1 & Fig. 48.1).

CLASSIFICATION OF ALVEOLAR BONE FRACTURE BASED ON THEIR LOCATION AND DISPLACEMENT

Class I—fracture of edentulous segment.
Class II—fracture of dentulous segment with little displacement.
Class III—fracture of dentulous segment with moderate to severe displacement.
Class IV—fracture of dentulous segment with multiple fracture lines.

A classification system for traumatic injuries of the teeth and its supporting structures was originally presented by

WHO based on the International Classification of Dental and Stomatological Diseases. This was later modified by Andreasen based on the anatomy, prognosis and treatment. This classification can be applied both to the primary and permanent dentition.

TABLE 48.1 Ellis and Davey's Classification of Injuries to the Anterior Teeth (1960)

Class I	Fracture of the crown confined to the *enamel* only
Class II	Fracture of the crown involving the *enamel* and substantial portion of *dentine* but without pulpal exposure
Class III	Fracture of the crown involving the enamel and substantial portion of *dentine* along *with pulpal* exposure
Class IV	Fractured tooth turned nonvital
Class V	Tooth lost due to trauma
Class VI	Fracture of the root (crown structure may or may not be lost)
Class VII	Traumatised tooth is displaced without fracture of crown or root
Class VIII	Fracture of crown en masse
Class IX	Fracture of deciduous teeth

ANDREASEN'S CLASSIFICATION

INJURIES TO THE DENTAL HARD TISSUES AND PULP (Fig. 48.2)

Enamel infraction/micro cracks

Micro cracks are incomplete fracture lines within the enamel without loss of tooth structure. Various *Craze lines* can be detected running parallel with the direction of enamel rods and ending at the dentinoenamel junction.

Uncomplicated crown fracture

This fracture is associated with loss of tooth substance. It involves fracture of enamel or enamel and dentin *without pulpal* involvement.

Complicated crown fracture

It is a fracture with loss of both enamel and dentine *and pulpal* involvement. The exposed pulp gives rise to sensitivity and pain.

Uncomplicated crown-root fracture

It is a fracture involving the enamel, dentine and root structure (cementum) *without pulpal involvement.*

Complicated crown-root fracture

It is a fracture involving the enamel, dentine and cementum *with pulp exposure.*

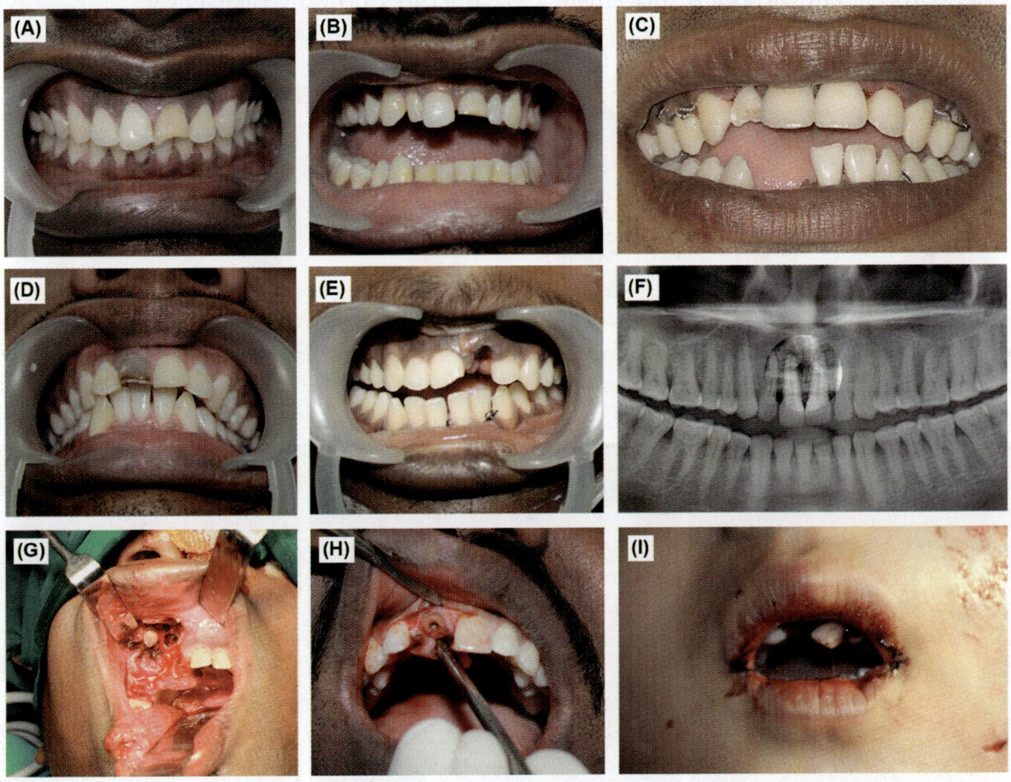

Figure 48.1 (A-I) Ellis and Davey's classification. A-Class I, B- Class II, C- Class III, D- Class IV, E-Class V, F-Class VI, G-Class VII, H-Class VIII, I- Class IX.

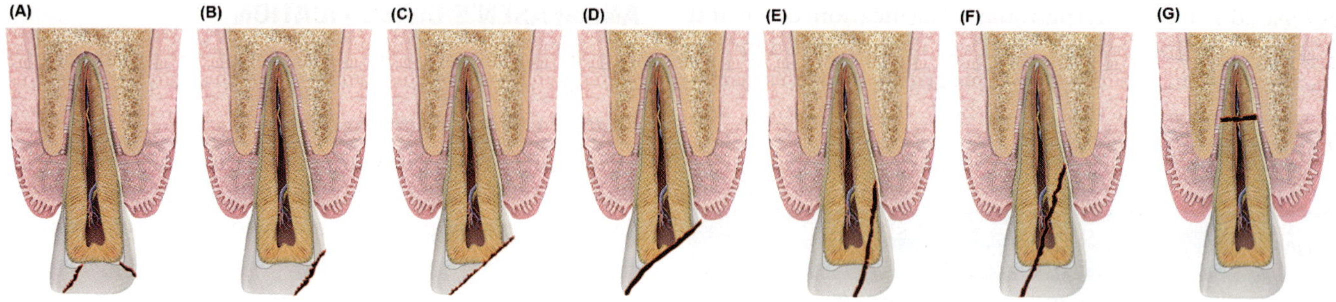

Figure 48.2 Injuries to the hard-dental tissue and pulp tissue. (**A**) Enamel infraction. (**B** and **C**) Uncomplicated crown fracture. (**D**) Complicated crown fracture. (**E**) Uncomplicated crown-root fracture. (**F**) Complicated crown-root fracture. (**G**) Root fracture.

Root fracture

It is a horizontal root fracture involving the dentine, cementum and pulp. This fracture is located within the alveolus and the tooth may be slightly extruded with tenderness on percussion.

INJURIES TO THE PERIODONTAL TISSUES (Figs. 48.3 and 48.4)

Concussion

A concussion is an injury to the supporting structures of the tooth without mobility or displacement of the tooth though the tooth is tender to touch and percussion.

Subluxation (loosening)

It is an injury to the supporting structures of the tooth with increased mobility of the tooth, but without displacement.

Intrusive luxation (central dislocation/intrusion)

It is an axial displacement of the tooth into the alveolar bone through the alveolar socket. Clinically, the crown appears shortened with bleeding from the gingiva. On percussion of the tooth, it is high and metallic, similar to that of an ankylosed tooth.

Extrusive luxation (partial avulsion/peripheral dislocation/extrusion)

It is partial or incomplete dislocation of the tooth out of the alveolar socket. The tooth appears elongated and mobile with bleeding from the gingiva.

Lateral luxation

It is movement of the tooth in any direction other than the vertical axis. It is often accompanied by comminution or fracture of the alveolar socket.

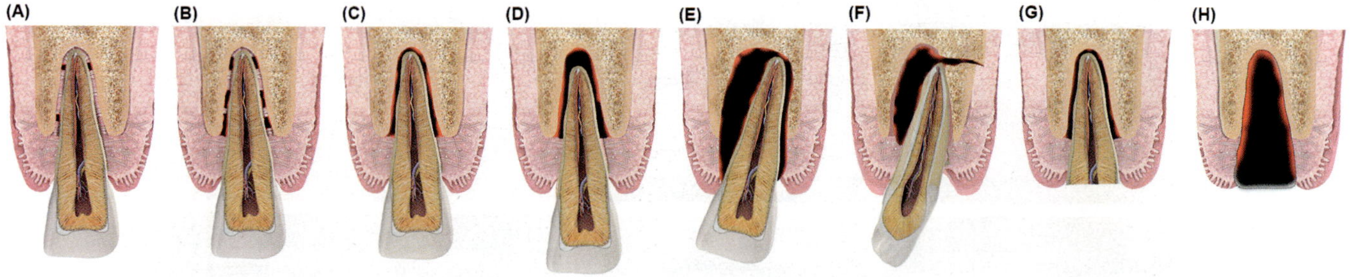

Figure 48.3 Periodontal tissue injuries. (**A**) Concussion. (**B**) Subluxation. (**C**) Intrusive luxation. (**D**) Extrusion. (**E** and **F**) Lateral luxation. (**G**) Retained root fracture and (**H**) Complete avulsion.

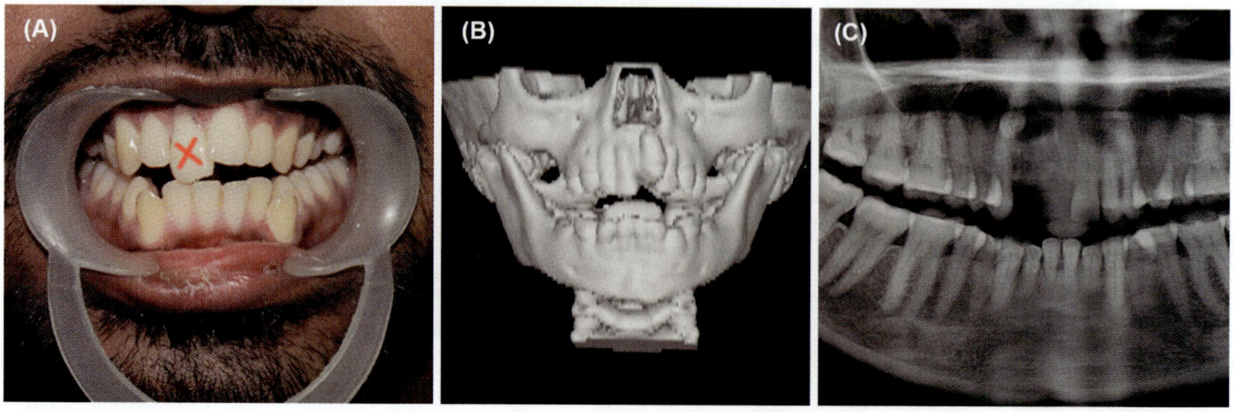

Figure 48.4 Periodontal injuries. (**A**) Extrusion. (**B**) Intrusion. (**C**) Intrusion of 12 and avulsion of 11.

Retained root fracture

It is a fracture with retention of the root segment and loss of the crown segment.

Exarticulation (complete avulsion)

It is the complete displacement of the tooth out of the alveolar socket with an empty bleeding socket.

INJURIES TO THE SUPPORTING BONE (Figs. 48.5 and 48.6)

Comminution of the tooth socket

It is crushing and comminution of the alveolar socket together with intrusive and lateral luxation.

Alveolar socket wall fracture

It is fracture of the alveolar socket confined to the buccal or lingual wall of the socket.

Fracture of the alveolar process

A fracture of the alveolar process with or without involvement of the tooth socket.

Fractures of the mandible or maxilla

Fracture involving the base of the mandible or maxilla with or without involvement of the alveolar socket.

INJURIES TO THE SOFT TISSUES (GINGIVA OR ORAL MUCOSA) (Fig. 48.7)

Laceration of gingiva or oral mucosa

Trauma by a sharp object giving rise to a shallow or deep mucosal tear in the oral mucosa.

Contusion of gingiva or mucosa

Trauma by a blunt object producing a bruise from a submucosal haemorrhage without a break in the mucosa.

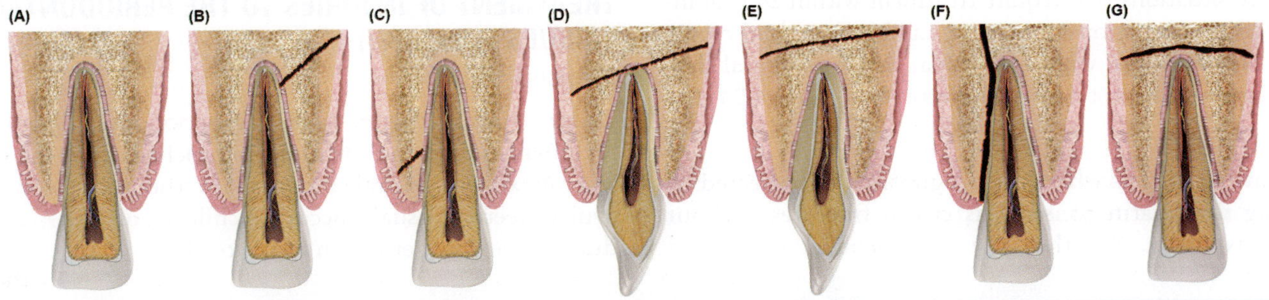

Figure 48.5 Injuries to the supporting bone. **(A)** Comminution of the alveolar socket. **(B and C)** Fracture of the alveolar socket wall. **(D and E)** Fracture of the alveolar process. **(F and G)** Fracture of maxilla and mandible.

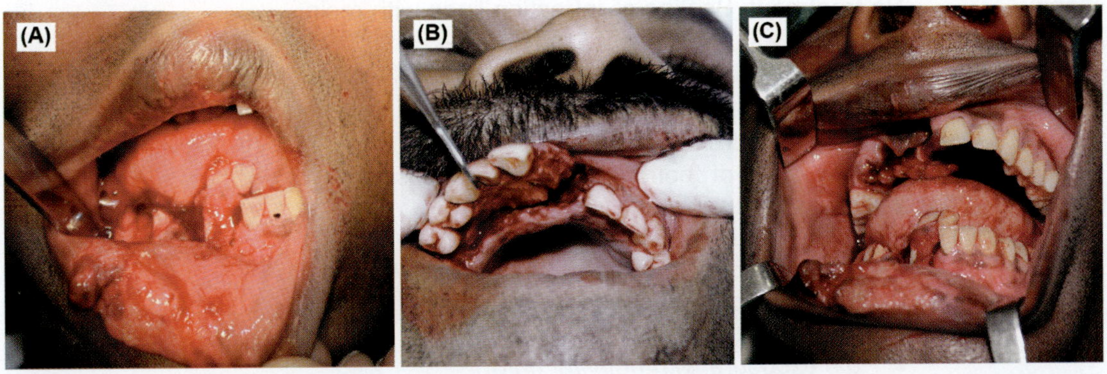

Figure 48.6 Alveolar bone fractures. **(A)** Mandibular dentoalveolar fracture. **(B)** Dentoalveolar fracture of the right maxilla. **(C)** Dentoalveolar fracture of maxilla and mandible.

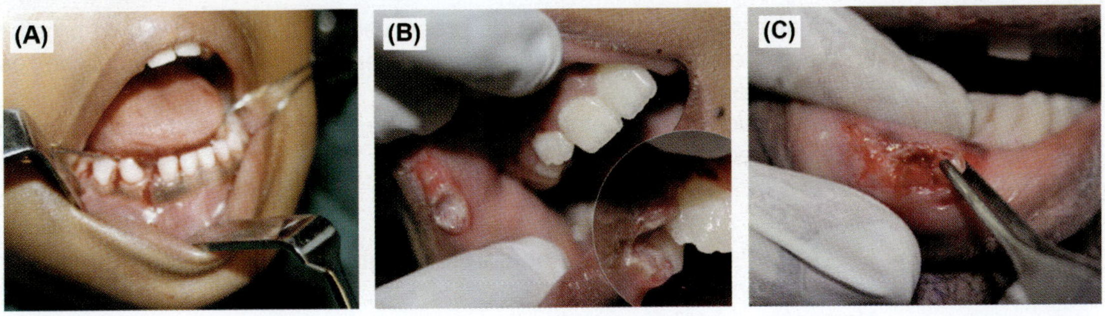

Figure 48.7 **(A)** Gingival tear and step deformity. **(B)** Laceration of upper lip. **(C)** Lower lip laceration.

Abrasion of gingiva or oral mucosa

A superficial injury caused by rubbing or scraping of the mucosa, presenting as a raw bleeding surface.

TREATMENT OF DENTOALVEOLAR INJURIES

GENERAL CONSIDERATIONS

The overall goal of treatment is to reposition the teeth and restore the functional state of teeth, bone and gingiva. The treatment priorities are as follows:

Acute treatment

These are situations that require treatment within a few hours such as tooth avulsion, extrusion, lateral luxation and alveolar fractures. Early repositioning and stabilisation produces excellent periodontal ligament repair.

Subacute treatment

These are situations that require treatment within 24 h of injury such as concussions, intrusions, subluxations and crown fractures with pulpal exposure. Pulpal and periodontal ligament responses are not adversely affected by a delay of 24 h.

Delayed treatment

These are situations where the prognosis is not affected by delaying the treatment, such as crown fractures without pulpal exposure. Whether the treatment is performed within a few or several hours, they appear to have the same prognosis.

The sequence of treatment for a dentoalveolar fracture is from an inside-to-outside approach, which includes bone, teeth and soft tissue.

TREATMENT OF INJURIES TO THE HARD DENTAL TISSUES AND PULP (Table 48.2)

The treatment of crown fractures is aimed at relieving the pulpal response initially followed by the final restoration of crown anatomy and occlusion.

The treatment of crown and root fractures includes reduction of the displaced coronal fragments and firm immobilisation by splinting for 2–3 months. The use of rigid fixation or extensive wiring is contraindicated as it can result in additional periodontal injury and affect healing.

TREATMENT OF INJURIES TO THE PERIODONTAL TISSUES (Table 48.3)

Avulsed tooth

Tooth avulsion occurs when the periodontal ligament attachment is torn and the tooth is 'expelled' from the socket. The maxillary central incisors are the most commonly avulsed teeth. It usually occurs in children of ages 7–10 years, due to continued eruption of the teeth.

TABLE 48.2 Management of Traumatically Injured Teeth and Pulp

Crown and Root Injury	Management
Crown infractions	No treatment. Sealing of infraction lines with resin
Crown fractures	• *Enamel only:* Smoothening of the sharp edges or restoration with composite • *Exposed dentin* • Calcium hydroxide base or glass ionomer liner • Restoration of tooth form with a composite • Relieve occlusion • *Pulp exposure with vital pulp* • Direct pulp capping with calcium hydroxide • Partial pulpotomy • Root canal therapy (RCT) • *Pulp exposure with nonvital pulp* • RCT with/without apexification • Definitive *restoration of crown fractures* includes composite restorations, full crown coverage and laminate veneers
Crown-root fractures	• Remaining root fragments can be preserved for a post and crown prosthesis • Fracture line above or slightly below the cervical margin, tooth can be restored with RCT and permanent restoration • Fracture involving more than one-3rd of the clinical root and vertical root fractures are indicated for extraction
Root fractures	• *Apical 3rd*—no treatment • *Middle 3rd*—splinting or extraction • *Cervical 3rd*—extraction of the coronal fragment and RCT for the remaining fragment or extraction of the tooth • *Vertical root fractures*—extraction

TABLE 48.3 Management of Traumatically Injured Periodontal Tissues

Periodontal Injuries	Management
Concussion	No treatment, occlusal grinding
Subluxation	Nonrigid splinting to the adjacent teeth for 7–10 days
Intrusive luxation	• Repositioning of the tooth and splinting • For immature tooth—allowed to re-erupt or orthodontic repositioning • Periodic vitality test
Extrusive luxation	• Repositioning and splinting with a nonrigid material, for 1–2 weeks • Periodic vitality test (Fig. 48.8)
Lateral luxation	Repositioning of tooth with concurrent compression forces over the labial and palatal bone plates and splinting
Avulsion (exarticulation)	• A true dental emergency • *The avulsed teeth should be reimplanted within 20 min of injury* • The tooth should be splinted, relieved from occlusion, with a soft diet for 2–3 weeks

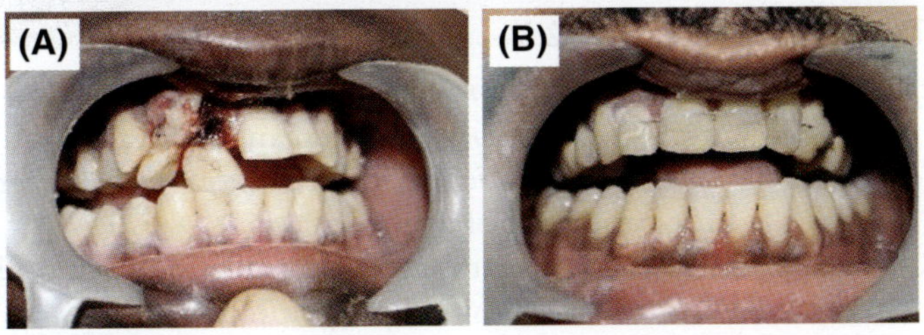

Figure 48.8 **(A)** Extruded 21 and 22. **(B)** The extruded teeth were replaced and stabilised using wire and composite.

The survival of an avulsed tooth is dependent on the vitality of the periodontal fibres on the root surface. Periodontal ligaments with extraoral exposure exceeding 15 min will have depleted cell metabolites. They become irreversibly necrotic with extraoral exposure exceeding 120 min. Hence treatment of an avulsed tooth is aimed at maintaining the cellular viability of the periodontal ligaments to achieve successful reattachment and decrease the chance of root resorption. The periodontal ligaments undergo regeneration approximately 3–4 weeks after replantation.

The goal of replanting the teeth after traumatic avulsion is to retain a viable pulp and periodontal ligament tissue to assist reattachment and avoid root resorption. *Replanting* the tooth within 15–20 min of avulsion prevents the loss of normal periodontal ligament cells and has a favourable long-term prognosis.

Management of avulsed tooth (Table 48.4)

At the accident site, emergency treatment and immediate replantation of the tooth should be attempted. The tooth should be gently rinsed with tap water and should not be scrubbed. The tooth is replanted and held in place either by finger pressure or by gently biting a cloth until they are brought to the emergency room. If replantation is not possible, the tooth should be placed in the best transport medium available. The transport medium recommended are as follows:

EXTRAORAL STORAGE MEDIA

- *Milk* is considered the ideal medium because of its availability. It prevents cell death and preserves periodontal viability for up to 6 h post avulsion
- *Saline*
- *Saliva*
- The *buccal vestibule* or under the tongue, unless there is a *risk of aspiration* or swallowing
- Water is the least favoured storage medium and is not recommended because of creation of a hypotonic environment, which leads to rapid cell breakdown and increased inflammation after replantation
- Transport containers with specialised cell culture media like ***Viaspan and Hanks' balanced salt solution (HBSS)*** are found to be highly effective in preserving the viability of the periodontal ligaments for a long duration. Viaspan has been used to transport organs, has a pH of 7.4, osmolality of 320 m OSM and the cells remain vital for 7 days
- **HBSS contents:**
  a. Glucose
  b. Sodium chloride
  c. Potassium chloride
  d. Calcium chloride
  e. Magnesium chloride
  f. Sodium phosphate
  g. Sodium bicarbonate
  h. Magnesium sulphate.
- Hanks' solution is available in the market as 'Save-A-Tooth' solution. Even depleted cells can be replenished in Hanks' solution. The tooth should be soaked in Hanks' solution for 30 min before replantation
- Other materials that can be used as a transport medium are contact lens solution, green tea, culture media (Dulbecco's storage medium), coconut water, egg white, probiotic solutions and ascorbic acid
- *Andreasen's* recommendation for replanting a permanent tooth:
  a. The avulsed tooth should not have advanced periodontal disease
  b. The alveolar socket must be reasonably intact to provide a seat for the avulsed tooth
  c. There should be no orthodontic considerations such as overcrowding of the teeth
  d. If the tooth is replanted within 30 min of avulsion, there is a good chance of successful replantation. For

TABLE 48.4 Summary of the Treatment of Avulsion

Treatment of Avulsion within 2 h
General Guidelines
• Minimal extraoral period • If possible replant at accident site itself • No removal of periodontal ligament • Transport in whole milk or Hank's solution • No removal of blood clot from socket • Analgesics, antibiotic coverage for 7–10 days and tetanus vaccination • Oral hygiene and chlorhexidine rinse • Splinting for 7–10 days
Closed Apex
• Soak in Hank's solution for 30 min • Replant the tooth and splinting for 7–14 days • At 7–14 days, the pulp is removed and the canal is filled with calcium hydroxide • After 6–12 months, the tooth is obturated with gutta-percha
Incomplete Apex
• Soak in Hank's solution for 30 min and in a 1 mg/20 mL doxycycline solution for 5 min • Replant and splint for 7–14 days • Fill the canal with calcium hydroxide, only if the pulp becomes necrotic
Treatment of Avulsion After 2 h
General Guidelines
• Minimal extraoral period, replant at the accident site if possible • No removal of periodontal ligament • Transport in whole milk or Hank's solution • No removal of blood clot from socket • Analgesics and antibiotic coverage for 7–10 days • Oral hygiene and chlorhexidine rinse • Tetanus vaccination • Splinting for 7–10 days
Closed or Incomplete Apex
• The periodontal ligament is removed either by scraping or soaking in a sodium hypochlorite solution for 30 min • Endodontic debridement, cleaning and shaping of the canal in the hand • The tooth is soaked in citric acid solution for 3 min—to open dentinal tubules and permit fibrous attachment • In 1% stannous fluoride solution for 5 min, and 1 mg/20 mL doxycycline solution for 5 min—to kill the bacteria and make the tooth more resistant to resorption • The canal is dried and obturated with gutta-percha • The tooth is replanted and splinted for 7–10 days

extraalveolar periods *greater than 2 h*, complications such as *root resorption* increases significantly

e. The stage of root development should also be assessed. In teeth with incomplete root formation, survival of the pulp tissue is possible if replanted *within 2 h* of avulsion.

AT THE EMERGENCY ROOM (Fig. 48.9)

The tooth is rinsed with saline without removing the remaining periodontal ligaments. The alveolar socket should be irrigated with saline without removing the blood clot. The tooth is replanted and the facial and lingual bony plates are compressed towards the tooth. A radiograph can be taken to verify proper positioning of the replanted tooth. The tooth should be relieved from occlusion.

ROOT MANAGEMENT

Preparation of the root depends on the stage of tooth maturity (open vs closed apex) and the dry time (duration of time after avulsion and before placement in a storage medium). A *dry time of up to 2 h* is considered optimal after which periodontal ligament cells are less likely to survive.

Tooth replanted within 2 h

Open apex—gently rinse off debris, soak in doxycycline for 5 min or cover with minocycline followed by replantation

Closed apex—the root should be rinsed with water or saline to get rid of debris and replanted as gently as possible.

Tooth replanted after 2 h

Closed apex—placed in *acid for 5 min* to remove the periodontal ligament, soaked in *fluoride* and replanted. Endodontic treatment (RCT) must be performed extraorally (refer Table 48.4 for treatment of avulsion)

Open apex—it is often treated as closed apex by extraoral root canal treatment followed by replantation.

Intrusive luxation/intrusion

Recommended treatments are as follows:

- Immature teeth are allowed to re-erupt
- Immediate repositioning of the tooth into the arch, but this is associated with high incidence of external root resorption and damage to the periodontal structures
- Splinting to the adjacent tooth
- Orthodontic repositioning of the tooth for a period of 3–4 weeks
- Root canal therapy for re-erupted tooth.

Splinting

A splint is a rigid or flexible aid that is used to support, protect and immobilise teeth that have been weakened, traumatised, replanted or fractured.

Splinting provides *stabilisation* of the traumatised teeth and prevents further damage to the pulp and periodontal tissue, allowing the attachment apparatus to regenerate.

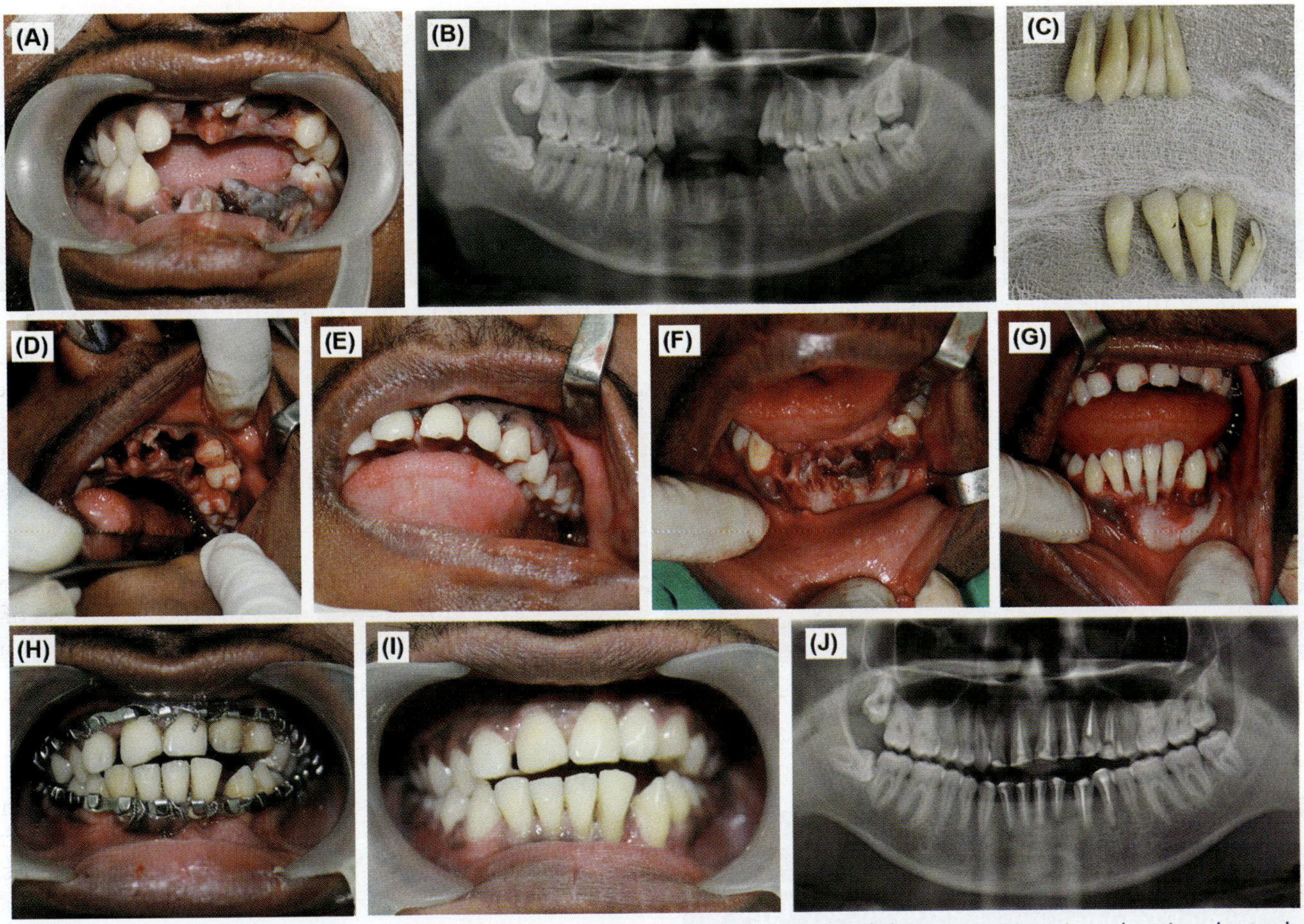

Figure 48.9 Management of avulsed upper and lower anteriors following trauma. (**A**) Preoperative view showing dentoalveolar fracture of upper and lower anteriors with missing teeth. (**B**) Preoperative OPG. (**C**) Avulsed teeth. (**D** and **E**) Replacement of the avulsed teeth in maxilla. (**F** and **G**) Replacement of avulsed tooth in mandible and bone grafts placed at the lower anteriors for additional support. (**H**) The teeth were stabilised with arch bars. (**I**) Postoperative view. (**J**) Postoperative OPG.

It is important that the splint should allow slight flexibility or physiologic mobility to accelerate the healing of the periodontally injured teeth. Rigid splints increase resorption and eventually tooth loss.

Indications:

- Periodontal tissue injuries (subluxation, luxation and avulsion)
- Alveolar wall and bone injuries
- Class IV root fractures

Contraindications:

- Injuries of primary tooth (luxation or avulsion)

Requirements for an acceptable splint:

- It should be simple to prepare and easy to place
- Enable physiological movement of tooth
- It should not cause further trauma to the injured tooth
- Ability to restore occlusion
- Easily removable.

Types of splint:

- **Rigid splints** (Fig. 48.10A–D)
  1. Suture splints
  2. Arch bar splints
  3. Acrylic splints
  4. Composite splints
- **Nonrigid/semi-rigid/flexible splints** (Fig. 48.11A–D)
  5. Orthodontic brackets and arches
  6. Wire and acid etched composite splints
  7. Fibre splints
  8. Titanium trauma splints (TTS).

The splints are categorised based on the possibility of physiological mobility of the tooth. A *rigid splint* does not permit any physiological mobility of the tooth and thereby increasing the possibility of complications such as ankylosis or external resorption.

In *nonrigid or semi-rigid splints*, there is the possibility of physiological mobility of the traumatised tooth, which is desirable for periodontal ligament healing, thereby reducing the possibility of complications.

Duration of splinting varies with the type of dental trauma. Generally, the splint is recommended for 7–10 days. In cases of root and alveolar bone fracture, longer periods of 2–4 months are recommended (Table 48.5). The commonly used splints are *Erich arch bars, interdental wiring such as figure-eight wiring and acid-etched resin splint.*

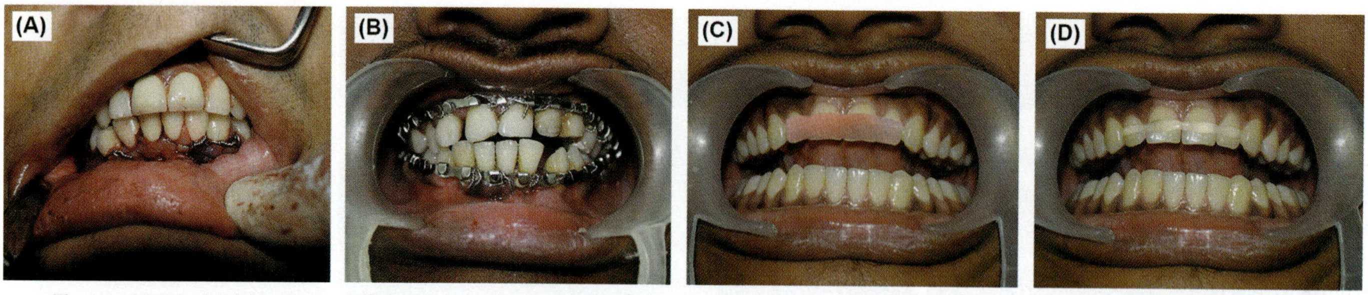

Figure 48.10 Rigid splints. (**A**) Suture and wire splints. (**B**) Arch bar splints. (**C**) Acrylic splints. (**D**) Composite splints.

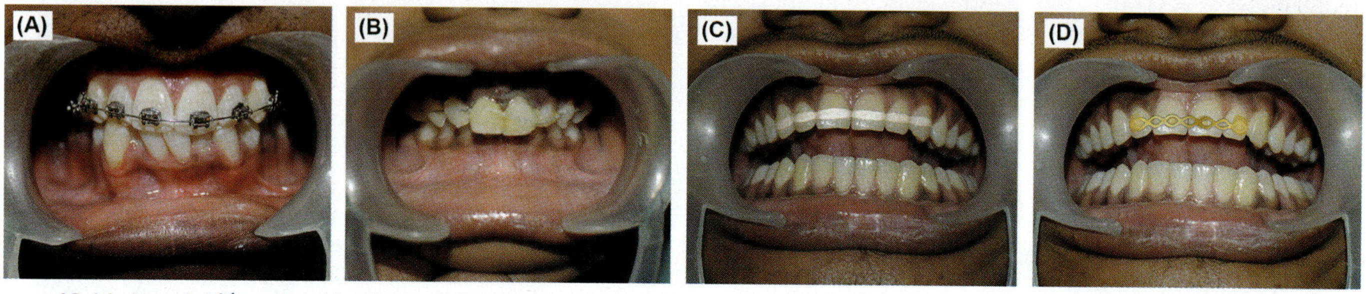

Figure 48.11 Nonrigid/semi-rigid splints. (**A**) Orthodontic brackets and arches. (**B**) Wire and composite splints. (**C**) Fibre splints. (**D**) Titanium trauma splints (TTS).

TABLE 48.5 Duration of Splinting Based on the Type of Trauma

Type of Trauma	Duration of Splinting	Type of Splint
Subluxation	2 weeks	Flexible
Extrusive luxation	2 weeks	Flexible
Avulsion	2 weeks	Flexible
Lateral luxation	4 weeks	Flexible
Intrusion	4–8 weeks	Flexible
Root fracture (middle 3rd)	4 weeks	Rigid
Fracture of the alveolar process	4 months	Rigid

Rigid splints

Wire and suture splints

In this type of splint, materials such as soft wire and surgical thread are used around the traumatised and neighbouring teeth. They are indicated for use in the mixed dentition stage with shorter periods of immobilisation. The disadvantages of this type of immobilisation are that the metal thins and breaks with chewing and also leads to gingivitis. Surgical sutures are used when there are no neighbouring teeth to which a splint can be fixed.

Arch bar splints

These are metal bars with hooks, which are fitted to the dental arch and ligated to the individual teeth using wires. Erich arch bar is most commonly used in jaw fractures. It is recommended only if adequate number of teeth are available for fixation. The disadvantage is that it may cause gingivitis or increased tooth mobility.

Acrylic splints

These splints are made from acrylic material and are indicated in cases of luxation of teeth in combination with alveolar bone fracture (e.g. Pfeiffer splint). This splint can be made either by direct or indirect method.

Composite splints/acid etch resin splint

It provides stabilisation of the teeth using a composite resin material. It is simple, efficient and provides excellent stabilisation. It is most commonly used for all types of dentoalveolar trauma (luxation, root fractures, avulsion and alveolar fractures). The disadvantage is that the composite material is brittle and can break when exposed to masticatory forces.

Semi-rigid splints (Fig. 48.11A–D)

It is indicated in traumatised teeth with no associated alveolar fractures, allowing physiological movement of the traumatised teeth.

Orthodontic splints

This splint involves orthodontic brackets and orthodontic wires for stabilisation. The brackets are placed in the middle 3rd of the labial surface of the tooth and connected by wires of 0.016 mm. The advantage of this splint is that it allows tooth movement along with stabilisation, especially in cases of intrusion.

Wire and composite splints

It is a modification of the composite technique, where an orthodontic wire and composite material is used, instead of a composite bridge for splinting. It is the most commonly used technique nowadays and can be used in all traumatic injuries. For rigid fixation, 24-gauge wire is preferred, whereas for semi-rigid fixation 28-gauge wire is indicated. The involved tooth is stabilised with two stable adjacent teeth to provide support. The labial surface is etched, dried, coated with bonding agent and light cured. The composite material is placed over the tooth and the wire is positioned and light cured. The only teeth that might not be suitable are those with artificial crowns or large fillings as they cannot be etched and bonded.

Fibre splints

Instead of wire, the materials that can be used are glass-ionomer fibre, fishing line, Ribbond splint and Kevlar fibre. It is indicated for all traumatic injuries except for alveolar fractures. Fibre splints are easy to apply and have a favourable outcome.

Titanium trauma splints (TTS)

A TTS is a more recent splint, made from pure titanium, 0.2 mm in thickness, and available in 52- and 100-mm lengths. It is a rhomboidal flexible mesh, which is fixed to the tooth in the same way as a wire-composite splint. The weakness of this splint is that it is very expensive in comparison with other splints.

Single-tooth fixation techniques

Techniques which were previously used are endosteal (transdental) pin fixation, amalgam splints, and the Maryland type of etched cast framework, which are considered as an unacceptable method of fixation and are not recommended.

Current recommendation for dentoalveolar trauma is to use a functional and flexible splint for luxation and avulsion, and a rigid splint for tooth luxation in combination with alveolar bone fracture and alveolar process fracture.

Follow-up of the splints:

After 1 week—splint is removed followed by endodontic treatment, if necessary

Three to four weeks—radiographic examination to examine root resorption or periradicular lesions

Six weeks—clinical and radiographic examination for pulp necrosis and root resorption

Three to six months—assessment of the pulpal and periodontal healing and complications.

TREATMENT OF FRACTURES TO THE SUPPORTING BONE/ALVEOLAR BONE (Table 48.6 & Fig. 48.12)

TREATMENT OF SOFT TISSUE INJURIES (GINGIVAL AND MUCOSAL INJURIES)

Management of gingival injuries depends on the presence or absence of injuries to the underlying structures (Table 48.7).

TREATMENT OF INJURIES TO THE PRIMARY DENTITION

Paediatric patients have a relatively large pulp chamber to tooth ratio and their poor coordination necessitates the management of dentoalveolar injuries with sedation. In paediatric patients, tooth displacements are more common than tooth fractures due to the relative resilience of surrounding bone.

Management of the primary dentition should be done by considering the presence of the permanent tooth bud lying underneath the primary tooth. Transmission of forces to the developing tooth bud can interfere with odontogenesis and cause enamel hypoplasia.

- Enamel and dentine fractures are treated with $Ca(OH)_2$, glass ionomer or composite resin
- Pulpal involvement is treated by Formocresol pulpotomy or Zinc oxide-eugenol pulpectomy
- For root fractures, the tooth fragments are removed or if only apical 3rd is present it can be allowed to resorb

TABLE 48.6 Management of Traumatic Injuries to the Alveolar Bone

Comminution of the alveolar bone	It is usually associated with lateral or intrusive luxation injuries. These fractures are reduced, tooth repositioned and splinted for 1–2 weeks
Fractures of the alveolar socket wall	• Fracture reduction by digital pressure • Repositioning of the tooth into occlusion • Rigid splinting for 4 weeks • Soft diet for 2 weeks
Fractures of the alveolar process	• Early reduction and stabilisation of the involved segments • Closed reduction by digital manipulation and immobilisation with rigid splint for 4 weeks • Open reduction if the alveolar segment or the involved teeth is notably displaced. The alveolar segment is stabilised with transosseous wire or small plates • Rigid splinting of the involved teeth using an arch bar for 4 weeks
Fractures of the maxilla and mandible	Generally, reduction and maxillomandibular fixation (MMF) with wires are done once the patient's condition is stable. Open reduction of the jaw can be done later. Discussed in Chapters 49 and 52

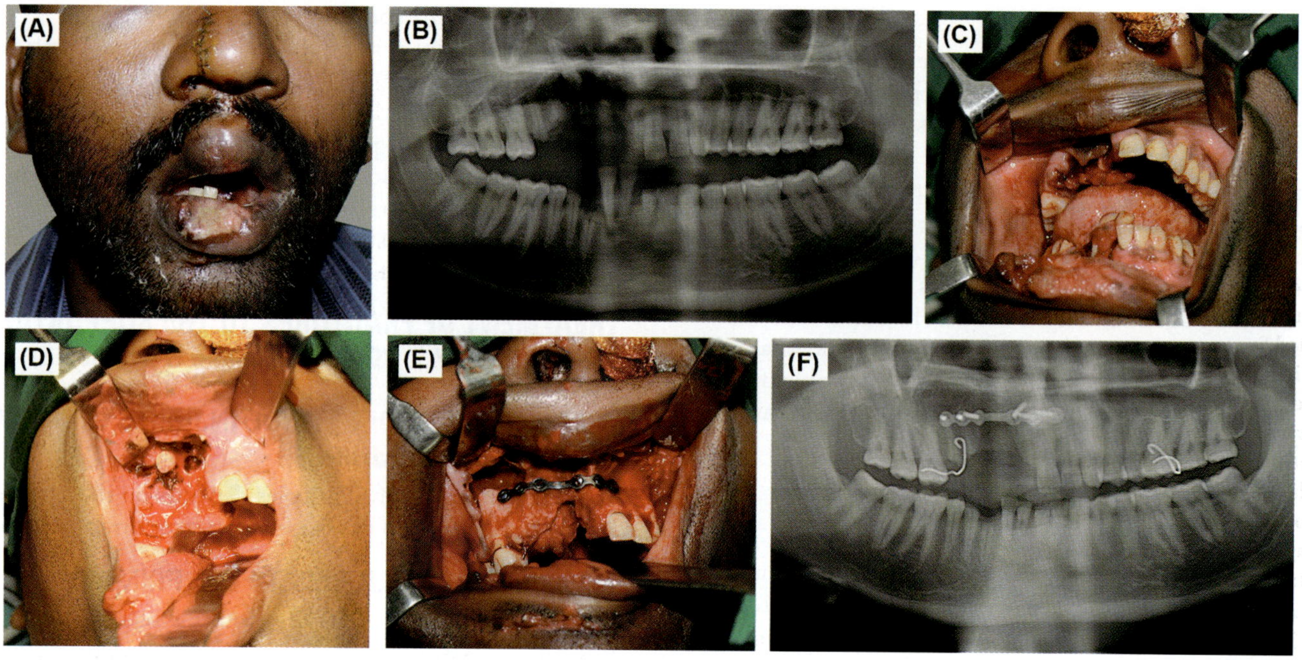

Figure 48.12 Management of dentoalveolar fracture. (**A**) Preoperative view showing swelling and abrasion of the upper and lower lip. (**B**) Preoperative OPG showing dentoalveolar fracture of right upper anteriors and lower anteriors with fractured 14,15,43,44, intruded 13, extruded 31,41, missing 11,12. Fracture line of the dentoalveolar segment extending from 44 to 32 region. (**C** and **D**) Intraoral view showing fractured alveolar segment with missing, fractured and extruded teeth. (**E**) The wound was debrided and the intruded teeth were removed. The alveolar segment was reduced and stabilised using miniplate. (**F**) Postoperative OPG showing reduced bone fragments with miniplate.

TABLE 48.7 Treatment of Gingival and Mucosal Injuries

Contusion	No Treatment
Abrasion	Cleaning to remove foreign material, oral hygiene maintenance
Lacerations	• Antibiotic coverage and tetanus prophylaxis • Cleaning and reapproximation of the tissue by sutures
Avulsive wounds	• Small avulsed areas without underlying injuries—should be left to granulate • A gross alveolar fracture associated with a luxated or displaced tooth—soft tissue flaps • Large areas of exposed bone—advancement soft tissue flaps

- In luxation and intrusion, the primary tooth is either realigned, removed or allowed to re-erupt (Refer to Chapter 56).

COMPLICATIONS FROM DENTOALVEOLAR INJURIES

- Pulpal complications:
  a. Pulp canal obliteration
  b. Pulp necrosis
  c. Internal root resorption
- Periodontal complications:
  a. Inflammatory root resorption
  b. Dentoalveolar ankylosis
- Infection and abscess
- Loss of space in the dental arch
- Ankylosis
- Resorption of root structure
- Loss of supporting bone.

Chapter 49

Fractures of the Mandible

OUTLINE

INTRODUCTION

Mandibular fractures ensue more frequently than any other fractures of the facial skeleton. It is the 2nd most common fracture of the maxillofacial bone secondary to the nose. It is because of its prominent position, inherent weak sites and lack of support to the bone and soft tissues. The mandibular bone is peculiar as it is the only mobile bone in the facial skeleton and plays a critical role in achieving the occlusion, aesthetics and function.

The major *causes* of mandibular fractures include motor vehicle accidents, interpersonal violence, falls and sports-related injuries. The energy required to fracture the mandible, which is a strong bone, ranges from 44.6 to 74.4 kg/m. The most prevalent fracture locations in the mandible are as follows: angle (30%), condyle (23%), symphysis (22%), body (18%), ramus (2%) and coronoid (1%) (Fig. 49.1). The location of the mandibular fracture depends on the mechanism of injury rather than the age or inherent characteristics of the mandible.

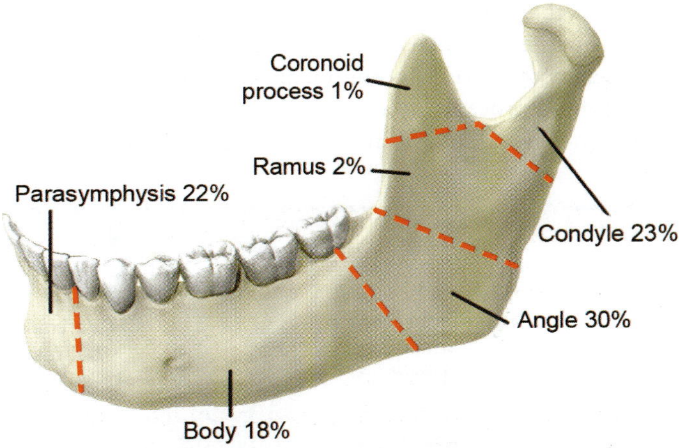

Figure 49.1 Regional occurrence of mandibular fracture.

FRACTURE PATTERNS

Mandibular injuries can occur as a result of direct or indirect trauma (Fig. 49.2).

Fractures of the mental region, canine and alveolar process region are often caused by direct trauma. For example, injuries associated with assault are more likely to receive a forceful lateral blow to the mandible resulting in body and angle fractures. Injuries and fractures of the condylar neck and temporomandibular joint (TMJ) are usually caused by indirect trauma. For example, an anterior blow directed towards the chin can result in bilateral condylar fractures.

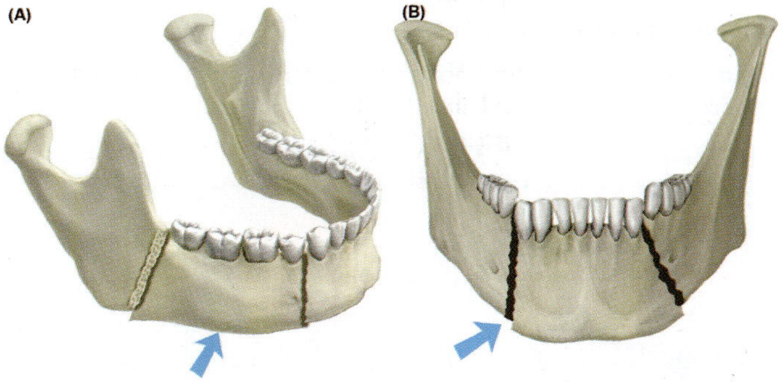

Figure 49.2 Fracture patterns (**A**) Direct trauma. Lateral blow to the mandible resulting in body and ipsilateral angle fracture. (**B**) Indirect trauma. Anterior blow to the chin resulting in bilateral condylar fracture.

APPLIED SURGICAL ANATOMY OF MANDIBLE

- The mandible is the only freely movable bone of the skull. The mandible ***develops*** bilaterally from the 1st brachial arch at the 6th week of Intrauterine life (IUL). At the 7th week, the body of mandible except the anterior part is formed through intramembranous ossification. The symphysis, part of ramus above the mandibular foramen, coronoid and condylar process develops through endochondral ossification. The right and left portions of the mandibular arch are joined at the symphysis region during the 1st year of life, generating a horseshoe-shaped skeletal component
- It is a ***corticocancellous bone*** with an outer cortical plate and central cancellous bone. The anterior lower border of the mandible has thick cortical bone, whereas the posterior lower border is relatively thin. The strength of the mandible lies in these dense cortical plates
- The ***shape of the mandible*** varies considerably with age and growth, whereas the teeth play a significant role in determining the mandibular height
- Each mandible consists of ***vertical and horizontal buttresses*** that allow the transmission of forces. The horizontal buttresses consist of the body and parasymphysis, whereas the vertical components consist of the condyle, coronoid process and ramus, which unite at the sigmoid notch (Fig. 49.3). The angle serves as the junction of the vertical and horizontal components. These lines of orientation of the *bony trabeculae (buttresses) correspond to the pathway of maximal pressure and tension*. The major advantages of these trajectories are that it helps in dissipation of forces from the body of mandible to condyle, thus preventing injury to the middle cranial fossa

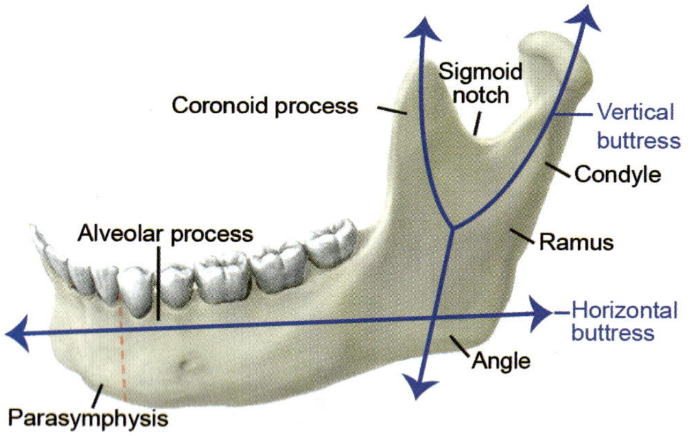

Figure 49.3 Vertical and horizontal buttresses of the mandible.

- **Muscle attachment and displacement of fracture:**

Muscles attached to the mandible considerably influence the direction and displacement of the fracture segments. The movement of the mandible is imparted by two groups of muscle: the *muscles of mastication* (temporalis, masseter, lateral pterygoid and medial pterygoid) *and the suprahyoid muscles* (digastric, mylohyoid, geniohyoid and stylohyoid) (Fig. 49.4 & Table 49.1).

a. ***Fracture at the symphysis and parasymphysis region:***
   - For fractures occurring at the midline along the symphysis region, the mylohyoid and geniohyoid muscles act as a stabilising force and resist displacement of the fracture fragments
   - However, if the fracture line of symphysis region is oblique, the pull of these muscles results in overriding of the fragments
   - When the fractures occurs at the parasymphysis region bilaterally, the fracture fragments are displaced posteriorly under the effect of genioglossus and geniohyoid muscles. This fracture may be associated with loss of tongue control and obstruction of the airway due to fall back of the tongue (Fig. 49.5)
   - The canine region is more prone to fracture as it has the maximum curvature in that region and longer root, making the bone weaker

b. ***Fracture of ramus and coronoid process:***
   Fractures of the ramus are controlled by the masseter muscle on the lateral aspect and medial pterygoid on the medial aspect, resulting in minimum displacement Similarly, fracture of the coronoid also results in minimal displacement as it is splinted by the tendons of the *temporalis* muscle

c. ***Fracture at the angle region:***
   Fractures at the angle of mandible are influenced by the *medial pterygoid and masseter muscles.* The force exerted by the medial pterygoid is greater resulting in upward,

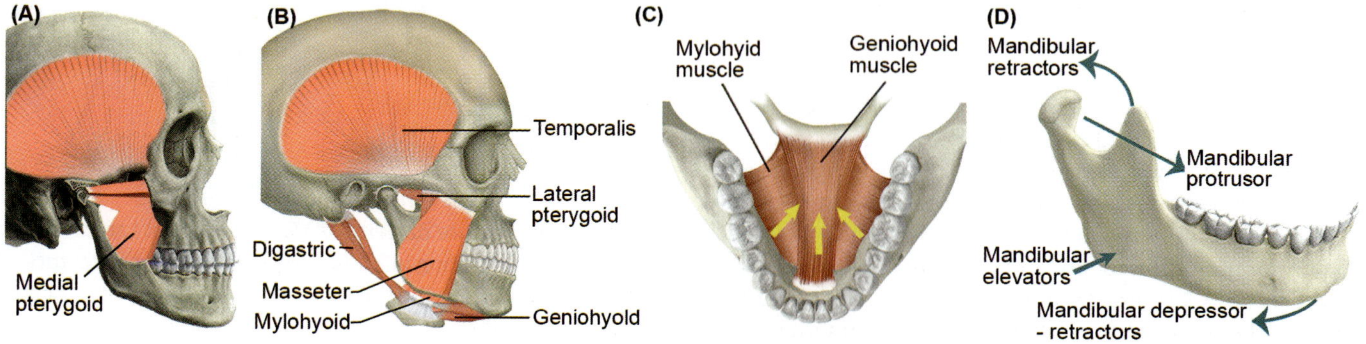

Figure 49.4 **(A–C)** Muscles of mastication and suprahyoid muscles with their attachment. **(D)** Actions of muscle on mandible.

TABLE 49.1 Muscles Involved and their Actions on Mandible

Mandibular retractors	Posterior part of temporalis muscle and deep part of masseter muscle
Mandibular protrusor	Lateral pterygoid muscle
Mandibular elevators	Masseter, medial pterygoid and anterior part of temporalis muscle
Mandibular depressor	Digastric, mylohyoid and geniohyoid muscle

forward and inward displacement of the posterior fragment of mandible

Angle fractures are classified as **(1) vertically favourable or unfavourable and (2) horizontally favourable or unfavourable** (Fig. 49.6)

This concept of favourable versus unfavourable fracture is also referred to as stable versus unstable fracture. This classification was based upon the direction of a fracture line and the effect of muscle action, as viewed on radiographs in a horizontal or vertical plane

Favourable Fractures—The fracture line is considered favourable when the muscle pull resists displacement of the fracture fragments

Unfavourable Fractures—An unfavourable fracture occurs when the muscle pull distracts the fractured fragments away from each other and results in its displacement

- ***Horizontally favourable:***
  When viewed in a horizontal plane (buccal aspect), the fracture line resists the upward displacing forces exerted by the masseter and temporalis muscles on the posterior fragment. The fracture line passes from the alveolar margin, downwards and forward to the lower border of the mandible (Fig. 49.6A)
- ***Horizontally unfavourable fracture:***
  When viewed in a horizontal plane (buccal aspect), the fracture line passes from the alveolar process downwards and backwards to the lower border causing displacement of the posterior segment (i.e. the fracture fragments will shift upwards and medially) (Fig. 49.6B). Horizontal fractures are best seen in lateral oblique and orthopantomogram (OPG). Muscles involved are masseter and temporalis
- ***Vertically favourable fracture:***
  When viewed in a vertical plane (superior aspect), the fracture line resists the medial pull of the medial pterygoid on the posterior fragment. The fracture line passes from the outer or buccal plate obliquely backwards to the lingual plate (Fig. 49.6C)

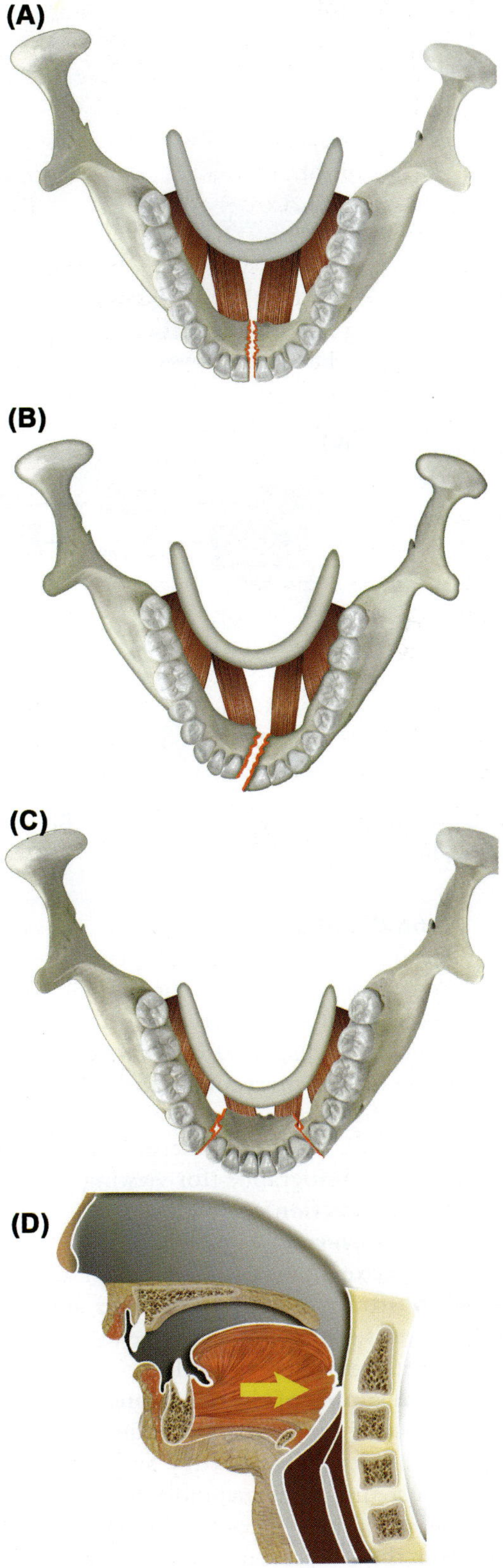

Figure 49.5 (**A**) Fracture in the midline of mandible without any displacement. (**B**) Oblique fracture line with overriding of the fragments. (**C** and **D**) Bilateral parasymphysis fracture with the tongue falling back posteriorly, obstructing the hypopharynx (airway).

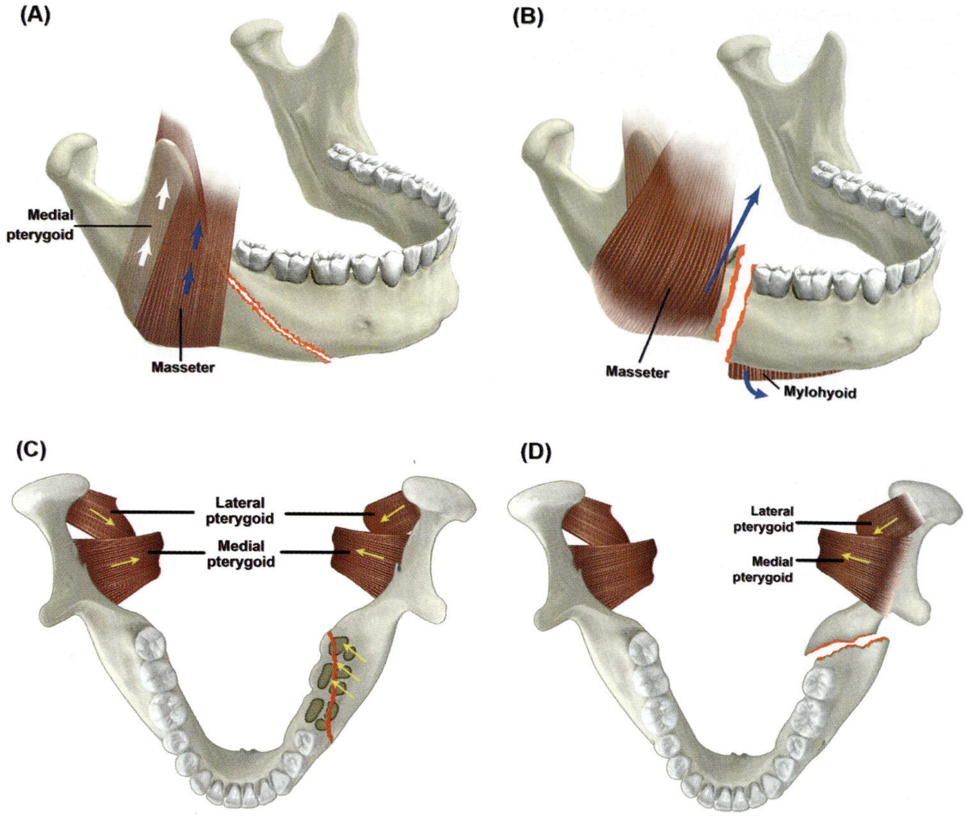

Figure 49.6 **(A)** Horizontally favourable fracture. **(B)** Horizontally unfavourable fracture. **(C)** Vertically favourable fracture. **(D)** Vertically unfavourable fracture.

- ***Vertically unfavourable fractures:***
  The fracture line runs obliquely forward from the buccal side towards the lingual plate. When viewed from the superior aspect, the posterior fragment is displaced lingually due to the pull of the medial pterygoid muscle. The separation of the fragments is in the buccolingual plane (Fig. 49.6D). Vertical fractures are best seen in occlusal radiographs (for viewing in the buccolingual direction)

d. ***Comminuted fractures:***
When this fracture involves the ramus or angle of mandible where strong muscle attachments are present, its displacement is minimal. This is due to sandwiching of the fragments between the muscles

- **Blood supply of the mandible:**
  The blood supply of the mandible is mainly from the inferior alveolar artery and the surrounding periosteum of the mandible. In younger patients, the mandible receives an *endosteal blood supply* from the inferior dental artery. In elderly patients, the inferior dental artery diminishes in size and eventually disappears. Thus, in the elderly, the *periosteal blood supply* gains importance in healing of fractures. Hence, open reduction in the elderly with elevation of the periosteum causes further deprivation of blood supply resulting in delayed union or nonunion
  Any rupture of lingual veins present medial to the angle fracture can result in a large *sublingual haematoma*
- **Nerve supply:**
  The *mandibular nerve* enters the bone at the mandibular foramen on the lingual side and continues through the mandible in the mandibular canal as the *inferior alveolar nerve.* It runs together with the arteries and veins. The inferior alveolar nerve exits the mandibular body between the 1st and 2nd premolars as the *mental nerve*, providing sensation to the lower lip (Fig. 49.7)
  Fractures of the body and the angle of the mandible between the mental foramen and mandibular foramen can cause injury to the inferior alveolar nerve, resulting in paraesthesia of the ipsilateral lip and chin
- **The teeth:**
  The presence of teeth is more crucial in determining the location of fracture. The relative areas of weakness in the mandible are the condylar process, mandibular angle with unerupted 3rd molars, canine tooth region with long dental roots and cysts. The teeth are also a potential source of infection for many mandibular fractures.

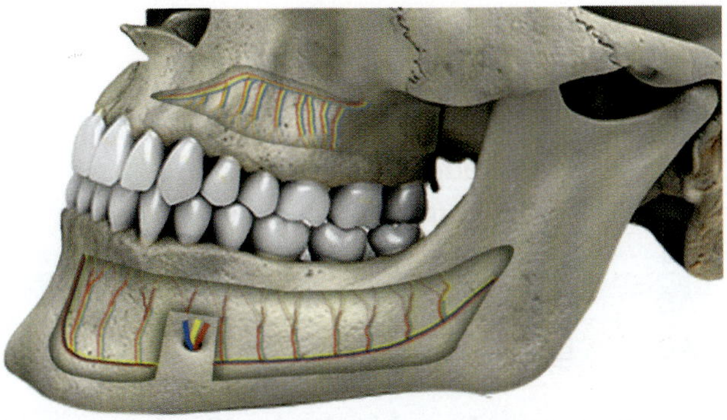

Figure 49.7 Nerve supply to the mandible and teeth.

CLASSIFICATION OF MANDIBULAR FRACTURE

Mandibular fractures have been classified as follows:

1. **Dorland's Medical Dictionary**—Different types of fracture:
   a. *Simple or closed*: A fracture that does not result in an open wound to the external environment, whether it be through the skin, mucosa or periodontal membrane
   b. *Compound or open*: A fracture in which an external wound involving skin, mucosa or periodontal membrane communicates with the break in the bone
   c. *Comminuted:* A fracture where the bone is shattered or crushed
   d. *Greenstick:* A fracture in which one cortex of the bone is broken and the other cortex is bent
   e. *Pathologic:* A fracture occurring from mild injury because of preexisting bone disease
   f. *Multiple:* A variety in which there are two or more lines of fracture on the same bone that are not communicating with each another
   g. *Impacted:* A fracture in which one fragment is firmly driven into the other
   h. *Atrophic:* A spontaneous fracture that occurs due to atrophy of the bone, such as in edentulous mandibles.
   i. *Indirect:* A fracture that occurs at a point distant from the site of injury
   j. *Complicated or complex:* A fracture in which there is considerable injury to the adjacent soft tissue or adjacent parts
2. **Dingman and Natvig classification** (Fig. 49.8):
   a. *Midline:* Fractures between central incisors
   b. *Symphysis:* Fractures occurring within the area of the mandibular midline
   c. *Parasymphyseal:* Fractures bounded by vertical lines distal to the canine teeth
   d. *Body:* From the distal of canine to a line coinciding with the alveolar border of the masseter muscle, usually including the 3rd molar (between the canine region and the angle)
   e. *Angle:* Triangular region bounded by the anterior border of the masseter muscle to the posterosuperior attachment of the masseter muscle (usually distal to the 3rd molar)
   f. *Ramus:* Bounded by the superior aspect of the angle to two lines forming an apex at the sigmoid notch
   g. *Condylar process:* Area of the condylar process superior to the ramus region
   h. *Coronoid process:* Includes the coronoid process of the mandible superior to the ramus region
   i. *Alveolar process:* The region that would normally contain teeth
3. **Kazanjian and Converse:**
   This classification is based on the presence or absence of teeth in relation to the line of fracture
   Class I: Presence of teeth on both sides of the fracture line
   Class II: Tooth present on only one side of the fracture line
   Class III: The patient is edentulous
4. **Kruger and Schilli:**
   A. Relation to the external environment
      a. Simple or closed
      b. Compound or open

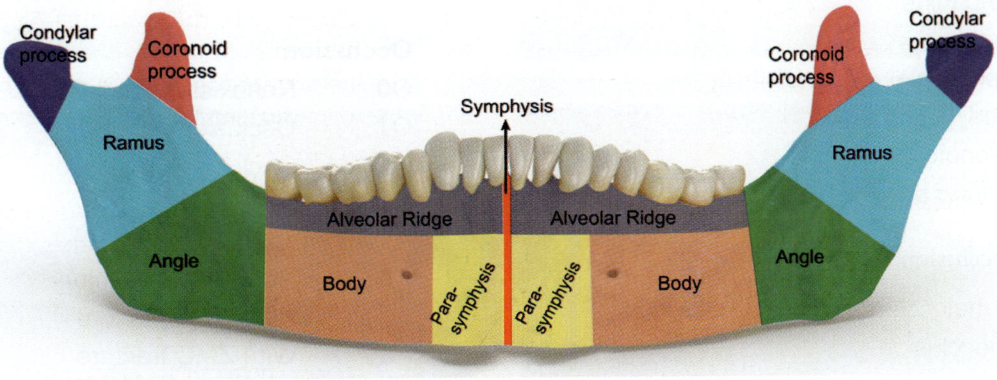

Figure 49.8 Dingman and Natvig classification.

B. Types of fractures:
   a. Incomplete
   b. Greenstick
   c. Complete
   d. Comminuted
C. Dentition of the jaw:
   a. Sufficiently dentulous jaw
   b. Edentulous or insufficiently dentulous jaw
   c. Primary and mixed dentition
D. Localisation:
   a. Fractures involving the symphysis region between the canines
   b. Fractures of the canine region
   c. Fractures involving the body of the mandible from the canine to the angle
   d. Fractures in the angle of mandible over the 3rd molar region
   e. Fractures involving the mandibular ramus between the angle and sigmoid notch
   f. Fractures of the coronoid process
   g. Fractures of the condylar process

5. **Spiessel classification:**

F	No. of fractures or fragments
L	Location of the fracture
O	Status of occlusion
S	Soft tissue involvement
A	Associated fractures

F: No. of fractures

F0	Incomplete fractures
F1	Single fractures
F2	Multiple fractures
F3	Comminuted fractures
F4	Fracture with bone defect

L: Location of fracture

L1	Precanine
L2	Canine
L3	Postcanine
L4	Angle
L5	Supraangle
L6	Condyle
L7	Coronoid
L8	Alveolar process

O: Status of occlusion

O0	No malocclusion
O1	Malocclusion
O2	Edentulous mandible

A: Associated fracture

A0	None
A1	Dentoalveolar fracture
A2	Nasal bone fracture
A3	Zygoma fracture
A4	Le Fort I
A5	Le Fort II
A6	Le Fort III

6. **Mandibular angle and body classification**—According to displacement and favourability of treatment:
   - Horizontally favourable
   - Horizontally unfavourable
   - Vertically favourable
   - Vertically unfavourable
7. **Passi and Malkunje (2017)**: They proposed a classification of mandibular fracture—FLOATIS, which covers all the required criteria.

Type of Fracture	
F0	Partial
F1	Unilateral
F2	Bilateral
F3	Multiple
F4	Comminuted
F5	Disarticulation

Location of Fracture	
L0	Alveolar process
L1	Symphysis
L2	Parasymphysis
L3	Body of mandible
L4	Angle of mandible
L5	Ramus of mandible
L6	Condyle of mandible
L7	Coronoid process
L8	Total avulsion of mandible/Disarticulation

Occlusion	
O0	Nonexistent occlusion
O1	Occlusion intact
O2	Occlusion deranged

Associated Injury	
A0	No associated injury
A1	With NOE fracture
A2	With ZMC fracture
A3	With Le Fort I, II, III fracture

Teeth in Line of Fracture	
T0	Without
T1	No infected teeth
T2	With infected teeth

Infection	
I0	Without infection
I1	With infection

Soft Tissue Component	
S0	Closed mandible fracture
S1	Fracture opened intraorally
S2	Fracture opened extraorally
S3	Fracture with soft tissue loss

CLINICAL EVALUATION

The patient should be evaluated for the following signs and symptoms (Fig. 49.9):

Extraoral examination:

- Swelling
- Haematoma and ecchymosis
- Lacerations
- Facial asymmetry
- Trismus
- Inability to chew/swallow
- Bone tenderness
- Crepitus
- Paraesthesia of the lower lip
- Pain
- Bleeding from the ear

Intraoral examination:

- Sublingual ecchymosis (Coleman's sign)
- Step deformity in the alveolus
- Mobility of fracture fragment across the fracture
- Limited mouth opening
- Inhibition of mandibular movements
- Deranged occlusion
- Open bite/crossbite
- Luxation/fracture of individual teeth
- Missing crowns, bridges or fillings, broken dentures.

EXTRAORAL EXAMINATION

- Swelling, ecchymosis, erythema, abrasion and lacerations present as indirect signs of injury. Laceration or contusion in chin may indicate symphysis fracture with or without bilateral condylar fracture

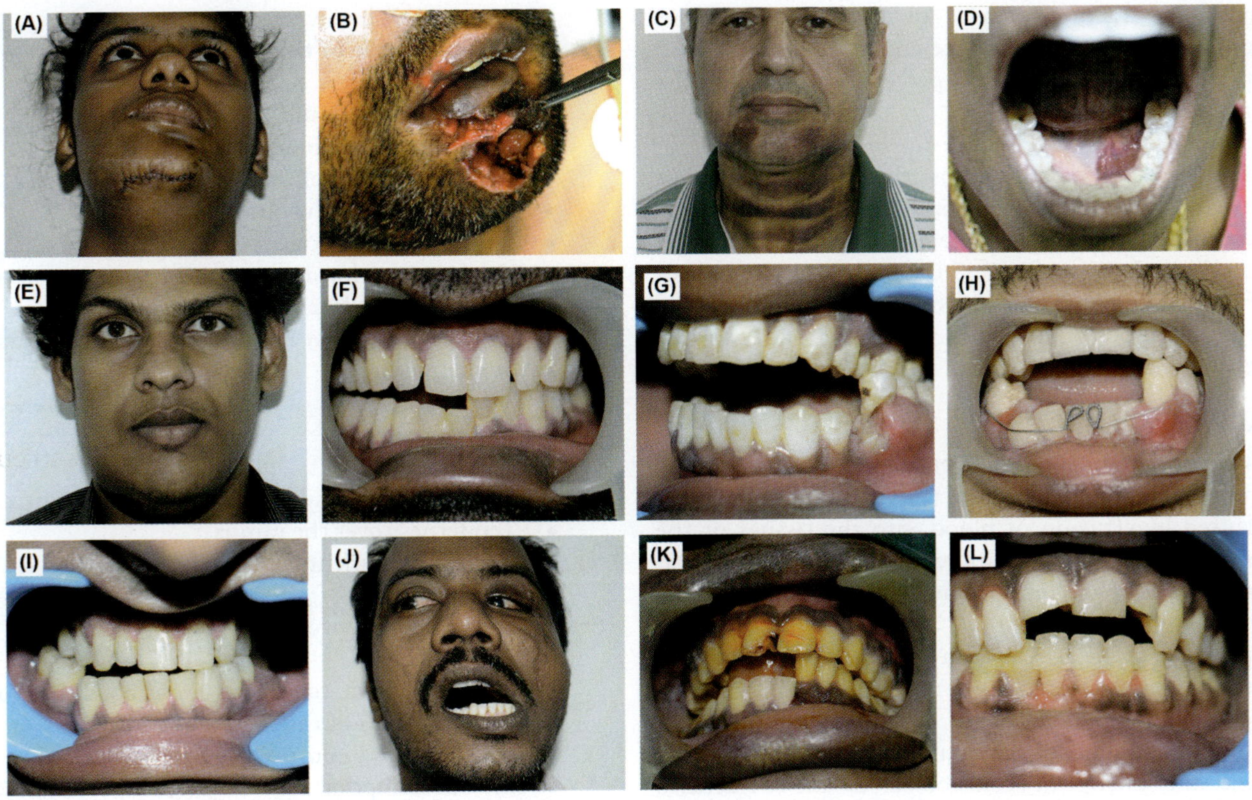

Figure 49.9 Clinical features: **(A)** Swelling, **(B)** Laceration, **(C)** Haematoma/ecchymosis, **(D)** Sublingual ecchymosis (Coleman's sign), **(E)** Facial asymmetry, **(F)** Inability to occlude the teeth, **(G)** Deranged occlusion, **(H)** Anterior open bite, **(I)** Posterior crossbite, **(J)** Limited mouth opening, **(K)** Step deformity at the alveolus, **(L)** Fracture of teeth.

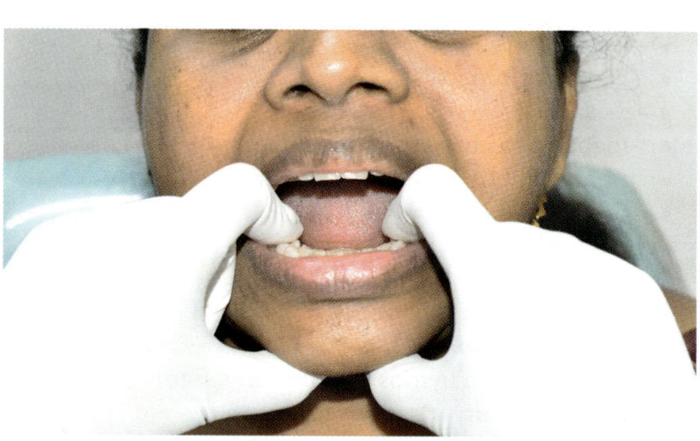

Figure 49.10 Bimanual palpation of mandible.

- *Facial deformity:* There may be obvious deformity in the bony contour of the mandible, and if considerable displacement has occurred, the patient is unable to approximate the anterior teeth together and the mouth remains in an open posture (open bite)
- Except angle, ramus and condyle regions, all fractures along the tooth-bearing areas are considered as compound. Saliva is a significant source of infection and is frequently observed drooling from the corners of the mouth
- Palpation should begin bilaterally in the condylar region and then continued downwards along the lower border of the mandible. Bone tenderness on palpation is pathognomonic of fracture, even in an undisplaced fracture. The movement of the fracture ends causes crepitus in displaced fractures, as well as a perceptible step deformity along the lower border
- *Bimanual palpation* (Fig. 49.10):

  The abnormal mobility across the fracture site can be elicited by bimanual palpation. The mandible is grasped on either side of the fracture line with the index finger on the occlusal surface and the thumb on the inferior border. The proximal and distal segments are moved in the anteroposterior and superoinferior direction to elicit the abnormal mobility.

INTRAORAL EXAMINATION

- ***Coleman's sign (sublingual haematoma)***—It is a pathognomonic sign for the body of the mandible fracture. It is caused by effusion of blood into the tissues of the floor of the mouth, raising the mucous membrane and producing a characteristic bluish swelling under the tongue
- Step defects at the alveolus can be seen in displaced fractures along with lacerations of the overlying mucosa and gingiva
- Malocclusion is one of the significant signs of mandibular fracture. Change in occlusion can be due to fractures involving the tooth, alveolar process, mandible or TMJ injury
- Mobility between the fracture segments can be elicited on palpation.

CLINICAL FEATURES OF MANDIBULAR FRACTURE AT VARIOUS SITES

Symphysis and parasymphysis fracture:

- Sublingual haematoma or ecchymosis in the floor of the mouth—Coleman's sign
- Tenderness over the bone
- Unilateral or posterior open bite
- Premature dental contact resulting in an inability to close the jaw
- Mobility of the bony fragment at the fracture site
- A retruded chin in bilateral parasymphyseal fracture
- Occasionally, loss of tongue control and airway obstruction occurs in bilateral parasymphyseal fracture
- They are commonly associated with fractures of one or both condyles

Fracture of the body of the mandible (molar and premolar regions):

- Swelling and bone tenderness
- Sublingual haematoma (Coleman's sign)
- Derangement of occlusion
- Premature contact of the distal fragment (ramus)
- Inability to open or close the jaw
- Paraesthesia of lower lip due to inferior alveolar nerve (IAN) involvement

Fracture of the angle of the mandible:

- Swelling
- Bone tenderness and crepitus
- Movement of segment at the fracture site
- Step deformity behind the last molar tooth
- Haematoma on the buccal/lingual mucosa
- Deranged occlusion
- Trismus to some degree
- Anterior open bite in bilateral angle fracture
- Ipsilateral open bite is more common in unilateral angle fracture
- The lateral aspect of the face appears flattened

Fracture of the ramus:

- Rare fracture
- Swelling and ecchymosis both extra and intraorally
- Tenderness over the ramus
- Painful movements of the mandible
- Severe trismus

Fracture of coronoid process:

- Rare fracture
- It results from reflex contracture of the powerful anterior fibres of the temporalis muscle
- The fractured coronoid is pulled upwards towards the infratemporal fossa by the temporalis muscle
- Tenderness over the anterior part of the ramus
- Limitation of mandibular movement.

RADIOGRAPHIC EXAMINATION

The radiographs are helpful in achieving a precise diagnosis and treatment plan. The following are the radiographs that are helpful in diagnosing mandibular fracture (Fig. 49.11 and Table 49.2):

a. Panoramic radiograph (OPG)
b. Lateral oblique radiograph
c. Posteroanterior radiograph
d. Occlusal view
e. Periapical view
f. Reverse Townes view
g. TMJ, including tomograms
h. Computed tomography (CT) scans.

MANAGEMENT OF MANDIBULAR FRACTURE

BIOMECHANICAL CONSIDERATIONS

Under function, the mandible exhibits *tensile forces (zones of tension) at the superior border and maximum compression at the inferior border* (Fig. 49.12A and B). In between the zones of tension and compression lies the neutral zone, where the forces are zero. The neutral zone of mandible lies approximately at the level of the inferior alveolar canal.

It would be ideal to apply rigid fixation at the zone of tension or the superior border of the mandible, but it is complicated by the presence of teeth, thin cortical bone and thin overlying soft tissue. As the neutral zone is located in the inferior alveolar canal, it is not an ideal location for hardware

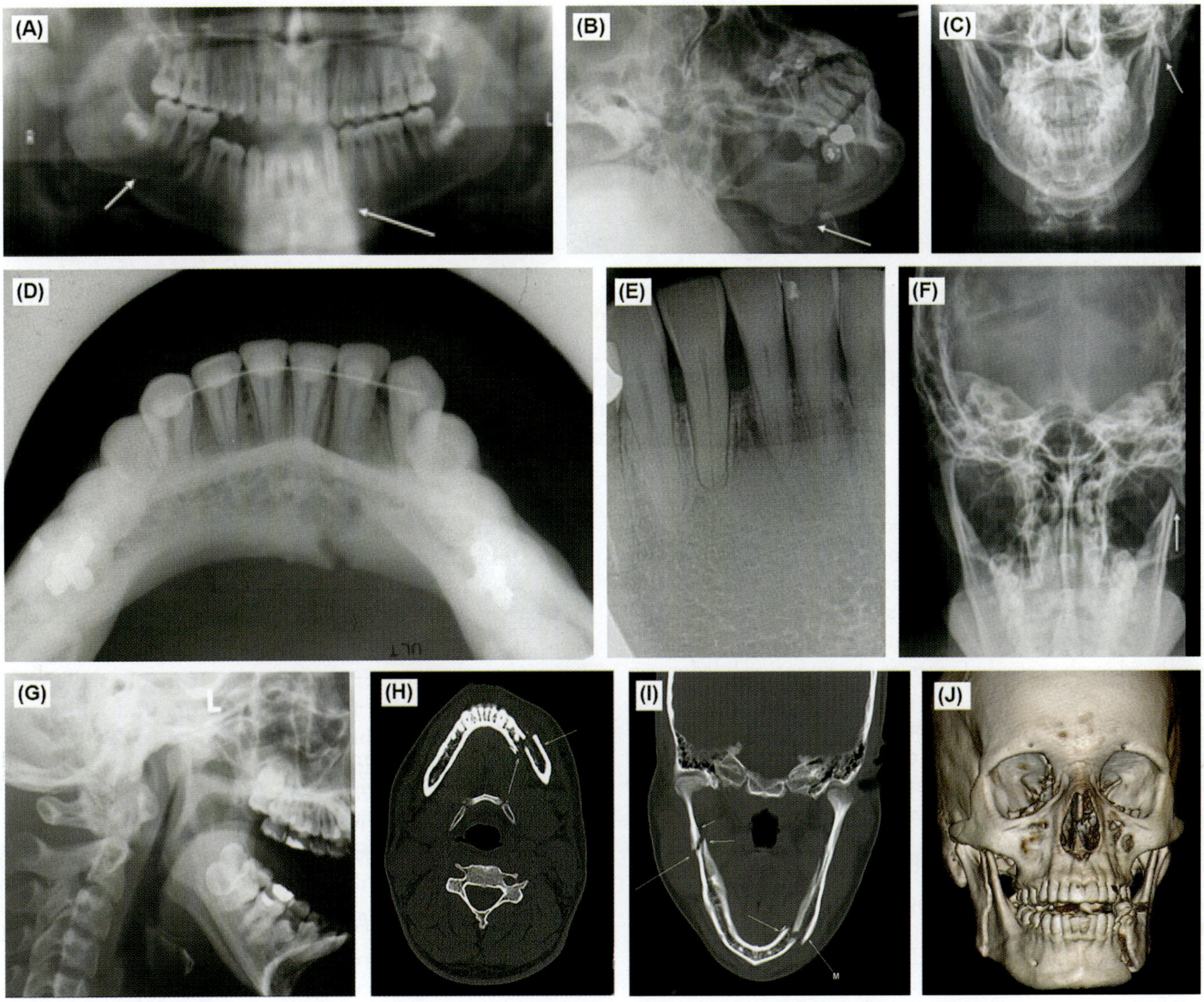

Figure 49.11 Radiographic evaluation of mandibular fracture. **(A)** OPG. **(B)** Lateral oblique radiograph. **(C)** Posteroanterior radiograph PA view **(D)** Mandibular occlusal view. **(E)** Periapical view. **(F)** Reverse Townes view. **(G)** TMJ, tomograms. **(H)** CT scan (axial view). **(I)** CT scans (coronal view). **(J)** CT scan 3D reconstruction.

TABLE 49.2 Radiographic Assessment for Mandible Fracture

Radiographs	Area Visualised
Panoramic radiograph (OPG)	Entire mandible
Lateral oblique radiograph	Ramus, angle and posterior body
Posteroanterior radiograph	Ramus, angle and body fractures (medial or lateral displacement)
Occlusal view	Medial and lateral position of body fractures, anteroposterior displacement in the symphysis
Periapical view	Nondisplaced linear fractures of the body, alveolar process and dental trauma
Reverse Townes view	Condyle and subcondylar region
TMJ, including tomograms	Condylar fractures (anterior displacement)
CT scans	Complete mandible Extent of fracture and degree of displacement can be assessed in CT scans

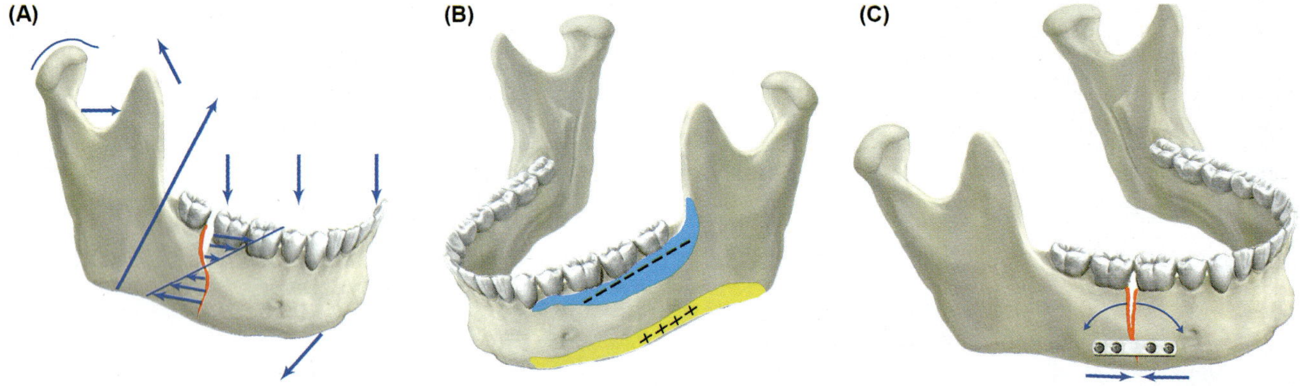

Figure 49.12 Zones of tension and compression. (**A**) Tensile forces along the superior border and compression along the lower border. (**B**) Tension zone marked in blue (−) and compression zones marked in yellow (+). (**C**) When compression plating is done at the lower border, the tensile forces at the superior border is exaggerated, resulting in the opening of the fracture.

fixation. Hence, the inferior border is biologically the ideal place for hardware fixation (49.12C). The inferior border is extremely stable with adequate soft tissue coverage and the dental structures usually does not extend to this area, but when compression plating is applied at the lower border, the tensile forces at the superior border can get exaggerated resulting in a gap between the fragments. To compensate for this lack of stability at the upper border, a tension band can be applied. The tension band could be a monocortical miniplate, lag screw or arch bar to resist the tensile forces.

GENERAL PRINCIPLES OF TREATMENT

The primary goals in treating mandibular fractures are aimed at:

- Restoration of the form and function of the mandible
- To achieve anatomic reduction
- Establishing the preinjury occlusion
- Stable fixation for healing
- Restoration of normal TMJ movements and function
- Avoidance of complications.

EMERGENCY MANAGEMENT (INITIAL/TEMPORARY STABILISATION)

Once the airway, breathing and circulation have been restored, the wounds must be sutured and the fracture must be initially stabilised. **Bridle wire** can be used to achieve the initial stabilisation of the fracture. It involves the manual reduction of dentate fracture fragments under local anaesthesia, followed by their stabilisation with a 26-gauge wire. Two healthy teeth adjacent to the fracture line are wrapped with the wire. The wire can be wrapped around a 2nd tooth if the adjacent tooth is mobile (Fig. 49.13).

Supportive bandages—Barrel bandages or four-tail bandage can be used temporarily to stabilise the mandibular fracture.

REDUCTION OF FRACTURE

Reduction of fracture is a method to restore the correct alignment of the fractured bony fragments. The two methods of reduction are:

- *Closed reduction* involves manual manipulation of the fractured bony fragments without surgical exposure of the fragments

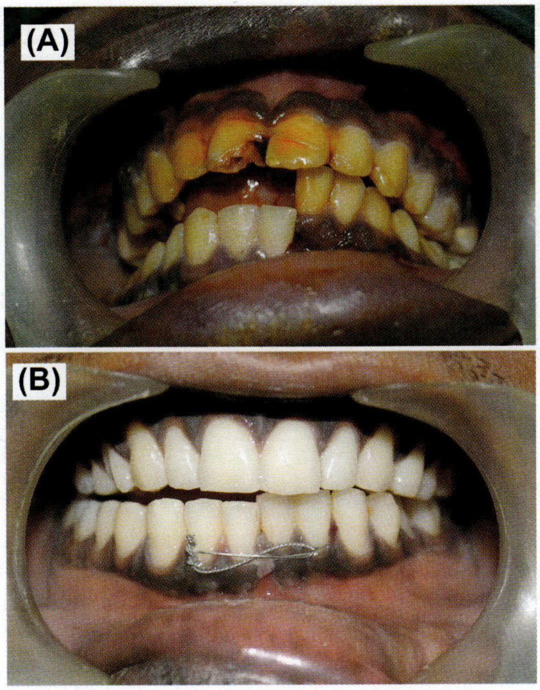

Figure 49.13 Bridle wire. (**A**) Intraoral view showing fracture at the symphysis region. (**B**) Emergency reduction of fracture and bridle wire wrapped around the fracture.

- *Open reduction* involves reduction of the fracture under direct vision by exposing the fracture fragments surgically.

Closed reduction

Indications of closed reduction

- Favourable fractures with full dentition
- Grossly comminuted fractures
- Undisplaced or minimally displaced fractures
- Fractures that are exposed due to loss of overlying soft tissue
- Edentulous mandibular fractures
- Mandibular fractures in children with developing dentition
- Infected fractures

Grossly comminuted fractures: Excellent blood supply of the face would facilitate the small fragments of the bones to coalesce and heal, whereas open reduction would jeopardise the vascular supply of the fragments

Fractures of the severely atrophic edentulous mandible: Open reduction requires stripping of the periosteum, which is the major source of blood supply to the edentulous mandible, leading to compromised healing

Lack of soft tissue coverage: It may lead to delay in bone union and infection of the plates and wires

Fractures in children: The open reduction procedure might pose a risk to the developing tooth buds

Infected fractures: It may cause delayed healing.

Advantages and disadvantages of closed reduction are described in Table 49.3.

TABLE 49.3 Advantages and Disadvantages of Closed Reduction

Advantages	Disadvantages
• Less-traumatic procedure • The vascularity of the trauma site is preserved • Less expensive • Shorter hospitalisation • Reduced risk of nerve injury and occlusal dysfunction	• Longer period of immobilisation leading to complications such as ankylosis • Requires intact dentition • Noncompliance of patient for IMF

Techniques of closed treatment (IMF/MMF)

Maxillomandibular fixation (MMF) is wiring the upper and lower arch bars together. It is a method for immobilising fractured mandibular segments by externally locking the occlusion, with the dentition serving as a point of stability. It aids in restoring the patient's preinjury occlusion and aids in the reduction and fixation of facial fractures.

A variety of MMF techniques are available (Fig. 49.14), which include:

a) Dental wiring
b) Arch bars
c) Intermaxillary fixation (IMF) screws
d) Splints
e) Suspension wires
f) External fixation

(Refer to Chapter 47.)

Period of intermaxillary fixation (immobilisation)

The duration of IMF is dependent on the type, location, number and severity of the mandibular fracture, the patient's age and general health, the presence of infection and the reduction technique.

- The average recommended immobilisation period for mandibular fractures is 3–6 weeks
- Treatment of edentulous mandibular fractures requires a longer period of IMF
- Age-related bone changes also contribute to the prolongation of the immobility period

  According to Killey and Kay, the period of immobilisation for fractures involving tooth-bearing areas is as follows:

- Young adult with angle fracture and tooth extracted from fracture line—3 weeks

  But if there are associated stipulations, the time can be extended as such:
  - Tooth retained in fracture line—add 1 week
  - Fracture at the symphysis—add 1 week
  - Age 40 years and above—add 1 week
  - Children and adolescents—subtract 1 week.

Applying this guide, the period of immobilisation can be calculated for fractures of lower jaw. For example, a fracture of symphysis in a 40-year-old patient where the

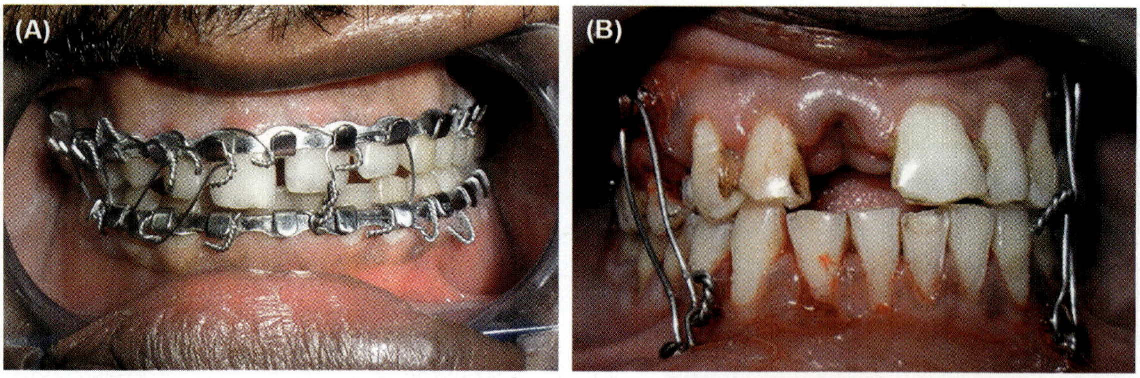

Figure 49.14 Techniques of closed reduction. (**A**) Arch bar and IMF, (**B**) IMF screws.

tooth in the fracture line is retained requires 6 weeks of immobilisation (i.e. basic 3 weeks + 1 week for less favourable site + 1 week for age + 1 week for tooth retained in the line of fracture).

Open reduction

Indications of open reduction:

- Displaced, unfavourable fractures
- Unstable fractures or those with rotation/angulation of fragment
- Multiple fractures of the facial bones
- Severely displaced edentulous mandibular fracture
- Edentulous maxilla opposing a mandibular fracture
- The presence of concomitant head injury
- Delayed treatment of displaced fractures
- Malunited mandibular fractures
- Cases failed by closed reduction
- Systemic conditions contraindicating IMF (epilepsy, alcoholism, diabetes, psychiatric disorders or severe disability).

Advantages and disadvantages of open reduction are described in Table 49.4.

TABLE 49.4 Advantages and Disadvantages of Open Reduction

Advantages	Disadvantages
• It allows direct visualisation and reduction of the fractured bone segments • Restoration of the patient's preinjury occlusion • Superior stabilisation of the fracture • Shorter period of bone healing • Early return to normal jaw function	• Potential for foreign body infections • Increased chance of morbidity due to compromised vascularity • Damage to the neurovascular structures

SURGICAL APPROACHES

Various factors, such as the location and level of the fracture, the presence of a laceration, the presence of additional fractures, the need for surgical exposure, the position of the nerve, cosmetic concerns and the type of fixation influence the choice of approach. For proper reduction and fixation of fractures, adequate exposure is necessary. The most frequently used techniques for treating mandibular fractures (Fig. 49.15) are:

- Intraoral approach/transoral
- Extraoral approach
  - Submental
  - Submandibular approach/Risdon's approach
  - Retromandibular approach
  - Preauricular approach
- Transbuccal approach
- Existing laceration

1. **Through existing laceration:**
   In certain fractures, the fracture fragment is accessed through preexisting lacerations. For adequate access to the fracture area, lacerations can be extended along *Langer's line* or *relaxed skin tension lines*.
2. **Intraoral approach** (Fig. 49.15E):
   Of all the approaches, the intraoral approach is commonly practiced for a vast majority of the mandible fractures
   Indications—Fractures of symphysis, parasymphysis, body and angle (superior border) of the mandible
   Advantages:
   - It is simple and precise
   - Less postoperative complications

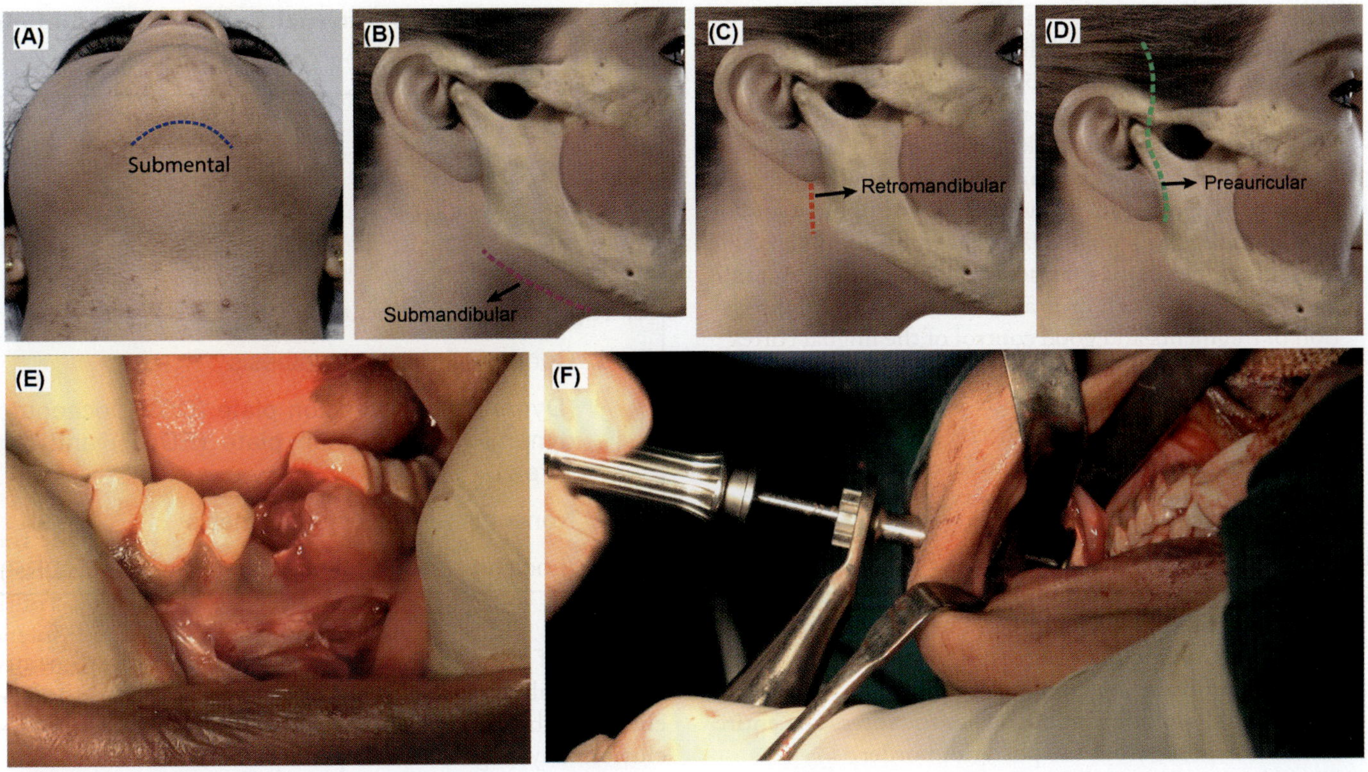

Figure 49.15 Surgical approaches for mandibular fractures: (A) Submental, (B) Submandibular, (C) Retromandibular, (D) Preauricular, (E) Intraoral approach, (F) Transbuccal approach.

- Less damage to the facial nerve branches
- No visible external scar
- Less intensity of pain as compared to other approaches

Technique:

Anterior mandibular fractures (symphysis and parasymphysis region):

- The vestibular region is infiltrated with local anaesthetic and vasoconstrictor
- The lower lip is everted and a curvilinear incision is placed using a no. 15 scalpel from canine to canine, leaving 10–15 mm of mucosa attached to the gingiva
- In the incisor region, the underlying mentalis muscle fibres are sharply incised in an oblique direction
- In the canine and premolar region, incision is placed more superiorly and oriented perpendicular to the bone, to prevent damage to the mental nerve branches
- Sufficient mentalis muscle should remain on the bone for sutures to be placed during closure
- Fracture site is identified, reduced and fixed with plates. The surgical wound is then irrigated and closed in layers
- The chin is covered by an adhesive bandage for supporting the mentalis muscle and to prevent drooping

Body, angle and ramus of the mandible:

- In the body region, the incision is placed 3–5 mm below the mucogingival junction to allow adequate tissue for closure
- Posteriorly, the incision is extended from the crest of the 2nd molar region along the external oblique ridge and laterally over the ascending ramus. The incision cuts through the buccinator muscle, buccopharyngeal fascia and periosteum of the mandible
- Usually, the incision is restricted till the occlusal plane to preclude herniation of buccal fat pad into the surgical site. The buccal artery and nerve are likewise spared
- With the help of retractors (Kocher clamp), the entire ramus and subcondylar region are exposed
- Fracture fragments are reduced and fixed. Single-layer closure is sufficient

3. **Submental approach:**

Indications—Anterior mandibular region (symphysis and parasymphysis) fractures.

Technique—The incision is made along the skin crease or following the curvature of the anterior mandible. Dissection involves the skin, subcutaneous tissue, platysma muscle and periosteum to reach the inferior border of the mandible. The wound closure is done in layers

4. **Submandibular approach/Risdon's approach:**
   Indications—Comminuted fractures and atrophic mandibular fractures involving the body and angle of the mandible. It is also indicated for fractures, which are not suitable by intraoral approach as it allows satisfactory manipulation of fragments and good control of the lingual cortex
   Technique—A skin incision of about 4–5 cm in length is placed 2–3 cm below the angle of the mandible. The incision is extended through the skin, subcutaneous tissue, platysma and superficial layer of the deep cervical fascia. Care is taken to preserve the marginal mandibular branch of the facial nerve. Facial vessels can be retracted or ligated and divided. The pterygomasseteric sling and the periosteum is then incised to expose the inferior border of the mandible. The wound is closed in layers to eliminate the dead space
5. **Retromandibular approach:**
   Indications—Ramus and subcondylar fractures. The entire ramus is exposed from the posterior border
   Technique—A vertical incision is made extending from just below the ear lobe towards the mandibular angle, parallel to the posterior border of the mandible. Incision is made through the skin and subcutaneous tissue, exposing the superficial musculoaponeurotic system (SMAS). An oblique incision is made through the SMAS and the parotid gland is identified. The parotid gland is bluntly dissected parallel to the direction of the facial nerve branches and towards the posterior border of the mandible. At the posterior border of the mandible, an incision is made through the pterygomasseteric sling and the masseter muscle is stripped off from the ramus. The wound re-approximation is done in layers and care is taken to close the parotid gland capsule tightly to prevent the formation of a salivary fistula
6. **Preauricular approach:**
   Indications—Condylar head and neck fractures. *Technique*—(refer to Chapter 50)
7. **Transbuccal approach:**
   Indications—Mandibular angle fracture
   It is an approach that combines the intraoral approach with an extraoral incision (small incision on the facial skin to insert the transbuccal trocar). Through the cannula, drilling and screw insertion is done at a right angle to the lateral mandibular surface.

FIXATION METHODS (INTERNAL FIXATION)

Open reduction and internal fixation (ORIF) refers to the surgical method of fixation by direct visualisation of the fractures and fixation using hardware-like stainless steel or titanium (refer to Chapter 47).

The basic systems of **internal fixation of mandibular fractures** include:

a. **Nonrigid fixation**
   Transosseous wiring
b. **Semirigid fixation**
   Noncompression miniplates
c. **Rigid fixation without IMF**
   i. Compression osteosynthesis
      (Dynamic compression plate (DCP), eccentric dynamic compression plate (EDCP) and lag screw)
   ii. Noncompression osteosynthesis
      (Locking plate, reconstruction plate and THORP)

Most of the nonrigid techniques require postoperative IMF for stability, whereas the semirigid and rigid techniques eliminate the need for postoperative IMF. If required, the occlusion may be guided with postoperative elastics.

NONRIGID FIXATION

Nonrigid fixation is the fixation that allows some *movement across the fracture line (interfragmentary motion)*. It serves only in approximating or realigning of the fracture fragments and preventing their displacement by the muscles of mastication. Healing of the fracture line occurs by secondary intention.

Transosseous wiring

It is wiring across the fracture line. It is commonly done for fractures involving the angle and symphysis region, either through the intraoral or extraoral approach. For minimally displaced angle fracture, transosseous wiring at the upper border of the mandible is preferred (Fig. 49.16). Transosseous wiring at the upper border of the mandible is recommended for mildly displaced angle fractures. With the methods and materials available today, *nonrigid fixation is no longer in use* (refer to Chapter 47).

SEMIRIGID FIXATION

Semirigid fixation refers to the fixation of the fracture fragments, with *some degree of rigidity*, which is not sufficient enough to withstand the masticatory forces.

Noncompression miniplates

Miniplates were originally designed by Champy with stainless steel.

Champy's line of osteosynthesis

Champy defined the *'ideal lines of osteosynthesis'* as the lines of maximum tensile stress, extending from the oblique ridge along the base of the alveolus to the mental foramen. He suggested

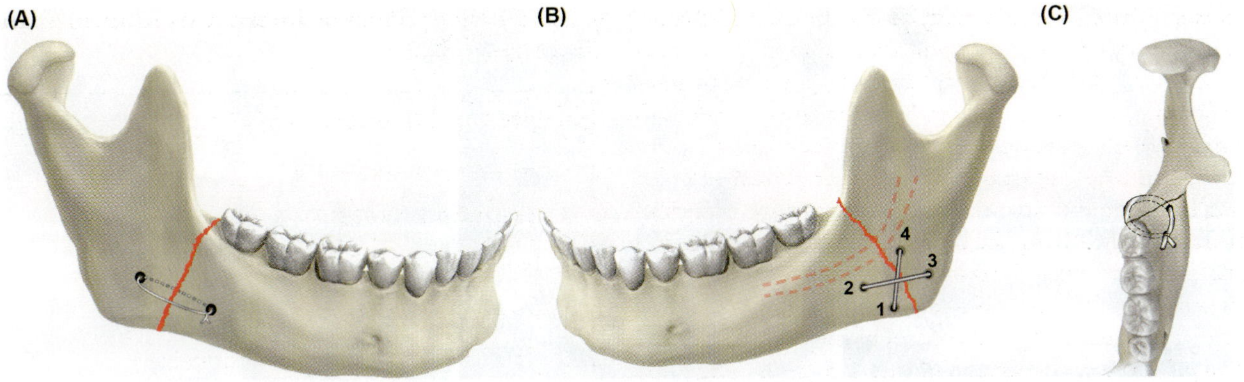

Figure 49.16 Nonrigid fixation—Transosseous wiring of angle fracture at various sites.

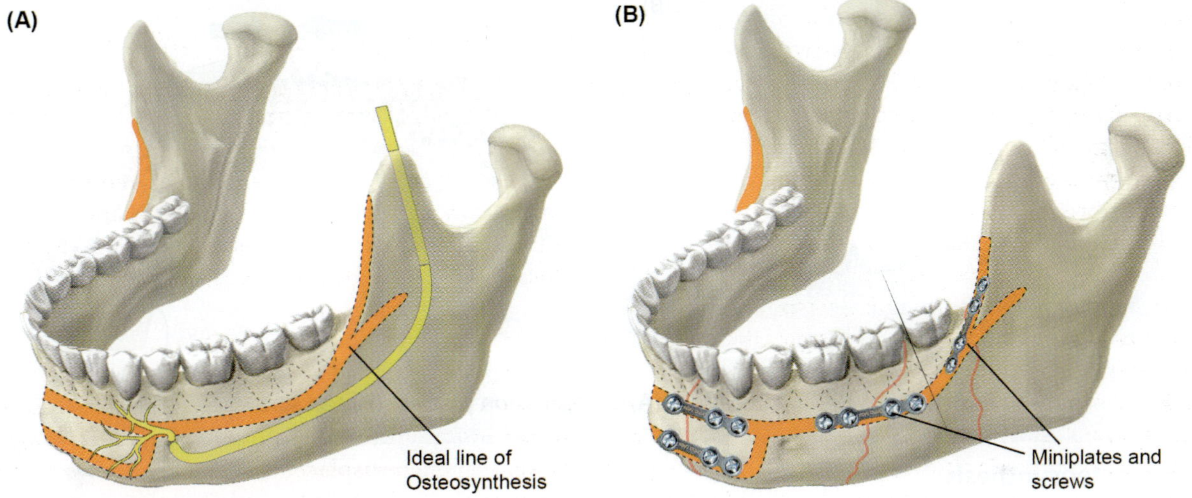

Figure 49.17 (**A**) Champy's line of osteosynthesis. (**B**) Miniplates along Champy's line.

that a single miniplate placed at the ideal lines of osteosynthesis is adequate to stabilise the mandibular fractures and achieve a predictable union (Fig. 49.17) (Table 49.5).

The superior border of the mandible experiences tensile force during function, while the inferior border experiences compression. The fragments are displaced due to the tensional forces along the upper border. Therefore, **Champy** created *monocortical, noncompression miniplates* that can be attached to the superior border. This method of fixation provides sufficient resistance to tensile forces and also promotes osteosynthesis (refer to Chapter 47).

TABLE 49.5 Areas of Plate Application (Fig. 49.18)

Location of Fracture	No. of Miniplates
Fractures anterior to mental foramen (symphysis to 1st premolar)	Two miniplates separated by 4–5 mm
Fractures posterior to the mental foramen (1st premolar to 3rd molar)	Single miniplate placed below the dental roots and above the inferior alveolar nerve
Fractures of the angle Region	Single miniplate on the superior border along the external oblique ridge

Noncompression miniplates

Noncompression miniplates are used along with self-tapping monocortical screws. Materials used are stainless steel or titanium.

- The length of the miniplates vary from 2 to 9 cm. The different lengths come in 2 holes, 4 holes, 5 holes, 6 holes, 8 holes to 16 holes with or without gap
- Plate size—1.5, 2.0 or 2.5 mm thickness
- Screw length—6, 8, 10 and 12 mm length
- Diameter of the screw—2 mm.

Most commonly used miniplates for mandibular fractures are 2 mm thick, 4-hole plates with gap and 8 mm screws.

RIGID FIXATION

Rigid fixation can be defined as 'any form of fixation that is applied directly to the bones and is strong enough to prevent *interfragmentary motion* across the fracture line'. The bone heals by *primary or direct bone union* without callus formation.

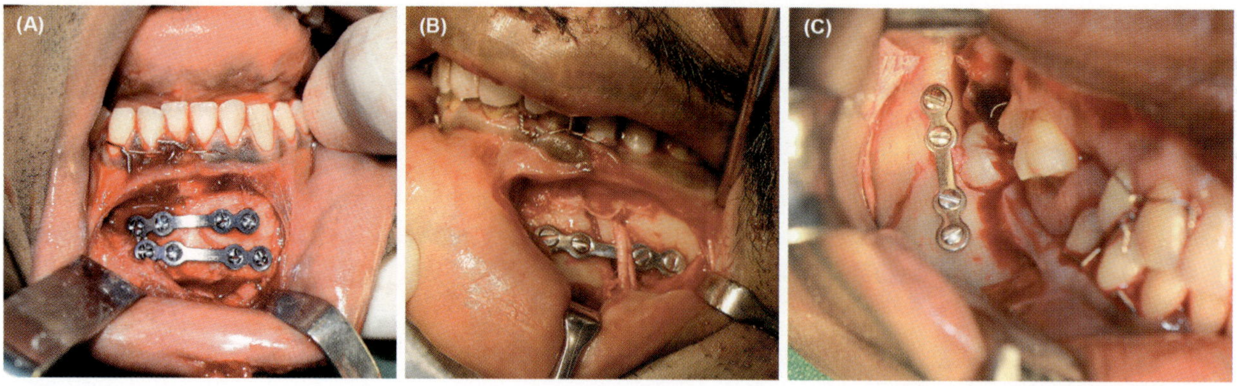

Figure 49.18 Semirigid fixation—Application of miniplates at different sites. (**A**) Symphysis region, (**B**) Body region, (**C**) Angle region.

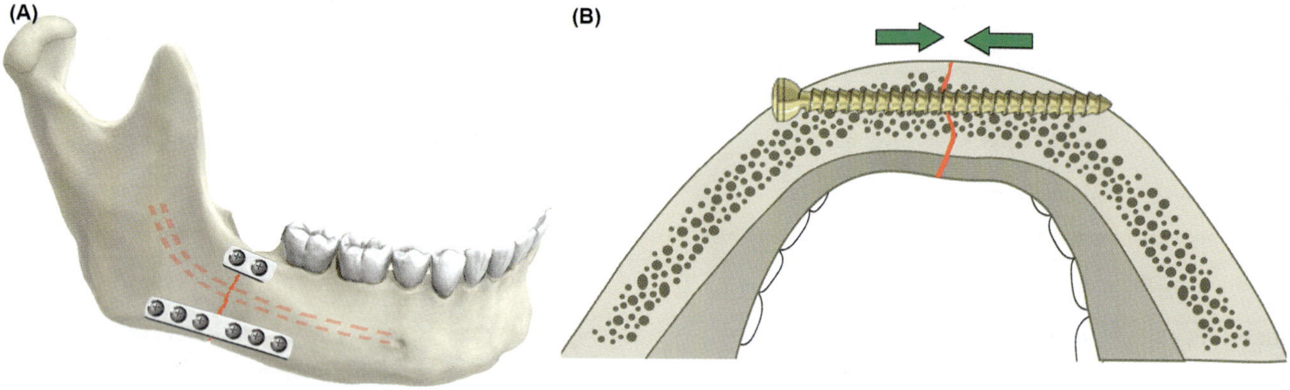

Figure 49.19 Rigid fixation. (**A**) Compression plating, (**B**) Lag screw.

Compression osteosynthesis

There is absolute stability across the fracture. Compression plates produce compression by *bringing the fractured margins closer together and compressing them* (Fig. 49.19). It also provides additional stability by increasing the frictional interlocking between them. It results in *zero movement between the fracture fragments* as well as complete immobility of the hardware against the bone.

Noncompression osteosynthesis

Reconstruction plate–The reconstruction plate is a load-bearing plate that carries the total functional load. The reconstruction plate's increased size increases its strength and stabilises the fragments against functional displacement (Fig. 49.20). In addition to the reconstruction of the mandibular defects, therefore used in load-bearing defects and gaps.

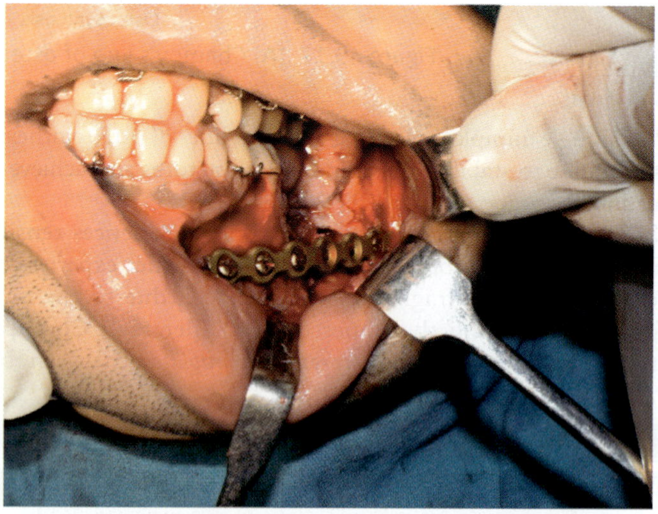

Figure 49.20 Rigid fixation with reconstruction plate.

MANAGEMENT OF MANDIBULAR FRACTURES BASED ON THE LOCATION (Table 49.6, Fig. 49.21)

MANAGEMENT OF TEETH IN LINE OF FRACTURE (Fig. 49.22)

Teeth in the line of fracture are a *potential source of infection* and may interfere with healing of the fracture due to the following reasons:

- The fracture becomes *compound* into the mouth with exposure of the periodontal ligament
- The *pulp* might become necrotic as a result of trauma to the teeth
- Preexisting pathological lesion of the teeth (e.g. apical granuloma).

The retention or removal of teeth has been a contentious issue for decades. When a tooth in the fracture line is structurally undamaged, potentially functional and not subluxated, it can be retained. Numerous authors have

TABLE 49.6 Management of Mandibular Fractures Based on the Location

Location	Treatment Options	Approach

Symphysis/ Parasymphysis fracture	• MMF with arch bars
	• Internal fixation (ORIF) by:
	  • Two 2.0-mm miniplates
	  • 3D plate
	  • Two lag screws
	  • Stronger plate at the lower border and arch bars
	  • Single reconstruction plate at the lower border
	  • Inferior locking plate and superior monocortical plate
	  • Arch bars can be used for temporary fixation
		Intraoral/extraoral if preexisting laceration or comminuted fractures (submental approach)

Body fracture	• Single four hole miniplate with gap at the lower border • Two miniplates at the superior border and the inferior border • Inferior stronger plate and arch bars • Inferior reconstruction plate • Mental nerve should be preserved	• Intraoral approach • Extraoral approach if the fracture is located along the posterior and inferior aspects of mandibular body
Angle fracture	• IMF (4–8 weeks) in undisplaced fractures • Single miniplate along the oblique ridge of the mandible • Single lag screw • Two 2.0 mm miniplates • Two 2.4 mm compression plate • A reconstruction plate in cases of significant comminution or poor bone stock with superior tension band	• Intraoral approach with or without transbuccal trocar instrument • Extraoral approach/Risdon's approach for comminuted and complex fractures
Ramus fracture	• Nondisplaced fractures—IMF (6–8 weeks) ORIF with • One 2.0-mm miniplate • Two 1.5/2.0-mm miniplate	Preauricular or submandibular approach
Coronoid fracture	• IMF for (4–6 weeks) • ORIF • Removal of the fragment in case of restricted mouth opening	Intraoral approach
Bilateral mandibular fractures (Fig. 49.21)	• ORIF with a locking reconstruction plate • Two miniplates at least on one side of the fracture	Intraoral/extraoral
Comminuted mandibular fracture	• Reconstruction plate with minimum of three or four screws on either side for the fragments • Multiple miniplates for the smaller fragments • Combination of reconstruction and miniplate • Bone grafts might be required in significant defects of the mandible • External fixation is considered for severe comminution, infection, significant bone or soft tissue defects	Intraoral/extraoral

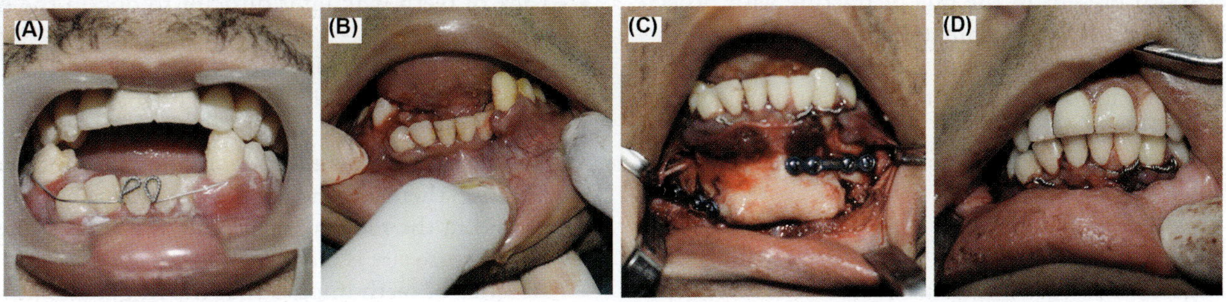

Figure 49.21 Case report—Management of bilateral parasymphysis fracture. (**A**) Intraoral view showing bilateral parasymphysis fracture and bridle wire in place. (**B**) Step deformity and mobility of the fragment. (**C**) Reduced and fixed fracture with miniplates. (**D**) Postoperative view with restored occlusion.

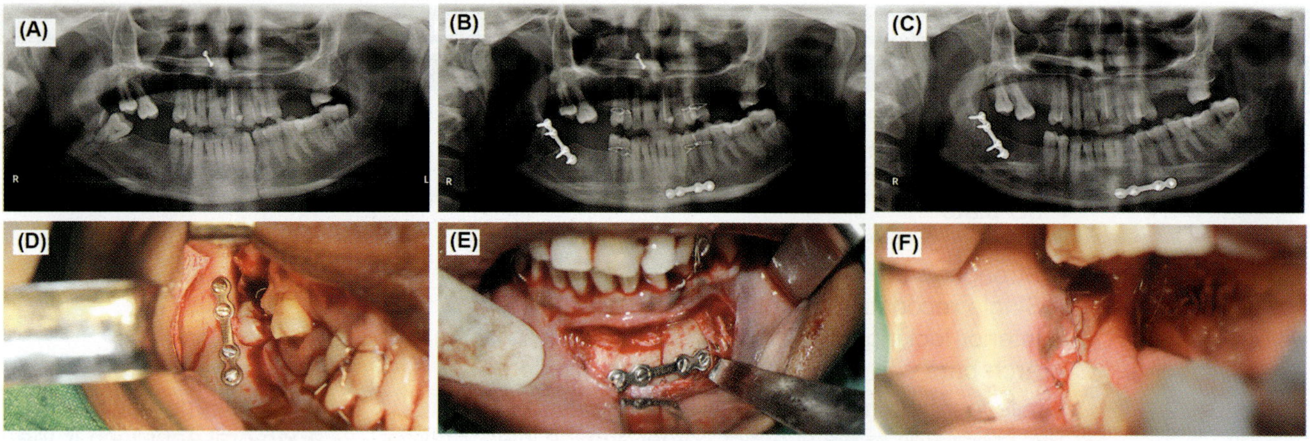

Figure 49.22 Management of teeth in line of fracture. (**A**) Preoperative OPG showing right angle fracture with 48 in the fracture line. (**B**) Immediate postoperative OPG. (**C**) Postoperative OPG after 1 year showing healed socket. (**D**) The right side angle fracture is reduced and fixed using 48 as guide. (**E**) Plating at the left side parasymphysis region. (**F**) The teeth in line of fracture was extracted and the socket closed.

TABLE 49.7 Indications for Removal of Teeth

Absolute Indications	Relative Indications
• Longitudinal/Vertical fracture involving the root • Dislocation or subluxation of the tooth from the socket • Presence of periapical infection • Grossly mobile • Interferes with fracture reduction • Infected fracture line • Root stumps • Acute pericoronitis	• Functionless teeth which would be eventually removed electively • Advanced caries • Advanced periodontal disease • Teeth which could be added to the existing denture

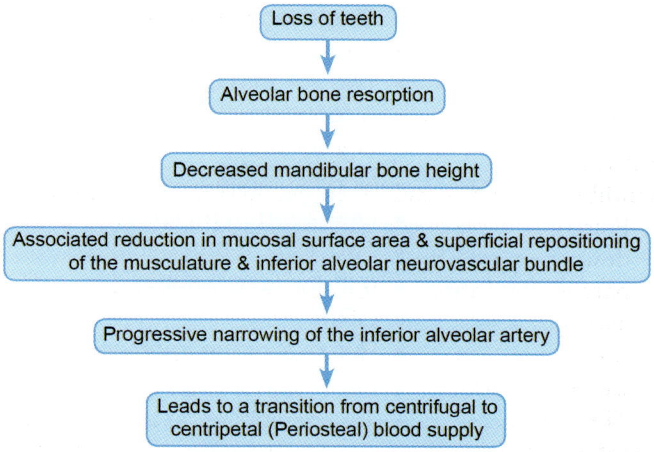

Flowchart 49.1 Pathological changes in an edentulous mandible.

recommended retaining teeth, provided they do not impede reduction, stabilisation and fixation of fractures.

According to *Killey and Kay*, indications for removal of teeth are described in Table 49.7.

Teeth which need to be retained in the fracture line

- Intact tooth present in the line of fracture with no evidence of mobility or inflammation
- A 2nd molar in the posterior segment of the fracture should be retained to prevent the superior displacement of the fracture segment.

It is critical to preserve the canine because it is the cornerstone of occlusion.

EDENTULOUS MANDIBULAR FRACTURE

The management of edentulous jaw fractures deserves special consideration due to the following ***age-related changes*** (Flowchart 49.1).

- Decreased endosteal or periosteal blood supply
- Impaired healing of the fracture
- Decreased osteogenesis
- Diminished surface area/lack of thick bone
- Other systemic comorbidities
- Poor baseline nutritional status
- Lack of teeth making it difficult to obtain the preinjury occlusion
- Increased risk for fibrous or nonunion
- Decrease in mandibular height/mandibular atrophy (<10 mm).

The ***advantage of the edentulous status*** of mandible are:

- Because there are no teeth, the fractures rarely compound in the mouth. As a result, the risk of infection at the fracture site is reduced
- Absence of teeth implies that the fragments need not be reduced to accurate occlusion. The inaccuracy in the reduction can be compensated by using dentures.

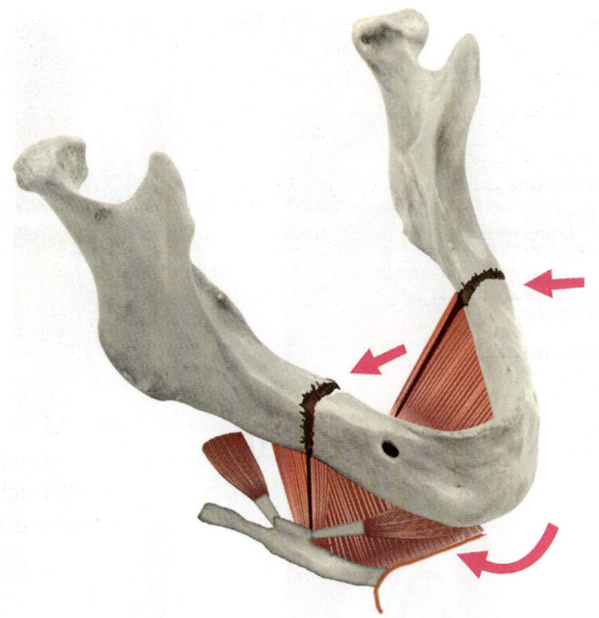

Figure 49.23 Fracture of edentulous mandible—Bucket handle fracture.

Fractures of edentulous mandible

Edentulous mandible are less resistant to fracture due to mandibular atrophy and its decreased physical size.

- Fractures of the edentulous mandible cause extreme downward and backward displacement of the anterior part of the mandible, producing a *'bucket-handle appearance* (Fig. 49.23)'
- It commonly occurs in bilateral fractures of the body of the edentulous mandible
- The digastric and the mylohyoid muscles are responsible for the downward and backward displacement of the fractured anterior segment. This displacement pulls the tongue posteriorly, resulting in airway obstruction.

OPG and CT scans can be used to diagnose and in planning the treatment of edentulous mandibular fracture.

Clinically

- Extraoral ecchymosis
- Mobility of the anterior mandible
- Intraoral ecchymosis in the floor of the mouth.

Classification (Table 49.8)

Cawood and Howell classification of edentulous jaws

Their classification is based on the resorption patterns of the alveolar bone following tooth extraction that occurs in the anterior or posterior direction.

Class I—Dentate
Class II—Postdental extraction
Class III—Broad alveolar process
Class IV—Knife-edge alveolar process
Class V—Flat ridge (loss of alveolar process)
Class VI—Submerged ridge (resorption into basal bone).

TABLE 49.8 Luhr Classification of Fractures of the Edentulous Atrophic Mandible

Class of Atrophy	Mandible Height at Fracture Site (mm)
I—Moderate atrophy	16–20
II—Significant atrophy	11–15
III—Extreme atrophy	<10

Management of edentulous mandibular fractures

Various treatment modalities have been used in the management of edentulous atrophic mandibular fractures, which include:

- **Closed reduction:**
  a. Gunning splints with circummandibular wires plus or minus IMF
  b. Existing dentures with circummandibular wiring
  c. External pin fixation
  d. Suspension wire fixation
  Advantages: Periosteal blood supply to the bone is maintained
  Disadvantages: Increased chance of infection
- **Open reduction with internal fixation:**
  According to *Bradley*, the major blood supply to the mandible is 'subperiosteal plexus', and reflection of periosteum in ORIF can seriously impair the vascular supply to the bone, resulting in nonunion. The various modalities are:
  - Miniplates (2.0 mm)
  - Reconstruction plate
  - Compression plates at the inferior and superior borders of the fracture
  - Simultaneous bone grafting and miniplate fixation
  - Titanium mesh and bone graft
  Advantages: Adequate fixation with no/minimum MMF
  Disadvantages: Delayed healing with loss in periosteal blood supply.

The management of the edentulous mandible is based on the degree of atrophy. An edentulous mandible with adequate ridge is usually treated with gunning splints. More rigid fixation is necessary for mandibles with bone height less than 15 mm. ORIF can be done with 2 mm miniplate or 2.4 mm reconstruction plate for edentulous mandibles of height less than 15 mm.

Gunning splints

Thomas Brain Gunning (1813-1889) was the 1st person to use gunning splints to immobilise edentulous or partially edentulous jaw segments. They resemble modified dentures in which the bite blocks are joined posteriorly and a feeding space is provided in the incisal area (Fig. 49.24). Attachment

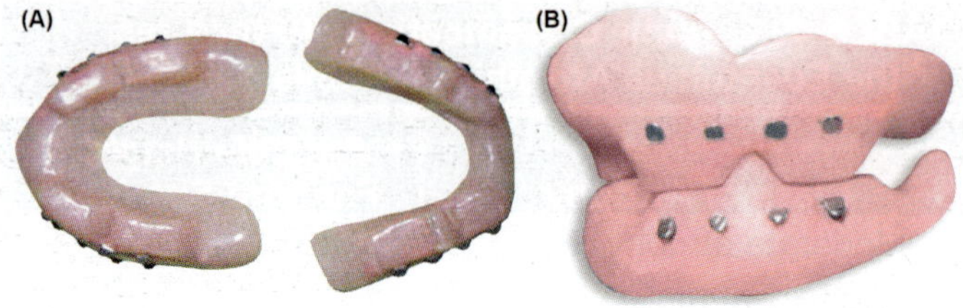

Figure 49.24 Gunning splints.

of arch bars or suspension brackets to bite blocks for immobilisation. Bone screws or circummolar or maxillary wires are used to secure it to the jaws. IMF uses wire loops or elastic bands to connect the two splints.

Advantages:

- Minimally invasive technique
- Can be used with the previously available dentures
- Does not require surgical exposure of the fracture site.

Disadvantages:

- Difficulty in maintenance of the oral hygiene
- Contraindicated for unfavourable fracture.

Construction of the gunning splint

The impression of the upper and lower jaw is taken and models are constructed. On these models, gunning splints are fabricated using acrylic resin and a trough in the anterior region. The buccal surfaces are fitted with IMF hooks for intermaxillary fixation. The fabricated gunning splints are secured to the fractured mandible using per-alveolar wiring or circumferential wiring.

Circumferential wiring for lower splint

By means of circumferential wires, the lower splint is attached to the reduced mandible. For this purpose, a curved awl is driven through the skin beneath the mandible and directed into the mouth on the lingual side of the bone. A 0.45 mm soft stainless steel wire is passed through the tip of the awl, and the instrument is withdrawn until it reaches the lower border of the mandible without piercing the skin (Fig. 49.25).

After that, the wire is taken along the lower border of the mandible onto the buccal surface of the mandible and pushed into the oral cavity and the wire is then disengaged from the awl. The wire should be applied as close to the bone as possible in order to *avoid any 'sawing' of the soft tissues*. The splints are provided with hooks or cleats on their buccal surface. These splints are attached by elastic bands or wire loops using these hooks or cleats to achieve intermaxillary fixation once they have been fastened to each jaw.

The patient's own denture can be utilised as a splint if it is available at the time of the fracture. At the end of the treatment, it is recommended to prescribe *antibiotics* to prevent any infection caused due to the passage of the wire.

Disadvantages

- Food stagnation between the splint and the mucosa
- Candida-induced stomatitis.

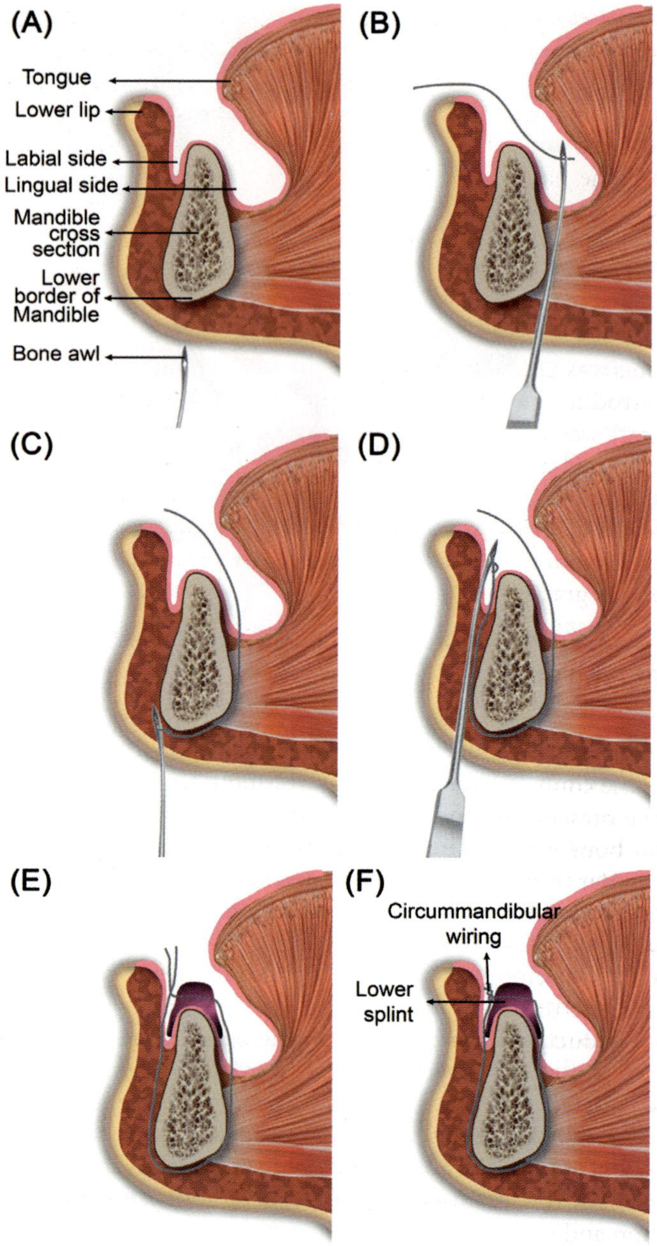

Figure 49.25 Circummandibular wiring. (**A**) A curved bone awl is passed from beneath the mandible and directed into the lingual side of the mouth. (**B**) A stainless steel wire is passed through the tip of the awl. (**C** and **D**) The instrument is withdrawn along the lingual side, lower border of the mandible into the buccal side. (**E** and **F**) The lower splint is adapted over the mandible and the circummandibular wire is secured around the splint.

Open reduction and internal fixation of edentulous mandible

The initial treatment strategies were directed towards minimal hardware with *miniplates*, which commonly get fractured under stress. *Locking systems* are available for over 10 years now. These systems had potential advantages in treating fractures of the atrophic mandible as the plate does not have to be perfectly adapted to the underlying bone.

Recently, the 2.0 mm miniplates have been widely used in atrophic mandibular fractures as the plate is thinner, easier to bend and adapt, and there is less likelihood that it will become palpable or exposed through the soft tissues. The lower height of the plate also decreases the risk of interference with denture wear. However, for larger and comminuted fractures, a *load-bearing reconstruction plate* is preferred.

Simultaneous bone grafting

This was used for ultrathin edentulous mandible and was 1st introduced by *Obwegeser* in the year 1973. Autogenous rib graft was the preferred graft. A 5 cm length of rib graft is obtained and is split into two pieces and placed on either side of the fracture site and they are stabilised using circumferential wires or plates. Bone morphogenetic proteins and tricalcium phosphate can be used as an alternative to autogenous grafts.

Advantage—The bone grafts aid in fracture healing.

PAEDIATRIC MANDIBULAR FRACTURE

The mandible is the 2nd most commonly fractured bone in children. The most common site of fracture in the mandible is the condyle followed by the symphysis region. In children, the presence of developing tooth buds makes the mandibular bone weaker and more susceptible to fracture. The mandibular fracture in paediatric patients can be managed in the following ways:

- Undisplaced fractures—Conservative management
- Fractures with minor displacement—MMF for 7–14 days
- Fractures with malocclusion and displacement—Closed reduction with cap splints secured by circummandibular wiring
- Fractures with severe displacement—Open reduction and internal fixation.

ORIF with plates may harm the tooth buds and the development of the jaw. Hence titanium miniplates are used for fixation and then removed after 3–12 months postoperatively. To avoid all these complications, biodegradable plates have been proposed. These plates do not interfere with growth and do not necessitate a 2nd procedure (refer to Chapter 56).

COMPLICATIONS OF MANDIBULAR FRACTURE (TABLE 49.9)

The most common complication of mandibular fractures is infection. Staphylococcus, streptococcus, bacteroides and gram-negative organisms are commonly involved. Infections are treated by removing the underlying cause, ensuring adequate drainage and administering the appropriate antibiotics. Penicillin G or Clindamycin is the preferred treatment for infections. In fractures that are unstable and infected, it may be necessary to replace the previously fixed plates with ones that are more rigid. Few cases require wound debridement and internal bone graft fixation.

TABLE 49.9 Complications of Mandibular Fracture

Complications During Treatment	Late Complications
• Incorrect position of the plate • Infection • Nerve damage • Displaced teeth and foreign bodies • Pulpitis • Gingival and periodontal complications • Drug reactions	• Malunion • Delayed and nonunion • TMJ derangement • Restricted mouth opening • Scar • Facial widening

Nonunion

Nonunion is the lack of osseous union between the fracture segments after the usual healing period. It can also be identified by mobility of the fragment in all planes. Nonunion may occur from a number of circumstances such as:

- Infection of the fracture site
- Inadequate reduction and immobilisation
- Unsatisfactory apposition of bone ends with interposition of soft tissue
- Excessive stripping of periosteum especially in comminuted and edentulous fractures
- Inadequate blood supply to the fractured site
- Loss of soft tissue as a result of severe trauma
- Patient's general condition, for example, osteoporosis, severe nutritional deficiency and disorder of calcium metabolism.

Radiographs demonstrate no evidence of healing and in later stages show rounding off and sclerosis of the bone ends, a condition referred to as *eburnation*.

Treatment involves re-surgery of the site with debridement of the soft tissue and nonviable bone, followed by stabilisation with internal fixation (reconstruction plate). If necessary bone grafting can be done.

Malunion

A fracture that has healed but is in a suboptimal position. Also known as misalignment of healed bone segments. Malunion can result from a complicated injury, a closed reduction, a patient with no complaints and when the surgeon fails to adhere to the fundamental principles of surgery. The healed bone may be shortened, rotated or bowed.

Additionally, nonunion is characterised by pain, abnormal mobility, joint degeneration and fragment instability. Malunion may result in malocclusion if a dentate portion is involved. After complete bony union, these malocclusions may be treated with orthodontics or osteotomies.

Delayed union

In roughly 3% of fractures, delayed union and nonunion are observed. The term 'delayed union' is difficult to define precisely due to considerations such as the patient's age and the location of the condition. The assumption must be made that the healing process has been disrupted. This is due to local factors including osteoporosis and nutritional deficiencies.

Management: In the short term, no active intervention is required for management. A fracture that has undergone fibrous union will frequently undergo slow bony consolidation during the subsequent 12 months after injury.

Fibrous union may be an acceptable outcome for an edentulous elderly patient. Individual prosthetic replacement of missing teeth is impractical in younger dentates if fracture site mobility persists, and nonunion must be accepted and treated at some point.

Nerve disorders

The most commonly injured nerves are the inferior alveolar nerve and its branches—mylohyoid, dental branches, incisive branch and the mental nerve. The motor dysfunction of the muscles of face or lips can result from trauma or from lacerations affecting the facial nerve, particularly, the marginal mandibular nerve. Over time, the vast majority of the sensory and motor functions associated with these nerves will return to normal. However, lacerations or loss of nerve tissue can result in permanent deficits.

Condylar Fractures

OUTLINE

INTRODUCTION

Condylar injuries deserve special consideration from the rest of the mandible because of its anatomical difference and healing potential. Condylar fractures are very common, constituting of about 10%–40% of all the mandibular fractures. The incidence of condylar fracture varies and is influenced by various factors such as age, geographic location and socioeconomic status of the population.

Motor vehicle accidents are the leading cause of condylar fracture, followed by work-related injuries, interpersonal violence, sporting accidents, and self-fall. Childbirth, orotracheal intubation, weight lifting, and whiplash injury are some of the less obvious causes.

SURGICAL ANATOMY

The mandibular condyle is a part of temporomandibular joint (TMJ), which deserves special attention due to its anatomic complexity and proximity to the craniofacial structures. TMJ is made of the following structures (Fig. 50.1, 50.2):

- Condyle of the mandible
- Squamous portion of the temporal bone
- Articular disc
- Ligaments.

Condyle and squamous portion of temporal bone

The mandible has two condylar processes on the superior portion of ramus. The condylar head is ovoid in shape, measuring around 15–20 mm mediolaterally and 8–10 mm anteroposteriorly. The condyle articulates with the glenoid fossa through the squamous part of the temporal bone. The squamous part of the temporal bone is a thin bone of approximately 2 mm in thickness; hence during trauma, the condylar processes may be driven into the middle cranial fossa.

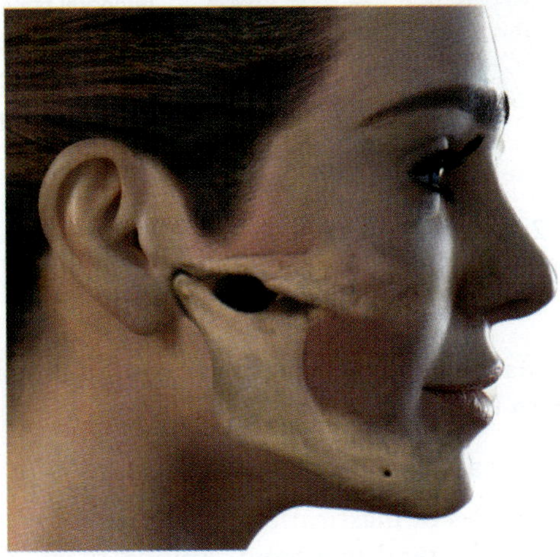

Figure 50.1 Relationship of condyle with glenoid fossa.

Articular disc

The squamous part of the temporal bone and the condyle are separated by a dense fibrous connective tissue called the articular disc. The disc is firmly anchored to the condyle by the medial and lateral ligaments and merges with the capsule at the periphery. The articular disc divides the TMJ space into superior and inferior compartments.

Temporomandibular joint capsule and ligaments

The capsule surrounds the TMJ and is attached to the neck of the mandible above the pterygoid fovea. The capsule is lined by the synovial membrane. This membrane produces synovial fluid for lubrication and nourishment of the joint.

The medial and lateral ligaments are also called as *collateral ligaments*. These ligaments connect the articular disc to the condyle. The lateral ligament also known as temporomandibular ligament which helps in stabilising the joint. The strength of the lateral ligament may be partly responsible for the fracture at the condylar neck just below the insertion of the ligament. In addition, there are two noncapsular

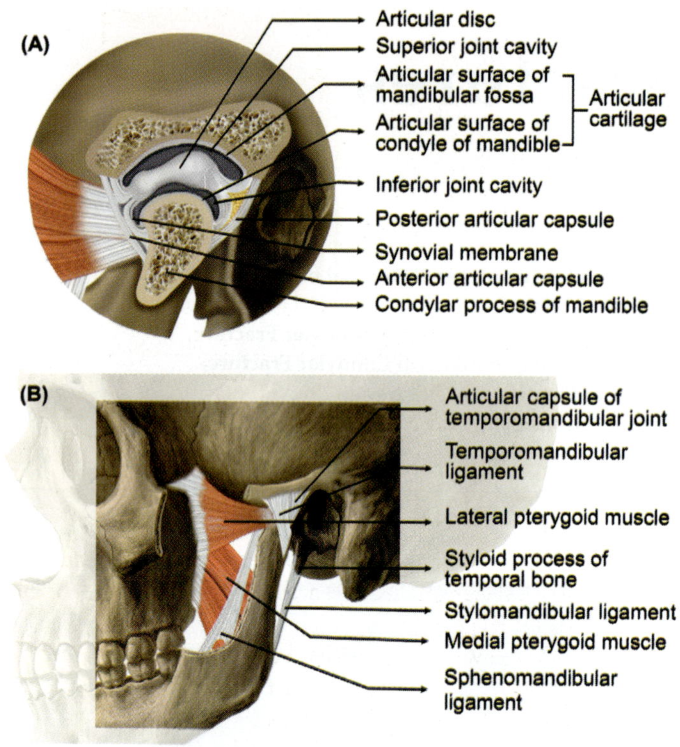

Figure 50.2 Anatomy of condyle. (**A**) Parts of TMJ. (**B**) TMJ capsule and its ligamentous attachment.

ligaments, namely, sphenomandibular and stylomandibular, which have a limited function.

Muscles of mastication

The four muscles of mastication are the masseter, temporalis, medial, and lateral pterygoid. Among them, the lateral pterygoid muscle attached to the neck of the condyle is responsible for the displacement in condylar fractures.

Vascularisation

The arterial supply to the TMJ is derived mainly from the terminal branches of external carotid artery: *Superficial temporal and maxillary artery*.

The condyle also receives blood supply from:

- Medullary bone supplied by inferior alveolar artery
- Overlying periosteum of the condyle
- Lateral pterygoid muscle attachment.

This blood supply helps in retaining the fractured condyle viable even after stripping of the periosteum during the surgical procedure.

The venous drainage starts in the retrodiscal plexus of the TMJ, which drains into the superficial temporal and maxillary veins that join to form the retromandibular vein, which in turn drains into the external jugular vein.

Innervation

The mandibular nerve provides the main nerve supply to the TMJ. Additional innervation is from the masseteric and deep temporal nerves. Auriculotemporal nerve is in direct contact with the medial aspect of condylar neck and capsule. During TMJ surgery, the nerve is vulnerable to damage and may result in postoperative complications.

Facial nerve

The facial nerve is responsible for the motor function of the muscles of facial expression. It transverses the face and divides into five terminal branches in the parotid gland. During surgeries (extraoral approaches) of the condylar fractures, these branches are likely to be damaged and should be kept in mind.

BIOMECHANICS OF CONDYLAR FRACTURE

The mandible is supported by condyles on both sides. While opening the mouth, two major movements, rotational and translational, occur in the TMJ. The mandible functions as a class III lever, with the TMJ acting as the fulcrum. The force (by muscles of mastication) is placed between the fulcrum and the load (teeth) (Fig. 50.3).

Mechanism of injury

1. Kinetic energy imparted by a subject falling on a static individual (Fig. 50.4A). It is an axial force transmitted to the condyle from the lower border of the mandible. Fractures occur at the site of injury and the condyle at a higher level
   - For example, trauma sustained from blows during sports, fighting
   - Industrial/work-related accidents.
2. Kinetic energy derived by a moving individual against a static subject (Fig. 50.4 B). Horizontal forces resulting in fracture, both at the site of impact and at the opposite side condyle
   - For example, 'Parade ground fracture'—fall of the victim owing to the sudden loss of consciousness in syncope
   - Fall during an epileptic attack

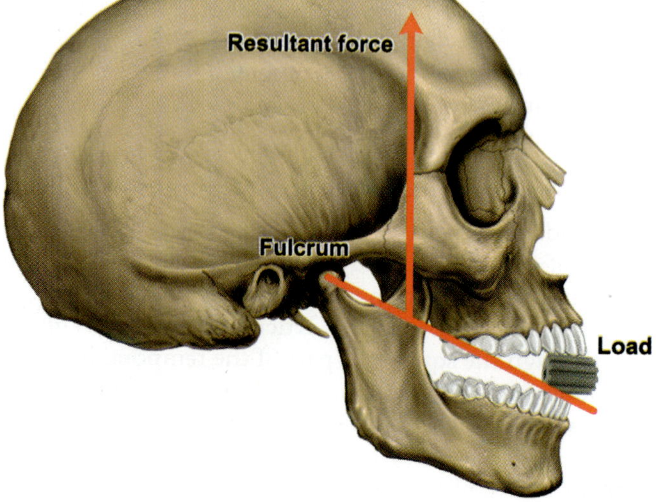

Figure 50.3 Mandible functions as class III lever.

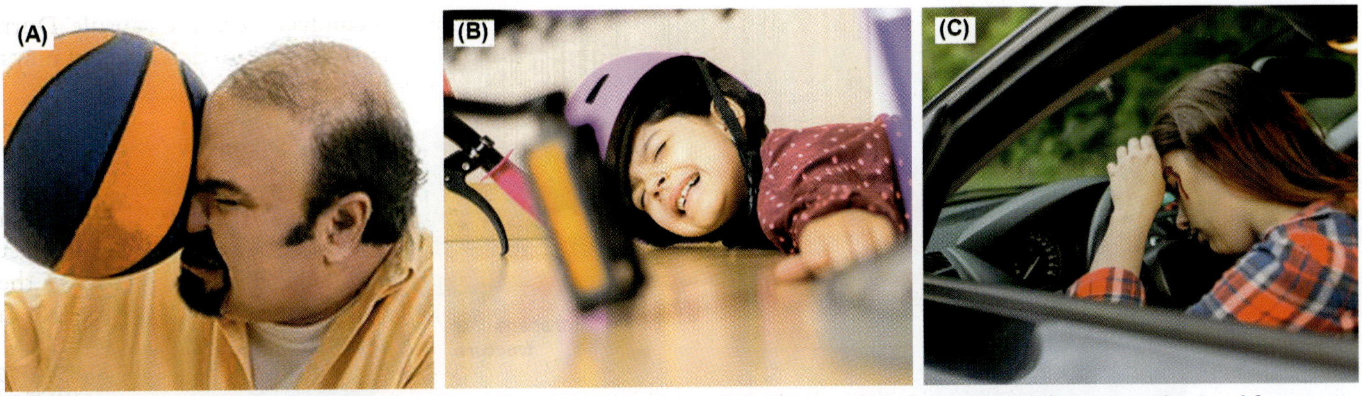

Figure 50.4 Mechanics of injury. (**A**) Trauma sustained by a subject falling on a static individual. (**B**) Trauma obtained from a moving individual against a static subject. (**C**) Trauma obtained from a combination of the above two forces.

3. Kinetic energy derived from a combination of the above two forces. It generally results in more severe injuries (Fig. 50.4C)
   - For example, road traffic accidents.

When an external force is applied to the mandible, it is generally distributed across the entire mandible. However, these forces can result in a fracture of the weak subcondylar region. This counter-coup fracture prevents displacement of the condyle into the middle cranial fossa during injuries.

CLASSIFICATION OF CONDYLAR FRACTURE

Condylar fractures are classified on the basis of anatomical site, displacement, fracture level and inclination of the fracture fragment.

1. **Common condylar fractures** (Fig. 50.5)
2. **Wassmund's classification (1934):**
   Type I: The angle between the condylar head and the long axis of the ramus is 10–45 degrees, with bone contact between the fragments (Fig. 50.6)
   Type II: The angle between the condylar head and the long axis of the ramus is 45–90 degrees, with slight bone contact between the fragments and tearing of the medial portion of the capsule
   Type III: Severe medial displacement of the condylar head with no contact between the bony fragments but confined within the glenoid fossa
   Type IV: Fractures where the condylar head articulates in a forward position to the articular eminence
   Type V: Vertical or oblique fractures through the head of the condyle
3. **Mac Lennan's classification (1952):**
   He described the difference between the simple 'bending' of the condylar process to displacement and dislocation
   Class I: No deviation (bending)
   Class II: Deviation (bending) at the fracture level
   Class III: Displacement (condylar head remains within fossa)
   Class IV: Dislocation (condylar head outside the fossa)

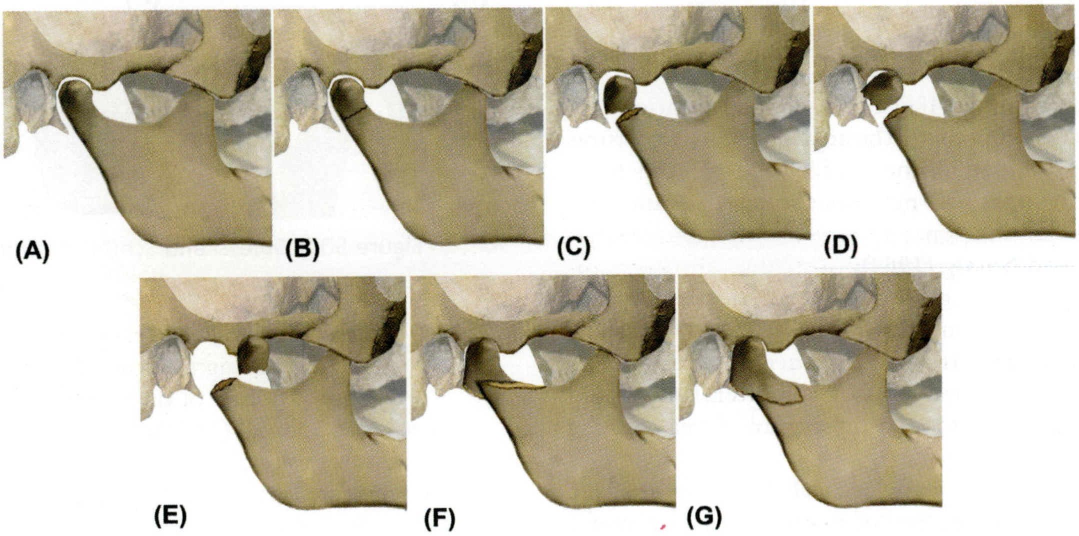

Figure 50.5 Common condylar fractures. (**A**) Normal condyle. (**B**) No displacement. (**C**) Deviation. (**D**) Displacement. (**E**) Dislocation. (**F**) Medial override. (**G**) Lateral override.

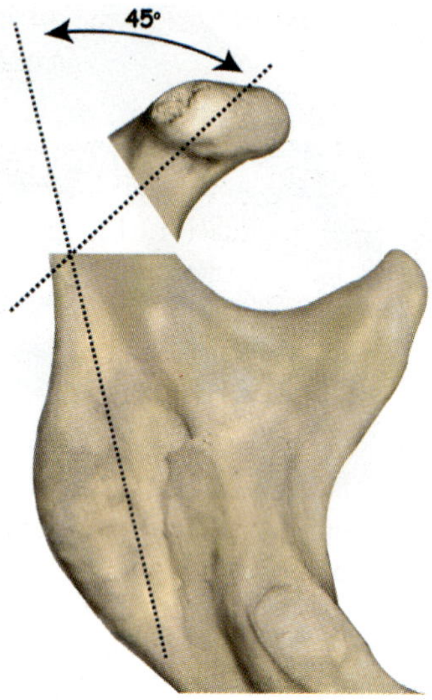

Figure 50.6 The angle between the ramus and the condylar head.

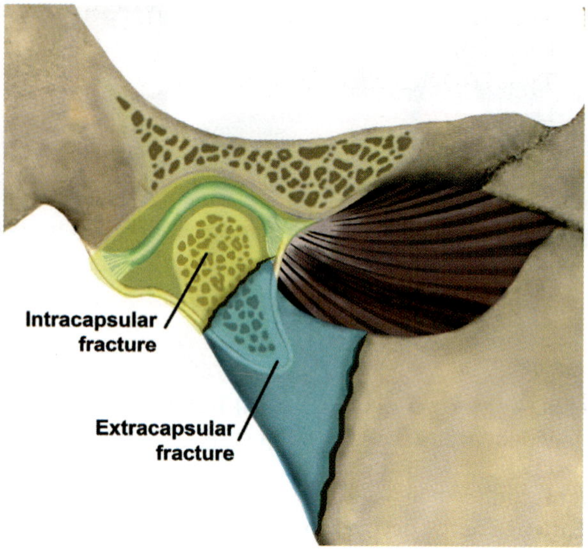

Figure 50.7 Intracapsular and extracapsular fractures.

No deviation is fracture without any displacement of the fragments

Fracture deviation is a simple angulation of the fracture segments without overlap or separation. For example, Greenstick fracture in children

Fracture displacement is characterised by the overlap of the fracture segments. The overlap may be anterior, posterior, lateral or medial. Medial displacement is most commonly seen because of the anteromedial pull of the lateral pterygoid muscle

Fracture dislocation is where the condylar head is completely outside the glenoid fossa and capsule

4. **Rowe and Killey (1955):**
   This classification is based on the relationship of capsule with the surrounding structures of the TMJ
   - Intracapsular or high condylar fracture (Fig. 50.7)
   - Extracapsular or low condylar or subcondylar fractures
   - Fractures that are associated with injury to the TMJ capsule, TMJ ligaments and articulating disk
   - Fractures involving the adjacent bony structures (e.g. fracture of the roof of the glenoid fossa or the tympanic plate of the external auditory meatus)
5. **Dingman and Natvig (1964):**
   It is based on the insertion of the lateral pterygoid muscle at the condylar neck
   - **High condylar neck fracture**: Fracture line is at or above the level of the lateral pterygoid attachment on the pterygoid fovea of the condyle
   - **Intermediate condylar neck fracture:** Fracture line is below the level of insertion of lateral pterygoid muscle

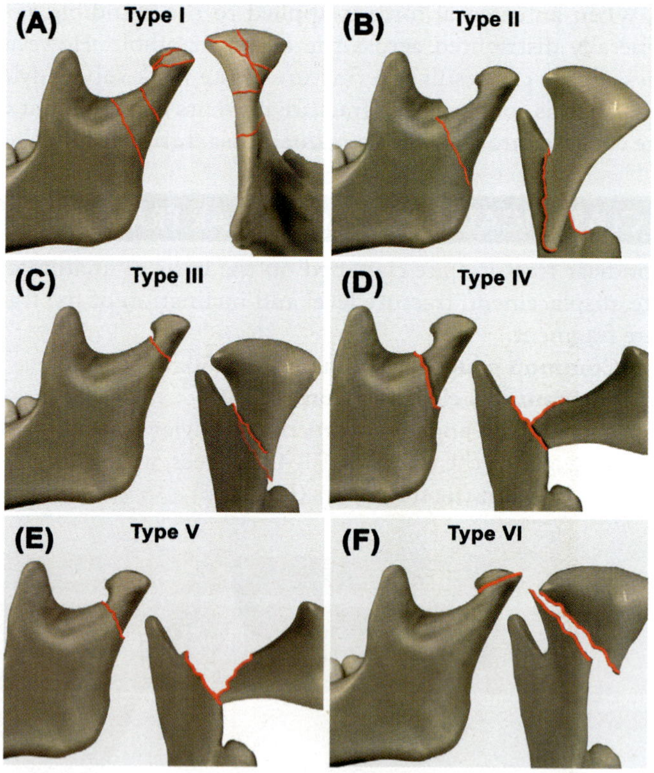

Figure 50.8 Spiessl and Schroll classification.

   - **Low condylar neck fracture**: Fracture begins at or below the sigmoid notch and extends to the posterior border of the mandibular ramus
6. **Spiessl and Schroll (1972):**
   The fractures were described based on the displacement of the fracture fragments (Fig. 50.8)

   Type I: Condylar neck fracture without Deviation/ Displacement

Type II: Low condylar neck fracture with Deviation/ Displacement

Type III: High condylar neck fracture with Deviation/ Displacement

- III a: Ventral
- III b: Medial
- III c: Lateral
- III d: Dorsal

Type IV: Low condylar neck fracture with dislocation

Type V: High condylar neck fracture with dislocation

Type VI: Intracapsular fracture of the condylar head

7. **Lindahl (1997):**

This classification system is highly complex but commonly used. It is based on the level of the fracture, the amount of displacement and the relationship of condylar head to the articulating fossa

1. Fracture level
   1a: Condylar head
   1b: Condylar neck
   1c: Subcondylar/condylar base
2. Deviation and displacement
   2a: Bending/Deviation with medial overlapping segments (Fig. 50.9A)
   2b: Bending/Deviation with lateral overlapping segments (Fig. 50.9B)
   2c: Bending/Displacement without overlapping (Fig. 50.9C)
   2d: Nondisplaced fracture without deviation (Fig. 50.9D)
3. Relation between condylar head and fossa
   3a: No dislocation
   3b: Slight dislocation (Fig. 50.9E)
   3c: Moderate dislocation (Fig. 50.9F)
   3d: Severe and/or complete dislocation (Fig. 50.9G)
4. Condylar head fracture
   4a: Horizontal
   4b: Vertical
   4c: Compression fracture

Lindahl's definition (Fig. 50.10)

- ***Condylar head fracture***–The fracture fragments are located within the joint capsule
- ***Condylar neck fracture***–The fracture is located inferior to the joint capsule and lateral pterygoid muscle attachment
- ***Subcondylar fracture***–The fracture line begins at the sigmoid notch and extends to the posterior aspect of the mandible

8. **Loukota et al., (2005):**

He proposed 'Line A', which is a perpendicular line that extends from the sigmoid notch to the mandibular ramus. This line identifies the structural anatomy of the mandible which is easily reproducible

- **Dicapitular fracture:** The fracture line starts in the articular surface and may extend outside the TMJ capsule (Fig. 50.11A–C)

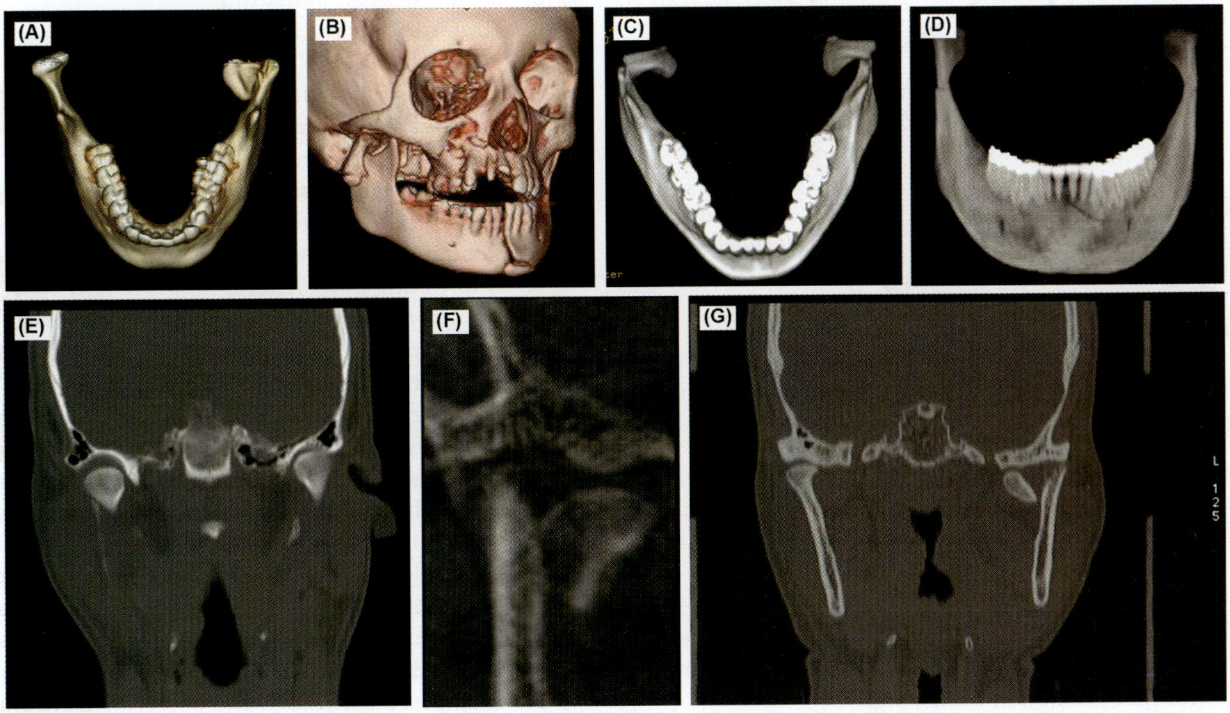

Figure 50.9 (**A**) Displaced condylar fragment with medial overlap. (**B**) Displaced condylar fragment with lateral overlap. (**C**) Deviated condylar fragment without overlapping. (**D**) Undisplaced condylar neck fracture. (**E**) Slight dislocation with increased joint space. (**F**) Moderate dislocation. (**G**) Severe dislocation with no contact.

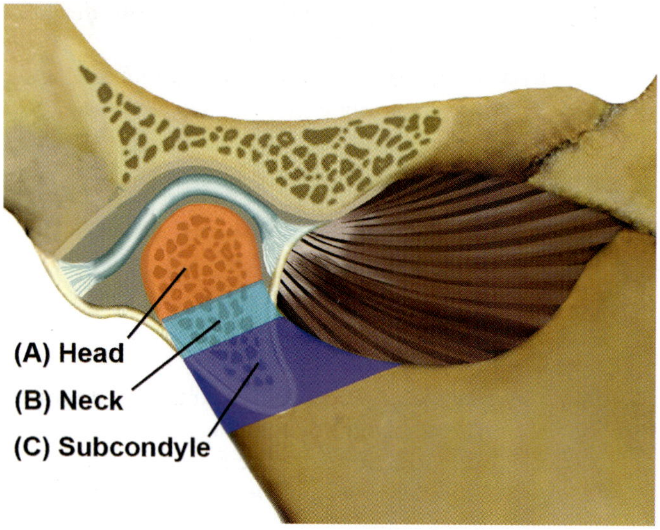

Figure 50.10 Lindahl's definition. (**A**) Condylar head. (**B**) Condylar neck. (**C**) Subcondyle.

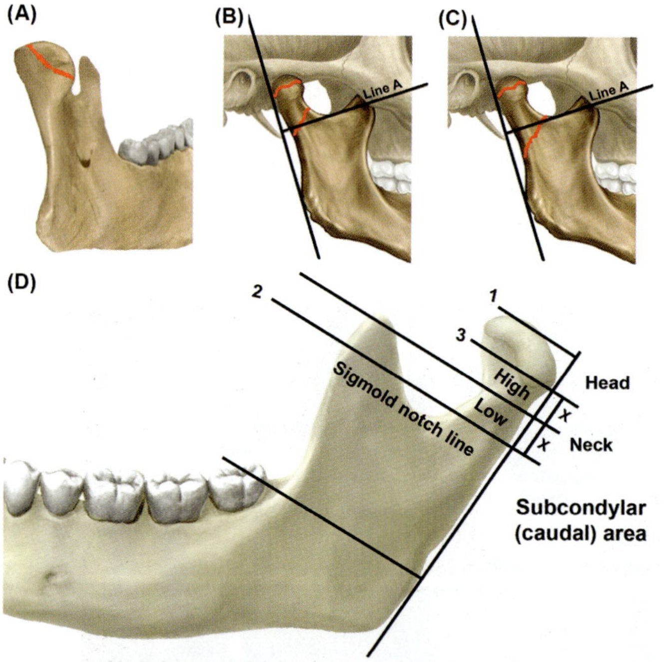

Figure 50.11 (**A**) Dicapitular fracture. (**B**) Condylar neck fracture. (**C**) Condylar base fracture. (**D**) AO classification.

- **Condylar neck:** The fracture line starts somewhere above Line A and runs above Line A for more than half of its length
- **Condylar base:** The fracture line extends behind the mandibular foramen and runs below Line A for more than half of its length
- **Minimal displacement**: Displacement of less than 10 degrees or overlap of the bone edges by less than 2 mm, or both

9. **Neff et al.,:**
   He published the comprehensive Arbeitsgemeinschaft für Osteosynthesefragen Craniomaxillofacial Surgery (AOCMF) classification of condylar process fractures. This system not only highlights the location of fracture but also the relationship of condyle with the adjacent structures (Fig. 50.11D)
   Condylar head: The reference line runs perpendicular to the posterior ramus below the lateral pole of the condylar head
   Condylar neck: The line running through the deepest point of sigmoid notch perpendicular to the ramus line is known as the sigmoid notch line. The area extending superiorly from the sigmoid notch line to the condylar head is the condylar neck
   Base of the condylar process: The area extending inferior to the sigmoid notch line.

CLINICAL FEATURES OF CONDYLAR FRACTURES

The signs and symptoms of condylar fractures are dependent on the amount of displacement of the fracture fragments.

General features of condylar fracture:

1. Swelling over the TMJ region
2. Contusions, abrasions, chin lacerations, ecchymosis and haematoma
3. Bleeding from external auditory canal indicating anterior tympanic plate fracture
4. Facial asymmetry
5. Tenderness on palpation
6. Crepitus over the affected joints
7. Malocclusion
8. Deviation of mandibular midline
9. Limited mouth opening
10. Associated dentoalveolar injuries

Clinical features of unilateral condylar fractures (Fig. 50.12)

1. Ipsilateral premature contact of the posterior teeth
2. Posterior open bite on the contralateral side
3. Shortening of ipsilateral ramus height
4. *Deviation of mandible towards the fractured side*
5. Reduced or no palpable condylar movements on the ipsilateral side
6. Hollowness over the condylar head region in case of condyle dislocation
7. Restricted lateral excursions and protrusions
8. Paraesthesia of lower lip due to pressure exerted by the haemorrhage on the mandibular division of trigeminal nerve
9. Cerebrospinal fluid (CSF) otorrhoea in condylar fractures associated with middle cranial fossa

Clinical features of bilateral condylar fractures (Fig. 50.13)

1. Premature contact of the posterior teeth bilaterally (posterior gag)
2. Anterior open bite
3. Bilateral loss of vertical height

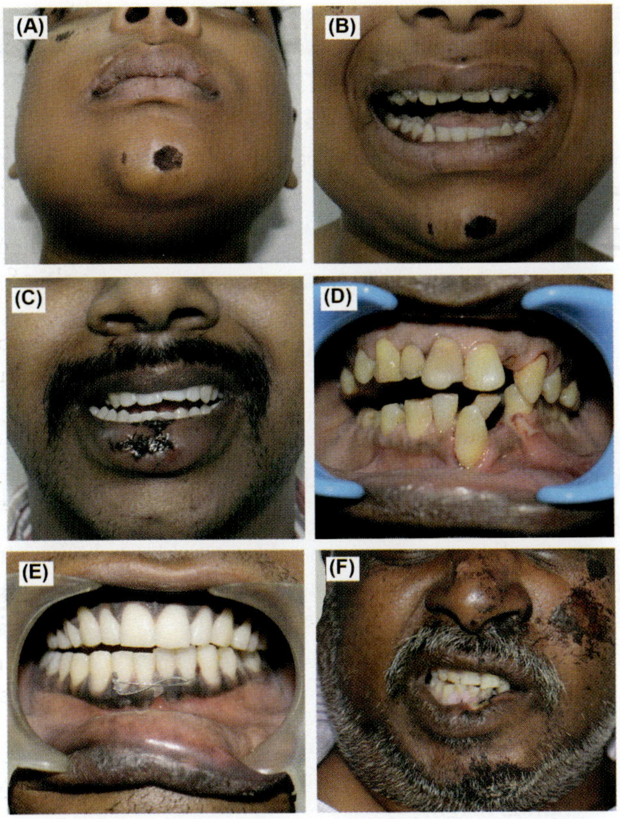

Figure 50.12 Clinical features of unilateral condylar fracture. (**A**) Swelling over the fractured site (right side). (**B**) Restricted mouth opening. (**C**) Deviation of mandible towards the fractured side (right side). (**D**) Premature contact of teeth on the affected side (left side). (**E**) Posterior open bite on the contralateral side (right side). (**F**) Paraesthesia of the lower lip.

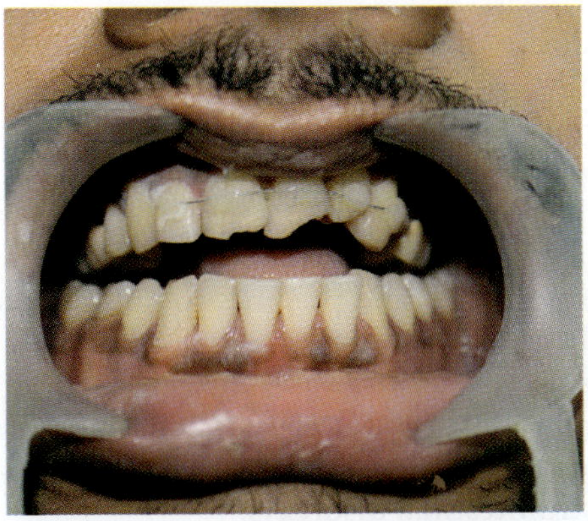

Figure 50.13 Clinical features of bilateral condylar fracture. Premature contact of the posterior teeth bilaterally with anterior open bite.

4. Little or no deviation in the midline
5. Restricted mouth opening.

Overall mandibular movement is usually restricted, as opposed to a unilateral fracture. Bilateral condylar fractures are frequently associated with symphysis or parasymphysis fractures.

Haemorrhage from the ear can result from laceration on the anterior wall of external auditory meatus or from the middle ear. It is important to distinguish the origin of the bleeding. Middle ear haemorrhage signifies fracture of the petrous temporal bone.

Ecchymosis of the skin just below the mastoid process is known as '*Battle's* sign'. This sign also occurs in fractures involving the skull base.

Displacement of the condyle from the fossa or overriding of the fractured condylar neck shortens the ramus on that side producing the *malocclusion*.

CSF *otorrhoea* occurs when the petrous part of the temporal bone is fractured in association with condylar fracture.

RADIOGRAPHIC INVESTIGATIONS

Imaging techniques help us in identifying the location, type, pattern and severity of the fracture, thereby assisting in deciding the treatment options (Fig. 50.14). Various views can be used to evaluate the condylar fractures which include:

- **Conventional radiography:**
  a. **Posteroanterior skull view (PA):**
  Represents proximal and distal fragments of the condyle in a mediolateral plane. It provides accurate details of the *ramus, angle and the body*. The symphysis and condyles are poorly displayed due to the superimposition by cervical spine and mastoid process
  b. **Lateral view:**
  This view is particularly helpful in assessing the fracture, dislocation and anterior displacement of the *condyle and TMJ region*, with limited access to medial and lateral displacement
  c. **Oblique view:**
  In this view, the *ramus, angle and body* are visualised well with limited details of condyle and symphysis region, due to superimposition of C2. The mandibular groove can often be mistaken for a cortical break
  d. **Reverse Townes view:**
  It is a PA view, with the patient having their cervical spine flexed and mouth open, hence providing excellent detail of *condylar neck fractures and medial or lateral displacement*
  e. **Orthopantomogram (OPG):**
  It provides images of the *entire mandible* in one-dimensional plane (anteroposterior). They are the most informative radiograph in detecting mandibular fracture in comparison to other X-ray views. It provides limited detail on the medial displacement of the condyle and is more prone to an artefact
  Thus, conventional X-ray for mandibular fractures is best restricted to trauma patients who can be ambulated or with isolated injuries

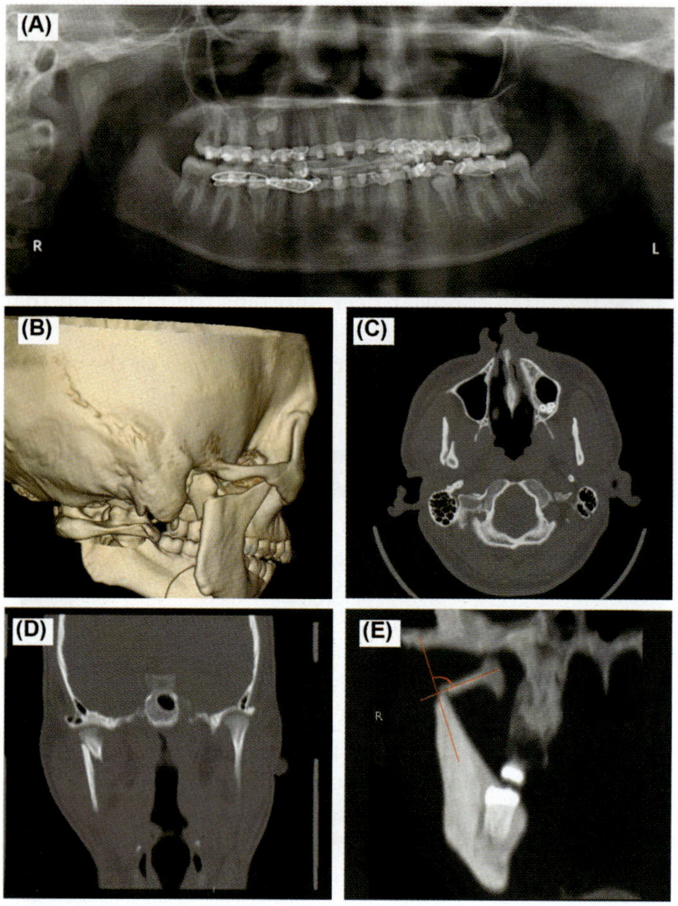

Figure 50.14 (**A**) OPG showing bilateral condylar neck fracture. (**B**) A 3D CT scan showing medially displaced right condyle and left body of mandible fracture. (**C**) Axial sections showing anteromedially displaced right condylar segment. (**D**) Coronal sections showing the anteromedial displacement of right condyle. (**E**) Fracture deviation measured in CT.

- **CT scans:**
  They are indicated in unstable patients with suspected mandibular fracture or when a fracture is likely and are not evident on conventional X-rays
- **Ultrasound:**
  Identifies *fractures with a step-deformity* but tough to diagnose nondisplaced fractures. It is particularly useful in unstable patients or *pregnant women*
- **Magnetic resonance imaging (MRI):**
  Yields excellent view of associated soft tissue injuries such as articular disc disruption, capsular tear, internal derangement and muscular injuries
  In summary, in an acutely injured patient, conventional X-rays *(lateral or reverse Townes view with OPG)* is sufficient for screening of fracture. If further diagnostic information is required then a CT scan or MRI may be indicated.

MANAGEMENT OF CONDYLAR FRACTURE

GENERAL PRINCIPLES IN TREATMENT OF CONDYLAR FRACTURES

There are three treatment methods advocated for condylar fractures:

1. *Conservative*: It involves immobilisation with intermaxillary fixation (IMF). The time duration for this treatment may range from 7 days to 4 weeks
2. *Functional*: It is the introduction of active physical movement to prevent the risk of ankylosis
3. *Surgical*: It includes direct reduction and fixation of the fragments using bone plates.

CLOSED REDUCTION/CONSERVATIVE MANAGEMENT

Closed reduction depends on the functional adaptation of the surrounding structures to achieve stable occlusion. It is not always possible to achieve an anatomical reduction in a closed method.

Indications:

- Nondisplaced or incomplete fractures
- Almost all condylar fractures in children
- Isolated intracapsular fractures
- Minimally displaced fracture without reduction in ramus height
- Fracture with a stable or reproducible occlusion
- Systemic risk of subjecting the patient to general anaesthesia

Method:

1. Observation and soft diet
2. Immobilisation [Maxillo-mandibular fixation (MMF)]

MMF can be achieved using:

a. Arch bars
b. Indirect interdental wiring (Eyelet or IVY loop)
c. IMF screws.

The period of immobilisation ranges from 2 to 6 weeks. The immobilisation period can be increased or decreased, based on the age of the patient, level of fracture and degree of displacement. Immobilisation also allows the initial union of fractured segments and prevents complications.

Contraindications to MMF:

- Seizure
- Compromised pulmonary function
- Psychiatric conditions
- Gastrointestinal disorders.

Advantages and disadvantages of closed reduction are given in Table 50.1.

Adaptation of mandible to fracture

When closed reduction is performed, following adaptations occur in order to facilitate the masticatory function:

i. *Neuromuscular adaptation*
ii. *Skeletal adaptation*
iii. *Dental adaptations.*

TABLE 50.1 Advantages and Disadvantages of Closed Reduction (MMF)

Advantages	Disadvantages

• Relatively safe treatment
• No injury to nerves and blood vessels
• No postoperative complications
• No tooth germ injury
	• Long period of IMF
	• Growth and functional disorders of the TMJ in children
	  • Contraindicated in medically compromised patients
	  • Imbalanced nutrition
	  • Poor oral hygiene maintenance
	• Mouth opening difficulty can occur after the release of IMF

i. Neuromuscular adaptations

Following the fracture of the condyle, a compensatory mechanism is triggered to protect the fractured site during biting. It comprises increased muscle activity on the nonfractured side and a decrease in the active force on the fractured side. These adaptations occur early and are short-termed.

ii. Skeletal adaptations

It is the development of a new temporomandibular articulation following the fracture. This adaptation begins immediately after injury and continues for many months afterward.

iii. Dental adaptations

Adaptations that occur within the dentoalveolar segment, along with skeletal adaptations. With closed treatment of condylar fractures, extrusion of the incisors and intrusion of the molars has been demonstrated.

Conservative treatment can be applied to all kinds of unilateral or bilateral fractures other than those with gross displacement (Fig. 50.15).

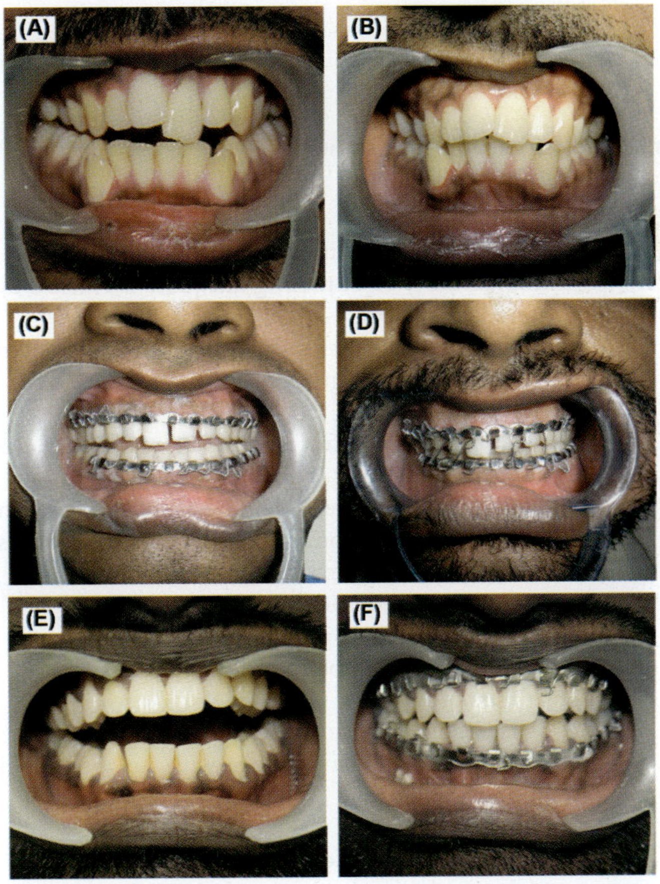

Figure 50.15 Conservative management with MMF. (**A**) Preoperative with left mandibular condyle fracture showing anterior and right lateral open bite. (**B**) Postoperative picture with restored occlusion. (**C–E**) Preoperative, bilateral condylar fracture with anterior open bite. (**D–F**) Postoperative MMF using arch bar and wires.

FUNCTIONAL THERAPY/REHABILITATION

Following the release of the IMF (closed reduction), an intense active physical therapy is crucial in restoring the mandibular movements. Functional treatment relies on *guiding elastics and active movements.*

Elastics

In case of persisting malocclusion and deviation even after the release of IMF, an arch bar with *guiding elastics* can be used to correct the occlusion. Initially, heavy elastics are placed, and then slowly shifted to light elastics. Elastics are recommended for a period of 2–4 weeks. Once the stable occlusion is achieved, the elastics can be discontinued, and the arch bar can be removed.

Active movements—Rehabilitation targets

- Maximum incisal opening > 40 mm
- Lateral excursive movements > 10 mm
- Protrusive excursive movements > 12 mm
- Full range of TMJ movements
- Stable occlusion.

OPEN REDUCTION AND INTERNAL FIXATION

The objective of open reduction and internal fixation (ORIF) is to achieve an adequate exposure of the condylar fragment, reduction to the normal relationship and stable fixation.

Surgical treatment/**ORIF is indicated** for adults with:

1. Bilateral condylar fractures
2. Gross condylar displacement > 45 degrees
3. Anatomic reduction of ramus height > 2 mm
4. Condylar fragments with an associated mid-face fracture
5. Unstable occlusion (periodontal disease, less teeth)

TABLE 50.2 Advantages and Disadvantages of Open Reduction

Advantages	Disadvantages
• Direct visualisation of the fragments • Reduction of displaced bony fragment to the most ideal anatomical site • Excellent stability • Rigid fixation • Early return to normal function • Prevents complications	• Difficulty of surgical access • Extraoral scars • Injury to the facial nerve • Aseptic necrosis of the condylar segment secondary to loss of periosteal blood supply during dissection • Parotid fistula • Postop infection

6. Condylar fracture for which adequate physiotherapy is impossible.

Indications of open reduction

1. **Zide and Kent (1983):**
   Absolute indications:
   - Condyle displaced into the middle cranial fossa
   - Impossibility of obtaining adequate occlusion by closed reduction
   - Lateral extracapsular displacement of the condyle
   - Invasion by a foreign body.

   Relative indications:
   - Bilateral condylar fractures in an edentulous patient where a splint is unavailable
   - Unilateral or bilateral condylar fractures when splinting is not recommended for medical reasons
   - Bilateral condylar fractures associated with:
     - Comminuted midfacial fractures
     - Retrognathia or prognathism
     - Open bite with periodontal problems
     - Loss of multiple teeth
     - Unstable occlusion due to orthodontics
   - Unilateral condylar fracture with an associated midface fracture.
2. **Mathes (1983):**
   Open reduction indication:
   - Malocclusion with centric relation
   - Fragment angulation more than 30 degrees
   - Bone gap more than 4–5 mm
   - Lateral override
   - Lack of contact of the fracture fragment

   Preferred for open reduction:
   - Low, dislocated subcondylar fracture
   - Low condylar fracture with multiple fractured mandible/maxillary/Le Fort fracture
   - Low condylar fracture with displacement of condylar head out of the glenoid fossa
   - Condylar fragment 14 degrees—medial tilt
   - Ramus shortening > 5%
   - Bilateral fracture with open bite
   - Malaligned gross fracture end
   - Fracture dislocation
   - Abnormal function, malocclusion.

Contraindications to open reduction and rigid fixation

Absolute contraindications:
- Condylar head fractures (at or above the ligamentous attachment)
- When medical illness add undue risk to general anaesthesia
- Good occlusion
- Acceptable mandibular movement

Relative contraindications:
- When a simpler method is effective
- Condylar neck fractures
- Obtunded neurologic status when there is no documented hope for improvement.

Advantages and disadvantages of open reduction are given in Table 50.2.

SURGICAL APPROACHES

The location of the fracture, the degree of displacement, and the type of internal fixation are the prime determinant in the selection of approach (Fig. 50.16). The various incisions used to approach the condylar fracture are:

1. Preauricular approach
2. Submandibular/Risdon approach
3. Retromandibular approach
4. Intraoral approach

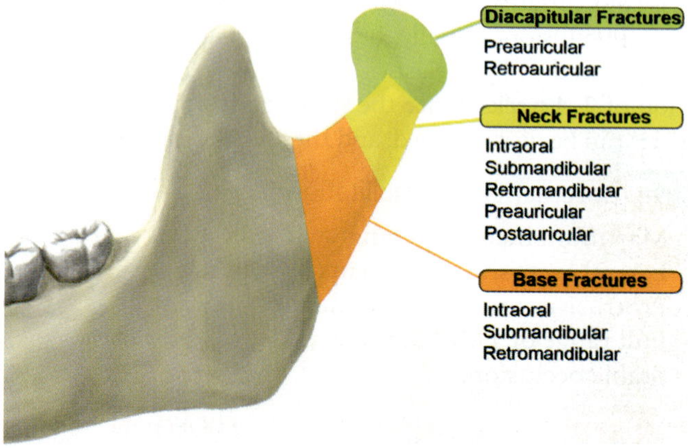

Figure 50.16 Location of fracture and the various approaches preferred.

5. Rhytidectomy
6. Bicoronal (bilateral condylar fracture along with frontal bone fracture).

Preauricular approach

It is the most standard and commonly used approach for TMJ region (Fig. 50.17).

Indications:
- High condylar fracture
- Anteromedially displaced condylar fragment
- Injured soft tissues of the TMJ

Advantages: It provides access to the superior most portion of the joint

Disadvantages:

However, the amount of ramus exposure is very limited hence rigid fixation using miniplate is difficult, especially when the fracture is inferior to the condyle neck

Anatomical structures involved:
- Superficial temporal artery
- Retromandibular vein
- Temporal branch of facial nerve
- Auriculotemporal nerve

Technique:
- The incision is made in the skin fold along the entire length of the ear, for about 3–4 cm from the inferior border of the tragus towards the external auditory canal
- Blunt dissection is done above the zygomatic arch to the level of the superficial layer of temporalis fascia and below the zygomatic arch along the external auditory meatus to the same depth
- Oblique incision is then made through the superficial layer of temporal fascia, from the root of zygomatic arch in front of the tragus towards the upper corner of the retracted flap. At the root of zygomatic arch, this incision is through both the superficial layer of temporalis fascia and the periosteum of the zygomatic arch
- Blunt dissection is done striping the periosteum from the lateral portion of the zygomatic arch and continued below the arch just superficial to the TMJ capsule. The dissected tissues are then retracted exposing the capsule
- The capsule is entered using scissors, just below the zygomatic arch exposing the interarticular joint space
- The fractured fragments are then reduced
- Closure—The inferior and the superior joint space are then sutured using a slowly resorbable or permanent suture to the joint capsule.

Intraoral endoscopic approach for condylar fracture

Fractures of the condylar base and low and middle parts of the condylar processes can be addressed through this technique. It requires special equipment such as a 90 degree angled screw driver and drill, Light intensive headlight, head clamp, angled endoscope and a special retractor with a fibreoptic light. Surgical access is obtained by extending the vestibular incision superiorly along the ascending ramus and dissection done exposing the fracture line. The fractured fragments are repositioned using endoscopes and fixed with miniplates. The intraoral mucosa is closed in the standard way.

Advantages:
- No visible scars
- Low risk of facial nerve damage
- Low risk of sialoceles and salivary fistulas

Disadvantages:
- Technically demanding procedure
- Requirement of special equipment
- Condylar head fractures cannot be repaired.

INTERNAL FIXATION

Following adequate exposure of the fractures site, the reduction of fragments can be achieved under direct vision. The vertical height of the posterior mandible is restored 1st by manual traction of the mandible. This is achieved by:
- Manual digital traction—The thumb finger is placed on the lower teeth and the mandible is pulled in an inferior and anterior direction.
- Bite block—A bite block placed on the fractured side molar region will result in inferior distraction of the mandible.
- Transosseous wire—A wire is passed on the posteroinferior border of the mandible and traction is applied in an interior and anterior traction.

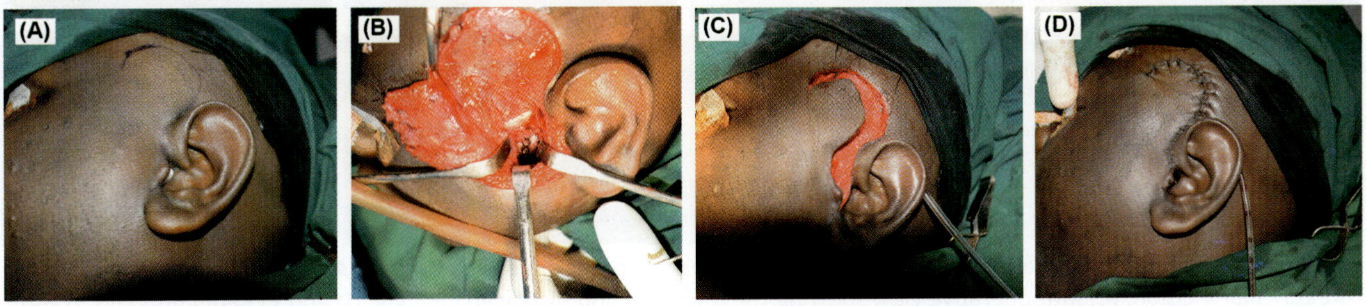

Figure 50.17 Preauricular approach. (**A**) Marking of preauricular incision. (**B**) Reduced and fixed condyle with miniplates. (**C** and **D**) Layer-wise closure of the incision.

Once the fractures are reduced, with the help of a clamp, the fragments are fixed using plates and screws. Internal fixation provides stability to the fracture fragments and also helps in healing of fractures.

Fixation techniques that are available are:

- Transosseous wire
- Lag screws
- K wires—Kirschner wire
- External fixation (bone pins)
- Rigid plates and screws
  - Dynamic compression plates 2.0
  - Miniplates 2.0
  - Locking plate 2.0
  - 3D plates
  - Bioresorbable plates.

Transosseous wire, Lag screws, K wires and Bone pins are explained in detail in Chapter 47.

Rigid plates and screws

Fixation of the condylar head is technically challenging as the fractures are intracapsular and the amount of space available for plates are limited. Few fractures could be associated with multiple small fragments and injury to the disc and capsule. Though there are many techniques available for fixation, currently, the majority of the rigid fixation uses titanium plates and screws. Bone plates provide both rigidity and stabilisation with an added advantage of easy application. Fixation can be in the form of single or two plates (Figs. 50.18 and 50.19).

Single plate—It is used in cases where the bone available for fixation is limited. A single heavier plate is used along the long axis of the condylar process. For example, high condylar fracture

Two plates—They are used for lower level fractures by placing plates along the anterior and posterior border in a triangular fashion.

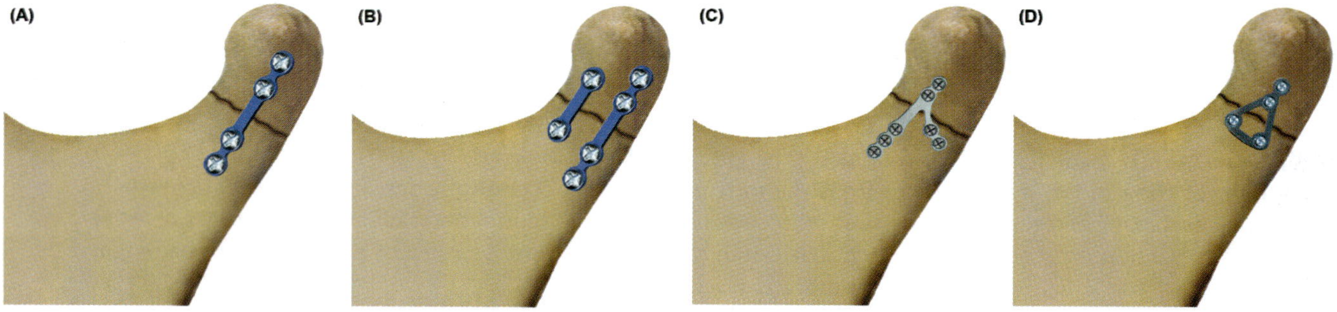

Figure 50.18 Plating of condyle. **(A)** Single-plate fixation. **(B)** Two-plate fixation. **(C)** Lambda plate. **(D)** Delta plate.

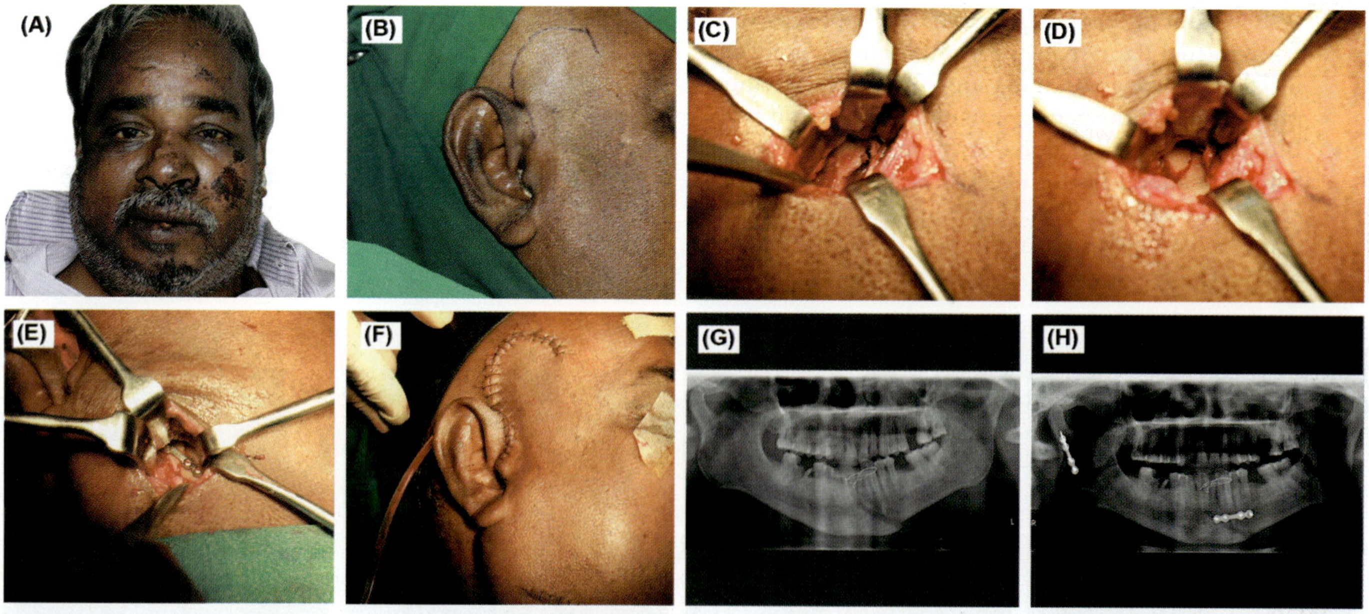

Figure 50.19 Case Report 1—Management of right condylar and left parasymphysis fracture. **(A)** Preoperative view. **(B)** Marking of preauricular incision. **(C)** Intraoperative view showing the fractured and displaced condyle. **(D and E)** Reduction and fixation of condyle with miniplate. **(F)** Closure of incision. **(G and H)** Pre- and postoperative OPG showing the left parasymphysis and right condylar fracture with miniplates.

MANAGEMENT OF UNILATERAL CONDYLAR FRACTURE (Box 50.1)

Displaced/dislocated unilateral condylar fracture

In displaced unilateral condylar fractures, management with closed reduction often results in ramus shortening and facial asymmetry. Fractures with a deviation of 10–45 degrees, or ramus shortening > 2 mm, should be treated with ORIF, irrespective of the level of the fracture.

BOX 50.1 Management of Unilateral Condylar Fracture

- **Unilateral intracapsular fractures** (condylar head)—Closed reduction with IMF for a period of 2–3 weeks
- **Unilateral extracapsular fractures** (neck and subcondyle)
  - Undisplaced fractures—Closed reduction using arch bar and IMF
  - Displaced/Dislocated fractures—ORIF

MANAGEMENT OF BILATERAL CONDYLAR FRACTURE (Box 50.2)

Bilateral extracapsular fracture

Conservative management of bilateral condylar fracture is *not recommended*, as it leaves behind a residual deformity due to the action of lateral pterygoid muscle. Surgical treatment provides better functional and morphological outcomes.

BOX 50.2 Management of Bilateral Condylar Fracture

- Bilateral intracapsular fractures (condylar head)—Closed reduction with IMF for a period of 3–4 weeks
- Bilateral extracapsular fracture—ORIF of one side
- Bilateral extracapsular fracture associated with other fractures (midface)—ORIF on both sides

According to Newman, '*if either condyle is displaced or dislocated, ORIF of at least one condyle is a treatment choice*'. Even though the fracture is bilateral, it is possible to achieve a good functional result with an ORIF of a unilateral condyle fracture. The advantages of open reduction of one side are that it reduces the degree of scarring on the face and decreases damage to the facial nerve, with a reduction in operating time. It also prevents the reduction of ramus height.

In patients with bilateral mandibular condyles associated with maxillary fractures, ORIF of the bilateral condyles is recommended. Because the mandible serves as a template for positioning the maxillary dental arches on the skull.

CONDYLAR FRACTURES IN CHILDREN

In the youngest age group (0–2 years)—necessitates active jaw function, which is helped by analgesics to prevent ankylosis.

In the 3–12 years age group—the treatment is completely functional for both unilateral and bilateral condylar fractures. IMF may be required for a period of 7–10 days in case of extreme pain. In significant fracture displacement with extensive soft tissue injury, a myofunctional interocclusal appliances may be used to prevent collapse of the ramus height.

In the 13–18 years age group— IMF for 2–3 weeks, and ORIF in situations of persistent gross occlusal disruptions or severely restricted jaw functions. (For detailed management of condylar fractures in children, refer to Chapter 56, page number 1045–1046.)

COMPLICATIONS FOLLOWING MANDIBULAR CONDYLAR FRACTURE

Despite the satisfactory results obtained with both closed and open reduction, the potential for complications exists (Table 50.3).

Malocclusion

It may result from alterations in the condyle's 'growth centre', incomplete reduction and inappropriate fixation. A properly timed elastics and physiotherapy can advert significant malocclusion. If the malocclusion still persists, occlusal

TABLE 50.3 Complications Following Mandibular Condylar Fracture

Early Complications	Late Complications
• Fracture of tympanic plate • Fracture of glenoid fossa with or without displacement of the condylar segments into the middle cranial fossa • Damage to the cranial nerves V and VII • Vascular injury	• Malocclusion • Nonunion and Malunion • Growth disorder and facial asymmetry • Condyle resorption • Temporomandibular derangement • Traumatic arthritis • Ankylosis • Facial nerve injury • Infection

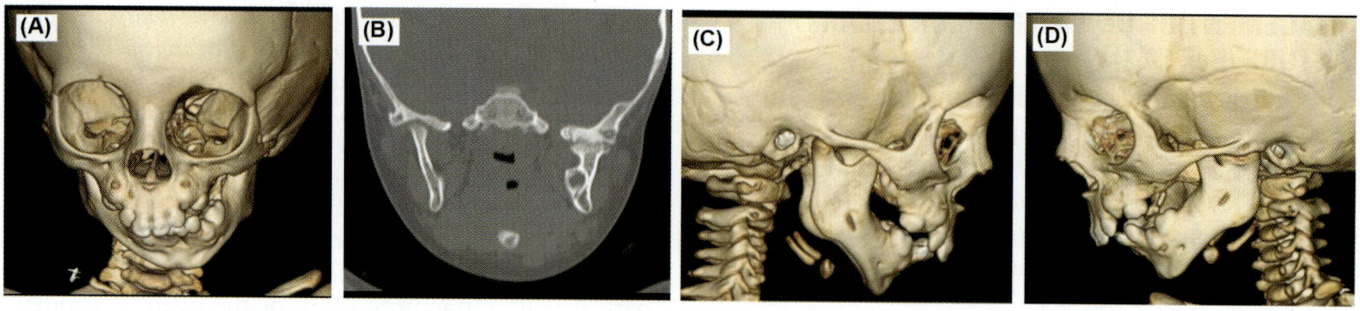

Figure 50.20 **(A–D)**: Left TMJ ankylosis in an 18-month-old child with history of trauma at the age of 8 months.

adjustment, orthodontics, orthognathic surgery or even re-surgery in severe cases may be required.

Growth disorder and facial asymmetry

The mandibular condyle, being the secondary growth centre, is influenced by the injuries of the soft tissue, adjacent muscle stiffness and scar, resulting in disrupted growth on the fractured side, whereas the unaffected side grows normally. This inequality of the growth of the mandible results in malocclusion, facial asymmetry and aesthetic deformity.

Condyle resorption

It is a change in the size and shape of the condyle. Excessive dissection and injury of the adjacent blood vessels during the surgery may cause condylar head resorption.

Temporomandibular joint dysfunction (internal derangement)

TMJ internal derangement following condylar fracture may result from direct trauma to the joint with disturbance in the position of the condyle-disc complex. This has been coined as *'condylar post fracture syndrome'*. It is prevented by early reduction and rigid fixation of the displaced bony fragments.

Traumatic arthritis

Traumatic arthritis occurs from the deformity of the joint due to the direct injury of the articular cartilage or fracture caused by trauma. Clinical symptoms include joint sound and pain, lock sensation and mouth opening limitation.

Hypomobility/Ankylosis

Ankylosis refers to abnormal immobility of the TMJ leading to significant or complete limitation of the mouth opening. It may interfere with speech, oral hygiene and maintenance of nutrition.

Factors that contribute to the formation of ankylosis include:

- Age of the patient
- Site and type of fracture
- Length of immobilisation
- Damage to the meniscus/articular disc.

A greater predisposition to the children below 10 years occurs (Fig. 50.20). Intracapsular fractures have a higher tendency for ankylosis. Ankylosis of TMJ is divided into two types: **True ankylosis** where ankylosis is attributable to the joint itself, whereas in **pseudoankylosis,** the causative factors are attributable to others except the joint.

Clinical manifestations of ankylosis:

- Deviation towards the affected side on mouth opening
- Reduced interincisal distance
- Anterior open bite in bilateral ankylosis patients
- Shortened ramus on the affected side
- Chin deviates towards the abnormal side
- Exaggerated antegonial notch on the affected side
- Flattened inferior border on the normal side
- Posterior cross bite on the affected side
- Angulated anterior teeth
- Almost nil mouth opening in bilateral cases.

If bilateral ankylosis occurs at growth stage, aesthetic disorder such as micrognathia and facial asymmetry may occur due to decreased mandibular growth.

Iatrogenic injury—facial nerve injury

Nerve injury occurs commonly during surgery. It generally takes 4–8 weeks for the nerve injury to recover. If the nerve injury is observed after the surgery, steroids can be administered to prevent permanent injury.

Infection

Postoperative infection can occur due to various factors such as fragment instability, the patient's systemic status, the degree of the fracture, foreign materials, and oral hygiene. Early treatment helps in minimising the complications associated with infection.

Chapter 51

Zygomaticomaxillary Complex Fracture

OUTLINE

INTRODUCTION

The zygomatic bone occupies a prominent position on the facial skeleton and is responsible for the anterior and lateral projection of the midface. The zygomaticomaxillary complex (ZMC) describes the skeletal unit formed by the maxillary and zygomatic bone. These bones articulate with each other, and any traumatic impact on one bone influences the other. This ZMC along with orbital bone is termed as 'orbitozygomaticomaxillary complex'.

Zygomatic fractures are the 2nd most common facial fractures after nasal bone fractures. Because of its multiple articulations, ZMC fractures are described using various names such as 'tripod, tetrapod or pentapod' fractures. ZMC fractures occurs most commonly due to motor vehicle accidents, assaults, industrial accidents and sports injuries. The left zygoma is most commonly affected because of the right-handed nature of individuals. ZMC fractures often result in cosmetic and functional deformities because of its prominent anatomical position and its proximity to vital structures such as orbit. Hence, proper restoration of the ZMC is essential for facial contour as well as ocular and mandibular functions.

ANATOMY OF ZYGOMATICOMAXILLARY COMPLEX

The zygomatic bone forms the major buttress of facial skeleton. The zygoma is a thick and strong bone. It is quadrilateral in shape, with an outer convex and an inner concave surface.

The ***zygoma has four processes***: *the temporal, orbital, maxillary and frontal* (Fig. 51.1A). These processes are significant in establishing the structural integrity of the lateral face. Fracture of zygomatic complex includes separation of four articulating sutures: *zygomaticofrontal, zygomaticotemporal, zygomaticomaxillary and zygomaticosphenoid sutures* (Fig. 51.1B).

Zygoma and orbit

The zygoma forms part of the floor and lateral surface of the orbit and plays a major role in protecting the globe and its associated soft tissues. The lateral wall of orbit has Whitnall's tubercle (a small bony elevation on the orbital surface of the zygomatic bone just behind the orbital margin and about 11 mm below the frontozygomatic suture) to which the suspensory ligament of Lockwood and lateral palpebral ligaments are attached. This suspensory ligament plays a major role in maintaining the horizontal axis of globe. A fracture above the Whitnall's tubercle causes inferior displacement of the zygoma as well as the Lockwood ligament. This displacement results in downward sloping of the palpebral fissure and the pupil known as antimongoloid slant (Fig. 51.2A). Hence, ZMC fractures greatly influences the structure and function of the orbit.

Zygoma and the mandible

The zygomatic arch is anatomically in close relationship with the coronoid process of the mandible. Thus, fracture involving the zygomatic arch may impede mandibular movement (trismus) either by impinging on the temporalis muscle or by obstructing the path of the coronoid process (Fig. 51.2B).

Zygoma and its muscle attachment

The muscles attached to the ZMC are masseter, temporalis and muscles of facial expression (e.g., zygomaticus major, zygomaticus minor and orbicularis oculi) (Fig. 51.2C). The

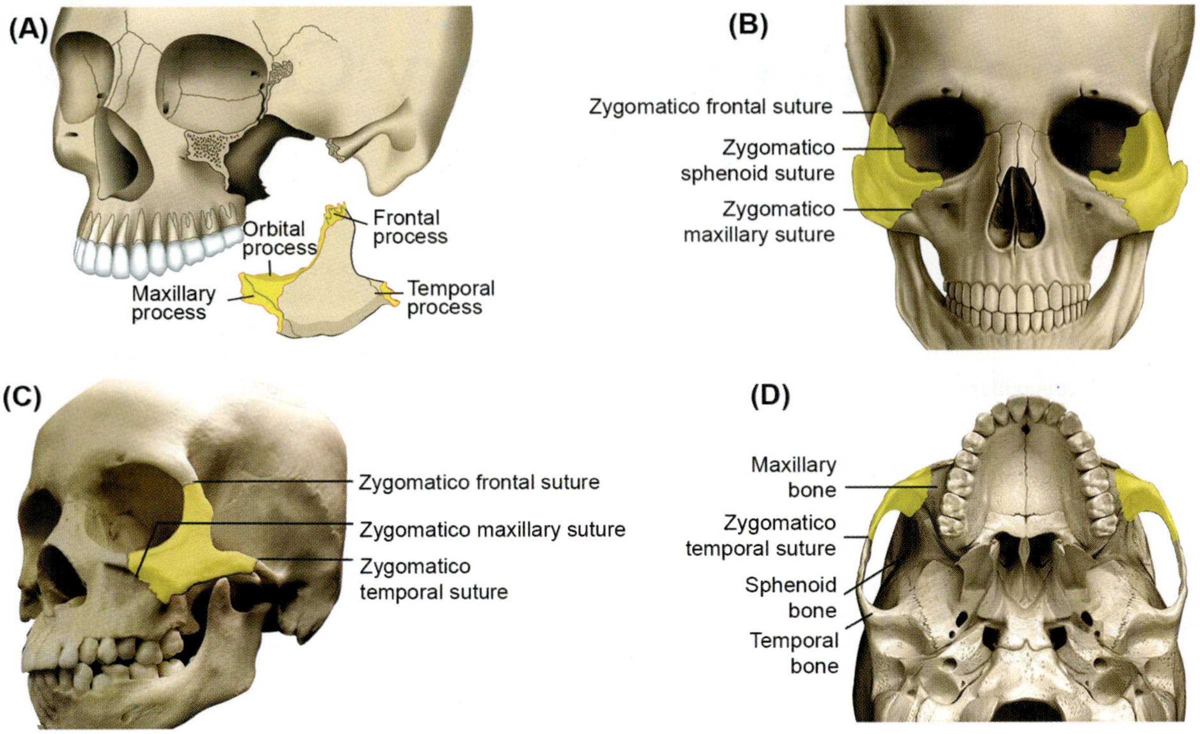

Figure 51.1 Anatomy of zygoma. (**A**) Articulations of zygoma with its processes. (**B** and **C**) Sutures involved in ZMC fractures. (**D**) Zygomatic arch.

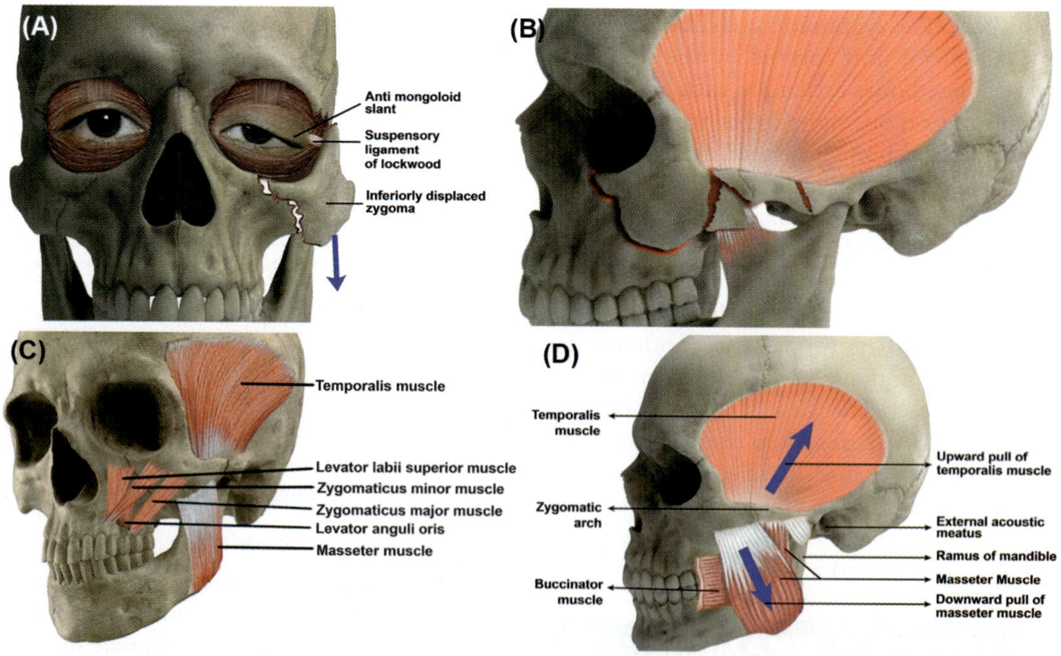

Figure 51.2 (**A**) Displacement of the zygoma and suspensory ligament of Lockwood producing antimongoloid slant. (**B**) Zygomatic arch impinging the temporalis and the coronoid process. (**C**) Zygoma and its muscle attachments. (**D**) Masseter exerting downward force on zygoma.

masseter displaces the zygoma downwards; hence, it has been considered as the main cause for the postreduction instability. Whereas the temporal fascia resists the downward displacement of the fractured zygoma (Fig. 51.2D).

The ***zygomatic arch*** plays a key role in re-establishing the sagittal and transverse width of the face. Zygomatic arch fractures produce depression of the malar eminence as well as trismus when the arch impinges the coronoid process (refer to page no. 976–978).

The ***nerves*** involved in ZMC are the *infraorbital and zygomatic nerves*. The infraorbital nerve runs along the infraorbital canal and exits into the face through the infraorbital foramen. The zygomatic nerve enters the orbit through the inferior orbital fissure and divides into two branches, the zygomaticofacial and zygomaticotemporal nerves. Paraesthesia of the face is a common sequence of ZMC fracture due to the involvement of these sensory nerves.

MECHANISM OF ZYGOMATICOMAXILLARY COMPLEX FRACTURES

In 1990, *Manson et al.* classified ZMC fractures based on the amount of energy dissipated by the facial bones secondary to traumatic force.

Low-energy fractures—They result in no or minimal displacement and without comminution of the articulations. These types of fractures are often seen at the zygomaticofrontal suture

Mid-energy fracture—They result in complete fracture of all articulations with mild-to-moderate displacement and comminution

High-energy fractures—They are associated with extreme displacement, comminution and segmentation of the bones.

FRACTURE PATTERNS

The zygomatic fractures involve three lines extending from the inferior orbital fissure in an anteromedial, superolateral and inferior direction.

- The 1st *line* extends from the inferior orbital fissure anteromedially along the orbital floor towards the infraorbital rim. It then extends from the infraorbital rim to the anterior surface of maxilla and inferiorly under the zygomaticomaxillary buttress (Fig. 51.3A)
- The 2nd *line* runs from the inferior orbital fissure inferiorly through the posterior aspect of maxilla and joins the fracture under the zygomaticomaxillary buttress (Fig. 51.3B)
- The 3rd *line* extends superiorly from the inferior orbital fissure along the lateral orbital wall of orbit separating the sphenozygomatic suture. It then extends superiorly, laterally and anteriorly to the lateral orbital rim separating the frontozygomatic suture (Fig. 51.3A)
- A ZMC fracture usually has an *additional fracture line* passing through the zygomatic arch, as the point of least resistance to fracture is usually at the middle of the zygomatic arch (Fig. 51.3C).

However, these fracture patterns may vary depending on the direction and magnitude of force, density of the adjacent bones and the soft tissue covering over the zygoma.

CLASSIFICATION OF ZYGOMATICOMAXILLARY COMPLEX FRACTURE

AXIS OF ROTATION

a. Vertical axis of rotation (Fig. 51.4A and B):
   Vertical axis is an imaginary line running through the frontozygomatic suture and the 1st molar tooth. Fractures along the vertical axis usually result in inward/*medial or outward/lateral displacement of the zygoma*
b. Horizontal axis of rotation (Fig. 51.4C and D):
   Horizontal axis is an imaginary line running through the infraorbital foramen and zygomatic arch. Fractures around the horizontal axis result in upward or downward movement of the broken segment.

Based on this classification, the stability of fractures after elevation can be demonstrated.

1. **Knight and Northwood classification (1961)**
   Group I: Undisplaced fractures
   Group II: Displaced arch fractures
   Group III: Unrotated body fractures

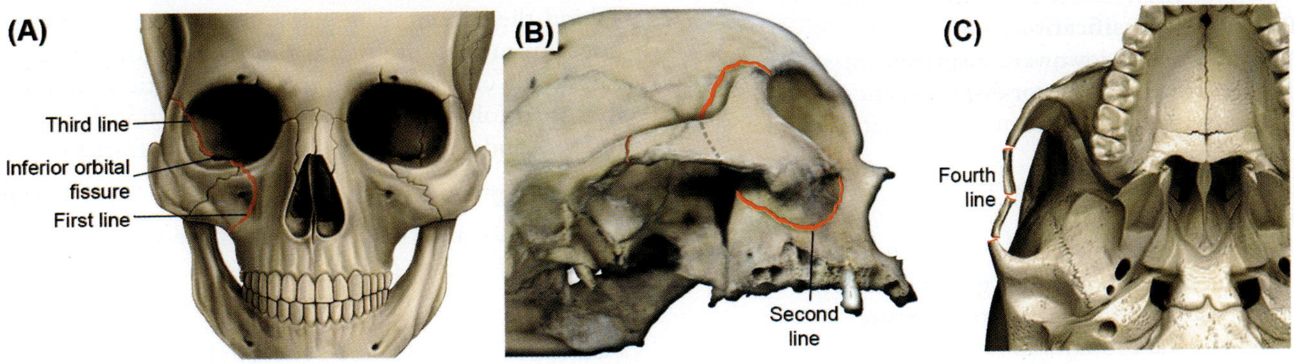

Figure 51.3 Fracture pattern of ZMC. (**A**) 1st and 3rd line. (**B**) 2nd line. (**C**) Additional fracture line.

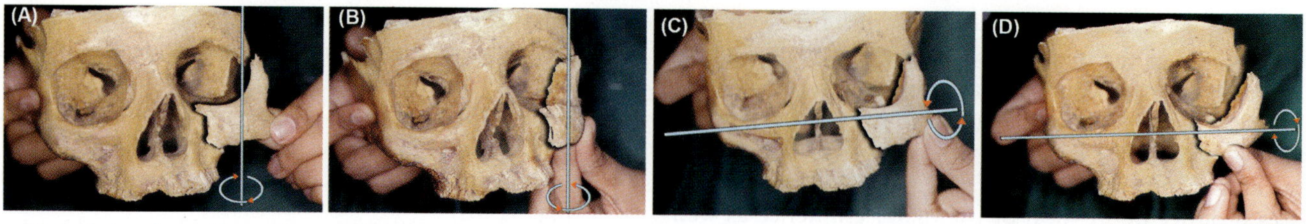

Figure 51.4 Axis of rotation. (**A** and **B**) Vertical axis of rotation. (**C** and **D**) Horizontal axis of rotation. (**A**) Medial displacement. (**B**) Lateral displacement. (**C**) Upward and outward displacement. (**D**) Down and inward displacement.

Group IV: Medially rotated body fractures
IVa. Outward at malar buttress
IVb. Inward at FZ suture
Group V: Laterally rotated body fractures
Va: Upward at the infraorbital margin
Vb: Outward at the FZ suture
Group VI: Comminuted fractures

2. **Rowe and Killey classification (1968)**
   Type I: No significant displacement
   Type II: Fracture of zygomatic arch
   Type III: Rotation around horizontal axis
   - Inward displacement of orbital rim
   - Outward displacement of orbital rim

   Type IV: Rotation around longitudinal axis
   - Medial displacement of frontal process of zygoma
   - Lateral displacement of frontal process of zygoma

   Type V: Displacement of the complex block
   - Medial
   - Inferior
   - Lateral

   Type VI: Displacement of orbital floor
   - Inferiorly
   - Superiorly

   Type VII: Displacement of orbital rim segment
   Type VIII: Complex comminuted fracture
3. **Larsen and Thomsen (1978)**
   Group A: *Stable fracture*—Fractures showing minimal or no displacement and hence requiring no intervention
   Group B: *Unstable fracture*—Fractures with great displacement and disruption at the frontozygomatic suture and comminuted fractures requiring reduction and fixation
   Group C: *Stable fracture*—Fractures of all other kinds, which required reduction but no fixation
4. **Poswillo's classification**
   A. Inward and downward displacement
   B. Inward and posterior displacement
   C. Outward displacement of zygomatic complex
   D. Comminution
   E. Fracture of arch alone
5. **Zing et al., (1992)**
   Type A: Incomplete low-energy zygomatic fractures with fracture of only one zygomatic pillar
   A1—isolated zygomatic arch fracture
   A2—lateral orbital wall fracture
   A3—infraorbital rim fracture
   Displacement of the malar prominence does not occur because of the intact remaining pillars
   Type B: Complete monofragment zygomatic fracture (tetrapod fracture)
   All the four articulations of zygomatic bone are fractured and displaced. It is the 'classic tripod fracture' but anatomically these are tetrapod fractures
   Type C: Multifragment zygomatic fracture. Same as type B, but with fragmentation of the body of zygoma
6. **Rowe and Williams (1985)**
   Type I—Fracture stable after elevation
   A. Arch only (medially displaced) (Fig. 51.5A)
   B. Rotation around a vertical axis (Fig. 51.5B and C)
   - Medially
   - Laterally

   Type II—Fractures unstable after elevation
   A. Arch only (inferiorly displaced) (Fig. 51.5D)
   B. Rotation around a horizontal axis (Fig. 51.5E)
   - Medially
   - Laterally

   C. Dislocations enbloc (Fig. 51.5F–H)
   - Inferiorly
   - Medially
   - Posterolaterally

   Type III—Comminuted fractures of the zygomatic complex (Fig. 51.5I).

CLINICAL ASSESSMENT

A thorough clinical examination of face, eye and occlusion is necessary to identify the fractures involving the ZMC. The zygoma is examined by placing the patient in a recumbent position or reclined in a chair with the surgeon standing behind the patient. The palpation is done using the index finger from the infraorbital rim through the lateral orbital rims, body of zygoma and to the zygomatic arch (Fig. 51.6). It is then followed by intraoral examination for zygomatic buttress and any associated dentoalveolar fractures.

Clinical signs and symptoms

The presence and the magnitude of the severity depends on the extent and type of injury (Table 51.1, Fig. 51.7).

Oedema

Oedema of the eyelids and periorbital region is the most common sign following orbital rim fracture, due to disruption of

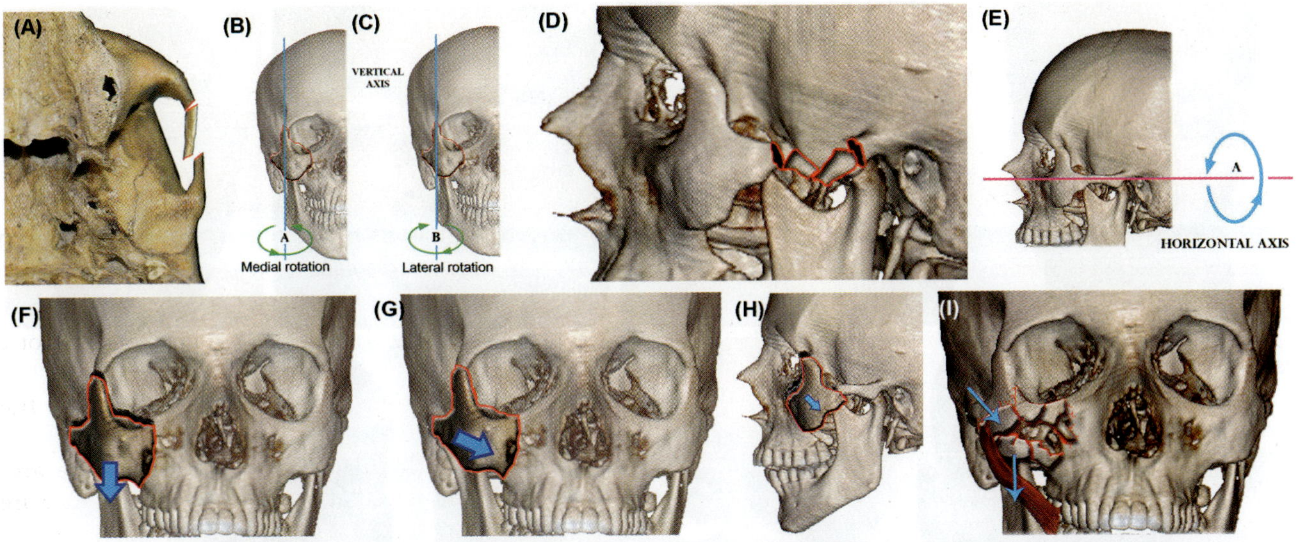

Figure 51.5 Rowe and Williams's classification. (**A–C**) Type I fracture. (**D–H**) Type 2 fracture. (**I**) Type 3 fracture.

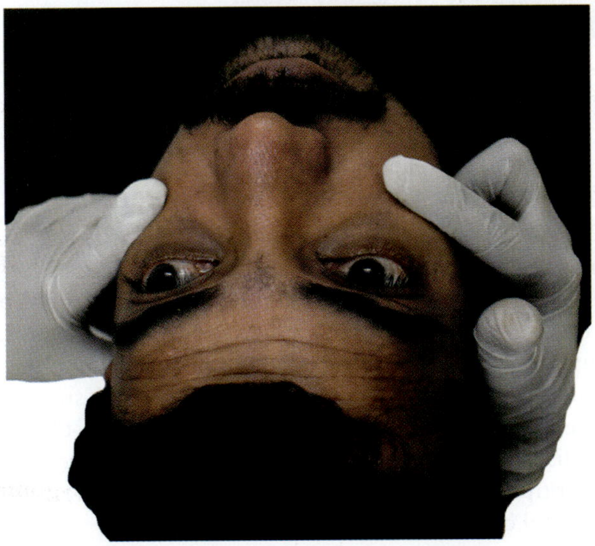

Figure 51.6 Clinical examination of zygoma.

the periosteum lining the bone. It can be localised to one area or generalised around the entire orbital area (Fig. 51.7A).

Subconjunctival ecchymosis

A frequent finding that occurs in orbital rim fractures due to disruption of periosteum lining the orbit. It appears as characteristically bright red colour across the transparent bulbar conjunctiva due to the absorption of atmospheric oxygen (Fig. 51.7B). However, its absence does not exclude orbital rim fracture.

Flattening of malar prominence

It is the most characteristic and striking feature of zygomatic injury. The body of zygoma provides a characteristic prominence to the face called the malar prominence. This prominence is lost in ZMC fractures resulting in flatness of

TABLE 51.1 Clinical Presentation of Zygomaticomaxillary Complex Fracture

Region	Signs and Symptoms
Soft tissue (facial asymmetry)	Periorbital oedema and ecchymosis Subconjunctival ecchymosis Chemosis Buccal sulcus haematoma
Bone deformity (facial asymmetry)	Flattening of malar prominence Step deformity—infraorbital margin/zygomatic buttress Crepitus Zygomatic arch depression
Eyes	Diplopia Enophthalmos Unequal pupillary levels Displacement of palpebral fissure (antimongoloid slant) Proptosis Epiphora Associated orbital floor fracture
Nerves	Infraorbital paraesthesia/anaesthesia Zygomaticotemporal paraesthesia Zygomaticofacial paraesthesia Alveolar nerve anaesthesia
Nasal	Epistaxis Nasal deformity (if fracture is continuous with nose)
Occlusal	Trismus (zygomatic arch fracture) Occlusal disturbance (if fracture extends into alveolar process)
Compartment syndromes	Superior orbital fissure syndrome Orbital apex syndrome

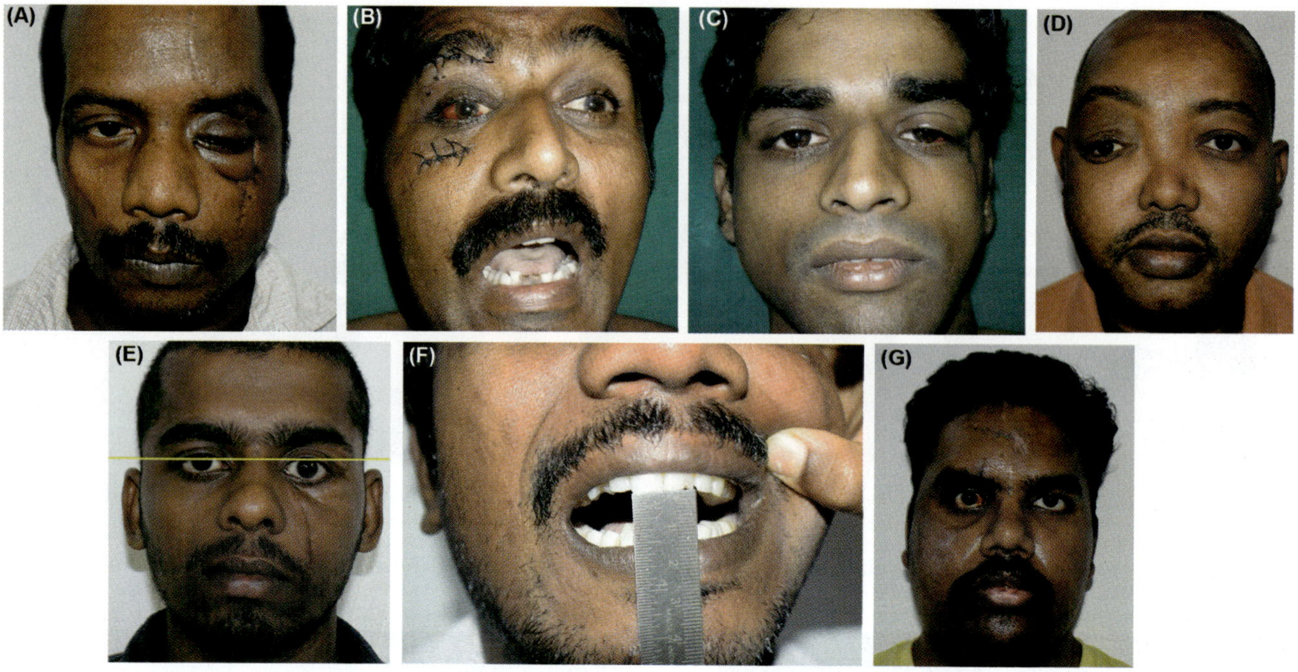

Figure 51.7 Clinical findings of ZMC fracture. **(A)** Periorbital oedema. **(B)** Subconjunctival ecchymosis. **(C)** Flattening of malar prominence. **(D)** Antimongoloid slant. **(E)** Unequal pupillary levels. **(F)** Trismus. **(G)** Enophthalmos.

cheek. In the presence of oedema, flattening may be difficult to discern, but by palpating the soft tissues with the index finger and comparing with the other side, it can be appreciated (Fig. 51.7C). Flattening of cheek can also be assessed by standing behind the patient and viewing from above, comparing the two sides of face (bird's eye and worm's view).

Air emphysema

Fracture of maxillary sinus with tearing of the mucosal lining allows air to escape into the facial soft tissue causing emphysema. It can be easily appreciated by alternatively rolling two fingers gently over the tissue, which produces a characteristic crackling sensation (crepitus). There is a potential for the spread of infection through the communication between the facial soft tissues and maxillary sinus. The emphysema usually disappears spontaneously without treatment in 2–4 days.

Displacement of the palpebral fissure

The Whitnall's tubercle (a bony elevation) is located 1 cm below the frontozygomatic suture and 4–5 mm posterior to the lateral orbital rim. The lateral canthal ligament and Lockwood's suspensory ligaments are attached to this Whitnall's tubercle. When the zygoma is fractured above the Whitnall's tubercle, the lateral palpebral ligament is also depressed, causing a downward slope to the palpebral fissure producing an *antimongoloid slant appearance* (downward slant of eyelid in a horizontal plane) (Fig. 51.7D). It is also called as *hooding of eye*. This depression of lower eyelid exposes more sclera and an apparent ectropion (everted eyelid). If the fracture line remains below Whitnall's tubercle, there is no alteration at the ocular level.

Unequal pupillary levels

The position of the globe in relation to the horizontal axis is maintained by Lockwood's suspensory ligament. The suspensory ligament is attached medially to the lacrimal bone and laterally to the Whitnall's tubercle. In ZMC fractures, the disruption of the orbital floor and lateral wall of the orbit produces displacement of Tenon's capsule and suspensory ligaments of the globe permitting depression of the globe. This displacement of globe is clinically manifested as unequal pupillary levels (Fig. 51.7E). This alteration in the globe level can also cause diplopia.

Epiphora

The lacrimal gland is located at the superior and outer edge of the orbital roof. Any injury to this lacrimal apparatus involving either puncta or passages can lead to continuous overflow of tears. But injury to the lacrimal gland following fracture of zygoma is a rare occurrence.

Infraorbital nerve paraesthesia

It is more common in displaced fractures than in undisplaced fractures. It occurs when the fracture through the orbital floor or the anterior maxilla causes tearing, shearing or compression of the infraorbital nerve along its canal or foramen. When the fracture line is lateral to the infraorbital groove and foramen, the infraorbital nerve is spared. Infraorbital nerve paraesthesia involves paraesthesia of the lower eyelid, upper lip and lateral aspect of the nose. Sometimes an altered sensitivity may be present in maxillary teeth and gingiva, due to disruption of the infraorbital nerve within its canal, where the middle and anterior superior alveolar nerves take origin. Recovery usually takes between 6 and 9 months.

Epistaxis

It is bleeding from the nose. It is observed due to the escape of pooled blood from the maxillary sinus following zygoma fracture.

Trismus

Trismus is restriction in mouth opening and lateral movements of the lower jaw. It is more common in isolated zygomatic arch fractures. This is because of the downward displacement of fractured zygoma or zygomatic arch impinging on the coronoid process causing (1) mechanical obstruction or (2) muscle spasm (temporalis muscle). Injury to the masseter can also lead to trismus (Fig. 51.7F).

Tenderness and step deformity

Digital palpation can reveal step deformity at the zygomatic buttress, frontozygomatic suture, infraorbital rim and zygomatic arch.

Flattening over the zygomatic arch

Direct injury to the lateral aspect of the face commonly fractures the zygomatic arch. Low force causes buckling of the arch, whereas heavy force causes transmission of force to the body of zygoma resulting in zygoma fracture. Clinically, arch fractures present as a dimple or depression over the lateral face.

Enophthalmos

The changes in the globe position resulting from ZMC fractures are exophthalmos and enophthalmos. Enophthalmos is defined as *retrodisplacement of the globe within the eye socket or recession of globe within the orbit.* Exophthalmos arises from posterior and medially displaced zygoma, whereas enophthalmos occurs from laterally and inferiorly displaced zygoma. Clinically, it is noted as a change in horizontal pupillary levels and decreased globe projection (Fig. 51.7G).

Enophthalmosis can be measured using Naugle's exophthalmometer, which utilises supraorbital rim as reference point. Hertel's exophthalmometer does not reflect the true position of the globe in displaced ZMC fractures, as it uses the orbital rim as reference point. However, CT evaluation is the most preferred modality for measuring Enophthalmosis. Surgical management includes restoration of orbital rims by reduction and fixation of ZMC fracture (refer to Chapter 53).

Diplopia

Diplopia is a very serious complication of the zygomatic fracture where the patient experiences blurred/double vision (refer to Chapter 53).

RADIOGRAPHIC EVALUATION

Radiographs helps in determining the type, location, magnitude and the direction of displacement of fractures (Fig. 51.8). The most commonly used radiographs for zygoma fracture are:

- Posteroanterior (PA) view of skull
- Caldwell projection/occipitofrontal view
- Waters view/occipitomental 37 degrees/Paranasal sinuses (PNS)
- Submentovertex view/jug handle view
- CT scan.

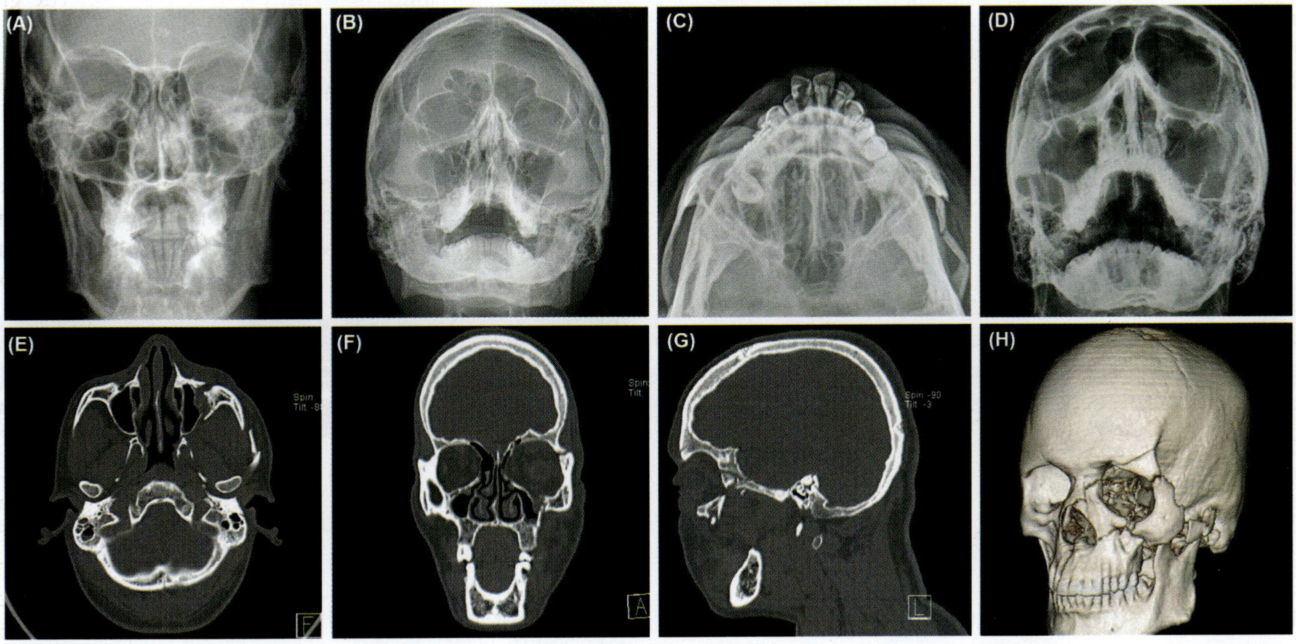

Figure 51.8 Radiographic evaluation. **(A)** PA view. **(B)** PNS/Waters view/occipitomental. **(C)** Submentovertex view. **(D)** Caldwell projection. **(E)** CT—Axial view. **(F)** CT— Coronal view. **(G)** CT—Sagittal view. **(H)** CT—3D reconstruction.

Caldwell's and Waters view provides a better view of paranasal and frontal sinus, apart from other structures such as orbit, zygomatic, nasal bone and coronoid process. Submentovertex is the single best view for the evaluation of zygomatic arch fracture. PA oblique view provides an excellent view of the zygoma, its arch and related structures such as infraorbital rim, orbital floor, lateral wall, zygomaticofrontal suture and maxillary sinus. CT scans accurately identify the fracture line, position and displacement of ZMC and zygomatic arch.

Plain radiographs were generally used in the identification of fractures. For further assessment and treatment planning, CT scans are considered to be the best radiographic assessment tool.

MANAGEMENT OF ZYGOMATICOMAXILLARY COMPLEX FRACTURE

Zygomatic fractures were 1st described by *Duverney*. A variety of methods ranging from conservative to surgical treatment (ORIF) have been suggested for treating ZMC fractures.

CONSERVATIVE TREATMENT

Conservative treatment is indicated for:

- Fractures with minimal or no displacement
- Medically compromised patients
- Elderly patients for whom invasive surgical procedures and a general anaesthesia are contraindicated.

Patients should be on a nonchew soft diet for 2–6 weeks, with close monitoring for displacement.

SURGICAL MANAGEMENT (OPEN REDUCTION AND FIXATION)

Indications for surgery include:

- Severely displaced fractures
- More than two fracture fragments
- Needs orbital reconstruction
- Cosmetic defects
- Functional disabilities
- Children associated with oculocardiac reflex

Steps in surgical management of ZMC fracture:

1. Prophylactic antibiotics
2. Anaesthesia
3. Clinical examination and forced duction test
4. Antiseptic preparation and globe protection
5. Surgical exposure (incision)
6. Surgical approaches (extraoral or intraoral)
7. Fracture reduction (direct or indirect)
8. Fixation
9. Orbital reconstruction
10. Assessment of ocular motility
11. Soft tissue closure.

SURGICAL EXPOSURE OF FRACTURE

Incisions are planned according to the fracture location and the amount of exposure needed for the surgery. Different areas in ZMC fracture are accessed through various incisions (Table 51.2).

TABLE 51.2 Surgical Exposure of Fracture

Site of Fracture	Incision
Frontozygomatic suture	Lateral eye brow incision and blepharoplasty (upper eyelid incision)
Zygomaticomaxillary buttress	Maxillary vestibular incision
Infraorbital rim and orbital floor	Transconjunctival incision Transcutaneous incisions (Subciliary, infraorbital incision)
Zygomaticotemporal region, Frontozygomatic suture and Sphenozygomatic suture (lateral wall of orbit)	Coronal incision

SURGICAL APPROACHES

The approaches for ZMC fracture reduction can be extraoral or intraoral (Table 51.3) (Fig. 51.9).

TABLE 51.3 Surgical Approaches for Zygomaticomaxillary Complex Fracture

Extraoral Approach	Intraoral Approach
1. Gillie's temporal approach 2. Percutaneous methods • Dingman's—lateral eyebrow • Poswillo's approach—stab incision 3. Endoscopic	1. Balasubramaniam's/ Keen's approach (upper buccal sulcus approach) 2. Quinn's procedure (lateral coronoid approach)

EXTRAORAL APPROACHES

Gillie's temporal approach

It was 1st introduced by Gillie in 1927 for the reduction of the zygomatic arch and ZMC fractures.

Advantages:

- It allows application of controlled force to disimpact the zygoma
- Quick and simple method
- Does not produce a visible scar
- Fewer complications.

The only contraindication is the possibility of a concomitant temporal bone fracture.

The temporalis muscle originates from the temporal fossa (temporal line) that runs vertically down the medial to the

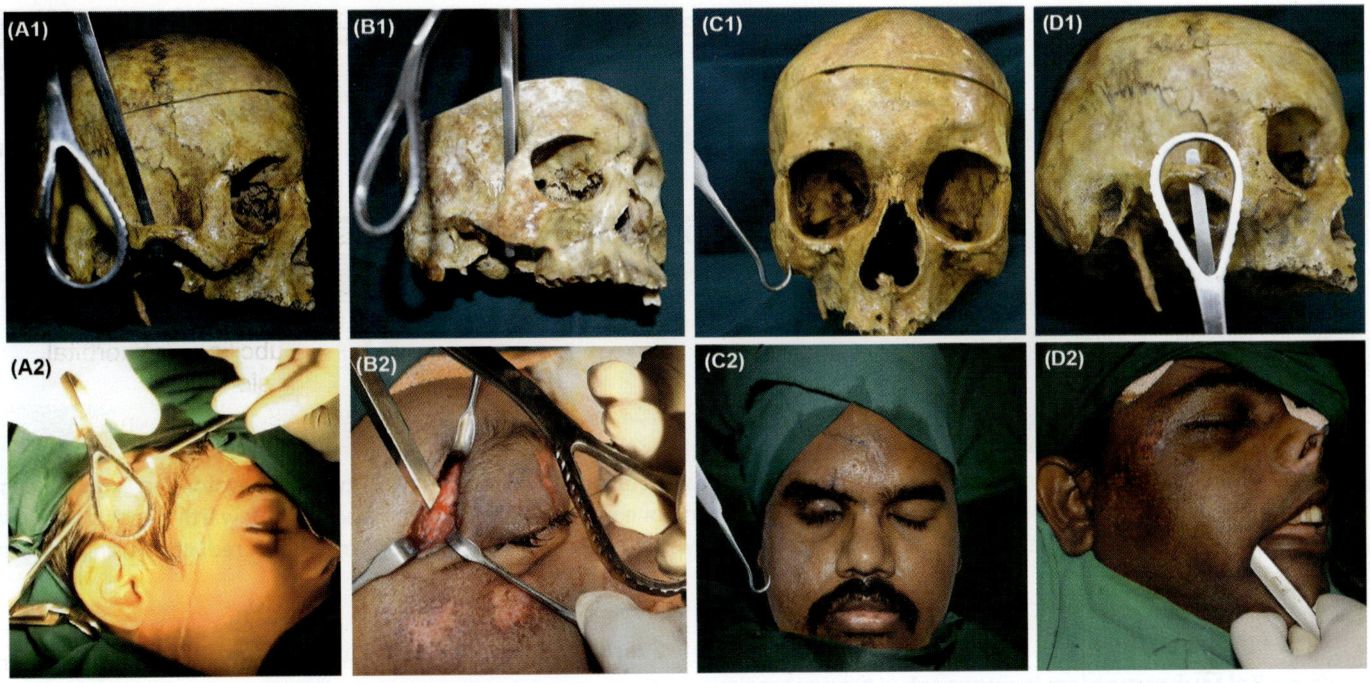

Figure 51.9 Surgical approaches to ZMC fractures. (**A1** and **A2**) Gillie's temporal approach. (**B1** and **B2**) Dingman's approach. (**C1** and **C2**) Percutaneous approach. (**D1** and **D2**) Keen's intraoral approach.

zygomatic arch and gets inserted into the anteromedial surface of the coronoid process of the mandible. The temporalis fascia is a dense fibrous sheet that surrounds the temporalis muscle. It originates from the same region of muscle and is attached inferiorly to the medial and lateral aspect of the zygomatic arch. This technique is based on the anatomical basis that *the plane between the fascia and the temporalis muscle offers direct access to the zygomatic arch and zygoma.*

Two types of **zygomatic elevators** are commonly used: ***Bristow's and Rowe's.***

Bristow's elevator—It has a single flat and elongated working tip attached to a handle and is used like a spatula for elevation.

Rowe's elevator—It has an additional arm which is attached to the working tip. It serves to:

(1) Provide the necessary counter traction during elevation (to relieve the fulcrum from the temporal bone)
(2) Evaluate the approximate depth of insertion of the working tip when inserted into the tissue.

Technique (Fig. 51.10)

A 2 cm temporal incision is made 2.5 cm superior and anterior to the helix, within the hairline, parallel to the anterior branch of the superficial temporal artery. The dissection is carried out through the skin, subcutaneous tissue and superficial temporal fascia. The superficial temporal fascia is then incised exposing the temporalis muscle. Howarth's elevator is inserted *below the temporalis fascia and above the temporalis muscle* to create a plane for the zygomatic elevator.

The zygoma elevator (Bristow's and Rowe's) is inserted into the plane created to reach the deeper surface of the zygomatic arch. Once the elevator is in position, the handle is elevated in anterior, superior and lateral direction to reduce the zygomatic arch. A back-and-forth motion is used to smoothen the collapsed arch. During elevation, an assistant must palpate the frontozygomatic suture and infraorbital rim while steadying the patients head against the elevator's pull. An audible crunch or crack often accompanies the elevation. Once adequate reduction has been accomplished, the elevator is withdrawn and the incision is closed in two layers.

Dingman's approach—lateral eyebrow

This technique is performed through a standard lateral eyebrow incision.

Advantages:

- Fracture at the orbital rim is visualised directly
- Fixation of fracture is done through the same incision

Disadvantages:

- Visible scar
- Requires 2nd incision for fixation of the orbital rim and floor

Technique:

A 2 cm incision is made on the lateral eyebrow parallel to hair follicles. Dissection is done through the skin, subcutaneous tissue and muscular layer. Another incision is made on the periosteum of the lateral wall of orbit and the fracture site identified. Howarth's elevator is then inserted behind the orbital rim into the temporal fossa. The elevator beneath the body of zygoma is lifted in an upward, forward and outward direction.

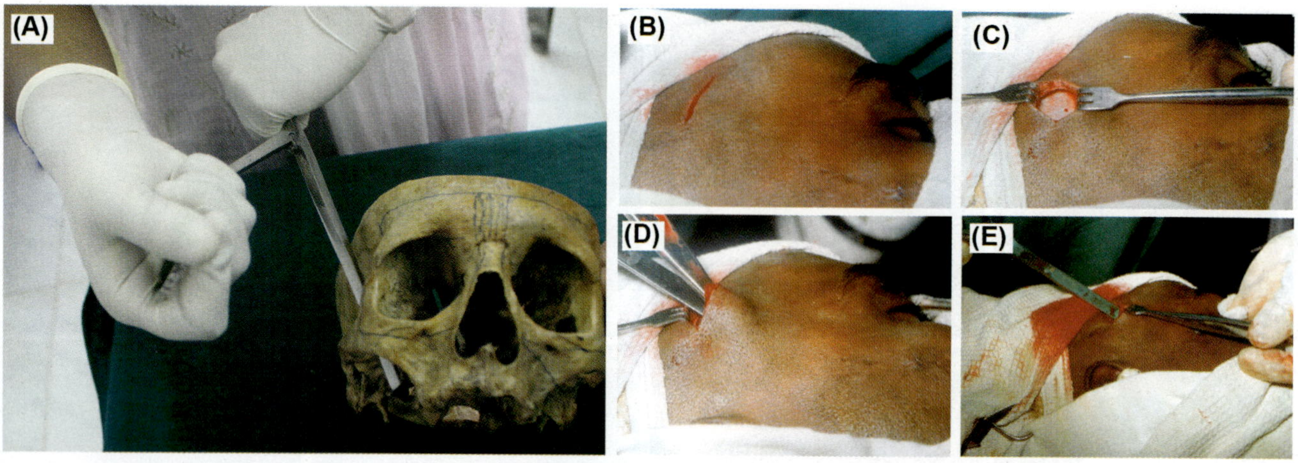

Figure 51.10 Gillie's temporal approach. (**A**) Illustration of Gillie's temporal approach using Rowe's zygoma elevator in a skull. (**B**) Temporal incision made 2.5 cm superior to the helix of ear. (**C**) Dissection done exposing the temporal fascia. (**D**) Howarth's periosteal elevator is inserted into the plane above the temporalis muscle and below the temporalis fascia. (**E**) Zygomatic arch reduction using elevator.

INTRAORAL APPROACHES

Keen's or Balasubramaniam's approach—transverse buccal sulcus

This approach uses a maxillary vestibular incision.

Advantages:

- No extraoral scar
- It offers more mechanical advantage than extraoral technique
- It can be used for both zygomatic arch and zygoma fracture

Technique (Fig. 51.11):

An incision of 1 cm is made in the maxillary buccal sulcus, just beneath the zygomatic buttress. The incision is extended through mucosa, submucosal and buccinator muscle. A periosteal elevator is used to dissect the soft tissues in a supraperiosteal plane to engage the infratemporal surface of the zygoma. An elevator is inserted and reduction is achieved with an upward, forward and outwardly directed force. It requires less force to elevate, as the force is directed entirely to the centre of the zygomatic body.

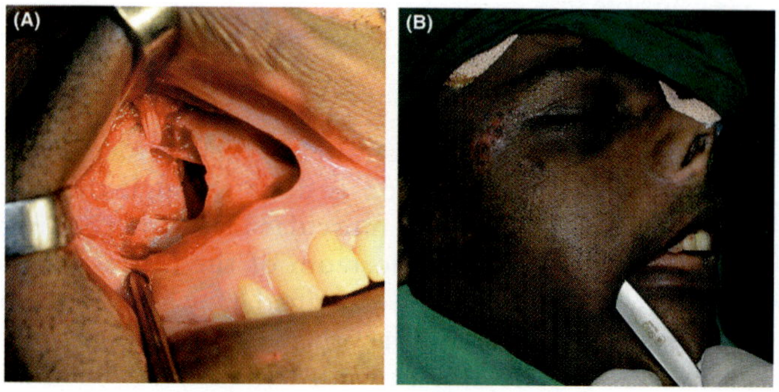

Figure 51.11 Keen's approach.

Quinn's procedure (lateral coronoid approach)

The incision is placed over the anterior border of ramus and the elevator is inserted supraperiosteally lateral to the coronoid process to reach the medial surface of the zygomatic arch. The arch is elevated in an ironing fashion.

REDUCTION OF FRACTURE

The aim of reduction is to replace the fractured and malpositioned bone into the correct anatomical position. Fracture reduction can be done either by direct or indirect method.

Direct reduction (open)

It involves reduction of fracture under direct visualisation (e.g. Coronal approach). It is indicated in:

- Severely displaced fracture
- Complex or comminuted fractures
- Stable reduction is doubtful
- Need for orbital reduction and reconstruction.

Indirect reduction

It is a blind technique where the fracture is reduced without exposure of the fracture site. It is the most commonly practiced method (e.g. Gilles reduction) for ZMC fractures. It is carried out by application of an instrument to the deeper aspect of the zygomatic bone through an incision remote from the fracture line.

The most commonly used instruments for reduction of zygoma are Bristow's elevator, Rowe's elevator, Stacey's bone hook and Carroll Girard's device (Fig. 51.12).

FIXATION TECHNIQUES

The objective of bone fixation is to maintain the reduced fragments in a stable position. The ***fixation sites*** can be any of these or a combination of the following sites:

- Frontozygomatic (FZ) suture
- Inferior orbital rim

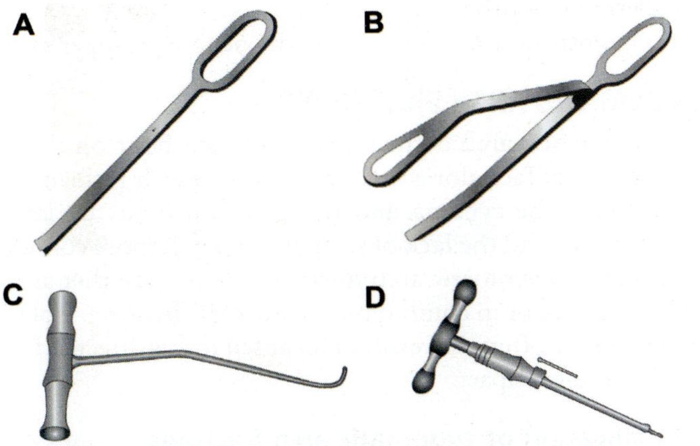

Figure 51.12 Zygoma elevators. (**A**) Bristow's elevator. (**B**) Rowe's elevator. (**C**) Stacey's bone hook. (**D**) Carroll Girard's device.

- Zygomaticosphenoid suture
- Zygomaticomaxillary (ZM) buttress
- Zygomatic arch.

Materials used for fixation

- Transosseous wiring
- K wire
- Lag screws
- Micro screws
- Miniplates
- Bioresorbable plates.

Miniplates or microplates has been considered to provide the best results with minimal complications. Low profile miniplates of size 1.5 mm or 2.0 mm are commonly used with 6 mm screws.

Fixation points (Fig. 51.13)

The number of fixation points is directly related to the stability required. Four different possibilities exist.

One-point fixation

Indication: Noncomminuted ZMC fracture without ocular symptoms

Site: Fixation at ZM or FZ suture.

Studies have shown that one-point fixation at the ZM buttress has more advantages than FZ, such as: absence of external scarring, ease of surgical access, adequate soft tissue cover and wider area of articulation. However, FZ may be used in fractures with comminuted ZM buttress.

Two-point fixation

Indication: Displaced fracture unstable after reduction

Site: Fixation at ZM buttress and FZ/IOR (infraorbital rim).

Three-point fixation/tripoding (Fig. 51.14)

Indication: Grossly displaced zygoma fracture.

Site: Fixation at the FZ, IOR and ZM buttress.

Many studies suggest that three-point fixation is more effective in establishing absolute clinical stability against displacing forces. Hence, three-point fixation is used as a standard treatment modality for the effective management of ZMC fractures.

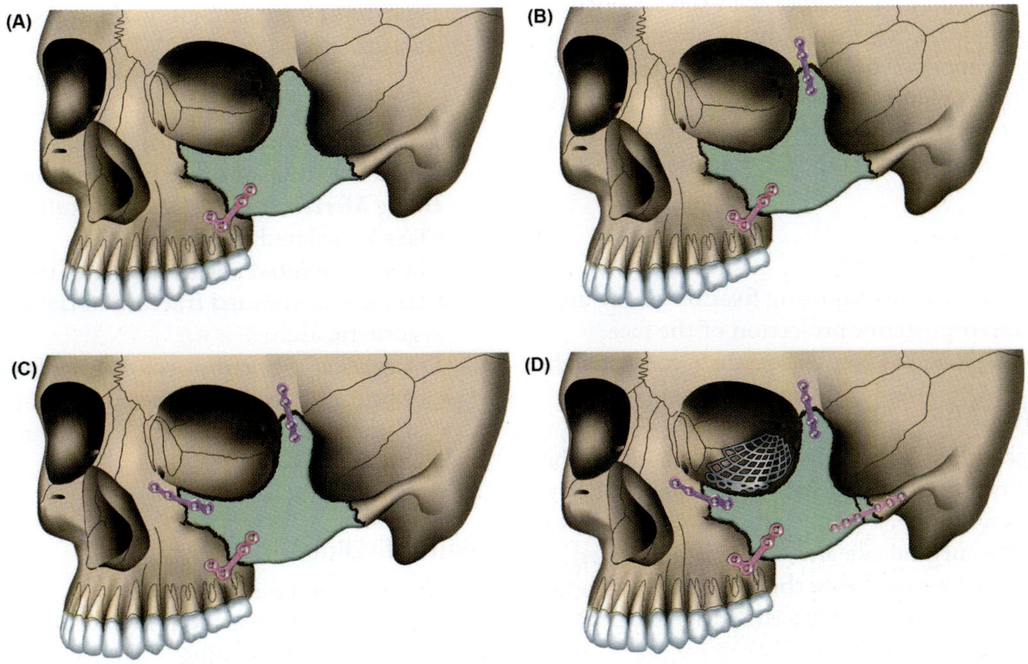

Figure 51.13 Fixation points for ZMC fracture. (**A**) One-point fixation. (**B**) Two-point fixation. (**C**) Three-point fixation. (**D**) Four-point fixation.

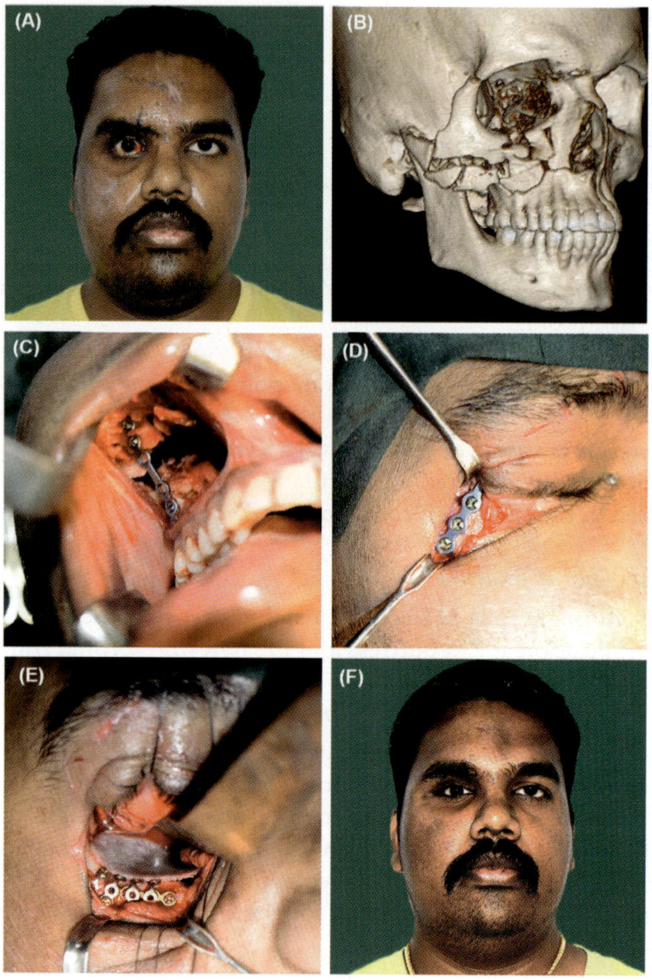

Figure 51.14 Three-point fixation of ZMC fracture. (**A**) Preoperative view showing right ZMC fracture with subconjunctival ecchymosis, enophthalmos, depressed malar prominence on the right side. (**B**) Preoperative CT scan showing fracture of right ZMC. (**C–E**) Three points of fixation at zygomatic buttress, frontozygomatic suture and orbital rim and floor, respectively. (**F**) Postoperative view with corrected ZMC fracture.

Four-point fixation/tetrapoding

Indication: Panfacial fractures requiring fixation of the arch to restore the anteroposterior projection of the face.

Site: Fixation at the FZ, IOR, ZM buttress and the zygomatic arch.

POSTOPERATIVE CARE

The following precautions have to be taken to maintain the postsurgical stability and to prevent soft tissue complications.

- Head end elevation
- Protection of the surgical site and eye. A tape labelled as 'Do not touch' can be pasted over the reduced zygoma for protection from the people around the patient. Ophthalmic ointments for eye protection
- Soft diet
- Nose blowing should be avoided
- Periodic ophthalmic assessment
- Physiotherapy to improve mouth opening postoperatively.

ZYGOMATIC ARCH FRACTURES

The zygomatic arch is the most prominent bone on the lateral aspect of face along with the external ear. It is formed by two bones: the zygoma and the temporal bone. Its lateral prominence and the lack of strength makes it more common to fracture. Zygomatic arch fractures can occur either as isolated fracture or in combination with ZMC fracture. Isolated fractures are often the result of localised forces directed laterally with low impact.

Classification of zygomatic arch fractures

1. ***Ozyazgen et al., (2007)***
   Type I—Isolated zygomatic arch fractures
   Type IA—Dual fracture
   Type IB—More than two fractures
   Type IB—V-shaped fracture
   Type IB—D-Displaced fracture
   Type II—Combined zygomatic arch fractures
   Type IIA—Single fracture
   Type IIB—Plural fracture
   Type IIB—R-Reduced
   Type IIB—D-Displaced
2. ***Yamamoto et al., (2007)***
   Classification of zygomatic arch fractures based on the degree of displacement and loss of bone contact in X-ray or CT scan (Fig. 51.15)
   Type I—No displacement
   Type II—Displacement with bone contact at all fracture lines
   Type III—Displacement without bone contact at one fracture line
   Type IV—Displacement without bone contact at two fracture lines
   Type V—Comminution or displacement without bone contact at three or more fracture lines
3. ***Honig Merten et al.,*** *(H–M classification)*
   Class I—Isolated tripod fracture
   Class II—Isolated stick fracture of the arch
   Class III—Combined fracture of the malar bone and the zygomatic arch
4. ***Fractures of zygomatic arch not involving the orbit***
   - Minimum or no displacement
   - Comminuted fractures
   - V-type fracture
   - W-type fracture.

Clinical findings

- Tenderness on palpation
- Depression over the arch (Fig. 51.16)
- Limited mouth opening
- Restricted lateral movements of mandible towards the injured side.

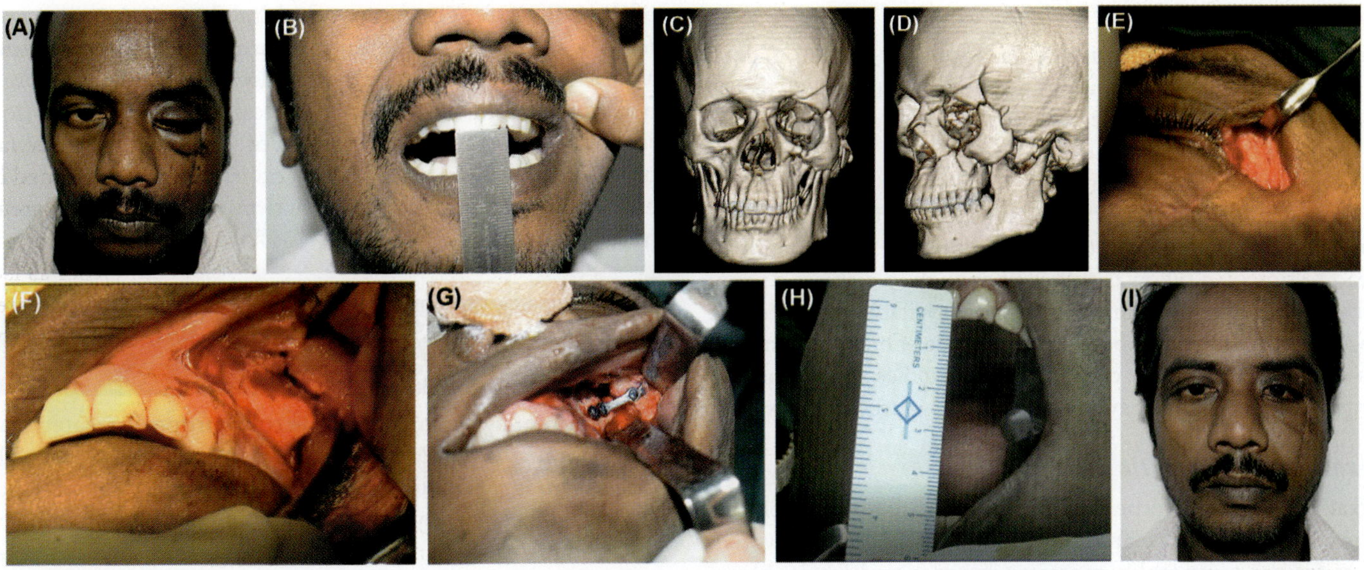

Figure 51.15 Management of ZMC fracture with trismus. (**A** and **B**) Preoperative view showing left ZMC fracture with trismus. (**C** and **D**) Preoperative CT scan showing inferiorly displaced ZMC fracture. (**E**) FZ suture exposed through lateral eyebrow incision. (**F** and **G**) Reduction and fixation of zygomatic buttress with miniplates. (**H**) Restored mouth opening. (**I**) Postoperative view.

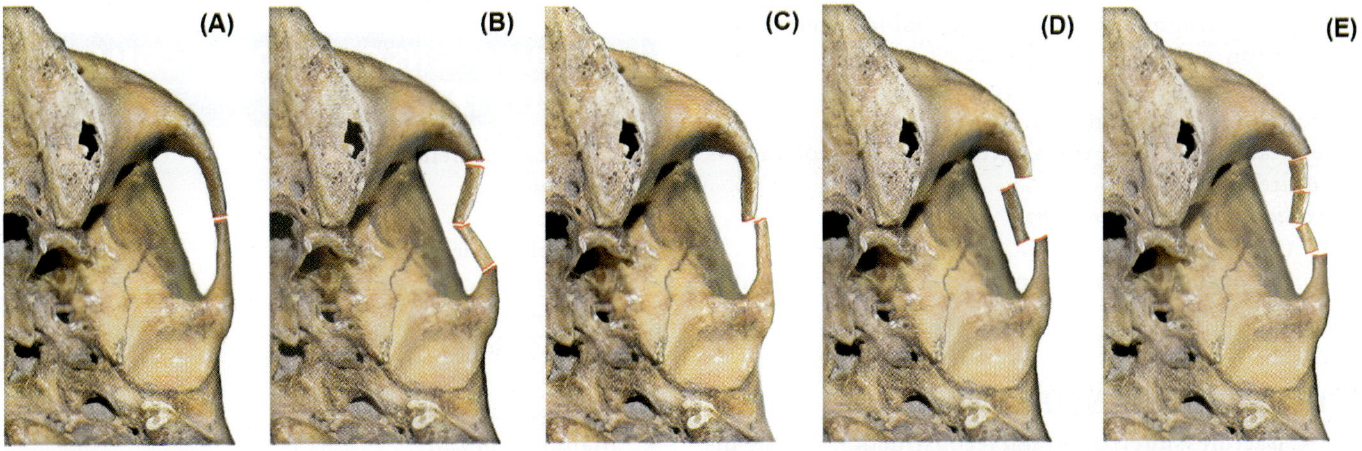

Figure 51.16 Yamamoto's classification of zygomatic arch fracture. (**A–E**) Type I, Type II, Type III, Type IV and Type V, respectively.

A severely depressed arch results in limited mouth opening due to (1) impingement of arch over the underlying temporalis muscle and/or (2) restriction of the forward movement of coronoid process.

Radiographic examination

The submentovertex/jug handle view provides the best representation of arch fracture. Loss of elephant trunk appearance is indicative of zygomatic arch fracture. CT scan remains the gold standard for three-dimensional assessment of fracture.

Management (Fig. 51.17)

If no cosmetic deformity and no functional deficit are apparent, the isolated fracture of the zygomatic arch can be observed without surgical treatment.

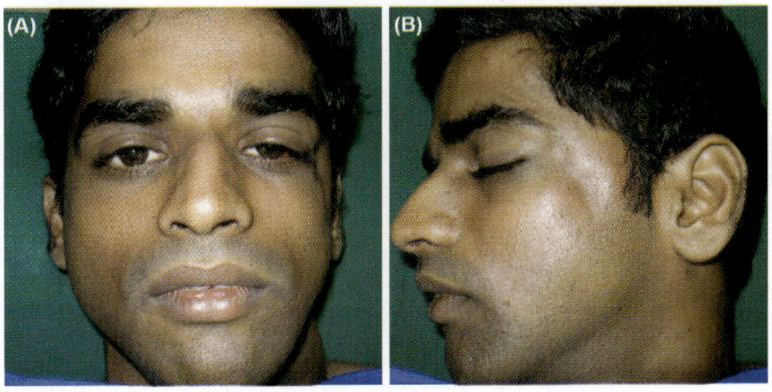

Figure 51.17 Zygomatic arch fracture. (**A** and **B**) Clinical picture showing depression in the left zygomatic arch area.

Reduction of zygomatic arch

Techniques that are commonly used for arch reduction are:

- Extraoral elevation (Gillie's method)
- Intraoral elevation (Keen's approach)
- Lateral brow technique
- Open reduction (coronal approach).

Following closed reduction of the arch fracture, the side of the head should be protected from injury. Even the weight of head resting on a pillow is sufficient enough to displace a properly reduced fracture. Many materials are available to protect the zygomatic arch that can be taped to the side of head. Commonly used materials are paper cups, metal eye patches and aluminum finger splints. Ideally, they should be left in place for 2–3 weeks.

Fixation of zygomatic arch

Fixation (ORIF) of the isolated arch fracture is rarely required, as most of the arch fractures are stable once elevated. Because the temporalis, masseter muscles and fascia, along with the adjacent soft tissues, splint the arch sufficiently to stabilise the fragments. The need for fixation of arch fractures varies with the location of the injury, number of fractures and the displacement of segments.

Indications for ORIF are:

- Fractures fragments that are unstable after closed reduction
- Multiple segment arch fracture
- Grossly displaced segments
- Re-establishment of the sagittal projection of face is required

Fixation can be performed by:

(1) Miniplate
(2) Spanning adaptation plate—for multifragmented arch
(3) Micro screw.

ORBITAL FLOOR RECONSTRUCTION

In ZMC fractures, internal orbital reconstruction may be indicated. Enophthalmos is the most common complication of ZMC fracture. The extent of orbital floor disruption varies from a linear crack to fragmentation of the entire floor. Many low energy ZMC fractures do not have herniation of periorbital contents, thus not necessitating the orbital floor reconstruction. If comminution of the orbital floor with prolapse of orbital soft tissues or if orbital volume is increased, orbital floor reconstruction should be performed (refer to Chapter 53).

MALUNITED ZYGOMATICOMAXILLARY COMPLEX FRACTURES

Malunion of zygoma can be due to improperly treated fracture or a neglected ZMC fracture that was not treated. The management of malunited zygoma fractures depends upon the type of deformity present, cosmetic or functional. Cosmetic deformities include facial asymmetry and altered globe position. They are managed by ZMC osteotomy with/without orbital floor reconstruction. Functional deficits present as restricted mouth opening, diplopia or paraesthesia. They can be corrected by ZMC osteotomy, coronoidectomy with/without orbital floor reconstruction.

COMPLICATIONS OF ZYGOMATICOMAXILLARY COMPLEX FRACTURE

- Oculocardiac reflex
- Ectropion
- Entropion
- Infraorbital nerve paraesthesia
- Implant infection, extrusion
- Persistent diplopia
- Enophthalmos
- Blindness
- Retrobulbar haemorrhage
- Malunion of ZMC
- Ankylosis of zygoma to coronoid.

Chapter
52

Fractures of the Maxilla

OUTLINE

INTRODUCTION

The mid-face is one of the most important parts of the face, both functionally and aesthetically. It plays an important role in voice resonance as well as ocular, olfactory, respiratory and digestive functions. Midfacial fractures result in distortion of the patient's appearance and also compromise the functions of mastication, speech, swallowing, vision and olfaction. The most common causes of midfacial fractures are motor vehicle accidents and assault. They are predominantly seen in the younger generation (20–40 years).

APPLIED ANATOMY OF THE MAXILLA

The maxilla forms the largest part of the middle 3rd of the face. It has a central body and four processes: frontal, zygomatic, alveolar and palatine process (Fig. 52.1A).

- *Frontal process*—Projects upwards to articulate with the maxillary process of the frontal bone, nasal bone anteriorly and the lacrimal bone posteriorly
- *Zygomatic process*—It is an extension from the body of the maxilla, forming the zygomaticomaxillary suture
- *Alveolar process*—It houses the dental arch with sockets and teeth
- *Palatine process*—It is a horizontal process that articulates with the opposite maxilla to form the palate.

The orbital or superior surface forms the floor and rim of the orbit. The body of the maxilla is hollowed out and contains the maxillary sinus.

Individually the facial bones are comparatively fragile, but when they are articulated to each other, they gain strength. This strength is often described as facial buttresses, which supports the facial skeleton. These buttresses are of two types, vertical and horizontal buttresses (Fig. 52.1B and C).

The *vertical buttresses* form the supporting pillars of the midface and are responsible for transmitting the masticatory forces to the skull base. The horizontal buttresses interconnect each other and provide support for the vertical buttress.

- *Vertical buttresses*: Nasomaxillary, zygomaticomaxillary and pterygomaxillary buttress
- *Horizontal buttresses*: Frontal bar, inferior orbital rims, maxillary alveolus and palate.

These buttresses help in fracture repair by providing bony structures for the insertion of osteosynthetic devices.

In midface fractures, the *maxilla is pulled downward and backward* by the internal and external pterygoid muscles, along an inclined plane resulting in gagging of posterior teeth. If extreme displacement of the maxilla occurs, the oral airway is occluded, where the soft palate meets the tongue.

The *blood supply to the maxilla* is via the internal maxillary artery together with the superior and posterior alveolar arteries supplying the hard and soft palates.

The *nerve supply* is through the maxillary nerve, a branch of trigeminal nerve. The maxillary nerve enters the maxilla via the maxillary foramen and runs through the maxilla in the infraorbital canal, giving off branches to supply the maxillary cheek and teeth. The infraorbital nerve exits the maxilla through the infraorbital foramen.

CLASSIFICATION OF MAXILLARY FRACTURES

RENE LE FORT (1901) CLASSIFICATION (Fig. 52.2A)

It is the most popular and widely used classification as it provides a simple and anatomically differentiated system.

Le Fort I fracture (Guerin or low-level fracture/floating maxilla)

- It is a horizontal fracture above the level of the nasal floor including the dental component (Fig. 52.2B and C)

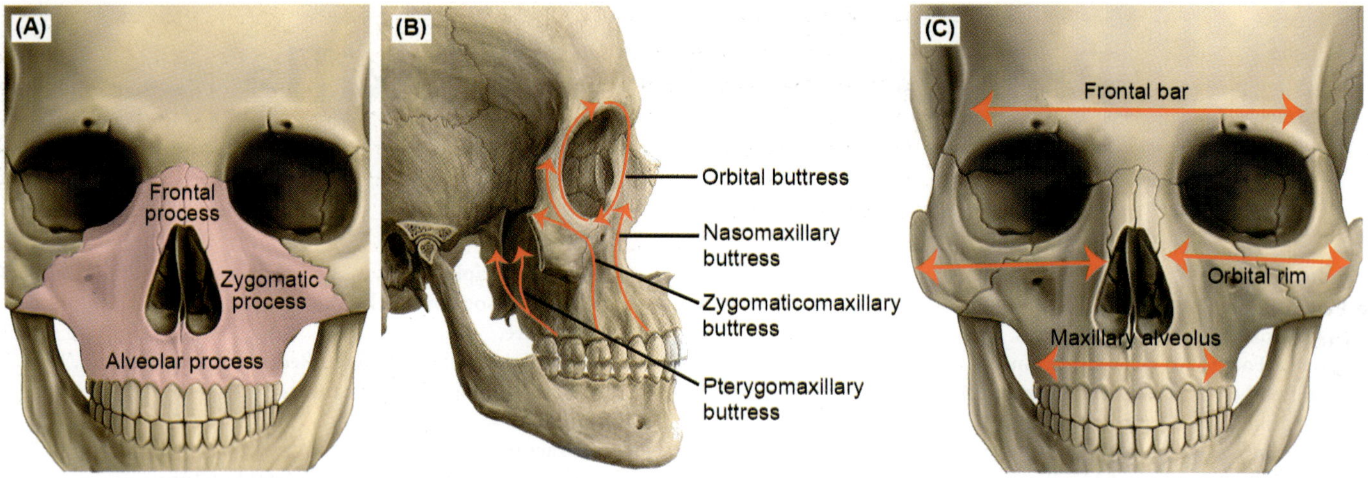

Figure 52.1 (**A**) Maxilla and its process. (**B** and **C**) Vertical and horizontal buttress of midface.

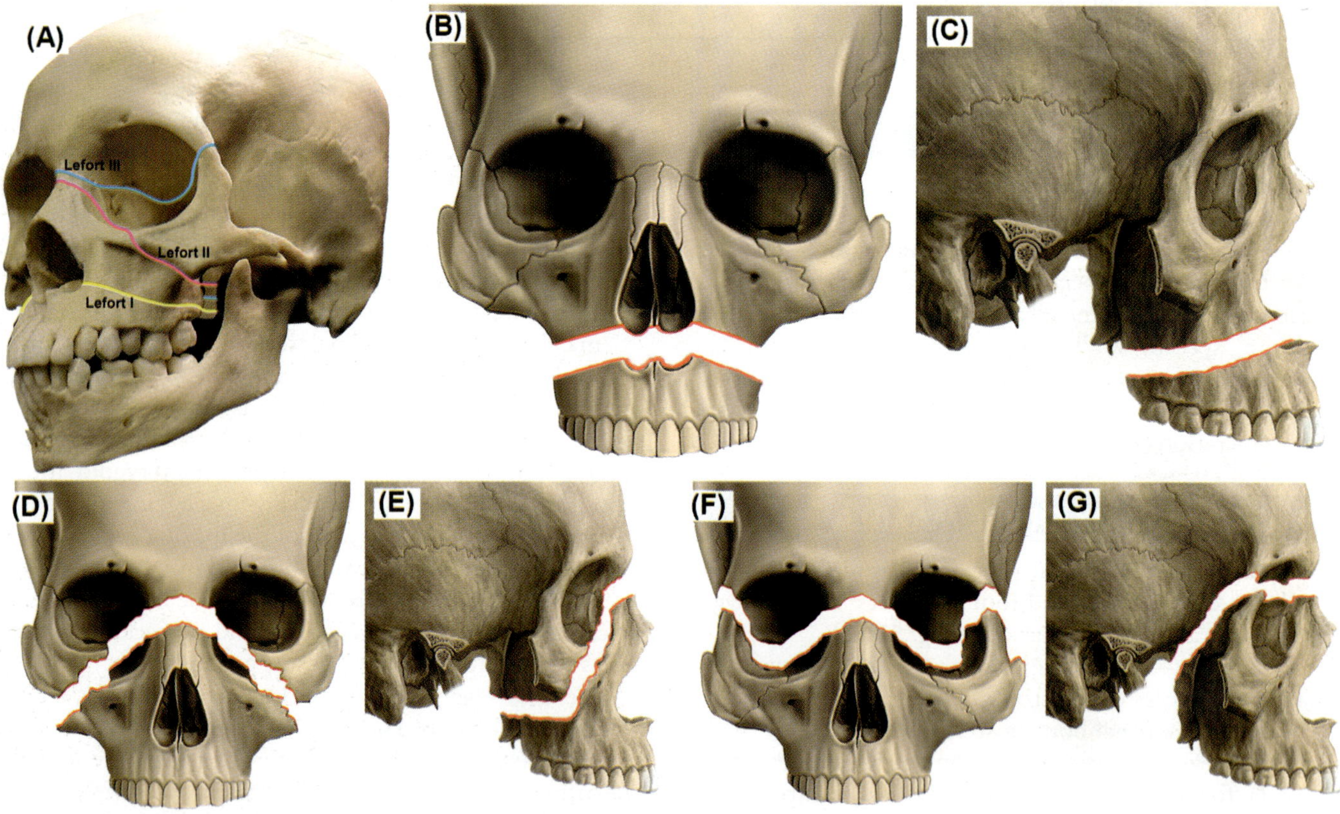

Figure 52.2 (**A**) Fracture levels of Le Fort I, II and III. (**B** and **C**) Le Fort I fracture. (**D** and **E**) Le Fort II fracture. (**F** and **G**) Le Fort III fracture.

- The *fracture line* extends backwards from the lateral margin of the anterior nasal aperture, below the zygomatic buttress and crosses the lower one-third of the pterygoid laminae. Posteriorly, the fracture line passes along the lateral wall of nose, lower part of septum and behind the tuberosity to join the fracture
- Thereby separating the whole complex of alveolar and palatal processes of the maxilla and lower parts of the pterygoid plates (just above the pterygomaxillary junction) from the skull base

Le Fort II fracture (pyramidal or subzygomatic)

- Le Fort II fracture is a pyramid-shaped fracture involving both maxilla (Fig. 52.2D and E)
- The *fracture line* runs from the middle area of the nasal bone or frontonasal junction crossing the frontal processes of the maxilla, into the medial wall of each

orbit, crosses the lacrimal bone behind the lacrimal sac—turns forwards to cross the infraorbital margin via the infraorbital foramen—extends downwards and backwards across the lateral wall of the antrum—below the zygomaticomaxillary suture and joins the pterygoid laminae at the middle one-third

- It separates the whole maxilla from the base of the skull via the nasal septum and may involve the floor of the anterior cranial fossa

Le Fort III fracture (suprazygomatic or craniofacial dysjunction)

- *Fracture line* extends from the frontonasal suture—transverses backwards, parallel with base of the skull, to full depth of the ethmoid bone including the cribriform plate. Within the orbit—the fracture passes below the optic foramen into the posterior limit of the inferior orbital fissure. From the base of the inferior orbital fissure, the fracture line extends in two directions:
  i. It runs backwards across the pterygomaxillary fissure to fracture the pterygoid laminae
  ii. Laterally across the lateral wall of the orbit, separating the zygomatic bone from the frontal bone. In addition, fracture of the zygomatic arch is an integral part of Le Fort III. In this way, the entire middle 3rd of the facial skeleton gets detached from the cranial base (Fig. 52.2F and G)
- It separates the zygomaticomaxillary complexes plus the nasal bones, palatal bones and most of the pterygoid plates from the rest of the cranium.

However, Le Fort fractures are very rarely encountered as pure forms in clinical practice. In most instances, the fracture lines combine in a quite unpredictable and asymmetric patterns.

MODIFIED LE FORT FRACTURES (MARCIANI 1993)

This classification system includes Le Fort, naso-orbito-ethmoid (NOE) and zygomaticomaxillary complex (ZMC) fractures (Fig. 52.3).

Le Fort I: Low maxillary fracture

I a: Low maxillary fracture/multiple segments

Le Fort II: Pyramidal fractures

II a: Pyramidal and nasal fractures

II b: Pyramidal and NOE fractures

Le Fort III: Craniofacial dysjunction

III a: Craniofacial dysjunction and nasal fractures

III b: Craniofacial dysjunction and NOE fractures

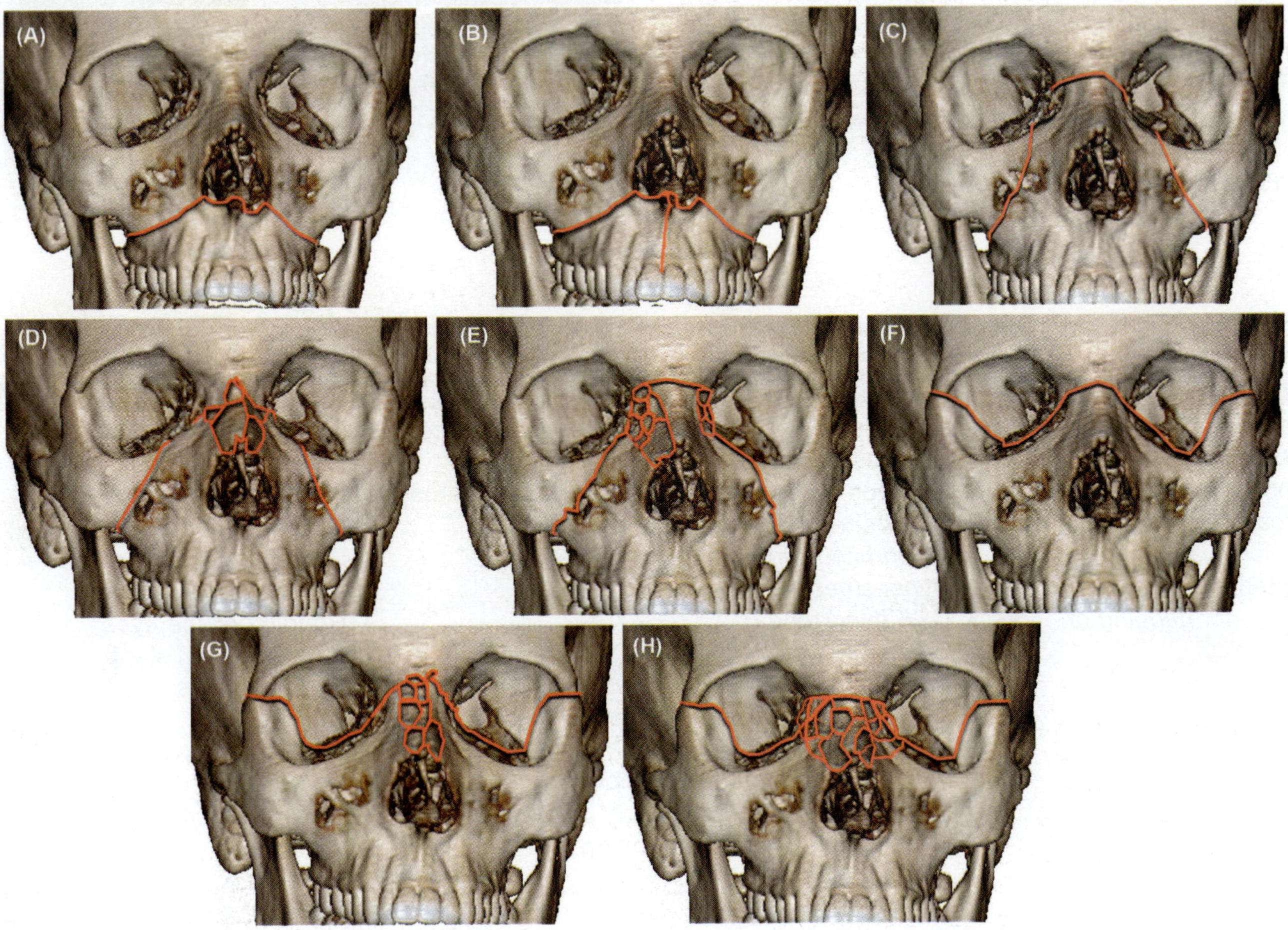

Figure 52.3 (**A–H**) Modified Le Fort fracture (Marciani 1993).

Le Fort IV: Le Fort II or III fractures and cranial base fractures
IV a: + supraorbital rim fractures
IV b: + supraorbital rim and anterior cranial fossa fractures
IV c: + anterior cranial fossa and orbital wall fractures

Frontal sinus fracture classification
I: Anterior wall fracture
II: Posterior wall fracture
III: Anterior and posterior wall fracture
IV: Frontal sinus fracture involving frontonasal ducts

Zygoma fracture classification
I: Undisplaced
II: Displaced
III: Comminuted.

ACCORDING TO ROWE AND WILLIAMS (1985)

A. **Fractures not involving the occlusion**
 I. **Central region**
  a. Fractures of the nasal bones and/or nasal septum
   - Lateral nasal injuries
   - Anterior nasal injuries
  b. Fractures of the frontal process of the maxilla
  c. Fractures of type (a) and (b) extending into the ethmoid bone (nasoethmoid)
  d. Fractures of type (a), (b) and (c), extending into the frontal bone (frontoorbitonasal dislocation)
 II. **Lateral region**:
  Fractures involving the zygomatic bone, arch and maxilla (ZMC) excluding the dentoalveolar component

B. **Fractures involving the occlusion**
 1. Dentoalveolar
 2. Subzygomatic
  a. Le Fort I (low level or Guerin)
  b. Le Fort II (pyramidal)
 3. Suprazygomatic/Le Fort III (high level or craniofacial dysjunction)
  a. Le Fort III with midline split
  b. Le Fort III with midline split + fracture of roof of orbit or frontal bone.

CLINICAL FINDINGS (Tables 52.1 and 52.2)

CLINICAL EXAMINATION OF MAXILLA

Maxillary fractures are examined for the site and level of mobility to distinguish between the Le Fort I, II and III fractures.

Step 1: Left palm is placed over the forehead, with the thumb over the right frontozygomatic junction, index finger over left frontozygomatic junction (Fig. 52.4A and B)

Step 2: The maxilla is grasped firmly with the right hand at the anterior portion of alveolus and not the teeth. The mobility of maxilla is checked at frontozygomatic (FZ) junction bilaterally (Fig. 52.4C and D)

TABLE 52.1 Comparison of Site of Mobility Evident in Different Fracture Levels

	Frontonasal Junction	Infraorbital Rim	Frontozygomatic Junction
Le Fort I	–	–	–
Le Fort II	+	+	–
Le Fort III	+	+	+

TABLE 52.2 Significant Clinical Features of Maxillary Fractures (Fig. 52.5)

Le Fort I Fracture	Le Fort II Fracture	Le Fort III Fracture
• Facial oedema • Ecchymosis of maxillary buccal sulcus • *Floating maxilla* • Malocclusion • Anterior open bite • *Posterior gagging of occlusion* • *Guerin sign* • Palatal fracture • *'Cracked-pot sound'* on percussion of the maxillary teeth	• Oedema of midface: *Moon-face appearance* • Depressed bridge of the nose—flat face • Raccoon eyes (bilateral circumorbital oedema) • Subconjunctival ecchymosis • *Infraorbital step deformity* • *Hypoesthesia of the cheek* • *CSF rhinorrhoea* • Epistaxis • Diplopia • *Mobility of midface detectable at nasal bridge and infraorbital margins* • Posterior gagging of occlusion • Midline or paramedian split of the palate • 'Cracked-pot' sound on tapping teeth	• Craniofacial dysjunction • *Panda face*—gross oedema of the face • *Dish-face deformity* • *Lengthening of the face* • Telecanthus • *Hooding of the eyes* • Antimongoloid slant • Enophthalmos • CSF leak • Posterior nasal bleed • Saddle nose deformity • *Mobility at the frontozygomatic suture* • *Fracture of zygomatic arch* • Posterior gagging of teeth with anterior open bite

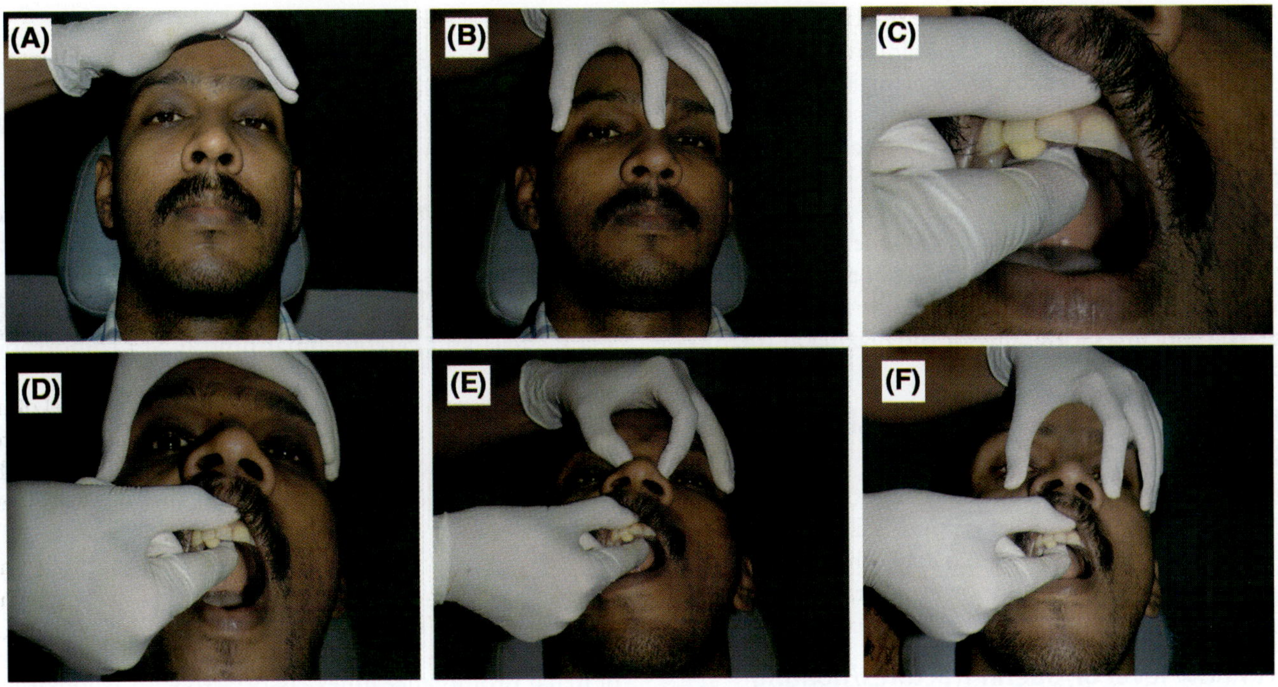

Figure 52.4 (**A–F**) Clinical examination of mobility of the maxilla at different levels.

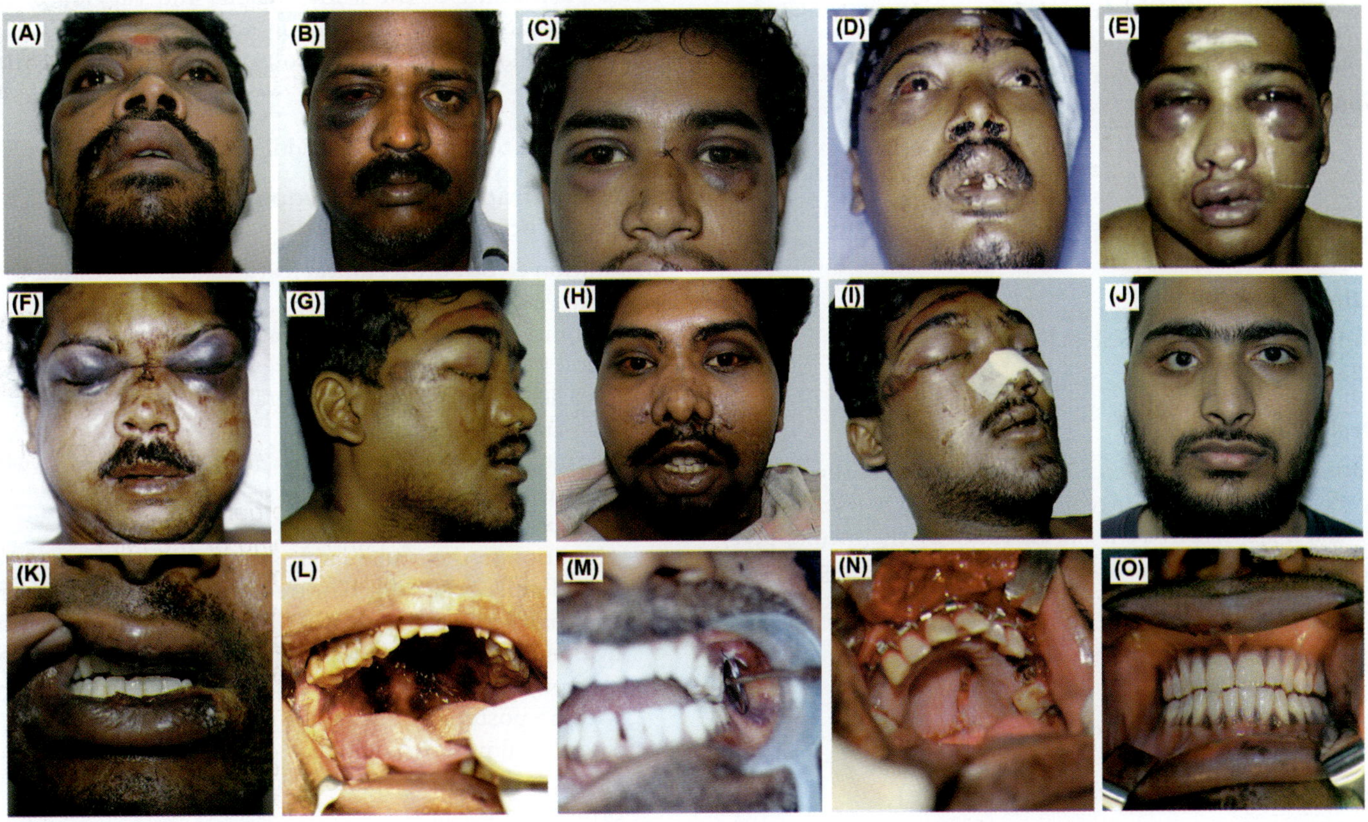

Figure 52.5 Clinical pictures of Le Fort fractures. (**A**) Swelling of upper lip—Le Fort I fracture. (**B**) Swelling over the right side of face. (**C**) Subconjunctival ecchymosis. (**D**) Nasal block. (**E**) Epistaxis. (**F**) Raccoons eye. (**G**) Dish-face deformity. (**H**) Depressed bridge of the nose. (**I**) CSF rhinorrhoea. (**J**) Enophthalmos. (**K**) Anterior open bite. (**L**) Palatal ecchymosis. (**M**) Buccal ecchymosis. (**N**) Palatal fracture. (**O**) Mild derangement in occlusion—Le Fort I fracture.

Step 3: The left thumb is placed over the frontonasal junction while the palm stabilises the cranium at the forehead and mobility of the maxillary segment is checked at the frontonasal junction. (Fig. 52.4E)

Step 4: The mobility of the maxillary segment is checked for at the frontonasal junction (Fig. 52.4E)

Step 5: Place two fingers of left hand one on each infraorbital rim, with the palm stabilising the cranium at the forehead and the concurrent mobility of the maxilla at the infraorbital rims is checked. (Fig. 52.4F)

Step 6: The concurrent mobility of the maxilla at the infraorbital rims is checked (Fig. 52.4F).

CLINICAL FINDINGS OF LE FORT I, II AND III FRACTURES

Swelling or gross oedema of the face, ecchymosis, nasal deformity, bleeding from the nose or nasal block, dish face deformity, retro positioning of maxilla with gagging on the posterior teeth, mobility of upper jaw and cracked-pot sound on the teeth are common to all levels of maxillary fractures.

Le Fort I (low level or Guerin fractures/floating maxilla)

Floating maxilla

Mobility of the dentulous segment of the maxilla. Palpation reveals tenderness and step deformity along the pyriform aperture, buccal sulcus and tuberosity regions.

Guerin sign

It is ecchymosis around the greater palatine foramen. It occurs due to fractures involving the palatine bone and dysjunction or fracture of pterygoid plate. It is a classic finding of Le Fort I fracture.

Palatal fracture

Midpalatal split is evident as linear mucosal tear in the midpalate region.

Occlusion

Undisplaced incomplete Le Fort I fractures usually cause no occlusal disturbance. In complete Le Fort I fractures, the *maxilla is pulled downward and backward* by the medial pterygoid muscle, along an inclined plane resulting in gagging of posterior teeth and anterior open bite. This posterior gagging of occlusion is a potential threat to airway.

Cracked-pot sound

It is heard on percussion of the maxillary teeth.

Le Fort II fractures (pyramidal fracture)

Mobility of maxilla

When maxillary alveolus is grasped anteriorly, the midfacial skeleton moves at the infraorbital margin and the nasal bridge.

Swelling

Bilateral periorbital oedema and circumorbital ecchymosis are described as **raccoon eyes or panda facies**. Gross and severe oedema of the middle 3rd of face is described as **'moon facies'**.

Subcutaneous emphysema

It is evident as crepitations on palpation of the swelling. It is due to the direct communication between the sinus cavities and the soft tissues of face.

Epistaxis and cerebrospinal fluid (CSF) rhinorrhoea are common.

Enophthalmos

Posterior displacement of the eyeball with limitation in ocular mobility can occur, as the fracture line involves the floor of the orbit.

Step deformity

Step deformity can be felt at the infraorbital rims or nasofrontal junction. Zygoma and its arch are intact and no loss of malar prominence unless associated with zygomaticomaxillary complex fractures.

Dish-face deformity

Retro-positioning of the whole maxilla and gagging of the occlusion can be seen creating an anterior open bite. This loss of maxillary prominence results in **dish-face deformity**.

Lengthening of face

It occurs due to separation of middle 3rd from the skull base.

Le Fort III fractures (suprazygomatic fracture or craniofacial dysjunction)

In addition to Le Fort II clinical features, it is associated with the following features:

- Mobility of the entire midfacial skeleton as a single unit felt at both the frontozygomatic region and nasal bridge. Step deformity palpable at lateral orbital rims, zygomatic arch and nasal bridge
- Characteristic raccoon eyes, *'dish-face'* deformity with lengthening of the face can be seen
- ***Hooding of eyes***
  Alteration in the ocular level as a result of the fracture of lateral wall of the orbit. The fracture line passes above the Whitnall's tubercle causing damage to the suspensory ligament of Lockwood that supports the globe of the eye
- Subconjunctival haemorrhage involving the entire eye with no posterior limit can be noticed
- Enophthalmos, hypoglobus, diplopia and telecanthus can occur due to fractures involving the medial wall and orbital floor
- ***Antimongoloid slant***
  The lateral palpebral ligament is attached to the zygomatic portion of the orbital rim. Inferior displacement of zygoma depresses the lateral palpebral ligament also,

causing a downward slope of the fissure (antimongoloid slant)
- *CSF rhinorrhoea* and CSF otorrhoea in associated skull base fractures
- Decreased mouth opening from zygomatic arch fractures
- Occlusion—deranged with severe anterior open bite, class III malocclusion, commonly associated with teeth or dentoalveolar fractures.

RADIOGRAPHIC INVESTIGATIONS

Plain radiographs include the Waters view (occipitomental view), a Caldwell view (PA view) and occasionally a Submentovertex view. Among the plain radiographs, occipitomental view provides a detailed evaluation of the facial skeleton.

McGregor and Campbell's line (1950)

They described a system for examining the occipitomental X-ray using four lines (Fig. 52.6A and B). These lines act as anatomical references to assess the facial bone injuries and also reduces the chance of failing to detect the fracture.

1. 1st line runs across the zygomaticofrontal sutures, the superior margin of the orbit and the frontal sinus
2. 2nd line passes through the zygomatic arch, zygomatic body, inferior orbital margin and nasal bone
3. 3rd line across the condyles, coronoid process and the maxillary sinus
4. 4th line across the mandibular ramus, occlusal plane
5. 5th line ***(Trapnell's line)*** across the inferior border of the mandible from angle to angle.

Dolan and Jacoby described three lines in occipitomental view, which can be used as an adjunct to Campbell's line (Fig. 52.6C).

1. The *orbital line*—It runs along the inner margins of the lateral, inferior and medial walls of the orbit, passing over the nasal arch to the opposite side
2. The *zygomatic line*—It runs along the superior margin of the zygomatic body and arch, lateral margin of the frontal process of zygoma, to the zygomaticofrontal suture
3. The *maxillary line*—It runs along the inferior margin of the zygomatic arch, inferior margin of the zygomatic body and buttress to the lateral wall of the maxillary sinus.

Computed tomography

Computed tomography (CT) scans can identify fractures that are difficult to identify in plain radiographs, and in addition, it accurately displays and localises the displaced bone fragments.

MANAGEMENT OF LE FORT FRACTURES

GENERAL PRINCIPLES

The aims of the treatment are as follows:

- Reconstruction of normal skeletal architecture and preservation of functions of the vital structures
- Re-establishing dental occlusion is the primary concern. The two areas of reference for reconstruction are cranium and dental occlusion
- To achieve adequate reduction followed by an adequate period of fixation to ensure stable union.

TIMING OF THE SURGERY

The timing of surgery is controversial. Immediate repair is recommended by a few authors for a stable patient. Generally, the fracture repair can be delayed for 7–14 days allowing oedema to subside for adequate manipulation of bones and soft tissues. Delaying surgery beyond 2 weeks is not encouraged due to the risk of fibrosis at the fracture site and subsequent difficulty to operate. Moreover, the results of delayed surgeries are not satisfactory, but if the patient is haemodynamically unstable, the time of surgery is delayed.

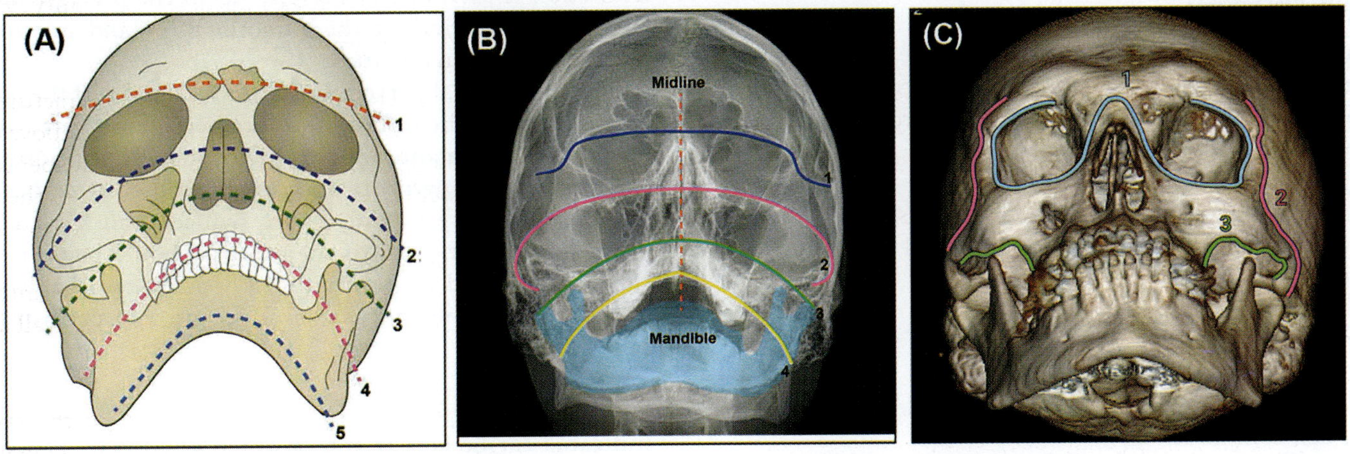

Figure 52.6 (**A** and **B**) McGregor and Campbell lines (1–4), Trapnell's line (5). (**C**) Dolan's line (1–3).

PROBLEMS ASSOCIATED WITH TREATMENT OF MIDDLE-3rd FRACTURE

1. Airway maintenance

The reduction of fractures of the middle 3rd requires general anaesthesia(GA), which can be administered through nasal intubation (Le Fort I), submental or tracheostomy (Le Fort II and III). Oral intubation can be indicated when there is extensive soft tissue injury to the nose and in emergency securing of airway.

2. Complexity of fractures

Le Fort fractures often does not present as a single-bone fracture. They present as a complex of fractures resulting in extremely complicated injury. Though occlusion is the main guide for reduction, establishment of occlusion provides only a relative position of mandible to maxilla. Hence it is necessary to achieve the vertical and transverse dimensions of the midface (facial form) by restoring the facial width, projection and height.

3. Associated facial bone fractures

Le Fort fractures not only involve the maxilla but also include fractures of the zygoma, orbit, frontal, nasal bone, and mandibular bones. The reorganisation of these multiple fragments into a skeletal framework is often a challenge to the surgeon. Generally, the outer framework is reconstructed 1st, followed by the central block (NOE) utilising the occlusion.

4. Fixation

Fixation requires an immobile point for support. As the lower jaw is movable, it is not possible to fix the fractured maxilla to the mandible. To avoid this, following accurate reduction of the lower jaw, the midface is fixed to a stable point, superior to the fracture (cranium) (e.g., circumzygomatic suspension for Le Fort I, where the zygoma is used as a stable bone).

SURGICAL APPROACHES FOR OPEN REDUCTION AND FIXATION

Various surgical approaches are available for the management of the maxillary fracture. The choice of approach depends on the site and extent of the fracture (Table 52.3).

TABLE 52.3 Surgical Approaches to the Midface and Upper Face Fractures

Incision/Approach	Indication/Fracture Location
Transoral/Intraoral approach • (Vestibular sulcus incision) • Midface degloving procedure	• Le Fort I, II, III fracture, Zygomatic buttress, nasal floor and septum • Le Fort I, II, III
Transcutaneous approach	
• Infraorbital, subciliary, subtarsal	• Orbital floor, medial and lateral wall fractures
• Lateral eyebrow incision	• Lateral orbital rim, FZ suture
• Glabella incision	• Frontal sinus and superior orbital walls, NOE region
• Coronal incision	• Frontal bone, nasal and NOE region
Transconjunctival incision	Orbital floor, medial and lateral orbital wall
Intranasal approach	Nasal septum and cartilage
Endoscopic approach	Maxillary sinus, frontal sinus, nasal bone, orbital floor

MAXILLARY VESTIBULAR APPROACH

It provides access to the entire midface skeleton from the zygomatic arch to the infraorbital rim and frontal process of the maxilla.

Advantages

- Hidden intraoral scar
- Procedure is relatively rapid and simple
- Few complications
- No nerve damage.

Technique

The incision is made approximately 3–5 mm above the mucogingival junction, leaving an unattached mucosa to facilitate closure. The length of incision depends on the area of interest and the extent of the surgical intervention. Posteriorly, the incision extends up to the 1st molar traversing the mucosa, fascial muscles and periosteum. Using periosteal elevators, the tissues are elevated in a subperiosteal plane. Dissection is extended posteriorly up to the pterygomaxillary fissure, superiorly to the infraorbital rim and anteriorly along the pyriform aperture.

The infraorbital nerve should be identified and the periosteum around the infraorbital foramen is completely dissected. The entire anterior part of the maxilla, infraorbital rim, zygoma and pyriform aperture is exposed after dissection. The fracture fragments are reduced and fixed with miniplates. The closure of the mucosa should begin from the posterior and proceed anteriorly using resorbable sutures through the mucosa, muscle and the periosteum (Fig. 52.7).

MIDFACE DEGLOVING INCISION

Indicated for Le Fort II and III fractures. It was popularised by Maniglia. The technique involves a wide maxillary

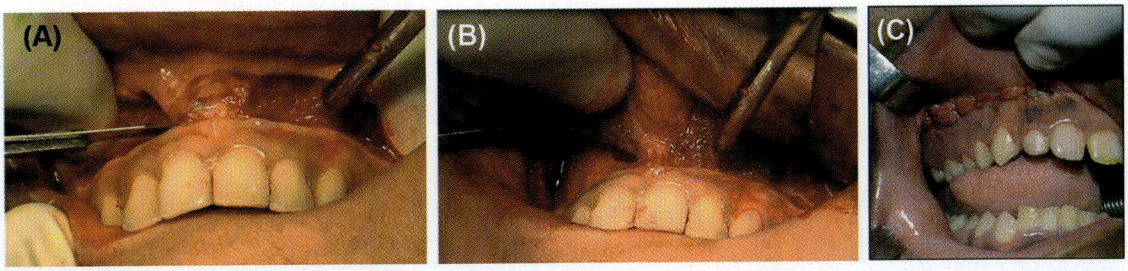

Figure 52.7 Maxillary vestibular approach. (**A**) Incision through the mucosa, facial muscles and periosteum. (**B**) Subperiosteal dissection of the anterior maxilla. (**C**) Closure of the incision.

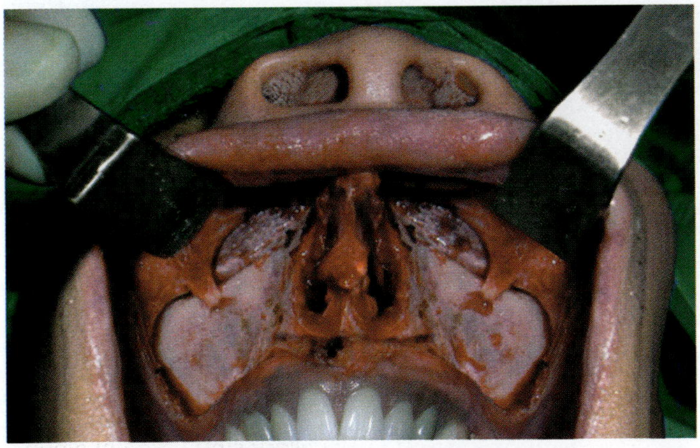

Figure 52.8 Midface degloving.

vestibular incision in combination with the release of soft tissue envelop around the pyriform margin and nasal skeleton. This approach allows access to the anterior surface of the maxilla, infraorbital rims, zygoma and the entire nasal skeleton (Fig. 52.8). This technique in combination with bicoronal approach favours exposing the whole facial skeleton.

REDUCTION OF MAXILLARY FRACTURES

Adequate and proper reduction of the maxillary fracture is required to achieve good dental occlusion. The fractured maxilla is usually displaced backwards and downwards; hence, the reduction should be done in a forward and upward direction. Reduction of the maxilla can be done using *Rowe's disimpaction and Hayton Williams's forceps* (Fig. 52.9). The disimpaction forceps aid in mobilising and freeing the maxilla completely by overcoming any bony interferences.

Rowe's disimpaction forceps are paired forceps with padded and unpadded blade. The unpadded blade is inserted into the nostril and the padded blade into the mouth and grips the palate. The surgeon should stand at the head of the operating table, grasping the handles of forceps and manipulation of the fragment is done. The manipulation should be deliberately rocking and rotating movements in sagittal and transverse planes. Once the fragment is mobile, forward traction is applied to correct any inferior displacement of the maxilla and also relieves 'gagging' of the posterior teeth. With this forceps, care is taken to avoid injury to the anterior teeth and palatal mucosa. Sometimes a combination of reduction with disimpaction forceps and direct manipulation at the fracture site might be required to achieve the dental occlusion.

In cases with palatal split, *Hayton Williams's forceps* can be used to apply traction from the buccal aspect of the alveolar process and cause medial compression till the two halves of the palate are approximated.

FIXATION OF MAXILLARY FRACTURES

Once adequate reduction of the fractured maxilla is obtained, it is necessary to do mandibulo-maxillary fixation (MMF) using arch bars or MMF screws, before proceeding to rigid internal fixation. The fixation methods can be broadly classified into two categories: Internal and External fixation (Table 52.4).

A. INTERNAL FIXATION (Fig. 52.10A–E)

Transosseous wiring

It is the direct wiring across the fracture line using a 26-gauge stainless steel wire that provides semirigid fixation.

Disadvantages:

- It does not prevent interfragmentary motion across the fracture
- Lack of adequate stabilisation impairs the normal healing process and may result in complications.

Miniplates and screws

They can be used effectively in a number of sites and produce more rapid immobilisation than the wiring techniques.

Advantages:

- Provides stable and anatomical reconstruction of the midface
- Avoids long period of IMF
- Allows early mobilisation
- Low risk of infection

Disadvantages:

- Cost of implant
- Implant removal
- Difficult surgical technique

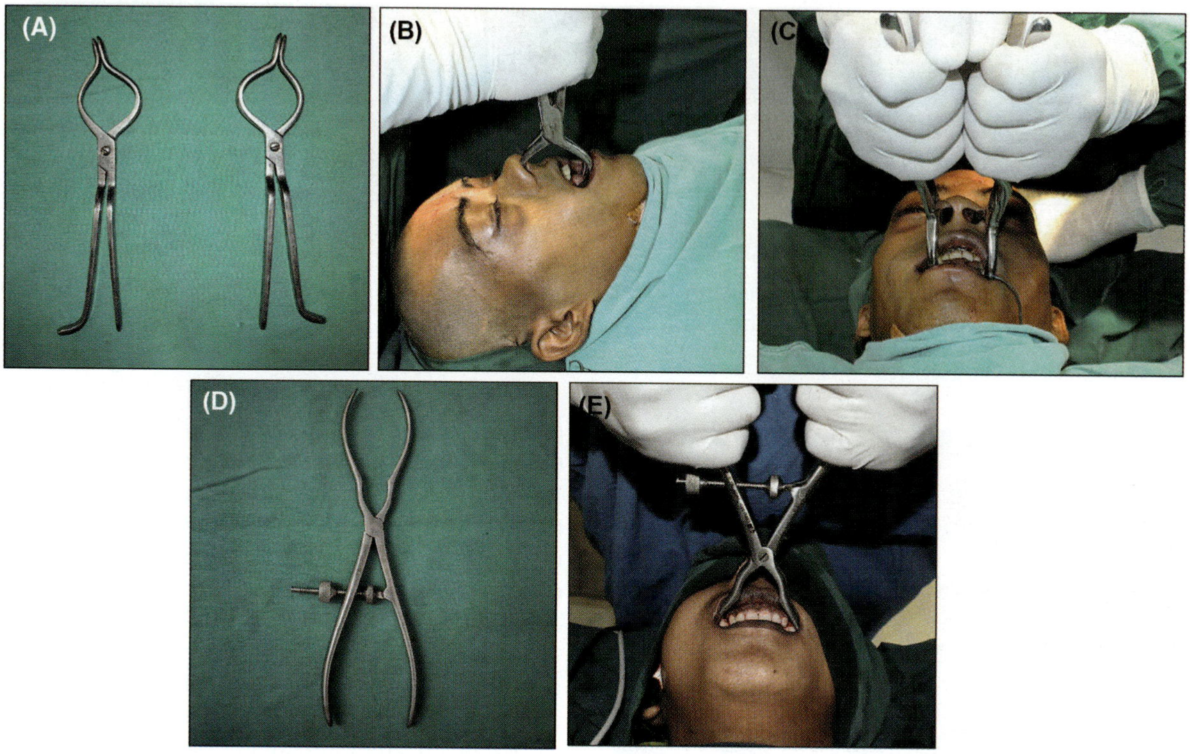

Figure 52.9 (**A**) Rowe's maxillary disimpaction forceps. (**B** and **C**) Closed reduction of the maxilla using Rowe's disimpaction forceps. (**D** and **E**) Hayton William's forceps.

TABLE 52.4 Methods of Maxillary Fracture Fixation/Immobilisation

A. ***Internal fixation*** (immobilisation within the tissues)
   1. **Direct osteosynthesis**
      a. Transosseous wiring
      b. Miniplates and screws
      c. Transfixation with Kirschner wire or Steinmann pins
   2. **Suspension wires**
      a. Frontal—central or lateral
      b. Circum-zygomatic
      c. Zygomatic
      d. Infraorbital
      e. Pyriform aperture
   3. **Support**
      a. Antral pack
      b. Antral balloon

B. ***External fixation*** (extraoral immobilisation)
   1. **Craniomandibular**
      a. Box-frame
      b. Halo-frame
      c. Plaster of Paris head cap
   2. **Craniomaxillary**
      a. Supraorbital pins
      b. Zygomatic pins
      c. Halo-frame

3. Transfixation with Kirschner wire or Steinmann pins

It is a less precise method of fixation where a Kirschner wire or Steinmann pin was passed externally from one zygoma to the other, transfixing the reduced fracture fragments. This method is largely outdated due to its inherent instability.

4. Suspension wires

It is sandwiching of the fractured midface between the mandible and the stable portion of the facial skeleton using wires. These wires are passed through the tissues with the aid of long curved needles, awls, or cannulae. The suspension wires were not able to produce rigid fixation as there were some anteroposterior movements of the fragments. The suspension wires are rarely used now and are indicated only for uncomplicated fractures or extremely communicated fractures in medically compromised patients.

5. Support

It is achieved by packing the maxillary sinus, or filling it with an inflatable balloon, which is not in use nowadays.

B. EXTERNAL FIXATION (Fig. 52.10F and G)

The mandible is fixed by a system of rods and universal joints to the cranial vault and the mobile middle 3rd is 'sandwiched' in between them. The facial frame acts as a scaffold which is suspended in front of the injured face. This rigid apparatus produces an accurate reduction and a firm

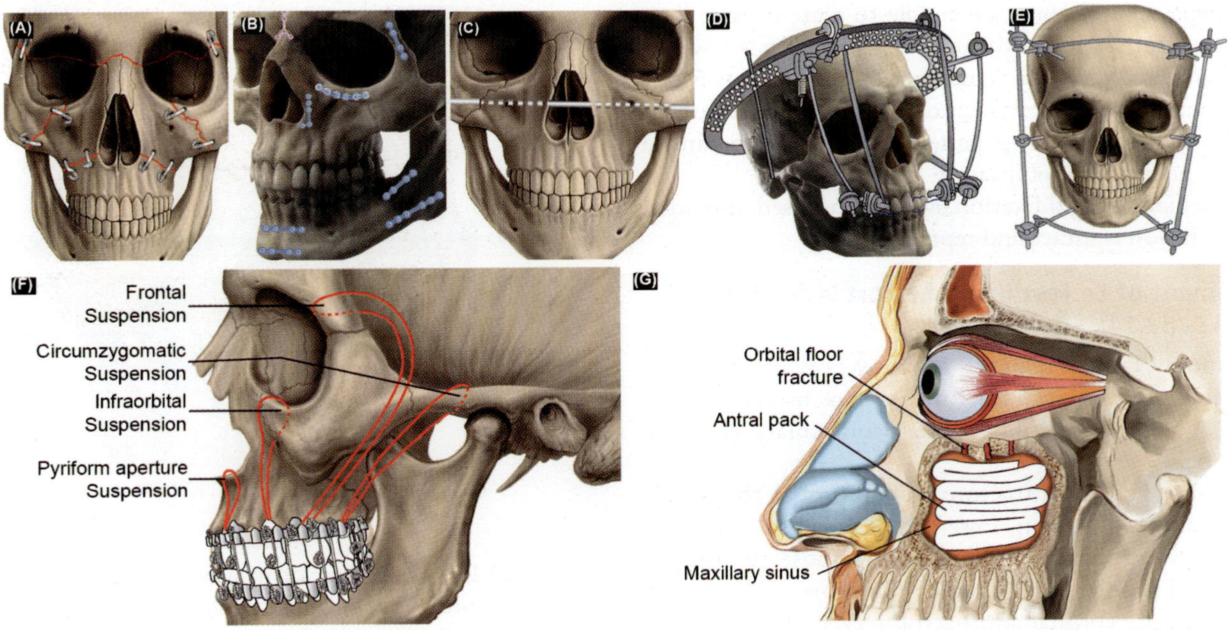

Figure 52.10 (**A**) Transosseous wiring. (**B**) Miniplates and screws. (**C**) Transfixation with Kirschner wire. (**D**) Suspension wires. (**E**) Maxilla sinus pack. (**F and G**) External fixation.

immobilisation of the numerous bony fragments. External fixation is rarely used today due to its large framework and patient compliance.

Management of Le Fort I fracture

- Early reduction and fixation within 7–10 days is preferable
- *Arch bars* are placed 1st in the maxilla and mandible. The fractured fragments are accessed through maxillary vestibular incision
- The maxilla is *reduced* using Rowe's disimpaction and Hayton Williams's forceps (Fig. 52.11)
- In difficult cases, such as impacted or incomplete maxillary fractures, reduction can be achieved by direct manipulation or byre-osteotomising the maxilla at the Le Fort I level
- After reduction of maxilla, *MMF* is established with the condyles seated in correct position; otherwise open bite might re-emerge after rigid fixation
- In case of *palatal fracture* without concurrent mandible fracture, the mandibular arch can be used to guide the width of the maxilla with arch bars and MMF
- In Le Fort fractures concurrent with *palatal and mandible fracture*, two options exist: (1) the mandible can be reconstructed 1st, followed by maxilla or (2) using maxillary splints prepared from model surgery to re-establish the occlusion
- Any deviated nasal septum is reduced into the nasal crest and secured to the anterior nasal spine through sutures
- For *uncomplicated Le Fort I fractures, fixation* with miniplates (1.5 or 2.0 mm plate) at pyriform rims and zygomatic buttresses is usually sufficient for stabilisation
- In case of more comminution and less bone contact between the fracture fragments, bone grafts should be considered

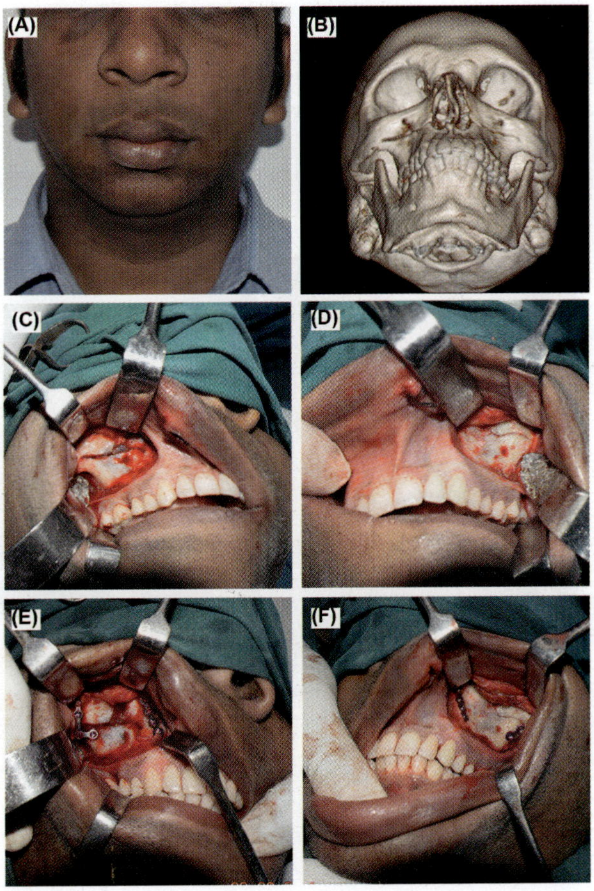

Figure 52.11 Case Report I—Management of Le Fort I fracture. (**A**) Preoperative view. (**B**) Preoperative CT showing Le Fort I fracture. (**C and D**) Intraoperative pictures exposing the fractured maxilla through maxillary vestibular incision. (**E and F**) The maxilla was reduced and fixed bilaterally with miniplates.

- *Comminuted fractures* not amenable to plate or wire fixation are treated with MMF and suspension for 4–6 weeks
- In *edentulous patient*, the same line of management is followed but if intraosseous fixation is not feasible, a custom acrylic occlusal splint or patient's own denture can be used to achieve immobilisation
- After achieving rigid fixation, MMF is released, provided the occlusion is intact and reproducible.

Management of Le Fort II and Le Fort III fracture
(Fig. 52.12– 52.14)

- Commonly, Le Fort II and III fractures present with combination of other facial fractures such as nasoorbitoethmoid, orbital floor and zygomaticomaxillary complex fractures
- *Access*—For Le Fort II fracture, in addition to the maxillary vestibular incision, lower eyelid incision and gull-wing incision might be required to expose the orbital floor and frontonasal junction. Le Fort III fractures might require coronal approach for FZ and frontonasal fixation in addition to intraoral and orbital incisions
- The *reduction* for Le Fort II and III fractures should be done in the same order as previously mentioned, either by using forceps or direct manipulation of fragments
- *Fixation*—Le Fort II fracture requires fixation at frontonasal suture region, bilateral infraorbital rims and also zygomaticomaxillary buttresses. However, in majority of the situations, fixation at the infraorbital rims and the zygomatic buttress is sufficient to achieve good results.

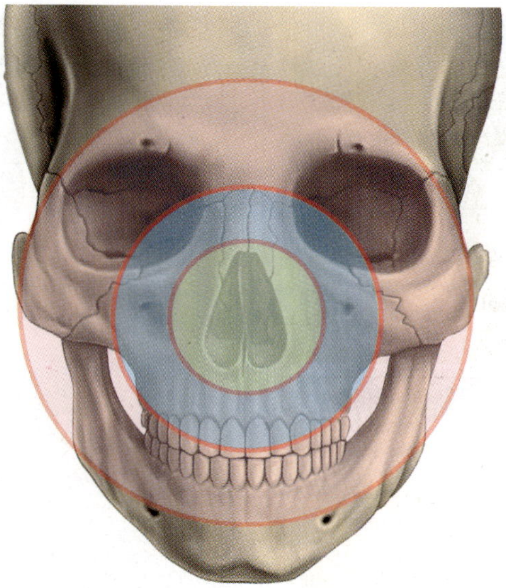

Figure 52.12 Sequencing of fixation for multiple fractures—from the outer circle (frontal, lateral orbital margin, zygoma), middle circle (maxilla) to the inner circle (nasal complex).

Most of the nasal fractures in Le Fort II fractures are managed by closed reduction

- Most often, Le Fort III fractures are a combination of bilateral zygomatic complex, nasal complex and Le Fort II fractures. Fixation of these complex fractures begins with the outer frame 1st to the central midface (orbital and nasal complex) (Fig. 52.12)

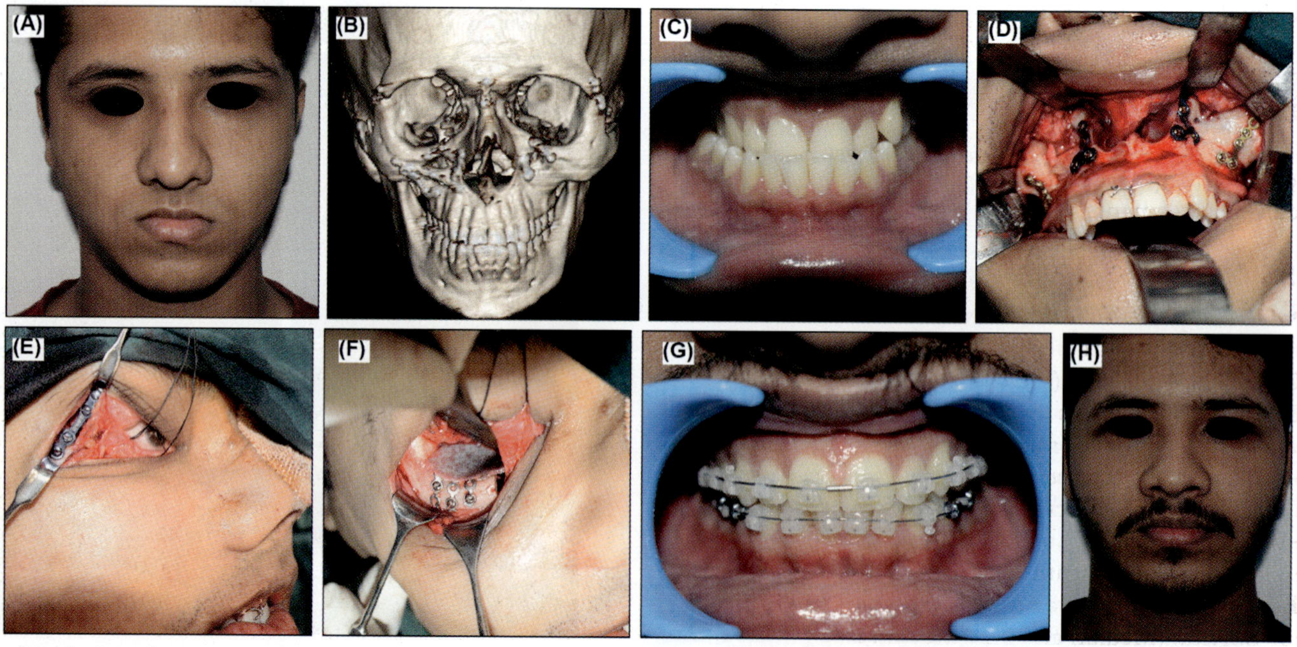

Figure 52.13 Case Report 2. Management of Le Fort III fracture. (**A**) Preoperative view with enophthalmos on the right eye. (**B**) Preoperative CT scan. (**C**) Intraoral view showing Class III malocclusion. (**D**) The fractured maxilla was reduced and fixed at the pyriform rim and zygomatic buttress. (**E**) Fixation at the FZ region. (**F**) Fixation at the orbital floor. (**G** and **H**) Postoperative view showing corrected enophthalmos and restored occlusion.

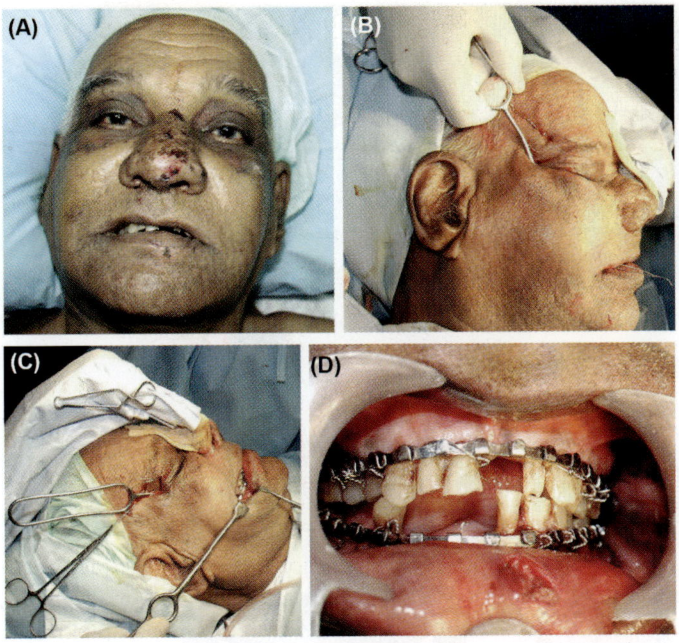

Figure 52.14 Case Report 3—Suspension wiring for aged patients. (**A**) Preoperative view. (**B**) Insertion of suspension wire at the FZ region. (**C**) Retrieval of suspension wire intraorally. (**D**) Suspension wire tied to the arch bar and MMF placed.

- Le Fort III fractures associated with other fractures (mandible) should be treated as panfacial fracture, following various sequences such as 'top-down' or 'bottom-up'
- The associated complications such as CSF rhinorrhoea, lacrimal obstruction require appropriate management.

PALATAL FRACTURES

Palatal fractures divide the alveolus sagittally or transversely and comminute the dentition, permitting rotation of the dentoalveolar segments.

HENDRICKSON CLASSIFICATION OF PALATAL FRACTURES (Fig. 52.15)

Type I: Alveolar fracture

I a: Anterior alveolus (incisor)

I b: Posterior alveolus (premolar, molar)

Type II: Sagittal fracture (midline split)

Type III: Para-sagittal fracture.

Type IV: Para-alveolar fracture.

Type V: Complex comminuted fracture.

Type VI: Transverse fracture.

Chen et al., classification (2008)

Type I—Sagittal (Median and Para median)

Type II—Transverse

Type III—Comminuted fractures.

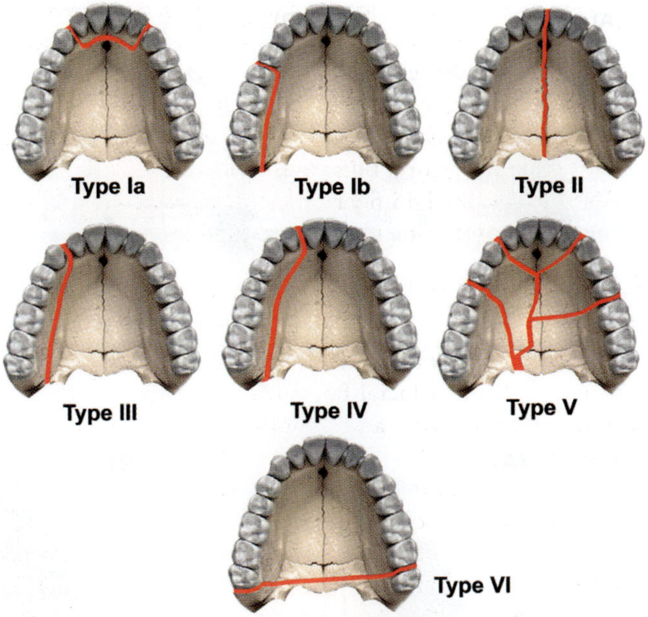

Figure 52.15 Hendrickson et al., classification of palatal fractures.

MANAGEMENT OF PALATAL FRACTURES

- Treatment of palatal fractures depends on the type of fracture, presence of dentition and associated facial fractures
- Previously, the palatal fractures were treated with closed reduction using splints. The dental segments were aligned with arch bar and wires and the reduction was stabilised with an acrylic splint. This technique was more cumbersome and less accurate
- For more accurate results and stability, open reduction and internal fixation (ORIF) were done. The problem with open reduction is the vascularity of maxilla. For a severely fractured maxilla, the blood flow is dependent on the ascending pharyngeal artery and palatal mucosa. Hence raising of a palatal flap should be done with caution
- Various options available for palatal fracture fixation include:
  a. Closed reduction (Fig. 52.16)
    - Transpalatal wires
    - Palatal splint secured with wires/arch bar
    - MMF with arch bars
  b. ORIF (Fig. 52.17)
    - Plating at palatal vault or anterior alveolar process
  c. External fixation (Fig. 52.18)
    - Locking plate
    - Transpalatal screw with wire
- In extremely comminuted palatal fractures, splints and IMF are recommended
- In edentulous patients with sagittal palatal fractures, who do not have the preexisting dentures, rigid fixation or splint is indicated.

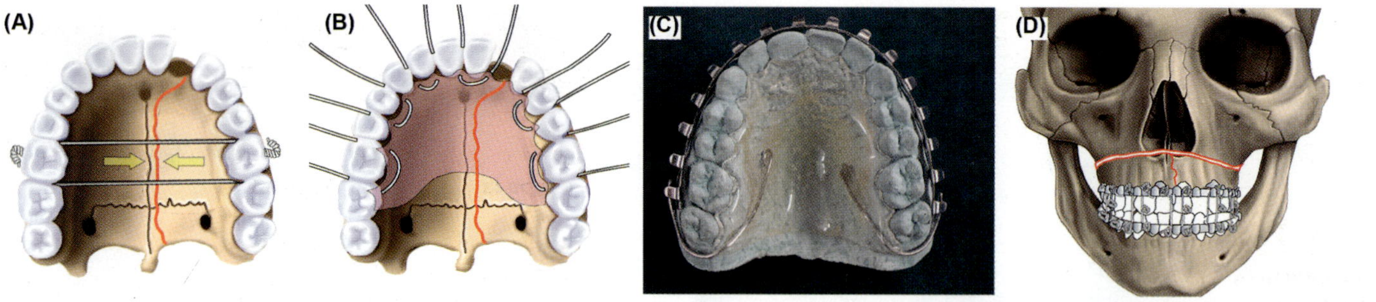

Figure 52.16 Treatment of palatal fracture. Closed reduction. (**A**) Transpalatal wiring. (**B**) Palatal splint with wires. (**C**) Palatal splint with arch bar. (**D**) MMF with arch bars.

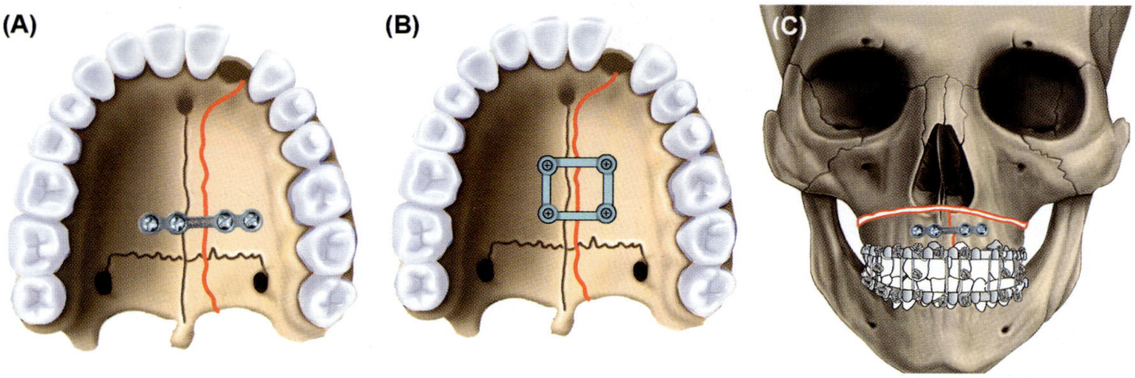

Figure 52.17 Open reduction and internal fixation. (**A** and **B**) Plating at the palatal vault. (**C**) Plating at the anterior alveolar process.

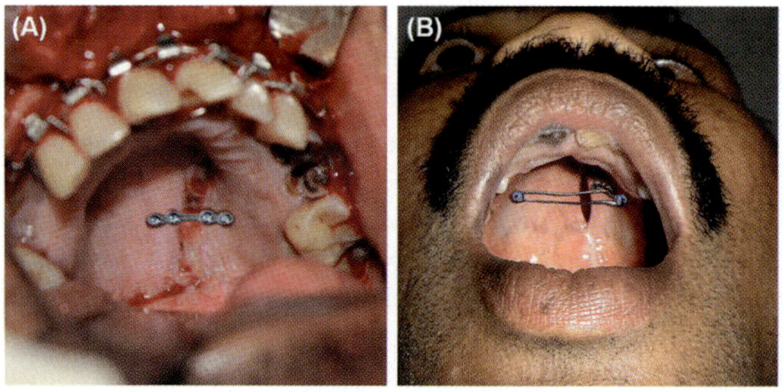

Figure 52.18 External fixation. (**A**) Locking plate fixation. (**B**) Transpalatal screw with wire.

COMPLICATIONS OF MAXILLARY FRACTURES

- Bleeding
- Enophthalmos
- Infection
- Diplopia
- Nonunion
- Mal-union
- Malocclusion
- Epiphora
- Scarring
- Sinusitis
- Foreign body reactions
- Maxillary hypoperfusion
- Wound dehiscence
- CSF leak
- Palatal fistula
- Nasal septal deviation
- Infraorbital paraesthesia
- Facial nerve paralysis

Chapter 53

Orbital Fractures

OUTLINE

INTRODUCTION

Orbital fractures are breaks in any of the bones surrounding the orbit/eye socket. Fractures involving the orbit are more common and are frequently associated with other injuries such as frontal sinus, naso-orbito-ethmoidal (NOE) complex, zygoma, Le Fort and skull fractures. Their proximity to the brain and eye, which could impede vision and/or globe position, necessitates meticulous consideration. Assaults, traffic collision, falls, sports, and industrial accidents are the most common causes of orbital injuries. Because of their complexity and proximity to vital structures, orbital fractures can provide challenge to surgeons.

ANATOMY

The orbit is a bony vault that protects the globe or eyeball.

The *bony orbit* is a quadrangular pyramid with a base and an apex. The *base* of the orbit that opens into the face has four borders (Fig. 53.1):

- **Roof**—It is formed by the frontal and the lesser wing of sphenoid bone
- **Floor**—It is formed by the maxilla, palatine and zygomatic bones
- **Medial wall**—It is formed by the maxilla, ethmoid, lacrimal and sphenoid bones
- **Lateral wall**—It is formed by the zygomatic and greater wing of sphenoid.

The *apex* contains the optic canal through which the bony orbit communicates with the middle cranial fossa.

Orbital cavities are symmetrical and comprise the eyes, ocular muscles, cranial nerves II, III, IV, V and VI, ciliary ganglion and short ciliary nerves, blood vessels, the lacrimal gland, palpebral and suspensory ligaments.

The **surface landmarks** in the orbital walls (Fig. 53.2) are:

Orbital floor—It is thin and shortest of all the walls, measuring 35–40 mm.

- *Infraorbital groove* that carries the infraorbital nerve and vessels
- At the posterior end is a raised plateau called the '*posterior medial bulge*', which acts as the limit of inferior dissection on the orbital floor

Medial wall of orbit—It has:

- *Lamina papyracea*—It is extremely thin (0.2–0.4 mm) and forms the largest section of the medial wall
- *Anterior and posterior ethmoidal foramen*
- *Lacrimal fossa or sac*—It is a concave depression on the lacrimal bone, housing the lacrimal sac and nasolacrimal duct (NLD)
- *Medial rectus muscle*

Lateral wall of orbit—strongest wall

- *Whitnall's tubercle*—It is a slight bony projection just behind (5 mm) the lateral orbital rim to which the lateral canthal tendon, inferior suspensory (Lockwood's) ligament and lateral rectus muscle are attached. Hence, it serves a critical role in the maintenance of eyelid contour
- *Zygomaticotemporal and Zygomaticofacial foramina*
- *Zygomatico-sphenoid suture and Fronto-sphenoid suture*

Orbital roof—It is a thin bone that separates the orbit from the anterior cranial fossa

- Laterally—lacrimal fossa
- Medially—trochlear fovea
- Supraorbital notch

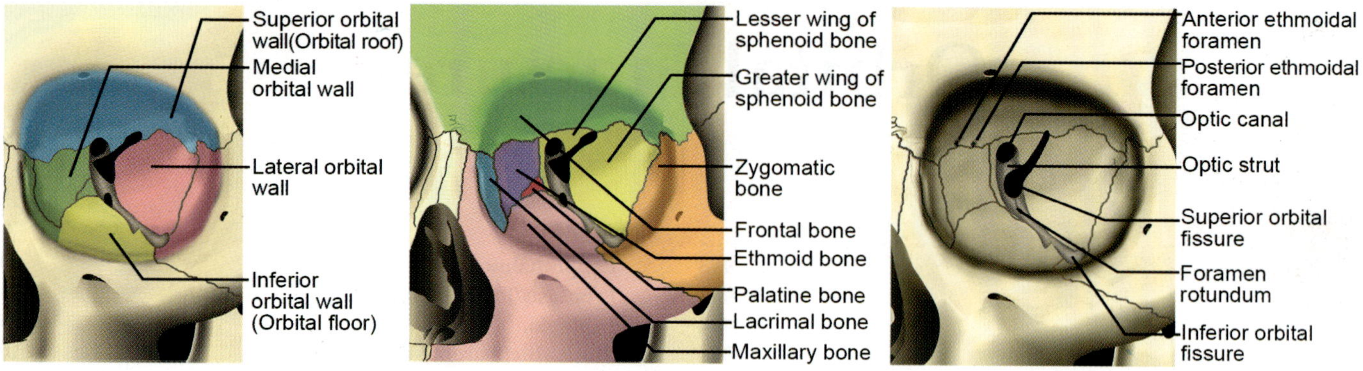

Figure 53.1 **(A)** Walls of the orbit. **(B)** Bones of the orbit. **(C)** Apex of the orbit.

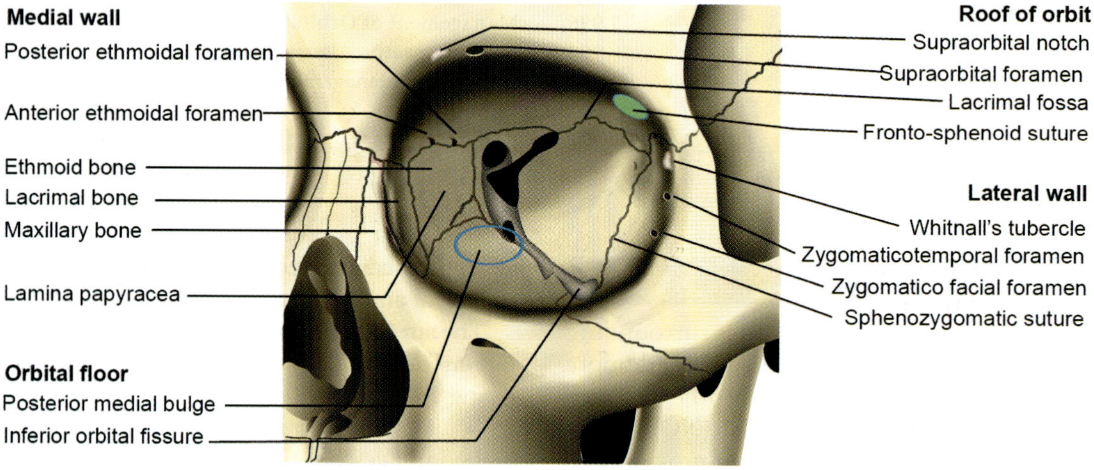

Figure 53.2 Surface landmarks of the orbital walls—orbital floor, medial wall, lateral wall and roof of the orbit.

FRACTURE PATTERNS

LINEAR FRACTURES

These are fractures where the periosteal attachment to the bone is maintained and does not result in a defect. Regardless, they have the potential to cause considerable enlargement of the orbit.

BLOWOUT AND BLOW-IN FRACTURES

It is a fracture that affects only one orbital wall. When an object strikes the eye, the force is transmitted into the orbital walls, causing the thinnest bones to break or buckle. This is referred as *'blowout'* fracture. Blowout fractures, which can be categorised as *'Pure'* or *'Impure'*, most commonly occur in the orbital floor. In pure blowout injury, the fracture involves only the orbital walls, leaving the orbital rim intact. The orbital rim and wall are both involved in an impure blowout.

BLOWOUT FRACTURES

Smith and Regan coined the term 'blowout fracture' in 1957. A blowout fracture involving the floor of orbit is often accompanied by displacement of the orbital contents (muscles, fat and connective tissue) into the maxillary sinus. The combined effects of displaced orbital tissues, increased orbital volume and fat necrosis result in enophthalmos (eyes sunken inside the orbit).

Children are more susceptible to a special type of fracture called *'trapdoor' or 'white-eye fracture'* due to the more elastic nature of the bones. During trauma, a hinged bone fragment is created that allows the soft tissues to evacuate from the orbit and then shut like a trapdoor. Because of the soft tissue entangled in the fracture segment, eye movements are severely constrained. This change in the motility of the eye/restriction of eye movements induces double vision.

The *mechanism* of blowout fracture has been explained by three theories (Fig. 53.3).

1. **The globe-to-orbital wall contact theory by Raymond Pfeiffer** (1943): A force delivered to the globe pushes it backward into the orbit, causing it to strike and fracture the bony walls. They stated that the 'displacement of the globe' directly causes fractures in the orbital walls
2. **Hydraulic theory or retropulsion theory or direct injury theory by Regan and Smith** (1957): Sudden compression and backward displacement of the globe

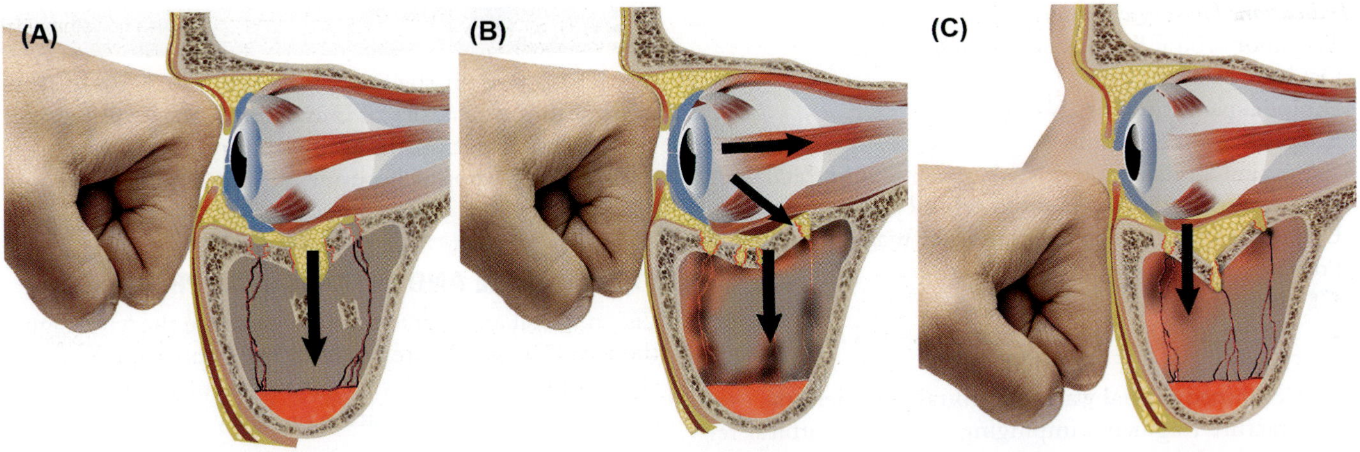

Figure 53.3 Mechanism of blowout fracture. (**A**) Globe to orbital wall contact. (**B**) Hydraulic theory. (**C**) Buckling theory.

raises the intraorbital pressure leading to fracture of the orbital floor, allowing the soft tissues of the floor to herniate into the maxillary sinus

3. **Buckling theory or transmission theory or indirect injury theory**: External force to inferior orbital rim is transmitted along the orbital walls causing a ripple effect, leading to fracture at the weakest point in the posteromedial region of the floor.

Clinical features

- Periorbital haematoma
- Subconjunctival ecchymosis
- Narrowing of palpebral fissure
- Step deformity of the orbital rim
- Diplopia
- Enophthalmos
- Restricted upward and downward movements of the eye
- Paraesthesia over the cheek.

Clinically significant enophthalmos (≥2 mm) occurs only when the bony orbital volume is increased by 1.5–2 mL.

Evaluation

- Visual acuity and pupillary response
- Ocular movements—Inferior rectus muscle entrapment
- Hertel exophthalmometer—Enophthalmos
- Forced duction test—Diplopia
- Muscle effort generation test—Diplopia.

Imaging

Plain X-rays—*Waters view and Lateral tomograms*—A polypoid mass (teardrop) protruding from the orbital floor into the maxillary antrum is a characteristic radiographic finding in blowout fractures of the orbital floor. This teardrop, often known as the *'hanging drop' sign/trapdoor entrapment*, exhibits herniated orbital contents, periorbital fat and inferior rectus muscle.

CT scans—They are the most accurate diagnostic aid in assessing the bony defect and also in measuring the orbital volume. Muscle entrapment in the fracture area and extensive prolapse of orbital adipose tissue into the maxillary sinus are two prominent CT signs of orbital floor fracture (Fig. 53.4).

Management of blowout fracture

A simple fracture with minimal or no double vision and no loss of orbital volume without affecting the function or aesthetics can be monitored and does not require surgical intervention. All other cases are managed surgically.

Immediate treatment involves:

- Ice pack
- Decongestants
- Avoidance of nose blowing
- Oral steroids.

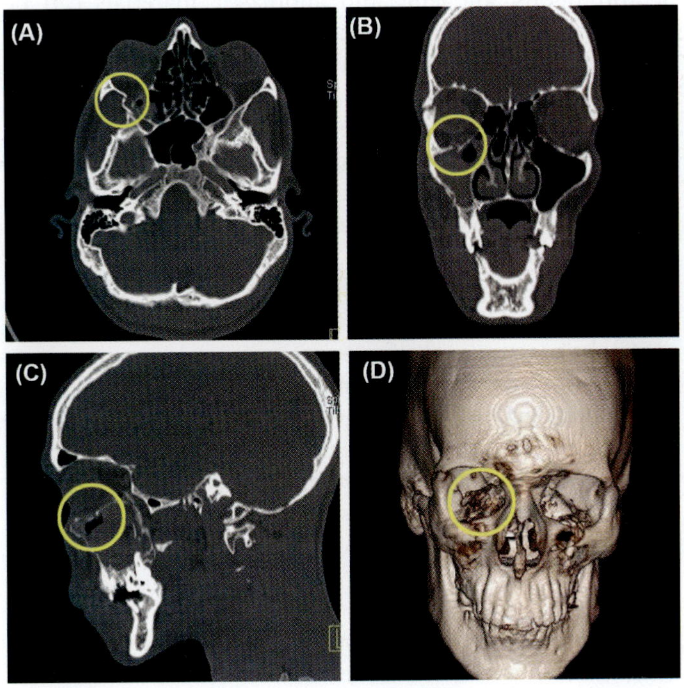

Figure 53.4 (A-D) CT pictures of orbital floor fracture.

***Indications for surgical intervention*:**
- Trapdoor orbital floor fracture in children
- Oculocardiac reflex
- Diplopia persisting for 2 weeks
- Enophthalmos (>2 mm)
- The orbital floor defect is more than half of the orbital floor
- Comminution/displacement in orbital floor or rim
- Displacement of orbital contents into maxillary sinus
- Positive forced duction test.
- **CT evidence of:**
  - Defects greater than 2 × 2 cm in orbital floor
  - Defects >50% of the orbital floor
  - Combined medial wall and orbital floor defects
  - Fracture fragments impinging on the periorbital region or globe
  - Increase in orbital volume of >10% (2.5 mL).

Timing of intervention/repair

Early intervention—The surgery should be performed in the acute phase of trauma (within the 1st 14 days).

Delayed surgery—A surgery performed between 3 weeks and 4 months after the trauma, the so-called grey period.

Late intervention—An intervention performed 4 and more months after the trauma.

Surgical management

The surgical approaches to the orbit include subciliary, transconjunctival, transantral and endoscopic approach. The primary objective of orbital reconstruction in blowout fractures is to restore the orbital walls, replace the prolapsed orbital contents to their appropriate position, and to eradicate any impinged or entrapped orbital soft tissues. A variety of autologous, allogenic and alloplastic materials can be used to reconstruct the orbital floor (discussed in materials used for orbital reconstruction in Table 53.2).

BLOW-IN FRACTURES

A blow-in fracture is an inwardly displaced fracture of the orbital rim or wall resulting in decreased orbital volume. These kinds of fractures are scarce. The most common clinical findings include:
- Proptosis—caused by decrease in orbital volume, restricted ocular motility and diplopia
- Globe rupture
- Superior orbital fissure syndrome
- Orbital nerve injury.

If the fractured segment is not significantly displaced, it does not require any treatment; nevertheless, fractures of the lateral orbital wall, regardless of the direction of displacement, necessitate surgery.

COMPLEX FRACTURES

These are extensive fractures affecting two or more orbital walls and are usually associated with other fractures such as zygoma, frontal sinus and Le Fort.

CLINICAL EXAMINATION

A brief history on the mechanism of injury, the direction of force and the nature of injury should be acquired before clinical examination. If needed, examination by an ophthalmologist should be done to rule out ocular injuries (Table 53.1).

VISION, PUPIL AND INTRAOCULAR PRESSURE

Vision, pupil and intraocular pressure are the 'vital signs' of the eye. The pupils are assessed for pupillary reflexes, size, shape and symmetry. An irregular pupil often points towards the site of a globe penetration or injury.

EXTRAOCULAR EYE MOVEMENTS

The movements of eyeball are controlled by the extraocular muscles. The eye movements are examined in different directions. Any restriction in the gaze aids in identifying the muscle involved. A forced duction test can be performed to identify the muscle entrapment.

ALTERATION OF GLOBE LEVEL

Fracture of the lateral orbital rim at the Whitnall's tubercle area results in alteration of the globe level.

DISPLACEMENT OF PALPEBRAL FISSURE

The lateral canthal ligament is attached to the Whitnall's tubercle, hence displacement of the lateral wall of orbit displaces the palpebral fissure along with it, culminating in an antimongoloid slant.

TABLE 53.1 Orbital/Ocular Injuries (Fig. 53.5)

Orbital Wall/ Bony Injuries	Ocular Injuries
• Circumorbital oedema and ecchymosis • Laceration • Step deformity • Mobility of fragment • Paraesthesia • Subconjunctival haemorrhage • CSF leak • Malar flattening	• Vision • Pupillary size, shape and symmetry • Diplopia • Extraocular eye movements • Alteration of globe level • Displacement of palpebral fissure • Retrobulbar haemorrhage • Enophthalmos • Exophthalmos/Proptosis • Ptosis • Traumatic optic neuropathy (TON) • Superior orbital fissure syndrome • Orbital apex syndrome

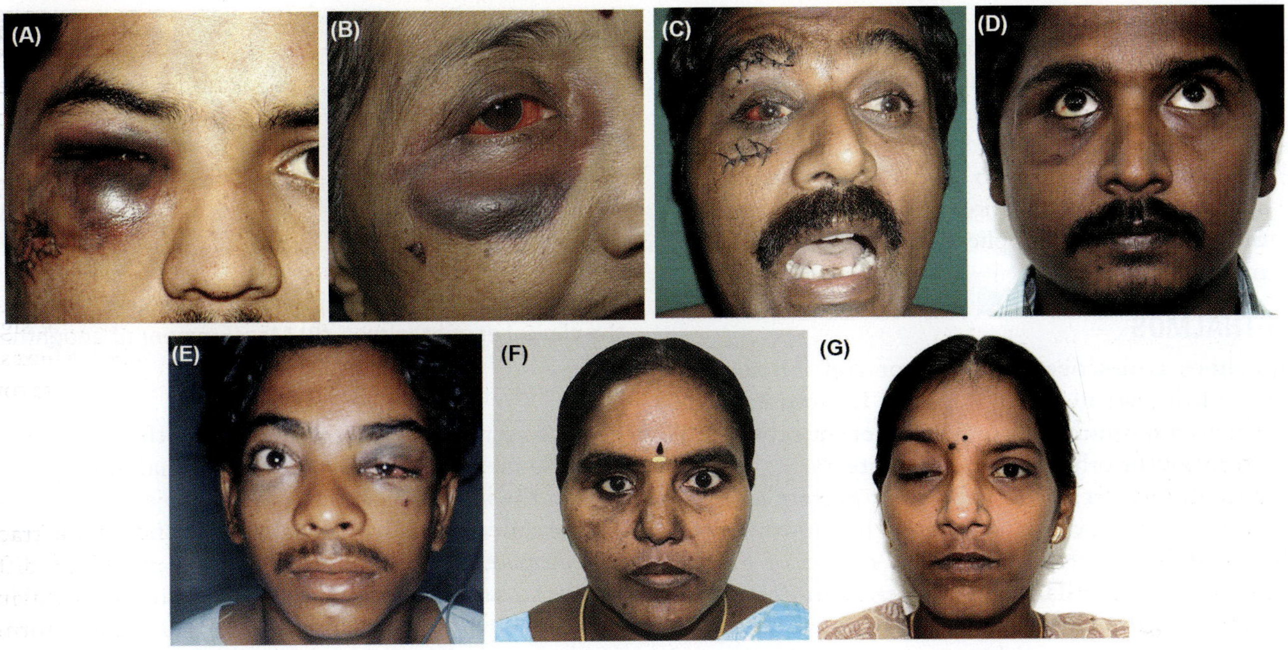

Figure 53.5 (**A**) Circumorbital oedema and ecchymosis. (**B**) Subconjunctival haemorrhage. (**C**) Laceration over the eyelid. (**D**) Restriction in the eye movements. (**E**) Altered globe level. (**F**) Enophthalmos. (**G**) Ptosis.

RETROBULBAR HAEMORRHAGE

Retrobulbar haematoma is a rare, rapidly progressive accumulation of blood in the retrobulbar space (Fig. 53.6). It is a sudden bleeding within a relatively closed compartment with lack of potential drainage pathways. It can lead to irreversible visual loss from damage to the optic nerve and/or retina.

Mechanism—It is caused by direct injury or forces transmitted to the globe by the displaced fracture segments, resulting in rupture of the infraorbital artery or anterior or posterior ethmoidal artery. The blood accumulation leads to elevation of intraorbital pressure (IOP) that results in central retinal artery compression or ischaemia of the optic nerve. Though rare, it is considered as a serious complication of all the orbital fractures.

Clinical features:

- Severe aching pain
- Progressive loss of vision
- Proptosis/exophthalmos
- Increased intraocular pressure
- Marked subconjunctival haemorrhage
- Gross eye swelling
- As vision is lost, pupil becomes fixed and dilated.

Management:

- The visual acuity, pupillary reaction and intraocular pressure should be recorded initially every 5 min
- In cases with spontaneous decompression, the vision recovers spontaneously and there is no need for emergency treatment
- However, if no spontaneous recovery occurs after 20 min and the loss of vision is progressive with

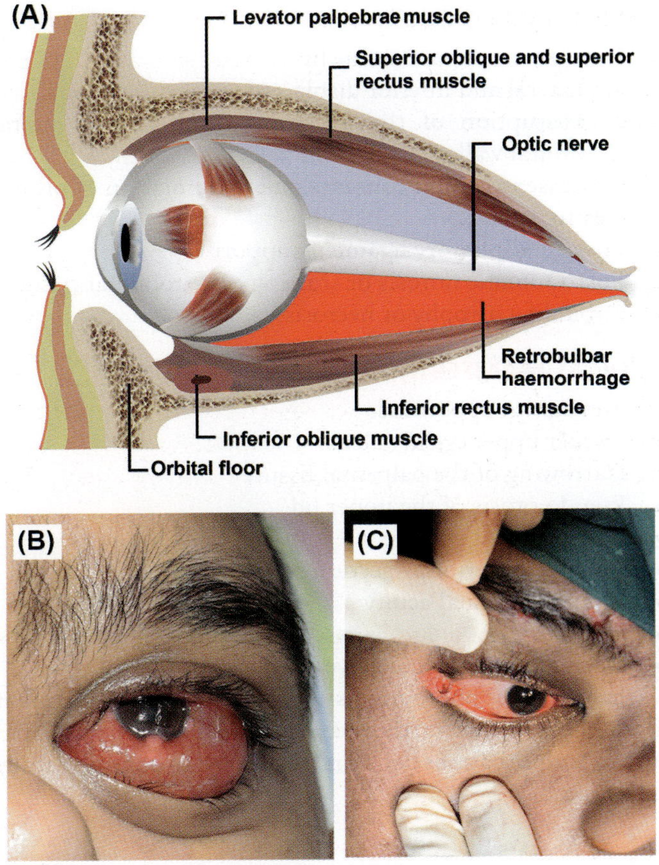

Figure 53.6 (**A**) Diagrammatic representation of retrobulbar haemorrhage. (**B**) Traumatic retrobulbar haemorrhage. (**C**) Lateral canthotomy.

elevated IOP, immediate intervention is required. The surgical management includes a *lateral canthotomy* with or without inferior cantholysis and *orbital decompression*. A small drain can be secured for 24–48 h for adequate drainage and prevent re-accumulation. Additional manoeuvres to lower the intraocular pressure include administration of intravenous mannitol or acetazolamide or application of various glaucoma medications.

ENOPHTHALMOS

Enophthalmos is described as posterior and inferior displacement of the eyeball within the orbit. It is caused by an increase in orbital volume due to fracture of the orbital wall and/or escape of the orbital soft tissue contents.

Enophthalmos can occur in *blowout fracture or Zygomaticomaxillary complex (ZMC) fracture*. In blowout fracture, the enophthalmos is due to the escape of orbital contents into the maxillary sinus, whereas in ZMC fracture, fracture of the lateral wall of the orbit causes displacement of the suspensory ligaments, leading to loss of support to the globe and subsequent enophthalmos.

Traumatic enophthalmos can be classified as immediate, early and late.

MECHANISM OF POSTTRAUMATIC ENOPHTHALMOS

- Increase in orbital volume by
  a. Lateral and inferior displacement of the zygoma
  b. Disruption of the inferior, medial and/or lateral orbital walls
- Decrease in orbital contents due to herniation of orbital soft tissues
- Loss of suspensory ligament support
- Posttraumatic fibrosis or scarring of retrobulbar tissues
- Orbital fat atrophy or necrosis.

CLINICAL MANIFESTATIONS

- Sunken eye appearance
- Deeper upper eyelid sulcus
- Narrowing of the palpebral fissure
- Pseudo ptosis of the upper lid
- Hypoglobus
- Reduced anterior projection of the globe
- Change in visual acuity
- Diplopia
- Decrease in extraocular eye movements.

Preoperative photographs are beneficial in treatment planning as well as for the record maintenance. More than 3 mm of enophthalmos deficit is considered to be aesthetically unacceptable.

MEASUREMENT OF ENOPHTHALMOS

An ***exophthalmometer*** (e.g. **Hertel, Naugle**) can be used to assess the globe projection (enophthalmos) using the lateral orbital rim as reference point (Fig. 53.7).

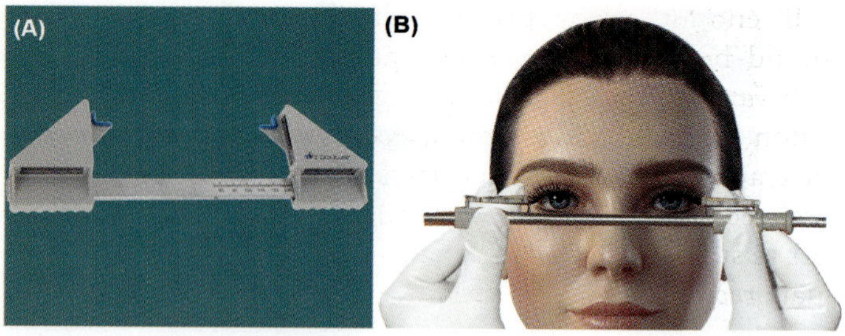

Figure 53.7 (**A**) Hertel exophthalmometer used for assessing the clinical enophthalmos. (**B**) Measurement of enophthalmos.

CT scan provides an excellent view of the orbital contents and also measures the degree of enophthalmos.

- On the injured side, the anterior projection of the eye is measured from the corneal apex to the orbital apex and compared to the uninjured side.

The status of the orbital soft tissues and the globe projection aid in the diagnosis of the enophthalmos. *Whitehouse* et al. found that a *1 cm^3 increase in orbital volume causes 0.8 mm of enophthalmos.*

MANAGEMENT OF POSTTRAUMATIC ENOPHTHALMOS

The main cause of posttraumatic enophthalmos is the displacement of the orbital wall due to an enlarged bony orbital cavity. Hence, enophthalmos correction is aimed at restoration of the orbital bony volume either by *reconstructing the internal orbit or by placing a material behind the globe and displacing the globe anteriorly*.

Grant et al. concepts to correct the posttraumatic orbital deformities are:

1. Mobilisation of the soft tissues in the area of fracture.
2. Repositioning of the orbital rim.
3. Reconstruction of the inner orbital wall and reattachment of the soft tissues to the proper location.

Orbital blowout and ZMC fractures are the most common aetiologies in causing *late enophthalmos*.

Deformity with orbital blowout fracture

The medial wall and orbital floor fracture with herniation of the orbital contents induce the increase in orbital volume in blowout fractures. It is corrected by reducing all the herniated orbital contents and placing for orbital defects. The grafts can be rigidly fixed to the orbital rim with micro screws or miniplates to prevent migration of the material.

Orbito-zygomatic deformity (ZMC fracture)

Displaced ZMC fractures produce a flattened malar area and displacement of the lateral orbital walls, which results in increased orbital volume and subsequent enophthalmos. The objective of enophthalmos correction is to reposition the zygoma and orbital rim to reconstruct the lateral orbital wall.

If enophthalmos persists, then orbital augmentation should be performed. Orbital augmentation can be done with various materials, such as glass beads, silicone sheets, Teflon beads, cartilage grafts, porous polythene sheets, hydroxyapatite, and metallic plates or mesh. A successful orbital reconstruction relies on complete mobilisation of the soft tissues, repositioning of the orbital segments, and adequate restoration of the orbital volume.

PROPTOSIS/EXOPHTHALMOS

It is an abnormally anteriorly positioned globe with respect to the bony orbit. It reflects a relative reduction in the size of the bony orbit.

DIPLOPIA

Diplopia is double vision or simultaneous perception of two images of a single object.

TYPES OF DIPLOPIA

Monocular or binocular (temporary or permanent).

Monocular diplopia—It is blurring of vision that occurs when one eye is closed and the other is open. It usually occurs due to intraocular pathologies like detached lens and hyphema, which require the immediate attention of an ophthalmologist.

Binocular diplopia—Blurring of vision occurs when the patient looks simultaneously with *both eyes*. The development of binocular diplopia following trauma can be due to soft tissue entrapment, neuromuscular injury, intraorbital oedema and change in orbital shape. Binocular diplopia can be temporary or permanent.

Temporary diplopia—Temporary diplopia is caused by a haematoma or oedema of the extraocular muscles which generally resolves in a few days (5–7 days).

Permanent diplopia—Paralysis or muscle entrapment within the fractured segments can cause permanent diplopia. This is a more serious cause of diplopia, which if left uncorrected can lead to permanent diplopia.

CAUSES OF TRAUMATIC DIPLOPIA

- Haematoma or oedema around the extraocular muscles
- Disruption of the inferior rectus or inferior oblique muscle attachment
- Orbital floor fracture with herniation of the periorbital fat into the maxillary sinus
- Neuromuscular injury resulting in paralysis of the muscle
- Fibrous tissue formation and adhesions between the periosteum, muscle or fat with the fractured bony margins
- Damage to the III, IV and VI cranial nerves.

DIPLOPIA SYMPTOMS

- One or both eyes not lining up (wandering eye)
- Blurred vision
- Pain on moving eyes
- Dizziness
- Fatigue.

TEST FOR DIPLOPIA (Fig. 53.8)

Finger gaze

A finger is held in front of the patient at a distance of an arm's length and moved in all directions as the patient's eyes follow the finger. Any double vision should be reported by

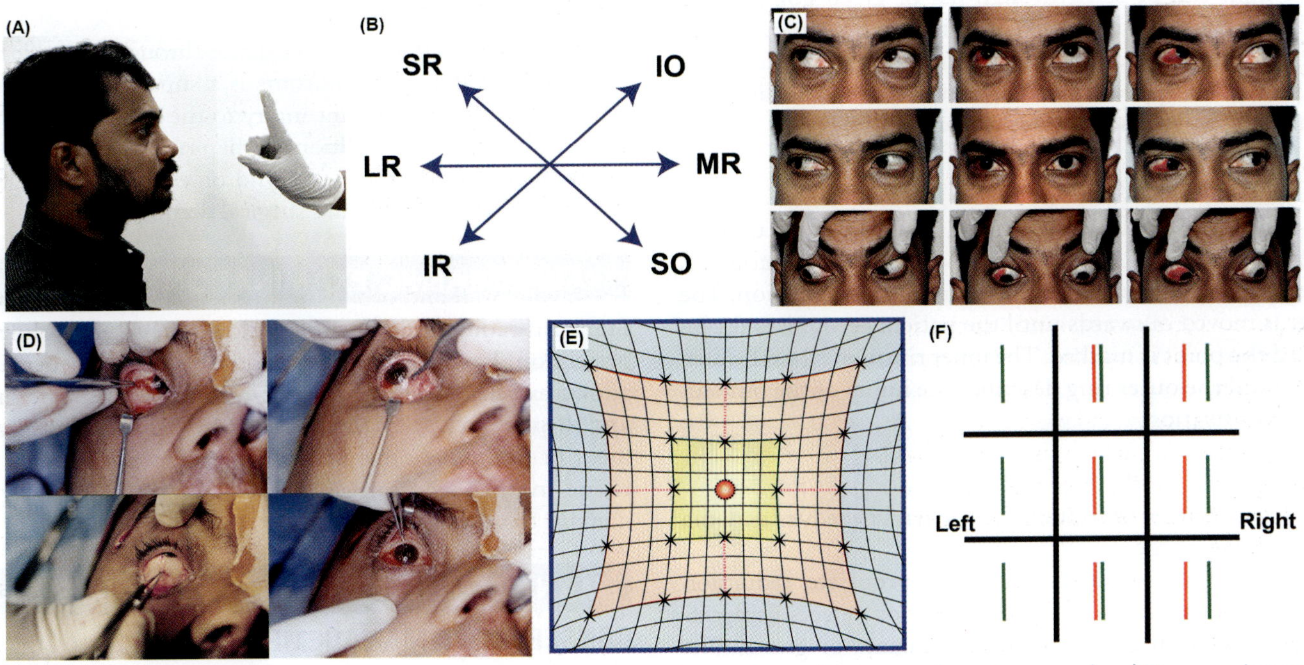

Figure 53.8 Tests for diplopia. (**A–C**) Finger gaze test to access the actions of extra oculomotor muscles (SR- superior rectus, SO- superior oblique, IR - inferior rectus, IO- inferior oblique). (**D**) Forced duction test. (**E**) Hess diplopia chart. (**F**) Diplopia chart.

the patient. Diplopia should be tested in all nine directions of gaze.

Forced duction test (traction test)

Diplopia caused due to oedema or haematoma of the extraocular muscles usually resolves in 5–7 days, but diplopia as a result of failure to rotate the eyes superiorly indicates paralysis (neurological) or entrapment (mechanical) of the muscle within the fractured segments. *Forced duction test is carried out to differentiate between these two causes (mechanical or neurological) of diplopia.*

Under topical anaesthesia, using a tissue holding forceps, the tendon of the inferior rectus muscle is grasped and the globe is manipulated through its entire range of motion (Fig. 53.8D). A failure to rotate the eyes superiorly indicates paralysis or entrapment of the muscle within the fractured segment in the orbital floor. Conversely, the absence of resistance can be due to a neurological deficit or a large nonrestrictive defect in the floor.

Hess diplopia chart (Lees screen)

Hess chart is used *to measure the degree of diplopia*. This test helps in identifying the nonfunctioning extraocular muscle. In this test, dissimilar images are projected on each eye at 1 meter distance with the patient wearing green or red goggles. This test also documents the range of ocular movements of both the affected and unaffected eye and its muscle limitations.

Diplopia chart

This is a simple tool for the diagnosis of diplopia. A vertical bar of light can be seen through red or green goggles at a fixed distance from the eye. The bar of light is moved into each direction of gaze, and the patient describes the image separation and appearance. It aids in detecting the direction of the gaze, where the diplopia is worst.

Field of binocular single vision

The field of binocular single vision (BSV) is a test used to describe the area of BSV and hence diplopia. The patient is seated at the perimeter with the chin central to fixation. The target is moved outwards until the patient recognises diplopia and the point is marked. The inner ring describes the area of BSV and the outer ring describes the limits of the binocular field of fixation.

MANAGEMENT OF DIPLOPIA

- Administration of steroids for 5–7 days to reduce oedema or haemorrhage
- Surgical management includes appropriate reduction and reconstruction of the orbital floor defects using reconstructive materials such as implants or grafts. The displaced soft tissues are carefully dissected from the line of fracture and restored to its original position.

PTOSIS (BLEPHAROPTOSIS)

Ptosis is defined as drooping or falling of the upper eyelid. It can decrease or even occlude the vision completely. A droopy eyelid/ptosis occurs when the muscle that elevates the eyelid (the levator palpebrae superioris) is weak from various reasons.

TRAUMATIC OPTIC NEUROPATHY

Traumatic optic neuropathy (TON) is an injury to the optic nerve secondary to trauma. It results in a visual loss that can be immediate or delayed. Treatment modalities include surgical decompression, high-dose steroids and observation. High-dose intravenous corticosteroids are more effective when administered within 8 h of injury. To mitigate the likelihood of neurotoxicity, a maximum daily dose of 1 g IV methylprednisolone has been recommended.

General guidelines for the use of high-dose corticosteroids are:

- Methylprednisolone 30 mg/kg over 30 min followed by methylprednisolone 15 mg/kg 2 h later
- It is continued at 15 mg/kg every 6 h for 24–48 h.

If visual function improves, corticosteroids are tapered. Patients who show deterioration or no response to corticosteroids can be treated by optic canal decompression.

SUPERIOR ORBITAL FISSURE SYNDROME

The cranial nerves III, IV, V and VI are injured when an orbital fracture extends to the superior orbital fissure. The symptoms include a combination of *ophthalmoplegia*, ptosis, proptosis, loss of corneal reflex and paraesthesia over the forehead. Treatment includes steroid administration and surgical decompression.

ORBITAL APEX SYNDROME

It is often due to a fracture that extends through the optic nerve canal. The orbital apex syndrome is a superior orbital fissure syndrome with concomitant injury to the optic nerve (CN II). There is blindness in addition to the features of the superior orbital fissure syndrome. Both syndromes can be managed by giving high-dose steroids and surgical decompression.

RADIOGRAPHIC EXAMINATION

Standard radiographs include Caldwell's projection, Waters projection, lateral projections, and oblique projections. CT allows excellent visualisation of orbital soft tissues, extent and displacement of fracture fragments as well as measurement of orbital volume. MRI is limited in determining soft tissue injuries, entrapment of muscles, and assessing the damage to the optic nerve.

MANAGEMENT OF ORBITAL FRACTURES

CONSERVATIVE MANAGEMENT

Conservative treatment is indicated when there is minimal or no displacement of the fractured bones, medically compromised or elderly patients for whom invasive surgical procedures and general anaesthesia are contraindicated.

SURGICAL MANAGEMENT

INDICATIONS FOR OPEN REDUCTION

- Severely displaced fractures
- Positive forced duction test
- Neuromuscular injuries
- Enophthalmos
- Unresolved diplopia
- Defects that are greater than half the surface area of the floor
- CT evidence of muscle entrapment
- CT evidence of periorbital disruption and prolapse of soft tissue into the antrum.

SURGICAL APPROACHES (Fig. 53.9)

1. Transcutaneous
   - Lynch
   - Lateral brow incision
   - Upper lid blepharoplasty
   - Subciliary
   - Subtarsal
   - Infraorbital
2. Transcaruncular
3. Transconjunctival

Subciliary incision

A series of incisions have been used to approach the inferior and lateral orbital rims. The most common approach to the orbital floor are subciliary, infraorbital and transconjunctival incisions.

The major difference between the subciliary, subtarsal and infraorbital incision is the level at which the incision is placed in the skin and the level of muscle that is transected.

Advantages

- Imperceptible scar
- It can be extended laterally for additional exposure of the lateral orbital rim.

Technique

The globe is protected by a simple tarsorrhaphy suture or scleral shell. The subciliary incision or blepharoplasty incision is a lower-lid incision made just below the eyelashes (approximately 2 mm) along the skin crease. The incision should be made only through the skin. The skin incision is followed by subcutaneous dissection towards the inferior orbital rim for approximately 4–6 mm. Dissection is then continued through the orbicularis muscle along the direction of the muscle to reach the periosteum over the orbital rim. A scalpel is used to make an incision on the periosteum 2–3 mm below the orbital rim. Subperiosteal dissection is done, exposing the inferior orbital rim, orbital floor and anterior surface of the maxilla. The fractured fragments are reduced and fixed. Closure is usually performed in two layers: periosteum and skin layer (Fig. 53.10).

PRIMARY RECONSTRUCTION OF ORBITAL FRACTURES

Orbital wall fractures can be linear, blowout or complex fractures.

Aesthetic deformities (enophthalmos) are the most prevalent consequence of *linear fractures*, whereas functional deformities are less common. The reconstruction of linear fractures

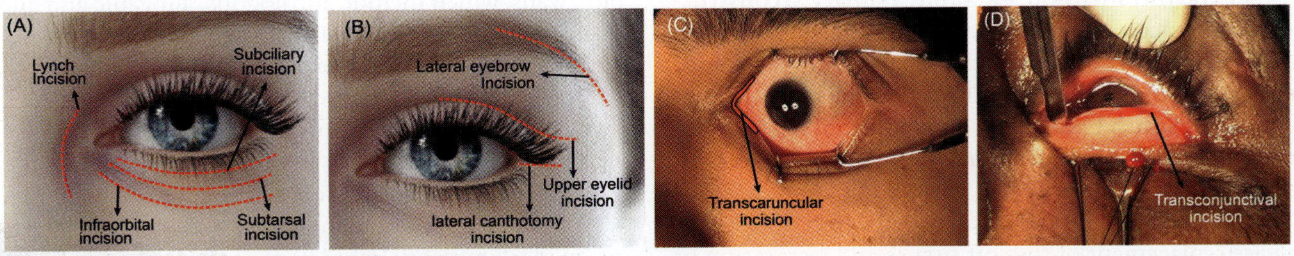

Figure 53.9 Surgical approaches to the orbit. **(A)** Lynch, subciliary, subtarsal and infraorbital incisions. **(B)** Lateral brow incision and upper eye lid incision. **(C)** Transcaruncular. **(D)** Transconjunctival.

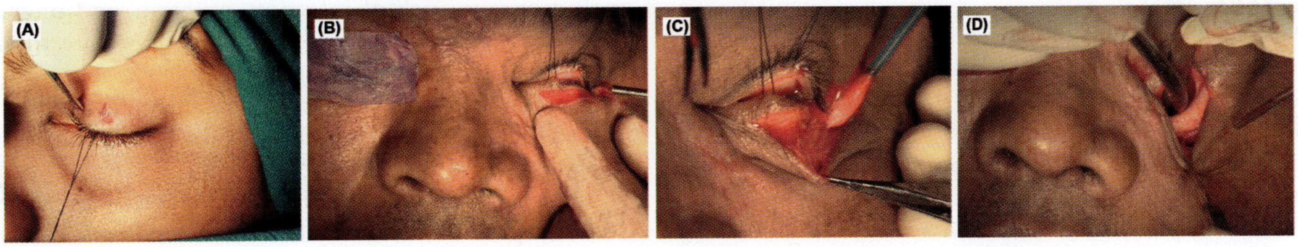

Figure 53.10 Subciliary incision. **(A)** Tarsorrhaphy suture. **(B)** Subciliary incision. **(C)** Dissection through the orbicularis muscle. **(D)** Incision over the periosteum and subperiosteal dissection exposing the bone.

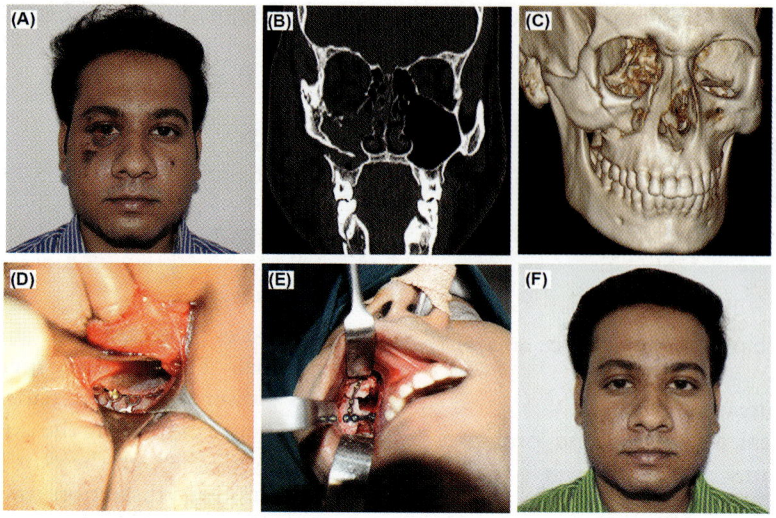

Figure 53.11 Case Report 1—Primary reconstruction of the orbital floor fracture with Medpor (implant). (**A**) Preoperative view. (**B** and **C**) CT scan showing fracture involving the right orbital floor and zygoma. (**D**) Orbital floor reconstruction with Medpor. (**E**) Zygomatic buttress fixation. (**F**) Postoperative view.

is aimed to restore the shape of the orbital walls and the orbital volume with a reconstructive material (graft).

In *blowout fractures*, functional deficits (such as diplopia) are more common than aesthetic deformities. The primary reconstruction of blowout fractures is aimed at restoring the mobility and function of globe along with elevation of prolapsed soft tissues from the sinuses using miniplates and graft (Fig. 53.11).

Isolated blowout fractures of the roof or medial wall do not contribute to the development of functional or cosmetic deformities. Hence, these defects are usually treated conservatively and monitored for several months.

Complex orbital fractures can occur alone or in conjunction with other fractures beyond the orbit. Primary reconstruction of these defects can be challenging due to its extent. It requires adequate exposure of the fracture, rigid fixation of the fractures outside the orbit, followed by reconstruction of the orbital walls with bone grafts or metallic mesh.

Principles to be followed in surgery during reconstruction of orbital floor:

- Complete exposure of the fracture and defect
- Precise replacement of the soft tissues and restoration of intraorbital volume
- Identification of the posterior limit in orbital floor and restoration of the posteromedial bulge of the orbit (Hammer's key area)
- Proper selection of reconstruction material based on the complexity of the defect.

SECONDARY RECONSTRUCTION (Fig. 53.12)

Delayed orbital reconstruction is sometimes necessary for:

- Inadequate primary reconstructions
- Orbital injuries that were missed
- Cosmetic deformities such as enophthalmos, telecanthus, contour abnormalities and eyelid deformities
- Functional deformities such as restricted ocular motility and diplopia.

Generally, secondary reconstruction is usually not undertaken until 6 months after the primary repair to allow for adequate healing and neuromuscular recovery. Secondary corrections are technically demanding due to fibrosis and contracture of soft tissues and distorted bony landmarks of the orbit.

RECONSTRUCTIVE MATERIALS USED FOR ORBITAL WALL FRACTURES

Numerous materials have been used to reconstruct the orbital walls, which include autologous, allogenic and alloplastic materials (Table 53.2) (Figs. 53.13 and 53.14).

Requirements of an ideal implant/graft:

- Simplicity of the shaping and adaptation
- Ability to support the orbital structures
- Rapid integration with the surrounding tissues
- Resistance to bacterial contamination
- Visualisation of implant on CT.

An ideal implant should be easy to insert and manipulate, inert, not prone to infection or extrusion, easily anchored to surrounding structures, and affordable. *Autogenous grafts* are preferable for large orbital defects as they are biocompatible with minimum risk of infection, rejection, and migration. Rib grafts and mandibular symphysis grafts are the most commonly used autogenous grafts.

The use of *Allografts* has significantly declined, this is due to its high resorption rate and the risk of transmitting disease.

In alloplasts, Titanium mesh is preferred as they are capable of osseointegration with low risk of infection. *Titanium-reinforced polyethylene implants* are the most recent implants as they are radiopaque and more rigid.

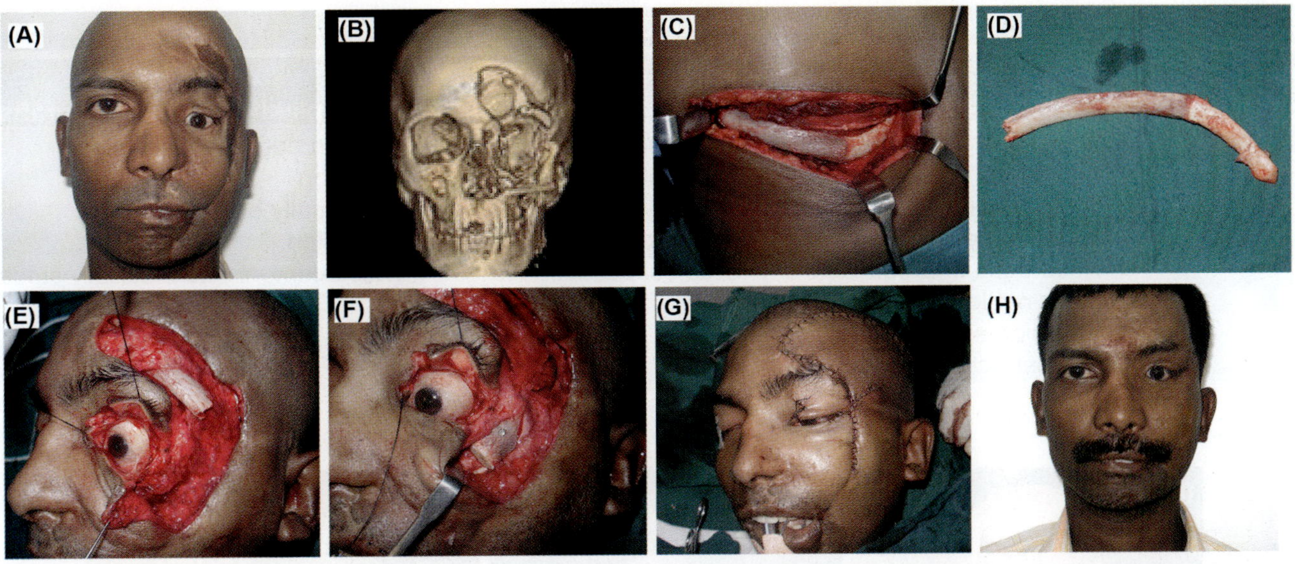

Figure 53.12 Case Report 2—Periorbital defect managed by secondary reconstruction with iliac bone graft. (**A**) Preoperative view. (**B**) Preoperative CT scan. (**C** and **D**) Iliac bone graft. (**E** and **F**) Reconstruction of the orbital defect with graft. (**G** and **H**) Postoperative view.

TABLE 53.2 Reconstructive Materials Available for Orbital Fractures

	Autologous Grafts	Allogeneic Materials (Allografts, Xenografts)	Alloplastic Materials/Exgrafts
Types	• Most favoured • Autogenous bone • Cartilage	Provides a structural framework for growth of host tissues (osteoinductive and/or osteoconductive)	• They are synthetic meterials, obtained from non-human or non-organic sources.
Examples	• Anterior iliac crest • Calvarium • Rib • Maxilla • Mandibular cortex • Cartilage- auricular	**Allografts:** • Lyophilised fascia/ Dura mater **Xenografts:** • Homologous bone • Homologous cartilage E.g. bovine and porcine pericardium	A. **Nonresorbable alloplasts** • Titanium mesh • Vitallium • Polymethylmethacrylate (PMMA) • Polyethylene • Silicon nitride • High-density porous polyethylene (Medpor) • Hydroxyapatite • Silicones and polytetrafluoroethylene (Teflon) B. **Resorbable alloplasts** • Polylactic • Polyglactin • Vicryl mesh/plate • *Polydioxanone plates (PDS)* • Gelatin film • Porous polyethylene implants (PE)
Advantages	• High-tissue compatibility • Relatively resistant to infection • Calvarial graft—radiopaque	• Do not require a 2nd operative site • Less operative time	• Elimination of donor-site morbidity • Decreased operative time • Multitude of sizes and shapes available • Easy to handle and cheap

Continued

TABLE 53.2 Reconstructive Materials Available for Orbital Fractures—cont'd

	Autologous Grafts	Allogeneic Materials (Allografts, Xenografts)	Alloplastic Materials/Exgrafts
Disadvantages	• 2nd surgical site and procedure • Patient morbidity • Increased operative time • Resorption unpredictable • Does not lead to high-precision anatomical reconstruction	• Antigenicity of the material • Viral contamination and transmission of infectious disease	• Foreign bodies reactions • Infection • Fibrotically encapsulated • Extrusion • Displacement into maxillary sinus

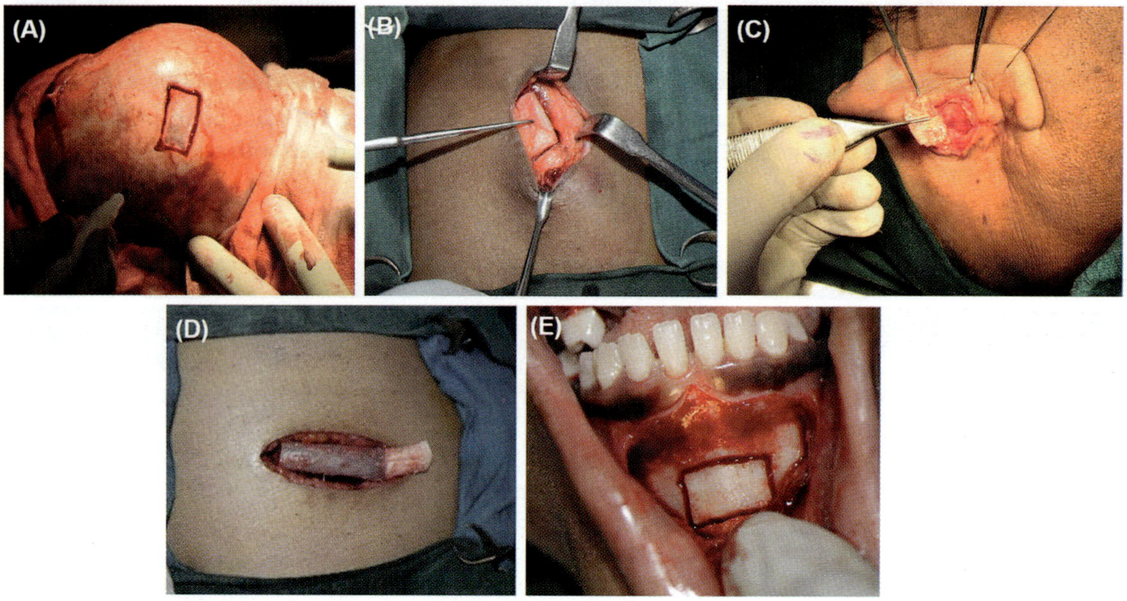

Figure 53.13 Autologous grafts. (**A**) Cranial vault bone. (**B**) Iliac bone. (**C**) Conchal cartilage. (**D**) Rib cartilage. (**E**) Mandible cortex.

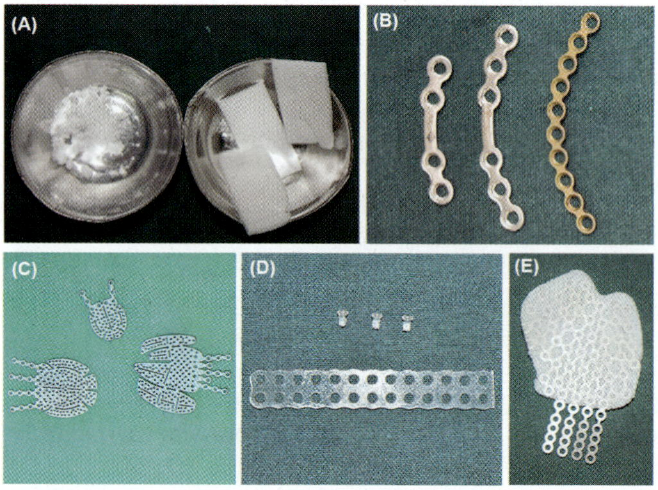

Figure 53.14 Alloplastic materials. (**A**) rhBMP-2. (**B**) Titanium miniplates. (**C**) Titanium mesh. (**D**) Absorbable miniplates and screws. (**E**) Medpor-porous polyethylene.

COMPLICATIONS

Complications associated in the management of orbital fractures may be categorised into immediate and delayed complications.

Immediate Complications	Delayed Complications
• Oculocardiac reflex-intraoperative • Oedema • Infection • Would dehiscence • Aberrant implant position • Extrusion of implants	• Persistent enophthalmos • Persistent diplopia with altered vision • Restricted ocular movement due to fibrosis and adhesion • Entropion/Ectropion • Hypertrophic scars/keloids

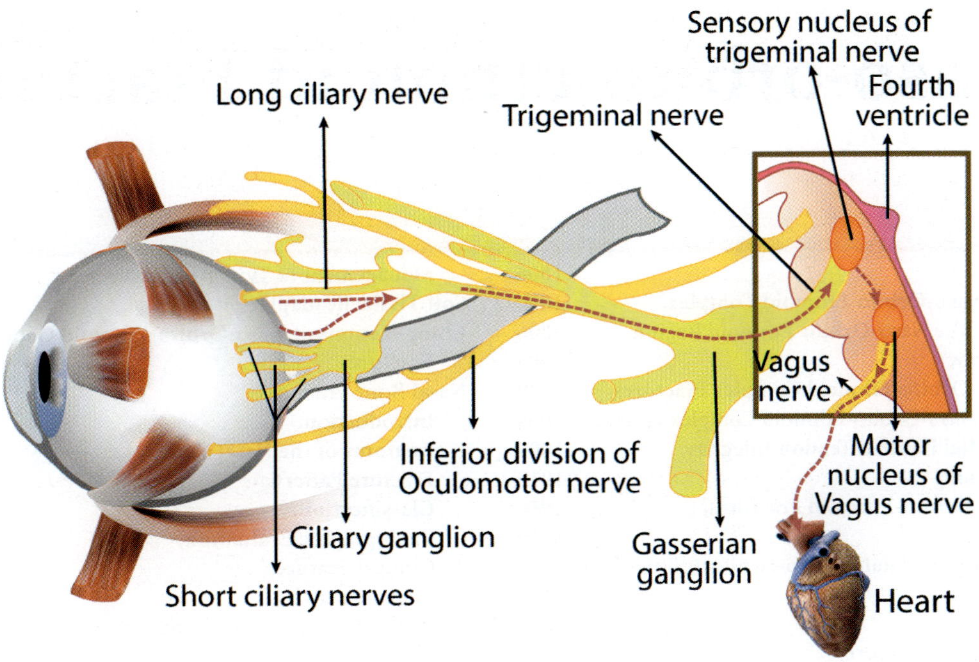

Figure 53.15 Oculocardiac reflex.

Oculocardiac reflex

The oculocardiac reflex (OCR) is defined as a decrease in heart rate that is induced due to pressure on the eyeball or sustained traction of extraocular muscles. The OCR also known as *Aschner phenomenon* is a triad of *bradycardia, nausea and syncope.* It is most typically encountered during orbital surgeries. Sustained traction on the extraocular muscles, ocular trauma or pressure over the globe may trigger an afferent signal via the trigeminal nerve that evokes an abrupt parasympathetic output of the vagus nerve, resulting in bradycardia and hypotension (Fig. 53.15 and Flowchart 53.1).

The classical findings of OCR are bradycardia, nausea, vomiting, vertigo, syncope, gastric hypermotility and orbital pain. The OCR can be managed by:

- Immediate cessation of the stimuli
- Avoiding sustained traction on extraocular movements
- Releasing the ocular pressure
- Using a regional nerve block in high-risk patients
- Increasing the depth of anaesthesia
- Atropine (10– 20 mcg/kg, IV) or Glycopyrrolate (10 mcg/kg, IV).

Fracture reduction and release of the muscle should be done *to avoid life-threatening cardiac arrhythmias* and *also to avoid ischaemic necrosis* of the muscle.

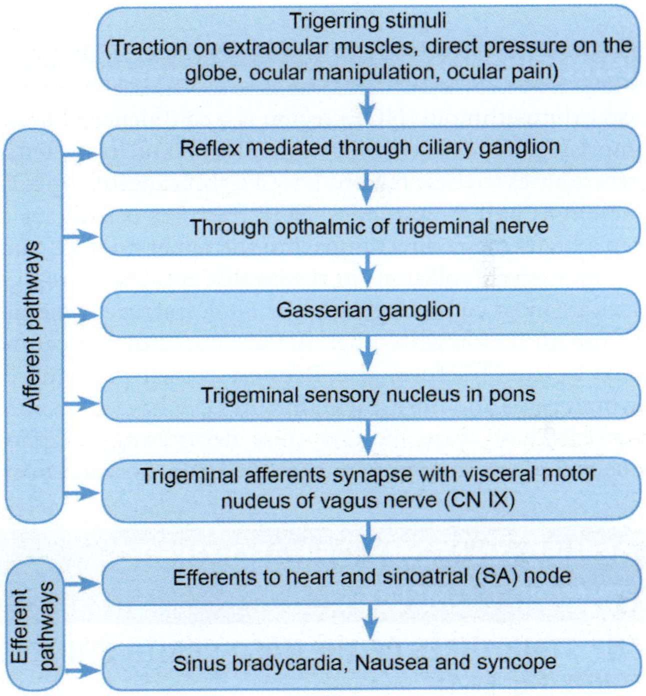

Flowchart 53.1 Mechanism of oculocardiac reflex.

Chapter 54

Naso-orbito-ethmoid Fracture

OUTLINE

INTRODUCTION

Naso-orbito-ethmoid (NOE) region is a confluence of bones comprising of the nose, orbit, ethmoid and skull base. Henceforth, injuries to these regions have a significant influence on function as well as aesthetics. NOE fractures usually result from a high-energy direct impact to the upper midface, such as in motorcycle collisions in road traffic accidents. Younger males are most commonly afflicted. NOE fractures generally occur in affiliation with other midface fractures, but can occur as isolated fractures also. Because of their proximity to the brain, eyes and nose, these fractures can have dire consequences. These fractures can cause devastating complications because of their proximity to the brain, eyes and nose.

APPLIED ANATOMY OF NASO-ORBITO-ETHMOID COMPLEX

BONY STRUCTURES OF THE NASO-ORBITO-ETHMOID REGION (Fig. 54.1)

The NOE region comprises of the central component of the face and is surrounded by the following bones:

- Anteriorly - the nasal bones and pyriform aperture
- Posteriorly - the lacrimal bone
- Superiorly - the frontal bone
- Inferiorly - the maxilla
- Medially - the ethmoid air cells
- Laterally - the orbit and its contents.

During trauma, the ethmoidal labyrinth present between the orbits acts as a shock absorber or a natural '*crumple zone*', this minimises the force dissipating into the orbit and cranial cavities.

SOFT TISSUE ANATOMY

MEDIAL CANTHAL LIGAMENT

- The medial canthal ligament (MCL) is a band of fibrous tissue, situated between the medial borders of the eyelids and the bones of the medial orbital wall. The medial canthal tendon (MCT) originates from the anterior and posterior lacrimal crest and frontal process of maxilla. It encloses the lacrimal sac and diverges to become the orbicularis muscle, tarsal plate and suspensory ligaments of eyelids
- Before inserting into the frontal process of maxilla, the medial canthal tendon splits into two limbs; the *anterior and posterior limb*, which encloses the lacrimal sac. The anterior horizontal limb is the strongest and is attached more firmly to the anterior lacrimal crest in the frontal process of maxilla
- The posterior limb is the weakest and is attached to the posterior lacrimal crest. It consists of the lacrimal fascia, the Horner's muscle and the areolar tissue. (Horner's muscle is a small extension of orbicularis oculi muscle.) The insertion of the posterior limb lacks strength, because of its weak fibres and small area of insertion. The underlying bone is also incapable of providing solid anchorage (Fig. 54.2)

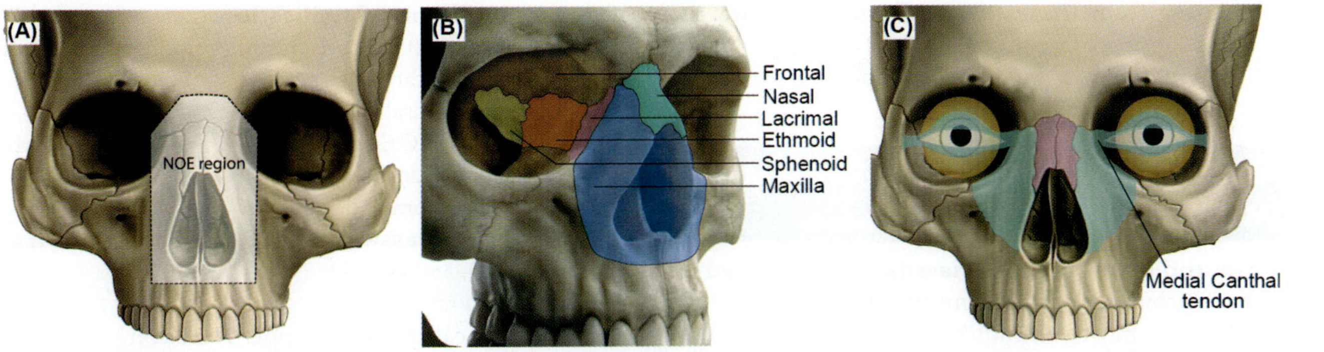

Figure 54.1 (**A**) Anatomy of NOE region. (**B**) Bony components of NOE region. (**C**) NOE region with its soft tissue attachments (medial canthal tendon).

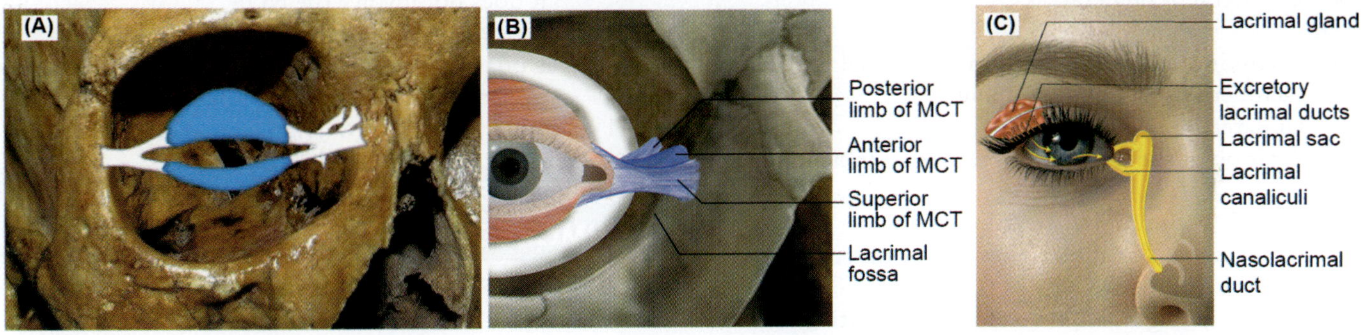

Figure 54.2 (**A** and **B**) Attachment of medial canthal tendon (MCT) (**C**) Lacrimal apparatus.

- The MCT plays a crucial role both functionally as well as cosmetically. It supports the eyelid, maintains the globe and holds the palpebral fissure. Separation of the MCT from the NOE area causes rounding of the palpebral fissure and telecanthus.

LACRIMAL APPARATUS (Fig. 54.2C)

The lacrimal apparatus is responsible for the drainage of lacrimal fluid from the eyes into the nose. It entails the following structures:

- Lacrimal gland
- Lacrimal canaliculi
- Lacrimal sac
- Nasolacrimal duct (NLD).

Lacrimal gland

It is an exocrine gland that secretes lacrimal fluid onto the surfaces of the conjunctiva and cornea of the eye. Lacrimal fluid helps to clean and lubricate the eyes, and tears are formed when it is produced in excess. The lacrimal gland is located within the lacrimal fossa, on the superior and lateral edge of the orbital roof. The gland is approximately 2 cm long and is divided into two main parts: orbital and palpebral.

Lacrimal canaliculi/canals

The lacrimal fluids from the surface of the eyes are drained into the lacrimal sac through the lacrimal canals. The lacrimal canals are small channels that lie in the medial corner of each eyelid, along with small openings called the puncta lacrimalia. These canaliculi are divided into superior and inferior ducts that drain into the lacrimal sac. Epiphora (excessive tearing) is caused by the obstruction or narrowing (stenosis) of the puncta.

Lacrimal sac

The lacrimal sac can be found in the lacrimal fossa, which is situated on the anterior portion of the medial wall of the orbit. The limbs of the MCT surround the lacrimal sac. The nasolacrimal duct is connected to the lacrimal sac and travels inferiorly within the bone to enter the nasal cavity. The lacrimal sac is continuous with the nasolacrimal duct. The nasolacrimal duct is responsible for transporting lacrimal fluid from the surface of the eye to the nasal cavity. This occurs via the lacrimal sac.

Nasolacrimal duct

The nasolacrimal duct drains the fluid into the inferior meatus of nose. The opening of the duct is guarded by *the valve of Hasner*.

Vascular supply to naso-orbito-ethmoid region

The branches of the internal and external carotid arteries supply the midface and nasal area. The anterior and posterior ethmoidal arteries from internal carotid artery and maxillary artery from the external carotid artery are the main arterial supply to the midface. The NOE region is innervated by ophthalmic and maxillary nerves, which are branches of the trigeminal nerve.

CLASSIFICATION OF NASO-ORBITO-ETHMOID COMPLEX FRACTURES

Markowitz and Manson (1991) classification are based on the fracture pattern, degree of comminution and MCT disruption. It is the most commonly used classification even now (Fig. 54.3).

Type I:

- Simple fracture with intact MCL attachment
- Unilateral or bilateral

Type II:

- Comminuted fracture with intact medial canthal attachment in the large fragment
- Unilateral or bilateral
- Fixation of the fracture segments is sufficient

Type III:

- Grossly comminuted fractures with the canthal attachment in a small fragment or completely avulsed tendon
- The bony fragments are so small for fixation and are reconstructed secondarily
- Transnasal wiring or resuspension of the canthus is required

Rowe and Williams classification:

- Isolated NOE and frontal region fracture without other midface fractures:
  - Unilateral/bilateral
- Isolated NOE and frontal region fracture with other midface fractures:
  - Unilateral/bilateral

Burstein et al., classification of paediatric NOE fractures (Fig. 54.4):

Type I fracture:

It is localised to the upper NOE complex and frontal bone, medial to superior orbital foramen

Type II fracture:

It involves half of the superior orbital wall, although it does not involve the NOE

Type III fracture:

It is bilateral and involves the superior orbital walls, upper NOE and bilateral frontal bones.

CLINICAL EVALUATION OF NASO-ORBITO-ETHMOID COMPLEX FRACTURES

The signs and symptoms of NOE fractures are given in Table 54.1.

The main indicators of NOE fracture include the following:

- Depressed nasal bridge as a result of loss in bony morphology

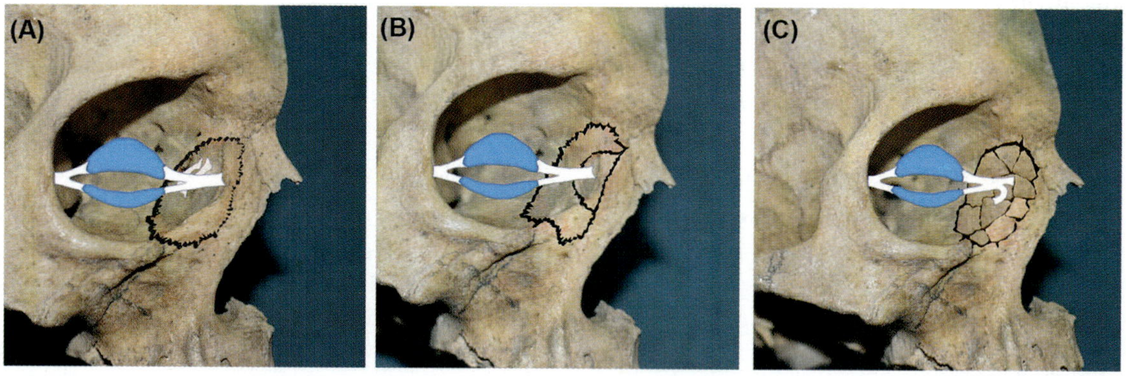

Figure 54.3 **(A)** Type I fracture. **(B)** Type II fracture. **(C)** Type III fracture.

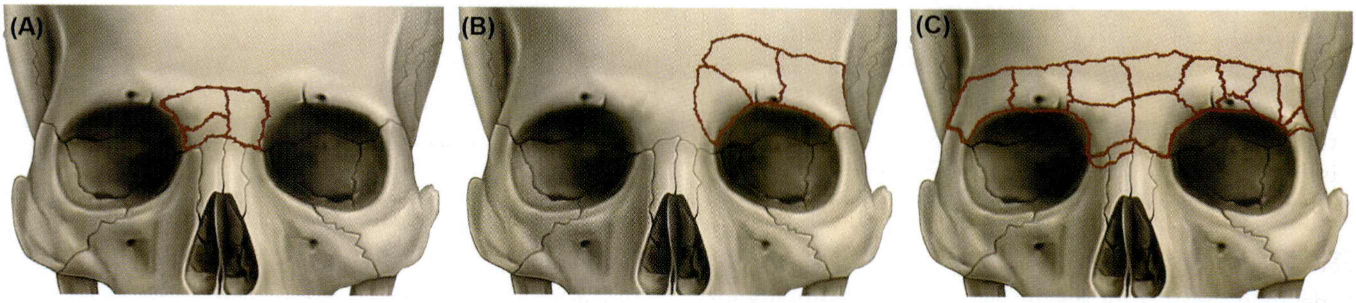

Figure 54.4 **(A–C)** Burstein's Type I, Type II and Type III fractures, respectively.

TABLE 54.1 Clinical Findings in NOE Fracture (Fig. 54.5)

Nasal Findings	Ocular Findings	Others
• Nasal deformity with crepitus • Flattened nasal bridge • Elevated nasal tip • Epistaxis • Hyposmia/anosmia • Nasal airway obstruction • Increased frontonasal angle giving a *pig snout* appearance • Nasolacrimal duct blockage	• Periorbital oedema • Telecanthus • Shortened palpebral fissures • Epiphora • Rounded medial canthal region • ICD >35 mm	• CSF rhinorrhoea • Paraesthesia of infraorbital, supratrochlear or supraorbital nerve • Meningitis • Sinusitis • Pneumocephalus

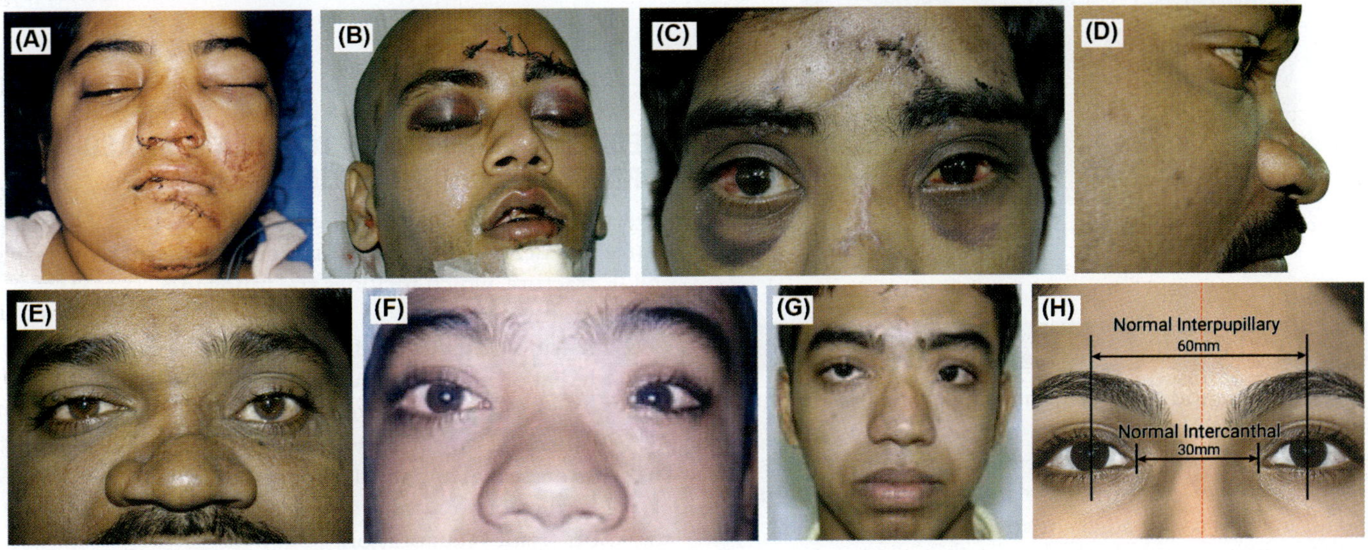

Figure 54.5 Clinical features. (**A**) Nasal deformity with epistaxis. (**B**) Periorbital ecchymosis. (**C**) Subconjunctival ecchymosis with flattened nasal bridge. (**D**) Flattened nasal bridge with elevated nasal tip. (**E**) Left eye orbital dystopia, hypoglobus and enophthalmos with supratarsal hooding. (**F**) Telecanthus and shortened palpebral fissures. (**G**) Rounded medial canthal region/epicanthal fold. (**H**) Normal intercanthal distance.

- The lateral displacement/detachment of MCT leads to *rounding of the medial palpebral fissure*, widening of the NOE region and transverse shortening of the palpebral aperture
- *Epiphora*—persistent tearing of eyes usually occurs due to obstruction of lacrimal apparatus at various levels
- *Traumatic telecanthus* or *pseudohypertelorism*. Telecanthus refers to increased intercanthal distance (>35 mm) due to the disruption of MCL attachment or widening of the fragments
- *Intercanthal distance (ICD):* It is the distance measured from one medial palpebral angle to the other or equal to the width of palpebral aperture. Normal ICD in females is 32 to 33 mm, whereas in males it is 33 to 34 mm approximately.

ASSESSMENT OF MEDIAL CANTHAL TENDON INTEGRITY

The detachment of MCL can be determined by the following tests:

Eyelid traction test/bowstring test (Fig. 54.6A)

The upper eyelid of the suspected orbit is grasped and pulled outwardly and laterally. If the MCL is intact, it will protrude through the skin like a subcutaneous bowstring. When the ligament is detached, there is no longer a bowstring that can be seen or felt.

Furness test

This test is performed by grasping the skin overlying the medial canthus with a small tissue forceps. A lack of resistance or detection of movement of the underlying bone at the tendon area is indicative of a fracture.

Bimanual test (Fig. 54.6B)

An instrument (e.g. Kelly's clamp) is placed high into the nose, with its tip directly beneath the MCT attachment. The presence of instability and crepitation at the tendon area, when the instrument is gently lifted, suggests a NOE fracture.

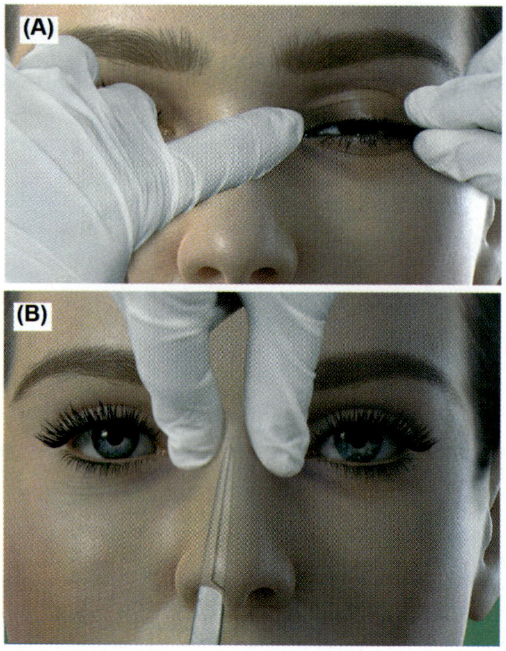

Figure 54.6 (**A**) Bowstring test. (**B**) Bimanual test.

RADIOGRAPHIC EVALUATION

- Occipitomental view (10 and 45 degrees) is helpful as initial screening tool
- CT scan examination is extremely significant in assessing the degree of fracture, displacement of NOE complex and injuries to the adjacent structures
- CT scan images in all planes (axial, coronal and sagittal) aid in accurate identification and assessment of the fracture pattern (Fig. 54.7).

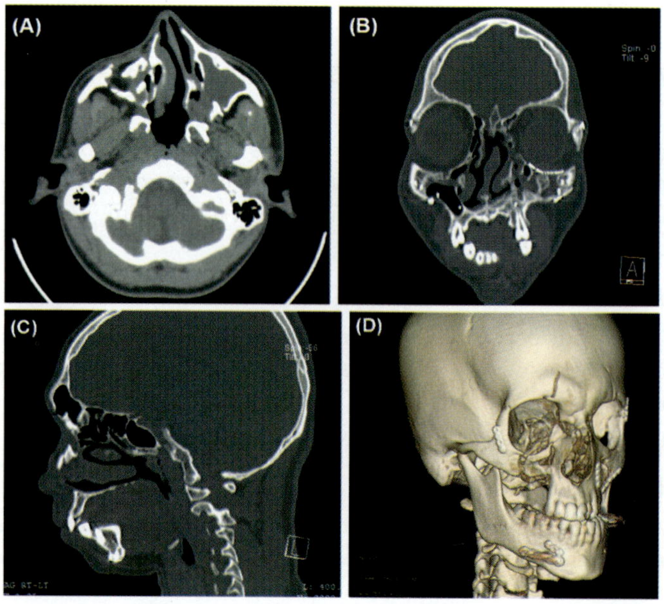

Figure 54.7 (**A**) Axial. (**B**) Coronal. (**C**) Sagittal. (**D**) 3D reconstruction.

MANAGEMENT OF NASO-ORBITO-ETHMOID FRACTURES

SURGICAL APPROACHES (Fig. 54.8)

A combination of surgical approaches is often required to adequately visualise, reduce and stabilise extensively comminuted fractures. For comprehensive surgical management, a coronal and lower eyelid incision is usually required.

- Existing laceration
- Glabella approach (a horizontal incision over the glabella region)
- Bicoronal approach
- Butterfly incision (combination of Gullwing and open sky incision)
- Vertical incision
- H-shaped incision.

SEQUENTIAL APPROACH TO ISOLATED NASO-ORBITO-ETHMOID FRACTURE

A systematic approach for the repair of isolated NOE fractures was described by *Ellis* to achieve successful reduction of NOE fracture, which includes the following:

1. Surgical exposure
2. Identification of the MCT and MCT-bearing bone
3. Medial orbital rim reduction and reconstruction
4. Reconstruction of the medial orbital wall
5. Transnasal canthopexy if required
6. Nasolacrimal apparatus repair
7. Nasal reconstruction (septal and nasal dorsum)
8. Soft tissue readaptation.

POINTS OF FIXATION

Fixation of the fractured segments helps in reestablishing the NOE segment to the surrounding bones. The fixation that is generally recommended for NOE complex fracture are three-point fixation (Fig. 54.9).

Three-point fixation at:

- *Frontal bone*—nasofrontal junction to the nasal complex
- *Pyriform aperture*—nasal complex to the maxillary buttress
- *Orbital rim*—nasal complex to the infraorbital rim.

Two-point fixation—fixation at any two of these sites.

One-point fixation—fixation at any one site.

Additional plates may be needed to further stabilise the comminuted fracture segments. Generally, fixation is done with 1.0-mm, 1.3-mm, 1.5-mm and 2.0-mm miniplates.

MANAGEMENT OF TYPE I FRACTURE

The Type I fractures are noncomminuted with intact MCL attachment and larger fracture segments. They are managed by open reduction and fixation, varying from 1, 2 or 3-point fixation (Fig. 54.10A). The goal is to achieve proper positioning of the frontal process of the maxilla and the MCT.

After gaining exposure, the central fragment (bone to which the MCT is attached) is located and checked for the

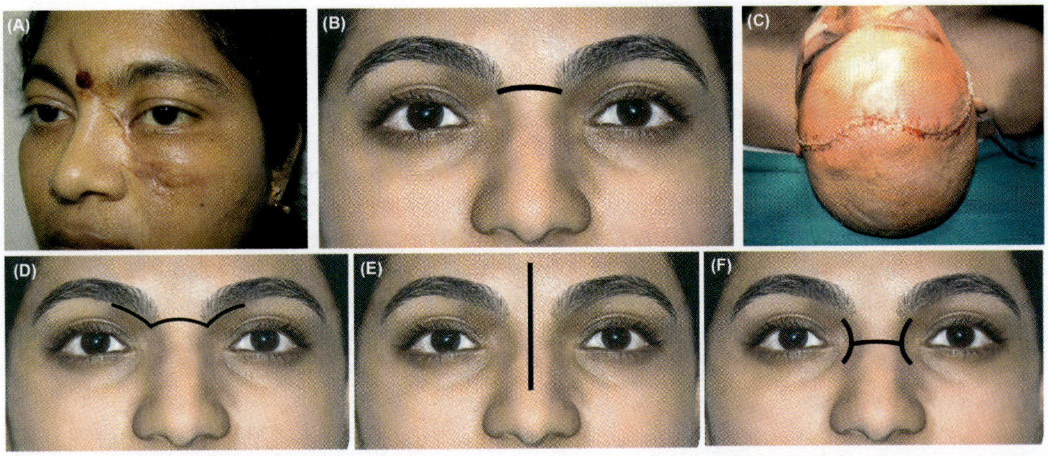

Figure 54.8 **(A)** Existing laceration. **(B)** Glabella incision. **(C)** Bicoronal incision. **(D)** Butterfly incision. **(E)** Vertical incision. **(F)** H-shaped incision.

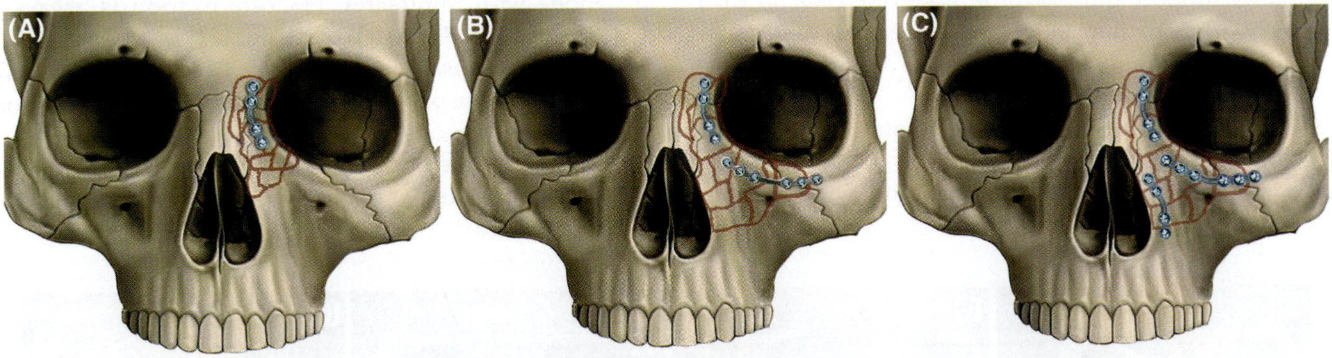

Figure 54.9 **(A)** One-point fixation. **(B)** Two-point fixation. **(C)** Three-point fixation.

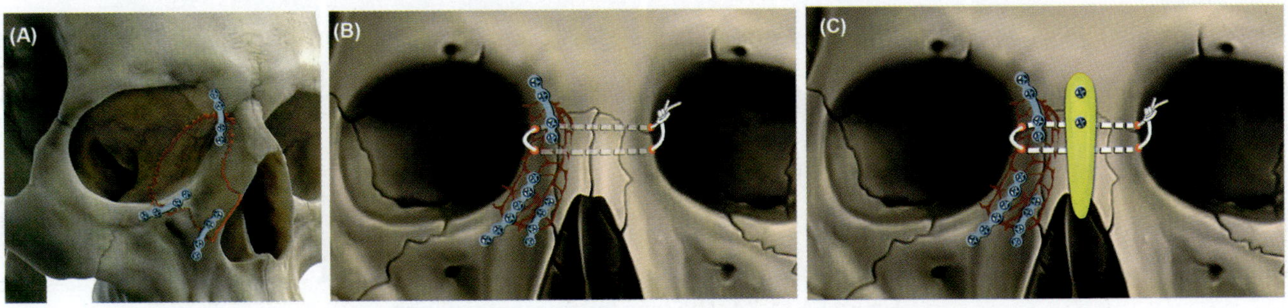

Figure 54.10 **(A)** Type I fracture fixation. **(B)** Type II fracture fixation. **(C)** Type III fracture fixation.

attachment of MCT and the supporting bony fragment. The bony fragment should be large enough to support direct plating (Table 54.2).

MANAGEMENT OF TYPE II FRACTURE

Type II fractures present with comminuted fracture fragments with intact MCT to the larger fragment. Type II fractures require open reduction and internal fixation (ORIF) with fixation at 2 or 3 points (Fig. 54.10B). In addition, transnasal wiring is needed for the stabilisation of the canthal-bearing segment.

MANAGEMENT OF TYPE III FRACTURE

Type III fractures involve extensive comminution of the osseous structure extending into the canthal tendon insertion or with an avulsed MCT. These fractures are difficult to reduce due to the small fracture fragments as well as poor direct access, requiring multiple surgical approaches. It can

TABLE 54.2 Management of NOE Fractures Based on the Type of Fracture

Type I	Type II	Type III
1, 2 or 3-point fixation	• 2 or 3-point fixation • Transnasal wiring	• 3-point exposure and fixation • Transnasal canthopexy • Bone grafts for nasal reconstruction • Lacrimal apparatus repair • Rule out Cerebrospinal fluid (CSF) leak and eye injuries

be managed by 3-point fixation with additional plates for further stabilisation of the comminuted fragments, transnasal wiring to stabilise the MCT and bone grafts to reestablish dorsal nasal support and nasal tip projection (Fig. 54.10C). Any soft tissue distortion should be corrected as well.

TRANSNASAL WIRING/CANTHOPEXY

When attempting to reposition the MCT, one of the methods that is utilised most frequently is known as transnasal wiring. It is recommended for fractures of Type I and Type II. During this procedure, a stainless steel wire is threaded through a hole that has been made in the fracture fragment that contains the MCT. The wire is then retrieved on the contralateral side, where it stabilises the fracture fragment by attaching it to the contralateral nasal bone or the contralateral MCL.

The steps involved in conventional transnasal wiring are (Figs. 54.11 and 54.12) as follows:

1. The fracture fragment with MCT is held with a forceps and two holes are drilled 4 to 5 mm apart using a burr
2. An artery forceps is used to pass the wire ends through these holes
3. Holes are drilled on the contralateral side with the help of a burr, spinal needle or bone awl
4. The two ends of the wire from the fracture fragment are pulled out on the contralateral normal side
5. The fracture fragment containing the MCT is reduced and its position is rechecked
6. The reduced fragment is then stabilised to the frontal bone with miniplates. Fracture fixation is always performed prior to MCT securing
7. The transnasal wire is then secured to a screw on the frontal bone of the contralateral side
8. It is always recommended to position the MCT, superior and posterior to the lacrimal fossa in order to avoid any malpositioning of the MCT.

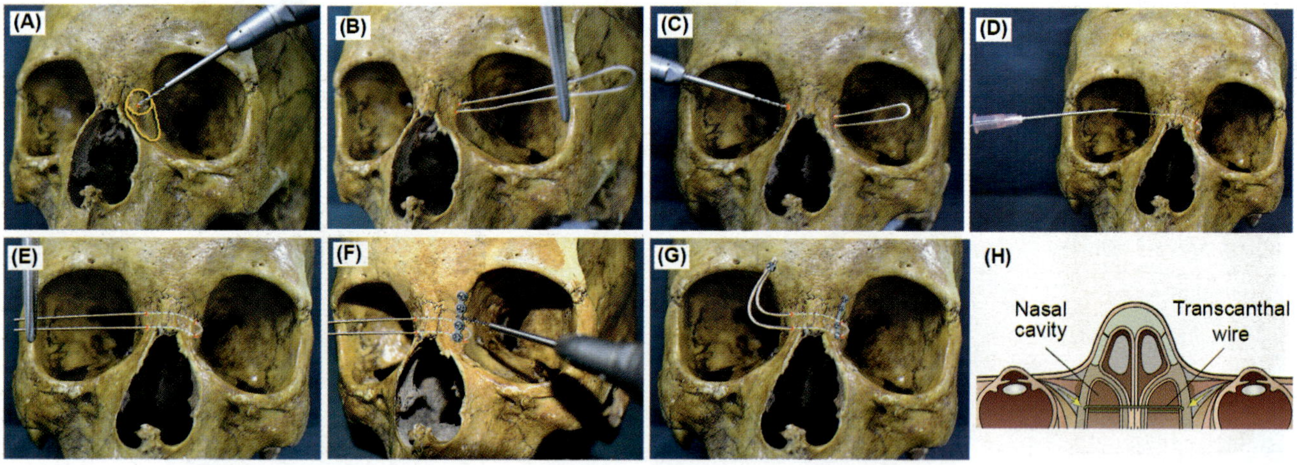

Figure 54.11 (**A–H**) Steps for transnasal wiring.

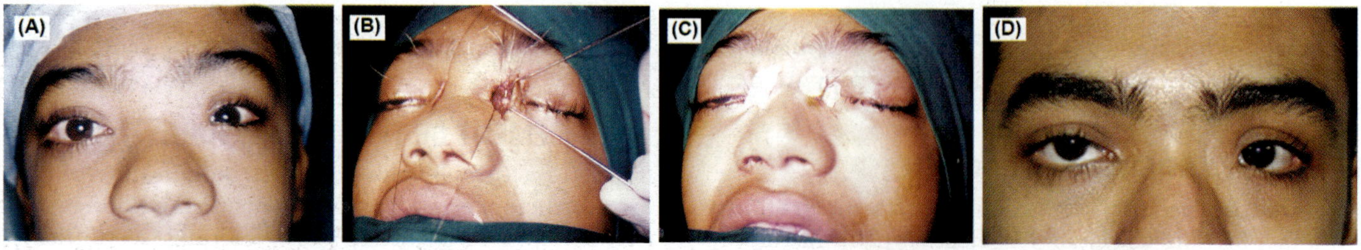

Figure 54.12 Transnasal wiring. (**A**) Preoperative view with telecanthus. (**B**) Transnasal wiring to reposition the left medial canthus. (**C**) Completed procedure with bolster dressing. (**D**) Postoperative view.

Disadvantages of the conventional transnasal wiring:

- An anterior migration of the medial canthus
- Deformation of the canthal bay
- Epiphora
- Inadequate reduction of the telecanthus
- Unnecessary involvement of the normal, unaffected medial orbital wall of the contralateral side.

OTHER METHODS TO STABILISE THE MEDIAL CANTHAL TENDON

- Figure of eight or modified Kessler's stitch using a 3-0 or 4-0 suture
- Anchor technique using a wire with barb or hook
- Miniplates (modified Y-plate).

Miniplate (modified Y-plate) (Fig. 54.13)

To overcome the disadvantages with conventional transnasal wiring, cantilevered *Y-plates* are used to reposition the displaced MCL. The Y-shaped miniplate is fixed on the lateral aspect of the nose, whose long arm is directed posteriorly into the orbit and the MCL is suspended to the long arm of the plate using 3-0 silk sutures or stainless-steel wires.

Y-plate facilitates in attaching the MCL more posteriorly to prevent anterior migration of the canthus.

Advantages of the cantilevered Y-plates

- Involves only the deformed side
- Acts as pseudolacrimal crest in comminuted fractures
- Provides a more anatomic, posteromedial attachment of the MCL
- Can also be used bilaterally
- Safe and simple method
- Can be combined with other grafts and fixations.

LACRIMAL SYSTEM MANAGEMENT

The lacrimal system is intimately related to the NOE region and is often affected in NOE fracture. The patency of the lacrimal system should be assessed at the time of surgical treatment. The lacrimal system damage is associated with the following symptoms:

- Epiphora
- Dacryocystitis
- Posttraumatic dacryostenosis
- Recurrent infections of the lacrimal pathways.

Epiphora—excessive watering of eyes due to obstruction of the nasolacrimal duct. It can be managed by lacrimal stenting or dacryocystorhinostomy (DCR). *Lacrimal stenting* is placing a plastic stent through the punctum and retrieving it from the nose. Stenting of the duct can be done using fine bore polyethylene or silicone tube (Fig. 54.14). *DCR* is a bypass procedure that creates an anastomosis between the lacrimal sac and the nasal mucosa via a bony ostium.

EPICANTHUS FOLD MANAGEMENT

Epicanthus or epicanthal fold is an abnormal skin fold at the medial canthus. It occurs with telecanthus in NOE fractures. The following are the techniques to correct the epicanthal fold:

- Z-plasty (Fig. 54.15)
- Y-V plasty
- Modified V-Y plasty
- V-W plasty.

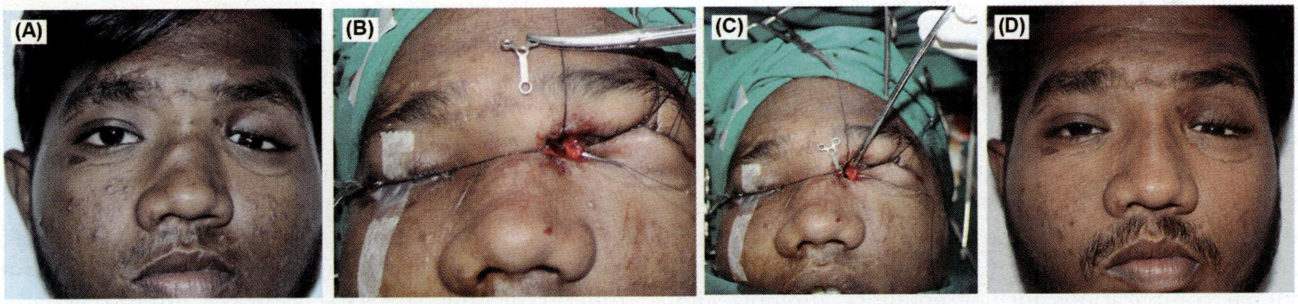

Figure 54.13 Canthopexy with Y-plate. (**A**) Preoperative view with telecanthus. (**B** and **C**) Securing of MCL to the Y-plate. (**D**) Postoperative view.

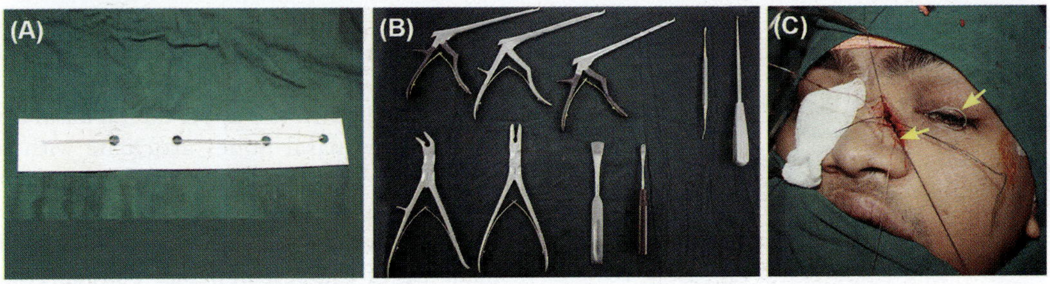

Figure 54.14 (**A**) Lacrimal stent. (**B**) Instruments required for stenting. (**C**) Intraoperative view of placing a plastic stent.

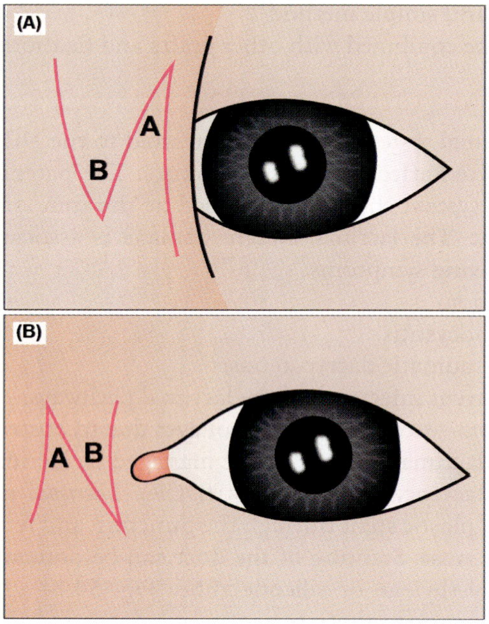

Figure 54.15 Z-plasty. (**A**) Marking of incision. (**B**) After Z-plasty.

SOFT TISSUE READAPTATION

Postoperatively, nasal bolster splint is required to reduce postoperative swelling and haematoma formation. It also helps to redrape the soft tissue to the underlying skeletal framework and prevents pseudotelecanthus. Bolsters are placed over the medial canthal region and should be retained for 1 to 2 weeks (Fig. 54.16). Inappropriate placement of the bolster can lead to skin necrosis. Intranasal packing can be used to keep the comminuted fragments stable while also controlling haemorrhage.

COMPLICATIONS OF NASO-ORBITO-ETHMOID COMPLEX FRACTURE

Incomplete management of the NOE complex fractures results in aesthetic as well as functional complications. The aesthetic complications include persistent telecanthus or depressed nasal bridge, which are difficult to correct secondarily. Hence, these should be addressed at the initial surgery. Functional complications include epiphora, diplopia and anosmia.

- Epiphora
- Persistent telecanthus

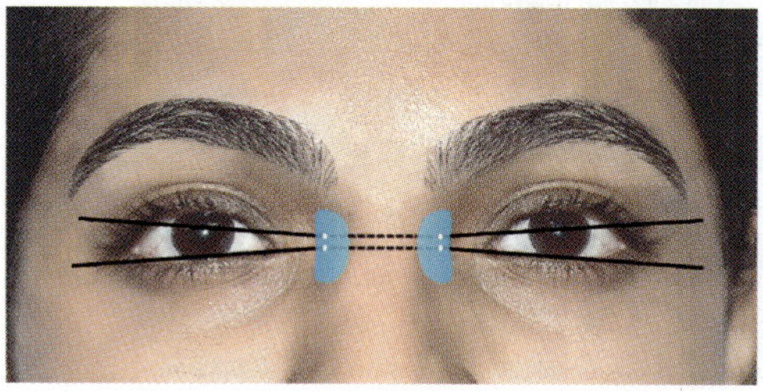
Figure 54.16 Bolster dressing placed over the medial canthal region.

- Nasal deformity
- Shortened palpebral fissure
- Unsightly scarring
- Enophthalmos and ocular dystopia
- Nasolacrimal injuries
- CSF leak and anosmia
- Meningitis
- Wound infection.

NASAL BONE FRACTURE

INTRODUCTION

Nose is the most exposed and prominent area of the face. Nasal bone is important for normal respiration, speech and smell perception. It is the most prominent feature of the face and is a distinguishing trait.

Nasal injuries are the commonest of the facial bone fractures due to its prominent positioning, relatively thin bone and comparatively smaller amount of force required to fracture it compared to other facial bones. They are more common in males when compared to females. Children are more protected from nasal fractures due to the greater cartilaginous portions of the nose than in adults. The major cause of nasal bone fractures are athletic injuries, interpersonal violence, falls and motor vehicle accidents.

Nasal injuries are not life threatening, but subsequently lead to aesthetic and functional deformities. Hence, management of nasal bone fractures should be aimed at optimising function and restoring aesthetics.

ANATOMY OF THE NASAL COMPLEX

The nasal bone is roughly pyramidal in shape and is composed of osseous and cartilaginous structures that support the skin, muscle, mucosa, nerves and vascular structures.

Osseous framework—it consists of nasal bones and nasal septum joined at the midline.

Cartilaginous framework—it consists of the lateral nasal cartilage, major alar cartilage, minor alar cartilage and cartilaginous portions of septum.

The ***nasal bones*** are rectangular bones that articulate with each other in the midline in the shape of a tent with the septum on the undersurface (Fig. 54.17A and B). They are thick and widest at the nasofrontal suture and thinner inferiorly below the intercanthal line. The nasal bones articulate:

- Superiorly with the frontal bone at the frontonasal suture
- Laterally with the frontal process of the maxilla at the nasomaxillary suture
- Inferiorly with the upper lateral nasal cartilages
- Medially, nasal bones articulate with its fellow of the opposite side at the internasal suture, which sits on the nasal septum.

The ***bony nasal septum*** is in the midline of the nose and is made up of the perpendicular plate of ethmoid and vomer bone posterosuperiorly, cartilaginous septum anteroinferiorly

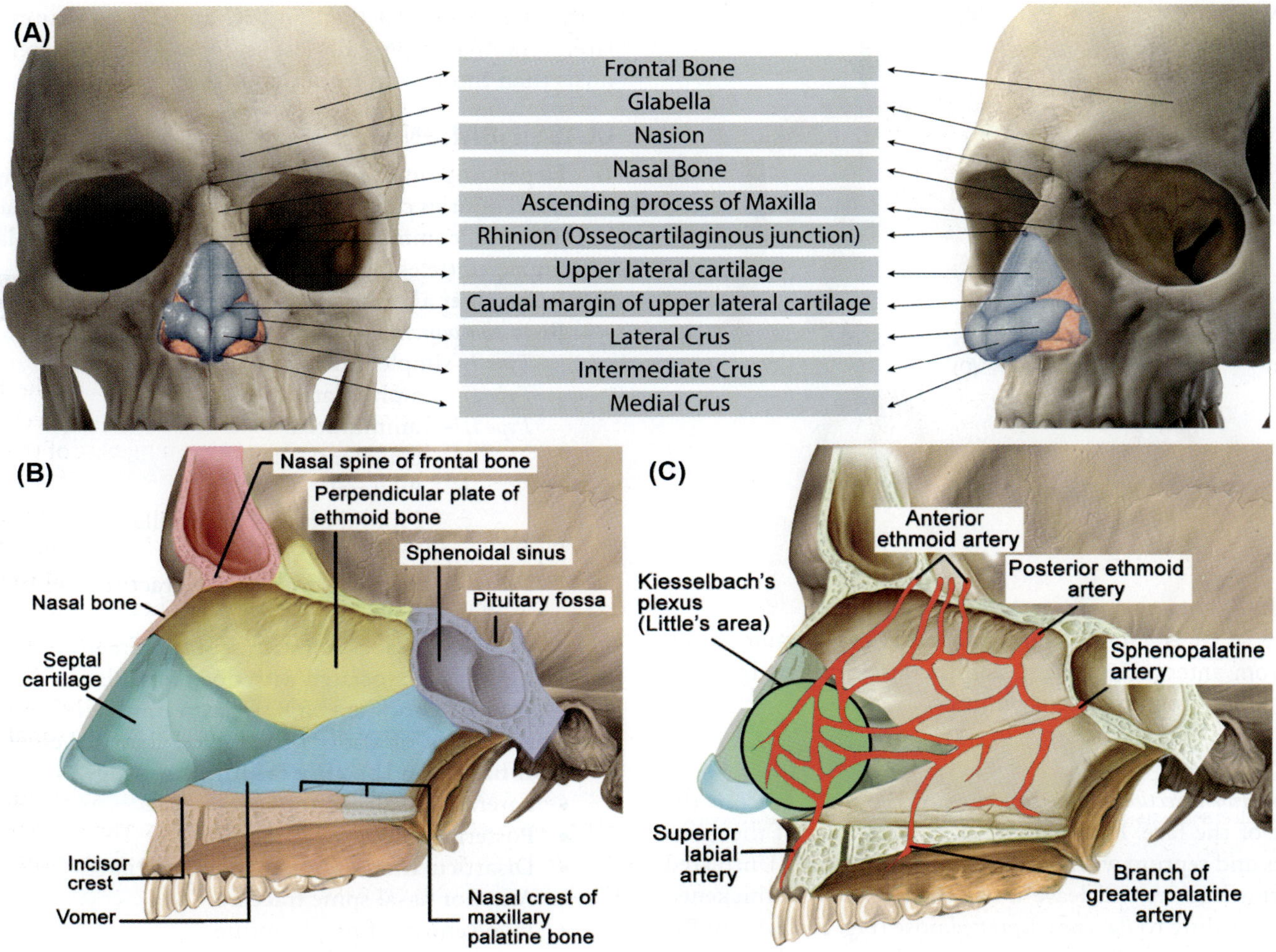

Figure 54.17 (**A**) Bony and cartilaginous structures of the nose. (**B**) Anatomy of nasal septum. (**C**) Kiesselbach's plexus.

and the vomer posteroinferiorly. The nasal septum provides the primary support to the nasal complex and separates the nasal cavity into two chambers (Fig. 54.17C).

The inferior portion of the nasal bone forms a 'lap joint' with the upper lateral cartilage of about 7–11 mm, made of solid fibrous union, which is referred to as the ***'Keystone' region***. Cottle's 'keystone' or K-area refers to the structural integrity of the nasal bones and upper lateral cartilage.

The lateral nasal cartilage is triangular and attached to the nasal bone superiorly and to the lateral crus of the major alar cartilage inferiorly.

The *major alar cartilages* are bilobed structures composed of *medial and lateral crura* with an intervening middle segment (intermediate crus) that plays an important role in the definition of the nasal tip. It lies below the upper lateral cartilage.

The inferior portion of the *cartilaginous part of the septum* (quadrilateral cartilage) lies in a bony groove at the nasal spine. The thick cartilaginous septum supports the majority of the nasal tip and prevents septal fractures.

The internal and external carotid arteries provide vascular supply to the nasal complex. The ophthalmic artery branch of the internal carotid supplies to both the internal nose via the anterior and posterior ethmoid vessels, and to the outer nose from the dorsal nasal artery and the external nasal artery.

The external carotid artery (ECA) provides the primary vasculature to the outer nose through the infraorbital, superior labial and angular arteries.

Kiesselbach's area or Little's area or Kiesselbach's triangle is a vascular network of five arteries that anastomose to form a plexus (Fig. 54.17D). It is located in the anterior nasal cavity and is the most common site of nasal bleed during fractures. The arteries involved are the following:

- Septal branch of superior labial artery
- Anterior ethmoidal artery
- Sphenopalatine artery
- Greater palatine artery
- Posterior ethmoidal artery.

Innervation to the nasal complex is primarily through the maxillary branch of trigeminal nerve.

FRACTURE PATTERN

The pattern of nasal bone fractures depends on variables such as the force, impact direction (anterior or lateral), nature of the striking object, patient's age and other host factors.

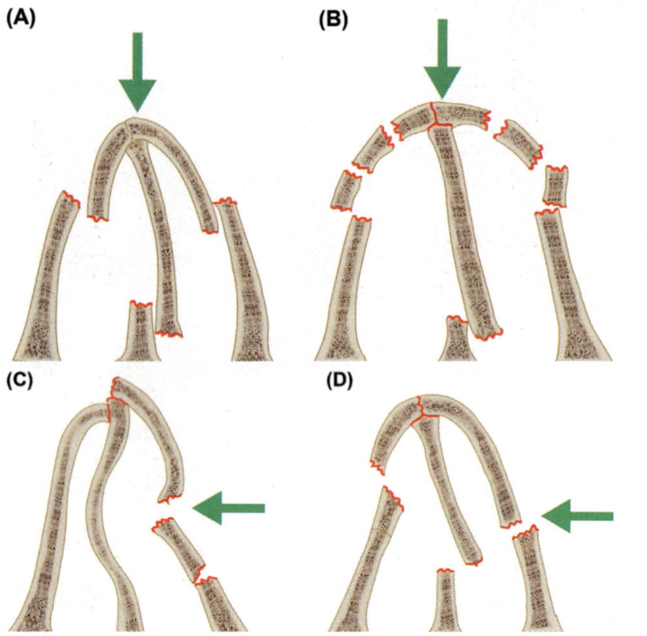

Figure 54.18 Fracture pattern. (**A** and **B**) Nasal fracture resulting from anterior impact. (**C** and **D**) Nasal fracture resulting from forces from the lateral direction.

Anterior direction: The direction of the force is from the front of the face. It results in severe flattening of the nasal bones and septum with flaring of the nasal width. Untreated anterior injuries will leave a flattened nose with thickened bridge leading to *flattened depressed* nose (Fig. 54.18A and B).

Lateral direction: The force is directed from the lateral side of face. They induce fracture and sinking of the ipsilateral nasal bone and septal fracture leading to deviation of the nasal pyramid. Untreated lateral types of injuries result in *deviation of the* nose to one side with probably a blockage of both nares (nostrils) (Fig. 54.18C and D). Fractures from lateral trauma are typically less severe and have a better prognosis than those from frontal injuries.

CLASSIFICATION

1. Depending on the trauma and individual anatomy, the nasal injuries can be of different types such as unilateral, bilateral, comminuted, depressed, open-book (splayed), impacted (telescoped) and greenstick (Fig. 54.19)
2. **Rohrich et al., (2000):**
   Bony component:
   Type I—simple unilateral
   Type II—simple bilateral
   Type III—comminuted:
      a. Unilateral
      b. Bilateral
      c. Frontal process of maxilla
   Septal component:
   Type IV—complex (nasal bone fractures with septal disruption):
      a. Associated with septal haematoma
      b. Associated with open nasal laceration
   Type V—associated NOE fracture/midface fracture
3. **Association of study of Internal fixation classification based on the clinical findings** (Fig. 54.20):
   - Laterally displaced fractures
   - Posteriorly depressed fractures
   - Disarticulation of upper lateral cartilage
   - Anterior nasal spine fracture
   - Involvement of nasal septum
4. **Based on the amount of impact**, the nasal bone fractures can be classified as:
   Class I: Low velocity trauma due to frontal or frontolateral force with a breach in the quadrilateral cartilage and displacement of the distal part of the nasal bone

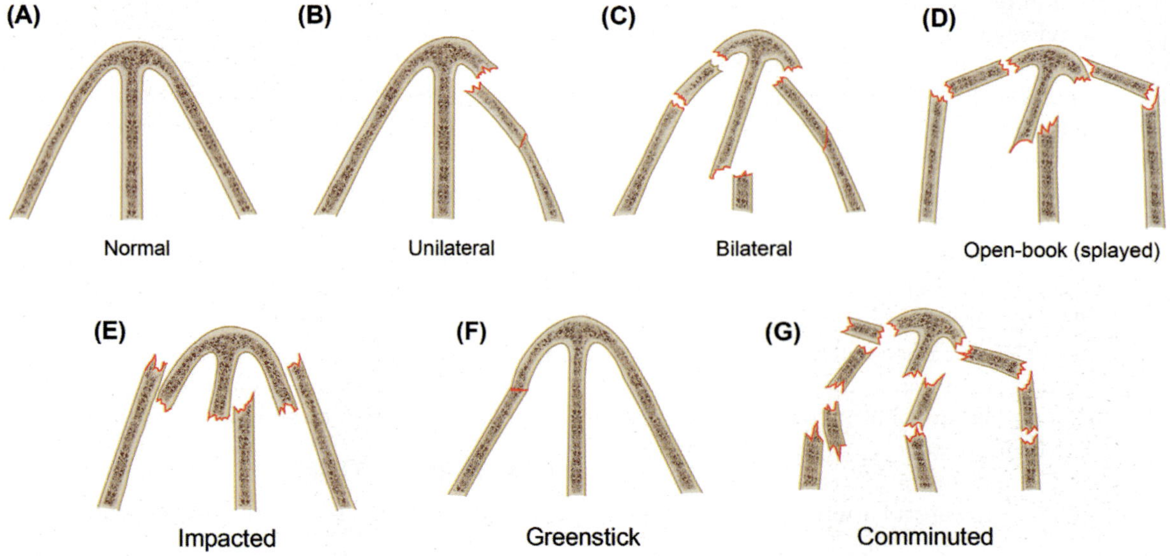

Figure 54.19 (**A–G**) Patterns of nasal bone fracture.

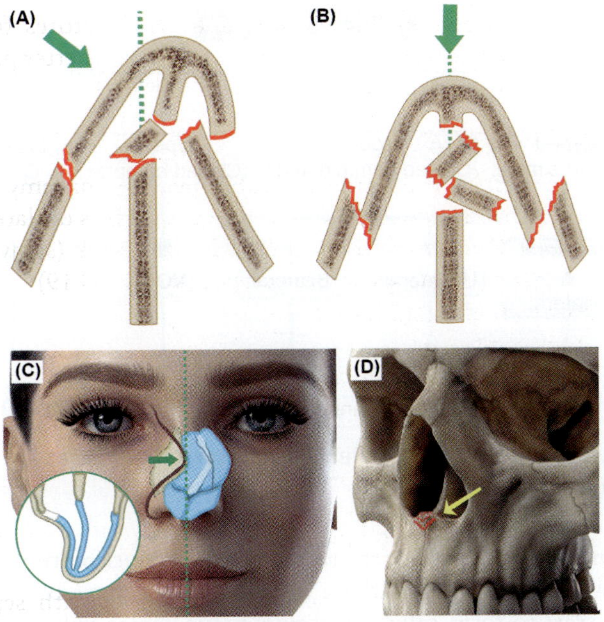

Figure 54.20 AO classification of nasal bone fracture. (**A**) Laterally displaced fractures. (**B**) Posteriorly depressed fractures. (**C**) Disarticulation of upper lateral cartilage. (**D**) Anterior nasal spine fracture.

Class II: Medium velocity lateral trauma with a breach in the root of the nasal bone and maxillary process of the frontal bone. The ethmoid labyrinth is intact

Class III: High velocity trauma. Fracture extends to the ethmoid labyrinth. Injury to the lacrimal sac and nasolacrimal duct may also be present.

RADIOGRAPHIC EVALUATION

Plain radiographic films, such as the lateral and Waters view, might be sufficient for determining the extent and displacement of nasal bone fractures; however, since the development of CT scans, plain radiographs have become less common in medical practice. CT scans are more helpful in providing complete visualisation and accurate details than other imaging methods (Fig. 54.21).

CLINICAL FEATURES

A detailed history and clinical examination are necessary to distinguish between the isolated nasal fractures and those associated with other injuries (Fig. 54.22). *History* should include the following:

- The mechanism and timing of injury
- Prior nasal trauma/surgery
- Brain injury symptoms
- Pretraumatic photographs.

Clinical signs and symptoms (Fig. 54.23)

- Pain and swelling of nasal region
- Flattening or other deformation of the shape of nose
- Widening of the nasal base.
- Crepitus—the crackling heard when broken bones are moved
- Saddle type depression of the nose
- A step-deformity may be palpated
- Anosmia.

Intranasally

- Septal haematomas
- Septal deviation

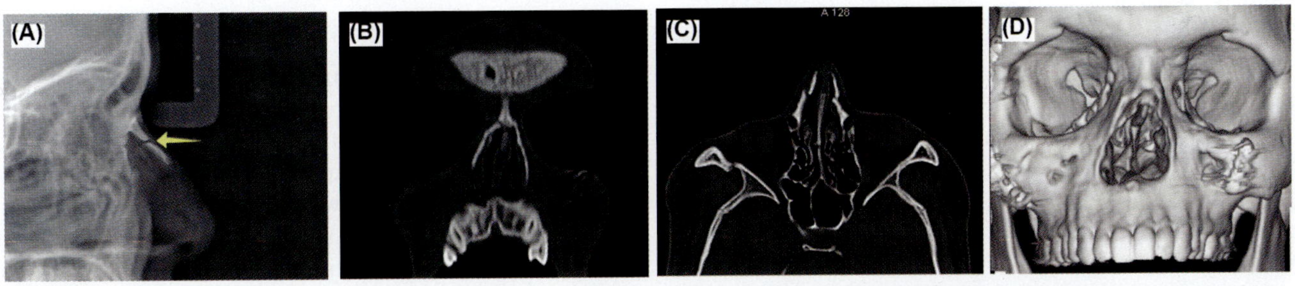

Figure 54.21 Various views showing nasal fracture. (**A**) Lateral skull. (**B–D**) CT scan (coronal, axial and 3D reconstruction).

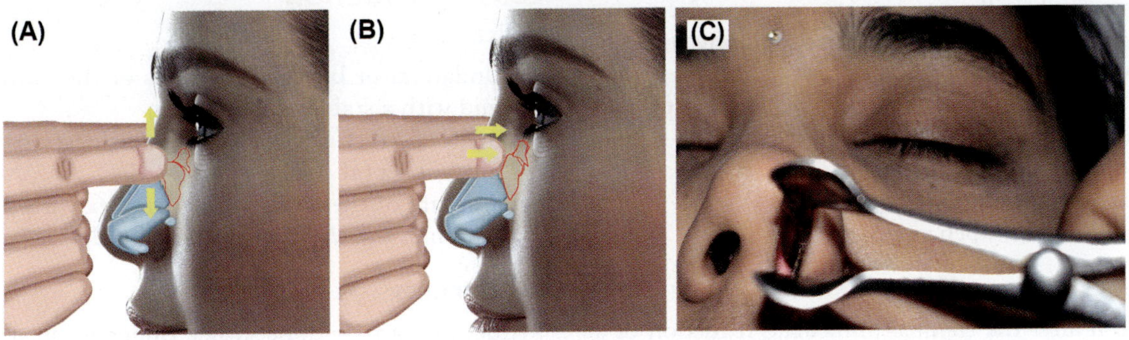

Figure 54.22 (**A** and **B**) Clinical examination of nose through bimanual digital palpation. (**C**) Intranasal examination using a nasal speculum.

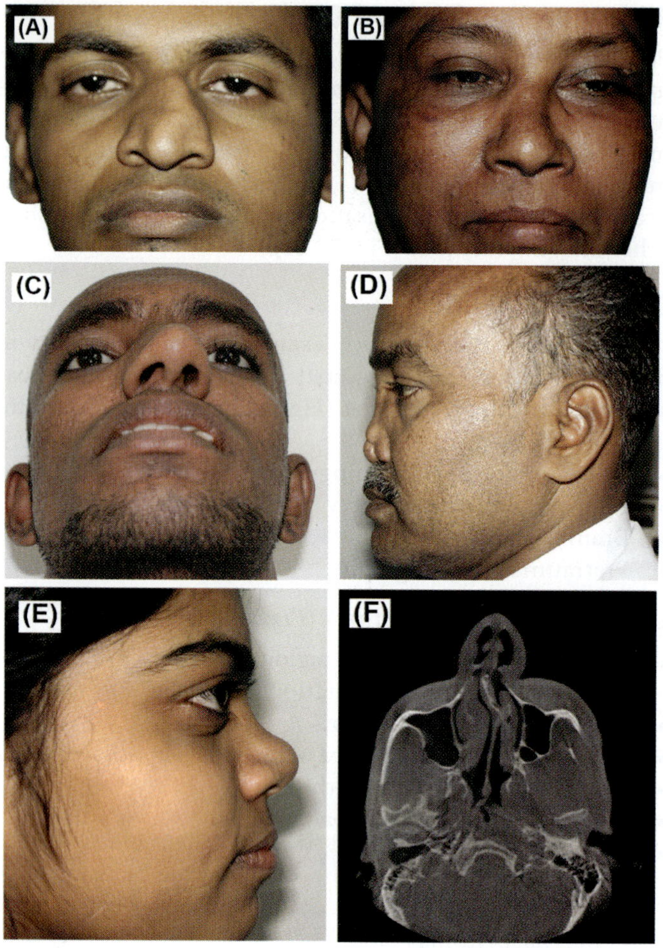

Figure 54.23 (**A**) Deformed nosed. (**B**) Nasal deviation. (**C**) Septal deviation. (**D**) Flattening of the nasal tip. (**E**) Saddle nose deformity. (**F**) Synechiae.

- Mucosal lacerations
- Epistaxis or bleeding from the nose
- CSF leaks
- Airway blockage.

MANAGEMENT

The goals of management of nasal bony injuries are to prevent the development of a posttraumatic nasal deformity, to restore proper nasal air flow, to prevent cosmetic deformity and to maintain proper nasal complex topography and projection (Flowchart 54.1).

There are three major aspects to be considered in providing appropriate treatment for nasal bone fractures:

A. Timing of surgery
B. Choice of appropriate anaesthesia
C. Surgical technique (open vs closed).

Timing of surgery

In the 1st 3–6 h after the trauma, immediate reduction of a fractured nose is recommended in order to prevent significant oedema from setting in. For nasal fractures ranging from mild

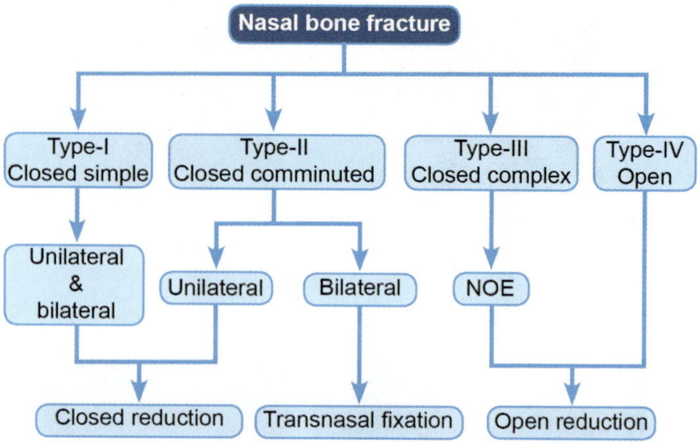

Flowchart 54.1 Management of nasal fractures based on the type of fracture.

to moderate in severity, the recommended reduction timing is between 5 and 7 days. After a week has passed, the adult bone will start to form callus or fibrous tissue, which will make it difficult to treat with closed reduction.

Choice of anaesthesia

Management of nasal fractures can be done with local anaesthesia, conscious sedation or general anaesthesia. Many authors have suggested that local anaesthesia is an effective, economical and well-tolerated treatment option for closed reduction of nasal fractures in adults. Paediatric patients and uncooperative patients are preferred to be treated with conscious sedation or general anesthesia. However, the most efficient method, and perhaps the most comfortable route, is to perform the repair under general anaesthesia.

Closed or open reduction

Reduction of nasal fractures can be done either by open or closed technique. Closed reduction is preferable for acute, simple and noncomminuted cases, and it is effective, safe and successful in the majority of cases. Open reduction is reserved for severe cases with significant nasal obstruction, septal deviation, loss of nasal septal support or fractures associated with other injuries that cannot be adequately reduced by closed reduction.

CLOSED REDUCTION

Indications

- Unilateral or bilateral fractures of the bony nasal pyramid with a stable nasal dorsum
- Bilateral fractures with minor dislocation without significant septal changes
- Fracture of the nasal septal complex with deviation less than half the width of the nasal bridge.

Instruments

Reduction can be done either under local anaesthesia or general anaesthesia using ***Walsham's and Asch's septal forceps*** (Fig. 54.24).

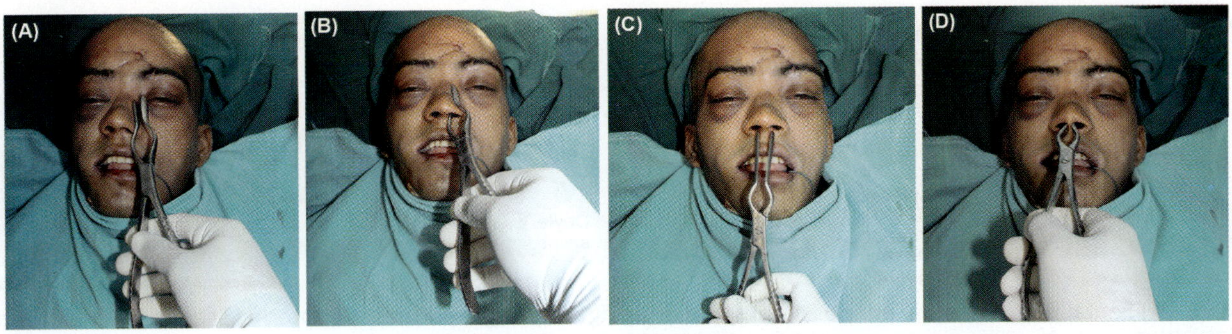

Figure 54.24 (**A** and **B**) Reduction of nasal bones using Walsham's forceps. (**C** and **D**) Reduction of nasal septum with Asch's forceps.

Technique

After inducing anaesthesia, the ***nasal bones are reduced*** into the midline position by using elevators and forceps. The unpadded blade of the Walsham's forceps is inserted into the nasal cavity underneath the nasal bones and the other padded blade is placed externally over the skin. The fractured fragments are secured between the blades, disimpacted and repositioned into their correct position by applying force.

For the *reduction of septal* fractures, Asch's forceps may be introduced with one blade in each nostril engaging the septum on either side reducing the fractured segment. Sometimes the cartilaginous septum may be dislocated from its anatomic position in the maxillary central groove. The septal cartilage can be grasped and repositioned into its groove. The lacrimal bones and the medial wall of the orbit on each side are compressed using digital pressure to reinstate the narrow bridge of the nose.

Majority of the nasal fractures treated with closed reduction require external stabilisation (nasal splints) with or without internal nasal packing. External nasal splints are removed in 7 to 10 days and internal nasal packs are usually removed after 1 to 3 days of surgery (Fig. 54.25).

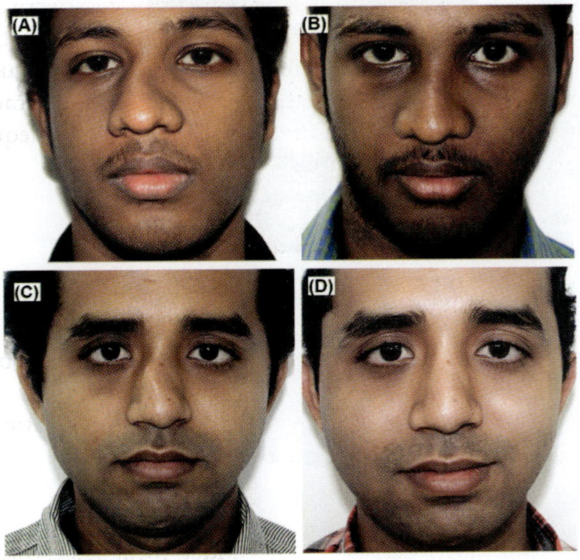

Figure 54.25 Preoperative (**A** and **C**) and postoperative (**B** and **D**) pictures of nasal reduction by closed technique.

OPEN REDUCTION

The open method allows for direct visualisation and precise reapproximation of the dislocated and fractured structures. Most of the open procedures are done when the nasal fracture is coupled with other fractures, and fractures that cannot be reduced by closed technique.

Indications

- Open/severe septal injuries
- Extensive fracture dislocation of nasal bones
- Deviation of the nasal pyramid greater than one half width of the nasal bridge
- Persistent deformity after closed reduction
- Severe loss of nasal support
- Associated orbital wall or ethmoid bone fractures
- Fractures presented 3 weeks or longer after injury.

Surgical approaches

There are various approaches to the reduction of nasal bones, which include the following:

- Existing laceration
- Coronal approach
- External rhinoplasty
- Transfixion incision.

Most commonly used approaches are through the bicoronal incision and through the existing laceration. Transfixion or hemitransfixion incisions are preferred for visualising and accessing the inferior and posterior septum.

Technique

After obtaining adequate access and exposure to the fractured segments, the septum and the nasal bones are reduced. The septum is considered as a crucial component in nasal fracture repair. The septum is commonly approached through a hemitransfixion incision on the side of dislocation and a mucoperichondrial flap is elevated.

The *displaced septum* is repositioned and fixed to the anterior nasal spine with a permanent suture or wires. For a *fractured and unstable septum*, an internal splint (Doyle/Silastic) is implanted and modified on the side of the septum and sutured.

The nasal bones are reduced using elevators, and if necessary, osteotomies are performed to facilitate reduction

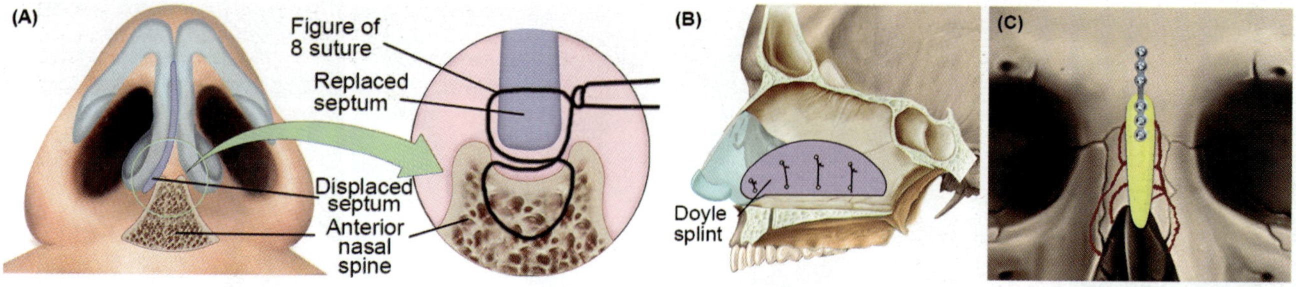

Figure 54.26 (**A**) Septal fixation to the anterior nasal spine using figure of eight sutures. (**B**) Internal silastic splint (Doyle's splint). (**C**) Bone or cartilage grafting.

of the fracture. The fixation of nasal fractures can be done using microplates, miniplates, absorbable plates and fibrin glue. In severe comminuted cases, bone grafts are required to reestablish nasal bone projection and nasal length (Fig. 54.26). Most commonly used grafts are split calvarial, rib, iliac and ear grafts.

METHODS OF IMMOBILISATION

Nasal pack and splints are required to maintain the stability of the comminuted fragments and prevent inward collapse of the bony fragments. Nasal packs also aid in controlling bleeding and prevents haematoma formation. Nasal splints can be (1) external splint or (2) internal splint (Table 54.3).

External splints are placed over the patient's nose (Fig. 54.27A–C).

Uses:

- It provides support and protection to the reduced bones
- Helps in adherence of skin to the underlying structures of the nose
- Elimination of dead space
- Reduces the overlying soft tissue oedema
- The plaster of Paris (POP) splint is the most widely used extranasal splint. It consists of eight layers of POP bandage that are sliced to create a strip of plaster across the bridge on either side of the nose along with

TABLE 54.3 Types of Nasal Splints

External Splints	Internal Splints
• Plaster of Paris (POP) • Thermoplastic splints • Collodium gauge and soft metal sheet • Polyvinyl siloxane • Aluminium nasal splints • Adhesive tapes/ Steri-Strips • Denver splint set	• Ribbon gauze with paraffin • Silastic splints • Silicone splint (Fig. 54.28) • Doyle's nasal splint • Bivalve nasal splint • Nasal elliptical septal button • Nasopore

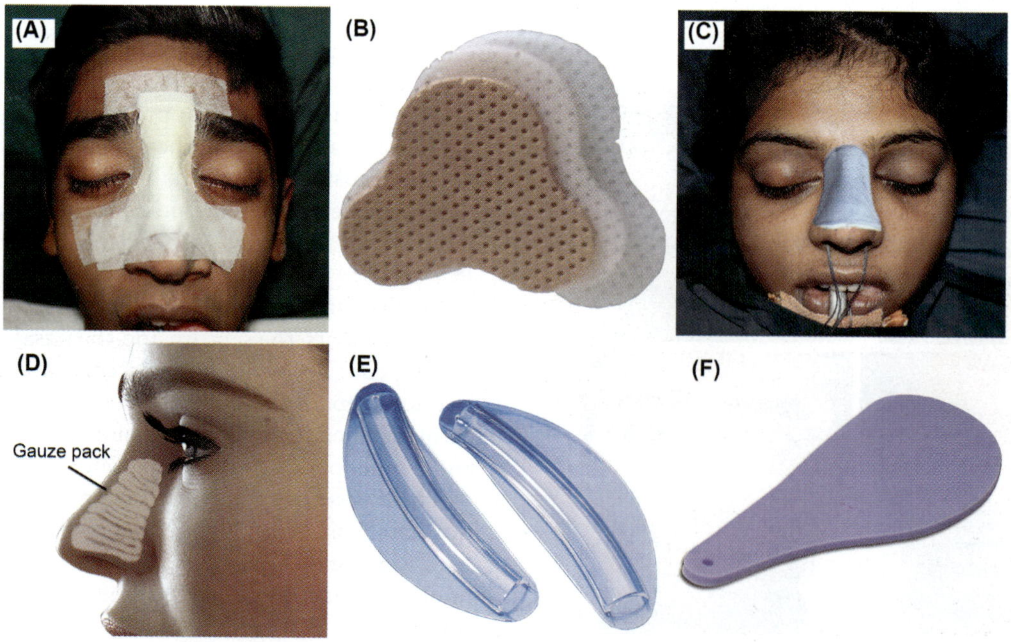

Figure 54.27 (**A–C**) External splints—plaster of Paris, thermoplastic splints and polyvinyl siloxane, respectively. (**D–F**) Internal splints—ribbon gauze pack, Doyle's nasal splint and silicone nasal splint.

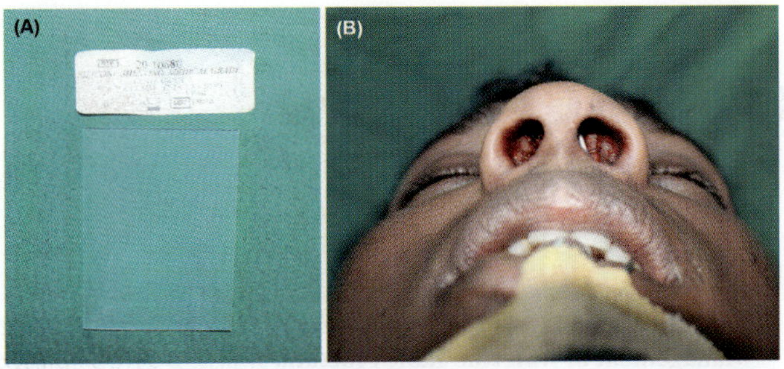

Figure 54.28 (**A**) Silicone sheet for intranasal splint. (**B**) Intranasal splinting with silicone sheet to support the septum.

frontal extension. This bandage should be applied when the POP is still wet and molded to the shape of the nose. The splint should not extend onto the soft part of the nose. The nasal splint is held in position by surgical tape externally. It should remain in position for 1 week. Antibiotic-impregnated gauze packing can be retained in each nostril for 1–5 days, depending on the mobility of the segments and the amount of bleeding.

Intranasal packing is placed inside the nostrils and should be placed prior to the external splint (Figs. 54.27D–F and 54.28).

Uses:

- It supports the septum and prevents synechiae formation
- It provides support to the fractured fragments and prevents their inward collapse.

Disadvantages:

- Inadequate anteroposterior support
- Difficulty in breathing through the nose
- Potential source of infection.

Use of ribbon gauze is the most standard method of providing intranasal support. Ribbon gauze of 12–15 cm length is taken and inserted into the nose in layers beginning from above downwards. Overpacking of the nose causes displacement of the reduced fractured segments.

TABLE 54.4 Complications of Nasal Fractures

Early Complications	Late Complications
• Epistaxis • Septal haematoma • CSF rhinorrhoea	• Nasal obstruction • Nasolacrimal duct injury • Avascular necrosis of nasal septal cartilage • Secondary nasal deformity • Saddle nose deformity • Synechiae (adhesion) • Septal perforation • Malunion

COMPLICATIONS OF NASAL FRACTURE

Problems arising from nasal fracture complications should be adequately recognised and treated (Table 54.4).

Septal haematoma is caused by collection of blood underneath the perichondrial layer of the nasal septum. It presents as a swelling and erythema in the dorsum, columella and nasal tip region, usually within the 1st 24–72 h and results in partial nasal obstruction. It is managed by *incision and drainage* and should be performed urgently under local or general anaesthesia (Fig. 54.29). Localised unilateral septal haematomas can be aspirated with a needle.

Epistaxis is another complication associated with nasal fractures. Haemostasis can be achieved by:

- Manual pressure for 10–20 min
- Chemical cautery with silver nitrate
- Local haemostatic agents
- Nasal packs.

CSF rhinorrhoea indicates fractures involving the posterior wall of frontal sinus or the cribriform plate. **Synechiae** are adhesions formed between the septum and the nasal mucosa.

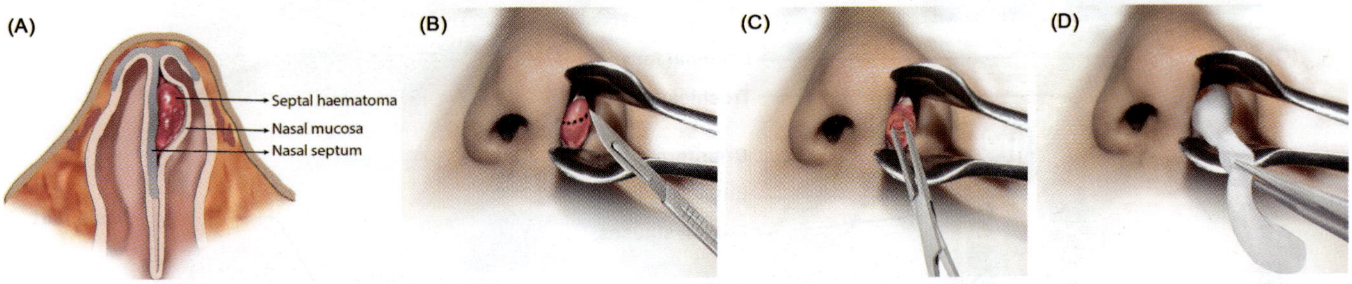

Figure 54.29 Incision and drainage of septal haematoma. (**A**) Septal haematoma. (**B**) Incision placed over the haematoma. (**C**) Drainage of haematoma. (**D**) Gauze pack in place.

Chapter 55

Frontal Bone Fractures

OUTLINE

INTRODUCTION

Fractures of frontal sinus are frequently associated with orbital, Naso-Orbito-Ethmoid (NOE), nasal and anterior cranial fossa injury. High-velocity automobile accidents and assaults are by far the most leading triggers of frontal sinus fractures. Because of the close proximity of the sinus to the brain, the trauma can be potentially fatal. Inappropriate treatment of frontal sinus fractures can culminate in sinusitis, brain abscess, encephalitis, etc.

APPLIED ANATOMY

The ***frontal bone*** forms the anterior part of the cranium, enclosing the brain. It is divided into two halves at birth, which generally fuses along the metopic suture by the end of 4th year of life. It articulates with 12 other cranial bones: 2 parietal bones, 2 zygomatic bone, 2 lacrimal bone, 2 maxillary bone, 2 nasal, the sphenoid and the ethmoid bone. A large vertical squamous portion and a horizontal orbital portion constitutes the frontal bone (Fig. 55.1).

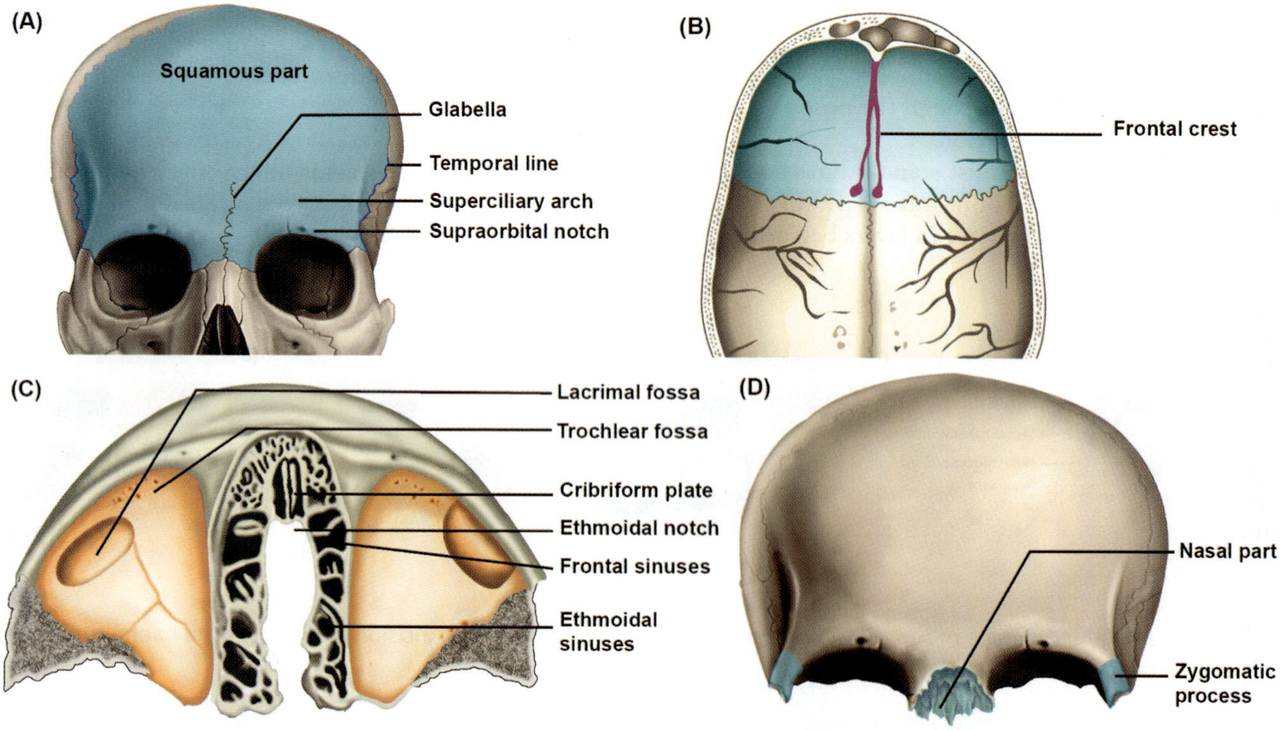

Figure 55.1 Parts of frontal bone. (**A**) Squamous part—external surface. (**B**) Squamous part—internal surface. (**C**) Orbital plates. (**D**) Nasal part and zygomatic process.

The ***squamous portion*** has a convex outer surface and forms the majority of forehead (Fig. 55.1A). It is composed of 2 layers of compact bone separated by cancellous bone (the diploe). The frontal sinus is located in the anterior region of the squamous frontal bone. The frontal eminence, superciliary arch and supraorbital borders are discernible on the outer surface. The anterior cranial fossa is formed by the concave inner surface (Fig. 55.1B). The nasal notch of the squamous part articulates with the nasal bone in the midline (Fig. 55.1C) and laterally with the zygomatic process of maxilla (Fig. 55.1C). At the supraorbital margin, the lower part of the squamous area continues with the orbital portion (Fig. 55.1D).

The ***orbital portion*** is a triangular curved plate of bone that extends horizontally backwards from the supraorbital margin, and forms the majority of the orbital roof and floor of anterior cranial fossa. The ethmoid notch is a median space between the two orbital plates that separates them. The ethmoid notch is filled by the cribriform plate of ethmoid bone (Fig. 55.1D).

The ***arterial supply*** to the frontal bone is by the supraorbital, anterior superficial temporal, anterior cerebral and middle meningeal arteries. The venous drainage is through the superficial temporal, supratrochlear, supraorbital, superior ophthalmic, frontal diploic and superior sagittal sinuses. The trigeminal nerve, specifically the supraorbital and supratrochlear nerves of the ophthalmic nerve, provides sensation to the forehead area.

The frontal bone has a *thick anterior table and a thinner posterior table*. The ***frontal sinus*** is located between the anterior and posterior tables (Fig. 55.2). The frontal sinus is a paired cavity in the frontal bone that communicates with the nasal cavity through the nasofrontal duct.

- The frontal sinus develops from one of these sites (primary pneumatisation): as a rudiment of ethmoid air cells, as an invagination of the frontal recess or from the superior middle meatus
- They are absent at birth, and secondary pneumatisation takes place between the age of 6 months and 2 years postnatally. It becomes well developed and can be identified radiographically by the age of 5–6 years. The pneumatisation is complete and the sinus reaches full size by around 12–16 years (Fig. 55.2)
- The intersinus septum divides the frontal sinus into right and left cavities, despite the fact that it appears to be a single sinus. Frontal sinus is of variable sizes and it may also be absent (agenesis) sometimes. The average dimensions of frontal sinus are as follows:
  a. Height: 32 mm
  b. Width: 26 mm
  c. Depth: 17 mm
  d. Surface area: 720 mm^2
- The *arterial supply* of the frontal sinus is by the supraorbital, supratrochlear and anterior ethmoidal artery, which are branches of the ophthalmic artery. Venous drainage is from the superior ophthalmic veins with additional drainage provided by the diploic veins and sagittal sinus

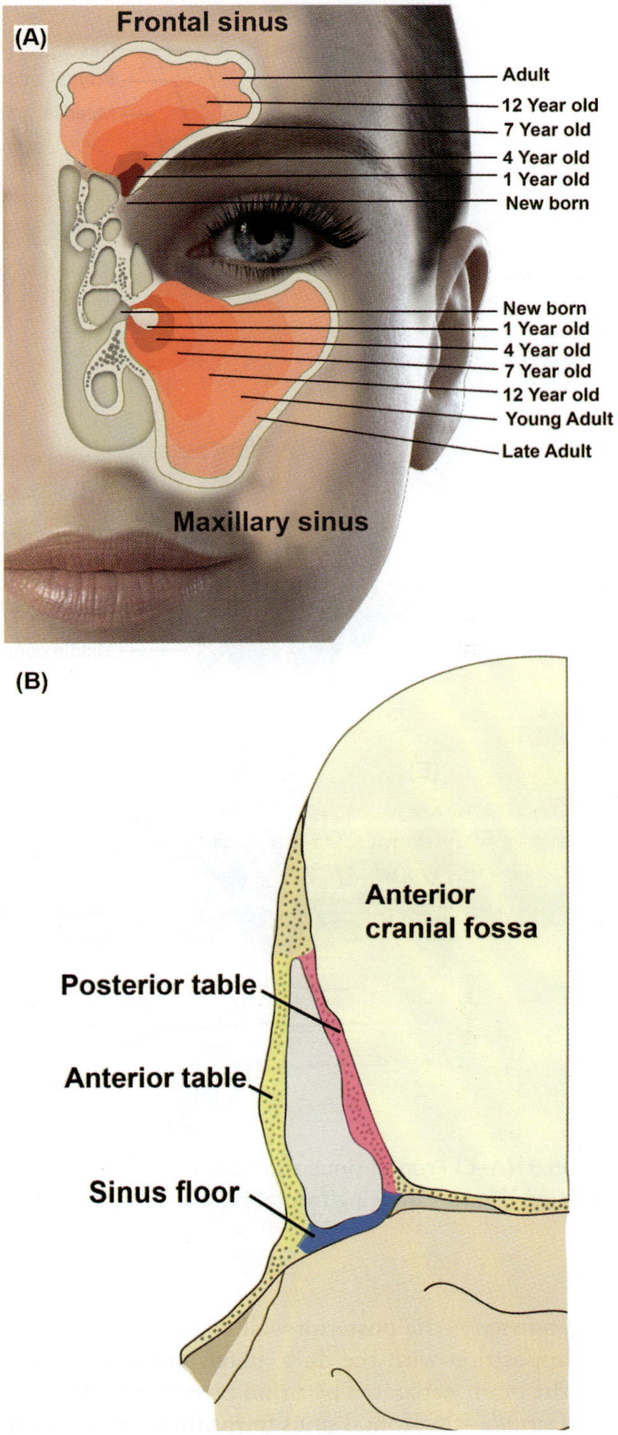

Figure 55.2 (**A**) Development of frontal sinus. (**B**) Lateral view of frontal sinus surrounded by a thick anterior table and thin posterior table with the floor of sinus forming the orbital roof.

- The frontal sinus is in close approximation to the anatomical structures, which is important in the management of its injury
  a. *Anteriorly*—it is guarded by the thick anterior table of frontal bone. The floor of sinus overlies the anterior ethmoidal sinus and nasal cavity (Fig. 55.3A and D)

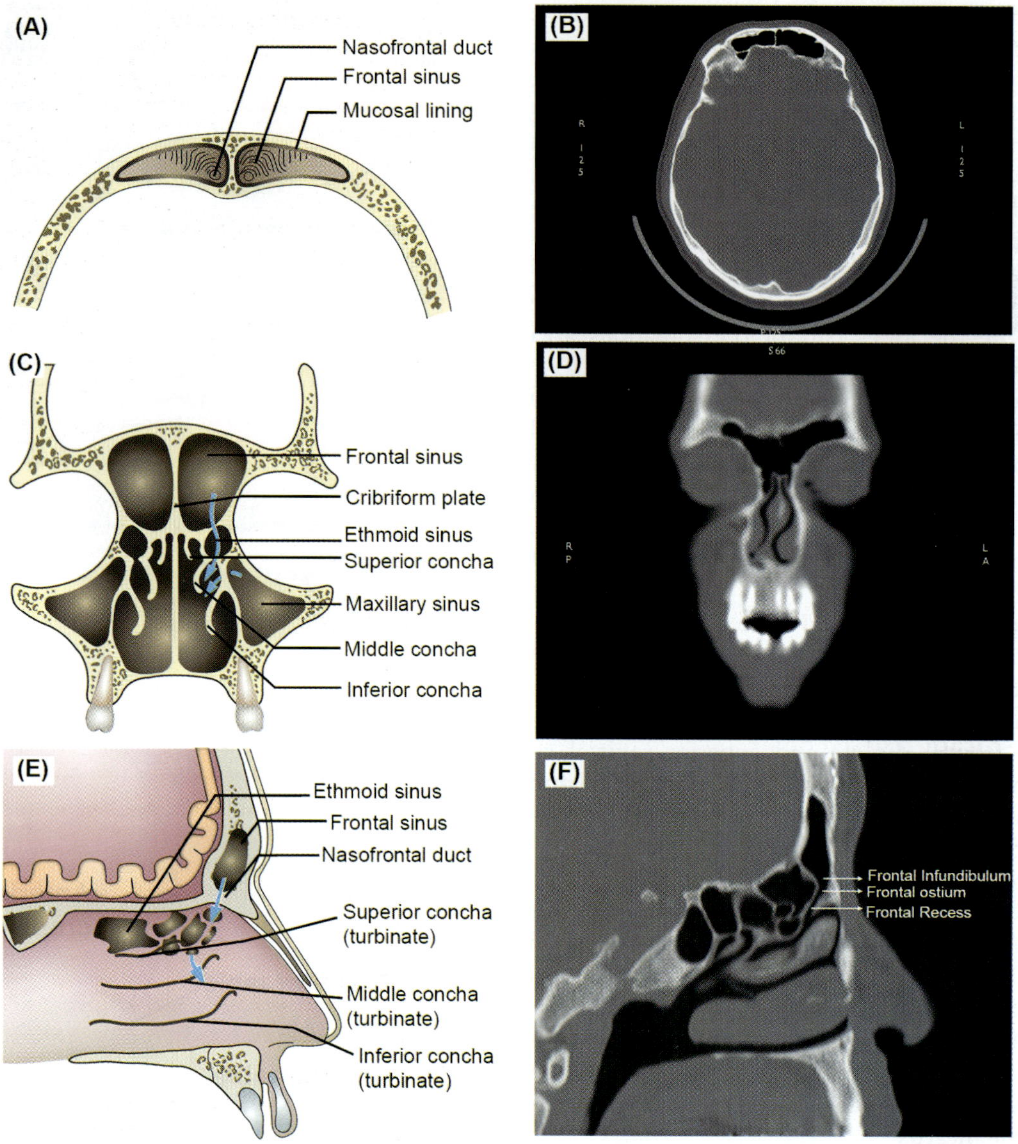

Figure 55.3 (**A–C**) Frontal sinus and nasofrontal duct in axial, coronal and sagittal view, respectively. (**D–F**) Axial, coronal and sagittal section CT scan showing frontal sinus and nasofrontal tract.

  b. *Posteriorly*—the posterior wall of the sinus is in close apposition with the dura mater and frontal lobe of the brain, separated by a thin posterior table
  c. *Laterally*—the frontal sinus forms the roof of the orbit
  d. *Medially*—posteromedially, the floor of the frontal sinus contains the opening of the *nasofrontal duct* (NFD)

- The frontal sinus drains into the anterior part of the middle meatus of nose either directly by a *NFD* or indirectly through the *frontal recess or ethmoidal infundibulum* (Fig. 55.3B and E)
- *Nasofrontal outflow tract (NFOT) or Frontal sinus outflow tract (FSOT)* is a funnel-shaped constriction that passes between the anterior wall of frontal sinus and anterior ethmoidal cells, with a highly variable course, for a few millimetres (2 cm) and terminates at the uncinate process in the nasal cavity. The duct usually lies in the posteromedial region of the floor of sinus (Fig. 55.3C and F).

FUNCTIONS OF FRONTAL SINUS

The mucosa of frontal sinus is lined by pseudostratified ciliated columnar epithelium with mucus-secreting glands. The venous drainage of the frontal sinus mucosa is through the ***foramina of Breschet*** present in the posterior wall of the sinus, which serves as a route of intracranial spread of infection. Interference with the drainage mechanism of the sinus or disease in the lining mucosa predisposes to sinusitis or mucocoele.

The various functions of the frontal sinus are as follows:
- Production and storage of mucus
- Resonator for voice
- Humidification and warming of inhaled air
- Accessory area of olfaction
- Conservation of heat
- Mechanical barrier to protect the brain and eyes.

CLASSIFICATION OF FRONTAL SINUS FRACTURES

The frontal bone is a prominent bone of the craniofacial skeletal framework that sustains trauma stress and protects vital structures. Before fracture, the anterior table can withstand between 350–1000 kg of strain. This is beyond the capacity of the other facial bones. The force of the frontal bone propagates, creating concomitant fractures in the orbit and nasoethmoid complex, which are weaker bones. Comminuted fractures of the outer and inner tables of the frontal bone can also cause cerebrospinal fluid (CSF) rhinorrhea due to dural tears. Fractures of the frontal sinus are often categorised according to location, extent of injury, frontonasal duct involvement and injury to the dura.

Gonty et al., classification based on *anatomic location and fracture pattern*:

Type I: Anterior table fracture:
  a. Isolated to anterior table
  b. Accompanied by supraorbital rim fracture
  c. Accompanied by nasoethmoidal complex fracture

Type II: Combination anterior and posterior table fracture:
  a. Linear fractures in:
    1. Transverse direction
    2. Vertical direction
  b. Comminuted fractures:
    1. Involving both tables
    2. Accompanied by NOE fracture

Type III: Posterior table fracture

Type IV: Through and through frontal sinus fracture

Classification based on *CT evaluation*:

Type 1—outside frontal sinus
Type 2—nondisplaced, involving one or both frontal sinus walls
Type 3—displaced anterior sinus wall, posterior wall intact or nondisplaced
Type 4—displaced anterior and posterior sinus wall
Type 5—displaced posterior sinus wall, anterior wall intact or nondisplaced.

CLINICAL EVALUATION OF FRONTAL SINUS FRACTURES

HISTORY

- Mechanism of injury
- Altered mental status
- Visual difficulties
- Possible skull fractures
- Numbness
- Pain
- Rhinorrhoea
- Sense of smell
- Previous history of nasal or sinus disease surgery.

TABLE 55.1 Clinical Findings of Frontal Sinus Fracture

Inspectory Findings	Palpatory Findings
• Forehead laceration • Frontal oedema • Forehead pain • Frontal bone depression/ flattening • Periorbital ecchymosis • CSF rhinorrhoea	• Step deformity at the supraorbital rim • Paraesthesia over the frontal region • Crepitation over the fractured segments and soft tissue emphysema • NFD injury • Neurological and ocular examination

PHYSICAL EXAMINATION (Table 55.1 and Fig. 55.4)

RADIOGRAPHIC EVALUATION

Plain radiographs that were previously used are as follows:
- Waters projections
- Reverse Townes projections
- Lateral skull films
- Tomograms.

The plain radiographs are of limited use nowadays with the advent of CT scans. CT scans can be utilised to detect frontal bone fractures, displacement of the fracture fragments and associated intracranial injuries. The different views of the CT scan are used in precise diagnosis of frontal sinus fracture (Fig. 55.5).
- *Axial view:* It imparts the location, severity and degree of comminution of anterior and posterior table fractures
- *Coronal view:* It imparts fractures involving the floor of the frontal sinus and orbital roof
- *Sagittal view:* This view evaluates the injury to the frontonasal duct
- *3D reconstruction*—external contour deformity.

The nasofrontal tract (NFT) can be evaluated in the axial, coronal and sagittal sections of CT scan.

MANAGEMENT OF FRONTAL SINUS FRACTURE

The management of frontal sinus fractures is aimed to create a safe sinus, restore facial contour and avoid short- and long-term complications (Flowchart 55.1). The management of the frontal sinus fractures is done by assessing the following anatomic parameters:
(a) Anterior table fracture
(b) Posterior table fracture

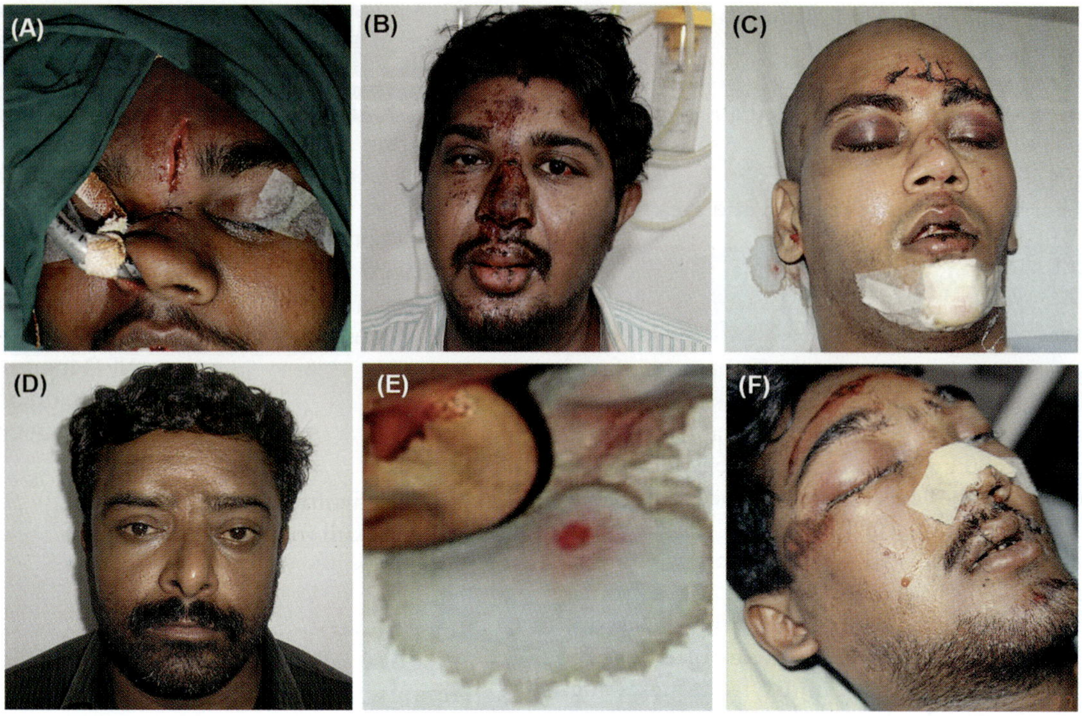

Figure 55.4 Clinical evaluation. (**A**) Forehead laceration. (**B**) Frontal oedema and ecchymosis. (**C**) Sutured laceration and periorbital ecchymosis. (**D**) Depressed frontal bone. (**E**) CSF otorrhoea. (**F**) Frontal and NOE fracture with CSF rhinorrhoea.

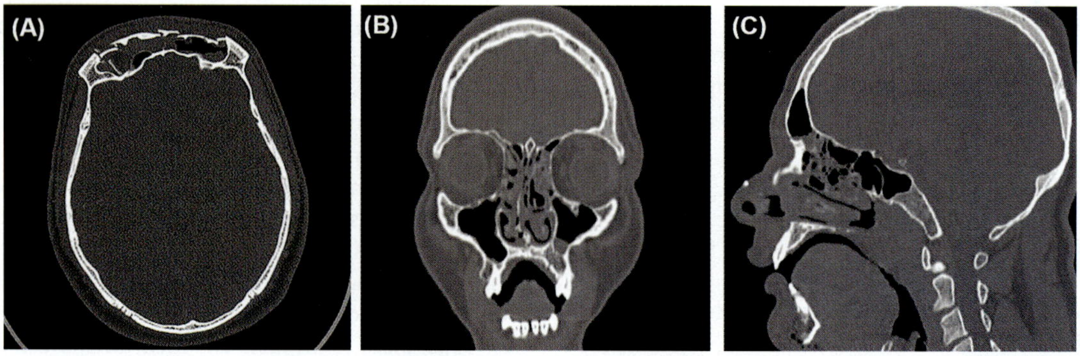

Figure 55.5 Radiographic evaluation. (**A**) Axial section CT scan showing fractures involving the anterior table of frontal sinus. (**B**) Coronal section CT scan showing fracture involving the floor of sinus and its communication with the nose. (**C**) Sagittal section CT scan shows fractures of the frontal bone with nasofrontal duct involvement.

(c) Nasofrontal duct involvement
(d) Dural tear (cerebrospinal fluid leak).

SURGICAL APPROACHES TO THE FRONTAL SINUS REGION

Adequate exposure is essential for accurate reduction and fixation of fractures, as well as for other adjuvant procedures. The frontal sinus can be approached through a number of incisions (Fig. 55.6):

- Existing lacerations
- Bicoronal incision
- Gullwing or eyeglass incisions
- Open-sky approach.

MANAGEMENT OF ANTERIOR TABLE FRACTURE

The anterior wall is highly susceptible to fracture because of its anterior position. Anterior table fractures can occur in isolation or in affiliation with other fractures such as NOE fracture, orbital or Le Fort II or III. Management of an anterior table fracture varies depending on the severity of displacement.

- Simple greenstick or nondisplaced anterior wall fractures do not require operative treatment
- Minimally displaced fractures can be managed through an *endoscopic reduction or recontouring* of the fractured anterior table
- The nasofrontal duct should be checked for patency in fractures that are minimally/moderately displaced. If the

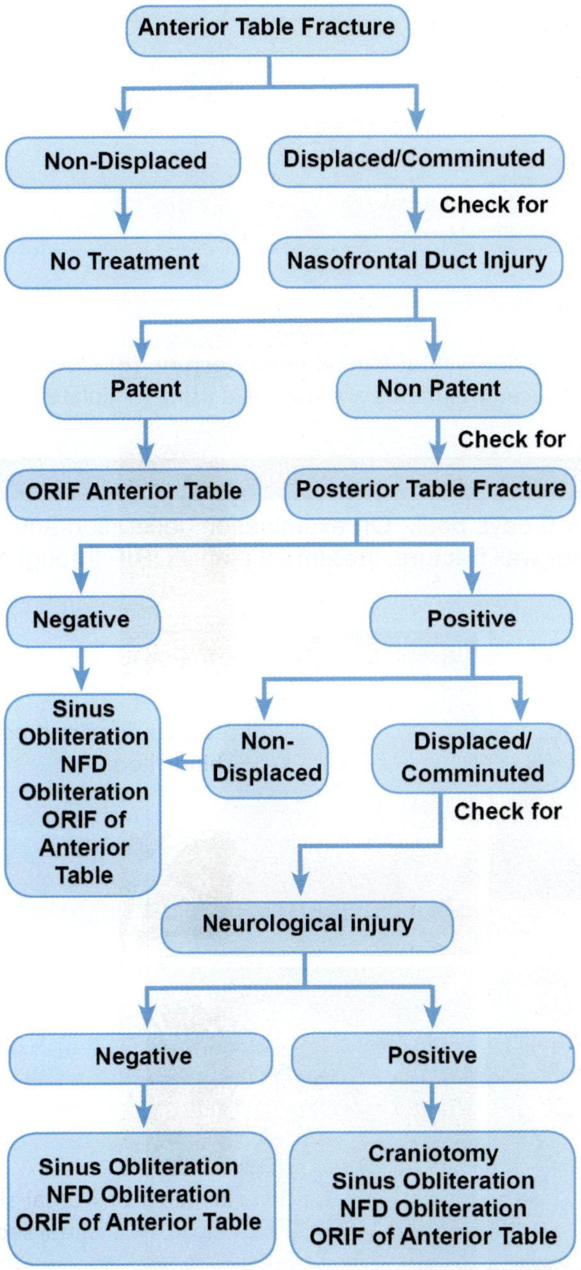

Flowchart 55.1 Algorithm for the management of frontal sinus fractures.

nasofrontal ducts are patent and the posterior wall is devoid of injury, then ***open reduction and internal fixation of the anterior table*** is recommended
- Sinus obliteration and Open reduction and internal fixation (ORIF) are recommended for severely displaced and complex anterior wall fractures with obstruction of the nasofrontal outflow tract, and no posterior wall involvement
- It should be treated as a posterior table fracture if the fracture is severely displaced and complicated, with obstruction of the NFD and posterior wall involvement.

OPEN REDUCTION AND INTERNAL FIXATION FOR ANTERIOR TABLE FRACTURE

Indications

- Anterior table fracture with cosmetic deformity
- No evidence of frontonasal duct injury
- No CSF rhinorrhoea
- Intact sinus lining.

Technique (Figs. 55.7 and 55.8 [Case 55.1])

The anterior wall of the frontal sinus is accessed and dissected, exposing the area of fracture, using a preexisting laceration or coronal incision. The fractured fragments are reduced by using a periosteal elevator, bone hook, or bur to pull them back to their original position. Miniplates, long-curved plates, titanium mesh, or biodegradable fixation are used to stabilise the organised and reduced fragments. The flaps are closed using sutures.

MANAGEMENT OF NASOFRONTAL DUCT INJURY

The nasofrontal ducts transmits the mucus produced by the frontal sinus into the nose. The outflow tract is obstructed when the nasofrontal ducts are disrupted, increasing the risk of mucocoele, sinusitis, meningitis and osteomyelitis. CT scans are used to evaluate nasofrontal duct obstruction. Using an angiocatheter and injecting a compatible fluid, the relative patency of the duct can be evaluated. Methylene blue, fluorescein, ethiodol, indigo carmine and Congo red are some of the fluids that can be administered. Ductal obstruction and/or sinus obliteration are used if the ducts are not patent.

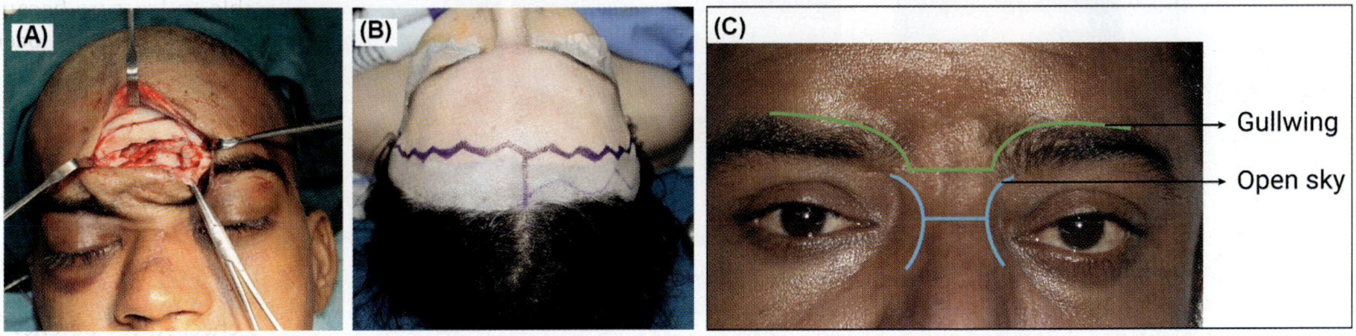

Figure 55.6 Surgical approaches. (A) Existing laceration. (B) Bicoronal incision. (C) Gullwing and open sky incision.

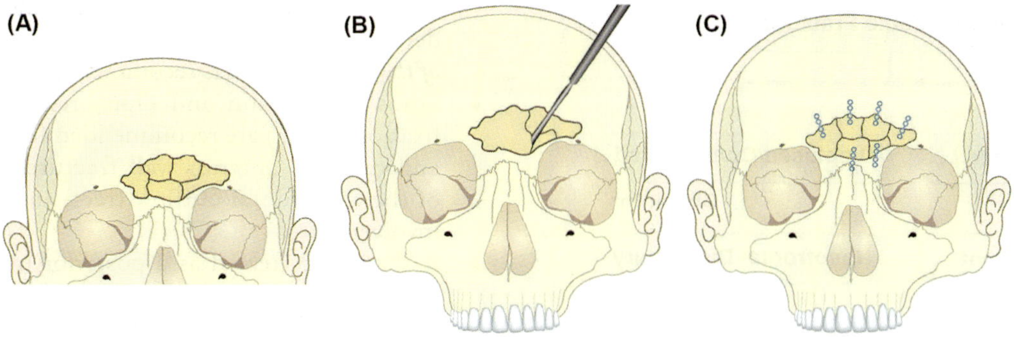

Figure 55.7 ORIF of anterior table fracture. (**A**) Fracture involving the anterior wall of frontal bone fracture. (**B**) Elevation and reduction of the fractured fragments using periosteal elevator. (**C**) The reduced fragments are stabilised using miniplates.

CASE 55.1 Anterior Wall of Frontal Sinus Fracture (Simple)

C/O unaesthetic appearance for past 3 days with history of RTA 5 days back. On examination, laceration and depression was found over the right frontal region suggesting anterior wall fracture. Treatment plan—ORIF through the pre-existing laceration.

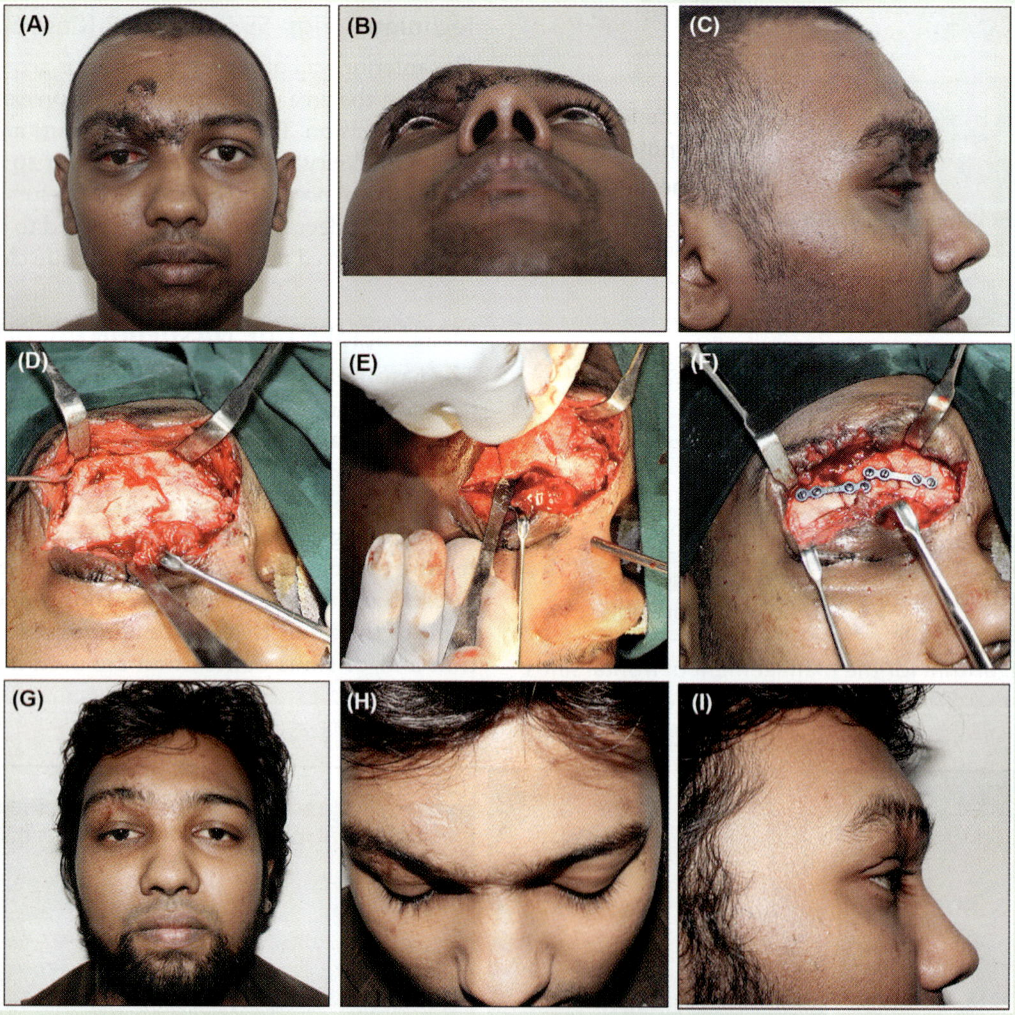

Figure 55.8 (**A**) Preoperative frontal view. (**B**) Worm's eye view showing depression over the right frontal region. (**C**) Lateral view. (**D**) Intraoperative picture showing the minimally displaced anterior wall segments. (**E**) Reduction of the fracture fragments through elevator. (**F**) Reduced and fixed fracture fragments with miniplates. (**G–I**) Postoperative picture after 5 months.

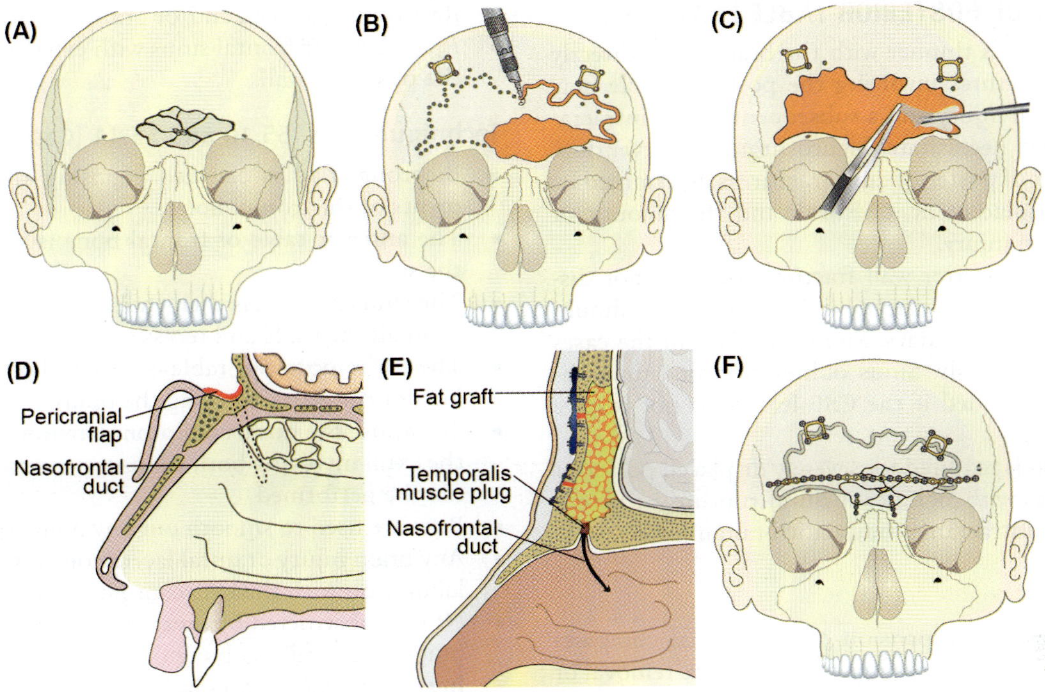

Figure 55.9 Frontal sinus obliteration. (**A**) Anterior wall fracture. (**B**) The anterior table is removed/osteotomised using bur. (**C**) Fontal sinus mucosa is completely removed using bur/elevator. (**D**) The NFT is obstructed with graft. (**E**) Frontal sinus obliteration with fat graft. (**F**) The anterior wall fragments are replaced and fixed with plates.

NASOFRONTAL DUCT OBSTRUCTION

NFD obstruction is sealing off the frontal sinus from the nasal contaminants by plugging the nasofrontal tract with another material. Access is obtained through the anterior table and the sinus mucosa is removed by curettage and surgical bur. The NFD is then obstructed with various materials such as *free temporal fascia, temporal muscle, bone graft, tensor fascia, autologous platelet gel and fibrin glue.*

FRONTAL SINUS OBLITERATION

By plugging the NFT and the functional sinus/dead space with another material, sinus obliteration separates the sinus from the nasal cavity. Obliteration of the sinuses entails the following:

- Complete removal of sinus mucosa
- Permanent occlusion of the nasofrontal outflow tract
- Obliteration of dead space/sinus cavity with materials.

Indications

- Nasofrontal duct injury from anterior table fracture
- Severely comminuted fractures of the anterior table
- Nonfunctional sinus resulting from severe injuries of the anterior and/or posterior table or significant mucosal disruption.

Technique

Obliteration of the sinus cavity is a procedure wherein the sinus lining is carefully removed, followed by filling up of the cavity with the appropriate chosen material. The steps involved are (Fig. 55.9) as follows:

- A bicoronal technique is used to approach the fracture site
- The sinus cavity is exposed once the fractured anterior wall is removed
- The lateral, posterior, inferior, orbital and ethmoidal portions of the sinus lining are removed from all walls
- By firmly impacting a wedge or plug of cancellous bone or other suitable material above the invaginated nasal mucosa, the frontonasal canal is completely blocked
- The entire sinus cavity is filled with materials followed by fixation of the anterior wall fragments (Table 55.2).

TABLE 55.2 Materials Used for Obliteration of Sinus Cavity

Autogenous Graft	Allografts	Alloplastic Materials
• Fat • Muscle • Bone • Fascia-pericranial flap • Adipose stem cells with growth factors	Lyophilised cartilage	• Methyl methacrylate • Hydroxyapatite cement • Proplast—Polytetrafluoroethylene • Bio-glass

MANAGEMENT OF POSTERIOR TABLE FRACTURE

The posterior table is thinner with the brain being directly adjacent to it. Fractures involving the posterior table may lead to intracranial injury and a subsequent rise in intracranial pressure that necessitates neurosurgical intervention. The management of posterior table fracture is determined by the degree of displacement, CSF leak and the amount of concomitant brain injury.

- Patients with posterior wall fractures that are not displaced or are mildly displaced but have a CSF leak should be monitored for 5–7 days. More than 50% of the cases resolve spontaneously. Sinus obliteration or cranialisation is recommended if the CSF leak does not resolve within 10 days
- Cranialisation is required for severely displaced posterior table fractures with significant dural rupture, recurrent CSF leak and intracranial traumatic brain injuries.

CRANIALISATION

Cranialisation involves expansion of the cranial compartment (brain) into the frontal sinus with complete removal of the posterior table, frontal sinus mucosa and obliteration of the sinus cavity using the cranial contents.

Indications

- Severely displaced and comminuted frontal sinus fractures with significant posterior table involvement and dural lacerations
- Recurrent CSF leak and/or brain injury
- *Pyocoele* of the frontal sinus with extensive destruction of the posterior wall.

Technique (Figs. 55.10 and 55.11 [Case 55.2])

- Bicoronal flap is elevated exposing the fractured segments of the frontal bone
- The anterior table of frontal bone is removed exposing the sinus
- The sinus mucosa is then entirely removed and debrided from all the walls and recesses
- The entire posterior table is removed or resected using a burr or rongeurs exposing the brain
- To expose the dura, craniotomy (removal of a portion of the skull involving both the anterior and posterior walls) may be performed
- Burs are used to smooth out any bony irregularities
- Any brain injury or dural lacerations are corrected in collaboration with the neurosurgical team
- NFD is obstructed by invagination of the nasal mucosa, plugs of cancellous bone or other material to achieve a **hermetic seal**. A vascularised galeal frontalis or pericranial flap is used to reinforce the floor. This isolates the cranium from the nasal cavity
- The cranial contents are permitted to herniate anteriorly into the frontal sinus region
- Miniplates/mesh are used to reconstruct the anterior table
- The coronal flap is then replaced and sutured.

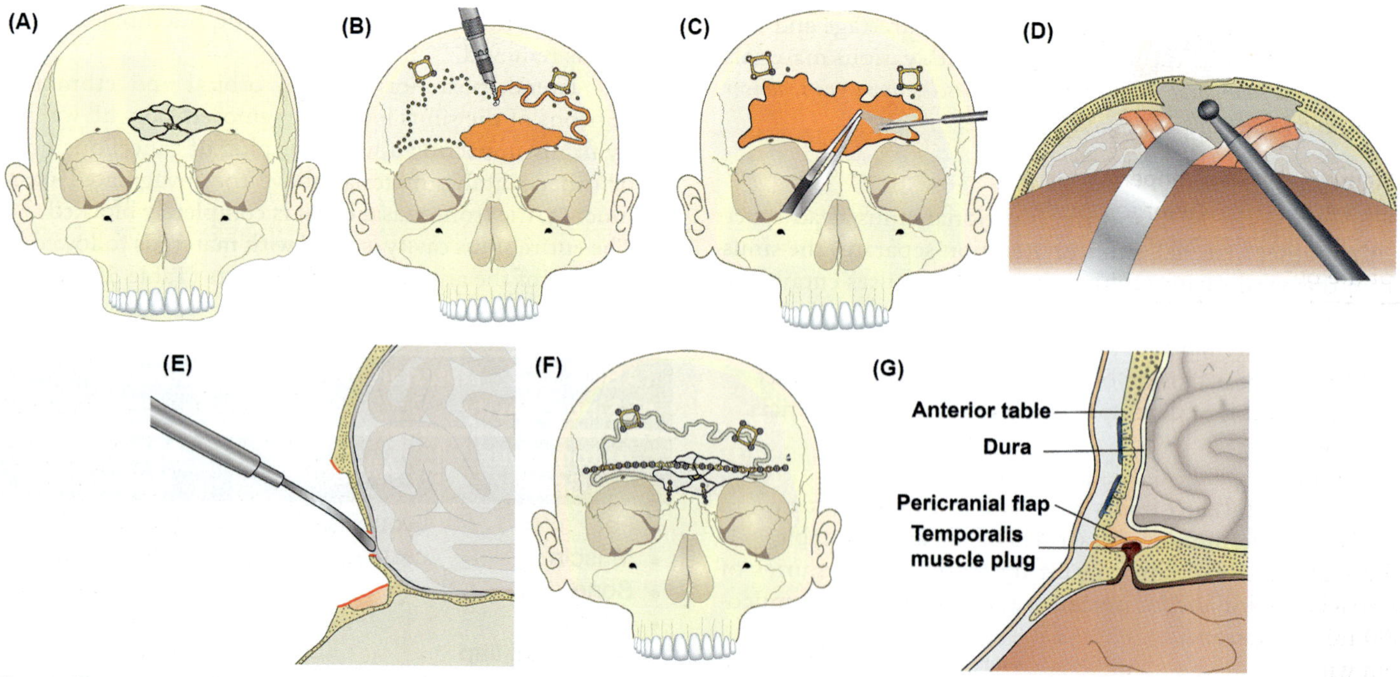

Figure 55.10 Cranialisation. (**A–C**) Frontal bone fracture, marking and removal of anterior wall and debridement of sinus mucosa. (**D**) Removal of posterior wall using bur. (**E**) NFD obstruction using bone chips and floor of the sinus is covered with pericranial flap. (**F**) Replacement and fixation of anterior wall of frontal bone. (**G**) Completed craniotomy.

CASE 55.2 Cranialisation of Frontal Sinus

A 24-year-old man reported with injuries due to assault, for which he was primarily treated elsewhere. The patient complains of pain and swelling in the forehead region with a history of nasal bleeding and CSF rhinorrhoea, which was resolved spontaneously. On examination, the patient had depression over forehead, periorbital ecchymosis, fracture of frontal sinus involving both the anterior and posterior walls and fracture and obstuction in the NFOT. Treatment plan—cranialisation and NFD obstruction, in coordination with neurosurgeon.

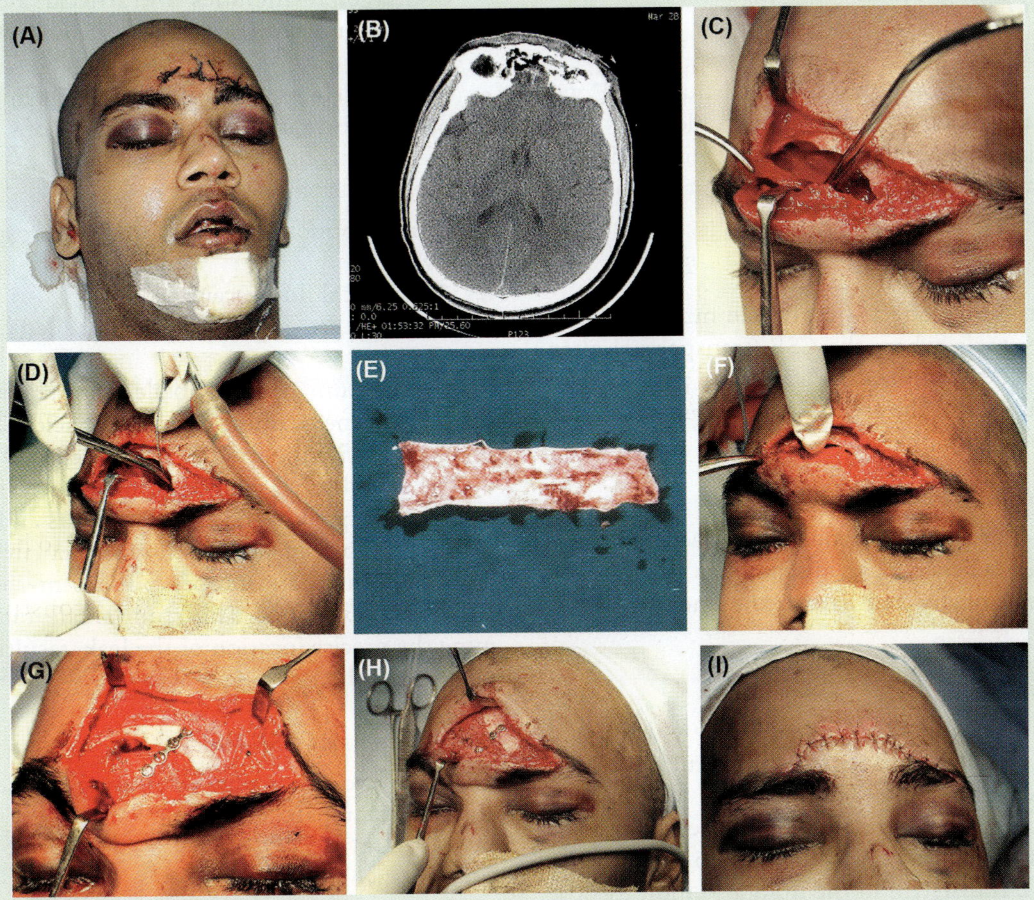

Figure 55.11 (**A**) Preoperative frontal view with depression in the glabella region and periorbital ecchymosis. (**B**) Axial CT showing fracture of anterior and posterior table. (**C**) Intraoperative view with exploration of the frontal sinus. (**D**) Removal of posterior wall. (**E**) Harvested fascia lata. (**F**) The sinus was obliterated with fascia lata and frontalis muscle. (**G** and **H**) Repositioning of the outer table and rigid fixation of the fragment with a long plate. (**I**) The frontalis muscle was redraped and closure done.

Cerebrospinal fluid (CSF)

CSF is a clear body fluid that exists in the subarachnoid space, which is the space between arachnoid mater and pia mater. It cushions and buffers the cortex.

Formation

The CSF production occurs at the choroid plexus in the ventricles of the brain at a rate of 20 mL/h approximating 500 mL daily, and circulates the entire central nervous system within the subarachnoid space. Cerebrospinal fluid is a colourless, clear fluid, typically devoid of cells and consisting of water, electrolytes, glucose, amino acids and various proteins.

CSF rhinorrhoea

CSF rhinorrhoea refers to leakage of CSF through the nose presenting as frank, clear or blood-stained nasal discharge. When patient is in the supine position, CSF rhinorrhoea manifests as postnasal drip giving a salty taste. Persistent CSF rhinorrhoea creates a nasofrontal communication, which poses the risk of spread of infection leading to life-threatening meningitis, brain abscess, etc.

Cause of CSF leak

CSF leakage can develop when the posterior table of the frontal sinus or the cribriform plate are fractured, and the dura mater is disrupted.

Clinical presentation

- Clear and watery drainage from the nose
- Salty postnasal drip
- Ear fullness or hearing loss
- Headache
- 'Reservoir sign' when taking a head up position from lying position.

Identification of CSF fluid

Halo or double ring or target sign

A filter paper is placed over the suspected fluid. CSF will transit farther than blood when mixed with blood or nasal discharge, resulting in an inner ring of blood encircled by an outer ring of clear CSF. It is called a target sign, double ring sign or halo effect.

Tramline sign

A characteristic tramline effect is created in mixed CSF rhinorrhoea and epistaxis, where the CSF (transparent) alternates with the dried blood, creating a tramline pattern. This finding may be absent in the reclining position due to CSF escape into the posterior pharynx.

Handkerchief/starch test

The CSF fluid is clear and nonviscous when placed on gauze or a handkerchief, whereas nasal discharge is unclear and viscous. CSF does not dry and harden the linen like nasal secretion does.

Chemical markers (Table 55.3)

Collecting 0.1 mL of fluid and comparing the glucose and chloride levels of this fluid with the patient's serum levels can confirm the presence of CSF.

The presence of CSF is indicated by high chloride and low glucose concentrations in fluid compared to serum. The presence of beta 2 transferrin in the fluid also indicates the existence of CSF.

Radiological evaluation

- A *high-resolution* CT scan is the best diagnostic imaging tool for detecting a CSF leak and confirm the site of abnormality. It also aids in determining the causative skull base defect, the origin, extent and degree of damage
- *CSF scintigraphy*—it involves injecting radioactive tracers like 99m Tc—human serum albumin, iodine131 human serum albumin, into the lumbar subarachnoid space, followed by a CT scan. Hotspots or areas of increased uptake indicate CSF leaks
- *CT cisternography*—it aids in identifying the precise location of a CSF leak in patients with active clear nasal drainage. It includes intrathecal administration of radiopaque contrast (metrizamide) followed by CT scanning
- MRI—it detects CSF leak in multiple imaging planes and offers information on the contents of CSF fistula.

TABLE 55.3 Chemical Markers for Identification of CSF

Glucose: *Glucose oxidase test strips*	Sensitive and specific marker of CSF. Colour change indicates presence of CSF mixed with nasal secretions
β2-Transferrin	Reliable marker of CSF
Beta-trace protein (β-TP)	2nd most common protein found in CSF after albumin

Nuclear medicine studies

Radio nucleotide tracers used for cerebrospinal fluid are as follows:

a. Intrathecal fluorescein
b. Radioactive iodine (I-131)-labelled serum albumin (RISA)
c. Technetium Tc-99m-labelled serum albumin
d. Diethylene triamine pentaacetic acid (DTPA)
e. Radioactive indium (In-111)-labelled DTPA.

The spinal canal is injected with nuclear isotopes. These isotopes escape into the nose or sinuses and are gathered on cotton pads placed into the nose as they circulate around the brain. The nuclear isotopes present in these pads are retrieved and examined. This study is safe, but it cannot determine the precise location of the leak, resulting in more false positive results.

Management of CSF leak

There are two major ways of treating CSF leak: conservative and surgical repair.

Conservative treatment

It is indicated for patients with linear fractures of the facial bones. It includes the following:

- Three days of complete bed rest
- Thirty degrees of head elevation
- Advising patient to avoid coughing, sneezing, nose blowing and straining
- Prophylactic antibiotics to prevent meningitis.

Surgical management

Indications for surgical management:

- Penetrating injury
- Intracranial haematoma
- Meningitis
- Herniation of brain tissue through the nose and ear
- Low probability of natural dural repair
- Persistent CSF leakage after 10 days of conservative management.

Surgical methods are classified into two groups: intracranial and extracranial approach.

Intracranial repair of CSF leak

Anterior fossa craniotomy is performed through a bicoronal incision, exposing the cranial contents.

The advantage of intracranial approach is the widely exposed operation field for convenient repair of CSF leakage and the possibility to repair the leakage site, even if the intracranial pressure (ICP) is high.

Extracranial techniques

Transfacial extracranial approach was considered as the main method in the past. However, nowadays, endonasal repair by endoscopic approach has emerged as the primary technique in repairing CSF leakage. The major advantages of endoscopic endonasal repair are a low risk of retraction injury to the brain cortex.

COMPLICATIONS OF FRONTAL SINUS FRACTURE

Frontal bone fractures involving the anterior and posterior tables as well as the frontal sinus may result in complications related to the sinus, intracranial, orbital or nasal structures (Table 55.4).

EARLY COMPLICATIONS

CSF LEAK

CSF leak is the most frequent and significant complication. CSF leak can be treated by bed rest, prophylactic antibiotic or lumbar drainage.

MENINGITIS

The most feared early complication is meningitis. Meningitis has a high morbidity and fatality rate, hence early diagnosis is crucial. Any signs of fever, nuchal rigidity or altered sensorium indicates meningitis. The immediate management includes a lumbar puncture and medical management with empirical antibiotics (ceftriaxone and ampicillin/sulfadiazine) with good CSF penetrance. Further, the draining CSF may be cultured for the microbial colonies and the sensitive drug identified.

TABLE 55.4 Complications of Frontal Sinus Fracture

Early Complications	Late Complications
• CSF leak • Meningitis • Pneumocephalus • Sinusitis • Diplopia • Paraesthesia	• Mucocoele or a mucopyocoele • Brain abscess • Osteomyelitis • Cosmetic defect • Headache

PNEUMOCEPHALUS

Pneumocephalus refers to air within the cranial cavity which can be found in any of the intracranial compartments: frontal, subdural or intracerebral locations. It is identified by *'Bruit-hydroaerique'* or *'cranial succession splash'* sign. On posture change, the patient hears a splashing sound that can be observed by auscultation of the head. Definitive treatment includes repair of the underlying dural tear and fistula.

FRONTAL SINUSITIS

It is more common in early postoperative period and patients may present with increased oedema, erythema, and generalised tenderness in the forehead and periorbital regions. Nasal decongestants used as a preventative measure serve to reduce mucosal inflammation and optimise sinus drainage and function.

LATE COMPLICATIONS (AFTER 6 MONTHS)

MUCOCOELE

A mucocoele is an expansive cyst in the ciliated mucosa that is filled with mucus generated by goblet cells. It may develop if the frontonasal duct is obstructed or if respiratory mucosa is wedged between fracture segments.

A mucocoele can induce bony expansion and erosion, and is capable of extending into the sinuses, orbit and cranium. Complete excision of the mucocoele (marsupialisation) with restoration of the nasofrontal outflow tract is a viable strategy. Mucopyocoeles are infected mucocoeles and are managed by antibiotics and surgical management.

BRAIN ABSCESS

Brain abscess is caused by infection spreading along the periarteriolar spaces of Virchow, the arterial supply of the brain parenchyma. It is rare and potentially fatal. It manifests as loss of appetite, fatigue, lethargy and personality changes. Treatment includes intravenous antibiotics, which can cross the blood–brain barrier and has high CSF penetrance.

OSTEOMYELITIS

It is a rare complication. Frontal bone osteomyelitis was called Pott's puffy tumour in the preantibiotic era. It is treated by complete surgical excision of the frontal bone, antimicrobial treatment with antibiotics and subsequent reconstruction at a later stage.

COSMETIC DEFECT

Lack of rigid fixation and subsequent bone loss results in cosmetic defects. Introduction of miniplate and microplate fixation and the use of primary bone grafts have resulted in the eradication of frontal contour defects.

Chapter 56

Panfacial and Paediatric Fractures

OUTLINE

PANFACIAL FRACTURES

INTRODUCTION

Markowitz and Manson described panfacial fractures as those that involve the upper (cranio-orbital), middle (orbito-zygomaticomaxillary) and lower (mandibular region) thirds of the face. Severe panfacial fractures lead to destruction of the bony framework resulting in complex facial deformities such as decreased facial height, increased facial width, enophthalmos and malocclusion. Sometimes, they can be associated with soft tissue injuries or other injuries, which can be potentially life threatening. It usually results from high-energy injuries such as motor vehicle collisions, assaults, sports-related accidents, industrial accidents and gunshot wounds (Fig. 56.1 and Table 56.1).

Panfacial fractures represent a combination of the following fractures: Le Fort I, Le Fort II, Le Fort III, frontal sinus, bilateral naso-orbito-ethmoid (NOE), bilateral zygoma, bilateral orbit, simple sagittal split of the palate, segmental mandibular body/parasymphyseal, condyle fractures.

Multiple displaced and comminuted fractures constitute panfacial fractures. Management of these fractures are often complex and the treatment must be individualised for each

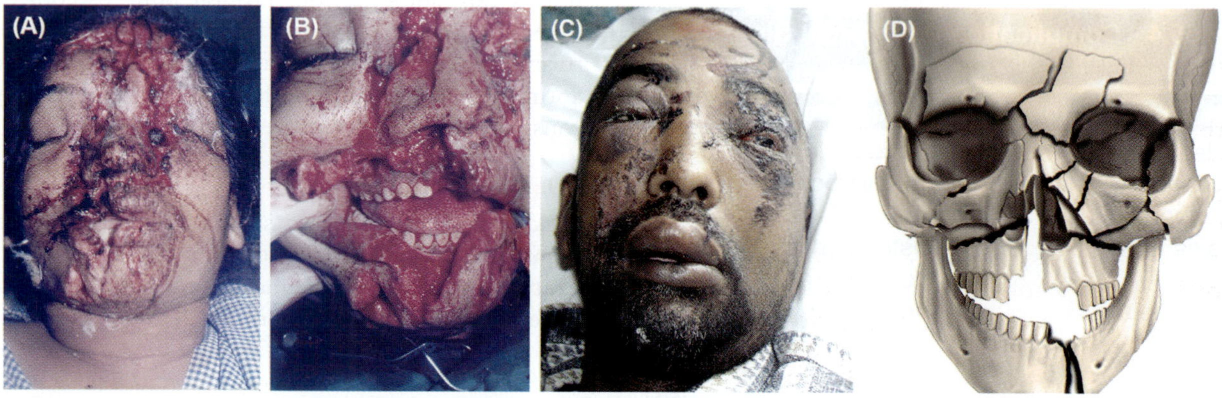

Figure 56.1 (**A–C**) Panfacial fracture. (**D**) Panfacial fracture involving multiple bones.

TABLE 56.1 Bony components Primarily Involved in Panfacial Fracture

Upper 3rd	Middle 3rd	Lower 3rd
• Frontal bone • Fronto-orbital region • Sphenoid sinus	• Orbit • Zygoma • Ethmoid • Nose • Maxilla	• Mandible

patient. These injuries can often be complicated by the concomitant injuries that require immediate attention and delay the early repair of fractures. However, with proper diagnosis, treatment planning, sequencing and technology have paved the way for more effective treatments resulting in better prognosis and patient satisfaction. The reestablishment of facial height, width and projection is crucial for the prevention of facial abnormalities as well as the individual's social well-being.

CLASSIFICATION

Scoring of severity of the injury is important for evaluating the prognosis of trauma patients.

The *abbreviated injury scale (AIS) and the injury severity score (ISS)* have been widely used scoring systems in the world. *Guerrissi* devised a *maxillofacial trauma scoring system* that aims to identify patients with potentially life-threatening maxillofacial injuries, and to quantify the severity of facial injuries according to the functional and aesthetic impact.

The *maxillofacial injury severity score (MFISS) method* combined AIS severity scores with three functional parameters: malocclusion (MO), limited mouth opening (LMO) and facial deformity (FD) (Table 56.2).

TABLE 56.2 Maxillofacial Injury Severity Score (MFISS)

Index	Scores	Description of Injury
LMO	1	• Mouth opening range 2–3.7 cm
	2	• Mouth opening range <2 cm
MO	1	• Mouth opening range <6 teeth in single jaw
	2	• Mouth opening range >6 teeth in single jaw
	3	• Malocclusion in both jaws
FD	1	• Open soft-tissue injury (<4 cm in length), without tissue defect • Fracture without displacement
	2	• Open soft-tissue injury (>4 cm in length) and tissue defect <2 cm^2 • Facial nerve branch injury • Fracture with displacement, fracture with bone defect < half side of single jaw
	3	• Open soft-tissue injury (>4 cm in length) and tissue defect >2 cm^2 • Facial nerve trunk injury • Bone defect > half side of single jaw, bone defect in both jaws

LMO, limited mouth opening; MO, malocclusion; FD, facial deformity.

ANATOMICAL CONSIDERATIONS

FACIAL BUTTRESSES

The facial bones are made of two different types of architectural structures: *dense rigid buttresses and laminar sheets.* The buttresses are dense cortical pillars, which provide the stability and structure to the face. The bones at the buttress area are generally thicker and help to counteract the masticatory forces. In addition to restoring the occlusion, proper reduction of these buttresses is essential to reconstruct the width, height and projection of the face. Sicher and Tandler (1928) were the first to describe buttresses as the key in reconstruction of the panfacial fractures (Fig. 56.2).

Two types of buttress: *vertical and horizontal buttresses.*

Vertical buttresses: form the vertical height of the face and forms the major bony support. They consist of the following:

- Nasomaxillary
- Zygomaticomaxillary
- Pterygomaxillary buttresses.

The *nasomaxillary buttress* includes the maxillary process of the frontal bone and the frontal process of the maxilla, extending lateral to the pyriform rim. The *zygomaticomaxillary buttress* is composed of the zygomatic process of the frontal bone, lateral orbital rim, lateral zygomatic body and zygomatic process of the maxilla. The *pterygomaxillary buttress* consists of the pterygoid plates of the sphenoid and maxillary tuberosities. The *condyle and the posterior mandibular ramus* both serve as buttresses and aids in establishing the posterior facial height.

The ***horizontal buttresses or anterior posterior buttresses*** provide cross stability and maintain the anteroposterior as well as the horizontal dimensions of the face. These include the following:

- Frontal
- Zygomatic
- Maxillary
- Mandibular

The *frontal buttress* is composed of the supraorbital rims and the glabellar region. The *zygomatic buttress* consists of the zygomatic arch, zygomatic body and infraorbital rim. It is immensely crucial in establishing the malar eminence and facial symmetry. *The maxillary and mandibular buttresses* are composed of the basal bone of their respective arches, which

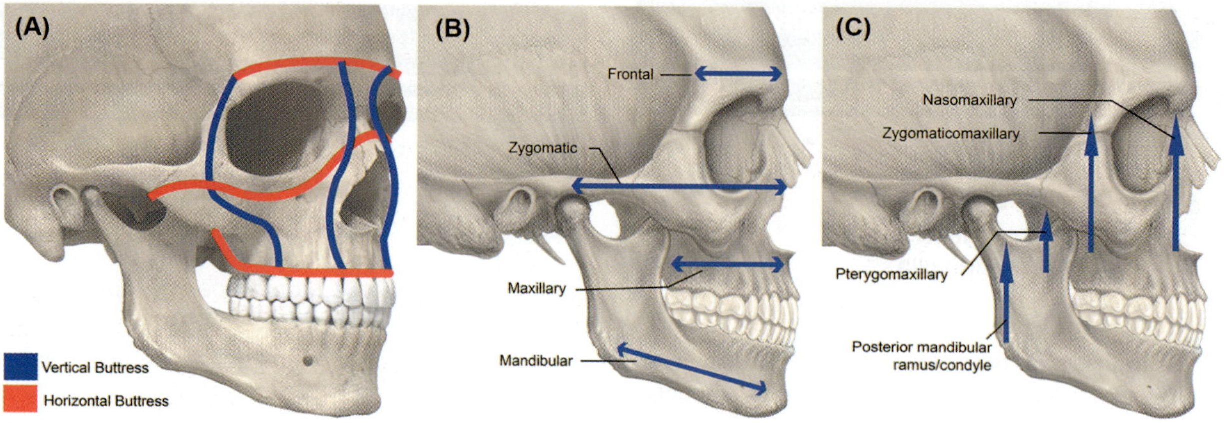

Figure 56.2 (**A**) Facial buttresses. (**B**) Horizontal buttresses. (**C**) Vertical buttresses.

plays a major role in maintaining the lower 3rd width and occlusal arch.

KEY ANATOMICAL LANDMARKS

In panfacial fractures, few landmarks aid in determining the proper positioning of the facial skeleton which includes: the dental arches, mandible, sphenozygomatic suture, maxillary buttress and the intercanthal region.

i. ***Dental arches:***
In fractures, if one of the dental arch is intact, it can be used as a guide to establish the occlusion
   - Le Fort fracture without midpalatal split, and intact maxillary arch can be used as a guide to align the mandibular arch
   - Fractures of maxilla associated with midpalatal split, mandible and condyle fractures are troublesome and can easily lead to widening of the entire facial complex. These situations can be corrected by any of the following methods:
     - Exposure and *fixation at the palatal fracture*. This is preferred in solitary midpalatal fracture without comminution. But in panfacial injuries, fixation at the palate should not be considered as the 1st step
     - A 2nd approach is the fabrication of *surgical splints* using dental models. Establishing a preinjury occlusion becomes increasingly challenging as the severity of the injury increases
     - The 3rd option is the primary *reconstruction of mandible*, as mandible can be anatomically reduced and fixed. The reconstructed mandible can be used as a guide in reducing maxilla

ii. ***The mandible:***
   - Anatomic reduction of mandible can be achieved at the symphysis and body region, as it allows direct visualisation of buccal and lingual surfaces and the inferior border. Reduction at both the buccal and the lingual cortex yields better results
   - It is necessary to treat bilateral subcondylar fractures in order to determine the posterior facial height and width

iii. ***Sphenozygomatic suture:***
   - The sphenozygomatic suture, present along the internal surface of the lateral orbital wall is the key landmark in the fixation of *ZMC fractures*. It also helps in proper positioning of the zygoma and its arch. However, relying solely on this suture as reference can result in errors
   - The sphenozygomatic suture is usually exposed along the internal surface of the lateral orbital wall. Fixation in this area is challenging due to its angulation. Hence once reduced, instead of sphenozygomatic suture the fixation is done along the frontozygomatic suture
   - The zygomatic buttress also forms another important landmark in establishing the proper reduction of the zygoma and/or maxilla

iv. ***Intercanthal region:***
The intercanthal distance is fairly constant in the adult facial skeleton and can be used to reestablish the midfacial width. Restoration of the proper intercanthal distance involves adequate reduction of the NOE complex

v. ***Other commonly used landmarks:***
Frontal bar, lateral orbital rim, frontozygomatic suture, infraorbital rim, zygomaticomaxillary buttress, curve along the pyriform aperture, inferior border of the mandible and the external oblique ridge (Fig. 56.3).

ASSESSMENT OF PANFACIAL FRACTURES

The initial assessment and management of patients presenting with panfacial fractures are similar to that of the other maxillofacial injuries and should follow the principles of Advanced Trauma Life Support (ATLS).

Primary survey of a patient with multiple injuries includes the assessment of Glasgow Coma Scale (GCS) score, airway compromise, orofacial haemorrhage, accompanying head injury, concomitant cervical spine injury and cardiovascular compromise. Before planning for craniofacial reconstruction,

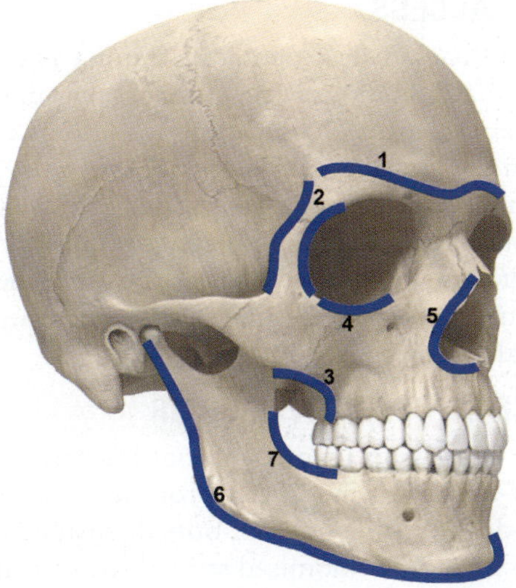

Figure 56.3 Commonly used landmarks to confirm proper bony reduction. (1) Frontal bar along the superior orbital rim and frontal bone. (2) Lateral orbital rim and frontozygomatic suture. (3) Curvature of the maxilla at the zygomaticomaxillary buttress. (4) Infraorbital rim contour. (5) Natural curve along the pyriform aperture. (6) Inferior border of the mandible. (7) External oblique ridge of mandible.

all other concomitant injuries must be ruled out and the patient should be stabilised. Maintenance of ***airway*** in a panfacial fracture is a crucial life-saving decision. Patients typically fall into two broad groups: (1) those whose injuries at the initial presentation requires a definitive airway, intubation and ICU care; and (2) those with facial injuries that are not airway threatening.

After completion of the primary survey, it is necessary to find other concomitant body injuries, as their presence may affect the treatment and subsequent rehabilitation. Radiographs and ***CT scan*** can be taken for assessment of the fracture (Fig. 56.4). An *OPG* (orthopantomogram), if possible, can be taken for full dental assessment or other factors that make the preinjury occlusion difficult.

CLINICAL EXAMINATION

The clinical findings in a panfacial trauma patient are a combination of signs and symptoms of various subunit fractures of the face. The most common signs and symptoms are elongated face, dish face deformity, bilateral raccoon's eyes, traumatic telecanthus and deranged occlusion. (Refer to respective Chapters 48–55 for signs and symptoms of individual fracture.)

MANAGEMENT OF PANFACIAL FRACTURES

MANAGEMENT PRINCIPLES

The aim of treatment for panfacial fractures is to restore the facial region to its preinjury form and function. The facial form should be restored in a *three-dimensional space* (anteroposterior projection, width and vertical height). It requires precise anatomic reconstitution of the craniofacial skeleton as well as the overlying soft tissues. Primary repair is the best way to restore the form and function and also prevent the development of posttraumatic deformities.

Bone grafting and soft tissue resuspension

Panfacial fractures with severely damaged areas or with comminution may necessitate *primary bone grafting*. Bone grafts are delayed only if the wound is infected.

Soft tissue loss should be managed with a free tissue transfer or composite free flap. It is advisable to prevent local tissue advancement across the defect area, as it creates secondary deformity that may be irreversible.

Even after restoring the skeletal form, failure to restore the correct *position of the soft tissue* can result in compromised results. For example:

- Medial canthal tendon (MCT) of the orbital region. It may contribute to lower eyelid retraction and scleral show
- Loss of support to the Superficial muscular aponeurotic system (SMAS) layer in the temporal region may contribute to temporal hollowing, which usually occurs in the coronal flap

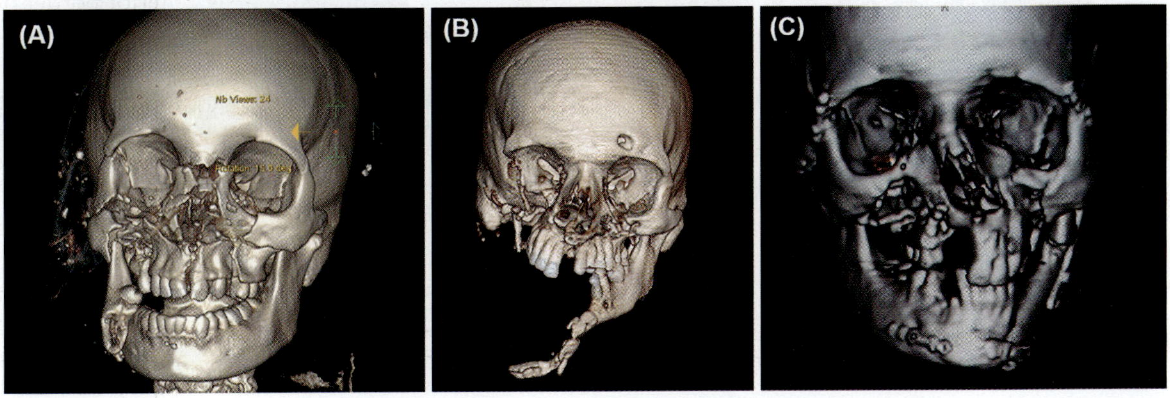

Figure 56.4 **(A–C)** CT scan of panfacial fractures.

Management of the soft tissue drape should be given attention to restore proper facial soft tissue support.

TIMING OF SURGERY

The upper and middle 3rd injuries usually result in considerable swelling. Reduction of swelling is important to unmask the underlying fractures and deformity. Depending on the severity of the damage and the patient's age, definitive treatment can be delayed by up to 2 weeks.

Beyond 7 days—internal healing and fibrosis occurs in the malpositioned area.

Beyond 2 weeks—accelerated callus formation occurs in the fractured site.

Mandibular fracture with airway threat should be treated within 24–48 h after injury. It is recommended to do surgery only when the patients are neurologically and systemically stable.

When soft tissue injuries are present along with panfacial trauma, it is ideal to utilise the golden hour to address both the soft tissue and the skeletal system at the same time. Sometimes, depending on the soft tissue injuries, it is recommended to close the soft tissue injuries early without reducing the fractures.

AIRWAY MANAGEMENT

Panfacial fractures necessitate a surgical airway for unrestricted access to the middle and lower face. For extensive injuries with airway compromise, intubation may be required. Intubation can be nasal, oral or submental intubation. In cases where prolonged intubation is anticipated, tracheostomy should be considered (Fig. 56.5).

SURGICAL ACCESS

Surgical approaches in a panfacial trauma patient should permit adequate access and exposure for anatomic reduction of the facial skeleton. The location and extent of exposure depends on the location and severity of the injury (Fig. 56.7). Greater fragmentation suggests greater difficulty attaining adequate stability, demanding better fixation, with or without bone grafting, and hence wider exposure. The following describes the fractures that can be accessed through the various surgical approaches (Table 56.3).

SEQUENCE OF OPERATIVE REPAIR

For proper management of panfacial fractures, various sequences of reduction have been proposed, such as bottom to up, top-down, inside-outside, outside-inside (Table 56.4). There have been no randomised studies to ascertain whether one approach is superior to the other. The most commonly used method for reduction in panfacial fracture is 'bottom-up and outside-in'.

Kelly et al. suggested reducing and stabilising the hard palate as a guide for mandible reconstruction. *Gruss and Phillips* advised reduction of the zygomatic arch and malar prominence as a 1st step, to reestablish the 'outer facial frame'. *Merville* suggested reduction of the frontozygomatic suture 1st, as it determines the facial width and projection and should proceed from 'top-bottom' sequence. As NOE fracture fragments are fragile, it is difficult to find a stable fixation point in the nasoethmoid-orbital area. Therefore, it is recommended for an 'outside-inside' sequence for reconstruction of panfacial fractures.

i. The *bottom-up approach* uses the mandible as a guide for fixing the rest of the face. 1st the occlusion is set by placing

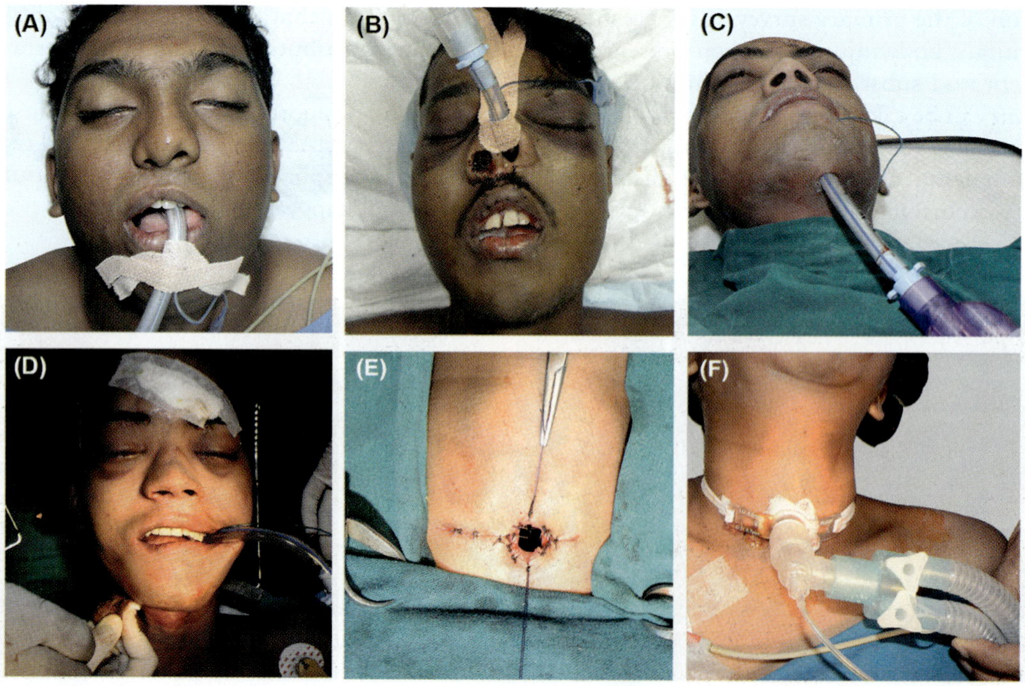

Figure 56.5 (**A**) Oral intubation. (**B**) Nasal intubation. (**C**) Submental intubation. (**D**) Retromolar intubation. (**E and F**) Tracheostomy.

TABLE 56.3 Surgical Approaches to the Facial Skeleton

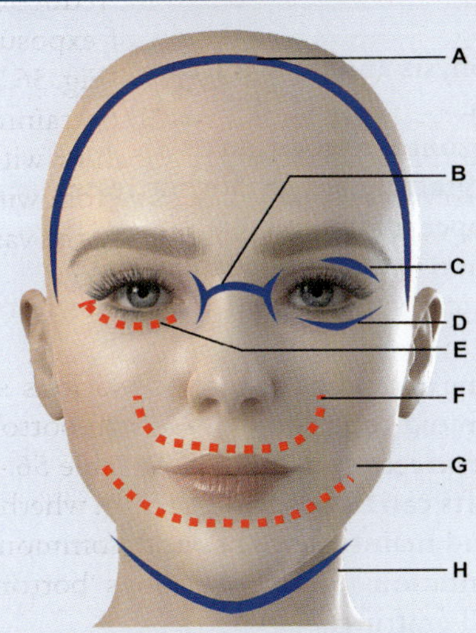

A - Coronal with preauricular extension
B - Paranasal
C - Superior tarsal crease
D - Subciliary
E - Transconjunctival with lateral canthotomy
F - Maxillary vestibule
G - Mandibular vestibule
H - Cervical crease

Incision/Approach	Location of Fracture
Coronal flap	Frontal sinus, supraorbital rim and orbital roof • Naso-orbitoethmoid and medial canthal tendon • Superior aspect of the medial and lateral orbital wall • Zygomatic arch • Mandibular condyle (with preauricular extension)
Subciliary and trans-conjunctival incision with lateral canthotomy	• Infraorbital rim, medial and lateral orbital wall, and orbital floor • Frontozygomatic suture • Lateral nasal region
Upper eyelid crease incision	• Superior and lateral regions of the orbit • Frontozygomatic suture
Perinasal incisions	• Naso-orbitoethmoid region, medial canthal tendon and nasolacrimal sac. These incisions are generally avoided because of the potential for significant scarring.
Maxillary vestibular incision	Maxilla and zygomaticomaxillary buttress
Mandibular vestibular incision	Mandible from the ramus to the symphysis
Cervical incisions (neck)	Mandible, except for high condylar neck fracture. It is also indicated for comminuted and complicated fractures.

TABLE 56.4 Sequencing in Panfacial Fracture

Bottom-Up	Top-Down
1. Repair of palatal fracture	1. Repair of frontal sinus fracture
2. Maxillomandibular fixation	2. Repair of bilateral ZMC fracture
3. Repair of condyle fracture	3. Repair of NOE fracture
4. Repair of mandible fracture (body/symphysis/ramus)	4. Repair of Le Fort fracture (palatal split)
5. Repair of ZMC and arch	5. Maxillomandibular fixation
6. Repair of frontal sinus fracture	6. Repair of bilateral subcondylar fractures
7. Repair of NOE fracture	7. Repair of mandible fracture (body/symphysis/ramus)
8. Repair of maxilla	

Maxillomandibular fixation (MMF) with the maxilla. It is followed by the reduction and fixation of ZMC complex fractures which allows for a more accurate repositioning of the upper midface. The maxilla is then fixed along the zygomaticomaxillary buttress. Lastly, the NOE complex is reduced and stabilised (Fig. 56.6)

ii. The '*top-down*' starts at the zygomatic region. Reduction begins at the sphenozygomatic suture which is fixed either inside the orbit or along the lateral aspect of the orbit. The zygomatic arch is then reduced and plated. Under projection of the midface can occur if the arches are not properly reduced. The zygoma is further reduced and fixated at the frontozygomatic suture. It is followed by the fixation of NOE complex. The maxilla is addressed next, using the zygomaticomaxillary buttress and pyriform rim as a guide. Maxillomandibular fixation can then be established followed by the reduction and fixation of the mandibular condyle and the symphysis/body/angle fractures (Fig. 56.7)

iii. Neither one of these techniques will achieve optimal results in every situation. Rather, a method that progresses from the known to the unknown is more accurate. For example, if there is a significant calvarial injury, it may be difficult to start from the cranium and proceed caudally. In this case, a sequence that starts from bottom to top may yield ideal outcomes, allowing the surgeon to

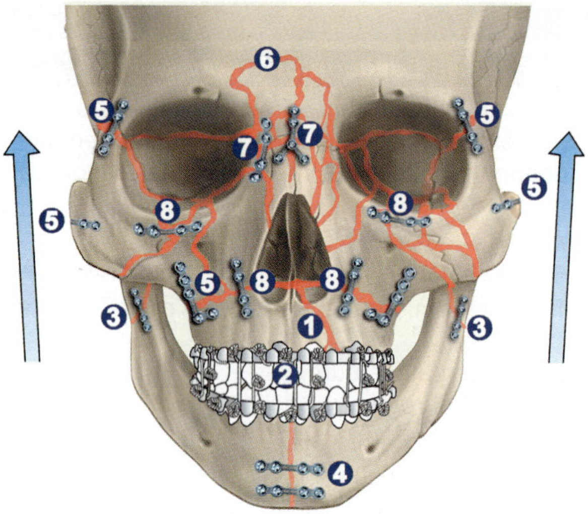

Figure 56.6 Bottom-up sequence. (1) Palatal fracture. (2) Intermaxillary fixation (IMF). (3) Condyle fracture. (4) Fractures of the mandible (5) ZMC (zygomaticomaxillary buttress and zygomatic arch and frontozygomatic (FZ) suture). (6) Frontal bone. (7 and 8) Orbital and NOE fractures.

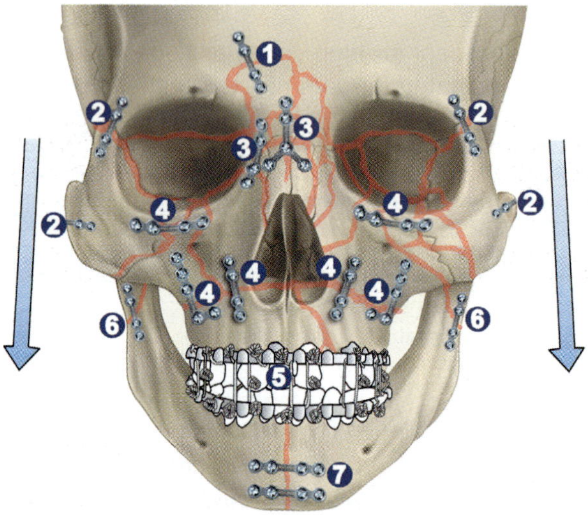

Figure 56.7 Top-down sequence. (1) Frontal bone. (2) Zygoma. (3) NOE fractures. (4) Infraorbital rim and zygomatic buttress. (5) IMF. (6) Condyle. (7) Mandible is reduced lastly at the symphysis and body region, respectively.

reconstruct the damaged cranial portion last. Conversely, if there is a significant comminution of the mandible, it may be appropriate to start from the cranium and proceed down (top to bottom). Thus, the panfacial trauma can be managed by both approaches with the use of known landmarks to achieve optimal results.

A summary of the systematic outline to panfacial fracture reconstruction is as follows:

A. Panfacial fractures—all or most levels of the facial skeleton
B. Mandible:
   i. Maxillomandibular fixation
   ii. Fixation of condylar region:
      - Unilateral (if there is significant displacement)
      - Bilateral fixation (for restoring vertical height of mandible)
   iii. Fixation of symphysis and body fractures
C. Zygomas and maxilla:
   i. Vertical and horizontal restoration
   ii. If required bone grafting to recreate buttresses
D. Reconstruction of upper midface:
   i. Orbital rim fixation (inferior and lateral rim):
      - Provides vertical support and forms the horizontal frame
      - Orbital volume should be restored
   ii. Naso-orbital-ethmoid complex:
      - Telecanthus correction
      - If needed grafts can be used
   iii. Establishment and maintenance of nasal patency
E. Implants and augmentation:
   i. Orbital floor/wall grafting:
      - Porous polyethylene
      - Split calvarial grafts
   ii. Nasal dorsal onlay grafting:
      - Calvarium, rib, alloplastic grafts
   iii. Other onlay grafts (malar eminence, frontal bar)
F. Soft tissue supports

Manson et al. sequencing of fracture:

Manson et al. described panfacial fractures as two facial halves separated by a fracture at the Le Fort I level (Fig. 56.8A)

- The *upper facial half* was divided into an upper unit, comprising the frontal bone with its supraorbital ridges and roof of orbits, and a midfacial unit
- The *lower facial half* was further divided into an upper occlusal level, comprising the maxillary and mandibular alveolar processes with their associated teeth as well as the palate, and a lower unit comprising the vertical ramus and horizontal basal mandible.

Killey and Kay sequencing of fracture:

They used three concentric rings as guide for fixation of panfacial fractures. Fixation begins from the outer circle (frontal, lateral orbital rim, zygoma), middle circle (maxilla) to the inner circle (nasal complex) (Fig. 56.8B).

SECONDARY RECONSTRUCTION OF PANFACIAL FRACTURES

Delayed repair of panfacial fractures occurs either due to severity of other injuries or comorbidities associated with trauma. These patients can have recurrent infections, enophthalmos, malocclusion, trismus, facial flattening or asymmetric widening. Bony malunion and soft tissue atrophy can occur if the surgery is delayed for more than 2- 3 weeks (Table 56.5).

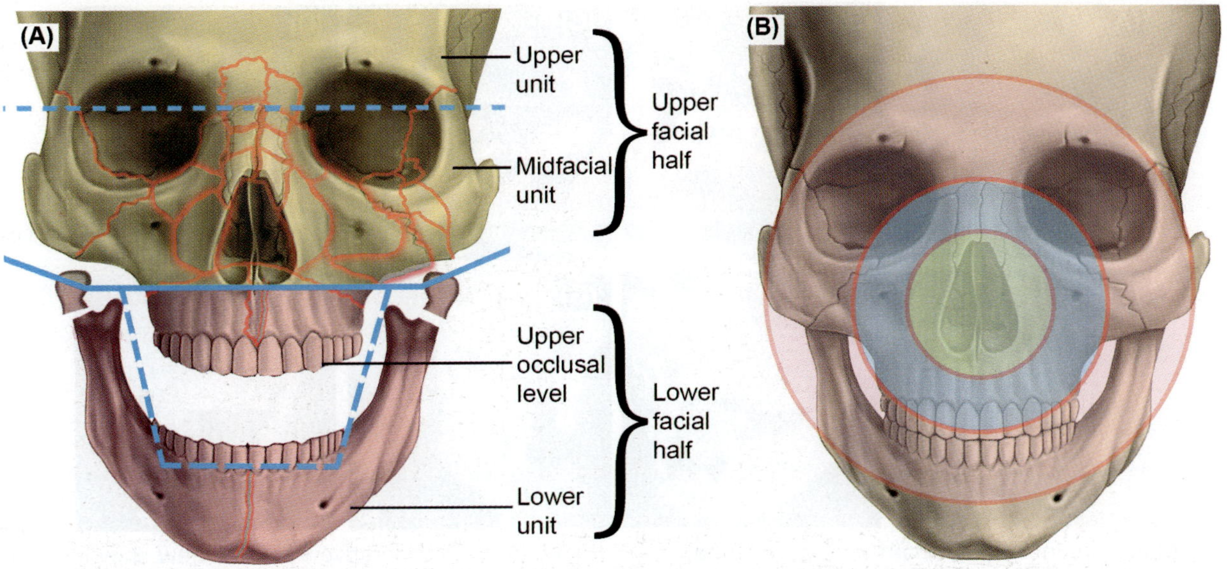

Figure 56.8 (**A**) Manson's division of panfacial fractures into two facial halves separated by a fracture at the Le Fort I level. (**B**) Killey and Kay sequencing of fracture.

TABLE 56.5 Classification of Panfacial Fracture According to Mandibular Fracture Patterns (Edward Ellis)

Type	Mandibular Fracture
I	Arch disruption
II	Angle/condyle
III	Arch disruption and angle/condyle

Planning for delayed treatment of panfacial fractures (greater than 4 weeks after injury) is very challenging. For treatment planning and to analyse the deformities, we require the following:

- CT scans
- Stereolithographic models for severely comminuted fractures
- Virtual surgical planning can guide us in free manipulation of the fracture fragments, as well as to custom plates
- Dental impression and models can be cut, realigned and articulated to reestablish the maxillary and mandibular arch form and the occlusion
- Surgical splints can also be fabricated to assist in surgery
- Severe cases might require orthognathic surgery/Le Fort I osteotomy to correct malocclusion.

Managing the panfacial fractures secondarily are difficult and may require additional osteotomies, grafts and custom made implants. *The goal is to establish the preinjury facial bony appearance—facial width, projection and height* (Table 56.6 and Fig. 56.9).

TABLE 56.6 Management of Panfacial Fractures

Type I	The occlusion was reestablished first before fixing the fragments.
Type II	The mandibular angle, ascending ramus or condyle region were repaired first.
Type III	Osteotomies of the malunited angle or condyle were done first. The mandibular arch was restored using a splint followed by reduction and stabilisation of the ramus or condyle.

COMPLICATIONS

Panfacial fractures are associated with many complications, but the most prevalent complication is widening of the facial complex. It is due to improperly reduced key areas. If the 1st area approached is fixed in an improper location, subsequent fragments will be reduced and fixed in an improper spatial arrangement, resulting in a series of errors and a widened facial complex. To prevent this, it is advisable to use stable segments, known landmarks and anatomic reduction in the management of panfacial fractures. In severe cases, a three-dimensional stereolithographic model can be made to recreate the fractures and for proper reduction and fixation of the fractures.

- Malocclusion
- Nonunion
- Infection
- Enophthalmos
- Asymmetry
- Mandibular hypomotility
- Soft tissue problem.

CONCLUSION

The management of panfacial fractures is extremely complex. However, with advances in technology and correct diagnosis, surgeons can implement an effective treatment plan for panfacial fractures.

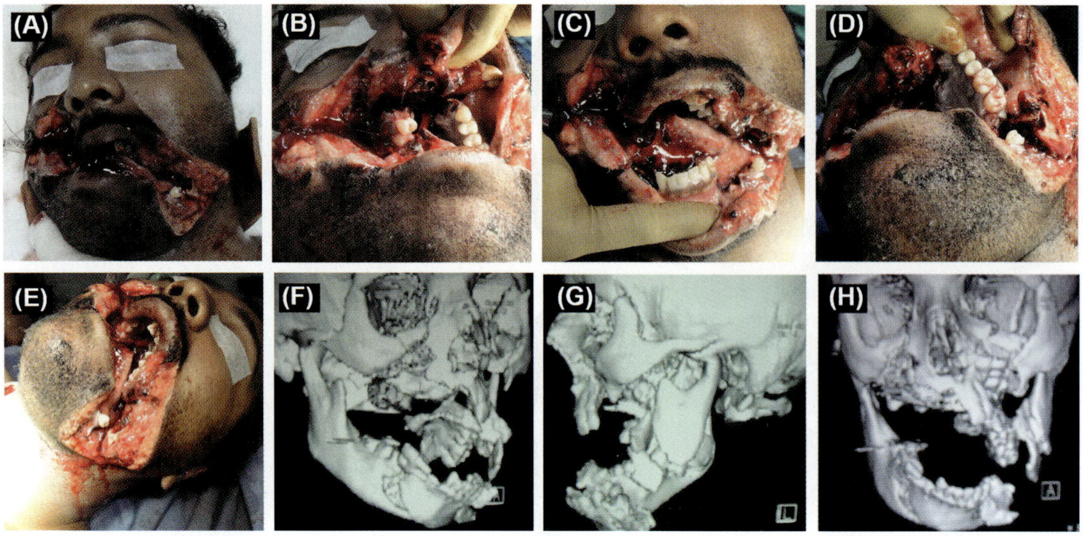

Figure 56.9 Management of panfacial fracture. (**A**) Preoperative view. (**B–E**) Preoperative intraoral view showing through and through lacerations on the right and left cheek and lips, comminuted maxilla involving the palate, and mandible fracture. (**F–H**) CT scan shows panfacial fracture involving the frontal, maxilla, zygoma, nasal bone and mandible, comminuted maxilla into multiple fragments, loss of bone in the left mandibular body.

PAEDIATRIC FACIAL FRACTURES

I. Anatomical considerations
II. Assessment of trauma in paediatric patients:
  a. Airway
  b. Breathing
  c. Circulation
  d. Disability
III. Diagnosis of facial fracture
IV. Management of paediatric facial fractures:
  a. Anterior cranial fracture (frontal and orbital roof fracture)
  b. NOE and nasal fracture
  c. Orbital fracture
  d. ZMC fracture
  e. Maxillary fracture
  f. Mandible fracture
  g. Condylar fracture
  h. Dentoalveolar fracture
V. Growth disturbance.

ANATOMICAL CONSIDERATIONS

The developmental anatomy of paediatric patients differs significantly from that of adults. At the time of birth, the cranium to face ratio is 8:1, which decreases to 4:1 at the age of 5 and becomes 2.5:1 in an adult. Thus, in infants, a *large cranium* protects the face. But as the child grows older this ratio decreases making the child more susceptible to fractures.

The most important consideration of a growing jaw is the presence of tooth and its development, which makes the surgical manipulation in the developing teeth area challenging.

The paediatric facial bone has a greater cancellous to cortical ratio, making the maxillofacial complex more *malleable*. Thus, greenstick fractures occur more frequently in children when compared to adults. Having more cancellous bone makes screw fixation of fractures less favourable. For these reasons, closed reduction has become the practical option for most paediatric facial fractures.

ASSESSMENT OF TRAUMA IN PAEDIATRIC PATIENTS

Emergency evaluation of an injured child must follow the ATLS protocol similar to adults. Shock and inadequate oxygen delivery to the tissues are the most common causes of mortality in injured children. The primary assessment should be aimed at resuscitating the severely injured child.

AIRWAY

Children's airways are smaller than those of adults. Hence, it is vital to conduct an airway assessment. The smaller airway increases the airway resistance and the ease of obstruction. The 1st priority in a maxillofacial trauma patient is the establishment and maintenance of a patent airway. The airway should be cleared from any secretions, foreign bodies, loose teeth or tissues.

BREATHING

After establishing the airway patency, status of breathing and adequate exchange of air (ventilation) should be evaluated by chest movements, pulse oximetry, arterial blood gas and chest X-ray. Adequate ventilation (oxygen administration) is maintained by high flow oxygen masks or ambu bag.

CIRCULATION

Hypovolaemia (blood loss) can be identified by increased heart rate, irregular pulse, pale skin tone and decreased urine output. Total blood volume in a child is approximately 80 mL/kg. Blood loss is compensated by initial intravenous fluid resuscitation of 20 mL/kg normal saline or ringer lactate for 15–20 min.

If required cross-matched blood can be transfused with initial bolus of 10–20 mL/kg.

DISABILITY

A rapid neurological assessment and presence of any life-threatening injuries should be identified. The level of consciousness and the severity of the injury can be assessed by the Glasgow Coma Scale (GCS) (Table 56.7).

EXPOSURE AND COMPLETE EXAMINATION OF THE PATIENT

Careful examination of the child is done to identify fractures and wounds throughout the body. The cervical spine should be stabilised with cervical collars.

The secondary survey involves a more comprehensive examination of injuries from head to toe.

DIAGNOSIS OF FACIAL FRACTURE

The mechanism of injury should be known by the clinician as it may indicate the type of force imparted over the facial skeleton.

Examination of facial injury involves both skeletal and soft tissue components. Soft tissue examination involves swelling, lacerations, abrasions, contusions and penetrating injuries. Skeletal examination includes palpation for step deformity, irregularities along the bony margin and mobility of the fragment. CT scans provide a rapid and accurate assessment of bony injuries.

MANAGEMENT OF PAEDIATRIC FACIAL FRACTURES

FRONTAL SINUS FRACTURE

Frontal sinus fractures are rare in children. Frontal sinus fractures are often associated with intracranial injury. Management is focused on treating the concomitant intracranial injury and preventing the long-term complications such as meningitis, Cerebrospinal fluid (CSF) leak, frontal sinusitis and other cosmetic deformities.

- Conservative management is recommended for undisplaced anterior or posterior table fractures without CSF leak
- Displaced frontal sinus fractures involving the anterior table require open reduction and internal fixation (ORIF). Fixation can be done using resorbable plates or titanium plates, which may require removal in the future
- Displaced fractures involving the posterior table may require cranialisation of the frontal sinus.

NASO-ORBITO-ETHMOID (NOE) AND NASAL BONE FRACTURE

The NOE complex involves the nasal bones, medial orbital wall and nasal projection of frontal bone. NOE fractures manifest as telecanthus and unstable medial canthal ligament and central bony fragment. Normal *intercanthal distance* in children is *22 mm* approximately. Surgical management is complex and is aimed in restoring the orbital volume, nasal contour, midface projection and intercanthal distance. To gain access to the NOE complex, a coronal incision is made and transnasal fixation is done with nonabsorbable sutures. Most of the paediatric NOE fractures require secondary intervention.

Nasal fractures in children:

Nasal fractures are uncommon in children due to the lack of projection and relative suppleness of the nasal bones. Nasal injuries in children should not be overlooked as it may impede the growth of the septum and nasomaxillary complex.

At the age of 8 years, the lateral walls almost reach 90% of their final size. By the age of 14, most of the anatomic components are completely grown with little difference.

It is crucial to treat children's nasal fractures, as undetected injuries can later result in deformities.

- Most of the fractures are treated by closed reduction as these injuries are often greenstick fractures
- Simple nasal fractures with adequate airflow are often approached with closed reduction and postoperative nasal packing
- A fractured and displaced nasal septum causing airway obstruction and growth disturbance can be treated by open reduction

TABLE 56.7 Paediatric Glasgow Coma Scale (GCS)

Eye Opening (E)	Verbal Response (V)	Motor Response (M)
Spontaneously = 4 To voice = 3 To pain = 2 None = 1	Age appropriate words, smiles = 5 Cries but consolable, irritable, uncooperative, inappropriate interaction = 4 Moaning, inconsistently consolable = 3 Inconsolable, agitated, unaware of the environment = 2 None = 1	Obeys commands = 6 Localising pain = 5 Withdrawal from pain = 4 Flexion to pain = 3 Extension to pain = 2 None = 1

Total GCS= E+V+M=15. GCS less than 8 indicates severe injury. The disability can be quickly assessed by AVPU.
A: Alert. **V:** Responds to **Vocal** stimuli. **P:** Responds only to **Painful** stimuli. **U: Unresponsive**.

- Secondary rhinoplasty may be needed to correct the post-traumatic deformities
- *Septal haematomas* are more common in paediatric nasal trauma. Untreated haematoma may lead to infection, septal destruction and long-term nasal deformity and airway obstruction.

The optimal age for septal surgery in children is 13–14 years old, when growth is complete.

ORBITAL FRACTURES

The orbital floor is extremely thin and any injury to the globe usually results in fracture of the orbital floor (blowout fracture). In children, the orbital floor bone is pliable and often tends to recoil, entrapping the inferior rectus muscle and associated periorbital tissues resulting in 'trap door' phenomenon. This entrapped orbital tissue leads to restriction of eye movements and diplopia. Ophthalmic consultation is necessary to rule out any associated ocular injuries. Fracture of orbital floor and muscle entrapment can be ruled out by CT imaging.

Diplopia, enophthalmos bigger than 2 mm, and orbital floor abnormalities greater than 1 cm in CT scans require surgical intervention. In children, surgery is best recommended between 7 and 10 days. Orbital floors can be reconstructed with autogenous materials or absorbable mesh.

Jordan et al., were the first to report 'white-eyed blowout fracture'. It is described as orbital blowout fracture in children with lack of external signs of injury. It may be associated with the following characteristics:

1) Discrete evidence of fracture on CT
2) Restriction in ocular movements
3) Minimal to no soft tissue trauma
4) Patients may present with bradycardia, or headache due to the oculocardiac reflex, mimicking intracranial injury.

White-eyed blowout fracture require immediate surgical intervention within 24 h.

ZYGOMATICOMAXILLARY COMPLEX (ZMC) FRACTURE

Though the ZMC fracture is uncommon in children, its incidence increases as they grow due to the development of sinuses and increased prominence of zygoma. Zygomatic fractures present with periorbital oedema, flattening of the malar eminence, and step deformities, trismus if the arch is fractured and displaced, and infraorbital nerve hypoaesthesia.

- Undisplaced or minimally displaced fractures are treated conservatively
- For significantly displaced or comminuted fractures ORIF is necessary to: (1) correct facial asymmetry, (2) restore normal mouth opening and (3) restore the globe position, eye movements and normal vision.

Surgical approaches can be vestibular (intraoral), lateral eyebrow, or to its potential for postoperative alopecia. A transconjunctival approach is well tolerated by the children. Though microplates provide adequate stability and fixation without compromising vital structures, bioresorbable plates may be used to avoid resurgery.

MAXILLARY FRACTURE

Midface fractures are less common in children. It is because of the protection provided by the mandible and cranium, absorbing most of the traumatic force, elastic nature of the bones and flexibility of the osseous suture lines. The midface of the children have fewer pneumatised paranasal sinuses and tooth buds in the developing jaws. Maxillary fractures present with mobility of maxilla, malocclusion and paraesthesia. Treatment should be aimed in restoring the occlusion and midface projection.

- Closed reduction by IMF with arch bars is difficult as the children have mixed dentition and the teeth might get avulsed. The erupted teeth might not provide adequate retention for arch bars, due to the weak and undeveloped roots
- Cap or occlusal splints secured with circumferential wires can be used for IMF for 2–3 weeks
- Skeletal fixation by ORIF is reserved for significantly displaced maxillary fractures. The presence of developing tooth buds limits the placement of plate and screws
- Resorbable plating systems have been preferred to avoid complications such as plate extrusion and growth restriction.

MANDIBLE FRACTURE

Mandible fractures are one of the most common paediatric facial fracture. The most common causes of fractures are motor vehicle accidents, sports-related injuries, falls and assaults. The presence of developing tooth buds make the mandibular bone weaker and more susceptible to fracture.

Anatomy of paediatric mandible:

- The mandible is a unique bone, forming a U-shaped construct
- The growth of mandible occurs in a superior and posterior direction, resulting in a concomitant downward and forward displacement of the mandibular body and symphysis
- The inferior alveolar nerve changes its position from the lingual inferior border to a more superior position as the child grows
- It has high osteogenic potential due to its rich blood supply from the inferior alveolar artery
- The medullary centre of the mandible becomes more thickened and calcified following permanent tooth eruption.

Physical examination includes pain on palpation over the fracture site, malocclusion, decreased mouth opening, deviation of jaw on opening, paraesthesia and intraoral lacerations or ecchymosis. OPG and CT scan remain the gold standard imaging for mandible fractures.

The treatment of mandibular fractures in children is aimed at restoring the facial form, occlusion and mandibular function. Proper management is critical in paediatric patients, as it may disrupt the growth and dental development.

- Most of the paediatric mandible fractures can be managed conservatively
- Children with mixed dentition have the capacity for spontaneous occlusal readjustments
- Mild malocclusions and minimally displaced fractures are kept under observation. Soft diets, physiotherapy, symptomatic pain treatment, and long-term follow-up are recommended for children
- Closed reduction for 2–3 weeks of MMF is used to treat mild to moderately displaced mandibular fractures. (IMF screws, cap splints, gunning splint or lingual splint.)
- Open reduction and internal fixation (ORIF) is indicated for severely displaced mandible fractures, patients where closed reduction is not feasible, or with an associated condylar fracture
- The intraoral approach is preferred as it eliminates scars and facial nerve injury
- Children with mixed dentition do not require a superior border plating and fixation with monocortical screws are sufficient. ORIF with plates may harm the tooth buds and the development of jaw. Hence, titanium miniplates were used for fixation and then removed after 3–12 months postoperatively. To avoid all these complications, biodegradable plates have been proposed. These plates do not interfere with growth and do not require secondary surgery for plate removal
- *Bioresorbable plates* provide reliable stability without major complications. They are safe, efficient with low infection rate (Fig. 56.10).

CONDYLAR FRACTURE IN CHILDREN

The most common sites of fracture in mandible are condyle (55%), parasymphysis (27%), body (9%) and angle (8%). In children, the mandibular condyles are short, stout and highly vascular with thin cortical plate, making the condyle susceptible to 'burst' type of fractures. The multiple small fragments and high osteogenicity within the joint space increases the risk of joint ankylosis.

Condylar fractures in children less than 3 years of age are at greater risk for growth disturbance. Inadequate or overtreatment may lead to growth retardation and mandibular hypomobility. The treatment should be aimed at: (1) preserving the mandible function and (2) maintenance of ramus height.

Conservative management with a brief period of IMF for 7–10 days, followed by active movement of the joint is recommended, for children <12 years (Table 56.8).

Permanent dentition stage:

In adolescents (13–17 years), the potential for major regeneration and remodelling is at a lesser degree. Open reduction should be considered in unilateral or bilateral condylar fractures with persistent malocclusion and dislocation after 7–10 days of intermaxillary fixation to avert progressive deformity (Figs. 56.11 and 56.12).

Indications for open reduction of condyle fracture:

- Displaced condyle into the middle cranial fossa
- Unacceptable occlusion after closed reduction
- Lateral extracapsular displacement of the condyle
- Bilateral fractures of the condyles with comminuted midface fractures
- Penetrating wound
- Invasion by a foreign body.

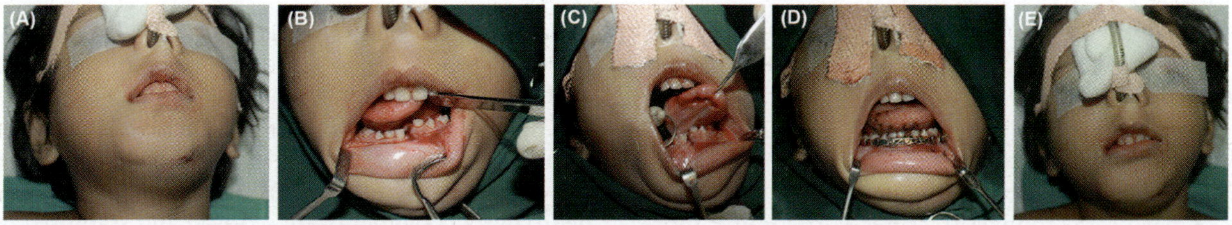

Figure 56.10 Closed reduction of left parasymphysis fracture. **(A)** Preoperative extraoral view with swelling over the chin region. **(B)** Preoperative intraoral view with fracture between the lower incisors. **(C)** Intraoral view with laceration involving the tongue. **(D)** The fracture was reduced and immobilised using arch bar. **(E)** Immediate postoperative view.

TABLE 56.8 Management of Condyle Fracture in Primary and Mixed Dentition (6–12 Years)

Fracture Pattern	Management
Unilateral condylar fractures—relatively normal opening and stable occlusion	Analgesics, soft diet for 5–7 days
Significant pain and severe malocclusion	Short period of immobilisation for 7–10 days
Bilateral subcondylar fractures—relatively normal opening and stable occlusion	Analgesics and soft diet for 7–10 days
Bilateral fractures with significant dislocation, malocclusion	• Immobilisation for 7–10 days followed by guiding elastics for 7–10 days • If malocclusion persists, open reduction should be considered

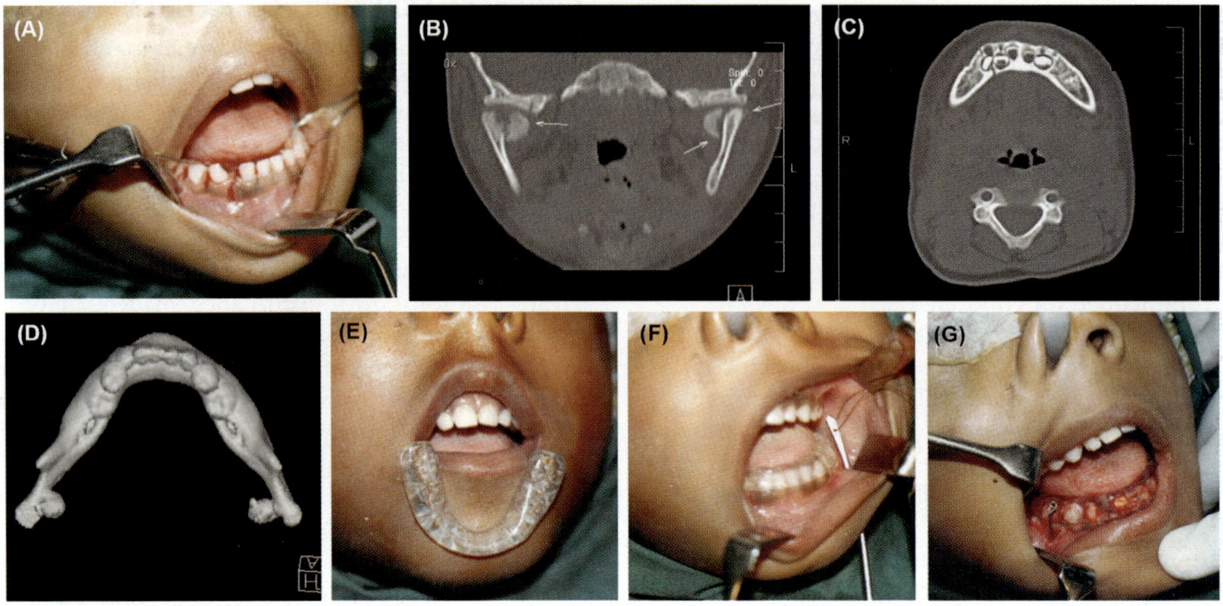

Figure 56.11 Bilateral mandibular condyle fracture. (**A**) Preoperative view showing gingival laceration and step deformity between the lateral incisor and canine. (**B–D**) Preoperative CT scan showing bilateral condyle fracture with medial displacement and right parasymphysis fracture. (**E–G**) The fracture was reduced and the cap splint was secured using circummandibular wiring.

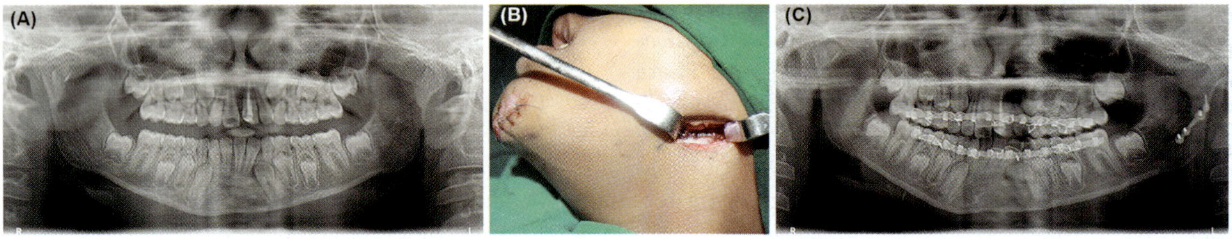

Figure 56.12 Open reduction of paediatric condyle fracture. (**A**) Preoperative OPG showing fracture involving the left condyle. (**B**) Intraoperative view showing reduced and fixed left condyle through Risdon's incision. (**C**) Postoperative OPG showing miniplate at the left condyle region.

Relative indications:

- Inability to tolerate IMF
- Severe airway obstruction
- Severely injured or disabled patients.

ORIF of paediatric condyle fractures is becoming more popular with the introduction of miniplates, microplates and resorbable plates.

DENTOALVEOLAR FRACTURE

Children up to 6 years have only primary dentition, 6–12 have mixed dentition, and those over 12 have permanent dentition. In children, trauma to the teeth can be divided into primary or secondary dentition (Table 56.9).

Generally, trauma to the primary dentition (fractured, luxated or avulsed teeth) is treated with extraction, unless it is necessary for space maintenance. Avulsed primary teeth are not preferred for replantation, as they might cause damage to the underlying permanent teeth. Less displaced teeth without occlusal interference can be left and monitored. Dentoalveolar fractures are usually reduced and stabilised with arch bar and wires.

Trauma to the permanent dentition are treated based on the degree of injury. Luxated or avulsed permanent teeth should be repositioned and reimplanted within 60 min and stabilised with bonded wires or arch bars. Fractures of the dentoalveolar segments are reduced and stabilised with arch bars or wires. Larger alveolar segments can be treated with plate and screw fixation (Figs. 56.13 and 56.14).

(Refer to Chapter 48 for further management of permanent teeth injuries).

GROWTH DISTURBANCE

In children, fractures may affect the growth and development of face. The most commonly affected areas of growth are the orbital region, nasomaxillary complex and condyle region.

Fractures involving the orbital region at a very young age can result in loss of orbital volume and periorbital tissue atrophy. After 6 years, the growth disturbance on the orbit decreases.

Injuries to the cartilaginous part of the nasomaxillary complex can affect the midface projection and elongation. These children require long-term follow-up.

TABLE 56.9 Management of Primary and Mixed Dentition Injuries

Type of Injury	Treatment
Crown Fractures	
Class I (enamel only)	Smoothen rough edges
Class II (enamel and dentin)	1. $Ca(OH)_2$ or glass ionomer liner over dentin 2. Composite resin restoration
Class III (pulpal involvement)	
• Vital pulp	1. Formocresol pulpotomy 2. Coronal coverage:
• Nonvital pulp	1. $Zn(OH)_2$—eugenol pulpectomy 2. Coronal coverage
Class IV (root fracture)	
• Apical 3rd	No treatment; follow-up
• Cervical 3rd	1. Remove tooth fragments 2. Allow apical 3rd to resorb if compromise to permanent tooth bud is expected
Luxations	
• Subluxation	Monitor/follow-up
• Lateral luxations	Realign/remove as needed
• Extrusion	Realign/remove as needed
• Intrusion	1. Allow to reerupt 4–6 week 2. Remove if in contact with permanent successor 3. Remove if infection presents

Condyle being the mandibular growth centre, fractures may result in growth anomalies such as malocclusion, facial asymmetry or Temporomandibular Joint (TMJ) arthritis. On the contrary, the ability of the children to remodel and spontaneous healing can result in condylar remodelling and complete recovery of the condylar injuries.

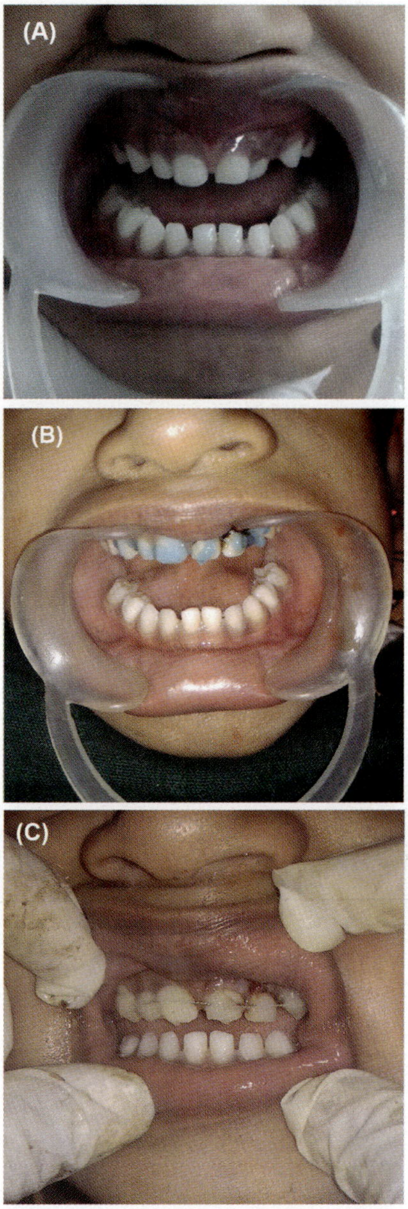

Figure 56.13 (**A**) Intruded and palatally displaced 62 in a 3-year-old child due to self-fall. (**B** and **C**) Teeth is reduced, etched and splinting done using wire and composite.

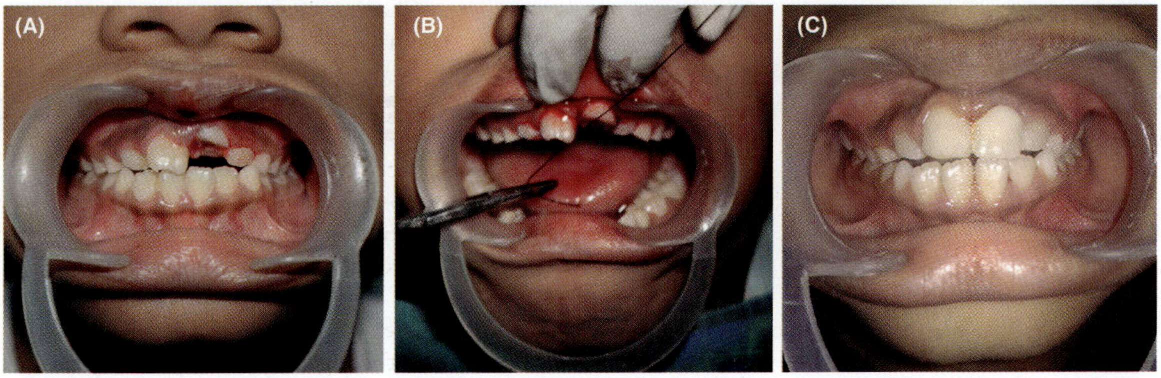

Figure 56.14 (**A**) Fractured and labially displaced 21. (**B**) The labially placed tooth was reduced and the gingiva sutured. (**C**) The fractured tooth was root canal treated and restored with crown.

Section XIV

Recent Advances

Chapter 57

Recent Advances in Oral and Maxillofacial Surgery

OUTLINE

RECENT ADVANCES IN RECENT ANATOMICAL DISCOVERIES

TUBARIAL SALIVARY GLAND

It is located in the lateral walls of the nasopharynx overlying the torus tubarius. On average, it is about 1.5 inches (3.81 cm) in length.

After visualisation by positron emission tomography (PET)/computed tomography (CT) with prostate-specific membrane antigen (PSMA) ligands, the presence of previously unnoticed bilateral macroscopic salivary gland locations in the human nasopharynx was suspected (Fig. 57.1).

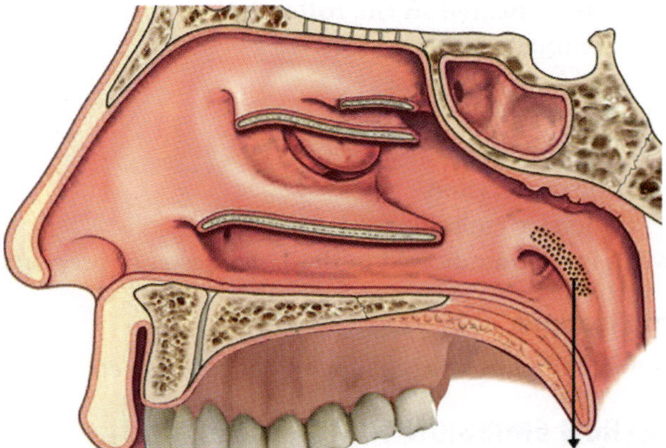

Figure 57.1 Schematic representation of region of the torus tubarius with overlying tubarial gland.

RECENT ADVANCES IN IMAGING

COMPUTED TOMOGRAPHY ANGIOGRAPHY

Computed tomography angiography (CTA) can assess arteries as small as 1 mm in diameter. Since it is volumetric, CTA allows three-dimensional visualisation of the vasculature to separate superimposed structures.

CTA or magnetic resonance imaging (MRI) is indicated to improve lesion characterisation and treatment guidance. In most cases, MRI protocols not only include conventional sequences but also contrast-enhanced magnetic resonance angiography (MRA), which improves the evaluation of the

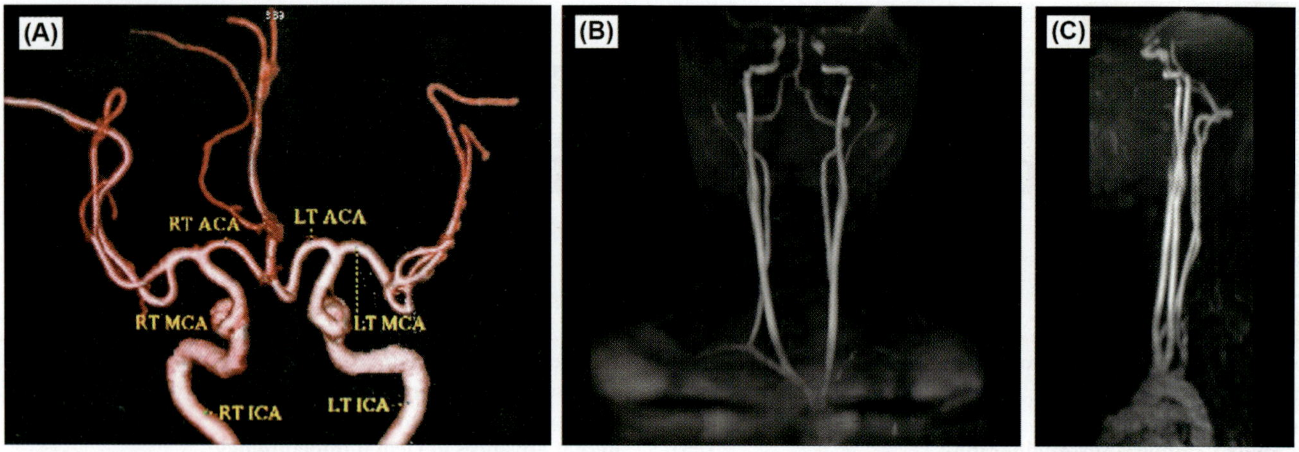

Figure 57.2 (**A**) Computed tomography angiography. (**B** and **C**) Magnetic resonance angiography.

vascular network and helps to characterise vascular malformations (Fig. 57.2A).

MAGNETIC RESONANCE ANGIOGRAPHY (MRA)

MRA encompasses several imaging techniques based on MRI, developed for studying the arterial and venous systems (Fig. 57.2B).

In comparison to traditional angiography, an MRA has the following advantages:

- Noninvasive
- High-resolution volumetric images
- It does not expose patients to ionising radiation
- The iodine-based contrast materials that are used for CT scanning are more likely to trigger an allergic reaction than the gadolinium-based contrast material, which is used for MRA.

MRA is indicated in the following:

1) Trigeminal neuralgia (TN)
2) Carotid artery disease
3) Cerebral stroke
4) Congenital heart disease
5) Aortic coarctation
6) Pulmonary embolism.

MRA is contraindicated in the 1st trimester of pregnancy.

Complications

Blisters, reddening of the skin, loss of hearing, etc.

POSITRON EMISSION TOMOGRAPHY (PET)

- It uses positron emission from particular radionuclides to produce detailed functional images within the body
- The PET method gives quantitative measurements, which makes it possible to track relative changes over time as a disease progresses or as a response to a certain stimulus
- The method is based on the detection of radioactivity emitted when a radioactive tracer is injected into a peripheral vein in minute quantities.

SINGLE-PHOTON EMISSION COMPUTED TOMOGRAPHY (SPECT)

- It is a nuclear imaging technique commonly employed in diagnostic medicine
- A radioactive tracer (also called a probe) is injected into the bloodstream and then taken up by certain tissues
- SPECT produces a 3D image of the distribution of the tracer by using a specialised nuclear medicine camera.

Indications

Encephalitis, detecting cerebrovascular disease, coronary artery disease.

Complications

Side effects include headache, GI distress, hypotension, chest discomfort, etc. (Refer to **Chapter 4** for SPECT, PET, CBCT.)

RECENT ADVANCES IN SURGICAL PLANNING

STEREOLITHOGRAPHY

Chuck Hull in 1984 coined the term ‘stereolithography’. It is a form of technology using 3D printing for creating models, prototypes, patterns and production of parts in layers using photopolymerisation. Photopolymerisation is a process, which causes linkage of chains of molecules in the presence of light, thereby forming polymers. These polymers form a body of a 3D solid structure (Fig. 57.3A and B).

Technique

It functions by focusing an ultraviolet (UV) laser on a photopolymer resin vat. The computer aids in manufacturing or computer-aided design software.

CAD/CAM is utilised for the UV laser to draw a preprogrammed design or shape the photopolymer resin vat. As photopolymers are sensitive to ultraviolet light, the resin is solidified photochemically and a single layer of the desired

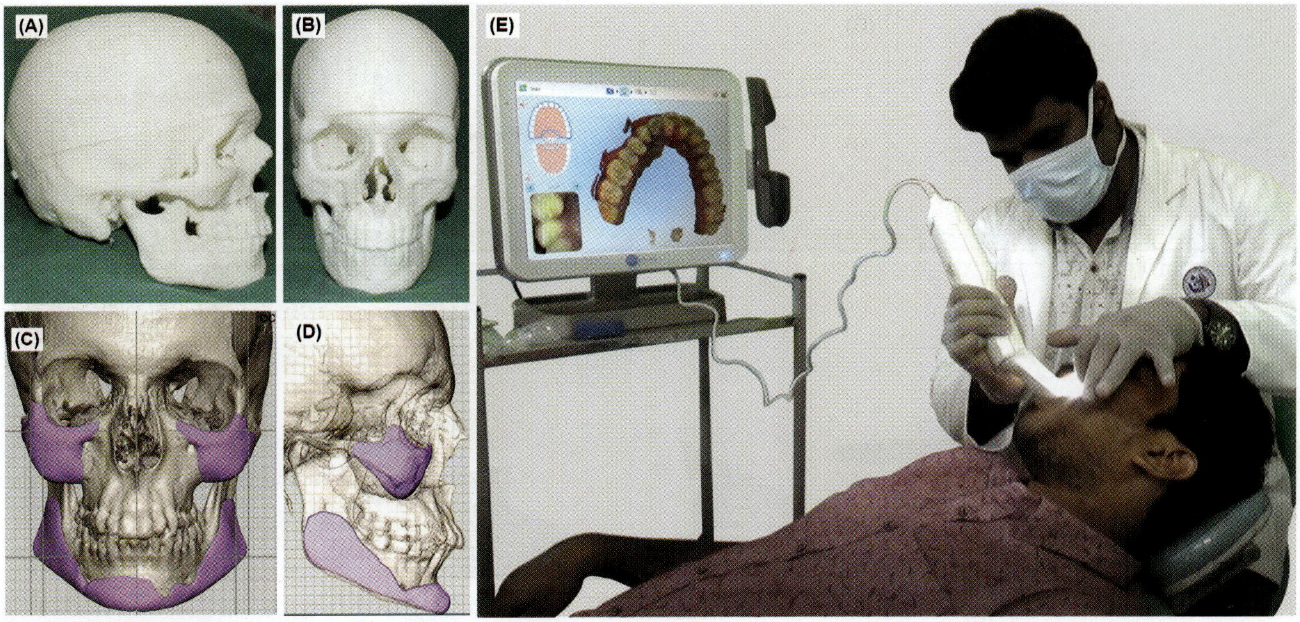

Figure 57.3 (**A** and **B**) Stereolithographic model. (**C** and **D**) Virtual planning software. (**E**) Stereophotogrammetry.

3D object is formed. The 3D object is completed by repeating this process for each layer of the design. The thickness varies from 0.05 to 0.15 mm for a single layer of the design. Modelling for medical purposes involves the use of CT or MRI.

Materials

Models are available in acrylic, polyurethane.

Uses

- To create accurate 3D models
- To create prototypes for products
- In medical modelling
- Complete replacement of temporomandibular joint (TMJ)
- In diagnosis of congenital craniofacial deformities
- Preoperative planning
- Designing implant
- Manufacture of implant
- Orofacial prosthesis
- For patient education and motivation.

Advantages

- Capable of producing any design
- High accuracy
- Quick
- Visualisation as a model
- Prefabrication of custom acrylic resin cranial implants.

Disadvantages

- Expensive
- Accuracy is influenced by multiple factors
- Brittle if made of acrylic.

VIRTUAL PLANNING IN ORTHOGNATHIC SURGERY

In the field of surgical planning, there has been remarkable progress. The intraoperative precision of maxillary repositioning in orthognathic surgery has been greatly improved by computer-assisted virtual surgical planning and the use of CAD–CAM produced splints (Fig. 57.3C and D).

STEREOPHOTOGRAMMETRY

Stereophotogrammetry (SPT) is a technique for calculating three-dimensional coordinates from a series of two-dimensional projections (Fig. 57.3E).

Uses

- Assessment of craniofacial growth and development
- Evaluation of facial soft tissues.

WAFERLESS ORTHOGNATHIC SURGERY

This procedure entails the creation of custom-fabricated cutting stents and patient-specific fixation implants that not only help accomplish the osteotomy but also fix the segment in the proper position without the need of an occlusal wafer.

RECENT ADVANCES IN ANAESTHESIA

LOCAL ANAESTHESIA (REFER CHAPTER 11)

ACCUPAL

- It is a cordless, handheld, compact device
- It inhibits pain by preconditioning the injection site with pressure and vibration
- Accupal integrates the pain gate theory in order to energise the dental tissue in and around the needle-insertion site (Fig. 57.4A).

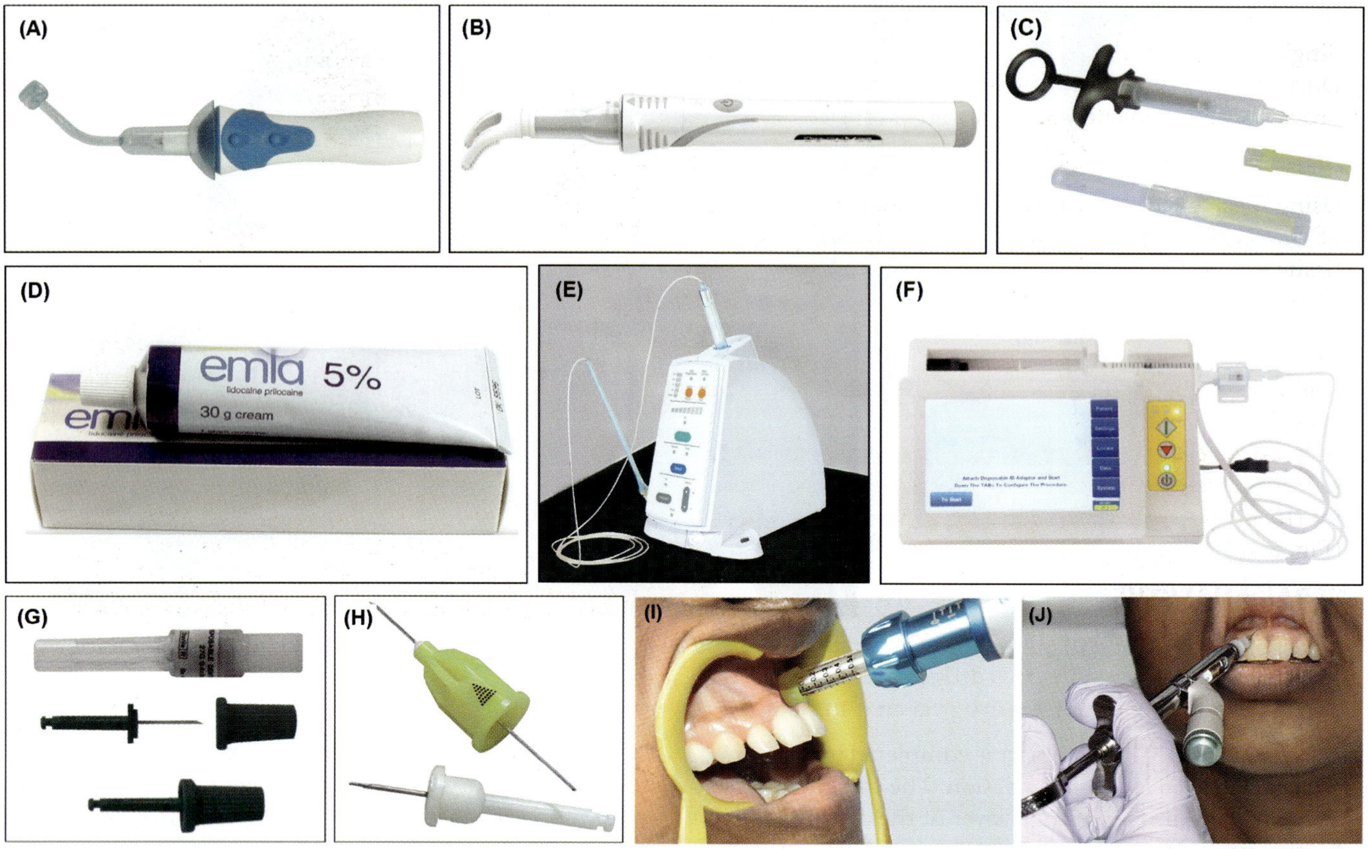

Figure 57.4 (**A**) Accupal. (**B**) Dental vibe. (**C**) Safety dental syringes. (**D**) Eutectic mixture of local anaesthetics (EMLA). (**E**) Computer-controlled local anaesthetic delivery (C-CLAD). (**F**) CompuFlo. (**G**) Stabident. (**H**) X-tip. (**I**) Jet injection. (**J**) VibraJect.

DENTAL VIBE

- It is a cordless, handheld and rechargeable device
- It produces micro-oscillations that are soothing, pulsating and percussive to the injection site
- When compared to a conventional approach, dental vibe remarkably lowered adolescent self-reported pain during local anaesthesia injection (Fig. 57.4B).

SAFETY DENTAL SYRINGES

- The needle has a protective sheath, which helps to prevent needle stick injuries (Fig. 57.4C)
- There are various safety dental syringes available such as:
  a. Ultra Safety Plus XL syringe
  b. UltraSafe syringe
  c. Hypo Safety syringe
  d. RevVac Safety syringe.

EUTECTIC MIXTURE OF LOCAL ANAESTHETICS

- It is an eutectic mixture of local anaesthetics (EMLA) containing lignocaine and prilocaine in the ratio of 1:1 by weight (Fig. 57.4D)
- Prior to painful procedures such as injections, venipuncture, etc., it is applied directly to the skin as a topical agent
- It should be applied 1 h prior to the procedure
- It is widely used in children.

COMPUTER-CONTROLLED LOCAL ANAESTHETIC DELIVERY

- This device aids in the controlled delivery of the anaesthetic and thereby reducing the pain during injection. (Fig. 57.4E)
- Advantages of computer-controlled local anaesthetic delivery (C-CLAD) devices are:
  i) Highly efficient than traditional syringes
  ii) It helps in controlling the speed of injection by administering the anaesthesia gradually.

COMPUFLO

It permits immediate, real-time measurement of fluid exit pressure at the needle tip.

This method of measuring fluid exit pressure at the needle tip is referred to as dynamic pressure sensing technology (Fig. 57.4F).

STABIDENT

- It is a device used for intraosseous anaesthesia
- *Disadvantage:* Anaesthesia cannot be administered to locations that are inaccessible (Fig. 57.4G).

X-TIP

- Single-step method
- During administration, a preliminary drill is set up to provide single-step entry and withdrawal (Fig. 57.4H).

JET INJECTION

- Using mechanical energy, under pressure, a thin column of the local anaesthetic solution is forced into the soft tissue without damaging it
- There is minimal or no pain (Fig. 57.4I).

VIBRAJECT

- It is a vibrating dental local anaesthetic attachment that uses the gate-control principle as its foundation
- It is operated by a battery and when attached to the barrel, it produces intense vibrations that are sensed by the patient, thereby reducing the pain perception (Fig. 57.4J).

GENERAL ANAESTHESIA

TARGET-CONTROLLED INFUSION SYSTEMS

- It administers intravenous (IV) drugs based on the pharmacokinetic behaviour of the drug via an infusion pump controlled by a computer
- Target-controlled infusion (TCI) systems are used to deliver i.v. sedation and general anaesthesia drugs such as propofol and opioids.

PATIENT-CONTROLLED ANALGESIA PUMP

- The objective of patient-controlled analgesia (PCA) is to provide pain relief at the patient's preferred dose and schedule by enabling them to administer a predetermined bolus dose of medication on-demand at the click of a button
- It is indicated for the management of acute, chronic, postsurgical and labour pain
- Drugs can be given intravenously, epidurally or transdermally
- Opioids and local anaesthetics are the most frequently used drugs
- PCA has been shown to be more effective than nonpatient opioid injections for pain management and to increase patient satisfaction.

Contraindications

1. Infections at the area of PCA placement
2. Allergic responses to the prescribed drug
3. Chronic renal failure
4. Sleep apnoea.

MODERN ANAESTHETIC WORKSTATION

It is intended to function as a full anaesthesia, respiratory gas delivery and monitoring system. In order to create an integrated anaesthesia care station, it integrates advanced ventilation characteristics, gas supply and agent vaporisation with patient monitoring and information management.

Workstation components include

1. Gas delivery and scavenging system
2. Vaporisers
3. Electronic flow meters
4. Ventilators
5. Monitors.

Significant components of the modern anaesthetic workstation include

Hypoxia guard

In order to prevent nitrous oxide from being accidentally delivered to the breathing circuit without oxygen or with an oxygen concentration less than 0.25, these systems have mechanically, pneumatically and electrically linked the nitrous oxide and oxygen flows. The knobs control the NO_2 and O_2 and are linked mechanically (Fig. 57.5).

Automated machine check

Manual inspection and testing of the machine to look for leaks and other malfunctions is frequently either not performed at all or only accomplished partially, but since modern machines are more advanced and sophisticated, the several conventional tests of machine check can perhaps be applied. The vast majority of contemporary anaesthesia delivery systems are capable of conducting their own self-tests and have the capacity to identify and report any faults that may occur. However, one must take note that not all faults or misconnections can be reported by these machines, and backup ventilation equipment such as manual resuscitators should be inspected and kept ready.

VIDEO LARYNGOSCOPE

It depicts an enlarged video image of structures of the airway (Fig. 57.6).

Advantages

1. Improved laryngeal visualisation
2. Less application of force than direct laryngoscopy
3. Less haemodynamic stress
4. Higher success rates.

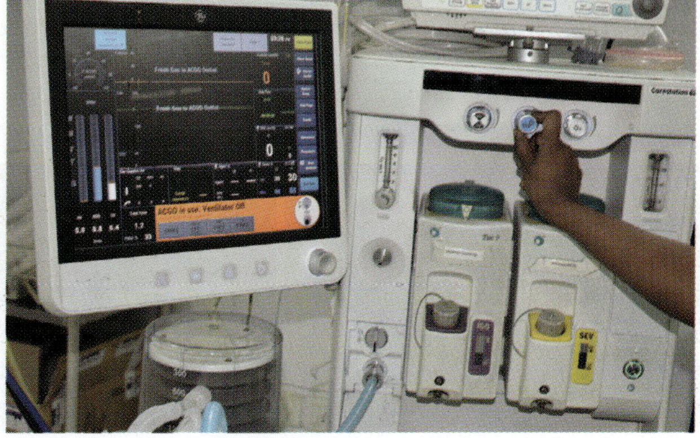

Figure 57.5 Hypoxia guard.

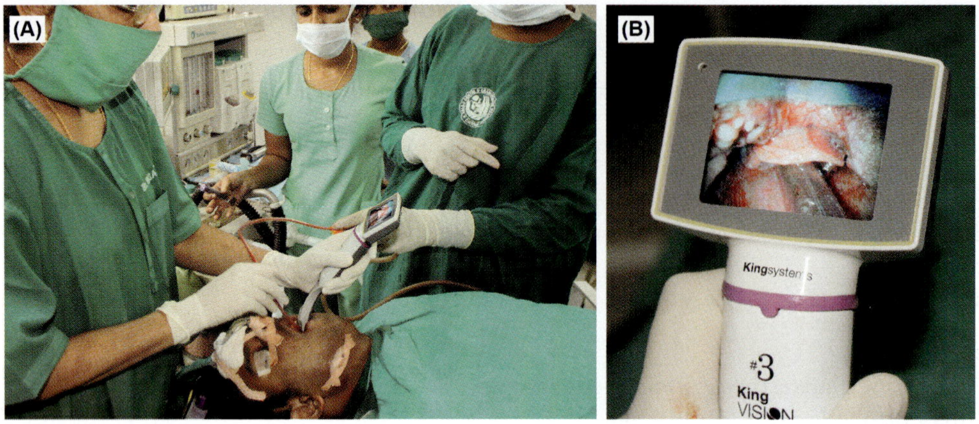

Figure 57.6 (**A** and **B**) Video laryngoscope.

Disadvantages

1. The view may be obstructed by fog as well as secretions
2. The inability to perceive depth
3. Longer processing time.

ENDOSCOPY

With the advancement in technology, minimally invasive surgeries are possible with endoscopes (Fig. 57.7).

Endoscope was 1st used by Takagi in 1918. The surgeon gets a clear view of the structures in and around the surgical field through a monitor.

Parts

Endoscope has the following parts:

- A rigid or flexible tube
- A light delivery system
- A lens system
- Videoscopes
- A pathway for the entry of medical instruments or manipulators
- Suction.

Uses

- Diagnosis
- Trauma surgery (e.g. condylar fracture)
- Orthognathic surgery
- Sialoendoscopy for sialolith removal ('basket approach' is used)
- Retrieval of foreign bodies
- Removal of implants displaced from their location (e.g. into the maxillary sinus)
- Biopsy
- Cauterise a bleeding vessel
- Surgeries of the maxillary sinus (functional endoscopic sinus surgery).

Advantages

- Minimally invasive
- Less chance of damage to vital structures
- Minimal scarring
- Accurate visualisation
- Better access than other approaches
- Faster healing
- Reduced hospital stay.

Disadvantages

- Expensive
- It needs technical skill and expertise
- Time-consuming in the early stages.

RECENT ADVANCES IN STERILISATION

LOW-TEMPERATURE STERILISATION

Surgical instruments and supplies that cannot tolerate steam sterilisers at high temperatures are typically sterilised using this method.

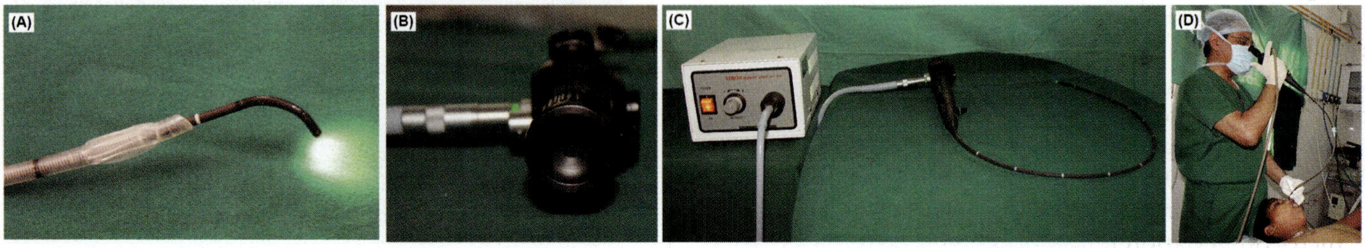

Figure 57.7 Fibreoptic endoscope.

Modern low-temperature sterilisation (LTS) processes include:

- Ethylene oxide (ETO)
- Hydrogen peroxide plasma
- Low-temperature steam and formaldehyde (LTSF)
- Gamma radiation
- Electron beam technology
- Liquid chemical sterilisation (LCS)
- Ozone (O_3).

TABLE TOP AUTOCLAVE

- Automatic pressure and high-temperature sterilisers
- It works with the help of steam medium
- Operating temperature: 121°C–134°C
- **Features:**
  a. High functionality, shock resistance and flexibility
  b. Easy to operate
  c. Outstanding performance
  d. Safety door lock system.

Refer to **Chapter 15,** Fig. 15.3.

RECENT ADVANCES IN EQUIPMENT AND MATERIAL USED IN ORAL AND MAXILLOFACIAL SURGERY

ROBOTIC SURGERY

Head and neck region is complex with many vital vessels and muscles crisscrossing each other. Surgical manipulation in this area requires adequate knowledge, skill and dexterity. Hence, the constant endeavour of maxillofacial surgeons was to develop a minimally invasive surgery (MIS) that can be well tolerated. It should provide rapid recovery with lower pain, better cosmetic results as well as minimal use of postoperative drugs. Robotic-assisted precision surgeries offer this type of MIS in several surgical specialties. With better options of automation and optics, the dexterity of the machines has drastically improved over the time. This new modality has been demonstrated to be safe, cost-effective, reliable as well as better in terms of outcome to be compared with time tested conventional modalities. Conventional surgical approaches require large surgical incisions and dissections, often including airways that culminate in major tissue inflammation, functional compromise and significant postoperative morbidity at least for a considerable period of time. The MIS employs latest video imaging as well as endoscopic technology and instrumentation to overcome certain limitations, which the head and neck surgeon often faces are:

- A limited range and restricted handling of instrumentation
- Training is often limited to 'line of sight' and surgeon comfortable with tissue in sight
- Increased deviation in normal anatomy
- Compromised 3D preoperative imaging.

McLeod and Melder designed and used transoral robotic surgery (TORS) for the 1st time in maxillofacial surgery to remove a vallecular cyst.

The FDA approved this treatment in 2009 for use in stage T1 and T2 oropharyngeal carcinoma. It has been most commonly employed for base of tongue lesions.

The unit has a vision cart, a surgical cart and surgeon's console. The surgical cart has multiple (usually four) robotic arms that can be operated from a console through a wireless remote, including one camera and others having precision surgical instruments. The vision cart has video-assisted visualisation with computer and optic enhancement, which is made up of light sources, insufflators and image control hardware. The surgeon's console has provision for two images, one for each eye, creating a 3D image to improve depth perception and accuracy. Attached provisions are hand manipulators, pedals for controlling optics, instrument arms, focus adjustments, etc (Fig. 57.8).

Advantages

The advantages of robotic-assisted head and neck surgery are as follows:

- **Enhanced visualisation:** The high-power camera and in-built optic system ensure an amplified visual picture, ensuring perception of high-quality images in real clinical situations
- **Elimination of physiologic tremors and scale motion:** The unit eliminates hand tremors, fulcrum effect of instruments, especially when insertion of endoscopes is involved. The torque, force and scale motion are greatly reduced, leading to better surgery, lower iatrogenic injury ensuring safer surgery
- **Multiarticulated instruments:** Simultaneous, coordinated handling of multiple instruments such as drills, suction and electrocautery units in a controlled environment
- **Fatigue reduction:** The unit instils confidence, reduces time of surgery owing to clear field, precision and accurate manipulation. All of these lead to reduced surgical time as well as fatigue reduction to the surgical team

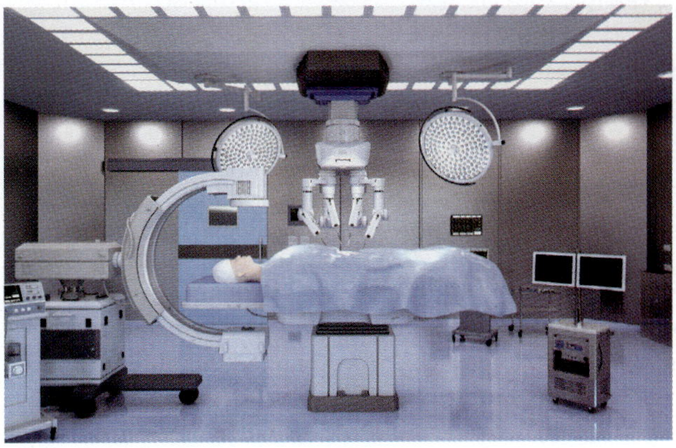

Figure 57.8 Robotic surgery.

- **Restore proper hand–eye coordination:** High-resolution camera and accurate robotic handling ensures proper hand–eye coordination
- **Telesurgery:** The modality ensures remote surgery as the surgeon's console can be kept away and the remaining unit can be connected through high-speed internet.

Disadvantages

The disadvantages of the system include the following:

- Absence of tactile sensation: In the course of surgery, it is mandatory to feel a resistance, a bone and so on to guide the surgery. Robotic system lacks this aspect, as the procedure is not performed by hand
- Equipment size and weight: The system is large and heavy; hence, mobility of instruments and careful handling is essential
- Cost of the device is enormous, so is the maintenance. Therefore, the cost of the surgery increases
- New technology and training periods are issues that need to be taken care of.

ROBOTIC SIALADENECTOMY

Through a modified face-lift approach, robotic sialadenectomy of the submandibular gland has been performed. Surgery was success when Virgilio et al. performed this surgery on five patients. He used three robotic arms, two operative arms and a facedown 30-degree endoscopic arm.

MICROSCOPIC SURGERY

ENDODONTIC SURGERY

Newer instruments utilised in microsurgery:

- Dental operating microscopes, ultrasonic tips, diamond-coated micromirrors, microsurgical scalpels
- Micromirrors are used to examine buccal and lingual walls of the retrocavity
- Microsurgical scalpels are useful for incising the intrasulcular areas and interproximal papillae dissection.

MICROPAROTIDECTOMY INCISION

It consists of preauricular and postauricular incisions that curve around the lobule and are subsequently joined (Fig. 57.9).

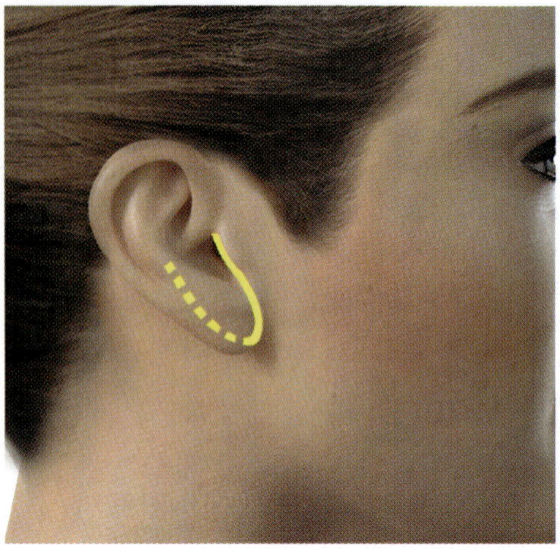

Figure 57.9 Microparotidectomy incision.

Advantages

- Minimally invasive
- Preservation of the facial nerve and its branches
- Preservation of the greater auricular nerve
- Lowering the risk of Frey's syndrome.

FACE TRANSPLANTATION

The goal of a face transplantation is to restore the appearance and function of severely damaged facial features.

Facial transplantation integrates microvascular techniques used in head/neck reconstruction with modern techniques used in orthognathic surgery, TMJ surgery, maxillofacial trauma repair, cosmetic facial surgery and facial nerve dissection. The need for lifelong immunosuppression increases the risk of death, chronic organ rejection, alternative surgery and economic burdens. Compliance and expectations for both cosmetic and functional outcomes must be considered when selecting patients.

Modern reconstructive techniques have significantly improved the ability to restore the patient's preexisting facial appearance and function.

LASERS IN ORAL SURGERY

'Laser' is an acronym for light amplification by stimulated emission of radiation. Lasers are intense, focused, parallel beams of electromagnetic energy of selective monochromatic wavelengths.

PROPERTIES OF LASER

- Laser light is **monochromatic** because it generates a beam of single wavelength, which is invisible if its wavelength is outside the visible part of the spectrum
- Each wave of light is **coherent** or identical in physical shape and size. This means the amplitude and the frequency of all the waves of photons are identical.

LASER PRODUCTION

- Light (electromagnetic wave) and its energy packets are called photons
- Photon on interaction with the stable atomic system will rise to a higher energised state. This is called absorption
- Now, this energised atomic state can emit a photon and decay to a more stable atomic state. This is called ***spontaneous emission***
- However, if a photon interacts with an atomic system that is already in an excited state, the decay of that system occurs, this results in the release of two photons: the original photon and the photon emitted by the decay of the system
- The two emitted photons are of equal wavelength and they are coordinated in time and space. This process is

called ***stimulated emission*** and is the underlying principle of laser physics

- The emitted wavelength is directly dependent on the specific lasing medium
- The laser optical resonating chamber consists of two mirrors. One is totally reflective, adding to the stimulated emission by reflection of the radiation, and the other is partially transmissive, which allows for escape of a specific wavelength of energy
- The emitted radiant energy is extremely intense and is also unidirectional or collimated (there is little divergence of the radiant energy beam). The beam is monochromatic (the wavelength of the photons is the same) and coherent (all waves being exactly in phase with each other in both time and space)
- If the laser beam is then passed through a lens, the emitted radiant energy can be focused to a very small beam diameter or spot size. There is little or no radiant energy wasted and this extremely small intense beam of energy is capable of cutting, coagulating or vaporising tissue
- The radiant energy of a laser must be absorbed by the target tissue and converted to heat. Laser energies of different wavelengths have specific absorptive characteristics in tissue
- The target tissue should be exposed to the laser energy for the briefest time, which would produce desired thermal effect. Different types of lasers (e.g. argon and CO_2) emit radiant energy of different wavelengths, hence they can be used only on specific types of tissue (Fig. 57.10, Box 57.1).

LASER PHYSICS

- Laser light is produced by a chain reaction of atoms
- For laser production, a source of energy and a laser medium are required
- The source of energy could be electrical, chemical or another light source
- The laser medium can be in solid, liquid or gaseous state.
- The lasers are named based on the laser medium used. For example, CO_2, argon and ruby
- Both the medium and the energy source are contained within the laser tube. The energy source excites the medium, thereby the atoms are charged to an excited state. The energised atoms interact with each other and return to the ground state emitting photons of identical wavelength (monochromatic)

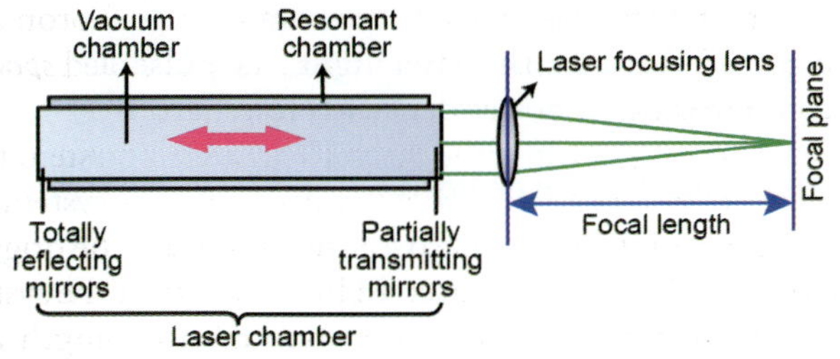

Figure 57.10 Laser chamber.

- The photons oscillate at the same wavelength, unidirectional and in parallel fashion (collimation)
- As the photons continue to travel within the laser chamber, they excite more atoms producing more photons. This process is called as amplification of the laser beam
- When the laser chamber is opened, the laser beam can be delivered as monochromatic, collimated beam. This property of coherence allows the laser to be focused to a precise point in a delivery system
- The laser could be delivered through:
  a. Fibre-optic cable
  b. Articulated arm
  c. Hollow wave guide
- Tissue delivery can be done through contact or noncontact mechanism (free beam).

LASER-TISSUE INTERACTION

- Each laser has a particular wavelength
- When laser is directed at a tissue, tissue components called chromospheres determine the tissue's inherent absorption capacity for a particular wavelength
- Each type of laser emits a different wavelength that absorbs differently depending on whether the target tissue is soft (mucosa) or hard (hydroxyapatite). The laser's efficiency depends on the tissue's ability to absorb or reflect the generated wavelength
- Unlike other soft-tissue lasers, the CO_2 laser's wavelength is absorbed by water rather than tissue pigments, making it unique. It is because the mucosa is 75%–90% water, it easily absorbs the CO_2 wavelength
- Haemoglobin has affinity for green and blue light of argon laser
- Four types of tissue reactions occur with laser (Fig. 57.11)
  a. Reflection
  b. Scattering
  c. Transmission
  d. Absorption
- Absorption and scattering are the most important of the tissue reactions
- The amount of selective tissue damage is determined by the amount of absorption, while the amount of peripheral tissue damage is determined by the amount of scattering
- The temperature effects of the laser on the tissue rely on the amount of temperature increase created by the laser energy.

Nonthermal reactions

The quantum energy of the laser photons is utilised to excite certain specific molecules called sensitisers. For example, dye molecules which predominantly accumulate in tumorous tissues will be excited on absorption of laser light. After transfer of internal energy, this excitation energy will be transmitted to oxygen molecules resulting in the formation of singlet radicals of oxygen, which are a cell toxin causing a purely phototoxic effect.

BOX 57.1 Classification of Lasers

1. *Based on ionising property*
   - *Ionising laser:* For example, xenon (308 nm), excimer (193–351 nm)—halide gases. Due to its DNA mutagenic property, they are not used in oral surgery
   - *Nonionising lasers:* For example, argon, CO_2. All lasers used in oral surgery belong to this group
2. *Based on visibility*
   a. *Visible spectrum:* Argon (blue green), ruby (red)
   b. *Invisible spectrum:* Nd:YAG (near-infrared)
3. *Based on state of laser medium*
   a. *Solid:* For example, ruby, Nd:YAG
   b. *Liquid:* Dye lasers
   c. *Gas:* For example, CO_2, argon
4. *Based on delivery system*
   a. *Noncontact* or free beam laser system with angled mirrors to direct the beam at 90 or 120 degrees, for example, CO_2
   b. *Contact laser:* Nd:YAG
   c. *Both contact and noncontact*-Hol:YAG
5. *Based on exposure time*
   Exposure time is 'the amount of time the operator keeps the laser light directed at the tissues'
   a. *Continuous wave:* No fluctuation of the beam with time, uniform flow of radiation
   b. *Pulsed wave:* Delivers photons in the form of single pulses or trains of pulses (rate = pulses/s)
   c. *Superpulsed:* Reaches higher peak powers per pulse decreasing lateral tissue damage
   d. *Ultrapulsed:* Increased pulse speed for precise tissue removal with less lateral tissue damage
   e. *Flash scanned:* Continuous wave in circular patterns using movable mirrors reducing the contact period and thus reducing lateral tissue damage
   f. *Q switch or quality switching:* All energy is concentrated to single intense pulses (bursts) of short duration, approximately 25 ns.
6. *Based on tissue interaction*
   a. *Soft tissue:* For example, diode laser
   b. *Hard tissue:* For example, excimer and erbium lasers are strongly absorbed by dental hard tissue
7. *Based on medium of laser*
   a. CO_2
   b. Ruby
   c. Argon
   d. Er:YAG
   e. Nd:YAG
   f. Hol:YAG
   g. KTP (modified version of Nd:YAG)
   h. Copper vapour
   i. Excimer
   j. HeNe (Helium–Neon)
   k. Alexandrite

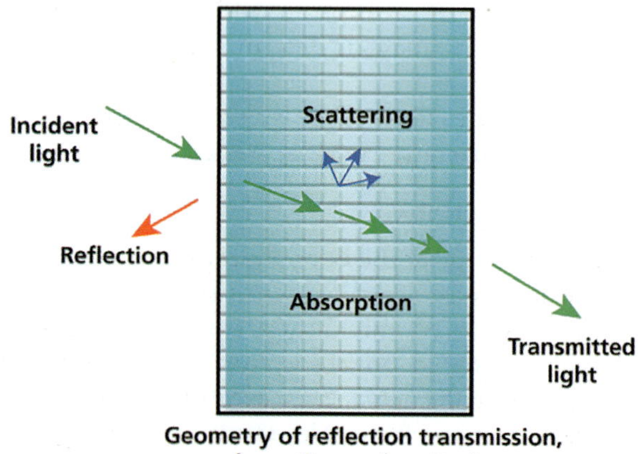

Figure 57.11 Laser-tissue reactions.

Thermal reactions

Medical lasers are used for cutting and coagulation. During coagulation, the tissue passes through various stages of thermal damage until vaporisation occurs at several 100°C.

The factors determining thermal reactions are as follows:

1. Wavelength-dependent penetration depth of the laser light
2. Thermal diffusion inside the tissues
3. Exposure time of the laser light, its pulse length and consequently its power density (Flowchart 57.1).

Ablative effect of laser light

The ablation of soft and hard tissues is reliant on the tissue's high absorption of laser light in order to reach the ablation threshold with only the initial fraction of the pulse energy. Shorter the pulse, the lower the ablation threshold.

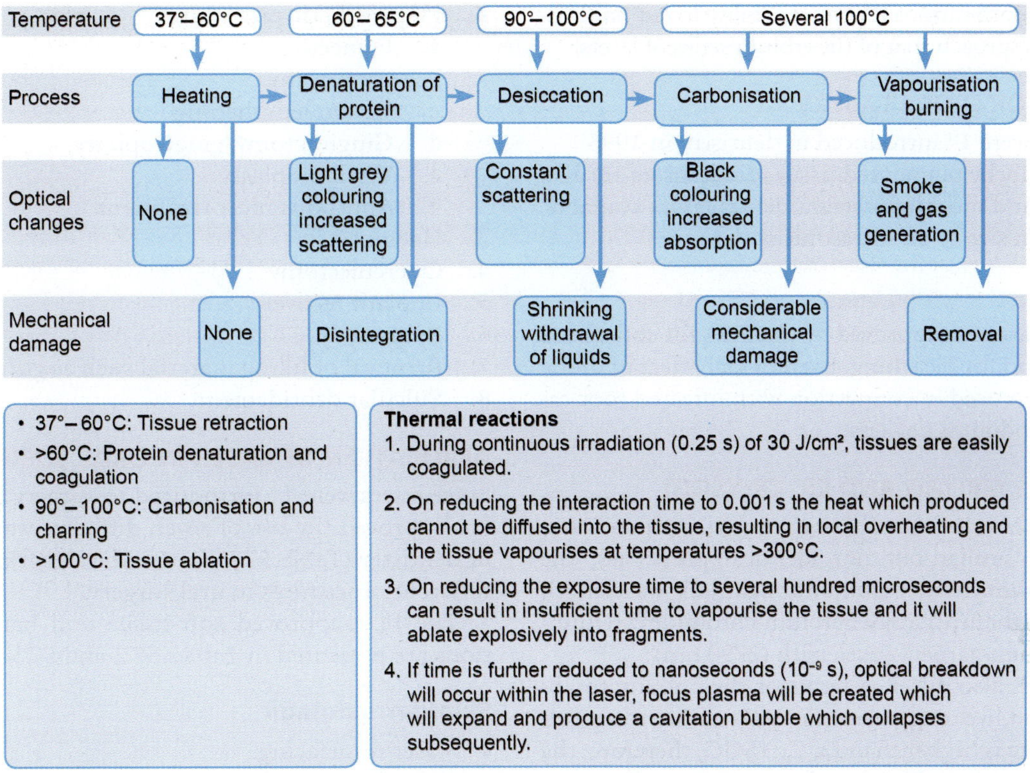

Flowchart 57.1 Changes of the optical, thermal and mechanical properties of tissues during laser irradiation.

The ablation process and the occurrence of tissue fragmentation start after 2 μs and continue for free-running lasers with a pulse length of up to 500 μs, until the pulse energy drops below the ablation threshold. The necrotic zone is wider than the theoretical penetration depth of the light as the remaining energy has the ability to penetrate tissue and even propagate by thermal diffusion.

CO_2 LASERS

- Developed in 1964
- Rays of the CO_2 laser with a wavelength of 10.6 μm are absorbed in water-based tissues, resulting in the vaporisation of intracellular and extracellular fluid and the disintegration of cells
- The CO_2 laser can be used in different modes, ranging from continuous wave to pulsed modes in the range of microseconds emitted at a defined frequency. Example:
  a. Excision of benign oral lesions such as papillomas, fibromas, haemangiomas, mucoceles, gingival overgrowth, mucosal frenula, aphthous ulcers, tongue-ties (ankyloglossia), and premalignant lesions such as oral leukoplakias and erythroleukoplakias
  b. Preprosthetic surgery
  c. Periodontal surgery
  d. Guided tissue regeneration
  e. Oral cancer resections
- Some studies have supported the use of the CO_2 laser for the surgical treatment of oral malignancies in the early stages (e.g. T1N0 and T2N0 carcinomas) or even more advanced stages of verrucous carcinoma
- Although its wavelength can be absorbed by hydroxyapatite, the CO_2 laser is primarily a soft-tissue laser.

Advantages

- Instant disinfection
- Nearly bloodless surgery
- Favourable wound healing
- Minimal scarring
- Decreased postoperative pain.

In animal models, a shorter pulse duration has resulted in a less extensive damage zone and earlier wound healing. Histopathologically, different thermal damage zones have been described with different laser modes. It has been speculated that delayed wound healing may be due to the extent of the lateral thermal damage zone.

ND:YAG LASERS

- Used in dentistry since 1990
- These lasers are absorbed by pigmented tissue; the darker the tissue, the more readily this wavelength is absorbed.

Uses

- Soft-tissue surgery in prosthetics, periodontics, cosmetic, paediatric and orthodontic procedures
- The FDA has also approved this wavelength for removing 1st-degree enamel caries. Although the Nd:YAG can remove

pigmented surface carious lesions, its ability to cut hard tissue does not approach that of the erbium series of lasers.

SEMICONDUCTOR DIODE LASERS

- Diode lasers were 1st introduced in dentistry in 1995
- Absorbed easily by pigmented tissue, diode lasers are also the smallest and most lightweight dental lasers available, comparable in size to an ultrasonic scaler unit.

Uses

- Diode lasers are also approved by the FDA for soft-tissue procedures and for bleaching. Bactericidal effect of diode lasers has been used in connection with infected root canals and periodontal pockets.

ERBIUM LASERS (ER:YAG AND ER, CR:YSGG)

- The erbium series of dental lasers consists of two wavelengths with similar but not identical properties, the Er:YAG (erbium:yttrium-aluminium-garnet) wavelength (2940 nm) and the Er, Cr:YSGG (erbium-chromium:yttrium-scallium-gallium-garnet) wavelength (2790 nm)
- The two lasers also differ in terms of their ability to absorb water and hydroxyapatite. Er:YAGs ability to absorb hydroxyapatite is higher than Er, Cr:YSGG; therefore, the laser drilling with Er:YAG resulted in greater mass removal of dentine and a smaller increase in pulpal temperature compared with the Er, Cr:YSGG
- The Er:YAG dental laser was 1st approved for caries removal and cavity preparation in 1997
- These wavelengths have a high affinity for hydroxyapatite in tooth structure and osseous structure and the highest water-absorption rate available for any dental wavelength.

Uses

- During class V gingival lesion or root caries, these wavelengths can be used to contour the soft tissue or to perform a gingivectomy that will expose the decay and remove the carious lesion without using infiltration or block analgesia
- Erbium wavelengths cannot coagulate and cauterise bleeding tissue as well as the CO_2 and Nd:YAG soft-tissue wavelengths. Therefore, they are not indicated for soft-tissue procedures except in procedures that do not require sealing off capillaries, for example, when preparing a bed for a soft-tissue graft
- These wavelengths are mainly used for hard-tissue procedures as to remove dental caries without the need for analgesia
- Er:YAG is considered superior to other wavelengths when performing procedures such as the removal of lipopolysaccharides from root surfaces without charring, melting or carbonising the root surfaces.

INDICATIONS IN ORAL SURGERY

1. Incision
   a. Biopsies (incisional/excisional)
   b. Abscess (incision and drainage)
2. Preprosthetic procedures
   a. Frenectomy
   b. Frenotomy
   c. Crown lengthening
   d. Gingivectomy/gingivoplasty
   e. Vestibuloplasty
   f. Aphthous ulcer treatment
3. Haemostasis
4. Operculectomy
5. Implant recovery
6. Pulpotomy
7. Removal of filling material such as gutta-percha or resin
8. Sulcular debridement.

APPLICATION OF LASER IN ORAL SURGERY

Since lasers were 1st introduced to surgery in 1970, the FDA has approved the use of seven different wavelengths for use in dentistry (Table 57.1). These wavelengths can be used for different procedures in oral surgery.

The FDA-approved soft-tissue and hard-tissue applications are presented in Tables 57.2 and 57.3.

Skin/dermatologic

- Laser resurfacing
- Laser blepharoplasty
- Laser treatment of tattoos, pigmentation disorders and various other vascular disorders, such as port-wine stains, facial telangiectasia, etc.
- Hair reduction by laser
- Nonablative laser rejuvenation of wrinkles.

Caries removal

Cavity removal can be accomplished with two currently available laser machines. Both lasers have the ability to remove decay (tooth caries) within a tooth and prepare the surrounding enamel cavity for bonded fillings. The major advantage over traditional methods is that the need for anaesthesia is greatly reduced or eliminated over the traditional methods. Laser energy dramatically reduces the bacterial level found in dental caries and has been demonstrated to enhance the tooth's ability to 'heal' in situations where case of 'deep cavities' had existed. However, there were several limitations in

TABLE 57.1 FDA-Approved Wavelength

Wavelength in Nanometres (nm)	Absorption
Nd:YAG 1064	Pigment
Diode 810–830	Pigment
Diode 980	Pigment
Er, Cr:YSGG 2790	Water
Er:YAG 2940	Water
CO_2 10,600	Water
Er:YAG 810–830	Water

TABLE 57.2 FDA-Approved Soft-Tissue Procedures

• Abscess incision and drainage
• Aphthous ulcer treatment
• Biopsies (incisional/excisional)
• Crown lengthening (soft tissue only)
• Haemostatic assistance
• Fibroma removal
• Frenectomy
• Frenotomy
• Gingival excision/incision
• Gingivectomy/gingivoplasty
• Operculectomy
• Oral papillectomy
• Tissue retraction for impression
• Vestibuloplasty
• Exposure of unerupted or partially erupted teeth
• Implant recovery
• Lesion (tumour) removal
• Leukoplakia
• Pulpotomy
• Pulpotomy as an adjunct to root canal therapy
• Removal of filling material, such as gutta-percha or resin, as an adjunct treatment during root canal retreatment
• Sulcular debridement (removal of diseased or inflamed soft tissue in the periodontal pocket) to improve clinical indices, including gingival index, gingival bleeding index, probe depth, attachment level and tooth mobility

TABLE 57.3 FDA-Approved Hard-Tissue Procedure

• Removal of caries
• Cavity preparation
• Etching of enamel
• Enameloplasty, excavation of pits and fissures for placement of sealants
• Cutting, shaving, contouring and resection of oral osseous tissue
• Apicoectomy
• Endodontics

caries removal using laser such as inability to adequately remove amalgam fillings, onlays and metal crowns.

Curing and teeth whitening

Lasers have become important in curing or hardening the bonding materials. Curing the filling and bonding material is less time-consuming. Teeth whitening can be done using special solutions, which are applied over the tooth surface in the dental office and activated by laser energy. Even colour changes of several shades are possible in a very short time. Dramatic changes can be seen in even the most difficult cases when laser treatment is combined with at-home tray-based whitening systems.

Dentinal hypersensitivity

The prevalence of treatment-resistant dentinal hypersensitivity has diminished considerably with the advent of desensitising agents. On the other hand, the placement of fillings using composites and inlays has brought a new reason for the very same. Gershman has proved that dentinal hypersensitivity can be successfully treated with laser therapy. Mild pulpitis requires higher doses when compared to common dentinal hypersensitivity and repeated treatments. Frequently, sensitivity due to abrasion can be treated in a single application.

Herpes simplex

Oral herpes (HSV1) is a common condition to be seen in the dental office. As with any HSV1 treatment, a treatment in the early prodromal stage is most successful. Immediate results can be seen, such as complete reduction in the pain level, and the blisters will disappear within a few days. Unlike Acyclovir, there are no side effects. It has also been proven that the laser therapy can even be used in the latent period between the attacks to reduce recurrence rate.

The therapeutic lasers provide beneficial response in the treatment of pain, inflammation, oedema and wound healing.

Mucositis

Mucositis is the major side effect in patients undergoing radiotherapy and/or chemoradiotherapy. Nutrition is troublesome and therapy regimens may have to be suboptimal for this reason. Although laser therapy is used to treat mucositis, using laser therapy before radiotherapy/chemotherapy will reduce the mucosal irritation.

Pain

Laser therapy can reduce or eliminate pain of various origins. Irradiating the operated area postoperatively before anaesthesia wears off will substantially eliminate the postoperative discomfort after surgery.

Paraesthesia

Paraesthesia may occur after some oral surgical procedures, especially in the mandibular region. Laser therapy has been used to eliminate or reduce such complications.

Temporomandibular joint

The treatment should be concentrated in the joint areas in case of arthritic cases, whereas in myogenic cases the muscular insertions and trigger points should be concentrated. Conventional treatment should also be used in addition to laser therapy to improve the treatment outcome.

Tinnitus/vertigo

Patients with Meniere's disease (tinnitus/vertigo) have tension in the masticatory, neck and trapezius muscles. Relaxation of the tension in these muscles and occlusal stabilisation procedures (occlusal adjustment, bite splint) will minimise or eliminate the symptoms of tinnitus and vertigo in these patients. Laser therapy has been proven to be a successful tool to promote muscular relaxation and pain relief in these patients.

Zoster

Herpes zoster in the course of the trigeminal nerve should be treated in its early phase. Some zoster attacks may be followed by a condition called postherpetic neuralgia that persists for years or even life-lasting. Laser therapy is an economical, non-invasive treatment method without any side effects.

Other uses

It can also be used in periodontal or gum procedures such as recontouring or reshaping gums, removing extra or diseased gum tissue due to the use of certain medications or periodontal disease, removing the bacteria in periodontal pockets to promote healing, tumour ablation, reducing the blood loss by sealing small blood vessels, for sealing lymph vessels to reduce swelling and the spread of tumour cells, to treat some skin conditions, including warts, moles, tattoos, birthmarks, scars and wrinkles.

Advantages

- Increased bone healing
- Reduced risk of infection
- Less need for anaesthesia or injections
- Less bleeding
- Less noise than the traditional dental drill
- Less postoperative pain
- Better results
- Ability to do more than one procedure in a single appointment.

Precaution

The only physical risk in laser therapy is the damage to the eyes, especially when using an invisible and collimated (parallel) beam. Care should be taken by using suitable protective goggles by the patient for extraoral therapy in the face. As all the therapeutic lasers are well above the ionising spectrum level, there is no risk of cancerous changes.

Side Effects

- *Temporary increase of pain in chronic conditions:* There could be a temporary acute exacerbation in chronic conditions causing pain
- *Tiredness after the treatment:* This could be due to pain relief where the pain previously has prevented a normal relaxation pattern
- *Redness and a feeling* of warmness in the irradiated area as a result of increased microcirculation.

SUTURE MATERIAL AND WOUND CLOSURE

POLYBUTESTER (NOVAFIL)

- It is a recent thermoplastic material
- It has unique stress-strain properties
- It is a copolymer composed of polytetramethylene ether glycol and polybutylene terephthalate and coated with polytribolate
- It has greater strength, elasticity and a lower coefficient of friction
- It has high level of knot security
- Due to its exceptional elastic property, it is beneficial in early stages of wound healing.

TAPES

- It is used for wound closure, reducing suture tension and enhancing the healing process once stitches are removed, various surgical adhesive tapes are utilised
- Quick and easy to perform
- Application of tape is painless
- Less prone to infections
- Used to close superficial lacerations
- A follow-up appointment to remove the tape is not required
- Scars from residual suture tracks are spared
- Use of tapes has certain limitations for closing wounds such as in an area under substantial tension
- Tapes are challenging to adhere on extremely convex surfaces, uneven wounds and areas of slack tissue
- They adhere poorly to moist surfaces, such as in oral mucosa
- These tapes are often composed of synthetic, reinforced material with a hypoallergenic adhesive and their pores are designed to allow skin to 'breathe'
- Modifications to tape-based wound closure include a zip-lock mechanism and clip attachment to bring wound edges together.

TISSUE ADHESIVES

- Tissue adhesives can be used to approximate wounds that do not need deep-layer closure or have significant tension on the edges
- It is typically used to heal superficial skin tears and for surface closure after sutures have secured the deeper layers
- Additionally it can also be used for bone graft attachment, sealing CSF leaks, dentoalveolar flaps closure, etc
- Tissue adhesives for surface closure are applied after a complete cleaning and haemostasis has been completed
- **Advantages:** (1) Painless and rapid (2) better aesthetic result since suture track scars are avoided
- **Disadvantages:** (1) Not suitable for areas of tension (2) minor risk of toxicity.

RECENT ADVANCES IN DENTAL IMPLANTOLOGY

COMPUTER-GUIDED IMPLANT TREATMENT

Refer Chapter 22, page no. 415–416.

ZYGOMA IMPLANT

Refer Chapter 22, page no. 426–427.

RECENT ADVANCES IN THE FIELD OF EXODONTIA

PIEZOELECTRIC SURGERY

Piezoelectric surgery is an innovative osteotomy and osteoplastic technique that uses piezoelectric ultrasonic vibrations. It can perform precise and safe osteotomies due to its characteristic micrometric and selective cuts that contrast with the traditional hard and soft tissue management methods with rotating instruments.

History

To overcome the limits of traditional instruments in oral bone surgery, Tomaso Vercellotti invented the piezosurgery instrument in 1988. Nerves, vessels and soft tissues are not injured by the microvibrations (60–200 mm/s), which are optimally adjusted to target only mineralised tissue.

Although ultrasonic osteotomies were 1st described more than 20 years ago by Horton et al., It was not until 2000 that Vercellotti et al. renewed this approach for nerve and soft tissue protecting surgery.

The innovation of this technique is mainly due to three major characteristics: (1) a micrometric cut of 60–200 μm, (2) a selective cut which works on hard tissues but not on soft tissues and (3) a relative blood free surgical field due to the air-water cavitation effect of the ultrasonic device.

Need for piezoelectric surgery

Rotating instruments are potentially injurious, due to the production of excessively high temperatures during osseous drilling, which can produce marginal osteonecrosis and impair bone regeneration. It is recommended to use a careful surgical technique to reduce the amount of frictional heating with saline irrigation.

Because of micrometric and selective cutting, this device works only on mineralised tissues, sparing soft tissues and their blood supply.

Principle

Microvibrations are created by the piezoelectric effect. Certain ceramics and crystals deform when an electric current is passed across them resulting in oscillation of the ultrasonic frequency.

Technique

The equipment consists of piezoelectric handpiece and foot switch that are connected to a main unit, which supplies power and has holders for handpiece and irrigation fluids. For the handpiece, several autoclavable tool tips called inserts are available. Some are coated with titanium or diamonds in various grades. The microvibrations that are created in the piezoelectric handpiece cause the inserts to move between 60 and 210 μm, providing the handpiece with power exceeding 5 W.

There is a peristaltic pump for cooling with a jet of solution that discharges from the insert with an adjustable flow of 0-60mL/min and removes debris from the cutting area. The settings for power and frequency modulation of the device can be selected on a control panel with a digital display and a keypad according to the planned task. The unit uses a frequency of 25–29 kHz. This adjustability prevents the insert from impacting the bone and avoids overheating while maintaining optimum cutting capacity.

The instrument was originally designed for augmentation in implant operations, including sinus lift and ridge expansion. For the cutting of bone in maxillofacial operations, the most efficient setting is boosted mode with maximum irrigation. The handpiece is guided over the bone firmly, but without excessive force. While cutting, it is important to pay attention to irrigation to avoid heating of the bone. After prolonged cutting, the handpiece will get warm and a short pause may be advisable to let the handpiece cool down (Fig. 57.12).

Advantages

- Because of its physical and mechanical properties, the definitive clinical advantage of piezoelectric bone surgery with regard to precision cutting lies in the sparing of vital neurovascular bundles and soft tissue. In addition, better visualisation of the surgical field ensures its great safety
- The usefulness of piezoelectric bone surgery during neurosurgical procedures is particularly relevant when there are anatomic difficulties because of poor intraoperative visibility or the presence of delicate anatomic structures
- The selective and thermally harmless nature of the piezosurgery instrument results in a low bleeding tendency
- The instrument can be used in operations requiring either local or general anaesthesia
- The precise nature of the instrument allows exact, clean and smooth cut geometries during surgery
- Postoperatively, excellent wound healing, with no nerve and soft tissue injuries, is observed
- It is apparent that the range of applications of piezosurgery is not limited to minor operations. Because of its highly selective and accurate nature, with its cutting effect exclusively targeting hard tissue, its use may be extended to more complex oral surgery cases as well as to other interdisciplinary problems.

Precautions

- It should, however, be noted that soft tissue structures, such as the mucous membrane of the maxillary sinus or

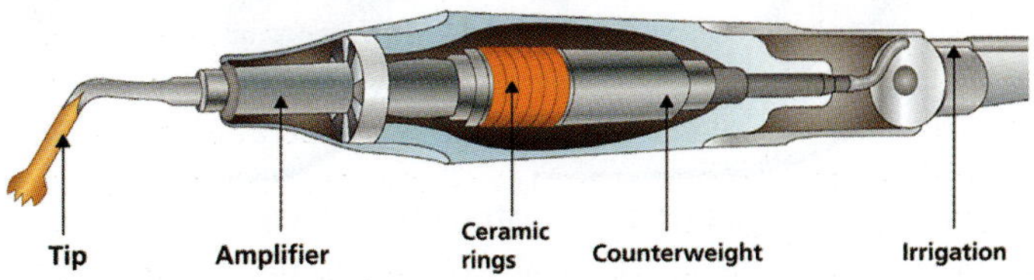

Figure 57.12 Piezoelectric unit.

a cyst follicle, may be perforated or injured by excessive mechanical force from the instrument tip. Careful operating technique remains critical

- Before the widespread use of piezosurgery for osteotomies, possible side effects such as thrombogenesis or impaired bony blood circulation need to be examined. One area for special concern is the poorly vascularised mandible where thrombosis of its intraosseous vessels may lead to obvious clinical problems.

PHYSICS FORCEPS

Dr. Richard Golden developed the physics forceps in 2004. They aid in the instrumentation for the extraction of teeth (Fig. 57.13).

Technique

Popularly referred to as the 'beak and bumper' technique. The 'beak' is placed on the palatal or lingual root of the tooth into the gingival sulcus, whereas the 'bumper' is positioned on the buccal or facial aspect at the mucogingival junction. After engaging the forceps, only wrist movement is made until resistance is felt. It is based on the 1st-class lever principle, thereby delivering a mechanical advantage. Constant, steady pressure is applied parallel to the long axis of the tooth with the wrist only using the bumper as a pivot or fulcrum (Fig. 57.14, Flowchart 57.2).

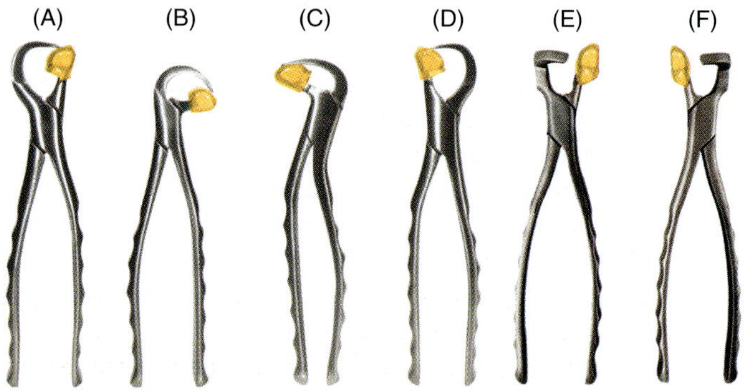

Figure 57.13 (**A**) Upper right posterior forceps. (**B**) Lower universal forceps. (**C**) Upper anterior forceps. (**D**) Upper left posterior forceps, (**E** and **F**) Right and left upper 3rd molar forceps.

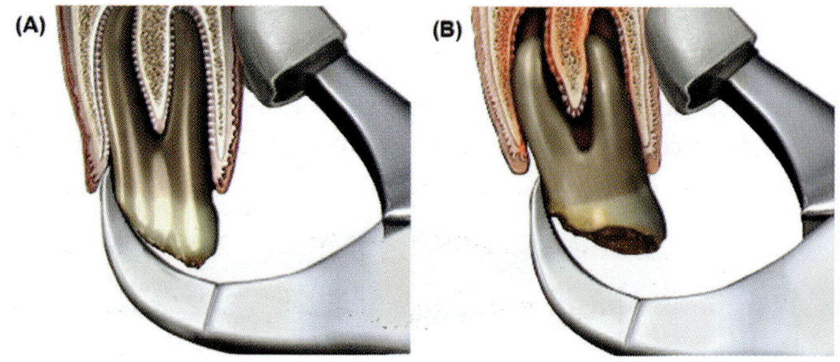

Figure 57.14 Diagrammatic illustration showing (**A**) placement of beak on the palatal root of the tooth into the gingival sulcus and the bumper end on the buccal aspect (**B**) application of constant steady force using wrist alone using the bumper as fulcrum.

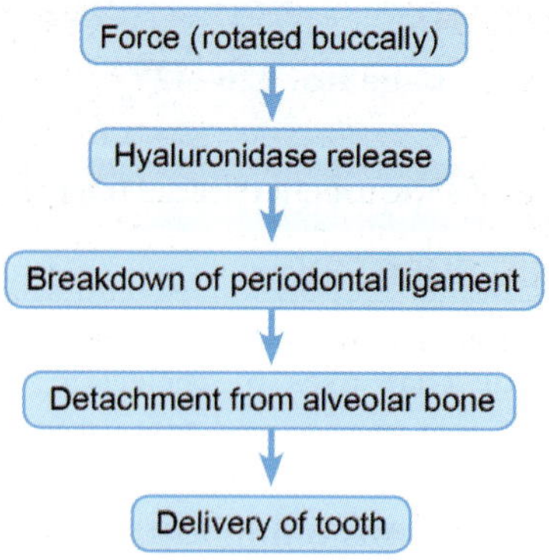

Flowchart 57.2 Mechanism of tooth extraction by physics forceps.

Uses

- Extractions of grossly decayed teeth
- Orthodontic extraction
- In cases of intentional tooth replantation
- For immediate implants.

Advantages

- Preserves the socket and alveolar bone
- Minimal trauma to surrounding soft tissues
- Reduces the duration of procedure
- Atraumatic extractions
- It eliminates complications such as root tip fractures
- Simple to use.

Disadvantages

- Expensive
- Cannot be used in conditions such as severe crowding
- Potential for being misused
- Damage to buccal plate.

LUXATOR PERIOTOMES

These are sharp slender instruments. When using Luxator Periotomes, they are inserted in between the tooth and the gingiva to perform their function. Because of this, it is easier to engage in a plane that uses a rotatory action that is both gentle and firm to strip the periodontal fibres. Rocking motion is performed continually while these fibres are being stripped; as well as in the widening of the socket. Force applied is significantly less.

EASY X-TRAC SYSTEM

Through the use of a screw, it engages the tooth root, which results in improved retention and control.

Removing the screw and the root can be done by applying equal amounts of force.

It allows immediate implantation after extraction, thus preventing posttraumatic swelling, rotary movements, etc.

BENEX TECHNIQUE

- This technique is mainly for single-rooted teeth below the marginal gingiva
- It works on the vertical pulling principle.

RECENT ADVANCES IN TREATMENT OF FRACTURES

In recent decades, the treatment of facial fractures has experienced numerous advancements. Computer-assisted presurgical planning, intraoperative navigation, computer-assisted design and incision procedures are all examples of technical developments.

FIXATION

RESORBABLE PLATES AND SCREWS

Resorbable plate systems combine the benefits of rigid internal fixation with the convenience of biodegradation, eliminating the need for removal and minimising interference with craniofacial growth.

Hence, it is reliable, efficient and adaptable enough to be used in a variety of maxillofacial sites. However, the resorbable plate may need to be refixed and rebent if bone segments are incorrectly reduced or repositioned.

The aim of internal fixation for skeletal fractures and osteotomies is to achieve undisturbed proper fracture healing. Although plates and screws are used for fixation, their need is only temporary, until the fracture union has occurred.

Titanium plates and screws are the gold standard for fixation in various craniofacial surgeries and their use in maxillofacial trauma surgery is well documented (Fig. 57.15).

Disadvantages inherent to rigid fixation system using plates

- Growth disturbances
- Migration of fixed plate
- Need for 2nd surgery for its removal
- Reduced compatibility with advanced imaging aids
- Long-term palpability
- Thermal sensitivity
- Malunion of the site
- Difficult in controlling the postoperative occlusion.

Consequences of not removing the plate

- Palpable or prominent hardware
- Loosening of fixed plates and screws

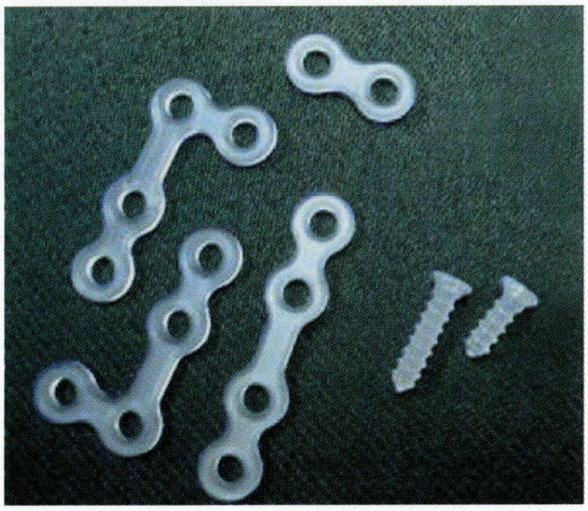

Figure 57.15 Bioresorbable plate and screws.

- Pain and infection
- Wound dehiscence in the surgical site
- Thermal sensitivity
- Plate migration.

In addition, studies have proven that rigid internal fixation adversely affects skeletal growth and development in growing children, which led to the development of biodegradable hardware that is strong, biocompatible, adaptable and provides enough stability to allow fracture healing and then resorbs quickly without a foreign body reaction.

Bioresorbable polymer science has evolved during the last 10 years and there has been a significant improvement in the mechanical properties of degradable plates and screws. Presently, these plates provide optimal strength and degradation time.

History of absorbable implants

The possibility of using biodegradable devices in bone surgery has been studied extensively for more than 50 years. The 1st clinical trials of the use of such materials in fracture surgery took place more than 40 years ago with disappointing results. As the stability of the devices was not adequate, the osteosynthesis did not result in rigid, functionally stable fixation.

Various researches around 1970s have resulted in major improvements. Implant fabrication was accomplished by melt moulding and extrusion of the polymer into pins and rods. In the late 1970s and early 1980s, more complex designs such as screws and small plates became possible.

Advances in polymer chemistry and material processing methods have improved the quality of biodegradable materials to the extent that its clinical use has become safe. Stability has been achieved and maintained for a sufficiently long time to allow normal bone healing to occur.

Chemical composition of absorbable implants

Alpha compounds such as polyglycolic acid (PGA), polylactic acid and polyesters polyparadioxanon are organic macromolecular compounds, which can be degraded and absorbed by the human body. They also have the chemical and physical properties, which are necessary for internal fixation devices.

Mechanism of action

Bioresorbable plate is converted into CO_2 and H_2O via bulk hydrolysis by the body and metabolised by the liver with the theoretical advantage of gradual degradation in order to reduce the risk of local inflammation and osteolysis. The foreign body reactions seen usually with the more rapidly degrading polymers such as PGA are not typically seen with these materials.

Features of this system

- Tensile and flexural strength are comparable to titanium plating system
- Easy to adapt with aid of heat pack at the surgical site
- Wide selection of implant sizes and shapes are available
- Convenient hex-drive breakaway delivery system, which simplifies screw placement

- No growth restriction and implant migration for paediatric craniofacial reconstruction
- It is resorbed completely, so no need for a 2nd surgery
- No late-stage inflammatory reaction.

Advantages of resorbable plates

- Small and compact
- Biocompatible
- Adaptable to the surgical site
- It possesses adequate stability to achieve bony union
- Subsequently resorbs in a timely fashion.

Titanium versus biodegradable plates

The biodegradable material is softer and weaker than titanium plates and it requires tapping to place the screws. Firm pressure and "tight" screw placement are preferable in titanium plates, but in the case of biodegradable screws, it only needs to be "finger tight," and care must be taken when inserting them into thin bone. Excessive torque should not be applied to avoid the breakage of the screw head. The resorbable plates and screws are not radiographically apparent; hence, postoperatively the radiolucent screw holes can be identified. These screw holes also serve as a measure of degradation time; if the hole is no longer detectable on a radiograph, it can be assumed that it has been resorbed.

The use of biodegradable materials in paediatric craniofacial surgery has been favourable, leading to their use in orthognathic and maxillofacial trauma surgery. Although resorbable plates and screws are biomechanically inferior to titanium, they appear to offer equivalent results when compared with similar metal fixation devices in an animal model. Two major differences are that a heating device is required to provide malleability, and the bone must be tapped prior to screw placement. The mandible and forehead have relatively flat and gently curved surfaces, which do not require enough bending, whereas in the zygoma and orbit, more complex shaping of the plates may be needed. The major concern is the performance of these materials when exposed to the functional demands of the maxillofacial skeleton.

Uses of biodegradable plates

- Fixation of fractures involving the tooth-bearing area of the mandible (as in children with unerupted permanent teeth)
- Bone-anchored method of maxillomandibular fixation
- Very low load-bearing fracture of the midface region
- Fixation of paediatric craniofacial osteotomy
- The use of resorbable plates and screws for fixation of paediatric facial fractures is well tolerated and effective. It helps in realignment and stable positioning of rapidly healing fracture segments while eliminating the need for the removal by 2nd surgery.

Selection of patient for the use of resorbable plates (Fig. 57.16)

The paediatric facial trauma patient invokes several different considerations that are not present in the adult. 1st, the paediatric population has the huge advantage of an accelerated healing in a very short time with very few complications, which is aided by the well-vascularised tissues of the face. 2nd, through the assistance of growth and an inherent ability to adapt, recovery of damaged orofacial tissues and function is much better than in the adult.

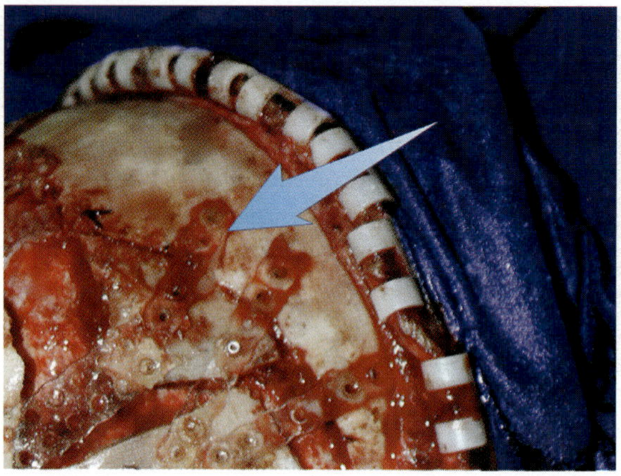

Figure 57.16 Fixation with bioresorbable plate.

Although they have various advantages, certain differences do exist in the paediatric facial trauma patient that must be considered. These include an appreciation of the unique characteristics and anatomy of the developing immature face, the different facial injury patterns that occur in the paediatric patient and the potential growth implications from traumatised facial structures, all of which necessitate long-term follow-up of these patients.

SELF-DRILLING SCREWS AND SELF-TAPPING SCREWS

Self-drilling screw has a drill-shaped cutting end and requires no predrilling. It provides various advantages over self-tapping screws, such as eliminating the need to drill the hole and preventing heat damage, which can lead to infection, screw loosening, osteomyelitis and nonunion. Additionally, it protects tooth roots and nerves from harm caused by drills and reduces complications associated with drill bit fracture (Fig. 57.17).

Self-tapping screw is the screw that is inserted into a pre-drilled hole without being tapped (Fig. 57.17).

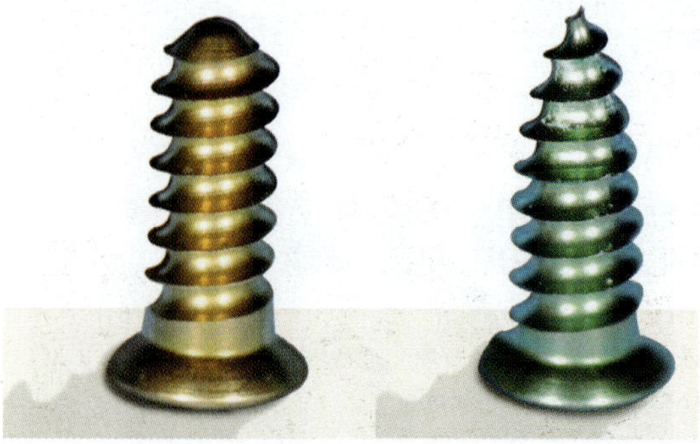

Figure 57.17 (**A**) Self-drilling screw. (**B**) Self-tapping screw.

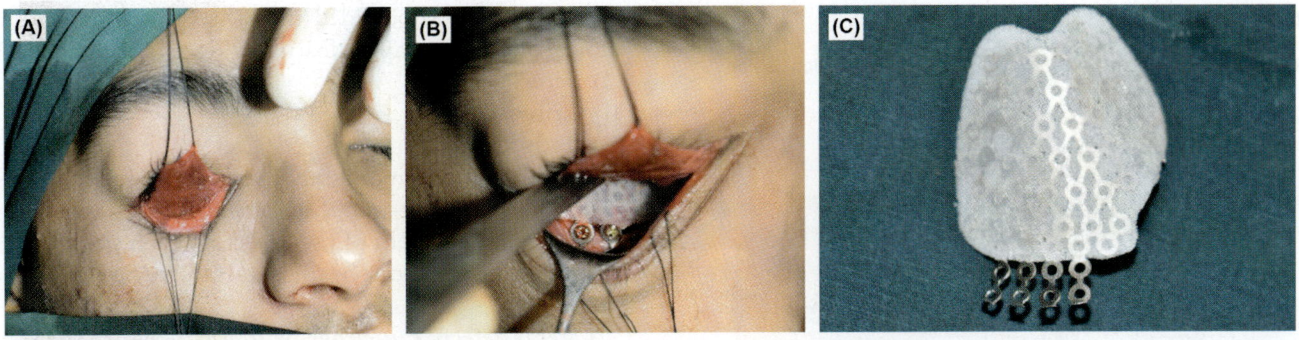

Figure 57.18 (**A** and **B**) Medial and orbital floor reconstruction with titanium MEDPOR mesh. (**C**) MEDPOR—porous polyethylene.

MULTIDIRECTIONAL FIXATION—TRILOCK PLATES

TriLock plates are a step forward in the technology of locking plates as it enables multidirectional fixation. Medartis in Basel, Switzerland, introduced the concept called TriLock technology. In terms of multidirectional and angular stable fixation, this constitutes a big step forward. The spherical three-point wedge locking makes a connection between the head of the screw and the plate hole that is stable in angle and axial plane. Within a range of 15 degrees, the locking can be modified as much as three times without compromising its stability.

ORBITAL FRACTURES

Advancement in three-dimensional printing allows actual prototyping of 3D models, creating an exact depiction of the patient's anatomy.

In case of orbital fracture, initially the patient's CT scan records are used as the basis for the creation of three-dimensional physical models.

Next, this model is used as a template and the porous polyethylene plate (MEDPOR) is layered on the ledges of the defect and precisely sized and trimmed ex vivo.

Surgeons are able to accomplish considerable aesthetic and therapeutic improvement by using a preshaped, custom-made prosthesis based on a 3D anatomical model. Anatomical models can be constructed using CT scan datasets. It is cost-effective and can be utilised for repairing severe fractures in the orbital floor (Fig. 57.18).

RECENT ADVANCES IN SOFT TISSUE RECONSTRUCTION

TISSUE EXPANDERS

Refer Chapter 33, page number 676.

TISSUE ENGINEERING APPROACHES FOR TEMPOROMANDIBULAR JOINT TISSUES

When surgical treatment of temporomandibular joint disease (TMD) is required, tissue engineering of the TMJ focuses on regenerative alternatives.

Tissue engineering has the potential to provide improved solutions in a number of areas, including those relating to disc replacement materials, structural degeneration and alternatives to total joint replacement (TJR).

Complex features such as the fossa and condyle can be restored by anatomically precise and osteoinductive scaffolds in tissue engineering. Engineered tissue devices may one day allow surgeons to repair the injured TMJ structures without the use of TJR devices completely. The most effective combination of cells, scaffold materials and growth factors is one of the obstacles that must be overcome when using this method.

Scaffolds provide a supportive structure that gives engineered tissues their shape and volume. Changing the pore size and porosity of the scaffold can alter its diffusional characteristics. Additionally, the mechanical and surface properties can be customized to meet the specific needs of the engineered material. The selection of scaffolds should correspond with scaffold degradation with matrix synthesis. Scaffolds can be impregnated with growth factors to promote rapid matrix synthesis in vivo. The engineering of tissue replacements for TMD patients is emerging as a viable strategy for giving biological remedies to these as-yet unsolvable challenges. Despite a lack of a commercially available tissue-engineered treatment for TMD, a number of studies have been conducted to create the necessary tools for engineering TMJ tissues.

GUIDED NERVE REGENERATION

Refer Chapter 40, page number 768.

RECENT ADVANCES IN BONE RECONSTRUCTION

DISTRACTION OSTEOGENESIS

TRANSPORT DISTRACTION OSTEOGENESIS

Transport distraction is the latest development in distraction osteogenesis, which uses osteogenesis and histogenesis from the residual host tissues. Refer Chapter 44, page number 846.

Transport distraction osteogenesis (TDO) can be described as the formation of bone and soft tissue in order to fill a defect. This is accomplished by repositioning a disc of bone and allowing formation of new tissues behind it until the disc docks the receiving host bone (Figs. 57.19).

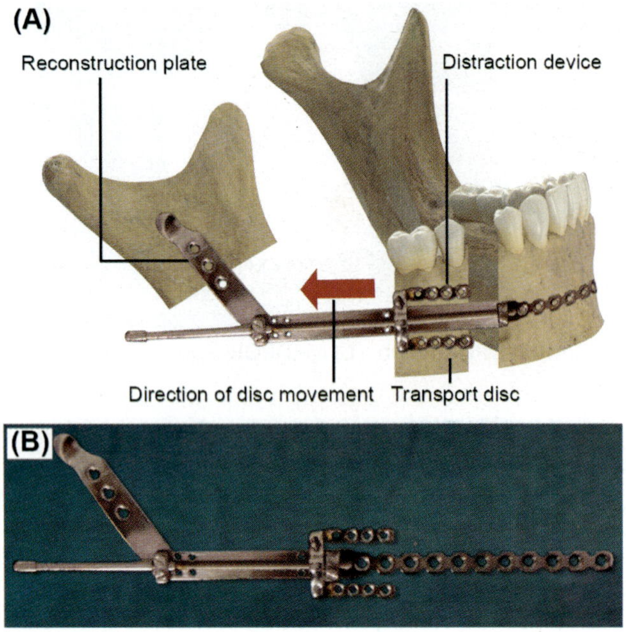

Figure 57.19 (**A**) Line diagram showing transport distraction osteogenesis (TDO) process in a mandible that requires reconstruction for a segmental defect. (**B**) TDO device.

TDO can be subdivided into three types depending on clinical and radiographic features (Fig. 57.20, Case 57.1):

I) Bifocal
II) Trifocal
III) Tetrafocal

Classification of mandibular segmental defects for reconstruction with TDO-*central and lateral defects*.

Based on the extent of the defect on each side of the midline, central defects can be divided into *symmetrical and asymmetrical*.

Lateral defects can either be *straight* when they are posterior to the 2nd premolar (involving only one mandibular vector) or *arched* when they are anterior to the 2nd premolar (involving more than one vector).

GRAFTS

TOOTH TRANSFORMER

Tooth Transformer (TT) is an innovative medical device that can quickly process and transform a patient's extracted tooth into bone graft material.

This procedure was previously performed manually (Fig. 57.21). Autogenous demineralised tooth graft, which contains BMP-2, ensures that the recipient site is completely compatible.

CASE 57.1 Multifocal Transport Distraction for Reconstruction of Mandible after Resection of Ameloblastoma

Indication: Loss of mandibular continuity after resection of ameloblastoma

Device: Herford plate-guided mandibular transport distractor

Vector: Univector

Osteotomy: Two transport discs created from the remaining mandibular ramus. One of the transport discs was fixed to the mandibular reconstruction plate and sectioned again to create a new transport disc in order to achieve the mandibular 'U' form

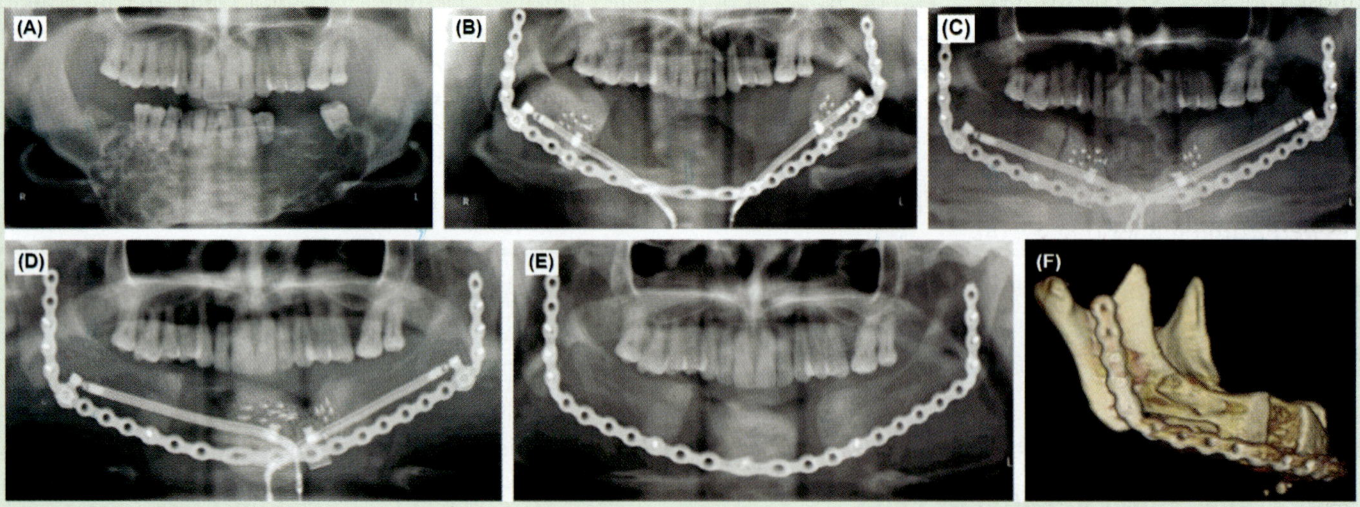

Figure 57.20 (**A**) OPG of the mandible before excision of the tumour. (**B**) After removal of the tumour and fixation of the reconstruction plate, two distractors were fixed bilaterally and two segments transported medially 1 mm per day. (**C**) The left-side fragment was fixed to the reconstruction plate and the same transport segment fragmented for the next stage distraction. (**D**) OPG of the mandible after completion of the distraction. (**E**) After removal of the distractors and fixing the fragments to the reconstruction plate. (**F**) CT after device removal.

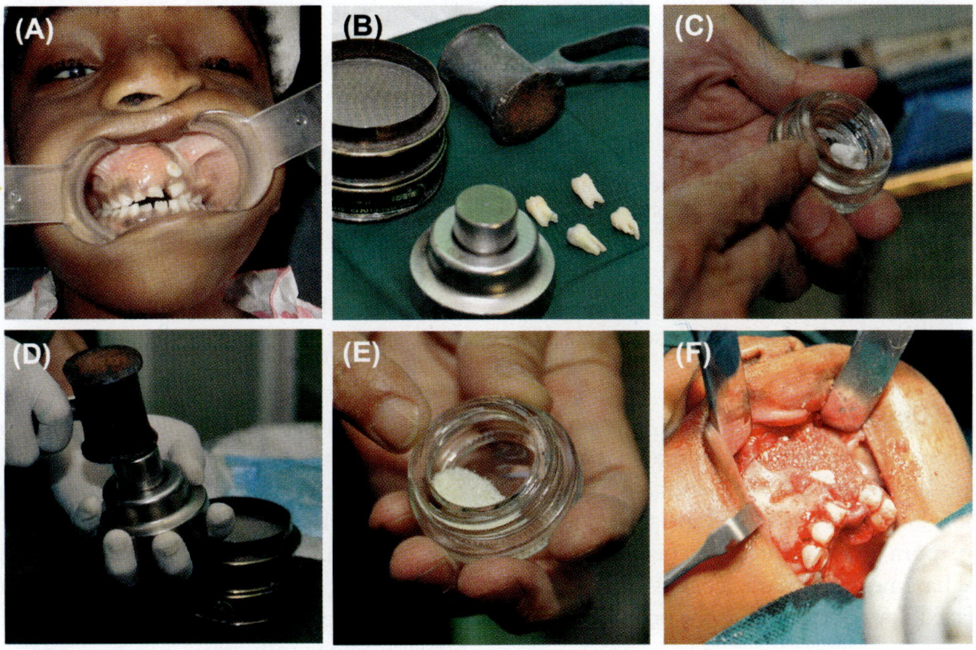

Figure 57.21 (**A**) Preoperative clinical photograph of the patient with alveolar cleft. (**B**) Extracted wisdom teeth with manual tooth grinding device with processing materials used to transform the tooth as graft. (**C**) Processed tooth. (**D**) Manually transforming the extracted tooth into bone graft material. (**E**) Bone graft material. (**F**) Alveolar socket filled with bone graft material.

ALLOPLASTIC IMPLANTS

The advent of the alloplastic implant has reduced many complications, which arise as a result of autografts and allografts. Alloplastic materials have numerous advantages, including no risk of immunologic reactions and graft rejection, reduced disease risk, simplified surgical procedure and an unrestricted supply of implant material. The selection of the proper alloplastic implant material must be done with utmost care because each implant type and material has unique properties. Cautious surgical techniques are essential in reducing the risk of infection and extrusion.

The major aesthetic areas of the facial skeleton such as the malar, midface area, nose and chin offer the structural configuration of the face. Based on the aesthetic necessity of the individual, the implantation procedures are carried out to achieve symmetry and balance.

Various alloplastic materials have been used in the earlier days for soft and bony augmentation, which include ivory, acrylics and precious metal remains (gold cleft palate implants, ivory nasal inlays, etc.).

Better knowledge about the host tissue and implant interface response has led to the improvement of bioactive implants. Proper surgical procedure influences both the short-term and long-term outcomes in the facial skeletal augmentation.

The success of an alloplastic implant material depends upon the following:

- Relation between the implant and the host
- The host reaction
- Location of the implant
- Technique used by the operator
- Function of the implant
- The implant material.

Ideal properties of an alloplastic material

Before the selection of the implant for the skeletal or soft-tissue augmentation, the surgeon should consider the qualities of the selected implant for the safety and durability of the placed implant.

- The material should be biocompatible with any type of tissue in the human body
- The material should be readily available either in blocks or precarved forms
- Sterilisation should be possible when necessary
- It should have better adaptability and flexibility to allow better adaptation between the host tissue–implant interfaces
- The material should have a natural feel when placed in the tissue
- It should have stability when placed and be resistant to migration from its position
- It should be porous enough to allow the tissue ingrowths
- It should not have shape memory, which may cause implant mobility, extrusion from its site or resorption
- It should be readily retrievable, if necessary
- It should be easy to shape and secure
- It should be reliable and safe
- It should be osteoconductive and allow ingrowth of calcified tissue
- It should have an appreciable colour match to the skin tissue when used in scanty tissue areas
- It should allow additional augmentation, if necessary.

Advantages

- Availability of material and simplification of operative procedure
- No need for tissue harvest
- Decreased duration of anaesthesia required
- Extensive range of compositions of synthetic material provides various combinations of strength, elasticity and durability to choose.

Types of alloplastic materials

The following are the different types of alloplastic materials used in the field of oral surgery.

Dimethylsiloxane (silicone)

Dimethylsiloxane (silicone) is a rubber implant material with or without polymer fabric. It has been used for various surgical applications. It is available both as a preformed template and can be customised using room temperature vulcanising silicone. This implant material has 'memory' characteristics and requires adaptation in the 'relaxed' state according to the bone contour.

Advantages

- It can be easily modified intraoperatively using a scalpel or scissors
- Easy fixation to the underlying tissues using a screw or suture
- Sterilisation is possible either by autoclave or by radiation without causing damage to the material
- Inert and does not cause surrounding tissue reaction.

Disadvantages

- Active bending of the material may cause extrusion or resorption of the bone
- Formation of a thin fibrous capsule only and there will be no ingrowth of the tissue.

Uses

Frontal, orbital, zygomatic, nasal, paranasal, nasal dorsum, chin, maxillary, malar, ear, parasymphyseal and mandibular deficiencies augmentation.

Polytetrafluoroethylene

- Polytetrafluoroethylene (PTFE) was initially promoted as Proplast. The material was banned due to its disintegration and foreign body response in TMJ reconstruction for replacement of the glenoid fossa
- Gore and associates marketed the material as Gore-Tex, which is considered as a polymer (microporous) of PTFE. It is then used for the augmentation of various soft-tissue and skeletal defects
- It can be obtained in the range of 1-, 2- and 4-mm sheets permitting modifications in shape and positioned beneath the soft tissues
- It has noninterconnected surface holes with 10–30 mm pore sizes which is favourable for tissue ingrowth, allowing fibrous tissue capsulation at a minimal level.

Advantages

- Gore-Tex causes very less foreign body response, forming a fibrous encapsulation
- Micropores allow some soft-tissue ingrowths, which offer some stability
- It should be removed easily if necessary.

Uses

Augmentation in areas of the face such as lips and nasolabial folds as a subdermal implantation.

Polyethylene (MEDPOR)

Polyethylene is a porous substance with increased tensile strength and sizes of the pores are in the range of 125–250 mm. This material can be shaped or customised to adapt in a required tissue space. The foreign body reaction is minimal and it results in the formation of a thin fibrous encapsulation. This fibrous capsule helps in the reduction of contraction. Carving and shaping is difficult, and despite its porosity, which allows for the ingrowth of soft tissue and vascular supply, it is not actually osteoconductive.

Uses

It has various uses and is being used in the augmentation of midface, chin and mandibular region.

Polyester

Biodegradable polyesters are polymers that are degraded in the body at physiologic pH from weeks to months. They are used for chin and nasal augmentation.

Acrylics

- Polymethylmethacrylate (PMMA)
- Hard-tissue replacement (HTR)
- Bioplant HTR.

Polymethylmethacrylate (PMMA)

PMMA resin is the material used as bone cement for joint prosthesis in orthopaedic surgery. The mixture of a monomer liquid and a polymer powder results in the formation of a rigid, almost translucent plastic by an exothermic reaction. Preoperatively, models are prepared and implants are fabricated using this model, for using in the operating theatre after sterilisation, thus avoiding surrounding tissue damage due to exothermic reaction during mixing. Impregnation of antibiotics into the mixture aids to avoid bacterial inoculation and related complications. Incorporation of the metal mesh provides additional strength and helps in reducing the risk of fracture.

Uses

Predominantly used in oral and cranial reconstruction procedures for full-thickness skull defects.

Disadvantages

- Unbearable odour and it releases teratogenic fumes. Cool irrigation must be applied to compensate for the high temperature during reaction

- It cannot be placed in opportunistic microorganisms residing areas because they have a higher affinity for this surface (e.g. oral cavity, paranasal sinuses, etc.).

Hard-tissue replacement (HTR)

HTR is obtained by the combination of polyhydroxyethylmethacrylate and PMMA.

HTR contains interconnecting pores and a coating of calcium hydroxide, thus giving negative charge for the material. It is hydrophilic and a very strong material. It was initially used for dental work in the earlier days and is currently available as a preformed implant material, which can be customised using CT scan illustrating the defect.

Uses

- Augmentation and filling of very large defects in the cranium and other regions
- Effective in preserving ridge height and width after tooth extraction, hence extensively used for ridge augmentation.

Bioplant HTR is a synthetic bone alloplast of a calcified copolymer (polyhydroxyethylmethacrylate and PMMA) and calcium hydroxide.

Calcium phosphate ceramics

- Hydroxyapatite and other calcium materials are well known for their interaction with each other and their ability to incorporate into living bone tissue (Fig. 57.22). Both porous and dense ceramic forms are used as implants
- They are fragile and easily breakable, although they are nonresorbable. They have excellent biocompatibility as well as they can bond to bone by natural cementing process
- They are osteoconductive and permit for tissue infiltration with lack of a fibrous encapsulation. However, it does not have the osteoinductive property
- Nonceramic forms are also available in the powder form that can be mixed during the operation to fill any defects in the bone.

Uses

Limited to mandibular ridge augmentation and as interposition grafts in facial osteotomies.

Disadvantage

Due to the lack of strength and propensity to fracture, it cannot be used in stress-bearing areas.

OSTEOACTIVE AGENTS

An osteoactive agent is defined as the material with potential to stimulate bone deposition. The osteoinduction phenomenon was 1st described by Urist and his coworkers. The bone matrix was found to stimulate bone formation when implanted within the muscle of many animal species. The specific extract from the bone was identified and the protein was named bone morphogenetic protein (BMP). They are differentiated as osteoinducers, osteopromotors or bioactive peptides.

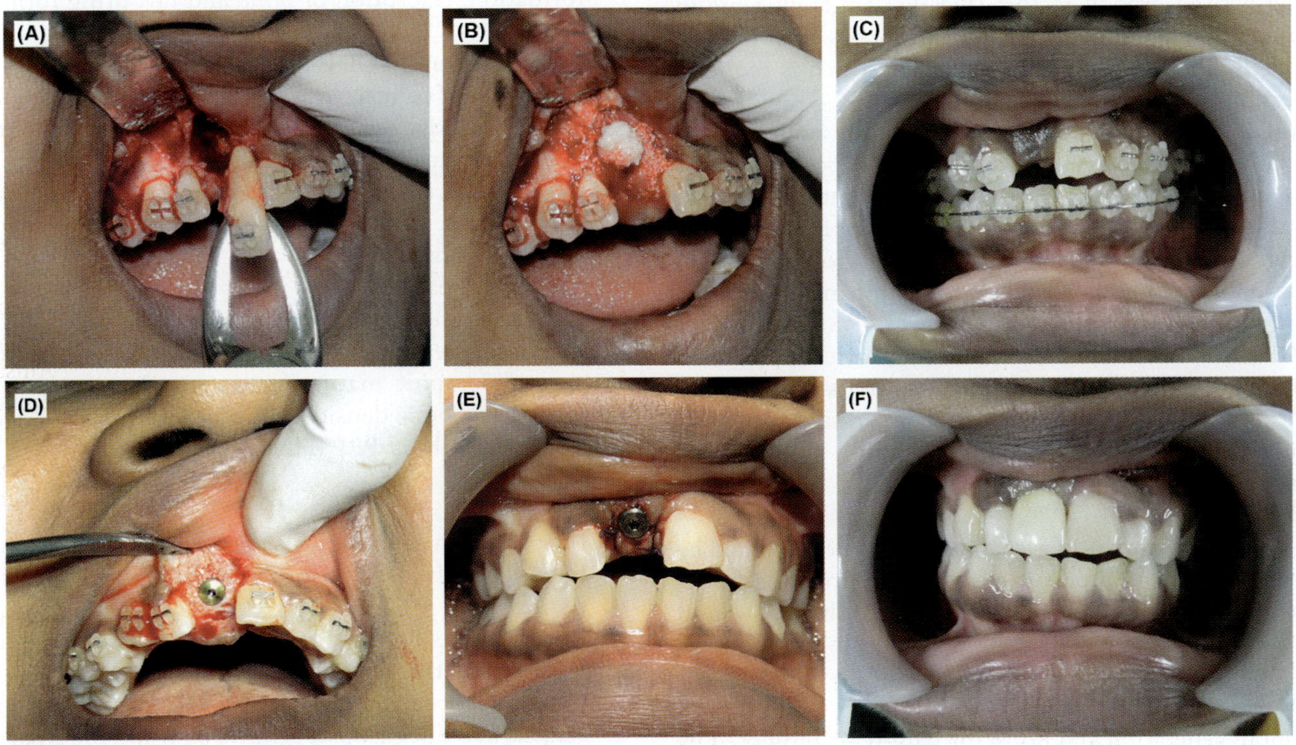

Figure 57.22 **(A)** Extraction of 11. **(B)** Complete filling of the extracted socket with Bio-Oss. **(C)** Wound closed. **(D and E)** Implant placement i.r.t. 11. **(F)** Postoperative view.

Transforming growth factor-β

Transforming growth factor beta (TGF-β) group proteins are grouped under osteopromotors, which have the ability for bone healing. The BMP family is found to include TGF-β. TGF-β has been found to be involved in all stages of bone healing.

- In the primary inflammatory phase, platelets release TGF-β resulting in the proliferation of mesenchymal cells
- It acts as a chemotactic factor for cells causing bone formation, stimulates angiogenesis and limits the activity of the osteoclast cells in the revascularisation phase
- At the commencement of osteogenesis phase, the TGF-β increases osteoblast mitoses. The regulation of osteoblast function results in the increase of bone matrix synthesis. TGF-β inhibits type II collagen; however, it promotes the type I collagen
- During the process of remodelling, they help in bone cell turnover
- At high concentrations, TGF-β suppresses osteoblastic proliferation and differentiation (biphasic effect).

TGF-β is considered to be more effective than BMP in conditions where bone healing is required rather than bone induction. The combination of BMP and TGF-β has been shown to improve the osteoinduction and osteopromotive properties of an alloplastic implant. The carrier media for TGF-β is still under progress unlike BMP.

Platelet-derived growth factor

Platelet-derived growth factors (PDGFs) are angiogenic in nature and aid in proliferation and chemotaxis of connective tissue cells including matrix deposition, which is required for bone healing.

Insulin-like growth factors (IGFs) have the ability to amplify bone cell mitosis and bone matrix deposition. Both PDGF and IGF have the ability to work together and produce the synergistic effect during the repair phases of bone healing. PGDF–IGF-saturated devices are used in cases of defects associated with dental implants for increased bone healing.

TGF-β and PDGF are the important growth factors of the platelets. Degranulation of the platelets results in the release of those factors, which are essential for the initiation of healing of graft.

Platelet-rich plasma

Platelet-rich plasma (PRP) is coagulated platelet prepared by centrifugation from a person's own blood, followed by sequestering and concentrating the platelets, the PGDF and TGF-β for clinical use.

Principle

Thrombin generation and fibrin formation are promoted by the adherence and aggregation of platelets at the site of vascular injury.

- Platelets release growth factors (PDGF, TGF-β), cytokines (PF4, CD40L), chemokines and active metabolites responsible for neoangiogenesis, tissue repair and regeneration
- Concentrating platelets in a fibrin clot or glue generates a higher dose of these healing proteins where it is applied
- Cell membrane receptors of cancellous bone grafts have the ability to respond to those growth factors as evidenced by monoclonal antibody assessment.

Mechanism of action

- Platelets release various growth factors such as PDGF, vascular endothelial growth factor, transforming growth factors β1 and β2 (TGF-β1 and TGF-β2), basic fibroblast growth factor and platelet-activating factor-4, which play a major role in wound healing
- These growth factors are responsible for the following early wound healing process
  a. Increase in cell mitosis
  b. Increase in production of collagen
  c. Attracting other cells to the injury site
  d. Vascular ingrowth initiation
  e. Cell differentiation initiation
- PDGF stimulates healing of connective tissue and helps in the activation of bone regeneration by initiating angiogenesis and stimulating macrophages
- TGF-β acts as a growth factor aid in the repair and regeneration of connective tissue as well as differentiation. It also acts as an effective inhibitor of osteoclast cells formation, resorption of bone and favouring formation of bone
- Both PDGF and TGF-β facilitate the following:
  a. Repair of connective tissue and regeneration of bone
  b. Trigger adjacent cells such as preosteoblasts for mitosis (increase in numbers)
  c. Induce preosteoblasts differentiation into mature osteoblasts, thus helping in the initiation of remodelling of bone
  d. Tissue healing
  e. Bone mineralisation.

Marx et al., reported their evidence of nearly three times higher radiographic maturation rate and increased histomorphometric bone density in grafts with PRP in comparison to grafts without PRP (Flowchart 57.3).

Uses

- PRP has been extensively used to support tissue healing
- It is clinically used to promote healing of bones and tissues
- Used in maxillofacial reconstruction and periodontal regenerative therapy
- Extraction socket healing: Use of PRP in extraction sockets aids in reducing postoperative pain and inflammation, though no systematic acceleration of osseous healing at the postextraction site could be demonstrated. Moreover,

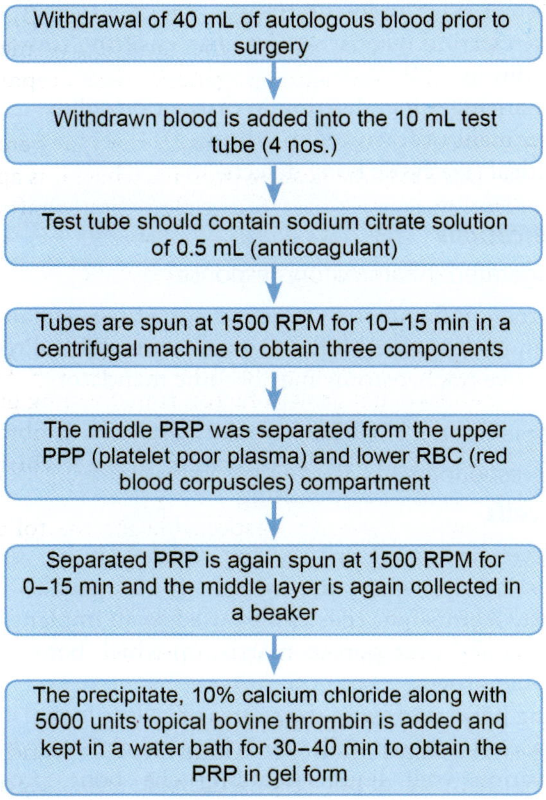

Flowchart 57.3 Preparation of platelet-rich plasma (PRP) gel.

lower rate of alveolar osteitis, less pain and denser radiographic bone healing were found when PRP was placed into 3rd molar extraction sockets

- Dental implants: PRP may be used to promote osseointegration and bone regeneration during the placement of dental implants
- Bone graft enhancer: When PRP is used along with particulate bone grafting materials, PRP acts as a biologic adhesive, which holds together the particles, making the graft material manipulation much easier. PRP may be used as an additive to nonvascularised bone grafts in alveolar cleft, critical size bony defects and mandibular continuity defects.

Bioactive polypeptides

The bioactive polypeptides may act as osteoinducers or osteoenhancers. P-15 and OSA-117MV are the two short amino acid chain peptides that have demonstrated the bone activity. P-15 polypeptide has a conformational arrangement known as the 'beta bend', which promotes bone induction and growth when used in some in vitro studies. The octenyl succinic anhydride (OSA) molecule is smaller than P-15 and was used in the treatment of osteoporosis where OSAs effect is concentrated in areas of high stress. Studies have started to explore the local effects of this peptide, and initial reports suggest that it may enhance the osteoinductive effect of demineralised bone matrix.

Recombinant bone morphogenetic proteins

BMPs are naturally occurring anabolic proteins in the body found in various tissues such as bone, cartilage, musculature and connective tissue.

BMP family

- BMPs are subfamily of TGF-β superfamily
- There are 20 different proteins but not all members have the capacity to induce bone (osteogenic potential)
- BMP-1 is a metalloprotease and does not possess osteogenic properties
- BMP-2 and 4 composed of one osteogenic group
- BMP-3 and 13 function as BMP antagonists
- BMP-5, 6, 7, 8, 9 and 10 form another osteogenic group.

BMP in bone

- BMPs are produced by osteoprogenitor cells, namely osteoblasts, chondrocytes and platelets
- BMPs induce chondrogenesis, osteogenesis, angiogenesis and extracellular matrix.

Recombinant Human Bone Morphogenetic Protein (rhBMP)
These are osteoinductive protein additives derived through recombinant tissue engineering technology that can induce de novo bone formation when they are implanted.

Osteoinductive properties of BMP

Implantation of rhBMP results in a complex series of cellular events:

1. Mesenchymal cell infiltration
2. Cartilage formation (in endochondral ossification)
3. Vascularisation
4. Bone formation
5. Bone remodelling along with population by haematopoietic bone marrow elements (Table 57.4).

The BMPs causes the mesenchymal cells to differentiate into bone and cartilage-forming mature cells.

TABLE 57.4 Overview of BMP Characteristics

Sub family	BMP	Involved in
1	BMP-2 BMP-4	• Bone and cartilage formation • Teeth and bone formation
2	BMP-5 BMP-6 BMP-7 BMP-8	• Cartilage development • Joints, liver • Renal development, kidney • Bone and cartilage formation
3	BMP-9 BMP-10	• CNS, liver, angiogenesis • Morphogenesis of the heart

History

- In 1979, Urist coined the term BMPs
- Hari Reddi et al., were the 1st to identify, isolate and purify the signals of BMP
- John Wozney and colleagues at Genetics Institute enabled the cloning of BMPs creating rhBMP which paved the way for its mass production.

Advantages

- They induce the formation of their own bone
- The bone formed functions and remodels in a way appropriate for the anatomic site and biomechanical environment in which it is placed
- More conducive to normal growth, tooth eruption, mechanical manipulation and osseointegration than other forms of grafts.

Need for a carrier or scaffold

BMPs can be rapidly eliminated by the body if it is not bound to a carrier. The ideal carrier must bind BMP until all the differentiation processes are complete and resorb in time to provide space for the developing bone to form. The currently used carrier is absorbable collagen sponge.

Clinical application in oral surgery

- rhBMP-2 and rhBMP-7 are the molecules that are in clinical use.
- Cleft alveolar bone grafting (Fig. 57.23)
- Sinus lift
- Alveolar ridge augmentations
- Postresection reconstruction after ensuring tumour-free condition
- Enhancing mineralisation in distraction callus
- Treatment of fractured malunion
- Critical size cystic bony defects.

Complications

i) Exaggerated inflammatory response

An extreme inflammatory reaction sometimes endangering life as in neck swelling following use in mandible. Preoperative elective tracheostomy may become mandatory.

ii) Ectopic bone formation

iii) Nonresponders

Stem cells

The developed tissue engineering technology has brought the possibilities, where the hybrids of biomaterials seeded with osteocompetent cells can be used as an implant. These 'hybrid grafts' were porous matrix, on which bone marrow cells could grow.

Using bone marrow as the source of cells is logical as bone marrow contains stem cells which have the ability to differentiate various cell lines, including the bone producing osteocompetent cells. Seeding of bone marrow cells into porous matrix enhances the osteogenic potential of the matrix as a hybrid. Another advantage of the tissue culturing technique is that bone marrow cells can be further expanded in numbers.

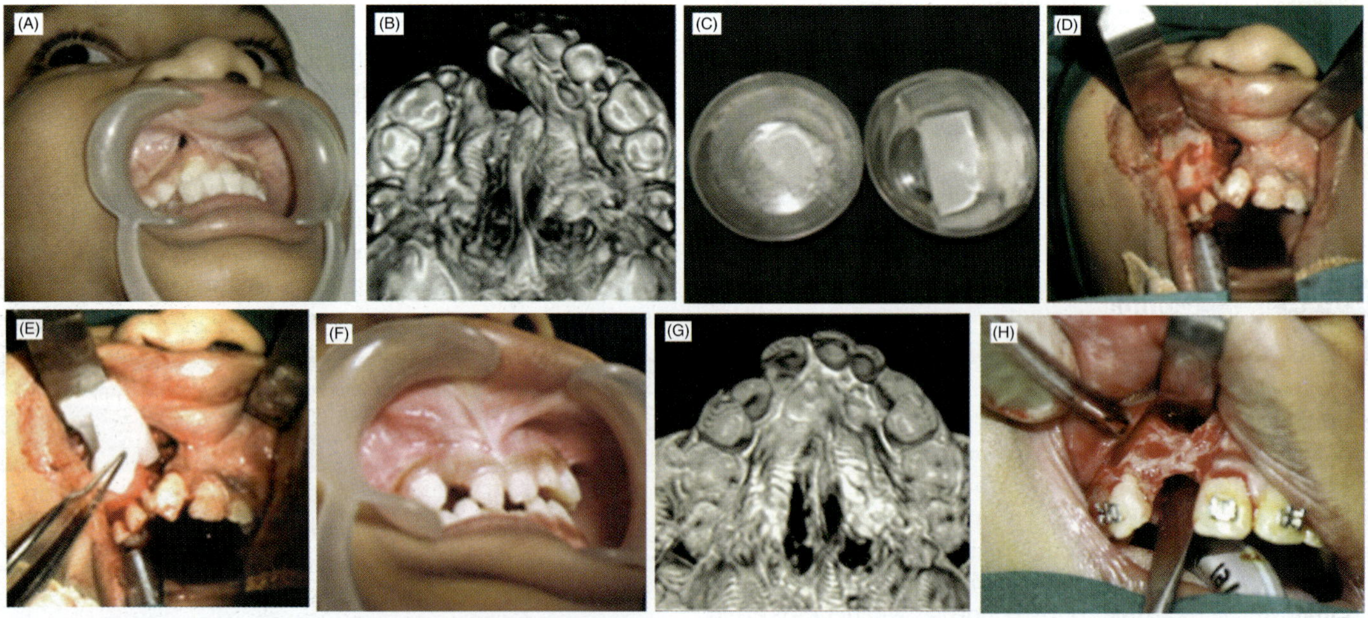

Figure 57.23 **(A)** Preoperative clinical photograph of the patient with unilateral alveolar cleft. **(B)** CT scan showing the alveolar cleft. **(C)** BMP powder and the absorbable collagen sponge prior to mixing. **(D)** Surgical exposure of the alveolar cleft. **(E)** Packing of the alveolar cleft with BMP. **(F)** Postoperative clinical photograph. **(G)** Postoperative 3D CT scan showing closure. **(H)** Regenerated new bone visible during implant placement.

These bone marrow-derived cells are influenced by dexamethasone and 1,25-dihydroxycholecalciferol and differentiate into bone cells. Human bone marrow cells have the ability to adhere to the porous coral matrices and matrices made of hydroxyapatite. The combination of coral scaffold and in vitro-expanded marrow stromal cells has been used as tissue-engineered artificial bone graft (hybrid grafts), which has been used to treat large segmental long bone defects leading to complete recorticalisation and medullary canal formation. The bone cells can be harvested using special devices, for example, suction trap, and could be used for the same individual at a later date by cryopreservation.

TEMPOROMANDIBULAR JOINT PROSTHESIS

Alloplastic TMJ prosthesis represents a safe and predictable way to restore TMJ-acquired defects. (Fig. 57.24; Tables 57.5–57.7).

TECHNIQUE

Stock prosthesis

1. The standard surgical technique with this type of prosthesis requires preauricular and submandibular or retromandibular approaches
2. Once exposure of the TMJ and mandibular ramus is achieved, a condylar osteotomy is done if necessary

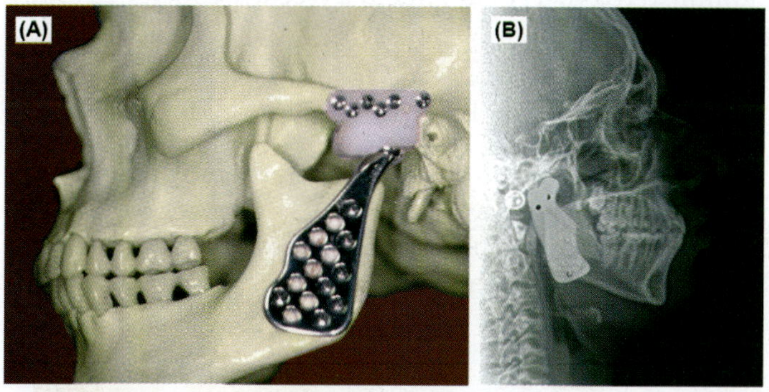

Figure 57.24 (**A** and **B**) Temporomandibular joint prosthesis.

TABLE 57.5 Indications and Contraindications of TMJ Prosthesis

Indications	Contraindications
• Congenital and developmental disorders (condylar agenesis, condylar hyperplasia) • Neoplasia • Severe degenerative disease • Posttraumatic deformities • Ankylosis • Previous failed autogenous or alloplastic reconstructions	• Growing patients • Uncontrolled systemic disease • Psychiatric instability • Active infection • Allergy to prosthetic components • Uncontrolled parafunction

TABLE 57.6 Advantages and Disadvantages of TMJ Prosthesis

Advantages	Disadvantages
• Decreased operating time • Immediate function/no need for postoperative MMF • No donor site • Patient-specific devices available • Simultaneous correction of malocclusions possible	• Cost • Possible need for replacement • No growth potential • Possible fixation failure • Wear

3. Approximately between 2 and 2.5 mm of space is required between the articular surface and the residual mandible to be able to fit the prosthetic parts
4. A large-barrelled bur or a reciprocating rasp is then used to flatten the articular eminence to adapt the fossa component

TABLE 57.7 Comparison Between Stock and Custom-Made Total TMJ Prosthesis

Stock Prosthesis	Custom-Made Prosthesis
• Make fit • Lower cost • Shorter treatment time frames • Removal of bone • More difficult to obtain primary stability • Potential micromovement • Placement versatility • Limited use for large or difficult anatomic defects • It has a fossa component of three sizes (small, medium, large) made completely of ultrahigh molecular weight polyethylene; three different lengths—45, 50 and 55 mm; and two different widths—standard and narrow	• Made to fit • Higher cost • Longer treatment time frames • No or minimal removal of bone • Easier to obtain primary stability • No micromovement • Less placement versatility • Excellent for large or difficult anatomic defects

5. After properly sizing it, the fossa component is implanted before fitting and placement of the mandibular ramus component is performed
6. Occlusion should be checked and layer-wise closure to be done.

Custom-made prosthesis

1. The process for construction of this type of device starts with a thin-cut maxillofacial CT scan that is used for the construction of a stereolithographic model
2. The surgeon approves the prosthetic design after a wax-up is done on the stereolithographic model
3. The fossa component has a titanium mesh backing with an ultrahigh molecular weight polyethylene-articulating surface
4. The mandibular component has a body made of machined alloyed titanium and a condylar head made of chrome–cobalt–molybdenum alloy
5. Preauricular and submandibular or retromandibular approaches are used to access the TMJ
6. Once these areas are exposed, the necessary planned osteotomies are performed. The fossa component is placed and secured 1st, followed by the mandibular component
7. Sterility is crucial to prevent contamination and potential infection of the prosthesis.

Complications

Complications with these types of reconstruction include:
- Hardware failure
- Infection
- Heterotopic bone formation.

RECENT ADVANCES IN TREATMENT OF OSTEORADIONECROSIS

The combination of pentoxifylline and tocopherol medications work together as effective antifibrotic agents and these drugs are readily available, affordable and well tolerated by the patient. This is also effective in the treatment of chronic septic osteoradionecrosis of the mandible (Refer to chapter 24).

Pentoxifylline is a derivative of the methylxanthine that has a negative effect on TNF-α. It increases erythrocyte flexibility, dilates blood vessels, inhibits inflammatory reactions and inhibits the proliferation of human dermal fibroblasts and the production of extracellular matrix in vivo and increases collagenase activity in vitro.

Tocopherol is given with pentoxifylline, which aids in reducing fibrosis by scavenging the reactive oxygen species that were generated during oxidative stress, protecting cell membranes against the peroxidation of lipids, and partially inhibiting TGF-β1 and the expression of procollagen genes.

Clodronate: It is a new generation bisphosphonate.

It reduces the number and activity of osteoclasts, thereby inhibiting bone resorption. By increasing bone production and decreasing fibroblast proliferation, it directly acts on osteoblastic cells.

RECENT ADVANCES IN TRIGEMINAL NEURALGIA

Minimally invasive neurolytic techniques, such as low-level laser therapy (LLLT) and ozone injection, have revolutionised the treatment of trigeminal neuralgia (TN) with the advent of newer technologies.

Vixotrigine and eslicarbazepine are potential new drugs for lowering the frequency and intensity of epileptic episodes.

VIXOTRIGINE

It is a sodium channel blocker that suppresses seizures or noxious stimuli by focusing on higher frequencies. It was found that giving TN patients a dose of 150 mg vixotrigine three times a day alleviated their pain.

ESLICARBAZEPINE

It is an antiepileptic medicine that belongs to the dibenzepine category and is the 3rd generation of the drug. The medication, which treats focal seizures by targeting voltage-gated sodium channels, has recently been given permission for use in adjunctive therapy. Dose of 200–1200 mg/day was administered to TN patients in a recently concluded study.

NEURAL PROLOTHERAPY

It is also referred to as perineural injection therapy (PIT) and it is one of the recent advancements in regenerative medicine. PIT targets pain-generating neurogenic inflammation in subcutaneous nerves.

The procedure entails injecting hypertonic dextrose saline with local anaesthetics into the trigger sites and typically takes multiple appointments.

NERVE COMBING

It is also known as internal neurolysis. It is a type of surgical approach that longitudinally divides the branches of the trigeminal nerve using a specific fibre knife based on preoperative locations of pain and intraoperative observation.

COMPLEMENTARY MEDICINE

In addition to typical conventional treatment, there are a number of complementary therapies that assist in TN pain reduction. Acupuncture, electroacupuncture and spinal regulation therapies are among them. Sound therapy, low-intensity and low-frequency acoustic ultrasound patches, vitamin B, vitamin C and biofeedback are some of the other complementary medicine techniques.

NEUROMODULATION

It is a new treatment option for TN patients, aiming to restore normal neurological function by either neural stimulation or inhibition. Several neuromodulation approaches have recently been investigated for the treatment of TN. Some of these are transcranial magnetic stimulation, motor cortex stimulation, deep brain stimulation, spinal cord stimulation, transcutaneous electrical nerve stimulation and peripheral nerve stimulation.

CARBON DIOXIDE LASER

Patients with drug-refractory TN have their peripheral nerves ablated with a CO_2 laser. Recently, it has been demonstrated to lower pain scores in TN and provide relief for up to a year.

OZONE INJECTION AROUND GASSERIAN GANGLION

Ozone and oxygen mixture gas was injected into the area around the Gasserian ganglion under C-arm X-ray guidance in an extensive retrospective research. Structural nerve injury before surgery was found to be associated with a lower clinical effect or a worse clinical outcome. Refractory TN patients can benefit from ozone injection around Gasserian ganglion (OIAGG), according to the results of the study.

LOW-LEVEL LASER THERAPY

It uses a single wavelength light source. It works on the concept that irradiation with monochromatic light may alter cell function. This method involves irradiating the area of interest followed by laser puncture at predetermined points along the path of the nerve.

RECENT ADVANCES IN ORTHOGNATHIC SURGERY

SURGERY-FIRST APPROACH (SFA)

In this surgical approach, orthognathic surgery is conducted without the need for presurgical orthodontic treatment. It is considered a paradigm change in contrast to the conventional orthognathic method. In 1991, Brachvogel et al., suggested a concept known as 'surgery-first and orthodontics 2nd' with the purpose of eliminating some of the drawbacks and complications associated with presurgical orthodontics. To shorten the time needed to complete orthodontic therapy, he asserted that the normalised soft tissues (lips, cheeks and tongue) allow the teeth to settle into better positions after surgery. Later, surgery-first approach (SFA) was proposed by Nagasaka et al. in 2003 (Fig. 57.25).

Indications

SFA requirements include the following:
- Normal to mild proclined or retroclined incisors
- Aligned or mild crowding

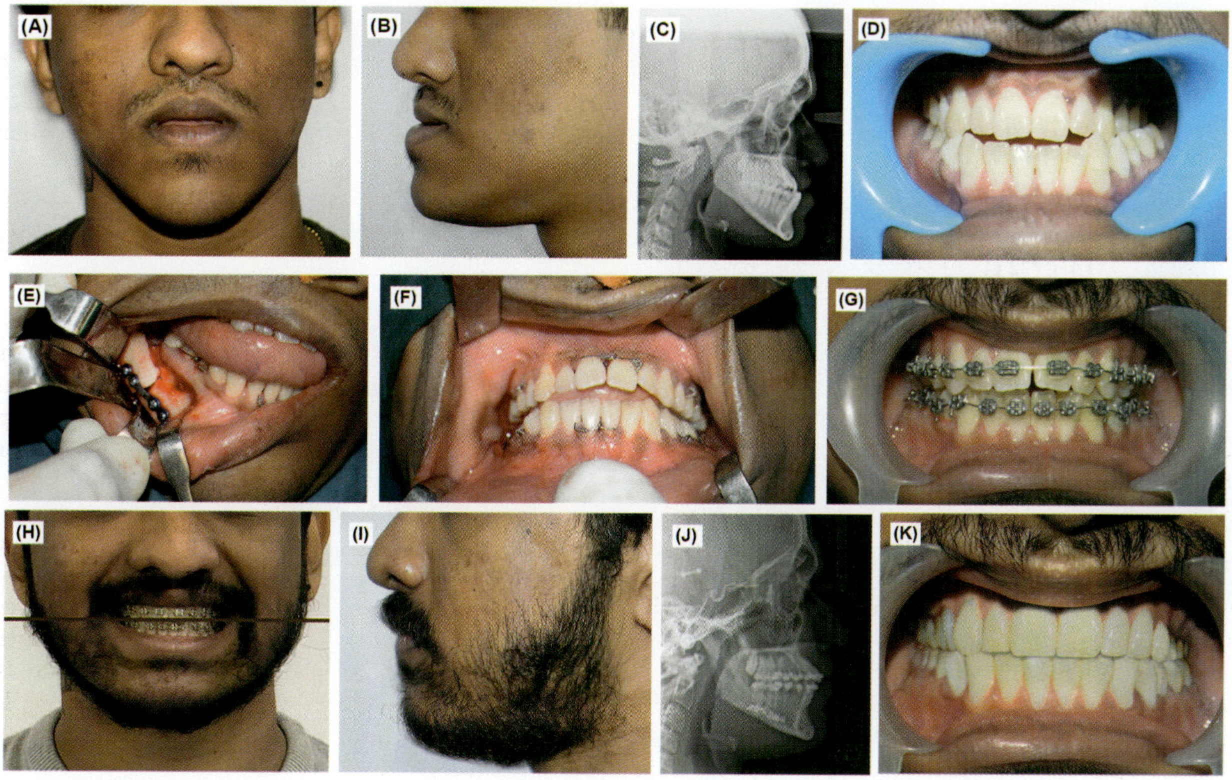

Figure 57.25 (**A** and **B**) Preoperative views showing mandibular anteroposterior excess and increased anterior lower facial height. (**C** and **D**) Preoperative lateral cephalogram and occlusal view. (**E** and **F**) Intraoperative showing BSSO. (**G**) Postsurgical orthodontic treatment for dental arch alignment. (**H–K**) Postoperative frontal and profile view, occlusion and lateral cephalogram. (Note: No occlusal cant present.)

- Minimal transverse discrepancy
- Flat to mild curve of Spee.

Most of the cases treated with this technique have been Class III malocclusion cases that met the above requirements.

Advantages

- Patient-centred approach
- Early improvement of facial aesthetics
- Patient's social life is not adversely affected
- Allowing for a shorter total treatment time
- Eliminating the necessity for an aggravated gross appearance during the presurgical orthodontic period.

Disadvantages

- Necessity for precise and knowledgeable decision-making concerning the likelihood of SFA
- 3rd molars cannot be extracted prior to surgery
- Possible requirement for a prolonged intermaxillary bone fixation
- Chewing problems shortly after surgery resulting from incomplete occlusion.

INDEX

C

D

E

M

N

O

P

Index

Q

R

U

V

W

X

Z